The Complete Directory
for
People with Chronic Illness

2015/16
Twelfth Edition

The Complete Directory
for
People with Chronic Illness

Condition Descriptions

Associations

Publications

Research Centers

Support Groups

Web Sites

A SEDGWICK PRESS Book

Grey House Publishing

PUBLISHER: Leslie Mackenzie
EDITORIAL DIRECTOR: Laura Mars

PRODUCTION MANAGER & COMPOSITION: Kristen Thatcher
MARKETING DIRECTOR: Jessica Moody

A Sedgewick Press Book
Grey House Publishing, Inc.
4919 Route 22
Amenia, NY 12501
518.789.8700
FAX 845.373.6390
www.greyhouse.com
e-mail: books@greyhouse.com

While every effort has been made to ensure the reliability of the information presented in this publication, Grey House Publishing neither guarantees the accuracy of the data contained herein nor assumes any responsibility for errors, omissions or discrepancies. Grey House accepts no payment for listing; inclusion in the publication of any organization, agency, institution, publication, service or individual does not imply endorsement of the editors or publisher.

Errors brought to the attention of the publisher and verified to the satisfaction of the publisher will be corrected in future editions.

First edition published 1994
Twelfth edition published 2015

The complete directory for people with chronic illness – 1994-2015
Printed in Canada

1053 p.; 27.5 cm
Other title: DCI
ISSN: 1080-7659

1. Chronic diseases – United States – Directories. 2. Chronic Diseases – Bibliography. 3. Chronic Disease – United States – Directories. 4. Social Support – United States – Directories. 5. Information Services – United States – Directories. 6. Rehabilitation – United States – Directories. I. Title: DCI.

RC108 .C645
616' .0025'73   96-640803

ISBN: 978-1-61925-548-7

Table of Contents

Table of Contents

Introduction

This is the twelfth edition of *The Complete Directory for People with Chronic Illness*. It offers a comprehensive overview of 90 specific chronic illnesses from Addison's to Wilson's Disease, from Allergies to Cancer. NEW to this edition is a chapter on Post-Traumatic Stress Disorder. Each chapter includes an easy-to-understand medical description, plus a wide range of condition-specific support services and information resources that deal with the variety of issues concerning those with a chronic illness, as well as those who support the chronic illness community.

Praise for previous editions:

"...this volume is among the most useful of directories, with its goal of helping people with long-term medical conditions find helpful resources."
—**Choice**

"...logically organized and offers an extensive range of information resources and support services."
—**Doody's Notes**

Surveys report that 125 million Americans currently suffer from a chronic illness. This number is expected to reach 157 million by the year 2020. The word "chronic" comes from the Greek word *chronos* meaning time. The Chronic Illness Alliance defines a chronic illness as one *...that is permanent or lasts a long time. It may get slowly worse over time ... or ... go away. It may cause permanent changes to the body (and) will certainly affect the person's quality of life.* The National Center for Health Statistics defines chronic illness as *one lasting 3 months or more.*

However you define chronic illness, this directory will prove invaluable in dealing with the many aspects of chronic disease. It includes associations, state agencies, libraries & resource centers, research centers, magazines, newsletters, audio & video, hot lines, support groups and valuable web sites. In addition to chapters dealing with specific medical conditions, this edition includes several chapters designed to help all those in the chronic illness community, including wish foundations, death and bereavement groups and medical homes – primary care settings in the community.

The Complete Directory for People with Chronic Illness is designed for both those dealing for the first time with the stress and crucial need-to-know issues that accompany chronic illness, as well as those already coping with chronic disease. ...How can I connect with others with diabetes? ...Which cancer treatment is best for me? ...What do I need to know about protecting my 2-year old, who was just diagnosed with a heart condition? ...Why is my partner angrier than our chronically ill child? You'll find answers to these questions and more in the pages of this edition.

In addition to resources crucial for people with chronic illness as they transition from diagnosis to home, work, and community life, this directory is also invaluable to hospital and medical center personnel, especially discharge planners, social service workers, and disability coordinators. *The Complete Directory for People with Chronic Illness* provides, in one source, comprehensive, critical, immediate information – from national associations to children's books. It's the perfect choice for both those who find navigating the Internet overwhelming (we've done it for you) along with those who feel comfortable surfing the Net (we provide valuable, specific web sites).

Following this Introduction are three valuable elements:

Chronic Illness-Body Systems Chart
This two-part table includes first a list of chronic illnesses and their relevant body systems, and then a list of body systems and the chronic illnesses that affect it.

Accepting & Coping with a Chronic Illness
This article discusses what you can expect from the time you are diagnosed with a chronic illness and during its duration, physically and emotionally.

Next Steps After Your Diagnosis
This informative article, with phone numbers and web sites, offers information and support in five steps: Take the Time you Need; Get the Support you Need; Talk with Your Doctor; Seek out Information; and Decide on a Treatment Plan.

Arrangement

The 90 chronic condition chapters are arranged alphabetically by name of the disorder. Each chapter begins with a brief description of the illness, written in layman's terms, with probable causes, symptoms and treatment options.

Following each description are disease-specific resources. Most chapters contain the following: National Associations; State Agencies; Libraries & Resource Centers; Magazines, Newsletters, Pamphlets; Research Centers; Books for Adults; Books for Children; Support Groups & Hotlines; Audio & Video Resources; Web Sites.

This reference work profiles 10,858 listings. This edition includes 7,488 fax numbers, 6,612 e-mails, 9,632 web sites, and 11,011 key executives. Brief descriptions and other details are included depending on the type of listing; Associations may include year founded and yearly dues, while Magazines may include frequency and number of pages.

In addition to the 90 chapters of chronic illnesses, *The Complete Directory for People with Chronic Illness* includes several supplemental chapters in the back of the book designed to provide value to individuals with chronic illness and their families: General Resources – information relevant to the general chronic illness community; Wish Foundations – organizations devoted to granting wishes of chronically and terminally ill individuals; and Death & Bereavement – support services for those who find themselves or a loved one close to death or grieving a loss.

Rounding out this directory are two indexes that allow users additional access to the information: Entry Name Index and Geographic Index.

The Complete Directory for People with Chronic Illness is also available for subscription on G.O.L.D. – Grey House OnLine Database. Subscribers to G.O.L.D. can access their subscription via the Internet and do customized searches that make finding information quicker and easier. Visit http://gold.greyhouse.com for more information.

Chronic Illness — Body Systems

The following chart lists the chronic illness and its body system(s) or disorder category. Chronic conditions not listed do not fall into a specific system(s). A cross-reference chart that lists the information in reverse follows — body system or disorder categories followed by chronic illnesses.

CHRONIC ILLNESS	BODY SYSTEM/DISORDER CATEGORY
Addison's Disease	Endocrine
Aging	Cells & Tissues
AIDS/HIV	Immune, Infectious Disease
Allergies	Immune
Alzheimer's Disease	Nervous
Amyotrophic Lateral Sclerosis	Nervous
Arthritis	Muscular, Skeletal
Asthma	Respiratory
Ataxia	Nervous
Attention Deficit Hyperactivity Disorder	Behavioral, Developmental
Autistic Spectrum Disorders	Behavioral, Developmental
Brain Tumors	Nervous
Carpal Tunnel Syndrome	Muscular, Skeletal, Nervous
Celiac Disease	Gastrointestinal
Cerebral Palsy	Nervous, Muscular
Chronic Fatigue Syndrome	Immune
Chronic Pain	Nervous
Cooley's Anemia (Thalassemia)	Blood
Congential Heart Disease	Cardiovascular
Crohn's Disease	Gastrointestinal
Cystic Fibrosis	Respiratory, Gastrointestinal
Diabetes Mellitus	Endocrine
Down Syndrome	Developmental
Eating Disorders (Anorexia Nervosa, Bulimia)	Behavioral
Endometriosis	Reproductive
Fabry Disease	Gastrointestinal
Fibromyalgia Syndrome	Muscular, Skeletal
Gastrointestinal Disorders	Gastrointestinal
Gaucher's Disease	Gastrointestinal
Growth Disorders	Developmental
Head Injuries	Nervous
Hearing Impairment	Sensory
Heart Disease	Cardiovascular
Hemophilia	Blood
Hepatitis	Infectious Disease
Hydrocephalus	Nervous
Hypertension	Cardiovascular
Impotence	Reproductive
Incontinence	Urinary
Infertility	Reproductive
Kidney Disease	Gastrointestinal

CHRONIC ILLNESS	BODY SYSTEM/DISORDER CATEGORY
Liver Disease	Gastrointestinal
Lung Disease	Respiratory
Lupus Erythematosus	Cells & Tissues
Mental Illness: General	Behavioral
Mental Illness: Depression	Behavioral
Mental Illness: Schizophrenia	Behavioral
Migraine	Cardiovascular, Nervous
Multiple Sclerosis	Nervous
Muscular Dystrophy	Nervous
Myasthenia Gravis	Nervous
Neurofibromatosis	Nervous, Dermatologic
Osteogenesis Imperfecta	Skeletal
Osteoporosis	Skeletal
Paget's Disease	Skeletal
Parkinson Disease	Nervous
Post-Polio Syndrome	Muscular, Skeletal
Post-Traumatic Stress Disorder	Nervous
Prader Willi Syndrome	Endocrine
Raynaud's Disease	Cardiovascular
Sarcoidosis	Cells & Tissues, Respiratory
Scleroderma	Cells & Tissues, Dermatologic
Scoliosis	Skeletal
Seizure Disorders	Nervous
Sexually Transmitted Diseases	Reproductive, Infectious Disease
Sickle Cell Disease	Blood
Sjogren's Syndrome	Cells & Tissues
Skin Disorders	Dermatologic
Sleep Disorders	Dermatologic
Spina Bifida	Nervous, Skeletal
Spinal Cord Injuries	Nervous
Stroke	Nervous
Substance Abuse	Behavioral
Tay Sachs Disease	Nervous
Thyroid Disease	Endorcrine
Tick-Borne Disease	Infectious Disease
Tourette Syndrome	Nervous
Tuberculosis	Respiratory, Infectious Disease
Tuberous Sclerosis	Nervous, Dermatologic
Turner Syndrome	Endocrine
Ulcerative Colitis	Gastrointestinal
Visual Impairment	Sensory
War Syndromes	Nervous
Wilson's Disease	Gastrointestinal

By Body System/Disorder Category

Behavioral
Attention Deficit Disorder; Autism; Eating Disorders; Mental Illness; Substance Abuse

Blood
Cooley's Anemia; Hemophilia; Sickle Cell Disease

Cardiovascular
Heart Disease; Hypertension; Migraine; Raynaud's Disease

Cells & Tissues
Aging; Lupus Erythematosus; Scleroderma; Sjogren's Syndrome

Dermatologic
Neurofibromatosis; Scleroderma; Skin Disorders; Tuberous Sclerosis

Developmental
Attention Deficit Disorder; Autism; Down Syndrome; Growth Disorders

Endocrine
Addison's Disease; Diabetes; Turner Syndrome

Gastrointestinal
Celiac Disease; Crohn's Disease; Cystic Fibrosis; Fabry Disease; Gastrointestinal Disorders; Gaucher's Disease; Kidney Disease; Liver Disease; Ulcerative Colitis

Immune
AIDS; Allergies; Chronic Fatigue Syndrome

Infectious Disease
AIDS; Hepatitis; Sexually Transmitted Diseases; Tick-Borne Disease; Tuberculosis

Muscular
Arthritis; Carpal Tunnel Syndrome; Cerebral Palsy; Fibromyalgia Syndrome; Post-Polio Syndrome

Nervous
Agent Orange Related Injuries; Alzheimer's Disease; Amyotrophic Lateral Sclerosis; Ataxia; Brain Tumors; Carpal Tunnel Syndrome; Cerebral Palsy; Charcot-Marie-Tooth Disorder; Chronic Pain; GulfWar Syndrome; Head Injuries; Hydrocephalus; Multiple Sclerosis; Muscular Dystrophy; Myasthenia Gravis; Neurofibromatosis; Parkinson Disease; Post-Traumatic Stress Disorder; Seizure Disorders; Spina Bifida; Spinal Cord Injuries; Stroke; Tourette Syndrome; Tuberous Sclerosis

Reproductive
Endometriosis; Impotence; Infertility; Sexually Transmitted Diseases

Respiratory
Asthma; Cystic Fibrosis; Lung Disease; Tuberculosis

Skeletal
Arthritis; Carpal Tunnel Syndrome; Fibromyalgia Syndrome; Osteognesis Imperfecta; Osteoporosis; Paget's Disease; Post-Polio Syndrome; Scoliosis; Spina Bifida

Sensory
Hearing Impairment; Visual Impairment

Urinary
Incontinence

Accepting and Coping with a Chronic Illness

Reactions to Illness

Reactions to learning of one's chronic illness are varied, but they are always powerful. Emotions may range from shock to relief, and everything in between. Even when symptoms have been present for a long time, the diagnosis can be upsetting.

While shock may be the first reaction to learning your diagnosis, denial is also common, as are anger and grief over the loss of health. Many people struggle to understand their condition, asking, "What does this mean? Is this a mistake? Is there a cure?" This sense of shock and denial is very common, but it does have a purpose. Dr. Kubler-Ross explains that the reaction may actually facilitate the individual's eventual acceptance of the news by allowing time to process the overwhelming information at a more comfortable pace.

While denial is natural, it can be unhealthy if it hinders your ability or willingness to care for yourself, comply with treatment, and establish treatment goals. An eventual acceptance of the condition is critical in taking control of the condition and effectively managing it.

Coping Techniques

With more than 100 million people having a chronic illness, it may be reassuring to know that many continue to lead fairly normal lives. Most people with chronic conditions learn to adapt psychologically and physically to their illness. Effectively managing a chronic condition is certainly a challenge but not impossible. Here are some suggestions for coping:

- **Learn all you can about your condition and treatment.** Becoming a student of your condition can be an important way to know what is going on with your body. Use as many sources as you can to gather information. Learn about your medications and watch for their side effects. Follow your physician's instructions and keep focused on the goal—getting to the point of effective disease management. Be sure to use trusted sources of medical information when doing your research—you may want to begin by talking to your medical team.
- **Build your medical team and develop good relationships with the team members.** You are a primary member of this team. Your physician may have the latest information on medical treatments, but a dietician will be able to provide you with nutritional information. A social worker will be able to direct you to support groups and community supports. If you are a diabetic you may want to make sure that you have an ophthalmologist and optometrist, a dentist and a podiatrist on your team. Build your team wisely based upon your research and try to coordinate your care with all the team members.
- **Be aware of your attitude and mental health.** It can directly impact your health and healing. Expect that there will be times when your mood is low and you may feel sad and hopeless. This is normal. Watch for the signs of depression and speak with your primary physician if you think you are depressed.
- **Build a support team and reach out.** Your medical team is not your only resource. Try joining a support group to talk about your concerns, problems and even things that are going well. By doing so you will not only be able to obtain additional information but you may be able to help someone else.
- **Gather information on local resources.** Many communities have agencies and services that can assist with managing day-to-day life. Some people with chronic conditions may need temporary assistance with transportation to the physician, help with the grocery shopping, errands or housekeeping, or even financial assistance paying for utilities. Being familiar with the agencies and services within your community will allow you to find and obtain assistance and additional support when it is needed.

- **Make those necessary lifestyle changes and be sure to include the entire family.** Lifestyle changes are never easy especially the ones that we feel "forced" to make because of a chronic condition. We all know those changes—changing your diet, quitting smoking, exercising, cutting out sugar. Studies have shown that individuals with chronic illness who make these changes are more likely to manage their illness successfully. Try including the family if at all possible. That way everyone will be adopting a healthier lifestyle.
- **Make those necessary legal and financial plans.** Discuss your situation with trusted individuals, legal counsel, and/or a financial advisor. These individuals can assist with plans that will best meet your individual needs. Doing this as early as possible will prevent additional stress during a crisis.

Conclusion

Upon learning of your diagnosis, you may have assumed the worst. A chronic condition presents challenges you have not planned for or may never have expected, but don't forget that you are in charge. There are many positive things you can do to maintain your health. Talk with your physician, friends, and family. Learn all you can do and enjoy each day as it comes.

Next Steps After Your Diagnosis: Finding Information and Support

Introduction

Your doctor* gave you a diagnosis that could change your life. This article can help you take the next steps.

Every person is different, of course, and every person's disease or condition will affect them differently. But research shows that after getting a diagnosis, many people have some of the same reactions and needs.

About this Article

Next Steps After Your Diagnosis offers general advice for people with almost any disease or condition. And it has tips to help you learn more about your specific problem and how it can be treated.

The information in this article is presented in a simple way to help you scan the material and read only what you need right now. Organizations, publications, and other resources are included if you would like to know more. The on-line version www.ahrq.gov/consumer/diaginfo.htm has many additional resources and their Internet links.

Five Basic Steps

This article describes five basic steps to help you cope with your diagnosis, make decisions, and get on with your life.

Step 1: Take the time you need.
Do not rush important decisions about your health. In most cases, you will have time to carefully examine your options and decide what is best for you.

Step 2: Get the support you need.
Look for support from family and friends, people who are going through the same thing you are, and those who have "been there." They can help you cope with your situation and make informed decisions.

* Your medical care might come from a doctor, nurse, physician assistant, or another kind of clinician or health care practitioner. To keep it simple, in this article we use the term "doctor" to refer to any of these professionals with whom you might interact.

Step 3: Talk with your doctor.

Good communication with your doctor can help you feel more satisfied with the care you receive. Research shows it can even have a positive effect on things such as symptoms and pain. Getting a "second opinion" may help you feel more confident about your care.

Step 4: Seek out information.

When learning about your health problem and its treatment, look for information that is based on a careful review of the latest scientific findings published in medical journals.

Step 5: Decide on a treatment plan.

Work with your doctor to decide on a treatment plan that best meets your needs.

As you take each step, remember this: Research shows that patients who are more involved in their health care tend to get better results and be more satisfied.

Step 1:
Take the time you need.

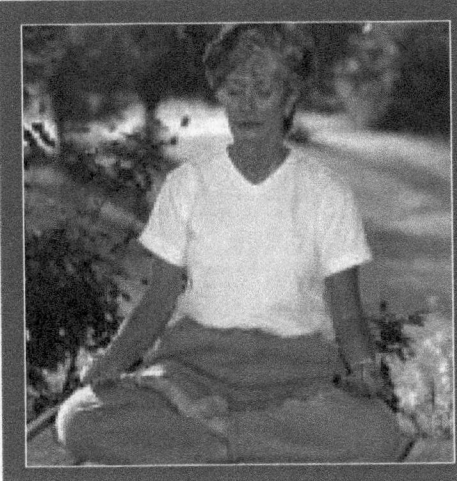

Take time to breathe. Don't panic, and don't feel pressured into making a rush decision.

Alexis, cancer survivor

A diagnosis can change your life in an instant.

Like so many other people in your situation, you might be feeling one or more of the following emotions after getting your diagnosis:

- Afraid
- Alone
- Angry
- Anxious
- Ashamed
- Confused
- Depressed
- Helpless
- In denial

- Numb
- Overwhelmed
- Panicky
- Powerless
- Relieved (that you finally know what's wrong)
- Sad
- Shocked
- Stressed

It is perfectly normal to have these feelings. It is also normal, and very common, to have trouble taking in and understanding information after you receive the news – especially if the diagnosis was a surprise. And it can be even harder to make decisions about treating or managing your disease or condition.

Take time to make your decisions.

No matter how the news of your diagnosis has affected you, do not rush into a decision. In most cases, you do not need to take action right away. Ask your doctor how much time you can safely take.

Taking the time you need to make decisions can help you:

- Feel less anxious and stressed.
- Avoid depression.
- Cope with your condition.
- Feel more in control of your situation.
- Play a key role in decisions about your treatment.

Step 2:
Get the support you need.

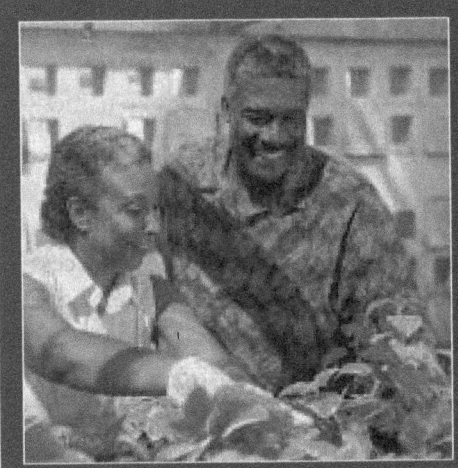

I was shocked when I was diagnosed with diabetes. The extra support I got from my friends and support group really helped me adjust to the new lifestyle I had to adopt.

Richard, person with diabetes

You do not have to go through it alone.

Sometimes the emotional side of illness can be just as hard to deal with as the physical side. You may have fears or concerns. You may feel overwhelmed. No matter what your situation, having other people to turn to will help you know you are not alone.

Here are the kinds of support you might want to seek:

▇ Family and friends.

Talking to family and friends you feel close to can help you cope with your illness or condition. Just knowing that someone is there can be a comfort.

Sometimes it is hard to ask for help. And sometimes your family and friends want to help, but they do not want to intrude, or they do not know how to ask or what to offer. Think about specific ways people can help you. One idea is to ask someone to come with you to a doctor's appointment to help ask questions, take notes, and talk with you afterward.

If you do not have family or friends who can provide support, other people or groups can.

■ Support or self-help groups.

Support groups are made up of people with the same disease or condition who get together to share information and concerns and to help one another. Support groups may or may not be led by experts. Self-help groups are similar to support groups but usually are led by the participants. The names "support group" and "self-help group" sometimes are used to refer to either kind.

Research on support groups shows that participants feel less anxious, experience less depression, have a better quality of life, and have more success coping with their disease or condition. Similar findings have been reported for self-help groups.

■ On-line support or self-help groups.

The Internet has support or self-help groups for people whose concerns and situations may be similar to yours. You can also find "message boards," where you can post questions and get answers. These on-line communities can help you connect with people who can give you support and provide information.

But be careful. Not every idea or treatment you come across in these groups will be scientifically proven to be safe and effective. If you read about something interesting and new, check it out with your doctor.

■ Counselor or therapist.

A good counselor or therapist can help you cope with sadness, depression, and feelings of being overwhelmed. If you think this kind of help might be right for you, ask your doctor or other health care professional to recommend someone in your area.

■ People like you.

You might want to meet and talk with someone in your own situation. Someone who has "been there" can talk about the real-life outcomes of their treatment choices as well as how they have learned to live with their disease or condition. Some advocacy or support groups can help you make this kind of contact.

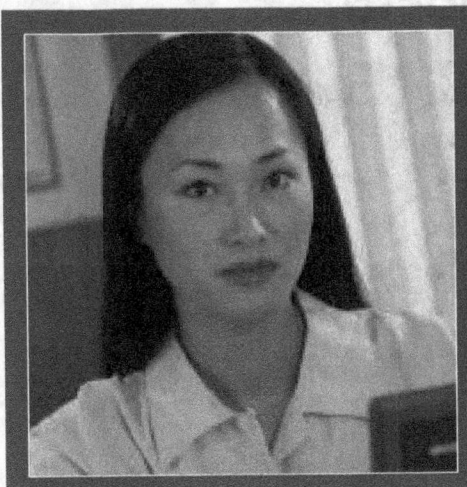

If only I had known what it would be like to live with the after-effects of this type of surgery, I might have chosen a different kind.

Susan, who underwent surgery for a digestive disease

Help is available.

Take advantage of the support that is available to you. See "Where to Find More Information" on page xxxiv for specific places to find support. An expanded list appears in the on-line version of this article at www.ahrq.gov/consumer/diaginfo.htm.

Step 3:
Talk with your doctor.

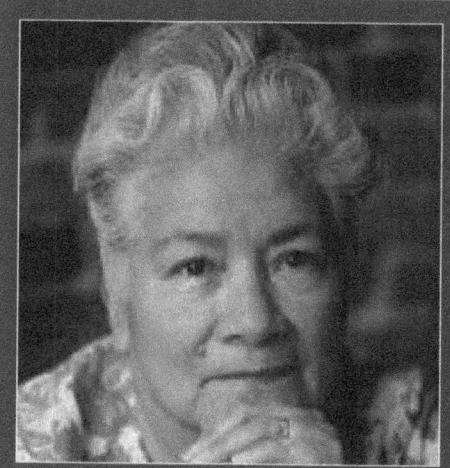

I had trouble under-standing what my doctor was telling me. The words were too technical, and there was too much to absorb. I finally asked her to slow down and keep it simple. That helped a lot.

Dana, person with heart disease

Your doctor is your partner in health care.

You probably have many questions about your disease or condition. The first person to ask is your doctor.

It is fine to seek more information from other sources; in fact, it is important to do so. But consider your doctor your partner in health care—someone who can discuss your situation with you, explain your options, and help you make decisions that are right for you.

It is not always easy to feel comfortable around doctors. But research has shown that good communication with your doctor can actually be good for your health. It can help you to:

- Feel more satisfied with the care you receive.

- Have better outcomes (end results), such as reduced pain and better recovery from symptoms.

Being an active member of your health care team also helps to reduce your chances of medical mistakes, and it helps you get high-quality care.

Of course, good communication is a two-way street. Here are some ways to help make the most of the time you spend with your doctor.

Prepare for your visit.

- Think about what you want to get out of your appointment. Write down all your questions and concerns. Some suggested questions are listed on page xxix.

- Prepare and bring to your doctor visit a list of all the medicines you take.

- Consider bringing along a trusted relative or friend. This person can help ask questions, take notes, and help you remember and understand everything once you leave the doctor's office.

Give information to your doctor.

- Do not wait to be asked.

- Tell your doctor everything he or she needs to know about your health— even the things that might make you feel embarrassed or uncomfortable.

- Tell your doctor how you are feeling—both physically and emotionally.

- Tell your doctor if you are feeling depressed or overwhelmed.

Get information from your doctor.

- Ask questions about anything that concerns you. Keep asking until you understand the answers. If you do not, your doctor may think you understand everything that is said.

- Ask your doctor to draw pictures if that will help you understand something.

- Take notes.

- Tape record your doctor visit, if that will be helpful to you. But first ask your doctor if this is okay.

- Ask your doctor to recommend resources such as Web sites, booklets, or tapes with more information about your disease or condition.

Also see "Ten Important Questions to Ask Your Doctor After a Diagnosis," on page xxvii.

Do not hesitate to seek a second opinion.

A second opinion is when another doctor examines your medical records and gives his or her views about your condition and how it should be treated. You might want a second opinion to:

- Be clear about what you have.
- Know all of your treatment choices.
- Have another doctor look at your choices with you.

It is not pushy or rude to want a second opinion. Most doctors will understand that you need more information before making important decisions about your health.

Check to see whether your health plan covers a second opinion. In some cases, health plans require second opinions.

Here are some ways to find a doctor for a second opinion:

- Ask your doctor. Request someone who does not work in the same office, because doctors who work together tend to share similar views.
- Contact your health plan or your local hospital, medical society, or medical school.
- Use the Doctor Finder on-line service of the American Medical Association at www.ama-assn.org.

Get information about next steps.

- Get the results of any tests or procedures. Discuss the meaning of these results with your doctor.
- Make sure you understand what will happen if you need surgery.
- Talk with your doctor about which hospital is best for your health care needs.

Finally, if you are not satisfied with your doctor, you can do two things: (1) talk with your doctor and try to work things out, and/or (2) switch doctors, if you are able to. It is very important to feel confident about your care.

To learn more, see "Where to Find More Information" on page xxxiv. The online version of this article includes additional resources.

Ten Important Questions to Ask Your Doctor After a Diagnosis

These 10 basic questions can help you understand your disease or condition, how it might be treated, and what you need to know and do before making treatment decisions.

1. What is the technical name of my disease or condition, and what does it mean in plain English?

   _____

2. What is my prognosis (outlook for the future)?

   _____

3. How soon do I need to make a decision about treatment?

   _____

4. Will I need any additional tests, and if so what kind and when?

   _____

5. What are my treatment options?

   _____

6. What are the pros and cons of my treatment options?

   _____

7. Is there a clinical trial (research study) that is right for me?
   (See page xxiv.)

   _____

8. Now that I have this diagnosis, what changes will I need to make in my daily life?

   _____

9. What organizations do you recommend for support and information?

   _____

10. What resources (booklets, Web sites, audiotapes, videos, DVDs, etc.) do you recommend for further information?

    _____

Step 4:
Seek out information.

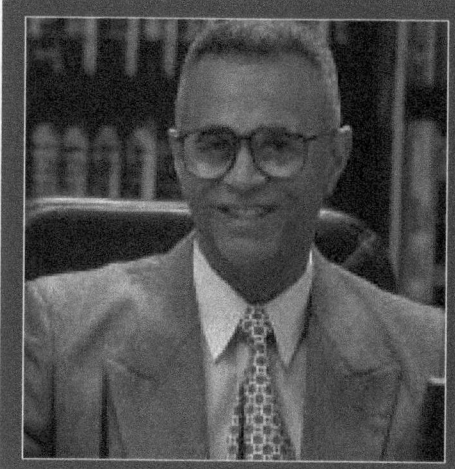

I'm really glad I took the time to research my options. It stopped me from jumping into a treatment that would have been completely wrong for me.

Seth, prostate cancer survivor

Now that you know your treatment options, you can learn which ones are backed up by the best scientific evidence. "Evidence-based" information— that is, information that is based on a careful review of the latest scientific findings in medical journals—can help you make decisions about the best possible treatments for you.

Evidence-based information comes from research on people like you.

Evidence-based information about treatments generally comes from two major types of scientific studies:

- **Clinical trials** are research studies on human volunteers to test new drugs or other treatments. Participants are randomly assigned to different treatment groups. Some get the research treatment, and others get a standard treatment or may be given a placebo (a medicine that has no effect), or no treatment. The results are compared to learn whether the new treatment is safe and effective.

- **Outcomes research** looks at the impact of treatments and other health care on health outcomes (end results) for patients and populations. End results include effects that people care about, such as changes in their quality of life.

Take advantage of the evidence-based information that is available.

Health information is everywhere—in books, newspapers, and magazines, and on the Internet, television, and radio. However, not all information is good information. Your best bets for sources of evidence-based information include the Federal Government, national nonprofit organizations, medical specialty groups, medical schools, and university medical centers.

Some resources are listed below, grouped by type of information. See "Where to Find More Information" on page xxxiv for additional ideas. The online version of Next Steps After Your Diagnosis lists many more, and includes links to Internet sites.

■ Information.

Information about your disease or condition and its treatment is available from many sources. Here are some of the most reliable:

- **healthfinder®**: www.healthfinder.gov/organizations/OrgListing.asp
  The healthfinder® site—sponsored by the U.S. Department of Health and Human Services—offers carefully selected health information Web sites from government agencies, clearinghouses, nonprofit groups, and universities.

- **Health Information Resource Database:**
  www.health.gov/nhic/#Referrals
  Sponsored by the National Health Information Center, this database includes 1,400 organizations and government offices that provide health information upon request. Information is also available over the telephone at 800-336-4797.

- **MEDLINEplus®**: www.nlm.nih.gov/medlineplus
  MedlinePlus® has extensive information from the National Institutes of Health and other trusted sources on over 650 diseases and conditions. The site includes many additional features.

- **National nonprofit groups** such as the American Heart Association, American Cancer Society, and American Diabetes Association can be valuable sources of reliable information. Many have chapters nationwide. Check your phone book for a local chapter in your community. The Health Information Resource Database (www.health.gov/nhic/#Referrals) can help you find national offices of nonprofit groups.

- **Health or medical libraries** run by government, hospitals, professional groups, and other reliable organizations often welcome consumers. For a list of libraries in your area, go to the MedlinePlus® "Find a Library" page at http://www.nlm.nih.gov/medlineplus/libraries.html.

Current medical research.

You can find the latest medical research in medical journals at your local health or medical library, and in some cases, on the Internet. Here are two major online sources of medical articles:

- **MEDLINE/PubMed®:** http://www.ncbi.nlm.nih.gov/entrez/query.fcgi PubMed® is the National Library of Medicine's database of references to more than 14 million articles published in 4,800 medical and scientific journals. All of the listings have information to help you find the articles at a health or medical library. Many listings also have short summaries of the article (abstracts), and some have links to the full article. The article might be free, or it might require a fee charged by the publisher.

- **PubMed Central:** http://www.pubmedcentral.nih.gov/ PubMed Central is the National Library of Medicine's database of journal articles that are available free of charge to users.

Clinical trials.

Perhaps you wonder whether there is a clinical trial that is right for you. Or you may want to learn about results from previous clinical trials that might be relevant to your situation. Here are two reliable resources:

- **ClinicalTrials.gov:** http://clinicaltrials.gov/ct/g ClinicalTrials.gov provides regularly updated information about federally and privately supported clinical research on people who volunteer to participate. The site has information about a trial's purpose, who may participate, locations, and phone numbers for more details. The site also describes the clinical trial process and includes news about recent clinical trial results.

- **Cochrane Collaboration:** www.cochrane.org The Cochrane Collaboration writes summaries ("reviews") about evidence from clinical trials to help people make informed decisions. You can search and read the review abstracts free of charge at http://www.cochrane.org/

reviews/index.htm. Or you can read plain-English consumer summaries of the reviews at www.informedhealthonline.org.

The full Cochrane reviews are available only by subscription. Check with your local medical or health library (see page xxxvi) [link back to library section in on-line version] to see whether you can access the full reviews there.

▬ Outcomes research.

Outcomes research provides research about benefits, risks, and outcomes (end results) of treatments so that patients and their doctors can make better informed decisions. The U.S. Agency for Healthcare Research and Quality (AHRQ) supports improvements in health outcomes through research, and sponsors products that result from research such as:

- **National Guideline Clearinghouse™:** www.guideline.gov
  The National Guideline Clearinghouse™ is a database of evidence-based clinical practice guidelines and related documents. Clinical practice guidelines are documents designed to help doctors and patients make decisions about appropriate health care for specific diseases or conditions. The clearinghouse was originally created by AHRQ in partnership with the American Medical Association and America's Health Insurance Plans.

Steer clear of deceptive ads and information.

While searching for information either on or off the Internet, beware of "miracle" treatments and cures. They can cost you money and your health, especially if you delay or refuse proper treatment. Here are some tip-offs that a product truly is too good to be true:

- Phrases such as "scientific breakthrough," "miraculous cure," "exclusive product," "secret formula," or "ancient ingredient."

- Claims that the product treats a wide range of ailments.

- Use of impressive-sounding medical terms. These often cover up a lack of good science behind the product.

- Case histories from consumers claiming "amazing" results.

- Claims that the product is available from only one source, and for a limited time only.

- Claims of a "money-back guarantee."
- Claims that others are trying to keep the product off the market.
- Ads that fail to list the company's name, address, or other contact information.

To learn more about finding evidence-based information, see "Where to Find More Information," page xxxiv. The on-line edition of this article has many additional resources.

Step 5:
Decide on a treatment plan.

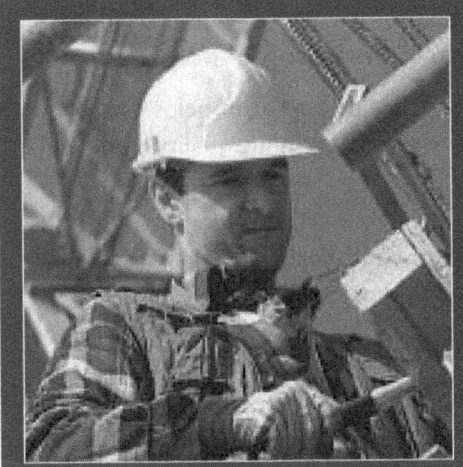

My doctor told me I had done one of the hardest but most important things a patient has to do: Face up to the diagnosis and make decisions. It feels good to be where I am now.

Bob, person with a
neurological disorder

At this point, you have learned about your disease or condition and how it can be treated or managed. Your information may have come from the following sources:

- Your doctor.

- Second opinions from one or more other doctors.

- Other people who are or were in the same situation as you.

- Information sources such as Web sites, health or medical libraries, and nonprofit groups.

Work with your doctor to make decisions.

When you are ready to make treatment decisions, you and your doctor can discuss:

- Which treatments have been found to work well, or not work well, for your particular condition.

- The pros and cons of each treatment option.

Make sure that your doctor knows your preferences and feelings about the different treatments – for example, whether you prefer medicine over surgery.

Once you and your doctor decide on one or more treatments that are right for you, you can work together to develop a treatment plan. This plan will include everything that will be done to treat or manage your disease or condition—including what you need to do to make the plan work.

Remember, being an active member of your health care team helps to reduce your chances of medical mistakes, and it helps you get high-quality care.

Take another deep breath.

You have taken important steps to cope with your diagnosis, make decisions, and get on with your life. Remember two things:

- Call on others for support as you need it.

- Make use of evidence-based information for any future health decisions.

Where to Find More Information

Get the support you need.

American Self-Help Group Clearinghouse
http://mentalhelp.net/selfhelp/

National Board for Certified Counselors (NBCC)
3 Terrace Way, Suite D
Greensboro, NC 27403-3660
336-547-0607.
www.nbcc.org

National Institute of Mental Health
Public Information and Communications Branch
6001 Executive Boulevard, Room 8184, MSC 9663
Bethesda, MD 20892-9663
Phone: 866-615-6464 (toll-free)
TTY: 301-443-8431
http://www.nimh.nih.gov/HealthInformation/GettingHelp.cfm

Talk to your doctor.

Be an Active Member of Your Health Care Team. Food and Drug Administration. 2004. http://www.fda.gov/cder/consumerinfo/active_member.htm. Phone: 888-INFO-FDA (888-463-6332).

Be Informed: Questions to Ask Your Doctor Before You Have Surgery. Agency for Healthcare Quality and Research. 1995. http://www.ahrq.gov/consumer/surgery.htm. Phone: 800-358-9295.

Five Steps to Safer Health Care. Agency for Healthcare Research and Quality. 2003. http://www.ahrq.gov/consumer/5steps.htm. Phone: 800-358-9295.

Getting a Second Opinion Before Surgery. Centers for Medicare & Medicaid Services. 2004. www.medicare.gov/Publications/Pubs/pdf/02173.pdf. Phone: 800-MEDICARE (800-633-4227).

How to Get a Second Opinion. National Women's Health Information Center. 2003. http://www.4woman.gov/pub/secondopinion.htm. Phone: 1-800-994-WOMAN.

Quick Tips – When Planning for Surgery. Agency for Healthcare Research and Quality. 2002. http://www.ahrq.gov/consumer/quicktips/tipsurgery.htm. Phone: 800-358-9295.

Quick Tips – When Talking with Your Doctor. Agency for Healthcare Research and Quality. 2002. http://www.ahrq.gov/consumer/quicktips/doctalk.htm. Phone: 800-358-9295.

Talking with Your Doctor: A Guide for Older People. National Institute on Aging. 2002. www.niapublications.org/pubs/talking/index.asp. Phone: 800-222-2225.

Seek out information.

2005 Toll-Free Numbers for Health Information. National Health Information Center. www.health.gov/nhic/pubs/tollfree.htm. Phone: 800-336-4797.

AARP Health Guide. AARP. 2004. www.aarp.org/health/healthguide. Phone: 888-OUR-AARP (888-687-2277).

HON Code of Conduct (HONcode) for Medical and Health Web Sites Health on the Net Foundation. http://www.hon.ch/HONcode/

How to Evaluate Health Information on the Internet: Questions and Answers. National Cancer Institute. 2003. http://cis.nci.nih.gov/fact/2_10.htm. Phone: 800-4-CANCER (800-422-6237).

How to Find Medical Information. National Institute of Arthritis and Musculoskeletal and Skin Diseases. 2001. http://www.niams.nih.gov/hi/topics/howto/howto.htm. Phone: 877-22-NIAMS (877-226-4267) (toll-free).

JAMA Patient Page: Health Information on the Internet. The Medem Network. http://www.medem.com/medlb/article_detaillb.cfm?article_ID=ZZZLJLLLTMC&sub_cat=603

National Guideline Clearinghouse™. Agency for Healthcare Research and Quality. http://www.guideline.gov/

NOAH: New York Online Access to Health. http://www.noah-health.org/

A User's Guide to Finding and Evaluating Health Information on the Web. Medical Library Association. 2003. http://www.mlanet.org/resources/userguide.html#1

Virtual Treatments Can Be Real-World Deceptions. Federal Trade Commission. 2001. http://www.ftc.gov/bcp/conline/pubs/alerts/mrclalrt.htm

Your Guide to Choosing Quality Health Care. Agency for Healthcare Research and Quality. 2002. http://www.ahrq.gov/consumer/qntool.htm. Phone: 800-358-9295.

AHRQ consumer publications:

20 Tips to Help Prevent Medical Errors—Practical tips and questions to ask. (AHRQ 00-P038)

20 Tips to Help Prevent Medical Errors in Children (AHRQ 02-P034)

Five Steps to Safer Health Care—Shorter version of 20 Tips. (AHRQ 03-M007)

Ways You Can Help Your Family Prevent Medical Errors!—Easy-to-read version, with drawings. (AHRQ 01-0017)

Your Guide to Choosing Quality Health Care—Based on research about the information people want and need when choosing health plans, doctors, treatments, hospitals, and long-term care. (AHRQ 99-012)

Improving Health Care Quality: A Guide for Patients and Their Families—Short version of *Your Guide to Choosing Quality Health Care*. (AHRQ 01-0004)

Quick Checks for Quality—Checklist to use when choosing health plans, doctors, treatments, hospitals, and long-term care. (AHRQ 99-R027)

Quick Tips:
　　When Getting Medical Tests (AHRQ 01-0040b)
　　When Getting a Prescription (AHRQ 01-0040c)
　　When Planning for Surgery (AHRQ 01-0040d)
　　When Talking with Your Doctor (AHRQ 01-0040a)

To order AHRQ publications:

For electronic copies of these publications, go to the AHRQ Web site at www.ahrq.gov/consumer

For print copies, contact the AHRQ Publications Clearinghouse at 800-358-9295.

Next Steps After Your Diagnosis. October 2012. Agency for Healthcare Research and Quality, Rockville, MD.
http://www.ahrq.gov/patients-consumers/diagnosis-treatment/diagnosis/diaginfo/index.html

Description

1 Addison's Disease

Addison's disease is a rare disorder that stems from the malfunction of the adrenal glands located on top of the kidneys. In this disease, there is a deficiency of hormones produced by the adrenal cortex, the gland's firm outer layer. Most often, Addison's disease results from destruction of the adrenal gland. This glandular destruction may result from unusual infections, malignant tumors, an autoimmune process or other rare disorders. At least half of all cases of Addison's disease result from patient's developing antibodies against their own adrenal tissue (autoimmune process).

There can be increased water excretion in the urine and lowered blood pressure, which can lead to severe dehydration and other major complications. The symptoms of Addison's disease increase with the progression of the disease. Early signs may include fatigue, loss of appetite, low blood pressure (hypotension), weakness and significant loss from the kidneys of water and minerals. Other symptoms may include darkened scars and skin folds, as well as dark freckles on the head and shoulders. In the later stages, nausea may develop, as well as dizziness, further dehydration, low blood sugar (hypoglycemia) and mental changes including confusion.

Patients who are treated early have an excellent prognosis, but it is imperative that treatment be instituted immediately and vigorously. In order to counteract the hormonal loss, physicians prescribe steroid hormone replacement therapy. Certain doses of hormones need to be increased during times of illness and surgery. Treatment should never be stopped, even for a day, without the advice of a physician. Persons on treatment should wear an alert bracelet to let emergency medical providers know of their diagnosis.

National Agencies & Associations

2 American Association of Endocrine Surgeons
11300 W. Olympic Blvd
Los Angeles, CA 90064
310-986-6452
Fax: 310-437-0585
e-mail: information@endocrinesurgery.org
www.endocrinesurgery.org
The American Association of Endocrine Surgeons (AAES) is dedicated to the advancement of the science and art of endocrine surgery.
Stacy Kent, Executive Director
Diana Munoz, Administrative Assistant

3 Endocrine Society
8401 Connecticut Avenue
Chevy Chase, MD 20815
301-941-0200
888-363-6274
Fax: 301-941-0259
e-mail: societyservices@endo-society.org
www.endo-society.org
Source of state-of-the-art research and clinical advancements in endocrinology and metabolism. Dedicated to promoting excellence in research education and clinical practice in the field of endocrinology. Prime advocate and integrative force for clinicians.
Teresa K. Woodruff, Ph.D., President
Richard J. Santen, M.D., President-Elect

4 Hypoparathyroidism Association
P.O. Box 2258
Idaho Falls, 83403
208-524-3857
866-213-0394
e-mail: jsanders@hypopara.org
www.hypopara.org
The HypoPARathyroidism Association is an non-profit patient organization working to improve lives touched by hypoparathyroidism, a rare medical disorder in which the parathyroid glands fail to produce sufficient amounts of the parathyroid hormone.
James Sanders, President
Julie Hunsaker, Vice-President

5 National Adrenal Diseases Foundation
505 Northern Boulevard
Great Neck, NY 11021
516-487-4992
Fax: 516-829-5710
e-mail: nadfsupport@nadf.us
www.nadf.us
Nonprofit organization dedicated to offer support information and research for individuals having diseases of the adrenal glands. Goals of the organization include assisting patients through informational and educational activities as well as support programs.
Paul Margulies, M.D., FACP, F, Medical Director
Melanie G Wong, Executive Director

6 National Institute of Diabetes & Digestive & Kidney Diseases
National Institutes of Health
31 Center Drive
Bethesda, MD 20892-2560
301-496-3583
800-860-8747
Fax: 703-738-4929
e-mail: ndic@info.niddk.nih.gov
www.diabetes.niddk.nih.gov
Conducts and supports research on many of the most serious diseases affecting public health. The Institute supports much of the clinical research on the diseases of internal medicine and related subspecialty fields as well as many basic science disciplines.
Griffin P. Rodgers, M.D., M.A.C.P., Director

7 Pediatric Endocrine Society
6728 Old McLean Vg. Dr.
McLean, VA 22101
703-556-9222
Fax: 703-556-8729
e-mail: info@pedsendo.org
www.pedsendo.org
The home for Pediatric Endocrinologists & those seeking care for Children with Endocrine Disorders.
Mitchell E. Geffner, President
Karen Rubin, Treasurer

Support Groups & Hotlines

8 National Health Information Center
PO Box 1133
Washington, DC 20013
310-565-4167
800-336-4797
Fax: 301-984-4256
e-mail: info@nhic.org
www.health.gov/nhic
Offers a nationwide information referral service, produces directories and resource guides.

Magazines

9 Endocrine News
Endocrine Society
2055 L Street NW
Washington, DC 20036
202-971-3636
888-363-6274
Fax: 202-971-3646
e-mail: societyservices@endo-society.org
www.endo-society.org
Endocrine News is the source of trends and insights for members of the endocrine community.
Monthly
Kelly E Mayo PhD, President
Scott Hunt, Executive Director

Newsletters

10 **Addison News**
6142 Territorial
Pleasant Lake, MI 49272   www2.dmci.net/users/hoffmanrj

11 **NADF News**
National Adrenal Diseases Foundation
505 Northern Boulevard   516-487-4992
Great Neck, NY 11021   Fax: 516-829-5710
                               e-mail: nadfsupport@nadf.us
                                       www.nadf.us
Contains information on the latest research, question and answer
column by an endocrinologist and helpful hints for those with Ad-
dison's Disease.
Quarterly Monthly
Melanie G Wong, Executive Director
Debbie Benish, Editor

Web Sites

12 **Healing Well**
                                       www.healingwell.com
An online health resource guide to medical news, chat, information and articles, newsgroups and message boards, books, disease-related web sites, medical directories, and more for patients,
friends, and family coping with disabling diseases, disorders, or
chronic illnesses.

13 **Health Finder**
                                       www.healthfinder.gov
A government Web site where you will find information and tools
to help you and those you care about stay healthy.

14 **Health Link USA**
                                       www.healthlinkusa.com
Discussion forum for treatments, symptoms and causes of 700
health conditions, diseases and topics.

15 **Helios Health**
                                       www.helioshealth.com
Online resource for your health information. Detailed information
about specific health topics, access to expert advice from our Medical Advisory Board, and up-to-date health news.

16 **Hormone Foundation**
                                       www.hormone.org
Educational resource for you, your loved ones, and your health
professionals on the prevention, treatment, and cure of hor-
mone-related conditions.

17 **MedicineNet**
                                       www.medicinenet.com
An online resource for consumers providing easy-to-read, authoritative medical and health information.

18 **Medscape**
                                       www.medscape.com
Search engine providing links to websites with information on illnesses, diseases and disorders.

19 **National Adrenal Disease Foundation**
                                       www.nadf.us
Non-profit organization dedicated to providing support, information and education to individuals having Addison's disease as well
as other diseases of the adrenal glands.

20 **WebMD**
                                       www.webmd.com
Provides credible information, supportive communities, and
in-depth reference material about health subjects. A source for
original and timely health information as well as material from
well known content providers.

Description

21

Aging

The elderly population in the United States is growing faster than any other segment of the population, and has done so since 1900. It is estimated that this trend will continue at least through the year 2050. In 2004, there were 36.3 million people in the U.S. One in eight persons is over 85 years, classified as 'old old.' By 2040, it is anticipated that one person in five will exceed 65 years of age, and the number of people over 85 will increase to four times their number today, representing the aging of the baby boomers.

Aging is not a disease, but part of the normal life cycle, and many seniors retain good health and live independently for long past the traditional age of retirement. In time, however, most will develop one or more chronic conditions; for those over 75 years of age, the most common conditions are hypertension, heart disease, hearing loss, arthritis, and cataracts. By the year 2030, 150 million Americans are expected to have a chronic condition, and 42 million will be limited in their ability to work or live independently. Treating this population will require many medical and nonmedical services, integrated to provide a comprehensive continuum of care. See also *Alzheimer's Disease.*

National Agencies & Associations

22

American Association of Retired Persons
601 E Street NW
Washington, DC 20049
888-687-2277
TTY: 877-434-7598
e-mail: member@aarp.org
www.aarp.org
AARP is the nation's leading organization for people age 50 and older. It serves their needs and interests through information and education, advocacy and community services provided by a network of local chapters and experienced volunteers.
Barry Rand, CEO
Robert G Romasco, President

23

Commission on Accreditation of Rehabilitation Services
6951 E Southpoint Road
Tucson, AZ 85756
520-325-1044
888-281-6531
Fax: 520-318-1129
carf.org
CARF reviews and grants accreditation services nationally and internationally at the request of a facility or program. Their standards are rigorous, so those services that meet them are among the best available.
Brian J. Boon, President/CEO
Amanda E. Birch, Adminsterator of Operations

24

Gerontological Society of America
1220 L Street NW
Washington, DC 20005
202-842-1275
Fax: 202-842-1150
e-mail: geron@geron.org
www.geron.org
Nonprofit professional organization with more than 5000 members in the field of aging. Provides researchers, educators, practitioners and policy makers with opportunities to understand, advance, integrate and use basic and applied research on aging populations.
Rita B. Effros, President
Suzanne R. Kunkel, Treasurer

25

Institute for Life Course and Aging
263 McCaul St.
Toronto, Ontario, M5T1W-3J1
416-978-0377
Fax: 416-978-4771
e-mail: aging@utoronto.ca
www.aging.utoronto.ca
The Institute is a research center under the auspices of the School of Graduate Studies at the University of Toronto.
Dr. Lynn McDonald, PhD., Director
Susan Murphy, Administration

26

International Federation on Aging
351 Christie Street
Toronto, Ontario, M6GC6-3C3
416-342-1655
Fax: 416-392-4157
e-mail: jbarratt@ifa-fiv.org
www.ifa-fiv.org
To inform, educate and promote policies and practice to improve the quality of life of older persons around the world.
Greg Shaw, Director, International & Corporate Rela
Dr. Jane Barratt, Secretory General

27

Leading Age
2519 Connecticut Avenue NW
Washington, DC 20008-1520
202-783-2242
Fax: 202-783-2255
e-mail: info@LeadingAge.org
www.leadingage.org/?
National association of more than 4 000 nonprofit nursing homes continuing care retirement communities independent living centers and community service providers serving more than 60,000 older Americans each year.
William L Minnix Jr, President and CEO
Katrinka Smith Sloan, COO and SVP Member Services

28

National Council on Aging
1901 L Street NW
Washington, DC 20036
202-479-1200
Fax: 202-479-0735
TTY: 202-479-6674
TDD: 202-479-6674
e-mail: info@ncoa.org
www.ncoa.org
The nation's first charitable organization dedicated to promoting the dignity, independence, well-being and contributions of older Americans. NCOA serves as a national voice and powerful advocate on behalf of older Americans.
James P Firman EdD, President/CEO
Jay Greenberg, Vice President

29

Problems of the Elderly Committee
1050 Connecticut Avenue
Washington, DC 20003-1019
202-662-1000
Fax: 202-662-1501
e-mail: crimjustice@abanet.org
www.abanet.org/crimjust
This Committee examines the issues that affect the elderly as victims of street crime, identity theft, financial exploitation and other crimes of which they are targets. The committee looks at issues arising from the aging prisons populations and the elders as perpetrators of crime, also.
Laurel G. Bellows, President
Robert M. Carlson, Chair Person

30

Senior Resource
4521 Campus Drive
Irvine, CA 92612
858-793-7901
877-793-7901
Fax: 858-792-9080
e-mail: questions@seniorresource.com
www.seniorresource.com
An agency that helps seniors to understand aging and gives different resources consisting of sociologic changes; metabolic changes; positive aging; and physical changes.
Bryan D Hatchell, Chair

31

US Administration on Aging
1 Massachusetts Avenue
Washington, DC 20001
202-619-0724
Fax: 202-357-3555
e-mail: aclinfo@acl.hhs.gov
www.aoa.gov
The Administration on Aging an agency in the US Department of Health and Human Services is one of the nation's largest providers

of home and community-based care for older persons and their caregivers.
Kathy Greenlee, Administrator
Sharon Lewis, Acting Principal Deputy

State Agencies & Associations

Alaska

32 **AARP Alaska State Office**
3601 C Street
Anchorage, AK 99503
866-227-7447
Fax: 907-341-2270
e-mail: ak@aarp.org
www.aarp.org/states/ak
AARP is a nonprofit nonpartisan membership organization for people age 50 and over. AARP is dedicated to enhancing the quality of life as one ages, in addition to facilitating social change and delivering value to members through information and advocacy.
Fred Jenkins, Development Director
George Hieronymus, AARP Alaska State President

Arizona

33 **AARP Arizona: Phoenix Collier Center**
Collier Center
201 E Washington Street
Phoenix, AZ 85004-2428
866-389-5649
Fax: 602-256-2928
e-mail: azaarp@aarp.org
www.aarp.org/states/az
AARP is a nonprofit nonpartisan membership organization for people age 50 and over. AARP is dedicated to enhancing the quality of life as one ages, in addition to facilitating social change and delivering value to members through information and advocacy.
Leonard J Kirschner PhD, Arizona AARP State President
David Mitchell, Arizona AARP State Director

Arkansas

34 **AARP Arkansas State Office: Little Rock**
1701 Centerview Drive
Little Rock, AR 72211
866-544-5379
Fax: 501-227-7710
e-mail: araarp@aarp.org
www.aarp.org/states/ar
AARP is a nonprofit nonpartisan membership organization for people age 50 and over. AARP is dedicated to enhancing the quality of life as one ages, in addition to facilitating social change and delivering value to members through information and advocacy.
Mary Dillard, Arkansas AARP State President
Pat Jones, Arkansas AARP State Media Relations

California

35 **AARP California State Office: Pasadena**
200 S Los Robles Avenue
Pasadena, CA 91101-2422
866-448-3615
Fax: 626-583-8500
e-mail: calosangeles@aarp.org
www.aarp.org/states/ca
AARP is a nonprofit nonpartisan membership organization for people age 50 and over. AARP is dedicated to enhancing the quality of life as one ages, in addition to facilitating social change and delivering value to members through information and advocacy.
Helen Russ, California AARP State President
Thomas A Porter, California AARP State Director

36 **AARP California State Office: Sacramento**
1415 L Street
Sacramento, CA 95814
866-448-3614
Fax: 916-446-2223
e-mail: casacramento@aarp.org
www.aarp.org/states/ca
AARP is a nonprofit nonpartisan membership organization for people age 50 and over. AARP is dedicated to enhancing the qual-

ity of life as one ages, in addition to facilitating social change and delivering value to members through information and advocacy.
Helen Russ, California State AARP President
Thomas A Porter, California State AARP Director

Colorado

37 **AARP Colorado State Office: Denver**
303 E 17th Avenue
Denver, CO 80203-5012
866-554-5376
Fax: 303-764-5999
e-mail: coaarp@aarp.org
www.aarp.org/states/co
AARP is a nonprofit nonpartisan membership organization for people age 50 and over. AARP is dedicated to enhancing the quality of life as one ages, in addition to facilitating social change and delivering value to members through information and advocacy.
Robert Martinez, Colorado AARP State President
Jon Looney, Colorado AARP State Director

Florida

38 **AARP Florida State Office: St. Petersburg**
400 Carillon Parkway
Saint Petersburg, FL 33716
866-595-7678
Fax: 727-369-5191
TTY: 727-561-9544
e-mail: flaarp@aarp.org
www.aarp.org/states/fl
AARP is a nonprofit nonpartisan membership organization for people age 50 and over. AARP is dedicated to enhancing the quality of life as one ages, in addition to facilitating social change and delivering value to members through information and advocacy.
Kathy Marma, Florida AARP State Media Relations
Thomas Thame MD, Florida AARP State Board of Directors

39 **Goodwill Industries-Suncoast**
Goodwill Industries-Suncoast
10596 Gandy Boulevard
St. Petersburg, FL 33702
727-523-1512
888-279-1988
Fax: 727-563-9300
TTY: 727-579-1068
e-mail: gw.marketing@goodwill-suncoast.org
www.goodwill-suncoast.org
A nonprofit, community-based organization whose mission is to help people achieve self-sufficiency through the dignity and power of work, serving people who are disadvantaged, disabled or elderly. The mission is accomplished through providing independent living skills, affordable housing, and training and placement in community employment.
Jay Mc Cloe, Director Resource Development

Georgia

40 **AARP Georgia: Atlanta**
999 Peachtree Street NE
Atlanta, GA 30309-4421
866-295-7281
Fax: 404-881-6997
e-mail: gaaarp@aarp.org
www.aarp.org/states/ga
AARP is a nonprofit nonpartisan membership organization for people age 50 and over. AARP is dedicated to enhancing the quality of life as one ages, in addition to facilitating social change and delivering value to members through information and advocacy.
Matthew McWilliams, Georgia AARP State Media Relations
Will Phillips, AARP Georgia Associate State Director

Hawaii

41 **AARP Hawaii State Office: Honolulu**
1132 Bishop Street
Honolulu, HI 96813
808-843-1906
866-295-7282
Fax: 808-843-1908
e-mail: oahuaarp@hawaii.rr.com
www.aarp.org/states/hi
AARP is a nonprofit nonpartisan membership organization for people age 50 and over. AARP is dedicated to enhancing the qual-

ity of life as one ages, in addition to facilitating social change and delivering value to members through information and advocacy.
Stuart TK Ho, AARP Hawaii Interim State President
Barbara Kim Stanton, Hawaii AARP State Director

Idaho

42 **AARP Idaho State Office: Meridian**
3830 E Gentry Way
Meridian, ID 83642   866-295-7284
                                        Fax: 208-288-4424
                                   e-mail: aarpid@aarp.org
                                   www.aarp.org/states/id
AARP is a nonprofit nonpartisan membership organization for people age 50 and over. AARP is dedicated to enhancing the quality of life as one ages, in addition to facilitating social change and delivering value to members through information and advocacy.
Cheryl Tussey, Idaho AARP State Media Relations
Jim Wordelman, AARP Idaho State Director

Illinois

43 **AARP Illinois State Office: Chicago**
222 N LaSalle Street
Chicago, IL 60601-1033   866-448-3613
                                        Fax: 312-372-2204
                                   e-mail: aarpil@aarp.org
                                   www.aarp.org/states/il
AARP is a nonprofit nonpartisan membership organization for people age 50 and over. AARP is dedicated to enhancing the quality of life as one ages, in addition to facilitating social change and delivering value to members through information and advocacy.
Evelyn Gooden, Illinois AARP State President
Gerardo Cardenas, Illinois AARP State Media Relations

Indiana

44 **AARP Indiana State Office: Indianapolis**
One N Capitol Avenue
Indianapolis, IN 46204-2025   866-448-3618
                                        Fax: 317-423-2211
                                   e-mail: inaarp@aarp.org
                                   www.aarp.org/states/in
AARP is a nonprofit nonpartisan membership organization for people age 50 and over. AARP is dedicated to enhancing the quality of life as one ages, in addition to facilitating social change and delivering value to members through information and advocacy.
Martin DeAgostino, Indiana AARP State Media Relations
June Lyle, AARP Indiana State Director

Iowa

45 **AARP Iowa State Office: Des Moines**
600 E Court Avenue
Des Moines, IA 50309   866-554-5378
                                        Fax: 515-244-7767
                                   e-mail: iaaarp@aarp.org
                                   www.aarp.org/states/ia
AARP is a nonprofit nonpartisan membership organization for people age 50 and over. AARP is dedicated to enhancing the quality of life as one ages, in addition to facilitating social change and delivering value to members through information and advocacy.
Ann Black, Iowa AARP State Media Relations
Bruce Koeppl, Iowa AARP State Director

Kansas

46 **AARP Kansas State Office: Topeka**
555 S Kansas
Topeka, KS 66603   866-448-3619
                                        Fax: 785-232-8259
                                   e-mail: ksaarp@aarp.org
                                   www.aarp.org/states/ks
AARP is a nonprofit nonpartisan membership organization for people age 50 and over. AARP is dedicated to enhancing the quality of life as one ages, in addition to facilitating social change and delivering value to members through information and advocacy.
Mary Tritsch, Kansas AARP State Media Relations
Maren Turner, Kansas AARP State Director

Kentucky

47 **AARP Kentucky State Office: Louisville**
10401 Linn Station Road
Louisville, KY 40223   866-295-7275
                                        Fax: 502-394-9918
                                   e-mail: kyaarp@aarp.org
                                   www.aarp.org/states/ky
AARP is a nonprofit nonpartisan membership organization for people age 50 and over. AARP is dedicated to enhancing the quality of life as one ages, in addition to facilitating social change and delivering value to members through information and advocacy.
Bill Harned, AARP Kentucky State President
Fred Smith, Executive Council Community Service

Louisiana

48 **AARP Louisiana State Office: Baton Rouge**
301 Main Street
Baton Rouge, LA 70825   866-448-3620
                                        Fax: 225-387-3400
                                   e-mail: la@aarp.org
                                   www.aarp.org/states/la
AARP is a nonprofit nonpartisan membership organization for people age 50 and over. AARP is dedicated to enhancing the quality of life as one ages, in addition to facilitating social change and delivering value to members through information and advocacy.
Earl A White, AARP Louisiana State President
Julia Kenny, AARP Louisiana State Director

Maine

49 **AARP Maine State Office: Portland**
1685 Congress Street
Portland, ME 04102   866-554-5380
                                        Fax: 207-775-5727
                                   e-mail: me@aarp.org
                                   www.aarp.org/states/me
AARP is a nonprofit nonpartisan membership organization for people age 50 and over. AARP is dedicated to enhancing the quality of life as one ages, in addition to facilitating social change and delivering value to members through information and advocacy.
Bruce Kinney, Maine AARP State Advocacy Coordinator
Phyllis Cohn, Maine AARP State Media Relations

Massachusetts

50 **AARP Massachusetts State Office: Boston**
1 Beacon Street
Boston, MA 02108   866-448-3621
                                        Fax: 617-723-4224
                                   e-mail: ma@aarp.org
                                   www.aarp.org/states/ma
AARP is a nonprofit nonpartisan membership organization for people age 50 and over. AARP is dedicated to enhancing the quality of life as one ages, in addition to facilitating social change and delivering value to members through information and advocacy.
Charlie Desmond, AARP Massachusetts State President
Claire Redmond, Executive Council Member

Michigan

51 **AARP Michigan State Office: Lansing**
309 N Washington Square
Lansing, MI 48933   866-227-7448
                                        Fax: 517-482-2794
                                        TTY: 877-434-7598
                                   e-mail: miaarp@aarp.org
                                   www.aarp.org/states/mi
AARP is a nonprofit nonpartisan membership organization for people age 50 and over. AARP is dedicated to enhancing the quality of life as one ages, in addition to facilitating social change and delivering value to members through information and advocacy.
Steve Gools, AARP Michigan State Director
Stepheni Schlinker, Michigan AARP State Media Relations

Minnesota

52 AARP Minnesota State Office: Saint Paul
30 E Seventh Street
Saint Paul, MN 55101
866-554-5381
Fax: 651-221-2636
e-mail: aarpmn@aarp.org
www.aarp.org/states/mn
AARP is a nonprofit nonpartisan membership organization for people age 50 and over. AARP is dedicated to enhancing the quality of life as one ages, in addition to facilitating social change and delivering value to members through information and advocacy.
Michele Kimball, AARP Minnesota State Director
Amy Gromer McDonough, AARP Minnesota State Media Relations

Missouri

53 AARP Missouri State Office: Kansas City
700 W 47th Street
Kansas City, MO 64112-1805
866-389-5627
Fax: 816-561-3107
e-mail: moaarp@aarp.org
www.aarp.org/states/mo
AARP is a nonprofit nonpartisan membership organization for people age 50 and over. AARP is dedicated to enhancing the quality of life as one ages, in addition to facilitating social change and delivering value to members through information and advocacy.
John McDonald, AARP Missouri State Director
Anita K Parran, AARP Missouri State Media Relations

Montana

54 AARP Montana State Office: Helena
30 W 14th Street
Helena, MT 59601
866-295-7278
Fax: 406-441-2230
e-mail: mtaarp@aarp.org
www.aarp.org/states/mt
AARP is a nonprofit nonpartisan membership organization for people age 50 and over. AARP is dedicated to enhancing the quality of life as one ages, in addition to facilitating social change and delivering value to members through information and advocacy.
Max Logan, AARP Montana Volunteer State President
Bob Bartholomew, AARP Montana State Director

Nebraska

55 AARP Nebraska State Office: Lincoln
301 S 13th Street
Lincoln, NE 68508
866-389-5651
Fax: 402-323-6908
e-mail: neaarp@aarp.org
www.aarp.org/states/ne
AARP is a nonprofit nonpartisan membership organization for people age 50 and over. AARP is dedicated to enhancing the quality of life as one ages, in addition to facilitating social change and delivering value to members through information and advocacy.
Sunny Andrews, AARP Nebraska State President
Devorah Lanner, AARP Nebraska State Media Relations

Nevada

56 AARP Nevada State Office: Las Vegas
5820 S Eastern Avenue
Las Vegas, NV 89119
866-389-5652
Fax: 702-938-3225
e-mail: nvaarp@aarp.org
www.aarp.org/states/nv
AARP is a nonprofit nonpartisan membership organization for people age 50 and over. AARP is dedicated to enhancing the quality of life as one ages, in addition to facilitating social change and delivering value to members through information and advocacy.
Deborah Moore, AARP Nevada Spokeswoman
Nancy Andersen, AARP Nevada State Volunteer Coordinator

New Hampshire

57 AARP New Hampshire State Office-Manchester
900 Elm Street
Manchester, NH 03101
866-542-8168
Fax: 603-629-0066
e-mail: nh@aarp.org
www.aarp.org/states/nh
AARP is a nonprofit nonpartisan membership organization for people age 50 and over. AARP is dedicated to enhancing the quality of life as one ages, in addition to facilitating social change and delivering value to members through information and advocacy.
Kelly Clark, AARP New Hampshire State Director
Jamie Bulen, AARP New Hampshire State Media Relations

New Jersey

58 AARP New Jersey State Office: Princeton
101 Rockingham Row
Princeton, NJ 08540
866-542-8165
Fax: 609-987-4634
e-mail: njaarp@aarp.org
www.aarp.org/states/nj
AARP is a nonprofit nonpartisan membership organization for people age 50 and over. AARP is dedicated to enhancing the quality of life as one ages, in addition to facilitating social change and delivering value to members through information and advocacy.
Sy Larson, AARP New Jersey State President
Jane Margesson, AARP New Jersey State Media Relations

New Mexico

59 AARP New Mexico State Office: Sante Fe
535 Cerrillos Road
Santa Fe, NM 87501
866-389-5636
Fax: 505-820-2889
e-mail: nmaarp@aarp.org
www.aarp.org/states/nm
AARP is a nonprofit nonpartisan membership organization for people age 50 and over. AARP is dedicated to enhancing the quality of life as one ages, in addition to facilitating social change and delivering value to members through information and advocacy.
Louis Sarabia, AARP New Mexico State President
Stan Cooper, AARP New Mexico State Director

New York

60 AARP New York State Office: Albany
1 Commerce Plaza
Albany, NY 12260
866-227-7442
Fax: 518-434-6949
e-mail: nyaarp@aarp.org
www.aarp.org
AARP is a nonprofit nonpartisan membership organization for people age 50 and over. AARP is dedicated to enhancing the quality of life as one ages, in addition to facilitating social change and delivering value to members through information and advocacy.
Marilyn Pinksy, State President

61 AARP New York State Office: New York City
780 3rd Avenue
New York, NY 10017
866-227-7442
Fax: 212-644-6390
e-mail: nyaarp@aarp.org
www.aarp.org/states/ny
AARP is a nonprofit nonpartisan membership organization for people age 50 and over. AARP is dedicated to enhancing the quality of life as one ages, in addition to facilitating social change and delivering value to members through information and advocacy.
Lois Aronstein, AARP New York State Director
Madeleine Moore, AARP New York State President

North Carolina

62   **AARP North Carolina State Office: Raleigh**
1511 Sunday Drive
Raleigh, NC 27607   866-389-5650
Fax: 919-755-9684
TTY: 919-508-0290
e-mail: ncaarp@aarp.org
www.aarp.org/states/nc
AARP is a nonprofit nonpartisan membership organization for people age 50 and over. AARP is dedicated to enhancing the quality of life as one ages, in addition to facilitating social change and delivering value to members through information and advocacy.
Diana D Hatch, AARP North Carolina State President
Bob Garner, Communications Director

North Dakota

63   **AARP North Dakota State Office: Bismarck**
107 W Main Avenue
Bismarck, ND 58501   866-554-5383
Fax: 701-255-2242
e-mail: ndaarp@aarp.org
www.aarp.org/states/nd
AARP is a nonprofit nonpartisan membership organization for people age 50 and over. AARP is dedicated to enhancing the quality of life as one ages, in addition to facilitating social change and delivering value to members through information and advocacy.
Betty Keegan, AARP North Dakota State President
Lyle Halvorson, AARP North Dakota State Media Relations

Ohio

64   **AARP Ohio State Office: Columbus**
17 S High Street
Columbus, OH 43215-3467   866-389-5653
Fax: 614-224-9801
e-mail: ohaarp@aarp.org
www.aarp.org/states/oh
AARP is a nonprofit nonpartisan membership organization for people age 50 and over. AARP is dedicated to enhancing the quality of life as one ages, in addition to facilitating social change and delivering value to members through information and advocacy.
Kathy Keller, AARP Ohio State Media Relations
Joanne Limbach, AARP Ohio State President

Oklahoma

65   **AARP Oklahoma State Office: Edmond**
126 N Bryant Avenue
Edmond, OK 73034   866-295-7277
Fax: 405-844-7772
e-mail: ok@aarp.org
www.aarp.org/states/ok
AARP is a nonprofit nonpartisan membership organization for people age 50 and over. AARP is dedicated to enhancing the quality of life as one ages, in addition to facilitating social change and delivering value to members through information and advocacy.
Robert Bristow, AARP Oklahoma State President
Marjorie Lyons, Executive Council Member

Oregon

66   **AARP Oregon State Office: Clackamas**
9200 SE Sunnybrook Boulevard
Clackamas, OR 97015-5762   866-554-5360
Fax: 503-652-9933
e-mail: oraarp@aarp.org
www.aarp.org/states/or
AARP is a nonprofit nonpartisan membership organization for people age 50 and over. AARP is dedicated to enhancing the quality of life as one ages, in addition to facilitating social change and delivering value to members through information and advocacy.
Ray Miao, AARP Oregon State President
Don Bruland, Director

Pennsylvania

67   **AARP Pennsylvania State Office: Harrisburg**
30 N 3rd Street
Harrisburg, PA 17101   866-389-5654
Fax: 717-236-4078
e-mail: sgardner@aarp.org
www.aarp.org/states/pa
AARP is a nonprofit nonpartisan membership organization for people age 50 and over. AARP is dedicated to enhancing the quality of life as one ages, in addition to facilitating social change and delivering value to members through information and advocacy.
J Shane Creamer, AARP Pennsylvania State President
Steve Gardner, AARP Pennsylvania State Media Relations

South Carolina

68   **AARP South Carolina Office: Columbia**
1201 Main Street
Columbia, SC 29201   866-389-5655
Fax: 803-251-4374
e-mail: scaarp@aarp.org
www.aarp.org/states/sc
AARP is a nonprofit nonpartisan membership organization for people age 50 and over. AARP is dedicated to enhancing the quality of life as one ages, in addition to facilitating social change and delivering value to members through information and advocacy.
Charles A Johnson, AARP SC State President
Patrick Cobb, AARP SC State Media Relations

Tennessee

69   **AARP Tennessee State Office: Nashville**
150 4th Avenue N
Nashville, TN 37219   866-295-7274
Fax: 615-313-8414
e-mail: tnaarp@aarp.org
www.aarp.org/states/tn
AARP is a nonprofit nonpartisan membership organization for people age 50 and over. AARP is dedicated to enhancing the quality of life as one ages, in addition to facilitating social change and delivering value to members through information and advocacy.
Margot Seay, AARP Tennessee State President
Rebecca Kelly, AARP Tennessee State Director

Texas

70   **AARP Texas State Office: Austin**
98 San Jacinto Boulevard
Austin, TX 78701   866-227-7443
Fax: 512-480-9799
e-mail: rayuso@aarp.org
www.aarp.org/states/tx
AARP is a nonprofit nonpartisan membership organization for people age 50 and over. AARP is dedicated to enhancing the quality of life as one ages, in addition to facilitating social change and delivering value to members through information and advocacy.
Rafael Ayuso, AARP Texas State Media Relations
Bob Jackson, AARP Texas State Director

Utah

71   **AARP Utah State Office: Midvale**
6975 Union Park Center
Midvale, UT 84047   866-448-3616
Fax: 801-561-2209
e-mail: utaarp@aarp.org
www.aarp.org/states/ut
AARP is a nonprofit nonpartisan membership organization for people age 50 and over. AARP is dedicated to enhancing the quality of life as one ages, in addition to facilitating social change and delivering value to members through information and advocacy.
Pat Gamble Hovey, Volunteer State President of AARP Utah
Ruby Hammel, Executive Council Advocacy Coordinator

72   AARP Vermont State Office: Montpelier
199 Main Street
Burlington, VT 05401   866-227-7451
                                       Fax: 802-651-9805
                                       e-mail: vtaarp@aarp.org
                                       www.aarp.org/states/vt
AARP is a nonprofit nonpartisan membership organization for
people age 50 and over. AARP is dedicated to enhancing the quality of life as one ages, in addition to facilitating social change and
delivering value to members through information and advocacy.
Nancy C Lang, AARP Vermont State President
Dave Reville, AARP Vermont State Media Relations

73   AARP Virginia State Office: Richmond
707 E Main Street
Richmond, VA 23219   866-542-8164
                                       Fax: 804-819-1923
                                       e-mail: vaaarp@aarp.org
                                       www.aarp.org/states/va
AARP is a nonprofit nonpartisan membership organization for
people age 50 and over. AARP is dedicated to enhancing the quality of life as one ages, in addition to facilitating social change and
delivering value to members through information and advocacy.
Bill Kallio, AARP Virginia State Director
Tony Hylton, AARP Virginia State Media Relations

74   AARP Washington State Office: Seattle
9750 3rd Avenue NE
Seattle, WA 98115   866-227-7457
                                       Fax: 206-517-9350
                                       e-mail: waaarp@aarp.org
                                       www.aarp.org/states/wa
AARP is a nonprofit nonpartisan membership organization for
people age 50 and over. AARP is dedicated to enhancing the quality of life as one ages, in addition to facilitating social change and
delivering value to members through information and advocacy.
John Barnett, AARP Washington State President
Doug Shadel, AARP Washington State Director

75   AARP West Virginia Office: Charleston
300 Summers Street
Charleston, WV 25301   866-227-7458
                                       Fax: 304-344-4633
                                       e-mail: wvaarp@aarp.org
                                       www.aarp.org/states/wv
AARP is a nonprofit nonpartisan membership organization for
people age 50 and over. AARP is dedicated to enhancing the quality of life as one ages, in addition to facilitating social change and
delivering value to members through information and advocacy.
Ruth Wagner, AARP West Virginia State President
Ginger Thomp McDaniel, AARP West Virginia State Media Relations

76   AARP Wisconsin State Office: Madison
222 W Washington Avenue
Madison, WI 53703   866-448-3611
                                       Fax: 608-251-7612
                                       e-mail: wistate@aarp.org
                                       www.aarp.org/states/wi
AARP is a nonprofit nonpartisan membership organization for
people age 50 and over. AARP is dedicated to enhancing the quality of life as one ages, in addition to facilitating social change and
delivering value to members through information and advocacy.
Ethel Percy Andrus, Founder
Albert W Majkrzak, AARP Wisconsin State President

77   AARP Wyoming State Office: Cheyenne
2020 Carey Avenue
Cheyenne, WY 82009   866-663-3290
                                       e-mail: wy@aarp.org
                                       www.aarp.org/states/wy
AARP is a nonprofit nonpartisan membership organization for
people age 50 and over. AARP is dedicated to enhancing the quality of life as one ages, in addition to facilitating social change and
delivering value to members through information and advocacy.
Les Engelter, AARP Wyoming State President
Joanne Bowlby, AARP Wyoming State Media Relations

Libraries & Resource Centers

78   Aging In America/Morningside House Nursing
1000 Pelham Pkwy South
Bronx, NY 10461   877-244-6469
                                       e-mail: admissiondept@aiamsh.org
                                       www.aginginamerica.org
Aging in America is a community-based, social service agency.
Morningside House is a provider of specialized medical, nursing
and rehabilitative services.
Dr William T Smith, President/CEO

Research Centers

79   Case Western Reserve University: Center on Aging and Health
10900 Euclid Avenue   216-368-4413
Cleveland, OH 44106   800-515-2774
                                       Fax: 216-368-3842
                                       e-mail: contact-cas@cwru.edu
                                       fpb.case.edu/Centers/UCAH
Research organization conducting supporting and facilitating re-
search into the chronically ill aged person.
Diana L Morris, PhD, RN, FAAN, F, Executive Director
Evelyn Duffy, DNP, ANP/GNP-BC,, Associate Director

80   Center for the Study of Aging
706 Madison Avenue   518-465-6927
Albany, NY 12208-3604   Fax: 518-462-1339
                                       e-mail: iapaas@aol.com
                                       www.centerforthestudyofaging.org
Not-for-profit educational and research center for social and medical research on aging health exercise lifelong health and fitness
and programs to improve the health and quality of life for older
men and women.
Sara Harris, Executive Director
Debra Treadgold, President

81   Columbia University Center for Geriatrics Gerontology
College of Physicians and Surgeons
630 West 168th Street   212-305-3595
New York, NY 10032   Fax: 212-305-1343
                                       e-mail: psadmissions@columbia.edu
                                       www.cumc.columbia.edu/dept/ps
Clinical research in geriatric/gerontology and long-term care.
Lee Goldman MD, Dean

82   Creighton University Center for Healthy Aging
2500 California Plaza   402-280-2700
Omaha, NE 68178   Fax: 402-280-4623
                                       e-mail: medadmissions@creighton.edu
                                       medicine.creighton.edu/CAAD
Focuses on human development, aging and health care for the el-
derly.
Robert W. Dunlay, M.D., Dean
Michael D. White, M.D., Associate Dean for Medical Education

83   Landon Center on Aging University of Kansas Medical Center
University of Kansas Medical Center
3901 Rainbow Boulevard   913-588-5000
Kansas City, KS 66160   800-766-3777
                                       Fax: 913-588-1201
                                       e-mail: rnudo@kumc.edu
                                       www2.kumc.edu/coa

Provides support for interdisciplinary research on the issue of age and aging.
Randolph J Nudo, Director
Linda Redford, Associate Director

84   Purdue University: Center for Research on Aging
1202 W. State Street   765-494-9692
W Lafayette, IN 47907-2055   Fax: 765-494-2180
                                    e-mail: calc@purdue.edu
                                    www.purdue.edu/aging
Social science research on aging health and health care delivery.
Kenneth F Ferraro, Director
David J Waters,, Assistant Director

85   Roy M and Phyllis Gough Huffington Center on Aging
Huffington Center on Aging
Baylor College of Medicine   713-798-5804
Houston, TX 77030   Fax: 713-798-6688
                                    e-mail: Gretchen@bcm.tmc.edu
                                    www.hcoa.org
Internal unit of Baylor College representing research into the biology of aging.
Robert E. Roush, Director
Nancy L Wilson, Assistant Director

86   University of Pennsylvania Institute on Aging
3615 Chestnut Street   215-898-3163
Philadelphia, PA 19104-2676   Fax: 215-573-5566
                                    e-mail: aging@mail.med.upenn.edu
                                    www.med.upenn.edu/aging
The mission of the IOA is to improve the health of the elderly by increasing the quality and quantity of clinical and basic research as well as educational programs focusing on normal aging and age-related diseases at the UPSM and across the entire Penn campus.
John Q Trojanowski, Acting Director
Steven E Arnold, Associate Director

Support Groups & Hotlines

87   Aging Support Group
Consultants for Aging Families
649 Remington Street   970-498-0730
Fort Collins, CO 80524   e-mail: nanceemc@aol.com
                                    www.fortnet.org/CAF
A source of support, guidance, and accurate, thorough information to help manage the needs and preferences of your older family members.
Nancy McCambridge, Director

88   Children of Aging Parents
PO Box 167   215-355-6611
Richboro, PA 18954   800-227-7294
                                    Fax: 215-355-6824
                                    e-mail: info@caps4caregivers.org
                                    www.caps4caregivers.org
A nonprofit, charitable organization that assists the nation's nearly 54 million caregivers of the elderly or chronically ill with reliable information, referrals and support, and to heighten public awareness.

89   National Health Information Center
PO Box 1133   310-565-4167
Washington, DC 20013-1133   800-336-4797
                                    Fax: 301-984-4256
                                    e-mail: info@nhic.org
                                    www.health.gov/nhic
A health information referral service sponsored by the Office of Disease Prevention and Health Promotion. NHIC puts health professionals and consumers who have health questions in touch with those organizations that are best able to provide answers.

Books

90   Activities for the Disabled, Elderly and Adults
Haworth Press

10 Alice Street   607-722-5857
Binghamton, NY 13904-1580   800-429-6784
                                    Fax: 607-722-0012
                                    www.haworthpress.com
Learn how to effectively plan and deliver activities for a growing number of older people with developmental disabilities. It aims to stimulate interest and continued support for recreation program development and implementation among developmental disability and aging service systems.
136 pages Hardcover
ISBN: 1-560240-92-X

91   Adult Children and Aging Parents
American Counseling Association
6101 Stevenson Ave.   703-823-9800
Alexandria, VA 22304-3302   800-347-6647
                                    Fax: 703-823-0252
                                    e-mail: webmaster@counseling.org
                                    www.counseling.org
Provides effective intervention strategies and suggestions for counselors who work with older persons, individually and with the family. Offers information on many vital topics such as Alzheimer's Disease, retirement, elder abuse and suicide.
216 pages
ISBN: 0-840354-48-7

92   Aging and Family Therapy
Haworth Press
10 Alice Street   607-722-5857
Binghamton, NY 13904-1580   800-429-6784
                                    Fax: 607-722-0012
                                    www.haworthpress.com
Here are creative strategies for use in therapy with older adults and their families. This book provides practitioners with information, insight, reference tools, and other sources that will contribute to more effective intervention with the elderly and their families.
244 pages Hardcover
ISBN: 0-866567-78-3

93   Aging and Our Families
Human Sciences Press
233 Spring Street   212-620-8000
New York, NY 10013-1522   800-221-9369
                                    www.springer.com
Handbook for family caregivers.
132 pages Paperback
ISBN: 0-898854-41-5

94   Caregivers' Roller Coaster
Loyola University Press
3441 N Ashland Avenue   773-281-1818
Chicago, IL 60657-1355   800-621-1008
                                    Fax: 773-281-0555
                                    e-mail: marketing@loyolapress.com
                                    www.loyolapress.com
A simply written self-help guide for caregivers of the frail elderly. Offers support for men and women, not trained professionals, who find themselves caring for aging family members in their own homes. Offers practical advice and information on Alzheimer's, Medicare, insurance and community services for the elderly.
150 pages
ISBN: 0-829407-45-6

95   Caring for Those You Love: A Guide to Compassionate Care for the Aged
Bethany Chaffin, author
Horizon Publishers & Distributors, Inc.
191 N 650 East   801-295-9451
Bountiful, UT 84010-3628   Fax: 801-298-1305
                                    e-mail: hpservice09@hotmail.com
                                    horizonpublishersbookstore.com
Includes helpful information on identifying the problems of the aged. It explains the best and most frequently used treatments prescribed for these problems, and tells how family members can help to meet the physical, emotional, and spiritual needs of aging parents and other loved ones.
108 pages
ISBN: 0-882902-70-9
Duane S Crowther, Owner/CEO
Jean D Crowther, Owner/CEO

96   Continuing Care Retirement Community Directory
American Assoc. of Homes & Services for the Aging
901 E Street NW
Washington, DC 20004-2037   800-508-9442
                                       Fax: 301-206-9789
A national consumer's directory of continuing care retirement communities. This directory is a vital tool for individuals searching and evaluating a community for themselves or a loved one.

97   Court-Related Needs of the Elderly and Persons with Disabilities
Commission on the Mentally Disabled
1800 M Street NW
Washington, DC 20036-5802   202-331-2240
                                       www.statejustice.org/
Report of the National Conference, examines the barriers of the judicial system impeding access for the elderly and persons with disabilities.

98   Creative Movements for Older Adults
Human Sciences Press
233 Spring Street   212-620-8000
New York, NY 10013-1522   800-221-9369
                                       www.springer.com
Exercises for the elderly.
172 pages Cloth
ISBN: 0-898854-14-8

99   Diagnosis and Treatment of Old Age
S Karger Publishers
26 W Avon Road   860-675-7834
Farmington, CT 06085-1162   800-828-5479
                                       Fax: 860-675-7302
                       www.karger.ch/company/karger.htm#10
These papers furnish a concise update on the diagnosis and treatment of Alzheimer's disease.
112 pages Hardcover
ISBN: 3-805548-44-3

100   Elder Care
Center For Public Representation
975 Bascom Mall   608-262-2240
Madison, WI 53706-0049   800-369-0388
                                       Fax: 608-251-1263
                                       law.wisc.edu
A compendium of alternatives for providing and financing long-term care. This practical guide provides the most comprehensive and comforting information to help navigate a number of consumer minefields.
224 pages
ISBN: 0-873371-13-5

101   Elderly in Modern Society
Vance Bibliographier
PO Box 229   217-762-3831
Monticello, IL 61856-0229
A bibliography of laws and human rights for the elderly.
15 pages
ISBN: 0-792001-10-9

102   Falling in Old Age
Reing Tideiksaar PhD, author
Springer Publishing Company
11 W 42nd Street   212-431-4370
New York, NY 10036   877-687-7476
                                       Fax: 212-941-7842
                              e-mail: cs@springerpub.com
                                       www.springerpub.com
This book provides an enormous body of fall-related research that has been organized by the author into easy, digestible information for geriatric health professionals. Extensively updated and revised for its second edition, the book has direct clinical applications and strategies for preventing and managing falls. It also contains new information on the physical, psychological, and social complications of falling.
412 pages Hardcover
ISBN: 0-826152-91-6

103   Family Carebook
CAREsource Program Development

505 Seattle Tower   206-625-9080
Seattle, WA 98101-3021
Guide to aging, the special needs of older adults, and the demands of providing care and support. Experts explain potential conflicts, planning opportunities and strategies for success.
475 pages Paperback
ISBN: 1-878866-12-5

104   From Theory to Therapy: The Development of Drugs for Alzheimer's Disease
Alzheimer's Association
225 N Michigan Avenue
Chicago, IL 60611-1696   800-272-3900
                                       Fax: 866-699-1246
                                       TDD: 312-335-8700
                                   e-mail: media@alz.org
                                       www.alz.org
Provides a layman's explanation of how experimental drugs are being developed and tested for Alzheimer's disease, and information about patient participation in clinical drug trials.

105   Geriatric Rehabilitation Preview
RTC on Aging
7601 E Imperial Highway
Downey, CA 90242-4155   310-940-7402
                              gero.usc.edu/RRTConAging
Covers research, training activities, and other issues pertaining to the rehabilitation of elderly persons with disabilities.

106   Health Care of the Aged
Abraham Monk, PhD, author
Haworth Press
10 Alice Street   607-722-5857
Binghamton, NY 13904-1580   800-429-6784
                                       Fax: 607-722-0012
                                       www.haworthpress.com
Focusing on the need for developing new service delivery models for the aged, this book examines fiscal, political, and social criteria influencing this challenge of the 1990s. The aged are caught in the sweeping changes currently occurring in the financing, organizing and delivery of human health care services.
183 pages Hardcover
ISBN: 1-560240-65-5

107   Healthy Aging: Good Investment & Together We Care: Helping Caregivers Find Supp.
National Council on Aging
1901 L Street NW   202-479-1200
Washington, DC 20036   800-677-1116
                                       Fax: 202-479-0735
                                       TDD: 202-479-6674
                                   e-mail: info@ncoa.org
                                       www.ncoa.org
Describes seven model programs that could be used in community-based organizations serving older adults.
2 Book Set
James P Firman, EdD, President/CEO

108   International Health Guide for Senior Citizen Travelers
Pilot Books
103 Cooper Street   516-422-2225
Babylon, NY 11702-2368   Fax: 516-669-4173
Covers essential pre-departure health planning such as advice on specific health concerns, disease prevention, specific travel problems, medical preparedness and assistance.
70 pages Paperback
ISBN: 0-875761-39-9
Anne Small, President

109   Living Well in a Nursing Home
Lynn Dickinson, Xenia Vosen, author
Hunter House Publishing
445 Park Avenue   646-291-8961
New York, NY 10022   800-266-5592
                                       Fax: 646-291-8962
                          e-mail: ordering@hunterhouse.com
                                       www.turnerpublishing.com

This book concentrates on the positive aspects of nursing homes, providing tips, support and reassurance.
256 pages Paperback
ISBN: 0-897934-60-2

110 Mentally Impaired Elderly
Ellen D Taira, author
Haworth Press
10 Alice Street   607-722-5857
Binghamton, NY 13904-1580   800-429-6784
                                              Fax: 607-722-0012
                                         www.haworthpress.com
Provides effective support and sensitive care for the most vulnerable segment of the elderly population, those with mental impairment.
191 171 pages
ISBN: 1-560241-68-1

111 Mirrored Lives
Greenwood Publishing Group, Inc/Praeger Publishers
130 Cremona Drive
Santa Barbara, CA 93117-6926   800-225-5800
                                              Fax: 877-231-6980
                                    e-mail: service@greenwood.com
                             www.abc-clio.com/ABC-CLIOGreenwood
Discusses geriatric decline connected to nonterminal illness in old age. Koch takes a sensitive but thorough look at the declining years of his father.
240 pages
ISBN: 0-275936-71-6

112 Nursing Home Information Services
925 15th Street NW   202-347-8800
Washington, DC 20005-2301
Lists acceptable nursing homes across the nation and provides information about their costs, admission requirements, standards and programs.

113 Nursing Home and You: Partners in Caring
American Assn. of Homes & Services for the Aging
901 E Street NW
Washington, DC 20004-2037   800-508-9442
                                              Fax: 301-206-9789
Offers information to nursing home staff and family members about caring for persons with Alzheimer's Disease.

114 Older Americans Information Directory
Grey House Publishing
4919 Route 22   518-789-8700
Amenia, NY 12501   800-562-2139
                                              Fax: 518-789-8700
                                    e-mail: books@greyhouse.com
                                         www.greyhouse.com
An invaluable resource that offers up-to-date information on the prevalent social, health and financial issues facing older Americans in the 21st century, as well as recreational and educational opportunities to enrich their lives.
1200 pages
ISBN: 1-592375-43-X
Leslie Mackenzie, Publisher

115 On Your Behalf
CAREsource Program Development
505 Seattle Tower   206-625-9080
Seattle, WA 98101
This book takes the mystery out of very important sets of legal options. It gives lay people as well as advisors, service providers, and caregivers the information they need to understand their options and the importance of individual choice.
16 pages Books & Video
ISBN: 1-878866-14-1

116 Physical Activity and the Aging
Human Kinetic Publishers
1607 N Market Street
Champaign, IL 61820-5076   800-747-4457
                                              Fax: 217-351-1549
                                    e-mail: info@hkusa.com
                                         www.humankinetics.com

North America's leading scholars examine the effects of aging on motor function, cardiovascular function, balance, the nervous system, changes in activity level, and possible reasons for activity level changes.
208 pages
ISBN: 0-873222-20-2

117 Planning for Long-Term Care
National Council on Aging
1901 L Street NW   202-479-1200
Washington, DC 20036   800-677-1116
                                              Fax: 202-479-0735
                                              TDD: 202-479-6674
                                         e-mail: info@ncoa.org
                                              www.ncoa.org
Identify the various long-term care resources within your family and in your community using this thorough and readable guide.
160 pages
James P Firman, EdD, President/CEO

118 Read Easy
CAREsource Program Development
505 Seattle Tower   206-625-9080
Seattle, WA 98101
If books, audio tapes and computers can spark the imagination of the young adult and the middle aged, why not seniors as well? All it takes is commitment to make quality library resources and programs accessible and user-friendly to older readers. Read Easy is an invaluable planning and operations guide, explaining senior needs to library professionals and librarianship principles to senior care professionals.
95 pages
ISBN: 1-878866-13-3

119 Resources for Elders with Disabilities
Resources for Rehabilitation
22 Bonad Road   781-368-9080
Winchester, MA 01890   Fax: 781-368-9096
                                         e-mail: info@rfr.org
                                              www.rfr.org
Provides information that enables elders, family members and other caregivers, and service providers to locate appropriate services. Includes information about rehabilitation, laws that affect elders with disabilities, and self-help groups. Published in large print.

ISBN: 0-929718-31-3

120 Senior Center Self: Assessment & National Accreditation Manual
National Council on Aging
1901 L Street NW   202-479-1200
Washington, DC 20036   800-677-1116
                                              Fax: 202-479-0735
                                              TDD: 2024796674
                                         e-mail: info@ncoa.org
                                              www.ncoa.org
Based upon compliance with standards (best practices) developed by the National Institutes of Senior Centers. This program was developed under the auspices of NCOA's National Institute of Senior Centers (NISC).
Book & CD Set
James P Firman, EdD, President/CEO

121 Senior Citizens and the Law
Center for Public Representation
PO Box 260049   608-251-4008
Madison, WI 53726-0049   800-369-0388
                                              Fax: 608-251-1263
An introduction to legal problems facing the elderly in Wisconsin. This edition discusses legal problems associated with Social Security, Medicare, SSI, guardianship and its alternatives, community-based services, probate, taxes, private health insurance and consumer protection.
176 pages
ISBN: 0-932622-29-1

122 Successful Models of Community Long Term Care Services for the Elderly
Haworth Press

10 Alice Street
Binghamton, NY 13904-1580

607-722-5857
800-429-6784
Fax: 607-722-0012
www.haworthpress.com

Experienced practitioners provide examples of successful community-based long term care service programs for the elderly.
174 pages
ISBN: 0-866569-87-9

123 Unloving Care
Harper Collins Publishers/Basic Books
195 Broadway
New York, NY 10007-5299

212-207-7000
800-242-7737
Fax: 212-207-7203
e-mail: tmpcorrections@harpercollins.com
www.harpercollins.com

A leading public health expert gives his account of the negative aspects of nursing homes.
305 pages
ISBN: 0-465088-81-3

Magazines

124 AARP Magazine
American Association of Retired Persons
601 East Street NW
Washington, DC 20049

202-434-3525
888-687-2277
TTY: 877-434-7598
e-mail: member@aarp.org
www.aarp.org

Celebrity interviews. Features on health and finance. Movie reviews and more. All with an eye toward the topics and issues you care about most.
A Barry Rand, CEO

125 Abstracts in Social Gerontology
National Council on Aging
1901 L Street NW
Washington, DC 20036

202-479-1200
800-677-1116
Fax: 202-479-0735
TDD: 202-479-6674
e-mail: info@ncoa.org
www.ncoa.org

Detailed abstracts are provided for recent major journal articles, books, reports and other materials on many facets of aging, including adult education, demography, family relations, institutional care and work attitudes.
Quarterly
James P Firman, EdD, President/CEO

126 Innovations
National Council on Aging
1901 L Street NW
Washington, DC 20036

202-479-1200
800-677-1116
Fax: 202-479-0735
TDD: 2024796674
e-mail: info@ncoa.org
www.ncoa.org

Explores significant developments in the field of aging through opinion articles, profiles and research summaries. Features articles on social trends, articles on specific aging programs and information on NCOA's activities. Members are free.
Quarterly
James P Firman, EdD, President/CEO

127 International Journal of Technology and Aging
Human Sciences Press
233 Spring Street
New York, NY 10013-1522

212-620-8000
800-221-9369
Fax: 212-463-0742
www.springer.com

Designed to serve health-care professionals, researchers, academicians and industries concerned with the convergence of two recent trends, the dramatic advances in technology and the rapidly growing elderly population.

128 Modern Maturity
AARP

601 E Street NW
Washington, DC 20049-0003

202-434-3525
800-424-3410
TTY: 877-434-7598
e-mail: member@aarp.org
www.aarp.org

Offers news and information of concern to those 50 and older. Features articles on current events, health, recreation, housing, family life, legislation and other issues.
6x Year

Newsletters

129 AARP Bulletin
American Association of Retired Persons
601 East Street NW
Washington, DC 20049

202-434-3525
888-687-2277
TTY: 877-434-7598
e-mail: member@aarp.org
www.aarp.org

Get daily news about the issues that matter to you.
Bill Novelli, AARP CEO

130 Best Practices
American Assoc. of Homes & Services for the Aging
2519 Connecticut Ave NW
Washington, DC 20008-1520

202-783-2242
Fax: 202-783-2255
e-mail: info@aahsa.org
www.aahsa.org

Keeps nonprofit aging service providers informed of new trends and developments in quality of care for older persons.

131 Bulletin
AARP
601 E Street NW
Washington, DC 20049

202-434-3525
800-424-3410
TTY: 877-434-7598
e-mail: member@aarp.org
www.aarp.org

Get daily news about the issues that matter to you.
11x Year

132 CAPSule
Children of Aging Parents
PO Box 167
Richboro, PA 18954-0167

215-355-6611
800-227-7294
Fax: 215-355-6824
e-mail: info@caps4caregivers.org
www.caps4caregivers.org

Newsletter devoted to assisting caregivers of the elderly.
12 pages Quarterly
Lenore Sherman, Executive Director
Karen Rosenberg, Director Senior Services

133 Capital Advantage
Capital Advantage Publishing
3708 Mount Diablo Blvd
Lafayette, CA 94549

925-299-1500
Fax: 925-299-1599
e-mail: sales@capitaladvantage.com
www.capitaladvantage.com

Publishes articles on all aspects of aging including legislation, innovative programs and services.
Monthly

134 Center for the Study of Aging Newsletter
University of Pennsylvania Center for Aging Study
3615 Chestnut Street
Philadelphia, PA 19104-4205

215-898-7801
Fax: 215-573-8684
e-mail: ageweb@mail.med.upenn.edu
www.med.upenn.edu/aging

News and information concerning the University and Center aging activities, programs and seminars.

135 Elderly Health Services Letter
American Business Publishing
3100 Highway 138
Wall Township, NJ 0771

732-681-1133

Information on trends and developments in the expanding field of health services for the elderly.
Monthly
Robert Jenkins, Publisher

136 **Geriatric Care News**
DRS Geriatric Publishing Company
7435 SE 71st Street   206-232-9689
Mercer Island, WA 98040-5314
Newsletter for the elderly and their families.
Monthly
Denise Schramke, Publisher

137 **Geriatrics**
7500 Old Oak Boulevard   440-243-8100
Cleveland, OH 44130-3343
Articles for physicians and laypersons relating to care of middle-aged and elderly persons.
Monthly

138 **Gerontology News**
Gerontological Society of America
1220 L Street NW   202-842-1275
Washington, DC 20005   Fax: 202-842-1150
e-mail: geron@geron.org
www.geron.org
It reports on policy issues, legislative actions, Society events, research results, and recently released major reports on aging. Regular features include Washington Updates; Research Highlights; Grants Available; New Resources and Reports; Data Updates; and Calls for Papers, Nominations, and Manuscripts.
Carol Ann Schutz, Executive Director

139 **Health After 50: Johns Hopkins Medical Letter**
Johns Hopkins Medical Institutions
550 Broadway   410-955-3182
Baltimore, MD 21205-2011   800-829-9170
e-mail: www.medjhu.edu
Health newsletter for people over 50.
10 pages Monthly
ISBN: 1-042188-2 -
Rodney Friedman, Publisher

140 **Lifelong Health and Fitness**
Center for the Study of Aging
706 Madison Avenue   518-465-4927
Albany, NY 12208-3604   Fax: 518-462-1339
e-mail: iapaas@aol.com
www.centerforthestudyofaging-albany.org
A quarterly newsletter published by the Center for the Study of Aging.
8 pages Quarterly
Sara Harris, Executive Director

141 **NCOA Week**
National Council on Aging
1901 L Street NW   202-479-1200
Washington, DC 20036   800-677-1116
Fax: 202-479-0735
TDD: 202-479-6674
e-mail: info@ncoa.org
www.ncoa.org
Breaking news of NCOA initiatives, crucial legislative and policy issues, research studies, developments in work and volunteering for older adults, benefits for seniors, trends in aging, grant opportunities, and more. Members only.
Weekly
James P Firman, EdD, President/CEO

142 **Senior Focus**
National Council on Aging
1901 L Street NW   202-479-1200
Washington, DC 20036   800-677-1116
Fax: 202-479-0735
TDD: 202-479-6674
e-mail: info@ncoa.org
www.ncoa.org

Timely, objective, and practical information on health and wellness, lifestyle, and financial issues for seniors and people who work with them.
Bi-Monthly
James P Firman, EdD, President/CEO

143 **Vital Aging Report**
National Council on Aging
1901 L Street NW   202-479-1200
Baltimore, MD   800-677-1116
Fax: 202-479-0735
TDD: 202-479-6674
e-mail: info@ncoa.org
www.ncoa.org
Packed with news about health and financial matters as well as United Senior's Health Council's innovative programs and research. The USHC is a program of the National Council on the Aging. Member price $17.50.
Quarterly
James P Firman, EdD, President/CEO

Pamphlets

144 **American Perceptions of Aging in the 21st Century**
National Council on Aging
1901 L Street NW   202-479-1200
Washington, DC 20036   800-677-1116
Fax: 202-479-0735
TDD: 2024796674
e-mail: info@ncoa.org
www.ncoa.org
There are many interesting and important findings related to aging in America as reported by over 3000 respondents. This chartbook is intended as a handy reference for scholars, the press and advocates.
James P Firman, EdD, President/CEO

145 **Care of the Elderly in America**
Vance Bibliographies
PO Box 229   217-762-3831
Monticello, IL 61856-0229
A bibliography of aged care in America.
11 pages
ISBN: 1-555905-59-5

146 **Exploring Care Options for a Relative with Alzheimer's Disease**
American Assoc. of Homes & Services for the Aging
2519 Connecticut Ave NW   202-783-2242
Washington, DC 20008-1520   800-508-9442
Fax: 202-783-2255
e-mail: www.aahsa.org
pub@aahsa.org

147 **Medicare Health Plan Choices: Consumer Update**
National Council on Aging
1901 L Street NW   202-479-1200
Washington, DC 20036   800-677-1116
Fax: 202-479-0735
TDD: 202-479-6744
e-mail: info@ncoa.org
www.ncoa.org
Annually updated report contains important information about options that are available to Medicare beneficiaries. Medicare is changing, Medigap premiums are going up, and many Medicare HMOs are dropping service to seniors. Pamphlets available in single copies or packs of 50.
James P Firman, EdD, President/CEO

148 **Nonprofit Housing and Care Options for Older People**
American Assoc. of Homes & Services for the Aging
901 E Street NW   800-508-9442
Washington, DC 20004-2037   Fax: 301-206-9789
Offers information on continuing care facilities, retirement communities and more for the elderly and relatives caring for Alzheimer's patients.

149 **Time Out!**
Alzheimer's Association

225 N Michigan Avenue
Chicago, IL 60611-1696
800-272-3900
Fax: 866-669-1246
TDD: 312-335-8700
e-mail: media@alz.org
www.alz.org

Details the Association's position supporting a national respite care policy and recommends actions for federal and state policy makers.
1991 14 pages

Audio & Video

150 **Aphasia: Struggling for Understanding**
Filmakers Library
3212 Duke Street
Alexandria, VA 22314-1798
212-808-4980
Fax: 212-808-4983
e-mail: sales@alexanderstreet.com
www.filmakers.com

What if your ability to speak or understand speech was taken away without warning, and you struggled to find words that just won't come? This film is about two people faced with the daunting task of learning to speak again, of regaining their humanity. DVD or VHS, Classroom Rental VHS also available for $65. 14 minutes in length.
DVD or VHS
Sue Oscar, Co-President

Web Sites

151 **Alliance for Aging Research**
www.agingresearch.org
Improving the health and independence of Americans as they age. Promotes medical and behavioral research into the aging process.

152 **American Association of Retired Persons**
www.aarp.org
AARP is the nation's leading organization for people age 50 and older. Information and education, advocacy, and community services provided by a network of local chapters and experienced volunteers throughout the country.

153 **American Society on Aging**
www.asaging.org
An association of diverse individuals bound together by a common goal: to support the commitment and enhance the knowledge and skills of those who seek to improve the quality of life of older adults and their families.

154 **Gerontological Society of America**
www.geron.org
Nonprofit professional organization with more than 5000 members in the field of aging. Provides researchers, educators, practitioners and policy makers with opportunities to understand, advance, integrate and use basic and applied research on aging to improve the quality of life as one ages.

155 **Healing Well**
www.healingwell.com
An online health resource guide to medical news, chat, information and articles, newsgroups and message boards, books, disease-related web sites, medical directories, and more for patients, friends, and family coping with disabling diseases, disorders, or chronic illnesses.

156 **Health Finder**
www.healthfinder.gov
Searchable, carefully developed web site offering information on over 1000 topics. Developed by the US Department of Health and Human Services, the site can be used in both English and Spanish.

157 **Healthlink USA**
www.healthlinkusa.com
Health information concerning treatment, cures, prevention, diagnosis, risk factors, research, support groups, email lists, personal stories and much more. Updated regularly.

158 **Helios Health**
www.helioshealth.com
Online resource for your health information. Detailed information about specific health topics, access to expert advice from our Medical Advisory Board, and up-to-date health news.

159 **MedicineNet**
www.medicinenet.com
An online resource for consumers providing easy-to-read, authoritative medical and health information.

160 **Medscape**
www.medscape.com
Medscape offers specialists, primary care physicians, and other health professionals the Web's most robust and integrated medical information and educational tools.

161 **National Council on Aging**
www.ncoa.org
Seniors Corner includes many resources and health related information on older Americans and their caregivers.

162 **National Institute of Aging**
www.nia.nih.gov
Conducts research on aging, behavioral and social research, neuroscience and neuropsychology, geriatrics, and clinical gerontology.

163 **Research Center**
www.resarch.aarp.org
Online center offering information on consumer issues, demographics, independent living and other items of interest to senior citizens.

164 **US Administration on Aging**
www.aoa.gov
An agency in the US Department of Health and Human Services, is one of the nation's largest providers of home and community-based care for older persons and their caregivers.

165 **WebMD**
www.webmd.com
WebMD provides valuable health information, tools for managing your health, and support to those who seek information.

Description

166 **AIDS/HIV**

AIDS, Acquired Immune Deficiency Syndrome, is an infectious disorder that suppresses the normal function of the human body's immune system. AIDS is a result of HIV (Human Immunodeficiency Virus) infection, which destroys the body's ability to fight infections. Specifically, the virus infects and later destroys T-cells, which are a part of the body's immune system that responds to invading organisms. This destructive process is slow and silent, which means that HIV can be contracted years before any symptoms appear. When enough T-cells have been destroyed, the body is invaded by organisms that wouldn't ordinarily be able to cause serious disease. An early symptom of HIV infection is usually an increasing number of infections. Weight loss, fever and night sweats are common. Certain cancers, especially lymphoma and Kaposi's sarcoma, also take advantage of the body's lowered resistance.

HIV transmission requires contact with body fluids and is usually spread from an infected person to a noninfected person by unprotected sexual intercourse, or by sharing needles. Mothers can give HIV infection to their children before and during childbirth and while breastfeeding.

Prevention of HIV infection is the best way to stop the AIDS epidemic. Unfortunately, progress on a vaccine has been disappointing, so avoiding contact with the virus is the primary method of prevention. Avoiding the riskier types of sexual intercourse will reduce one's risk, as will the use of a condom duringvaginal and anal sex. Injecting drug users should not share needles. The use of needle exchange programs has decreased the spread of HIV infection. Women with HIV are encouraged to avoid pregnancy. If pregnant, HIV positive women should stay on medicine directed against HIV and should not breastfeed. Today, infants born to HIV women are treated with medication immediately after birth and this has greatly reduced the incidence of vertical transmission of the infection from mother to child. Until anti-HIV drugs became available, infected persons usually had a rapid downhill course. Today, combination drug treatment can offer most infected persons a long period of relatively good health. However, the treatment regimen is often complex and expensive, involving three or four drugs which must be taken several times a day. Since skipping doses encourages growth of virus that is resistant to the drugs, it is very important to take the drugs exactly as directed.

National Agencies & Associations

167 **AIDS Coalition of Cape Breton**
150 Bentinck Street 902-567-1766
Sydney, Nova Scotia, B1P-6H1 Fax: 902-567-1766
e-mail: christineporter@accb.ns.ca
www.aidscoalitionofcapebreton.ca/index.h

Provides support and advocacy services for PLW HIV/AIDS (people living with HIV/AIDS). Services provided deal with social, legal, ethical and spiritual issues.
Christine Porter, Executive Director
Jo-Anne Rolls, PHA Program Coordinator

168 **AIDS Committee of Durham**
22 King Street West 905-576-1445
Oshawa, Ontario, L1H-1A3 877-361-8750
Fax: 905-576-4610
e-mail: info@aidsdurham.com
www.aidsdurham.com

To provide HIV/AIDS related services to the infected or affected and the general community in the region of Durham.
Doug Willoughby, President
Todd Shearing, Vice President

169 **AIDS Committee of London**
#30-186 King Street 519-434-1601
London, Ontario, N6A-3C1 866-920-1601
Fax: 519-434-1843
e-mail: info@hivaidsconnection.ca
www.aidslondon.com

Is a community-based, charitable organization providing HIV-related services to people living with and concerned about HIV/AIDS in London and area.
Brian Lester, Executive Director
Elizabeth Lam, Office Manager

170 **AIDS Committee of Ottawa**
251 Bank Street 613-238-5014
Ottawa, Ontario, K2P-1X3 Fax: 613-238-3425
e-mail: info@aco-cso.ca
www.aco-cso.ca

Works to empower people living with HIV/AIDS and the PLWHA (persons living with HIV/AID) community in Ottawa through promoting the well being and quality of life of those living with, or close affected by HIV/AIDS.
Kathleen Cummings, Executive Director
Elysia Sugden, Office Administrator

171 **AIDS Committee of Toronto**
399 Church Street 416-340-2437
Toronto, Ontario, M5B-2J6 Fax: 416-340-8224
www.actoronto.org

Delivers responsive, effective, and valued community-based HIV support services and education, prevention, outreach and fundraising programs that promote health, well-being, worth and rights of individuals and communities living with, affected by and at risk for HIV/AIDS, and increase awareness of HIV/AIDS.
Richard Willett, Co Chair
Hazelle Palmer, Executive Director

172 **AIDS Committee of York Region**
194 Eagle Street E 905-953-0248
Newmarket, Ontario, L3Y-1J6 800-243-7717
Fax: 905-953-1372
e-mail: edacyr@bellnet.ca
www.acyr.org

The AIDS Committee of York Region envisions an informed and compassionate society, which is supportive of people living with HIV/AIDS who are striving to overcome social and service challenges, working with them towards a healthy and empowered lifestyle.
Radha Bhardwaj, Acting Executive Director
Vibhuti Mehra, Executive Assistant/ Office Manager

173 **AIDS Network**
600 Williamson Street 608-252-6540
Madison, WI 53703 800-486-6276
Fax: 608-252-6559
TTY: 608-441-3542
e-mail: info@aidsnetwork.org
www.aidsnetwork.org

Provides critical AIDS care and prevention services. Sustained in these efforts by the resources expertise and passion of hundreds of volunteers and donors.
Mary Vasquez, President
Lana Chute, Vice President

174   AIDS New Brunswick
65 Brunswick Street   506-459-7518
Fredericton, NB, E3B-1G5   800-561-4009
                                        Fax: 888-501-6301
                                    e-mail: info@aidsnb.com
                                            www.aidsnb.com
A provincial organization committed to facilitating community-based responses to the issues of HIV/AIDS. The aim is to promote and support the health and well-being of persons living with
and affected by HIV/AIDS and to reduce the spread of HIV/AIDS
in New Brunswick.
Stephen Alexander, Executive Director
Keri Ann Scott, Operation Coordinator

175   AIDS Niagara
Normandy Resource Center   905-984-8684
St. Catharines, Ontario, L2R-3C9   800-773-9843
                                        Fax: 905-988-1921
                                 e-mail: info@aidsniagara.com
                                         www.aidsniagara.com
AIDS Niagara is dedicated to improving the quality of life for
those infected and/or affected by HIV/AIDS.
Ash Shihora, Director
Francis Gregotski, Vice Chair

176   AIDS PEI
375 University Avenue   902-566-2437
Charlottetown, PE, C1A-4N4   Fax: 902-626-3400
                                    e-mail: info@aidspei.com
                                            www.aidspei.com
To create a supportive environment for Persons Living with
AIDS/HIV, to increase public understanding of the impact of
HIV/AIDS, and to reduce the incidence of HIV/AIDS in Prince
Edward Island.
Leslie Labobe, Director
Mike Chipman, Chairperson

177   AIDS Thunder Bay
574 Memorial Avenue   807-345-1516
Thunder Bay, Ontario, P7B 3-3Z2   800-488-5840
                                        Fax: 807-345-2505
                              e-mail: info@aidsthunderbay.org
                                      www.aidsthunderbay.org
Provide quality, compassionate support, education and advocacy
around HIV and AIDS, and related issues.
Dennis Eeles, President
Brent Trudel, Vice President

178   AIDS Treatment Data Network
57 Willoughby St.   347- 47- 740
Brooklyn, New York, NY 11201   TTY: 212-925-9560
                               e-mail: info@housingworks.org
                                         www.housingworks.org
The Network is a national independent community-based
not-for-profit organization that provides treatment access and ad-
vocacy, case management, supportive counseling and English and
Spanish language information services to men women and
children with HIV.
Natacha Baron, Associate Medical Director
Dr. Priya Parasher, Dental Director

179   AIDS United
1424 K Street, NW   202-408-4848
Washington, DC 20005   Fax: 202-408-1818
                                            www.aidsunited.org
National organization dedicated to the development analysis culti-
vation and encouragement of sound policies and programs in response to the HIV epidemic. We do this through the dissemination
of information and the building and use of advocacy.
Vignetta Charles, Ph.D., Senior Vice President
Michael Kaplan, President, CEO

180   AIDS.ORG
P.O. Box 69491
Los Angeles, CA 90069   323-656-6036
                                                www.aids.org
The mission of AIDS.ORG is to help prevent HIV infections and to
improve the lives of those affected by HIV and AIDS by providing

education and facilitating the free and open exchange of knowl-
edge at any easy-to-find centralized Web site.
Peter Dobson, Director
Alain Berrebi, Executive Director

181   AIDSinfo
PO Box 4780   1 3-1 3-5 28
Rockville, MD 20849-6303   800-448-0440
                                        Fax: 301-315-2818
                                        TTY: 888-480-3739
                            e-mail: contactus@aidsinfo.nih.gov
                                         www.aidsinfo.nih.gov
AIDSinfo is a U.S. Department of Health and Human Services
(DHHS) project that offers the latest federally approved information on HIV/AIDS clinical research, treatment and prevention, and
medical practice guidelines for people living with HIV/AIDS,
their families and friends, health care providers, scientists, and
researchers.

**182   ANKORS: Kootenay & Boundary HIV/AIDS and Hepatitis C
        Support Services**
101 Baker Street   250-505-5506
Nelson, BC, V1L-4H1   800-421-2437
                                        Fax: 250-505-5507
                               e-mail: information@ankors.bc.ca
                                            www.ankors.bc.ca
ANKORS' mission is to respond to the evolving needs of those liv-
ing with and affected by HIV/AIDS and Hepatitis C.
Cheryl Dowden, Executive Director
Gary Dalton, Community Care Team

183   Access AIDS Network
111 Elm Street   705-688-0500
Sudbury, Ontario, P3C-1T3   800-465-2437
                                        Fax: 705-688-0423
                        e-mail: aaninfo@reseauaccessnetwork.com
                                     www.accessaidsnetwork.com
A non-profit, community-based charitable organization, commit-
ted to promoting wellness, education, harm and risk reduction.
Richard Rainville, Executive Director
Christine Coutu, Clerical Intake Worker

184   Alberta Reappraising AIDS Society
Box 61037   403-289-6609
Calgary, Alberta, T2N-4S6   Fax: 403-206-7717
                                    e-mail: aras@aras.ab.ca
                                            www.aras.ab.ca
Promote critical discussion of the HIV/AIDS dogma.
David Crowe, President
Roger Swan, Treasurer

185   American Autoimmune Related Diseases Association
22100 Gratiot Avenue   586-776-3900
Eastpointe, MI 48021   800-598-4668
                                        Fax: 586-776-3903
                                    e-mail: aarda@aarda.org
                                            www.aarda.org
Awareness, education, referrals for patients with any type of auto-
immune disease.
Virginia T. Ladd, President/Executive Director
Stanley M. Finger, Chairman

186   American Civil Liberties Union AIDS Project
125 Broad Street   212-549-2500
New York, NY 10004   e-mail: media@aclu.org
                        www.aclu.org/HIVAIDS/HIVAIDSMain.cfm
Offers legislative and employment information public awareness
materials and support for persons with HIV/AIDS and their
families.
Susan Herman, President
Anthony D. Romero, Executive Director

187   American Federation of Teachers HIV/AIDS Education Project
555 New Jersey Avenue NW
Washington, DC 20001-2029   202-879-4400
                                                www.aft.org
A group of education professionals with the main purpose of their
work being the education and public awareness of HIV and AIDS.
Randi Weingarten, President
Lorretta Johnson, Secretary-treasurer

188   American Foundation for AIDS Research
120 Wall Street   212-806-1600
New York, NY 10005-3908   800-342-2437
                                                            Fax: 212-806-1601
                                                            TTY: 800-243-7889
                                             e-mail: kevin.frost@amfar.org
                                                            www.amfar.org
Supports research in basic clinical prevention and public policy
and publishes the HIV/AIDS Treatment Directory.
Kenneth Cole, Chairman
Patricia J. Matson, Vice Chairman

**189   Asian & Pacific Islander Wellness Center Community HIV/AIDS
         Services**
730 Polk Street   415-292-3400
San Francisco, CA 94109   Fax: 415-292-3404
                                                            TTY: 415-292-3410
                                             e-mail: info@apiwellness.org
                                                            www.apiwellness.org
HIV Care Services is the only integrated HIV services program targeting A&PIs in Northern California. Integrates primary care with
psychiatric mental health HIV treatment psychosocial support
and, in response to evolving needs, targeted HIV prevention.
Lin Lin, President
Bart Akoki, Vice President

190   Asian and Pacific Island Wellness Center
730 Polk Street   415-292-3400
San Francisco, CA 94109   Fax: 415-292-3404
                                                            TTY: 415-292-3410
                                             e-mail: info@apiwellness.org
                                                            www.apiwellness.org
Our mission is to educate support empower and advocate for Asian
and Pacific Islander communities - particularly A&PIs living with
or at-risk for HIV/AIDS.
Lin Lin, President
Bart Akoki, Vice President

191   Better Existence with HIV
1244 W. Thorndale   773-293-4740
Chicago, IL 60660   Fax: 773-293-4750
                                                            www.behiv.org
Private not-for-profit AIDS service organization. Only compre-
hensive AIDS service provider in all northern Cook County. Effec-
tively combines direct service and prevention programs.
Eric Nelson, Executive Director
Julie Supple, Director of Programs

192   Black Coalition for AIDS Prevention
20 Victoria Street   416-977-9955
Toronto, M5C-2N8   Fax: 416-977-7664
                                             e-mail: blackcap@black-cap.com
                                                            www.black-cap.com
A volunteer-driven, charitable, not-for-profit, community-based
organization. Works in partnership with organizations and individuals who support in principle and practice our mission, philosophy
and activities.
Angela Robertson, Chair
Trevor Grey, Co-Chair

193   British Columbia Persons with AIDS Society
1107 Seymour Street   604-893-2200
Vancouver, BC, V6B-5S8   800-994-2437
                                                            Fax: 604-893-2251
                                             e-mail: info@positivelivingbc.org
                                                            www.positivelivingbc.org
Exists to enable persons living with AIDS and HIV disease to em-
power themselves through mutual support and collective action.
John Bishop, Chair
Claudette Cardinal, Vice chair

194   CDC National Prevention Information Network (NPIN)
PO Box 6003   301-519-0459
Rockville, MD 20849-6003   1 8-0 4-8 04
                                                            Fax: 888-282-7681
                                                            TTY: 888-480-3739
                                             e-mail: info@cdcnpin.org
                                                            www.cdcnpin.org
The CDC National Prevention Information Network (NPIN) is the
U.S. reference, referral, and distribution service for information

on HIV/AIDS, sexually transmitted diseases (STD's), and tuberculosis (TB). NPIN produces, collects, catalogs, processes, stocks,
and disseminates materials and information on HIV/AIDS, STD's,
and TB to organizations and people working in those disease fields
in international, national, state, and local settings.

195   Canadian Foundation for AIDS Research
200 Wellington Street West   416-361-6281
Toronto, Ontario, M5V-3B8   800-563-2873
                                                            Fax: 416-361-5736
                                                            www.canfar.ca
A national charitable foundation whose goal is to raise awareness
in order to generate funds for research into all aspects of HIV infec-
tion and AIDS.
Andrew M Pringle, Chair
Salah J. Bachir, Deputy Chair

196   Central Alberta AIDS Network Society
4611-50th Avenue   403-346-8858
Red Deer, AB T4N-3Z9   877-346-8858
                                                            Fax: 403-346-2352
                                             e-mail: Info@caans.org
                                                            www.caans.org
Central Alberta AIDS Network Society is a local charity and a
Turning Point agency that offers support to individuals who are in-
fected or affected by HIV/AIDS and provides prevention and edu-
cation throughout Central Alberta.
Jennifer Vanderschae, Executive Director
Alma , Health Promotion Coordinator

197   Children Affected by AIDS Foundation
6033 W Century Boulevard   310-258-0850
Los Angeles, CA 90045   Fax: 310-258-0851
                                             e-mail: caaf@caaf4kids.org
                                                            www.caaf4kids.org
The mission of the Children Affected by AIDS Foundation
(CAAF) is to make a positive difference in the lives of children in-
fected with HIV and affected by AIDS. CAAF accomplishes this
by helping meet their diverse, special needs, advocating and
educating.
Jayne Harkness, President
Joe Christina, Founder, Vice President

198   Children's AIDS Fund
PO Box 16433   703-433-1560
Washington, DC 20041   866-829-1560
                                                            Fax: 703-433-1561
                                             e-mail: info@childrensaidsfund.org
                                                            www.childrensaidsfund.org
The Children's AIDS Fund works to limit suffering of children and
their families caused by HIV disease by providing care services
resourced referrals and education.
Anita Smith, President

199   Clinical Focus on Primary Immune Deficiency Diseases
Immune Deficiency Foundation
40 W Chesapeake Avenue   410-321-6647
Towson, MD 21204   800-296-4433
                                                            Fax: 410-321-9165
                                             e-mail: info@primaryimmune.org
                                                            www.primaryimmune.org
Educational monograph is designed specifically for health care
professionals and focuses on topics relevant to primary immune
deficiency diseases.
Marcia Boyle, President & Founder
John Seymour, Vice Chair

200   Committee of Ten Thousand
236 Massachusetts Avenue NE   202-543-0988
Washington, DC 20002   800-488-2688
                                                            Fax: 202-543-6720
                                             e-mail: cott-dc@earthlink.net
                                                            www.cott1.org
Represents people with hemophilia who contracted HIV/AIDS and
Hepatitis C from tainted factory concentrates in the 1970s and
1980s. The only national advocacy and support agency for this se-
riously disabled community.
Corey S Dubin, President
Mary Lou Murphy, Co-Vice President

201 Continuum
255 Golden Gate Avenue
San Francisco, CA 94102

415-437-2900
Fax: 415-437-2550
TTY: 415-861-1399
e-mail: anne@continuumhiv.org
web.mac.com/tenderloinhealth

Empower and dignify the lives of underserved people with HIV and AIDS providing innovative health and human services that establish community, and reduce the rate of HIV infection.
Colm Hegarty, Director Development & Public Relations
Chiquita T Tuttle, Interim Executive Director

202 Deaf AIDS Project Family Service Foundation
Family Service Foundation
5301 76th Avenue
Landover Hills, MD 20784

301-459-2121
866-935-4658
Fax: 301-459-0675
TTY: 301-731-2116
e-mail: ssoulier@fsfinc.org
www.deafnonprofit.net/dap

The AIDS Administration established in 1987 as a division of the Maryland Department of Health and Mental Hygiene leads public health initiatives regarding HIV (Human Immunodeficiency Virus), the virus that causes AIDS.

203 Elizabeth Glaser Pediatric AIDS Foundation
1140 Connecticut Avenue NW
Washington, DC 20036

202-296-9165
888-499-4673
Fax: 202-296-9185
e-mail: info@pedaids.org
www.pedaids.org

Creates a future of hope for children and families worldwide by eradicating pediatric AIDS providing care and treatment to people with HIV/AIDS and accelerating the discovery of new treatments for other serious and life-threatening pediatric illnesses.
Charles Lyons, President/CEO
Susie Zeegan, Co-Founder

204 Farha Foundation
576, Sainte-Catherine Street E
Montreal, QC, H2L-2E1

514-270-4900
Fax: 514-270-5363
e-mail: farha@farha.qc.ca
www.farha.qc.ca

A fundraising organization, committed to help men, women and children living with HIV/AIDS.
Nancy Farha, Executive Director
Lucille Valade, Event Manager

205 Foundation for Children with AIDS
6221 Blue Grass Avenue
Harrisburg, PA 17112-2331

717-489-0206
888-683-8323
Fax: 717-489-0214
e-mail: info@AFCAids.org
www.helpchildrenwithaids.org

A national nonprofit organization founded to improve the quality of life for drug-effected and HIV-infected children and their families. The foundation raises funds for family and community-based services for children and their families affected by HIV.
Nick Cassino, President
Robert Maynard, Vice President

206 HIV West Yellowhead Services
Box 2427
Jasper, Alberta, T0E-1E0

780-852-5274
877-291-8811
Fax: 780-852-5273
e-mail: hivdirector@incentre.net
www.hivwestyellowhead.com

Encourage a positive, healthy lifestyle and provide accurate information to the people living and working in the region.
Allan Bearns, Chair
Nancy Taylor, Vice Chair

207 HIV/Hepatitis C in Prison (HIP) Committee
California Prison Focus
San Francisco, CA 94103

510-665-1935
e-mail: contact@prisons.org
www.prisons.org/hivin.htm

The HIV/HCV in Prison Committee of California Prison Focus works on behalf of prisoners to fight for consistent access to quality medical care including access to all new HIV and hepatitis C medications, diagnostic testing and combination therapies.
Michelle Foy, Contact
Judy Greenspan, Contact

208 Health Information Network
PO Box 30762
Seattle, WA 98113

206-784-5655
Fax: 206-784-3240
www.healthinfonetwork.org

Offers information public awareness and support for women with HIV/AIDS and the public in general.
Kathi Knowles, Executive Director

209 Health Information Network for Women and AIDS
Positive Women's Network
2817 Rockefeller Avenue
Everett, WA 98201

425-259-9899
888-651-8931
Fax: 425-259-9880
www.pwnetwork.org

A partnership of women living with and affected by HIV/AIDS supports women in making informed choices about HIV/AIDS and health.
Rhea Reynolds, President
Tayah E. H. Renfro, Vice President

210 Heart Touch™ Project
3400 Airport Avenue
Santa Monica, CA 90405

310-391-2558
Fax: 310-391-2168
e-mail: executive@hearttouch.org
www.hearttouch.org

Non-profit educational and service organization devoted to the delivery of compassionate and healing touch to home or hospital-bound men women and children.
Patrick Callahan, Executive Director
Jennifer Noguera, Director of Programs

211 Immune Deficiency Foundation
40 W Chesapeake Avenue
Towson, MD 21204-4841

410-321-6647
800-296-4433
Fax: 410-321-9165
e-mail: info@primaryimmune.org
www.primaryimmune.org

The only national charitable organization aimed at fighting the primary immune deficiency diseases. The founders included parents of children with primary immune deficiency immunologists who treat immune deficient patients and other individuals with an immune deficiency.
Marcia Boyle, President & Founder
John Seymour, Vice Chair

212 International Council of AIDS Service Organization
65 Wellesley Street E
Toronto Ontario, M4Y 1-1G7

416-921-0018
Fax: 416-921-9979
e-mail: icaso@icaso.org
www.icaso.org

A global network of non-governmental and community-based organizations.
Mary Ann Torres, Executive Director
Margaret Quish, Financial Manager

213 Life Force: Women Fighting AIDS
57 Willoughby Street
Brooklyn, NY 11201-4300

718-797-0937
Fax: 718-797-4011
e-mail: info@lifeforceinc.org
www.lifeforceinc.org

A support network offering prevention education awareness risk reduction workshops and support for woman with HIV/AIDS.
Sayida Self, Program Director
Linney Smith, Executive Director

214 Living Positive
9912-106 Street
Edmonton, Alberta, T5K-1C5

780-488-5768
800-210-9561
Fax: 780-702-8211
www.edmlivingpositive.ca

Dedicated to providing emotional, spiritual and psychological support to all those living with HIV.
Lance Hansen, Director
Deborah Norris, Chairperson

215 Medical Library Association
65 E Wacker Place
Chicago, IL 60601-7246

312-419-9094
Fax: 312-419-8950
e-mail: info@mlahq.org
www.mlahq.org

Non-profit educational organization of more than 1,100 institutions and 3,600 individual members in the health sciences information field, committed to educating health information professionals, supporting health information research and promoting access to information.
Ruth Holst, President
Carla J Funk, Executive Director

216 Multifaith Works
1401 East Jefferson Street
Seattle, WA 98122

206-324-1520
Fax: 206-324-2041
e-mail: info@rosehedge.org
www.multifaith.org

Non-profit non-denominational organization that provides housing and supportive services to people living with AIDS or other life-threatening illness and community education on issues of human diversity.
Paul Binder, President
Anthony Radovich, Secretary

217 NAMES Project Foundation AIDS Memorial Quilt
AIDS Memorial Quilt
204 14th Street NW
Atlanta, GA 30318-5304

404-688-5500
Fax: 404-688-5552
e-mail: info@aidsquilt.org
www.aidsquilt.org

International non-governmental non-profit organization that is the custodian of the AIDS Memorial Quilt a poignant memorial and powerful tool for use in preventing new HIV infections.
Robert Bush, Chair
Tom Gertz, Vice Chair

218 National AIDS Fund
1424 K Street, N.W
Washington, DC 20005-1511

202-408-4848
888-234-AIDS
Fax: 202-408-1818
www.aidsfund.org

The National AIDS Fund is one of America's largest philanthropic organizations dedicated to eliminating HIV/AIDS as a major health and social problem. The Fund's primary purpose is channeling critical resources to community-based organizations to fight HIV.
Mark Ishaug, President & CEO
Douglas Brooks, Senior Vice President

219 National AIDS Treatment Advocacy Project
580 Broadway
New York, NY 10012

212-219-0106
888-26N-ATAP
Fax: 212-219-8473
e-mail: info@natap.org
www.natap.org

Educate by sending out literature e-mail lists and give forums on how to prevent HIV or how to live with it.
Jules Levin, Executive Director
Jose Ernesto Nunez, Executive Assistant

220 National Coalition on Immune System Disorders
1090 Vermont Avenue NW
Washington, DC 20005-4953

202-371-8090
800-438-2996
Fax: 202-371-1945

Professional and lay organizations with a primary interest in the immune system and its diseases.
Robert R Humphreys, Executive Director

221 National Hospice & Palliative Care Organization (NHPCO)
1731 King Street
Alexandria, VA 22314

703-837-1500
800-646-6460
Fax: 703-837-1233
e-mail: nhpco_info@nhpco.org
www.nhpco.org

The nation's only advocate for terminally ill patients and their families. Founded in 1978, the NHPCO is the only organization devoted to hospice in the United States. Support is included from state hospice organizations, patients, families, communities, provider program members and professional/volunteer members.

Represents hospice care interests to Congress, regulatory agencies, courts, voluntary organizations and the public.
Donald Schumacher, President/CEO
Samira Beckwith, Treasurer

222 National Minority AIDS Education Training Center
Howard University
1840 7th Street NW
Washington, DC 20001-3029

202-865-8146
Fax: 202-667-1382
e-mail: gdowner@howard.edu
www.aetcnmc.org/index

Located at Howard University as a HIV/AIDS training and technical resource for providers of minority HIV-infected patients throughout the country. The NMAETC receives 100% of its funding through the MAI Initiative.
Goulda Downe PhD RD, Principal Investigator
David Luckett, Deputy Director

223 National Native American AIDS Prevention Center
720 S Colorado Boulevard
Denver, CO 80246

720-382-2244
Fax: 720-382-2248
e-mail: information@nnaapc.org
www.nnaapc.org

To address the impact of HIV/AIDS on American Indians Alaska Natives and Native Hawaiians through culturally appropriate advocacy research education and policy development in support of healthy Indigenous people.
D Shane Barnett, Chairperson
Mary Helen Deer, Vice Chairperson

224 National Prevention Information Network CDC NPIN
PO Box 6003
Rockville, MD 20849-6003

301-519-0459
1 8-0 4-8 04
Fax: 888-282-7681
TTY: 888-480-3739
e-mail: info@cdcnpin.org
www.cdcnpin.org

The CDC National Prevention Information Network (NPIN) is the U.S. reference referral and distribution service for information on HIV/AIDS, sexually transmitted diseases (STDs) and tuberculosis (TB).
Jay Laudato, Executive Director

225 National Prison Project/ACLU AIDS in Prison Project
125 Broad Street
New York, NY 10004

212-549-2500
e-mail: media@aclu.org
www.aclu.org

National Prison Project seeks to create constitutional conditions of confinement and strengthen prisoners' rights through class action litigation and public education. Our policy priorities include reducing prison overcrowding and improving prisoner medical care.
Susan N Herman, President
Anthony Romero, Executive Director

226 New England AIDS Education and Training Center
38 Chauncy Street
Boston, MA 02111-3318

617-262-5657
Fax: 617-262-5667
e-mail: aidsed@neaetc.org
www.neaetc.org

Our goal is to increase the number of health care providers effectively trained to counsel diagnose treat and manage the care of individuals with HIV infection and to assist in the prevention of high risk behavior which may lead to infection.
James Meenaghan, Project Manager
Helene Bednarsh, Director

227 North Bay Aids Committee
269 Main Street W
North Bay, Ontario, P1B2T-2T8

705-497-3560
800-387-3701
Fax: 705-497-7850
e-mail: acnba@efni.com
www.aidsnorthbay.com

To assist and support all persons infected or affected by HIV/AIDS and to limit the spread of the virus through education and outreach strategies.
Stacey L Mayhall, Executive Director
Kirk Titmus, Board Chair

228   Ontario HIV Treatment Network
1300 Yonge Street   416-642-6486
Toronto, Ontario, M41X3   877-743-6486
                                                Fax: 416-640-4245
                                          e-mail: info@ohtn.on.ca
                                                  www.ohtn.on.ca
To optimize the quality of life of people living with HIV in Ontario
and to promote excellence and innovation in treatment, research,
education and prevention through a collaborative network of excellence representing consumers, providers, researchers and other
stakeholders.
David Hoe, President
Claire Kendell, Vice President

229   Pediatric AIDS Foundation
11150 Santa Monica Boulevard   310-314-1459
Los Angeles, CA 90025-3092   Fax: 310-314-1469
                                        e-mail: info@pedaids.org
                                                 www.pedaids.org
A national nonprofit organization confronting medical problems
unique to children infected with HIV/AIDS. The foundation funds
critically needed pediatric AIDS research and provides help to
hospitals that serve the needs of children with HIV/AIDS.
Charles Lyons, President/CEO
Susie Zeegan, Co-Founder

230   Peel HIV/AIDS Network
160 Traders Boulevard E   905-361-0523
Mississauga, Ontario, L4Z 3-4K1   866-896-8700
                                                Fax: 905-361-1004
                                          e-mail: info@phan.ca
                                                  www.phan.ca
Committed to serving people living with and affected by
HIV/AIDS and to limit the spread of the virus through support edu-
cation advocacy and volunteerism.
Tania Fernandes, Board Co Chair
Sanya Khan, Board Secretary

231   Project Inform
1375 Mission Street   415-558-8669
San Francisco, CA 94103   800-822-7422
                                                Fax: 415-558-0684
                              e-mail: support@projectforum.org
                         www.projectforum.org/HIVhealth/infoline
HIV Health Infoline has provided HIV treatment and access to care
information, free of charge, to people living with HIV, their providers and support networks. Staffed by highly trained volunteers,
the Infoline has the personal experiences and outside connections
to answer questions about living healthfully with HIV.
Dana Van Gorder, Executive Director
Michael Allerton, President

232   Resources and Services Database Centers for Disease Control
Centers for Disease Control
1600 Clifton Road   800-232-4636
Atlanta, GA 30333   877-242-9760
                                                Fax: 301-562-1050
                                              TTY: (888) 232-63
                                       e-mail: info@hivatwork.org
                                                 www.brta-lrta.org
Describes more than 16 000 organizations that provide HIV and
AIDS prevention education and social services. These include
public health departments community and social service organizations hospitals and clinics.

233   The AIDS Network
140 King Street East   905-528-0854
Hamilton, ON, L8N-1B2   866-563-0563
                                                Fax: 905-528-6311
                                       e-mail: info@aidsnetwork.ca
                                                 www.aidsnetwork.ca
Ruthann Tucker, Executive Director
Roxanne Ali, Director Program Services

234   Toronto People with AIDS Foundation
200 Gerard Street E   416-506-1400
Toronto, Ontario, M5A-2E6   Fax: 416-506-1404
                                       e-mail: info@pwatoronto.org
                                                 www.pwatoronto.org

The Toronto People with AIDS Foundation exists to promote the
health and well-being of all people living with HIV/AIDS by providing accessible, direct, and practical support services.
Cory Garlough, President
Brian Fior, Vice president

235   UNICEF USA
125 Maiden Lane   212-686-5522
New York, NY 10038   800-486-4233
                                                Fax: 212-779-1679
                               e-mail: information@unicefusa.org
                                                 www.unicefusa.org
Supports child survival protection and development worldwide
through education advocacy and fundraising for AIDS and other
conditions.
Caryl M Stern, President and CEO
Edward G Lloyd, Executive Vice President and CFO

236   Well Project
112 Krog Street NE   404-474-3152
Atlanta, GA 30307   888-616-9355
                                       e-mail: info@thewellproject.org
                                                 www.thewellproject.org
The Well Project is a not for profit corporation and an initiative
conceived developed and administered by HIV+ women and those
who are affected by this disease. Our Founder Dawn Averitt Bridge
was diagnosed with HIV in 1988.
Dawn Averitt Bridge, Founder & Board President
Richard Averitt, CO Founder

237   Women Alive
1301 N. Willowbrook Avenue   310-605-1365
Compton, CA 90222   800-554-4876
                                                Fax: 310-605-1366
                                       e-mail: info@women-alive.org
                                                 www.women-alive.org
Coalition of, by and for women living with HIV/AIDS. Created
ways to help women connect with each other, bring others out of
isolation, exchange information about HIV treatments and take
charge of their lives.
Alfredia Thomas, President
Carrie Broadus, Executive Director

238   Women's AIDS Network Women and Children's Service Program
Women and Children's Service Program
4 North Broad street
Trenton, NJ 08608   415-864-4376
                                                 www.njwan.org
Marylou Freund, President
Deborah Walker McCall, Associate Dean

State Agencies & Associations

Alabama

239   Alabama Department of Public Health
201 Monroe Street   334-206-5364
Montgomery, AL 36104-3000   800-228-0469
                                                Fax: 334-206-2092
                                                 www.adph.org/aids
Offers health education and risk education activities including
compiling a state community resource directory.
Danna Cargill, Office Manager
Jane B Cheeks, Division Director

Alaska

240   Alaska Department of Health and Social Services: AIDS/STD Program
3601 C Street   907-269-8000
Anchorage, AK 99503-0249   800-478-0084
                                                Fax: 907-562-7802
                              e-mail: mollie_cross@health.state.ak.us
                                        www.epi.hss.state.ak.us/hivstd
The HIV/STD Program addresses public health issues and activi-
ties with the goal of preventing sexually transmitted diseases
(STDs) and HIV infection in Alaska as well as their impact on

health. AIDS program offers education to providers and organizations.
John Middaug PhD, Chief Dept of Public Health/Epidemiology
Mollie Cross, Prevention Community Planning Group

Arizona

241 Arizona Department of Health Services
150 N 18th Avenue 602-542-1025
Phoenix, AZ 85007 800-334-1540
Fax: 602-542-0883
www.azdhs.gov

Provides HIV and AIDS seropositive surveillance case investigation and analysis and AIDS health education and training for the public.
Margery Sheridan, Division Chief
Will Humble, Interim Director

242 Body Positive HIV and AIDS Research and Re Southwest Center for HIV/AIDS
1144 E McDowell Road 602-307-5330
Phoenix, AZ 85006 Fax: 602-307-5021
e-mail: cweiner@phoenixbodypositive.org
http://swhiv.org/

Body Positive is a non-profit organization created by and for people infected and affected by HIV, that provides the community with the knowledge, resources and collective strength necessary for individuals to live long and well with HIV and to prevent the spread of the disease.
Ken Gabel, Chair
jessica Fotinoes, Vice Chair

243 Tucson Interfaith HIV/AIDS Network (TIHAN)
2660 North 1st avenue 520-299-6647
Tucson, AZ 85719 Fax: 520-784-0620
e-mail: friends@tihan.org
www.tihan.org

Serving interfaith communities of Tucson through compassionate care education training and spiritual support so that we can make more people aware of the health crisis which affects all of us. Also provide non-medical in-home help.
david Cormier, Treasurer
Catherine Davis, President

Arkansas

244 Arkansas Department of Health AIDS Prevention Program
AIDS Prevention Program
4815 West Markham Street 501-661-2000
Little Rock, AR 72205 800-462-0599
www.healthyarkansas.com

Provides educational materials such as pamphlets and films conducts HIV and AIDS research and operates a speakers bureau.
Dr. Clark fincher, President
Paul Halverson, Director

California

245 Aids, Medicine and Miracles
3288 21st Street 415-252-7111
San Francisco, CA 94110-2423 Fax: 415-252-7117
e-mail: amminfo@aidsmedicineandmiracles.org
www.aidsmedicineandmiracles.org

Provides culturally sensitive counseling and education to stop the spread of HIV infection, and to help people face the emotional, psychological and social changes of living with HIV disease.
Gregg Cassin, Chair
Daniel Ramos, Secretary

246 California Collaborative Treatment Group CCTG Data Center
CCTG Data Center
3900 Fifth Avenue 619-543-5006
San Diego, CA 92103-1910 Fax: 619-298-1359
e-mail: rhaubrich@ucsd.edu
www.cctg.ucsd.edu

The CCTG is a multi-center clinical trials organization founded by Dr. Allen McCutchan in 1986. The primary mission of the CCTG is

to improve the scientific basis for HIV patient care and HIV prevention. CCTG develops treatment protocols and drug therapies.
Richard Haub MD, Investigator/Professor of Medicine
Allen McCutc MD, Investigator/Professor of Medicine

247 California Department of Health Services Office of Aids
Office of Aids
PO Box 997377, 916-445-4171
Sacramento, CA 95899 800-458-5231
Fax: 916-440-7404
www.dhs.ca.gov/aids

Works to develop strategies and implement programs for education and prevention testing and counseling supportive care and treatment and research to control the spread of HIV infection.
David Maxwell-Jolly, Director

248 Los Angeles County Department of Health Services
AIDS Programs
600 S Commonwealth Avenue 213-351-8000
Los Angeles, CA 90005 800-243-7889
Fax: 213-738-0825
e-mail: aids@ph.lacounty.org
www.lapublichealth.org

Responsible for planning coordinating and implementing county wide HIV/AIDS efforts.
Charles L Henry, Director
Raymond H Johnson, Chief of Staff

249 San Francisco AIDS Foundation (SFAF)
1035 Market Street 415-487-3000
San Francisco, CA 94103 800-367-AIDS
Fax: 415-487-8079
TTY: 415-487-3012
TDD: 415-487-8099
e-mail: info@aidslifecycle.org
www.sfaf.org

SFAF provides confidential array of services-including financial benefits counseling client advocacy housing assistance HIV prevention efforts and needle exchange.
Neil Giuliano, CEO
Nancy Durlester, VP Development

250 San Francisco Area AIDS Education and Training Center
UCSF Box 1365
50 Beale Street 415-597-9168
San Francisco, CA 94105-1365 Fax: 415-597-9386
e-mail: sfaetc@ucsf.edu
http://www.sfaetc.ucsf.edu/

Helps to improve the care of people living with HIV and AIDS by supporting state-of-the-art clinical consultation education and training for health care professionals and organizations in Sa Francisco San Mateo and Marin counties.
Jacqueline Tulsky, Medical Director
Ronald H Goldschmidt, Director

Colorado

251 CO Center for AIDS Research: University Colorado Health Sciences Center/CFAR
Division of Infectious Diseases
4200 E 9th Avenue 303-315-7233
Denver, CO 80262 Fax: 303-315-8681
e-mail: colorado.cfar@uchsc.edu
www.uchsc.edu/ccfar

Describes forms and patterns of use of complimentary and alternative medicine (CAM) for the treatment of HIV/AIDS.
Edward N Janoff MD, CFAR Director
Kristin Jones, CFAR Administrator

252 Mountain-Plains AIDS Education and Training Center (MPAETC)
12631 E 17th Avenue 303-724-0867
Aurora, CO 80045 Fax: 303-724-0875
e-mail: info@mpaetc.org
www.mpaetc.org

One of 12 regional AETCs funded nationwide by a grant from the U.S. Health Resources and Services Administration through the Ryan White Comprehensive AIDS Resources Emergency (CARE)

Act. Provides educational programs about HIV infection for healthcare providers.
Beth Mullin Rotach, Director
Lucy Bradley-Springe, Principal Investigator

Connecticut

253 Connecticut Department of Health Services AIDS Programs
AIDS Programs
410 Capitol Avenue   860-509-8000
Hartford, CT 06134   800-842-0038
                            Fax: 860-509-7853
                e-mail: webmaster.dph@ct.gov
                            www.dph.state.ct.us
Operates a speakers bureau provides training workshops seminars and counseling services conducts meetings and offers information and referral services.
Rosa M Biaggi, Director
William Gerrish, Communications

254 Northwestern Connecticut AIDS Project
100 Migeon Avenue   860-482-1596
Torrington, CT 06790-0985   800-381-2437
                            Fax: 860-482-3606
                    e-mail: general@nwctaids.org
                www.freewebs.com/nwctaidsproject
A nonprofit organization offering support and a variety of services to people with AIDS and their loved ones. Provides education to all segments of the public about AIDS prevention and treatment.
Patricia Lafayette, Executive Director
Demetria McMilliAn, Program Director Client Services

Delaware

255 Delaware Department of Health and Social Services
Division of Public Health, HIV/STD Program
417 Federal Street   302-744-4700
Dover, DE 19901   888-459-2943
                            Fax: 302-739-6659
                    e-mail: dhssinfo@state.de.us
                www.dhss.delaware.gov/dhss/dph/index.htm
Provides HIV counseling and testing prevention education and AIDS surveillance and studies.
Jamie Rivera, Director

District of Columbia

256 Washington DC Department of Health HIV/AIDS Administration
HIV/AIDS Administration
899 North Capitol Street NE
Washington, DC 20002   202-442-5955
                            www.doh.dc.gov
Mission is to reduce the incidence of HIV/AIDS and number of deaths related to HIV/AIDS in the District of Columbia by the application of sound public health practices and initiatives through HIV disease surveillance tracking, monitoring, and intervention.
Mohammed Akhter, Director

Florida

257 Florida Department of Health Bureau of HIV/AIDS
Bureau of HIV/AIDS
4052 Bald Cypress Way   850- 24- 414
Tallahassee, FL 32399-1715 Fax: 850- 24- 444
                e-mail: DiseaseControl@doh.state.fl.us
                            www.doh.state.fl.us
Making voluntary HIV testing a routine part of medical care implementing new models for diagnosing HIV infections outside medical settings preventing new infections by working with persons diagnosed with HIV and their partners.
Tom Liberti, Bureau Chief
Janell Clemons, Administrative Assistant

258 Positive Voices
9526 NE 2nd Ave   786-873-8576
Miami, FL 33138   888-POS-CONN
                            Fax: 786-623-0701
                e-mail: email@positiveconnections.org
                            www.positiveconnections.org

The Center for Positive Connections is a non-profit community based organization that is run for those infected our community. Our mission is to provide educational emotional holistic and social support at all individuals living with HIV/AIDS.
Dr. David Newman, President
Rec Ken Furguson, Vice President

Georgia

259 Georgia Department of Human Resources: Division of Public Health
AIDS Section
2 Peachtree Street NW   404-657-2700
Atlanta, GA 30303   800-551-2728
                            Fax: 404-657-3100
                e-mail: gdphinfo@dhr.ga.us
                            http://health.state.ga.us
Provides technical support and assistance to the Public Health Districts to prevent STD and HIV infection ensuring the availability of quality STD/HIV prevention and treatment by improving quality assurance guidelines and methods by providing appropriate training.
Katheryn K. Cheek, Board Chair
James W Curran, Dean

Hawaii

260 Hawaii Department of Health: Communicable Disease Division
AIDS/Sexually Transmitted Diseases Control Branch
1250 Punchbowl St   80 - 5 - 44
Honolulu, HI 96813-2317   Fax: 80 - 5 - 44
                e-mail: janice.okubo@doh.hawaii.gov
                www.hawaii.gov/health/about/admin
Offers research education surveillance and testing components. AIDS information and guidelines about the placement of infants children and adolescents who test positive for HIV in nursery or school settings are also available.
Chiyome Fuki MD, Director
Loretta Fuddy, Deputy Director

Idaho

261 Idaho Department of Health and Welfare The STD/AIDS Program
The STD/AIDS Program
450 W State Street 1st Floor   208-334-6527
Boise, ID 83720-0036   Fax: 208-332-7346
                e-mail: apsportal@dhw.idaho.gov
                www.healthandwelfare.idaho.gov
Program receives federal funding to support testing treatment and prevention services for Idaho's reportable sexually transmitted infections.
Richard Roberge, Chairman
Janet Penfold, Vice Chair

Illinois

262 AIDS Legal Council of Chicago
180 N Michigan Avenue   312-427-8990
Chicago, IL 60601   866-506-3038
                            Fax: 312-427-8419
                    e-mail: info@aidslegal.com
                            www.aidslegal.com
Legal advice and services for persons who are HIV positive or have AIDS and their companions families etc.
Todd A Solomon, President
Dr. Matthew Feldhaus, Vice President

263 Chicago Department of Health
333 S State Street   312-747-9884
Chicago, IL 60604   Fax: 312-747-9765
                            TTY: 312-747-2374
                e-mail: publichealth@cdph.org
                            www.cityofchicago.org
Offers educational services audiovisual materials surveillance of HIV and AIDS counseling and referrals.
Carolyn Lopez, President
Bechara Choucair, Commissioner

264 **Illinois Department of Public Health: Division of Infectious Diseases**
535 W Jefferson Street
Springfield, IL 62761
217-782-4977
Fax: 217-782-3987
TTY: 800-547-0466
www.idph.state.il.us

Administers the AIDS Drug Assistance Program (ADAP). Currently nearly 3 300 clients use ADAP services each month accessing 10 000 prescriptions. Client approved for ADAP must re-apply on an annual basis in order to continue to receive services.
Damon Arnold, Director
Randy J Dunn, State Superintendent of Education

265 **Test Positive Aware Network (TPAN)**
5537 N Broadway Street
Chicago, IL 60640-1405
773-989-9400
Fax: 773-989-9494
e-mail: tpan@tpan.com
www.tpan.com

Empowers people living with HIV through peer-led programming support services information dissemination and advocacy. Provides services to the broader community to increase HIV knowledge and sensitivity and to reduce the risk of infection.
Bill Farrand, CEO/Dierctor of Client Services
Thomas Hart, President

Kansas

266 **Kansas Department of Health & Environment Epidemiology & Disease Prevention: HIV**
1000 SW Jackson
Topeka, KS 66612-1274
785-296-1500
Fax: 785-368-6368
e-mail: info@kdheks.gov
www.kdheks.gov

Conducts surveillance of HIV/AIDS in Kansas. Conducts Prevention Program with training for counselors and educators partial funding of counseling test sites and distribution of educational materials. Provides medications and primary care.
Sam Brownback, Governer
Robert Moser, Secretary

Louisiana

267 **Louisiana Department of Health & Hospitals : Office of Public Health**
Louisiana AIDS Prevention/Surveillance Program
628 N 4th Street
Baton Rouge, LA 70821-0629
22 - 3 - 80
Fax: 22 - 3 - 80
e-mail: avis.richard-griffin@la.gov
http://www.dhh.louisiana.gov/offices/?id

The HIV/AIDS Program was established in 1985 to provide leadership policy development and technical assistance including HIV/AIDS education prevention and services to parish health units and community based organizations throughout the state.
William Clark, Medical Director
William Hineman, Director/Program Manager II

Maine

268 **Maine Bureau of Health: Division of Disease Control**
HIV/STD Program
286 Water Street
Augusta, ME 04333
207-287-8016
800-821-5821
Fax: 207-287-3498
TTY: 800-606-0215
e-mail: chris.zukas-lessard@maine.gov
www.maine.gov/dhhs/boh/index.htm

Provides technical assistance to state agencies and private organizations regarding AIDS education and policy development.
Chris Zukas-Lessard, Deputy Director
Dora Anne Mills, Director

Massachusetts

269 **Massachusetts Department of Health HIV/AIDS Bureau**
HIV/AIDS Bureau
250 Washington Street
Boston, MA 02108
617-624-6000
800-235-2331
Fax: 617-624-5399
TTY: 617-437-1672
www.mass.gov/dph

Assisting in preventing the spread of the HIV epidemic and the development of appropriate cost-effective health and support services which will maintain patients in the least restrictive setting.
Kevin Cranston, Director
John Auerbach, Commissioner Department of Public Health

270 **New England AIDS Education & Training Center (NEHEC)**
38 Chauncy Street
Boston, MA 02215-3318
617-262-5657
Fax: 617-262-5667
e-mail: aidsed@neaetc.org
www.neaetc.org

The New England HIV Education Consortium (NEHEC), a HRSA minority AIDS initiative program, is a training and education program serving all six states in the New England region. The principal goal of NEHEC is to address the HIV-related training, educational, and support needs of the full, spectrum of providers as they provide state-of-the-art, quality and compassionate care to individuals living with HIV/AIDS.
Donna M Gallagher RNC/MS/ANP, Principal Investigator/Project Director
Barry Sandberg MS/MPA, Assistant Director/Administrator

Michigan

271 **Michigan Department of Community Health HIV/AIDS Prevention & Intervention Secti**
HIV/AIDS Prevention & Intervention Section
201 Townsend avenue
Lansing, MI 48913
17 -73 -740
888-826-6565
Fax: 517-241-5911
www.michigan.gov/mdch

Gives general public and high-risk education grants supporting educational materials programs and a hotline.
James K haven, Director Division HIV/AIDS-STD
Nick Lyon, Deputy Director

Minnesota

272 **Minnesota Department of Health: AIDS/STD Prevention Service**
Office of Infectious Diseases
P.O. Box 64975
Minneapolis, MN 55164-9272
651-201-5000
877-925-4189
Fax: 612-623-5743
e-mail: indepcweb@health.state.mn.us
www.health.state.mn.us

This division is to prevent death and disability from HIV and other sexually transmitted diseases by providing statewide leadership regarding the prevention of transmission and the availability of health and supportive services for infected persons.
Harry Hull, Director

Mississippi

273 **Mississippi Department of Public Health: STD/HIV Prevention Program**
570 E Woodrow Wilson Drive
Jackson, MS 39216
601-576-7400
866-458-4948
Fax: 601-576-7909
www.msdh.state.ms.us

Funds two statewide hotlines one for the general public and one for the gay community. Both offer health education and risk reduction activities of the Program include baseline evaluation of public knowledge about AIDS through surveys.
Joy Sennett, Director Communicable Disease Office

Missouri

274 **Missouri Department of Health: Bureau of AIDS Prevention**
912 Wildwood
Jefferson City, MO 65102-0570
573-751-6400
866-628-9891
Fax: 573-751-6010
e-mail: info@dhss.mo.gov
www.dhss.mo.gov

Human Immunodeficiency Virus (HIV) disease and infection and Acquired Immunodeficiency Syndrome (AIDS) surveillance monitors and analyzes data on the number of people infected with HIV and/or AIDS and identifies and tracks trends in disease incidence.
Margaret T Donnelly, Director
Bret Fischer, Director

Montana

275 Montana Deptartment of Health And Human Services
STD & HIV Prevention Program
1400 Broadway   406-444-4540
Helena, MT 59620   800-233-6668
                                        Fax: 406-444-1861
                                        www.dphhs.state.mt.us
This program receives a Federal grant through the Centers for Disease Control to carry out a health education/risk reduction program to detect and prevent the spread of HIV infection through a number of services.
Jane Smilie, Acting Administrator
Anna Whiting Sorrell, Director

Nevada

276 Nevada Department of Human Resources: Health Program Section
4126 Technology Way   775-684-4000
Carson City, NV 89706-2009   Fax: 775-684-4010
                                        e-mail: nvdhr@dhhs.nv.gov
                                        www.dhhs.nv.gov
Provides HIV counseling and testing a speakers bureau information and referrals resource materials including AIDS video recordings and education.
Harold Cook, Administrator
Mike Wilden, Director

277 TBAN
6955 N. Durango Dr. Ste   702-608- 247
Las Vegas, NV 89149-8333   Fax: 702-870-2474
                                        www.tban.com/
TBAN formerly The Tampa AIDS Network (TAN) is a community organization which provides prevention education emotional and physical support services and advocacy on behalf of all persons affected by HIV disease.
Mike Gardinear, President
Joe Russo, Treasurer

New Hampshire

278 New Hampshire Department of Health and Human Services
Division of Public Health Services
129 Pleasant Street   603-271-4502
Concord, NH 03301-4604   800-852-3345
                                        Fax: 603-271-4934
                                        TTY: 800-735-2964
                                        TDD: 8007352964
                                        www.dhhs.state.nh.us
HIV/AIDS Program receives both state and Federal funding pertaining to AIDS education risk reduction testing and surveillance.
Joyce J Welch, Program Coordinator
James Fredyma, Director

New Jersey

279 New Jersey Department of Health: Division of AIDS Prevention & Control
Division of HIV/AIDS Service (DHAS)
Po Box 360   609-292-7837
Trenton, NJ 08625-0360   800-367-6543
                                        www.state.nj.us/health
Serves to coordinate and direct primary HIV activities within the Department networking with other divisions and agencies to provide information and care programs to populations in need.
Laurence E Ganges, Assistant Commissioner
John Fasanella, Director

280 New Jersey Woman AIDS Network
4 North Broad Street   609-695-1200
Trenton, NJ 08608   800-747-1108
                                        Fax: 609-695-1201
                                        e-mail: office@njwan.org
                                        www.njwan.org
A leader in identifying issues facing women with HIV/AIDS educating service providers advocating for appropriate policies and building a multicultural women and HIV/AIDS movement.
Patryce Burgess, Interim Executive Director
Adrienne Smith, Program Coordinator

New Mexico

281 New Mexico Health Department: Public Health Division
HIV/AIDS/STD Prevention & Services Bureau
1190 S Saint Francis Drive   505-827-2613
Santa Fe, NM 87502-4182   800-545-2437
                                        Fax: 505-827-2530
                                        www.health.state.nm.us
Provides training programs and HIV education to the general public and professionals risk reduction information AIDS school curriculums classroom presentation information and an AIDS hotline.
Don Maestas, Director

New York

282 New York Department of Health, Office of Public Health: AIDS Institute
AIDS Institute
Empire State Plaza   518-474-9866
Albany, NY 12237-0001   866-881-2809
                                        Fax: 518-473-8814
                                        e-mail: hivpubs@health.state.ny.us
                                        www.health.state.ny.us
Awards grants and maintains relationships with regional AIDS service groups, crisis intervention, psychosocial counseling and legal, financial and housing assistance. The Institute also offers preventive education, risk reduction education, HIV counseling and testing and patient care.
Wendy V. Gould, Coordinator Educational Materials

North Carolina

283 North Carolina Department of Health & Natural Resources
HIV/STD Prevention & Care
2001 Mail Service Center   919-855-4800
Raleigh, NC 27699-1902   Fax: 919-870-4829
                                        e-mail: hivstdprevention@ncmail.net
                                        www.ncpublichealth.com
Oversee the AIDS surveillance program HIV counseling testing partner notification health education risk reduction and public information efforts in North Carolina.
Rebecca King, Chief
Jeffrey Engel, Director

Ohio

284 Ohio Department of Health: Division of Preventive Medicine
HIV/AIDS Surveillance Division
246 N High Street   614-466-3543
Columbus, OH 43215-0118   800-777-4775
                                        Fax: 614-644-1909
                                        TTY: 800-332-AIDS
                                        e-mail: Surveillance@odh.ohio.gov
                                        www.odh.ohio.gov
Consists of AIDS surveillance seroprevalence programs, health care worker education, health education and risk reduction projects.
John R. Kasich, Governor
Theodore E. Wymyslo, M.D., Director

Oklahoma

285 Oklahoma Department of Health: AIDS Division
1000 NE 10th   405-271-5600
Oklahoma City, OK 73117-1207   800-522-0203
                                        Fax: 405-271-5149
                                        www.health.state.ok.us

Provides prevention-related services and funding to the network of AIDS service delivery organizations, both public and private in Oklahoma. The Division provides services and training and certification of AIDS educators, surveillance, and seroprevalence staff.
Rocky D McElvany, Interim Commissioner of Health
Ken Feagins, Director

Oregon

286 Oregon Department of Human Resources Health Division HIV Program
Health Division, HIV Program
800 NE Oregon Street   971-673-1222
Portland, OR 97232   800-777-2437
                                            Fax: 971-673-1299
                                            TTY: 971-673-0372
                        e-mail: health.webmaster@state.or.us
                                        www.oregon.gov/DHS/ph
HIV Program includes training workshops for AIDS trainers curriculum development or revision and an AIDS hotline through Cascade AIDS Project.
Veda Latin, HST Program Manager
Mitch Zahn, HIV Prevention Manager

Pennsylvania

287 Pennsylvania Department of Health: Bureau of HIV/AIDS
Division of HIV/AIDS
8th Floor West   717-783-4677
Harrisburg, PA 17120   877-PA -EALT
                                            Fax: 717-772-6975
                          e-mail: c-hivepi@state.pa.us
                                        www.portal.state.pa.us
The purpose of the Division of HIV/AIDS is to develop and implement a multi-dimensional coordinated strategy to prevent disease and change high-risk behaviors as well as provide resources and direction for sustaining preventive behavior and avoiding infection.
Janice P Kopelman MSW LSW, Director

288 Philadelphia Department of Public Health: AIDS Program
AIDS Activities Coordinating Office (AACO)
1101 Market Street   215-685-5600
Philadelphia, PA 19107   800-985-AIDS
                                            Fax: 215-685-5293
                                        www.phila.gov/health
Administers federal state and city funded HIV/AIDS programs in Philadelphia through collaborative service contracts with community-based organizations.
Marla Gold MD, Program Coordinator
Nan Feyler, Chief of Staff

Rhode Island

289 Rhode Island Department of Health: Division of Disease Prevention & Control
Office of AIDS/HIV
3 Capitol Hill   401-222-5960
Providence, RI 02908   800-381-AIDS
                                            Fax: 401-222-2488
                                        www.health.state.ri.us
Provides health education and risk reduction activities through its AIDS program. Services include professional conferences, providing assistance for in-service programs, presentation of two courses and organization of an AIDS minority program. Also, provides public health services in HIV/AIDS and Viral Hepatitis. The office develops policies, funds community programs and conducts surveillances.
Paul G. Loberti, Chief Administrator
Lucille Minuto, Assistant Administrator

South Carolina

290 South Carolina Department of Health & Environmental Control
Bureau of Preventive Health Services
2600 Bull Street
Columbia, SC 29201   803-898-3432
                                        www.scdhec.net

Provides services to prevent the spread of sexually transmitted diseases (STD's) and HIV infection to reduce associated illness and death and to provide care and support resources for persons with HIV disease.
Jeff Jones MD, Director

Tennessee

291 Tennessee Department of Health: AIDS Program
Cordell Hull Building, 4th Floor
425 Fifth Avenue N   615-741-3111
Nashville, TN 37243   Fax: 615-741-2491
                                        e-mail: tn.health@tn.gov
                                            health.state.tn.us
Provides HIV/STD education and information, as well as collecting monitoring and distributing data. Provides assistance to individuals, and intervention and treatment services.
Bill Haslam, Governor
John J. Dreyzehner, MD, MPH, Commissioner

Texas

292 AIDS Outreach Center (AOC)
400 North Beach Street   817-335-1994
Fort Worth, TX 76111   Fax: 817-335-3617
                                        e-mail: info@aoc.org
                                            www.aoc.org
The staff and volunteers of the AIDS Outreach Center (AOC) provide a wide range of social services, outreach activities, testing and counseling, prevention education programs and public policy advocacy for men, women and children living with HIV, and their loved ones.
Shannon Hilgart, Executive Director
Michelle Barefield, Director of Prevention, Education and Ou

293 Houston Department of Health and Human Services: Bureau of HIV Prevention
8000 N Stadium Drive   713-794-9020
Houston, TX 77054-1823   Fax: 713-798-0830
                                            TTY: 713-794-9092
                                        www.houstontx.gov/health
Coordinates sexually transmitted disease surveillance, seroprevalence, contract tracing partner notification, public information, minority initiatives and health evaluation/risk reduction.
Stephen L Williams, Director

294 Texas Department of Health: Bureau of HIV and STD Prevention
HIV/STD Division
PO Box 149347   512-458-7111
Austin, TX 78756-3199   888-963-7111
                                            TTY: 800-735-2989
                                            TDD: 512-458-7708
                                        www.dshs.state.tx.us
Mission is to prevent, treat, and/or control the spread of HIV, STD, and other communicable diseases to protect the health of the citizens of Texas.
David Lakey, Commissioner

Utah

295 Utah Department of Health: Bureau of Communicable Disease Control
Division of Epidemiology & Laboratory Services
288 N 1460 W   801-538-6129
Salt Lake City, UT 84114-2105   800-537-1046
                                            Fax: 801-538-9923
                                        e-mail: rrolfs@utah.gov
                                        www.health.utah.gov/cdc
Secures and distributes funds for AIDS prevention services, provides educational programs and counseling to the general public, AIDS service organizations, health workers and groups at risk.
Teresa Garrett , MS, RN, Division Director, Chief Public Health N
Tamara Hampton, Administrative Assistant

Vermont

296   Vermont Department of Health: Health Surveillance HIV/AIDS/STD/TB Program
108 Cherry Street
Burlington, VT 05402-0070
802-863-7200
800-464-4343
Fax: 802-865-7754
TTY: 802-863-7235
www.healthvermont.gov
Provides health education and risk reduction activities nurses and other professional training, AIDS presentations, educational and media campaigns and counseling and referrals.
Rod Copeland PhD, Director HIV/AIDS Program

Virginia

297   Virginia Department of Health: Division of HIV, STD, and Pharmacy Services
109 Governor Street
Richmond, VA 23219
804-786-6267
800-533-4148
Fax: 804-786-7528
e-mail: hiv-stdhotline@vdh.virginia.gov.
www.vdh.virginia.gov
Supports local health departments and community-based organizations in the prevention, surveillance and treatment of HIV and other STD's, including their complications, through provision of education, information, and health care services.
Casey Riley, Director
Ashley Carter, HIV/STD Data and Statistics

Washington

298   Northwest AIDS Education and Training Center (AETC)
901 Boren Avenue
Seattle, WA 98104
206-685-0198
Fax: 206-221-4945
e-mail: mfa4@u.washington.edu
http://depts.washington.edu/nwaetc/
Located at the University of Washington, offering HIV treatment education, clinical consultation, capacity building and technical assistance to health care professionals and agencies in Washington, Alaska, Montana, Idaho, and Oregon.
Mary Annese, MPA, Evaluator
Laurie Conratt MBA, Director

299   Washington Department of Health: Division of HIV/AIDS Prevention Services
HIV Client Services
PO Box 47840
Olympia, WA 98504-7840
360-236-3434
877-376-9316
Fax: 360-236-3400
e-mail: brown.mcdonald@doh.wa.gov
www.doh.wa.gov/cfh/HIV_AIDS/Prev_Edu
Provides information and referrals to local, state and national resources relating to HIV/AIDS provides informational and educational materials to individuals, agencies and organizations and actively works with print and broadcast media to promote HIV/AIDS awareness.
Paul Brown, HIV Data Manager
Brown McDonald, HIV Prevention Services Manager

West Virginia

300   West Virginia Department of Health & Human Resources
HIV/AIDS & STD Program
One Davis Square
Charleston, WV 25301-3715
304-558-0684
800-352-6513
Fax: 304-558-1130
e-mail: wvdhhrsecretary@wvdhhr.org
www.wvdhhr.org
Provides the AIDS-related services in 15 public health HIV-counseling and testing centers which offer by appointment confidential or anonymous testing.
Martha Yeage Walker, Secretary

Wisconsin

301   Wisconsin Department of Health and Social Services: Division of Health
HIV/AIDS/Hepatitis Program

1 West Wilson Street
Madison, WI 53703
608-266-1865
877-865-3432
Fax: 608-267-2832
TTY: 888-701-1251
e-mail: DHSwebmaster@wisconsin.gov
www.dhs.wisconsin.gov
Coordinates counseling and testing sites activities and services to HIV-infected persons, produces a report that contains information and recommendations for health care workers, emergency medical technicians and food service workers.
Seth Foldy, Administrator and State Health Officer
Thomas Sieger, Deputy Administrator

Wyoming

302   Wyoming Department of Health HIV/AIDS/Hepatitis Program
HIV/AIDS/Hepatitis Program
401 Hathaway Building
Cheyenne, WY 82002-0001
307-777-7656
866-571-0944
Fax: 307-777-7439
www.health.wyo.gov
100 percent federally funded and responsible for the solicitation development and implementation of community AIDS prevention initiatives.
Thomas O. Forslund, Director and State Health Officer
Lee Clabbots, Deputy Director

Foundations

303   National Hemophilia Foundation
116 West 32nd Street
New York, NY 10001
212-328-3700
800-42H-ANDI
Fax: 212-328-3777
e-mail: handi@hemophilia.org
www.hemophilia.org
The National Hemophilia Foundation is dedicated to finding better treatments and cures for bleeding and clotting disorders and to preventing the complications of these disorders through education, advocacy and research.
Jorge De la Riva, Chair
Ken Trader, Vice Chair

Libraries & Resource Centers

304   AIDS Library of Philadelphia
1233 Locust Street
Philadelphia, PA 19107
215-985-4851
Fax: 215-985-4492
e-mail: library@aidslibrary.org
www.aidslibrary.org
Improving access to health and support services, preventing HIV transmission, and raising the public awareness of HIV/AIDS related issues.
Allie Frase, Collection Management Librarian
Ben Remsen, Public Services

305   National Library of Medicine
8600 Rockville Pike
Bethesda, MD 20894
301-594-5983
888-346-3656
Fax: 301-402-1384
TDD: 800-735-2258
e-mail: custserv@nlm.nih.gov
www.nlm.nih.gov/
The National Library of Medicine (NLM), on the campus of the National Institutes of Health in Bethesda, Maryland, is the world's largest medical library. The Library collects materials in all areas of biomedicine and health care, as well as works on biomedical aspects of technology, the humanities, and the physical, life, and social sciences.
Dr Donald Lindberg, Director
Betsy L Humphreys, Deputy Director

Research Centers

306 **CDC National Prevention Information Network (NPIN)**
PO Box 6003   404-679-3860
Rockville, MD 20849-6003   800-458-5231
                                                            Fax: 888-282-7681
                                                            TTY: 800-243-7012
                                                            e-mail: info@cdcnpin.org
                                                            www.cdcnpin.org

The CDC National Prevention Information Network (NPIN) is the U.S. reference, referral, and distribution service for information on HIV/AIDS, sexually transmitted diseases (STDs), and tuberculosis (TB). NPIN produces, collects, catalogs, processes, stocks, and disseminates materials and information on HIV/AIDS, STDs, and TB to organizations and people working in those disease fields in international, national, state, and local settings.
Kevin Fetnton, director
hazel D. Dean, Deputy Director

Alabama

307 **Centers for AIDS Research: University of Alabama at Birmingham**
BBRB 256
Birmingham, AL 35294-1150   205-934-4011
                                                            http://www.uab.edu

Provides expertise, resources, and services not otherwise readily obtained through traditional funding mechanisms.
Robert P. Kimberly, Director
Cheryl A. Perry, Deputy Director

308 **General Clinical Research Center: UAB**
Room 907 Medical Education Building   205-934-4852
Birmingham, AL 35294   e-mail: ccts@uab.edu
                                                            www.ccts.uab.org

AIDS and genetics research.
Burt Nabors, MD, Director
Stuart Frank, Co-Principal Investigator

309 **University of Alabama at Birmingham: National Cooperative Drug/AIDS**
UAB Center for AIDS Research
BBRB 256
Birmingham, AL 35294-1150   205-934-4011
                                                            http://www.uab.edu

Robert P. Kimberly, Director
Cheryl A. Perry, Deputy Director

California

310 **AIDS Clinical Trials Unit CARES Clinic**
CARES Clinic
2315 Stocktown blvd.   916-734-2011
Sacramento, CA 95817   800-2 U- DAV
                                                            Fax: 916-325-1955
                                                            e-mail: actu@ucdavis.edu
                                                            www.ucdmc.ucdavis.edu/actu

The ACTU at Davis Medical Center is dedicated to offering the latest in research clinical trials to HIV/AIDS patients throughout Northern Central California.
Thomas S. Nesbitt, Vice Chancellor
david A Acosta, Associate Vice Chancellor

311 **Adult Research Opportunities**
220 Dickinson Street   619-543-8080
San Diego, CA 92103-8208   Fax: 619-543-5066
                                                            www.avrctrials.org

A university-based nonprofit clinical trials unit. Conduct's patient-oriented research and educational programs on HIV and other chronic infections. Studies have pioneered the development of treatments that continue to change the course of the HIV epidemic.
Constance Benson, Director
Richard S Garfein, Professor and Chairman

312 **Center for AIDS Prevention Studies AIDS Research Institute University of C**
AIDS Research Institute, University of California

50 Beale Street   415-597-9100
San Francisco, CA 94105   Fax: 415-597-9213
                                                            e-mail: CAPS.Web@ucsf.edu
                                                            www.caps.ucsf.edu

The mission of the Center for AIDS Prevention Studies is to conduct domestic and international research to prevent the acquisition of HIV and to optimize health outcomes among HIV-infected individuals.
Stephen F Morin, Director
Susan Kegeles, Co-Director

313 **Center for Interdisciplinary Research in Immunology and Diseases at UCLA**
UCLA School of Medicine
924 Westwood Blvd. #545
Los Angeles, CA 90095   310-825-6373
                                                            dgsom.healthsciences.ucla.edu

Research into immunology and blood disorders with special focus on AIDS and HIV infections.
Albert Glover, Director, Academic Affairs

314 **Centers for AIDS Research: North-Central California**
UC Davis, Division of Infectious Diseases
4150 V Street   916-734-8033
Sacramento, CA 95817   Fax: 916-734-7766
                                                            e-mail: nccfar@ucdavis.edu
                                                            www.ucdmc.ucdavis.edu/nccfar

Provides expertise resources and services not otherwise readily obtained through more traditional funding mechanisms.
Richard B Pollard, Division Chief
Krystin E Cheung, Director

315 **Centers for AIDS Research: USCD Center for AIDS Research**
Center for AIDS Research
9500 Gilman Drive   858-534-5545
La Jolla, CA 92093-0716   Fax: 858-822-5840
                                                            e-mail: cfar@ucsd.edu
                                                            cfar.ucsd.edu

Provides expertise resources and services and services not otherwise readily obtained through traditional funding mechanisms.
Douglas Richman, Director
Kim Schafer, Administrative Director

316 **Centers for AIDS Research: University of California, Los Angeles**
UCLA AIDS Institute
10940 Wilshire Blvd.   310-794-4419
Los Angeles, CA 90024-1678   Fax: 310-794-3955
                                                            e-mail: ebayrd@mednet.ucla.edu
                                                            www.uclaaidsinstitute.org

Provides expertise, resources, and services not otherwise readily obtained through traditional funding mechanisms.
Irvin S.Y. Chen, Director
Dr. Thomas Coates, Associate Director

317 **City of Hope National Medical Center Drug Discover/AIDS Group**
City of Hope
1500 E Duarte Road
Duarte, CA 91010   626-256-4673
                                                            www.cityofhope.org

Developmental research into the treatment of AIDS.
Michael A Friedman MD, CEO
Robert Stone, President

318 **Kaiser Foundation Research Institute**
2000 Broadway
Oakland, CA 94612   510-891-3400
                                                            www.dor.kaiser.org

Tracy A Lieu, Director
Alyce Adams, Health Care Delivery and policy

319 **Stanford University General Clinical Research Center**
GCRC Administration
300 Pasteur Drive   650-723-4000
Stanford, CA 94305-5251   Fax: 650-725-6698
                                                            e-mail: gcrcstanford@stanford.edu
                                                            www.med.stanford.edu/gcrc

The Stanford General Clinical Research Center (GCRC) is the major clinical research facility for Stanford University School of Medicine. With patient care units in Stanford University Hospital

and Lucile Packard Children's Hospital the center plays a crucial role in the school's bench-to-bedside research mission.
Ellen Jo Baron, Director
Branimir I Sikic, Program Director

320   Stanford University National Cooperative Drug Discovery/AIDS Group
School of Medicine
300 Pasteur Drive
Stanford, CA 94305
650-723-4000
Fax: 650-725-6698
e-mail: gcrcstanford@stanford.edu
www.med.stanford.edu
Ellen Jo Baron, Director
Branimir I Sikic, Program Director

321   UCLA AIDS Clinical Research Center
1399 S Roxbury Drive
Los Angeles, CA 90035
310-557-2273
Fax: 310-557-3450
www.uclacarecenter.org
Dr.A Eugene, Chancellor
David T Feinberg, President

322   UCSD Antiviral Research Center
220 Dickinson Street
San Diego, CA 92103-8208
619-543-8080
Fax: 619-543-5066
www.avrctrials.org
Develops treatment protocols and drug therapies and recruits research volunteers for AIDS studies and HIV related disorders.
Jill Kunkel, Director
Michael Giancola, Screening Co-ordinator

323   USC Internal Medicine
1520 San Pablo Street
Los Angeles, CA 90033-1034
800-872-2273
Fax: 213-224-6687
www.usc.edu/health/internal
Research into internal medicine with specialties in cardiovascular endocrinology and diabetes gastrointestinal and liver disease geriatric medicine hematology infectious diseases nephrology oncology pulmonary and critical care and rheumatology and immunology.
Alexandra Levine, Head

324   University of California San Francisco Center for AIDS Prevention
Center for AIDS Prevention Studies (CAPS)
50 Beale Street
San Francisco, CA 94105-3411
415-597-9100
Fax: 415-597-9213
e-mail: CAPS.web@ucsf.edu
www.caps.ucsf.edu
The mission of the Center for AIDS Prevention Studies is to conduct domestic and international research to prevent the acquisition of HIV and to optimize health outcomes among HIV- infected individuals.
Stephen F Morin, Director
Susan Kegeles, Co-Director

325   University of California: Institute of Health Policy Studies
513 Parnassus Avenue
San Francisco, CA 94143-410
415-476-9000
Fax: 415-476-0705
e-mail: claire.brindis@ucsf.edu
www.ihps.medschool.ucsf.edu
Health policy and AIDS research.
Susan Desmond-Hellman, Chancellor
Phillip R. Lee, director

Colorado

326   Centers for AIDS Research: University of Colorado Health Sciences Center
Colorado Center for AIDS Research
4200 East 9th Avenue
Denver, CO 80262
303-315-7233
Fax: 303-315-8681
e-mail: colorado.cfar@uchsc.edu
www.uchsc.edu/ccfar
Describes forms and patterns of use of complimentary and alternative medicine (CAM) for the treatment of HIV/AIDS.
Robert T. Schooley, Director

District of Columbia

327   George Washington National Cooperative: Drug Discovery/AIDS Treatment
Department of Pharmacology & Physiology
2300 Eye Street NW
Washington, DC 20037-2336
202-994-3541
Fax: 202-994-2870
e-mail: phmsmc@gwumc.edu
www.gwumc.edu/pharm
Studies and researches natural products and synthetic anti-AIDS agents.
Susan Ceryak, Associate Research Professor
Jian-Zhong Guo, Associate Research Professor

328   Whitman Walker Clinic AIDS/Medical Services Programs
1701 14th Street NW
Washington, DC 20009-3840
202-745-7000
Fax: 202-745-0238
e-mail: info@wwc.org
www.wwc.org
A non-profit community-based health organization serving the Washington D.C. metropolitan region. Established by and for the gay and lesbian community our clinic is comprised of diverse volunteers and staff who provide or facilitate the delivery of high quality comprehensive accessible health care and community services. Especially committed to ending the suffering of all those infected and affected by HIV/AIDS.
Adam Falcone, Chair
June Crenshaw, Vice Chair

Florida

329   Department of Epidemiology and Health Policy Research: University of Florida
1329 SW 16th Street
Gainesville, FL 32608
352-265-8035
Fax: 352-265-8047
e-mail: rdarbelles.ichp.ufl.edu
www.ichp.ufl.edu
Studies into child and adolescent health financing and organization of health care delivery systems community health chronic conditions transition from pediatric to adult health care access to health care for vulnerable populations quality of life and outcomes research.
Clifford J Crook, Chair
John C Bierly, Program Assistant

330   Tampa Bay Research Institute
10900 Roosevelt Boulevard N
Saint Petersburg, FL 33716-2308
727-576-6675
Fax: 727-577-9862
e-mail: development@tampabayresearch.org
www.tampabayresearch.org
TBRI is the first independent biomedical research organization of its kind in Florida. Our scientists dedicate their lives work to conquering chronic and infectious diseases while gaining a better understanding of the immune system.
Clifford J Crook, Chair
John C Bierly, Program Assistant

331   University of South Florida Center for HIV Education and Research
13301 Bruce B Downs Boulevard
Tampa, FL 33612-3807
813-974-4430
866-352-2382
Fax: 813-974-8451
e-mail: Contact@FCAETC.org
www.usfcenter.org
Serves health care professionals throughout Florida by providing education and information on the transmission control treatment and prevention of HIV and AIDS and by conducting related research and community outreach.
jeffery beal, Director
Debbie Cestaro, Project Co-ordinator

Georgia

332   AIDS School Health Education Database Centers for Disease Control
Centers for Disease Control

1600 Clifton Road
Atlanta, GA 30333

404-639-3534
800-232-4636
TTY: 888-232-6348
e-mail: cdcinfo@cdc.gov
www.cdc.gov

An information awareness resource produced by the Division of Adolescent and School Health. The database offers descriptions of various educational resources for professionals relevant to the education of children and youth about HIV infection and AIDS.
Thomas R. Frieden, Director
Ileana Arias, Principal Deputy Director

333   Center for AIDS Research: Emory University Rollins School of Public Health
1518 Clifton Road NE
Atlanta, GA 30322-4201

404-727-2924
Fax: 404-727-9853
e-mail: cfar@emory.edu
www.cfar.emory.edu

Provides expertise resources and services not otherwise readily obtained through more traditional funding mechanisms.
James W Curran, Director
Carlos del Rio, Co-Director for Clinical Science

334   Educational Materials Database Centers for Disease Control
Centers for Disease Control
1600 Clifton Road
Atlanta, GA 30333-4201

404-639-3534
800-232-4636
TTY: 888-232-6348
e-mail: cdcinfo@cdc.gov
www.cdc.gov

An information awareness resource produced by the Division of Adolescent and School Health. The database offers descriptions of various educational resources for professionals relevant to the education of children and youth about HIV infection and AIDS.
Thomas R. Frieden, Director
Ileana Arias, Principal Deputy Director

335   Emory University: National Cooperative Drug Discovery for AIDS Treatment
Emory Healthcare Pediatrics Department
201 Dowman Drive
Atlanta, GA 30322

404-727-6123
Fax: 404-727-5737
www.pediatrics.emory.edu

Barbara J Stoll MD, Professor, Chair
James W Wagner, President

336   Funding Database Centers for Disease Control
Centers for Disease Control
1600 Clifton Road
Atlanta, GA 30329

404-639-3534
800-232-4636
TTY: 888-232-6348
e-mail: cdcinfo@cdc.gov
www.cdc.gov

A listing of HIV and AIDS related funding opportunities for community-based and HIV and AIDS service organizations.
Thomas Friedman MD, Director
Harold Jaffe, MD, MA, Associate Director of Science

Illinois

337   Clinical Research Center Northwestern Center for Clinical Researc
Northwestern Center for Clinical Research
ÿ633 Clark Street,
Chicago, IL 60611

312-503-8649
e-mail: nucats@northwestern.edu
www.nucats.northwestern.edu

Colleen De Luca, Associate Director, Administration
Philip Greenland, Director

Indiana

338   Purdue University Center for AIDS Research
School of Pharmacy and Pharmaceutical Sciences
575 Stadium Mall Drive
W Lafayette, IN 47907-2091

765-494-1361
Fax: 765-494-7880
e-mail: oss@pharmacy.purdue.edu
www.pharmacy.purdue.edu

Steve Byrn, Department Head
Stanley L Hem, Associate Department Head

Maryland

339   Center for AIDS Research: Johns Hopkins University School of Medicine
733 N. Broadway
Baltimore, MD 21205-2196

410-955-3182
www.hopkinsmedicine.org/aidsresearch

Provides expertise resources and services not otherwise readily obtained through more traditional funding mechanisms.
Ronald R Peterson, ,President, JHH/HS
Edward D Miller, MD, Dean, CEO

340   Johns Hopkins University: Center for Communication Programs
Johns Hopkins Bloomberg School of Public Health
111 Market Place
Baltimore, MD 21202

410-659-6300
Fax: 410-659-6266
e-mail: info@jhuccp.org
www.jhuccp.org

Health communications family planning and AIDS prevention research.
Susan Krenn, Director
James bon tempo, Associate Director of Communican Science

341   University of Maryland Center for Research, Grants & Contracts
Family Studies Depatrment
1142 School of Public Health
College Park, MD 20742

301-405-3672
Fax: 301-314-9161
e-mail: fmst@umd.edu
www.hhp.umd.edu/FMST

Erin McClure, Co-ordinator
Doris Richardson, business Manager

342   University of Maryland Center for Studies Family Studies Depatrment
1142 School of Public Health
College Park, MD 20742

301-405-3672
Fax: 301-314-9161
e-mail: fmsc@umd.edu
www.sph.umd.edu/fmsc

Erin McClure, Co-ordinator
Doris Richardson, business Manager

343   University of Maryland: Medical Biotechnology Center
701 E. PRATT ST,ÿ
Baltimore, MD 21202-1513

410-706-8802
Fax: 410-706-8184
e-mail: ÿhill@UMCES.edu
www.umbi.umd.edu

Offers research into AIDS and HIV infection including vaccine development.
W Jonathan Lederer, Director
Kadir Aslan, Assistant Professor

Massachusetts

344   Center for AIDS Research: Harvard Medical School, Division of AIDS
The Landmark Buiding
104 Mt. Auburn Street
Cambridge, MA 02138

617-384-9039
Fax: 617-495-8231
e-mail: aids@hms.harvard.edu
aids.med.harvard.edu/cfar.htm

Provides expertise resources and services not otherwise readily obtained through traditional funding mechanisms.
Bruce Walker, Director
Myron Essex, Associate Director

345   Center for Blood Research Harvard Medical School/CBR
Harvard Medical School/CBR
200 Longwood Avenue
Boston, MA 02115

617-278-3140
Fax: 617-278-3131
e-mail: kirchhausen@crystal.harvard.edu
www.idi.harvard.edu

Offers research into blood disorders including multidisciplinary studies on AIDS and hemophilia cancer and diabetes research as well.
Fredrick Alt, President/ Director
Stephen Carriuolo, Financial Manager

346 Centers for AIDS Research: University of Massachusetts Medical School
364 Plantation Streetÿ
Worcester, MA 01605
508-856-3159
e-mail: publicaffairs@umassmed.edu
www.umassmed.edu/cfar
Provides expertise, resources, and services not otherwise readily obtained through traditional funding mechanisms.
celia Schiffer, Director
Shan Lu, Co-Director

347 Dana Farber Cancer Institute National Drug Discovery Group for AIDS Treatment
Dana-Farber Cancer Institute
450 Brookline Avenue
Boston, MA 02215-5450
617-632-3000
800-408-3324
TTY: 617-632-5330
TDD: 617-632-5330
e-mail: dana-farbercontactus@dfci.harvard.edu
www.dana-farber.org
Edward Benz, President and CEO
Dorthy E Puhy, Executive Vice President and COO

348 Developmental Medicine Center Children's Hospital Boston
Children's Hospital Boston
300 Longwood Avenue
Boston, MA 02115
617-355-6000
Fax: 617-730-0633
TTY: 617-730-0152
www.childrenshospital.org
Studies developmental effects of infants at risk and development effects of congenital HIV infection.
James Mandell, CEO
Sandra Fenwick, President, COO

Michigan

349 University of Michigan: National Cooperative Drug/AIDS Group
School of Dentistry
1011 N University Avenue
Ann Arbor, MI 48109-1078
734-763-6933
Fax: 734-763-3453
e-mail: paulk@umich.edu
www.dent.umich.edu
Focuses on the design of new drugs to fight AIDS.
John C Drach PhD, Director
Paul H Krebsbach, Department Chair

350 Wayne State University Center for Health Research
College of Nursing
Center for Health Research
Detroit, MI 48202
313-577-4082
888-837- 08
Fax: 313-577-6949
e-mail: nursinginfo@wayne.edu
www.nursing.wayne.edu/CHR
Facilitates interdisciplinary health research across diverse settings where nursing is practiced and healthcare is provided.
Nancy T Artinian, Director
Barbara K Redman, Dean

New York

351 Aaron Diamond AIDS Research Center
455 First Avenue
New York, NY 10016
212-448-5000
Fax: 212-725-1126
e-mail: webinfo@adarc.org
www.adarc.org
Committed to finding solutions to end the AIDS epidemic. In the decade and a half since HIV was identified researchers have learned more about this virus than about any other in history.
David Ho, Director & CEO
Gerald Friedland MD, Chairman

352 Centers for AIDS Research: Albert Einstein College of Medicine
Albert Einstein College of Medicine
Jack and Pearl Resnick Campus
Bronx, NY 10461
718-430-2000
Fax: 718-430-2374
e-mail: information@einstein.yu.edu
www.aecom.yu.edu/cfar
Provides consultation and support to the medical and research community in the scientific evaluation of CAM therapies.
Allen M Spiegel MD, Dean
Matthew Scharff MD, CFAR Investigator

353 Centers for AIDS Research: Columbia University College of Physicians
Center for AIDS Research
630 W 168th Street
New York, NY 10032
212-305-1296
e-mail: jka8@columbia.edu
www.cumc.columbia.edu
Provides a comprehensive framework for training educational programs and research which addresses health promotion disease prevention symptom management and quality of life for individuals with HIV. The goal of the Center is to create innovative research and service approaches for the prevention and management of HIV. This objective is fulfilled through research program development and program evaluations.
Lee Goldman MD, Executive Vice President
Lee Bollinger, JD, President of the University

354 Centers for AIDS Research: NYU School of Medicine
522 First Avenue
New York, NY 10016
212-263-8527
e-mail: zinszh01@med.nyu.edu
www.hivinfosource.org/hivis/cfar
Provides expertise resources and services not otherwise readily obtained through traditional funding mechanisms.
Derya Unutmanz MD, Director
David levy, Associate Dean

355 General Clinical Research Center Mount Sinai School of Medicine
Mount Sinai School of Medicine
One Gustave L Levy Place
New York, NY 10029-6574
212-241-6500
Fax: 212-348-5811
e-mail: hugh.sampson@mssm.edu
www.mssm.edu/gcrc
Focuses on AIDS education and prevention.
Dennis S Charney, Executive Vice President
Kennith Davis, President

356 HIV Center for Clinical and Behavioral Studies
1051 Riverside Drive
New York, NY 10032
212-543-5969
Fax: 212-543-6003
e-mail: whiteme@pi.cpmc.comlumbia.edu
www.hivcenternyc.org
Interdisciplinary research center that investigates the behavioral causes and consequences of HIV/AIDS. Focusing on the intersections of HIV infection gender and sexuality; treatment strategies for infected populations; and innovative dissemination of scientific findings.
Anke A Ehrhardt, Director
Heino F L Meyer-Bahlbur, Associate Director

357 Institute for Clinical Research Weill Cornell Medical College
Weill Cornell Medical College
1300 York Avenue
New York, NY 10065
212-746-5454
Fax: 212-746-8970
e-mail: cto@med.cornell.edu
www.med.cornell.edu
The mission of the ICR is to support, advance and promote clinical and translational research enterprises at WCMC. As part of Research and Sponsored Programs (RASP) the ICR streamlines the clinical research process and offers a wide range of services, resources and training.
David J Skorton MD, President of the University
Michelle A Lewis, MS, Director (Research and Sponsored Program

358 SUNY at Buffalo National Cooperative Drug Discovery Group for AIDS Treatment
Department of Biochemistry
140 Farber Hall
Buffalo, NY 14214-3000
716-829-2727
Fax: 716-829-2725
e-mail: jluck@buffalo.edu
www.buffalo.edu
Kenneth M Blumenthal, Professor and Chairman
Elizabeth O'Brocta, Assistant to the Chairman

359 Spellman Center for HIV Related Disease The Spellman Center
The Spellman Center
415 W Fifty-First Street
New York, NY 10019
212-459-8130
www.stclaresny.org
David Kaufman, Director

360   State University of New York: SUNY Stony HIV Treatment Development Center
Center for Infectious Diseases
101 Nicolls Road   631-444-4000
Stony Brook, NY 11794-5120   Fax: 631-444-2493
e-mail: rsteigbigel@notes.cc.sunysb.edu
www.stonybrookmedicalcenter.org
Human immunodeficiency virus research.
Joyce Klien, Director
Laura Coppola, Assistant Director

North Carolina

361   Centers for AIDS Research: Univeristy of North Carolina at Chapel Hill
UNC Center For AIDS Research
Lineberger Cancer Center   919-966-8645
Chapel Hill, NC 27599   e-mail: cfar@med.unc.edu
cfar.med.unc.edu
Administrative and shared research support to synergistically enhance and coordinate high quality AIDS research projects.
Ronald Swanstrom, Director
Myron S Cohen, Associate Director

Ohio

362   Centers for AIDS Research: Case Western University
Department of Medicine
Division of Infectious Diseases   216-368-0271
Cleveland, OH 44106-5029   Fax: 216-368-3055
e-mail: mxl6@case.edu
www.clevelandactu.org
Provides administrative and shared research support to enhance and coordinate high quality AIDS research projects.
Michael M Lederman, Co-Director
Jonathan Karn, Associate Director

Pennsylvania

363   Centers for AIDS Research: University of Pennsylvania
Penn Center for AIDS Research
295 John Morgan Building   215-573-7354
Philadelphia, PA 19104-6140   Fax: 215-573-7356
e-mail: oliviere@mail.med.upenn.edu
www.med.upenn.edu
Also the Children's Hospital and the Wistar Institute provides important services and research for high quality projects.
James A Hoxie, Director
Ronald G Collman, Co-Director

364   Temple University Clinical Research Center Office of Clinical Research
Office of Clinical Research
Medical Education and Research Buil   215-707-7000
Philadelphia, PA 19140   Fax: 215-201-2684
e-mail: tusm@temple.edu
www.temple.edu/medicine
CRC Unit provides space to perform clinical research on 4 West of Temple University Hospital. The CRC Unit has the potential for three rooms for inpatient/outpatient studies and an additional room for outpatient studies.
Antonio Giorgio MD, President

365   Thomas Jefferson University: Center for Research in Medical Education
Jefferson Medical College
1020 Walnut Street   215-955-6000
Philadelphia, PA 19107   Fax: 215-923-7583
e-mail: Joseph.Gonnella@jefferson.edu
www.jefferson.edu/jmc
Joseph Gonne MD, Director
Robert L Barchi MD, President

Rhode Island

366   Centers for AIDS Research: Brown University
The Miriam Hospital

CFAR/RISE Building   401-793-4068
Providence, RI 02906   Fax: 401-793-4704
e-mail: vgodleski@lifespan.org
www.lifespan.org/cfar
Provides expertise resources and services not otherwise readily obtained through traditional funding mechanisms.
Charles C J Carpenter, Director
Susan Cu-Uvin, HIV and Women Core Co-Director

South Carolina

367   Medical University of South Carolina Health Services Administration
Medical University of South Carolina
171 Ashley Avenue   843-792-1414
Charleston, SC 29425   800-424-6872
Fax: 843-792-2601
www.musc.edu
Devoted to public health policy and health care management including AIDS research.
Raymond S Greenburg, President
Dr. Mark Sothman, Vice President

Tennessee

368   Centers for AIDS Research: Vanderbilt University Medical Center
Division of Infectious Disease
1161 21st Avenue S   615-322-8972
Nashville, TN 37232-2582   e-mail: richard.daquila@vanderbilt.edu
www.mc.vanderbilt.edu/cfar
Provides expertise resources and services not otherwise readily obtained through more traditional funding mechanisms.
Richard D' Aquila, Director
G Fatima Lima Ph.D., Associate Director

Texas

369   Centers for AIDS Research: Baylor College of Medicine
Department of Molecular Virology & Microbiology
One Baylor Plaza   713-798-3006
Houston, TX 77030   Fax: 713-798-5019
e-mail: jbutel@bcm.edu
www.bcm.edu/cfar
A research center that is a branch of the Centers for AIDS Research.
Janet S Butel, Director
William T Shearer, Co-Director

Vermont

370   University of Vermont: Office of Health Promotion Research
1 S Prospect Street   802-656-4187
Burlington, VT 05401   Fax: 802-656-8826
e-mail: ohpr@uvm.edu
www.uvm.edu/~ohpr
Research done into public policy and human health including AIDS information and evaluation.
Anne L Dorwaldt, Assistant Director
Rachael Chicoine, AAS, Research Project Assistant

Washington

371   Centers for AIDS Research: University of Washington, Harborview Medical Center
Center For AIDS & STDs
325 Ninth Avenue   206-744-4239
Seattle, WA 98104-2499   Fax: 206-744-3693
e-mail: worthy@u.washington.edu
www.depts.washington.edu/cfas
Provides administrative and shared research support to synergistically enhance and coordinate high quality AIDS research projects. CFARs accomplish this through core facilities that provide expertise resource and services not otherwise readily obtained through more traditional funding mechanisms.
King K Holmes, Director
Mary Fielder, Assistant to the Director

372   HIV Prevention Trials Unit University of Washington/Seattle HPTU Si
University of Washington/Seattle HPTU Site
Cabrini Medical Tower 901 Boren Av   206-520-3800
Seattle, WA 98104   Fax: 206-520-3801
e-mail: hptu@u.washington.edu
www.depts.washington.edu
A worldwide collaborative clinical trials network established by the National Institutes of Health (NIH) to evaluate the safety and efficacy of non-vaccine prevention interventions alone or in combination using HIV incidence as the primary endpoint.
Connie Celum, Principal Investigator

Support Groups & Hotlines

373   AEGIS AIDS Education Global Information System
PO Box 184   949-495-1952
San Juan Capistrano, CA 92693   Fax: 949-443-1755
e-mail: comments@aegis.org
www.aegis.org
A not-for-profit, tax-exempt, educational corpoation that adds more than 3000 documents each month. Reach more than 10 million users annually, including: the US Federal Government, US Educational Institutions, and Nonprofit organizations both here and abroad.
Vanessa Robison, President
Sister Mary Elizabeth, Assistant Operations Director

374   AIDS Alabama
3521 7th Avenue S   205-324-9822
Birmingham, AL 35222   800-592-2437
Fax: 205-324-9311
e-mail: maryanne@aidsalabama.org
www.aidsalabama.org
Devotes its energy and resources statewide to helping people with HIV/AIDS live healthy, independent lives and works to prevent the spread of HIV. It is our goal to provide housing for those with HIV in the Birmingham area, secure and administer grants for care of persons with HIV statewide, and specialize in targeted prevention education programs.
Elaine Cottle, Executive Director

375   AIDS Hotline of Central New York
AIDS Community Resources
627 W Genesee Street   315-475-2430
Syracuse, NY 13204   800-475-2430
Fax: 315-472-6515
e-mail: information@aidscommunityresources.com
www.aidscommunityresources.com
A not-for-profit, community-based organization providing prevention, education and support services to those infected with and affected by HIV/AIDS Serves Cayuga, Herkimer, Jefferson, Lewis, Madison, Oneida, Onondaga, Oswego and St. Lawrences counties in New York State.
Michael Crinnin, Executive Director

376   AIDS Support Group of Cape Cod
428 S Street   508-778-1957
Hyannis, MA 02610   866-990-2437
Fax: 508-778-4501
e-mail: info@asgcc.org
www.asgcc.org
Our mission is to provide services that maintain and enhance the quality of life for persons living with HIV and AIDS on Cape Cod and Martha's Vineyard and to provide health education, prevention and harm reduction outreach via timely and accurate information about HIV/AIDS, STIs and viral hepatitis.
Krystin St. Onge, Interim Director

377   AIDSinfo
US Department of Health and Human Services
PO Box 6303   301-315-2816
Rockville, MD 20849-6303   800-448-0440
Fax: 301-315-2818
TTY: 888-480-3739
e-mail: contactus@aidsinfo.nih.gov
www.aidsinfo.nih.gov
Offers the latest federally approved information on HIV/AIDS clinical research, treatment and prevention, and medical practice

guidelines for people living with HIV/AIDS, their families and friends, health care providers, scientists, and researchers.

378   Alaskan Statewide AIDS Helpline
1057 W Fireweed   907-263-2050
Anchorage, AK 99503   800-478-AIDS
Fax: 907-263-2051
www.alaskanaids.org
A key collaborator within the state of Alaska in the provision of supportive services to persons living with HIV/AIDS and their families and in the elimination of the transmission of HIV infection and its stigma.
Heather Davis, Executive Director
Maureen Suttman, Client Resource Services

379   BABES Network-YWCA
1118 Fifth Ave   206-720-5566
Seattle, WA 98101   888-292-1912
Fax: 206-720-5901
e-mail: the_staff@babesnetwork.org
www.babesnetwork.org
A peer-based program, a sisterhood of women facing HIV together. Reduces isolation, promotes self-empowerment, enhances quality of life and serves the needs of women facing HIV and their families through peer support, advocacy, education and outreach
Rhonda Kimm, Advocacy Coordinator
Amelia Vader, Program Manager

380   COMPASS Program
c/o Institute for Urban Family Health
16 East 16th Street   212-924-7744
New York, NY 10003   Fax: 212-691-4610
e-mail: info@institute2000.org
www.institute2000.org/health/rwp.htm
Medical services include HIV testing and specialized HIV medical care for adults in addition to women's health services including gynecology, PAP tests, family planning and birth control methods. Mental health services includes individual, couples, and family counseling and psychiatric evaluations and monitoring.
Neil Calman MD/ABFP/FAAFP, President/Chief Executive Officer
Weston Willett, Chief Information Officer

381   Cascade AIDS Project Hotline
200 SW Fifth Avenue   503-223-5907
Portland, OR 97204   Fax: 503-223-6437
e-mail: info@cascadeaids.org
www.cascadeaids.org
Provides HIV prevention and services information by phone and internet to youth and adults across Orgeon and the Northwest.
Charles Washington, President
warren Jimanez, Vice President

382   Dunshee House
303-17th Avenue East   206-322-2437
Seattle, WA 98112   Fax: 206-322-1779
e-mail: josh@dunsheehouse.org
www.dunsheehouse.org
A non-profit organization, builds community and cultivates powerful, healthy lives by providing emotional support and personal development services to those affected by HIV/AIDS, the Queer communities, and those who love them.
Michael Kann, President
Adrienne Miller, Vice President

383   HEAL
Sidney Hillman Family Pracitce
16 E 16th Street   212-924-7744
New York, NY 10003-3105   e-mail: healweb@thorup.com
www.thorup.com/HEAL
The Health Education AIDS Liaison provides alternative and holistic support groups and resources for people with HIV.

384   HIV/AIDS Prevention Program
Centers for Disease Control and Prevention
1600 Clifton Road   404-639-3534
Atlanta, GA 30333   800-232-4636
TTY: 888-232-6348
e-mail: cdcinfo@cdc.gov
www.cdc.gov

An information awareness resource produced by the Division of Adolescent and School Health. The database offers descriptions of various educational resources for professionals relevant to the education of children and youth about HIV infection and AIDS.
Thomas R. Frieden, Director
Ileana Arias, Principal Deputy Director

385 Immunization Division Centers for Disease Control
1600 Clifton Road   404-639-3534
Atlanta, GA 30333-2303   800-232-4636
                                                        TTY: 888-232-6348
                                                        e-mail: cdcinfo@cdc.gov
                                                        www.cdc.gov

An information awareness resource produced by the Division of Adolescent and School Health. The database offers descriptions of various educational resources for professionals relevant to the education of children and youth about HIV infection and AIDS.
Thomas R. Frieden, Director
Ileana Arias, Principal Deputy Director

386 King County Crisis Clinic
9725 3rdÿAvenue NE   206-461-3210
Seattle, WA 98115   866-427-4747
                                                        Fax: 206-461-8368
                                                        TDD: 206-461-3219
                                                        e-mail: info@crisisclinic.org
                                                        www.crisisclinic.org

A non-profit organization, we offer an array of support services available to everyone in King County, Washington.
Kathleen Southwick, Executive Director
Susan Gemmel, Director

387 Minnesota AIDS Project AIDSLine
1400 Park Avenue   612-341-2060
Minneapolis, MN 55404   800-248-7321
                                                        Fax: 612-341-4057
                                                        TTY: 888-820-2437
                                                        e-mail: mapaidsline@mnaidsproject.org
                                                        www.mnaidsproject.org

A statewide, toll-free information and referral service that can answer your questions about HIV and connect you to resources that can help
Bill Tiedmann, Executive Director

388 National Health Information Center
PO Box 1133   310-565-4167
Washington, DC 20013-1133   800-336-4797
                                                        Fax: 301-984-4256
                                                        e-mail: info@nhic.org
                                                        www.health.gov/nhic

A health information referral service sponsored by the Office of Disease Prevention and Health Promotion. NHIC puts health professionals and consumers who have health questions in touch with those organizations that are best able to provide answers.

389 Project Inform Hotline
273 Ninth Street   415-558-8669
San Francisco, CA 94103-2621   800-822-7422
                                                        Fax: 415-558-0684
                                                        e-mail: web@projectinform.org
                                                        www.projectinform.org

Represents HIV-positive people in the development of treatments and a cure, supports individuals to make informed choices about their HIV health, advocates for quality health care to respond to HIV and related conditions, and promotes medical strategies that prevent new infections.
Christopher Esposito, President
Ferdinand Garcia, Vice President

Books

390 ABC of AIDS
Michael W. Adler, author
BMJ Publishing Group

PO Box 281   800-2FO-NBMJ
Annapolis, MD 20701-0281   Fax: 800-2FA-XBMJ
                                                        e-mail: bmjpg@pmds.com
                                                        ww.bmjpg.com

118 pages Paperback
ISBN: 0-727915-03-7

391 AIDS & HIV Related Diseases
Harper Collins Publishers
195 Broadway   212-207-7000
New York, NY 10007   e-mail: tmpcorrections@harpercollins.com
                                                        www.harpercollins.com

An education guide for professionals and the public which covers such topics as: Understanding HIV and its effect on the immune system; HIV transmission; The history of AIDS and HIV; HIV testing; The natural course of an HIV infection; Medical treatment and those who administer them; The people who have AIDS; AIDS education.
1996 246 pages
ISBN: 0-306450-85-2

392 AIDS & Other Manifestations of HIV Infection
Academic Press (Elsevier)
1183 Westline Indus Drive
St Louis, MO 63146   800-545-2522
                                                        Fax: 800-535-9935
                                                        e-mail: usbkinfo@elsevier.com
                                                        www.elsevier.com

An essential reference resource providing a comprehensive overview of the biological properties of this etiologic viral agent, its clinicopathological manifestations, the epidemiology of its infection, and present and future therapeutic options.
2004-4th Edi 1000 pages
ISBN: 0-127640-51-7
Gary Wormser, Editor

393 AIDS Alert
American Health Consultants
3525 Piedmont Road   404-262-5476
Atlanta, GA 30355   800-688-2421
                                                        Fax: 800-284-3291
                                                        www.ahcmedia.com

The definitive source of AIDS news and advice for health care professionals. Covers up-to-the-minute developments and guidance on the entire spectrum of AIDS challenges, including treatment, education, precaustion, screening, diagnosis and policy.

394 AIDS and HIV Related Diseases
Josh Powell, author
Plenum Publishing Corporation
233 Spring Street   212-620-8000
New York, NY 10013   800-221-9369
                                                        Fax: 212-463-0742
                                                        e-mail: books@plenum.com
                                                        www.springer.com

An education guide for professionals and the public which covers such topics as: Understanding HIV and its effect on the immune system; HIV transmission; The history of AIDS and HIV; HIV testing; The natural course of an HIV infection; Medical treatment and those who administer them; The people who have AIDS; AIDS education.
1996 243 pages
ISBN: 0-306450-85-2

395 AIDS and Persons with Developmental Disabilities
Commission on the Mentally Disabled
1800 M Street NW   202-331-2240
Washington, DC 20036
A discussion of federal and state laws that defines the rights and responsibilities of individuals with disabilities and service providers with respect to HIV infection.

396 AIDS in the Twenty-First Century: Disease and Globalization
Tony Barnett, Alan Whiteside, author
Palgrave Macmillan

175 Fifth Avenue
New York, NY 10010

212-982-3900
800-221-7945
Fax: 212-777-6359
e-mail: authors@palgrave.com
www.palgrave.com

Presents compelling data and research which reveals the shocking social and economic impact of HIV/AIDS on a global scale
432 pages
ISBN: 1-403900-05-0

397 AIDS, Revised Edition
Alan E. Nourse, M.D., author

Franklin Watts c/o Grolier
90 Old Sherman Tpke
Danbury, CT 06816

203-797-3500
800-621-1115
Fax: 203-797-6986
www.grolier.com

This bestselling book has been updated with the latest findings and research into the AIDS epidemic. Includes new statistical information and findings on HIV and AIDS.
144 pages
ISBN: 0-531106-62-4

398 AIDS: A Communication Perspective
Lawrence Erlbaum Associates Publishers
10 Industrial Avenue
Mahwah, NJ 07430-2262

201-236-9500
Fax: 201-236-6396
www.erlbaum.com

ISBN: 0-805809-98-8

399 AIDS: Distinguishing Between Fact and Opinion
Teresa Opheim, author

Greenhaven Press
PO Box 9187
Farmington Hills, MI 48333-9187

800-877-GALE
Fax: 800-414-5043
solutions.cengage.com/greenhaven/

For beginning debaters, reports and classroom use this book offers three debates: Can AIDS be spread by casual contact? Should the Food and Drug Administration make AIDS drugs more available? Is AIDS a moral issue?.
36 pages
ISBN: 0-899086-33-0

400 AIDS: How it Works in the Body
Lorna Greenberg, author

Franklin Watts
96 Leonard Street
London EC2A 4XD,
For readers ages 9-12

www.wattspub.co.uk

64 pages School Binding

401 AIDS: Trading Fears for Facts: A Guide for Young People
Karen Hein, Theresa Foy Digernimo, author

Consumer Reports Books
101 Truman Avenue
Yonkers, NY 10703-1057

www.consumerreports.org

Listed for young adult readers.
232 pages Paperback
ISBN: 0-890437-21-1

402 Amfar AIDS Handbook: The Complete Guide to Understanding HIV and AIDS
Darrell Ward, author

W.W. Norton & Company, Inc.
500 Fifth Avenue
New York, NY 10110

212-354-5500
Fax: 212-869-0856
in.norton.com

Gives a greater understanding of HIV/Aids. The causes and effects, what new treatment options are being developed.
360 pages
ISBN: 0-393316-36-X

403 Black Death: AIDS in Africa
Susan Hunter, author

Macmillan

175 Fifth Avenue
New York, NY 10010

646-307-5151
us.macmillian.com

The untold story of AIDS in Africa, home to 80 percent of the 40 million people in the world currently infected with HIV. Brings the staggering statistics to life and paints for the first time a stunning picture of the most important political issue today.
256 pages
ISBN: 1-403967-17-2

404 Children and the AIDS Virus: A Book for Children, Parents, and Teachers
Rosmarie Hausherr, author

Clarion Books
For readers ages 4-8.
48 pages Library Binding
ISBN: 0-899198-34-1

405 Community Service Delivery for Children with HIV Infection and Families
Geneva, Woodruff & Christopher Hanson, author

South Shore Mental Health Center
500 Victory Road
Quincy, MA 02171

617-847-1950
800-852-2844
Fax: 617-786-9894
e-mail: contactus@ssmh.org
www.ssmh.org

A manual providing guidelines for developing community-based, family-centered services for children with HIV infection and their families. Describes how services can be planned and delivered using guiding principles and practices of transagency case management.

406 Coping When You or a Friend is HIV-Positive
Pat Kelly, author

Hazelden Publishing & Educational Services
15251 Pleasant Valley Rd
Center City, MN 55012-0176

651-213-4200
800-328-9000
Fax: 651-213-4793
e-mail: info@hazelden.org
www.hazelden.org

Provides compassionate counsel for teens who have been diagnosed with the virus.
136 pages Paperback
ISBN: 1-568381-77-8

407 Dancing Against the Darkness: A Journey Through America in the Age of AIDS
Steven Petrow, author

Rowman & Littlefield Publishing Group
4501 Forbes Blvd.
Lanham, MD 20706

301-459-3366
800-462-6420
Fax: 301-429-5748
e-mail: custserv@rowman.com
www.lexingtonbooks.com

218 pages Hardcover
ISBN: 0-669243-09-4

408 Everything You Need to Know About AIDS
Katherine White, author

Rosen Publishing Group
29 E 21st Street
New York, NY 10010

212-777-3017
800-237-9932
Fax: 888-436-4643
e-mail: customerservice@rosenpub.com
www.rosenpublishing.com

Without proper information, our teens remain at risk for AIDS. This volume presents balanced information on the disease and on safer sex precautions, in a language that readers can understand.
64 pages Library Binding
ISBN: 0-823933-14-8
Barbara Taylor, Author

409 Everything You Need to Know About Being HIV Positive
Amy Shire, author

Rosen Publishing Group

29 E 21st Street
New York, NY 10010

212-777-3017
800-237-9932
Fax: 888-436-4643
e-mail: customerservice@rosenpub.com
www.rosenpublishing.com

To teens who need to understand what thier options are when living with HIV on a day-to-day basis. This book explains the facts about HIV.
Hardcover
ISBN: 0-823926-14-1
Amy Shire, Author

410   Everything You Need to Know When a Parent has AIDS
Barbara Hermie Draimin, author

Rosen Publishing Group
29 E 21st Street
New York, NY 10010

212-777-3017
800-237-9932
Fax: 888-436-4643
e-mail: customerservice@rosenpub.com
www.rosenpublishing.com

More and more teens have a parent who has AIDS. Teens must learn where they can turn for help in dealing with this difficult situation. By presenting stories of teens in the same situation, this book helps readers deal with their anger and grief.
64 pages Library Binding
ISBN: 0-823916-90-1
Barbara Hermie Draimin DSW, Author

411   Global AIDS: Myths and Facts, Tools for Fighting the AIDS Pandemic
Alexander Irwin, Joyce Millen, author

South End Press
7 Brookline Street
Cambridge, MA 02139-4146

718-874-0089
e-mail: info@southendpress.org
www.southendpress.org

10 myths about HIV/AIDS treatment and prevention while calling for an international movement to fight the disease.
296 pages
ISBN: 0-896086-73-9

412   Guide to Living With HIV Infection
John G. Bartlett, Ann K. Finkbeiner, author

John's Hopkins University Press
2715 N Charles Street
Baltimore, MD 21218-4363

410-516-6900
800-537-5487
Fax: 410-516-6968
e-mail: webmaster@jhupress.jhu.edu
www.press.jhu.edu

The most complete source of medical, emotional, social, and practical advice available for those infected with HIV and their loved ones. Provides essential information for making decisions about treatment and testing in a world transformed by new research and pharmacotherapy.
1996 408 pages Paperback
ISBN: 0-801884-85-6

413   Invisible People: How the U.S. Has Slept Through the Global AIDS Pandemic
Greg Behrman, author

Free Press Publishing Co.
1010 W Cass St
Tampa, FL 33606-1307

813-254-5888

368 pages
ISBN: 0-743257-55-3

414   Living Well With HIV and AIDS
Allen L Gifford MD, Kate Loring RN, author

Bull Publishing Company
PO Box 1377
Boulder, CO 80306

303-545-6350
800-676-2855
Fax: 303-545-6354
www.bullpub.com

Offers the latest information based on the HIV care guidelines from the Department of Health & Human Services and the Center for Disease Control. Disscuses a shift in treatments emphasis to the ways of managing side effects such as lypodystrophy, redistri-

bution of body fat, cardiac risks, and concerns with vulnerability to other ailments called comorbidities
2005 328 pages Papberback
ISBN: 0-923521-86-8

415   Living on the Edge
Michael Kelly, author

HarperCollins Canada Limited/Order Department
1995 Markham Road
Ontario, Canada M1 B 5M8,

800-387-0117
Fax: 800-668-5788

A gritty, honest, biographical account of one young man's experience from the original diagnosis via the development of the illness, how Michael has learned to live with his illness and how it has affected him and all his friends who support him.
160 pages
ISBN: 0-551027-49-5

416   Local AIDS Sercices: The National Directory
US Conference of Mayors
1620 I Street NW
Washington, DC 20006

202-293-7330
Fax: 202-293-2352
e-mail: info@usmayors.org
www.usmayors.org

2,500 organizations that provide various information and services for AIDS coordinates and other health-related professionals.

417   Lynda Madaras Talks to Teens About AIDS
Lynda Madaras, author

Waterfront Books
98 Brookes Avenue
Burlington, VT 05401

802-658-7477
800-639-6063
e-mail: helpkids@waterfrontbooks.com
www.waterfrontbooks.com

An informative book about the HIV virus and AIDS.
128 pages

418   Night Kites
M.E. Kerr, author

HarperCollins Children's Books
1350 Ave of the Americas
New York, NY 10019

212-261-6500
www.harperchildrens.com

For young adults.
224 pages Paperback
ISBN: 0-064470-35-0

419   No Longer Immune: A Counselor's Guide to AIDS
American Counseling Association
6101 Stevenson Ave.
Alexandria, VA 22304

703-823-9800
800-347-6647
Fax: 703-823-0252
e-mail: webmaster@counseling.org
www.counseling.org

Covers a broad range of issues such as working with specific populations, handling pre- and posttesting situations, coping with fear, grief and survivor guilt, preventing caregiver burnout and dealing with countertransference.
295 pages Paperback
ISBN: 1-556200-64-1

420   Parent Education Program-HIV/AIDS: A Challenge to Us All
Pediatric AIDS Foundation
1140 Connecticut Ave, NW
Washington, DC 20036-3092

202-296-9165
800-499-4673
Fax: 202-296-9185
e-mail: info@pedcids.org
www.pedaids.org

This parent meeting kit with a guide book and two videos will help any adult set up a parent meeting on the subject of AIDS. This kit provides accurate information to parents about HIV/AIDS, allows parents to voice concerns and fears, gives examples of appropriate answers to your child's questions about HIV/AIDS and replaces fear with knowledge and compassion.

421   Predicting AIDS and Other Epidemics
Christopher Lampton, author

Franklin Watts

96 Leonard Street
London EC2A 4XD,
www.wattspub.co.uk
144 pages S & L Binding

422 Scarlet Letters
AIDS Project Los Angeles
The David Geffen Center
Los Angeles, CA 90005
213-201-1600
e-mail: info@apla.org
www.apla.org
A bilingual (Spanidh/English) journal targeted at HIV prevention providers in the U.S. The Scarlet Letters features opinion pieces and research-based essays by invited HIV/STD prevention experts.

423 Teen Guide to AIDS Prevention
Alan E. Nourse, author
Franklin Watts
96 Leonard Street
London EC2A 4XD,
www.wattspub.co.uk
For young adult readers.
61 pages S & L Binding

424 We Have AIDS
Elaine Landau, author
Franklin Watts
96 Leonard Street
London EC2A 4XD,
www.wattspub.co.uk
For young adult readers.
S & L Binding

425 What Is AIDS?
Anna Forbes, author
The Rosen Publishing Group
PowerKids Press
New York, NY 10010
212-777-3017
800-237-9932
Fax: 888-436-4643
e-mail: customerservice@rosenpub.com
www.rosenpublishing.com
For reader levels ages 4-8.
1st Edition 24 pages Hardcover

426 Women & AIDS
Diane Richardson, author
Methuen
35 Hospital Fields Road
York, YO10 4DZ,
190-462-4730
Fax: 190-462-4733
www.methuen.co.uk
The first sourcebook to provide the information women need by identifying the most accurate sources and providing valuable statistical data.
183 pages Paperback
ISBN: 0-416017-51-7

427 Women and AIDS: A Practical Guide for Those Who Help Others
Continuum Publishing Corporation
370 Lexington Avenue
New York, NY 10017-6503
212-532-3650
Tailored to women, this book grapples with attitudes and realities of AIDS.

428 Women and Aids: Coping and Caring
Plenum Publishing Corportation
233 Spring Street
New York, NY 10013-1522
212-620-8000
800-221-9369
Fax: 212-463-0742
e-mail: info@plenum.com
www.springer.com
1996 263 pages
ISBN: 0-306452-58-8
Ann O'Leary, Editor

429 You Have HIV: A Day at a Time
Lynn S. Baker, author
W.B. Saunders Company
www.elsevierhealth.com
258 pages paperback
ISBN: 0-721636-06-3

Children's Books

430 AIDS Overview Series
Lucent Books
Thomson Gale
Farmington Hills, MI 48333-9187
800-877-4253
Fax: 800-414-5043
e-mail: gale.customerservice@thomson.com
www.gale.com/lucent
A straightforward account that teaches young adults all about the growing problem of AIDS.
1998 112 pages
ISBN: 1-560061-93-6

431 AIDS Awareness Library
Rosen Publishing Group
29 E 21st Street
New York, NY 10010
800-237-9932
Fax: 888-436-4643
e-mail: customerservice@rosepub.com
www.rosenpublishing.com
For reader levels ages 4-8.
1996 24 pages
ISBN: 0-823974-06-1

432 AIDS To the Point: Confronting Youth Issues
Diana L. Hynson, author
Abingdon Press
201 8th Avenue S
Nashville, TN 37202-0801
615-749-6347
800-251-3320
Fax: 615-749-6577
www.abingdonpress.com
A resource that offers a practical means of talking with teens, individually or in a group, about AIDS. This volume offers teaching articles, ready-to-go programs for teens, leader's guides, worship resources, facts and figures, where to go for help and a section exclusively in Spanish. This is a volume in the To The Point: Confronting Youth Issues series of books.
96 pages Paperback
ISBN: 0-687782-20-1

433 AIDS: How it Works in the Body
Franklin Watts Grolier
90 Old Sherman Turnpike
Danbury, CT 06816-0001
203-797-3500
Fax: 203-797-6986
www.grolier.com
Focuses on the physiological effects AIDS has on the body, explains the causes of the disease, how the immune system works to defend the body and how the HIV virus affects the immune system.
64 pages Grades 5-7
ISBN: 0-531200-74-4

434 AIDS: Trading Fears for Facts a Guide for Teens
Consumer Reports Books
9180 La Saint Drive
Fairfield, OH 45014
914-378-2567
Fax: 914-378-2907
www.consumerreports.com
Written specifically for teenage readers and filled with illustrations, this book includes the current facts about AIDS, discusses how the virus is transmitted and precautions that should be taken.

435 AIDS: Trading Fears for Facts: A Guide for Young People
Consumer Reports Books
9180 La Saint Drive
Fairfield, OH 45014
914-378-2567
Fax: 914-378-2907
www.consumerreports.com
Written specifically for teenage readers and filled with illustrations, this book includes the current facts about AIDS, discusses how the virus is transmitted and precautions that should be taken.
1993
ISBN: 0-890432-62-4

436 Dancing Against the Darkness: A Journey Through America in the Age of AIDS
Heath Publishing
125 Spring Street
Lexington, MA 02421-7801
617-822-6650

A professional in the field, this author has chosen people across the nation to interview and use as examples for how the AIDS epidemic has struck America and what kind of lives it has affected.
Grades 7-12

437   Everything You Need to Know When a Parent Has AIDS
Barbara Hermie Draimin, DSW, author
Rosen Publishing Group
29 E. 21st Street   212-777-3017
New York, NY 10010   800-237-9932
                                                      Fax: 888-436-4643
                              e-mail: customerservice@rosepub.com
                                          www.rosenpublishing.com
For reader levels ages 4-8.

ISBN: 0-823916-90-1

438   Impact of AIDS
Franklin Watts Grolier
90 Old Sherman Turnpike   203-797-3500
Danbury, CT 06816-0001   800-621-1115
                                                      Fax: 203-797-6986
                                                      www.grolier.com
Examines the effects of the HIV infection and discusses the efforts in finding a cure for AIDS.
64 pages Grades 5-7
ISBN: 0-531172-25-2

439   Night Kites
Harper Collins
195 Broadway   212-207-7000
New York, NY 10007   e-mail: tmpcorrections@harpercollins.com
                                          www.harpercollins.com
This book focuses on two brothers, one of whom is homosexual and how they interact in the face of AIDS and the intolerance of homosexuality among the many people they know.
Grades 8-12

440   Our Immune System
Sara LeBien, author
Immune Deficiency Foundation
110 West Road   410-321-6647
Towson, MD 21204-4841   800-296-4433
                                                      Fax: 410-321-9165
                                    e-mail: idf@primaryimmune.org
                                          www.primaryimmune.org
This storybook educates children about primary immunodeficiency diseases through delightful, eye-catching illustrations. The characters explain how the immune system works and describe the treatments for pediatric patients. Children will understand their own bodies and be better prepared to deal with their own primary immunodeficiency.
G. Richard Barr, Chairman
Marcia Boyle, Founder, Chairperson

441   Predicting AIDS and Other Epidemics
Franklin Watts Grolier
90 Old Sherman Turnpike   203-797-3500
Danbury, CT 06816-0001   800-621-1115
                                                      Fax: 203-797-6986
                                                      www.grolier.com
Surveys the efforts of scientists and researchers to predict the spread of epidemic diseases, including AIDS.
128 pages Grades 7-12
ISBN: 0-531107-85-0

442   Problem of AIDS
Franklin Watts Grolier
90 Old Sherman Turnpike   203-797-3500
Danbury, CT 06816-0001   800-621-1115
                                                      Fax: 203-797-6986
                                                      www.grolier.com
Part of the Let's Talk About series, this book addresses the questions and answers children and young adults have about AIDS.
32 pages Grades 3-5
ISBN: 0-531171-91-4

443   Teen Guide to AIDS Prevention
Franklin Watts Grolier

90 Old Sherman Turnpike   203-797-3500
Danbury, CT 06816-0001   800-621-1115
                                                      Fax: 203-797-6986
                                                      www.grolier.com
Directly addresses the questions and fears of teenagers by explaining clearly and simply what AIDS is, how it is spread, and the preventive measures young persons should take.
64 pages Grades 9-12
ISBN: 0-531109-66-6

444   We Have AIDS
Franklin Watts Grolier
90 Old Sherman Turnpike   203-797-3500
Danbury, CT 06816-0001   800-621-1115
                                                      Fax: 203-797-6986
                                                      www.grolier.com
This book goes beyond statistics and facts and focuses on the personal side of the disease. Offers source notes, a bibliography and an index.
128 pages
ISBN: 0-531108-98-8

445   What's a Virus, Anyway? The Kid's Book About AIDS
Waterfront Books
98 Brookes Avenue   802-658-7477
Burlington, VT 05401-3326
A simple introduction to help adults talk with children about the subject of AIDS.
67 pages

Magazines

446   AIDS Alert
American Health Consultants
3525 Piedmont Road   404-262-5476
Atlanta, GA 30355   800-688-2421
                                                      Fax: 404-262-5560
                                                      www.ahcmedia.com
Covers up-to-the-minute developments and guidance on the entire spectrum of AIDS challenges, including treatment, education, precautions, screening, diagnosis and policy.

447   AIDS Clinical Care
New England Journal of Medicine
860 Winter Street   781-893-4610
Waltham, MA 02451-1413   800-322-2303
                                                      Fax: 781-893-3800
                                          e-mail: nejcust@mms.org
                                                      www.massmed.org
Up to date information specifically targeted at physicians with AIDS patients.
Monthly

448   AIDS: A Year In Review
Lippincott Williams & Wilkins
16522 Hunters Green Pkwy   301-223-2300
Hagerstown, MD 21740   800-638-3030
                                                      Fax: 301-223-2400
                                          e-mail: orders@lww.com
                                                      www.lww.com
An interdisciplinary journal providing a synthesis of AIDS-related information from all relevant clinical and basic sciences.

449   AIDS: International Monthly Journal
Lippincott Williams & Wilkins
16522 Hunters Green Pkwy   301-223-2300
Hagerstown, MD 21740   800-638-3030
                                                      Fax: 301-223-2400
                                          e-mail: orders@lww.com
                                                      www.lww.com
An interdisciplinary journal providing a synthesis of AIDS-related information from all relevant clinical and basic sciences.

450   AIDS: The Disease State Management Resource
American Health Consultants
PO Box 550669   404-262-5476
Atlanta, GA 30355   800-688-2421
                                                      Fax: 800-284-3291
                                                      www.ahcmedia.com

Covers up-to-the-minute developments and guidance on the entire spectrum of AIDS challenges, including treatment, education, precautions, screening, diagnosis and policy.

451 Critical Path AIDS Project
2062 Lombard Street
Philadelphia, PA 19146-1315   215-545-2212
                                     www.critpath.org
Articles and reprints on experimental treatments and alternative therapies, and a listing of Philadelphia-area resources.
Monthly

452 Institute on Health Care for the Poor and Underserved at Meharry Medical College
Sage Publications
1005 DB Todd Boulevard   615-327-6819
Nashville, TN 37208   800-669-1269
                                     Fax: 615-327-6362
                                     e-mail: vbrennan@mmc.edu
Offers health care and public health policy research focusing on poor and underserved populations.
100 pages 4x a year
Dr. Amy Cato, Director
Dr. Virginia Brennan, Editor

453 Journal of Acquired Immune Deficiency Syndrome
Lippincott Williams & Wilkins
16522 Hunters Green Pkwy   301-223-2300
Hagerstown, MD 21740-2601   800-638-3030
                                     Fax: 301-223-2400
                                     e-mail: orders@lww.com
                                     www.lww.com
An interdisciplinary journal providing a synthesis of AIDS-related information from all relevant clinical and basic sciences.
Monthly
ISBN: 0-894925-5 -
William A Hazeltine, Editor

454 Journal of the Medical Library Association
Medical Library Association
65 E Wacker Place   312-419-9094
Chicago, IL 60601-7246   Fax: 312-419-8950
                                     e-mail: info@mlahq.org
                                     www.mlahq.org
An international, peer-reviewed journal that aims to advance the practice and research knowledgebase of health science librarianship.
Quarterly
Carla J Funk, Executive Director
Elizabeth Lund, Publications Director

455 POZ Magazine
POZ Publishing
462 Seventh Avenue   212-242-2163
New York, NY 10018-7424   Fax: 212-675-8505
                                     e-mail: poz-editor@poz.com
                                     www.poz.com
A magazine for people living with, and affected by, HIV/AIDS.
60 pages BiMonthly
Regan Hofmann, Editor in Chief
Jennifer Morton, Managing Editor

456 Risky Business
San Francisco AIDS Foundation Materials Dept.
333 Valencia Street   415-861-3397
San Francisco, CA 94103-3547
A comic book style magazine providing accurate information about AIDS using humor and real-life situations. Contains stories that stress the importance of knowing how AIDS is transmitted and prevented.

457 Straight Talk: A Magazine for Teens About AIDS
Custom Publishing Division of Rodale Press
33 E Minor Street   610-967-5171
Emmaus, PA 18098-0001
A lively magazine that includes articles about teens with AIDS, teens involved in peer education and teens at risk for getting infected. Good information is presented in an interesting format for young adults.

458 Washington Update
Committee of Ten Thousand
500 Belmont Street   508-587-2512
Brockton, MA 02301   e-mail: cott-dc@earthlink.net
                                     www.cott1.org
Is a primer on government related issues of importance to COTT's constituency. From health care legislation, to regulatory affairs to Administration policy for chronic diseases. A hands-on journal for grass roots health care advocacy in our Nation's capital.
Bi-Monthly
John Rider, Contact

Newsletters

459 AIDS Alert
American Health Consulants
3525 Piedmont Road   404-262-5476
Atlanta, GA 30355   800-688-2421
                                     Fax: 404-262-5560
                         e-mail: customerservice@ahcpub.com
                                     www.ahcmedia.com
Covers up-to-the-minute developments and guidance on the entire spectrum of AIDS challenges, including treatment, education, precautions, screening, diagnosis and policy.

460 AIDS Link
University of Cincinnati-Medical Center Info.
231 Bethesda Avenue   513-558-5661
Cincinnati, OH 45267-0001   Fax: 513-558-3136
                                     medcenter.uc.edu/
Aimed at healthcare professionals working with HIV/AIDS inflicted patients.
Rebecca Atterrin, Editor

461 AIDS News
Northern California Chapter of the NHF
7700 Edgewater Drive   510-568-6243
Oakland, CA 94621-3023
Provides current information for people who need to cope mentally and physically with the issues of virus infection and transmission. Provides answers to questions about AIDS, ARC, HIV infection and transmission prevention.
BiMonthly

462 AIDS Policy and Law
LRP Publications
747 Dresher Road
Horsham, PA 19044-0980   www.lrp.com
A report on AIDS policy and law developments from the courts, NIH, federal and state AIDS agencies and advocacy organizations.
24 year

463 AIDS Treatment Data Network
611 Broadway   212-260-8868
New York, NY 10012   800-734-7104
                                     Fax: 212-260-8869
                                     www.atdn.org
Information bulletins covering new treatments, clinical trials, and more.

464 AIDS Treatment News
ATN Publications
PO Box 411256
San Francisco, CA 94141-1256   800-873-2812
                                     www.atnonline.org
Reports on the developments in treatments for HIV disease and related infections. Also covers issues relating to research.
BiMonthly

465 AIDS Update
Dallas Gay Alliance
PO Box 190812   214-528-4233
Dallas, TX 75219-0812   Fax: 214-521-6424
                                     e-mail: info@dgla.org
                                     www.divanet.com/dgla/
Includes general information on AIDS issues and treatments.

466 AIDS Weekly Plus
Charles Henderson

Po Box 5528
Atlanta, GA 31107-0528   e-mail: info@hendersonnet.atl.ga.us
All aspects of AIDS epidemic coverage, including research, treatments, vaccine development, political and public policy.
46 year

467   AIDS/STD News Report
CD Publications
2222 Sedwick Drive   301-588-6380
Durham, NC 27713   800-666-6380
                                       Fax: 301-588-6385
                              e-mail: info@cdpublications.com
                                       www.cdpublications.com
Formerly AIDS News Alert, provides grant listings from federal, private, and corporate sources; proposal writing tips; updates on successful programs, and the latest news on AIDS/STD federal/state legislation, research, and successful programs.

468   APICHA News
Asian & Pacific Islander Coalition on HIV/AIDS
400 Broadway   212-334-7940
New York, NY 10013   866-274-2429
                                       Fax: 212-334-7956
                              e-mail: apicha@apicha.org
                                       www.apicha.org
Provides information on prevention education, client services and advocacy for Asians and Pacific Islanders.
Quarterly
Therese R Rodriguez, CEO

469   APLA Update
AIDS Project Los Angeles
3550 Wilshire Boulevard
Los Angeles, CA 90010   213-201-1600
                                       www.apla.org
Presents news about AIDS and programs of AIDS Project Los Angeles to people affected by the disease.
20 pages

470   BETA
San Francisco AIDS Foundation
1035 Market Street   415-487-3000
San Francisco, CA 94103   e-mail: feedback@sfaf.org
                                       www.sfaf.org
Medical information.
Quarterly

471   Being Alive
Being Alive People with HIV/AIDS Action Coalition
7531 Santa Monica Blvd   323-874-4322
West Hollywood, CA 90046   Fax: 323-969-8753
                              e-mail: info@beingalivela.org
                                       www.beingalivela.org
Medical updates, plus information on AIDS advocacy, a calendar of local events and listings of AIDS support groups.

472   Being Alive Newsletter
Being Alive-People with HIV/AIDS Action Coalition
7531 Santa Monica Blvd   323-874-4322
West Hollywood, CA 90040   Fax: 323-969-8753
                              e-mail: kevin@beingalivela.org
                                       www.beingalivela.org
A regularly-published source of information and education for our peers living with HIV/AIDS and for the greater community. Standing articles cover timely issues such as HIV/AIDS treatment options, mental health, substance abuse, nutrition, advocacy, community referrals, and a variety of other topics. Additionally, we feature information on Being Alive events alongside other relevant community events.
Quarterly
Kevin Kurth, Executive Director/Editor

473   CORPUS
AIDS Project Los Angeles
The David Geffen Center
Los Angeles, CA 90005   213-201-1600
                              e-mail: info@apla.org
                                       www.apla.org

A journal that uses art, cultural criticism, poetry, short stories and humor to reveal the challenges of HIV prevention in gay and bisexual communities.
Annually
Craig E Thompson, Executive Director

474   COTT News
Committee on Ten Thousand
500 Belmont Street
Brockton, MA 02301   508-587-2512
                                       www.cott1.org
A range of information, reportage and viewpoints regarding issues and events of importance to grass roots health care advocacy and support.
John Rider, Contact

475   Center for AIDS Prevention Studies
AIDS Research Institute
550 16th Street   415-476-6288
San Francisco, CA 94158   Fax: 415-597-9213
                              e-mail: capsweb@psg.ucsf.edu
                                       www.caps.ucsf.edu
Local, national, and international interdisciplinary research.

476   Community Health Funding Report
CD Publications
2222 Sedwick Drive   301-588-6380
Durham, NC 27713-4571   800-666-6380
                                       Fax: 301-588-6385
                              e-mail: info@cdpublications.com
                                       www.cdpublications.com
Covers grants for AIDS and sexually transmitted disease related programs from federal and private sources. Includes news on national and local issues affecting AIDS and STD's and case studies of successful fundraising programs. This biweekly newsletter describes changes in funding streams for community based health programs, including AIDS programs. It lists available federal and private grant opportunities, along with Washington News Medicare/Medicaid.
18 pages BiMonthly
Mike Gerecht, Publisher
Amy Bernstein, Editor

477   Cott Washington Update
Committee of Ten Thousand
236 Massachusetts Ave NE   202-543-0988
Washington, DC 20002-4971   800-488-2688
                                       Fax: 202-543-6720
                                       www.cott1.org
Offers legislative updates, information on clinical trials, therapies, book reviews, business and politics, a readers forum and resources pertaining to HIV/AIDS.
10 pages Monthly
Corey Dubin, President
Dave Cavenaugh, Government Relations

478   FOCUS
UCSF AIDS Health Project
1930 Market Street   415-476-3902
San Francisco, CA 94102   TTY: 415-476-3587
                              e-mail: ahpinfo@ucsf.edu
                                       www.ucsf-ahp.org
Reviews the counseling aspects of AIDS: how HIV-related counseling is affected by the medical, epidemiological, and social realities of AIDS, as well as the emotional response to the disease. It is written for mental health and health care providers working on the front lines and is of interest to researchers, policy makers, and program administrators.
10x/year
James W Dilley MD, Executive Director

479   Gay Men's Health Crisis
119 West 24th Street
New York, NY 10011   212-367-1000
                                       www.gmhc.org
Not-for-profit, voluteer-supported and community-based organization committed to national leadership in the fight against AIDS.

480   HIV Counselor PERSPECTIVES
UCSF AIDS Health Project

1930 Market Street
San Francisco, CA 94102

415-476-3902
TTY: 415-476-3587
e-mail: ahpinfo@ucsf.edu
www.ucsf-ahp.org

An educational resource for HIV antibody test counselors, prevention case managers, and other health and mental health professionals, particularly those working in brief counseling venues.
4 year
James W Dilley MD, Executive Director

481 HIV Frontline
Center for AIDS Prevention Studies
University of California
San Francisco, CA 94158

415-476-6288
Fax: 415-597-9213
e-mail: CAPSweb@psg.ucsf.edu
www.caps.ucsf.edu

Monthly newsletter aimed at mental health and healthcare professionals who counsel people living with HIV/AIDS.
Monthly
Dr. Leon McKusick

482 IDF Advocate
Immune Deficiency Foundation
110 West Road
Towson, MD 21204

800-296-4433
e-mail: idf@primaryimmune.org
www.primaryimmune.org

Mailed to patients, family members, physicians, nurses, industry, government and interested individuals.
3x/year
Marcia Boyle, President/Founder

483 Immune Deficiency Foundation Newsletter
Immune Deficiency Foundation
110 West Road
Towson, MD 21204-4841

410-321-6647
800-296-4433
Fax: 410-321-9165
e-mail: idf@primaryimmune.org
www.primaryimmune.org

Offers medical updates and technology news on the latest services, products and treatments for persons with immune diseases.
Tamara Brown, Medical Programs Manager

484 In Focus
Project Inform
273 Ninth Street
San Francisco, CA 94103-2461

415-558-8669
877-435-7443
Fax: 415-558-0684
e-mail: web@projectinform.org
www.projectinform.org

The organizational newsletter of Project Inform.
20+ pages 3x/year
Skip Emerson, Executive Assistant

485 Just Kids
3 Corners
5th Avenue
New York, NY 10014

212-634-4879

Covers medical and social issues faced by HIV-positive children, teens and their parents.
Annual

486 MLA News
Medical Library Association
65 East Wacker Place
Chicago, IL 60601-7246

312-419-9094
Fax: 312-419-8950
e-mail: info@mlahq.org
www.mlanet.org

Keeps you at the forefront of association matters and the profession as a whole. Regular departments include calendar, continuing education, employment opportunities, international news, Internet resources, personals, professional development, and technology. Columns include consumer health, expert searching, hospital librarianship, leadership and management, and new members. Members only.
Jean P Shipman, President

487 NMAC Update
National Minority AIDS Council

1931 13th Street, NW
Washington, DC 20009-4389

202-483-6622
Fax: 202-483-1135
www.nmac.org

A newsletter reporting on public policy issues and information on subjects in organizational management.
BiMonthly

488 OUTReach
The San Francisco AID Foundation
1035 Market Street
San Francisco, CA 94103

415-487-3000
Fax: 415-487-8009
TDD: 415-487-8099
e-mail: feedback@sfaf.org
www.sfaf.org

Features concise articles on a wide range of HIV/AIDS topics.

489 PAACNOTES
101 W Grand Avenue
Chicago, IL 60610-4272

312-222-1326
800-243-3059

A news journal of the Physicians Coalition for AIDS Care featuring articles on clinical management, scientific research and a diverse range of legal, ethical and economic issues directly affecting the care of persons with HIV disease.

490 PWA Rag
Prisoners With AIDS Rights Advocacy Group
1626 Wilcox Avenue
Loa Angeles, CA 90028

770-946-9346
e-mail: RAGNEWS@aol.com
www.hometown.aol.com

Contains articles, treatment updates, and resources for prisoners.

491 Positive Living
APLA
3550 Wilshire Boulevard
Los Angeles, CA 90010

213-201-1600
800-922-2438

Monthly

492 Positive Outlook
2655 Swann Avenue
Tampa, FL 33609

813-877-5696

Focuses on local people and issues in West Central Florida.
Quarterly

493 Positive Social Support Newsletter
Lambda Center
4228 Wisconsin Avenue NW
Washington, DC 20016

202-965-8434
877-252-6232
e-mail: contact@lambcenter.com
www.thelambdacenter.com

Sponsored by and for people with HIV.

494 Positive Voice Newsletter
National Association of People with AIDS (NAPWA)
8401 Colesville Road
Silverspring, MD 20910

240-247-0880
866-846-9366
Fax: 240-247-0574
e-mail: info@napwa.org
www.napwa.org

Frank J Oldham Jr, President/CEO
Peter Kronenberg, VP Communications/Editor

495 Positive Woman
PO Box 34372
Washington, DC 20043-4372

202-898-0372

Provides medical information, including alternative and holistic therapies for HIV-positive women.
BiMonthly

496 Positively Aware
Test Positive Aware Network
5537 N Broadway Street
Chicago, IL 60640

773-989-9400
Fax: 773-989-9494
e-mail: tpan@tpan.com
www.tpan.com

An internationally known and respected magazine devoted to HIV treatment, wellness, and optimum quality of life for those living with HIV, as well as those who care for them.
Bi-monthly
Jeff Berry, Publications Director

497 RAP* Time
Rural Center for AIDS/STD Prevention
Indiana University   812-855-7974
Bloomington, IN 47405-3085   800-566-8644
                                                    Fax: 812-855-3936
                                        e-mail: aids@indiana.edu
                                              www.indiana.edu/~aids/
Summarizes current research concerning HIV/STD prevention,
particularly in rural settings.
William L Yarber HSD, Senior Director

498 STEP Perspective
Seattle Treatment Exchange Project
750 3rd Avenue   206-329-4857
New York, NY 10017-5711   800-869-7837
                                        e-mail: info@stepproject.org
                                              www.thebody.com
Updates on treatments for HIV and related diseases condensed
from journals, conferences and databases by the scientific review
committee.

499 Seasons
National Native American AIDS Prevention Center
1031 33rd Street   510-444-2051
Denver, CO 80205-2011   Fax: 510-444-1593
                                        e-mail: information@nnaape.org
                                              www.nnaapc.org
Features articles and artwork by Native Americans impacted by
HIV/AIDS.
Quarterly

500 Treatment Issues
Dep of Medical Info   212-337-1950
New York, NY 10011-3601
The gay men's health crisis newsletter of experimental AIDS ther-
apies.
10x Year

501 Up Front Drug Information
5701 Biscayne Boulevard   305-757-2566
Miami, FL 33137-2601
Provides information on drugs and drug referrals.

502 Walk Talk
AIDS Coalition Silicon Valley
Walk For AIDS Silicon Vly   408-451-WALK
San Jose, CA 95154   Fax: 408-248-7423
                                        e-mail: info@walkforaids.org
The AIDS Coalition Silicon Valley Newsletter highlighting Walk
for AIDS Silicon Valley fundraising events, issues and articles
about HIV/AIDS service providers in the County.

503 Wisconsin AIDS Update
Wisconsin AIDS/HIV Program, Department of Health
1 West Wilson Street   608-266-1865
Madison, WI 50703-0309   888-701-1251
                                        e-mail: webmaildph@dhfs.state.wi.us
                                              www.dhs.wisconsin.gov
Includes epidemiological and clinical care articles, selections
from the most important current abstracts in ATIN and a statewide
list of events and resources.
Quarterly

504 World/Mundo
PO Box 11535   415-658-6930
Oakland, CA 94611-0535
Contains letters, advice, events calendar, and information on sup-
port groups in Northern California.

Pamphlets

505 AIDS Medicines in Development
Pharmaceutical Research & Manufacturers of America
950 F Street NW   202-835-3400
Washington, DC 20004   Fax: 202-835-3414
                                              www.phrma.org
An annual chart of antivirals, as well as information on diagnostics
and vaccines.

506 AIDS and Hemophilia: Protecting Yourself and Others
Hemophilia Council of California: Bay Area Office
7700 Edgewater Drive   510-568-7074
Oakland, CA 94621   Fax: 510-568-2048
                                        e-mail: hccoak@aol.com
Lori Drake, Mental Health Counselor/Health Educator

507 AIDS, the Law & You
AIDS Action Committee
75 Amory Street   617-437-6200
Boston, MA 02119-5145   800-424-2634
                                                    Fax: 617-437-6445
                                        e-mail: webmaster@aac.org
                                              www.aac.org
Discusses legal protection against AIDS-related discrimination,
HIV testing and the law.

**508 Americans with Disabilities Act: What it Means for People with
AIDS**
American Civil Liberties Union AIDS Project
125 Broad Street
New York, NY 10004-6503   212-549-2500
                                              www.aclu.org

509 Basics of HIV Disease: Questions and Answers
National Hemophilia Foundation
7 Penn Plaza   212-328-3700
New York, NY 10001-3212   800-424-2634
                                                    Fax: 212-328-3777
                                        e-mail: handi@hemophilia.org
                                              www.hemophilia.org
This publication contains basic information about hemophilia and
HIV disease.
1992 28 pages
Alan Kinniburgh, PhD, CEO

510 Be Smart About HIV
American Red Cross
8550 Arlington Blvd.   703-584-8400
Fairfax, VA 22031-3100   Fax: 703-312-8738
                                              www.redcross.org
This brochure offers very simple and informative information on
the HIV virus, in both English and Spanish.
1996
Sandra L Mertz, Product Manager

511 Children with AIDS: Guidelines for Parents and Caregivers
AIDS Task Force of Central New York
627 W Genesee Street   315-415-2430
Syracuse, NY 13204-2347
Offers general information on AIDS, diet and feeding, household
chores, and coping with the illness.

512 Clinical Focus
Immune Deficiency Foundation
110 West Road   410-321-6647
Towson, MD 21204-4841   800-296-4433
                                                    Fax: 410-321-9165
                                        e-mail: info@primaryimmune.org
                                              www.primaryimmune.org
Biannual publication for medical professionals covering current
issues and information regarding clinical approaches to primary
immune deficiencies.
BiAnnual
Marcia Boyle, Founder/Chair

513 Clinical Focus on Primary Immune Deficiency Diseases
Immune Deficiency Foundation
40 W Chesapeake Avenue   410-321-6647
Towson, MD 21204-4841   800-296-4433
                                                    Fax: 410-321-9165
                                        e-mail: info@primaryimmune.org
                                              www.primaryimmune.org
educational mongraph is designed specifically for health care professionals and focuses on topics relevant to primary immune deficiency diseases.
Marcia Boyle, Founder/Chair

514 Clinical Presentation of the Primary Immunodeficiency Diseases
Immune Deficiency Foundation

40 W Chesapeake Avenue
Towson, MD 21204-4841

410-321-6647
800-296-4433
Fax: 410-321-9165
e-mail: info@primaryimmune.org
www.primaryimmune.org

A primer for physicians.
Tamara Brown, Medical Programs Manager

515 Clinical Trials: Talking it Over
NIAID, Office of Communications
200 Independence Avn, SW
Washington, DC 20201-0001

301-496-5717
877-696-6775
www.hhs.gov

Educational pamphlet pertaining to clinical trials.
Sylvia M. Burwell, HHS Secretary
Mary K. Wakefield, HHS Acting Deputy Secretary

516 Condoms and Sexually Transmitted Diseases, Especially AIDS
Department of Health and Human Services
Nat Institutes of Health
Bethesda, MD 20892-0001

202-673-7700

Offers information on condoms and how various forms of protection can be used to prevent sexually transmitted diseases, especially HIV/AIDS.

517 Eating Defensively: Food Safety Advice for Persons with AIDS
AIDSinfo
PO Box 4780
Rockville, MD 20849-6303

301-315-2816
800-448-0440
Fax: 301-315-2818
TTY: 888-480-3739
e-mail: ContactUs@aidsinfo.nih.gov
www.aidsinfo.nih.gov

The food safety advice in this brochure is intended to help persons with HIV infection to reduce the risk of food poisoning, thereby avoiding an illness that could worsen their condition or even cause death.
1992

518 HIV Infection and AIDS
NAID Office of Communications
31 Center Drive
Bethesda, MD 20892-0001

301-496-1653
Fax: 301-402-0779
e-mail: bettends@ficod.fic.nih.gov
www.grants.nih.gov

Offers information on transmission, treatment, early symptoms, diagnosis, prevention and research.

519 HIV and AIDS During Pregnancy
March of Dimes
233 Park Avenue South
New York, NY 10003

212-353-8353
Fax: 212-254-3518
e-mail: NY639@marchofdimes.com
www.marchdofdimes.com

520 HIV/AIDS in the Workplace
New York Business Group on Health
386 Park Avenue S
New York, NY 10016-8804

212-252-7440
e-mail: nybgh@nybgh.org
www.nybgh.org

Offers information on federal law and state law regarding HIV/AIDS in the workplace, universal risks, health insurance and other business costs.

521 Hope for Children with AIDS
Pediatric AIDS Foundation
16130 Ventura Blvd.
Los Angeles, CA 91436-3092

818-338-6361
888-499-4673
Fax: 818-906-6951
e-mail: info@pedaids.org
www.pedaids.org

A brochure offering information on the latest research and advances in the area of pediatric AIDS.

522 How to Keep an Infusion Log
Immune Deficiency Foundation
110 West Road
Towson, MD 21204

800-296-4433
e-mail: info@primaryimmune.org
www.primaryimmune.org

This brochure explains the value of keeping an immune globulin infusion log, as well as practical information on how to set up your personal records.
Marci Boyle, President/Founder

523 IDF Guide for Nurses on Immune Globulin Therapy for Primary Immunodeficiency
Immune Deficiency Foundation
110 West Road
Towson, MD 21204

800-296-4433
e-mail: info@primaryimmune.org
www.primaryimmune.org

This guide provides direction for nurses to administer immune globulin replacement therapy in the safest and most effective way. Information includes: clinical uses for immune globulin replacement therapy; product selection and characteristics; infusions, complications and adverse events of IVIG and SCIG; concomitant medications; nursing interventions and responsibilities and helpful references and resources.
Marcia Boyle, President/Founder

524 IDF Patient and Family Handbook
Immune Deficiency Foundation
110 West Road
Towson, MD 21204

800-296-4433
e-mail: info@primaryimmune.org
www.primaryimmune.org

For patients and family members, contains information about the diagnosis and treatment of primary immunodeficiency diseases, the immune system, specific diseases, therapies, general care, health insurance and issues specific to adult, adolescent and pediatric patients.
R Michael Blaese MD, Editor
E. Richard Stiehm MD, Editor

525 Immune Deficiency Foundation
110 West Road
Towson, MD 21204

800-296-4433
e-mail: info@primaryimmune.org
www.primaryimmune.org

Your partner for living with primary immune deficiency diseases. This brochure describes the IDF and its activities and services.

526 Infections Linked to AIDS
NAID Office of Communications
31 Center Drive
Bethesda, MD 20892-0001

301-496-5717
www.hhs.gov

Offers information on infections related to HIV/AIDS and referral numbers of where to receive help.

527 Our Immune System
Sara LeBien, author
Immune Deficiency Foundation
110 West Road
Towson, MD 21204-4841

410-321-6647
800-296-4433
Fax: 410-321-9165
e-mail: info@primaryimmune.org
www.primaryimmune.org

This storybook educates children about primary immunodeficiency diseases through delightful, eye-catching illustrations. The characters explain how the immune system works and describe the treatments for pediatric patients. Children will understand their own bodies and be better prepared to deal with their own primary immunodeficiency.
Marcia Boyle, President & Founder
Sarah Rose, Chief Financial Officer

528 Taking the HIV (AIDS) Test: How to Help Yourself
NAID Office of Communications
31 Center Drive
Bethesda, MD 20892-0001

301-496-5717

Offers information on the AIDS test, how it works, how it can help and should it be taken.

529 Teeens, Sexually Transmitted Diseases & HIV/AIDS
4 Brighton Road
West Sussex, RH13 5BA UK,

e-mail: info@avert.org
www.avert.org

Designed for teens, and contains information on what STD's are, how to avoid becoming infected, safer sex, how to spot symptoms of STD's, STD treatment, information about HIV/AIDS, information about testing and treatment, and advice helplines.

530   Testing Positive for HIV
NAID Office of Communications
31 Center Drive   301-496-5717
Bethesda, MD 20892-0001
Information on what a positive HIV test means, how not to spread the disease to others, and various health and dieting tips.

531   Testing for HIV Infection
American Red Cross
1616 Fort Myer Drive   703-312-8724
Arlington, VA 22209-3100   Fax: 703-312-8738
1996
Sandra L Mertz, Product Manager

532   Women, Sex, and HIV
American Red Cross
1616 Fort Myer Drive   703-312-8724
Arlington, VA 22209-3100   Fax: 703-312-8738
1992
Sandra L Mertz, Product Manager

533   Your Job and HIV: Are There Risks?
American Red Cross
1616 Fort Myer Drive   703-312-8724
Arlington, VA 22209-3100   Fax: 703-312-8738
1992
Sandra L Mertz, Product Manager

Audio & Video

534   AIDS Work: Six Healthcare Workers Face the AIDS Crisis
Fanlight Productions
32 Court Street   718-488-8900
Brooklyn, NY 11201   800-876-1710
                                          Fax: 718-488-8642
                                  e-mail: info@fanlight.com
                                          www.fanlight.com
Two physicians and four nurses reflect on several decades of combined experiences in caring for patients with HIV/AIDS. They discuss facing fear, frustration, burnout and grief as they struggle to deliver compassionate care, as well as the rewards of caring for this population. This inspirational program is invaluable for stress management programs, and in preparing students and new workers for the realities they will face.
VHS
ISBN: 1-572952-20-2
Steve Guy, Producer

535   Does Anyone Die of AIDS Anymore?
Louise Hogarth, author
Fanlight Productions
32 Court Street   718-488-8900
Brooklyn, NY 11201   800-876-1710
                                          Fax: 718-488-8642
                                  e-mail: info@fanlight.com
                                          www.fanlight.com
The answer to this disturbing film's title question is a resounding yes! Despite the much-hyped advances in treatment which, for some patients, have transformed HIV from a death sentence to a chronic illness, tens of thousands of people are still dying of AIDS in the United States. And tens of thousands more will die, even in this rich and medically advanced nation, because of ignorance and denial which have resulted in a 'third wave' of HIV infection.
26 Minutes
ISBN: 1-572958-48-0
Gregory A. Freeman, Author
Louise Hogarth, Producer

536   Roger's Story: For Cori
Howard Shepps, author
Fanlight Productions

32 Court Street   718-488-8900
Brooklyn, NY 11201   800-876-1710
                                          Fax: 718-488-8642
                                  e-mail: info@fanlight.com
                                          www.fanlight.com
Forty-four year-old Roger shares the harrowing story of his 20-year struggle against heroin, and his recent diagnosis with AIDS.
1989 28 Minutes
ISBN: 1-572950-47-1

537   Too Little, Too Late
Micki Dickoff, author
Fanlight Productions
32 Court Street   718-488-8900
Brooklyn, NY 11201   800-876-1710
                                          Fax: 718-488-8642
                                  e-mail: info@fanlight.com
                                          www.fanlight.com
In this moving video, family members of people with AIDS share their pain and frustration, as well as the solace they have derived from having been able to help their loved one to a peaceful death.
1987 49 Minutes
ISBN: 1-572950-27-7

538   Undetectable: The New Face of AIDS
Jay Corcoran, author
Fanlight Productions
32 Court Street   718-488-8900
Brooklyn, NY 11201   800-876-1710
                                          Fax: 718-488-8642
                                  e-mail: info@fanlight.com
                                          www.fanlight.com
This gripping documentary follows six women and men, straight and gay, of different ethnic and cultural backgrounds, over a three-year period as they deal for the first time with hope. Though the new multi-drug therapies for HIV disease offer a possible reprieve from what was once a death sentence, those who are lucky enough to respond to the drugs nonetheless face both a grueling treatment regimen, and the complex physical and psychological challenges of rebuilding their lives.
2001 56 Minutes
ISBN: 1-572958-45-6

Web Sites

539   AIDS United
                                          www.aidsunited.org
To end the AIDS epidemic in the United States. We will achieve this goal through national, regional and local policy/advocacy, strategic grantmaking, and organizational capacity building. With partners throughout the country, we will work to ensure that people living with and affected by HIV/AIDS have access to the prevention and care services they need and deserve.

540   AIDS.ORG
                                                www.aids.org
The mission of AIDS.ORG is to help prevent HIV infections and to improve the lives of those affected by HIV and AIDS by providing education and facilitating the free and open exchange of knowledge at any easy-to-find centralized website.

541   Children Affected by AIDS Foundation
                                          keepachildalive.org
There mission is to realize the end of AIDS for children and families, by combating the physical, social and economic impacts of HIV.

542   Committee of Ten Thousand
                                                www.cott1.org
A grass-roots, peer-led, education, advocacy and support organization for persons with HIV disease. Dedicated to the belief that persons with HIV/AIDS and all chronic diseases can lead productive and healthy lives

543   HIV/Hepatitis C in Prison (HIP) Committee
                                    www.prisons.org/hivin.htm

Fighting for consistent access to quality medical care including access to all new HIV and Hepatitis C medications, diagnostic testing and combination therapies.

544   Healing Well

www.healingwell.com

A social network and support community for patients, caregivers, and families coping with the daily struggles of diseases, disorders and chronic illness.

545   Health Finder

www.healthfinder.gov

Searchable, carefully developed web site offering information on over 1000 topics. Developed by the US Department of Health and Human Services, the site can be used in both English and Spanish.

546   Healthlink USA

www.healthlinkusa.com

Health information concerning treatment, cures, prevention, diagnosis, risk factors, research, support groups, email lists, personal stories and much more. Updated regularly.

547   Helios Health

www.helioshealth.com

Online resource for your health information. Detailed information about specific health topics, access to expert advice from our Medical Advisory Board, and up-to-date health news.

548   Immune Deficiency Foundation

www.primaryimmune.org

The national patient organization dedicated to improving the diagnosis, treatment and quality of life of persons with primary immunodeficiency diseases through advocacy, education and research.

549   MedicineNet

www.medicinenet.com

An online resource for consumers providing easy-to-read, authoritative medical and health information.

550   Medscape

www.medscape.com

Medscape offers specialists, primary care physicians, and other health professionals the Web's most robust and integrated medical information and educational tools.

551   National AIDS Information Clearinghouse

www.cdc.gov

Provides information and materials for employers on national, state and local resources related to HIV/AIDS in the workplace.

552   National Minority AIDS Education Training

www.nmaetc.org

Located at Howard University, as a HIV/AIDS training and technical resource for providers of minority HIV-infected patients throughout the country. The NMAETC receives 100% of its funding through the MAI Initiative. The NMAETC in collaboration with other HRSA funded programs seeks to influence health care professionals who treat minority HIV-infected patients.

553   New England AIDS Education & Training Ctr.

www.neaetc.org

One of eleven regional education centers funded by the Ryan White CARE Act and sponsored regionally by the Office of Community Programs at the University of Massachusetts Medical Center. The AETC Program is administered by Health Resources and Services Administration (HRSA) HIV/AIDS bureau.

554   People with AIDS Health Group

www.Aidsinfonyc.org

PWA is a non-profit buyers club organized to assist people with AIDS in obtaining medications — as well as provide support groups committed to the self-empowerment of people living with AIDS. They offer three programs: Treatment Education and Support, Advocacy and Public Policy, and Early Treatment Access.

555   San Francisco Area AIDS Education Center

www.ucsf.edu/sfaetc

Helps to improve the care of people living with HIV and AIDS by supporting state-of-the-art clinical consultation, education, and training for health care professionals and organizations in San Francisco, San Mateo, and Marin counties.

556   Smart & Strong

www.smartstrong.com

A healthcare education company that supports providers and empowers HIV positive patients through publications, seminars and innovative educational programs.

557   WebMD

www.webmd.com

Provides credible information, supportive communities, and in-depth reference material about health subjects. A source for original and timely health information as well as material from well known content providers.

Description

558 # Allergies

Allergy means altered reactivity. Allergies are usually characterized by a hypersensitivity to substances, such as pollens, pet dander, certain foods, some medications and molds. Such substances (allergens) can trigger an allergic response in susceptible individuals. Symptoms of allergies may present in a wide spectrum ranging from the mild sneezing, runny nose and congestion of hayfever to life-threatening reactions, known as anaphylaxis. Additional allergic reactions include itchy, watery eyes, skin rashes and asthma. More severe symptoms may include a tingling sensation in the mouth, swelling of the tongue and throat, difficulty breathing, hives, vomiting abdominal cramps, diarrhea, drop in blood pressure, loss of consciousness, and cardiovascular collapse leading to death. Allergic symptoms typically appear within minutes to two hours after the person has been exposed to the allergen.

Approximately 35 million people suffer from allergies in the United States. The cause of allergies is unclear, although there may be a genetic link in some people.

Treatment for allergies depends upon the specific substance, beginning with avoidance. Strict avoidance of the allergy-causing food is the only way to avoid a food allergy reaction. There are no medications that cure food allergies. Most people outgrow their food allergies, although peanuts, nuts, fish and shellfish are often considered life-long allergies.

For non-food allergies, medications such as antihistamines and inhaled bronchodilators, as well as allergy shots to reduce the allergic response, may be prescribed by doctors. Epinephrine, also called adrenaline, is the medication of choice for controlling a severe reaction. Individuals at risk of an anaphylactic reaction should have a bracelet or necklace with that information. Those who are allergic to insect stings should carry and use a pre-filled syringe of epinephrine (epipen) for prompt self-treatment.

National Agencies & Associations

559 **Allergy & Asthma Network Mothers of Asthmatics**
8201 Greensboro Drive   703-641-9595
Fairfax, VA 22102   800-878-4403
                              Fax: 703-288-5271
                         e-mail: info@aanma.org
                          www.breatherville.org
Leading nonprofit membership organization dedicated to eliminating suffering and death due to asthma, allergies and related conditions through education, advocacy, community outreach and research.
Michael Amato, Founder/President
Maria Marchiano, Board

560 **Allergy Asthma Information Association**
295 The West Mall   416-621-4571
Toronto, Ontario, M9C4z-4Z4   800-611-7011
                              Fax: 416-621-5034
                         e-mail: admin@aaia.ca
                                 www.aaia.ca

To develop societal awareness of the seriousness of allergic disease, including asthma, and to enable allergic individuals, their families and caregivers, to increase control over allergy symptoms by providing leadership in information, education, advocacy, in partnership with health care professionals, business, industry and government.
Sharon Van Gyzan, Chair
Louis Isabella, Treasurer

561 **American Academy of Allergy, Asthma & Immunology**
555 East Wells Street   414-272-6071
Milwaukee, WI 53202-3823   800-822-2762
                              Fax: 414-272-6070
                         e-mail: info@aaaai.org
                                www.aaaai.org
Strives to serve the public through information on asthma and allergies, as well as referrals to allergists. Also offers pollen and mold statistics from the Committee on Pollen & Molds.
Kay Whalen, Executive Director
Marianne Canter, Director of Communications

562 **American Academy of Environmental Medicine**
6505 E Central Avenue   316-684-5500
Wichita, KS 67206   Fax: 316-684-5709
              e-mail: administrator@aaemonline.org
                                www.aaem.com
Offers names of Clinical Ecologists and Allergy Specialists in the United States.
Amy L Dean, President
Jennifer Armstrong, Secretary

563 **American College of Allergy, Asthma & Immunology**
85 West Algonquin Road   847-427-1200
Arlington Heights, IL 60005   Fax: 847-427-1294
                         e-mail: mail@acaai.org
                                www.acaai.org
This association focuses its attention on research and public awareness of allergies. Distributes informational brochures and pamphlets, offers referrals and counseling services, as well as patient care.
Richard W Webber, President
James L Sublet, Vice President

564 **American Dietetic Association**
120 South Riverside Plaza   312-899-0040
Chicago, IL 60606-6995   800-877-1600
                              Fax: 312-899-1979
                     e-mail: media@eatright.org
                               www.eatright.org
Offers information and support to allergy sufferers. Serves the public through the promotion of optimal nutrition, health, and well-being.
Patricia M Babjak, CEO
Judith Rodriguez, President

565 **Association of Birth Defect Children Birth Defect Research for Children**
976 Lake Baldwin Lane   407-566-8304
Celebration, FL 32814   e-mail: staff@birthdefects.org
                             www.birthdefects.org
Offers informational packets on childhood asthma and prevention.
Betty Mekdeci, Contact

566 **Asthma and Allergy Foundation of America**
8201 Corporate Drive   202-466-7643
Landover, MD 20785   800-727-8462
                              Fax: 202-466-8940
                         e-mail: info@aafa.org
                                 www.aafa.org
Nonprofit patient organization dedicated to improving the quality of life for people with asthma and allergies and their caregivers, through education, advocacy and research.
Lynn Hanessian, Chair
Michael Abu Carrick, Vice Chair

567 **Canadian Society of Allergy and Clinical Immunology**
PO BOX 51045   613-986-5869
Orleans, K1S-5N8   Fax: 613-730-1116
                    e-mail: csaci@royalcollege.ca
                                 www.csaci.ca

Is the advancement of the knowledge and practice of allergy, clinical immunology, and asthma for optimal patient care.
Dr Paul Keith, President
Dr.Sandy Kapur, Vice President

568   Eczema Association for Science and Education
4460 Redwwod Highway   415-499-3474
San Rafael, CA 94903-1953   800-818-7546
                                   e-mail: info@nationaleczema.org
                                        www.nationaleczema.org
Offers resources and information for allergy patients.
Jamie Hubber, Chair
Susan Tofte, Secretary

569   Food Allergy and Anaphylaxis Network
7925 Jones Branch Dr.
McLean, VA 22102-3309
                                              800-929-4040
                                         Fax: 703-691-2713
                                   e-mail: faan@foodallergy.org
                                          www.foodallergy.org
Increases public awareness about food allergies and anaphylaxis advances research and provides education, emotional support and coping strategies to patients; serves as the communication link between the food industry, the government and the airline industry.
John L Lehr, CEO
George Dahlman, Vice President of Advocacy & Government

570   Immune Deficiency Foundation
40 W Chesapeake Avenue   410-321-6647
Towson, MD 21204-4841   800-296-4433
                                         Fax: 410-321-9165
                                   e-mail: idf@primaryimmune.org
                                          www.primaryimmune.org
The national patient organization dedicated to improving the diagnosis treatment and quality of life of persons with primary immunodeficiency diseases through advocacy education and research.
Marcia Boyle, President & Founder
John Seymour PhD LMFT, Vice Chair

571   National Institute of Allergy and Infectious Diseases
NIAID Office of Communications and Public Liason
6610 Rockledge Drive   301-496-5717
Bethesda, MD 20892-6612   866-284-4107
                                         Fax: 301-402-3573
                                         TDD: 800-877-8339
                                   e-mail: clane@niaid.nih.gov
                                            www.niaid.nih.gov
Conducts and supports research on allergies; focused on understanding what happens to the body during the allergic process. Educates patients and health care workers in controlling allergic disease; offers various research centers that conduct and evaluate educational programs focused on methods to control allergic diseases.
Anthony S Fauci, MD, Director

State Agencies & Associations

California

572   Asthma and Allergy Foundation of America: Southern California Chapter
5900 Wilshire Boulevard   323-937-7859
Los Angeles, CA 90036   800-624-0044
                                         Fax: 323-937-7815
                                 e-mail: Breathingmatters@aafa-ca.org
                             http://www.aafa.org/display.cfm?id=10&su
Dedicated to controlling and curing asthma and allergic diseases through education, a network of support groups, the support of research and specialized training, increasing public awareness and providing medication and treatment to the under served. Program highlights include the Breathmobile, asthma camps and air power games for children.
Michael Ingram, Executive Director

District of Columbia

573   Food Safety and Inspection Service
U.S. Dep of Agriculture   202-720-9113
Washington, DC 20250   e-mail: fsis.webmaster@usda.gov
                                             www.fsis.usda.gov
The Food Safety and Inspection Service (FSIS) is the public health agency in the U.S. Department of Agriculture responsible for ensuring that the nation's commercial supply of meat, poultry, and egg products is safe, wholesome, and correctly labeled and packaged.
Steven A. Fisher, Chief Financial Officer
Janet B. Stevens, PMP, Chief Information Officer

574   National Institute for Occupational Safety and Health
395 E Street, SW   202-245-0625
Washington, DC 20201   800-232-4636
                                         Fax: 513-533-8347
                                         TTY: 888-232-6348
                                           www.cdc.gov/niosh/
The National Institute for Occupational Safety and Health (NIOSH) is the U.S. federal agency that conducts research and makes recommendations to prevent worker injury and illness.
John Howard, MD, Director
Frank Hearl, PE, Chief of Staff

575   National Institute of Food and Agriculture
Waterfront Centre
Washington, DC 20024   e-mail: sonny@nifa.usda.gov
                                              nifa.usda.gov
National Institute of Food and Agriculture (NIFA) provides leadership and funding for programs that advance agriculture-related sciences.
r. Sonny Ramaswamy, Director
Meryl Broussard, Associate Director for Programs

Florida

576   Asthma and Allergy Foundation of America: Florida Chapter
200 Orangewood Drive   727-738-1146
Dunedin, FL 34698   Fax: 727-736-4484
                                 e-mail: cherylsmall@aafaflorida.org
                                                www.aafa.org
Works to serve its community through programs, advocacy, education, research and national involvement.
John Little, Executive Director

Georgia

577   Agency for Toxic Substances and Disease Registry
4770 Buford Hwy NE
Atlanta, GA 30341   800-232-4636
                                         TTY: 888-232-6348
                                             www.atsdr.cdc.gov
The Agency for Toxic Substances and Disease Registry (ATSDR), based in Atlanta, Georgia, is a federal public health agency of the U.S. Department of Health and Human Services. ATSDR serves the public by using the best science, taking responsive public health actions, and providing trusted health information to prevent harmful exposures and diseases related to toxic substances.
Patrick Breysse, PhD, CIH, Director
Donna Knutson, PhD, Acting Deputy Director

578   Division of Adolescent and School Health
4770 Buford Hwy, NE
Atlanta, GA 30341   800-232-4636
                                         TTY: 888-232-6348
                                        www.cdc.gov/HealthyYouth
CDC promotes the health and well-being of children and adolescents to enable them to become healthy and productive adults.

Maryland

579   Agency for Healthcare Research and Quality
540 Gaither Road
Rockville, MD 20850   301-427-1364
                                           www.ahrq.gov/index.html
The Agency for Healthcare Research and Quality's (AHRQ) mission is to produce evidence to make health care safer, higher quality, more accessible, equitable, and affordable, and to work within

the U.S. Department of Health and Human Services and with other partners to make sure that the evidence is understood and used.
Richard G. Kronick, PhD, Director, Director
Sharon B. Arnold, PhD, Deputy Director

580   Asthma and Allergy Foundation of America: Maryland/Greater Washington, DC
1498 Reisterstown Rdÿ   410-484-2054
Baltimore, MD 21208   800-727-9333
                                          Fax: 410-484-2043
                                      e-mail: aafamd@rcn.com
                                             www.aafa-md.org
Serves the state of Maryland, District of Columbia and Northern Virginia areas. Dedicated to helping asthma and allergy sufferers successfully manage and control their disease through the education, referrals and research. Major activities include accredited child care provider course, school liaison, asthma camp, patient assistance, college scholarships for high school seniors and professional education courses. Breathmobile, Mobile Asthma Clinic, visiting schools in the city of Baltimore.
Susan Sweitzer, Executive Director

581   Centers for Medicare & Medicaid Services
7500 Security Boulevard   410-786-3000
Baltimore, MD 21244   877-267-2323
                                          TTY: 866-226-1819
                               e-mail: Mandy.Cohen@cms.hhs.gov
                                                www.cms.gov
US federal agency which administers Medicare, Medicaid, and the State Children's Health Insurance Program.
Dr. Mandy Cohen, M.D., MPH, Chief of Staff
Timothy P. Love, Chief Operating Officer

582   National Center for Complementary and Integrative Health
9000 Rockville Pike
Bethesda, MD 20892   888-644-6226
                                          TTY: 866-464-3615
                                e-mail: nccih-info@mail.nih.gov
                                               nccih.nih.gov
The National Center for Complementary and Integrative Health (NCCIH) is the Federal Government's lead agency for scientific research on the diverse medical and health care systems, practices, and products that are not generally considered part of conventional medicine.
Josephine P. Briggs, M.D., Director
David Shurtleff, Ph.D., Deputy Director

583   National Human Genome Research Institute
Building 31, Room 4B09   301-402-0911
Bethesda, MD 20892   Fax: 301-402-2218
                                              www.genome.gov
The National Human Genome Research Institute began as the National Center for Human Genome Research (NCHGR), which was established in 1989 to carry out the role of the National Institutes of Health (NIH) in the International Human Genome Project (HGP).
Eric D. Green, M.D., Ph.D., Director
Lawrence Brody, Ph.D., Director, Division of Genomics & Society

584   National Institute of Biomedical Imaging and Bioengineering
9000 Rockville Pike   301-496-8859
Bethesda, MD 20892   e-mail: info@nibib.nih.gov
                                              www.nibib.nih.gov
The mission of the National Institute of Biomedical Imaging and Bioengineering (NIBIB) is to improve health by leading the development and accelerating the application of biomedical technologies.
Roderic I. Pettigrew, Ph.D., M.D., Director
Marcella Canada, Administrative Officer

585   National Institute of General Medical Sciences
45 Center Drive MSC 6200   301-496-7301
Bethesda, MD 20892   e-mail: info@nigms.nih.gov
                                              www.nigms.nih.gov
The National Institute of General Medical Sciences (NIGMS) supports basic research that increases understanding of biological processes and lays the foundation for advances in disease diagnosis, treatment and prevention.
Jon R. Lorsch, Ph.D., Director
Judith H. Greenberg, Ph.D., Deputy Director

586   U.S. Food and Drug Administration
10903 New Hampshire Ave   301-796-8240
Silver Spring, MD 20993   888-463-6332
                                                www.fda.gov
FDA is responsible for protecting the public health by assuring the safety, efficacy and security of human and veterinary drugs, biological products, medical devices, our nation's food supply, cosmetics, and products that emit radiation.
Stephen Ostroff, M.D., Acting Commissioner
James Tyler, Chief Financial Officer

Massachusetts

587   Asthma and Allergy Foundation of America: New England Chapter
109 Highland Ave.   781-444-7778
Needham, MA 02494   877-227-8462
                                          Fax: 781-444-7718
                                          TTY: 877-227-8462
                                   e-mail: aafane@aafane.org
                                    www.asthmaandallergies.org
Serves Massachusetts, Rhode Island, Connecticut, Maine, New Hampshire and Vermont. Program highlights include speakers and exhibits, telephone information and referrals, tobacco control program, scholarship essay contest for high school juniors, advocacy for safer environments and training programs for school, daycare and health professionals.
Debbie Saryan, Executive Director
Sharon Schumack, Health Education Coordinator

Michigan

588   Asthma and Allergy Foundation of America: Michigan Chapter
2075 Walnut Lake Rd   248-406-4254
West Bloomfield, MI 48323-8768   888-444-0333
                                          Fax: 248-757-2102
                                  e-mail: aafamich@sbcglobal.net
                                             www.aafamich.org
Serves the state of Michigan through public forums, work place educational programs, patient advocacy, Asthma Camp and telephone referrals and information.
Kathleen Felice Slonager, Executive Director
Dr. Rola Bokhari-Panza, President

Missouri

589   Asthma and Allergy Foundation of America: St. Louis Chapter
1500 S Big Bend   314-645-2422
St. Louis, MO 63117   Fax: 314-692-2022
                                     e-mail: aafa@aafastl.org
                                             www.aafastl.org
This chapter has provided children who suffer from asthma and allergies with life saving medications, equipment and educational and emotional support. The founders of the St. Louis chapter identified the apparent need in their community to help children effectively manage their asthma through the provision of medical resources, equipment and education.
Joy Kreiger, Executive Director

North Carolina

590   National Institute of Environmental Health Sciences
111 T.W. Alexander Drive   919-541-4580
Research Triangle Park, NC 27709   e-mail: carroll1@niehs.nih.gov
                                             www.niehs.nih.gov
The mission of the NIEHS is to discover how the environment affects people in order to promote healthier lives.
Linda S. Birnbaum, Ph.D., Director
Richard Woychik, Ph.D., Deputy Director

Oregon

591   Asthma and Allergy Foundation of America: Oregon Chapter
14530 SW 144th Avenue   503-524-2232
Tigard, OR 97224-1445   Fax: 208-474-6839
                                   e-mail: hensches@teleport.com
Serving the state of Oregon.
Sandra L Henschel, Executive Director

592   Asthma and Allergy Foundation of America: Southern Pennsylvania Chapter
470 Sentry Parkway East   610-397-1540
Blue Bell, NJ 19422   Fax: 856-224-5893
e-mail: aafasepa@verizon.net
http://www.aafa.org/

In the process of establishing a vital, new program that will aid children with chronic asthma. Many parents, some who are without medical insurance, are unaware of the availability of a medical support system that can help their children. The Children at Risk program will enable parents to have their children evaluated and also receive a free one month supply of medication. Parents will also receive information regarding available options for follow up care and prescription coverage.
Marijo Washburn, Executive Director

Texas

593   Asthma and Allergy Foundation of America: North Texas Chapter
3904 Justin Drive   817-297-3132
Ft. Worth, TX 76244   888-932-2232
Fax: 817-297-6564
e-mail: info@aafatexas.org
www.aafatexas.org

Offers many educational programs and services that touch patients, caregivers, physicians and allied health professionals, including: child care provider education programs, school nurse and respiratory therapist education programs, work site allergy education programs, spacer and peak flow meter distribution to those in need, a toll free hotline, prescription assistance information, free educational materials in English and Spanish, an electronic newsletter, professional education, etc.
Laura Steves, Executive Director

Washington

594   Asthma and Allergy Foundation of America: Washington State Chapter
108 S Jackson Street   206-368-2866
Seattle, WA 98104   800-778-2232
Fax: 206-368-2941
e-mail: aafawa@aafawa.org
www.aafawa.org

Program highlights include trainings for health care professionals on asthma and allergy management, working collaboratively with other local and regional agencies to improve the quality of life for those affected by asthma and allergies, organizing health fairs and other public events and providing educational materials and products.
Penny Nelson, Executive Director

Research Centers

595   Columbus Children's Research Institute
700 Children's Drive   614-722-2000
Columbus, OH 43205   Fax: 614- 35- 079
e-mail: John.Barnard@NationwideChildrens.org
www.nationwidechildrens.org

Research institute dedicated to enhancing the health of children by engaging in the high quality cutting-edge research according to the highest scientific and ethical standards.
John A Barnard, Research Institute President
Steve Allen MD, CEO

596   Creighton University Allergic Disease Center
601 N 30th Street   402-280-4403
Omaha, NE 68131-0001   Fax: 402-280-4803
e-mail: casalej@creighton.edu
medicine.creighton.edu/allergy/homepage.

Robert G Townley, Investigator
Thomas B Casale, Chief

597   Institute for Rehabilitation and Research
21720 Kingsland Blvd.
Katy, TX 77450   800-447-3422
Fax: 713-874-1798
e-mail: tirr.referrals@memorialhermann.org
www.tirr.memorialhermann.org

Carl Josehart, Chief Executive Officer
Gerard E. Francisco, Chief Medical Officer

598   Mayo Clinic and Foundation: Division of Allergic Diseases
Department of Immunology
200 First Street SW   507-284-2511
Rochester, MN 55905   Fax: 507-284-0161
TTY: 507-284-9786
e-mail: lee.theresa@mayo.edu
www.mayoclinic.org

Provides a focus for research into the causes prevention and management of allergic diseases.
John H Noseworthy MD, President
William C Rupp MD, Vice President, CEO

599   National Jewish Center for Immunology and Respiratory Medicine
Goodman Building Room 611   303-398-1287
Denver, CO 80206   800-423-8891
Fax: 303-398-1806
www.nationaljewish.org

Basic and clinical research into the causes and treatments of asthmatic disorders.
Tom Gart, Chairman
Michael Salem, President & CEO

600   Research Institute of Palo Alto Medical Foundation
795 El Camino Real
Palo Alto, CA 94301-2302   650-326-8120
www.pamf.org/research

Clinical and general medical sciences research including allergy and immunology disorders.
Jane Risser, Director
Andrea Norcia, Assistant Director

601   Scripps Research Institute
10550 N Torrey Pines Road
La Jolla, CA 92037   858-784-1000
www.scripps.edu

William Burfitt, President
Alex Bruner, Executive Vice President and Chief Opera

602   Texas Children's Allergy and Immunology Clinic
Clinical Care Center
6701 Fannin Street   832-824-1000
Houston, TX 77030   800-364-5437
Fax: 832-825-3072
e-mail: pediai@texaschildrenshospital.org
www.texaschildrenshospital.org

Mark A Wallace, President & CEO
Mark W Kline MD, Physician In Chief

603   University of Florida: General Clinical Research Center
University of Florida
1600 SW Archer Road   352-273-5500
Gainesville, FL 32610-0322   888-635-0763
Fax: 352-273-5541
e-mail: thomprd@ufl.edu
www.med.ufl.edu

Studies on allergies and immunology.
Robert Thompson, Program Director

604   University of Kansas Allergy and Immunology Clinic
University of Kansas Medical Center
3901 Rainbow Boulevard   913-588-5000
Kansas City, KS 66160   TTY: 913-588-7963
TDD: 913-588-7963
e-mail: dstechsc@kumc.edu
www.kumc.edu

This service provides complete evaluation of patients with allergic diseases such as rhinitis and asthma immunological deficiencies food and drug intolerances and autoimmune dysfunctions.
Barbara F Atkinson MD, Executive Vice Chancellor
Shelley Gebar, RN, MHA, Chief of Staff

605   University of Michigan Montgomery: John M. Sheldon Allergy Society
Alllergy & Clinical Immunology
24 Frank Lloyd Wright Drive   734-232-2154
Ann Arbor, MI 48106-0380   Fax: 734-647-6263
                                    e-mail: echoreed@med.umich.edu
                                    www.med.umich.edu/sheldonsociety
Travis A Miller, President

606   University of Texas Southwestern Medical Center at Dallas
University of Texas Southwestern Medical Center
5323 Harry Hines Boulevard   214-648-3111
Dallas, TX 75390   Fax: 214-648-9119
                                    e-mail: news@utsouthwestern.edu
                                    www.utsouthwestern.edu
Immunodermatology department researching allergies and immune disorders.
Daniel K Podolsky MD, President

607   Warren Grant Magnuson Clinical Center
National Institute of Health
9000 Rockville Pike   301-496-2563
Bethesda, MD 20892   800-411-1222
                                    Fax: 301-402-2984
                                    TTY: 866-411-1010
                                    e-mail: prpl@mail.cc.nih.gov
                                    www.cc.nih.gov
Established in 1953 as the research hospital of the National Institutes of Health. Designed so that patient care facilities are close to research laboratories so new findings of basic and clinical scientists can be quickly applied to the treatment of patients. Upon referral by physicians, patients are admitted to NIH clinical studies.
Michael J Klag MD, Chair
David K Henderson MD, Clinical Director

Support Groups & Hotlines

608   ASTHMA Hotline
American Academy of Allergy, Asthma and Immunology
2275 East Bayshore Road   650-328-3123
Palo Alto, CA 53202   800-822-2762
                                    Fax: 650-321-4457
                                    www.aaai.org
Referral line offering information on allergy and asthma treatments, referrals to an allergy/immunology specialist, lay organization or support groups across the country.

609   National Health Information Center
PO Box 1133   310-565-4167
Washington, DC 20013-1133   800-336-4797
                                    Fax: 301-984-4256
                                    e-mail: info@nhic.org
                                    www.health.gov/nhic
A health information referral service sponsored by the Office of Disease Prevention and Health Promotion. NHIC puts health professionals and consumers who have health questions in touch with those organizations that are best able to provide answers.

Books

610   Allergies A to Z
Facts on File
132 W 31st Street   212-967-8800
New York, NY 10001   800-322-8755
                                    Fax: 800-678-3633
                                    e-mail: custserv@factsonfile.com
                                    www.infobasepublishing.com
This vital resource for the one in five Americans who suffer from alleries provides reliable, up-to-date information on every aspect of this condition.
Paperback

611   Allergy Alerts from Living with Allergies
American Allergy Association
PO Box 7273   650-322-1663
Menlo Park, CA 94026-7273
These alerts cover a wide range of areas from dyes in medications to medication interactions, food additives like sulfites, spelt, situations that could trigger asthma, problems with collagen and even fabric softeners.

612   Allergy Plants that Cause Sneezing and Wheezing
Asthma and Allergy Foundation of America
8201 Corporate Drive   202-466-7643
Landover, MD 20785-2330   800-727-8462
                                    Fax: 202-466-8940
                                    e-mail: info@aafa.org
                                    www.aafa.org
Destined to be displayed on coffee tables, the spectacular photographs in this book actually show allergy sufferers what causes their sneezing and wheezing.
64 pages Paperback

613   Complete Book of Children's Allergies
Allergy Central Products
1620-D Satellite Blvd   203-438-9580
Duluth, GA 30097-4053   800-422-3878
                                    Fax: 203-431-8963
                                    www.allergycontrol.com
Major childhood allergies, recommendations for treatment.
Softcover

614   Cooking for the Allergic Child
Allergy Central Products
1620-D Satellite Blvd   203-438-9580
Duluth, GA 30097-4053   800-442-3878
                                    Fax: 203-431-8963
                                    www.allergycontrol.com
More than 300 recipes with nutrients analysis.
Softcover

615   Diets to Help Gluten and Wheat Allergy
HarperCollins Canada Limited/Order Department
1995 Markham Road
Scarborough, M1B 5M8,   800-387-0117
                                    Fax: 800-668-5788
This book offers sound and practical advice on gluten allergy wheat sensitivity and Celiac disease.
96 pages
ISBN: 0-722529-10-4

616   Food Allergy: A Primer for People
Asthma and Allergy Foundation of America
8201 Corporate Drive   202-466-7643
Landover, MD 20785-2330   800-727-8462
                                    Fax: 202-466-8940
                                    e-mail: info@aafa.org
                                    www.aafa.org
Food allergies demystified.
66 pages Hardcover

617   Human Exposure Assessment for Airborne Pollutants: Advances & Opportunity
National Academies Press
500 5th Street NW   202-334-3313
Washington, DC 20001   888-624-8373
                                    Fax: 202-334-2451
                                    e-mail: customer_service@nap.edu
                                    www.nap.edu
Explores the need for strategies to address indoor and outdoor exposures and examines the methods and tools available for finding out where and when significant exposures occur.
344 pages
ISBN: 0-309042-84-0
Sandy Adams, Publishing Operations Director
Dottie Lewis, Publishing Services Director

618   Indoor Allergens: Assessing & Controlling Adverse Health Effects
National Academies Press
500 5th Street NW   202-334-3313
Washington, DC 20055   888-624-8373
                                    Fax: 202-334-2793
                                    e-mail: customer_service@nap.edu
                                    www.nap.edu
This comprehensive and practical volume will be important to allergists and other health care providers; public health professionals; specialists in building design, construction, and maintenance;

faculty and students in public health; and interested allergy patients.
350 pages
ISBN: 0-309048-31-6
Andrew M. Pope, Author
Roy Patterson, Author

619 Infant Formulas for Allergic Infants and Dietetic Concerns for Toddlers
American Allergy Association
PO Box 7273   650-322-1663
Menlo Park, CA 94026-7273
Offers information on reliable food labels, evaluations of infant formulas, FDA labeling requirements under the new law and more.

620 New Food Labels
American Allergy Association
PO Box 7273   650-322-1663
Menlo Park, CA 94026-7273
Offers clear-cut and precise information on new label word definitions.

621 Pollen Times: By State, By Month
American Allergy Association
PO Box 7273   650-322-1663
Menlo Park, CA 94026-7273
A comprehensive guide offering information on how to plan vacations while avoiding pollen problems.

622 Traveling with Allergies: Prepare and Avoid Problems
American Allergy Association
PO Box 7273   650-322-1663
Menlo Park, CA 94026-7273
Prepare for travel, recognize and minimize the risk, sidestep smoke, food allergies, pollen, mold, dander, weather and emergencies.

Children's Books

623 All About Allergies
Dutton Children's Books
375 Hudson Street   212-366-2000
New York, NY 10014-3658   Fax: 212-366-2262
                                    www.pengiunputnam.com
1993 64 pages
ISBN: 0-525674-10-1

624 Allergies
Franklin Watts Grolier
90 Old Sherman Turnpike   203-797-3500
Danbury, CT 06816-0001   800-621-1115
                                    Fax: 203-797-3197
                                    www.grolier.com
Covers the major types of allergies, including those of the respiratory and gastrointestinal tracts.
112 pages Grades 7-12
ISBN: 0-531125-16-5

625 Living with Allergies
Franklin Watts Grolier
90 Old Sherman Turnpike   203-797-3500
Danbury, CT 06816-0001   800-621-1115
                                    Fax: 203-797-3197
                                    www.grolier.com
Shows how people with allergies are able to overcome their handicap to lead full and productive lives.
32 pages Grades 5-7
ISBN: 0-531108-57-0

Magazines

626 Allergy & Asthma Today
Allergy and Asthma Network Mothers of Asthmatics
8229 Boone Boulevard
Vienna, VA 22182
                                    800-878-4403
                                    Fax: 703-288-5271
                                    e-mail: info@aanma.org
                                    aanma.site-ym.com

The practical, family-friendly magazine for people living with asthma, allergies and other respiratory conditions. Award-winning and medically reviewed, packed with news and real-life inspiration and success stories, the ultimate resource for patients, families and healthcare providers.
40 pages Quarterly
Laurie Ross, Managing Editor

Newsletters

627 Advice From Your Allergist
American College of Allergy & Immunology
85 W Algonguin Road
Alrlington Heights, IL 60005   847-359-2800
                                    www.allergy.mcg.edu
Offers information on the effects, triggers and causes of allergies including house dust, pets, hay fever, hives and exercise.

628 Food Allergy News
Food Allergy and Anaphylaxis Network
7925 Jones Branch Dr.   703-691-3179
McLean, VA 22102-2208   800-929-4040
                                    Fax: 703-691-2713
                                    e-mail: faan@foodallergy.org
                                    www.foodallergy.org
Contains allergy free recipes, practical tips such as birthday party, trick-or-treating and travel tips, a dietitian's column, medical information and product information.
12 pages BiMonthly
James R. Baker, Jr., MD, CEO
Donna McKelvey, Senior VP and Chief Development Officer

629 MA Report
Allergy and Asthma Network/Mothers of Asthmatics
8229 Boone Boulevard   703-641-9595
Vienna, VA 22182   800-878-4403
                                    Fax: 703-288-5271
                                    e-mail: editor@aanma.org
                                    www.allergyasthmanetwork.org
Provides up-to-date medical news, emotional support and practical strategies for overcoming asthma and allergies.
8 pages 8x Year
Mary McGowan, Executive Director
Nancy Sander, Editor-in-Chief

Pamphlets

630 Allergic Diseases
National Institute of Allergy & Infectious Disease
31 Center Drive   301-496-3204
Bethesda, MD 20892-2520   Fax: 301-480-4137
                                    e-mail: domingug@mail.nih.gov
                                    www.niaid.nih.gov
Offers information on allergies, who gets them, diagnosis and treatments for various types of allergic diseases.

631 Allergies and You
American Lung Association
1740 Broadway   212-315-8700
New York, NY 10019-4315
Answers basic questions about allergy, particularly as it relates to asthma.

632 Eating Without Packet
American Allergy Association
PO Box 7273   650-322-1663
Menlo Park, CA 94026-7273
Twelve information sheets describing the most common food allergens, specific problems with common foods and supplements, and the facts on milk ingredient labeling, milk allergies, and milk sensitivity. Included in the packet is a 16-page handbook, Understanding Calcium and Osteoporosis.

633 FAAN Flashbacks
Food Allergy and Anaphylaxis Network

7925 Jones Branch Dr.
McLean, VA 22102-2208

703-691-3179
800-929-4040
Fax: 703-691-2713
e-mail: faan@foodallergy.org
www.foodallergy.org

Series of reprints on specific topics of Food Allergy News. Specific pamphlets offer information on wheat, milk, soy, egg, fish, peanuts, managing food allergy in schools and anaphylaxis.
James R. Baker, Jr., MD, CEO
Donna McKelvey, Senior VP and Chief Development Officer

634 Food Allergy and Atopic Dermatitis
Food Allergy and Anaphylaxis Network
7925 Jones Branch Dr.
McLean, VA 22102-2208

703-691-3179
800-929-4040
Fax: 703-691-2713
e-mail: faan@foodallergy.org
www.foodallergy.org

The purpose of this booklet is to provide tips and other sources of information to help parents raise a child who is afflicted with atopic dermatitis.
12 pages
James R. Baker, Jr., MD, CEO
Donna McKelvey, Senior VP and Chief Development Officer

635 Guide to Gluten-Free Diets
American Allergy Association
PO Box 7273
Menlo Park, CA 94026-7273

650-322-1663

Offers information on safe substitutes for baking and cooking. Differentiates celiac disease from wheat allergy. Sources of gluten in diet with warnings on when to check with the manufacturer.

636 Helpful Hints for the Allergic Patient
American Academy of Allergy, Asthma and Immunology
555 East Wells Street
Milwaukee, WI 53202-3889

414-272-6071
800-822-2762
Fax: 414-272-6070
www.aaaai.org

An informational brochure good for someone who has just been diagnosed with allergies.
8 pages

637 Just One Little Bite Can Hurt! Important Facts About Anaphylaxis
Food Allergy and Anaphylaxis Network
7925 Jones Branch Dr.
McLean, VA 22102-2208

703-691-3179
800-929-4040
Fax: 703-691-2713
e-mail: faan@foodallergy.org
www.foodallergy.org

Offers information on what anaphylaxis is, what the patient should do if they have a reaction and important medical safety tips regarding the illness.
8 pages Booklet
James R. Baker, Jr., MD, CEO
Donna McKelvey, Senior VP and Chief Development Officer

638 Nutrition Guide to Food Allergies
Food Allergy and Anaphylaxis Network
7925 Jones Branch Dr.
McLean, VA 22102-2208

703-691-3179
800-929-4040
Fax: 703-691-2713
e-mail: faan@foodallergy.org
www.foodallergy.org

Offers answers to the most commonly asked questions about food allergies, common allergy causing foods and resources for the patient.
24 pages
James R. Baker, Jr., MD, CEO
Donna McKelvey, Senior VP and Chief Development Officer

639 Something in the Air: Airborne Allergens
National Institute of Allergy & Infectious Disease
9000 Rockville Pike
Bethesda, MD 20892-0001

301-496-5717
www.niaid.nih.gov

Offers information on the symptoms to airborne substances, pollen, mold, dust, animal, chemical allergies and treatments for them.

Audio & Video

640 Alexander, the Elephant Who Couldn't Eat Peanuts
Food Allergy and Anaphylaxis Network
7925 Jones Branch Dr.
McLean, VA 22102-3309

800-929-4040
Fax: 703-691-2713
www.foodallergy.org

Helps children cope with their own allergies and teach other children about tolerance. Both videos combine colorful animation with interviews of real-life children with food allergies who talk about their experiences.
James R. Baker, Jr., MD, CEO
Donna McKelvey, Senior VP and Chief Development Officer

641 Allergic Rhinitis
American Academy of Allergy, Asthma and Immunology
555 East Wells Street
Milwaukee, WI 53202-3889

414-272-6071
800-822-2762
Fax: 414-272-6070
www.aaaai.org

Allergic rhinitis, often called hay fever, affects the quality of life of millions of Americans. This video covers the causes and symptoms of seasonal and chronic allergic rhinitis, as well as environmental controls and treatments.
10-13 minutes

642 Allergic Rhinitis: Nothing to Sneeze At!
Asthma and Allergy Foundation of America
8201 Corporate Drive
Landover, MD 20785-2330

202-466-7643
800-727-8462
Fax: 202-466-8940
e-mail: info@aafa.org
www.aafa.org

The basics of allergic rhinitis, with a touch of humor. Common allergens, environmental control, skin testing and immunotherapy medications.
Videotape

643 Allergic Skin Reactions
American Academy of Allergy, Asthma and Immunology
555 East Wells Street
Milwaukee, WI 53202-3889

414-272-6071
800-822-2762
Fax: 414-272-6070
www.aaaai.org

In some people, allergy symptoms include itching redness, rashes, or hives. This video describes the symptoms, triggers, and treatment for common skin reactions such as dermatitis, hives and angioedema.
10-13 minutes

644 An Overview of Allergy
American College of Allergy & Immunology
800 E NW Highway
Palatine, IL 60067-6580

847-359-2800

Strengthen relationships with patients by providing them with the essential information they need.

645 Sinusitis and Sinus Surgery
Milner-Fenwick
119 Lakefront Drive
Hunt Valley, MD 21030-3100

410-252-1700
800-432-8433
Fax: 410-252-6316
e-mail: mail@milner-fenwick.com
www.milner-fenwick.com

Discusses sinusitis symptoms, causes, evaluation and treatments. Animation depicts how sinuses function and how irritants, allergies, colds or structural abnormalities cause sinus blockages. Also explains the role of medical therapy and irrigation in managing acute sinusitis.
14 minutes
Dolores McKee, Advertising Director

Web Sites

646 American College of Allergy, Asthma & Immunology

www.acaai.org

51

The American College of Allergy, Asthma and Immunology, established in 1942, is a professional association of more than 6,000 Allergists/Immunologists and allied health professionals. Promotes excellence in the practice of the subspecialty of allergy and immunology.

647   American Lung Association

www.lung.org

The leading organization working to save lives by improving lung health and preventing lung disease through Education, Advocacy and Research.

648   Asthma and Allergy Foundation of America

www.aafa.org

The leading patient organization for people with asthma and allergies, and the oldest asthma and allergy patient group in the world. Dedicated to improving the quality of life for people with asthma and allergic disease through education, advocacy and research.

649   Birth Defect Research for Children

www.birthdefects.org

Provides parents and expectant parents with information about birth defects and support services for their children

650   Food Allergy and Anaphylaxis Network

www.foodallergy.org

To raise public awareness, to provide advocacy and education, and to advance research on behalf of all those affected by food allergies and anaphylaxis.

651   Healing Well

www.healingwell.com

A social network and support community for patients, caregivers, and families coping with the daily struggles of diseases, disorders and chronic illness.

652   Health Finder

www.healthfinder.gov

Government website where individuals can find information and tools to hel you and those you care about stay healthy.

653   Healthlink USA

www.healthlinkusa.com

Health information concerning treatment, cures, prevention, diagnosis, risk factors, research, support groups, email lists, personal stories and much more. Updated regularly.

654   Helios Health

www.helioshealth.com

Online resource for your health information. Detailed information about specific health topics, access to expert advice from our Medical Advisory Board, and up-to-date health news.

655   Immune Deficiency Foundation

www.primaryimmune.org

National patient organization dedicated to improving the diagnosis, treatment and quality of life of persons with primary immunodeficiency diseases through advocacy, education and research.

656   MedicineNet

www.medicinenet.com

An online resource for consumers providing easy-to-read, authoritative medical and health information.

657   Medscape

www.medscape.com

Medscape offers specialists, primary care physicians, and other health professionals the Web's most robust and integrated medical information and educational tools.

658   WebMD

www.webmd.com

Provides credible information, supportive communities, and in-depth reference material about health subjects. A source for original and timely health information as well as material from well known content providers.

Description

659   Alzheimer's Disease

Alzheimer's disease is a degenerative neurologic disease that attacks the brain and impairs memory, thinking faculties and behavior. As the most common form of dementing illness, it afflicts 4 million adults and is twice as common in women as in men. It primarily affects older people.

In spite of diligent research, the cause of Alzheimer's disease is unknown. The disease runs in families in about 15 to 20 percent of cases, although the remainder may have some genetic component. There are multiple symptoms of Alzheimer's disease, the most pronounced being gradual memory loss. Other symptoms include the inability to perform routine tasks, loss of language skills, disorientation and personality changes. The diagnosis is largely based on an interview with the patient and family members and an examination of the patient, although brain imaging tests and blood tests may add helpful information.

The brain's cells communicate with each other through various chemicals called neurotransmitters. In Alzheimer's disease, levels of the neurotransmitter acetylcholine are decreased. Recently-released drugs which enhance the transmission of acetylcholine can cause at least limited improvement in memory during the early stages of Alzheimer's disease. A new drug, memantine, has been developed to slow the progression of advanced disease.

An extract of Ginkgo biloba may also slow memory loss and other symptoms. Some research suggests that certain activities that involve using the brain, such as reading and doing crossword puzzles, seem to reduce the risk. Because Alzheimer's disease severely affects both the patient and the family, proper planning, as well as medical and social programs tailored to the individual and to family members are essential. A well-structured and safe living environment is the best way to preserve the welfare and dignity of the person with Alzheimer's disease. See also *Aging*.

National Agencies & Associations

660   Alzheimer Society of Canada
20 Eglinton Avenue W   416-488-8772
Toronto, Ontario, M4R-1K8   800-618-8816
                                Fax: 416-322-6656
                          e-mail: info@alzheimer.ca
                                www.alzheimer.ca

Identified, develops and facilitates national priorities that enable its members to effectively alleviate the personal and social consequences of Alzheimer's disease and related disorders, promotes research and leads the search for a cure.
Richard Nakoneczny, President

661   Alzheimer's Disease Education and Referral Center
PO Box 8250   301-495-3311
Silver Spring, MD 20907-8250   800-222-2225
                                Fax: 301-495-3334
                          e-mail: niaic@nia.nih.gov
                          www.nia.nih.gov/alzheimers

A service of the National Institute on Aging the center distributes information on Alzheimer's disease on current research activities and on services available to patients and family members. Offers a free list of publications available upon request.

662   Alzheimer's Disease and Related Disorders Association
International Conference on Alzheimer's Disease
Montrose Avenue and Simonds Drive   847-324-0356
Chicago, IL 60613-7633   800-272-3900
                                Fax: 866-699-1246
                                TTY: 312-335-5886
                          e-mail: chicagowalk@alz.org
                                www.alz.org

Dedicated to research for the prevention cure and treatment of Alzheimer's disease and related disorders and to providing support and assistance to the afflicted patients and their families.
Harry Johns, President and CEO
Rachel Cleaveland, Local Contact

663   Benjamin B Greenfield National Alzheimer's Center
Montrose Avenue and Simonds Drive   847-324-0356
Chicago, IL 60613-7633   800-272-3900
                                Fax: 866-699-1238
                                TTY: 312-335-5886
                                TDD: 312-335-8700
                          e-mail: chicagowalk@alz.org
                                www.alz.org

Located at the national Alzheimer's Association in Chicago this library offers a sizable collection of videos on a variety of subjects that may interest the Alzheimer's patient family members and caregivers.
Edward Berube, Chair
Rachel Cleaveland, Local Contact

664   Interior Alzheimer Society
#217, 1889 Springfield Road   250-762-3312
Kelowna, BC, V1Y-5V5   Fax: 250-762-3312
                          e-mail: ias@silk.net
                          www.alzheimer-society.ca

A registered, independent, charitable non-profit society that was founded in 1981. Mission is to support, educate, and advocate for all those affected by Alzheimer disease in the Central Okanagan area of British Columbia: the patients, caregivers, patients' families and the community.

665   John Douglas French Alzheimer's Foundation
11620 Wilshire Boulevard   323-930-6228
Los Angeles, CA 90025-1781   800-477-2243
                                Fax: 310-479-0516
                          e-mail: bwelch@alz.org
                                www.jdfaf.org

Provides seed money for promising research including the cause cure and prevention of Alzheimer's disease. Also gives funding to scientists who might not otherwise be funded.
Michael M Minchin Jr, President
Brian Welch, Local Contact

State Agencies & Associations

Alabama

666   Alzheimer's Association: North Alabama Chapter
4747 Bob Wallace Avenue SW   256-880-1575
Huntsville, AL 35805-4872   800-272-3900
                                Fax: 256-880-8596
                          e-mail: cwhite2@alz.org
                                www.alz.org

Al Wiggins, Chair
Courtney White, Local Contact

667   Alzheimer's Association: Southeast Alabama Chapter
PO Box 609   334-677-6799
Dothan, AL 36302   800-272-3900
                                Fax: 334-671-3715
                                www.alz.org

Kay Jones, Executive Director

668 Alzheimer's Association: Southwest Alabama Chapter
PO Box 9272
Mobile, AL 36691
334-660-5661
800-272-3900
Fax: 334-660-5667
www.alz.org

Bunnie Sutton, Executive Director

Alaska

669 Alzheimer's Disease Resource Agency of Alaska
1750 Abbott Road
Anchorage, AK 99507
907-561-3313
800-272-3900
Fax: 907-561-3315
e-mail: dnobre@alzalaska.org
www.alz.org

Jackie Brunton, President
Debbie Newsham, Vice President

Arizona

670 Alzheimer's Association: Desert Southwest Chapter
1028 E McDowell Road
Phoenix, AZ 85006-2622
602-528-0545
800-272-3900
Fax: 602-528-0546
e-mail: deborah.schaus@alz.org
www.alz.org

Serving the state of Arizona and Southern Nevada offices in Phoenix, Tucson, Sun City, Prescott and Las Vegas.
Deborah Schaus, Executive Director
Dawn Boeck, Development Assistant

671 Alzheimer's Association: Northern Arizona
225 Grove Avenue
Prescott, AZ 86301-2911
928-771-9257
800-272-3900
Fax: 520-771-9297
e-mail: pwinkels@alz.org
www.alz.org

Don Connell, Regional Director
Patty Winkels, Local Contact

672 Alzheimer's Association: Northern Nevada
225 Grove Avenue
Prescott, AZ 86301
928-771-9257
800-272-3900
Fax: 520-771-9297
e-mail: pwinkels@alz.org
www.alz.org

Meg Fenzi, Regional Director
Patty Winkels, Local Contact

673 Alzheimer's Association: Southern Arizona
5132 East Pima Street
Tucson, AZ 85712
520-322-6601
800-272-3900
Fax: 520-322-6739
e-mail: kraach@alz.org
www.alz.org

Tormay Newman, Director
Kelly Raach, Local Contact

674 Alzheimer's Association: Southern Arizona Region
3003 S Country Club Road
Tucson, AZ 85713
520-322-6601
800-272-3900
Fax: 520-322-6739
e-mail: kraach@alz.org
www.alz.org

Heriberto Contreras, Regional Director
Kelly Raach, Local Contact

Arkansas

675 Alzheimer's Arkansas Programs and Services
400 President Clinton Ave
Little Rock, AR 72205
501-265-0027
800-272-3900
Fax: 501-227-6303
e-mail: sdavis@alz.org
www.alz.org

Phyllis Watkins, Executive Director
Susie Davis, Local Contact

676 Alzheimer's Association: Western Arkansas Chapter
121 Riverfront Drive
Fort Smith, AR 72901-3454
479-426-5541
800-272-3900
Fax: 479-782-3185
e-mail: sdavis@alz.org
www.alz.org

Rebecca Freeman, Executive Director
Susie Davis, Local Contact

California

677 Alzheimer's Association San Diego/Imperial Chapter
6632 Convoy Court
San Diego, CA 92111
858-966-3319
800-272-3900
Fax: 858-492-4406
e-mail: walksandiego@alz.org
www.alz.org

The leading voluntary health organization in Alzheimer care, support and research. The mission is to eliminate Alzheimer's disease through the advancement of research; to provide and enhance care and support for all affected; to advocate for policy change; and to reduce the risk of dementia through the promotion of brain health.
Lisa Bruner, Executive Director
Shelita Weinfield, Local Contact

678 Alzheimer's Association: California Central Chapter: Ventura County Office
80 North Wood Road
Camarillo, CA 93010
80 - 4 - 60
800-272-3900
Fax: 805-485-4767
e-mail: nfeatherston@centralcoastalz.org
www.alz.org

The local chapter of the National Alzheimer's Association. The chapter stands by people with Alzheimer's disease, their families and professional caregivers through the following programs and services: a telephone help line, support groups, respite grants.
Norma Featherston, Area Director
Carol Swinney, Office Manager

679 Alzheimer's Association: Greater Sacramento
11th St. & N St.
Sacramento, CA 95814
916-930-9080
800-272-3900
Fax: 916-930-9085
e-mail: estone@alz.org
www.alz.org

Mary Gillon MPA, Regional Director
Erin Stone, Local Contact

680 Alzheimer's Association: Greater North Valley Chapter
1000 Woodland Ave
Chico, CA 95928-3148
530-895-9661
800-272-3900
Fax: 530-872-7470
e-mail: swatroba@alz.org
www.alz.org

Herb Williams, President
Suzanne Watroba, Local Contact

681 Alzheimer's Association: Los Angeles Chapter
133 N Sunol Drive
Los Angeles, CA 90063-5017
323-930-6228
800-272-3900
Fax: 323-938-1036
e-mail: bwelch@alz.org
www.alz.org

Earl Greinetz, President
Brian Welch, Local Contact

682 Alzheimer's Association: Monterey County Chapter
5 Custom House Plaza
Monterey, CA 93940-5337
831-647-9890
800-272-3900
Fax: 831-655-9241
e-mail: janderson@alz.org
www.alz.org

Herb Williams, President
Joy Anderson, Local Contact

683 Alzheimer's Association: North Bay Chapter
4340 Redwood Highway   415-472-4340
San Rafael, CA 94903   800-272-3900
                                Fax: 415-472-4350
                          e-mail: info@alznorcal.org
                                         www.alz.org
Provides a continuum of services for Alzheimer's families, education and referral in Marin, Sonoma and Napa counties. To provide leadership and to eliminate Alzheimer's disease through the advancement of research while enhancing care and support services.
Herb Williams, President
Eduardo Salaz, Vice President

684 Alzheimer's Association: Orange County Chapter
17771 Cowan   949-955-9000
Irvine, CA 92614   800-272-3900
                                Fax: 949-757-3700
                          e-mail: helpoc@alz.org
                                         www.alz.org
Dedicated to providing services, education and advocacy for individuals, families and the community affected by Alzheimer's disease and related memory disorders. Services include: 24/7 help line, support groups, family orientation program and care managers.
Norma Castellano, Program Specialist
Bobbie Babbage, Family Services Coordinator

685 Alzheimer's Association: Riverside/San Bernardino Counties Chapter
5900 Wilshire Boulevard   323-930-6228
Los Angeles, CA 90036   800-272-3900
                                Fax: 323-938-1036
                          e-mail: bwelch@alz.org
                                         www.alz.org
Help line, support groups, information and education for caregivers and community.
400 Members
Earl Greinetz, President
Brian Welch, Local Contact

686 Alzheimer's Association: San Francisco Bay Area Chapter
1060 La Avenida   650-962-8111
Mountain View, CA 94043   800-272-3900
                                Fax: 650-962-9644
                          e-mail: info@alznorcal.org
                                         www.alz.org

Herb Williams, President
Eduardo Salaz, Vice President

687 Alzheimer's Association: Santa Barbara Central Coast Chapter
3400 Calle Real   805-892-4259
Santa Barbara, CA 93105-8820   800-272-3900
                                Fax: 805-892-4250
                          e-mail: gbolton@alz.org
                                         www.alz.org
The Alzheimer's Association California Central Coast Chapter serves families caring for people with Alzheimer's disease and related dementia throughout San Luis Obispo, Santa Barbara and Ventura Counties, offering a variety of educational and supportive programs.
Rhonda Spiegel, Executive Director
Genny Bolton, Local Contact

688 Alzheimer's Association: Santa Cruz County Chapter
1777-A Capitola Road   831-464-9982
Santa Cruz, CA 95062   800-272-3900
                                Fax: 831-464-8930
                          e-mail: info@alznorcal.org
                                         www.alz.org

Herb Williams, President
Eduardo Salaz, Vice President

Colorado

689 Alzheimer's Association: Greater Grand Junction Area Chapter
2232 N 7th Street   970-256-1274
Grand Junction, CO 81501   800-272-3900
                                Fax: 970-256-0569
                   e-mail: walktoendalzWS@alzco.org
                                         www.alz.org

Linda Mitchell, President/CEO
Lisa Miller, Local Contact

690 Alzheimer's Association: Rocky Mountain Chapter
455 Sherman Street   303-813-1669
Denver, CO 80203   800-272-3900
                                Fax: 303-813-1670
                          e-mail: jlorentz@alz.org
                                         www.alz.org

Linda Mitchell, President/CEO
Jill Lorentz, Local Contact

691 American Homes for the Aging: Western
5010 Aspen Drive   303-795-5465
Littleton, CO 80123   Fax: 303-794-0487
Part of the national association representing retirement communities, nursing homes and community services for the elderly.

Connecticut

692 Alzheimer's Association: Connecticut Chapter
99 Trinity Street   860-956-9560
Hartford, CT 06106   800-272-3900
                                Fax: 860-956-9590
                          e-mail: walkhelpct@alz.org
                                         www.alz.org
Works with all individuals and family members affected by Alzheimer's disease and related disorders; ensures humane systems of care and support and promotes research efforts to treat and cure Alzheimer's disease.
Christopher Rupp, Chairman
Daniel P Finke, Treasurer

693 Alzheimer's Association: South Central Connecticut Chapter
2911 Dixwell Avenue   203-230-1777
Hamden, CT 06518   800-272-3900
                                Fax: 203-230-1712
                                         www.alz.org

Patricia Clark, Executive Director

Delaware

694 Alzheimer's Association: Delaware Chapter
240 N James Street   302-633-4420
Newport, DE 19804   800-272-3900
                                Fax: 302-633-4494
                    e-mail: Wendy.Campbell@alz.org
                                         www.alz.org

Wendy L Campbell, President
Theresa Haenn, Vice President Development

District of Columbia

695 Alzheimer's Association: Greater Washington DC Chapter
2524 Pensylvania Avenue Southeast   703-359-4440
Washington, DC 20020   800-272-3900
                                Fax: 202-483-4164
                        e-mail: alzwalknca@alz.org
                                         www.alz.org
Help line-telephone referral support groups, caregiver education, respite services. We have three offices serving DC and surrounding Maryland counties.

Abigail Reinecker, Local Contact

Florida

696 Alzheimer's Association: Broward County Chapter
201 E Sample Road   800-861-7826
Deerfield Beach, FL 33407   800-272-3900
                                      Fax: 954-786-1538
                       e-mail: barbara.grasch@alz.org
                                      www.alz.org

Barbara Grasch, Director of Program Services
Ellen Brown, CEO

697 Alzheimer's Association: East Central Florida Chapter
Wickham Road   407-951-7992
Melbourne, FL 32935   800-272-3900
                                      Fax: 407-729-8044
                             e-mail: jgiovanni@alz.org
                                      www.alz.org

Joan Giovanni, Local Contact

698 Alzheimer's Association: Florida Gulf Coast Chapter
9365 US Highway 19 N   727-578-2558
Pinellas Park, FL 33782   800-272-3900
                                      Fax: 727-578-2286
                          e-mail: milnel@alzflgulf.org
                                      www.alz.org
Provides information and services to families and professionals
dealing with memory related disorders.
Gloria JT Smith, President/CEO
Paul Anderson, Vice President Finance

699 Alzheimer's Association: Greater Miami Chapter
501 Marlins Way   305-891-6228
Miami, FL 33125   800-272-3900
                                      Fax: 305-751-5551
                             e-mail: snewman@alz.org
                                      www.alz.org

Reni Rizzo, Community Education Coordinator
Sharon Newman, Local Contact

700 Alzheimer's Association: Greater Orlando Area Chapter
Ampitheatre at 300 Robinson St., Do   407-951-7992
Orlando, FL 32801   800-272-3900
                                      Fax: 407-228-4201
                             e-mail: jgiovanni@alz.org
                                      www.alz.org

Stu Gaines, Chair
Joan Giovanni, Local Contact

701 Alzheimer's Association: Greater Palm Beach Area Chapter
600 N Congress Avenue   561-478-3120
Delray Beach, FL 33445   800-272-3900
                                      Fax: 561-278-4910
                                      www.alz.org

702 Alzheimer's Association: Northeast Florida
4237 Salisbury Rd   904-281-9077
Jacksonville, FL 32216   800-272-3900
                                      Fax: 866-281-9078
                              e-mail: mdrinks@alz.org
                                      www.alz.org

Michelle Drinks, Local Contact

703 Alzheimer's Association: Northern Central Florida Chapter
1001 NW 34th St   904-281-9077
Gainesville, FL 32605   800-272-3900
                                      Fax: 352-372-2038
                              e-mail: mdrinks@alz.org
                                      www.alz.org

Michelle Drinks, Local Contact
Tish Sheesley, CEO

704 Alzheimer's Association: Northwest Florida Chapter
119 Hollywood Boulevard   850-302-0581
Ft. Walton Beach, FL 32548   800-272-3900
                                      Fax: 850-302-0583
                                      www.alz.org

705 Alzheimer's Association: Southwest Florida Chapter
4075 Tamiami   941-235-7470
Port Charlotte, FL 33952   800-272-3900
                                      Fax: 941-235-7473
                                      www.alz.org

706 Alzheimer's Association: Tampa Bay Chapter
601 N Old Coachman Rd   727-259-2317
Clearwater, FL 33765   800-272-3900
                                      Fax: 941-380-5701
                          e-mail: farinasr@alzflgulf.org
                                      www.alz.org

Gloria JT Smith, President/CEO
Rachel Farinas, Local Contact

707 Alzheimer's Association: Volusia/Flagler Branch
111 N Frederick Avenue   407-951-7992
Daytona Beach, FL 32114-5126   800-272-3900
                                      Fax: 386-238-8293
                             e-mail: jgiovanni@alz.org
                                      www.alz.org

Joan Giovanni, Local Contact

708 Alzheimer's Association: West Central Florida Chapter
PO Box 2070   813-848-8888
New Port Richey, FL 34656-2070   800-272-3900
                                      Fax: 813-849-6124
                                      www.alz.org

Georgia

709 Alzheimer's Association: Atlanta Chapter
1925 Century Boulevard   404-728-6066
Atlanta, GA 30345-4021   800-272-3900
                                      Fax: 404-636-9768
                             e-mail: rrotunda@alz.org
                                      www.alz.org

Bennett Watts, Chair
Robyn Rotunda, Local Contact

710 Alzheimer's Association: Augusta Chapter
1899 Central Avenue   706-731-9060
Augusta, GA 30904-5755   800-272-3900
                                      Fax: 706-731-9099
                           e-mail: kim.franklin@alz.org
                                      www.alz.org

Bennett Watts, Chair
Bruce Flechter, Treasurer

711 Alzheimer's Association: Central Georgia Chapter
277 Martin Luther King Jr Boulevard   478-746-7050
Macon, GA 31201-3498   800-272-3900
                                      Fax: 478-746-6679
                           e-mail: kim.franklin@alz.org
                                      www.alz.org

Bennett Watts, Chair
Bruce Flechter, Treasurer

712 Alzheimer's Association: Greater Columbus Chapter
5900 River Road   706-327-6838
Columbus, GA 31904-0185   800-272-3900
                                      Fax: 706-494-0533
                              e-mail: cvogler@alz.org
                                      www.alz.org

Bennett Watts, Chair
Christina Vogler, Local Contact

713 Alzheimer's Association: Greater Georgia Chapter
1925 Century Boulevard   404-728-6066
Atlanta, GA 30345-4021   800-272-3900
                                      Fax: 404-636-9768
                             e-mail: rrotunda@alz.org
                                      www.alz.org

Bennett Watts, Chair
Robyn Rotunda, Local Contact

714 Alzheimer's Association: Southeast Georgia Chapter
201 Television Circle   912-920-2231
Savannah, GA 31406   800-272-3900
Fax: 912-921-7960
e-mail: dheddendorf@alz.org
www.alz.org

Deborah Heddendorf, Local Contact

715 Alzheimer's Association: Southwest Georgia Chapter
1512-1 Gillionville Road   229-388-8219
Albany, GA 31707   800-272-3900
Fax: 229-888-2620
e-mail: dphillips@alz.org
www.alz.org

Maggie Keenan, Office Volunteer
Dan Phillips, Local Contact

Hawaii

716 Alzheimer's Association: Honolulu Chapter
1050 Ala Moana Boulevard   808-591-2771
Honolulu, HI 96814   800-272-3900
Fax: 808-591-9071
e-mail: ebatalon@alz.org
www.alz.org

Eric Batalon, Local Contact
Chris Shirai, Chairman

717 Alzheimer's Association: West Hawaii Chapter
PO Box 390247   808-591-2771
Kailua Kona, HI 96739-0247   800-272-3900
Fax: 808-322-0008
e-mail: ebatalon@alz.org
www.alz.org

Eric Batalon, Local Contact

Idaho

718 Alzheimer's Association: Greater Idaho Chapter
1111 S Orchard   208-384-1788
Boise, ID 83705-2878   800-272-3900
Fax: 208-385-7191
e-mail: suzette.albers-tunnell@alz.org
www.alz.org

Suzette Albers-Tunne, Executive Director

719 Alzheimer's Association: Northern Idaho Chapter
2003 Kootenai Health Way   208-666-2996
Coeur D Alene, ID 83814   800-272-3900
Fax: 509-473-3389
e-mail: pchristo@alz.org
www.alz.org

PJ Christo, Outreach Coordinator
Joel Loiacono, Executive Director

Illinois

720 Alzheimer's Association: Central Illinois Chapter
606 W Glen Avenue   309-681-1100
Peoria, IL 61614-4831   800-272-3900
Fax: 309-681-1101
e-mail: kgabbert@alz.org
www.alz.org

Nikki Vulgaris, Executive Director
Kari Gabbert, Local Contact

721 Alzheimer's Association: East Central Illinois Chapter
303 N. Hershey   217-351-1726
Bloomington, IL 61704-7337   800-272-3900
Fax: 217-351-2161
www.alz.org

Provides information, support, and referral services to families and individuals facing Alzheimer's disease. Includes newsletter, support groups, and education.

722 Alzheimer's Association: Four Rivers Chapter
401 N Wall Street   815-936-0464
Kankakee, IL 60901   800-272-3900
Fax: 815-936-9363
www.alz.org

723 Alzheimer's Association: Greater Illinois Chapter
4709 Golf Road   847-933-2413
Skokie, IL 60076-1260   800-272-3900
Fax: 847-933-2417
e-mail: info@alz.org
www.alz.org

724 Alzheimer's Association: Greater Illinois Chapter: Carbondale Office
402 E Plaza Drive   618-985-1095
Carterville, IL 62918-1429   800-272-3900
Fax: 618-457-7830
e-mail: GI.Chapter@alz.org
www.alz.org

Jill Schoenborn, Coordinator Outreach & Development

725 Alzheimer's Association: Land of Lincoln Chapter
South Second Street & Southwind Roa   217-801-9352
Springfield, IL 62703-4833   800-272-3900
Fax: 217-726-5185
e-mail: tarnold@alz.org
www.alz.org

Jane Field, Office Manager
Tina Arnold, Local Contact

726 American Homes for the Aging: Midwest Regional Office
911 N Elm Street   630-323-6755
Hinsdale, IL 60521-3641   800-272-3900
Fax: 630-325-0749
www.alz.org

Regional office of the AHA, a national professional association of nonprofit nursing homes, retirement communities and homes for the aging.

Indiana

727 Alzheimer's Association: Central Indiana Chapter
601 W. New York Street   317-575-9620
Indianapolis, IN 46202-1816   800-272-3900
Fax: 317-582-0669
e-mail: IndianaWalk@alz.org
www.alz.org

Heather Allen Hershberger, Executive Director
Leslie Bush, Local Contact

728 Alzheimer's Association: Northern Indiana Chapter
922 E Colfax Avenue   57 - 2 - 41
S Bend, IN 46617-3112   800-272-3900
Fax: 57 - 2 - 42
e-mail: AlzServicesNI@sbcglobal.net
www.alz.org

Iowa

729 Alzheimer's Association: Big Sioux Chapter
401 Gordon Drive   712-279-5802
Sioux City, IA 51101-3716   800-272-3900
Fax: 712-277-8076
e-mail: tschroeder@alz.org
www.alz.org

Kim McCormick, Executive Director
Terri Schroeder, Local Contact

730 Alzheimer's Association: East Central Iowa Chapter
1570 42nd Street NE   319-294-9699
Cedar Rapids, IA 52402   800-272-3900
Fax: 319-294-0068
e-mail: amiller2@alz.org
www.alz.org

Kelly Hauer, Executive Director
Abbey Miller, Local Contact

731 Alzheimer's Association: Greater Iowa Chapter
1730 28th Street
W Des Moines, IA 50266
515-440-2722
800-272-3900
Fax: 515-440-6385
e-mail: Carol.Sipfle@alz.org
www.alz.org

Carol Sipfle, Executive Director
Holly Bradford, Finance Director

732 Alzheimer's Association: Heart of Iowa Chapter
3915 Mortensen Road
Ames, IA 50014-7259
515-440-6383
800-272-3900
Fax: 515-292-0125
e-mail: cmathany@alz.org
www.alz.org

Chantelle Mathany, Local Contact

733 Greater Iowa Chapter Alzheimer's Association Quadcity Office
736 Federal Street
Davenport, IA 52803-5750
563-324-1022
800-272-3900
Fax: 563-324-6267
e-mail: Jerry.Schroeder@alz.org
www.alz.org

Jerry Schroeder, Program Specialist
Julie Seier, Community Relations Coordinator

Kansas

734 Alzheimer's Association: Heart of America Chapter
3846 W 75th Street
Prairie Village, KS 66208-4126
913-831-3888
800-272-3900
Fax: 913-831-1916
e-mail: jan.horn@alz.org
www.alz.org

Debra R Brook, Executive Director
Michelle Niedens, Education Director

735 Alzheimer's Association: Sunflower Chapter
347 S Laura
Wichita, KS 67211-4109
316-267-7333
800-272-3900
Fax: 316-267-6369
e-mail: lbelton@alz.org
www.alz.org

Marsha Hills, Executive Director
Lanette Belton, Local Contact

Kentucky

736 Alzheimer's Association: Lexington/ Bluegrass Chapter
465 E High Street
Lexington, KY 40507
859-266-5283
800-272-3900
Fax: 859-268-4764
e-mail: amber.lakin@alz.org
www.alz.org

Debbie Lacy Goodman, VP Awareness & Community Relations
Amber Lakin, Local Contact

737 Alzheimer's Association: Louisville Chapter
6100 Dutchmans Lane
Louisville, KY 40205
502-451-4266
800-272-3900
Fax: 502-456-2701
e-mail: wvogel@alz.org
www.alz.org

Teri Shirk, Chapter President & CEO
Whitney Vogel, Local Contact

Louisiana

738 Alzheimer's Association: Northeast/Central Louisiana Chapter
2300 Sycamore
Monroe, LA 71201
318-861-8680
800-272-3900
Fax: 318-998-7360
e-mail: dhayes@alz.org
www.alz.org

Debbie Hayes, Local Contact

739 Alzheimer's Association: Greater New Orleans Chapter
DePaul Hospital

1040 Calhoun Street
New Orleans, LA 70118-5999
504-648-4084
800-272-3900
Fax: 504-895-0493
e-mail: charrell@alz.org
www.alz.org

Chet Harrell, Local Contact

740 Alzheimer's Services of the Capital Area
3772 N Boulevard
Baton Rouge, LA 70806
225-334-7494
800-548-1211
Fax: 225-387-3664
e-mail: info@alzbr.org
www.alzbr.org

The mission of Alzheimer's Services of the Capital Area is to provide education and support services to memory impaired individuals as well as caregivers and professionals; and to enhance community awareness of Alzheimer's disease and related disorders.
Barbara Auten, Executive Director

Maine

741 Alzheimer's Association: Maine Chapter
383 U.S. Route 1
Scarborough, ME 04074-2419
207-772-0115
800-272-3900
Fax: 207-289-3705
e-mail: laurie.trenholm@alz.org
www.alz.org

Joy Heptner, Executive Director
Liz Weaver, Program Director

742 Maine Alzheimer's Care Center
154 Dresden Avenue
Gardiner, ME 04345
207-626-1770

Maryland

743 Alzheimer's Association: Central Maryland Chapter
1850 York Road
Timonium, MD 21093-5122
410-561-9099
800-272-3900
Fax: 410-561-3433
e-mail: info.maryland@alz.org
www.alz.org

Cass Naugle, Executive Director
Teri Bennett, Helpline Coordinator

744 Alzheimer's Association: Eastern Shore Chapter
909 Progress Circle
Salisbury, MD 21804
410-543-1163
800-272-3900
Fax: 410-546-0184
e-mail: dmagarelli@alz.org
www.alz.org

Cass Naugle, Executive Director
Damian Magarelli, Local Contact

745 Alzheimer's Association: Western Maryland Chapter
101 Clarke Pl.
Frederick, MD 21701
301-696-0315
800-272-3900
Fax: 301-696-9061
e-mail: kweddle@alz.org
www.alz.org

To eliminate Alzheimer's disease through the advancement of research and to enhance care and support for individuals their families and caregivers.
Cathy Hanson, Program Coordinator
Kristen Weddle, Local Contact

Massachusetts

746 Alzheimer's Association: Massachusetts Chapter
311 Arsenal Street
Watertown, MA 02472
617-868-6718
800-272-3900
Fax: 617-868-6720
www.alz.org

Nonprofit, national, voluntary health organization dedicated to Alzheimer research and care. Provides 24 hour help line, support

groups, a wanderers prevention program early stage patient programs, family educators, professional training, and advocacy.
James Wessle MBA, President & CEO
Betsy Fitzgerald-Cam, Vice President Communications

747 Alzheimer's Association: Western Regional Office: Massachusetts Chapter
264 Cottage Street   413-787-1113
Springfield, MA 01104   800-272-3900
                                      Fax: 413-787-1109
                                      www.alz.org
Nonprofit organization serving family and professional caregivers in seven counties in southwest Michigan. Provides information on Alzheimer's and other diseases, educational programs, resource libraries. Train-the-trainer agency referral, autopsy liaison, and other services.
Marcia McKen Med, Manager
Annie Clattenburg, Coordinator Administrative Services

Michigan

748 Alzheimer's Association: East Central Michigan Chapter
G-3287 Beecher Road   810-720-2791
Flint, MI 48503   800-272-3900
                                      Fax: 810-720-3040
                                      www.alz.org

749 Alzheimer's Association: Greater Michigan Chapter
20300 Civic Center Drive   248-351-0280
Southfield, MI 48076   800-272-3900
                                      Fax: 248-351-0417
                                      www.alz.org
A national network of chapters, is the largest national voluntary health organization committed to finding a cure for Alzheimer's and helping those affected by the disease. Provides a wide range of services and programs for Alzheimer's and other dementia patients for their families and for the general public.

750 Alzheimer's Association: Greater Michigan Chapter: Upper Peninsula Region
1420 Pine Street   906-228-3910
Marquette, MI 49855-4521   800-272-3900
                                      Fax: 906-228-2455
                                      TTY: 877-204-6924
                                      e-mail: ralmen@alz.org
                                      www.alz.org
Pamela Parkkila, Director
Ruth Almen, Local Contact

751 Alzheimer's Association: Michigan Great Lakes Chapter: West Shore Region
1740 Village Drive   734-475-7043
Muskegon, MI 49442-5546   800-272-3900
                                      Fax: 231-780-1494
                                      e-mail: mglcwalk@alz.org
                                      www.alz.org
Providing caregiver support groups a help line informational materials community education and a quarterly newsletter.
Barb Betts, Program Coordinator
Stephanie Barnhill, Local Contact

752 Alzheimer's Association: Mid-Michigan Chapter
4604 N Saginaw Road   989-839-9910
Midland, MI 48640   800-272-3900
                                      Fax: 989-839-5910
                                      TTY: 877-204-6924
                                      e-mail: boneill@alz.org
                                      www.alz.org
Dawn Spicer, Director
Betty O'Neill, Local Contact

753 Alzheimer's Association: Northeast Michigan Chapter
526 W Chisholm St   989-356-4087
Alpena, MI 49707   800-272-3900
                                      Fax: 989-354-7879
                                      e-mail: sruetz@alz.org
                                      www.alz.org

Shawn Ruetz, Local Contact

754 Alzheimer's Association: Northwest Michigan Chapter
921 W. 11th. Street   616-459-4558
Traverse City, MI 49864   800-272-3900
                                      Fax: 231-922-1584
                                      e-mail: sruetz@alz.org
                                      www.alz.org

Shawn Ruetz, Local Contact

Minnesota

755 Alzheimer's Association: Minnesota/Dakotas
1 Twins Way   952-830-0512
Minneapolis, MN 55403   800-272-3900
                                      Fax: 952-830-0513
                                      e-mail: mnnd-walk@alz.org
                                      www.alz.org
Mary Birchard, Executive Director
Libby Wilhelmy, Local Contact

Mississippi

756 Alzheimer's Association: Mississippi Chapter
1900 Dunbarton Drive   601-987-0020
Jackson, MS 39216   800-272-3900
                                      Fax: 601-987-9020
                                      e-mail: rruello@alz.org
                                      www.alz.org
Barb Dobrosky, Program Director
Rachel Ruello, Local Contact

757 Alzheimer's Foundation of the South: Mississippi Division
PO Box 2394   228-867-6251
Gulfport, MS 39503   800-272-3900
                                      Fax: 228-864-8843
                                      e-mail: alzms@cs.com
                                      www.alz.org
Rosemary Hudgins, Executive Director

Missouri

758 Alzheimer's Association: Mid-Missouri Chapter
2400 Bluff Creek Drive   573-443-8665
Columbia, MO 65201   800-272-3900
                                      Fax: 573-499-9701
                                      e-mail: cbaker@alz.org
                                      www.alz.org
Linda Newkirk, Executive Director
Chris Baker, Local Contact

759 Alzheimer's Association: Northwest Missouri-Chapter
10th and Faraon   816-364-4467
St. Joseph, MO 64502-1241   800-272-3900
                                      Fax: 816-364-2553
                                      e-mail: brenda.gregg@alz.org
                                      www.alz.org

760 Alzheimer's Association: Southwest Missouri Chapter
1500 S Glenstone   417-886-2199
Springfield, MO 65804   800-272-3900
                                      Fax: 417-886-0337
                                      e-mail: nreed@alz.org
                                      www.alz.org
Rebecca Argilagos, President/CEO
Nate Reed, Local Contact

761 Alzheimer's Association: St. Louis Chapter
700 Clark Avenue   314-801-0465
Saint Louis, MO 63102-3214   800-272-3900
                                      Fax: 314-432-3824
                                      e-mail: stlwalksupport@alz.org
                                      www.alz.org
Joan D'Ambrose, President
Alyssa Vorhies, Local Contact

Montana

762   Alzheimer's Association: Greater Billings Area Chapter
2100 South Shiloh Road   406-252-3053
Billings, MT 59101   800-272-3900
                                      Fax: 406-252-2933
                                      e-mail: sshannon@alz.org
                                      www.alz.org

Kelly Donovan, President
Sharon Shannon, Local Contact

Nebraska

763   Alzheimer's Association: Great Plains Chap ter
1500 S. 70th St   402-420-2540
Lincoln, NE 68506   800-272-3900
                                      e-mail: mfeit@alz.org
                                      www.alz.org

The Alzheimer's Association of the Great Plains is dedicated to supporting those with Alzheimer's disease and their families and friends through specialized programs and services, educating families, communities, and health professionals about Alzheimer's disease.
Karen Noel, President/CEO
Mark Feit, Local Contact

764   Alzheimer's Association: Lincoln/Greater Nebraska Chapter
1500 S. 70th St.   402-420-2540
Lincoln, NE 68506   800-272-3900
                                      Fax: 402-420-2541
                                      e-mail: mfeit@alz.org
                                      www.alz.org

Karen Noel, President/CEO
Mark Feit, Local Contact

765   Alzheimer's Association: Omaha/Eastern Nebraska Chapter
3220 Farnam St   402-502-4301
Omaha, NE 68131-2167   800-272-3900
                                      Fax: 402-502-7001
                                      e-mail: cenoviso@alz.org
                                      www.alz.org

Duane Gross, President and CEO
Cathy Enoviso, Local Contact

Nevada

766   Alzheimer's Association: Northern Nevada Chapter
1301 Cordone Avenue   775-786-8061
Reno, NV 89502-6362   800-272-3900
                                      Fax: 775-786-1920
                                      e-mail: info@alznorcal.org
                                      www.alz.org

Herb Williams, President
Eduardo Salaz, Vice President

767   Alzheimer's Association: Southern Nevada Chapter
5190 S Valley View Boulevard   702-248-2770
Las Vegas, NV 89118-6062   800-272-3900
                                      Fax: 702-248-2771
                                      e-mail: achavez@alz.org
                                      www.alz.org

Luis Carrillo, Regional Director
Albert Chavez, Local Contact

New Hampshire

768   Alzheimer's Association of Vermont and New Hampshire
10 Ferry Street   603-226-5868
Concord, NH 03301-5004   800-272-3900
                                      Fax: 603-225-8126
                                      www.alz.org

Robbie Nicol, Chair
Robert Dowd, First Vice Chair

New Jersey

769   Alzheimer's Association: Greater New Jersey Chapter
400 Morris Avenue   973-586-4300
Denville, NJ 07834   800-272-3900
                                      Fax: 973-586-4342
                                      www.alz.org

Provides programs and services to individuals with Alzheimer's disease, their families and caregivers, including education and training, support groups, a toll free telephone help line and respite assistance.

770   Alzheimer's Association: South Jersey Chapter
3 Eves Drive   856-797-1212
Marlton, NJ 08053   800-272-3900
                                      Fax: 609-784-8486
                                      e-mail: Wendy.Campbell@alz.org
                                      www.alz.org

Wendy L Campbell, President & CEO
Theresa Haenn, Vice President Development

New Mexico

771   Alzheimer's Association: New Mexico Chapter
9500 Montgomery Boulevard NE   505-266-4473
Albuquerque, NM 87111   800-272-3900
                                      Fax: 505-266-0108
                                      e-mail: nlawrie@alz.org
                                      www.alz.org

Agnes Vallejos, Executive Director
Nika Lawrie, Local Contact

New York

772   Alzheimer's Association: Sullivan/Delaware Chapter
PO Box 911   941-794-3774
Monticello, NY 12701   800-272-3900
                                      www.alz.org

773   Alzheimer's Association: Central New York Chapter
441 W Kirkpatrick Street   315-472-4201
Syracuse, NY 13204-1361   800-272-3900
                                      Fax: 315-472-4206
                                      e-mail: gfletcher@alz.org
                                      www.alz.org

Larry Malfitano, President
Grant Fletcher, Local Contact

774   Alzheimer's Association: Hudson Valley/ Rockland/Westchester NY Chapter
2 Jefferson Plaza   845-471-2655
Poughkeepsie, NY 12601-4027   800-272-3900
                                      Fax: 845-471-8960
                                      e-mail: info@alzhudsonvalley.org
                                      www.alz.org

Elaine Sproat, President & CEO
Meg Boyce, Director of Programs & Services

775   Alzheimer's Association: Long Island Chapter
3281 Veterans Memorial Highway   631-580-5100
Ronkonkoma, NY 11779-3521   800-272-3900
                                      Fax: 631-580-3100
                                      e-mail: Info@alzheimersli.org
                                      www.alz.org

Voluntary health agency that provides care and consultation, information and referral, education, national safe return program and support groups to individuals with Alzheimer's, their families and/or caregivers.
Mary Ann Malack-Ragona, Executive Director/CEO
Linda Cody, Director of Development

776   Alzheimer's Association: New York City Chapter
360 Lexington Avenue   646-744-2900
New York, NY 10017   800-272-3900
                                      Fax: 212-490-6037
                                      e-mail: helpline@alznyc.org
                                      www.alz.org/nyc

Lou-Ellen Barkan, President/CEO
Jed A. Levine, Executive Vice President

777 Alzheimer's Association: Northeastern New York Chapter
4 Pine West Plaza   518-867-4999
Albany, NY 12205-2083   800-272-3900
                                     Fax: 518-867-4997
                                  e-mail: infoeny@alz.org
                                             www.alz.org
Regional affiliate of national association. Works to educate and
support families, while raising funds in support of research.
Paul A Wajda, Chair
Warren E Garling, Vice Chair

778 Alzheimer's Association: Putnam County Chapter
Robin Hill Corporate Park
15 Mount Ebo Road S   845-278-0343
Brewster, NY 10509-2164   800-272-3900
                            e-mail: info@alzhudsonvalley.org
                                             www.alz.org
Stuart Greif, Program Development Specialist

779 Alzheimer's Association: Rochester Chapter
85 Adams Street   585-760-5472
Rochester, NY 14608   800-272-3900
                                     Fax: 585-760-5401
                               e-mail: rochesterwalk@alz.org
                                             www.alz.org
Chris Lacey, Local Contact
Judy Lemoncelli, Local Contact

780 Alzheimer's Association: Southern Tier Chapter
401 Hayes Avenue   607-785-7852
Endicott, NY 13760-5421   800-272-3900
                                     Fax: 607-785-4004
                                 e-mail: alzcny@alzcny.org
                                             www.alz.org
L Jane Hudreck, Regional Director

781 Alzheimer's Association: Western New York Chapter
2805 Wehrle Drive   716-626-0600
Williamsville, NY 14421   800-272-3900
                                     Fax: 717-626-2255
                            e-mail: Donna.McKenzie@alz.org˜
                                             www.alz.org
David Cascio, President
Linda Sabo, Executive Director

782 Alzheimer's Foundation of Staten Island
789 Post Avenue   718-667-7110
Staten Island, NY 10310-6427   877-574-7068
                                     Fax: 718-667-8431
                               e-mail: info@sialzheimers.org
                                       www.sialzheimers.org
Not-for-profit health and human services organization, serving
people with Alzheimer's disease and related dementias.
Leilani Joven Pelletie, Executive Director
David Cascio, President

North Carolina

783 Alzheimer's Association: Eastern North Carolina Chapter
1305 Navaho Dr.   919-832-3732
Raleigh, NC 27609   800-272-3900
                                     Fax: 919-832-7989
                                e-mail: awatkins@alznc.org
                                             www.alz.org
Dedicated to providing program services education for patients,
families and professional caregivers, advocacy and research.
Alice Watkins, Executive Director
Rita Bhan, Developmental Director

784 Alzheimer's Association: Western North Car olina Chapter
3800 Shamrock Drive   704-532-7390
Charlotte, NC 28215   800-272-3900
                                     Fax: 704-532-5421
                                 e-mail: infonc@alz.org
                                             www.alz.org
A nonprofit voluntary organization dedicated to improving the
quality of life for those with Alzheimer's and their families
through a broad range of programs, including patient and family

services, education, advocacy and support of research through
national programs.
Beth Croom MA, Director of Programs/Education
Teresa Hoover, Program Associate/Helpline Coordinator

North Dakota

785 Alzheimer's Association: Fargo/Moorhead Regional Center
5225 31st Ave South   701-277-9757
Fargo, ND 58104   800-272-3900
                                     Fax: 701-277-9785
                              e-mail: traie.dockter@alz.org
                                             www.alz.org
Gretchen Dobervich, Regional Center Director
Traie Dockter, Local Contact

Ohio

786 Alzheimer's Association: Canton Chapter
408 Ninth St. SW
Canton, OH 44707   800-272-3900
                                     Fax: 330-996-7757
                                 e-mail: geoachl@alz.org
                                             www.alz.org
Pam Schuellerman, Executive Director
Andy Junn, Development Director

787 Alzheimer's Association: Central Ohio Chapter
330 Huntington Park Lane   614-442-2014
Columbus, OH 43215-2112   800-272-3900
                                     Fax: 614-457-6634
                                  e-mail: jsega@alz.org
                                             www.alz.org
Kenneth Strong, Executive Director
Jennifer Monroe-Sega, Local Contact

788 Alzheimer's Association: Clark/Champaign, Miami Valley Chapter
1700 S. Patterson Blvd.   937-291-3332
Dayton, OH 45409-2620   800-272-3900
                                     Fax: 937-323-9259
                           e-mail: walkmiamivalley@alz.org
                                             www.alz.org
Judy Turner, Executive Director
Marie McLaughlin, Local Contact

789 Alzheimer's Association: Cleveland Area Chapter
23215 Commerce Park Drive   216-721-8457
Beachwood, OH 44122-1013   800-272-3900
                                     Fax: 216-831-8585
                               e-mail: helpline@alzclv.org
                                             www.alz.org
Nancy B Udelson, Executive Director
Robert Bazzarelli, President

790 Alzheimer's Association: Greater Cincinnati Chapter
720 E. Pete Rose Way   513-721-4284
Cincinnati, OH 45202-1742   800-272-3900
                                     Fax: 513-345-8446
                               e-mail: diana.bosse@alz.org
                                             www.alz.org
Committed to support education, advocacy and research on behalf
of those affected by Alzheimer's disease.
Clarissa Rentz, Executive Director
Diana Bosse, Local Contact

791 Alzheimer's Association: Greater East Ohio Chapter: Greater Youngstown Office
3695B Boardman-Canfield Rd   330-533-3300
Canfield, OH 44406-0321   800-272-3900
                                     Fax: 330-533-3307
                                 e-mail: geoachl@alz.org
                                             www.alz.org
Pam Schuellerman, Executive Director
Andy Junn, Development Director

792 Alzheimer's Association: Miami Valley Chapter
1700 S. Patterson Blvd.   937-291-3332
Dayton, OH 45409-3661   800-272-3900
                                          Fax: 937-291-0463
                             e-mail: walkmiamivalley@alz.org
                                                  www.alz.org

Judy Turner, Executive Director
Marie McLaughlin, Local Contact

793 Alzheimer's Association: Northwest Ohio Chapter
75 N. Main St.   419-537-1999
Mansfield, OH 44902-7906   800-272-3900
                                          Fax: 419-522-5318
                                   e-mail: nvargas@alz.org
                                                  www.alz.org
Voluntary health organization committed to finding a cure for Alzheimer's and helping those affected by the disease.
Michael Malone, President
Nick Vargas, Local Contact

794 Alzheimer's Association: West Central Ohio Chapter
200 East High Street   419-537-1999
Lima, OH 45801-3468   800-272-3900
                                          Fax: 419-222-6212
                                 e-mail: tschindler@alz.org
                                                  www.alz.org
A voluntary health agency providing information Alzheimer's disease and related dementias, serving 7 counties: Allen, Auglaize, Hancock, Hardin, Mercer, Putnam and Van Wert. Offers support group meetings in each county and provides a toll-free help line.
Salli Bollin, Executive Director
Toni Schindler, Local Contact

Oklahoma

795 Alzheimer's Association: Oklahoma Chapter
2448 E. 81st Street   918-392-5012
Tulsa, OK 74137-7804   800-272-3900
                                          Fax: 918-481-7745
                                          TTY: 800-493-1411
                                 e-mail: shauptman@alz.org
                                                  www.alz.org
Dedicated to serving Alzheimer's patients, their families, and caregivers through education, outreach, programs, support services and public advocacy.
Judi A Ver Hoef, President/CEO
Sarah Hauptam, Local Contact

Oregon

796 Alzheimer's Association: Columbia-Willamet Chapter
1940 North Victory Boulevard   503-416-0209
Portland, OR 97217-1610   800-272-3900
                                          Fax: 503-413-6909
                                 e-mail: kara.busick@alz.org
                                                  www.alz.org

Judy McKellar, Executive Director
Kara Busick, Local Contact

797 Alzheimer's Association: Cascade/Coast Chapter
100 Day Island Road   503-416-0209
Eugene, OR 97401   800-272-3900
                                          Fax: 541-345-5797
                                 e-mail: kara.busick@alz.org
                                                  www.alz.org

Judy Clarke, Vice President
Kara Busick, Local Contact

798 Alzheimer's Association: Mary's Peak Chapter
1925 NW Circle Boulevard   541-752-1012
Corvallis, OR 97330-1312   800-272-3900
                                          Fax: 541-757-1395
                                                  www.alz.org

799 Alzheimer's Association: Mid-Willamette Chapter
PO Box 12768   503-371-7728
Salem, OR 97309-0768   800-272-3900
                                          Fax: 503-571-9842
                                 e-mail: midwillamatte@alz.org
                                                  www.alz.org

Pennsylvania

800 Alzheimer's Association: Delaware Valley Chapter
1 Citizens Bank Way   215-561-2919
Philadelphia, PA 19148   800-272-3900
                                          Fax: 215-561-4663
                                 e-mail: keely.boyle@alz.org
                                                  www.alz.org

Wendy L Campbell, President
Keely Boyle, Local Contact

801 Alzheimer's Association: Greater Pennsylvania Chapter: SW Regional Office
Landmarks Building, 100 Station   412-261-5040
Pittsburgh, PA 15219   800-272-3900
                                          Fax: 412-471-2722
                                   e-mail: mlong@alz.org
                                                  www.alz.org
Education training, information, support groups, free newsletter, telephone support, services to caregivers and diagnosed individuals, as well as professionals.
Diane Balcom, President/CEO
Mellisa Long, Local Contact

802 Alzheimer's Association: Greater Mid-Ohio
1100 Liberty Avenue   412-261-5040
Pittsburgh, PA 15222   800-272-3900
                                          Fax: 412-471-2722
                                   e-mail: mlong@alz.org
                                                  www.alz.org
Education training information support groups free newsletter telephone support services to caregivers and diagnosed individuals as well as professionals.
Bob LeRoy, President/CEO
Mellisa Long, Local Contact

803 Alzheimer's Association: Laurel Mountains Chapter
194 Donohoe Road   412-261-5040
Greensburg, PA 15601-1095   800-272-3900
                                          Fax: 724-837-4567
                                  e-mail: aspreng@alz.org
                                                  www.alz.org

Abby Spreng, Local Contact

804 Alzheimer's Association: Northeast Pennsylvania Chapter
63 North Franklin Street   717-822-4278
Wilkes Barre, PA 18701   800-272-3900
                                          Fax: 717-822-9915
                                                  www.alz.org

805 Alzheimer's Association: Northwest Pennsylvania Chapter
726 West Bayfront Parkway   814-456-9200
Erie, PA 16507   800-272-3900
                                          Fax: 814-454-0414
                                   e-mail: ahurd@alz.org
                                                  www.alz.org

Bob LeRoy, President/CEO
Amanda Hurd, Local Contact

806 Alzheimer's Association: South Central Pennsylvania Chapter
3544 North Progress Avenue   717-651-5020
Harrisburg, PA 17110   800-272-3900
                                          Fax: 717-651-5066
                                 e-mail: tchambers@alz.org
                                                  www.alz.org
Bob LeRoy, President/CEO
Tiffani Chambers, Local Contact

Rhode Island

807 Alzheimer's Association: Rhode Island Chapter
245 Waterman Avenue   401-421-0008
Providence, RI 02906   800-272-3900
                                          Fax: 401-941-8988
                             e-mail: Donna.McGowan@alz.org
                                                  www.alz.org

Elizabeth Morancy, Executive Director
Marge Angilly, Program Director

South Carolina

808   **Alzheimer's Association: Low Country Chapter**
20 Patriots Point Road   843-571-2641
Charleston, SC 29464   800-272-3900
                                          Fax: 843-571-6020
                                     e-mail: kalmstedt@alz.org
                                                  www.alz.org

Ashton Houghton, VP of Development & Communications
Kim Almstedt, Local Contact

809   **Alzheimer's Association: Mid-State South Carolina Chapter**
3223 Sunset Blvd   803-791-3430
W Columbia, SC 29169-7044   800-272-3900
                                          Fax: 803-791-8388
                                                  www.alz.org

Adelle Stanley, Program Director
Lynee Moore, Director of Development

810   **Alzheimer's Association: Upstate South Carolina Chapter**
3027 MLK Jr. Blvd   864-224-3045
Anderson, SC 29625-5528   800-272-3900
                                          Fax: 864-225-1387
                                     e-mail: kwilliams@alz.org
                                                  www.alz.org

Cindy Alewine, President/CEO
Kimberly Williams, Local Contact

Tennessee

811   **Alzheimer's Association: Eastern Tennessee Chapter**
1600 World's Fair Park Drive   865-200-6668
Knoxville, TN 37916   800-272-3900
                                          Fax: 865-544-6249
                                      e-mail: jim.ward@alz.org
                                                  www.alz.org

Janice Wade-Whitehea, Executive Director
Jim Ward, Local Contact

812   **Alzheimer's Association: Highland Rim Chapter**
201 W Lincoln Street   931-455-3345
Tullahoma, TN 37388-1004   800-272-3900
                                          Fax: 931-455-5396
                                       e-mail: swood@alz.org
                                                  www.alz.org

George Jensen, Chair
Sarah Wood, Local Contact

813   **Alzheimer's Association: Memphis Area Office**
500 North Pine Lake Drive   901-565-0011
Memphis, TN 38134   800-272-3900
                                          Fax: 901-565-9550
                                      e-mail: sgraham@alz.org
                                                  www.alz.org

George Jensen, Chair
Susan Graham, Local Contact

814   **Alzheimer's Association: Middle Tennessee Chapter**
4205 Hillsboro Pike   615-292-4938
Nashville, TN 37215-2859   800-272-3900
                                          Fax: 615-386-9768
                                     e-mail: ajackson1@alz.org
                                                  www.alz.org

George Jensen, Chair
Andrew Jackson, Local Contact

815   **Alzheimer's Association: Northeast Tennessee Chapter**
207 North Boone Street   423-928-4080
Johnson City, TN 37604   800-272-3900
                                          Fax: 423-928-1152
                                  e-mail: tracey.kendall@alz.org
                                                  www.alz.org

Provide support, education, advocacy and research to those af-
fected by Alzheimer's disease and their families.
George Jensen, Chair
Bruce Duncan, Vice Chair

816   **Alzheimer's Association: Southeast Tennessee Chapter**
7625 Hamilton Park Drive   423-265-3600
Chattanooga, TN 37421   800-272-3900
                                          Fax: 423-265-3611
                                      e-mail: clowery@alz.org
                                                  www.alz.org

George Jensen, Chair
Cindy Lowery, Local Contact

Texas

817   **Alzheimer's Alliance: Texarkana Area**
104 Cypress   903-223-8021
Texarkana, TX 75503-7812   877-312-8536
                                          Fax: 903-792-1792
                             e-mail: lindanickersonalz@cableone.net
                                            www.alztexark.org

Linda Nickerson, Executive Director
Fran Long, Program Director

818   **Alzheimer's Association: Capital of Texas Chapter**
3520 Executive Center Drive   512-241-0420
Austin, TX 78731   800-272-3900
                                          Fax: 512-241-0430
                                    e-mail: Annie.lagow@alz.org
                                                  www.alz.org

The Alzheimer Association Greater Austin Chapter is dedicated to
providing leadership to enhance care and support services for individuals and their families while promoting the advancement of research eliminate Alzheimer's disease.
Daniel Hamilton, Chair
Annie LaGow, Local Contact

819   **Alzheimer's Association: El Paso Chapter**
4687 N Mesa   915-544-1799
El Paso, TX 79912-1147   800-272-3900
                                          Fax: 915-544-8746
                                   e-mail: susie.gorman@alz.org
                                                  www.alz.org

Mitch Moss, Chair
Susie Gorman, Local Contact

820   **Alzheimer's Association: Greater Beaumont Area Chapter**
8750 Phelan Blvd.   409-833-1613
Beaumont, TX 77706   800-272-3900
                                          Fax: 713-314-1315
                                       e-mail: walk@alztex.org
                                                  www.alz.org

Richard Elbein, Chief Executive Officer
Clarissa Urban, Local Contact

821   **Alzheimer's Association: Greater Dallas Chapter**
4144 N Central Expressway   214-540-2413
Dallas, TX 75204-4228   800-272-3900
                                          Fax: 214-827-2064
                                        e-mail: dhill@alz.org
                                                  www.alz.org

Provides support and assistance to persons affected by Alzhei-
mer's disease and related dementias and their families and care-
givers. Serving Collin, Cooke, Dallas, Deaton, Ellis, Fanning,
Grayson, Hunt, Kaufmau, Navarro and Rockwall counties.
John R Gilchrist Jr, Executive Director
Jack Broyles, Chairman

822   **Alzheimer's Association: Greater East Texas Chapter**
2900 Raguet   713-314-1343
Nacogdoches, TX 75962   800-272-3900
                                          Fax: 936-569-0514
                                       e-mail: walk@alztex.org
                                                  www.alz.org

Phil King, Chief Financial Officer
Jessica Abad-Serpas, Local Contact

823   Alzheimer's Association: Greater Wichita Falls Chapter
901 Indiana   940-767-8800
Wichita Falls, TX 76301-3206   800-272-3900
                                            Fax: 940-322-6259
                                 e-mail: patty.taylor@alz.org
                                                    www.alz.org

Theresa Hocker, Executive Director
Patty Taylor, Local Contact

824   Alzheimer's Association: Houston and Southeast Texas Chapter
400 Hamilton Street   713-314-1340
Houston, TX 77002   800-272-3900
                                            Fax: 713-314-1315
                                   e-mail: walk@alztex.org
                                                    www.alz.org

Richard Elbein, CEO
Rasheeda Daugherty, Local Contact

825   Alzheimer's Association: Northeast Texas Chapter
211 Winchester   903-509-8323
Tyler, TX 75701-8732   800-272-3900
                                            Fax: 903-509-8373
                               e-mail: jana@alzalliance.org
                                                    www.alz.org

Jana Humphrey, Executive Director
Sherlon Spurling, Client Services Coordinator

826   Alzheimer's Association: Rio Grande Valley Region
222 E Van Buren   956-440-0636
Harlingen, TX 78550   800-272-3900
                                            Fax: 956-440-9290
                                                    www.alz.org

A nonprofit organization designed to educate and support individuals with Alzheimer's, their families and caregivers.

827   Alzheimer's Association: STAR Chapter, Midland Region
4400 N Big Spring   432-570-9191
Midland, TX 79705   800-272-3900
                                            Fax: 432-683-2345
                                 e-mail: derdwurm@alz.org
                                                    www.alz.org

Mitch Moss, Chair
Debbie Erdwurm, Local Contact

828   Alzheimer's Association: South Central Texas
7400 Louis Pasteur Drive   210-822-6449
San Antonio, TX 78229   800-272-3900
                                            Fax: 210-824-8069
                                e-mail: bbenavidez@alz.org
                                                    www.alz.org

Mitch Moss, Chair
Belinda Benavides, Local Contact

829   Alzheimer's Association: Tarrant County Chapter
101 Summit Avenue   817-336-4949
Fort Worth, TX 76102   800-272-3900
                                            Fax: 817-336-4966
                              e-mail: lyn.downing@alz.org
                                                    www.alz.org

Offers support to those afflicted with Alzheimer's disease and their families through education, support groups, case management, telephone help line and referral to services (i.e. long term care, adult daycare, medical assistance, legal assistance etc.).
Theresa Hocker, Executive Director
Lyn Downing, Local Contact

Utah

830   Alzheimer's Association: Utah Chapter
296 E. Murray Park Ave   801-265-1944
Salt Lake City, UT 84107   800-272-3900
                                            Fax: 801-269-1226
                                  e-mail: Emartini@alz.org
                                                    www.alz.org

Nick Sussman, Program Director
Elaine Martini, Local Contact

Vermont

831   Alzheimer's Association: Vermont Chapter
300 Cornerstone Drive   802-316-3839
Williston, VT 05495-1139   800-272-3900
                                            Fax: 802-229-5231
                       e-mail: ashley.witzenberger@alz.org
                                                    www.alz.org

Randy Brock, President and Chair
Ashley Witzenberg, Director of Development

Virginia

832   Alzheimer's Association: Central Virginia Chapter
1160 Pepsi Place   434-973-6122
Charlottesville, VA 22901   800-272-3900
                                            Fax: 434-973-4224
                                  e-mail: alzcwva@alz.org
                                                    www.alz.org

Sue Friedman, President and CEO
Brian Phelps, Chair

833   Alzheimer's Association: Greater Richmond Chapter
4600 Cox Road   804-967-2580
Glen Allen, VA 23060   800-272-3900
                                            Fax: 804-967-2588
                             e-mail: sherry.peterson@alz.org
                                                    www.alz.org

Alzheimer's Association provides support and services to those with Alzheimer's and their families services include: help line, support groups, educational programs for family and professional caregivers, monthly newsletter, lending library, and a speakers
Sherry Peterson, CEO
Marry Ann Johnson, Program Director

834   Alzheimer's Association: National Capital Area Chapter
3701 Pender Drive   703-359-4440
Fairfax, VA 22030   800-272-3900
                                            Fax: 703-359-4441
                          e-mail: Danielle.Otsuka@alz.org
                                                    www.alz.org

Provides support and services to those diagnosed with Alzheimer's disease and related disorders and their families. Services include information on the disease, care options, caregiving techniques and research, support groups, education and training, and advocacy.
Matthew B Aaron, Chair
Danielle Otsuka, Director of Development

835   Alzheimer's Association: Piedmont-Valley Area Chapter
1160 Pepsi Place   434-973-6122
Charlottesville, VA 22901   800-272-3900
                                            Fax: 434-973-4224
                                  e-mail: mhanson@alz.org
                                                    www.alz.org

Sue Friedman, President and CEO
Mary Pat Hanson, Local Contact

836   Alzheimer's Association: Roanoke Salem Chapter
3959 Electric Rd   540-345-7600
Roanoke, VA 24018   800-272-3900
                                            Fax: 540-345-7900
                                  e-mail: mhanson@alz.org
                                                    www.alz.org

Sue Friedman, President and CEO
Mary Pat Hanson, Local Contact

837   Alzheimer's Association: Southeastern Virginia Chapter
6350 Center Drive   757-459-2405
Norfolk, VA 23502   800-272-3900
                                            Fax: 757-461-7902
                                 e-mail: InfoSEVA@alz.org
                                                    www.alz.org

Provides support to people with Alzheimer's disease or related dementia and their families; educates professionals and the public about Alzheimer's disease and related dementia; supports research into causes, improved diagnosis, therapies and cures.
Gino V Colombara, Executive Director
Patricia Far Lacey, Director of Education & Family Services

838 Alzheimer's Association: Southside Virginia Chapter
120 S Hill Avenue   434-447-3963
S Hill, VA 23970-0310   800-272-3900
Fax: 434-447-9024
e-mail: gino.colombara@alz.org
www.alz.org

Gino V Colombara, Executive Director
June Rainey, Education & Family Services Coordinator

Washington

839 Alzheimer's Association: Inland Northwest Chapter
800 N. Howard St.   509-473-3390
Spokane, WA 99201   800-272-3900
Fax: 509-473-3389
e-mail: sdruffel@alz.org
www.alz.org

Joel Loiacono, Executive Director
Sandi Druffel, Local Contact

840 Alzheimer's Association: Western & Central Washington Chapter
100 W. Harrison St   206-529-3898
Seattle, WA 98119   800-272-3900
Fax: 206-363-5700
e-mail: walk@alzwa.org
www.alz.org

Nancy Dapper, Executive Director
Justine Stevens, Local Contact

West Virginia

841 Alzheimer's Association: Greater Mid-Ohio Valley Chapter
1920 Park Ave.   304-865-6775
Parkersburg, WV 26101   800-272-3900
e-mail: wendy.hamilton@alz.org
www.alz.org

Jane Marks, Executive Director
Wendy Hamilton, Local Contact

842 Alzheimer's Association: N Central West Virginia Chapter
1299 Pineview Drive   304-599-1159
Morgantown, WV 26505-4543   800-272-3900
Fax: 304-291-2577
e-mail: wvinfo@alz.org
www.alz.org

Jane Marks, Executive Director
Jane Siers, Development Director

843 Alzheimer's Association: South West Virginia Chapter
601 Morris St.   304-343-2717
Charleston, WV 25301   800-272-3900
Fax: 304-343-2723
e-mail: kford@alz.org
www.alz.org

Jane Marks, Executive Director
Kaarmin Ford, Local Contact

Wisconsin

844 Alzheimer's Association: Greater Wisconsin Chapter
La Crosse & Second Streets   608-784-5011
La Crosse, WI 54601   800-272-3900
Fax: 608-784-4428
e-mail: bwilliams@alz.org
www.alz.org

To eliminate Alzheimer's disease through the advancement of research; to provide and enhance care and support for all affected; and to reduce the risk of dementia through the promotion of brain health.
Brad Beckman, President
Brett Williams, Local Contact

845 Alzheimer's Association: Indianhead Chapter
Carson Park Dr   715-345-2969
Eau Claire, WI 54703-5996   800-272-3900
Fax: 715-345-2969
e-mail: kdavies@alz.org
www.alz.org

Mary B Bouche, Executive Director
Kathy Davies, Local Contact

846 Alzheimer's Association: Lake Superior Chapter
US Highway 2 East   715-392-3255
Ashland, WI 54806-1652   800-272-3900
Fax: 715-682-6561
e-mail: fcarlson@alz.org
www.alz.org

Kim Kinner, Executive Director
Freda Carlson, Local Contact

847 Alzheimer's Association: Midstate Wisconsin Chapter
1800 S Central Ave   715-845-7440
Marshfield, WI 54449   800-272-3900
Fax: 715-387-5727
e-mail: aswatek@alz.org
www.alz.org

848 Alzheimer's Association: North Central Wisconsin Chapter
1205 Lincoln St   715-362-7779
Rhinelander, WI 54501   800-272-3900
Fax: 715-362-1879
e-mail: jstpierre@alz.org
www.alz.org

Kim Kinner, Executive Director
Julie St. Pierre, Local Contact

849 Alzheimer's Association: Northeast Wisconsin Chapter
1265 Lombardi Ave   920-469-2110
Green Bay, WI 54304   800-272-3900
Fax: 920-498-2203
e-mail: bbartlett@alz.org
www.alz.org

Kim Kinner, Executive Director
Beverly Bartlett, Local Contact

850 Alzheimer's Association: South Central Wisconsin Chapter
1 John Nolen Drive   608-203-8502
Madison, WI 53703   800-272-3900
Fax: 608-232-3407
e-mail: ehilker@alz.org
www.alz.org

Provides support and assistance to the families of those impacted by Alzheimer's and related dementias, including educational programs, support groups, information and referral and advocacy.
150 Members
Paul Rusk, Executive Director
Emily Hilker, Local Contact

851 Alzheimer's Association: Southeast Wisconsin Chapter
2900 North Menomonee River Parkway   414-479-8800
Milwaukee, WI 53222   800-272-3900
Fax: 414-479-8819
TTY: 414-479-8466
e-mail: slatona@alz.org
www.alz.org

To eliminate Alzheimer's disease through advancement of research and to enhance care and support for individuals, their families and caregivers. Individual consultation over the phone or in person. Extensive library of educational materials for loan or purchase.
Kendra Albers, Special Events Manager
Shelby LaTona, Development Coordinato

Wyoming

852 Alzheimer's Wyoming
900 Werner Court   307-265-7960
Casper, WY 82602   Fax: 307-265-7960
e-mail: alzawy@tribcsp.com
www.alzheimerswyoming.org

Alzheimer's Affiliation of Wyoming is an independent organization that makes presentations about Alzheimer's Disease; assists

Alzheimer support groups; provides funds for respite care; maintains a lending library; refers patients and their families to services.
Mary Hein, Executive Director

Foundations

853 Long Island Alzheimers Foundation
5 Channel Drive · · · · · · · · · · · · · · · · · · 516-767-6856
Port Washington, NY 11050 · · · · · · · Fax: 516-767-6864
e-mail: info@liaf.org
www.liaf.org
To help lighten the burden and improve the quality of life for those suffering with Alzheimer's disease and related dementias, their caregivers and their families.
Fred Jenny, Executive Director
Sean Phillips, Director of Development

Research Centers

854 Aging and Alzheimer's Disease Center Oregon Health Sciences University
Oregon Health Sciences University
3181 SW Sam Jackson Park Road · · · · · · · 503-494-8311
Portland, OR 97239-3098 · · · · · · · Fax: 503-494-6695
e-mail: kaye@ohsu.edu
www.ohsu.edu/research/alzheimers
Researches causes and consequences of Alzheimer's disease and ways of clinical services. Publishes a newsletter twice a year.
Jeffrey Kaye, Director
Joan Benedict, Administrative Coordinator

855 Alzheimer's Disease Center Emory University/VA Medical Center
201 Dowman Drive · · · · · · · · · · · · · · · · 404-727-6069
Atlanta, GA 30322 · · · · · · · · · · · · Fax: 404-286-55
e-mail: emoryadrc@emory.edu
www.med.emory.edu/ADRC
Researchers work to translate advances into improved care and diagnosis for Alzheimer's patients.
Allan Levey, Director
Stuart Zola, Co-Director

856 Alzheimer's Disease Center Kentucky University
Sanders-Brown Center on Aging
1030 South Broadway · · · · · · · · · · · · · · 859-257-1412
Lexington, KY 40504-0230 · · · · · · · Fax: 859-323-2866
e-mail: rdavi3@email.uky.edu
/www.mc.uky.edu/coa
Researchers work to translate advances into improved care and diagnosis for Alzheimer's patients.
Linda J. Van Eldik, Ph.D., Director
Vince J Kellen, Chief Information Officer

857 Alzheimer's Disease Center Mayo Clinic Mayo Medical School
Mayo Medical School
200 First Street SW · · · · · · · · · · · · · · · 507-284-2511
Rochester, MN 55905 · · · · · · · · · · Fax: 507-538-0161
TDD: 507-2849786
e-mail: mayoADC@mayo.edu
www.mayoclinic.com
Researchers work to translate advances into improved care and diagnosis for Alzheimer's patients.
John H Noseworhty MD, President
William C Rupp MD, Vice President, CEO

858 Alzheimer's Disease Center Pennsylvania University School of Medicine
Ralston House
3615 Chestnut Street · · · · · · · · · · · · · · 215-662-7810
Philadelphia, PA 19104 · · · · · · · · · Fax: 215-662-7812
e-mail: jason.karlawish@uphs.upenn.edu
www.pennadc.org
Researchers work to translate advances into improved care and diagnosis for Alzheimer's patients.
John Q Trojanowski, Director

859 Alzheimer's Disease Center: Boston University
Boston University School of Medicine

72 E Concord Street · · · · · · · · · · · · · · · 617-638-5426
Boston, MA 02118 · · · · · · · · · · · · · · · 888-458-2823
Fax: 617-414-1197
e-mail: buad@bu.edu
www.bu.edu/alzresearch
Researchers work to translate advances into improved care and diagnosis for Alzheimer's patients.
Neil W Kowall, Director
Richard Fine, Associate Director

860 Alzheimer's Disease Center: Johns Hopkins University School of Medicine
Johns Hopkins University Department of Pathology
720 Rutland Avenue · · · · · · · · · · · · · · · 410-502-5164
Baltimore, MD 21205 · · · · · · · · · · Fax: 410-955-9777
e-mail: edelman1@jhmi.edu
www.alzresearch.org
Researchers work to translate advances into improved care and diagnosis for Alzheimer's patients.
Marilyn Albert, Director
Philip Wong, Associate Director

861 Alzheimer's Disease Center: University of California, Davis
4860 Y Street · · · · · · · · · · · · · · · · · · · 916-734-5496
Sacramento, CA 95817 · · · · · · e-mail: wjjagust@lbl.gov
alzheimer.ucdavis.edu/
Researchers work to translate advances into improved care and diagnosis for Alzheimer's patients.
Charles DeCarli MD, Clinical Core Director

862 Alzheimer's Disease Center: University of Alabama at Birmingham
1720 7th Avenue S · · · · · · · · · · · · · · · · 205-934-3847
Birmingham, AL 35294-0017 · · · · · Fax: 205-975-7365
e-mail: adbrain@uab.edu
www.main.uab.edu/adc
Researchers work to translate advances into improved care and diagnosis for Alzheimer's patients.
Daniel C Marson, Director
J Michael Wyss, Associate Director

863 Alzheimer's Disease Center: Washington University
1660 S Columbian Way · · · · · · · · · · · · · 206-764-2069
Seattle, WA 98108-1597 · · · · · · · · · · · · 800-317-5382
Fax: 206-768-5456
e-mail: wamble@u.washington.edu
www.depts.washington.edu/adrcweb
Researchers work to translate advances into improved care and diagnosis for Alzheimer's patients.
Sydney Lewis, Education and Outreach Coordinator
Nancy Brown, Lead Psychometrist and Autopsy Coordinat

864 Alzheimer's Disease Research Center Washington University School of Medicine
Washington University School of Medicine
4488 Forest Park Avenue · · · · · · · · · · · · 314-286-2683
St Louis, MO 63108 · · · · · · · · · · · Fax: 314-286-2763
e-mail: morrisj@abraxas.wustl.edu
www.adrc.wustl.edu
Researchers work to translate advances into improved care diagnosis and treatment for Alzheimer's patients.
John Morris, Director
Virginia D Buckles, Executive Director

865 Alzheimer's Disease Research Center Duke University
Bryan ADRC
2200 W Main Street Suite A200 · · · · · · · · 919-668-0820
Durham, NC 27705 · · · · · · · · · · · · · · · 866-444-2372
e-mail: kwe@duke.edu
adrc.mc.duke.edu
Researchers work to translate advances into improved care and diagnosis for Alzheimer's patients.
Kathleen A Welsh-Bohmer, Director
James Robert Burke, Associate Director

866 Cognitive Neurology and Alzheimer's Disease Center
CNADC

320 E Superior Street
Chicago, IL 60611
312-908-9339
Fax: 312-908-8789
e-mail: CNADC-Admin@northwestern.edu
www.brain.northwestern.edu
Researchers work to translate advances into improved care and diagnosis for Alzheimer's patients.
Megan Atchu, MA, Research Administrator
Kevin Connolly, Business Administrator

867 **Cornell University: Winifred Masterson Burke Medical Research-Dementia**
1300 York Avenue
New York, NY 10065
212-746-5454
Fax: 212-821-0576
e-mail: publicaffairs@med.cornell.edu
www.med.cornell.edu
Clinical and basic studies in metabolic aspects of the nervous system especially Alzheimer's disease.
David J Skorton MD, President
Thomas H Blair lll, Senior Director Administrator

868 **Duke University Center for the Study of Aging and Human Development**
Duke University
Box 3003
Durham, NC 27710
919-660-7500
Fax: 919-668-0453
e-mail: webmaster@geri.duke.edu
www.geri.duke.edu
Basic and clinical research into geriatrics and gerontology focusing on a number of chronic diseases in the elderly including osteoporosis cancer heart disease infectious diseases Alzheimer's disease and other disorders leading to dysmobility.
Harvey Jay Cohen MD, Director
Linda K George, Associate Director

869 **Duke University Clinical Research Institute**
Headquarters
2400 Pratt Street
Durham, NC 27705
919-668-8700
www.dcri.duke.edu
Multidisciplinary clinical research into the cause and prevention of human diseases such as Alzheimer's.
Robert A Harrington, Director
Elizabeth Be Reed, Chief Operating Officer

870 **Indiana University Center for Aging Research**
The Center for Aging Research
1050 Wishard Blvd
Indianapolis, IN 46202-2872
317-630-6083
Fax: 317-423-5695
e-mail: nnienaber@regenstrief.org
www.medicine.iupui.edu/iucar/?
Researchers work to translate advances into improved care and diagnosis for Alzheimer's patients.
Christopher Callahan, Director
Douglas K Miller, Associate Director

871 **Indiana University: Human Genetics Center of Medical & Molecular Genetics**
School of Medicine
340 West 10th Street
Indianapolis, IN 46202-3082
317-274-8157
e-mail: kcornett@iupui.edu
www.medicine.iu.edu
Comprised of a core group of scientists with primary appointments in the Department and a group of molecular biologists from other departments who hold joint appointments in Medical and Molecular Genetics.
D Craig Brater MD, Dean
John F. Fitzgerald, MD, MBA, Executive Associate Dean

872 **Institute for Basic Research in Developmental Disabilities**
1050 Forest Hill Road
Staten Island, NY 10314-0001
718-494-0600
866- 94- 973
TTY: 866- 933-488
e-mail: ibr@opwdd.ny.gov
www.opwdd.ny.gov/institute-for-basic-res
James F Moran, Acting Commissioner

873 **Long Island Alzheimers Foundation**
5 Channel Drive
Port Washington, NY 11050
516-767-6856
Fax: 516-767-6856
e-mail: info@liaf.org
www.liaf.org
Researchers work to translate advances into improved care and diagnosis for Alzheimer's patients.
Fred Jenny, Executive Director
Anna Maria Warmuz, Executive Assistant

874 **Massachusetts Alzheimers Disease Research Center**
Massachusetts ADRC
16th Street
Charlestown, MA 02129
617-726-3987
Fax: 617-724-1480
www.madrc.org
Multi-institutional consortium of Harvard affiliated facilities encompasses five Core units: an Administrative Core a Clinical Core a Database Management and Statistics Core a Neuropathology Core and an Education and Information Transfer Core. The ADRC also supports four specific research projects funded for 3-5 years and annually designates three or four pilot research projects that are funded for 1 year.
John H Growdon, Clinic Director
Bradley T Hyman, Center Director

875 **Medical College of Georgia Alzheimers Research Center**
1120 15th Street
Augusta, GA 30912
706-721-0211
Fax: 706-721-7063
e-mail: jbuccafu@mcg.edu
www.mcg.edu/centers/alz
Clinical and basic research of Alzheimer's disease.
Jerry Buccaf MD, Director
J Warren Beach, Member

876 **Michigan Alzheimer's Disease Research Center**
University of Michigan
2101 Commonwealth Blvd.,
Ann Arbor, MI 48105-0316
734-936-4000
e-mail: sgilman@umich.edu
www.med.umich.edu/alzheimers
Researchers work to translate advances into improved care and diagnosis for Alzheimer's patients.
Sid Gilman MD, Director
Bruno Giordani Ph.D., Core Director

877 **Mount Sinai School of Medicine: Alzheimers Disease Research Center**
Alzheimer's Disease Research Center
One Gustave L Levy Place
New York, NY 10029-6574
212-241-6696
Fax: 212-369-2344
e-mail: mary.sano@mssm.edu
www.mssm.edu
Focuses on Alzheimer's disease research.
Mary Sano, Director
Samuel Gandy, Associate Director

878 **Neurosciences Institute of the Neurosciences Research Program**
The Neurosciences Institute
10640 John Jay Hopkins Drive
San Diego, CA 92121
858-626-2000
Fax: 858-626-2099
e-mail: info@nsi.edu
www.nsi.edu
Nonprofit organization focusing on Alzheimer's and related disorders.
Gerald M Edelman, President

879 **Ohio State University Neuroscience Program**
1835 Neil Avenue
Columbus, OH 43210
614-292-8185
Fax: 614-921-44
www.psy.ohio-state.edu
Specializes in brain disorders such as Alzheimer's disease.
Richard Petty, Chair
Scott Burch, Behavioral Neurosciences Area Assistant

880 **Taub Institute for Research on Alzheimers Disease and the Aging Brain**
630 West 168th Street
New York, NY 10032
212-305-1818
Fax: 212-342-2849
e-mail: taubinstitute@columbia.edu
www.alzheimercenter.org

Researchers work to translate advances into improved care and diagnosis for Alzheimer's patients.
Michael L Shelanski, Co-Director
Richard Mayeux MD, Co-Director

881 The Alzheimer's Disease & Memory Disorders Center
ADMDC
One Baylor Plaza   713-798-5971
Houston, TX 77030   Fax: 713-798-7434
e-mail: neurons@bcm.edu
www.bcm.edu/neurology/admdc
Researchers work to translate advances into improved care and diagnosis for Alzheimer's Disease and other memory disorders.
Eli M Mizrahi, Chair, Department of Neurology
Keith Davis, Department Administrator

882 The Sam and Rose Stein Institute for Research on the Aging
University of California San Diego
9500 Gilman Drive   858-534-6299
La Jolla, CA 92093-0664   Fax: 858-534-5475
e-mail: steininstitute@ucsd.edu
www.sira.ucsd.edu
Research on aging and Alzheimer's disease.
Debra Kaine, Director
Maureen Halp MS, Executive Director

883 University Alzheimer Center University of Alabama at Birmingham
University of Alabama at Birmingham
1530 3rd Avenue S   205-934-4011
Birmingham, AL 35294-1150   800-333-6543
Fax: 205-975-7365
TTY: 205-934-4642
e-mail: adbrain@uab.edu
main.uab.edu
Researchers work to translate advances into improved care and diagnosis for Alzheimer's patients.
Dr. Carol Garrison, President
Kristen N Burdick, Director of Executive Affairs

884 University Alzheimer Center UHC: Case Western Reserve University
12200 Fairhill Road   216-844-6400
Cleveland, OH 44120   Fax: 216-844-6446
e-mail: Kathy.Shaw@Case.Edu
www.ohioalzcenter.org
Researchers work to translate advances into improved care and diagnosis for Alzheimer's patients.
Alan Lerner, Co-Director
Kathleen A Smyth, Administrator

885 University of Chicago Dept of Neurology University of Chicago Hospital
University of Chicago Hospital
5841 S Maryland Avenue   773-702-6390
Chicago, IL 60637-1470   Fax: 773-702-9076
e-mail: cgomez@neurology.bsd.uchicago.edu
neurology.uchicago.edu
Covers Translational Neuroscience Research and research programs in neuroimmunology neuromuscular disease and neurovirology provided the initial foundation and brought national recognition.
Kenneth Goodell, Senior Executive Administrator
Judith Maratea, Administrative Assistant

886 University of Illinois Health Services Research
University of Illinois College of Medicine
1601 Parkview Avenue   815-395-0600
Rockford, IL 61107   Fax: 815-395-5887
e-mail: prrockford@uic.edu
www.uirockford.com
A unit of the University of Illinois College of Medicine at Rockford serves faculty students health care providers human services agencies and other community organizations throughout Illinois with demographic health social and economic data. The skills data and resources available to faculty and students at the college are also available to individuals and organizations needing assistance.
Joann Glacken, Research Support Services

887 University of Maryland: Division of Infectious Diseases
UM Baltimore Department of Medicine
655 West Baltimore Street   410-706-7410
Baltimore, MD 21201   Fax: 410-706-0235
e-mail: rredfield@ihv.umaryland.edu
www.medschool.umaryland.edu
Focuses research on elderly studies including drug use treatments and infectious diseases of the aged.
E. Albert Reece, Vice President
Richard Pierson III MD, Senior Associate Dean for Academic Affai

888 University of Miami: Center on Aging Center on Aging
Center on Aging
1695 NW 9th Avenue   305-355-9080
Miami, FL 33136   Fax: 305-355-9076
e-mail: ajaret@med.miami.edu
centeronaging.med.miami.edu
Focuses on aged disorders such as Alzheimer's research.
Sara J Czaja, Co-Director
Charles B. Nemeroff, M.D., Ph.D, Director

889 Yeshiva University: Resnick Gerontology Center
Albert Einstein College of Medicine
Jack and Pearl Resnick Campus   718-920-6722
Bronx, NY 10467   866-633-8255
Fax: 718-655-9672
e-mail: ljacobs@aecom.yu.edu
www.aecom.yu.edu
Alzheimer's disease and other dementia studies.
Allen M Spiegel MD, Dean
Amy R Ehrlich, Geriatrics Fellowship Program Director

Support Groups & Hotlines

890 Alzheimer's Association Autopsy Assistance Network
Alzheimer s Association
Western/Central Washington Chapter   206-363-5500
Seattle, WA 98125   800-848-7097
Fax: 206-363-5700
e-mail: rowena.rye@alz.org
http://alzwa.org/resources6.htm
The primary purposes of the Autopsy Assistance Network are: to provide families with information regarding autopsy; to assist in obtaining a confirmed diagnosis; provide tissue for Alzheimer's disease research; and establish diagnosis for purpose of clinical and epidemiological studies.
Nancy Dapper, Executive Director
Rowena Rye, Community Resources

891 Alzheimer's Support Group
Columbus Health Rehabilitation Center
2100 Midway Street   812-372-8447
Columbus, IN 47201   Fax: 812-375-5117
www.columbushrc.com/
The skilled Nursing Center includes a separate unit dedicated to the care of residents with Alzheimer's disease and other forms of dementia. The Alzheimer's program is designed to celebrate the spirit of their residents, striving to offer a comfortable and compassionate environment that emphasizes positive life experiences and active involvement in a daily routine.
Mike Spencer, Executive Director

892 National Health Information Center
PO Box 1133   310-565-4167
Washington, DC 20013   800-336-4797
Fax: 301-984-4256
e-mail: info@nhic.org
www.health.gov/nhic
Offers a nationwide information referral service, produces directories and resource guides.

Books

893 36-Hour Day
Hachette Book Group USA

3 Center Plaza
Boston, MA 02108

800-759-0190
Fax: 800-331-1664
e-mail: webmaster@hbgusa.com
www.hachettebookgroup.com

A family guide to caring for persons with Alzheimer's disease, related dementing illnesses, and memory loss later in life.
1999
ISBN: 0-446618-76-2
Nancy L. Mace M.A., Author
Peter V. Rabins M.D., M.P.H., Author

894 Alzheimer Early Stages
Daniel Kuhn MSW, author
Hunter House Publishers
424 Church Street
Nashville, TN 37219

615-255-2665
800-266-5592
Fax: 615-255-5081
e-mail: ordering@hunterhouse.com
www.turnerpublishing.com

First steps in caring and treatments. This book is for family members and friends of those recently diagnosed with Alzheimer's Disase.
288 pages Paperback
ISBN: 0-897933-97-4

895 Alzheimer's Disease
Springer Publishing Company
11 West 42nd Street
New York, NY 10036-3955

212-431-4370
877-687-7476
Fax: 212-941-7842
e-mail: cs@springerpub.com
www.springerpub.com

This volume presents the latest research and findings on Alzheimer's disease.
1996 224 pages Softcover
ISBN: 0-826196-22-5
Annette Imperati, Marketing Director

896 Alzheimer's Disease Orientation Kit
Alzheimer's Association
225 North Michigan Avenue
Chicago, IL 60601-1696

312-335-8700
800-272-3900
Fax: 866-699-1246
TDD: 312-335-5886
e-mail: info@alz.org
www.alz.org

A collection of materials developed to familiarize the audience with Alzheimer's disease and its effects on the patient and family. Includes the Orientation to Alzheimer's Disease videotape, Learning Guide and Caregiver Packet.

897 Alzheimer's Disease: A Guide to Federal Programs
Alzheimer's Disease Education & Referral Center
31 Center Drive
Bethesda, MD 20892-8250

800-438-4380
Fax: 301-495-3334
e-mail: niaic@nia.nih.gov
www.nia.nih.gov/alzheimers

Directory of Alzheimer's disease programs sponsored by federal agencies. Lists agency by agency, it provides locations and telephone numbers for multisite activities and demonstration programs and lists information resources.

898 Alzheimer's Disease: Activity-Focused Care
Butterworth-Heinemann
3255 Bell Helicopter
Fort Worth, TX 76118

817-280-2011
800-366-2665
Fax: 817-280-2321
www.bh.com

Information for professional and family caregivers on activity-focused care for Alzheimer's patients.
436 pages
ISBN: 0-750699-08-6

899 Alzheimer's Disease: Advances in Neurology
Raven Press

1185 Ave of the Americas
New York, NY 10036-2601

212-930-9500
800-777-2295
304 pages
ISBN: 0-781700-81-7

900 Alzheimer's Disease: Questions and Answers
Merit Publishing International
5840 Corporate Way
West Palm Beach, FL 33407

561-697-1116
Fax: 561-477-4961
e-mail: meritpi@aol.com
www.meritpublishing.com

Answers questions about Alzheimer's, explains what it is, how it is diagnosed, causes, and how if affects functions of the brain.
1999
ISBN: 1-873413-52-1
Gene Evans, President
Martin Garrido, VP

901 Alzheimer's Disease: Thesaurus
Alzheimer's Disease Education & Referral Center
31 Center Drive
Bethesda, MD 20892-8250

800-438-4380
Fax: 301-495-3334
e-mail: niaic@nia.nih.gov
www.nia.nih.gov/alzheimers

To help librarians and others to save time and money when searing online for books, journal articles, videos and other materials related to Alzheimer's disease.
140 pages

902 Alzheimer's Disease: Treatment and Family Stress: Directions for Research
Superintendent of Documents
PO Box 371954
Pittsburgh, PA 15250-7954

202-512-2250

Presents a collection of papers giving current information on research investigations that increase the understanding of the nature and consequences of family caregiving.
486 pages

903 Alzheimer's, Stroke and 29 Other Neurological Disorders Sourcebook
Omnigraphics
PO Box 8002
Aston, PA 19014-3993

610-461-3548
800-234-1340
Fax: 610-532-9001
e-mail: customerservice@omnigraphics.com
www.omnigraphics.com

Provides vital information for the nontechnical reader focusing on Alzheimer's disease, stroke and various neurological disorders. Answers thousands of questions related to afflications of the central nervous system with each chapter reviwing a particular disorder and offers in-depth discussions.

ISBN: 0-780806-66-2
Georgiann Lauginiger, Customer Service Manager

904 Care That Works: A Relationship Approach to Persons with Dementia
John's Hopkins University Press
2715 N Charles Street
Baltimore, MD 21218-4319

410-516-6900
800-537-5487
Fax: 410-516-6998
www.press.jhu.edu

Focuses on building and improving the relationship between the caregiver and the person with Alzheimer's.
272 pages
ISBN: 0-801860-26-1
Jitka M. Zgola, Author

905 Care of Alzheimer's Patients: A Manual for Nursing Home Staff
Lisa P Gwyther, author
Alzheimer's Association
225 North Michigan Avenue
Chicago, IL 60601-1696

312-335-8700
800-272-3900
Fax: 866-699-1246
TDD: 312-335-5886
e-mail: info@alz.org
www.alz.org

A care guide for nursing home staff. A useful resource for any caregiver or professional.
122 pages
Lisa P. Gwyther, Author

906 Caregiver Helpbook
Legacy Health System
1015 NW 22nd Avenue   503-413-6778
Portland, OR 97210   Fax: 503-413-6911
                    e-mail: kshannon@lhs.org
                    www.legacyhealth.org
A helpful guide with useful self care tools for family caregivers of frail or ill older adults.
300 pages Paperback
ISBN: 0-937915-54-6
Kathy Shannon, Manager/Caregiver

907 Caring for Alzheimer's Patients: A Guide for Family & Healthcare Providers
Plenum Publishing Corporation
233 Spring Street   212-620-8460
New York, NY 10013-1522   800-221-9369
                    Fax: 212-463-0742
                    e-mail: books@plenum.com
Consists of five organizations that furnish information and resources concerning Alzheimer's Disease support groups and hospitals.
308 pages
ISBN: 0-306431-99-8

908 Complete Guide to Alzheimer's Proofing Your Home
Purdue University Press
509 Harrison Street   765-494-2038
West Lafayette, IN 47907-2025 800-247-6553
                    Fax: 765-496-2442
                    e-mail: pupress@purdue.edu
                    www.thepress.purdue.edu
Guide on how to modify homes of Alzheimer's patients to facilitate caregiving.
496 pages Paperback
ISBN: 1-557532-02-8
Mark Warner, Author

909 Confronting Alzheimer's Disease
American Assoc. of Homes and Services for Aging
2519 Connecticut Ave NW   202-783-2242
Washington, DC 20008-2008   Fax: 202-783-2255
                    www.aahsa.org
A resource for administrators, professional caregivers and families dealing with Alzheimer's disease and related disorders.
225 pages

910 Court-Related Needs of the Elderly and Persons with Disabilities
Commission on the Mentally Disabled
1800 M Street NW   202-331-2240
Washington, DC 20036
Report of the National Conference, examines the barriers of the judicial system impeding access for the elderly and persons with disabilities.

911 Developing Support Groups for Individuals with Early-Stage Alzheimer's Disease
Robyn Yale, author
Health Professions Press
PO Box 10624   410-337-9585
Baltimore, MD 21285-0624   888-337-8808
                    Fax: 410-337-8539
                    www.healthpropress.com
This one-of-a-kind, step-by-step guidebook has been used as a national and international model to meet the needs of people just diagnosed with Alzheimer's disease. Clinical and administrative issues include selecting group participants, training facilitators and managing unique group topics, interactions and dynamics.
256 pages Paperback
ISBN: 1-878812-62-2
Robyn Yale, Author

912 Directory of Alzheimer's Disease Treatment Facilities & Home Health Care
Oryx Press

4041 N Central Avenue   602-265-2651
Phoenix, AZ 85012-3397   800-279-4663
                    www.oryxpress.com
A compilation of 1,500 specialized facilities with day care, residential care, diagnosis and treatment facilities.

913 Ginny: A Love Remembered
Iowa State Press
2121 State Street   515-292-0155
Ames, IA 50014   800-862-6657
                    Fax: 515-292-3348
                    e-mail: orders@iowastatepress.com
                    iowastatepress.com
This book tells the story of midwest cartoonist Bob Artley's life with his beloved wife and their 10 year battle together against Alzheimer's disease, which finally claimed her.
278 pages Hardcover
ISBN: 0-813821-04-5
Brad Nobiling, Credit Manager

914 Hospice Alternative
Harper Collins Publishers/Basic Books
10 E 53rd Street   212-207-7057
New York, NY 10022-5299   800-242-7737
                    Fax: 212-207-7203
An account of the hospice experience. An innovative and humane way of caring for the terminally ill.
256 pages
ISBN: 0-465030-61-0

915 Hospice Care for Patients with Advanced Progressive Dementia
Springer Publishing Company
536 Broadway   212-431-4370
New York, NY 10012   877-687-7476
                    Fax: 212-941-7842
                    e-mail: marketing@springerpub.com
                    www.springerpub.com
Discusses adpating hospice care for terminally ill patients with dementia. Topics include infections, eating difficulties, and providing palliative care.
320 pages Hardcover
ISBN: 0-826111-62-9
Annette Imperati, Marketing Director

916 I'm Just Not Myself Anymore: A Family Guide to Alzheimer's Disease
Northwestern University Press
633 Clark Street   312-503-8649
Evanston, IL 60208-4210   Fax: 847-491-8150
                    e-mail: nupress@nwu.edu
                    www.northwestern.edu
1993 283 pages Paperback
ISBN: 1-880416-72-7

917 Interventions for Alzheimer's Disease: A Caregiver's Complete Reference
Ruth M Tappen, author
Health Professions Press
PO Box 10624   410-337-9585
Baltimore, MD 21285-0624   888-337-8808
                    Fax: 410-337-8539
                    www.healthpropress.com
For professionals who plan, administer or provide services to Alzheimer's patients.
256 pages Paperback
ISBN: 1-878812-39-4

918 Key Elements of Dementia Care
Alzheimer's Association
225 North Michigan Avenue   312-335-8700
Chicago, IL 60601-1696   800-272-3900
                    Fax: 866-699-1246
                    TDD: 312-335-5886
                    e-mail: info@alz.org
                    www.alz.org
Defines, describes, and illustrates dementia-capable care throughout the range of residential care settings.
1997 90 pages

919 Nursing Home and You: Partners in Caring for a Relative with Alzheimer's Disease

American Assn. of Homes & Services for the Aging
901 E Street NW
Washington, DC 20004-2037

202-783-2242
800-508-9442
Fax: 202-783-2255

Offers suggestions for families of nursing home residents on how to work with staff to foster smooth transitions.
32 pages

920 Occupational Therapy Practice Guidelines for Adults with Alzheimer's Disease

American Occupational Therapy Association
4720 Montgomery Lane
Bethesda, MD 20814-1220

301-652-2682
Fax: 240-762-5150
TDD: 800-377-8555
www.aota.org

21 pages
ISBN: 1-569001-46-4

921 Positive Interactions Program of Activities for People with Alzheimer's
Sylvia Nissenboim, author

Health Professions Press
PO Box 10624
Baltimore, MD 21285-0624

410-337-9585
888-337-8808
Fax: 410-337-8539
www.healthpropress.com

All interactions focus on preventing individual dignity and providing opportunities to experience meaningful involvement and satisfaction. Works in a variety of settings and promotes the OBRA quality of care guidelines.
176 pages 1997
ISBN: 1-878812-40-8
Christine Vroman, Editor
Sylvia Nissenboim, Author/Editor

922 Rethinking Alzheimer's Care
Sam Fazio, Dorothy Seman, author

Health Professions Press
PO Box 10624
Baltimore, MD 21285-0624

410-337-9585
888-337-8808
Fax: 410-337-8539
www.healthpropress.com

Appropriate for all settings providing long-term care, adult day services, or assisted living, this fresh and humanistic approach to Alzheimer's care will encourage caregivers to rethink the disease experience and explore its possibilities, instead of its limitations.
200 pages Paperback
ISBN: 1-878812-62-9
Jane Stansell, Editor
Sam Fazio, Author/Editor

923 Speaking Our Minds: Personal Reflections from Individuals with Alzheimer's

WH Freeman and Company
41 Madison Avenue
New York, NY 10010

212-576-9400
888-330-8477
Fax: 212-689-2383
www.macmillanhighered.com/

Personal reflections of people with Alzheimer's disease.
161 pages Hardcover
ISBN: 0-716732-24-6

924 The Comfort of Home for Alheimer's Disease A Guide for Caregivers
M. Meyer, M. Mittelman, P. Derr, C. Epstein, author

CareTrust Publications LLC
PO Box 10283
Portland, OR 97296-0283

800-565-1533
Fax: 415-673-2005
e-mail: sales@comfortofhome.com
www.comfortofhome.com

Walks readers through all Alzheimer's stages and cover the basics from understanding the difference between AD and normal aging, to coping with the behavioral symptoms that come with the diminishing reasoning skills. Additionally, Comfort talks about how to provide safe physical care around other medical conditions the Alzheimer's sufferer may have, due to normal aging. Not the least of all, Comfort provides self-care tips for the caregivers to remain emotionally and mentally healthy.
2008 288 pages
ISBN: 0-978790-30-8

925 Therapeutic Interventions in Alzheimer's

Aspen Publishers
7201 McKinney Circle
Frederick, MD 21705-0990

301-698-7100
800-638-8437
Fax: 301-695-7931
e-mail: customerservice@aspenpub.com
www.aspenpub.com

A program of functional skills for activities of daily living.
197 pages

926 Time for Alzheimer's: A True Story

Emerald Ink Publishing
7141 Office City Drive
Houston, TX 77087-3722

800-324-5663
www.emeraldink.com

Based on the author's personal experience in caring for her mother.
139 pages
ISBN: 1-885373-13-3

927 Understanding Alzheimer's Disease

University Press of Mississippi
3825 Ridgewood Road
Jackson, MS 39211-6492

601-432-6205
800-737-7788
Fax: 601-432-6217
e-mail: press@ihl.state.ms.us
www.upress.state.ms.us

Aimed at people with Alzheimer's, family members, caregivers, health care and human service professionals. Describes Alzheimer's from early to advanced stages. Discusses the care of AD patients, ideas to help families care for the AD patient at home, reviews treatments for the psychiatric, behavioral and cognitive effects of AD and describes research efforts to better understand AD and develop effective therapies. Price $28 Hardcover, $12 Paperback.
1996 150 pages
ISBN: 0-878059-11-3
Neal R. Cutler, M.D., Author
John J. Sramek, Pharm.D., Author

928 When We Become the Parent to Our Parents

MEA Productions
55 Binks Hill Road
Plymouth, NH 03264

603-536-2641
Fax: 603-536-4851
e-mail: mc.allen@juno.com
www.maryemmallen.blogspot.com

Experiences of a woman who cared for her mother and aunt, both Alzheimer's patients.
62 pages
ISBN: 0-965167-51-8
Mary Emma Allen, Author

Children's Books

929 Grandpa Doesn't Know It's Me
Donna Guthrie, author

Alzheimer's Association
225 North Michigan Avenue
Chicago, IL 60601-1696

312-335-8700
800-272-3900
Fax: 866-699-1246
TDD: 312-335-5886
e-mail: info@alz.org
www.alz.org

Geared to the concerns of a young child who has a relative with Alzheimer's disease.
26 pages
Donna Guthrie, Author

930 Grandpa's Music: A Story About Alzheimer's
Alison Acheson, author

Albert Whitman & Company

250 S. Northwest Highway
Park Ridge, IL 60068-2723
847-232-2800
800-255-7675
Fax: 847-581-0039
e-mail: mail@whitmanco.com
www.albertwhitman.com

Children's book using text and illustrations to show the effects of Alzheimer's disease.

ISBN: 0-807530-52-8
Alison Acheson, Author
Joe Campbell, Customer Service

931 Just for Children: Helping You Understand Alzheimer's Disease
Alzheimer's Association
225 North Michigan Avenue
Chicago, IL 60601-1676
312-335-8700
800-272-3900
Fax: 866-699-1246
TDD: 312-335-5886
e-mail: info@alz.org
www.alz.org

Information about Alzheimer's disease written especially for children.
1997 2 pages Pack of 100

932 Let's Talk About When Someone You Love Has Alzheimer's Disease
Rosen Publishing Group's PowerKids Press
29 E 21st Street
New York, NY 10010
212-777-3017
800-237-9932
Fax: 888-436-4643
e-mail: customerservice@rosenpub.com
www.rosenpublishing.com

This book sensitively helps children cope with this unsettling disease.

ISBN: 0-823923-06-1
Elizabeth Weitzman, Author

933 Through Tara's Eyes: Helping Children Cope with Alzheimer's Disease
American Health Assistance Foundation
22512 Gateway Center Dr.
Clarksburg, MD 20871
301-948-3244
800-437-2423
Fax: 301-258-9454
e-mail: info@brightfocus.org
www.brightfocus.org

Told from the perspective of Tara who has a grandmother with Alzheimer's disease but does not know anything is wrong with her grandmother.
36 pages

934 What's Wrong with Grandma? A Family Experience with Alzheimer's
Margaret Shawver, author
Prometheus Books
59 John Glenn Drive
Amherst, NY 14228-2197
716-691-0133
800-421-0351
Fax: 716-691-0137
e-mail: marketing@prometheusbooks.com
www.prometheusbooks.com

The story of a family's struggle with Alzheimer's disease as told by the youngest child.
62 pages Paperback
ISBN: 1-159011-74-2
Margaret Shawver, Author

935 Window of Time
Associated Publishers Group
1501 Country Hospital Rd
Nashville, TN 37218
615-254-2450
800-327-5113
Fax: 615-254-2405
e-mail: vlill@apgbooks.com
www.apgbooks.com

Illustrated book about the relationship between a grandfather with Alzheimer's and his grandson.
28 pages
ISBN: 0-963633-51-1

Magazines

936 Alzheimer Disease and Associated Disorders: An International Journal
Raven Press
1185 Ave of the Americas
New York, NY 10036-2601
212-930-9500
800-777-2295
journals.lww.com

A leading international forum for reports of new research findings and new approaches to diagnosis and treatments. Contributions are offered from all scientific and medical fields.
Quarterly
ISBN: 0-89303H- -
Charles DeCarli, MD, Editor-in-Chief

937 Mature Health
Haymarket Group, Ltd.
45 W 34th Street
New York, NY 10001-3073
212-239-0855

Magazine featuring articles on health aspects of aging, as well as articles on recreation and leisure.

938 Research & Practice
Alzheimer's Association
225 North Michigan Avenue
Chicago, IL 60601-1696
312-335-8700
800-272-3900
Fax: 866-699-1246
TDD: 312-335-5886
e-mail: info@alz.org
www.alz.org

Provides practical information for healthcare professionals on the current status of prominent areas of Alzheimer research.
Quarterly
ISBN: 2-909342-84-0

Newsletters

939 Advances: Progress in Alzheimer Research and Care
Alzheimer's Association
225 North Michigan Avenue
Chicago, IL 60601-1696
312-335-8700
800-272-3900
Fax: 866-699-1246
TDD: 312-335-5886
e-mail: info@alz.org
www.alz.org

Provides information related to research and caregiving.
Quarterly

940 Aging and Alzheimer's Disease Center Newsletter
Oregon Health Sciences University
3181 SW Sam Jackson
Portland, OR 97201-3098
503-494-6976
Fax: 503-494-7499
e-mail: kaye@ohsu.edu
www.ohsu.edu/som-alzheimers

Researches causes and consequences of Alzheimer's disease and ways of clinical services.
2x Year
Jeffrey Kaye, Director

941 Alzheimer Disease and Associated Disorders
Charles Decarli, author
Lippincott Williams & Wilkins
16522 Hunters Green Pkwy
Hagerstown, MD 21740
301-223-2300
800-638-3030
Fax: 301-223-2398
e-mail: orders@lww.com
www.lww.com

A leading international forum for reports of new research findings and new approaches to diagnosis and treatment.
Quarterly Journal
Charles DeCarli MD, Editor

942 Alzheimer's Association: Tarrant County Chapter
2630 West Freeway
Fort Worth, TX 76102
817-336-4949
800-471-4422
Fax: 817-336-4966
e-mail: info@alz.org
www.alz.org/northcentraltexas

Newsletter for those afflicted with Alzheimer's disease. Includes education, support groups, case management, telephone helpline and referral to services (i.e. long term care, adult daycare, medical assistance, legal assistance, etc.).
8 pages
Theresa Hocker, Executive Director
Susanna Luk-Jones, Director Services

943   LIAFLine Newsletter
Long Island Alzheimers Foundation
5 Channel Drive   516-767-6856
Port Washington, NY 11050   Fax: 516-767-6864
                                                    e-mail: info@liaf.org
                                                        www.liaf.org

It is intended for caregivers, service providers and anyone interested in Alzheimer's Disease or the Foundation.
Fred Jenny, Executive Director

Pamphlets

944   10 Warning Signs of Alzheimer's Disease
Alzheimer's Association
225 N Michigan Avenue   312-335-8700
Chicago, IL 60601-7633   800-272-3900
                                                    Fax: 866-699-1246
                                                   TDD: 866-403-3073
                                                   e-mail: info@alz.org
                                                        www.alz.org

Contains a list of symptoms and answers to the most frequently asked questions.
Pack of 100
Harry Johns, President/CEO

945   Alzheimer's Disease
National Institutes of Health
9000 Rockville Pike   301-496-4000
Bethesda, MD 20892-0001   TTY: 301-402-9612
                                          e-mail: NIHinfo@od.nih.gov
                                                        www.nih.gov

Contains information on the diagnosis and treatment of Alzheimer's and on research that offers hope for the future. Included is a list of sources of help for both the patient and the family.

946   Alzheimer's Disease: The Basics
Alzheimer's Association
225 N Michigan Avenue   312-335-8700
Chicago, IL 60601-7633   800-272-3900
                                                    Fax: 866-699-1246
                                                   TDD: 312-335-5886
                                                   e-mail: info@alz.org
                                                        www.alz.org

Symptoms, diagnosis, treatments and more
32 pages
Harry Johns, President/CEO

947   Behaviors
Alzheimer's Association
225 N Michigan Avenue   312-335-8700
Chicago, IL 60601-7633   800-272-3900
                                                    Fax: 866-699-1246
                                                   TDD: 312-335-5886
                                                   e-mail: info@alz.org
                                                        www.alz.org

The most common behaviors and how to manage them.
12 pages
Harry Johns, President/CEO

948   Caregiver Stress
Alzheimer's Association
225 N Michigan Avenue   312-335-8700
Chicago, IL 60601-7633   800-272-3900
                                                    Fax: 866-699-1246
                                                   TDD: 312-335-5886
                                                   e-mail: info@alz.org
                                                        www.alz.org

Symptoms of caregiver stress and ways you can become a healthy caregiver.
6 pages
Harry Johns, President/CEO

949   Caring for Alzheimer's Patients
Human Sciences Press
233 Spring Street   212-620-8000
New York, NY 10013-1522   800-221-9369
This handbook is designed for families, friends, and health-care professionals coping with the myriad of problems encountered by those afflicted with Alzheimer's disease.
308 pages Cloth

950   Dementia Care Practice Recommendations Phases 1 and 2
Alzheimer's Association
225 N Michigan Avenue   312-335-8700
Chicago, IL 60601-7633   800-272-3900
                                                    Fax: 866-699-1246
                                                   TDD: 312-335-5886
                                                   e-mail: info@alz.org
                                                        www.alz.org

Covers fundamentals of dementia care and six key care practice areas: food and fluid consumption, pain management, social engagement, resident wandering, falls and physical restraint-free care.
32 pages
Harry Johns, President/CEO

951   Early-Onset Alzheimer's: I'M Too Young to Have Alzheimer's Disease
Alzheimer's Association
225 N Michigan Avenue   312-335-8700
Chicago, IL 60601-7633   800-272-3900
                                                    Fax: 866-699-1246
                                                   TDD: 312-335-5886
                                                   e-mail: info@alz.org
                                                        www.alz.org

Addresses unique challenges for diagnosed individuals who are younger than 65
12 pages
Harry Johns, President/CEO

952   Early-Stage Alzheimer's: If You Have Alzheimer's Disease What You Should Know
Alzheimer's Association
225 N Michigan Avenue   312-335-8700
Chicago, IL 60601-7633   800-272-3900
                                                    Fax: 866-699-1246
                                                   TDD: 312-335-5886
                                                   e-mail: info@alz.org
                                                        www.alz.org

Coping strategies and tips for living with Alzheimer's
16 pages
Harry Johns, President/CEO

953   Home Safety for People with Alzheimer's Disease
Alzheimer's Disease Education & Referral Center
31 Center Drive   301-495-3311
Bethesda, MD 20892   800-438-4380
                                                    Fax: 301-495-3334
                                          e-mail: adear@nia.nih.gov
                                                        www.nia.nih.gov

For those who provide in-home care for people with Alzheimer's disease or related disorders. The goal is to improve home safety by identifying potential problems in the home and offering possible solutions to help prevent accidents.
32 pages

954   If You Have Alzheimer's Disease: What You Should Know, What You Should Do
Alzheimer's Association
225 North Michigan Avenue
Chicago, IL 60611-1696   800-272-3900
                                                    Fax: 866-699-1246
                                                   TDD: 312-335-8700
                                                   e-mail: media@alz.org
                                                        www.alz.org

Guide for the person with Alzheimer's disease. Includes suggestions of things to do that will help the person cope.
1994 Pack of 100

955   Just for Teens: Helping You Understand Alzheimer's Disease
Alzheimer's Association

225 North Michigan Avenue
Chicago, IL 60611-1696

800-272-3900
Fax: 866-699-1246
TDD: 312-335-8700
e-mail: media@alz.org
www.alz.org

Information about Alzheimer's disease aimed at teenagers.
Pack of 100

956   Late Stage Care
Alzheimer's Association
225 North Michigan Avenue
Chicago, IL 60611-1696

800-272-3900
Fax: 866-699-1246
TDD: 312-335-8700
e-mail: media@alz.org
www.alz.org

Suggestions for coping with caregiving problems that commonly occur late in the progression of Alzheimer's disease.
Pack of 100

957   Legal Plans
Alzheimer's Association
225 N Michigan Avenue
Chicago, IL 60601-7633

312-335-8700
800-272-3900
Fax: 866-699-1246
TDD: 312-335-5886
e-mail: info@alz.org
www.alz.org

Covers legal documents and how to find a lawyer.
16 pages
Harry Johns, President/CEO

958   MedicAlert & Alzheimer's Association Safe Return
Alzheimer's Association
225 N Michigan Avenue
Chicago, IL 60601-7633

312-335-8700
800-272-3900
Fax: 866-699-1246
TDD: 312-335-5886
e-mail: info@alz.org
www.alz.org

Enroll in the nationwide emergency response program that provides help when a person with dementia wanders or has a medical emergency.
1 pages
Harry Johns, President/CEO

959   Money Matters
Alzheimer's Association
225 N Michigan Avenue
Chicago, IL 60601-7633

312-335-8700
800-272-3900
Fax: 866-699-1246
TDD: 312-335-5886
e-mail: info@alz.org
www.alz.org

Identifies care costs and how to pay for them.
28 pages
Harry Johns, President/CEO

960   National Public Policy Program to Conquer Alzheimer's Disease
Alzheimer's Association
225 North Michigan Avenue
Chicago, IL 60611-1676

312-335-8700
800-272-3900
Fax: 866-699-1246
TDD: 312-335-5886
e-mail: info@alz.org
www.alz.org

Summary of the Association's public policy goals, objectives and policies.
1997-Present 12 pages

961   Nutrition Screening Initiative
Nutrition Screening Initiative
2626 Pennsylvania Ave NW
Washington, DC 20037-1618

202-625-1662
e-mail: nsi@gmmb.com
www.cafp.org

Offers information on nutrition pertaining to older Americans and illnesses such as Alzheimer's disease.

962   Partnering with Your Doctor: A Guide for Persons with Memory Problems
Alzheimer's Association
225 N Michigan Avenue
Chicago, IL 60601-7633

312-335-8700
800-272-3900
Fax: 866-699-1246
TDD: 312-335-5886
e-mail: info@alz.org
www.alz.org

Tips on working with your doctor to get the best care.
20 pages
Harry Johns, President/CEO

963   Phase 3: Dementia Care Practice Recommendations
Alzheimer's Association
225 N Michigan Avenue
Chicago, IL 60601-7633

312-335-8700
800-272-3900
Fax: 866-699-1246
TDD: 312-335-5886
e-mail: info@alz.org
www.alz.org

Covers minimizing physical, emotional and spiritual distress; maximizing well-being; snsuring communication with the resident, family and care team.
28 pages
Harry Johns, President/CEO

964   Practice Recommendations for Home Care Professionals
Alzheimer's Association
225 N Michigan Avenue
Chicago, IL 60601-7633

312-335-8700
800-272-3900
Fax: 866-699-1246
TDD: 312-335-5886
e-mail: info@alz.org
www.alz.org

Covers concrete, evidence-based practice suggestions for addressing issues unique to people with dementia living in the community.
68 pages
Harry Johns, President/CEO

965   Report of the Panel on Alzheimer's Disease
National Clearinghouse for Alcohol and Drug Abuse
PO Box 2345
Rockville, MD 20857

800-729-6686
www.health.org

52 pages

966   Respite Care Guide
Alzheimer's Association
225 N Michigan Avenue
Chicago, IL 60601-7633

312-335-8700
800-272-3900
Fax: 866-699-1246
TDD: 312-335-5886
e-mail: info@alz.org
www.alz.org

Find help when you need a break from caregiving.
19 pages
Harry Johns, President/CEO

967   Steps to Diagnosis
Alzheimer's Association
225 North Michigan Avenue
Chicago, IL 60611-1696

800-272-3900
Fax: 866-699-1246
TDD: 312-335-8700
e-mail: media@alz.org
www.alz.org

Educates individuals and their families on the importance of seeking a diagnosis, and the various test completed to obtain an accurate diagnosis.

968   Steps to Enhancing Communication
Alzheimer's Association
225 North Michigan Avenue
Chicago, IL 60611-1696

800-272-3900
Fax: 866-699-1246
TDD: 312-335-8700
e-mail: media@alz.org
www.alz.org

Offers caregivers techniques for improving their approach to listening to and communication with the individual with Alzheimer's disease.
1996 Pack of 100

969 **Tax Credits and Deductions**
Alzheimer's Association
225 N Michigan Avenue 312-335-8700
Chicago, IL 60601-7633 800-272-3900
Fax: 866-669-1246
TDD: 321-335-5886
e-mail: info@alz.org
www.alz.org

Outlines caregiving tax deductions and credits.
3 pages
Harry Johns, President/CEO

970 **Terms & Tips: An Alzheimer Care Handbook**
Marjorie Brandenburg, author
Alzheimer's Association
225 North Michigan Avenue
Chicago, IL 60611-1696 800-272-3900
Fax: 866-699-1246
TDD: 312-335-8700
e-mail: media@alz.org
www.alz.org

Offers an explanation for over 250 terms and offers practical caregiver ideas and tips. Primarily for people with dementia and their caregivers, family members, and all providers of hands-on assistance.
1995 84 pages

971 **Treatments for Alzheimer's Disease**
Alzheimer's Association
225 N Michigan Avenue 312-335-8700
Chicago, IL 60601-7633 800-272-3900
Fax: 866-699-1246
TDD: 312-335-5886
e-mail: info@alz.org
www.alz.org

Information about FDA-approved drugs.
3 pages
Harry Johns, President/CEO

972 **Useful Information on Alzheimer's Disease**
National Clearinghouse for Alcohol and Drug Abuse
PO Box 2345
Rockville, MD 20857-0001 800-729-6686
e-mail: www.webmaster@health.org
www.health.org

24 pages

973 **You Are One of Us: Clergy/Church Connections to Alzheimer Families**
Alzheimer's Disease Education & Referral Center
31 Center Drive 301-495-3311
Bethesda, MD 20892-8250 800-438-4380
Fax: 301-495-3334
e-mail: adear@nia.nih.gov
www.nia.nih.gov/alzheimers
Describes how clergy and church members can help families by including patients and their relatives in church activities, visiting patients and developing church programs that support family caregivers.

Audio & Video

974 **Alzheimer's Association Caregiver Resources**
Alzheimer's Association
225 N. Michigan Ave. 312-335-8700
Chicago, IL 60601 800-848-7097
Fax: 866-699-1246
TDD: 312-335-5886
e-mail: info@alz.org
http://alzwa.org/resources6.htm
A variety of numerous resources, materials and publications providing information for assisting those with Alzheimer's Disease including a documentation guide, informational fact sheets on top-

ics such as bathing, dressing, eating and dealing with grief, in addition resources on long term care options and a newsletter.
Nancy Dapper, Executive Director
Rowena Rye, Community Resources

975 **Alzheimer's Association Dementia Care Conference**
Alzheimer's Association
225 North Michigan Avenue 312-335-5790
Chicago, IL 60601-7633 800-272-3900
Fax: 866-699-1246
TDD: 312-335-8700
e-mail: careconference@alz.org
www.alz.org/careconference/
Selected sessions from the conference discussing topics such as assisted living preconference, sexuality, intimacy and lifestyle changes, and activity intensive changing approaches to Alzheimer care.
Marisol Sukhu, Hotel/Events Information
Sheryl Trotz, Continuing Education & Presentations

976 **Alzheimer's Association Safe Return Police Training Video**
Alzheimer's Association Massachusetts Chapter
225 N. Michigan Ave. 617-868-6718
Chicago, IL 60601 800-548-2111
Fax: 617-868-6720
e-mail: communications@alzmass.org
www.alzmass.org/
An educational package designed to help police officers recognize and respond appropriately to Alzheimer patients who may need assistance. Kit includes 1 videotape and 3 print pieces.
James Wessler, President/Chief Executive Officer
Betsy Fitzgerald, Director of Communications

977 **Alzheimer's Association: Waves of Stone Video and Documentary**
Alzheimer's Association Rhode Island Chapter
245 Waterman Street 401-421-3900
Providence, RI 02906 800-272-3900
Fax: 401-421-0115
e-mail: info@alz.org
http://www.alz-ri.org/Videoshtm.htm
PBS documentary on Alzheimer's disease that discusses both scientific research and caregiver issues.
1994 57 minutes
Elizabeth Morancy, Executive Director
Rita St Pierre, Program Director

978 **Another Home for Mom**
Lori Hope, author
Fanlight Productions
32 Court Street 718-488-8900
Brooklyn, NY 11201-1731 800-876-1710
Fax: 718-488-8642
e-mail: info@fanlight.com
www.fanlight.com
A gentle documentary following one couple as they confront the decision of whether to place the husbands mother, who has Alzheimer's disease, in a nursing home.
1989 27 Minutes
ISBN: 1-572950-77-3

979 **Caring...Sharing: The Alzheimer's Caregiver**
Fanflight Productions
32 Court Street 718-488-8900
Brooklyn, NY 11201 800-876-1710
Fax: 718-488-8642
e-mail: info@fanlight.com
www.fanlight.com
Examines what it means to be a caregiver. This program will be invaluable for any person or group involved in the care of the elderly.
38 minutes
ISBN: 1-572951-22-2
Hal Kirn, Producer

980 **For Those Who Take Care: An Alzheimer's Disease Training Program for Nurses**
Alzheimer's Disease Education & Referral Center

31 Center Drive
Bethesda, MD 20892-8250
301-495-3311
800-438-4380
Fax: 301-495-3334
e-mail: adear@nia.nih.gov
www.nia.nih.gov/alzheimers

Guide for training nursing assistants and nurses' aides in long term care facilities, adult day care and private homes. Manual, text and student handouts. Produced by the University of Kentucky.

Web Sites

981 Alzheimer Research Forum

www.alzforum.org

The web's most dynamic scientific community dedicated to understanding alzheimer's disease and related disorders.

982 Alzheimer Support

www.alzheimersupport.com

Serves Alzheimer's sufferers and their loved ones by reporting the latest news in research and treatment, making hard-to-find, recommended nutritional supplements available at manufacturer-direct low prices, and, most importantly, donating profits from each purchase to fund Alzheimer's medical research.

983 Alzheimer's Association

www.alz.org

The leading, global voluntary health organization in Alzheimer care and support, and the largest private, nonprofit funder of Alzheimer research.

984 Alzheimer's Disease International

www.alz.co.uk/adi

The international federation of 73 Alzheimer associations around the world, in relations with the World Health Organization.

985 Healing Well

www.healingwell.com

A social network and support community for patients, caregivers, and families coping with the daily struggles of diseases, disorders and chronic illness.

986 Health Finder

www.healthfinder.gov

A government website where individuals can find information and tools to help you and those you care about stay healthy.

987 Healthlink USA

www.healthlinkusa.com

Health information concerning treatment, cures, prevention, diagnosis, risk factors, research, support groups, email lists, personal stories and much more. Updated regularly.

988 Helios Health

www.helioshealth.com

Online resource for your health information. Detailed information about specific health topics, access to expert advice from our Medical Advisory Board, and up-to-date health news.

989 MEDLINEplus Health Information

www.nlm.nih.gov/medlineplus

MedlinePlus is the National Institutes of Health's Web site for patients and their families and friends.

990 MedicineNet

www.medicinenet.com

An online resource for consumers providing easy-to-read, authoritative medical and health information.

991 Medscape

www.medscape.com

Medscape offers specialists, primary care physicians, and other health professionals the Web's most robust and integrated medical information and educational tools.

992 Neurology Channel

www.healthcommunities.com

Find clearly explained, medically accurate information regarding conditions, including an overview, symptoms, causes, diagnostic procedures and treatment options. On this site it is possible to ask questions and get information from a neurologist and connect to people who have similar health interests.

993 WebMD

www.webmd.com

Provides credible information, supportive communities, and in-depth reference material about health subjects. A source for original and timely health information as well as material from well known content providers.

Description

994 Amyotrophic Lateral Sclerosis

Amyotrophic Lateral Sclerosis, ALS, also called Lou Gehrig's disease, is a neurological disorder that affects the motor nerves in the brain and spinal cord. The cause of ALS is unknown. It is marked by progressive muscle weakness.

Initial symptoms may be subtle, but early signs of ALS can include twitching and cramping of muscles (particularly in the hands and feet), as well as difficulty in swallowing. As the disorder progresses, use of legs and arms, breathing, speaking, and swallowing become increasingly difficult.

Although the physical symptoms of ALS are most debilitating, the disease does not seem to impair intellectual functioning, although recent research indicates a significant number of people with ALS who have cognitive defects. Voluntary eye movement (blinking) and the senses also remain unaffected.

Currently, there is no cure for ALS. A regime of physical therapy and psychological support can help patients and their families.

National Agencies & Associations

995 ALS Association National Office
1275 K Street NW
Washington, DC 20005

818-880-9007
800-782-4747
Fax: 818-880-9006
e-mail: alsinfo@alsa-national.org
www.alsa.org

National nonprofit voluntary health organization dedicated solely to the fight against amytrophic lateral sclerosis. Its mission: to find a cure for and improve living with ALS. The four fronts of battle are: encouraging identifying funding and monitor
Jane H Gilbert, President/CEO
Lucie Bruijn PhD, Chief Scientist

996 American Association of Neuromuscular & Electrodiagnostic Medicine
2621 Superior Drive NW
Rochester, MN 55901

507-288-0100
Fax: 507-288-1225
e-mail: aanem@aanem.org
www.aanem.org

The American Association of Neuromuscular & Electrodiagnostic Medicine (AANEM) is a nonprofit membership association dedicated to the advancement of neuromuscular, musculoskeletal, and electrodiagnostic medicine.
Vincent J. Tranchitella, MD, President
Shirlyn A. Adkins, JD, Executive Director

997 The International Alliance of ALS/MND Associations
1333 Race St.
Philadelphia, PA 19107

215-568-2462
Fax: 215-543-3366
e-mail: alliance@als-mnd.org
www.alsmndalliance.org

The International Alliance of ALS/MND Associations was founded in 1992 to provide an international community for individual ALS/MND associations from around the world.
Carol Birks, Chairwoman
Rachel Patterson, General Manager

State Agencies & Associations

Arizona

998 Arizona Chapter of the ALS Association
4643 E Thomas Road
Phoenix, AZ 85018

602-297-3800
866-350-2572
Fax: 602-297-3804
e-mail: ken@alsaz.org
webaz.alsa.org

This chapter provides newsletters and other information to help patients and their families find sources of supplies, referrals or counseling as needed. Provides monthly support meetings, public awareness information and fundraising.
Ken Brissa, President
Taryn Norley, Executive Director

California

999 ALS Association: Bay Area Chapter
565 Commercial Street
San Francisco, CA 94111

415-904-2572
800-209-0433
Fax: 415-904-2573
e-mail: fightALS@alsabayarea.org
www.webaz.alsa.org

ALS Association chapters are multifaceted grass roots organizations that carry out ALSA's mission and strategic goals at the community level. The chapter, with supporting services from the national office, actively pursues the association's goals.
Fred Fisher, Executive Director
Madelon M Thomson, Director Patient/Family Services

1000 ALS Association: Greater Los Angeles Chapter
28720 Roadside Drive
Agoura Hills, CA 91301

818-865-8067
866-750-2572
Fax: 818-865-8066
e-mail: webmaster@alsala.org
www.alsala.org

ALS Association chapters are multifaceted grass-roots organizations that carry out ALSA's mission and strategic goals at the community level. The chapter — with supporting services from the National Office — actively pursues the Association's goals.
Cameron Ward, Chairman
Barbara Frova, Vice Chair

1001 ALS Association: Greater Sacramento Chapter
2717 Cottage Way
Sacramento, CA 95825

916-979-9265
Fax: 916-979-9271
e-mail: lou@alssac.org
www.alssac.org

ALS Association chapters are multifaceted grass roots organizations that carry out ALSA's mission and strategic goals at the community level. The chapter, with supporting services from the national office, actively pursues the association's goals.
Scott Ehlen, President
Richard Kline, Vice President

1002 ALS Association: Greater San Diego CIO
7920 Silverton
San Diego, CA 92126-6350

858-271-5547
Fax: 858-271-5687
e-mail: info@alsasd.com
www.alsasd.com

ALS Association chapters are multifaceted grass-roots organizations that carry out ALSA's mission and strategic goals at the community level. The chapter — with supporting services from the National Office — actively pursues the Association's goals.
Jane Mitchell, Chairman
John Fieberg, Vice Chairman

1003 Orange County Chapter of the ALS Association
1232 Village Way
Santa Ana, CA 92705-2334

714-285-1088
Fax: 714-285-0305
e-mail: information@alsaoc.org
weboc.alsa.org

Provides information to ALS patients families and caregivers; offers support groups, information and referrals, a loan closet and public awareness information.
Mark Hershey, President
Chad Kessler, Vice President

Colorado

1004 ALS Association: Rocky Mountain Chapter
7403 Church Ranch Blvd.   303-832-2322
Westminster, CO 80021   866-ALS-3211
                                       Fax: 303-832-3365
                                e-mail: info@alsaco.org
                                       www.alscolorado.org
The ALS Association chapters are multifaceted grass-roots orga-
nizations that carry out ALSA's mission and strategic goals at the
community level. The chapter — with supporting services from the
National Office — actively pursues the Association's goals.
Pam Rush-Negri, Executive Director
Leslie Ryan, Patient Services Director

Connecticut

1005 Connecticut Chapter of the ALS Association
4 Oxford Road   203-874-5050
Milford, CT 06460   877-257-2281
                                       Fax: 203-874-7070
                                e-mail: Lauren@alsact.org
                                       www.alsact.org
The central source in Connecticut for services and education of
ALS patients, families and caregivers. Provides ALS patients with
information concerning medical care and facilities, support
groups, daily living aids and other services.
Lauren D'Alessandro, Executive Director
Chris Capobianco, President

District of Columbia

1006 ALS Association: National Capital Area Chapter
7507 Standish Place   301-978-9855
Rockville, MD 20855   Fax: 301-978-9854
                                e-mail: info@ALSinfo.org
                                       www.alsinfo.org
Offers patient referrals, informational newsletters and brochures,
patient support groups and meetings and fund raising for research
into finding cures and treatments for ALS.
Ronnie Gunnerson, Executive Director
Wilson Krahnke, President

Florida

1007 ALS Association: Florida Chapter
3242 Parkside Center Circle   813-637-9000
Tampa, FL 33619   888-257-1717
                                       Fax: 813-637-9010
                                e-mail: cbright@als-florida.org
                                       webfl.alsa.org
ALS Association chapters are multifaceted grass-roots organiza-
tions that carry out ALSA's mission and strategic goals at the com-
munity level. The chapter — with supporting services from the
National Office — actively pursues the Association's goals.
Nancy Baily, President

1008 ALS Association: Florida Chapter East Coast Regional Office
5005 W Laurel Street   813-637-9000
Tampa, FL 33607   888-257-1717
                                       Fax: 813-637-9010
                                e-mail: office@als-florida.org
                                       webfl.alsa.org
ALS Association chapters are multifaceted grass-roots organiza-
tions that carry out ALSA's mission and strategic goals at the com-
munity level. The chapter — with supporting services from the
National Office — actively pursues the Association's goals.
Nancy Baily, President

Georgia

1009 ALS Association of Georgia
1955 Cliff Valley Way   404-636-9909
Atlanta, GA 30329   888-636-9940
                                       Fax: 404-636-9949
                                e-mail: info@alsaga.org
                                       www.alsaga.org

Offers meetings, local support groups, patient support equipment
loan and research for persons suffering from ALS.
Kent Murphy, Chair
Candace Wood, Executive Director

Illinois

1010 Lois Insolia ALS Center at Northwestern Memorial Hospital
5550 West Touhyu   847-679-3311
Skokie, IL 60077   888-ALS-1107
                                       Fax: 847-679-9109
                                e-mail: info@lesturnerals.org
                                       www.lesturnerals.org
Utilizes a multidisciplinary approach in treating ALS. Trained specialists provide diagnostic, rehabilitative and supportive services
that focus on assessment, care planning and education. Patients
and loved ones are encouraged to attend the support groups offered. Provides in-home visits by ALS nurse consultants and social
worker, support groups, a lending bank of equipment, and grant
programs for financial aid.
Teepu Siddique MD, Director

Indiana

1011 ALS Association: Indiana Chapter
6525 E 82nd Street   317-915-9888
Indianapolis, IN 46250   888-508-3232
                                       Fax: 317-573-9889
                                e-mail: jlewellen@alsaindiana.org
                                       webin.alsa.org
ALS Association chapters are multifaceted grass-roots organiza-
tions that carry out ALSA's mission and strategic goals at the com-
munity level. The chapter — with supporting services from the
National Office — actively pursues the Association's goals.
Melissa Pershing, Executive Director
Abbie Vollmar, Director of Patient Services

Kansas

1012 ALS Association: Keith Worthington Chapter
6950 Squibb Rd   913-648-2062
Mission, KS 66202   800-878-2062
                                       Fax: 913-642-2431
                                e-mail: bcooper@alsa-midwest.org
                                       www.alsa-midwest.org
ALS Association chapters are multifaceted grass-roots organiza-
tions that carry out ALSA's mission and strategic goals at the com-
munity level. The chapter — with supporting services from the
National Office — actively pursues the Association's goals.
Beckie Cooper, Executive Director
Sally Dwyer, Program Director

**1013 ALS Association: Keith Worthington Chapter Central/Western
Kansas Branch**
526 South Market   316-612-0188
Wichita, KS 67202   800-878-2062
                                       Fax: 316-612-8768
                                e-mail: kwille@alsa-midwest.org
                                       www.alsa-midwest.org
ALS Association chapters are multifaceted grass-roots organiza-
tions that carry out ALSA's mission and strategic goals at the com-
munity level. The chapter — with supporting services from the
National Office — actively pursues the Association's goals.
Kathleen Willie, Awareness and Development

Kentucky

1014 ALS Association: Kentucky CIO
2807 Amsterdam Road   85 - 3 - 13
Villa Hills, KY 41017   800-406-7702
                                       Fax: 85 - 3 - 19
                                e-mail: mbacon@alsaky.org
                                       webky.alsa.org
ALS Association chapters are multifaceted grass-roots organiza-
tions that carry out ALSA's mission and strategic goals at the com-
munity level. The chapter — with supporting services from the
National Office — actively pursues the Association's goals.
Mary Bacon, Executive Director
Jennifer Lepa, Administrative Coordinator

Massachusetts

1015 ALS Association: Massachusetts Chapter, Wakefield Office
7 Lincoln Street
Wakefield, MA 01880-3021
781-245-2133
800-258-3323
Fax: 781-245-5414
e-mail: info@als-ma.org
www.webma.alsa.org/site/PageServer?pagen
Offers informational brochures and newsletters to promote public awareness, support groups and meetings for patients and their families, and referral information for members in the Massachusetts area.
Rick J Arrowood

Michigan

1016 ALS Association: Michigan Chapter
24359 Northwestern Highway
Southfield, MI 48075
648-354-6100
800-882-5764
Fax: 248-354-6440
e-mail: sueb@alsofmi.org
www.alsofmichigan.org
ALS Association chapters are multi-faceted grass-roots organizations that carry out ALSA's mission. and strategic goals at the community level. The chapter — with supporting services from the National Office — actively pursues the Association's goals.
Sue Burstein-Kahn, Executive Director
Lisa Alteri, President

1017 ALS Association: West Michigan Chapter
678 Front Street
Grand Rapids, MI 49504
616-459-1900
800-387-7121
Fax: 616-459-4522
e-mail: stacey@alsa-michigan.org
webmi.alsa.org
ALS Association chapters are multi-faceted grass-roots organizations that carry out ALSA's mission. and strategic goals at the community level. The chapter — with supporting services from the National Office — actively pursues the Association's goals.
Stacey Orsted, Executive Director
Katee Stahl, Administrative Assistant

Minnesota

1018 ALS Association: Minnesota Chapter
333 N Washington Avenue
Minneapolis, MN 55401
612-672-0484
888-672-0484
Fax: 612-672-9110
e-mail: info@alsmn.org
webmi.alsa.org
ALS Association chapters are multifaceted grass-roots organizations that carry out ALSA's mission and strategic goals at the community level. The chapter — with supporting services from the National Office — actively pursues the Association's goals.
Sue Spaulding, Executive Director
Sandy Judge, Development Director

Missouri

1019 ALS Association: Keith Worthington Chapter Central Missouri Branch Office
2025 E. Chestnut Expressway
Springfield, MO 65802
417-886-5003
888-386-1200
Fax: 417-886-5003
e-mail: springfield@alsa-midwest.org
www.alsa-midwest.org
ALS Association chapters are multifaceted grass-roots organizations that carry out ALSA's mission and strategic goals at the community level. The chapter — with supporting services from the National Office — actively pursues the Association's goals.
Paul Blackwell, Services Staff
Valerie Gustin, Awareness and Development

1020 ALS Association: St. Louis Regional Chapter
2258 Weldon Parkway
Saint Louis, MO 63146
314-432-7257
888-873-8539
Fax: 314-432-2991
e-mail: mhill@alsastl.org
webstl.alsa.org
A chapter serving the Eastern Missouri and Southern Illinois regions dedicated solely to finding the cause and cure of ALS through research, patient support, information and referrals and public awareness.
Maureen Barber-Hill, President
Richard Palank, Board Chair

Nebraska

1021 ALS Association: Keith Worthington Chapter Nebraska Branch Office
10730 Pacific at Shaker Place
Omaha, NE 68114
402-991-8788
866-762-6361
Fax: 402-991-3690
e-mail: nebraska@alsa-midwest.org
www.alsa-midwest.org
ALS Association chapters are multifaceted grass-roots organizations that carry out ALSA's mission and strategic goals at the community level. The chapter — with supporting services from the National Office — actively pursues the Association's goals.
Shannon Todd, Services Staff
Sherrie Hanneman, Awareness and Development

New Hampshire

1022 ALS Association: Northern New England Chapter
The Champlain Mill
10 Ferry Street
Concord, NH 03301
603-226-8855
866-257-6663
Fax: 603-226-8890
e-mail: executive.director@alsanne.org
www.alsanne.org
ALS Association chapters are multifaceted grass-roots organizations that carry out ALSA's mission and strategic goals at the community level. The chapter — with supporting services from the National Office — actively pursues the Association's goals.
Kathleen L Phillips, Executive Director
Christine Richards, Patient Services Director

New Mexico

1023 ALS Association: New Mexico CIO
PO Box 16495
Albuquerque, NM 87191-6495
505-323-6348
e-mail: als@alsanm.org
www.alsa-nm.org
ALS Association chapters are multifaceted grass-roots organizations that carry out ALSA's mission and strategic goals at the community level. The chapter — with supporting services from the National Office — actively pursues the Association's goals.
Chuck Borgman, President
Terie Baker, Executive Director

New York

1024 ALS Association: Greater New York Chapter
42 Broadway
New York, NY 10004
212-619-1400
800-672-8857
Fax: 212-619-7409
e-mail: als@als-ny.org
www.als-ny.org
ALS Association chapters are multifaceted grass-roots organizations that carry out ALSA's mission and strategic goals at the community level. The chapter — with supporting services from the National Office — actively pursues the Association's goals.
Richard Rose, Chairman
Wendy Schriber, Vice Chairman

1025 ALS Association: Upstate New York CIO
890 7th N Street
Liverpool, NY 13088
315-413-0121
866-499-7257
Fax: 315-413-0508
e-mail: info@alsaupstateny.org
webuny.alsa.org
ALS Association chapters are multifaceted grass-roots organizations that carry out ALSA's mission and strategic goals at the community level. The chapter — with supporting services from the National Office — actively pursues the Association's goals.
Katharine Loomis, Executive Director
Shiann Atuegbu, Patient Services Coordinator

Ohio

1026 ALS Association: Northeast Ohio Chapter
6155 Rockside Road
Independence, OH 44131

216-592-2572
888-592-2572
Fax: 216-592-2575
e-mail: alsa@alsaohio.org
webnoh.alsa.org

Offers telephone consultation services, support groups, caregivers support groups, equipment loan bank and a 24 hour telephone answering service for persons with ALS.
Mary Wilson Wheelock, Executive Director
Fred M DeGrandis, President

1027 ALS Association: Western Ohio Chapter
1170 Old Henderson Road
Columbus, OH 43220

614-273-2572
866-273-2572
Fax: 614-273-2573
e-mail: alsohio@alsohio.org
webcsoh.alsa.org

Offers telephone consultation services, support groups, caregivers support groups, equipment loan bank and a 24 hour telephone answering service for persons with ALS.
Marlin Seymour, Executive Director
Yvonne Dressman, Care Coordinatorÿ

Oregon

1028 ALS Association: Oregon & SW Washington CIO
700 NE Multnomah
Portland, OR 97232

503-238-5559
800-681-9851
Fax: 503-296-5590
e-mail: info@alsa-or.org
webor.alsa.org

The ALS Association chapters are multifaceted grass-roots organizations that carry out ALSA's mission and strategic goals at the community level. The chapter — with supporting services from the National Office — actively pursues the Association's goals.
Lance Christian, Executive Director
Aubrey McCauley, Development Director

Pennsylvania

1029 ALS Association: Greater Philadelphia Chapter
321 Norristown Road
Ambler, PA 19002

215-643-5434
877-434-7441
Fax: 215-643-9307
e-mail: alsassoc@alsphiladelphia.org
www.alsphiladelphia.org

To lead the fight to treat and cure ALS through global research and nationwide advocacy while also empowering people with Lou Gehrig's Disease and their families to live fuller lives by providing them with compassionate care and support.
Joan Borowsky, Development Coordinator
Jeffrey Cline, Chief Development Officerÿ

1030 ALS Association: Western Pennsylvania Chapter
416 Lincoln Avenue
Pittsburgh, PA 15209

412-821-3254
800-967-9296
Fax: 412-821-3549
e-mail: mbernarding@alswp.org
webwpawv.alsa.org

The mission of this chapter is to provide services and education to ALS patients, families and caregivers through medical information, support groups, assisting health care providers and providing communication devices.
Michael Bernarding, Executive Director
Marie Folino, Patient Services Director

South Carolina

1031 ALS Association: Jim (Catfish) Hunter Chapter
120-101 Penmarc Drive
Raleigh, NC 27603

919-755-9001
877-568-4347
Fax: 919-755-0910
e-mail: jerry@catfishchapter.org
www.catfishchapter.org

ALS association chapters are multifaceted grass roots organizations that carry out ALSA's mission and strategic goals at the community level. The chapter, with supporting services from the national office, actively pursues the association's goals.
Jerry Dawson RN BSN, President & CEO
Megan Gardner, Executive Director

Tennessee

1032 ALS Association: Middle Tennessee Chapter
522 E Iris Drive
Nashville, TN 37204

61 - 3 - 55
877-216-5551
Fax: 615-331-5796
e-mail: cheri.sanders@alstn.org
webtn.alsa.org

ALS Association chapters are multifaceted grass-roots organizations that carry out ALSA's mission and strategic goals at the community level. The chapter — with supporting services from the National Office — actively pursues the Association's goals.
Cheri Sanders, Executive Director
Patty Lane, Patient Services Coordinator

Texas

1033 ALS Association: Greater Houston CIO
PO Box 271561
Houston, TX 77277-1561

713-942-2572
866-788-2572
Fax: 218-497-2572
e-mail: linda.richardson@alsa-houston.org
www.alsa-houston.org

ALS Association chapters are multi-faceted grass roots organizations that carry out ALSA's mission and strategic goals at the community level. he chapter — with supporting services from the National Office — actively pursues the Association's goals.
Linda Richardson, President
Georgia Mclain, Patient Services

1034 ALS Association: North Texas Chapter
1231 Greenway Drive
Irving, TX 75038

972-714-0088
877-714-0088
Fax: 972-714-0066
e-mail: a.reid@alsanorthtexas.org
webntx.alsa.org

ALS Association chapters are multi-faceted grass roots organizations that carry out ALSA's mission and strategic goals at the community level. he chapter — with supporting services from the National Office — actively pursues the Association's goals.
David Chayer, Executive Director
Bonnie Walsh, Development Director

1035 ALS Association: South Texas Chapter
8600 Wurzbach
San Antonio, TX 78240

210-733-5204
877-257-4673
Fax: 210-733-5206
e-mail: Information@alsasotx.org
www.alsasotx.org

ALS Association chapters are multi-faceted grass roots organizations that carry out ALSA's mission and strategic goals at the community level. he chapter — with supporting services from the National Office — actively pursues the Association's goals.
Bonnie Walsh, Executive Director
Julia Dyer, Development Associate

Washington

1036 ALS Association: Evergreen Chapter
19115 68th Avenue
Kent, WA 98032

425-656-1650
866-786-7257
Fax: 425-656-1649
e-mail: BeckyMooreED@alsa-ec.org
webwa.alsa.org

The ALS Association chapters are multifaceted grass-roots organizations that carry out ALSA's mission and strategic goals at the community level. The chapter — with supporting services from the National Office — actively pursues the Association's goals.
Rebecca Moore, Executive Director
Sonja Zimmer, Patient Services Director

1037 ALS Association: Oregon & SW Washington CIO
700 NE Multnomah
Portland, OR 97232
503-238-5559
800-681-9851
Fax: 503-296-5590
e-mail: info@alsa-or.org
webor.alsa.org

The ALS Association chapters are multifaceted grass-roots organizations that carry out ALSA's mission and strategic goals at the community level. The chapter — with supporting services from the National Office — actively pursues the Association's goals.
Cindy Burdell, Director
Lance Christian, Executive Director

Wisconsin

1038 ALS Association: Southeast Wisconsin Chapter
2505 N 124th Street
Brookfield, WI 53005
262-784-5257
Fax: 262-784-5260
e-mail: info@alsawi.org
webwi.alsa.org

Begun in 1987 as a support group this chapter is managed by a Board of Directors from all walks of life and disciplines. All members share a dedication to carry out the mission of Hope Through Research and Support Through Caring. The goal is to help ALS
Melanie Roach-Bekos, Executive Director
Linda Lehmann, Office Manager

Research Centers

1039 ALS Center at UCSF
350 Parnassus Avenue
San Francisco, CA 94117
415-353-2108
Fax: 415-353-2524
e-mail: alscenter@ucsf.edu
www.neurology2.ucsf.edu

Research serves as a cornerstone for our patient programs allowing us to translate the most recent advancement in therapies drug development and clinical management into care for our patients.
Catherine Lomen-Hoer, Director
Carolyn Rodriguez, Clinical Coordinator

1040 ALS Clinic at Penn Neurological Institute ALS Association Greater Philadelphia Cha
ALS Association Greater Philadelphia Chapter
321 Norristown Road
Ambler, PA 19002
215-643-5434
Fax: 215-643-9307
e-mail: brenda@alsphiladelphia.org
www.pennhealth.com/als

A multidisciplinary center for the evaluation and treatment of amyotrophic lateral sclerosis (ALS) and related disorders.
Brenda Edelm LCSW BCD, Director of Patient Services
Lauren Elman, Associate Medical Director

1041 ALS Clinical Department of Neurology
College of Medicine of the University of Vermont
89 Beaumont Avenue
Burlington, VT 05405-3456
802-656-2154
Fax: 802-656-8577
e-mail: Rup.Tandan@uvm.edu
www.med.uvm.edu

Clinical care facility for ALS patients.
Daniel Mark Fogel, President
Robert Cioffi, Chair

1042 Center for ALS and Related Diorders The Cleveland Clinic DepartmentOf Neurol
The Cleveland Clinic DepartmentOf Neurology
9500 Euclid Avenue
Cleveland, OH 44195-5227
216-444-5538
800-223-2273
Fax: 216-445-4653
TTY: 216-444-0261
e-mail: andrewd@ccf.org
my.clevelandclinic.org

Clinical care and research facility for ALS patients.
Erik P Pioro, Director
Kathleen M Kelly, ALS Clinical Coordinator

1043 Les Turner Research Laboratory Northwestern University Medical School
Northwestern University Medical School
5550 W Touhy Avenue
Skokie, IL 60077
847-679-3311
888-ALS-1107
Fax: 847-679-9109
e-mail: info@lesturnerals.org
www.lesturnerals.org

Scientists and researchers dedicate their time to discover what causes ALS and find a cure for the disease. The international team of scientists at the Laboratory are internationally recognized for their accomplishments in the field of ALS research.
Harvey Gaffen, President
Wendy Abrams, Executive Director

1044 Mayo Clinic: Department of Neurology
200 First Street SW
Rochester, MN 55905
507-284-2511
Fax: 507-284-0161
TDD: 507-284-9786
www.mayo.edu

Ongoing research and treatment for ALS.
John H Noseworthy MD, President
William C Rupp, MD, Vice President, CEO

1045 Motor Neuron Disease Clinic University of Connecticut Health Center
University of Connecticut Health Center
263 Farmington Avenue
Farmington, CT 06030
860-679-2000
Fax: 860-679-1454
TTY: 860-679-2242
www.uchc.edu

Francisco L. Borges, Chairman
Sanford Cloud Jr., Chair

1046 Motor Neuron Disease Program University of Michigan Health System
University of Michigan Health System
1500 E Medical Center Drive
Ann Arbor, MI 48109-316
734-936-6641
Fax: 734-153-53
www.med.umich.edu

Regional clinic that is dedicated to the diagnosis of Amyotrophic Lateral Sclerosis and improving the well-being of patients who have this disease.
Ora Hirsh Pescovitz MD, Vice President
Douglas L Strong, CEO

1047 Neuromuscular and ALS Center The Clinical Academic Building
The Clinical Academic Building
125 Patterson Street
New Brunswick, NJ 08901
732-235-7331
Fax: 732-235-7344
e-mail: nmalsweb@umdnj.edu
www2.umdnj.edu/nmalsweb

A multidisciplinary program for the diagnosis evaluation and long-term management of a host of neuromuscular diseases found in adults.
Jerry Belsh MD, Director
Annmarie Coyne-West, Patient Care Coordinator

1048 New England Medical Center: ALS Laboratory
800 Washington Street
Boston, MA 02111-1533
617-636-5000
Fax: 617-636-8568
www.tuftsmedicalcenter.org

Specializes in Amyotrophic Lateral Sclerosis research.
Ellen Zane, President, CEO
Margret Vosburgh, Chief Operating Officer

1049 Solomon Park Research Institute
12815 NE 124th Street
Kirkland, WA 98034
425-650-2020
800-470-1817
Fax: 425-650-2028
e-mail: pclapshaw@soloman.org
www.solomon.org

Amyotrophic lateral sclerosis research.
Patric Clapshaw, Director
Sheila Dunagan, Office Manager

1050 Stem Cell Research Program University of Wisconsin-Madison
University of Wisconsin-Madison
1500 Highland Avenue
Madison, WI 53705-2280
608-890-0173
Fax: 608- 26- 526
e-mail: gilbert@waisman.wisc.edu
www.waisman.wisc.edu/scrp

The mission of this program is to understand the molecular mechanisms responsible for the proliferation and differentiation of stem cells and assess their safety and efficacy following transplantation into various disease models.
Jacalyn McHugh, Research Program Manager
Anita Bhattacharyya, Principal Ivestigator

1051 Virginia Mason Medical Center Neuroscience Institute
Virginia Mason Medical Center
1100 9th Avenue   206-341-1900
Seattle, WA 98101   888-862-2737
                                                  www.virginiamason.org

Clinical care and research.
Gary Kaplan, Chairman, CEO

Support Groups & Hotlines

1052 ALS Association Free Standing Support Groups
ALS Association National Office
27001 Agoura Road   818-880-9007
Calabasas Hills, CA 91301-5104   800-782-4747
                                                  Fax: 818-880-9006
                                        e-mail: alsinfo@alsa-national.org
                                                  www.alsa.org
We know of support groups in Alabama, California, Florida, Illinois, New York, Oklahoma, Oregon, Puerto Rico, Utah and Virginia.
Gary Leo, President
Sondi Scheck, VP Operations/Administration

1053 American Society of Human Genetics
9650 Rockville Pike   301-634-7000
Bethesda, MD 20814-3998   Fax: 301-634-7001
                                      e-mail: estrass@genetics.faseb.org
                                                  www.faseb.org
This society will locate a genetic counselor in various areas across the United States for persons with ALS.

1054 Amyotrophic Lateral Sclerosis Toll Free Hotline
ALS Association
27001 Agoura Road   818-880-9007
Calabasas Hills, CA 91301-5104   800-782-4747
                                                  Fax: 818-880-9006
                                        e-mail: alsinfo@alsanational.org
                                                  www.alsa.org
Informs individuals with ALS and their families of services available through the ALS Association.
Gary Leo, President
Sondi Scheck, VP Operations/Administration

1055 Les Turner Amyotrophic Lateral Sclerosis Foundation
5550 West Touhy   847-679-3311
Skokie, IL 60077   888-257-1107
                                                  Fax: 847-679-9109
                                       e-mail: info@lesturnerals.org
                                                  www.lesturnerals.org
Support groups offer patients and family members a chance to not feel alone and frustrated in coping with ALS and offers them the support of professionals as well as others who are experiencing similar problems.
Claire Owen, Director Patient Services

1056 National Health Information Center
PO Box 1133   310-565-4167
Washington, DC 20013   800-336-4797
                                                  Fax: 301-984-4256
                                          e-mail: info@nhic.org
                                                  www.health.gov/nhic
Offers a nationwide information referral service, produces directories and resource guides.

Books

1057 Amyotrophic Lateral Sclerosis: Guide for Patients and Families
Hiroshi Mitsumoto MD, author
Demos Medical Publishing

11 W 42nd Street   212-683-0072
New York, NY 10036   800-532-8663
                                       e-mail: support@demosmedical.com
                                                  www.demosmedpub.com
Covers every aspect of the management of ALS, from clinical features of the disease, to diagnosis, to an overview of symptom management. Major sections deal with medical and rehabilitative management, living with ALS, managing advanced disease, end-of-life issues and resources that can provide support and assistance in this time of need.
450 pages
ISBN: 1-932603-72-7

1058 Complete Bedside Companion: No-Nonsense Advice to Caring for the Seriously Ill
Rodger McFarlane, Philip Bashe, author
Simon & Shuster
1230 Ave of the Americas   212-698-7094
New York, NY 10020   Fax: 212-698-7171
                                        www.simonandschuster.com
Offers warmth, encouragement, and the medical, legal, financial, and emotional advice you need when caring for an ailing loved one.
1999 544 pages
ISBN: 0-684843-19-6

1059 Easy-to-Swallow, Easy-to-Chew Cookbook
Donna L Weihofen, JoAnne Robbins, Paula A Sullivan, author
Wiley Publishers
111 River Street   201-748-6000
Hoboken, NJ 07030-5774   Fax: 201-748-6088
                                          e-mail: info@wiley.com
                                                  www.wiley.com
Presents a collection of more than 150 nutritious recipes that make eating enjoyable and satisfying for anyone who has difficulty chewing or swallowing. Also shares helpful tips and techniques to make eating easier for the elderly and those with such as Parkinson's, AIDS, or head and neck cancers.
256 pages
ISBN: 0-471200-74-1

1060 Journeys with ALS
DLRC Press
PO Box 61661   757-473-1130
Virginia Beach, VA 23466   800-776-0560
                                    e-mail: mary@davidlawrence.com
Compiled by an ALS patient, this book contains 33 first person journeys with ALS. Some are hopeful, some are sad, a few are angry. All are powerful, real-life examples of people doing their best to cope, often with humor and high spirits.
1998
ISBN: 1-880731-58-4

1061 Learning to Fall: the Blessings of an Imperfect Life
Philip Simmons, author
Random House
1745 Broadway
New York, NY 10019   www.randomhouse.com
Philip Simmons was just thirty-five years old in 1993 when he learned that he had ALS, or Lou Gehrig's disease, and was told he had less than five years to live. As a young husband and father, and at the start of a promising literary career, he suddenly had to learn the art of dying. Nine years later, he has succeeded, against the odds, in learning the art of living.
176 pages
Philip Simmons, Author

1062 Life on Wheels: for the Active Wheelchair User
Gary Karp, author
O'Reilly Media
1005 Gravenstein Hwgy N   707-827-7000
Sebastopol, CA 95472   800-998-9938
                                                  Fax: 707-829-0104
                                         e-mail: orders@oreilly.com
                                                  www.oreilly.com
For people who want to take charge of their life experience. Describes medical issues (paralysis, circulation, rehab, cure research); day-to-day living (exercise, skin, bowel and bladder, sexuality, home access, maintaining a wheelchair); and social is-

sues (self-image, adjustement, friends, family, cultural attitudes, activism)
565 pages
ISBN: 1-565922-53-2
Gary Karp, Author

1063 Non Chew Cookbook
Wilson Publishing Company
5708 Nicollet Avenue S
Minneapolis, MN 55419   800-843-2409
                                e-mail: nonchew@excite.com
                                www.nonchewcookbook.com
Soft food recipes good for the whole family.

1064 Realities in Coping with Progressive Neuromuscular Diseases
Charles Press Publishers
2037 Chestnut Street   215-561-2786
Philadelphia, PA 19103   Fax: 215-600-1248
                                e-mail: mail@charlespresspub.com
                                www.charlespresspub.com
Focuses on this fundamental question by bringing together the work of 51 eminent authorities on neurology, nursing, psychology, social work, psychiarty, respiratory therapy, pastoral care and other related disciplines.
248 pages Hardcover only
ISBN: 0-914783-20-3

Newsletters

1065 ALS Today
Les Turner ALS Foundation
5550 West Touhy   847-679-3311
Skokie, IL 60077   888-257-1107
                                Fax: 847-679-9109
                                e-mail: info@lesturnerals.org
                                www.lesturnerals.org
Offers information on clinical trials, medical updates, recipes, resources and support groups available from the foundation.
3 per year

1066 LINK
ALS Association
27001 Agoura Road   818-880-9007
Calabasas Hills, CA 91301-5104   800-782-4747
                                Fax: 818-880-9006
                                e-mail: alsinfo@alsa-national.org
                                www.alsa.org
Offers information on a national level to all patients and chapter members of the ALS Association. Medical updates, loan equipment, resources, hotlines, support groups and news of charity and fundraising events are included as well.

1067 Massachusetts Chapter of the ALS Association Newsletter
Massachusetts Chapter of the ALS Association
315 Norwood Park S.   781-255-8884
Norwood, MA 02062-3021   800-258-3323
                                Fax: 781-255-8811
                                e-mail: info@als-ma.org
                                webma.alsa.org
Offers information on activities, events, charity and fundraising activities, resources and more for members.
BiMonthly
Ginny DelVecchio, President

1068 Peach Lines
ALS Association of Georgia
3795 Manor House Drive   770-642-7962
Marietta, GA 30062-5147
Chapter newsletter offering information on support groups, meetings, hotlines, resources and reviews the newest technology and daily living aids for persons with ALS in the Georgia area.
BiMonthly

1069 Reaching Out
Orange County Chapter of the ALS Association
16787 Beach Boulevard   949-587-9700
Huntington Beach, CA 92647-4848

Offers information on support groups, meetings, charity events, fundraising activities and more for ALS members in the Orange County area.
BiMonthly

1070 South Texas Chapter of the ALS Association Newsletter
8600 Wurzbach Road   210-493-1311
San Antonio, TX 78240   877-714-0088
                                webtx.alsa.org
Offers chapter information on events, charities, memorials, tributes and resources for persons with ALS and their families.
BiMonthly

1071 ALS News & Views
Western Pennsylvania Chapter-ALS Association
1323 Forbes Avenue   412-261-5940
Pittsburgh, PA 15219-4725
Offers information on resources, medical articles, events, charities, fundraising activities and more for patients with ALS, families and caregivers in the western Pennsylvania region.
8 pages BiMonthly
Rita Patchan, Editor

Pamphlets

1072 Basic Home Care for ALS Patients
ALS Association
1275 K Street NW   202-407-8580
Washington, DC 20005   800-782-4747
                                Fax: 202-289-6801
                                e-mail: alsinfo@alsa-national.org
                                www.alsa.org
Provides basic information about home care for people affected by ALS. This booklet is intended as an introductory guide and should be used along with professional medical care from one's physician, nurse and social worker.
Jane H Gilbert, President/CEO

1073 Maintaining Good Nutrition with ALS
ALS Association
1275 K Street NW   202-407-8580
Washington, DC 20005   800-782-4747
                                Fax: 202-289-6801
                                e-mail: alsinfo@alsa-national.org
                                www.alsa.org
Helps people with ALS overcome the obstacles to eating well. Discusses the importance of nutrition to people with ALS and makes suggestions for dealing with various eating problems.
Jane H Gilbert, President/CEO

Audio & Video

1074 Driving Force: A Story of Life
Production House
811 St. John's   847-433-3172
Highland Park, IL 60035   Fax: 847-433-9383
Inspiring video featuring Dr. Frank de Leon Jones, a pychiatrist and ALS patient. Despite his disease and the need for continuous medical ventilation, Dr. de Leon Jones continues his challenging medical practice and physical education responsibilities. This is a film of courage, persistence and love of life. It offers poignant messages for ALS patients, family and caregivers as well as healthcare providers. Available in VHS or DVD.
Howie Samuelson, Executive Director

1075 Living with ALS: Adapting to Breathing Changes/Use of Non Invasive Ventilation
ALS Association
1275 K Street NW   202-407-8580
Washington, DC 20005   800-782-4747
                                Fax: 202-289-6801
                                e-mail: alsinfo@alsa-national.org
                                www.alsa.org
Describes how ALS impacts this vital body function and what can be done to help the person with ALS.
Jane H Gilbert, President/CEO

1076   Living with ALS: Adjusting to Swallowing Difficulties & Good Nutrition
ALS Association
1275 K Street NW   202-407-8580
Washington, DC 20005   800-782-4747
                                               Fax: 202-289-6801
                           e-mail: alsinfo@alsa-national.org
                                                    www.alsa.org
In this video we look at the impact of ALS on swallowing and one's ability to maintain good nutrition. Health care professionals provide guidelines and tips for diet changes and for decision-making regarding a feeding tube; patients and their families share their own experiences and demonstrate their ingenuity in adapting to the changes that weakened swallowing muscles and structures can cause.
2003
Jane H Gilbert, President/CEO

1077   Living with ALS: Communication Solutions & Symptom Management
ALS Association
1275 K Street NW   202-407-8580
Washington, DC 20005   800-782-4747
                                               Fax: 202-289-6801
                           e-mail: alsinfo@alsa-national.org
                                                    www.alsa.org
Companion video to Living with ALS Manual #3 and 5
Jane H Gilbert, President/CEO

1078   Living with ALS: Mobility, Activities of Daily Living, Home Adaptions
ALS Association
1275 K Street NW   202-407-8580
Washington, DC 10005   800-782-4747
                                               Fax: 202-289-6801
                           e-mail: alsinfo@alsa-national.org
                                                    www.alsa.org
This first video, Functioning When Your Mobility is Affected, covers a range of mobility issues that occur with ALS. Our goal is to help you maximize your mobility, independence, safety and comfort. Health care professionals, persons with ALS and their families not only provide information in this video, but also demonstrate equipment and techniques that can help you maximize your function.
Jane H Gilbert, President/CEO

1079   Ventilation: Decision Making Process
Les Turner ALS Foundation
5550 West Touhy   847-679-3311
Skokie, IL 60077   888-257-1107
                                               Fax: 847-679-9109
                                 e-mail: info@lesturnerals.org
                                              www.lesturnerals.org
Designed for ALS patients, their family members and health professionals. Includes interviews with three ventilator dependent ALS patients, family members and the medical staff from Lois Insolia ALS Center at Northwestern University Medical School. Available for loan to ALS patients.
20 Minutes

Web Sites

1080   Healing Well
                                            www.healingwell.com
A social network and support community for patients, caregivers, and families coping with the daily struggles of diseases, disorders and chronic illness.

1081   Health Finder
                                              www.healthfinder.gov
A government web site where individuals can find information and tools to help you and those you care about stay healthy.

1082   Healthlink USA
                                            www.healthlinkusa.com
Health information concerning treatment, cures, prevention, diagnosis, risk factors, research, support groups, email lists, personal stories and much more. Updated regularly.

1083   Helios Health
                                              www.helioshealth.com
Online resource for your health information. Detailed information about specific health topics, access to expert advice from our Medical Advisory Board, and up-to-date health news.

1084   MedWebPlus
                                              www.medwebplus.com
An independently run site related to everything medical and a few things that aren't.

1085   MedicineNet
                                               www.medicinenet.com
An online resource for consumers providing easy-to-read, authoritative medical and health information.

1086   Medscape
                                                 www.medscape.com
Medscape offers specialists, primary care physicians, and other health professionals the Web's most robust and integrated medical information and educational tools.

1087   Neurology Channel
                                           www.healthcommunities.com
Find clearly explained, medically accurate information regarding conditions, including an overview, symptoms, causes, diagnostic procedures and treatment options. On this site it is possible to ask questions and get information from a neurologist and connect to people who have similar health interests.

1088   WebMD
                                                   www.webmd.com
Provides credible information, supportive communities, and in-depth reference material about health subjects. A source for original and timely health information as well as material from well known content providers.

Description

1089 Arthritis

Arthritis is a nonspecific term meaning inflammation of one or more joints. There are over 100 kinds of arthritis, many of them associated with illnesses of other body systems, such as the skin, gut, or liver. Most cases of arthritis are chronic and involve multiple joints. The three most common are rheumatoid arthritis (RA), osteoarthritis (OA), sometimes called degenerative joint disease, and gouty arthritis, or gout. Juvenile Rheumatoid Arthritis (JRA) affects children.

Rheumatoid arthritis may strike either sex at any age, but typically affects women in the early adult years. It is marked by considerable inflammation, commonly of the hands and feet. RA may also involve the knee, elbow, shoulder, ankle and neck, as well as other body systems in addition to the joints. Osteoarthritis tends to occur later in life, related to repeated wear and tear most commonly on weight-bearing joints, such as the hip and knee. Osteoarthritis often occurs earlier in people who have injured their joints in sports. Gout, which typically affects men in midlife, reflects a disorder in the body's metabolism of uric acid. Its most common feature is excruciating pain in the big toe.

Joints affected by arthritis are typically painful, stiff, and swollen. Nonspecific treatment may be used for arthritis of any sort. This includes the nonsteroidal anti-inflammatory drugs (NSAIDs) and aspirin. Steroids can be injected into the knee in OA and be indicated in an oral form for RA. Severe casesof rheumatoid arthritis are generally treated with more specific drugs that attempt to alter the body's immune system. Gouty arthritis responds to drugs that alter the production and metabolism of uric acid. For any kind of arthritis, local application of heat and cold, as well as physical therapy, are often helpful. In certain cases, joint surgery is recommended.

National Agencies & Associations

1090 American Juvenile Arthritis Organization Arthritis Foundation
Arthritis Foundation
PO Box 7669   404-872-7100
Atlanta, GA 30357-0669   800-283-7800
                                         Fax: 404-872-9559
                                  e-mail: help@arthritis.org
                                         www.arthritis.org
A council established by the Arthritis Foundation which serves the special needs of young people with arthritis and their families. Provides information, inspiration and advocacy by identifying the needs of children with arthritis and speaks out on their behalf.
David E Shuey, Chair
John H Klippel MD, President & CEO

1091 Arthritis & Autoimmunity Research Centre (AARC) Foundation
190 Elizabeth Street   416-340-3843
Toronto, Ontario, M5G-2C4   Fax: 416-340-3453
                          e-mail: aarc.foundation@aarcf-uhn.ca
                                       uhn.info@uhn.on.ca
Increase awareness of this large family of diseases, which affects over four million Canadians.
Gerri Grant, Executive Director
Pippa Shaddick, Development Manager

1092 Arthritis Foundation
PO Box 7669   404-872-7100
Atlanta, GA 30335-669   800-283-7800
                                         Fax: 404-872-0457
                                  e-mail: help@arthritis.org
                                         www.arthritis.org
A nonprofit organization that depends on volunteers to provide services to help people with arthritis. Supports research to find ways to cure and prevent arthritis and provides services to improve the quality of life for those affected by arthritis. Provides help through information, referrals, speakers bureaus, forums, self-help courses, and various support groups and programs nationwide.
David E Shuey, Chairman, CEO

1093 Arthritis Society
393 University Avenue   416-979-7228
Toronto Ontario, M5G 1-1E6   800-321-1433
                                         Fax: 416-979-8366
                                     e-mail: info@arthritis.ca
                                         www.arthritis.ca
Promoting evaluating and funding research in the areas of causes prevention treatment and cures of arthritis.
Janet Yale, CEO/President
Derek Rodrigues, Chief Financial Officer (CFO)

1094 Myositis Association
1737 King Street   70 -29 -485
Alexandria, VA 22314   800-821-7356
                                         Fax: 70 -53 -675
                                   e-mail: tma@myositis.org
                                         www.myositis.org
Involves swelling of the muscles. It is an inflammatory myopathies that is a disease of the muscle where there is swelling and loss of muscle.
Bob Goldberg, Executive Director
Theresa R Curry, Communications Manager

1095 National Arthritis and Musculoskeletal & Skin Diseases Information Clearinghouse
National Institutes of Health
31 Center Drive - MSC 2350   301-496-8190
Bethesda, MD 20892-2350   Fax: 301-480-2814
                              e-mail: niamsinfo@mail.nih.gov
                                         www.niams.nih.gov
Our mission is to support research into the causes treatment and prevention of arthritis and musculoskeletal and skin diseases, the training of basic and clinical scientists to carry out this research and the dissemination of information on research programs.
Stephen I Katz MD PhD, Director
Robert H Carter, Deputy Director

1096 National Institute of Arthritis and Musculoskeletal and Skin Disease (NIAMS)
1 AMS Circle   301-495-4484
Bethesda, MD 20892   877-226-4267
                                         Fax: 301-718-6366
                                         TTY: 301-565-2966
                              e-mail: niamsinfo@mail.nih.gov
                                         www.niams.nih.gov
The NIAMS Information Clearinghouse provides information about various forms of arthritis and rheumatic disease and bone, muscle, and skin diseases. It distributes patient and professional education materials and refers people to other sources of information.
Stephen I Katz MD, PhD, Director
Robert H Carter, Deputy Director

State Agencies & Associations

Alabama

1097 Alabama Chapter of the Arthritis Foundation
2700 Hwy 280 E   205-979-5700
Birmingham, AL 35223-3775   800-879-7896
                                         Fax: 205-979-4172
                                 e-mail: info.al@arthritis.org
                                         www.arthritis.org

Founded in 1948 this chapter affects thousands of lives through programs services information and referrals public and professional education and more for residents of Alabama. Research is a great priority of the chapter which supports the advancement
Kristin Whitehurst, Regional VP
Lisa Hemphill, Regional Development Director

Arizona

1098 Arthritis Foundation: Central Arizona Chapter
1313 E. Osborn Road   602-264-7679
Phoenix, AZ 85014   800-477-7679
                                    Fax: 602-264-0563
                              e-mail: info.caz@arthritis.org
                                       www.arthritis.org
A nonprofit health agency serving the needs of Arizona residents with arthritis. This chapter provides arthritis self-help courses, aquatic programs, foundation clubs, a juvenile arthritis parent group, exercise programs and informational brochures.
Warren Rizzo, Chair
Robert Leslie, Vice Chair

Arkansas

1099 Arthritis Foundation: Arkansas Chapter
6213 Father Tribou Street   501-664-7242
Little Rock, AR 72205-3002   800-482-8858
                                    Fax: 501-664-6588
                               e-mail: info.ar@arthritis.org
                                       www.arthritis.org

Carla Davis, Secretary
Diane Denham, VP Finance/Administration

California

1100 Arthritis Foundation: Northern California Chapter
657 Mission Street   415-356-1230
San Francisco, CA 94105-4120   800-464-6240
                                    Fax: 415-356-1240
                              e-mail: info.nca@arthritis.org
                                       www.arthritis.org
Offers research into the causes of arthritis and more effective treatments; serves people in California with arthritis through information and referral services, exercise programs, self-help courses, education and other activities.
PJ Handelhand, President
Deborah Jackson, Senior VP

1101 Arthritis Foundation: San Diego Area Chapter
9089 Clairemont Mesa Boulevard   858-492-1090
San Diego, CA 92123-1288   800-422-8885
                                    Fax: 858-492-9248
                               e-mail: info.sd@arthritis.org
                                       www.arthritis.org
Offers various programs and services including professional seminars, a speakers bureau, public forums, exercise classes, patient and family support groups, arthritis self-help courses and medical research to the residents of the San Diego area living with arthritis.
Veronica Braun, President
Sandra Hayhurst, Director Health Promotion

1102 Arthritis Foundation: Southern California Chapter
800 W 6th Street   323-954-5750
Los Angeles, CA 90017-3775   800-954-2873
                                    Fax: 323-954-5790
                              e-mail: info.sac@arthritis.org
                                       www.arthritis.org

Cynthia Callihan, Administrative Assistant
Christeen Amloian, Assistant Controller

Colorado

1103 Arthritis Foundation: Rocky Mountain Chapter
2280 S Albion Street   303-756-8622
Denver, CO 80222-4906   800-475-6447
                                    Fax: 303-759-4349
                               e-mail: info.rm@arthritis.org
                                       www.arthritis.org

Serves Colorado, Montana, and Wyoming and is dedicated to finding solutions to over 100 forms of arthritis which affect 43 millions of people nationwide.
Kristie Archer, Programs Coordinator
Laura Rosseisen, President

Connecticut

1104 Arthritis Foundation: Southern New England Chapter
35 Cold Spring Road   860-563-1177
Rocky Hill, CT 06067   800-541-8350
                                    Fax: 860-563-6018
                              e-mail: info.sne@arthritis.org
                                       www.arthritis.org
A resource center for persons in Southern New England, Connecticut, Maine and Vermont with arthritis. Offers self-help courses, exercise programs, aquatic programs, Dial-A-Doctor help line, and physician referrals.
Stephen Evangelista, CEO
Gail Campbell, CFO

District of Columbia

1105 Arthritis Foundation: Metropolitan Washington Chapter
2011 Pennsylvania Avenue NW   202-537-6800
Washington, DC 20006   Fax: 202-537-6859
                              e-mail: info.mwa@arthritis.org
                                       www.arthritis.org
The mission of the Arthritis Foundation is to improve lives through leadership in the prevention control and cure of arthritis and related conditions.
Calaneet Balas, President/CEO
Jacquelyn Hair, Director of Operations

Florida

1106 Arthritis Foundation: Florida Chapter, Gulf Coast Branch
3816 W Linebaugh Avenue   813-968-7000
Tampa, FL 33618   800-850-9455
                                    Fax: 941-795-0348
                              e-mail: info.fl.b4@arthritis.org
                                       www.arthritis.org
Dedicated to improving the quality of life for those in the seven county area of Pinellas, Pasco, Citrus, Levy, Hillsborough, Hernando and Polk, who have one or more of over 100 conditions that comprise the disease known as arthritis. Provides patient education and referral services.
Alexa Simpkins, Events Coordinator
Alvi McConahay, Regional Executive Director

Georgia

1107 Arthritis Foundation: Georgia Chapter
2790 Peachtree Road   404-237-8771
Atlanta, GA 30305   800-933-7023
                                    Fax: 404-237-8153
                               e-mail: info.ga@arthritis.org
                                       www.arthritis.org
A statewide health organization dedicated to reducing the devastating effects of arthritis by offering programs for people with arthritis and their families, information and educational services for people with arthritis, medical professionals and the general public.
Andrea Collins, Vice President Mission Delivery
Christina Lennon, VP Resource Development

Illinois

1108 Arthritis Foundation: Greater Chicago Chapter
35 E Wacker Drive   312-372-2080
Chicago, IL 60601   800-795-0096
                                    Fax: 312-372-2081
                               e-mail: info.gc@arthritis.org
                                       www.arthritis.org
Offers self-help courses, wellness workshops, educational seminars, aquatic programs, brochures and publications for persons with arthritis in the state of Illinois.
Roxanne Bartol, Information Systems Coordinator
Tom Fite, President

1109 Arthritis Foundation: Greater Illinois Chapter
2621 N Knoxville Avenue   309-682-6600
Peoria, IL 61604-3623   Fax: 309-682-6732
e-mail: greaterillinois@arthritis.org
www.arthritis.org

Craig Rogers, Area Director

Indiana

1110 Arthritis Foundation: Indiana Chapter
615 N Alabama   317-879-0321
Indianapolis, IN 46204   800-783-2342
Fax: 317-876-5608
e-mail: info.in@arthritis.org
www.arthritis.org

Offers programs and services for the arthritis community of Indiana.
Jenny Conder, Area Vice President
BJ Farrell, Director of Development

Iowa

1111 Arthritis Foundation: Iowa Chapter
2600 72nd Street   515-278-0636
Des Moines, IA 50322-4724   866-378-0636
Fax: 515-278-2603
e-mail: info.ia@arthritis.org
www.arthritis.org

Julie Dalrymple, Program Coordinator
Doyle Monsma CFRE, President/CEO

Kansas

1112 Arthritis Foundation: Kansas Chapter
1999 N Amidon Avenue   316-263-0116
Wichita, KS 67203-2122   800-362-1108
Fax: 316-263-3260
e-mail: info.ks@arthritis.org
www.arthritis.org

Serves 103 counties and is governed by the Volunteer Board of Directors elected from throughout the state. Services offered include water exercise classes, arthritis support groups, children's summer camp, loan closet of hospital equipment and self-help programs.
Dennis Bender, Area VP
Valerie Fairchild, Program Director

Kentucky

1113 Arthritis Foundation: Kentucky Chapter
2908 Brownsboro Road   502-585-1866
Louisville, KY 40206   800-633-5335
Fax: 502-585-1657
e-mail: myoung@arthritis.org
www.arthritis.org

Serves residents of 117 counties in Kentucky and the counties of Floyd and Clark in Indiana. This chapter is a resource center for funding research education programs for health professionals, community education and support services for people with arthritis.
Barbara Perez, President/CEO
Annette Beach, Annual Giving Coordinator

Maryland

1114 Arthritis Foundation: Maryland Chapter
9505 Reisterstown Road   410-654-6570
Owings Mills, MD 21117   800-365-3811
Fax: 410-654-9270
e-mail: info.md@arthritis.org
www.arthritis.org

This chapter supports research both locally and nationally to help find causes better treatments and ways to prevent the many forms of arthritis. Offers various educational booklets and brochures, a referral service for physician referrals, and other support services.
Barbara Newhouse, CEO
Gail Norman, COO

Massachusetts

1115 Arthritis Foundation: Massachusetts Chapter
29 Crafts Street   617-244-1800
Newton, MA 02458-1287   800-766-9449
Fax: 617-558-7686
e-mail: info.ma@arthritis.org
www.arthritis.org

Offers essential information research programs and services for the close to one million Massachusetts residents with arthritis.
Suha Bekdash, Administrative Assistant
Carmen Quinonez, Finance Manager

Michigan

1116 Arthritis Foundation: Michigan Chapter Chapter and Metro Detroit
1050 Wilshire Drive   248-649-2891
Troy, MI 48084-1564   800-968-3030
Fax: 248-649-2895
e-mail: info.mi@arthritis.org
www.arthritis.org

Supports research to prevent, control, and cure arthritis and related diseases. The Foundation also helps improve the lives of people with arthritis and their families by offering self-help classes, exercise programs, support groups, information and referrals.
Mary Sue Langen, Development Manager
Michelle Glazier, President/CEO

Minnesota

1117 Arthritis Foundation: North Central Chapter
1876 Minnehaha Avenue West   651-644-4108
Saint Paul, MN 55104   800-333-1380
Fax: 651-644-4219
e-mail: info.mn@arthritis.org
www.arthritis.org

A nonprofit organization providing programs and services to anyone affected by arthritis in the Minnesota area. Offers aquatic programs support groups juvenile arthritis support groups, research, grants program and information and referrals.
Chris Davis, Community Development Coordinator
Deb Cassidy, Assistant to the President

Mississippi

1118 Arthritis Foundation: Mississippi Chapter
731 Avignon Drive   601-853-7556
Ridgeland, MS 39157   Fax: 601-853-7516
e-mail: cbaker@arthritis.org
www.arthritis.org

Many Mississippians volunteer their services to help the chapter with fund raising and program support. Programs include land and water based exercise classes, and support groups, direct assistance to needy individuals to purchase arthritis medications and services.
Cynthia Baker, Development Specialist
Pamela Snow, Programs~Director

Missouri

1119 Arthritis Foundation: Eastern Missouri Chapter
9433 Olive Boulevard   314-991-9333
Saint Louis, MO 63132   800-406-2491
Fax: 314-991-4020
e-mail: info.emo@arthritis.org
www.arthritis.org

Jan Bignall, Director of Development
Karen Shoulders, Director of Programs

1120 Arthritis Foundation: Western Missouri, Greater Kansas City
1900 W 75th Street   913-262-2233
Prairie Village, KS 66208   888-719-5670
Fax: 91 -26 -228
e-mail: info.wmo@arthritis.org
www.arthritis.org

The only organization in the area representing the National Office in support of its international research program and in providing

services throughout the bi-state area. Offers a wide range of services and programs to deal with the needs of persons with arthritis.
Sherri Hayes, Director of Operations
Alyson Watkins, Special Events Coordinator

Nebraska

1121 Arthritis Foundation: Nebraska Chapter
600 N 93rd Street   402-330-6130
Omaha, NE 68114   800-642-5292
                                     Fax: 402-330-6167
                           e-mail: mpuccioni@arthritis.org
                                       www.arthritis.org
For close to 40 years the Arthritis Foundation has been the source for help and hope to the 263 000 Nebraskans and residents of Pottawattamie County Iowa with arthritis. Provides a wide variety of services designed to help people better cope with arthritis.
Cindy Doerr, Program Director/Editor
Marzia Pucci Shields, Executive Director

New Jersey

1122 Arthritis Foundation: New Jersey Chapter
555 Route 1 South   732-283-4300
Iselin, NJ 08830   888-467-3112
                                     Fax: 732-283-4633
                              e-mail: info.nj@arthritis.org
                                       www.arthritis.org
Offers various programs for the residents of New Jersey including support groups, self-help courses, water exercise and arthritis fitness classes and informational public forums.
Linda Gruskiewicz, President & CEO
Tanya Barbarics, Director

New York

1123 Arthritis Foundation: Central New York Chapter
3300 Monroe Avenue   585-264-1480
Rochester, NY 14618   Fax: 585-264-1517
                             e-mail: info@uny@arthritis.org
                                       www.arthritis.org
Melinda Merante, Executive Director
Nicole Mau, Director

1124 Arthritis Foundation: Long Island Chapter
501 Walt Whitman Road   631-427-8272
Melville, NY 11747-2189   Fax: 631-427-3546
                              e-mail: into.li@arthritis.org
                                       www.arthritis.org
The mission of the Arthritis Foundation is to fund research to find the cause and cures for arthritis and to improve the quality of life for those affected. There is a wide range of programs available for patients.
Patrick T McAsey, President
Roshane Gillespie, Program Secretary

1125 Arthritis Foundation: New York Chapter
122 E 42nd Street   212-984-8700
New York, NY 10168-1898   Fax: 212-878-5960
                              e-mail: nfo.ny@arthritis.org
                                       www.arthritis.org
Offers land exercise programs warm water resources and programs, self-help groups and courses, events and activities video clinics, peer support and a lending library to arthritis sufferers in the New York area.
Suzanne Bliss, President CEO

1126 Arthritis Foundation: Rockland/Orange Unit
Helen Hayes Hospital
Route 9W   845-947-3000
W Haverstraw, NY 10993   Fax: 845-429-9602
                          e-mail: ameyerowitz@arthritis.org
                                       www.arthritis.org
Aviva Meyerowitz, Community Outreach Coordinator
Beatrice Jasanya, Community Outreach Coordinator

North Carolina

1127 Arthritis Foundation: Carolinas Chapter
4530 Park Road   704-529-5166
Charlotte, NC 28209   800-365-3811
                                     Fax: 704-529-0626
                             e-mail: info.car@arthritis.org
                                       www.arthritis.org
Barbara Newhouse, President CEO
Candy Fuller, Community Development Coordinator

Ohio

1128 Arthritis Foundation: Central Ohio Chapter
3740 Ridge Mill Drive   614-876-8200
Hilliard, OH 43026   Fax: 614-876-8363
                             e-mail: info.coh@arthritis.org
                                       www.arthritis.org
Offers information and referral services, self-help courses, aquatics program equipment loans, clinics, home assessment and continuing education to help more than 350,000 people in Central Ohio, including over 5,000 children affected with the 100 types of arthritis
Stephanie Houck, Director of Special Events
David Painter, Director of Outreach

1129 Arthritis Foundation: Northeastern Ohio Chapter
4630 Richmond Road   216-831-7000
Cleveland, OH 44128-5525   800-245-2275
                                     Fax: 216-831-1764
                            e-mail: info.neoh@arthritis.org
                                       www.arthritis.org
Barb Cvelbar, Director of Health Promotion
Cheryl Carter, Director of Development

1130 Arthritis Foundation: Northwestern Ohio Chapter
35 E Wacker Drive   31 -37 -208
Chicago, IL 60601   800-735-0096
                                     Fax: 31 -37 -208
                              e-mail: info.gc@arthritis.org
                                       www.arthritis.org
Tom Fite, CEO

1131 Arthritis Foundation: Ohio River Valley Chapter
7124 Miami Avenue   513-271-4545
Cincinnati, OH 45243   800-383-6843
                                     Fax: 513-271-4703
                             e-mail: info.orv@arthritis.org
                                       www.arthritis.org
Barbara Perez, President/CEO
Edith Nixon, Chair

1132 Arthritis Foundation; Great Lakes Region, Northeastern Ohio
4630 Richmond Road   216-831-7000
Cleveland, OH 44128-5525   800-245-2275
                                     Fax: 216-831-1764
                            e-mail: info.neoh@arthritis.org
                                       www.arthritis.org
Mary L Kudasick, Regional VP

Oklahoma

1133 Arthritis Foundation: Oklahoma Chapter
710 W. Wilshire Blvd   405-936-3366
Oklahoma City, OK 73116   800-627-5486
                                     Fax: 405-936-0617
                              e-mail: info.ok@arthritis.org
                                       www.arthritis.org
Sherri O'Neil, Executive Director
Sherri Harris, Director Special Events

Pennsylvania

1134 Arthritis Foundation: Central Pennsylvania Chapter
3544 North Progress Avenue   717-763-0900
Harrisburg, PA 17110   800-776-0746
                                     Fax: 717-763-0903
                             e-mail: info.cpa@arthritis.org
                                       www.arthritis.org

Serves 28 counties in the central Pennsylvania area. More than 441,233 persons in the chapter area are affected with one of the forms of arthritis seriously enough to require medical care. The chapter offers research services, professional education and training, parent and community services and public health education.
Douglas Knepp, Interim Executive Director

Rhode Island

1135 Arthritis Foundation: Southern New England Chapter
35 Cold Spring Road   860-563-1177
Rocky Hill, CT 06067   800-541-8350
Fax: 860-563-6018
e-mail: info.sne@arthritis.org
www.arthritis.org
Offers programs and services for persons in the Rhode Island area who are living with arthritis.
Stephen Evangelista, CEO
Gail Campbell, CFO

Tennessee

1136 Arthritis Foundation: Southeast Region
421 Great Circle Road   615-254-6795
Nashville, TN 37228   800-454-4662
Fax: 615-254-8316
e-mail: info.tn@arthritis.org
www.arthritis.org
This chapter serves the residents of Tennessee by offering arthritis support through Life Improvement Series Classes, exercise programs, educational programs, free information, public forums and seminars.
David Popen Esq, CEO

Texas

1137 Arthritis Foundation: North Texas Chapter
4300 Macarthur   214-826-4361
Dallas, TX 75209-6524   800-442-6653
Fax: 214-824-5842
e-mail: info.ntx@arthritis.org
www.arthritis.org
With over 1.5 million people in the North Texas Chapter area with arthritis, the chapter's mission is to improve lives through leadership in the prevention, control and cure of arthritis and related diseases.
Carla Brandt, CFO/COO
Jane Hynes, Director Administration/Info Systems

Utah

1138 Arthritis Foundation: Utah/Idaho Chapter
448 E 400 S   801-536-0990
Salt Lake City, UT 84111   800-444-4993
Fax: 801-536-0991
e-mail: info.utid@arthritis.org
www.arthritis.org
A nonprofit organization serving individuals with arthritis and their families in Utah and Idaho by providing invaluable services, programs and activities.
Lisa B Fall, President
Leslie Nelson, Program Director

Vermont

1139 Arthritis Foundation: Northern New England Chapter
6 Chenell Drive   603-224-9322
Concord, NH 03301   800-639-2113
Fax: 603-224-3778
e-mail: info.sne@arthritis.org
www.arthritis.org

Stephen Evangelista, CEO
Margaret Duffy, Regional Program Director

Virginia

1140 Arthritis Foundation: Virginia Chapter
3805 Cutshaw Avenue   804-359-1700
Richmond, VA 23230   800-456-4687
Fax: 804-359-4900
e-mail: info.va@arthritis.org
www.arthritis.org
Founded in 1954 this chapter is a nonprofit voluntary health organization dedicated to finding the cause prevention and cure for the entire group of diseases called arthritis. Offered classes books and information to better manage arthritis.
Angela Courtney, Vice President Community Development
C Annie Magnant, President

Washington

1141 Arthritis Foundation: Washington/Alaska Chapter
3876 Bridge Way N   206-547-2707
Seattle, WA 98103   800-746-1821
Fax: 206-547-2707
e-mail: tzuehl@arthritis.org
www.arthritis.org
Offers arthritis help lines and information lines for residents of Washington state. Provides self-help courses arthritis aquatic programs and resources for persons living with various forms of arthritis.
Barbara Osen, North Puget Sound Branch Director
Kim Mellen, Campaign Coordinator

Wisconsin

1142 Arthritis Foundation: Wisconsin Chapter Foundation
1650 S 108th Street   414-321-3933
W Allis, WI 53214-4021   800-242-9945
Fax: 414-321-0365
e-mail: info@wi@arthritis.org
www.arthritis.org
Statewide programs offered. Including aquatics exercise programs, support groups, self-help courses, professional education, public education seminars, advocacy counsel, juvenile arthritis support programs and children's camp information and referral help.

Libraries & Resource Centers

1143 New York Chapter of the Arthritis Foundation
122 East 42nd Street   212-984-8700
New York, NY 10168-1898   Fax: 212-878-5960
e-mail: info.ny@arthritis.org
www.arthritis.org
Offers people with arthritis, their families and all those with an interest in the rheumatic diseases, information on how to live every day to its fullest, even when affected by a chronic disease.

Research Centers

1144 Affiliated Children's Arthritis Centers of New England
New England Medical Center
750 Washington Street   617-636-7285
Boston, MA 02111-1533   Fax: 617-350-8388
Research organization comprised of a network of 15 territory pediatric centers throughout New England and based at the Floating Hospital of New England Medical Center.
Jane G Schaller MD, Coordinator

1145 Arthritis and Musculoskeletal Center: UAB Shelby Interdisciplinary Biomedical Rese
Shelby Interdisciplinary Biomedical Research Bldg
1825 University Boulevard   205-934-0245
Birmingham, AL 35294-2182   Fax: 205-934-1564
e-mail: rpk@uab.edu
www.main.uab.edu/amc
Arthritis and related rheumatic disorders are studied.
Robert Kimbe MD, Director
Jennifer A Croker, Executive Administrator

1146 Boston University Arthritis Center
580 Harrison Avenue
Boston, MA 02118

617-638-4590
Fax: 617-638-5226
e-mail: mikyork@bu.edu
www.bumc.bu.edu

The research efforts of the Rheumatology Section relate to basic biologic mechanisms in the pathogenesis of scleroderma vasculitis amyloidosis osteoarthritis and systemic lupus erythematosus. There are concordant research efforts in clinical investigation of these disorders including testing of novel therapies.
Karen H Antman, Dean
Paul Monach, Associate Fellowship Program Director

1147 Boston University Medical Campus General Clinical Research Center
72 E Concord Street
Boston, MA 02118

617-638-4542
Fax: 617-638-8890
e-mail: jkopp@bu.edu
www.ctsi.bu.edu

Integral unit of the University Hospital specializing in arthritis and connective tissue studies.
Courtney Alpert, Administrative Coordinator
Janice Kopp, Executive Director

1148 Brigham and Women's Orthopedica and Arthritis Center
Brigham and Women's Hospital
75 Francis Street
Boston, MA 02115

617-732-5500
800-BWH-9999
TTY: 617-732-6458
www.brighamandwomens.org

Research studies into arthritis and rheumatic diseases.
Matthew Lian MD, Director

1149 Central Missouri Regional Arthritis Center Stephen's College Campus
Stephen's College Campus
1205 University Ave
Columbia, MO 65211

573-882-8097
888-702-8818
Fax: 573-884-5509
TDD: 0
e-mail: phelpsam@missouri.edu
marrtc.missouri.edu

Research into arthritis and rheumatic diseases.
Liz ÿ Raine, MPH, CHES,, Health Educator
ÿBeth Richards ,BS,TRS, Director

1150 Department of Pediatrics, Division of Rheumatology
Duke University School of Medicine
T909 Children's Health Center
Durham, NC 27710-1

919-684-6575
Fax: 919-684-6616
rheum.pediatrics.duke.edu

Clinical and laboratory pediatric rheumatoid studies.
Laura Schanberg MD, Cochairman
Egla Rabinovich MD, Co-Chairman

1151 Hahnemann University Hospital, Orthopedic Wellness Center
Hahnemann University Hospital
230 N Broad St
Philadelphia, PA 19102-1511

215-762-7000
Fax: 215-762-8109
www.hahnemannhospital.com

Research activity at Hahnemann University into the areas of arthritis.
Dr. Arnold Berman, Director

1152 Medical University of South Carolina
96 Jonathan Lucas Street
Charleston, SC 29403

843-792-1991
800-424-MUSC
Fax: 843-792-7121
www.muschealth.com

Offers basic and clinical research on various types of arthritis.
Richard M Silver, Division Director/Professor
Gary S Gilkeson, Vice Chairman Research

1153 Medical University of South Carolina: Division of Rheumatology & Immunology
96 Jonathan Lucas Street
Charleston, SC 29403

843-792-1991
Fax: 843-792-7121
www.musc.edu

Offers basic and clinical research on various types of arthritis.
Richard M Silver, Division Director/Professor
Gary S Gilkeson, Vice Chairman Research

1154 Multipurpose Arthritis and Musculoskeletal Disease Center
School of Medicine Rheumatology Division
545 Barnhill Drive
Indianapolis, IN 46202

317- 27- 843
Fax: 317-274-1437
medicine.iupui.edu

The mission of this center is to pursue major biomedical research interests relevant to the rheumatic diseases. Current areas of emphasis include articular cartilage biology pathogenesis and treatment of various forms of amyloidosis the pathogenesis of dermatomyositis and immunologic and biochemical markers of cartilage breakdown and repair.
Bernetta Hartman, Executive Assistant to the Chairman
Martin Friedman, ÿVP Medicine Specialties Division, IUHP

1155 Oklahoma Medical Research Foundation
825 NE 13th Street
Oklahoma City, OK 73104-5005

405-271-6673
800-522-0211
Fax: 405-271-OMRF
e-mail: contact@omrf.org
www.omrf.ouhsc.edu

Focuses on arthritis and muscoloskeletal disease research.
Dr Paul Kincade, Head of OMRF's Immunobiology
Philip M Silverman PhD, Member

1156 Rehabilitation Institute of Chicago
345 E Superior Street
Chicago, IL 60611

312-238-1000
800-354-7342
TTY: 312-238-1059
www.ric.org

Expertise in treating a range of conditions from the most complex conditions including cerebral palsy spinal cord injury stroke and traumatic brain injury to the more common such as arthritis chronic pain and sports injuries.
Edward B Case, Executive Vice President and Chief Finan
Joanne C Smith, President and Chief Executive Officer

1157 Rosalind Russell Medical Research Center for Arthritis at UCSF
350 Parnassus Avenue
San Francisco, CA 94117

415-476-1141
Fax: 415-476-3526
e-mail: rrac@medicine.ucsf.edu
www.rosalindrussellcenter.ucsf.edu

Arthritis research and its probable causes.
Ephraim P Engelman MD, Director
David Wofsy, Associate Director

1158 University of Michigan: Orthopaedic Research Laboratories
University of Michigan Mott Hospital
109 Zina Pitcher Place
Ann Arbor, MI 48109-2200

734-936-7417
Fax: 734-647-0003
www.orl.med.umich.edu

Develops and studies the causes and treatments for arthritis including new devices and assistive aids.
Dr SA Goldstein, Director

1159 Warren Grant Magnuson Clinical Center
National Institute of Health
9000 Rockville Pike
Bethesda, MD 20892

301-496-2563
800-411-1222
Fax: 301-480-9793
TTY: 866-411-1010
e-mail: prpl@mail.cc.nih.gov
www.clinicalcenter.nih.gov

Established in 1953 as the research hospital of the National Institutes of Health. Designed so that patient care facilities are close to research laboratories so new findings of basic and clinical scientists can be quickly applied to the treatment of patients. Upon referral by physicians, patients are admitted to NIH clinical studies.
John Gallin, Director
David Henderson, Deputy Director for Clinical Care

Support Groups & Hotlines

1160 Arthritis Foundation Information Hotline
1330 W. Peachtree Street
Atlanta, GA 30309-0669
404-872-7100
e-mail: contactus@arthritis.org
www.arthritis.org

Offers information and referrals, counseling, physicians information and more to persons living with arthritis.
John H Klippel, President/CEO

1161 Kids on the Block Arthritis Programs
Arthritis Foundation
PO Box 19000
Atlanta, GA 31126-1000
404-872-7100
800-283-7800
Fax: 404-872-0457

State and local programs that use puppetry to help children understand what it is like for children and adults who have arthritis.

1162 National Health Information Center
PO Box 1133
Washington, DC 20013
310-565-4167
800-336-4797
Fax: 301-984-4256
e-mail: info@nhic.org
www.health.gov/nhic

Offers a nationwide information referral service, produces directories and resource guides.

Books

1163 250 Tips for Making Life with Arthritis Easier
Arthritis Foundation Distribution Center
PO Box 6996
Alpharetta, GA 30023-6996
800-207-8633
Fax: 770-442-9742
www.arthritis.com

Learn about helpful services you didn't know were available through you bank, post office, phone company, grocery store, and other businesses you frequent.
88 pages

1164 Arthritis 101: Questions You Have, Answers You Need
Arthritis Foundation Distribution Center
PO Box 6996
Alpharetta, GA 30009-6996
800-207-8633
Fax: 770-442-9742
www.arthritis.com

Expert reviewers answer questions about basic arthritis facts, treatments, research, surgery and more. Also, specific information about six common conditions: rheumatoid arthritis, osteoarthritis, osteoporosis, fibromyalgia, lupus and gout.
144 pages

1165 Arthritis Helpbook: A Tested Self-Management Program for Coping
Kate Lorig and James Fries, author
Da Capo Press
Order Department
Jackson, TN 38301
800-343-4499
Fax: 800-351-5073
www.perseusbooksgroup.com/dacapo

This book teaches people proven techniques to reduce pain and increase dexterity, build a calcium-rich diet and maintain a healthy weight, design an exercise program that matches their needs, find tips and gadgets that solve common problems, overcome fatigue, depression, and other troubling feelings associated with these health issues, and learn about all available arthritis medications and surgeries.
2006 288 pages 6th Edition
ISBN: 0-201409-63-1

1166 Arthritis Self-Help Products
Aids for Arthritis
35 Wakefield Drive
Medford, NJ 08055-3204
609-654-6918
Fax: 609-654-8631
e-mail: aidsforarthritis@gmail.com
www.aidsforarthritis.com

Offers lists of arthritis self-help devices.

1167 Arthritis Self-Management
RA Rapaport Publishing
150 W 22nd Street
New York, NY 10011-2421
212-989-0200
800-234-0923
Fax: 212-989-4786
e-mail: editor@arthritis-self-mgmt.com
www.arthritisselfmanagement.com

Publishes practical, how to information, focusing on the day-to-day and long term aspects of arthritis in a positive and up-beat style. Gives subscribers up-to-date news, facts and advice to help them mai tain their wellness and make informed decisions regarding their health.
48+ pages Bi-Monthly
Christine Martin Grove, Editor
Ingrid Strauch, Editor

1168 Arthritis: What Exercises Work
Dava Sobel, Arthur C Klein, author
MacMillan
175 5th Avenue
New York, NY 10010
212-674-5151
800-221-7945
Fax: 212-420-9314
e-mail: customerservice@mpsvirginia.com
us.macmillan.com

The right exercises for your kind of arthritis, pain-level, age, occupation, and hobbies. The most effective exercises for arthritis available anywhere, supported by medical doctors and backed by the latest research.
200 pages
ISBN: 0-312130-25-1

1169 Arthritis: Your Complete Exercise Guide
Human Kinetics Press
1607 N Market Street
Champaign, IL 61820-5076
217-351-1549
800-873-6759
Fax: 217-351-2674
e-mail: ce@hkusa.com
www.humankinetics.com

1993 152 pages Paperback
ISBN: 0-873223-92-6
Steve Ruhlig, Marketing Director

1170 Bone Up on Arthritis
Arthritis Foundation
PO Box 6996
Alpharetta, GA 30009-6996
800-207-8633
Fax: 770-442-9742
www.arthritis.com

A self-help education packet designed for home-study use, this program can improve your pain and function levels by teaching proven self-help techniques.
w/Audio Tapes

1171 Clinical Care in the Rheumatic Disease
Arthritis Foundation Distribution Center
PO Box 6996
Alpharetta, GA 30023-6996
800-207-8633
Fax: 770-442-9742
www.arthritis.com

This book was written for all health professionals caring for people with rheumatic diseases and for students in these disciplines.
224 pages

1172 Educational Rights for Children with Arthritis: A Parents Manual
AJAO
1314 Spring Street NW
Atlanta, GA 30309-2810
404-872-7100
www.arthritis.org/

A self-instructional manual helping parents to identify and obtain school services needed by their child with arthritis. Covers laws and special services, explores strategies for working with school personnel and stresses good communication and advocacy techniques.

1173 Exercise Beats Arthritis
Bull Publishing Company

PO Box 1377
Boulder, CO 80306

303-545-6350
800-676-2855
Fax: 303-545-6354
www.bullpub.com

Easy-to-follow program will help arthritis sufferers of all ages manage the problems of living with this condition. In depth look at minimizing the pain and limitations of arthritis, keep their joints mobile, increase muscle strength, strengthen bones and ligaments, perform daily tasks more easily.
1998 144 pages
ISBN: 0-923521-45-3
Valerie Sayce, Author
Ian Fraser, Author

1174   Help Yourself Cookbook
Arthritis Foundation
PO Box 6996
Alpharetta, GA 30023-6996

800-207-8633
Fax: 770-442-9742
www.arthritis.com

158 pages

1175   Living With Rheumatoid Arthritis
John's Hopkins University Press
2715 N Charles Street
Baltimore, MD 21218-4319

410-516-6900
800-537-5487
Fax: 410-516-6968
www.press.jhu.edu

This book offers practical and usable answers to the questions of everyday life. The authors provide clear explanations of the causes, diagnosis and treatment of the disease and why medication, joint protection, physical activity and good nutrition are essential components of care.
1993 312 pages Paperback
ISBN: 0-801871-47-6
Tammi L. Shlotzhauer, M.D, Author

1176   Personal Guide to Living Well with Fibromyalgia
Arthritis Foundation Distribution Center
PO Box 6996
Alpharetta, GA 30023-6996

800-207-8633
Fax: 770-442-9742
www.arthritis.com

With this guide you'll learn the latest information about fibromyalgia, what researchers have uncovered about its causes, and an overview of the best treatment options available. Helpful worksheets and tables allow you to manage your condition and document your progress.
224 pages

1177   Primer on the Rheumatic Diseases
John H Klippel, author
Springer Publishing
233 Spring Street
New York, NY 0013

212-460-1500
Fax: 212-460-1575
e-mail: service-ny@springer.com
www.springer.com

Designed to provide up-to-date information about the najor clinical syndromes. One of the most prestigious and comprehensive texts on arthritis and related diseases, including osteoarthritis, rheumatoid arthritis, osteoporosis, lupus, and more than one hundred others.
724 pages
ISBN: 0-387356-64-8
J.H. Klippel, Author
J.H. Stone, Author

1178   Toward Healthy Living: A Wellness Journal
Arthritis Foundation Distribution Center
PO Box 6996
Alpharetta, GA 30023-6996

800-207-8633
Fax: 770-442-9742
www.arthritis.com

This spiral-bound journal has ample pages where you can record your thoughts, plus scales to monitor your mood and pain. Throughout the book you will also find wisdom from a variety of famous and ordinary people - those who live with chronic ilness, and those whose life lessons can help you gain a more positive outlook on daily living.
144 pages

1179   Understanding Juvenile Rheumatoid Arthritis
American Juvenile Arthritis Organization
PO Box 19000
Atlanta, GA 31126-1000

800-283-7800

A manual for health professionals to use in teaching children with JRA and their families about disease management and self-care.
372 pages

1180   We Can: A Guide for Parents of Children with Arthritis
AJAO
1330 W Peachtree Strt NW
Atlanta, GA 30309-2904

404-872-7100
www.arthritis.org/

Offers parents tips for daily living and practical points for helping their child toward independent adulthood.

Children's Books

1181   Arthritis
Franklin Watts Grolier
90 Old Sherman Turnpike
Danbury, CT 06816-0001

203-797-3500
800-621-1115
Fax: 203-797-3197
www.grolier.com

This book offers a clear explanation of the various forms and effects of the disease of arthritis and what treatments are available.
96 pages Grades 7-12
ISBN: 0-531108-01-5

1182   JRA and Me
American Juvenile Arthritis Organization
PO Box 19000
Atlanta, GA 31126-1000

800-283-7800

A workbook for school-aged children who have juvenile arthritis. This book offers a variety of educational games, puzzles and worksheets to teach children about their illness and how to take care of themselves.
57 pages

1183   Living with Arthritis
Franklin Watts Grolier
90 Old Sherman Turnpike
Danbury, CT 06816-0001

203-797-3500
800-621-1115
Fax: 203-797-3197
www.grolier.com

Shows how people with arthritis can overcome their pain and lead productive, full lives.
32 pages Grades 5-7

1184   Yard Sale Coloring Book
American Juvenile Arthritis Organization
PO Box 19000
Atlanta, GA 31126-1000

800-283-7800

A coloring/activity book based on a Kids on the Block script, written for third and fourth grade students. It can be used with Kids on the Block performances, as a stand-alone piece or with a free lesson plan packet.

Magazines

1185   Arthritis Today
Arthritis Foundation
1330 W Peachtree Strt NW
Atlanta, GA 30309-2922

404-872-7100
800-933-0032
Fax: 404-872-9559
www.arthritis.org

The authoritative and respected source of information for persons with arthritis, their families and health professionals who manage their care. As the official magazine of the Arthritis Foundation, it is backed by the Foundation's experience of 44 years and leadership in the fight against arthritis. This magazine gives its readers the advice, information and inspiration they need to live better with arthritis.
Monthly

Newsletters

1186 AJAO Newsletter
American Juvenile Arthritis Organization
1330 W Peachtree Strt NW
Atlanta, GA 31126-2904
404-872-7100
www.arthritis.org/answers
Offers information and updates about the organization's activities
and events. Legislative information, medical updates, camp information and more for children living with arthritis.
Quarterly
Janet Austin MEd, Editor

1187 Arthritis Accent
Arthritis Foundation Southern N.E. Chapter
35 Cold Spring Road
Rocky Hill, CT 06067-3166
860-563-1177
800-541-8350
Fax: 860-563-6018
e-mail: sevangel@arthritis.org
www.arthritis.org
Information on chapter events and activities.
Quarterly

1188 Arthritis Foundation of Illinois
Greater Chicago Chapter
35 E Wacker Drive
Chicago, IL 60601
312-372-2080
800-735-0096
Fax: 312-372-2081
e-mail: info.gc@arthritis.org
www.arthritis.org
Illinois serves the 2,511,000 adults and 13,100 children affected
by arthritis in the area.
Marilynn J Cason, Chairman

1189 Arthritis Foundation: Newsletter of Nebraska Chapter
600 North 93rd Street
Omaha, NE 68114
402-330-6130
800-642-5292
Fax: 402-330-6167
e-mail: mpuccioni@arthritis.org
www.arthritis.org
Contains information on research, medication, different types of
arthritis and features on oustanding volunteers.
3x Year
Cindy Doerr, Program Director/Editor

1190 Arthritis Foundation: Southern Arizona Chapter
6464 E Grant Road
Tucson, AZ 85715
520-290-9090
800-444-5426
Offers updated information and news on chapter activities and
events for persons with arthritis.
Monthly
Richard M Brown EdD, CFRE, President

1191 Arthritis News
Arthritis Foundation - WI Chapter
10427 W Lincoln Avenue
West Allis, WI 53227
414-321-3933
800-333-1380
Fax: 414-321-0365
e-mail: info.wi@arthritis.org
www.arthritis.org
Offers information on activities, events, medical research, information and referrals to persons living in the Wisconsin area that are
afflicted with arthritis.
Quarterly
Judy Haugsland, CEO

1192 Arthritis Observer
Rocky Mountain Chapter of the Arthritis Foundation
2280 S Albion Street
Denver, CO 80222-4906
303-756-8622
888-391-9389
Fax: 303-759-4349
e-mail: info.m@arthritis.org
www.arthritis.org
Offers chapter information and educational programs to the community as well as updates on fund-raising events, resources, publications and medical updates for the arthritis community.
Quarterly

1193 Arthritis Reporter
New York Chapter of the Arthritis Foundation

122 E 42nd Street
New York, NY 10168-0002
212-984-8700
Fax: 212-878-5960
e-mail: IMontecino@arthritis.org
www.arthritis.org
Chapter newsletter offering information on upcoming events, ac-
tivities and groups for the arthritis community.
Quarterly
Ingrid Montecino, President and CEO

1194 Arthritis Update of Rhode Island
Arthritis Foundation Rhode Island Office
Airport Office Park
Warwick, RI 02886
401-739-3773
Fax: 401-739-8990
e-mail: sevangel@arthritis.org
www.arthritis.org
Offers information, activities, events and updates on the chapter.
Quarterly
Stephen Evangelista, Chief Executive Officer
Gail Campbell, Chief Financial Officer

1195 Arthritis Volunteer
Tennessee Chapter of the Arthritis Foundation
1719 W End Avenue
Nashville, TN 37203-5123
615-320-7626
Fax: 615-329-3982
Keeps members up-to-date on arthritis developments and on pro-
grams, services and special events in Tennessee.
Quarterly

1196 Factor Fax
Arthritis Foundation: Northeast California Chapter
3040 Explorer Drive
Sacramento, CA 95827
916-368-5599
800-571-3456
Fax: 916-368-5596
e-mail: info.neca@arthritis.org
www.arthritis.org
Offers information on all of the chapter's activites, events and resources for the arthritis community of central California.
Patrick Dunlap, VP Events/Programs/Services
Edward Kelley, Motion Coordinator

1197 Focus
Arthritis Foundation: Central Ohio Chapter
3740 Ridge Mill Drive
Hilliard, OH 43026-9231
614-876-8200
Fax: 614-876-8363
www.arthritis.org
Offers updated information on arthritis as well as news of the ser-
vices and activities of the chapter.
Quarterly
Irene Baird, President

1198 Health Points
TyH Publications
12005 Saguaro Blvd
Fountain Hills, AZ 85268
480-837-7590
800-801-1406
e-mail: customerservice@e-tyh.com
www.e-tyh.com
National newsletter with articles on complementary therapy, latest
nutrition news, disability issues and much more. Focus is on
fibromyalgia, chronic fatigue, arthritis and chronic pain.
Quarterly

1199 News Across Our Horizons
Northern & Southern New England Chapter
35 Cold Spring Road
Rocky Hill, CT 06060
860-563-1177
800-541-8350
Fax: 860-563-6018
e-mail: info.sne@arthritis.org
www.arthritis.org
Chapter newsletter offering information on programs, activities
and events of the foundation, medical and research articles and resources for persons with arthritis.

1200 Newsletter of the Central Pennsylvania Chapter
Central Pennsylvania Chapter/Arthritis Foundation
Foster Plaza #11
Pittsburgh, PA 15220-5459
412-566-1645
800-776-0746
Fax: 412-539-1182
e-mail: info.cpa@arthritis.org
www.arthritis.org

Offers information on activities and events of the Chapter.
Quarterly

1201 Spectrum
Michigan Chapter of the Arthritis Foundation
1050 Wilshire Drive   248-649-2891
Troy, MI 48084-1564   800-968-3030
                                  Fax: 248-649-2895
                          e-mail: info.mi@arthritis.org
                                      www.arthritis.org
Promotes various activities and programs and provides current information about arthritis.

1202 Volunteer Voice
Kentucky Chapter of the Arthritis Foundation
410 W Chestnut Street   502-893-9771
Louisville, KY 40202-2368   800-633-5335
Newsletter offering information and updates on chapter activities, events, camps, juvenile programs and government/legislative information.

Pamphlets

1203 Americans with Disabilities Act Resource Manual
Arthritis Foundation
PO Box 7669   404-872-7100
Atlanta, GA 30357-0669   800-283-7800
                                  Fax: 404-872-0457

1204 Ankylosing Spondylitis
Arthritis Foundation
PO Box 7669   404-872-7100
Atlanta, GA 30357-0669   800-283-7800
                                  Fax: 404-872-0457

1205 Arthritis Answers: Basic Information About Arthritis
Arthritis Foundation
PO Box 7669   404-872-7100
Atlanta, GA 30357-0669   800-283-7800
                                  Fax: 404-872-0457

1206 Arthritis Foundation Services
Arthritis Foundation
PO Box 7669   404-872-7100
Atlanta, GA 30357-0669   800-283-7800
                                  Fax: 404-872-0457

1207 Arthritis Information: Advocacy and Government Affairs
Arthritis Foundation
PO Box 7669   404-872-7100
Atlanta, GA 30357-0669   800-283-7800
                                  Fax: 404-872-0457

1208 Arthritis Information: Children
Arthritis Foundation
PO Box 7669   404-872-7100
Atlanta, GA 30357-0669   800-283-7800
                                  Fax: 404-872-0457
List of materials for children with arthritis, their families and the health professionals who care for them.

1209 Arthritis and Diet Information Package
NAMSIC/National Institutes of Health
1 AMS Circle   301-495-4484
Bethesda, MD 20892-0001   877-226-4267
                                  Fax: 301-718-6366
                                  TTY: 301-565-2966
                     e-mail: niamsinfo@mail.nih.gov
                                      www.nih.gov/niams/
Offers information on nutrition and diet pertaining to the arthritis community.
16 pages

1210 Arthritis and Employment: You Can Get the Job You Want
Arthritis Foundation
1330 W Peachtree Strt NW   404-872-7100
Atlanta, GA 30309-0669   800-283-7800
                                  Fax: 404-872-0457
                                      www.arthritis.org
Free brochures offered by Arthritis Foundation.

1211 Arthritis and Inflammatory Bowel Disease
Arthritis Foundation
PO Box 7669   404-872-7100
Atlanta, GA 30357-0669   800-283-7800
                                  Fax: 404-872-0457

1212 Arthritis and Pregnancy
Arthritis Foundation
1330 W Peachtree Strt NW   404-872-7100
Atlanta, GA 30309-0669   800-283-7800
                                  Fax: 404-872-0457
                                      www.arthritis.org
How arthritis affects pregnancy, managing pregnancy and a new baby.
Mary Anne Dunkin, Writer

1213 Arthritis and Vocational Rehabilitation
Arthritis Foundation
2970 Peachtree Road NW   404-237-8771
Atlanta, GA 30305   800-933-7023
                                  Fax: 404-237-8153
                          e-mail: info.ga@arthritis.org
                                      www.arthritis.org

1214 Arthritis in Children Information Package
NAMSIC/National Institutes of Health
1 AMS Circle   301-495-4484
Bethesda, MD 20892-0001   877-226-4267
                                  Fax: 301-718-6366
                                  TTY: 301-565-2966
                     e-mail: niamsinfo@mail.nih.gov
                                      www.nih.gov/niams/

1215 Arthritis in Children and La Artritis Infantojuvenil
American Juvenile Arthritis Organization
PO Box 19000
Atlanta, GA 31126-1000   800-283-7800
A medical information booklet about juvenile rheumatoid arthritis. This booklet is written for parents or other adults and includes details about different forms of JRA, medications, therapies and coping issues.

1216 Arthritis on the Job: You Can Work With It
Arthritis Foundation
PO Box 7669   404-872-7100
Atlanta, GA 30357-0669   800-283-7800
                                  Fax: 404-872-0457

1217 Arthritis: Do You Know?
Arthritis Foundation
PO Box 7669   404-872-7100
Atlanta, GA 30357-0669   800-283-7800
                                  Fax: 404-872-0457
A brief overview of arthritis and the services of the Arthritis Foundation.

1218 Aspirin and Other Nonsteroidal Anti-Inflamatory Drugs
Arthritis Foundation
8600 Rockville Pike   404-872-7100
Bethesda, MD 20894-0669   888-346-3656
                                  Fax: 404-872-0457
                        e-mail: info@ncbi.nlm.nih.gov
                                      www.ncbi.nlm.nih.gov
A book on hypersensitivity to aspirin and other non steroidal anti-inflammatory drugs (NSAIDs) manifestation.
AL1 de Weck, Author
PM Gamboa, Author

1219 Back Pain
Arthritis Foundation
PO Box 7669   404-872-7100
Atlanta, GA 30357-0669   800-283-7800
                                  Fax: 404-872-0457

1220 Behcet's Disease
Arthritis Foundation
1330 W Peachtree Strt NW   404-872-7100
Atlanta, GA 30309-0669   800-283-7800
                                  Fax: 404-872-0457
                                      www.arthritis.org

Beh‡et's disease, also called Beh‡et's syndrome, is a rare disorder that causes seemingly unrelated symptoms in different parts of the body, including mouth sores, genital sores, eye inflammation, and skin rashes and lesions.

1221 Bursitis, Tendionitis and Other Soft Tissue Rheumatic Syndromes
Arthritis Foundation
PO Box 7669   404-872-7100
Atlanta, GA 30357-0669   800-283-7800
                                Fax: 404-872-0457

1222 CPPD Crystal Deposition Disease
Arthritis Foundation
1330 W Peachtree Strt NW   404-872-7100
Atlanta, GA 30309-0669   800-283-7800
                                Fax: 404-872-0457
                                www.arthritis.org
Calcium pyrophosphate dihydrate crystal deposition disease (CPPD) occurs when these crystals form deposits in the joint and surrounding tissues.

1223 Corticosteriod Medications
Arthritis Foundation
1330 W Peachtree Strt NW   404-872-7100
Atlanta, GA 30309-0669   800-283-7800
                                Fax: 404-872-0457
                                www.arthritis.org
Corticosteroids (glucocorticoids) are medications that mimic the effects of the hormone cortisol, which helps reduce inflammation in the body.

1224 Diet and Arthritis
Arthritis Foundation
PO Box 7669   404-872-7100
Atlanta, GA 30357-0669   800-283-7800
                                Fax: 404-872-0457

1225 Ehlers-Danlos Syndrome
Arthritis Foundation
1330 W Peachtree Strt NW   404-872-7100
Atlanta, GA 30309-0669   800-283-7800
                                Fax: 404-872-0457
                                www.arthritis.org
Ehlers-Danlos syndrome (EDS) is a collection of genetic disorders that affect connective tissue.

1226 Exercise and Your Arthritis
Arthritis Foundation
PO Box 7669   404-872-7100
Atlanta, GA 30357-0669   800-283-7800
                                Fax: 404-872-0457
Types of exercise for people with arthritis and how to do them.

1227 Family
Arthritis Foundation
PO Box 7669   404-872-7100
Atlanta, GA 30357-0669   800-283-7800
                                Fax: 404-872-0457
Effects of arthritis on family life and ways to cope.

1228 Family: Making the Difference
Arthritis Foundation
PO Box 7669   404-872-7100
Atlanta, GA 30357-0669   800-283-7800
                                Fax: 404-872-0457

1229 Gold Treatment
Arthritis Foundation
PO Box 7669   404-872-7100
Atlanta, GA 30357-0669   800-283-7800
                                Fax: 404-872-0457

1230 Gout
Arthritis Foundation
1330 W Peachtree Strt NW   404-872-7100
Atlanta, GA 30309-0669   800-283-7800
                                Fax: 404-872-0457
                                www.arthritis.org
Gout is a form of inflammatory arthritis that develops in some people who have high levels of uric acid in the blood.

1231 Guide to Effective Volunteer Lobbying
Arthritis Foundation
PO Box 7669   404-872-7100
Atlanta, GA 30357-0669   800-283-7800
                                Fax: 404-872-0457

1232 Health, Life and Disability Insurance for People with Arthritis
Arthritis Foundation
PO Box 7669   404-872-7100
Atlanta, GA 30357-0669   800-283-7800
                                Fax: 404-872-0457
Information about these three types of insurance.

1233 Hydroxychloroquine
Arthritis Foundation
PO Box 7669   404-872-7100
Atlanta, GA 30357-0669   800-283-7800
                                Fax: 404-872-0457

1234 Individuals with Arthritis
Mainstream
1030 5th Street NW   202-898-1400
Washington, DC 20001-2504
Mainstreaming individuals with arthritis into the workplace.
12 pages

1235 Juvenile Dermatomyositis
Arthritis Foundation
1330 W Peachtree Strt NW   404-872-7100
Atlanta, GA 30309-0669   800-283-7800
                                Fax: 404-872-0457
                                www.arthritis.org
Juvenile dermatomyositis (JDM) is an inflammatory disease that causes muscle weakness and a skin rash on the eyelids and knuckles.

1236 Living and Loving: Information About Sexuality and Intimacy
Arthritis Foundation
PO Box 7669   404-872-7100
Atlanta, GA 30357-0669   800-283-7800
                                Fax: 404-872-0457

1237 Managing Your Activities
Arthritis Foundation
PO Box 7669   404-872-7100
Atlanta, GA 30357-0669   800-283-7800
                                Fax: 404-872-0457

1238 Managing Your Fatigue
Arthritis Foundation
PO Box 7669   404-872-7100
Atlanta, GA 30357-0669   800-283-7800
                                Fax: 404-872-0457

1239 Managing Your Health Care
Arthritis Foundation
PO Box 7669   404-872-7100
Atlanta, GA 30357-0669   800-283-7800
                                Fax: 404-872-0457

1240 Managing Your Pain
Arthritis Foundation
1330 W Peachtree Strt NW   404-872-7100
Atlanta, GA 30309-0669   800-283-7800
                                Fax: 404-872-0457
                                www.arthritis.org
Complimentary health lecture by Arthiritis Foundation.

1241 Managing Your Stress
Arthritis Foundation
1330 W Peachtree Strt NW   404-872-7100
Atlanta, GA 30309-0669   800-283-7800
                                Fax: 404-872-0457
                                www.arthritis.org
Complimentary health lecture by Arthiritis Foundation.

1242 Methotrexate
Arthritis Foundation
1330 W Peachtree Strt NW   404-872-7100
Atlanta, GA 30309-0669   800-283-7800
                                Fax: 404-872-0457
                                www.arthritis.org

Methotrexate is one of the most effective and widely used medications for treating rheumatoid arthritis (RA).

1243 Myositis
Arthritis Foundation
1330 W Peachtree Strt NW
Atlanta, GA 30309-0669
404-872-7100
800-283-7800
Fax: 404-872-0457
www.arthritis.org
Myositis is a term meaning inflammation in the muscles. There are several types of myositis, the most common being polymyositis and dermatomyositis.

1244 Osteoarthritis
Arthritis Foundation
1330 W Peachtree Strt NW
Atlanta, GA 30309-0669
404-872-7100
800-283-7800
Fax: 404-872-0457
www.arthritis.org
Osteoarthritis (OA) is the most common chronic condition of the joints.

1245 Osteonecrosis
Arthritis Foundation
1330 W Peachtree Strt NW
Atlanta, GA 30309-0669
404-872-7100
800-283-7800
Fax: 404-872-0457
www.arthritis.org
Osteoporosis drugs called bisphosphonates have been linked with the development of osteonecrosis (bone death) in the jaw.

1246 Overcoming Rheumatoid Arthritis
Michigan Chapter of the Arthritis Foundation
1050 Wilshire Drive
Troy, MI 48084-1564
248-649-2891
800-968-3030
Fax: 248-649-2895
e-mail: info.mi@arthritis.org
www.arthritis.org
Provides extensive information about the disease and treatment, with an emphasis on what you can do for yourself.

1247 Penicillamine
Arthritis Foundation
PO Box 7669
Atlanta, GA 30357-0669
404-872-7100
800-283-7800
Fax: 404-872-0457

1248 Polyarteritis Nodosa and Wegener's Granulomatosis
Arthritis Foundation
PO Box 7669
Atlanta, GA 30357-0669
404-872-7100
800-283-7800
Fax: 404-872-0457

1249 Polymyalgia Rheumatica and Giant Cell Arthritis
Arthritis Foundation
PO Box 7669
Atlanta, GA 30357-0669
404-872-7100
800-283-7800
Fax: 404-872-0457

1250 Pseudoxanthoma Elasticum Fact Sheet
Arthritis Foundation
PO Box 7669
Atlanta, GA 30357-0669
404-872-7100
800-283-7800
Fax: 404-872-0457

1251 Psoriatic Arthritis Information Package
NAMSIC/National Institutes of Health
1 AMS Circle
Bethesda, MD 20892-0001
301-495-4484
877-226-4267
Fax: 301-718-6366
TTY: 301-565-2966
e-mail: niamsinfo@mail.nih.gov
www.nih.gov/niams/

1252 Q&A's About Arthritis and Rheumatic Disease
NIH/National Institutes of Health
1 AMS Circle
Bethesda, MD 20892-0001
301-495-4484
877-226-4267
Fax: 301-718-6366
TTY: 301-565-2969
e-mail: niamsinfo@mail.nih.gov
www.nih.gov/niams

This pamphlet offers information, technical articles and research on arthritis and related disorders. Also included are referral organizations to help patients uncover more information.

1253 Reflex Sympathetic Dystrophy Syndrome Fact Sheet
Arthritis Foundation
PO Box 7669
Atlanta, GA 30357-0669
404-872-7100
800-283-7800
Fax: 404-872-0457
www.arthritis.org
Reactive arthritis is an inflammatory type of arthritis which affects the joints, and may affect the eyes, skin and urinary tract (bladder, vagina, urethra).

1254 Reiter's Syndrome
Arthritis Foundation
1330 W Peachtree Strt NW
Atlanta, GA 30309-0669
404-872-7100
800-283-7800
Fax: 404-872-0457

1255 Rheumatoid Arthritis Information Package
NAMSIC/National Institutes of Health
1 AMS Circle
Bethesda, MD 20892-0001
301-495-4484
877-226-4267
Fax: 301-718-6366
TTY: 301-565-2966
e-mail: niamsinfo@mail.nih.gov
www.nih.gov/niams
Offers an introduction and definition of rheumatoid arthritis, treatments, causes, objectives, daily living, resources and medical information.

1256 Surgery: Information to Consider
Arthritis Foundation
PO Box 7669
Atlanta, GA 30357-0669
404-872-7100
800-283-7800
Fax: 404-872-0457

1257 Thinking About Tomorrow: A Career Guide for Teens with Arthritis
Arthritis Foundation
PO Box 7669
Atlanta, GA 30357-0669
404-872-7100
800-283-7800
Fax: 404-872-0457

1258 When Your Student Has Arthritis: A Guide for Teachers
Arthritis Foundation
PO Box 7669
Atlanta, GA 30357-0669
404-872-7100
800-283-7800
Fax: 404-872-0457
A medical information booklet written for teachers or other adults who have arthritis. The booklet describes different forms of juvenile arthritis, how arthritis might affect the child at school, and how to help the child work around these problems.

Audio & Video

1259 FIT Video
Arthritis Foundation
550 Pharr Road
Altlanta, GA 30023-6996
404-237-8771
800-933-7023
Fax: 404-237-8153
e-mail: info.ga@arthritis.org
www.arthritis.org

1260 In Control
Arthritis Foundation
1330 W Peachtree Strt NW
Atlanta, GA 30309-2922
404-872-7100
800-283-7800
Fax: 404-872-0457
An excellent at-home program which includes video, audio cassettes and the Arthritis Helpbook. Provides tools to help meet the challenges of arthritis.

1261 PACE I
Arthritis Foundation
PO Box 6996
Alpharetta, GA 30023-6996
800-207-8633

1262 PACE II
Arthritis Foundation
PO Box 6996
Alpharetta, GA 30023-6996   800-207-8633
                                         Fax: 770-442-9742
                                         www.arthritis.com

1263 Pathways to Better Living
Arthritis Foundation
PO Box 6996
Alpharetta, GA 30023-6996   800-207-8633
                                         Fax: 770-442-9742
                                         www.arthritis.com

1264 Pool Exercise Program
Arthritis Foundation Distribution Center
PO Box 6996
Alpharetta, GA 30023-6996   800-207-8633
                                         Fax: 770-442-9742
                                         www.arthritis.com

This video features water exercises that will help you increase and maintain joint flexibility, strengthen and tone muscles, and increase endurance. All exercises are performed in water at chest level. No swimming skills are necessary.

Web Sites

1265 American Juvenile Arthritis Organization
                                         www.arthritis.com
Serves the special needs of young people with arthritis and their families. Provides information, inspiration and advocacy.

1266 Arthritis Foundation
                                         www.arthritis.org
Provide services to help through information, referrals, speakers bureaus, forums, self-help courses, and various support groups and programs nationwide.

1267 Healing Well
                                         www.healingwell.com
An online health resource guide to medical news, chat, information and articles, newsgroups and message boards, books, disease-related web sites, medical directories, and more for patients, friends, and family coping with disabling diseases, disorders, or chronic illnesses.

1268 Health Finder
                                         www.healthfinder.gov
Searchable, carefully developed web site offering information on over 1000 topics. Developed by the US Department of Health and Human Services, the site can be used in both English and Spanish.

1269 Healthlink USA
                                         www.healthlinkusa.com
Health information concerning treatment, cures, prevention, diagnosis, risk factors, research, support groups, email lists, personal stories and much more. Updated regularly.

1270 Helios Health
                                         www.helioshealth.com
Online resource for your health information. Detailed information about specific health topics, access to expert advice from our Medical Advisory Board, and up-to-date health news.

1271 MedicineNet
                                         www.medicinenet.com
An online resource for consumers providing easy-to-read, authoritative medical and health information.

1272 Medscape
                                         www.medscape.com
Medscape offers specialists, primary care physicians, and other health professionals the Web's most robust and integrated medical information and educational tools.

1273 National Arthritis & Musculoskeletal & Skin Diseases Information Clearinghouse
                                         www.niams.nih.gov
The mission of the National Institute of Arthritis and Musculoskeletal and Skin Diseases is to support research into the causes, treatment, and prevention of arthritis and musculoskeletal and skin diseases; the training of basic and clinical scientists to carry out this research; and the dissemination of information on research progress in these diseases.

1274 WebMD
                                         www.webmd.com
Provides credible information, supportive communities, and in-depth reference material about health subjects. A source for original and timely health information as well as material from well known content providers.

Description

1275 Asthma

Asthma is a respiratory disorder that causes shortness of breath, wheezing, coughing and chest tightness. About 12 million people in the U.S. have asthma, and its incidence is increasing. It is the leading cause of hospitalization for children; however, some children with asthma will outgrow the disorder by the time they are teenagers or adults. Asthma ranges from mild illness to life-threatening episodes.

Numerous environmental factors trigger an asthma attack including allergies, infections, exercise, cold weather and stress. Treatment consists of avoiding or minimizing factors that cause an asthma attack, for example pet dander and pollen.

In addition, several medications are used to relieve asthma symptoms by opening lung airways, known as bronchodilation. Many of these drugs can be inhaled so that they work directly on the lungs. Inhaled steroids may be used for long-term control. Research and new therapies are being directed at trying to find medications that will prevent asthma from occurring. See also *Lung Disease*.

National Agencies & Associations

1276 Allergy & Asthma Network Mothers of Asthmatics
2751 Prosperity Avenue   703-641-9595
Fairfax, VA 22031   800-878-4403
Fax: 30 -40 -298
e-mail: info@aanma.org
www.breatherville.org
A national nonprofit network of families with a desire to overcome allergies and asthma by producing the most accurate timely practical and livable alternatives to suffering.
Nancy Sander, Founder/President
Hiwote Aberra, Database/Member Services Coordinator

1277 American Academy of Allergy, Asthma & Immunology
555 East Wells Street   414-272-6071
Milwaukee, WI 53202-3823   800-822-2762
Fax: 414-272-6070
e-mail: info@aaaai.org
www.aaaai.org
Strives to serve the public through information on asthma and allergies, as well as referrals to allergists. Also offers pollen and mold statistics from the Committee on Pollen & Molds.
Thomas B Casale, Executive Vice President
Kay A Walen, Executive Director

1278 American Lung Association
1301 Pennsylvania Avenue NW   202-785-3355
Washington, DC 20004   800-LUN-GUSA
Fax: 202-452-1805
e-mail: info@lungusa.org
www.lungusa.org
The mission of the American Lung Association is to prevent lung disease and promote lung health. Founded in 1904 to fight tuberculosis, the American Lung Association today fights disease in all its forms, with special emphasis on asthma, tobacco control and environmental health.
Charles Dean O'Conner, President, CEO
Don Awerkamp, Director

1279 Association of Birth Defect Children Birth Defect Research for Children
800 Celebration Avenue   407-566-8304
Celebration, FL 34747   Fax: 407-566-8341
e-mail: staff@birthdefects.org
www.birthdefects.org
Non-profit organization that provides parents and expectant parents with information about birth defects and support services for their children. Sponsors the National Birth Defect Registry, a research project that studies associations between birth defects and genetics.
Betty Mekdeci, Executive Director
John Bragg, Administrative Assistant

1280 Asthma Society of Canada
124 Merton Street   416-787-4050
Toronto, Ontario, M4S 2-6K1   866-787-4050
Fax: 416-787-5807
e-mail: info@asthma.ca
www.asthma.ca
A national registered healthcare charity, operating within a civil society business structure.
Dr. Robert Oliphant, President, CEO
Zhen Liu, Office Manager

1281 Asthma and Allergy Information Association
8201 Coprorate Drive   202-466-7643
Lanover, MD 20785   800-727-8462
Fax: 202-466-8940
e-mail: info@aafa.org
www.aafa.org
A not-for-profit organization, is the leading patient organization for people with asthma and allergies, and the oldest asthma and allergy patient group in the world. AAFA provides practical information, community based services and support through a national network of chapters and support groups. AAFA develops health education, organizes state and national advocacy efforts and funds research to find better treatments and cures.
Christopher Cole, Chair

1282 National Advisory Allergic and Infectious Disease Council
6610 Rockledge Drive   301-496-2644
Bethesda, MD 20892-6612   866-284-4107
Fax: 301-402-7123
TDD: 800-877-8339
e-mail: ocpostoffice@niaid.nih.gov
www.niaid.nih.gov/Pages/default.aspx
The National Institute of Allergy and Infectious Diseases (NIAID) conducts and supports basic and applied research to better understand treat and ultimately prevent infectious immunologic and allergic diseases.
Anthony S Fauci MD, Director
H Clifford Lane MD, Acting Deputy Director

State Agencies & Associations

Alaska

1283 Asthma and Allergy Foundation of America: Alaska Chapter
PO Box 201927   907-696-4810
Anchorage, AK 99520-1927   Fax: 907-696-4810
e-mail: aafaalaska@gci.net
www.aafaalaska.com
Formed in April, 2001, the AAFA Alaska chapter is moving quickly to provide educational programs and information about asthma and allergies through classes, workshops and educational materials. Focused not only on reaching children and adults with asthma information, but also health care professionals, caregivers, childcare providers and school personnel.
Suzi Jackson, Executive Director
Kathleen Bell, RN, Secretary

California

1284 Asthma and Allergy Foundation of America: Southern California Chapter
3435 Wilshire Boulevard 323-937-7859
Los Angeles, CA 90036 800-624-0044
Fax: 323-937-7815
e-mail: aafasocal@aol.com
www.aafasocal.com
Dedicated to controlling and curing asthma and allergic diseases through education, a network of support groups, the support of research and specialized training, increasing public awareness and providing medication and treatment to the under served. Program highlights include the Breathmobile, asthma camps and air power games for children.
Francene Lifson, Executive Director

District of Columbia

1285 Administration for Children and Families
370 L'Enfant Promenade
Washington, DC 20447 www.acf.hhs.gov
The Administration for Children & Families (ACF) is a division of the U.S. Department of Health & Human Services (HHS). ACF promotes the economic and social well-being of families, children, individuals and communities.
Mark Greenberg, Acting Assistant Secretary
Jeff Hild, Chief of Staff

1286 Asthma and Allergy Foundation of America: Washington Chapter
1233 20th Street 206-368-2866
Washington, DC 20036 800-727-8462
Fax: 206-368-2941
e-mail: Info@aafa.org
www.aafa.org
Program highlights include trainings for health care professionals on asthma and allergy management, working collaboratively with other local and regional agencies to improve the quality of life for those affected by asthma and allergies, organizing health seminars and education programs.
Mary Brasle, Director of Programs and Services
Amy Patterson, Director Administration/Governance

1287 National Institute for Occupational Safety and Health
395 E Street, SW 202-245-0625
Washington, DC 20201 800-232-4636
Fax: 513-533-8347
TTY: 888-232-6348
www.cdc.gov/niosh/
The National Institute for Occupational Safety and Health (NIOSH) is the U.S. federal agency that conducts research and makes recommendations to prevent worker injury and illness.
John Howard, MD, Director
Frank Hearl, PE, Chief of Staff

Georgia

1288 Agency for Toxic Substances and Disease Registry
4770 Buford Hwy NE
Atlanta, GA 30341 800-232-4636
TTY: 888-232-6348
www.atsdr.cdc.gov
The Agency for Toxic Substances and Disease Registry (ATSDR), based in Atlanta, Georgia, is a federal public health agency of the U.S. Department of Health and Human Services. ATSDR serves the public by using the best science, taking responsive public health actions, and providing trusted health information to prevent harmful exposures and diseases related to toxic substances.
Patrick Breysse, PhD, CIH, Director
Donna Knutson, PhD, Acting Deputy Director

1289 Division of Adolescent and School Health
4770 Buford Hwy, NE
Atlanta, GA 30341 800-232-4636
TTY: 888-232-6348
www.cdc.gov/HealthyYouth
CDC promotes the health and well-being of children and adolescents to enable them to become healthy and productive adults.

Maryland

1290 Agency for Healthcare Research and Quality
540 Gaither Road
Rockville, MD 20850 301-427-1364
www.ahrq.gov/index.html
The Agency for Healthcare Research and Quality's (AHRQ) mission is to produce evidence to make health care safer, higher quality, more accessible, equitable, and affordable, and to work within the U.S. Department of Health and Human Services and with other partners to make sure that the evidence is understood and used.
Richard G. Kronick, PhD, Director, Director
Sharon B. Arnold, PhD, Deputy Director

1291 Centers for Medicare and Medicaid Services
7500 Security Boulevard 410-786-3000
Baltimore, MD 21244 877-267-2323
TTY: 866-226-1819
e-mail: Mandy.Cohen@cms.hhs.gov
www.cms.gov
US federal agency which administers Medicare, Medicaid, and the State Children's Health Insurance Program.
Dr. Mandy Cohen, M.D., MPH, Chief of Staff
Timothy P. Love, Chief Operating Officer

1292 National Center for Complementary and Integrative Health
9000 Rockville Pike
Bethesda, MD 20892 888-644-6226
TTY: 866-464-3615
e-mail: nccih-info@mail.nih.gov
nccih.nih.gov
The National Center for Complementary and Integrative Health (NCCIH) is the Federal Government's lead agency for scientific research on the diverse medical and health care systems, practices, and products that are not generally considered part of conventional medicine.
Josephine P. Briggs, M.D., Director
David Shurtleff, Ph.D., Deputy Director

1293 National Human Genome Research Institute
Building 31, Room 4B09 301-402-0911
Bethesda, MD 20892 Fax: 301-402-2218
www.genome.gov
The National Human Genome Research Institute began as the National Center for Human Genome Research (NCHGR), which was established in 1989 to carry out the role of the National Institutes of Health (NIH) in the International Human Genome Project (HGP).
Eric D. Green, M.D., Ph.D., Director
Lawrence Brody, Ph.D., Director, Division of Genomics & Society

1294 National Institute of Biomedical Imaging and Bioengineering
9000 Rockville Pike 301-496-8859
Bethesda, MD 20892 e-mail: info@nibib.nih.gov
www.nibib.nih.gov
The mission of the National Institute of Biomedical Imaging and Bioengineering (NIBIB) is to improve health by leading the development and accelerating the application of biomedical technologies.
Roderic I. Pettigrew, Ph.D., M.D., Director
Marcella Canada, Administrative Officer

1295 National Institute of General Medical Sciences
45 Center Drive MSC 6200 301-496-7301
Bethesda, MD 20892 e-mail: info@nigms.nih.gov
www.nigms.nih.gov
The National Institute of General Medical Sciences (NIGMS) supports basic research that increases understanding of biological processes and lays the foundation for advances in disease diagnosis, treatment and prevention.
Jon R. Lorsch, Ph.D., Director
Judith H. Greenberg, Ph.D., Deputy Director

1296 National Institute of Nursing Research
31 Center Drive 301-496-0207
Bethesda, MD 20892 Fax: 301-496-8845
e-mail: info@ninr.nih.gov
www.ninr.nih.gov

The mission of the National Institute of Nursing Research (NINR) is to promote and improve the health of individuals, families, communities, and populations.

Patricia A. Grady, Institute Director
Dr. Ann R. Knebel, Deputy Director

1297   U.S. Food and Drug Administration
10903 New Hampshire Ave   301-796-8240
Silver Spring, MD 20993   888-463-6332
                                        www.fda.gov
FDA is responsible for protecting the public health by assuring the safety, efficacy and security of human and veterinary drugs, biological products, medical devices, our nation's food supply, cosmetics, and products that emit radiation.

Stephen Ostroff, M.D., Acting Commissioner
James Tyler, Chief Financial Officer

Massachusetts

1298   Asthma and Allergy Foundation of America: New England Chapter
220 Boylston Street   617-965-7771
Chestnut Hill, MA 02467   877-227-8462
                                   Fax: 617-965-8886
                                   TTY: 877-227-8462
                  e-mail: info@asthmaandallergies.org
                            www.asthmaandallergies.org
Serves Massachusetts, Rhode Island, Connecticut, Maine, New Hampshire and Vermont. Program highlights include speakers and exhibits, telephone information and referrals, tobacco control program, scholarship essay contest for high school juniors, advocacy for safer environments and training programs for school, daycare and health professionals.

Patricia Goldman, Executive Director
Sharon Schumack, Health Education Coordinator

Michigan

1299   Asthma and Allergy Foundation of America: Michigan Chapter
2075 Walnut Lake Road   248-406-4254
West Bloomfield, MI 48323-8768   888-444-0333
                                   Fax: 248-757-2102
                     e-mail: aafamich@sbcglobal.net
                                   www.aafamich.org
Serves the state of Michigan through public forums, work place educational programs, patient advocacy, Asthma Camp and telephone referrals and information.

Karen Katz, Executive Director
Dr. Rola Bokhari-Panza, President

Missouri

1300   Asthma and Allergy Foundation of America: Greater Kansas City Chapter
9140 Ward Parkway   816-333-6608
Kansas City, MO 64114   888-542-8252
                                   Fax: 816-333-6684
                           e-mail: info@aafakc.org
                                   www.aafakc.org
Provides college scholarships, Family Asthma Education Day, adult discussion groups, Superkids Asthma Day Camp for grades 1-5, professional education, ACT, health fair participation, breathing machine, peak flow meter and spacer distribution programs. They also have a quarterly newsletter, an asthma action line, emergency medication assistance, assistance to local school districts, free educational materials, seminars for work site clinicians and daycare workers and the smoke-free dining group.

Noel Albert, Executive Director

1301   Asthma and Allergy Foundation of America: St. Louis Chapter
1500 South Big Bend   314-645-2422
St. Louis, MO 63117   Fax: 314-692-2022
                            e-mail: aafa@aafastl.org
                                   www.aafastl.org/
The Asthma and Allergy Foundation of America (AAFA), St. Louis Chapter, was founded in 1981 by a group of volunteer board-certified allergists, including Dr. Phillip Korenblat of Washington University and Dr. Raymond Slavin of St. Louis University. AAFA St. Louis provides services to the community in

helping children effectively manage their asthma through the provision of medical resources, equipment and education.

H. James Wedner, M.D., ÿPresident
Bill Reichhardt, Vice President

New Jersey

1302   Asthma and Allergy Foundation of America: Southeast Pennsylvania Chapter
32 Caspertown Street   856-224-9547
Gibbstown, NJ 08027   Fax: 856-224-5893
                         e-mail: aafasepa@prodigy.net
                                   www.aafa.org
In the process of establishing a vital, new program that will aid children with chronic asthma. Many parents, some who are without medical insurance coverage, are unaware of the availability of a medical support system that can help their children. The Children at Risk program will enable parents to have their children evaluated and also receive a free one month supply of medication. Parents will also receive information regarding available options for follow up care and prescription coverage.

Lynn Hanessian, Chair
Michele Abu Carrick ,LICSW, Co-Chair, Governance

North Carolina

1303   National Institute of Environmental Health Sciences
111 T.W. Alexander Drive   919-541-4580
Research Triangle Park, NC 27709 e-mail: carroll1@niehs.nih.gov
                                   www.niehs.nih.gov
The mission of the NIEHS is to discover how the environment affects people in order to promote healthier lives.

Linda S. Birnbaum, Ph.D., Director
Richard Woychik, Ph.D., Deputy Director

Oregon

1304   Asthma and Allergy Foundation of America: Oregon Chapter
14530 Southwest 144th Avenue   503-579-8375
Tigard, OR 97224-1445   Fax: 208-474-6839
                        e-mail: hensches@teleport.com

Serving the state of Oregon.

Sandra L Henschel, President

Texas

1305   Asthma and Allergy Foundation of America
9101 Quarter Horse Lane   817-297-3132
Fort Worth, TX 76123   888-933-AAFA
                                   Fax: 817-563-5696
                          e-mail: info@aafatexas.org
                                   www.aafatexas.org
Offers many educational programs and services that touch patients, caregivers, physicians and allied health professionals, including: child care provider education programs, school nurse and respiratory therapist education programs, and work site allergy education.

Joan Hart, Executive Director
Jim Rosenthal, President

1306   Asthma and Allergy Foundation of America: North Texas Chapter
3904 Justin Drive   817-297-3132
Ft. Worth, TX 76244   888-933-AAFA
                                   Fax: 817-563-5696
                        e-mail: aafantx@hotmail.com
                                   www.aafatexas.org
Offers many educational programs and services that touch patients. caregivers, physicians and allied health professionals, including: child care provider education programs, school nurse and respiratory therapist education programs, work site allergy education programs, spacer and peak flow meter distribution to those in need, a toll free hotline, prescription assistance information, free educational materials in English and Spanish, an electronic newsletter, professional education, etc.

Jim Roseenthal, President
Stephen J Apaliski MD, VP Publications

1307 National Science Foundation
4201 Wilson Blvd
Arlington, VA 22230

703-292-5111
TDD: 703-292-5090
e-mail: info@nsf.gov
www.nsf.gov

NSF is the only federal agency whose mission includes support for all fields of fundamental science and engineering, except for medical sciences.
France A. Cçrdova, Director
Richard O. Buckius, Chief Operating Officer

Foundations

1308 Asthma and Allergy Foundation of America
1233 20th Street NW
Washington, DC 20036

202-466-7643
800-727-8462
Fax: 202-668-40
e-mail: info@aafa.org
www.aafa.org

AAFA provides practical information, community based services and support through a national network of chapters and support groups. AAFA develops health education, organizes state and national advocacy efforts and funds research to find better treatments and cures
William McLin, Executive Director

Research Centers

1309 Brigham and Women's Hospital: Rheumatology Immunology, and Allergy Division
75 Francis Street
Boston, MA 02115

61 -73 -550
Fax: 617-525-1001
TTY: 617-732-6458
www.brighamandwomens.org

Internationally renowned for excellence in clinical care clinical investigation and basic research. A faculty of 36 board certified rheumatologists and allergists provide eldtive urgent and emergency consultations as necessary.
Michael B Brenner MD, Division Chief
Jonathan S Coblyn, Clinical Director Rheumatology

1310 Childrens Hospital Immunology Division Children's Hospital
Children's Hospital
300 Longwood Avenue
Boston, MA 02115

61 -35 -600
www.childrenshospital.org

Organizational research unit of the Children's Hospital that focuses on the causes prevention and treatments of asthma infections and allergies.
Dr. James Mandell, CEO
Sandra Fenwick, President & COO

1311 Clinical Immunology, Allergy, and Rheumatology
Tulane Medical School
1700 Perdido Street
New Orleans, LA 70112-1210

504-988-5187
Fax: 504-988-3686
e-mail: medsch@tulane.edu
www.som.tulane.edu/medciar

Mauel Lopez MD, Director

1312 Duke Asthma, Allergy and Airway Center
4309 Medical Park Drive
Durham, NC 27704

919-620-7300
www.aaac.duhs.duke.edu/

Raffeal Rau, President
Dr Monica Kraft, Director

1313 Johns Hopkins University: Asthma and Allergy Center
5501 Hopkins Bayview Circle
Baltimore, MD 21224-6801

410-550-2101
Fax: 410-550-3256
e-mail: jhuallergy@jhmi.edu
www.hopkinsmedicine.org/allergy

Studies of allergic diseases and individuals with allergic disease pulmonary diseases and diseases involving inflammation and immunological processes.
Bruce S Bochner, Director
Peter S Creticos, Clinical Director

1314 National Jewish Division of Immunology
National Jewish Medical and Research Center
1400 Jackson Street
Denver, CO 80206-2762

303-398-1337
80 -42 -889
Fax: 303-270-2125
e-mail: harbeckr@njc.org
www.njc.org

The only medical center in the country whose research and patient care resources are dedicated to respiratory and immunologic diseases.
John Cambier, Chairman
Ronald J Harbeck, Medical Director

1315 Northwestern University: Division of Allergy and Immunology
The Feinberg School of Medicine
251 East Huron Street
Chicago, IL 60611

312-926-6895
Fax: 312-926-6905
e-mail: rpschleimer@northwestern.edu
www.medicine.northwestern.edu

A referral center of local regional and national stature.~ Areas of clinical excellence include asthma allergic bronchopulmonary aspergillosis idiopathic anaphylaxis drug allergy occupational immunologic lung disease and allergen immunotherapy.
Douglas E Vaughan MD, Chair
James Foody MD, Vice Chair Clinical Affairs

1316 University of Virginia: General Clinical Research Center
University of Virginia Health System
2515 Lee Street
Charlottesville, VA 22908-0787

434-924-2394
Fax: 434-924-9960
e-mail: gcrc@virginia.edu
www.healthsystem.virginia.edu/

Focuses on asthmatic disorders.
Arthur Garso Jr MD MPH, Principal Investigator
Eugene J Barrett, Program Director

1317 University of Wisconsin: Asthma, Allergy and Pulmonary Research Center
600 Highland Avenue
Madison, WI 53792-2454

608-263-6400
Fax: 608-263-6401
www.medicine.wisc.edu

Sheri L Lawrence, MBA, Administrator
Sharon Gehl, MBA, Associate Administrator

Support Groups & Hotlines

1318 Allergy & Asthma Networks Hotline
Allergy and Asthma Network/Mothers of Asthmatics
2751 Prosperity Avenue
Fairfax, VA 22031

703-641-9595
800-878-4403
Fax: 703-573-7794
www.breatherville.org

Mary McGowan, Executive Director
Michael Amato, Chair

1319 Asthma and Allergy Foundation of America
1233 20th Street NW
Washington, DC 20036

202-466-7643
Fax: 202-466-8940
e-mail: info@aafa.org
www.aafa.org

The foundation was formed to alleviate suffering and loss from asthma and allergy disorders. The foundation offers a nationwide network of chapters and support groups and provides education and emotional support for persons with allergies and asthma. Also funds research for improved treatments and ultimately a cure.

1320 National Health Information Center
PO Box 1133
Washington, DC 20013

310-565-4167
800-336-4797
Fax: 301-984-4256
e-mail: info@nhic.org
www.health.gov/nhic

Offers a nationwide information referral service, produces directories and resource guides.

1321 Physician Referral and Information Line
American Academy of Allergy Asthma and Immunology
555 East Wells Street
Milwaukee, WI 53202-3889
414-272-6071
800-822-2762
Fax: 414-272-6070
www.aaaai.org
Referral line offering information on allergy and asthma, referral to an allergy/immunology specialist.

1322 Support for Asthmatic Youth
Asthma and Allergy Foundation of America
1080 Glen Cove Avenue
Glen Head, NY 11545-1565
516-625-5735
Fax: 516-625-2976
A network of educational/support groups for adolescents between the ages of 9 and 17. All meetings are free and feature guest speakers, informational programs, games and other fun activities.
Renee Theodorakis MA, Director Adolescent Services

Books

1323 Asthma Care Training for Kids
Asthma and Allergy Foundation of America
8201 Corporate Drive
Landover, MD 20785
202-466-7643
Fax: 202-466-8940
e-mail: info@aafa.org
www.aafa.org
Designed to help children ages 7-12 and their parents take charge of their asthma. In a series of three action filled sessions, children and their parents meet separately with their peers to learn about asthma management.

1324 Asthma Organizer
Allergy and Asthma Network/Mothers of Asthmatics
2751 Prosperity Avenue
Fairfax, VA 22031-4397
703-641-9595
800-878-4403
Fax: 703-573-7794
www.mothersofasthmatics.org
Includes daily symptom diary and forms to track medications, office visits and updates to your personal management plan. Information on peak flow monitoring, managing asthma at school, understanding asthma activators, and allergy-proofing also included. Available in Spanish.
Loose Leaf
Mary McGowan, Executive Director

1325 Asthma Resources Directory
Allergy and Asthma Network/Mothers of Asthmatics
2751 Prosperity Avenue
Fairfax, VA 22031-4397
703-641-9595
800-878-4403
Fax: 703-573-7794
www.mothersofasthmatics.org
Comprehensive listings of thousands of products, services, and resources for allergy and asthma questions.
Mary McGowan, Executive Director

1326 Asthma Self-Help Book
Asthma and Allergy Foundation of America
8201 Corporate Drive
Landover, MD 20785
202-466-7643
Fax: 202-466-8940
e-mail: info@aafa.org
www.aafa.org
A thorough, practical look at asthma that includes information from the National Heart, Lung and Blood Institute's 1991 Asthma Guidelines.

1327 Asthma in the School: Improving Control with Peak Flow Monitoring
Asthma and Allergy Foundation of America
8201 Corporate Drive
Landover, MD 20785
202-466-7643
Fax: 202-466-8940
e-mail: info@aafa.org
www.aafa.org
Comprehensive and practical guide to help the school nurse monitor and assist students with asthma.

1328 Asthma in the Workplace
John H Dekker & Sons
2941 Clydon Street SW
Grand Rapids, MI 49509
616-538-5160
Fax: 616-538-0720
1993 664 pages
ISBN: 0-824787-99-4

1329 Asthma: The Complete Guide
Asthma and Allergy Foundation of America
8201 Corporate Drive
Landover, MD 20785-2330
202-466-7643
800-727-8462
Fax: 202-466-8940
e-mail: info@aafa.org
www.aafa.org
An excellent self-management guide for asthma and allergy patients and their families.
357 pages Paperback

1330 Breathing Disorders: Your Complete Exercise Guide
Human Kinetics
1607 N Market Street
Champaign, IL 61820-5076
217-351-1549
800-873-6759
Fax: 217-351-2674
e-mail: ce@hkusa.com
www.humankinetics.com
1993 144 pages Paperback
ISBN: 0-873224-26-4
Steve Ruhlig, Marketing Director

1331 Bronchial Asthma: Principles of Diagnosis and Treatment
Humana Press
999 Riverview Drive
Totowa, NJ 07512
973-256-1699
Fax: 973-256-8341
e-mail: humana@humanapr.com
www.springer.com
2001 496 pages
ISBN: 0-896038-61-0

1332 Children with Asthma: A Manual for Parents
Allergy Control Products
1620-D Satellite Blvd
Duluth, GA 30097-0793
203-438-9580
800-422-3878
Fax: 203-431-8963
www.allergycontrol.com
Known as the asthma bible, this second edition is sprinkled with anecdotes by patients and their parents.
296 pages Paperback

1333 Conquering Asthma
Michael Newhouse, MD, author
B.C Decker, Inc.
50 King Street E, Floor 2
Ontario, Canada L8N 3K7,
905-522-7017
800-568-7281
Fax: 905-522-7839
e-mail: info@bcdecker.com
www.bcdecker.com
This text shows asthmatics how to live a healthier and happier life hardly aware that they have asthma.
1998 107 pages Paperback
ISBN: 1-896998-01-1

1334 Coping with Asthma
Rosen Publishing Group
29 E 21st Street
New York, NY 10010
212-777-3017
800-237-9932
Fax: 888-436-4643
e-mail: customerservice@rosenpub.com
www.rosenpublishing.com
This book prepares students by explaining to them the dangers of asthma, a condition which, when properly treated, is completely manageable.
ISBN: 0-823929-69-8
Carolyn Simpson, Author

1335 Understanding Asthma
Phil Lieberman, MD, author
University Press of Mississippi

3825 Ridgewood Road
Jackson, MS 39211-6492
601-432-6205
800-737-7788
Fax: 601-432-6217
e-mail: kburgess@ihl.state.ms.us
www.upress.state.ms.us

A guide to how the disease behaves and how the latest therapies work.
1999 120 pages Paperback
ISBN: 1-578061-42-3
Phil Lieberman, M.D., Author

Children's Books

1336 All About Asthma
Asthma and Allergy Foundation of America
8201 Corporate Drive
Landover, MD 20785-2330
202-466-7643
800-727-8462
Fax: 202-466-8940
e-mail: info@aafa.org
www.aafa.org

Written by a 10-year-old with asthma, this cleverly illustrated book explains causes and symptoms, and ways to control asthma to lead a normal life.
39 pages Paperback

1337 Asthma
Franklin Watts Grolier
90 Old Sherman Turnpike
Danbury, CT 06816-0001
203-797-3500
800-621-1115
Fax: 203-797-3197
www.grolier.com

This book offers vital information on causes and treatments, plus advice on how to prevent flare-ups.
96 pages Grades 7-12
ISBN: 0-531106-97-7

1338 Asthma Challenge
Asthma and Allergy Foundation of America
8201 Corporate Drive
Landover, MD 20785
202-466-7643
Fax: 202-466-8940
e-mail: info@aafa.org
www.aafa.org

An exciting new team game for large or small groups. Custom designed, full color, stand up board and two sets of pretested question cards. Teens and adults win AAFA Bucks as they test their knowledge in categories like Sneezes and Wheezes and Asthma Nuts and Bolts.

1339 Best of Superstuff Activity Booklet
American Lung Association
1740 Broadway
New York, NY 10019-4315
212-315-8700

For young children with asthma featuring a series of activities designed to help youngsters cope with asthma.
32 pages Ages 6-8

1340 Bronkie the Bronchiasaurus
Asthma and Allergy Foundation of America
8201 Corporate Drive
Landover, MD 20785-2330
202-466-7643
800-727-8462
Fax: 202-466-8940
e-mail: info@aafa.org
www.aafa.org

A Super Nintendo role-playing adventure in which players manage the asthma of two dinosaurs. They must avoid triggers, maintain their peak-flow and take daily medications. Only then can they use their strongest defense - the powerful breath blast. Designed for ages 7 to 15.

1341 Childhood Asthma: Learning to Manage
Asthma and Allergy Foundation of America
8201 Corporate Drive
Landover, MD 20785-2330
202-466-7643
800-727-8462
Fax: 202-466-8940
e-mail: info@aafa.org
www.aafa.org

Self-paced, entertaining activity books for home use featuring practical guidelines for managing childhood asthma with a focus on using peak flow meters.

1342 Clubhouse Kids Learn About Asthma
Asthma and Allergy Foundation of America
8201 Corporate Drive
Landover, MD 20785-2330
202-466-7643
800-727-8462
Fax: 202-466-8940
e-mail: info@aafa.org
www.aafa.org

Interactive CD-ROM helps children ages 4-12 learn about asthma at their own pace. Sound, animation and game-like features draw players into the life of Janie, who has just been diagnosed with asthma.

1343 I'm a Meter Reader
Allergy and Asthma Network/Mothers of Asthmatics
2751 Prosperity Avenue
Fairfax, VA 22031-4397
703-641-9595
800-878-4403
Fax: 703-573-7794
www.mothersofasthmatics.org

Provides expert advice on how a peak flow meter can help detect when an asthma attack can occur in an easy to understand format with colorful illustrations. Available in Spanish. Companion video, I'm a Meter Reader, available as part of a set for $12.00.
Ages 4-9
Mary McGowan, Executive Director
Nancy Sander, Editor-in-Chief

1344 Let's Talk About Having Asthma
Rosen Publishing Group's PowerKids Press
29 E 21st Street
New York, NY 10010
212-777-3017
800-237-9932
Fax: 888-436-4643
e-mail: customerservice@rosenpub.com
www.rosenpublishing.com

This book talks about the cause and treatments for asthma as well as the precautions sufferers should take. Recommended for grades K-4.

ISBN: 0-823950-32-8

1345 Lion Who Had Asthma
Asthma and Allergy Foundation of America
8201 Corporate Drive
Landover, MD 20785-2330
202-466-7643
800-727-8462
Fax: 202-466-8940
e-mail: Info@aafa.org
www.aafa.org

A beautifully illustrated book that encourages preschoolers to use their imaginations and take their asthma medications.
24 pages Hardcover

1346 Luke Has Asthma Too!
Allergy Control Products
PO Box 793
Ridgefield, CT 06877-0793
800-422-3878
Fax: 203-431-8963

This gentle book will make for good reading with children, whether they have asthma or not.

1347 Scorpions
Harper & Row
10 E 53rd Street
New York, NY 10022-5299
212-207-7000
www.harpercollins.com

This novel, while not wholly dedicated to examining the ramifications of asthma on a child's life, does incorporate the theme into a compelling narrative.
Grades 6-9
Walter Dean Myers, Author

1348 So You Have Asthma Too!
Allergy and Asthma Network/Mothers of Asthmatics
2751 Prosperity Avenue
Fairfax, VA 22031-4397
703-641-9595
800-878-4403
Fax: 703-573-7794
www.mothersofasthmatics.org

A children's illustrated book, offering a clear description and understanding of childhood asthma. Available in Spanish. Also see

companion video, SO YOU HAVE ASTHMA TOO!, available as part of a set for $12.00.
Mary McGowan, Executive Director
Nancy Sander, Editor-in-Chief

1349 Winning Over Asthma
Asthma and Allergy Foundation of America
8201 Corporate Drive
Landover, MD 20785-2330

202-466-7643
800-727-8462
Fax: 202-466-8940
e-mail: Info@aafa.org
www.aafa.org

Simple coloring book explains asthma through a story about five-year-old Graham.
30 pages Paperback

Magazines

1350 Controlling Asthma
American Lung Association
1740 Broadway
New York, NY 10019-4315

212-315-8700

For parents of children with asthma, this newsmagazine tells how parents can help their child deal with the many problems presented by asthma.
16 pages

1351 Starting Strong-Staying Strong: A Resource Guide for Educational Support Groups
Asthma and Allergy Foundation of America
8201 Corporate Drive
Landover, MD 20785

202-466-7643
800-727-8462
Fax: 202-466-8940
e-mail: info@aafa.org
www.aafa.org

A resource guide to help educational support groups get organized, publicize and remain successful. Great for people who want to start an asthma or allergy support group and for existing group leaders who want to strengthen their programs. Filled with stories of success and struggle from other group leaders, medical advisors and group members across the country. A companion CD-ROM provides additional tips.
Guide + CD-ROM
William McLin, Executive Director
Mike Tringale, Director Marketing/Communications

Newsletters

1352 Advance
Asthma and Allergy Foundation of America
8201 Corporate Drive
Landover, MD 20785-2330

202-466-7643
800-727-8462
Fax: 202-466-8940
e-mail: Info@aafa.org
www.aafa.org

A bi-monthly , 8 page newsletter for patients and their families filled with timely and useful information about managing asthma and allergies.
BiMonthly

1353 Allergy & Asthma ADVOCATE Newsletter
American Academy of Allergy, Asthma and Immunology
555 East Wells Street
Milwaukee, WI 53202

414-272-6071
800-822-2762
Fax: 414-272-6070
www.aaaai.org

Offers tips and medical information on allergies and asthma via articles written by allied health and physician AAAAI members.
6 pages Quarterly

1354 BReATHE
Asthma and Allergy Foundation of America
8201 Corporate Drive
Landover, MD 20785

800-727-8462
e-mail: info@aafa.org
www.aafa.org

E-newsletter filled with information on how to control asthma and allergies, with stories from patients who are living life without limits.
Bi-Monthly
William McLin, President/CEO
Angel Waldron, Sr Manager Marketing/Communications

1355 FreshAAIR
Asthma and Allergy Foundation of America
8201 Corporate Drive
Landover, MD 20785

202-466-7643
800-727-8462
Fax: 202-466-8940
e-mail: info@aafa.org
www.aafa.org

Filled with information about asthma, seasonal allergies, food allergies, back-to-school tips for parents, educational materials and more.
Bi-Monthly
William McLin, President/CEO
Angel Waldron, Sr Manager Marketing/Communications

1356 Leaders Link
Asthma and Allergy Foundation of America
8201 Corporate Drive
Landover, MD 20785

800-727-8462
e-mail: info@aafa.org
www.aafa.org

Provides useful and timely insights on how to plan and lead asthma and allergy support group meetings, how to keep your support group active and strong, and useful ideas from other support groups.
Bi-Monthly
William McLin, President/CEO
Angel Waldron, Sr Manager Marketing/Communications

1357 MA Report
Allergy and Asthma Network/Mothers of Asthmatics
2751 Prosperity Avenue
Fairfax, VA 22031-4397

703-641-9595
800-878-4403
Fax: 703-573-7794
www.mothersofasthmatics.org

Offers information on medical breakthroughs, patient care, public awareness, activities and events focusing on the allergy and asthma patient. This newsletter keeps a patient fully informed with medical articles written by experts in the field.
Monthly
Mary McGowan, Executive Director
Nancy Sander, Editor-in-Chief

Pamphlets

1358 About Asthma
American Lung Association
1740 Broadway
New York, NY 10019-4315

212-315-8700

A popular style pamphlet explaining symptoms, treatment and more for persons with asthma.
16 pages

1359 Adverse Reactions to Foods
American Academy of Allergy, Asthma and Immunology
555 East Wells Street
Milwaukee, WI 53202-3889

414-272-6071
800-822-2762
Fax: 414-272-6070
www.aaaai.org

A patient's guide to problem foods, food additives, diagnosis, and treatment.

1360 Allergies and You
American Lung Association
1740 Broadway
New York, NY 10019-4315

212-315-8700

Answers basic questions about allergy, particularly as it relates to asthma.

1361 Allergies to Animals
American Academy of Allergy, Asthma and Immunology

555 East Wells Street
Milwaukee, WI 53202-3889

414-272-6071
800-822-2762
Fax: 414-272-6070
www.aaaai.org

1362 Allergy & Asthma
American Academy of Allergy, Asthma and Immunology
555 East Wells Street
Milwaukee, WI 53202-3889

414-272-6071
800-822-2762
Fax: 414-272-6070
www.aaaai.org

An informational brochure discussing major topics of allerges and asthma.

1363 Allergy and Asthma: An Informational Brochure
American Academy of Allergy, Asthma and Immunology
555 East Wells Street
Milwaukee, WI 53202-3889

414-272-6071
800-822-2762
Fax: 414-272-6070
www.aaaai.org

Offers information on asthma, its symptoms, causes, diagnosis and treatments.

1364 Anaphylaxis
American Academy of Allergy, Asthma and Immunology
555 East Wells Street
Milwaukee, WI 53202-3889

414-272-6071
800-822-2762
Fax: 414-272-6070
www.aaaai.org

1365 Asthma Alert
American Lung Association
1740 Broadway
New York, NY 10019-4315

212-315-8700

Quick reference folders with information on asthma, the symptoms and what to do in an emergency.

1366 Asthma Handbook
American Lung Association
1740 Broadway
New York, NY 10019-4315

212-315-8700

Explains asthma, gives self-care methods for handling it and helps patients work more effectively with their doctor.
28 pages

1367 Asthma Lifelines
American Lung Association
1740 Broadway
New York, NY 10019-4315

212-315-8700

Promotional brochure providing descriptions of ALA asthma education materials.
12 pages

1368 Asthma and Allergies in Seniors
American Academy of Allergy, Asthma and Immunology
555 East Wells Street
Milwaukee, WI 53202

414-272-6071
800-822-2762
Fax: 414-272-6070
www.aaaai.org

1369 Asthma and Pregnancy
American Academy of Allergy, Asthma and Immunology
555 East Wells Street
Milwaukee, WI 53202-3889

414-272-6071
800-822-2762
Fax: 414-272-6070
www.aaaai.org

1370 Asthma and the School Child
American Academy of Allergy, Asthma and Immunology
555 East Wells Street
Milwaukee, WI 53202-3889

414-272-6071
800-822-2762
Fax: 414-272-6070
www.aaaai.org

1371 Atopic Dermatitis
American Academy of Allergy, Asthma and Immunology
555 East Wells Street
Milwaukee, WI 53202-3889

414-272-6071
800-822-2762
Fax: 414-272-6070
www.aaaai.org

This brochure offers information on symptoms, diagnosi, treatment, and prognosis.

1372 Being Close
National Jewish Center for Immunology
1400 Jackson Street
Denver, CO 80206-2762

303-388-4461

A booklet offering information to patients suffering from a respiratory disorder such as emphysema, asthma or tuberculosis, that discusses sexual problems and feelings.

1373 Childhood Asthma
American Academy of Allergy, Asthma and Immunology
555 East Wells Street
Milwaukee, WI 53202-3889

414-272-6071
800-822-2762
Fax: 414-272-6070
www.aaaai.org

1374 Childhood Asthma: A Guide for Parents
Asthma and Allergy Foundation of America
8201 Corporate Drive
Landover, MD 20785-2330

202-466-7643
800-727-8462
Fax: 202-466-8940
e-mail: Info@aafa.org
www.aafa.org

This colorful booklet helps parents learn all about asthma in children.
32 pages

1375 Childhood Asthma: A Matter of Control
American Lung Association
1740 Broadway
New York, NY 10019-4315

212-315-8700

A guide for parents of children with asthma, this booklet covers topics such as identifying asthma signs and symptoms as well as controlling the condition.
28 pages

1376 Consumer Guide to Health Care Plans
American Academy of Allergy, Asthma and Immunology
555 East Wells Street
Milwaukee, WI 53202-3889

414-272-6071
800-822-2762
Fax: 414-272-6070
www.aaaai.org

Gives answers to some commonly asked questions on health care.

1377 Efficacy of Asthma Education, Selected Abstracts
American Lung Association
1740 Broadway
New York, NY 10019-4315

212-315-8700

Abstracts documenting the efficacy of asthma education programs for physicians and other health professionals.

1378 Exercise-Induced Asthma & Bronchospasm
American Academy of Allergy, Asthma and Immunology
555 East Wells Street
Milwaukee, WI 53202-3889

414-272-6071
800-822-2762
Fax: 414-272-6070
www.aaaai.org

This brochure covers testing, treatment, and other advice on how to deal with exercise-induced asthma.

1379 Facts About Asthma
American Lung Association
1740 Broadway
New York, NY 10019-4315

212-315-8700

Primary public information leaflet on asthma.
12 pages

1380 Facts About Peak Flow Meters
American Lung Association
1740 Broadway
New York, NY 10019-4315

212-315-8700

Discusses the use of a peak flow meter for adults and children with asthma.
8 pages

1381 Healthy Breathing
National Jewish Center for Immunology
1400 Jackson Street
Denver, CO 80206-2762

303-388-4461

Offers patients with lung or respiratory disorders information on exercise and healthy breathing.

1382 Helping Others Breathe Easier
Allergy and Asthma Network/Mothers of Asthmatics
2751 Prosperity Avenue   703-641-9595
Fairfax, VA 22031-4397   800-878-4403
                                   Fax: 703-573-7794
                          www.mothersofasthmatics.org
Offers information on educational resources, support groups and the Network for persons afflicted with asthma or allergic disorders.
Mary McGowan, Executive Director
Nancy Sander, Editor-in-Chief

1383 Home Control of Allergies and Asthma
American Lung Association
1740 Broadway   212-315-8700
New York, NY 10019-4315
Discusses substances in the home that may trigger asthma and allergy problems and offers suggestions for controlling them.
12 pages

1384 Immunitherapy
American Academy of Allergy, Asthma and Immunology
555 East Wells Street   414-272-6071
Milwaukee, WI 53202-3889   800-822-2762
                                   Fax: 414-272-6070
                                        www.aaaai.org
This brochure offers information on administration, benefits, and potential side effects of immune therapy.

1385 Inhaled Medications for Asthma
American Academy of Allergy, Asthma and Immunology
555 East Wells Street   414-272-6071
Milwaukee, WI 53202-3889   800-822-2762
                                   Fax: 414-272-6070
                                        www.aaaai.org
This brochure gives helpful information on classes of inhaled medication, types of inhalation devices, spacers and holding chambers, how proper training is necessary.

1386 Latex Allergy
American Academy of Allergy, Asthma and Immunology
555 East Wells Street   414-272-6071
Milwaukee, WI 53202-3889   800-822-2762
                                   Fax: 414-272-6070
                                        www.aaaai.org

1387 Making the Most of Your Next Doctor Visit
American Academy of Allergy, Asthma and Immunology
555 East Wells Street   414-272-6071
Milwaukee, WI 53202-3889   800-822-2762
                                   Fax: 414-272-6070
                                        www.aaaai.org
A personal asthma management monitor. Includes personal tracking charts to help you along.
10 pages

1388 Many Faces of Asthma
American Lung Association
1740 Broadway   212-315-8700
New York, NY 10019-4315
Provides an overview of asthma as a major public health problem, describes what happens during asthma attacks and explains how asthma is treated and managed.
12 pages

1389 Nocturnal Asthma
National Jewish Center for Immunology
1400 Jackson Street   303-388-4461
Denver, CO 80206-2762
Offers information to patients about how to understand and manage asthma at night.

1390 Occupational Asthma
American Academy of Allergy, Asthma and Immunology
555 East Wells Street   414-272-6071
Milwaukee, WI 53202-3889   800-822-2762
                                   Fax: 414-272-6070
                                        www.aaaai.org

This brochure also contains a list of most common agents theat cause occupational asthma and who is at risk.

1391 Occupational Asthma: Lung Hazards on the Job
American Lung Association
1740 Broadway   212-315-8700
New York, NY 10019-4315
Discusses occupational asthma, a form of asthma in which airways overreact to various irritants in the workplace.

1392 Outpatient Treatment of Asthma
American Academy of Allergy, Asthma and Immunology
555 East Wells Street   414-272-6071
Milwaukee, WI 53202-3889   800-822-2762
                                   Fax: 414-272-6070
                                        www.aaaai.org

1393 Peak Flow Meter: A Thermometer for Asthma
American Academy of Allergy, Asthma and Immunology
555 East Wells Street   414-272-6071
Milwaukee, WI 53202-3889   800-822-2762
                                   Fax: 414-272-6070
                                        www.aaaai.org

1394 Pollen and Spores Around the World
American Academy of Allergy, Asthma and Immunology
555 East Wells Street   414-272-6071
Milwaukee, WI 53202-3889   800-822-2762
                                   Fax: 414-272-6070
                                        www.aaaai.org
Multi-paged brochure offering graphes and tables of pollen levels and different times of the year in different parts of the country.
10 pages

1395 Removing House Dust and Other Allergic Irritants From Your Home
American Academy of Allergy, Asthma and Immunology
555 East Wells Street   414-272-6071
Milwaukee, WI 53202-3889   800-822-2762
                                   Fax: 414-272-6070
                                        www.aaaai.org
This brochure covers some good ideas on how to reduce dust in the home.

1396 Role of the Allergist & Clinical Immunologist in Patient Care
American Academy of Allergy, Asthma and Immunology
555 East Wells Street   414-272-6071
Milwaukee, WI 53202-3889   800-822-2762
                                   Fax: 414-272-6070
                                        www.aaaai.org
An informational brochure containing definitions and addresses for further information.

1397 School Information Packet
Allergy and Asthma Network/Mothers of Asthmatics
2751 Prosperity Avenue   703-641-9595
Fairfax, VA 22031-4397   800-878-4403
                                   Fax: 703-573-7794
                          www.mothersofasthmatics.org
Practical, medical, and legal information for school administrators and parents of students with asthma.
Mary McGowan, Executive Director
Nancy Sander, Editor-in-Chief

1398 Standards for the Diagnosis and Care of Patients with Asthma
American Lung Association
1740 Broadway   212-315-8700
New York, NY 10019-4315
Standards developed by the American Thoracic Society, the medical section of the ALA. For physicians.
24 pages

1399 Student Asthma Action Card
Asthma and Allergy Foundation of America
8201 Corporate Drive   202-466-7643
Landover, MD 20785-2330   800-727-8462
                                   Fax: 202-466-8940
                          e-mail: Info@aafa.org
                                        www.aafa.org

Indispensable tool for familiarizing school personnel with asthma triggers, daily medications and emergency directions for each of their students with asthma.

1400 Superstuff
American Lung Association
1740 Broadway   212-315-8700
New York, NY 10019-4315
Kit specifically designed to help the elementary schoolchild with asthma to learn how to manage the condition. The kit contains teaching tools, puzzles, riddles, stories and games.

1401 Teens Talk to Teens About Asthma
Asthma and Allergy Foundation of America
8201 Corporate Drive   202-466-7643
Landover, MD 20785-2330   800-727-8462
                                            Fax: 202-466-8940
                                         e-mail: Info@aafa.org
                                              www.aafa.org
Quotes and thoughts from teens capture the essence of what it feels like to have asthma.

1402 There are Solutions for the Student with Asthma
American Lung Association
1740 Broadway   212-315-8700
New York, NY 10017
Leaflet telling how parents and school personnel can work together to make life easier for children with asthma.
4 pages

1403 Tips to Remember
American Academy of Allergy, Asthma and Immunology
611 E Wells Street   414-272-6071
Milwaukee, WI 53202-3889
A set of 23 tip sheets offering information on various topics including allergy and asthma treatments, pregnancy and asthma, animal allergies, sinusitis and more.

1404 Tips to Remember Brochures
American Academy of Allergy, Asthma and Immunology
555 East Wells Street   414-272-6071
Milwaukee, WI 53202-3889   800-822-2762
                                            Fax: 414-272-6070
                                              www.aaaai.org
Thirty three colorful brochures offered on numerous topics in allergy, asthma, and immunology.

1405 Triggers of Asthma
American Academy of Allergy, Asthma and Immunology
555 East Wells Street   414-272-6071
Milwaukee, WI 53202-3889   800-822-2762
                                            Fax: 414-272-6070
                                              www.aaaai.org
This brochure gives helpful information on what will cause an asthma attack.

1406 Understanding Asthma
National Jewish Center for Immunology
1400 Jackson Street   303-388-4461
Denver, CO 80206
Offers a brief introduction to asthma and then goes into the physiology of asthma, the triggers of asthma, and diagnosis and monitoring of asthma.
27 pages

1407 Understanding Immunology
National Jewish Center for Immunology
1400 Jackson Street   303-388-4461
Denver, CO 80206-2762
Offers information to patients and the public on the body's defenses. Explains how immunity develops, the basics of immunologic medicine and coping with respiratory disorders.

1408 Understanding Your Child with Asthma
National Jewish Center for Immunology
1400 Jackson Street   303-388-4461
Denver, CO 80206-2762   800-222-5264
Offers information on patient care, research, education and adult programs offered by the Association.

1409 Understanding the Pollen and Mold Season
American Academy of Allergy, Asthma and Immunology
555 East Wells Street   414-272-6071
Milwaukee, WI 53202-3889   800-822-2762
                                            Fax: 414-272-6070
                                              www.aaaai.org

1410 Unproven Methods in Diagnosing and Treating Allergies
Asthma and Allergy Foundation of America
8201 Corporate Drive   202-466-7643
Landover, MD 20785-2330   800-727-8462
                                            Fax: 202-466-8940
                                         e-mail: Info@aafa.org
                                              www.aafa.org

1411 Use of Steroids for Asthma and Allergies
American Academy of Allergy, Asthma and Immunology
555 East Wells Street   414-272-6071
Milwaukee, WI 53202-3889   800-822-2762
                                            Fax: 414-272-6070
                                              www.aaaai.org

1412 What Every Patient Should Know About Asthma & Allergy Medications
American Academy of Allergy, Asthma and Immunology
555 East Wells Street   414-272-6071
Milwaukee, WI 53202-3889   800-822-2762
                                            Fax: 414-272-6070
                                              www.aaaai.org

1413 What is an Allergic Reaction?
American Academy of Allergy, Asthma and Immunology
555 East Wells Street   414-272-6071
Milwaukee, WI 53202-3889   800-822-2762
                                            Fax: 414-272-6070
                                              www.aaaai.org
This brochure gives helpful information on what will cause an allergic reaction.

1414 Your Child and Asthma
National Jewish Center for Immunology
1400 Jackson Street   303-388-4461
Denver, CO 80206-2762
A booklet offering information to parents and family about their child with asthma. Offers information on diagnosis, treatments, triggers and family concerns.

Audio & Video

1415 Asthma Handbook Slides
American Lung Association
1740 Broadway   212-315-8700
New York, NY 10019-4315
Slides and script based on The Asthma Handbook for asthma patients and others.
Film

1416 Asthma Management
American Academy of Allergy, Asthma and Immunology
555 East Wells Street   414-272-6071
Milwaukee, WI 53202-3889   800-822-2762
                                            Fax: 414-272-6070
                                              www.aaaai.org
Although there is currently no cure for asthma, attacks can be controlled by appropriate asthma management. This video describes what happens during an asthma attack, how your allergists diagnoses asthma, and ways your allergist can help you to manage your condition.
10-13 minutes

1417 Asthma and the Athlete
American Academy of Allergy, Asthma and Immunology
555 East Wells Street   414-272-6071
Milwaukee, WI 53202   800-822-2762
                                            Fax: 414-272-6070
                                              www.aaaai.org
In the past, people with asthma were sometimes discouraged from exercising. Today we know that everyone, including asthmatics, can benefit from physical activity. This video details which exer-

cises are best for those with asthma, and how an allergist can help asthmatic athletes to properly manage and treat their disease.
10-13 minutes

1418 Environmental Control Measures
American Academy of Allergy, Asthma and Immunology
555 East Wells Street   414-272-6071
Milwaukee, WI 53202-3889   800-822-2762
                                     Fax: 414-272-6070
                                          www.aaaai.org
By conrtolling your environment, you can reduce your exposure to substances called allergens that trigger your allergic symptoms. This program depicts common outdoor and indoor allergens, methods an allergist uses to diagnose which substances you're allergic to, and how to reduce your exposure to allergic triggers.
10-13 minutes

1419 I'm a Meter Reader
Allergy and Asthma Network/Mothers of Asthmatics
2751 Prosperity Avenue   703-641-9595
Fairfax, VA 22031-4397   800-878-4403
                                     Fax: 703-573-7794
                                www.mothersofasthmatics.org
Provides expert advice on how a peak flow meter can help detect when an asthma attack can occur in an easy to understand format. Companion book, I'm a Meter Reader, available as part of a set for $12.00.
Video
Mary McGowan, Executive Director
Nancy Sander, Editor-in-Chief

1420 Immunotherapy
American Academy of Allergy, Asthma and Immunology
555 East Wells Street   414-272-6071
Milwaukee, WI 53202-3889   800-822-2762
                                     Fax: 414-272-6070
                                          www.aaaai.org
Immunotherapy, of allergy shots, is a long-term allergy and asthma treatment program that helps control allergic symptoms and reduces the need for medications. Learn more about immunotherapy through this video, which includes information on allergy testing and how your allergist determines if immunotherapy is right for you.
10-13 minutes

1421 Managing Asthma in School: An Action Plan
Asthma and Allergy Foundation of America
8201 Corporate Drive   202-466-7643
Landover, MD 20785-2330   800-727-8462
                                     Fax: 202-466-8940
                                   e-mail: Info@aafa.org
                                           www.aafa.org
Gives the basics of asthma and a plan for school nurses, parents and physicians to work together.
14 minutes

1422 Managing Childhood Asthma
American Lung Association
Box 596-COL   212-245-8000
New York, NY 10001   800-586-4872
                                     Fax: 312-440-9374
                                e-mail: webmaster@ala.org
                                            www.ala.org
What parents need to know to manage asthma. 22 minutes.
Video

1423 Pharmacologic Therapy of Pediatric Asthma
American Lung Association
1740 Broadway   212-315-8700
New York, NY 10019-4315
A Learning Resource Program developed by a joint committee of the American Thoracic Society and the ALA.
Film

1424 Regular Kid
American Lung Association
1740 Broadway   212-315-8700
New York, NY 10019-4315
This film shows how families and children cope with asthma problems. Proven asthma management strategies are presented through

the experiences of four children with asthma, ranging in age from toddler to teenager.
Film

1425 So You Have Asthma Too!
Allergy and Asthma Network/Mothers of Asthmatics
2751 Prosperity Avenue   703-641-9595
Fairfax, VA 22031-4397   800-878-4403
                                     Fax: 703-573-7794
                                www.mothersofasthmatics.org
Offers a clear description and understanding of childhood asthma.
Video
Mary McGowan, Executive Director
Nancy Sander, Editor-in-Chief

1426 Stinging Insect Allergy
American Academy of Allergy, Asthma and Immunology
555 East Wells Street   414-272-6071
Milwaukee, WI 53202-3889   800-822-2762
                                     Fax: 414-272-6070
                                          www.aaaai.org
Although many people are afraid of stinging insects such as bees, the stings of these insects actually cause some people to have serious allergic reactions. This video tells how to recognize and avoid stinging insects, what to do if you are stung and how to identify symptoms of an allergic reaction and get medical help.
10-13 minutes

1427 Understanding Allergic Reactions
American Academy of Allergy, Asthma and Immunology
555 East Wells Street   414-272-6071
Milwaukee, WI 53202-3889   800-822-2762
                                     Fax: 414-272-6070
                                          www.aaaai.org
During an allergic reaction, your body responds to a substance generally considered harmless to most people. This video portrays what happens in you body's immune system during an allergic reaction, how to avoid allergic substances, and methods your allergist uses to treat your allergies.
10-13 minutes

1428 What School Personnel Should Know About Asthma
American Lung Association
1740 Broadway   212-315-8700
New York, NY 10019-4315
Professionally produced videotape discussing the triggers, symptoms and management of childhood asthma.
Videotape

1429 You're in Charge: Teens with Asthma
Asthma and Allergy Foundation of America
8201 Corporate Drive   202-466-7643
Landover, MD 20785-2330   800-727-8462
                                     Fax: 202-466-8940
                                   e-mail: Info@aafa.org
                                           www.aafa.org
Designed for young adults dealing with the daily challenges of asthma management. Teens share their experiences and use of peak flow meters and prescribed medications.
10 minutes

Web Sites

1430 American Academy of Allergy, Asthma and Immunology
                                          www.aaaai.org
The largest professional medical organization devoted to the allergy/immunology specialty. Represents asthma specialists, clinical immunologists, allied health professionals and others with a special interest in the research and treatment of allergic disease.

1431 American College of Allergy, Asthma and Immunology
                                          www.acaai.org
A professional association of more than 5,000 allergists/immunologists and allied health professionals whose mission is to promote excellence in the practice of the subspecialty of allergy and immunology.

1432 American Lung Association
                                           www.lung.org

To save lives by improving lung health and preventing lung disease.

1433   Asthma and Allergy Foundation of America

e-mail: Info@aafa.org
www.aafa.org

Dedicated to improving the quality of life for people with asthma and allergic diseases through education, advocacy and research.

1434   Gazoontite

www.gazoontite.com

Provides links to websites involving asthma and also asthma-related products, such as books and guides.

1435   Healingwell

www.healingwell.com

A social network and support community for patients, caregivers, and families coping with the daily struggles of diseases, disorders and chronic illness.

1436   Health Finder

www.healthfinder.gov

A government web site where individuals can find information and tools to help you and those you care about stay healthy.

1437   Healthlink USA

www.healthlinkusa.com

Health information concerning treatment, cures, prevention, diagnosis, risk factors, research, support groups, email lists, personal stories and much more. Updated regularly.

1438   Helios Health

www.helioshealth.com

Online resource for your health information. Detailed information about specific health topics, access to expert advice from our Medical Advisory Board, and up-to-date health news.

1439   MedicineNet

www.medicinenet.com

An online resource for consumers providing easy-to-read, authoritative medical and health information.

1440   Medscape

www.medscape.com

Medscape offers specialists, primary care physicians, and other health professionals the Web's most robust and integrated medical information and educational tools.

1441   WebMD

www.webmd.com

Provides credible information, supportive communities, and in-depth reference material about health subjects. A source for original and timely health information as well as material from well known content providers.

Description

1442 **Ataxia**

Ataxia refers to a group of diseases that cause failure of muscular coordination, resulting in a staggered gait, the inability to stand or sit straight and the inability to make smooth, voluntary movements. All ataxias involve deterioration of the cerebellum and/or the brain and spinal structures that communicate with it. Conditions that are associated with ataxia may be hereditary or sporadic.

The most common hereditary ataxia is Friedreich's ataxia, which typically begins between 5 and 15 years of age. At first there is gait unsteadiness and slurred speech which progresses to weakness of the extremities. Some patients develop spinal deformity or cardiac problems. Other, less common hereditary ataxias generally begin during adult life. Sporadic cases also begin in adulthood and may be due to toxins, such as alcohol, or may be of unknown cause. Sporadic cases are often a symptom of some other disease, such as multiple sclerosis, stroke, or vitamin deficiencies. Although essentially all patients will become wheelchair-dependent at some point, the outlook for long-term survival is good.

Treatment for any of the ataxias is aimed at the underlying cause, but often supportive, with physical therapy, assistive devices, psychological support, career counseling and treatment of complications. Genetic counseling is appropriate for those with the hereditary forms and their families.

National Agencies & Associations

1443 **International Parkinson and Movement Disorder Society**
555 East Wells Street 414-276-2145
Milwaukee, WI 53202 Fax: 414-276-3349
e-mail: info@movementdisorders.org
www.movementdisorders.org
The International Parkinson and Movement Disorder Society (MDS) is a professional society of clinicians, scientists, and other healthcare professionals who are interested in Parkinson's disease, related neurodegenerative and neurodevelopmental disorders, hyperkinetic movement disorders, and abnormalities in muscle tone and motor control.
Matthew B. Stern, MD, President
Anne McGhiey, CAE, Executive Director

1444 **National Ataxia Foundation**
2600 Fernbrook Lane
Minneapolis, MN 55447 763-553-0020
Fax: 763-553-0167
e-mail: naf@ataxia.org
www.ataxia.org
The National Ataxia Foundation is dedicated to improving the lives of persons affected by ataxia through support education and research.
Michael Parent, Executive Director
Susan Hagen, Patient Services Director

1445 **National Health Information Center**
PO Box 1133
Washington, DC 20013 310-565-4167
800-336-4797
Fax: 301-984-4256
e-mail: info@nhic.org
www.health.gov/nhic
Offers a nationwide information referral service, produces directories and resource guides.

Support Groups & Hotlines

Alabama

1446 **Alabama Ambassador: National Ataxia Foundation**
123 Leigh Ann Road 256-828-4858
Hazel Green, AL 35750 e-mail: diannebw@aol.com
www.ataxia.org
Ambassadors are often in areas not served by a support group or chapter.
Dianne Blaine-Williamson, NAF Ambassador

1447 **Alabama Support Group: National Ataxia Foundation**
16 Oaks Circle 205-531-2514
Birmingham, AL 35244 e-mail: donnellyB6132@aol.com
www.ataxia.org
Becky Donnelly, Group Contact

Arizona

1448 **Phoenix Area Support Group: National Ataxi a Foundation**
2322 W Sagebrush Drive 480-726-3579
Chandler, AZ 85224-2155 e-mail: rtg22@cox.net
www.ataxia.org
Rita Garcia, Director

1449 **Tucson Support Group: National Ataxia Foundation**
7665 E Placita Luna Preciosa 520-885-8326
Tucson, AZ 85710 e-mail: bbeck15@cox.net
www.ataxia.org
Bart Beck, Director

California

1450 **California Ambassador: National Ataxia Foundation**
315 W Alamos 559-281-9188
Clovis, CA 93612 e-mail: mike betchel@yahoo.com
www.ataxia.org
Mike Betchel, NAF Ambassador

1451 **Los Angeles Support Group: National Ataxia Foundation**
339 W Palmer 818-246-5758
Glendale, CA 91204 e-mail: harryluther@sbcglobal.net
www.ataxia.org
Sid Luther, President

1452 **Northern California Support Group: National Ataxia Foundation**
26840 Eldridge Avenue 510-783-3190
Hayward, CA 94544 e-mail: rsisbig@aol.com
www.ataxia.com
Deborah Ominctin, Leader

1453 **Orange County Support Group: National Ataxia Foundation**
829 W Gary Ave 323-788-7751
Montebello, CA 90640 e-mail: dnavar@ucla.edu
www.ataxia.org
Daniel Navar, Group Leader

1454 **San Diego Support Group: National Ataxia Foundation**
2087 Granite Hills Drive 619-447-3753
El Cajon, CA 92019 e-mail: sdasg@cox.net
www.ataxia.org
Earl McLaughlin, Group Leader

Colorado

1455 **Denver Support Group: National Ataxia Foundation**
5902 W Maplewood Drive 303-973-8035
Littleton, CO 80123 e-mail: tom_sathre@acm.org
www.ataxia.org
Tom Sathre, Group Leader

Florida

1456 **Florida Ambassador: National Ataxia Foundation**
302 Beach Drive 850-654-2817
Destin, FL 30541 e-mail: csugars@cox.net
www.ataxia.org

Ambassadors are often in areas not served by a support group or chapter.
Christina Sugars, NAF Ambassador

1457   Northwest Florida Support Group: National Ataxia Foundation
54 Troon Terrace   904-273-4644
Ponte Vedra, FL 32082-3321   e-mail: jmcgranepvb@bellsouth.net
www.ataxia.org

June McGrane, Group Leader

1458   West Central FL Support Group: National Ataxia Foundation
9753 Elm Way   813-453-1084
Tampa, FL 33635   e-mail: flataxia@yahoo.com
www.ataxia.org

Crystal Frohna, Group Leader

Georgia

1459   Georgia Support Group: National Ataxia Foundation
320 Peters Street   404-822-7451
Savannah, GA 30313   e-mail: rookssgj@yahoo.com
www.ataxia.org

Greg Rooks, Group Leader

Illinois

1460   Chicago Area Support Group: National Ataxia Foundation
410 W Mahogany Ct   847-496-7544
Palatine, IL 60067   e-mail: caasg2@aol.com
www.ataxia.org

Craig Lisack, Group Leader

1461   Chicago Metro Support Group: National Ataxia Foundation
5633 N Kenmore   773-334-1667
Chicago, IL 60660   e-mail: cmarsh34@ameritech.net
www.ataxia.org

Chris Marsh, Group Leader

Indiana

1462   Southern Indiana Support Group: National Ataxia Foundation
1102 Ridgewood Drive   812-630-4783
Huntingburg, IN 47542   e-mail: monicasfaith@insightbb.com
www.ataxia.org

Monica Smith, Group Leader

Louisiana

1463   Louisiana Support Group: National Ataxia Foundation
2250 Gause Blvd   985-643-0783
Slidell, LA 70431   e-mail: ataxia1@earthlink.net
www.ataxia.org

Charlene Danielson, President
Camille Daglio, Vice-President

Maine

1464   Maine Support Group: National Ataxia Foundation
PO Box 113
Bowdoinham, ME 04008   e-mail: rollins@gwi.net
www.ataxia.org

Kelly Rollins, Group Leader

Maryland

1465   Chesapeake Area Support Group: National Ataxia Foundation
3200 Baker Circle   301-644-1836
Adamstown, MD 21710-9666   e-mail: carljlauter@erols.com
www.ataxia.org

Carl J Lauter, Group Leader

Massachusetts

1466   New England Area Support Group: National Ataxia Foundation
45 Juliette Street
Andover, MA 01810   978-475-8072
www.ataxia.org

Donna Gorzela, Group Leader

Michigan

1467   Detroit Support Group: National Ataxia Foundation
20217 Wyoming   313-736-2827
Detroit, MI 48221   e-mail: tinyt48221@yahoo.cpom
www.ataxia.org

Tanya Tunstul, Group Leader

Minnesota

1468   Minnesota Ambassador: National Ataxia Foundation
5179 Meadow Drive SE   504-282-7127
Rochester, MN 55904   e-mail: logoetz@gmail.com
www.ataxia.org

Lori Goetzman, NAF Ambassador

1469   Twin Cities Area Support Group: National Ataxia Foundation
2549 32nd Avenue S   612-724-3487
Minneapolis, MN 55406   e-mail: lschultz@bitstream.net
www.ataxia.org

Lenore Healy Schultz, Group Leader

Mississippi

1470   Mississippi Area Support Group: National Ataxia Foundation
PO Box 17005
Hattisburg, MS 39404   e-mail: daglio1@bellsouth.net
www.ataxia.org

Camille Daglio, Group Leader

Missouri

1471   Kansas City Support Group: National Ataxia Foundation
17700 E 17th Terrace Court S
Independence, MO 64057   816-257-2428
www.ataxia.org

Lois Goodman, Group Leader

1472   Mid Missouri Support Group: National Ataxia Foundation
1609 Cocoa Court   573-474-7232
Columbia, MO 65202   e-mail: rogercooley@localnet.com
www.ataxia.org

Roger Cooley, Contact

New York

1473   Central NY Area Support Group: National Ataxia Foundation
2849 Bingley Road
Cazenovia, NY 13035   e-mail: johnsons@summitsolutions.net
www.ataxia.org

Linda Johnson, President

1474   New York Ambassador National Ataxia Foundation
36 W Redoubt Rd   763-553-0020
Fishkill, NY 12524   e-mail: vrabsolutely@aol.com
www.ataxia.org

Valerie Ruggiero, NAF Ambassador

1475   Tri-State Area Support Group: National Ataxia Foundation
Northgate 6C   212-844-8711
Bronxville, NY 10708   e-mail: markmeghan@aol.com
www.ataxia.org

Mark Mitchell, Group Leader

Ohio

1476   Central Ohio Support Group: National Ataxia Foundation
7852 Country Court   440-255-8284
Mentor, OH 44060   e-mail: wurbanski@oh.rr.com
www.ataxia.org

Cecilia Urbanski, Group Leader

1477   North East Ohio Support Group National Ataxia Foundation
PO Box 148   440-693-4454
Mesopotamia, OH 44439   e-mail: kakah@windstream.net
www.ataxia.org

Joe Miller, President

1478 Ohio Ambassador: National Ataxia Foundation
1283 Westfield SW
North Canton, OH 44720
330-499-4060
e-mail: jkardos@juno.com
www.ataxia.org

James Kardos, NAF Ambassador

Oklahoma

1479 Oklahoma Ambassador: National Ataxia Foundation
5700 SE Hazel Road
Bartlesville, OK 74006
918-331-9530
e-mail: droopydog36@hotmail.com
www.ataxia.org

Darrell Owens, NAF Ambassador

Oregon

1480 Willamette Valley Support Group: National Ataxia Foundation
Albany General Hospital
Albany, OR 97321
541-812-4162
Fax: 541-812-4614
e-mail: malindam@samhealth.org
www.ataxia.org

Malinda Moore, President

South Carolina

1481 Carolinas Support Group: National Ataxia National Ataxia Foundation
1305 Cely Road
Easley, SC 29642
864-220-3395
e-mail: cecerussell@hotmail.com
www.ataxia.org

Cece Russell, Group Leader

Texas

1482 Houston Support Group: National Ataxia Foundation
9405 Highway 6 S
Houston, TX 77083
281-693-1826
e-mail: angelahcloud@aol.com
www.ataxia.org

Angela Cloud, Group Leader

1483 North Texas Support Group: National Ataxia Foundation
7 Wentworth Court
Trophy Club, TX 76262
e-mail: cheve11e@sbcglobal.net
www.ataxia.org

David Henry Jr, Group Leader

1484 Texas Ambassador: National Ataxia Foundation
356 Las Brisas Blvd
Seguin, TX 78155-0193
830-557-6050
e-mail: acemom@peoplepc.com
www.ataxia.org

Charlene Danielsonÿ, President
Camilie Daglio, Vice-President

Utah

1485 Utah Support Group: National Ataxia Foundation
Moran Eye Clinic
Salt Lake City, UT 84132
801-585-2213
e-mail: julia.kleinschmidt@hsc.utah.edu
www.ataxia.org

Dr Julia Kleinschmidt, Group Leader

Washington

1486 Seattle Support Group: National Ataxia Foundation
14104 107th Avenue
Kirkland, WA 98034
425-823-6239
e-mail: ataxiaseattle@comcast.net
www.ataxia.org/chapters/Seattle/default.
Milly Lewendon, Group Leader

1487 Washington Ambassador National Ataxia Foundation
PO Box 19045
Spokane, WA 99219
509-482-8501
www.ataxia.org

Linda Jacoy, Ambassador

Books

1488 Directory of National Genetic Voluntary Organizations
Genetic Alliance
4301 Connecticut Ave NW
Washington, DC 20008-2369
202-966-5557
800-336-4363
Fax: 202-966-8553
e-mail: info@genticalliance.org
www.genticalliance.org
Lists hundreds of organizations and associations dealing with genetic conditions.

1489 Hereditary Ataxia: Guidebook for Managing Speech & Swallowing
National Ataxia Foundation
2600 Fernbrook Lane N
Minneapolis, MN 55447-4752
763-553-0020
Fax: 763-553-0167
e-mail: naf@ataxia.org
www.ataxia.org

1490 Living with Ataxia
National Ataxia Foundation
2600 Fernbrook Lane N
Minneapolis, MN 55447-4752
763-553-0020
Fax: 763-553-0167
e-mail: naf@ataxia.org
www.ataxia.org
Compassionate resource for people who have or may be at risk of having ataxia, and for their families. This book explains the nature and causes of ataxia, the basic genetics that underlie many kinds of ataxia, discusses medical management of ataxia, provides practical advice for everyday living, points the way to many useful resources and assures that living a good life is an entirely reasonable aspiration, even with ataxia.
112 pages

1491 Ten Years to Live
National Ataxia Foundation
2600 Fernbrook Lane N
Minneapolis, MN 55447-4752
763-553-0020
Fax: 763-553-0167
e-mail: naf@ataxia.org
www.ataxia.org
Struggles of the Schut family with hereditary ataxia.

ISBN: 0-962716-63-1

Newsletters

1492 Alert
Alliance of Genetic Support Groups
4301 Connecticut Ave NW
Washington, DC 20008-2304
301-652-5553
800-336-4363
e-mail: alliance@capaccess.org
www.medhelp.org/www/agsg2.htm
Functions as a vehicle of communication between the Alliance and its constituency. Provides timely and useful information on genetics research.
Monthly

1493 GENES Information Services
Genetic Network of the Empire State
Empire State Plaza
Albany, NY 12201
518-474-7148
Fax: 518-474-8590

1494 Generations
National Ataxia Foundation
2600 Fernbrook Lane N
Minneapolis, MN 55447-4752
763-553-0020
Fax: 763-553-0167
e-mail: naf@ataxia.org
www.ataxia.org
Provides the latest in ataxia research, information on coping, reference material, updates on chapters and support groups and personal stories on living with ataxia. With a readership of more than 25,000, this publication is distributed throughout the US and the world. This publication is for ataxia families, the medical community, ataxia researchers and interested individuals. This publication is free to NAF members.
Quarterly

1495 Genexus
Great Plains Genetic Service Network
The University of Iowa · 319-356-2674
Iowa City, IA 52242 · Fax: 319-356-3347

1496 Great Lakes Genetic News
Great Lakes Regional Genetics Group
1500 Highland Avenue · 608-266-2907
Madison, WI 53705-2274 · Fax: 608-263-3496

1497 MARGIN
Mid-Atlantic Regional Human Genetics Network
260 S Broad Street · 215-456-7910
Philadelphia, PA 19102-5021 · Fax: 215-456-7911

1498 MSRGSN Newsletter
Mountain States Regional Genetics Service Network
4300 Cherry Creek Drive S · 303-692-2423
Denver, CO 80246 · Fax: 303-782-5576
e-mail: joyce.hooker@state.co.us
www.mostgene.org

8-12 pages
Joyce Hooker, Coordinator

1499 NERG News
New England Regional Genetics Group
PO Box 670 · 207-839-5324
Mount Desert, ME 04660-0670 · Fax: 207-839-8637

1500 SERGG
Southeast Regional Genetics Group
PO Box 1642 · 404-778-8551
Decatur, GA 30031-1642 · Fax: 404-778-8562
e-mail: mlane@sergginc.org
sergginc.org

Pamphlets

1501 Alliance Brochure
Genetic Alliance
4301 Connecticut Ave NW · 202-966-5557
Washington, DC 20008-2304 · Fax: 202-966-8553
e-mail: info@geneticalliance.org
www.geneticalliance.org
Explains the services and programs offered by the alliance.

1502 Ataxia Fact Sheet
National Ataxia Foundation
2600 Fernbrook Lane N · 763-553-0020
Minneapolis, MN 55447-4752 · Fax: 763-553-0167
e-mail: naf@ataxia.org
www.ataxia.org
Describes ataxia as a symptom and its association with other medical problems as well as the hereditary types.

1503 Familial Spastic Paraplegia
National Ataxia Foundation
2600 Fernbrook Lane N · 763-553-0020
Minneapolis, MN 55447-4752 · Fax: 763-553-0167
e-mail: naf@ataxia.org
www.ataxia.org
Defines this disorder and notes symptoms, causes and treatments.

1504 Frenkel's Exercises
National Ataxia Foundation
2600 Fernbrook Lane N · 763-553-0020
Minneapolis, MN 55447-4752 · Fax: 763-553-0167
e-mail: naf@ataxia.org
www.ataxia.org
Describes an exercise program designed for those with ataxia.

1505 Friedrich's Ataxia
National Ataxia Foundation
2600 Fernbrook Lane N · 763-553-0020
Minneapolis, MN 55447-4752 · Fax: 763-553-0167
e-mail: naf@ataxia.org
www.ataxia.org
Describes symptoms, diagnosis, genetics and hints on coping.

1506 Gene Testing for Ataxia
National Ataxia Foundation
2600 Fernbrook Lane N · 763-553-0020
Minneapolis, MN 55447-4752 · Fax: 763-553-0167
e-mail: naf@ataxia.org
www.ataxia.org
Describes the latest information about who should consider it and where to have it done.

1507 Health Insurance
National Ataxia Foundation
2600 Fernbrook Lane N · 763-553-0020
Minneapolis, MN 55447-4752 · Fax: 763-553-0167
e-mail: naf@ataxia.org
www.ataxia.org
Offers health insurance advice for persons with ataxia.

1508 Hereditary Ataxia: Brochure
National Ataxia Foundation
2600 Fernbrook Lane N · 763-553-0020
Minneapolis, MN 55447-4752 · Fax: 763-553-0167
e-mail: naf@ataxia.org
www.ataxia.org
Describes recessive and dominant ataxias, information on how hereditary ataxia is transmitted and explanations of the NAF's role in education, service and prevention.

1509 Hereditary Ataxia: Fact Sheets
National Ataxia Foundation
2600 Fernbrook Lane N · 763-553-0020
Minneapolis, MN 55447-4752 · Fax: 763-553-0167
e-mail: naf@ataxia.org
www.ataxia.org
Various ataxia fact sheets relating to specific forms of hereditary ataxia. Individual ataxia fact sheets include Friederich's ataxia and specific forms of spinocerebellar ataxias (SCAs).

1510 Incorporating Consumers into Regional Genetics Networks
Genetic Alliance
4301 Connecticut Ave NW · 202-966-5557
Washington, DC 20008-2304 · Fax: 202-966-8553
e-mail: info@geneticalliance.org
www.geneticalliance.org

1511 Informed Consent: Participation In Genetic Research Studies
Genetic Alliance
4301 Connecticut Ave NW · 202-966-5557
Washington, DC 20008-2304 · Fax: 202-966-8553
e-mail: info@genticalliance.org
www.geneticalliance.org
This booklet explains the nature of genetic research with its benefits and risks.

1512 Pen-Pal Directory
National Ataxia Foundation
2600 Fernbrook Lane N · 763-553-0020
Minneapolis, MN 55447-4752 · Fax: 763-553-0167
e-mail: naf@ataxia.org
www.ataxia.org
National, state and international directory of others who are affected by ataxia. Available to NAF Pen-Pal members only. Application available.

1513 Students with Friedreich's Ataxia
National Ataxia Foundation
2600 Fernbrook Lane N · 763-553-0020
Minneapolis, MN 55447-4752 · Fax: 763-553-0167
e-mail: naf@ataxia.org
www.ataxia.org
Worksheet for teachers, parents and others who need to understand the physical constraints of ataxia.

Audio & Video

1514 Together...There Is Hope
National Ataxia Foundation
2600 Fernbrook Lane N · 763-553-0020
Minneapolis, MN 55447-4752 · Fax: 763-553-0167
e-mail: naf@ataxia.org
www.ataxia.org

Video discussing ataxias genetic patterns of inheritance and the National Ataxia Foundation and its research efforts.

Web Sites

1515 Healing Well

www.healingwell.com

An online health resource guide to medical news, chat, information and articles, newsgroups and message boards, books, disease-related web sites, medical directories, and more for patients, friends, and family coping with disabling diseases, disorders, or chronic illnesses.

1516 Health Finder

www.healthfinder.gov

Searchable, carefully developed web site offering information on over 1000 topics. Developed by the US Department of Health and Human Services, the site can be used in both English and Spanish.

1517 Healthlink USA

www.healthlinkusa.com

Health information concerning treatment, cures, prevention, diagnosis, risk factors, research, support groups, email lists, personal stories and much more. Updated regularly.

1518 Helios Health

www.helioshealth.com

Online resource for your health information. Detailed information about specific health topics, access to expert advice from our Medical Advisory Board, and up-to-date health news.

1519 MedicineNet

www.medicinenet.com

An online resource for consumers providing easy-to-read, authoritative medical and health information.

1520 Medscape

www.medscape.com

Medscape offers specialists, primary care physicians, and other health professionals the Web's most robust and integrated medical information and educational tools.

1521 National Ataxia Foundation

e-mail: naf@ataxia.org
www.ataxia.org

Information on ataxia, ataxia research, listing of chapters and support groups and related links. Researchers may download NAF's ataxia reserch application guidelines and forms. Exerpts of articles in NAF's quarterly news publication, Generations. Online registration for NAF's annual membership meetings. Caladar of events on NAF activities. This site is for ataxia familes, the medical community, ataxia reserachers and interested individuals.
William P. Sweeney, President
Camille Daglio, Vice President

1522 WebMD

www.webmd.com

Provides credible information, supportive communities, and in-depth reference material about health subjects. A source for original and timely health information as well as material from well known content providers.

Description

1523 Attention Deficit Hyperactivity Disorder

Attention Deficit-Hyperactivity Disorder, ADHD, and Attention Deficit Disorder, ADD, are neurologically based disorders. ADHD primarily affects children, with 2 to 4 percent of the school-age population in the United States having some symptoms. In about 25 percent of attention deficit cases, hyperactivity is not present, and it is thus labeled ADD. ADHD's three major symptoms are distractibility, impulsivity and hyperactivity. The dominant symptom of ADD is day dreaming or tuning out. ADHD is seen 10 times more frequently in boys than girls. Studies show that 90 percent have academic problems or are underachievers, although these difficulties may not begin until the middle school years.

While studies suggest that about 50 percent of children with these disorders will improve at puberty, both ADHD and ADD can exist throughout a lifetime and, in fact, may first be diagnosed in teen or adult years.

Often, an affected individual experiences difficulties that can impact learning, peer relations, family life, and self-esteem. These difficulties may manifest themselves through angry outbursts, self-imposed social isolation, blaming others, a quickness to fight, and a high sensitivity to criticism.

Treatment of ADHD and ADD include: education programs with resource or tutorial help; psychological programs to improve self-esteem and help families and individuals deal with associated stress; and medical therapy. Treatment must be individualized to address both intrinsic characteristics of the child and relevant environmental factors, and be coordinated with a variety of interventions within the school, home and community.

Many professionals agree that medication, when appropriate, combined with counseling, best controls symptoms. Stimulant medications, including the new longer active agents, are the drugs of choice. To identify children with this disorder and to develop the most appropriate treatment plan, parents will need to consult with a psychiatrist, pediatric neurologist, or pediatrician.

National Agencies & Associations

1524 Children & Adults with Attention Deficit Disorders
8181 Professional Place
Landover, MD 20785

301-306-7070
800-233-4050
Fax: 301-306-7090
www.chadd.org

CHADD's primary objectives are: to provide a support network for parents and caregivers; to provide a forum for continuing education; to be a community resource and disseminate accurate evidence-based information about AD/HD to parents, educators and adults.
E Clarke Ross, CEO
Ruth Hughes, Chief Program Officer Community Service

1525 Council for Exceptional Children
2900 Crystal Drive
Arlington, VA 22202-3557

703-620-3660
88 -23 -773
Fax: 703-264-9494
TTY: 866-915-5000
e-mail: service@cec.sped.org
www.cec.sped.org

Advocates appropriate policies standards and development for individuals with special needs. Provides professional development for special educators.
Bruce Ramirez, Executive Director
Joan Melner, Assistant Executive Director

1526 Feingold Association of the US
37 Shell Road
Rocky Point, NY 11778

631-369-9340
800-321-3287
Fax: 631-369-2988
e-mail: help@feingold.org
www.feingold.org

Helps families of children with learning and behavior problems including attention deficit disorder. Also helps chemically-sensitive and salicylate-sensitive adults. Program is based upon a diet which primarily eliminates certain synthetic food additives.

1527 Learning Disabilities Association of America
4156 Library Road
Pittsburgh, PA 15234-1349

412-341-1515
888-300-6710
Fax: 412-344-0224
e-mail: info@LDAAmerica.org
www.ldaamerica.org

An information and referral center for parents and professionals dealing with learning disabilities.
Barbara Lefler, Director of Affiliate Services
Patricia Lillie, President

1528 National Center for Learning Disabilities
381 Park Avenue S
New York, NY 10016-8806

212-545-7510
888-575-7373
Fax: 212-545-9665
www.ncld.org

One of the foremost nonprofit organizations committed to improving the lives of the estimated one in ten children with learning disabilities raising public awareness and understanding.
James H Wendorf, Executive Director
Sheldon H Horowitz EdD, Director/Professional Services

1529 National Dissemination Center for Children with Disabilities
1825 Connecticut Avenue NW
Washington, DC 20009

800-695-0285
Fax: 202-884-8441
TTY: 202-884-8200
e-mail: nichcy@aed.org
www.nichcy.org

Publishes free, fact filled newsletters. Arranges workshops. Advises parents on the laws entitling children with disabilities to special education and other services.
Dr Suzanne Ripley, Contact

Libraries & Resource Centers

1530 HEATH Resource Center
George Washington University
2134 G Street NW
Washington, DC 20052-0001

202-973-0904
800-544-3284
Fax: 202-994-3365
e-mail: askheath@gwu.edu
http://www.heath.gwu.edu/

The HEATH Resource Center of The George Washington University, Graduate School of Education and Human Development, is the national clearinghouse on postsecondary education for individuals with disabilities.
Dr Lynda West, Principal Investigator
Dr Joel Gomez, Co-Principal Investigator

Support Groups & Hotlines

1531 Attention Deficit Information Network
475 Hillside Ave   617-455-9895
Needham, MA 02194
Offers support and information to families of children with attention deficit disorder, adults with ADD and professionals through an international network of 60 parent and adult chapters.

1532 National Federation of Families for Children's Mental Health
9605 Medical Center Drive   240-403-1901
Rockville, MD 20850   Fax: 240-403-1909
                                    e-mail: ffcmh@ffcmh.org
                                            www.ffcmh.org
Provides advocacy at the national level for the rights of children and youth with emotional, behavioral and mental health challenges and their families; provides leadership and technical assistance to a nation-wide network of family run organizations; and collaborates with family run and other child serving organizations to transform mental health care in America.
Sandra Spencer, Executive Director
Andrea Barnes, Policy & Research Assistant

1533 National Health Information Center
PO Box 1133   310-565-4167
Washington, DC 20013-1133   800-336-4797
                                        Fax: 301-984-4256
                                    e-mail: info@nhic.org
                                         www.health.gov/nhic
A health information referral service sponsored by the Office of Disease Prevention and Health Promotion. Puts health professionals and consumers who have health questions in touch with those organizations that are best able to provide answers.

Books

1534 ADHD Parenting Handbook: Practical Advice for Parents from Parents
Colleen Alexander-Roberts, author

Taylor Trade Publishing
4501 Forbes Boulevard   301-459-3366
Lanham, MD 20706   Fax: 301-429-5743
                                    e-mail: custserv@nbnbooks.com
                                            www.rlpgtrade.com
A compilation of practical advice and tips for handling day-to-day activities that routinely become problematic for ADHD children, such as getting dressed for school, going to bed, performing chores, completing homework, and playing with other children.
Paperback
ISBN: 0-878338-62-4

1535 ADHD in Schools: Assessment and Intervention Strategies
George J DuPaul, Gary Stoner, author

Guilford Publications
370 Seventh Avenue
New York, NY 10001   800-365-7006
                                        Fax: 212-966-6708
                                    e-mail: info@guilford.com
                                            www.guilford.com
Provides essential guidance for school-based professionals meeting the challenges of ADHD at any grade level. Comprehensive and practical, includes several reproducible assessment tools and handouts.
330 pages Paperback
ISBN: 1-593850-89-0

1536 ADHD: Handbook for Diagnosis & Treatment
Western Psychological Services
12031 Wilshire Boulevard   310-478-2061
Los Angeles, CA 90025-1201   800-648-8857
                                        Fax: 310-478-7838
                                            www.wpspublish.com
This second edition helps clinicians diagnose and treat Attention Deficit Hyperactivity Disorder. Written by an internationally recognized authority in the field, it covers the history of ADHD, its primary symptoms, associated conditions, developmental course

and outcome, and family context. A workbook companion manual is also available.
700 pages

1537 Attention Deficit Disorder: A Different Perception
Underwood-Miller
708 Westover Drive
Lancaster, PA 17601-1242   717-285-2255
                                        www.vance.hw.nl/dbase/publisher
1993 180 pages Paperback
ISBN: 0-887331-56-4

1538 Attention Deficit Disorder: Learning Disabilities
Random House
25 Van Zant Street   410-848-1900
East Norwalk, CT 06855-1726   800-726-0600
                                        Fax: 800-214-1438
                                            www.randomhouse.com
Realities, myths, and controversial treatments. Section I tries to dispel the myths and discusses proven treatments for ADHD and LD. Section II explains how the scientific community evaluates new treatment methods, and Section III summarizes alternative treatments and discusses scientific evidence pertaining to its usefulness.
256 pages
ISBN: 0-385469-31-4

1539 Attention Deficit Hyperactivity Disorder: What Every Parent Wants to Know
Paul H Brookes Publishing Company
PO Box 10624   301-337-9580
Baltimore, MD 21285-0624   800-638-3775
                                        Fax: 410-337-8539
                                    e-mail: custserv@brookspublishing.com
                                            www.brookespublishing.com
1993 320 pages Paperback
ISBN: 1-557661-41-3
Dante Washington, Customer Service Representative

1540 Coping with ADD/ADHD
Rosen Publishing Group
29 E 21st Street   212-777-3017
New York, NY 10010-6209   800-237-9932
                                        Fax: 888-436-4643
                                    e-mail: customerservice@rosenpub.com
                                            www.rosenpublishing.com
At least 3.5 million American youngsters suffer from ADD. This book defines the syndrome and provides specific information about treatment and counseling.
150 pages Hardcover
ISBN: 0-823931-96-X

1541 Helping Your ADD Child With or Without Hyperactivity
John F Taylor PhD, author

Random House Inc.
Dep of Library Marketing   800-733-3000
New York, NY 10017   800-726-0600
                                        Fax: 212-940-7381
                                    e-mail: crownpublicity@randomhouse.com
                                            www.randomhouse.com
Inside this book you will find step-by-step tools for helping your ADD or ADHD child. From extensive screening for spotting the initial signs to the pros and cons of nutritional, psychological, and drug treatments.
2001
ISBN: 0-761527-56-7

1542 Hyperactive Children Grown Up
Gabrielle Weiss, Lily Trokenberg Hechtman, author

Guilford Publications
370 Seventh Avenue
New York, NY 10001   800-365-7006
                                        Fax: 212-966-6708
                                    e-mail: info@guilford.com
                                            www.guilford.com
Reports findings on the etiology, treatment, and outcome of attention deficits and hyperactivity at all stages of development.
473 pages Paperback
ISBN: 0-898625-96-7

1543 **LD Child and the ADHD Child**
Suzanne H Stevens, author
John F Blair Publishing
1406 Plaza Drive   336-768-1374
Winston-Salem, NC 27103   800-222-9796
                                                         Fax: 336-768-9194
                                                e-mail: blairpub@aol.com
                                                         www.blairpub.com
Helps parents raise their LD and/or ADHD children so that they,
too, can grow up to be okay-so that they will be happy, well-ad-
justed, and successful adults despite the learning and behavior pat-
terns that make them different.
Paperback
ISBN: 0-895871-42-8

1544 **Managing Attention Deficit Hyperactivity Disorder in Children:**
Sam Goldstein, Michael Goldstein, author
Wiley Publishing
111 River Street   201-748-6000
Hoboken, NJ 07030-5774   Fax: 201-748-6088
                                                   e-mail: info@wiley.com
                                                         www.wiley.com
A proven approach to the diagnosis and management of one of the
most challenging childhood disorders. In this book the authors describe a proven multidisciplinary approach to the diagnosis and
treatment of childhood ADHD, developed at the prestigous Neurology, Learning and Behavior Center in Salt Lake City.
1998 896 pages
ISBN: 0-471121-58-9

1545 **Maybe You Know My Kid: A Parent's Guide to Identifying
ADHD**
Birch Lane Press
120 Enterprise Avenue S
Secaucus, NJ 07094-1902   800-447-2665
The author writes about her family experiences with their son, David, who has attention deficit disorder. Contains a comprehensive
review of important issues plus descriptions of some helpful management techniques.
222 pages

1546 **Medications for Attention Disorders and Related Medical
Problems**
Specialty Press
300 NW 70th Avenue   954-792-8100
Plantation, FL 33317   800-233-9273
                                                         Fax: 954-792-8545
                                        e-mail: sales@addwarehouse.com
                                                     www.addwarehouse.com
A comprehensive handbook covering the history, characteristics,
and causes of ADHD. The equal importance of appropriate academic programming, counseling, and medication are stressed
throughout.
415 pages Hardcover

1547 **Parents Helping Parents: A Directory of Support Groups for
ADD**
CibaGelgy, Pharmaceuticals Division
1400 Parkmoor Avenue   408-727-5775
San Jose, CA 95126   855-727-5775
                                                         Fax: 408-286-1116
                                                                 www.php.com

1548 **Parents' Hyperactivity Handbook: Helping the Fidgety Child**
Plenum Press
233 Spring Street   212-460-1550
New York, NY 10013-1578   800-777-4643
                                                         Fax: 212-460-1575
                                                e-mail: support@apress.com
                                                            www.springer.com

1993 306 pages
ISBN: 0-306444-65-8

1549 **Rethinking Attention Deficit Disorders**
Miriam Cherkes-Julkowski, author
Brookline Books

8 Trumbull Rd   413-584-0184
Northampton, MA 01060   800-666-2665
                                                         Fax: 413-584-6184
                                                           brooklinebks.com
Gives the classroom teacher useful information that provides ideas
and strategies for working with children suffering from ADD.
1997 Paperback
ISBN: 1-571290-37-0

1550 **The New ADD in Adults Workbook**
Lynn Weiss, PhD, author
Taylor Trade Publishing
4501 Forbes Boulevard   301-459-3366
Lanham, MD 20706   Fax: 301-429-5743
                                           e-mail: custserv@nbnbooks.com
                                                          www.rlpgtrade.com
Not only touches on and dispels the most recent clinical findings,
but also emphasizes the bigger perspective, focusing on the em-
powerment and diversity issues facing all of us on the A.D.D. continuum today. Persuades readers to work through their challenges
with practical, prescriptive exercises and insights.
Paperback
ISBN: 0-878338-50-0

1551 **You Mean I'm Not Lazy, Stupid or Crazy?**
Tyrell & Jerem Press
PO Box 20089
Cincinnati, OH 45220-0089   800-622-6611
A new self-help book is the first written by ADD adults for ADD
adults. This comprehensive guide provides accurate information,
practical how-tos and moral support.

1552 **Attention Deficit/Hyperactivity Disorder**
Guilford Publications
370 Seventh Avenue   212-431-9800
New York, NY 10012-4068   800-365-7006
                                                         Fax: 212-966-6708
                                                           www.guilford.com
A second edition that is the handbook on the diagnosis and treatment of ADHD in the 1990s. A companion workbook is also available with forms that may be photocopied.
747 pages Hardcover
ISBN: 0-898624-43-6

Children's Books

1553 **Self-Control Games & Workbook**
Western Psychological Services
12031 Wilshire Boulevard   310-478-2061
Los Angeles, CA 90025-1201   800-648-8857
                                                         Fax: 310-478-7838
This game is designed to teach self-control in academic and social
situations. Addresses a total of 24 impulsive, inattentive and hyperactive behaviors. The companion workbook reinforces the use
of positive self-statements, and problem-solving techniques,
instead of expressing anger.
Game

1554 **Shelley, the Hyperactive Turtle**
Deborah Moss, author
Woodbine House
6510 Bells Mill Road
Bethesda, MD 20817   800-843-7323
                                                         Fax: 301-897-5838
                                          e-mail: info@woodbinehouse.com
                                                       www.woodbinehouse.com
Reassures young children who are going through the diagnostic
process or who are having problems behaving at school or making
friends because of AD/HD.
20 pages
ISBN: 1-890627-75-1

Magazines

1555 **Attention**
Children & Adults with Attention Deficit Disorder

8181 Professional Place
Landover, MD 20785-7221

301-306-7070
800-233-4050
Fax: 301-306-7090
TTY: 301-429-0641

Quarterly

Newsletters

1556 ADHD Report
Guilford Publications
370 Seventh Avenue
New York, NY 10001

800-365-7006
Fax: 212-966-6708
e-mail: info@guilford.com
www.guilford.com

Examines the nature, diagnosis, and outcomes associated with the disorder, and provides a single reliable guide to the latest developments in the fields of clinical management and education. Includes research findings, as well as ongoing coverage of ADHD in the news.
16 pages BiMonthly

1557 Chadder
Children & Adults with Attention Deficit Disorder
8181 Professional Place
Landover, MD 20785-7221

301-306-7070
800-233-4050
Fax: 301-306-7090
TTY: 301-429-0641

Quarterly

1558 Challenge
Challenge
PO Box 488
West Newbury, MA 01985-0688

978-462-0495
800-233-2322

National newsletter on ADD/ADHD that carries interviews with nationally-known scientists, as well as physicians, psychologists, social workers, educators, and other practitioners in the field of ADHD.
12 pages BiMonthly
Jean C Harrison, Executive Director

1559 Pure Facts
Feingold Association of the US
PO Box 6550
Alexandria, VA 22306-0550

703-768-3287

Monthly newsletter with articles on nutrition and behavior and lists of approved brand-name foods.

Pamphlets

1560 ADHD
Learning Disabilities Association of America
4156 Library Road
Pittsburgh, PA 15234-1349

412-341-1515
888-300-6710
Fax: 412-344-0224
e-mail: info@ldaamerica.org
www.ldaamerica.org

A booklet for parents offering information on Attention Deficit Hyperactivity Disorders and learning disabilities.

1561 Attention Deficit Disorders and Hyperactivity
Council for Exceptional Children
2900 Crystal Drive
Arlington, VA 22202

703-620-3660
888-232-7733
Fax: 703-264-9494
TTY: 866-915-5000
e-mail: service@cec.sped.org
www.cec.sped.org

Published by the Council for Exceptional Children.

1562 COGREHAB
Life Science Associates
1 Fennimore Road
Bayport, NY 11705-2115

631-472-2111
Fax: 631-472-8146
e-mail: lifesciassoc@pipeline.com
lifesciassoc.home.pipeline.com

Divided into six groups for diagnosis and treatment of attention, memory and perceptual disorders to be used by and under the guidance of a professional.
$95 - $1,950

1563 Fact Sheet: Attention Deficit Hyperactivity Disorder
Learning Disabilities Association of America
4156 Library Road
Pittsburgh, PA 15234-1349

412-341-1515
888-300-6710
Fax: 412-344-0224
e-mail: info@ldaamerica.org
www.ldaamerica.org

A pamphlet offering factual information on ADHD.

1564 Helping Adolescents with ADHD and Learning Disabilities
Learning Disabilities Association of America
4156 Library Road
Pittsburgh, PA 15234-1349

412-341-1515
888-300-6710
Fax: 412-344-0224
e-mail: info@ldaamerica.org
www.ldaamerica.org

Audio & Video

1565 ADD Stepping Out of the Dark
ADD Videos
PO Box 622
New Paltz, NY 12561-0622

845-255-3612
Fax: 845-883-6452

A powerful, effective video, ideal for health professionals, educators and parents providing a visual montage designed to promote an understanding and awareness of attention deficit disorder. Based on actual accounts of those who have ADD, including a neurologist, an office worker, and parents of children with ADD. The video allows the viewer to feel the frustration and lack of attention that ADD brings to many.
Video
Lenae Madonna, Producer
Sheila Buckley, Executive Director

1566 ADHD in Adults
Guilford Publications
370 Seventh Avenue
New York, NY 10001-4068

212-431-9800
800-365-7006
Fax: 212-966-6708
e-mail: info@guilford.com
www.guilford.com

This program integrates information on ADHD with the actual experiences of four adults who suffer from the disorder. Representing a range of professions, from a lawyer to a mother working at home, each candidly discusses the impact of ADHD on his or her daily life. These interviews are augmented by comments from family members and other clinicians who treat adults with ADHD.
Video

1567 ADHD in the Classroom: Strategies for Teachers
Rusell A Barkley, author
Guilford Publications
370 Seventh Avenue
New York, NY 10001

800-365-7006
Fax: 212-966-6708
e-mail: info@guilford.com
www.guilford.com

Designed to help teachers create a learning environment that is responsive to the needs of all students, including those with ADHD.

1568 ADHD: What Do We Know?
Guilford Publications
370 Seventh Avenue
New York, NY 10001-4068

212-431-9800
800-365-7006
Fax: 212-966-6708
e-mail: info@guilford.com
www.guilford.com

An introduction for teachers and special education practitioners, school psychologists and parents of ADHD children. Topics outlined in this video include the causes and prevalence of ADHD, ways children with ADHD behave, other conditions that may accompany ADHD and long-term prospects for children with ADHD.
Video

1569 Around the Clock
Guilford Publications
370 Seventh Avenue   212-431-9800
New York, NY 10001-4068   800-365-7006
                                   Fax: 212-966-6708
                                  e-mail: info@guilford.com
                                   www.guilford.com
This videotape provides both professionals and parents a helpful
look at how the difficulties facing parents of ADHD children can
be handled.

1570 Attention Deficit Disorder
Pro-Ed, Inc.
8700 Shoal Creek Blvd   512-451-3246
Austin, TX 78757-6897   800-897-3202
                                   Fax: 800-397-7633
                                  e-mail: info@proedinc.com
                                   www.proedinc.com/
A video and book providing helpful suggestions for both home and
classroom management of students with attention deficit disorder.
216 pages Paperback
ISBN: 0-890797-42-0
Krista Anderson, Technical Advisor
Matt Synatschk, Books & Materials Permissions Editor

1571 Educating Inattentive Children
Western Psychological Services
12031 Wilshire Boulevard
Los Angeles, CA 90025-1201   800-648-8857
                                   Fax: 310-478-7838
An excellent resource for teachers who encounter inattention and
hyperactivity in the classroom. It helps teachers distinguish deliberate misbehavior from the incompetent, nonpurposeful behavior
of the inattentive child.
Video

1572 It's Just Attention Disorder
Western Psychological Services
12031 Wilshire Boulevard   310-478-2061
Los Angeles, CA 90025-1201   800-648-8857
                                   Fax: 310-478-7838
This ground-breaking videotape takes the critical first steps in
treating attention-deficit disorder: it enlists the inattentive or hy-
peractive child as an active participant in his or her treatment.
Video

1573 Why Won't My Child Pay Attention?
Western Psychological Services
12031 Wilshire Boulevard   310-478-2061
Los Angeles, CA 90025-1201   800-648-8857
                                   Fax: 310-478-7838
Practical and reassuring videotape, noted child psychologist tells
parents about two of the most common and complex problems of
childhood: inattention and hyperactivity.
Video

Web Sites

1574 Attention Deficit Information Network
                              www.addinfonetwork.com
Offers support and information to families of children and adults
with ADD and to professionals.

1575 Healing Well
                                 www.healingwell.com
A social network and support community for patients, caregivers,
and families coping with the daily struggles of diseases, disorders
and chronic illness.

1576 Health Finder
                                  www.healthfinder.gov
A government web site, where individuals can find information
and tools to help you and those you care about stay healthy.

1577 Healthlink USA
                                 www.healthlinkusa.com
Health information concerning treatment, cures, prevention, diagnosis, risk factors, research, support groups, email lists, personal
stories and much more. Updated regularly.

1578 Helios Health
                                  www.helioshealth.com
Online resource for your health information. Detailed information
about specific health topics, access to expert advice from our Medical Advisory Board, and up-to-date health news.

1579 MedicineNet
                                  www.medicinenet.com
An online resource for consumers providing easy-to-read, authoritative medical and health information.

1580 Medscape
                                    www.medscape.com
Medscape offers specialists, primary care physicians, and other
health professionals the Web's most robust and integrated medical
information and educational tools.

1581 WebMD
                                     www.webmd.com
Provides credible information, supportive communities, and
in-depth reference material about health subjects. A source for
original and timely health information as well as material from
well known content providers.

Description

1582 Autistic Spectrum Disorders

Autistic Spectrum Disorders, ASD, includes (from most to least severe) autism, high-functioning autism (HFA), Asperger's syndrome, and PDD-NOS (pervasive development disorder — not otherwise specified). ASD typically appear during the first three years of life. Autism involves severe impairment of social and communication development. HFA symptoms are less severe, but include delayed language development. Asperger's is similar to HFA, but with no speech delay. PPD-NOS describes autistic categories that do not fit into any of the above. ASD affects behavior, communication, social interaction and other neurological functions.

ASD has numerous symptoms, all of which reduce the child's ability to communicate and interact. Many autistic children have abnormal social relationships, impaired understanding, and uneven intellectual development with mental retardation in most cases. They may exhibit repetitive movement (i.e., rocking, spinning, and hand twisting), avoid making eye contact, and have impaired verbal skills. Occasionally, children with ASD will have decreased sensitivity to pain, and have abnormal responses to light, touch and sound. The disorder can include self-injury and bizarre behavior.

ASD is two to four times more common in boys than in girls. It is found in people of all ethnic backgrounds, and throughout the world. In 2009, nine in 1000 children were diagnosed with ASD, up from one in 500 just six years ago.

In some cases, ASD may be linked to damage to the brain or nervous system. Studies of twins with autism point to a possible genetic link. ASD has been associated with the following risk factors: pre- and perinatal birth complications; prenatal infections with certain viruses; abnormalities of the brain detected with a CT scan or MRI (although no specific defects in the brain structure have been consistently identified). More recently, usual childhood vaccines, environmental toxins, and pollutants are being questioned to explain the sharp rise in ASD cases in recent decades, but researchers have been unable to confirm these findings.

Although there are no known cures for ASD, experts advocate early and intense behavioral, developmental and speech therapy. Medications may alleviate some of the accompanying behavior problems, but provide minimal help for the disorder itself and are generally not used. There is strong emphasis on early diagnosis, early intervention, and individualized educational programs to provide the opportunity for maximum development for the child with Autistic Spectrum Disorder.

National Agencies & Associations

1583 ARRISE
9238 Parklane Avenue
Franklin Park, IL 60131-2836
847-451-2740

Provides information about autism.

1584 Autism Research Institute
4182 Adams Avenue
San Diego, CA 92116-2536
619-281-7165
866-366-3361
Fax: 619-563-6840
www.autism.com
A clearinghouse for research on autism and related disorders of learning and behavior. Conducts and compiles research findings to provide people with the latest research available.
Stephen M Edelson PhD, Director

1585 Autism Services Center
929 Fourth Avenue
Huntington, WV 25701-0507
304-525-8014
Fax: 304-525-8026
www.autismservicescenter.org
Provides educational information to the public and professional communities on autism provides case management activities and referrals for persons afflicted with autism and their families.
Ruth Christ Sullivan, Founder and Executive Director

1586 Autism Society of America
4740 East-West Hwy
Bethesda, MD 20814
301-657-0881
800-328-8476
Fax: 301-657-0869
e-mail: info@autism-society.org
www.autism-society.org
A national charitable organization with the mission of providing as much information as possible about autism and the various options, approaches, methods and systems available to parents of children with autism, family members and professionals.
Lee Grossman, President/CEO
Barbara Newhouse, Chief Operating Officer

1587 Autism Treatment Center of America
2080 S Undermountain Road
Sheffield, MA 01257
413-229-2100
877-766-7473
Fax: 413-229-3202
e-mail: correspondence@option.org
www.autismtreatmentcenter.org
Since 1983 the Autism Treatment Center of America has provided innovative training programs for parents and professionals caring for children challenged by Autism Autism Spectrum Disorders Pervasive Developmental Disorder (PDD) and other developmental disorders.
Barry Neil Kaufman, Co-Founder/Co-Creator Son-Rise Program
Bryn Hogan, Director Son-Rise Program

1588 Autism Treatment Center of America: Son-Rise Program
2080 South Undermountain Road
Sheffield, MA 01257
413-229-2100
877-766-7473
Fax: 413-229-3202
e-mail: correspondence@option.org
www.son-rise.org
Since 1983, the Autism Treatment Center of America has provided innovative training programs for parents and professionals caring for children challenged by Autism, Autism Spectrum Disorders, Pervasive Developmental Disorder (PDD) and other developmental difficulties. The Son-Rise Program teaches a specific yet comprehensive system of treatment and education designed to help families and caregivers enable their children to dramatically improve in all areas of learning.
Sean Fitzgerald, Assistant Director Son-Rise Program
Barry Neil Kaufman, Co-Founder

1589 Community Services for Autistic Adults & Children
8615 E Village Avenue
Montgomery Village, MD 20886
240-912-2220
Fax: 301-926-9384
e-mail: csaac@csaac.org
www.csaac.org
The Community Services for Autistic Adults & Children is a non-profit organization dedicated to helping those with autism. Since 1979 CSAAC has served over 150 individuals and helped people with autism find housing, employment and other community services.
Ian Paregol, Executive Director
Don Rodrick, Chief Financial Officer

1590 National Institute of Neurological Disorders and Stroke
NIH Neurological Institute   301-496-5751
Bethesda, MD 20824   800-352-9424
Fax: 301-402-2186
TTY: 301-468-5981
www.ninds.nih.gov

The mission of NINDS is to reduce the burden of neurological disease - a burden borne by every age group, by every segment of society, by people all over the world.
Story C Landis, PhD, Director
Walter J Koroshetz, Deputy Director

State Agencies & Associations

Alabama

1591 Autism Society of Alabama
Birmingham, AL 35243   205-951-1364
877-4AU-TISM
Fax: 205-967-8244
e-mail: info@autism-alabama.org
www.autism-alabama.org

Ryan Thomas, President
Jennifer Muller, Executive Director

1592 Autism Society of North Alabama
PO Box 2902   256-776-0505
Huntsville, AL 35801   e-mail: sherron@northalabamaautism.org
www.northalabamaautism.org

Teresa White, President
Carol Wright, Vice President

Arizona

1593 Autism Society of Pima County
PO Box 44156   520-770-1541
Tucson, AZ 85733-4156   Fax: 520-319-5979
e-mail: az-pimacounty@autismsocietyofamerica.org
www.tucsonautism.org

Peter Earhart, President
Stephanie Hill, Vice President

California

1594 Autism Society of California
PO Box 15247   562-943-3335
Long Beach, CA 90815-0600   800-700-0037
e-mail: brubin698@earthlink.net
www.autismsocietyca.org

Dean Wilson, President
Gregory Fletcher, First Vice President

Colorado

1595 Autism Society of Colorado
550 S Wadsworth Boulevard   720-214-0794
Lakewood, CO 80226-4169   Fax: 720-274-2744
e-mail: co-colorado@autismsocietyofamerica.org
www.autismcolorado.org

Betty Lehman, Executive Director
Lorri Park, Programs Director

Connecticut

1596 Autism Society of Connecticut
PO Box 1404
Guilford, CT 06437   888-453-4975
www.autismsocietyofct.org

Delaware

1597 Autism Society of Delaware
924 Old Harmony Road   302-224-6020
Newark, DE 19713   Fax: 302-224-6017
e-mail: delautism@delautism.org
www.delautism.org

Theda Ellis, Executive Director
Kim Siegel, Development Director

District of Columbia

1598 Autism Society of District Columbia
5167 7th Street NE   202-561-5300
Washington, DC 20011-2624   Fax: 202-561-8634
e-mail: dc-washington@autismsocietyofamerica.org
www.autism-society.org/chapter130
Scott Badesch, President/ChiefÿExecutive Officer
John Dabrowski, Chief Financial Officer

Florida

1599 Autism Society of Greater Orlando
4743 Hearthside Drive   407-855-0235
Orlando, FL 32837-5445   e-mail: contact@asgo.org~
www.asgo.org

Donna Lorman, President
Marzena Batignani, Vice President

Georgia

1600 Autism Society of Greater Georgia
PO Box 3707   770-904-4474
Suwanee, GA 30024   Fax: 770-904-4476
www.asaga.com

Steve Doran, President
Cindy Pike, Executive Director

Hawaii

1601 Autism Society of Hawaii
PO Box 2995   808-282-3676
Honolulu, HI 96802-2995   e-mail: naomig122@hotmail.com
www.autismhi.org

William Bolman, President
ÿJessica Wong-Sumida, M.A., J.D., Executive Director

Idaho

1602 Autism Society of Treasure Valley
PO Box 44831   208-336-5676
Boise, ID 83711-9404   Fax: 202-884-5582
e-mail: Autism.asatvc@yahoo.com
www.asatvc.org

Illinois

1603 Autism Society of Illinois
2200 S Main Street   630-691-1270
Lombard, IL 60148-5366   888-691-1270
Fax: 630-932-5620
e-mail: info@autismillinois.org
www.autismillinois.org

Karen McDonough, Executive Director
Kym Bills, President

Indiana

1604 Autism Society of Indiana
4740 Kingsway Drive   317-695-0252
Indianapolis, IN 46205-0252   Fax: 317-815-0859
e-mail: info@inautism.org
www.autismsocietyofindiana.org

Joshua Carr, President
Kylee Hope, Vice-President

Iowa

1605 Autism Society of Iowa
4549 Waterford Drive   515-327-9075
W Des Moines, IA 50265-2059   888-722-4799
Fax: 319-557-1169
e-mail: autism50ia@aol.com
www.autismia.org

James Ball, Ed.D., BCBA-D, Executive Chair
Ron E. Simmons, Vice Chair

Kansas

1606 Autism Society of Kansas Autism Society of America
Autism Society of America
PO Box 860984   913-706-0042
Shawnee, KS 66286-2325   Fax: 316-943-3292
e-mail: ks-johnsoncounty@autismsocietyofamerica.
www.autismsocietyoftheheartland.org

Bill Robinso, President
DeeDee Velasquez-Per, Board Member

Kentucky

1607 Autism Chapter of Bluegrass Chapter
243 Shady Lane
Lexington, KY 40503-2034   859-299-9000
www.asbg.org

Sara Spragens, President

1608 Autism Society of Western Kentucky
230 Second Street Suite 206   270-826-0510
Henderson, KY 42419-1647   e-mail: nboyett1956@yahoo.com
www.autism.org

Nancy Boyett, President

Louisiana

1609 Autism Society of Louisiana
5430 S Woodchase Court
Baton Rouge, LA 70808   800-955-3760
e-mail: pjmanco@cox.net
www.lastateautism.org

Pat Giamanco, President

Maine

1610 Autism Society of Maine
72B Main Street
Winthrop, ME 04364-1406   800-273-5200
Fax: 207-377-9434
e-mail: nancy@asmonline.org
www.asmonline.org

Kim Humphrey, President
Lynda Mazzola, Vice President

Maryland

1611 Autism Society of Baltimore-Chesapeake
PO Box 10822   410-655-7933
Parkville, MD 21234   e-mail: info@baltimoreautismsociety.org
www.baltimoreautismsociety.org

Debbie Page, Co-President:
Kay Holman, Vice-President:

Massachusetts

1612 Autism Society of Massachusetts
20 Alice Agnew Drive   877-622-2884
Attleboro Falls, MA 2763-2108   Fax: 774-643-6331
e-mail: asamasschapter@hotmail.com
www.nationalautismassociation.org

Jo Pike, Co-Founder President/Executive Director
Laura Bono, Founding Board Member

Michigan

1613 Autism Society of Michigan
1213 Center Street   517-882-2800
Lansing, MI 48906-5338   800-223-6722
Fax: 517-862-2816
e-mail: mi-michigan@autismsocietyofamerica.org
www.autism-mi.org

Kathy Johnson, President
Penny Bearden, Vice President

Minnesota

1614 Autism Society of Minnesota
2380 Wycliff Street   651-647-1083
St Paul, MN 55114-1257   Fax: 651-642-1230
e-mail: info@ausm.org
www.ausm.org

Pam Erickson, Executive Director
Laurie Dixon, Associate Director

Missouri

1615 Autism Society of Gateway Chapter
7777 Bonhomme Avenue   314-863-0077
St Louis, MO 63105   Fax: 314-863-7494
e-mail: PegiSues@aol.com
www.autism-society.org

Pegi Price, President
James Ball, Ed.D., BCBA-D, Executive Chair

Nebraska

1616 Autism Society of Nebraska
1672 Van Dorn Street   402-472-4346
Lincoln, NE 68502   877-375-0120
e-mail: autismsociety@autismnebraska.org
www.autismnebraska.org

Shawn Neff, President
Georgann Albin, Executive Director

Nevada

1617 Autism Society of Northern Nevada
3490 Southampton Drive   775-786-9315
Reno, NV 89509-8911   Fax: 775-786-0984
www.autism-society.org/chapter547

Paul Deane, Vice President
Dinah Deane, President

New Hampshire

1618 Autism Society of New Hampshire
PO Box 68   603-679-2424
Concord, NH 03302-0068   Fax: 301-657-0869
e-mail: info@nhautism.com
www.nhautism.com

Stacey Shannon, President

New Jersey

1619 Autism Society of Southwest New Jersey
10 Shadow Oak Court   856-722-8518
Mount Laurel, NJ 08054-2113   e-mail: CMedo@aol.com
www.autism-society.org

New Mexico

1620 Autism Society of New Mexico
PO Box 30955   505-332-0306
Albuquerque, NM 87190   e-mail: nmautism@nmautismsociety.org
www.nmautismsociety.org

Sarah Baca, Executive Director
Sharon Esch, President

New York

1621 Autism Society of Albany
PO Box 3487   518-355-2191
Schenectady, NY 12303   Fax: 518-355-2191
e-mail: info@albanyautism.org
www.albanyautism.org

Gordon Zuckerman, President
Jenny DeBellis, Treasurer

North Carolina

1622 Autism Society of North Carolina
505 Oberlin Road
Raleigh, NC 27605-1345
919-743-0204
800-442-2762
Fax: 919-743-0208
e-mail: info@autismsociety-nc.org
www.autismsociety-nc.org

Scott Badesch, Chief Executive Officer
David Laxton, Director Communications

North Dakota

1623 Autism Society of North Dakota
628 6th Avenue
Alice, ND 58031
701-281-8254
e-mail: Jocelyn@AutismND.org
www.AutismND.org

Kris Wallman, President
Renie Chadwell, Vice President

Ohio

1624 Autism Society of Greater Cincinnati
PO Box 58385
Cincinnati, OH 45258
513-561-2300
Fax: 513-561-4748
e-mail: asgc@cinci.rr.com
www.autismcincy.org

Kay Brown, President
Sue Radabaugh, Vice President

1625 Autism Society of Ohio Tri-County Chapter
1749 S Raccoon Road
Austintown, OH 44515
330-720-2066
www.triautism.com

Terry Chapin, President
Jack Campbell, Vice President

Oklahoma

1626 Autism Society of Central Oklahoma
PO Box 720103
Norman, OK 73070
405-370-3220
e-mail: ASOCO-owner@yahoogroups.com
www.asofok.org

Jeremy Rand, Contact

Oregon

1627 Autism Society of Oregon
PO Box 396
Marylhurst, OR 97036-0396
503-636-1676
888-288-4761
Fax: 503-636-1696
e-mail: info@oregonautism.com
www.oregonautism.com

Jenny Schoonbee, President
Genevieve Athens, Executive Director

Pennsylvania

1628 Autism Society of Greater Harrisburg
PO Box 101
Enola, PA 17025-0856
717-732-8400
800-277-2425
e-mail: georgia.rackley@verizon.net
www.autismharrisburg.com

Georgia Rackley, President
Sherry Christian, Vice President

Rhode Island

1629 Autism Society of Rhode Island
PO Box 16603
Rumford, RI 02916
401-595-3241
e-mail: LRego@asa-ri.org
www.asa-ri.org

Lisa Rego, President
Claudia Swiader, Vice President

South Carolina

1630 Autism Society of South Carolina
806 Twelfth Street
W Columbia, SC 29169
803-750-6988
800-438-4790
Fax: 703-750-8121
e-mail: scas@scautism.org
www.scautism.org

Craig Stoxen, President & CEO
Tim Conroy, Chief Operating Officer & Vice President

South Dakota

1631 Autism Society of Black Hills
521 7th Street
Rapid City, SD 57701-4347
605-737-0377
e-mail: sheritony@rap.midco.net
www.autismsd.com

Sandy Burns, President
Sheri Perkins

Tennessee

1632 Autism Society of East Tennessee
PO Box 30015
Knoxville, TN 37930
865-824-2897
Fax: 865-824-2896
e-mail: asaetc@gmail.com
www.asaetc.org

Mike Manfredo, President
Roddey M. Coe, Vice President

Texas

1633 Autism Society of Dallas
10503 Metric Drive
Dallas, TX 75243
214-208-0792
e-mail: autismsociety_dallas@yahoo.com
www.autism-society.org

Carolyn Garver, Contact
Pamela Lane, President

Vermont

1634 Autism Society of Vermont Autism Society of America
Autism Society of America
PO Box 978
White River Junction, VT 05001-0978
800-559-7398
e-mail: vt-vermont@autismsocietyofamerica.org
www.autism-info.org

Virginia

1635 Autism Society of Northern Virginia
PO Box 1334
Vienna, VA 22183-1334
703-495-8444
Fax: 703-571-8138
e-mail: info@asanv.org
www.asanv.org

Kymberly S DeLoatche, Executive Director
Christopher Waddell, President

Washington

1636 Autism Society of Washington
P. O. Box 503
Olympia, WA 98507
888-279-4968
Fax: 253-503-1157
e-mail: info@autismsocietyofwa.org
www.autismsocietyofwa.org

Jeffrey Foster, President
Teresa McCann, Vice-President

West Virginia

1637 Autism Socity of West Virginia
PO Box 1024
Wayne, WV 25570
304-272-9834
e-mail: wv-westvirginia@autismsocietyofamerica.o
www.aswv.org

Kim Farley, President
Ginny Gattlieb, 1st VP

1638 Autism Society of Wisconsin
1477 Kenwood Drive
Menasha, WI 54952
920-558-4602
888-428-8476
Fax: 920-553-0034
e-mail: asw@asw4autism.org
www.asw4autism.org

Nancy Alar, President
Dale Prahl, Vice President

Libraries & Resource Centers

1639 Autism Services Center
Keith Albee Building
929 4th Avenue
Huntington, WV 25710
304-525-8014
Fax: 304-525-8026
www.autismservicescenter.org
Serves people with autism, other developmental disabilities and those who care for and about them.
John Fields, Director
Mike Grady, Chief Executive Officer

1640 Emory Autism Resource Center
Emory University School of Medicine
Justin Tyler Traux Building
Atlanta, GA 30322-0001
404-727-8350
Fax: 404-727-3969
e-mail: michael.j.morrier@emory.edu
www.psychiatry.emory.edu/PROGRAMS/autism
The Emory Autism Resource Center is a component of the Department of Psychiatry and Behavioral Sciences of Emory University's School of Medicine. It is the only Georgia resource that provides a comprehensive continuum of services specially designed to meet the needs of children and adults with autism and their families.
Gail G McGee, PhD, Director
Michael J Morrier, MA, Asst Director Research Manager

1641 Indiana Resource Center for Autism (IRCA)
Indiana Institute on Disability & Community
Indiana University-Bloomington
Bloomington, IN 47408-2696
812-855-6508
800-825-4733
Fax: 812-855-9630
TTY: 812-855-9396
e-mail: prattc@indiana.edu
www.iidc.indiana.edu/irca
The Indiana Resource Center for Autism staff conduct outreach training and consultations, engage in research, and develop and disseminate information focused on building the capacity of local communities, organizations, agencies, and families to support children and adults across the autism spectrum in typical work, school, home, and community settings.
Dr Cathy Pratt PhD, Director

Research Centers

1642 Center for Neurodevelopmental Studies
5430 W Glenn Drive
Glendale, AZ 85301
623-915-0345
800-352-3792
Fax: 623-937-5425
e-mail: admin@ccnsaz.org
www.thechildrenscenteraz.org
Effective treatment methods for autism and developmental disabilities are subjects researched and studied at the Center.
Lorna Jean King, Founder
Kent Rideout, Executive Director

1643 Division TEACCH University of North Carolina at Chapel H
University of North Carolina at Chapel Hill
100 Renee Lynne Court
Carrboro, NC 27510-6305
919-966-5156
Fax: 919-966-4003
e-mail: teacch@unc.edu
www.teacch.com
This organization is the division for the treatment and education of Autistic and related communication handicapped children.
Catherine Jones, Office Manager/Parent Intake Coordinator
Elaine Coonrod, Clinical Director

1644 Institute for Basic Research in Developmental Disabilities
1050 Forest Hill Road
Staten Island, NY 10314-6356
718-494-0600
Fax: 718-494-0833
www.health.gov/NHIC/
Conducts research into neurodegenerative diseases, Alzheimer's disease, developmental disabilities, fragile X syndrome, Down's syndrome, autism, epilepsy and basic science issues underlying all developmental disabilities.

1645 Institute on Communication and Inclusion at Syracuse University
University of Syracuse
370 Huntington Hall
Syracuse, NY 13244-2340
315-443-9379
Fax: 315-443-2274
e-mail: icistaff@syr.edu
http://ici.syr.edu
College offering facilitated learning research into communication with persons who have autism or severe disabilities. Offers books videos and public awareness information on the research projects.
Douglas Biklen, Dean

1646 National Alliance for Autism Research
1 East 33rd Street
New York, NY 10016
212-252-8584
Fax: 212-252-8676
e-mail: contactus@autismspeaks.org
www.autismspeaks.org
The National Alliance for Autism Research has merged with Autism Speaks to further reach for the goal of finding the causes the best prevention and treatments and a cure for autism.
Peter H Bell, Executive Vice President
Mark Roithmayr, President

1647 State University of New York Health Sciences Center
SUNY Downstate Medical Center
450 Clarkson Avenue
Brooklyn, NY 11203-2098
718-270-1000
Fax: 718-270-1271
e-mail: health@downstate.edu
www.downstate.edu/
Child psychiatry research programs.
John C Larosa, President

1648 The West Virginia Autism Training Center Marshall University
Marshall University
1 John Marshall Drive
Huntington, WV 25755
304-696-2332
800-344-5115
e-mail: wvatc@marshall.edu
www.marshall.edu/coe/atc
The Autism Training Center was established through the efforts of parents of children with autism throughout West Virginia to provide education training and treatment programs for West Virginians who have Autism Pervasive Developmental Disorder (NOS) or Asperger's Disorder and have been formally registered with the Center.

Support Groups & Hotlines

1649 Autism Society of America
4340 East-West Highway
Bethesda, MD 20814
301-657-0881
800-328-8476
www.autism-society.org
Exists to improve the lives of all affected by autism by increasing public awareness about the day-to-day issues faced by people in the spectrum, advocating for apporopriate services for individuals across the lifespan, and providing the latest information regarding treatment, education, research and advocacy.
Lee Grossman, President/CEO
John Dabrowski, Chief Financial Officer

1650 Genetic Alliance
4301 Connecticut Avenue NW
Washington, DC 20008-2369
202-966-5557
800-336-4363
Fax: 202-668-8533
e-mail: info@geneticalliance.org
www.geneticalliance.org
A nonprofit health advocacy organization committed to transforming through genetics and promoting an environment of openness centered on the health of individuals, families and communities.
Sharon Terry, President/CEO

1651 National Autism Hotline Autism Services Center
Keith Albee Building
929 4th Avenue   304-525-8014
Huntington, WV 25710   Fax: 304-525-8026
                                www.autismservicescenter.org
Serving people with autism, other developmental disabilities anf
those who care for and about them.
Mike Grady, CEO, Autism Services Center
Derek Hyman, President & Treasurerÿ

1652 National Health Information Center
PO Box 1133   310-565-4167
Washington, DC 20013-1133   800-336-4797
                                              Fax: 301-984-4256
                                              e-mail: info@nhic.org
                                              www.health.gov/nhic
A health information referral service sponsored by the Office of
Disease Prevention and Health Promotion. Puts health profession-
als and consumers who have health questions in touch with those
organizations that are best able to provide answers.

Books

1653 A Miracle to Believe In
Option Indigo Press
2080 S Undermountain Road   413-229-2100
Sheffield, MA 01257   800-714-2779
                                              Fax: 413-229-8931
                                              optioninstitutestore.org/?
A group of people from all walks of life come together and are
transformed as they reach out, under the direction of the
Kaufmans, to help a little boy the medical world had given up as
hopeless.
379 pages
ISBN: 0-440201-08-2
Bears Kaufman, Founder
Samahria Kaufman, Founder

**1654 A Parent's Guide to Asperger's Syndrome & High-Functioning
Autism**
Guilford Press
370 Seventh Avenue
New York, NY 10001   800-365-7006
                                              Fax: 212-966-6708
                                              e-mail: info@guilford.com
                                              www.guilford.com
For parents of children on the higher end of the autistic spectrum.
All educators, the authors provide the basic on diagnosis, causes,
and treatment.
2002 278 pages
ISBN: 1-572307-67-6

**1655 Activities for Developing Pre-Skill Concepts In Children with
Autism**
Toni Flowers, author
Autism Society of North Carolina Bookstore
505 Oberlin Road   919-743-0204
Raleigh, NC 27605-1345   800-442-2762
                                              Fax: 919-743-0208
                                              e-mail: info@autismsociety-nc.org
                                              www.autismsociety-nc.org
Chapters include auditory development, concept development, so-
cial development and visual-motor integration.

1656 Asperger Syndrome or High-Functioning Autism?
Eric Schopler, Gary B Mesibov, Linda J Kunce, author
Springer Publishing
233 Spring Street
New York, NY 10013   212-460-1550
                                              800-777-4643
                                              Fax: 212-460-1575
                                              e-mail: support@apress.com
                                              www.springer.com
The precise relationship between high-functioning autism and
Asperger Syndrome is still a subject of debate. Leaders in the field
provide a general overview of the disorder and present diverse

opinions on diagnosis and assessment-neuropsychological is-
sues-treatment, and related conditions.
428 pages Hardcover
ISBN: 0-306457-45-3

1657 Asperger's Syndrome: A Guide for Parents and Professionals
Taylor & Francis
325 Chestnut Street
Philadelphia, PA 19106   215-625-8900
                                              www.tonyattwood.com
Offers insight into the identification and treatment of children on
the higher functioning end of ASD.
201 pages
ISBN: 1-853025-77-1

1658 Autism Society of North Carolina Bookstore
505 Oberlin Road   919-743-0204
Raleigh, NC 27605-1345   800-442-2762
                                              Fax: 919-743-0208
                                              e-mail: info@autismaociety-nc.org
                                              www.autismsociety-nc.org
Offers one of the largest selections of books about autism.

1659 Autism Through the Lifespan: The Eden Model
Woodbine House
6510 Bells Mill Road   301-897-3570
Bethesda, MD 20817-1636   800-843-7323
                                              Fax: 301-897-5838
Presents Eden's comprehensive model for helping children and
adults with autism, offering services that extend over their entire
lifespan. An overview of what is known about autism today, discussions about Eden's approach to behavior modification, placement and treatment, curriculum from early childhood to adulthood,
staffing issues, integration, decision making, and parental roles.
Also contains dozens of examples and case histories that illustrate
the program's successes.
1998 383 pages Paperback
ISBN: 0-933149-28-x

1660 Autism Treatment Guide
Elizabeth King Gerlach, author
Autism Society of North Carolina Bookstore
505 Oberlin Road   919-743-0204
Raleigh, NC 27605-1345   800-442-2762
                                              Fax: 919-743-0208
                                              e-mail: info@autismsociety-nc.org
                                              www.autismsociety-nc.org
This 3rd edition offers many of the most current findings in treatments fo autism spectrum disorder. First published in 1993 and updated regularly, this concise handbook provides hundres of
resource listings and suggested readings pertaining to ASD. This
is a must-have reference book for parents and professionals
2003 157 pages Softcover

1661 Autism and Asperger Syndrome Preparing for Adulthood
Autism Society of North Carolina Bookstore
505 Oberlin Road   919-743-0204
Raleigh, NC 27605-1345   800-442-2762
                                              Fax: 919-743-0208
                                              e-mail: info@autismsociety-nc.org
                                              www.autismsociety-nc.org
Chapters include topics such as what becomes of adults with ASD,
interventions for ASD, problems af communication, social functioning in adulthood, sterotyped, ritualistic, and obsessional behaviors, secondary education, post-secondary education, finding
and coping with employment, pyschiatric disturbances in adulthood, leagal issues, sexual relationships and marriage, and
enhancing independence.
2004 388 pages Softcover

1662 Autism in Adolescents and Adults
Eric Schopler, Gary B Mesibov, author
Springer Publishing
233 Spring Street
New York, NY 10013   121-460-1500
                                              800-777-4643
                                              Fax: 212-460-1575
                                              e-mail: support@apress.com
                                              www.springer.com
456 pages Hardcover
ISBN: 0-306410-57-4

1663 Autism...Nature, Diagnosis and Treatment
Guilford Press
370 Seventh Avenue
New York, NY 10001
Fax: 212-966-6708
e-mail: info@guilford.com
www.guilford.com
Covers perspectives, issues, neurobiological issues and new directions in diagnosis and treatment.
417 pages
ISBN: 0-898627-24-9

1664 Autism: Explaining the Enigma
Uta Frith, author
Wiley Publishing
111 River Street
201-748-6000
Hoboken, NJ 07030-5774
Fax: 201-748-6088
e-mail: info@wiley.com
www.wiley.com
Includes a new chapter outlining recent developments in neuropsycgological research, and overviews one of the most important theoretical and practical consequences of Frith's original insights into this puzzling condition.
264 pages
ISBN: 0-631229-01-8

1665 Autism: Identification, Education and Treatment
Dianne Zager, author
Lawrence Earlbaum Associates
198 Madison Avenue
201-258-2200
New York, NY 10016
800-926-6579
Fax: 201-236-0072
global.oup.com/academic
Chapters include medical treatments, early intervention and communication development in autism.
2005 608 pages
ISBN: 0-805845-79-8

1666 Autism: The Facts
Simon Baron-Cohen, Patrick Bolton, author
Oxford University Press
2001 Evans Road
Cary, NC 27513
800-445-9714
Fax: 919-677-1303
e-mail: custserv.us@oup.com
www.oup-usa.org
Explains in a clear, straightforward manner what is known about the condition. Written first and foremost as a guide for parents, but required reading for interested professionals, it covers the recognition and diagnosis of autism, its biological and physiological causes, and the various treatments and educational techniques available.
128 pages
ISBN: 0-192623-27-3

1667 Autistic Adults at Bittersweet Farms
Haworth Press
10 Alice Street
607-722-5857
Binghamton, NY 13904-1580
800-429-6784
Fax: 607-722-0012
www.haworthpress.com
A touching view of an inspirational residential care program for autistic adolescents and adults.
205 pages Paperback
ISBN: 1-560240-57-0

1668 Beyond Gentle Teaching
J.J McGee and F.J Menolascino, author
Springer
233 Spring Street
212-460-1500
New York, NY 10013
800-777-4643
Fax: 212-460-1575
e-mail: support@apress.com
www.springer.com

252 pages Hardcover
ISBN: 0-306438-56-1

1669 Biology of the Autistic Syndromes
Christopher Gillberg and Mary Coleman, author
Blackwell Publishing, Inc.
Commerce Place
317-572-3994
Malden, MA 02148
800-862-6657
Fax: 781-388-8210
www.blackwellpublishing.com
Autism is not a disease but a syndrome of different diseases. In this completely reworked and updated 3rd edition, the authors adress the difficulties this presents for clinical diagnosis with diagnostic aids and clear guidlines for medical evaluation. This is an essential text text for clinicians and will also be of interest to parents of autistic children.
2000 340 pages
ISBN: 1-898683-22-0

1670 Children with Autism
Woodbine House
6510 Bells Mill Road
Bethesda, MD 20817
800-843-7323
e-mail: info@woodbinehouse.com
www.woodbinehouse.com
A must-have reference if for the both the new parent coping with a child's recent diagnosis and one who's an experienced advocate. Available online only.
368 pages Paperback

1671 Communication Unbound: How Facilitated Communication Is Challenging Views
Teachers College Press
1234 Amsterdam Avenue
212-678-3929
New York, NY 10027
Fax: 212-678-4149
e-mail: tcpress@tc.columbia.edu
www.teacherscollegepress.com
Addresses the ways in which we receive persons with autism in our society, our community and our lives.
1993 221 pages

1672 Diagnosis Autism: Now What? 10 Steps to Improve Treatment Outcomes
Lawrence P Kaplan, PhD, author
Autism Society of North Carolina Bookstore
505 Oberlin Road
919-743-0204
Raleigh, NC 27605-1345
800-442-2762
Fax: 919-743-0208
e-mail: info@autismsociety-nc.org
www.autismsociety-nc.org
This practical guide was written to help parents of children with autism spectrum disorder form successful pediatric partnerships with physicians and other healthcare practitioners involved in their child's diagnosis and treatment. Containing chrts and worksheets, sample questions, research resources, and numerous planning strategies, this guide will aid parents and caregivers as they strive to build collaborative relationships with their child's case management team.
2005

1673 Effective Teaching Methods for Autistic Children
Rosalind C Oppenheim, author
Charles C Thomas Publisher
2600 S 1st Street
217-789-8980
Springfield, IL 62704-4730
800-258-8980
Fax: 217-789-9130
e-mail: books@ccthomas.com
www.ccthomas.com
The Rimland School for Autistic Children in Evanston, Illinois, with a Foreward by Bernard Rimland. This enlightening monograph is seven chapters detailing the specific problems encountered in teaching autistic children. Anecdotal reports of seven such children bring to light the need for special training and provide an insight into their handling. Related research is reviewed and discussed.
1974 116 pages Paperback
ISBN: 0-398028-58-3

1674 Encounters with Autistic States
Jason Aronson

P.O.Box 15556
York, PA 17405-7100

646-415-2561
800-782-0015
Fax: 201-840-7242
e-mail: mail@aronson.com
www.aronson.com

Dr. Victor examines the myths that cloud an understanding of this disorder and describes the meanings of its specific behavioral symptoms.
Hardcover
ISBN: 0-765700-62-

1675 Handbook of Autism and Pervasive Developmental Disorders
Autism Society of North Carolina Bookstore
4340 East-West Hwy
Bethesda, MD 20814-1345

301-657-0881
Fax: 919-743-0208
e-mail: info@autism-society.org
www.autism-society.org

A list of contributors address such topics as characteristics of autistic syndromes and interventions.
2005 1317 pages 2 volumes

1676 Helping Children with Autism Learn: Treatment Approaches for Parents
Bryna Siegel, author
Oxford University Press
2001 Evans Road
Cary, NC 27513

800-445-9714
Fax: 919-677-1303
e-mail: custserv.us@oup.com
www.oup.com

512 pages
ISBN: 0-195325-06-0

1677 Hidden Child: The Linwood Method for Reaching the Autistic Child
Woodbine House
6510 Bells Mill Road
Bethesda, MD 20817-1636

301-897-3570
800-537-3394
Fax: 301-897-5838
e-mail: info@woodbinehouse.com
www.woodbinehouse.com

Chronicle of the Linwood Children's Center's successful treatment program for autistic children.
286 pages Paperback
ISBN: 0-933149-06-9

1678 I'm Not Autistic on the Typewriter
TASH
11201 Greenwood Avenue N
Seattle, WA 98133-8612

206-361-8870

An introduction to the facilitated communication training method.

1679 Keys to Parenting the Child with Autism
Marlene Targ Brill, M.Ed, author
Barrons Educational Series, Inc.
250 Wireless Boulevard
Hauppauge, NY 11788

800-645-3476
Fax: 631-434-3723
e-mail: barrons@barronseduc.com
www.barronseduc.com

This book explains what autism is and how it is diagnosed.
2001 224 pages
ISBN: 0-764112-92-9

1680 Let Community Employment Be the Goal for Individuals with Autism
Autism Society of North Carolina Bookstore
505 Oberlin Road
Raleigh, NC 27605-1345

919-743-0204
800-442-2762
Fax: 919-743-0208
e-mail: info@autismsociaty-nc.org
www.autismsociety-nc.org

A guide designed for people who are responsible for preparing individuals with autism to enter the work force.
1993 66 pages Booklet

1681 Let Me Hear Your Voice A Family's Triumph Over Autism
Catherine Maurice, author
Autism Society of North Carolina Bookstore

505 Oberlin Road
Raleigh, NC 27605-1345

919-743-0204
800-442-2762
Fax: 919-743-0208
e-mail: info@autismsociety-nc.org
www.autismsociety-nc.org

The Maurice family's second and third children were diagnosed with autism. This book recounts their experience with a home program using behavior therapy.
1993 371 pages Softcover
ISBN: 0-679408-63-0

1682 Management of Autistic Behavior
Pro-Ed, Inc.
8700 Shoal Creek Blvd
Austin, TX 78757-6897

512-451-3246
800-897-3202
Fax: 800-397-7633
e-mail: info@proedinc.com
www.proedinc.com

Comprehensive and practical book that tells what works best with specific problems.
450 pages Paperback
ISBN: 0-890791-96-1
Lindy Jordaan, Marketing Coordinator

1683 Navigating the Social World: A Curriculum for Individuals with Asperger's Syndrome
Jeanette McAfee, author
Future Horizons
721 W Abram Street
Arlington, TX 76013

800-489-0727
Fax: 817-277-2270
www.fhautism.com

Addresses the most urgent problems facing those with Asperger's Syndrome, high-functioning autism, and related disorders.
387 pages
ISBN: 1-885477-82-1
Ellen Notbohm, Author
Jed Baker, Author

1684 Neurobiology of Autism
Johns Hopkins University Press
2715 N Charles Street
Baltimore, MD 21218-4319

410-516-6936
Fax: 410-516-6998
www.jhupbooks.com

This book discusses recent advances in scientific research that point to a neurobiological basis for autism and examines the clinical implications of this research.
272 pages
ISBN: 0-801856-80-9

1685 News from the Border: A Mother's Memoir of Her Autistic Son
Houghton Mifflin Company/Order Processing
222 Berkeley Street
Boston, MA 02116

617-351-5000
800-225-3362
www.hmco.com

A searingly honest account of the author's family experiences with autism. Raising an autistic child is the central, ongoing drama of her married life and this riveting account of acceptance and coping.
1993 384 pages Cloth

1686 Pervasive Developmental Disorders: Finding a Diagnosis and Getting Help
O'Reilly & Associates
1005 Gravenstein Hgwy N
Sebastopol, CA 95472-3858

707-827-7019
800-889-8969
Fax: 707-824-8268
e-mail: orders@oreilly.com
www.oreilly.com

Published for parents and patients with PDD-NOS and atypical PDD.
Paperback
ISBN: 1-565925-30-0

1687 Please Don't Say Hello
Human Sciences Press
233 Spring Street
New York, NY 10013-1522

212-620-8000

Paul and his family moved into a new neighborhood. Paul's brother was autistic. The children thought that Eddie was retarded until

they learned that there were skills that he could do better than they could.
1976 47 pages Paperback
ISBN: 0-898851-99-8

1688 Psychoeducational Profile (PEP-3): TEACCH Individualized Psychoeducational Assessm
Autism Society of North Carolina Bookstore
505 Oberlin Road   919-743-0204
Raleigh, NC 27605-1345   800-442-2762
                                                      Fax: 919-743-0208
e-mail: info@autismsociety-nc.org
www.autismsociety-nc.org
This is the revised edition of Psychoeducational Profile, a widely recognized assessment tool used to identify the learning strengths and weaknesses of children with autism spectrum disorder (ASD). Developed by Division TEACCH clinicians, this instrument has been updated in several ways, including improved psychometric properties, revised function domains, new items and sub-tests, within-group comparison data, and the addition of key documentation.
2005

1689 Raising a Child with Autism: A Guide to Applied Behavior Analysis for Parents
Taylor & Francis
325 Chestnut Street   215-625-8900
Philadelphia, PA 19106   Fax: 215-625-2940
Applied behavior analysis activities that parents can use with ASD children. Inlcuded is helpful guidance for toilet training, daily living, and increasing communication and sibling interaction.
173 pages
ISBN: 1-853029-10-6

1690 Reaching the Autistic Child: A Parent Training Program
Martin Kozloff, author
Brookline Books/Lumen Editions
8 Trumbull Rd   413-584-0184
Northampton, MA 01060   800-666-2665
                                                      Fax: 413-584-6184
www.brooklinebooks.com
Detailed case studies of social and behavioral change in autistic children and their families show parents how to implement the principles for improved socialization and behavior.
1998 Softcover
ISBN: 1-571290-56-7

1691 Record Book for Individuals with Autism Spectrum Disorders
Marci Wheeler and Cathy Pratt, PhD, author
Autism Society of North Carolina Bookstore
505 Oberlin Road   919-743-0204
Raleigh, NC 27605-1345   800-442-2762
                                                      Fax: 919-743-0208
e-mail: info@autismsociety-nc.org
www.autismsociety-nc.org
This valuable resource provides a method for organizing and documenting information that will help parents track their child's development. This record book is divided into several categories, including: developmental and family history, sleeping and eating patterns, medical history, education history, behavior problems, skill development, and vital information. The book contains reproducible pages that will help parents keep important information up to date.
2000 44 pages Spiral Bound

1692 Riddle of Autism: A Psychological Analysis
Jason Aronson
P.O.Box 15556   646-415-2561
York, PA 17405-7100   800-782-0015
                                                      Fax: 201-840-7242
e-mail: mail@aronson.com
www.aronson.com
Dr. Victor examines the myths that cloud an understanding of this disorder and describes the meanings of its specific behavioral symptoms.
356 pages Softcover
ISBN: 1-568215-73-8

1693 Siblings of Children with Autism: A Guide for Families
Woodbine House

6510 Bells Mill Road   301-897-3570
Bethesda, MD 20817   800-537-3394
                                                      Fax: 301-897-5838
e-mail: info@woodbinehouse.com
www.woodbinehouse.com
Resource for families with autistic children and nonautistic siblings examines the perceptions, needs, compromises, and inevitable stresses that brothers and sisters face.
160 pages
ISBN: 1-890627-29-1

1694 TEACCH Transition Assessment Profile
Autism Society of North Carolina Bookstore
505 Oberlin Road   919-743-0204
Raleigh, NC 27605-1345   800-442-2762
                                                      Fax: 919-743-0208
e-mail: info@autismsociety-nc.org
www.autismsociety-nc.org
This new assessment profile is a major revision of the AAPEP. This comprehensive test was developed for older children and adolescents with autism spectrum disorder, particularly those who have transition needs. This assessment tool is structured to satisfy those provisions in the 2004 Individuals with Disabilities Education Act, which requires that adolescents be evaluated and also provided with a transition plan.
2007 Kit

1695 Targeting Autism: What We Know, Don't Know and Can Do to Help Young Children
University of California Press
1445 Lower Ferry Road   205-978-5000
Ewing, NJ 08618   800-777-4726
                                                      Fax: 800-999-1958
www.ucpress.com
Provides strong overviews of current work being done with autism and addresses the diferent life cycles of children with the condition through preschool, elementary school, and adolescence.
240 pages
ISBN: 0-520234-80-4

1696 Tasks Galore for the Real World
Laurie Eckenrode, Pat Fennell, and Kathy Hearsey, author
Autism Society of North Carolina Bookstore
505 Oberlin Road   919-743-0204
Raleigh, NC 27605-1345   800-442-2762
                                                      Fax: 919-743-0208
e-mail: info@autismsociety-nc.org
www.autismsociety-nc.org
These visually structured tasks are strategies that translate complex, everyday life skills into simpler, meaningful learning situations. The myriad of ideas in this guide will be valuable to anyone developing functional, daily living goals for a child or client.
2004

1697 Teach Me Language: A Language Manual for Children with Autism
Sabrina Freeman, PhD and Lorelei Dake, BA, author
Autism Society of North Carolina Bookstore
505 Oberlin Road   919-743-0204
Raleigh, NC 27605-1345   800-442-2762
                                                      Fax: 919-743-0208
e-mail: info@autismsociety-nc.org
www.autismsociety-nc.org
This book contains behaviorally based exercises and drills that adress common language weaknesses in children and incorporate professional speech pathology methods. These exercises were designed for children who are attentive, able to follow simple directions, have learned the basics of low-level language, and are visual learners. The activities and exercises are appropriate for children and young adults ages 5-18.
1997 410 pages Spiral Bound

1698 Teaching Children with Autism: Strategies to Enhance Communication and Socializing
Kathleen Ann Quill, author
Thomson Delmar Learning

Attn: Order Fullfillment
Florence, KY 41022

800-347-7707
Fax: 800-487-8488
www.delmarlearning.com

This book describes teaching strategies and instructional adaptations which promote communication and socialization in children with autism. It offers specific strategies that capitalize on the individual strengths and learning styles of the autistic child.
1996
ISBN: 0-827362-69-2

1699   Teaching Community Skills and Behaviors to Students with Autism or Related Problems
Indiana Resource Center for Autism
1905 North Range Rd
Bloomington, IN 47408-2696

812-855-6508
Fax: 812-855-9630
TTY: 812-855-9396
e-mail: iidc@indiana.edu
www.iidc.indiana.edu/irca/fmain1.html

Emphasizing the needs of the person with autism and the philosophy of community integration, this book cover the process of successful community-based teaching.
1988 117 pages

1700   The Autism Sourcebook
Karen Siff Exkorn, author
Autism Society of North Carolina Bookstore
505 Oberlin Road
Raleigh, NC 27605-1345

919-743-0204
800-442-2762
Fax: 919-743-0208
e-mail: www.autismsociety-nc.org
www.autismsociety-nc.org

This comprehensive handbook is for parents of newly diagnosed children who are looking for information about ASD, its diagnosis, treatment options, and practical strategies in one in-depth text.
2005

1701   The Everything Parent's Guide to Children with Autism
Adelle Jameson Tilton, author
Autism Society of North Carolina Bookstore
505 Oberlin Road
Raleigh, NC 27605-1345

919-743-0204
800-442-2762
Fax: 919-743-0208
e-mail: info@autismsociety-nc.org
www.autismsociety-nc.org

This book offers a wealth of information and reassuring advice for parents of newly diagnosed children. It is filled with hundreds of helpful tips, unique insights, and real-life situations, this is an essential guide for parents and family members.
2004 285 pages Softcover

1702   Understanding the Nature of Autism A Guide to the Autism Spectrum Disorders
Janice E Janzen, author
Autism Society of North Carolina Bookstore
505 Oberlin Road
Raleigh, NC 27605-1345

919-743-0204
800-442-2762
Fax: 919-743-0208
e-mail: info@autismsociety-nc.org
www.autismsociety-nc.org

Straightforward and comprehensive information that can be used by parents and professionals to develop curricula and programs for children with autism spectrum disorder. This important resource is a standard text used by educators, parents, and caregivers.
2003 508 pages Softcover

1703   When Snow Turns to Rain
Woodbine House
6510 Bells Mill Road
Bethesda, MD 20817-1636

301-897-3570
800-537-3394
Fax: 301-897-5838
e-mail: info@woodbinehouse.com
www.woodbinehouse.com

A gripping personal account of one family's experiences with autism. Chronicles a family's journey from parental bliss to devastation, as they learn that their son has autism. This book delves into diagnosis, treatments and attitudes toward persons with autism.
1993 250 pages Paperback
ISBN: 0-933149-63-8

1704   Autism Spectrum Disorders: The Complete Guide
Chantal Sicile-Kira, author
Autism Society of North Carolina Bookstore
505 Oberlin Road
Raleigh, NC 27605-1345

919-743-0204
800-442-2762
Fax: 919-743-0208
e-mail: info@autismsociety-nc.org
www.autismsociety-nc.org

This reference guide was written to help parents, professionals, and other members of the community learn more about autism spectrum disorder, and it presents a thorough overview of the disorder, from diagnosis through adulthood.
2004 360 pages Softcover

Children's Books

1705   Joey and Sam
Illana Katz and Edward Ritvo, MD, author
Autism Society of North Carolina Bookstore
505 Oberlin Road
Raleigh, NC 27605-1345

919-743-0204
800-442-2762
Fax: 919-743-0208
e-mail: ASNC@aol.com

A unique and invaluable tool for teaching children about others who are different. This awrd-winning and heartwarming sibling storybook examines the similarities and differences in behavior and educational experiences of two brothers, one of whom has autism.
1993 Softcover
ISBN: 1-882388-00-3

1706   Russell is Extra Special
Charles A Amenta III. MD, author
Autism Society of North Carolina Bookstore
505 Oberlin Road
Raleigh, NC 27605-1345

919-743-0204
800-442-2762
Fax: 919-743-0208
e-mail: info@autismsociety-nc.org
www.autismsociety-nc.org

A sensitive portrayal of an autistic boy written by his father.
Hardcover

1707   Wild Boy of Aveyron
Harlan Lane, author
Harvard University Press
79 Garden Street
Cambridge, MA 02138

617-495-2600
800-405-1619
Fax: 617-495-5898
e-mail: contact_HUP@harvard.edu
www.hup.harvard.edu

A dramatic account of a wild boy of nature and a young French doctor who shaped the modern education of retarded, deaf, and preschool children.
368 pages
ISBN: 0-674953-00-2

Newsletters

1708   Autism Research Review International
Autism Research Institute
4182 Adams Avenue
San Diego, CA 92116-2536

619-281-7165
Fax: 619-563-6840
www.autismresearchchinstitute.com

A quarterly newsletter published by the Autism Research Institute.
8 pages Quarterly
Dr. Bernard Rimland, Director

Pamphlets

1709   Avoiding Unfortunate Situations
Autism Society of North Carolina Bookstore

505 Oberlin Road
Raleigh, NC 27605-1345

919-743-0204
800-442-2762
Fax: 919-743-0208
e-mail: info@autismsociety-nc.org
www.autismsociety-nc.org

A collection of tips and information from and about people with autism and other developmental disabilities and their encounters with law enforcement agencies.

1710 Developing a Functional and Longitudinal Individual Plan
Nancy Dalrymple, author

Autism Society of North Carolina Bookstore
1905 North Range Rd
Bloomington, IN 47408-1345

812-855-6508
800-442-2762
Fax: 812-855-9630
e-mail: iidc@indiana.edu
www.iidc.indiana.edu

It is the author's view that a functional, longitudinal approach should be taken when educating persons with autism spectrum disorder, and that the developmentof an individualized plan should incorporate school, home, and community. This guide discusses the importance of defining strengths, striving for independent functioning, and determining which activitiesshould recieve priority in the areas of self-care, social and leisure activities, and employment.
1989 11 pages Booklet

1711 Enabling Communication in Children with Autism

Autism Society of North Carolina Bookstore
505 Oberlin Road
Raleigh, NC 27605-1345

919-743-0204
800-442-2762
Fax: 919-743-0208
e-mail: info@autismsociety-nc.org
www.autismsociety-nc.org

Based on a 2 year research project, the goal of this book is to help teachers develop more communication-enabling enviroments for children with atuism spectrum disorder who use little or no speech. The authors illustrate many communication-enabling strategies, including the minimal speech approach, proximal communication, prompting, and multipointing.
2001 207 pages Softcover

1712 Job Seeker Involvment in Securing Employment
Nancy Kalina, author

Indiana Resource Center for Autism
1905 North Range Rd
Bloomington, IN 47408-2696

812-855-6508
Fax: 812-855-9630
TTY: 812-855-9396
e-mail: iidc@indiana.edu
www.iidc.indiana.edu/irca/fmain1.html

A walk through the job development process, from identifying job options and writing a resume to negotiating workplace supports with a potential employer. Each step provides opportunities for the peronal with autism, or another disability, to become actively involved in their job search process.
1997 22 pages

1713 Learning to be Independent and Responsible
Nancy Dalrymple, author

Indiana Resource Center for Autism
1905 North Range Rd
Bloomington, IN 47408-2696

812-855-6508
Fax: 812-855-9630
TTY: 812-855-9396
e-mail: iidc@indiana.edu
www.iidc.indiana.edu/irca/fmain1.html

People with autism build trust in people and environments through successful interactions. Individualized, supportive programs, utilizing positive instructional and environmental supports that lead to increased opportunities, chouse, and motivation are described in this booklet.
1989 11 pages

1714 Parents as Trainers of Legislators, Other Parents and Researchers

Autism Services Center
101 Richmond Street
Huntington, WV 25702-1513

304-525-8014
Fax: 304-525-8026

Reprint offering information on parents of autistic children that learn early in their child's life how little professionals know about autism.

1715 Sex, Sexuality, and the Autism Specrtum
Wendy Lawson, author

Autism Society of North Carolina Bookstore
505 Oberlin Road
Raleigh, NC 27605-1345

919-743-0204
800-442-2762
Fax: 919-743-0208
e-mail: info@autismsociety-nc.org
www.autismsociety-nc.org

The author, a psychologist, who has Aspergers Syndrome, presents her unique perspective on sexuality and interpersonal relationships. Filled with honest insights and positive advice, this is a valuable guide for persons with ASD and the people who live and work with them.
2005 175 pages Softcover

1716 Son-Rise Method

Option Institute
2080 S Undermountain Road
Sheffield, MA 01257-9643

413-229-2100
Fax: 413-229-8931
e-mail: information@son-rise.org
www.autismtreatmentcenter.org

Describes a program Barry and Samahria Kaufman developed to help heal their once-autistic son.

1717 What Is Autism

Autism Society of America
4340 East-West Hwy
Bethesda, MD 20814-3065

301-657-0881
800-328-8476
Fax: 301-657-0869
e-mail: info@autism-society.org
www.autism-society.org

Offers a definition and introduction to autism, produces a wide range of autism information written for various audiences. Offers a quarterly magazine, national conference, nationwide chapter network and many other resources.

Audio & Video

1718 A Sense of Belonging: Including Students with Autism in their School Community

Indiana Resource Center for Autism
1905 North Range Rd
Bloomington, IN 47408-2696

812-855-6508
Fax: 812-855-9630
TTY: 812-855-9396
e-mail: iidc@indiana.edu
www.iidc.indiana.edu/irca/fmain1.html

Highlights the efforts of two elementary and one middle school in Indiana in teaching students with autism in general education settings. Comments from parents, school administrators, classmates, and educators illustrate the role they each played in supporting students with autism in becoming active learners in their school community. Includes practical strategies for teaching the student with autism.
1997 20 minutes

1719 Autism: A Strange, Silent World

Filmakers Library
3212 Duke Street
Alexandria, VA 22314

212-808-4980
Fax: 212-808-4983
e-mail: sales@alexanderstreet.com
www.academicvideostore.com

A comprehensive view of autism by focusing on three children of different ages, with very different behaviors. Also introduces us to a remarkable group of parents, teachers and therapists who strive to maximize
VHS/DVD
Sue Oscar, Co-President
Linda Gottesman, Co-President

1720 Autism: A World Apart
Karen Cunninghame, author

Fanlight Productions

32 Court Street
Brooklyn, NY 11201-1731

718-488-8900
800-876-1710
Fax: 718-488-8642
e-mail: info@fanlight.com
www.fanlight.com

In this documentary, three families show us what the textbooks and studies cannot, what it's like to live with autism day after day, raise and love children who may be withdrawn and violent and unable to make personal connections with their families.
DVD
ISBN: 1-572959-50-9

1721   Developing IEPs Under the New Idea Regulations
LRP Publications
360 Hiatt Drive
Palm Beach Gardens, FL 33418-2247

800-341-7874
Fax: 215-784-9639
e-mail: custserve@lrp.com
www.lrp.com

A practical, step-by-step approach makes it easy to understand the legal and educational issues surrounding IEPs.
26 minutes

1722   Discipline Under the New Idea: Practical Methods and Procedures
LRP Publications
360 Hiatt Drive
Palm Beach Gardens, FL 33418-2247

800-341-7874
Fax: 215-784-9639
e-mail: custserve@lrp.com
www.lrp.com

Provides practical explanation of the discipline methods and procedures school officials are permitted to use for students with disabilities.
26 minutes

1723   Embracing Play: Teaching Your Child with Autism
Woodbine House
6510 Bells Mill Road
Bethesda, MD 20817

301-897-3570
800-537-3394
Fax: 301-897-5838
e-mail: info@woodbinehouse.com
www.woodbinehouse.com

Guide for parents who incorporate applied behavior analysis with their child.
1993 47 minutes

1724   Functional Behavioral Assessments: How to Do Them Right!
LRP Publications
360 Hiatt Drive
Palm Beach Gardens, FL 33418-2247

800-341-7874
Fax: 215-784-9639
e-mail: custserve@lrp.com
www.lrp.com

Assist you in understanding why a behavior problem has occured, so you can maximize the effectiveness of a planned intervention.
18 minutes

1725   Getting Started with Facilitated Communication
Syracuse University, Facilitated Communication Ins
370 Huntington Hall
Syracuse, NY 13244-2340

315-443-9379
Fax: 315-443-9218
e-mail: fcstaff@syr.edu
soeweb.syr.edu/thefci/

Describes in detail how to help individuals with autism and/or severe communication difficulties to get started with facilitated communication.
Videotape

1726   Going to School with Facilitated Communication
Syracuse University, School of Education
805 S Krouse
Syracuse, NY 13244-0001

315-443-2693

A video in which students with autism and/or severe disabilities illustrate the use of facilitated communication focusing on basic principles fostering facilitated communication.
Videotape

1727   I Want My Little Boy Back
Autism Treatment Center of America

2080 S Undermountain Road
Sheffield, MA 01257

413-229-2100
800-714-2779
Fax: 413-229-8931
e-mail: information@son-risc.org
www.autismtreatmentcenter.org

This BBC documentary follows an English family with a child with autism before, during, and after their time at the Son-Rise Program. It uniquely captures the heart of the Son-Rise Program and is extremely useful in understanding the program's techniques.
Lauren Astor, Public Relations Manager

1728   I'm Not Autistic on the Typewriter
Syracuse University, School of Education
805 S Krouse
Syracuse, NY 13244-0001

315-443-2693

A video introducing facilitated communication, a method by which persons with autism express themselves.
Videotape

1729   Invisible Wall: Autism
PRIMEDIA/Films Media Group
Films for Hum. & Science
Princeton, NJ 08543

800-257-5126
Fax: 609-671-0266
e-mail: custserv@filmsmediagroup.com
www.films.com/

It features interviews with Ivar Lovaas, the creator of applied behavior analysis therapy.
2001 52 minutes
Dean B Nelson, Chairman & President
Kevin Neary, Chief Financial Officer

1730   Public Schools and Students with Autism: Components of a Defensible Program
LRP Publications
360 Hiatt Drive
Palm Beach Gardens, FL 33418-2247

800-341-7874
Fax: 215-784-9639
e-mail: custserve@lrp.com
www.lrp.com

This video assists you in understanding transition planning, documentation of student progress and proven strategies you can implement in your program.
13 minutes

1731   Standards and Inclusion: Can We Have Both?
LRP Publications
360 Hiatt Drive
Palm Beach Gardens, FL 33418-2247

800-341-7874
Fax: 215-784-9639
e-mail: custserve@lrp.com
www.lrp.com

Addresses the critical issues educators face when supporting students with disabilities in inclusive settings. Through dynamic, powerful presentations by two inclusion experts.
40 minutes

1732   Understanding Autism
Suzanne Newman, author
Fanlight Productions
32 Court Street
Brooklyn, NY 11201-1731

718-488-8900
800-876-1710
Fax: 718-488-8642
e-mail: info@fanlight.com
www.fanlight.com

Parents of children with autism discuss the nature and symptoms of this lifelong disability and outlines a treatment program based on behavior modification principles.
1993 19 Minutes
ISBN: 1-572951-00-1

Web Sites

1733   Autism Research Institute

www.autism.com/ari/

A clearinghouse for research on autism and related disorders of learning and behavior. Conducts and compiles research findings to provide people with the latest research available.

1734 Autism Resources

www.autism-resources.com

Provides information and links regarding the developmental disabilities autism and Asperger's Syndrome.

1735 Autism Society of America

4340 East-West Hwy   301-657-0881
Bethesda, MD 20814   800-328-8476
e-mail: info@autism-society.org
www.autism-society.org

Exists to improve the lives of all affected by autism by increasing public awareness about the day-to-day issues faced by people on the spectrum, advocating for appropriate services for individuals across the lifespan, and providing the latest information regarding treatment, education, research and advocacy.

James Ball, Executive Chair
Anne Holmes, Vice Chair

1736 Autism Treatment Center of America

www.autismtreatment.com

The worldwide teaching center for The Son-Rise Program , a powerful and effective treatment for children and adults challenged by Autism, Autism Spectrum Disorders, Pervasive Developmental Disorder (PDD) , Asperger's Syndrome, and other developmental difficulties.

1737 Community Services for Autistic Adults & Children

www.csaac.org

A private, non-profit agency which provides direct services to children and adults with autism across the lifespan. CSAAC's mission is to enable individuals with autism to reach their highest potential and contribute as confident individuals to their community.

1738 Healing Well

www.healingwell.com

A social network and support community for patients, caregivers, and families coping with the daily struggles of diseases, disorders and chronic illness.

1739 Health Finder

www.healthfinder.gov

A government web site there individuals can find information and tools to help you and those you care about stay healthy.

1740 Healthlink USA

www.healthlinkusa.com

Health information concerning treatment, cures, prevention, diagnosis, risk factors, research, support groups, email lists, personal stories and much more. Updated regularly.

1741 Helios Health

www.helioshealth.com

Online resource for your health information. Detailed information about specific health topics, access to expert advice from our Medical Advisory Board, and up-to-date health news.

1742 MedicineNet

www.medicinenet.com

An online resource for consumers providing easy-to-read, authoritative medical and health information.

1743 Medscape

www.medscape.com

Medscape offers specialists, primary care physicians, and other health professionals the Web's most robust and integrated medical information and educational tools.

1744 National Alliance for Autism Research

www.naar.org

The first organization in the United States dedicated to funding and accelerating biomedical research focusing on autism spectrum disorders.

1745 National Institute of Mental Health

www.nimh.nih.gov

Mission is to transform the understanding and treatment of mental illnesses through basic and clinical research, paving the way for prevention, recovery, and cure.

1746 Son Rise Program

www.autismtreatmentcenter.org

A powerful and effective treatment for children and adults challenged by Autism, Autism Spectrum Disorders, Pervasive Developmental Disorder (PDD) , Asperger's Syndrome, and other developmental difficulties.

1747 WebMD

www.webmd.com

Provides credible information, supportive communities, and in-depth reference material about health subjects. A source for original and timely health information as well as material from well known content providers.

Description

1748 Birth Defects

Birth defects, or congenital abnormalities, occur in 3 to 4 percent of newborns and can include structural defects of the heart, major blood vessels, kidneys, urinary tract, gastrointestinal tract, skeleton and nervous system. The incidence of specific abnormalities varies with the type of defect. These defects may be single or several defects may occur together, often known as a syndrome.

Although in many instances the cause of the defect is unknown, genetic factors may cause many single malformations and syndromes. Some syndromes, such as Down syndrome, result from chromosomal abnormalities. Factors during the pregnancy can sometimes result in defects, such as taking certain drugs (Coumadin, Dilantin), maternal illness (diabetes), and various infections (German measles, Rubella).

Prior to birth, ultrasound evaluation of the fetus and testing of the amniotic fluid surrounding it can identify some defects. If a defect is identified and is serious, parents can decide how or if they wish the pregnancy to proceed. Other abnormalities may not be identified until birth. Treatment and outcome vary greatly, depending on the type and severity of the defect. Parents and other family members need honest information and emotional support when caring for a child born with congenital defects. If genetic factors are suspected, the parents should receive genetic counseling. See also *Spina Bifida and Congenital Heart Disease*.

National Agencies & Associations

1749 Birth Defect Research for Children

800 Celebration Avenue   407-566-8304
Celebration, FL 34747   Fax: 407-566-8341
e-mail: staff@birthdefects.org.
www.birthdefects.org

A nonprofit organization that provides information about birth defects of all kinds to parents and professionals. Offers a library of medical books and files of information on less common categories of birth defects and is involved in research to discover causes and prevention.
Betty Mekdeci, Executive Director
John Bragg, Administrative Assistant

1750 CAPP National Parent Resource Center

95 Berkeley Street   617-482-2915
Boston, MA 02116   800-331-0688
Fax: 617-695-2939
e-mail: cec@cec.sped.org
www.cec.sped.org

A parent-run resource system designed to further the needs and goals of family-centered community-based coordinated care for children with special health needs and their families. Offers written materials, training packages, workshops and presentations.
Marilyn Friend, President
Mark Innocenti, Associate Director

1751 Cleft Palate Foundation

1504 E Franklin Street   919-933-9044
Chapel Hill, NC 27514-2820   800-24C-LEFT
Fax: 919-933-9604
e-mail: info@cleftline.org
www.cleftline.org

Major services are provided through CLEFTLINE, a 24 hour toll free hotline for anyone affected by a facial birth defect. We provide free educational materials referrals to local treatment and support groups and hope.
Nancy C Smythe, Executive Director
Samantha Jennings MSW, Family Services Director

1752 Cornelia de Lange Syndrome Foundation

302 W Main Street   860-676-8166
Avon, CT 06001   800-223-8355
Fax: 860-676-8337
e-mail: info@cdlsusa.org
www.cdlsusa.org

Provides information about birth defects caused by Cornelia de Lange Syndrome.
Liana Garcia-Fresher, Executive Director
Barbara Koontz, Information Coordinator

1753 Easter Seals

233 South Wacker Drive   312-726-6200
Chicago, IL 60606   800-221-6827
Fax: 312-726-1494
TTY: 312-726-4258
e-mail: info@easter-seals.org
www.easter-seals.org

Provides services to children and adults with disabilities as well as support to their families.
Reenie Kavalor, VP Medical/Rehabilitation Services
Stephen F Rossman, Chair

1754 Federation for Children with Special Needs

1135 Tremont Street   617-236-7210
Boston, MA 02120   800-331-0688
Fax: 617-572-2094
e-mail: fcsninfo@fcsn.org
www.fcsn.org

A center for parents and parent organizations to work together on behalf of children with special needs.
Deborah Allen, Director
Peter Brenna CPA, Board of Director

1755 March of Dimes Birth Defects Foundation

1275 Mamaroneck Avenue
White Plains, NY 10605   914-997-4488
www.marchofdimes.com

Our mission is to improve the health of babies by preventing birth defects premature birth and infant mortality. The March of Dimes carries out this mission through programs of research community services education and advocacy to save babies' lives.

1756 National Early Childhood Technical Assistance Center

Campus Box 8040 UNC-CH   919-962-2001
Chapel Hill, NC 27599-8040   Fax: 919-966-7463
TDD: 919-843-3269
e-mail: nectac@unc.edu
www.nectac.org

Assists states and other designated governing jurisdictions as they develop multidisciplinary, coordinated and comprehensive services for children with special needs.
Lynn Kahn, Director
Beverly Payne-Betts, Administrative Assistant

1757 National Foundation for Facial Reconstruction

333 East 30th Street   212-263-6656
New York, NY 10016   Fax: 212-263-7534
e-mail: info@nffr.org
www.nffr.org

The National Foundation for Facial Reconstruction addresses the plight of children with a facial disfigurement by supporting state of the art treatment, innovative research, psychosocial support and medical training that inspires a new generation of pediatric doctors.
Whitney Burnett, Executive Director
Michele B Golombuski, MS, Associate Executive Director

1758 Parent Professional Advocacy League

45 Bromfield Street   617-542-7860
Boston, MA 02108   866-815-8122
Fax: 617-542-7832
e-mail: info@ppal.net
www.ppal.net

An organization of families of children with mental emotional or behavioral needs and concerned professionals. PALS support groups are run in many areas across the country.
Earl N. "Ski Stuck, Chair
Anne Metzger, Treasurer

Research Centers

1759 Boston University Center for Human Genetics
715 Albany Street
Boston, MA 02118-2394

617-638-4640
Fax: 617-638-7092
e-mail: amilunski@bu.edu
www.bumc.bu.edu
Offers research into genetic disorders and growth disorders.
Dr Karen H Antman, Dean
Jeff Milunsky, Co-Director

1760 California Teratogen Information Service UC San Diego School of Medicine Dept of
UC San Diego School of Medicine Dept of Pediatrics
9500 Gilman Drive
La Jolla, CA 92093-828

619-294-6291
800-532-3749
Fax: 619-220-0228
e-mail: ctispregnancy@ucsd.edu
www.ctispregnancy.org
Statewide service operated by the California Teratogen Information Service (CTIS) and Clinical Research Program. Our goal is to promote healthy pregnancies through education and research.
Kenneth Lyon Jones MD, Medical Director
Christina D Chambers, Program Director

1761 Department of Reproductive Genetics: Magee Women's Hospital
200 Lothrop Street
Pittsburgh, PA 15213-2582

412-647-8748
800-533-8762
Fax: 412-641-1032
e-mail: dbrucha@mail.magee.edu
www.upmc.com
Obstetrical and gynecological teaching unit of the University of Pittsburgh School of Medicine. A full-service women's hospital and now has expanded to include a range of services for women and men.
W Allen Hogge, Clinical Investigator
Jie Hu, Assistant Investigator

1762 Division Of Developmental and Behavioral Pediatrics
Children's Hospital Medical Center of Cincinnati
3333 Burnet Avenue
Cincinnati, OH 45229-3039

513-636-4200
800-344-2462
TTY: 513-636-4900
www.cincinnatichildrens.org
The Division of Developmental and Behavioral Pediatrics provides services for infants children and adolescents from birth to age 21 who are experiencing developmental or behavioral problems.
David J Schonfeld, Director
Matthew W Zurad, Business Director

1763 Georgetown University Child Development Center
Box 571485
Washington, DC 20057-1485

202-687-5000
Fax: 202-687-8899
e-mail: gucdc@georgetown.edu
www.gucchd.georgetown.edu
The mission of the GUCCHD is to bring together policy, research and clinical practice for the betterment of individuals and families, especially children youth and those with special needs including: development disabilities and special health care needs, mental health needs, young children and those in the child welfare system.
John De Gioia, President
Neal Horen, Co-Director Training and Technical Assis

1764 Louisiana State University Genetics Section of Pediatrics
200 Clay Avenue
New Orleans, LA 70118

504-896-9524
Fax: 504-894-3997
e-mail: ylacas@lsuhsc.edu
www.medschool.lsuhsc.edu

Yves Lacassie, Section Head
Mary Camille Fournet, Research Associate

1765 New England Regional Genetics Group
PO Box 920288
Needham, MA 02492

781-444-0126
Fax: 781-444-0127
e-mail: mfgnergg@verizon.net
www.nergg.org
Human genetic services and educational planning pertaining to birth defects.
Mary-Frances Garber, Executive Director
Cindy Ingham, Co-Director

1766 Teratology OTIS
1295 N Martin
Tucson, AZ 85721-202

520-626-3547
866-626-6847
e-mail: contactus@otispregnancy.org
www.otispregnancy.org
Teratology Information Services are comprehensive and multidisciplinary resources for medical consultation on prenatal exposures. TIS interpret information regarding known and potential reproductive risks into risk assessments that are communicated to individuals of reproductive age and health care providers.
Dee Quinn, Executive Director
Lori Wolfe, President

1767 Thomas Jefferson University: Daniel Baugh Institute
329 Jefferson Alumni Hall
1020 Locust Street
Philadelphia, PA 19107

215-503-7823
Fax: 215-503-2636
e-mail: James.Schwaber@mail.dbi.tju.edu
www.dbi.tju.edu
Cares for both out and in-patients with complex problems involving a wide variety of infectious diseases. The Division has an active clinical research program bringing state-of-the-art treatments to patients.
James Schwaber, Director
Boris N Kholodenko, Director Computational Cell Biology

1768 University of Illinois at Chicago Craniofacial Center
College of Medicine
180 DENT M/C 588
Chicago, IL 60612

312-996-7546
Fax: 312-413-1157
e-mail: dreisber@uic.edu
www.uic.edu
David J Reisberg, Director

1769 University of Iowa Birth Defects and Genetic Disorders Unit
Iowa Registry for Congenital/Inherited Disorders
100 Oakdale Campus
Iowa City, IA 52242-5000

319-335-3500
866-274-4237
Fax: 319-335-4030
e-mail: ircid@uiowa.edu
www.uiowa.edu
Established through the joint efforts of the University of Iowa the Iowa Department of Public Health and the Iowa Department of Human Services to monitor birth defects in the state.
Paul A Romitti, Director
Kim Keppler-Noreuil, Clinical Director for Birth Defects

1770 University of Miami: Mailman Center for Child Development
1601 NW 12th Avenue
Miami, FL 33136-6820

305-243-6801
Fax: 305-243-5978
TTY: 305-243-5937
TDD: 305-243-5937
www.pediatrics.med.miami.edu
Focuses on birth defects and children's illnesses.
Dr Robert Stempfel Jr, Director

1771 Wayne State University: CS Mott Center for Human Growth and Development
275 E Hancock Street
Detroit, MI 48201

313-577-1485
Fax: 313-577-8554
home.med.wayne.edu
Human growth and development disorders.
Dr Robert Sokol, Director
Valerie M Parisi, Dean

1772 Wichita Medical Research & Education Foundation
3306 E Central Avenue
Wichita, KS 67208-3104

316-686-7172
Fax: 316-687-0033
e-mail: info@wichitamedicalresearch.org
www.wichitamedicalresearch.org

The Wichita Medical Research Foundation promotes research for the development of new medical skills and knowledge which serve patients from Wichita and throughout Kansas.
Peggy L Johnson, Executive Director/COO
William Hendry PhD, President

Support Groups & Hotlines

1773 CUNY: Teratogen Information Service
People
1219 N Forest Road 716-634-8132
Williamsville, NY 14221-3292 888-773-0753
Fax: 716-634-3889
www.people-inc.org

Mary Ann Kedron, Ph.D.ÿ, Chairperson
Joseph J. Abdallah, Vice Chairperson

1774 Connecticut Pregnancy Exposure Information Service
UConn Health Partners
Division of Human Genetics 860-523-6419
West Hartford, CT 06119 800-325-5391
humangenetics.uchc.edu
Provides up-to-date information on all types of exposures during pregnancy or breastfeeding for Connecticut residents or women who have Connecticut physicians.
Philip E Austin, President
James F Abromaitis, Commissioner

1775 Illinois Teratogen Information Service (IT IS)
680 N Lake Shore Drive 312-981-4354
Chicago, IL 60611 800-252-4847
e-mail: itis@fetal-exposure.org
www.fetal-exposure.org
A free statewide service that is financially supported by the Illinois Department of Public Health. Provides information regarding all types of exposures during pregnancy, and is available to women who are pregnant or planning a pregnancy, fathers, physicians, and other health care providers in the State of Illinois
Kristen L Dieter MS/CGC, Genetic Counselor/Coordinator ITIS
Eugene Pergament MD/Ph.D, Medical Geneticist

1776 Indiana Teratogen Information Service
Indiana University Medical Center
975 W Walnut Street
Indianapolis, IN 46202 317-274-2241
www.genetics.medicine.iu.edu
A telephone inquiry service that provides central, up-to-date, information from computersized sources, professional articles and expert consultants
David D Weaver MD, Director

1777 Missouri Teratogen Information Service
University of Missouri Health Care
1 Hospital Drive 573-882-7299
Columbia, MO 65212-1 Fax: 573-882-1593
e-mail: umhs-muhealth@missouri.edu
www.muhealth.org/
The Missouri Teratogen Information Services (MOTIS) helps promote healthy pregnancies by providing, counseling, education and information.
James Ross, Chief Executive Officer
James C Poehling, Chief Operating Officer

1778 National Health Information Center
PO Box 1133 310-565-4167
Washington, DC 20013-1133 800-336-4797
Fax: 301-984-4256
e-mail: info@nhic.org
www.health.gov/nhic
A health information referral service sponsored by the Office of Disease Prevention and Health Promotion. Puts health professionals and consumers who have health questions in touch with those organizations that are best able to provide answers.

1779 Nebraska Information Service
University of Nebraska Medical Center
985440 Nebraska Medical Center 402-559-5071
Omaha, NE 68198-5440 Fax: 402-559-7248

Teratogen Information Project
Beth Conover APRN, MS, Genetic Counselor
Kathleen Caldwell, Project Assistant

1780 New Jersey Pregnancy Risk Information Service
254 Easton Avenue 732-745-6659
New Brunswick, NJ 8901-1766
DebraLynn Day Salvatore, Medical Director

1781 PALS Support Groups
Parent/Professional Advocacy League
45 Bromfield Street 617-542-7860
Boston, MA 02108 866-815-8122
Fax: 617-542-7832
e-mail: info@ppal.net
ppal.net
Promotes a strong voice for families of children and adolescents with mental health needs. Advocates for supports, treatment and policies that enale families to live in their communities in an environment of stability and respect.
Lisa Lambert, Executive Director
Christopher Anselmo, Project Coordinator

1782 Pregnancy Healthline: Pennsylvania Hospital
8th & Spruce Streets 215-829-3601
Philadelphia, PA 19107
Betsy Schick-Boschetto MSN

1783 Pregnancy Risk Line
Utah Department of Health
PO Box 141010 801-328-2229
Salt Lake City, UT 84114-1010 800-822-2229
www.health.utah.gov/prl
Provides vaulable information to women who are pregnant, considering becoming pregnant, or breastfeeding, and to their healthcare providers.

1784 Pregnancy Safety Hotline
Western Pennsylvania Hospital
4800 Friendship Avenue
Pittsburgh, PA 15224-1722 412-687-7233
www.wphs.org

Michael Kerr MS

1785 Teratogen Information Services
University of Florida Health Science Center
PO Box 100296
Gainesville, FL 32610-0296 352-392-3050
www.health.ufl.edu

Donna H Poynor MA

1786 Teratogen and Birth Defects Information Project
University of South Dakota
414 E Clark Street 605-677-5011
Vermillion, SD 57069-2307 877-269-6837
Fax: 605-677-6534
e-mail: urelations@usd.edu
www.usd.edu

James Abbott, University President
Rod Parry, Dean of the Medical School

1787 University of Iowa Teratogen Information Service
University of Iowa Teratogen
200 Hakins Drive 319-353-7877
Iowa City, IA 52242 800-777-8442
www.uihealthcare.com
Donna Katen Bahensky, Chief Executive Officer
Anne Madenrice, Chief Operations Officer

1788 University of Nebraska Medical Center Tera Togen Project
Genetic Medicine-Munroe-Meyer Institute
985430 Nebraska Medical Center 402-559-6800
Omaha, NE 68198-5430 800-656-3937
Fax: 402-559-6688
e-mail: gbschaef@unmc.edu
www.unmc.edu/dept/mmi/
The section of Genetic Medicine provides comprehensive services for a variety of patients and their families. Direct services include diagnosis, interpretation of risks, supportive counseling, and suggestions/referrals for further management. The department partic-

ipates in clinics, inpatient consultation, and the Teratogen Information Project.
G Bradley Schaefer MD/FAAP/FACMG, Director Genetics Department

1789 Vermont Pregnancy Risk Information Service
Vermont Regional Genetics Center
1 Mill Street
Burlington, VT 05401-1530   800-932-4609
Alan E Guttmacher MD

Books

1790 Bendectin Report
976 Lake Baldwin Lane   407-895-0802
Orlando, FL 32814   800-313-2232
e-mail: staff@birthdefects.org
www.birthdefects.org
Report on research connecting the anti-nausea medication, Bendectin, with birth defects. Includes latest judicial opinion confirming $24 million judgment in a Bendectin case.
90 pages

1791 Dursban Report
976 Lake Baldwin Lane   407-895-0802
Orlando, FL 32814   800-313-2232
e-mail: staff@birthdefects.org
www.birthdefects.org
Report on research and latest EPA findings on Dursban and health problems, including MCS and birth defects.
90 pages

1792 Environmental Birth Defect Digest
976 Lake Baldwin Lane   407-895-0802
Orlando, FL 32814   800-313-2232
e-mail: staff@birthdefects.org
www.birthdefects.org
Compendium of research briefs from the world medical literature, plus original articles covering birth defects associated with medications, radiation, chemicals, toxic sites, dioxin, pesticides, lead, mercury, Bendectin, aspartame and more.
42 pages

1793 Understanding Birth Defects
Franklin Watts Grolier
90 Old Sherman Turnpike   203-797-3500
Danbury, CT 06816-0001   800-621-1115
Fax: 203-797-3197
www.grolier.com
What birth defects are, their genetic and environmental origins and what can be done to help, plus the problems of low birth weight are discussed.
128 pages
ISBN: 0-531109-55-0

Children's Books

1794 Don't Feel Sorry for Paul
JB Lippincott
530 Walnut Street   215-521-8300
Philadelphia, PA 19105   Fax: 215-521-8902
www.ilkins.com
Paul is seven and was born with deformities of both hands and feet. Paul must wear a prosthesis on both feet so that he can walk. He has a third prosthesis for his right hand. The third prosthesis has a pair of hooks Paul uses as fingers.
94 pages Hardcover
ISBN: 0-397315-88-0

1795 God, the Universe and Hot Fudge Sundaes
Houghton, Mifflin & Company
222 Berkeley Street
Boston, MA 02116-3107   617-351-5000
www.hmco.com

Newsletters

1796 Birth Defect News
Birth Defect Research for Children
976 Lake Baldwin Lane   407-895-0802
Celebration, FL 32814   e-mail: staff@birthdefects.org
www.birthdefects.org

8 pages Quarterly
Betty Mekdeci, Executive Director

1797 NewsLine
Federation for Children with Special Needs
95 Berkeley Street   617-482-2915
Boston, MA 02116-6230   800-331-0688
Offers information for parents and families on resources, medical updates, activities, fund-raising events and association news for their disabled children.
Quarterly

1798 PAL News
Parent Professional Advocacy League
95 Berkeley Street   617-482-2915
Boston, MA 02116-6264   800-331-0688
Offers information on medical and technological updates in the area of research on birth defects, support groups and family resources for persons with disabled children.
Quarterly

Pamphlets

1799 After School...Then What? The Transition to Adulthood
Federation for Children with Special Needs
95 Berkeley Street   617-482-2915
Boston, MA 02116-6230   800-331-0688
Preparing for the transition after high school for children with special needs.

1800 Agent Orange and Birth Defects
976 Lake Baldwin Lane   407-895-0802
Orlando, FL 32814   800-313-2232
e-mail: staff@birthdefects.org
www.birthdefects.org
Research booklet, including the latest findings from the National Birth Defect Registry and government research connecting Agent Orange to birth defects.
42 pages

1801 Birth Defects & Genetics: The Genetics Revolution
March of Dimes Birth
1275 Mamaroneck Avenueÿ   914-997-4488
White Plains, NY 10605   Fax: 212-254-3518
e-mail: NY639@marchofdimes.com
www.marchofdimes.com
Offers information on genetic testing and what it means to the patient and family members.

1802 Childhood Illnesses in Pregnancy: Chicken Pox & Fifth Disease
March of Dimes
1275 Mamaroneck Avenueÿ   914-997-4488
White Plains, NY 10605   Fax: 212-254-3518
e-mail: NY639@marchofdimes.com
www.marchofdimes.com
Located on the March of Dimes website.

1803 Cleft Lip & Palate
March of Dimes
1275 Mamaroneck Avenueÿ   914-997-4488
White Plains, NY 10605   Fax: 212-254-3518
e-mail: NY639@marchofdimes.com
www.marchofdimes.com
Located on March of Dimes website.

1804 Club Foot and Other Foot Deformities
March of Dimes
1275 Mamaroneck Avenueÿ   914-997-4488
White Plains, NY 10605   Fax: 212-254-3518
e-mail: NY639@marchofdimes.com
www.marchofdimes.com
Located on the March of Dimes website.

1805 Genetic Counseling
March of Dimes
1275 Mamaroneck Avenueÿ   914-997-4488
White Plains, NY 10605   Fax: 212-254-3518
e-mail: NY639@marchofdimes.com
www.marchofdimes.com
Located on the March of Dimes website.

1806 Gulf War and Birth Defects
930 Woodcock Road   407-225-7035
Orlando, FL 32812   800-313-2232
www.birthdefects.org
Information booklet on recent data from the National Birth Defect Registry and other research related to Gulf War exposures and birth defects.
30 pages

1807 How to Find More About Your Child's Birth Defect or Disability
Association for Birth Defect Children
5400 Diplomat Circle
Orlando, FL 32810-5603   800-922-9234
www.birthdefects.org
An informational fact sheet that encourages parents who have a child with a birth defect or disability to become the expert on the child's disability with some suggestions on how to educate themselves.

1808 Low Birthweight
March of Dimes
1275 Mamaroneck Avenue   914-997-4488
White Plains, NY 10605   Fax: 212-254-3518
e-mail: NY639@marchofdimes.com
www.marchofdimes.com
Fact Sheets: one or two page review written for the general public.

1809 PKU Quick Reference and Fact Sheet
March of Dimes
1275 Mamaroneck Avenue   914-997-4488
White Plains, NY 10605   Fax: 212-254-3518
e-mail: NY639@marchofdimes.com
www.marchofdimes.com
Phenylketonuria (PKU) is an inherited disorder that affects the way the body is able to process food. If left untreated, it causes mental retardation. How PKU is passed on and how it is treated are outlined.

1810 Teaching Social Skills to Youngsters with Disabilities
Federation for Children with Special Needs
95 Berkeley Street   617-482-2915
Boston, MA 02116-6230   800-331-0688
Explains the importance of instruction and training to learn appropriate social behavior.

1811 Toxoplasmosis
March of Dimes
1275 Mamaroneck Avenue   914-997-4488
White Plains, NY 10605   Fax: 212-254-3518
e-mail: NY639@marchofdimes.com
www.marchofdimes.com
Fact Sheets: one or two page review written for the general public.

Audio & Video

1812 Genetics and Inherited Traits
March of Dimes
1275 Mamaroneck Avenue   914-997-4488
White Plains, NY 10605   Fax: 212-254-3518
e-mail: NY639@marchofdimes.com
www.marchofdimes.com
Fact Sheets: one or two page review written for the general public.

1813 Why My Child
5400 Diplomat Circle   407-629-1466
Orlando, FL 32810-5603   800-313-2232
www.birthdefects.org
A 9 1/2 minute video that explores the feelings every parent has when their child is born with a birth defect. Emmy-award-winning producer, Karen Dorsett, has created a compelling video that begins with the parents' question, Why my child? and follows through to concerns about links between birth defects and environmental exposures to drugs, pesticides, dioxin, radiation, hazardous wastes, etc.

Web Sites

1814 Association for Birth Defect Children
www.birthdefects.org
Provides parents and expectant parents with information about birth defects and support services for their children.

1815 Healing Well
www.healingwell.com
A social network and support community for patients, caregivers, and families coping with the daily struggles of diseases, disorders and chronic illness.

1816 Health Finder
www.healthfinder.gov
A government web site where individuals can find information and tools to help you and those you care about stay healthy.

1817 Healthlink USA
www.healthlinkusa.com
Health information concerning treatment, cures, prevention, diagnosis, risk factors, research, support groups, email lists, personal stories and much more. Updated regularly.

1818 Helios Health
www.helioshealth.com
Online resource for your health information. Detailed information about specific health topics, access to expert advice from our Medical Advisory Board, and up-to-date health news.

1819 March of Dimes Birth Defects Foundation
www.marchofdimes.com
Help moms have full-term pregnancies and research the problems that threaten the health of babies.

1820 MedicineNet
www.medicinenet.com
An online resource for consumers providing easy-to-read, authoritative medical and health information.

1821 Medscape
www.medscape.com
Medscape offers specialists, primary care physicians, and other health professionals the Web's most robust and integrated medical information and educational tools.

1822 WebMD
www.webmd.com
Provides credible information, supportive communities, and in-depth reference material about health subjects. A source for original and timely health information as well as material from well known content providers.

Description

1823 Brain Tumors

Brain tumors are either primary (originate in the brain) or metastatic (travel from other cancer sites). About 29,000 people in the United States are diagnosed with primary brain tumors each year; approximately 50 percent of those are benign (noncancerous). Cancerous brain tumors originating in the brain make up roughly 2 percent of all cancers. They may occur at any age but are most common in early adult and middle life. Metastatic brain tumors (those that spread from other cancers) occur in 20 to 40 percent of all cancers.

There are many different types of brain tumors, each with a distinctive appearance under the microscope and a characteristic pattern of onset, progression, location and response to treatment. Depending on the exact site and rate of growth of the tumor, symptoms may include change in personality, moodiness, impaired vision and hearing, headaches, nausea, vomiting, seizures, lethargy and a varying degree of weakness. Some cancers have a genetic basis. In most cases, the cause of an individual's brain tumor is not known.

The treatment of brain tumors, as in many other cancers, consists of a combination of surgical removal, chemotherapy and radiation therapy. Steroids reduce swelling, and antiseizure medication is commonly given. If the disease or its treatment has caused damage to the brain's functioning, the patient may also need physical therapy, speech therapy, or general supportive care. The prognosis depends on the patient's age and on the location, extent and precise type of the tumor. See also *Head Injuries*.

National Agencies & Associations

1824 American Brain Tumor Association
2720 River Road
Des Plaines, IL 60018-4117
847-827-9910
800-886-2282
Fax: 847-827-9918
e-mail: info@abta.org
www.abta.org

Services includes over 40 publications which address brain tumors their treatment and coping with the disease. Materials address brain tumors in all age groups. Provide free social service consultations and a mentorship program for new brain tumor support groups.
Elizabeth M Wilson, Executive Director
Geri Jo Duda RN, Patient Services

1825 Brain Tumor Society
55 Chapel Street
Newton, MA 02458
617-924-9997
800-770-8287
Fax: 617-924-9998
e-mail: info@braintumor.org
www.braintumor.org

Exists to find a cure for brain tumors and strives to improve the quality of life of brain tumor patients and their families. Disseminates educational information and provides access to psycho-social support and raises funds.
N Paul TonThat, Chief Executive Officer
Carrie Treadwell, Director of Research

1826 National Brain Tumor Foundation
22 Battery Street
San Francisco, CA 94111-5520
415-834-9970
800-934-2873
Fax: 415-834-9980
e-mail: info@braintumor.org
www.braintumor.org

Nonprofit health organization which raises funds for research and provides information and support to patients, their family members and friends and health professionals. Sponsors national and regional conferences, patient and caregiver programs.
Harriet Patt MPH, Director of Patient Services
N. Paul TonThat, Executive Director

1827 National Brain Tumor Society
22 Battery Street
San Francisco, CA 94111-5520
415-834-9970
800-934-2873
Fax: 415-834-9980
e-mail: info@braintumor.org
www.braintumor.org

Nonprofit health organization which raises funds for research and provides information and support to patients, their family members and friends and health professionals. Sponsors national and regional conferences, patient and caregiver programs.
Gerogre Gellert, Chief Medical Officer
N. Paul TonThat, Executive Director

1828 National Institute of Neurological Disorders and Stroke
NIH Neurological Institute
Bethesda, MD 20824
301-496-5751
800-352-9424
Fax: 301-402-2186
TTY: 301-468-5981
www.ninds.nih.gov

The mission of NINDS is to reduce the burden of neurological disease - a burden borne by every age group, by every segment of society, by people all over the world.
Story C Landis, PhD, Director
Walter J Koroshetz, Deputy Director

Foundations

1829 Brain Tumor Foundation for Children
6065 Roswell Road NE
Atlanta, GA 30328
404-252-4107
Fax: 404-252-4108
e-mail: bfc@bellsouth.net
www.braintumorkids.org

Provides information and emotional support for families of children with brain tumors. They also raise funds for brain tumor research and provide a telephone network system of parents who offer emotional support.
Rick Sauers, Chairman/Co-Founder
R Hal Meeks, Jr, President

1830 Children's Brain Tumor Foundation
274 Madison Avenue
New York, NY 10016
212-448-9494
866-228-HOPE
Fax: 212-448-1022
e-mail: info@cbtf.org
www.cbtf.org

Children's Brain Tumor Foundation (CBTF) is a national organization whose mission is to improve the treatment, quality of life and long-term outlook for children with brain and spinal cord tumors through research, support, education, and advocacy to families and survivors. CBTF provides research and quality of life grants, offers information and support via our toll free line, written educational material, meet the unique needs of childhood brain tumor survivors.
Robert Budlow, President
Joseph B Fay, Executive Director

1831 Pediatric Brain Tumor Foundation
302 Ridgefield Court
Asheville, NC 28806
828-665-6891
800-253-6530
Fax: 828-655-6894
e-mail: pbtfus@pbtfus.org
www.pbtfus.org

Dedicated to finding the cause and cure of childhood brain tumors through the support of medical research. Increases public awareness, aids in early detection and treatment, supports a national database on all primary brain tumors. Helps to provide hope and

emotional support for the thousands of children and families affected by this life threatening disease.
Michael Traynor, President
Glenn Wilcox, Vice President

Research Centers

1832 Brain Research Center Children s Hospital National Medical Cen
Children s Hospital National Medical Center
111 Michigan Avenue NW   202-476-3000
Washington, DC 20010   800-884-5433
                                        Fax: 202-884-5226
                                     e-mail: tbear@cnmc.org
                                        www.dcchildrens.com

Edwin K Zechman Jr, President
Mark L Batshaw, Chief Medical Officer

1833 Brain Research Foundation
111 W Washington Street   312-759-5150
Chicago, IL 60602   Fax: 312-759-5151
                                     e-mail: info@theBRF.org
                                           www.thebrf.org
Supports cutting-edge neuroscience research that will lead to novel treatments and prevention of neurological disease and disorders in children and adults. Deliver this commitment through seed grants, which provide early stage fundinf for innovative research projects, as well as educational programs for researchers and the general public.
Nathan Hansom, President
Terre A Constantine PhD, Executive Director

1834 Brain Tissue Resource Center McLean Hospital
McLean Hospital
115 Mill Street   617-855-2000
Belmont, MA 02478   800-272-4622
                                        Fax: 617-855-3199
                              e-mail: mcleaninfo@mclean.harvard.edu
                                       www.brainbank.mclean.org
A centralized resource for the collection and distribution of human brain specimens for brain research.
Francine M Benes, Director
Edward D Bird, Director Emeritus

1835 Central Brain Tumor Registry of the US
244 E Ogden avenue   630-655-4786
Hinsdale, IL 60521   Fax: 630-655-1756
                                     e-mail: cbtrus@aol.com
                                           www.cbtrus.org
Nonprofit resource for gathering and distributing current statistics on all primary brain tumors for the entire US. Includes data on benign borderline and malignant primary brain tumors.
Carol Kruchko, President /Administrator
Jeri Dolan, Executive Administrator

1836 University of California, San Francisco Brain Tumor Research Center
Department of Neurological Surgery
505 Parnassus Avenue   415-353-7500
San Francisco, CA 94143-0112   Fax: 415-353-2889
                              e-mail: garritye@neurosurg.ucsf.edu
                                       www.neurosurgery.ucsf.edu
Continuously funded by grants from the National Institutes of Health Since 1072, the Brain Tumor Research Center at UCSF is internationally recognized as a major research and treatment center for adults and children with tumors of the brain and spinal cord. This center emphasizes translational research into the biology and behavior of brain tumors - research in which scientists and health care clinicians work in partnership to translate laboratory findings of new or improved forms of therapy.
Charles B Wilson, Director
Michael Gillis, Administrative Director

Support Groups & Hotlines

Alabama

1837 Pediatric Brain Tumor Support Group
Children's Hospital

1600 7th Avenue S   205-939-9090
Birmingham, AL 35233-1785
Groups for parents and siblings of brain tumor patients. Related to Children's Hospital of Alabama. Babysitting available.
Paula Teague

Arizona

1838 Arizona Brain Tumor Support Group
Barrow Neurological Ins of St. Joe's Hospital
350 W Thomas Road
Phoenix, AZ 85013   623-205-6446
                                    www.braintumorfoundation.org
Lanette Veres, Director

1839 Southern Arizona Brain Tumor Support Group
Arizona Cancer Cetner
1515 N Campbell Avenue   520-694-4605
Tucson, AZ   e-mail: mdrozdoff@umcaz.edu
                                    www.braintumorfoundation.org
Marsha Drozdoff, Contact

California

1840 Bereavement Group for Children
The Center for Attitudinal Healing
33 Buchanan Drive
Sausalito, CA 94965   415-331-6161
                                          www.braintumor.org
Jimmy Pete, Contact

1841 Brain Tumor Society
National Brain Tumor Society
22 Battery Street   415-834-9970
San Francisco, CA 94111-5520   800-770-8287
                                        Fax: 415-834-9980
                                    e-mail: info@braintumor.org
                                          www.braintumor.org
N Paul TonThat, Executive Director

1842 Brain Tumor Support Group: Duarte
City of Hope National Medical Center
55 Chapel Street   617-924-9997
Newton, MA 02458   Fax: 617-924-9998
                                          www.braintumor.org
Help you learn more about brain tumors including symptoms, treatment options, and considerations for caregivers.
Heather Ducksworth, Contact

1843 Brain Tumor Support Group: Fresno
Cancer Center at St. Agnes
7130 N Millbrook Avenue   559-450-5528
Fresno, CA 93720   e-mail: karen.kennedy@samc.com
                                          www.braintumor.org
Karen Kennedy, Contact

1844 Brain Tumor Support Group: Fullerton
St. Jude Medical Plaza
2151 N Harbor Blvd   714-446-7182
Fullerton, CA 92835   e-mail: kathy.pearson@stjoe.org
                                          www.braintumor.org
Kathy Pearson RN, Contact

1845 Brain Tumor Support Group: Newport Beach
Hoag Hospital
Advanced Technology Pavilion   949-764-6036
Newport Beach, CA 92663   e-mail: lberberet@hoaghospital.org
                                          www.braintumor.org
Lori Berberet RN, Contact

1846 Brain Tumor Support Group: Orange
UC Irvine-Chao Family Comprehensive Cancer Center
101 The City Drive   714-456-8609
Orange, CA 92868   e-mail: bakerd@uci.edu
                                          www.braintumor.org
N. Paul TonThat, Chief Executive Officer
Michele Rhee, Director of Program Initiatives

1847 Brain Tumor Support Group: Redding
American Cancer Society

3290 Bechelli Lane
Redding, CA 96002 530-222-1058
www.braintumor.org

1848 Brain Tumor Support Group: Sacramento
UC Davis Ambulatory Care Center
4860 Y Street 916-734-5613
Sacramento, CA 95817 e-mail: kksmith@ucdavis.edu
www.braintumor.org

Karen Smith RN, Contact
Carolyn Guadagnolo LCSW, Contact

1849 Brain Tumor Support Group: San Diego
Kaiser's Pt Loma Medical Facility
3250 Fordham
San Diego, CA 92117 619-515-9908
www.braintumor.org

Connie Campbell, Contact

1850 Brain Tumor Support Group: San Francisco
UCSF
521 Parnassus Avenue 415-990-4461
San Francisco, CA 94143 e-mail: mlovely@braintumor.org
www.braintumor.org

Sharon Lamb RN, Contact
Mary Lovely RN, Contact

1851 Brain Tumor Support Group: Santa Barbara
Cancer Center of Santa Barbara
300 W Pueblo Street
Santa Barbara, CA 93105 805-563-5852
www.braintumor.org

Rosario Campuzano, Contact

1852 Brain Tumor Support Group: Stanford
Stanford Cancer Center
875 Blake Wilbur Drive 415-990-4461
Stanford, CA 94305 e-mail: mlovely@braintumor.org
www.braintumor.org

Joanie Taylor RN, Contact
Sharon Lamb RN, Contact

1853 Brain Tumor Support Group: Westlake Village
The Wellness Community
530 Hampshire Road
Westlake Village, CA 91361 805-379-4777
www.braintumor.org

Rebecca Dekker MFT, Contact

1854 Brain Tumor/Pituitary Patient Support Group
John Wayne Cancer Institute
2200 Santa Monica Blvd 949-515-9595
Santa Monica, CA 90404 e-mail: pituitarybuddy@hotmail.com
www.braintumor.org

Sharmyn McGraw, Contact

1855 Children Living with Illness
The Center for Attitudinal Healing
33 Buchanan Drive 415-331-6161
Sausalito, CA 94965 Fax: 415-331-4545
www.healingcenter.org

Don Goewey, Executive Director

1856 Glendale Adventist Medical Center Brain Tumor Support Group
Cancer Services
381 Merrill Avenue
Glendale, CA 91026 818-409-3530
www.braintumor.org

Connie Munoz LCSW, Contact

1857 Heads Up!
Northridge Hospital Medical Center
18300 Roscoe Blvd 818-885-8500
Northridge, CA 91325 e-mail: robert.salazar@chw.edu
www.braintumor.org

Wanda Martin, Contact
Robert Salazar, Additional Contact

1858 Neuro-Oncology Information and Support Group
Sister Mary Pia Regional Cancer Center

1800 N California Street
Stockton, CA 95204-6019 209-467-6550
www.stjosephscares.org
For patients and family members living with primary and metastatic brain tumors as well as spinal cord tumors. Free child care and refreshments are provided.
Jim Linderman

1859 Neuroscience Institute Brain Tumor Hotline
Hospital of the Good Samaritan
637 Lucas Avenue
Los Angeles, CA 90017-1912 800-762-1692
e-mail: info@goodsam.org
www.goodsam.org

Diana Selover, LCSW

1860 Patient Services
22 Battery Street 415-834-9970
San Francisco, CA 94111-5520 800-934-2873
Fax: 415-834-9980
e-mail: info@braintumor.org
www.braintumor.org

Quickly access brain tumor information and resources.
12 pages
George Gellert, Chief Medical Officer
N. Paul TonThat, Executive Director

1861 Peninsula Support & Education Group for Parents of Children with Brain Tumors
Parents Helping Parents
1400 Parkmoor Avenue 408-727-5775
San Jose, CA 95126-3222 855-727-5775
Fax: 408- 28- 111
e-mail: info@php.com
www.php.com

A comprehensive family resource center providing information, training, guidance and support to families of children with special needs and the professionals who serve them.
Suzanne Cistulli, Chair
Robert Badagliacco, Treasurer

1862 Support Group for Caregivers of Brain Tumor Patients
UCLA Medical Center
200 UCLA Medical Plaza 310-206-6731
Los Angeles, CA 90095 e-mail: cabe@mednet.ucla.edu
Cheryl Abe LCSW, Clinical Social Worker
Pamela Hoff LCSW, Clinical Social Worker

1863 Vital Options International
4419 Coldwater Canyon Avenue 818-508-5657
Studio City, CA 91604-1479 Fax: 818-788-5260
e-mail: info@vitaloptions.org
www.vitaloptions.org
A not-for-profit cancer communications, support, and advocacy organization with a mission, to facilitate a global cancer dialogue.
Selma R Schimmel, CEO/Founder
Juliana Lee, Production Manager

1864 Wellness Community Cancer Support Groups
San Francisco/East Bay
3276 Mc Nutt Avenue 925-933-0107
Walnut Creek, CA 94597 e-mail: emaslan@yahoo.com
www.braintumor.org

Erika Maslan MFCC, Contact

1865 Wellness Community: South Bay Cities
109 W Torrance Blvd
Redondo Beach, CA 90277 www.braintumor.org
Tom May, Contact

1866 Wellness Community: West Los Angeles
2716 Ocean Park Blvd
Santa Monica, CA 90405 www.braintumor.org

1867 Support Group for Parents of Children with Brain Tumors
Oakland Children's Hospital
747 52nd Street 510-428-3885
Oakland, CA 800-400-PEDS
www.kidsfirst.org

Trish Murphy

Colorado

1868 Brain Tumor Resource and Vital Encouragement
Childrens Hospital
1056 19th Avenue   303-861-8888
Denver, CO   e-mail: webmaster@tchden.org
www.tchden.org
Pediatric focus. Education and support. Retreats for parents of
brain tumor patients.
Jim Shmerling, DHA, FACHE, President & CEO

1869 Colorado Brain Tumor Support Group
Swedish Medical Center   303-806-7420
Englewood, CO 80113   e-mail: lgibson@thecni.org
www.braintumorfoundation.org
Lorre Gibson, Contact

Connecticut

1870 Connecticut Brain Tumor Support Group
20 York Street   203-785-7528
New Haven, CT 06510   Fax: 203-688-2395
www.braintumorfoundation.org
Angela Thomas LCSW, Contact

Delaware

1871 Pediatric Brain Tumor Support Group
Ronald McDonald House
PO Box 269   302-661-4077
Wilmington, DE 19899-3629   e-mail: izienberg@kidshealth.org
www.kidshealth.org
Niel Izienberg MD, Chief Executive Officer and Founder

District of Columbia

1872 National Health Information Center
PO Box 1133   310-565-4167
Washington, DC 20013-1133   800-336-4797
Fax: 301-984-4256
e-mail: info@nhic.org
www.health.gov/nhic
A health information referral service sponsored by the Office of
Disease Prevention and Health Promotion. Puts health profession-
als and consumers who have health questions in touch with those
organizations that are best able to provide answers.

1873 Washington DC Metropolitan Area Support Group
George Washington University
2150 Pennsylvania Aveneu NW   202-994-4035
Washington, DC 20037-3201
Margaret Fiore, RN

Florida

1874 Angels in the Sun Brain Tumor Support Group
Wellness Community
3900 Clark Road
Sarasota, FL 34233   941-921-5539
www.braintumorfoundation.org
John Kleinbaum, Program Director

1875 Brain Tumor Support Group
Miami Children's Hospital Foundation
3000 SW 62nd Avenue   305-662-8386
Miami, FL 33155   e-mail: maria.penate@mch.com
Maria Penate RN, Facilitator
Raquel Pasaron, Facilitator

1876 Florida Brain Tumor Association
PO Box 770182   954-755-4307
Coral Springs, FL 33077-0182 e-mail: sshetsky@fbta.info
www.fbta.info
Provides hope, support and education to brain tumor survivors,
their families and friends; conquers brain tumors by funding re-
search into their causes and cures; and enriches the quality of life
of those touched by brain tumors
Sheryl Shetsky, President
Gary L Kornfeld, VP

1877 Florida Brain Tumor Support Group
Healthpark Medical Ctr, Meeting Rm
Ft Meyers, FL 33919   239-433-4396
www.braintumorfoundation.org
Dona Ross, Contact

1878 Florida Brain Tumor Support Group: Deerfield Beach
North Broward Medical Center   954-755-4307
Deerfield Beach, FL 33441   e-mail: sshetsky@fbta.info
www.fbta.info
Sheryl Shetsky, President
Gary L Kornfeld, VP

1879 Hollywood Area Brain Tumor Support Group
Memorial Regional Hospital   954-265-4725
Hollywood, FL 33021   e-mail: csurloff@mhs.net
www.floridabraintumor.com
Sheryl Shetsky, Founder & President
Gary L. Kornfeld, Vice President

1880 Sarasota Area Brain Tumor Support Group
Institute of Advanced Medicine
5880 Rand Avenue
Sarasota, FL   e-mail: sposin@fbta.info
www.fbta.info
Sheryl R Shetsky, President
Gary L Kornfeld, VP

1881 West Palm Beach Area Brain Tumor Support Group
Good Samaritan Medical Center
West Palm Beach, FL 33401   561-655-5511
www.fbta.info
Sheryl R Shetsky, President
Gary L Kornfeld, VP

Georgia

1882 All Ages Support Group
Brain Tumor Foundation for Children
6065 Roswell Road NE   404-252-4107
Atlanta, GA 30328-4015   Fax: 404-252-4108
e-mail: info@braintumorkids.org
www.braintumorkids.org/
Patient Support Group Activities includes bowling, fishing, craft
parties, picnics, sporting events, holiday parties, etc. These activities, social events and more are provided for children of all ages
and their families.
Mary Campbell, Executive Director
R Hal Meeks Jr, President

1883 Emory Brain Tumor Support Group
Emory Clinic
Department of Neurosurgery
Atlanta, GA 30322   404-778-3091
www.neurosurgery.emory.edu/btsg/index
Meets the first Thursday of each month with the purpose of provid-
ing an opportunity for information-sharing and suport for brain tu-
mor patients, as well as their family, friends and caregivers.
Maxine Brown, Contact

1884 Hearts and Minds
Piedmont Hospital
1968 Peachtree Road NW   404-373-5202
Atlanta, GA   Fax: 404-605-5000
www.piedmonthospital.org
H.M McFarling, M.D, Chairman
Leslie A. Donahue, President & CEO

1885 SBTF Brain Tumor Support Group
PO Box 422471   404-843-3700
Atlanta, GA 30342   e-mail: info@sbtf.org
www.sbtf.org
To improve the quality of life for brain tumor patients and their
families.
Costas Hadjipanayis, President
Jennifer Kee Giliberto, Vice President

Illinois

1886 Brain Tumor Support Group
Northwestern Memorial Hospital
675 N St. Clair   312-695-8143
Chicago, IL 60611   312-695-0990
e-mail: mmaher@nmff.org
www.cancer.northwestern.edu

Steven Rosen, Director
Leonidas Platanias, MD, PhD, Deputy Director

1887 Parents of Children with Brain Tumors PCBT
Children's Memorial Hospital
2300 Children's Plaza   773-880-4316
Chicago, IL 60614
Meets quarterly and publishes a monthly newsletter. Library available at meetings (at CMH). Educational speakers and family functions.
Gina Baldacci LCSW, Contact

Indiana

1888 Brain Tumor Support Group
Community Hospital East
1500 North Ritter Avenue   317-355-1411
Indianapolis, IN 46219   e-mail: m.w.kemf@att.net
www.ecommunity.com/east

Michael Kemf, Facilitator
Marsha Cline, Facilitator

1889 Primary Brain Cancer Support Group
Women's Cancer Center at Lutheran Hospital
7950 W Jefferson Boulevard   260-435-7959
Fort Wayne, IN 46804
Linda Jordan RN, Contact

Iowa

1890 Iowa Brain Tumor Support Group
University of Iowa Hospitals
Iowa City, IA 52242   319-356-2557
Lori Roetlin, Contact
Sue May, Additional Contact

1891 Neurological Center of Iowa
Iowa Clinic
5950 University Avenue   515-875-9100
Des Moines, IA 50266-1418   Fax: 515-241-6090
www.iowaclinic.com/
Networks people in similar situations.
Mark A. Reece, Chairman of the Board
Steven A. Keller, Chair Patient Care Committee

1892 Quad Cities Brain Tumor Support Group
Genesis Medical Center
1401 W Central Park   563-421-1907
Davenport, IA 52804   e-mail: ided@genesishealth.com
Deb Ide, Contact

Kansas

1893 Gray Matters Support: Kansas City
24050 W 57th Street
Shawnee, KS 66226   e-mail: graymatters2007@yahoo.com
Debbie Stephenson, Contact

1894 Headstrong Brain Tumor Support Group
Victory in the Valley
3755 E Douglas   316-682-7400
Wichita, KS 67218   e-mail: info@victoryinthevalley.com
www.victoryinthevalley.org

Cary Cozby, Golf Pro & CEO
Tim Farrell, President, RST Ventures, Inc

Kentucky

1895 Meningioma/Benign Brain Tumor Support Group
Michael Quinlan Brain Tumor Foundation

4012 Dupont Circle   502-896-1701
Louisville, KY 40207
Kathy Quinlan-Thompson, Contact

1896 Wellness Community: Kentucky
1717 Dixie Highway
Fort Wright, KY 41011   859-331-5568
www.cancersupportcincinnati.org

Rick Bryan, Executive Director
Gail Lauleÿ, Office Manager

Louisiana

1897 Brain Tumor Support Group
3939 Houma Boulevard, Doctor's Row   504-835-5715
Metairie, LA 70005   e-mail: gmom224@cox.net
www.braintumor.org
Meets on the third Sunday of each month at 1:30 p.m., call to confirm.
Gayle Johnson, Contact Person

Maine

1898 Brain Tumor Support Group of Maine
Maine Medical Center
22 Bramhall Street   207-871-4527
Portland, ME 04102
Meets on the second Tuesday of each month from 7:00 to 9:00 p.m.
Nancy Fortier LCSW, Contact

Maryland

1899 Brain Tumor Networking Group
10628 Falls Road
Lutherville, MD 21022   410-832-2719
www.loyolamedicine.org

Ronald Petrocelli, Chairÿ
Michael Cathey, Vice Chair

1900 Brain Tumor Support Group: Maryland
NIH Clinical Research Center
9000 Rockville Pike   301-496-6380
Bethesda, MD 20892   e-mail: garrenn@mail.nih.gov
www.braintumor.org

Nancy Garren, Contact

1901 Brainiacs
Perryville Library   410-459-8157
Perryville, MD 21903
Liz Carrino, Contact

1902 Johns Hopkins Brain Tumor Education Group
Weinberg Building   410-502-2789
Baltimore, MD 21231
Liz Carrino, Contact

1903 Washington DC Metropolitan Area Brain Tumor Support Group
George Washington Ambulatory Center
I & 22nd Street   301-371-8660
Middletown, MD 21769
Lionel Chaiken, Contact
Jeff Schanz, Contact

Massachusetts

1904 Brain Tumor Patient and Caregiver Support Group
Dana Farber Cancer Institute
Boston, MA 02115   617-632-3634
Nancy Tharler LICSW, Contact

1905 Brain Tumor Support Group: Lahey
Lahey Clinic Medical Center
41 Mall Road
Burlington, MA 01805   617-726-1061
www.lahey.org

Michele Lucas MSW LICSW, Contact

1906 Brain Tumor Support Group: Worcester
UMass Memorial Medical Center-University Campus

55 Lake Avenue N
Worcester, MA 01655
508-334-7595
Fax: 800-697-2593
e-mail: ellen.sharenow@umassmemorial.org
www.braintumor.org
Ellen Sharenow PhD, Contact

1907 Neurological Support Group of St. Luke's Hospital
101 Page Street
508-997-1515
New Bedford, MA 02740-3464
Diane Robinson RN

1908 Parent Education/Support Group
Dana Farber Cancer Institute
44 Binney Street
617-632-3301
Boston, MA 2115
800-525-5068
e-mail: dana.farbercontactus@dfci.harvard.edu
www.dfci.harvard.edu
For parents of children with brain tumors. Please call for schedule.
Beverly Lavalley Run, Facilitator
Edward Benz Jr, President

Michigan

1909 Brain Tumor Networking Club
Gilda's Club Metro Detroit
3517 Rochester Road
248-577-0800
Royal Oak, MI 48073
Fax: 248-577-0898
Kristen Bernat, Contact

1910 Brain Tumor Support Group for Patients & Families
University of Michigan Medical Center
1500 E Medical Center Drive
734-936-9071
Ann Arbor, MI 48109-0316
Christina Crandall, Contact
Kathy Wilson, Contact

1911 Brain Tumor Support Group: Ann Arbor
St Joseph Mercy Hospital, Cancer Care Center
5301 E Huron River Drive
Ann Arbor, MI 48106
734-712-3658
www.sjmh.com
Paula Nedela RN, Contact

1912 Brain Tumor Support Group: West Bloomfield
Henry Ford Hospital
6777 W Maple
313-916-1796
West Bloomfield, MI 48322
Sandy Remer RN, Contact

Missouri

1913 Brain Cancer Support Group
St John's Hospital
Main Hospital
417-820-3157
Springfield, MO 65804
e-mail: laura.flowers@mercy.net
Laura Flowers, Contact

1914 Brain Tumor Support Group: Kansas City
St Luke's Hospital of Kansas City
4321 Washington Suite 4000
816-932-6015
Kansas City, MO 64111
Michelle Martin, Contact

1915 Brain Tumor Support and Networking Group
Wellness Community of Greater St. Louis
1058 Old Des Peres Road
314-238-2000
Saint Louis, MO 63131
e-mail: info@wellnesscommunitystl.org
www.wellnesscommunitystl.org/
Mitchell L Baris, Chair of the Board
Mary Jane Pieroni, CPA, Treasurer

Montana

1916 Cancer Patient/Caregiver Support Group
Wellness Community
1820 W Lincoln Street
406-582-1600
Bozeman, MT 59715
e-mail: twcmontana@qwest.net
Becky Robideaux, Contact

New Hampshire

1917 Brain Injury/Brain Tumor Support Group
Frisbie Memorial Hospital
Carol Mitchell LMSW, Contact
Rochester, NH 03867

New Jersey

1918 Brain Tumor Support Group: New Jersey
90 Bergen Street
973-972-1164
Newark, NJ 07103
e-mail: mcclamls@umdnj.edu
LaDawn McClamb, Contact

1919 Brain Tumor Support Group: Toms River
Community Medical Center
99 Highway 37 W
732-557-8270
Toms River, NJ 08755
e-mail: slaniado@sbhcs.com
Sherry Laniado LCSW, Contact

1920 Central New Jersey Brain Tumor Support Group
St. Luke's Roman Catholic Church
300 Clinton Avenue
732-321-7000
North Plainfield, NJ 07063
Patty Anthony RN, Contact
Virginia Shrodo, Contact

New Mexico

1921 People Living Through Cancer Support Groups
3411 Candelaria NE
505-242-3263
Albuquerque, NM 87107
888-441-4439
Fax: 505-242-6756
e-mail: info@pltc.org
www.pltc.org
A not for profit organization that connects and supports cancer survivors and caregivers by transforming shared individual experiences into enduring hope.
Beth Brown, Executive Director
Mary Ellen Kurucz, Program Director

New York

1922 Brain Tumor Support Group for Patients and Families
Albany Medical Center
Office of NY Oncology/Hematology
845-338-4820
Albany, NY 12208-3412
e-mail: eehauser@gmail.com
www.braintumor.org/patients-family-frien
Emilie Hauser, Contact

1923 Brain Tumor Support Group: Long Island
230 Main St. Emma Clark Library
516-747-8749
Setauket, NY
Billie Wilczek

1924 Long Island Brain Tumor Support Group
Old Bethpage Public Library
999 Old Country Road
516-996-3705
Plainview, NY 11803
Bob Crescenzo, Contact

1925 Mount Sinai Medical Center Brain Tumor Support Group
Ruttenberg Care Center-Guggenheim Pavilion
1190 Fifth Ave
212-717-3527
New York, NY 10029
Kathleen Maloney-Lutz RN, Contact

1926 New York Brain Tumor Support Group
525 E 68th Street
212-746-3986
New York, NY 10021
e-mail: wem9011@nyp.org
www.braintumor.org
Wendy Mitchell LMSW, Contact

North Carolina

1927 Brain Tumor Support Group: Raleigh Area
Raleigh Community Hospital
3400 Wake Forest Road
Raleigh, NC 27609-7373
919-846-0923
www.raleighcommunity.com

143

Lectures, educational materials, and newsletter. Home and hospital visitation.
Louise Clark, Director

1928 Duke Pediatric Brain Tumor Family Support Program
Preston Robert Tisch Brain Tumor Center
Duke University Medical Center   919-684-5301
Durham, NC 27710   Fax: 919-684-6674
                    e-mail: korpi001@mc.duke.edu
                                www.cancer.duke.edu/btc/
Darell D. Binger, MD, PhD, Director
Allan H Friedman MD, Deputy Director

1929 Preston Robert Tisch Brain Tumor Center at Duke
Cornucopia Cancer Support Center
5517 Durham Chapel Hill Blvd   919-668-6178
Durham, NC 27707   e-mail: stephanie.english@duke.edu
                                        www.cancer.duke.edu
Stephanie English MSW LCSW, Contact

Ohio

1930 Brain Tumor Support Group: Cincinnati
Wellness Community
4918 Cooper Road   513-791-4060
Cincinnati, OH 45242   Fax: 513-791-8239

1931 Southwest Ohio Brain Tumor Support Group
Kettering Medical Center
3535 Southern Boulevard   937-298-3399
Kettering, OH 45429-1221   e-mail: jean.ruppert@kmcnetwork.org
Ronald Petrocelli, M.D., Chair
Michael Cathey, Vice Chair

1932 Support Group for Parents of Children with Brain Tumors
Cincinnati Childrens Hospital Medical Center
Childrens Hospital Medical Center   513-636-4200
Cincinnati, OH 45229-3039   800-344-2462
                    www.cincinnatichildrens.org/default.htm
Thomas Boat, Director
Stephen Daniels, Associate Chair

Oregon

1933 Brain Tumor Education & Support Group
Legacy Good Samaritan Hospital Cancer Center
1130 NW 22nd Ave   503-413-7921
Portland, OR 97210
Wendy Talbot MSW LCSW, Contact
Selma Annala RT CLC, Contact

1934 Central Oregon Brain Tumor Support Group
900 SW 23rd Place   541-350-7243
Redmond, OR 97756   e-mail: rgklug@crestviewcable.com
Rubyanne Klug, Contact

Pennsylvania

1935 Brain Tumor Community Group
Lancaster General Health Campus
Wellness Conference Room   800-860-9949
Lancaster, PA 17601
Christine Burfete RN, Contact

1936 Brain Tumor Support Group: Johnstown
John P Murtha Neuroscience and Pain Institute
1450 Scalp Avenue   814-534-3797
Johnstown, PA 15904   e-mail: dlehew@conemaugh.org
                                        www.braintumor.org
N. Paul TonThat, Chief Executive Officer
Michele Rhee, Director of Program Initiatives

1937 Brain Tumor Support Group: Philadelphia
University of PA Hospital-Neurological Institute
3400 Spruce Street   215-615-5240
Philadelphia, PA 19104
Alisha Amendt MSN CRNP, Contact
Arbena Merolli MSW, Contact

1938 Brain Tumor Support Group: Pittsburgh
Cancer Caring Center

4117 Liberty Avenue   412-622-1212
Pittsburgh, PA 15224   e-mail: indo@cancercaring.org

1939 Delware Valley Brain Tumor Support Group at Jefferson
Jefferson Health System
Bluemle Life Sciences Building   215-955-4429
Philadelphia, PA 19107
Ann Marie DiBona RN, Contact
Janis Haaf RN, Contact

1940 Pediatric Cancer Foundation of the Lehigh Valley
Camelot for Children
2354 W Emmaus Avenue   610-393-9215
Allentown, PA 18103
Nicole Ronco, Contact

Rhode Island

1941 Brain Tumor Support Group: Providence
Brown University Campus
BioMedical Center   401-789-0126
Providence, RI 02912
Judy Allenson, Contact
Betty Bentley, Contact

1942 Rhode Island Brain & Spine Tumor Foundation
Bethany Home
229 Medway Street   401-272-4177
Providence, RI 02906   e-mail: ribstf@gmail.com
Colin Shaw, Contact

South Carolina

1943 Brain Tumor Support Group: Charleston
Hollings Cancer Center
86 Jonathon Lucas Street   843-792-8257
Charleston, SC 29445   e-mail: lizzic@musc.edu
                                        www.braintumor.org
Christa Lizzi RN, Contact

1944 Brain Tumor Support Group: Florence
Florence Neurosurgery and Spine
1204 E Cheves Street   843-206-1910
Florence, SC 29506   e-mail: info@florenceneurosurgery.com
                                        www.braintumor.org

South Dakota

1945 Cancer Support Group
Sanford Cancer Cetner Oncology Clinic
1020 W 18th Street
Sioux Falls, SD 57104   605-328-8000
            www.lls.org/aboutlls/chapters/mn/patient
Sue Halbritter RN NP, Contact

Tennessee

1946 Cancer Support Group: Knoxville
Wellness Community of East Tennessee
2230 Sutherland Avenue   865-546-4661
Knoxville, TN 37919   Fax: 865-522-0938
            e-mail: info@wellnesscommunitytn.org
                                www.cancersupportet.org
Christi Branscom, President
Beth Lee, Secretary

1947 Cancer Support Group: Nashville
Gilda's Club Nashville
1707 Division Street   615-329-1124
Nashville, TN 37203   e-mail: info@gildasclubnashville.org

1948 Memphis Regional Brain Tumor Survivors Group
Methodist University Hospital
1265 Union Ave   904-757-0806
Memphis, TN 38104   e-mail: cherrywel2@comcast.net
Cherry Welborn, Contact

Texas

1949 Brain Tumor Support Group: El Paso
Rio Grande Cancer Foundation
10460 Vista Del Sol Drive   915-562-7660
El Paso, TX 79925   e-mail: juttar@rgcf.org
Jutta Ramirez, Contact
Robert Lefferts, Contact

1950 Central Texas Brain Tumor Support Group
Brain and Spine Center at Brackenridge Hospital
274 Madison Avenue   512-636-1578
New York, NY 10016   866-228-4673
                                         e-mail: info@cbtf.org
                                         www.cbtf.org
Contains practical information to sort out the complexities of medical procedures, interruptions in school and social life, and uncertainty about the future.
Thomas Lewman, Contact

1951 Houston Area Brain Tumor Network
MD Anderson Cancer Center Brain & Spine Center
1515 Holcombe Blvd   713-794-1777
Houston, TX 77030   e-mail: spanju@mdanderson.org
Mark Anderson, Contact
Suki Panju, Contact

1952 South Texas Brain Tumor Foundation Support Group
San Antonio Employees Federal Credit Union
6000 NW Loop 410   210-670-9323
San Antonio, TX 78201
Susie Soriano, Contact

Utah

1953 Cancer Wellness House
59 S 1100 E   801-236-2294
Salt Lake City, UT 84102
Karen Elliott

Virginia

1954 Brain Tumor Support Group: Richmond
St Mary's Hospital
Education Center   877-284-3905
Richmond, VA 23226   e-mail: curebt@hotmail.com
                                         www.abta.org
Ronald Petrocelli, M.D., Chair
Michael Cathey, Vice Chair

1955 Valley Brain Tumor Support Group
Rehab2Health
Shenandoah Memorial Hospital   540-984-4921
Woodstock, VA 22664   e-mail: vbtsg@shentel.net
Valorie Hockman, Contact

Washington

1956 Brain Cancer Support Group: Port Orchard
2186 Yukon Harbor Rd SE   360-536-5042
Port Orchard, WA 98366   e-mail: ideas56@msn.com
Victoria Tierney MA RC, Contact

1957 Brain Cancer Support Group: Seattle
Northwest Hospital
Professional Building   206-297-2500
Seattle, WA 98133

1958 Virginia Mason Brain Tumor Support Group
1201 Terry Avenue   206-223-7552
Seattle, WA 98111
Michelle Handler RN, Contact

1959 Wenatchee Valley Brain Tumor Support Group
Wellness Place
1610 Fifth Street   509-679-9574
Wenatchee, WA 98801   e-mail: hastings9@charter.net
Jeff Hastings, Contact
Mary Lowe, Contact

West Virginia

1960 Brain Tumor Support Group: Southern West Virginia
First Presbyterian Church
16 Broad Street   304-744-0393
Charleston, WV 25301-2487
Jeri McDonald

Wisconsin

1961 Brain Tumor Support Group: John Sierzant Lutheran Hospital, Gunderson Clinic
1836 S Avenue   608-791-9862
LaCrosse, WI
Esther Lindeman RN

1962 LODAT: Brain Tumor Support Group
Children's Hospital of Wisconsin
Room 888
Milwaukee, WI   414-962-8984
                                         www.braintumor.org
Living One Day At a Time is a parent support group for families of chidren with cancer. Monthly newsletter, informational meetings, social activities for families, and bereavement support.
Frances Swigart

Books

1963 Brain Tumor Resource Directory
National Brain Tumor Foundation
1517 North Point Street   617-924-9997
San Francisco, CA 94123-5520   800-934-2873
                                         Fax: 617-924-9998
                                         e-mail: nbtf@braintumor.org
                                         www.braintumor.org
Help you learn more about brain tumors including symptoms, treatment options, and considerations for caregivers.
Rob Tufel, Director Patient Services

1964 Death Be Not Proud: A Memoir
Harper Collins
10 E 53rd Street
New York, NY 10022   212-207-7000
                                         www.harpercollins.com
The father of a young man diagnosed with glioblastoma multiforme wrote this 50-year-old classic.

ISBN: 0-060929-89-8

1965 Resource Guide for Parents of Children with Brain and Spinal Cord Tumors
Children's Brain Tumor Foundation
274 Madison Avenue   212-448-9494
New York, NY 10016   866-228-4673
                                         Fax: 212-448-1022
                                         e-mail: info@cbtf.org
                                         www.cbtf.org
Contains practical information to sort out the complexities of medical procedures, interruptions in school and social life, and uncertainty about the future.
Robert Budlow, President
Joseph B Fay, Executive Director

1966 Support Group Directory
National Brain Tumor Foundation
1517 North Point Street   617-924-9997
San Francisco, CA 94123-5520   800-934-2873
                                         Fax: 617-924-9998
                                         e-mail: nbtf@braintumor.org
                                         www.braintumor.org
Help you learn more about brain tumors including symptoms, treatment options, and considerations for caregivers.
Rob Tufel, Director Patient Services

1967 That's Unacceptable: Surviving a Brain Tumor: My Personal Story
Rebecca L Libutti, author
Krystal Publishing

PO Box 221
Martinsville, NJ 08836

908-889-6038
800-833-9327
Fax: 908-889-6038
e-mail: RLibutti@aol.com
www.krystalpublishing.com

Written by a ten-year survivor of glioblastoma multiforme, the book's title was the author's first response to the initial discouragement she received about pursuing aggressive treatment.
198 pages Paperback
RL Libutti

1968 The Essential Guide to Brain Tumors
National Brain Tumor Foundation
1517 North Point Street
San Francisco, CA 94123-5520

617-924-9997
800-934-2873
Fax: 617-924-9998
e-mail: nbtf@braintumor.org
www.braintumor.org

Help you learn more about brain tumors including symptoms, treatment options, and considerations for caregivers.
80 pages
Rob Tufel, Director Patient Services

1969 Understanding and Coping with Your Child's Brain Tumor
National Brain Tumor Foundation
1517 North Point Street
San Francisco, CA 94123-5520

617-924-9997
800-934-2873
Fax: 617-924-9998
e-mail: nbtf@braintumor.org
www.braintumor.org

Help you learn more about brain tumors including symptoms, treatment options, and considerations for caregivers.
52 pages
Rob Tufel, Director Patient Services

Children's Books

1970 My Name is Buddy
Dave Bauer, author
National Brain Tumor Foundation
1517 North Point Street
San Francisco, CA 94123-5520

617-924-9997
800-934-2873
Fax: 617-924-9998
e-mail: nbtf@braintumor.org
www.braintumor.org

Help you learn more about brain tumors including symptoms, treatment options, and considerations for caregivers.
Rob Tufel, Director Patient Services

Newsletters

1971 Butterfly Bulletin
Brain Tumor Foundation for Children
6065 Roswell Road NE
Atlanta, GA 30328-4015

404-252-4107
Fax: 404-252-4108
e-mail: info@braintumorkids.org
www.braintumorkids.org

Reporting on news and events of the Brain Tumor Foundation for Children.
Quarterly
Rick Sauers, Chairman/Co-Founder
R Hal Meeks, Jr, President

1972 Caring Hand
Pediatric Brain Tumor Foundation
302 Ridgefield Court
Asheville, NC 28806

828-665-6891
800-253-6530
Fax: 828-655-6894
e-mail: pbtfus@pbtfus.org
www.curethekids.org

The Pediatric Brain Tumor Foundation works to eliminate the challenges of childhood brain tumors. As the world's largest nonprofit source of funding for pediatric brain tumor research, our mission is to cure the kids.
Michael Traynor, President
Glenn Wilcox, Vice President

1973 Childhood Brain Tumor Foundation Newsletter
Childhood Brain Tumor Foundation
20312 Watkins Meadow Dr
Germantown, MD 20876-4259

310-515-2900
877-217-4166
Fax: 301-515-2900
e-mail: cbtf@childhoodbraintumor.org
www.childhoodbraintumor.org

It is a volunteer-run organization driven to help educate families whose children have been diagnosed with brain tumors. Our mission is to provide grant funding for researchers to further the cause to find a cure

1974 Helping Hand
Pediatric Brain Tumor Foundation
302 Ridgefield Court
Asheville, NC 28806

828-665-6891
800-253-6530
Fax: 828-655-6894
e-mail: pbtfus@pbtfus.org
www.curethekids.org

The Pediatric Brain Tumor Foundation works to eliminate the challenges of childhood brain tumors. As the world's largest nonprofit source of funding for pediatric brain tumor research, our mission is to cure the kids.
Michael Traynor, President
Glenn Wilcox, Vice President

1975 Message Line Newsletter
American Brain Tumor Association
8550 W. Bryn Mawr Ave.
Chicago, IL 60631-4117

773-577-8750
800-886-2282
Fax: 773-577-8738
e-mail: info@abta.org
www.abta.org

Describes research advances and announces updates to publications.
TriAnnual
Elizabeth Wilson, Executive Director
Geri Jo Duda, RN, Patient Services

1976 SEARCH
National Brain Tumor Foundation
1517 North Point Street
San Francisco, CA 94123-5520

617-924-9997
800-934-2873
Fax: 617-924-9998
e-mail: nbtf@braintumor.org
www.braintumor.org

Help you learn more about brain tumors including symptoms, treatment options, and considerations for caregivers.
Quarterly
Rob Tufel, Director Patient Services

1977 TLC (Tips for Living And Coping)
American Brain Tumor Association
8550 W. Bryn Mawr Ave.
Chicago, IL 60018-4117

773-577-8750
800-886-2282
Fax: 773-577-8738
e-mail: info@abta.org
www.abta.org

E-bulletin of news, research and development finds, support and treatment information.

ISBN: 0-944093-37-X
Elizabeth Wilson, Executive Director
Geri Jo Duda, RN, Patient Services

Pamphlets

1978 Clinical Trial Fact Sheet
National Brain Tumor Foundation
1517 North Point Street
San Francisco, CA 94123-5520

617-924-9997
800-934-2873
Fax: 617-924-9998
e-mail: nbtf@braintumor.org
www.braintumor.org

Help you learn more about brain tumors including symptoms, treatment options, and considerations for caregivers.

1979 Coping with Your Loved One's Brain Tumor
National Brain Tumor Foundation

1517 North Point Street
San Francisco, CA 94123-5520

617-924-9997
800-934-2873
Fax: 617-924-9998
e-mail: nbtf@braintumor.org
www.braintumor.org

Help you learn more about brain tumors including symptoms, treatment options, and considerations for caregivers.
12 pages Booklet

1980 Dictionary for Brain Tumor Patients
American Brain Tumor Association
8550 W. Bryn Mawr Ave.
Chicago, IL 60631-4117

773-577-8750
800-886-2282
Fax: 773-577-8738
e-mail: info@abta.org
www.abta.org

Offers a dictionary of terms used in the diagnosis and everday living with brain tumors.
Paperback
ISBN: 0-944093-27-2
Elizabeth Wilson, Executive Director
Geri Jo Duda, RN, Patient Services

1981 Ependymoma
American Brain Tumor Association
8550 W. Bryn Mawr Ave.
Chicago, IL 60631-4117

773-577-8750
800-886-2282
Fax: 773-577-8738
e-mail: info@abta.org
www.abta.org

ISBN: 0-944093-40-X
Elizabeth Wilson, Executive Director
Geri Jo Duda, RN, Patient Services

1982 Glioblastoma Multiforme and Anaplastic Astrocytoma
American Brain Tumor Association
8550 W. Bryn Mawr Ave.
Chicago, IL 60631-4117

773-577-8750
800-886-2282
Fax: 773-577-8738
e-mail: info@abta.org
www.abta.org

ISBN: 0-944093-36-1
Elizabeth Wilson, Executive Director
Geri Jo Duda, RN, Patient Services

1983 Living with A Brain Tumor
American Brain Tumor Association
8550 W. Bryn Mawr Ave.
Chicago, IL 60631-4117

773-577-8750
800-886-2282
Fax: 773-577-8738
e-mail: info@abta.org
www.abta.org

A guide for brain tumor patients.
2004
ISBN: 0-944093-54-X
Elizabeth Wilson, Executive Director
Geri Jo Duda, RN, Patient Services

1984 Medulloblastoma
American Brain Tumor Association
8550 W. Bryn Mawr Ave.
Chicago, IL 60631-4117

773-577-8750
800-886-2282
Fax: 773-577-8738
e-mail: info@abta.org
www.abta.org

Paperback
ISBN: 0-944093-33-7
Elizabeth Wilson, Executive Director
Geri Jo Duda, RN, Patient Services

1985 Meningioma
American Brain Tumor Association

8550 W. Bryn Mawr Ave.
Chicago, IL 60631-4117

773-577-8750
800-886-2282
Fax: 773-577-8738
e-mail: info@abta.org
www.abta.org

ISBN: 0-944093-23-X
Elizabeth Wilson, Executive Director
Geri Jo Duda, RN, Patient Services

1986 Metastatic Brain Tumors
American Brain Tumor Association
8550 W. Bryn Mawr Ave.
Chicago, IL 60631-4117

773-577-8750
800-886-2282
Fax: 773-577-8738
e-mail: info@abta.org
www.abta.org

ISBN: 0-944093-26-4
Elizabeth Wilson, Executive Director
Geri Jo Duda, RN, Patient Services

1987 Oligodendroglioma and Mixed Glioma
American Brain Tumor Association
8550 W. Bryn Mawr Ave.
Chicago, IL 60631-4117

773-577-8750
800-886-2282
Fax: 773-577-8738
e-mail: info@abta.org
www.abta.org

Pamphlet
ISBN: 0-944093-43-4
Elizabeth Wilson, Executive Director
Geri Jo Duda, RN, Patient Services

1988 Organizing a Support Group
American Brain Tumor Association
8550 W. Bryn Mawr Ave.
Chicago, IL 60631-4117

773-577-8750
800-886-2282
Fax: 773-577-8738
e-mail: info@abta.org
www.abta.org

Elizabeth Wilson, Executive Director
Geri Jo Duda, RN, Patient Services

1989 Pituitary Tumors
American Brain Tumor Association
8550 W. Bryn Mawr Ave.
Chicago, IL 60631-4117

773-577-8750
800-886-2282
Fax: 773-577-8738
e-mail: info@abta.org
www.abta.org

Pamphlet
ISBN: 0-944093-44-2
Elizabeth Wilson, Executive Director
Geri Jo Duda, RN, Patient Services

1990 Primer of Brain Tumors
American Brain Tumor Association
8550 W. Bryn Mawr Ave.
Chicago, IL 60631-4117

773-577-8750
800-886-2282
Fax: 773-577-8738
e-mail: info@abta.org
www.abta.org

A patient's reference manual offering information on brain tumors.

ISBN: 0-944093-35-3
Elizabeth Wilson, Executive Director
Geri Jo Duda, RN, Patient Services

1991 Radiation Therapy of Brain Tumors: A Basic Guide
American Brain Tumor Association
8550 W. Bryn Mawr Ave.
Chicago, IL 60631-4117

773-577-8750
800-886-2282
Fax: 773-577-8738
e-mail: info@abta.org
www.abta.org

ISBN: 0-944093-28-0
Elizabeth Wilson, Executive Director
Geri Jo Duda, RN, Patient Services

1992 Returning to Work: Strategies for Brain Tumor Patients
National Brain Tumor Foundation
1517 North Point Street
San Francisco, CA 94123-5520

617-924-9997
800-934-2873
Fax: 617-924-9998
e-mail: nbtf@braintumor.org
www.braintumor.org

Help you learn more about brain tumors including symptoms, treatment options, and considerations for caregivers.
16 pages Brochure
Rob Tufel, Director Patient Services

1993 Stereotactic Radiosurgery
American Brain Tumor Association
8550 W. Bryn Mawr Ave.
Chicago, IL 60631-4117

773-577-8750
800-886-2282
Fax: 773-577-8738
e-mail: info@abta.org
www.abta.org

ISBN: 0-944093-42-6
Elizabeth Wilson, Executive Director
Geri Jo Duda, RN, Patient Services

1994 Understanding Brain Tumors: Glioblastoma Multiforme
National Brain Tumor Foundation
1517 North Point Street
San Francisco, CA 94123-5520

617-924-9997
800-934-2873
Fax: 617-924-9998
e-mail: nbtf@braintumor.org
www.braintumor.org

Help you learn more about brain tumors including symptoms, treatment options, and considerations for caregivers.
16 pages
Rob Tufel, Director Patient Services

1995 Using A Medical Library
American Brain Tumor Association
8550 W. Bryn Mawr Ave.
Chicago, IL 60631-4117

773-577-8750
800-886-2282
Fax: 773-577-8738
e-mail: info@abta.org
www.abta.org

Elizabeth Wilson, Executive Director
Geri Jo Duda, RN, Patient Services

1996 What You Need to Know About Brain Tumors
National Cancer Institute
9609 Medical Center Drive
Bethesda, MD 20892-0001

301-435-3848
800-422-6237
www.cancer.gov

Offers factual information about brain tumors, possible causes, primary and secondary tumors, symptoms, diagnosis, treatment, side effects, followup care, support and medical terms.

1997 When Your Child Returns to School
American Brain Tumor Association
8550 W. Bryn Mawr Ave.
Chicago, IL 60631-4117

773-577-8750
800-886-2282
Fax: 773-577-8738
e-mail: info@abta.org
www.abta.org

Guides parents and teachers through a successful return to school when a child has had a brain tumor.
Paperback
ISBN: 0-944093-21-3
Elizabeth Wilson, Executive Director
Geri Jo Duda, RN, Patient Services

Audio & Video

1998 Conference Audiotapes
National Brain Tumor Foundation
1517 North Point Street
San Francisco, CA 94123-5520

617-924-9997
800-934-2873
Fax: 617-924-9998
e-mail: nbtf@braintumor.org
www.braintumor.org

Help you learn more about brain tumors including symptoms, treatment options, and considerations for caregivers.
Rob Tufel, Director Patient Services

1999 Strategies for Healing
National Brain Tumor Foundation
1517 North Point Street
San Francisco, CA 94123

617-924-9997
800-934-2873
Fax: 617-924-9998
e-mail: nbtf@braintumor.org
www.braintumor.org

Help you learn more about brain tumors including symptoms, treatment options, and considerations for caregivers.
Rob Tufel, Director Patient Services

Web Sites

2000 American Brain Tumor Association
www.abta.org

Provide free social service consultations; a mentorship program for new brain tumor support group leaders; a nationwide database of established support groups; the Connections pen-pal program; networking with organizations that provide services to patients and families; a resource listing of physicians offering investgative treatments.

2001 Brain Tumor Society
124 Watertown Street
Watertown, MA 02472

617-924-9997
800-770-8287
Fax: 617-924-9998
e-mail: info@tbts.org
braintumor.org

Disseminates educational information and provides access to psycho-social support and raises funds to advance carefully selected scientific research projects, improve clinical care and find a cure.

2002 Healing Well
www.healingwell.com

An online health resource guide to medical news, chat, information and articles, newsgroups and message boards, books, disease-related web sites, medical directories, and more for patients, friends, and family coping with disabling diseases, disorders, or chronic illnesses.

2003 Health Finder
www.healthfinder.gov

Searchable, carefully developed web site offering information on over 1000 topics. Developed by the US Department of Health and Human Services, the site can be used in both English and Spanish.

2004 Healthlink USA
www.healthlinkusa.com

Health information concerning treatment, cures, prevention, diagnosis, risk factors, research, support groups, email lists, personal stories and much more. Updated regularly.

2005 Helios Health
www.helioshealth.com

Online resource for your health information. Detailed information about specific health topics, access to expert advice from our Medical Advisory Board, and up-to-date health news.

2006 MedicineNet
www.medicinenet.com

An online resource for consumers providing easy-to-read, authoritative medical and health information.

2007 Medscape
www.medscape.com

Medscape offers specialists, primary care physicians, and other health professionals the Web's most robust and integrated medical information and educational tools.

2008 National Brain Tumor Foundation
braintumor.org

Disseminates educational information and provides access to psycho-social support and raises funds to advance carefully selected scientific research projects, improve clinical care and find a cure.

2009   Pediatric Brain Tumor Foundation of the US

www.curethekids.org

Goal is to create an awareness about this growing disease among children and adults so that fundraising programs may continue to expand in increased laboratory research.

2010   WebMD

www.webmd.com

Provides credible information, supportive communities, and in-depth reference material about health subjects. A source for original and timely health information as well as material from well known content providers.

Description

Cancer

Cancer is a general term for more than 100 diseases characterized by abnormal or uncontrolled growth of cells. The resulting mass, or disease, can invade and destroy surrounding normal tissue. Cancer cells from the tumor can also spread (metastasize) through the blood or lymph (plasmatic fluid) to start new cancers in other parts of the body. In 2010, about 1,529,560 new cancer cases were diagnosed, and about 569,490 Americans died from their disease. Cancer is the second leading cause of death in the U.S., exceeded only by heart disease. Although these figures seem bleak, most cancers are potentially curable if detected at an early stage. Cancer, also called a malignancy (from Latin, meaning bad), can be either a solid tumor (carcinoma), such as lung cancer, or a disorder of blood cell formation, such as leukemia.

Cancer is caused by an interplay of internal and external factors, individually or in combination. Abnormal genes can cause multiple changes that affect cell growth. Environmental factors, such as cigarette smoke, (also called a carcinogen – causing cancer) and exposure to radiation, play a role. Many cancers can be prevented by health awareness. For example, 90 percent of the over one million skin cancers that will be diagnosed this year could be drastically reduced by protection from solar rays. Lung cancer, one of the most prevalent and hazardous cancers could be drastically reduced by eliminating tobacco use. The American Cancer Society estimates that 30 percent of all cancer deaths are related to cigarette smoking.

Cancer treatment may be curative – removes the tumor in the hope that it will not reoccur, or palliative – prolongs life and minimize discomfort when a cure is not possible. A treatment program typically includes a combination of surgery, radiation therapy, and chemotherapy. Immunotherapy is the newest form of treatment and uses agents known as biologic-response modifiers (BRM), to alter the immune system in its response to malignant growth. Brief descriptions of the more common cancers follow.

Brain Cancer

Brain cancer occurs at varying rates but overall it comprises approximately 5.6 cases per 100,000 populations each year. They are most common in early or middle adult life and incidence in the elderly population is increasing. Overall incidence is about equal in males and females.

The seriousness of brain tumors is determined by their size, location, and rate of growth. While brain cancer does not normally spread to others areas, many other cancers have the propensity of spreading throughout the nervous system and producing metastatic tumors in the brain. In adults, these tumors are most commonly from cancer of the lung, breast, or skin (melanoma). Symptoms include headaches, seizures, behavior problems, changes in eating or sleeping habits, lethargy and clumsiness. See also Brain Tumors.

Breast Cancer

Breast cancer is the most common malignant tumor in women in the western hemisphere. Approximately 207,090 new cases of breast cancer in women were diagnosed in 2010. As many as one in nine women will develop breast cancer during her lifetime. Incidence of breast cancer increases under the following conditions: age; (two-thirds of cases develop after age 55); a close relative (mother, sister) with breast cancer; a previous history of breast cancer; a previous history of breast cancer; exposure to radiation. Other risk factors include not having children, early onset of menstruation, and estrogen replacement therapy.

Early detection can be lifesaving. Many breast cancers are self-diagnosed. More than 80 percent of breast cancers occur as a painless mass. Monthly breast self-examination for women of all ages is crucial. The American Cancer Society recommends that women aged 20-39 have a clinical breast examination performed every three years. Depending on the presence of known risk factors, patients should undergo mammography either yearly or every other year between 40 and 50 years, and yearly after age 50.

Warning signs that can aid women in detecting breast cancer include lumps, swelling, skin irritation, tenderness of the nipple, and dimpling of the skin. Treatments vary, depending on when the cancer is discovered and whether it has spread. Research has shown that the traditional radical mastectomy (removal of the entire breast) canoften be replaced by lumpectomy (removal of just the tumor), coupled with radiation therapy. Chemotherapy or hormonal manipulation is also prescribed in some cases. The five year survival rate for localized (not spread) breast cancer has improved in recent years from 78 percent to 97 percent.

Colon and Rectal Cancer

In western countries, colon and rectal (colorectal) cancer account for more new cases of cancer per year than any other anatomic site except the lung. The incidence begins to rise at age 40 and peaks at age 60 to 75. Incidence of colorectal cancer increases in people who eat low-fiber diets that are high in animal protein, fat, and refined carbohydrates.

Symptoms vary, depending on the location and size of the tumor. Vague signs include weight loss, reduced appetite, and general malaise. More specific signs include rectal bleeding, blood in the stool, or a change in bowel habits.

A digital rectal examination and testing the stool for the

presence of blood are important screening tests. Flexible sigmoidoscopy in which the doctor inserts a thin, flexible tube into the rectum shows tumors in 60 percent of cases. A colonoscopy is performed when a tumor is believed to be higher up the colon. These procedures are used to visualize abnormalities and take tissue samples (biopsy).

Treatment consists of surgical removal of the tumor, followed by radiotherapy and/or chemotherapy.

Leukemia

Leukemia is a disorder characterized by uncontrolled growth of abnormal and immature white or red blood cells, and is divided into acute and chronic forms. Although leukemia is often thought of as a childhood disease, it strikes 10 times as many adults as children. New treatment, especially for acute leukemia in children has resulted in dramatic improvements in the 5- year survival rates. Today, the likelihood of disease remission is greater than 95 percent, with 30 percent chance of the disease reappearing.

Warning signs of leukemia are related to the disruption of the different cells in the blood: weakness and fatigue are caused by anemia (decreased red blood cells); easy bruising and hemorrhages (e.g. nosebleeds) from reduced clotting cells (platelets); and repeated infections from abnormal white cells. Generalized symptoms include weight loss and malaise.

Treatment for leukemia includes chemotherapy with a wide variety of anticancer drugs. Transfusions restore red cells and platelets, and frequent infections are treated with antibiotics. Bone marrow transplants, in which new blood cells are provided, are one of the most recent and successful advances in the treatment of this disease.

Liver Cancer

Liver cancer comprises only about 0.6 percent of all cancers diagnosed in the United States. Risk include hepatitis B infection, hepatitis C infection, and exposure to any agent that causes liver damage, including alcohol. The remaining patients have no underlying liver disorder.

Symptoms include abdominal pain, weight loss, and a mass on the upper right side of the abdomen. The outlook for patients with liver cancer is usually grim. Surgery provides the best hope, but is suitable in only a few cases. Most experts remain wary of the benefit of liver transplantation. See also Liver Disease.

Lung Cancer

Lung cancer is one of the most prevalent cancers with an estimated 170,000 new cases each year. The frequency is increasing rapidly. Originally a disease that primarily affected men older than 60, lung cancer has become the second most common cause of cancer in women.

Cigarette smoking and exposure to industrial substances, such as asbestos, are strongly linked to lung cancer. Recent research has shown that exposure to secondhand smoke increases the risk for this disease.

Warning signs of lung cancer are persistent coughing, shortness of breath, sputum streaked with blood, chest pain, and reoccurring pneumonia or bronchitis. Early detection is difficult, as symptoms do not appear until the disease is in advanced stages. Treatment includes surgical removal of the lung if the cancer has not spread (metastasized) and/or chemotherapy and radiation therapy. Survival rates depend on tumor size, location, and whether or not the disease has spread. Because lung cancer is so difficult to treat, public health efforts are focused on prevention. See also Lung Disease.

Oral Cancer

Oral cancer represents approximately 2 percent of all newly diagnosed cancers, and 1.5 percent of cancer deaths. Incidence is more than twice as high in men as in women, and is most frequently found in men over age 40. Risk factors include cigarette, pipe, and cigar smoking, as well as the use of chewing tobacco and excessive intake of alcohol.

Oral cancer symptoms include a sore that bleeds easily, or a lump, thickening, or persistent red or white patch in the mouth. Difficulties in chewing and swallowing are symptoms of progressive disease.

Oral cancer can affect any part of the mouth, and primary care physicians and dentists often detect the disease during routine check-ups. Treatment consists of surgical removal (frequently disfiguring), radiation therapy, or a combination of both.

Ovarian Cancer

Ovarian cancer develops in 1 in 70 women and accounts for 4 percent of cancers in women. Despite its low incidence, it is the cause of more deaths in women than any other female reproductive cancer. Incidence rates are highest in the industrialized nations.

Risk factors include prior history of breast cancer and not having had children. Women who become pregnant at an early age, who have early menopause, and who use oral contraceptives are at less risk.

Ovarian cancer symptoms usually do not appear until the disease is well developed. The most common sign is an enlarging abdomen from of accumulated fluid; digestive disturbance such as discomfort, gas and distention, may also occur.

Often an abdominal mass is discovered during a routine pelvic examination in women who are symptom free. Therefore, women age 18 or older, or earlier if they are sexually active should have annual check-ups. (The Pap smear detects cervical cancer, not ovarian cancer.) Once diagnosed, 78 percent of ovarian cancer patients survive longer than one year and more than 52 percent survive longer than five years. If the disease is diagnosed before it has spread to the other parts of the body, the five-year survival rate is 95 percent.

Treatment includes surgical removal, followed by varying combinations of chemotherapy. As in all cancers, early detection is the key to effective therapy.

Pancreatic Cancer

Pancreatic cancer is one of the most dangerous cancers because it is difficult to detect and responds poorly to anticancer therapy. The incidence of this tumor has been increasing during the 21st century with 43,140 cases diagnosed in 2010. Men are affected more commonly than women, and the average age of diagnosis is from 55 to 65 years.

There is an increased incidence in those who smoke, consume a fatty diet and, to a lesser extent, who are diabetics. Chronic inflammation of the pancreas, especially among alcoholics, is also a predisposing cause.

Pancreatic cancer runs a particularly silent course, with no symptoms until it has significant advanced. The overall 5- year survival rate for patients with pancreatic cancer is less than 5 percent. Surgery is the mainstay of therapy, but only is appropriate for 15 percent of patients; radiation and/or chemotherapy are often part of treatment.

Prostate Cancer

Approximately 1 in 6 men will develop prostate cancer by 85. Incidencerates are higher among blacks and increases with age.

Early prostate cancer is symptom free. Pain and difficulty urinating, are late signs of prostate cancer. More than 50 percent of patients have a nodule that can be felt by a digital examination.

The American Cancer Society recommends that beginning at age 50, the digital rectal examination and PSA (prostatespecific antigen) blood test should be performed annually to men with a life expectancy of at least 10 years, due to the slow growth of prostate cancer. African- American males, who are at a greater risk of developing prostate cancer, should start screening at age 45, as should men with a close relative (father, brother) was diagnosed with prostate cancer at a young age.

Surgery, radiation and hormones are all used to treat prostate cancer, depending on age and health of the patient and how far the disease has progressed.

Skin Cancer

There are over one million cases of skin cancer that are diagnosed each year. The vast majority of these cases, called basal cell or squamous cell cancers, appear on ar-

eas that are most exposed to the sun and are highly curable. Melanoma is the most serious skin cancer and accounts for 4 percent of cases. Diagnosis of melanomas has more than doubled since the mid-70s and is estimated now to develop in 1 of 50 Americans. Similar to the more benign skin cancers, melanoma develops as the result of excessive exposure to the sun and has a higher incidence among those who work outdoors. Persons with fair complexions are at particular risk.

The warning signs of skin cancer include a persistent skin lesion, especially those that change in the size, color or shape. Other signs include scaliness, oozing, bleeding, pain or spread of pigmentation.

Prevention plays a key role in the development of melanoma, especially avoiding the sun's ultraviolet rays between 10 a.m. and 3 p.m. Sunscreens and protective clothing should be worn by those who spend the majority of their time outside, those who easily sunburn, and all children. In addition, early detection is critical because, despite advances in treatment, including the use of biologic response modifiers, melanoma is difficult to cure.

Stomach Cancer

Stomach (or gastric) cancer is most common among those living in northern areas of the U.S., and poor African-American populations. Its incidence increases with age; more than 75 percent of patients are over 50 years of age.

Diet and infection are believed to play a role in the development of stomach cancer. It is also more common in persons with vitamin B12 deficiency (pernicious anemia). Other causes are under investigation.

Symptoms of stomach cancer are usually vague, and include indigestion, abdominal discomfort, bloating, heartburn, and weight loss.

Removal of the tumor when possible offers the only hope of cure. The prognosis is good if the tumor is limited, but most patients are not diagnosed until their disease has spread.

Testicular Cancer

Cancer of the testes accounts for approximately 1 percent of all male cancers. However, unlike most cancers, testicular cancer usually occurs in the 15 to 40 age group; with the average age at diagnosis is 32 years.

The cause of testicular cancer is uncertain, but the incidence is increased in men with cogenital crytorochidism (a failure of one or both testes to descend). Some researchers believe that getting an infection with a virus, such as mumps, may play a role.

Fortunately, testicular cancer is one of the most curable of all cancers, In order to discover it early, men must perform self examination at regular intervals to feel for local abnormal growths such as lumps or nodules. Pain in the scrotal sac can also occur, although more than 90 percent of patients have a painless, solid testicular swelling.

Treatment of testicular cancer may include surgical removal, radiation, and chemotherapy.

Urinary Tract Cancer

Urinary tract cancers comprise about 9 percent of new cancer cases each year in men and 4 percent in women. The two most common urinary tract cancers are of the bladder and kidney.

Overall, the incidence rate is three times greater among men than women, and usually occurs in patients who are 40-70 years of age. Smoking is the greatest risk factor, with smokers having twice the incidence of nonsmokers. African-Americans, those living in urban areas, and workers exposed to dye, rubber, or leather are also at higher risk.

Common symptoms of bladder cancer include microscopic or observable blood in the urine and painful, increased, and urgent urination. Pain the lower back may also be present. Bladder cancer may be treated by surgical removal of the tumor combined with chemotherapy.

Risk factors for kidney (renal) cancer are cigarette smoking (most important) and obesity in women. Symptoms are similar to those in bladder cancer and may also include weight loss, nausea, and vomiting.

Total removal of the cancerous kidney is the treatment of choice and is used in nearly 90 percent of cases; radiation therapy and chemotherapy are relatively ineffective. Biologic response modifiers are promising but must responses are limited in duration.

Uterine and Cervical Cancer

The overall incidence of cervical cancer has decreased over the past 40 years, due mainly to regular checkups and the use of the Pap smear test for early detection. Risk factors include intercourse at an early age, cigarette smoking, multiple sex partners, and history of a sexually transmitted disease. Infection with the virus that causes genital warts (HPV), is responsible for half of all cases of cervical cancer.

Warning signs include bleeding outside the normal menstrual cycle or after menopause. Cervical cancer in most patients is treated with surgery, radiation, or a combination of both. Due to a recently developed vaccine that is 100 percent effective against HPV, the rates of cervical cancer have sharply decreased.

The American Cancer Society recommends that all women who are, or have been, sexually annual Pap test and pelvic examination. After three or more consecutive satisfactory examinations with normal findings, the Pap test may be performed less frequently, after being discussed with your health care provider.

Uterine cancer has been increasing since the 1970s. Risk factors include obesity, diabetes, high blood pressure, late onset of menopause, and estrogen-only hormone replacement therapy. Symptoms for most women include some form of abnormal bleeding from the uterus.

Treatment for uterine and cervical cancers include surgery, radiation therapy, hormone therapy and, occasionally, chemotherapy.

National Agencies & Associations

2011   American Bone Marrow Donor Registry
PO Box 8841
Mandeville, LA 70470-8841
985-626-1749
800-745-2452
Fax: 985-626-7414
e-mail: jakabmdr@bellsouth.net
www.abmdr.org
A registry of bone marrow donors. Provides information on donor searches and recruitment.

2012   American Cancer Society
1599 Clifton Road NE
Atlanta, GA 30329-4250
404-320-3333
800-ACS-2345
TTY: 800-228-4327
www.cancer.org
A nationwide community based voluntary health organization dedicated to eliminating cancer as a major health problem by preventing saving lives and diminishing suffering through research education advocacy and services. Provides free printed materials.
Stephen F Sener, President
J. Lenard Lichtenfeld, MD, MACP, Deputy Chief Medical Officer

2013   American Prostate Society
10 East Lee St.
Baltimore, MD 21202-3117
410-837-3735
877-859-3735
Fax: 410-837-8510
e-mail: ameripros@mindspring.com
www.americanprostatesociety.com
The only organization dedicated exclusively to using existing medical capabilities to reduce death due to prostate cancer and to reduce unnecessary or ineffective prostate therapies for prostate growth.

2014   American Society of Colon and Rectal Surgeons
85 W Algonquin Road
Arlington Heights, IL 60005-4460
847-290-9184
Fax: 847-290-9203
e-mail: ascrs@fascrs.org
www.fascrs.org
ASCRS Represents more than 1000 board certified colon and rectal surgeons and other surgeons dedicated to advancing and promoting the science and practice of the treatment of patients with cancer and other diseases affecting the colon and related areas.
David Beck MD, President
Steven Wexner MD, President Elect

2015   Americas Association for the Care of the Children
P.O. Box 2154
Boulder, CO 80306-2154
303-527-2742
www.aaccchildren.net
Carries out a variety of programs to promote the health of children. Publishes educational materials on child health of interest to parents, educators and health professionals.
Judi Jackson, President
Doreen Trees, Vice President

2016   Association for Research of Childhood Cancer
PO Box 251
Buffalo, NY 14225-0251
716-681-4433
e-mail: president@arocc.org
www.arocc.org

A nonprofit organization staffed by volunteers and formed in 1971 by parents who had lost children to pediatric cancer. Charter members raise funds by various projects in order to provide seed money to various pediatric research centers.
Anne O'Donnell, President

2017 Association for the Cure of Cancer of the Prostate
1250 4th Street   310-570-4700
Santa Monica, CA 90401   800-757-4700
                                    Fax: 310-570-4701
                                  e-mail: info@pcf.org
                                         www.pcf.org
Goal is to find better treatments and a cure for recurrent prostate cancer. Pursues the mission by reaching out to individuals corporations and others to harness society's resources - both financial and human - to fight this deadly disease.
Mike Milken, Founder/Chairman
Neil DeFeo, Chairman, President and CEO

2018 Bone Marrow Foundation
30 E End Avenue   212-838-3029
New York, NY 10128   800-365-1336
                                    Fax: 21 -22 -008
                          e-mail: theBMF@BoneMarrow.org
                                     cmgm.stanford.edu
Goal is to improve the quality of life for bone marrow and stem cell transplant patients and their families by providing financial aid education and emotional support.
Christina Merrill, Founder and Executive Director
Lee Kozer, Director

2019 Breast Cancer Action
55 New Montgomery Street   415-243-9301
San Francisco, CA 94105   877-2ST-OPBC
                                    Fax: 415-243-3996
                              e-mail: info@bcaction.org
                                      www.bcaction.org
Breast Cancer Action carries the voices of people affected by breast cancer to inspire and compel the changes necessary to end the breast cancer epidemic.
Joyce Bichier, Deputy Director
Lori Baralt, Secretary

2020 Breast Cancer Society of Canada
420 East Street North Sarnia   519-336-0746
Sarnia, N7T6Y-6Y5   800-567-8767
                                    Fax: 519-336-5725
                                  e-mail: bcsc@bcsc.ca
                                         www.bcsc.ca
Is a registered charitable organization established in 1991 in Point Edwards Ontario. Our mandate is to fund vital Canadian research into improving the detection, prevention and treatment of breast cancer as well as to ultimately find a cure and create awareness through education.
Marsha Davidson, Executive Director
Raelene Peseski, Presidentÿ

2021 Burger King Cancer Caring Center
4117 Liberty Avenue   412-622-1212
Pittsburgh, PA 15224   Fax: 412-622-1216
                              e-mail: info@cancercaring.org
                                     www.cancercaring.org
Provides a wide variety of support services to cancer patients their families and friends including support groups, education classes, personal counseling and telephone help line.
Rebecca Whitlinger, Executive Director
Stephanie Samolovitch, MSW, LSW, Director Support Services

2022 Canadian Breast Cancer Network (CBCN)
300-331 Cooper Street   613-230-3044
Ottawa, Ontario, K2P-0G5   800-685-8820
                                    Fax: 613-230-4424
                                  e-mail: cbcn@cbcn.ca
                                         www.cbcn.ca
Is a survivor-directed, national network of organizations and individuals. CBCN is a national link between all groups and individuals concerned about breast cancer, and represents the concerns of all Canadians affected by breast cancer and those at risk.
Jackie Manthorne, CEO
Chantale Lavoie, Program Coordinator

2023 Canadian Cancer Society
55 St Clair Avenue West   416-961-7223
Toronto, M4V 2-3B1   Fax: 416-961-4189
                                  e-mail: info@cancer.ca
                                         www.cancer.ca
A national community-based organization of volunteers whose mission is the eradication of cancer and the enhancement of the quality of life of people living with cancer.
Peter Goodhand, President/CEO

2024 CancerCare
Public Information Associates
275 7th Avenue   212-302-2400
New York, NY 10001   800-813-4673
                                    Fax: 212-712-8495
                              e-mail: info@cancercare.org
                                      www.cancercare.org
National nonprofit organization that provides free, professional support services for anyone affected by a cancer diagnosis.
Helen H Miller LCSW, Executive Director
John Rutigliano, Chief Operating Officer

2025 Candlelighters Childhood Cancer Foundation
10400 Connecticut Avenue   301-962-3520
Kensington, MD 20895   800-366-2223
                                    Fax: 301-962-3521
                                 e-mail: staff@acco.org
                                   www.candlelighters.org
Founded by parents of children with cancer. Candlelighters helps families of pediatric and adolescent cancer patients cope with the educational and emotional needs of the disease. The organization is the largest distributor of free childhood cancer books and other materials.
Ruth Hoffman MPH, Executive Director
Amber Masso, Program Director

2026 Colon Cancer Canada
5915 Leslie Street   416-785-0449
Toronto, On, M2H-1J8   888-571-8547
                                    Fax: 416-785-0450
                          e-mail: info@coloncancercanada.ca
                                  www.coloncancercanada.ca
Raise public awareness for this deadly disease and to raise money for vital research.
Bunnie Schwartz, Co-Founder & President
Leah Archambault, Executive Officer Coordinator

2027 Colorectal Cancer Association of Canada
5 Place Ville Marie   514-875-7745
Montreal, QC, H3B-2G2   Fax: 514-875-7746
                              e-mail: admin@ccac-accc.ca
                                      www.ccac-accc.ca
Non-profit organization dedicated to improving the quality of life of patients and increasing awareness of the disease.
Barry D Stein, President
Heidi Watts, Program Director

2028 ENCORE YWCA-National Board
YWCA-National Board
726 Broadway   212-614-2827
New York, NY 10003-9502   800-953-7587
The YWCA's discussion and exercise program for women who have had breast cancer surgery. Designed to restore physical strength and emotional well-being.

2029 Foundation for Dignity
37 S 20th Street   215-567-2828
Philadelphia, PA 19103
Offers counseling and seminars concerning the employment rights of cancer patients and for human services workers. The society offers an extensive list of publications dealing with all aspects of cancer prevention and care.
Barbara Hoffman, Staff Attorney

2030 International Association of Laryngectomees
American Cancer Society

PO Box 691060
Stockton, CA 95269-1060

757-888-0324
866-425-3678
Fax: 209-472-0516
e-mail: ialhq@larynxlink.com
www.theial.com

Consists of local clubs worldwide that provides services and information to patients who have undergone laryngectomies and their families. Members are given information on first aid, postoperative care, rehabilitation, esophageal speech and other speech alternatives. Directories of speech instructors and self-care supplies for the surgical site are distributed.

Jack Henslee, Executive Director

2031   Leukemia and Lymphoma Society
1311 Mamaroneck Avenue
White Plains, NY 10605

914-949-5213
800-955-4572
Fax: 914-949-6691
www.lls.org

The Leukemia and Lymphoma Society is the world's largest voluntary health organization dedicated to funding blood cancer research education and patient services.

Timothy S. Durst, Chair of the Board
James H. Davis, PhD, JD, Vice Chair

2032   Make Today Count
1235 E Cherokee
Springfield, MO 65804-2263

417-885-3324
800-432-2273
Fax: 417-888-7426
smsu.edu/nursing/community

An organization that helps patients and their families cope with cancer and other serious diseases and improve their quality of life.

Connie Gores, Director
Chris Anderson, Executive Administrative Assistant

2033   National Alliance of Breast Cancer Organizations
9 E 37th Street
New York, NY 10016

888-806-2226
Fax: 212-689-1213
e-mail: nabcoinfo@aol.com
www.nabco.org

A network of breast cancer organizations that provides information assistance and referral to anyone with questions about breast cancer and acts as a voice for the interests and concerns of breast cancer survivors and women at risk.

2034   National Cancer Institute
9609 Medical Center Drive
Bethesda, MD 20892-8322

800-422-6237
e-mail: cancergovstaff@mail.nih.gov
www.cancer.gov

One of the largest organizations dealing solely with cancer in its many forms. Offers educational information public awareness research grants and more for patients their families and health care professionals. Information specialists answer cancer-related questions by phone, LiveHelp instant messaging, and e-mail.

Deborah Pearson RN MPH, Chief Public Inquiries Office

2035   National Cancer Institute of Canada
10 Alcorn Avenue
Toronto, Ontario, M4V-3B1

416-961-7223
Fax: 416-961-4189
e-mail: research@cancer.ca
www.ncic.cancer.ca

Was formed through a joint initiative of the Department of National Health and Welfare and the Canadian Cancer Society.

Dr Elizabeth Eisenhauer, President

2036   National Coalition for Cancer Survivorship
1010 Wayne Avenue
Silver Spring, MD 20910

301-650-9127
888-650-9127
Fax: 301-565-9670
e-mail: info@canceradvocacy.org
www.canceradvocacy.org

Survivor led advocacy organization working exclusively on behalf of people with all types of cancer and their families. Dedicated to assuring quality and care for all Americans.

Thomas P Sellers, President/CEO

2037   National Foundation for Cancer Research
4600 EW Highway
Bethesda, MD 20814

301-654-1250
800-321-2873
Fax: 301-654-5824
e-mail: info@nfcr.org
www.nfcr.org

Contracts with major universities for basic science cancer research in the fields of biophysics, theoretical physics and biochemistry.

William Potter, President
David M Sotsky, Director

2038   National Hospice & Palliative Care Organization (NHPCO)
1731 King Street
Alexandria, VA 22314

703-837-1500
800-658-8898
Fax: 703-837-1233
e-mail: nhpcoinfo@nhpco.org
www.nhpco.org

The nation's only advocate for terminally ill patients and their families. Founded in 1978, the NHPCO is the only organization devoted to hospice in the United States. Support is included from state hospice organizations, patients, families, communities, provider program members and professional/volunteer members. Represents hospice care interests to Congress, regulatory agencies, courts, voluntary organizations and the public.

J. Donald Schumacher, PsyD, President & CEO
Galen Miller, PhD, Executive Vice President

2039   National Institute on Aging Information Center
31 Center Drive MSC 2292
Bethesda, MD 20892

301-496-1752
800-222-2225
Fax: 301-496-1072
TTY: 800-222-4225
www.nih.gov/nia

Concerned with the health problems of older Americans. The Center offers free printed materials including fact sheets about going to the hospital and about prostate problems.

Richard J Hodes MD, Director
Linda Addiso Hardy, Lead Extraml Support Asst

2040   National Kidney and Urologic Diseases Information Clearinghouse
31 Center Drive, MSC 2560
Bethesda, MD 20892-2560

301-496-3583
800-891-5390
Fax: 301-907-8906
e-mail: nkudic@info.niddk.nih.gov
www.www2.niddk.nih.gov

A service of the Federal Government's National Institute for Diabetes and Digestive and Kidney Diseases. Offers free information about benign prostate enlargement and other non-cancerous urinary tract problems.

Griffin P Rodgers, Director

2041   National Marrow Donor Program
3001 Broadway Street NE
Minneapolis, MN 55413-1763

612-627-5800
800-627-7692
www.marrow.org

Created to improve the effectiveness of the search for bone marrow donors so that a greater number of bone marrow transplants can be carried out.

Jeffrey W Chell MD, CEO
Patricia A Coppo MS, COO

2042   National Ovarian Cancer Coalition
2501 Oak Lawn Avenue
Dallas, TX 75219

214-273-4200
888-OVA-RIAN
Fax: 561-393-7275
e-mail: NOCC@ovarian.org
www.ovarian.org

Our mission is to raise awareness about ovarian cancer and to promote education about this disease. By dispelling myths and misunderstandings the coalition is committed to improve the overall survival rate and quality of life for women with ovarian cancer.

Elizabeth Isham Cory, President
David Barley, CEO

2043 **New Brunswick Innovation Foundation**
440 King Street, Suite 602
Fredericton, NB, E3B-5H8
506-452-2884
877-554-6668
Fax: 506-452-2886
e-mail: info@nbif.ca
www.nbif.ca
An independent corporation, has the mission to contribute to building the province's innovation capacity.
Alfred W Lacey, President/CEO

2044 **Rethink Breast Cancer**
215 Spadina Avenue
Toronto, M5T 2-2C7
416-920-0980
Fax: 416-920-5798
e-mail: hello@rethinkbreastcancer.com
www.rethinkbreastcancer.com
Is a charity helping young people who are concerned about and affected by breast cancer through innovative breast cancer education, research and support programs.
MJ DeCoteau MA, Executive Director

2045 **Skin Cancer Foundation**
149 Madison Avenue
New York, NY 10016-8728
212-725-5176
800-754-6490
Fax: 212-725-5751
e-mail: info@skincancer.org
www.skincancer.org
Conducts public and medical education programs to help reduce skin cancer. Major goals are to increase public awareness of the importance of taking protective measures against the damaging rays of the sun and to teach people how to recognize the early signs.
Perry Robins MD, President

2046 **Support for People with Oral and Head and Neck Cancer**
PO Box 53
Locust Valley, NY 11560-0053
516-759-5333
800-377-0928
Fax: 516-671-8794
e-mail: info@spohnc.org
www.spohnc.org
Nonprofit organization founded in 1991 to address the broad emotional physical and humanistic needs of oral and head and neck cancer patients.
Nancy E Leupold, President/Founder
James J. Sciubba DMD, PhD, Vice President

2047 **Y-ME National Breast Cancer Organization**
135 S LaSalle Street
Chicago, IL 60603
312-986-8338
800-221-2141
Fax: 312-294-8597
e-mail: askyme@y-me.org
www.y-me.org
Provides support information and education to anyone touched by breast cancer. Support and information are available 24 hours through the National Breast Cancer Hotline which is staffed by breast cancer survivors who are trained peer counselors.
Cindy Geoghegan, CEO
Ginny Finn, Executive Director

State Agencies & Associations

Alabama

2048 **American Cancer Society: Alabama**
1100 Ireland Way
Birmingham, AL 35205
205-879-2242
Fax: 205-930-8895
e-mail: scarlet.thompson@cancer.org
www.cancer.org/docroot/com/com_0.asp
The American Cancer Society is the nationwide community-based voluntary health organization dedicated to eliminating cancer as a major health problem by preventing cancer, saving lives and diminishing suffering from cancer, through research and education.
Scarlet Thom (205-930-8889), Media/Public Relations Alabama

2049 **Leukemia and Lymphoma Society: Alabama Chapter**
Leukemia Society of America
100 Chase Park S
Birmingham, AL 35244
205-989-0098
888-560-9700
Fax: 205-989-0099
www.lls.org/aboutlls/chapters/al/

Dedicated to finding cures for leukemia and related cancers and to improving the quality of life for patients and their families.
Melanie Mooney, Executive Director
Kate McLean, Campaign Coordinator, Special Events

Alaska

2050 **American Cancer Society: Alaska**
3851 Piper Street
Anchorage, AK 99508
907-277-8696
Fax: 907-263-2073
e-mail: leslie.jones@cancer.org
www.cancer.org
The American Cancer Society is the nationwide community-based voluntary health organization dedicated to eliminating cancer as a major health problem by preventing cancer saving lives and diminishing suffering from cancer through research and education.
Leslie Jones, Media/Public Relations Alaska

Arizona

2051 **American Cancer Society: Arizona**
4212 N 16th Street
Phoenix, AZ 85016
602-224-0524
800-227-2345
Fax: 602-778-7699
e-mail: meg.kondrich@cancer.org
www.cancer.org
The American Cancer Society is the nationwide community-based voluntary health organization dedicated to eliminating cancer as a major health problem by preventing cancer saving lives, and diminishing suffering from cancer through research and education.
Meg Kondrich, Media/Public Relations Arizona

2052 **International Holistic Center**
PO Box 15103
Phoenix, AZ 85060-5103
928-771-2826
e-mail: ihcinc@cox.net
www.holisticresources.org
Provides information and referrals concerning holistic health care in Arizona and beyond.
Stan Kalson, President

2053 **Leukemia and Lymphoma Society: Mountain States Chapter**
Leukemia Society of America
3877 N 7th Street
Phoenix, AZ 85014
602-567-7600
800-568-1372
Fax: 602-567-7601
www.leukemia-lymphoma.org
Dedicated to finding cures for leukemia and related cancers and to improving the quality of life for patients and their families. Serves New Mexico and the Greater El Paso, TX area.
Tim Metzer, Executive Director

Arkansas

2054 **American Cancer Society: Arkansas**
901 N University
Little Rock, AR 72207
501-664-3480
Fax: 501-603-5223
e-mail: jodie.spears@cancer.org
www.cancer.org
The American Cancer Society is the nationwide community-based voluntary health organization dedicated to eliminating cancer as a major health problem by preventing cancer, saving lives, and diminishing suffering from cancer, through research and education.
Jodie Spears, Media/Public Relations Arkansas

2055 **Health Resource**
933 Faulkner Street
Conway, AR 72034
501-329-5272
800-949-0090
Fax: 501-329-9489
e-mail: research@thehealthresource.com
www.thehealthresource.com
A medical information service which provides clients with an individualized, in depth research report on his or her specific health problem. Reports include latest treatment options, mainstream, experimental and alternative and top specialists.
Janice Guthrie, Director/Researcher
Shirley Effinger, Researcher

California

2056 **American Cancer Society Santa Clara County / Silicon Valley / Central Coast Region**
747 Camden Avenue   408-871-1062
Campbell, CA 95008   Fax: 408-871-2993
e-mail: angie.carrillo@cancer.org
www.cancer.org
The American Cancer Society is the nationwide community-based voluntary health organization dedicated to eliminating cancer as a major health problem by preventing cancer, saving lives and diminishing suffering from cancer, through research and education.
Angie Carillo, Media/Public Relations Silicon Valley

2057 **American Cancer Society: Central Los Angeles**
3333 Wilshire Boulevard   213-386-6102
Los Angeles, CA 90010   Fax: 213-480-0806
e-mail: katherine.spangle@cancer.org
www.cancer.org
The American Cancer Society is the nationwide community-based voluntary health organization dedicated to eliminating cancer as a major health problem by preventing cancer, saving lives, and diminishing suffering from cancer, through research and education.
Katie Spangle, Media/Public Relations Los Angeles Area

2058 **American Cancer Society: East Bay/Metro Region**
1700 Webster Street   510-832-7012
Oakland, CA 94612   Fax: 510-763-8826
e-mail: patty.guinto@cancer.org
www.cancer.org
The American Cancer Society is the nationwide community-based voluntary health organization dedicated to eliminating cancer as a major health problem by preventing cancer, saving lives, and diminishing suffering from cancer, through research and education.
Patty Guinto, Media/Public Relations East Bay Area

2059 **American Cancer Society: Fresno/Madera Counties**
2222 W Shaw Avenue   559-451-0722
Fresno, CA 93711   Fax: 559-451-0744
e-mail: erica.jones@cancer.org
www.cancer.org
The American Cancer Society is the nationwide community-based voluntary health organization dedicated to eliminating cancer as a major health problem by preventing cancer, saving lives, and diminishing suffering from cancer, through research and education.
Erica Jones, Media/Public Relations Fresno CA

2060 **American Cancer Society: Inland Empire**
6355 Riverside Ave   951-683-6415
Riverside, CA 92506   Fax: 951-682-6804
e-mail: beckie.mooreflati@cancer.org
www.cancer.org
The American Cancer Society is the nationwide community-based voluntary health organization dedicated to eliminating cancer as a major health problem by preventing cancer, saving lives, and diminishing suffering from cancer, through research and education.
Beckie Moore, Media/Public Relations Riverside Region

2061 **American Cancer Society: Orange County**
1940 E Deere Avenue   949-261-9446
Santa Ana, CA 92705-5718   Fax: 949-261-9419
e-mail: jennifer.horspool@cancer.org
www.cancer.org
The American Cancer Society is the nationwide community-based voluntary health organization dedicated to eliminating cancer as a major health problem by preventing cancer, saving lives, and diminishing suffering from cancer, through research and education.
Jennifer Horton, Media/Public Relations Orange County

2062 **American Cancer Society: Sacramento County**
1765 Challenge Way   916-446-7933
Sacramento, CA 95815   Fax: 916-64 -977
e-mail: maria.robinson@cancer.org
www.cancer.org
The American Cancer Society is the nationwide community-based voluntary health organization dedicated to eliminating cancer as a major health problem by preventing cancer, saving lives, and diminishing suffering from cancer, through research and education.
Maria Robinson, Media/Public Relations Sacramento County

2063 **American Cancer Society: San Diego County**
2655 Camino Del Rio N   619-299-4200
San Diego, CA 92108   800-227-2345
Fax: 619-296-0928
e-mail: robin.brown@cancer.org
www.cancer.org
The American Cancer Society is the nationwide community-based voluntary health organization dedicated to eliminating cancer as a major health problem by preventing cancer, saving lives, and diminishing suffering from cancer, through research and education.
Robin Brown, Media/Public Relations San Diego CA

2064 **American Cancer Society: San Francisco County**
201 Mission Street   415-394-7100
San Francisco, CA 94105   Fax: 415-495-1877
e-mail: patty.guinto@cancer.org
www.cancer.org
The American Cancer Society is the nationwide community-based voluntary health organization dedicated to eliminating cancer as a major health problem by preventing cancer, saving lives, and diminishing suffering from cancer, through research and education.
Patty Guinto, Media/Public Relations San Francisco

2065 **American Cancer Society: Santa Maria Valley**
426 E Barcellus   805-922-2354
Santa Maria, CA 93454   Fax: 805-925-1424
e-mail: jeb.baird@cancer.org
www.cancer.org
The American Cancer Society is the nationwide community-based voluntary health organization dedicated to eliminating cancer as a major health problem by preventing cancer, saving lives and diminishing suffering from cancer, through research and education.
Jeb Baird, Media/Public Relations Santa Maria

2066 **American Cancer Society: Sonoma County**
1451 Guerneville Road   707-545-6720
Santa Rosa, CA 95403   Fax: 707-545-3179
e-mail: angie.carrillo@cancer.org
www.cancer.org
The American Cancer Society is the nationwide community-based voluntary health organization dedicated to eliminating cancer as a major health problem by preventing cancer, saving lives, and diminishing suffering from cancer, through research and education.
Angie Carillo, Media/Public Relations Central Coast

2067 **Cancer Control Society and Cancer Book House**
2043 N Berendo Street   213-663-7801
Los Angeles, CA 90027   Fax: 323-663-7757
www.cancercontrolsociety.com
An informational organization offering books, films, videos, clinic tours and lists of patients with cancer.
Lorraine Rosenthal, Co-Founder
Frank Cousineau, President

2068 **City of Hope National Medical Center Beckman Research Institute**
Beckman Research Institute
1500 E Duarte Road   626-256-4673
Duarte, CA 91010   800-826-4673
e-mail: tpogue@coh.org
www.cityofhope.org
City of Hope is an innovative biomedical research, treatment and educational institution dedicated to the prevention and cure of cancer and other life-threatening illness.
Stephen J Foreman, Chair

2069 **Leukemia & Lymphoma Society: Orange, Riverside, And San Bernadino Counties**
2020 E 1st Street   714-881-0610
Santa Ana, CA 92705   888-535-9300
Fax: 714-881-0616
www.leukemia-lymphoma.org
Dedicated to finding cures for leukemia and related cancers and to improving the quality of life for patients and their families.

2070 **Leukemia and Lymphoma Society: San Diego/Hawaii Chapter**
Leukemia Society of America

9150 Chesapeake Dr
San Diego, CA 92123
858-277-1800
888-535-9300
Fax: 858-277-1748
www.leukemia.org

Dedicated to finding cures for leukemia and related cancers and to improving the quality of life for patients and their families.
Keith Turner, Executive Director

2071 Leukemia and Lymphoma Society: Greater Sacramento Area Chapter
Leukemia Society of America
4604 Roseville Road
North Highlands, CA 95660
916-348-1793
Fax: 916-348-7864
www.leukemia.org

Dedicated to finding cures for leukemia and related cancers and to improving the quality of life for patients and their families.
Tracy Latino, Executive Director

2072 Leukemia and Lymphoma Society: Greater Los Angeles Chapter
Leukemia Society of America
6033 W Century Boulevard
Los Angeles, CA 90045
310-342-5800
Fax: 310-342-5801
www.leukemia-lymphoma.org

Dedicated to finding cures for leukemia and related cancers and to improving the quality of life for patients and their families.
Donna Lynch, Executive Director

2073 Leukemia and Lymphoma Society: Northern California Chapter
Leukemia Society of America
1390 Market Street
San Francisco, CA 94102
415-625-1100
Fax: 415-625-1155
e-mail: supportservices@lls.org
www.lls.org

Dedicated to finding cures for leukemia and related cancers and to improving the quality of life for patients and their families.

2074 Leukemia and Lymphoma Society: Orange, Riverside, And San Bernadino Counties
2020 E 1st Street
Santa Ana, CA 92705
714-881-0610
888-535-9300
Fax: 714-881-0616
www.lls.org

Dedicated to finding cures for leukemia and related cancers and to improving the quality of life for patients and their families.

2075 Leukemia and Lymphoma Society: Tri-County Chapter
Leukemia Society of America
2020 E 1st Street
Santa Ana, CA 92705
714-881-0610
888-535-9300
Fax: 714-881-0616
www.leukemia-lymphoma.org

Dedicated to finding cures for leukemia and related cancers and to improving the quality of life for patients and their families.
John Walter, President & CEO
Louis J DeGennaro, Chief Mission Officer

2076 National Health Federation
PO Box 688
Monrovia, CA 91017
626-357-2181
Fax: 626-303-0642
e-mail: contact-us@thenhf.com
www.thenhf.com

A nonprofit consumer-oriented organization devoted to health matters. Dedicated to preserving freedom of choice in health care issues, prevention of diseases and the promotion of wellness.
Scott Tips, President
Sylvia Provenza, Vice-President

2077 Regional Cancer Foundation
1200 Gough Street
San Francisco, CA 94109
415-775-9956
Fax: 415-346-8652
e-mail: mail@regionalcancerfoundation.org
www.regionalcancerfoundation.org

This foundation offers, at no charge, a second opinion consultation to individuals diagnosed with cancer. The patient and a family member or friend meet with an interdisciplinary panel of local cancer specialists with expertise in radiation therapy, chemotherapy, and cancer treatment plans.
William Gillis, CEO
Arhur J Inerfield, Chairman

2078 Rose Kushner Breast Cancer Advisory Center
PO Box 757
Malaga Cove, CA 90274
301-897-3445
Fax: 301-897-3444
e-mail: lkkushner@yahoo.com
www.rkbcac.org

Provides a mail service offering referrals to health professionals as well as information about detection, diagnosis, treatment and physical and psychological rehabilitation for patients with breast cancer.

Colorado

2079 American Cancer Society: Colorado
2255 S Oneida Street
Denver, CO 80224
303-758-2030
Fax: 303-759-1615
e-mail: lynda.solomon@cancer.org
www.cancer.org

The American Cancer Society is the nationwide community-based voluntary health organization dedicated to eliminating cancer as a major health problem by preventing cancer, saving lives and diminishing suffering from cancer, through research and education.
Lynda Solomo, Media/Public Relations Colorado
Joel Quevill, Media/Public Relations Colorado

Connecticut

2080 American Cancer Society: Connecticut
Meriden Executive Park
Meriden, CT 06450
203-379-4700
Fax: 203-379-5060
e-mail: simone.upsey@cancer.org
www.cancer.org

The American Cancer Society is the nationwide community-based voluntary health organization dedicated to eliminating cancer as a major health problem by preventing cancer, saving lives and diminishing suffering from cancer, through research and education.
Simone Upsey, Media/Public Relations NH/MS/NL Counties
Christian Me, Media/Public Relations LF/FF Counties

2081 Leukemia and Lymphoma Society: Connecticut Chapter
Leukemia Society of America
321 Research Parkway
Meriden, CT 06450
203-379-0445
888-282-9465
Fax: 203-379-0451
www.lls.org/aboutlls/chapters/ct/

Founded in 1949 to help serve and educate the communities and residents who have been touched by leukemia, lymphoma, multiple myeloma and Hodgkin's disease.
Jean Montano, Executive Director
Dina Mariani, Deputy Executive Director

2082 Leukemia and Lymphoma Society: Fairfield County Chapter
Leukemia Society of America
25 Third Street
Stamford, CT 06905
203-967-8326
Fax: 203-325-8559
www.lls.org

Dedicated to finding cures for leukemia and related cancers and to improving the quality of life for patients and their families.

Delaware

2083 American Cancer Society: Delaware
92 Reads Way
New Castle, DE 19720
302-324-4427
Fax: 302-324-4233
e-mail: dawn.ward@cancer.org
www.cancer.org

The American Cancer Society is the nationwide community-based voluntary health organization dedicated to eliminating cancer as a major health problem by preventing cancer, saving lives, and diminishing suffering from cancer, through research and education.
Dawn Ward, Media/Public Relations Delaware

2084 Leukemia and Lymphoma Society: Delaware Chapter
Leukemia Society of America
100 W 10th Street
Wilmington, DE 19801
302-661-7300
800-220-1617
Fax: 302-661-0363
www.leukemia-lymphoma.org

Our mission is to cure leukemia, lymphoma, Hodgkin's disease and myeloma and to improve the quality of life of patients and their families.
Timothy S Durst, Chairman
James Davis, Vice-Chair

District of Columbia

2085 American Cancer Society: District of Columbia
1875 Connecticut Avenue NW   202-483-2600
Washington, DC 20009   Fax: 202-483-1174
e-mail: angela.collins@cancer.org
www.cancer.org
The American Cancer Society is the nationwide community-based voluntary health organization dedicated to eliminating cancer as a major health problem by preventing cancer, saving lives, and diminishing suffering from cancer, through research and education.
Angela Colli, Media/Public Relations Washington DC

2086 American Institute for Cancer Research
1759 R Street NW   202-328-7744
Washington, DC 20009   800-843-8114
Fax: 202-328-7226
e-mail: aicrweb@aicr.org
www.aicr.org
Not-for-profit research and educational organization. Provides grants for research into the causes, development, prevention and treatment of cancer through diet and nutrition. Offers publications, research results, conferences and various public services.

2087 Center for Science in the Public Interest
1220 L Street N.W.   202-332-9110
Washington, DC 20005   Fax: 202-265-4954
e-mail: cspi@cspinet.org
www.cspinet.org
The nation's leading consumer group concerned with food and nutrition issues. Focuses on diseases that result from consuming too many calories, too much fat, sodium and sugar such as cancer and heart disease.
Don Allen, Director of Finance
Tom Gegax, Board of Directors

Florida

2088 American Cancer Society: Florida
2006 W Kennedy Boulevard   813-254-3630
Tampa, FL 33606   Fax: 813-349-4431
e-mail: cynthia.dunlap@cancer.org
www.cancer.org
The American Cancer Society is the nationwide community-based voluntary health organization dedicated to eliminating cancer as a major health problem by preventing cancer, saving lives, and diminishing suffering from cancer, through research and education.
C. Dunlap, Media/Public Relations Tampa Region
Kristen Redd, Media/Public Relations Tampa Region

2089 Leukemia & Lymphoma Society: Suncoast Chapter
3507 E Frontage Road   813-963-6461
Tampa, FL 33607   800-436-6889
Fax: 813-963-1306
www.lls.org
Serves patients with leukemia, lymphoma, multiple myeloma and Hodgkin's disease in Charlotte, Citrus, Collier, DeSoto, Hardee, Hernando, Hillsborough, Lee, Manatee, Pasco, Pinellas and Sarasota counties.

2090 Leukemia and Lymphoma Society: Southern Florida Chapter
Leukemia Society of America
3325 Hollywood Boulevard   954-961-3234
Hallandale, FL 33021   Fax: 954-961-7376
www.lls.org
Dedicated to finding cures for leukemia and related cancers and to improving the quality of life for patients and their families.

2091 Leukemia and Lymphoma Society: Central Florida Chapter
Leukemia Society of America
3319 Maguire Boulevard   407-898-0733
Orlando, FL 32803-3720   Fax: 407-896-8645
www.lls.org

Dedicated to finding cures for leukemia and related cancers and to improving the quality of life for patients and their families.

2092 Leukemia and Lymphoma Society: Northern Florida Chapter
Leukemia Society of America
9143 Phillips Highway   904-538-0721
Jacksonville, FL 32256   800-868-0072
Fax: 904-538-9245
www.lls.org
Dedicated to finding cures for leukemia and related cancers and to improving the quality of life for patients and their families.

2093 Leukemia and Lymphoma Society: Palm Beach Area Chapter
Leukemia Society of America
4360 Northlake Boulevard   561-775-9954
Palm Beach Gardens, FL 33410   888-478-8550
Fax: 561-775-0930
www.lls.org
Dedicated to finding cures for leukemia and related cancers and to improving the quality of life for patients and their families.

Georgia

2094 American Cancer Society: Georgia
50 Williams Street   404-315-1123
Atlanta, GA 30303   Fax: 404-315-9348
e-mail: elissa.mccrary@cancer.org
www.cancer.org
The American Cancer Society is the nationwide community-based voluntary health organization dedicated to eliminating cancer as a major health problem by preventing cancer, saving lives, and diminishing suffering from cancer, through research and education.
E. McCrary, Media/Public Relations Georgia

2095 Kidscope
2045 Peachtree Road
Atlanta, GA 30309   404-892-1437
www.kidscope.org
A nonprofit organization formed to help families and children better understand the effects from cancer in a parent. The name can also be read as Kids Cope - one of the goals being to improve the chances that a child will successfully cope with the diagnosis.
H Elizabeth King PhD, Board Member
Carol Webb PhD, Board Member

2096 Leukemia and Lymphoma Society: Georgia Chapter
Leukemia Society of America
3715 Northside Parkway   404-720-7900
Atlanta, GA 30327   800-399-7312
Fax: 404-720-7878
e-mail: dick.brown@lls.org
www.leukemia-lymphoma.org
Dedicated to finding cures for leukemia and related cancers and to improving the quality of life for patients and their families.
Dick Brown, Executive Director
Maureen Quin Davidson, Director TNT

Hawaii

2097 American Cancer Society: Hawaii
2370 Nuuanu Avenue   808-595-7544
Honolulu, HI 96817   800-ACS-2345
Fax: 808-595-7545
TTY: 866-228-4327
e-mail: milton.hirata@cancer.org
www.cancer.org
The American Cancer Society is the nationwide community-based voluntary health organization dedicated to eliminating cancer as a major health problem by preventing cancer, saving lives, and diminishing suffering from cancer, through research and education.
Milton Hirata, Media Relations Contact - Hawaii

Idaho

2098 American Cancer Society: Idaho
2676 Vista Avenue
Boise, ID 83705
208-345-2184
800-ACS-2345
Fax: 208-343-9922
TTY: 866-228-4327
e-mail: jim.ryan@cancer.org
www.cancer.org
The American Cancer Society is the nationwide community-based voluntary health organization dedicated to eliminating cancer as a major health problem by preventing cancer, saving lives, and diminishing suffering from cancer, through research and education.
Jim Ryan, Media Relations Contact - Idaho

Illinois

2099 American Cancer Society: Illinois
225 N Michigan Avenue
Chicago, IL 60601
312-372-0471
800-ACS-2345
Fax: 312-372-0910
TTY: 866-228-4327
e-mail: melissa.leeb@cancer.org
www.cancer.org
The American Cancer Society is the nationwide community-based voluntary health organization dedicated to eliminating cancer as a major health problem by preventing cancer, saving lives, and diminishing suffering from cancer, through research and education.
Melissa Leeb, Media Relations Contact - Illinois

2100 Leukemia and Lymphoma Society: Illinois Chapter
Leukemia Society of America
651 W Washington Boulevard
Chicago, IL 60661
312-651-7350
800-742-6595
Fax: 312-463-0980
e-mail: pam.swenk@lls.org
www.lls.org
Dedicated to finding cures for leukemia and related cancers and to improving the quality of life for patients and their families.
Pam Swenk, Executive Director
Jennifer Hufnagel, Director Donor Development

Indiana

2101 American Cancer Society: Indiana
5635 W 96th Street
Indianapolis, IN 46278
317-344-7800
800-ACS-2345
Fax: 317-344-7810
TTY: 866-228-4327
e-mail: leslie.smith@cancer.org
www.cancer.org
The American Cancer Society is the nationwide community-based voluntary health organization dedicated to eliminating cancer as a major health problem by preventing cancer, saving lives, and diminishing suffering from cancer, through research and education.
Leslie Smith Babione, Media Relations Contact - Indianapolis
Katie Burton, Media/Public Relations Indiana

2102 Leukemia and Lymphoma Society: Indiana Chapter
Leukemia Society of America
941 E 86th Street
Indianapolis, IN 46240
317-726-2270
800-846-7764
Fax: 317-726-2280
e-mail: amy.kwas@lls.org
www.lls.org
Dedicated to finding cures for leukemia and related cancers and to improving the quality of life for patients and their families.
Amy Kwas, Executive Director
Sarah Moore, Deputy Executive Director

Iowa

2103 American Cancer Society: Iowa
8364 Hickman Road
Des Moines, IA 50325
515-253-0147
800-ACS-2345
Fax: 515-253-0806
TTY: 866-228-4327
e-mail: chaarles.reed@cancer.org
www.cancer.org
The American Cancer Society is the nationwide community-based voluntary health organization dedicated to eliminating cancer as a major health problem by preventing cancer, saving lives, and diminishing suffering from cancer, through research and education.
Chuck Reed, Media Relations Contact - Iowa

2104 People Against Cancer
604 E Street
Otho, IA 50569-0010
515-972-4444
800-662-2326
Fax: 515-972-4415
e-mail: info@PeopleAgainstCancer.net
www.peopleagainstcancer.com
A nonprofit grassroots organization whose mission is to find the best cancer therapy for people with cancer worldwide.
Frank Wiewel, Executive Director

Kansas

2105 American Cancer Society: Kansas City
6700 Antioch
Merriam, KS 66024
913-432-3277
800-ACS-2345
Fax: 913-432-1732
TTY: 866-228-4327
e-mail: christine.winter@cancer.org
www.cancer.org
The American Cancer Society is the nationwide community-based voluntary health organization dedicated to eliminating cancer as a major health problem by preventing cancer, saving lives, and diminishing suffering from cancer, through research and education.
Christine Winter, Media Relations Contact

2106 Leukemia and Lymphoma Society: Mid-America Chapter
Leukemia Society of America
6811 W 63rd Street
Shawnee Mission, KS 66202
913-262-1515
800-256-1075
Fax: 913-262-2167
e-mail: janna.lacock@lls.org
www.lls.org
Dedicated to finding cures for leukemia and related cancers and to improving the quality of life for patients and their families.
Janna LaCock, Executive Director
Jill Ring, Development Director

2107 Leukemia and Lymphona Society: Kansas Chapter
Leukemia Society of America
300 N Main
Wichita, KS 67202
316-266-4050
800-779-2417
Fax: 316-266-4960
e-mail: kelly.gerstenkorn@lls.org
www.lls.org/ks
Cure leukemia, lymphoma, Hodgkin's disease and myeloma and improve the quality of life for patients and their families.
Timothy S Durst, Chairman
James Davis, Vice-Chair

Kentucky

2108 American Cancer Society: Kentucky
701 W Muhammad Ali Boulevard
Louisville, KY 40203
502-584-6782
800-ACS-2345
Fax: 502-584-6767
TTY: 866-228-4327
e-mail: doug.dressman@cancer.org
www.cancer.org
The American Cancer Society is the nationwide community-based voluntary health organization dedicated to eliminating cancer as a major health problem by preventing cancer, saving lives, and diminishing suffering from cancer, through research and education.
Doug Dressman, Executive Director-Louisville

2109 Leukemia and Lymphoma Society: Kentucky Chapter
Leukemia Society of America
600 E Main Street
Louisville, KY 40202-2661
502-584-8490
800-955-2566
Fax: 502-589-5316
e-mail: karyl.ferman@lls.org
www.lls.org
Founded in 1975 to serve Kentucky and Southern Indiana residents touched by leukemia and its related cancers. Goal is to find a cure

for leukemia and its related cancers and to improve the quality of life for patients and their families.
Karyl D Ferman, Executive Director
Katie Anderson, Director Team in Training

Louisiana

2110   American Cancer Society: Louisiana
2605 River Road   504-469-0021
New Orleans, LA 70121   800-ACS-2345
                                            Fax: 504-219-2290
                                            TTY: 866-228-4327
                         e-mail: jewel.m.bush@cancer.org
                                               www.cancer.org
The American Cancer Society is the nationwide community-based voluntary health organization dedicated to eliminating cancer as a major health problem by preventing cancer, saving lives, and diminishing suffering from cancer, through research and education.
Jewel M Bush, Media Relations Contact

Maine

2111   American Cancer Society: Maine
1 Bowdoin Mill Island   207-373-3700
Topsham, ME 04086   800-ACS-2345
                                            Fax: 207-725-6680
                                            TTY: 866-228-4327
                        e-mail: susan.clifford@cancer.org
                                               www.cancer.org
The American Cancer Society is the nationwide community-based voluntary health organization dedicated to eliminating cancer as a major health problem by preventing cancer, saving lives, and diminishing suffering from cancer, through research and education.
Susan Clifford, Media Relations Contact - Maine

Maryland

2112   American Cancer Society: Maryland
8219 Town Center Drive   410-931-6850
Baltimore, MD 21236   800-ACS-2345
                                            Fax: 410-931-6875
                                            TTY: 866-228-4327
                          e-mail: dawn.ward@cancer.org
                                               www.cancer.org
The American Cancer Society is the nationwide community-based voluntary health organization dedicated to eliminating cancer as a major health problem by preventing cancer, saving lives, and diminishing suffering from cancer, through research and education.
Dawn Ward, Media Relations Contact - Baltimore Area

2113   Leukemia and Lymphoma Society: Maryland Chapter
Leukemia Society of America
11350 McCormick Road   410-527-0220
Hunt Valley, MD 21031-2001   800-242-4572
                                            Fax: 410-527-0510
                        e-mail: sharon.yateman@lls.org
                                                  www.lls.org
Dedicated to finding cures for leukemia and related cancers and to improving the quality of life for patients and their families.
Sharon E Yateman, Executive Director
Allyson Yospe, Deputy Executive Director

Massachusetts

2114   American Cancer Society: Boston
18 Tremont Street   617-556-7400
Boston, MA 02108   800-ACS-2345
                                            Fax: 617-263-6825
                                            TTY: 866-228-4327
                       e-mail: kate.langstone@cancer.org
                                               www.cancer.org
The American Cancer Society is the nationwide community-based voluntary health organization dedicated to eliminating cancer as a major health problem by preventing cancer, saving lives, and diminishing suffering from cancer, through research and education.
Kate Langstone, Media Relations Contact - Boston Area

2115   American Cancer Society: Central New England Region-Weston MA
9 Riverside Road   781-894-6633
Weston, MA 02493   800-ACS-2345
                                            Fax: 781-314-2699
                                            TTY: 866-228-4327
                    e-mail: jessica.saporetti@cancer.org
                                               www.cancer.org
The American Cancer Society is the nationwide community-based voluntary health organization dedicated to eliminating cancer as a major health problem by preventing cancer, saving lives, and diminishing suffering from cancer, through research and education.
Jessica Saporetti, Media Relations Contact

Michigan

2116   Leukemia and Lymphoma Society: Michigan Chapter
1421 E 12 Mile Road   248-581-3900
Madison Heights, MI 48071   800-456-5413
                                            Fax: 248-581-3901
                         e-mail: peggy.shriver@lls.org
                                                  www.lls.org
Peggy Shriver, Executive Director
Robin R Rhea, Director Operations

Minnesota

2117   American Cancer Society: Duluth
130 W Superior Street   218-727-7439
Duluth, MN 55802   800-ACS-2345
                                            Fax: 218-727-8069
                                            TTY: 866-228-4327
                         e-mail: janis.rannow@cancer.org
                                               www.cancer.org
The American Cancer Society is the nationwide community-based voluntary health organization dedicated to eliminating cancer as a major health problem by preventing cancer, saving lives, and diminishing suffering from cancer, through research and education.
Janis Rannow, Media Relations Contact

2118   American Cancer Society: Mendota Heights Mendota Heights
Mendota Heights
2520 Pilot Knob Road   651-255-8100
Mendota Heights, MN 55120   800-ACS-2345
                                            Fax: 651-255-8133
                                            TTY: 866-228-4327
                          e-mail: lou.harvin@cancer.org
                                               www.cancer.org
The American Cancer Society is the nationwide community-based voluntary health organization dedicated to eliminating cancer as a major health problem by preventing cancer, saving lives, and diminishing suffering from cancer, through research and education.
Lou Harvin, Media Relations Contact
Janis Rannow, Media Relations Contact

2119   American Cancer Society: Rochester
2900 43 Street NW   507-287-2044
Rochester, MN 55901   800-ACS-2345
                                            Fax: 507-287-2178
                                            TTY: 866-228-4327
                         e-mail: janis.rannow@cancer.org
                                               www.cancer.org
The American Cancer Society is the nationwide community-based voluntary health organization dedicated to eliminating cancer as a major health problem by preventing cancer, saving lives, and diminishing suffering from cancer, through research and education.
Janis Rannow, Media Relations Contact

2120   American Cancer Society: Saint Cloud
3721 23rd Street S   320-255-0220
Saint Cloud, MN 56301   800-239-7028
                                            Fax: 320-255-5517
                                            TTY: 866-228-4327
                         e-mail: janis.rannow@cancer.org
                                               www.cancer.org
The American Cancer Society is the nationwide community-based voluntary health organization dedicated to eliminating cancer as a major health problem by preventing cancer, saving lives, and diminishing suffering from cancer, through research and education.
Janis Rannow, Media Relations Contact

2121 Leukemia and Lymphoma Society: Minnesota Chapter
5217 Wayzata Boulevard 763-852-3000
Golden Valley, MN 55426 888-220-4440
Fax: 763-852-3001
e-mail: Murray.Schmidt@lls.org
www.lls.org

Murray Schmidt, Executive Director
Vickie Shaw, Deputy Executive Director

Mississippi

2122 American Cancer Society: Jackson
1380 Livingston Lane 601-362-8874
Jackson, MS 39213 800-ACS-2345
Fax: 601-362-8876
TTY: 866-228-4327
e-mail: kelly.lindsay@cancer.org
www.cancer.org

The American Cancer Society is the nationwide community-based voluntary health organization dedicated to eliminating cancer as a major health problem by preventing cancer, saving lives, and diminishing suffering from cancer, through research and education.
Kelly Lindsay, Media Relations Contact

2123 Leukemia and Lymphoma Society: Mississippi Chapter
408 Fontaine Place 601-956-7447
Ridgeland, MS 39157 877-538-5364
Fax: 601-956-6957
e-mail: Travis.Lee@lls.org
www.lls.org

Travis Lee, Campaign Director Team in Training
Natalie Michael, Campaign Director Team in Training

Missouri

2124 American Cancer Society: Saint Louis
4207 Lindell Boulevard 314-286-8100
Saint Louis, MO 63108 800-ACS-2345
Fax: 314-286-8160
TTY: 866-228-4327
e-mail: christine.winter@cancer.org
www.cancer.org

The American Cancer Society is the nationwide community-based voluntary health organization dedicated to eliminating cancer as a major health problem by preventing cancer, saving lives, and diminishing suffering from cancer, through research and education.
Christine Winter, Media Relations Contact

Montana

2125 American Cancer Society: Montana
3550 Mullan Road 406-542-2191
Missoula, MT 59808 800-ACS-2345
Fax: 406-327-0146
TTY: 866-228-4327
e-mail: jim.ryan@cancer.org
www.cancer.org

The American Cancer Society is the nationwide community-based voluntary health organization dedicated to eliminating cancer as a major health problem by preventing cancer, saving lives, and diminishing suffering from cancer, through research and education.
Jim Ryan, Media Relations Contact

Nebraska

2126 American Cancer Society: Nebraska
9850 Nicholas Street 402-393-5800
Omaha, NE 68114 800-ACS-2345
Fax: 402-393-7790
TTY: 866-228-4327
e-mail: mike.lefler@cancer.org
www.cancer.org

The American Cancer Society is the nationwide community-based voluntary health organization dedicated to eliminating cancer as a major health problem by preventing cancer, saving lives, and diminishing suffering from cancer, through research and education.
Mike Lefler, Media Relations Contact

2127 Leukemia and Lymphoma Society: Nebraska Chapter
10832 Old Mill Road 402-344-2242
Omaha, NE 68154 888-847-4974
Fax: 402-344-2422
e-mail: pattie.gorham@lls.org
www.lls.org

Pattie Gorham, Executive Director
Tonya Schroeder, Patient Services Manager - Portland Area

Nevada

2128 American Cancer Society: Nevada
6165 S Rainbow Boulevard 702-798-6877
Las Vegas, NV 89118 800-ACS-2345
Fax: 702-798-0530
TTY: 866-228-4327
e-mail: paulette.anderson@cancer.org
www.cancer.org

The American Cancer Society is the nationwide community-based voluntary health organization dedicated to eliminating cancer as a major health problem by preventing cancer, saving lives, and diminishing suffering from cancer, through research and education.
Paulette Anderson, Media Relations Contact

New Hampshire

2129 American Cancer Society: New Hampshire Gail Singer Memorial Building
Gail Singer Memorial Building
2 Commerce Drive 603-472-8899
Bedford, NH 03110 800-ACS-2345
Fax: 603-472-7093
TTY: 866-228-4327
e-mail: peter.davies@cancer.org
www.cancer.org

The American Cancer Society is the nationwide community-based voluntary health organization dedicated to eliminating cancer as a major health problem by preventing cancer, saving lives, and diminishing suffering from cancer, through research and education.
Peter Davies, Media Relations Contact

2130 New Hampshire Cancer Pain Initiative
125 Airport Road 603-225-0900
Concord, NH 03301 e-mail: info@nhpain.org.
www.nhpain.org

Made up of concerned people who have joined together to promote the alleviation of cancer pain through education, research and advisory activities.

New Jersey

2131 American Cancer Society: New Jersey
2600 US Highway 1 732-297-8000
N Brunswick, NJ 08902 800-ACS-2345
Fax: 732-297-9043
TTY: 866-228-4327
e-mail: marjorie.kaplan@cancer.org
www.cancer.org

The American Cancer Society is the nationwide community-based voluntary health organization dedicated to eliminating cancer as a major health problem by preventing cancer, saving lives, and diminishing suffering from cancer, through research and education.
Marjorie Kaplan, Media Relations Contact

2132 CanHelp
PO Box 1678
Livingston, NJ 07039 800-364-2341
Fax: 888-800-0201
e-mail: joan@canhelp.com
www.canhelp.com

Offers reports for cancer patients on orthodox and alternative therapies and coaching/counseling to help with treatment decision-making and coping.
Patrick M McGrady, Founder
Joan Runfola LCSW, Director

2133 Leukemia and Lymphoma Society: Northern New Jersey Chapter
Leukemia Society of America

116 South Euclid Avenue
Westfield, NJ 07090
908-654-9445
Fax: 908-654-9496
e-mail: gina.panas@lls.org
www.lls.org
Dedicated to finding cures for leukemia and related cancers and to improving the quality of life for patients and their families.

2134   Leukemia and Lymphoma Society: Southern New Jersey Chapter
Leukemia Society of America
216 Haddon Avenue
Westmont, NJ 08108-2811
856-869-0200
888-920-8557
Fax: 856-869-7383
e-mail: gina.panas@lls.org
www.lls.org
Dedicated to finding cures for leukemia and related cancers and to improving the quality of life for patients and their families.

New Mexico

2135   American Cancer Society: New Mexico
10501 Montgomery Boulevard NE
Albuquerque, NM 87111
505-260-2105
800-ACS-2345
Fax: 505-266-9513
TTY: 866-228-4327
e-mail: john.weisgerber@cancer.org
www.cancer.org
The American Cancer Society is the nationwide community-based voluntary health organization dedicated to eliminating cancer as a major health problem by preventing cancer, saving lives, and diminishing suffering from cancer, through research and education.
John Weisgerber, Media Relations Contact

2136   Leukemia and Lymphoma Society: Mountain States Chapter
Leukemia Society of America
3411 Candelaria NE
Albuquerque, NM 87107
505-872-0141
888-286-7846
Fax: 505-872-2480
e-mail: gina.panas@lls.org
www.lls.org
Dedicated to finding cures for leukemia and related cancers and to improving the quality of life for patients and their families. Serves New Mexico and the Greater El Paso, TX area.
Deborah Hoffman, Executive Director
Mikki Aronoff, Patient Services Manager - Portland Area

New York

2137   American Cancer Society: Central New York Region/East Syracuse
6725 Lyons Street
E Syracuse, NY 13057
315-437-7025
800-ACS-2345
Fax: 315-437-8233
TTY: 866-228-4327
e-mail: kim.mcmahon@cancer.org
www.cancer.org
The American Cancer Society is the nationwide community-based voluntary health organization dedicated to eliminating cancer as a major health problem by preventing cancer, saving lives, and diminishing suffering from cancer, through research and education.
Kim McMahon, Media Relations Contact

2138   American Cancer Society: Long Island
75 Davids Drive
Hauppauge, NY 11788
631-436-7070
800-ACS-2345
Fax: 631-436-5380
TTY: 866-228-4327
e-mail: jennifer.cucurullo@cancer.org
www.cancer.org
The American Cancer Society is the nationwide community-based voluntary health organization dedicated to eliminating cancer as a major health problem by preventing cancer, saving lives, and diminishing suffering from cancer, through research and education.
Jennifer Cucurullo, Media Relations Contact

2139   American Cancer Society: New York City
132 W 32nd Street
New York, NY 10001-3983
212-586-8700
800-ACS-2345
Fax: 212-237-3855
TTY: 866-228-4327
e-mail: jennifer.cucurullo@cancer.org
www.cancer.org
The American Cancer Society is the nationwide community-based voluntary health organization dedicated to eliminating cancer as a major health problem by preventing cancer, saving lives, and diminishing suffering from cancer, through research and education.
Jennifer Cucurullo, Media Relations Contact

2140   American Cancer Society: Queens Region / Rego Park
97-99 Queens Boulevard
Rego Park, NY 11374
718-263-2224
800-ACS-2345
Fax: 718-261-0758
TTY: 866-228-4327
e-mail: jennifer.cucurullo@cancer.org
www.cancer.org
The American Cancer Society is the nationwide community-based voluntary health organization dedicated to eliminating cancer as a major health problem by preventing cancer, saving lives, and diminishing suffering from cancer, through research and education.
Jennifer Cucurullo, Media Relations Contact

2141   American Cancer Society: Westchester Region/White Plains
2 Lyon Place
White Plains, NY 10601
914-949-4800
800-ACS-2345
Fax: 914-397-8851
TTY: 866-228-4327
e-mail: jennifer.cucurullo@cancer.org
www.cancer.org
The American Cancer Society is the nationwide community-based voluntary health organization dedicated to eliminating cancer as a major health problem by preventing cancer, saving lives, and diminishing suffering from cancer, through research and education.
Jennifer Cucurullo, Media Relations Contact

2142   Foundation for Advancement in Cancer Therapy
Old Chelsea Station
New York, NY 10113
212-741-2790
www.fact-ltd.org
Distributes information on cancer prevention and nontoxic therapies for cancer.
Ruth Sackman, President/Co-founder
James H Davis, Vice Chair

2143   Leukemia & Lymphoma Society Chapter: New York City
475 Park Avenue S
New York, NY 10016
212-376-7100
800-955-4572
Fax: 212-448-9214
e-mail: ossom@lls.org
www.leukemia-lymphoma.org
Dedicated to finding cures for leukemia and related cancers and to improving the quality of life for patients and their families. Educational materials, support services and financial aid available. Volunteer opportunities.
Michael Osso, Executive Director
Sara Lipsky, Deputy Executive Director

2144   Leukemia & Lymphoma Society: Westchester/ Hudson Valley Chapter
1311 Mamaroneck Avenue
White Plains, NY 10605
914-949-0084
Fax: 914-949-0391
www.lls.org/wch
Mission is to cure leukemia, lymphoma, Hodgkin's disease and myeloma, and to improve the quality of life of patients and their families.
Dennis P Chillemi, Executive Director
Diandra Kodl, Deputy Executive Director

2145   Leukemia and Lymphoma Society Chapter: New York City
475 Park Avenue S
New York, NY 10016
212-376-7100
800-955-4572
Fax: 212-448-9214
e-mail: ossom@lls.org
www.leukemia-lymphoma.org
Dedicated to finding cures for leukemia and related cancers and to improving the quality of life for patients and their families. Educa-

tional materials, support services and financial aid available. Volunteer opportunities.
Michael Osso, Executive Director
Sara Lipsky, Deputy Executive Director

2146 Leukemia and Lymphoma Society: Central New York Chapter
Leukemia Society of America
401 N Salina Street
Syracuse, NY 13203
315-471-1050
800-690-8944
Fax: 315-471-6434
e-mail: chip.lockwood@lls.org
www.lls.org
Dedicated to finding cures for leukemia and related cancers and to improving the quality of life for patients and their families.
Chip Lockwood, Executive Director
Kristen Duggleby, Campaign Director Donor Relations

2147 Leukemia and Lymphoma Society: Long Island Chapter
Leukemia Society of America
555 Broadhollow Road
Melville, NY 11747
631-752-8500
Fax: 631-752-9066
e-mail: tammy.philic@lls.org
www.lls.org
Established to serve Long Islanders with leukemia, lymphoma, Hodgkin's disease and myeloma, their families and friends.
Tammy Philie, Executive Director
Nicole Kowaleski, Deputy Executive Director

2148 Leukemia and Lymphoma Society: Upstate New York Chapter
Leukemia Society of America
5 Computer Drive W
Albany, NY 12205
518-438-3583
866-255-3583
Fax: 518-438-6431
e-mail: Maureen.Thornton@lls.org
www.lls.org
Dedicated to finding cures for leukemia and related cancers and to improving the quality of life for patients and their families.
Maureen O'Brien-Thor, Executive Director
Raechel Hunt, Patient Services Manager - Portland Area

2149 Leukemia and Lymphoma Society: Western New York & Finger Lakes Chapter
Leukemia Society of America
4053 Maple Road
Amherst, NY 14226
716-834-2578
800-784-2368
Fax: 716-837-0335
e-mail: nancy.hails@lls.org
www.lls.org
Dedicated to finding cures for leukemia and related cancers and to improving the quality of life for patients and their families.
Nancy Hails, Executive Director
Luann Burgio, Deputy Executive Director

North Carolina

2150 American Cancer Society: North Carolina
8300 Health Park
Raleigh, NC 27615
919-334-5218
800-ACS-2345
Fax: 919-841-1422
TTY: 866-228-4327
e-mail: jbright@cancer.org
www.cancer.org
The American Cancer Society is the nationwide community-based voluntary health organization dedicated to eliminating cancer as a major health problem by preventing cancer, saving lives, and diminishing suffering from cancer, through research and education.
Jeff Bright, Media Relations Contact

2151 Leukemia and Lymphoma Society: Eastern North Carolina Chapter
Flagship Building
401 Harrison Oaks Boulevard
Cary, NC 27513
919-677-3993
800-936-9337
Fax: 919-677-3992
e-mail: tiffany.armstrong@lls.org
www.lls.org

Tiffany Armstrong, Executive Director
Loreal Massiah, Patient Services Manager - Portland Area

2152 Leukemia and Lymphoma Society: North Carolina Chapter
Leukemia Society of America
5950 Fairview Road
Charlotte, NC 28210
704-998-5012
800-888-9934
Fax: 704-998-5010
www.lls.org
Dedicated to finding cures for leukemia and related cancers and to improving the quality of life for patients and their families.
Tiffany Armstrong, Executive Director
Loreal Massiah, Patient Services Manager - Portland Area

North Dakota

2153 American Cancer Society: North Dakota
4646 Amber Valley Parkway
Fargo, ND 58104
701-232-1385
800-ACS-2345
Fax: 701-232-1109
TTY: 866-228-4327
e-mail: jim.ryan@cancer.org
www.cancer.org
The American Cancer Society is the nationwide community-based voluntary health organization dedicated to eliminating cancer as a major health problem by preventing cancer, saving lives, and diminishing suffering from cancer, through research and education.
Jim Ryan, Media Relations Contact

Ohio

2154 American Cancer Society: Ohio
870 Michigan Avenue
Columbus, OH 43215
888-227-6446
Fax: 877-227-2838
TTY: 866-228-4327
e-mail: robert.paschen@cancer.org
www.cancer.org
The American Cancer Society is the nationwide community-based voluntary health organization dedicated to eliminating cancer as a major health problem by preventing cancer, saving lives, and diminishing suffering from cancer, through research and education.
Robert Paschen, Media Relations Contact

2155 Leukemia and Lymphoma Society: Central Ohio Chapter
Leukemia Society of America
2225 City Gate Drive
Columbus, OH 43219
614-476-7194
800-686-CURE
Fax: 614-476-7189
e-mail: phil.tanner@lls.org
www.lls.org
Dedicated to finding cures for leukemia and related cancers and to improving the quality of life for patients and their families.
Phil Tanner, Executive Director
Dan Swisher, Office Manager

2156 Leukemia and Lymphoma Society: Northern Ohio Chapter
Leukemia Society of America
23297 Commerce Park
Cleveland, OH 44122
216-910-1200
800-589-5721
Fax: 216-910-1201
e-mail: frank.canning@lls.org
www.lls.org
Dedicated to finding cures for leukemia and related cancers and to improving the quality of life for patients and their families.
Frank Canning, Field Director
Nancy Toghill, Office Manager

2157 Leukemia and Lymphoma Society: Southern Ohio Chapter
Leukemia Society of America
4370 Glendale Milford Rd
Cincinnati, OH 45242
513-698-2828
Fax: 513-361-2109
e-mail: michelle.steed@lls.org
www.lls.org
Dedicated to finding cures for leukemia and related cancers and to improving the quality of life for patients and their families. This chapter serves a 22-county geographic area.
Michelle Steed, Executive Director
Gene Fisher, Operations Director

Oklahoma

2158 American Cancer Society: Oklahoma
6525 N Meridian   405-843-9888
Oklahoma City, OK 73116   800-ACS-2345
                                         Fax: 405-848-0795
                                         TTY: 866-228-4327
                e-mail: christina.lindholm@cancer.org
                                         www.cancer.org
The American Cancer Society is the nationwide community-based
voluntary health organization dedicated to eliminating cancer as a
major health problem by preventing cancer, saving lives, and diminishing suffering from cancer, through research and education.
Christina Li, Media/Public Relations

2159 Leukemia and Lymphoma Society: Oklahoma Chapter
Leukemia Society of America
500 N Broadway   405-943-8888
Oklahoma City, OK 73102   888-828-4572
                                         Fax: 405-943-8355
                       e-mail: sherry.martin@lls.org
                                         www.lls.org
Dedicated to finding cures for leukemia and related cancers and to
improving the quality of life for patients and their families.
Sherry Marti MSW LCSW, Patient Services Manager - Portland Area
Jill Hull, Campaign Director Team in Training

Oregon

2160 American Cancer Society: Oregon
330 SW Curry Street   503-295-6422
Portland, OR 97239   800-ACS-2345
                                         Fax: 503-228-1062
                                         TTY: 866-228-4327
              e-mail: gretchen.rosenberger@cancer.org
                                         www.cancer.org
The American Cancer Society is the nationwide community-based
voluntary health organization dedicated to eliminating cancer as a
major health problem by preventing cancer, saving lives, and diminishing suffering from cancer, through research and education.
Gretchen Rosenberger, Media Relations Contact

2161 Leukemia and Lymphoma Society: Oregon Chapter
Leukemia Society of America
9320 SW Barbur Boulevard   503-245-9866
Portland, OR 97219   800-466-6572
                                         Fax: 503-245-9865
                      e-mail: Sarah.Varner@lls.org
                                         www.lls.org
Dedicated to finding cures for leukemia and related cancers and to
improving the quality of life for patients and their families.
Sarah Varner, Executive Director
Sue Sumpter, Patient Services Manager - Portland Area

Pennsylvania

2162 American Cancer Society: Harrisburg Capital Area Unit
Capital Area Unit
3211 N Front Street   215-985-5336
Harrisburg, PA 17110   888-227-5445
                                         Fax: 717-231-5784
                                         TTY: 866-228-4327
                      e-mail: john.held@cancer.org
                                         www.cancer.org
The American Cancer Society is the nationwide community-based
voluntary health organization dedicated to eliminating cancer as a
major health problem by preventing cancer, saving lives, and di-
minishing suffering from cancer, through research and education.
Colleen Fitz, Media Relations Contact
John Held, Media Relations Contact

2163 American Cancer Society: Philadelphia
1626 Locust Street   215-985-5336
Philadelphia, PA 19103   888-227-5445
                                         Fax: 215-985-5406
                                         TTY: 866-228-4327
                      e-mail: john.held@cancer.org
                                         www.cancer.org
The American Cancer Society is the nationwide community-based
voluntary health organization dedicated to eliminating cancer as a

major health problem by preventing cancer, saving lives, and di-
minishing suffering from cancer, through research and education.
John Held, Media Relations Contact
Colleen Fitz, Media/Public Relations

2164 American Cancer Society: Pittsburgh
320 Bilmar Drive   215-985-5336
Pittsburgh, PA 15205   888-227-5445
                                         Fax: 412-919-1101
                                         TTY: 866-228-4327
                      e-mail: dcatena@cancer.org
                                         www.cancer.org
The American Cancer Society is the nationwide community-based
voluntary health organization dedicated to eliminating cancer as a
major health problem by preventing cancer, saving lives, and diminishing suffering from cancer, through research and education.
Dan Catena, Media Relations Contact

**2165 Leukemia and Lymphoma Society: Central Pennsylvania
Chapter**
800 Corporate Circle   717-652-6520
Harrisburg, PA 17110   800-822-2873
                                         Fax: 717-652-8614
                      e-mail: beth.mihmet@lls.org
                                         www.lls.org
Elizabeth Mihmet, Executive Director
Danielle Bubnis, Patient Services Manager

**2166 Leukemia and Lymphoma Society: Eastern Pennsylvania
Chapter**
555 N Lane   610-238-0360
Conshohocken, PA 19428   800-482-CURE
                                         Fax: 484-530-0833
                      e-mail: ursula.raczak@lls.org
                                         www.lls.org
Lydia Hernandez-Vele, Executive Director
Ursula Raczak, Deputy Executive Director

**2167 Leukemia and Lymphoma Society: Western Pennsylvania/West
Virginia Chapter**
Leukemia Society of America
333 E Carson Street   412-395-2873
Pittsburgh, PA 15219-1439   800-726-2873
                                         Fax: 412-395-2888
                      e-mail: massaric@lls.org
                                         www.lls.org
Tina Massari, Executive Director
Jeanne Caliguiri, Development Director

Rhode Island

2168 American Cancer Society: Rhode Island
931 Jefferson Boulevard   401-722-8480
Warwick, RI 02886   800-ACS-2345
                                         Fax: 401-421-0535
                                         TTY: 866-228-4327
              e-mail: jim.beardsworth@cancer.org
                                         www.cancer.org
The American Cancer Society is the nationwide community-based
voluntary health organization dedicated to eliminating cancer as a
major health problem by preventing cancer, saving lives, and diminishing suffering from cancer, through research and education.
Jim Beardsworth, Media Relations Contact

2169 Leukemia and Lymphoma Society: Rhode Island Chapter
1210 Pontiac Avenue   401-943-8888
Cranston, RI 02920   Fax: 401-943-1377
                      e-mail: koconisb@lls.org
                                         www.lls.org
Bill Koconis, Executive Director
Gloria Hincapie, Patient Services Manager

South Carolina

2170 American Cancer Society: South Carolina
128 Stonemark Lane
Columbia, SC 29210
803-750-1693
800-ACS-2345
Fax: 803-750-4000
TTY: 866-228-4327
e-mail: mjwardle@cancer.org
www.cancer.org
The American Cancer Society is the nationwide community-based voluntary health organization dedicated to eliminating cancer as a major health problem by preventing cancer, saving lives, and diminishing suffering from cancer, through research and education.
Mary Jane Wardle, Media Relations Contact

2171 Leukemia and Lymphoma Society: South Carolina Chapter
1247 Lake Murray Boulevard
Irmo, SC 29063
803-749-4299
Fax: 803-749-4088
www.lls.org

2172 Leukemia and Lymphoma Society: South/West
107 Westpark Boulevard
Columbia, SC 29210
803-731-4060
Fax: 803-731-4066
e-mail: paul.jeter@lls.org
www.lls.org

Paul Jeter, Executive Director
Cassandra Wineglass, Patient Services Manager

South Dakota

2173 American Cancer Society: South Dakota
4904 S Technopolis Drive
Sioux Falls, SD 57106
605-361-8277
800-ACS-2345
Fax: 605-361-8537
TTY: 866-228-4327
e-mail: charlotte.hofer@cancer.org
www.cancer.org
The American Cancer Society is the nationwide community-based voluntary health organization dedicated to eliminating cancer as a major health problem by preventing cancer, saving lives, and diminishing suffering from cancer, through research and education.
Charlotte Ho, Media Relations Contact

Tennessee

2174 American Cancer Society: Tennessee
2000 Charlotte Avenue
Nashville, TN 37203
615-327-0991
800-ACS-2345
Fax: 615-341-7335
TTY: 866-228-4327
e-mail: brian.gillespie@cancer.org
www.cancer.org
The American Cancer Society is the nationwide community-based voluntary health organization dedicated to eliminating cancer as a major health problem by preventing cancer, saving lives, and diminishing suffering from cancer, through research and education.
Brian Gillespie, Media Relations Contact

2175 Leukemia & Lymphoma Society: Tennessee Chapter
404 BNA Drive
Nashville, TN 37217
615-331-2980
800-332-2980
Fax: 615-331-2941
e-mail: winslowm@tn.leukemia-lymphoma.org
www.leukemia-lymphoma.org
Founded in 1982 to better serve the needs of Tennesseans. Offers contribution funded community services, family support groups, free educational materials and financial assistance for those affected by leukemia, Hodgkin's disease, myeloma and lymphomas.
Colleen Grady, Executive Director
Mary Winslow, Patient Services Manager

Texas

2176 American Cancer Society: Texas
2433 Ridgepoint Drive
Austin, TX 78754
512-919-1800
800-ACS-2345
Fax: 512-919-1846
TTY: 866-228-4327
e-mail: justine.hall@cancer.org
www.cancer.org

The American Cancer Society is the nationwide community-based voluntary health organization dedicated to eliminating cancer as a major health problem by preventing cancer, saving lives, and diminishing suffering from cancer, through research and education.
Justin Hall, Media Relations Contact

2177 Leukemia and Lymphoma Society: North Texas Chapter
Leukemia Society of America
8111 LBJ Freeway
Dallas, TX 75251
972-239-0959
800-800-6702
Fax: 972-239-0892
e-mail: Tina.Garcia@lls.org
www.lls.org
Dedicated to finding cures for leukemia and related cancers and to improving the quality of life for patients and their families.
Tina Garcia, Executive Director
Sarah Bayley, Donor Development Director

2178 Leukemia and Lymphoma Society: South/West Texas Chapter
Leukemia Society of America
431 Isom Road
San Antonio, TX 78216-4170
210-377-1775
800-683-2458
Fax: 210-344-3717
www.lls.org
Dedicated to finding cures for leukemia and related cancers and to improving the quality of life for patients and their families.
Jon Walter, President/CEO
Jimmy Nangle, CFO

2179 Leukemia and Lymphoma Society: Texas Gulf Coast Chapter
Leukemia Society of America
5005 Mitchelldale
Houston, TX 77092
713-680-8088
Fax: 713-683-9504
e-mail: BillieSue.Parris@lls.org
www.lls.org
Dedicated to finding cures for leukemia and related cancers and to improving the quality of life for patients and their families.
Billie Sue Parris, Executive Director
Jane Thompson, Office Manager

Utah

2180 American Cancer Society: Utah
941 E 3300 S
Salt Lake City, UT 84106
801-483-1500
800-ACS-2345
Fax: 801-483-1558
TTY: 866-228-4327
e-mail: patricia.monsoor@cancer.org
www.cancer.org
The American Cancer Society is the nationwide community-based voluntary health organization dedicated to eliminating cancer as a major health problem by preventing cancer, saving lives, and diminishing suffering from cancer, through research and education.
Patricia Monsoor, Media Relations Contact

Vermont

2181 American Cancer Society: Vermont
121 Connor Way
Williston, VT 05495
802-872-6300
800-ACS-2345
Fax: 802-872-6399
TTY: 866-228-4327
e-mail: chris.falk@cancer.org
www.cancer.org

The American Cancer Society is the nationwide community-based voluntary health organization dedicated to eliminating cancer as a major health problem by preventing cancer, saving lives, and diminishing suffering from cancer, through research and education.
Chris Falk, Media Relations Contact

Virginia

2182 American Cancer Society: Virginia
4240 Park Place Court
Glen Allen, VA 23060
804-527-3700
800-ACS-2345
Fax: 804-527-3797
TTY: 866-228-4327
e-mail: domenick.casuccio@cancer.org
www.cancer.org

The American Cancer Society is the nationwide community-based voluntary health organization dedicated to eliminating cancer as a major health problem by preventing cancer, saving lives, and diminishing suffering from cancer, through research and education.
Domenick Casuccio, Media Relations Contact

2183 Arlin J Brown Information Center
PO Box 251
Fort Belvoir, VA 22060-0251   540-752-9511
An information clearinghouse on types of cancer health methods and nontoxic cancer therapies.

2184 Leukemia and Lymophoma Society: National Capital Area Chapter
Leukemia Society of America
5845 Richmond Highway   703-399-2900
Alexandria, VA 22303   Fax: 703-399-2901
e-mail: donna.mckelvey@lls.org
www.lls.org
Serves the greater Washington DC metropolitan area including Northern Virginia Prince George's and Montgomery counties.
Gabrielle Urquhart, Executive Director
Beth Gorman, Deputy Director

Washington

2185 American Cancer Society: Washington
728 134th Street SW   425-741-8949
Everett, WA 98204   Fax: 425-741-9638
e-mail: liz.lamb-ferro@cancer.org
www.cancer.org
The American Cancer Society is the nationwide community-based voluntary health organization dedicated to eliminating cancer as a major health problem by preventing cancer, saving lives, and diminishing suffering from cancer, through research and education.
Liz Lamb-Ferro, Media Relations Contact

2186 Washington Leukemia and Lymphoma Society: Alaska Chapter
Leukemia Society of America
530 Dexter Avenue N   206-628-0777
Seattle, WA 98109   888-345-4572
Fax: 206-292-9791
e-mail: wachapter@lls.org
www.leukemia-lymphoma.org
Dedicated to finding cures for leukemia and related cancers and to improving the quality of life for patients and their families.
Anne Gillingham, Executive Director
Kimberly Conn, Deputy Executive Director

West Virginia

2187 American Cancer Society: West Virginia
301 RHL Boulevard   304-746-9950
Charleston, WV 25309   800-ACS-2345
Fax: 304-746-9962
TTY: 866-228-4327
e-mail: amy.wentz@cancer.org
www.cancer.org
The American Cancer Society is the nationwide community-based voluntary health organization dedicated to eliminating cancer as a major health problem by preventing cancer, saving lives, and diminishing suffering from cancer, through research and education.
Amy Wentz Berner, Media Relations Contact

Wisconsin

2188 American Cancer Society: Wisconsin
N19 W24350 Riverwood Drive   262-523-5500
Waukesha, WI 53188   800-ACS-2345
Fax: 262-523-5533
TTY: 866-228-4327
e-mail: peter.balistrieri@cancer.org
www.acscan.org/action/wi
The American Cancer Society is the nationwide community-based voluntary health organization dedicated to eliminating cancer as a major health problem by preventing cancer, saving lives, and diminishing suffering from cancer, through research and education.
Peter Balistrieri, Media Relations Contact
Christopher Hansen, President, ACS CAN

2189 Leukemia and Lymphoma Society: Wisconsin Chapter
Leukemia Society of America
200 S Executive Drive   262-790-4701
Brookfield, WI 53005   800-261-7399
Fax: 262-790-4706
e-mail: bede.barthpotter@lls.org
www.lls.org
Founded in 1963 to serve Wisconsites touched by leukemia, lymphoma, Hodgkin's disease and myeloma.
Bede Barth Potter, Executive Director
Karen Ropel, Deputy Executive Director

Wyoming

2190 American Cancer Society: Wyoming
333 S Beech Street   307-577-4892
Casper, WY 82601   800-ACS-2345
Fax: 307-234-0926
TTY: 866-228-4327
e-mail: joel.quevillon@cancer.org
www.acscan.org
The American Cancer Society is the nationwide community-based voluntary health organization dedicated to eliminating cancer as a major health problem by preventing cancer, saving lives, and diminishing suffering from cancer, through research and education.
John R Seffrin, CEO,ACS
Christopher Hansen, President, ACS CAN

Foundations

2191 Chemotherapy Foundation
183 Madison Avenue   212-213-9292
New York, NY 10016   Fax: 212-133-31
www.chemotherapyfoundation.com
The Chemotherapy Foundation is dedicated to developing more effective methods of treatment for the control and cure of cancer. They provide educational materials and provide funds for innovative chemotherapy research, and sponsor professional and public educational symposia.
Shirley Cox, Executive Director
Franco Muggia, Chairman & Medical Director

2192 Dermatology Foundation
1560 Sherman Avenue   847-328-2256
Evanston, IL 60201-4808   Fax: 847-328-0509
e-mail: dfgen@dermatologyfoundation.org
www.dermfnd.org

The Foundation focuses on funding research that will advance patient care, and help develop and retain tomorrow's teachers and clinical leaders in the specialty.
Sandra Rahn Benz, Executive Director
James H Davis, Vice Chair

2193 National Children's Cancer Society
One South Memorial Drive   314-241-1600
Saint Louis, MO 63102   800-882-6227
Fax: 314-241-1996
e-mail: krudd@children-cancer.org
www.children-cancer.org
Our mission is to improve the quality of life for children with cancer and their families worldwide. We serve as a financial, emotional, educational, and medical resource for those in need, at every stage of their illness and recovery. The NCCS provides direct financial assistance to families for expenses not covered by insurance during their treatment; including transportation, lodging, gas money, medical assistance, health insurance premiums, and phone cards.
Mark Slocomb, Chairman
Mark Stolze, President/CEO

Libraries & Resource Centers

2194 Cancer Federation
PO Box 1298   951-849-4325
Banning, CA 92220   Fax: 951-849-0156
e-mail: info@cancerfed.org
www.cancerfed.com

The Federation is a not-for-profit organization that provides information, counseling, educational materials and meetings for the cancer patients, their families and friends. Also, they fund research and scholarships.
John Steinbacher, Executive Director

2195 **Cancer Information Service**
National Cancer Institute
6116 Executive Boulevard   301-435-3848
Bethesda, MD 20892-8322   800-422-6237
                                           TTY: 800-332-8615
                                           http://cis.nci.nih.gov/

Kramer Barnett, Director
Adamson Kristin, Administrative Resource Center

2196 **Patient Advocates for Advanced Cancer Treatments (PAACT)**
PO Box 141695   616-453-1477
Grand Rapids, MI 49514-1695   Fax: 616-453-1846
                                   e-mail: paact@paactusa.org
                                           www.paactusa.org
Provides support and advocacy for prostate cancer patients, their families, and the general public at risk. Information relative to the advancements in the detection, diagnosis, evaluation, and treatment of prostate cancer. Information, referrals, phone help, conferences, newsletter.
Richard H. Profit, President
Saleem Durvesh, Executive Marketing Director

Research Centers

2197 **Purdue Cancer Center Purdue University**
Purdue University
201 S University Street   765-494-9129
W Lafayette, IN 47907-2064   Fax: 765-494-9193
                                e-mail: cancerresearch@purdue.edu
                                           www.cancer.purdue.edu
Provide a forum for 75 of Purdue's best and brightest scientists to collaborate across campus and nationwide to prevent cancer to ease its detection and to cure it.
Timothy Ratliff, Director
Andrea Gregory-Kreps, Operations Manager

Alabama

2198 **Birmingham VA Medical Center: Research and Development**
700 S 19th Street   205-933-8101
Birmingham, AL 35233   866-487-4243
                                           Fax: 205-933-4484
                                           www.birmingham.va.gov
An acute tertiary care facility with particularly strong programs in both medicine and surgery and~serves as the primary referral center for the state. We provide health care services to eligible veterans in the VA Southeast Network .
Steven L Keller, Acting Chairman
Rica Lewis-Payton, Medical Center Director

2199 **Breast Cancer Resource Foundation of Alabama**
PO Box 531225   205-996-5463
Birmingham, AL 35253   Fax: 205-975-2432
                                   e-mail: jgalbrea@uab.edu
                                           www.bcrfa.org
Dedicated to finding a cure for breast cancer.
Dianne Mooney, President
Jennifer Galbreath, Program Director

2200 **University of Alabama At Birmingham Comprehensive Cancer Center**
UAB Comprehensive Cancer Center
1802 6th Avenue S   205-934-5077
Birmingham, AL 35294-3300   800-UAB-0933
                                   e-mail: info@ccc.uab.edu
                                           www3.ccc.uab.edu
The Center provides advanced cancer care research and education based on stringent peer-reviewed data.
Edward E Partridge, Director and Associate Director for Comm
Kirby I Bland, Deputy Director

Arizona

2201 **Southwest Association for Education in Biomedical Research**
PO Box 210101   520-621-3931
Tucson, AZ 85721-0101   Fax: 520-621-3355
                                e-mail: swaebr@ahsc.arizona.edu
                                           www.swaebr.org
The mission of the Southwest Association for Education in Biomedical Research is to develop and implement a strong proactive campaign to educate school children as well as the general public in the vital role biomedical research plays in their everyday lives.
Charles Atkinson, President

2202 **University of Arizona Cancer Center**
1515 N Campbell Avenue   520-626-5279
Tucson, AZ 85724-1454   800-327-2873
                                           www.azcc.arizona.edu
Comprehensive cancer center for diagnosis treatment and prevention.
David S Alberts, Director
Paola Villar Werstler, Director Of Development

California

2203 **Burnham Institute Cancer Center The Burnham Institute for Medical Resear**
The Burnham Institute for Medical Research
10901 N Torrey Pines Road   858-646-3100
La Jolla, CA 92037   Fax: 858-646-3199
                                e-mail: info@sanfordburnham.org
                                           www.sanfordburnham.org
Known for world-class capabilities in stem cell research and drug discovery technologies. Dedicated to revealing the fundamental molecular causes of disease and devising the innovative therapies of tomorrow.
Kristiina Vuori, President & CEO
Gary Raisl, Executive VP,CFO,Treasurer

2204 **Cancer Prevention Institute of California**
2201 Walnut Avenue   510-608-5000
Fremont, CA 94538-2334   800-511-2300
                                           Fax: 510-608-5095
                                           www.cpic.org
The North California Cancer Center is dedicated to understanding the causes prevention and detection of cancer and to improving the quality of life for individuals living with cancer.
Reed Goertler, Chief Operations Officer
Sally Glaser PhD, CEO

2205 **City of Hope Comprehensive Cancer Research Center**
1500 E Duarte Road   626-256-4673
Duarte, CA 91010   800-256-4673
                                           Fax: 626-930-5394
                                   e-mail: tkronitis@coh.org
                                           www.cityofhope.org
Excellence in biomedical research patient-centered medical care and community outreach.
Theodore G Krontiris MD, Director
Richard Jove, Deputy Director

2206 **Geraldine Brush Cancer Research Institute California Pacific Medical Center**
California Pacific Medical Center
2333 Clay Street #201   415-600-6000
San Francisco, CA 94115   e-mail: cpmcadmin@sutterhealth.org
                                           www.cpmc.org

Martin Brotman, President
Robert Tomasello, Chairman

2207 **Ida and Joseph Friend Cancer Resource Center**
1600 Divisadero St.   415-885-3693
San Francisco, CA 94143-981   800-444-2559
                                           Fax: 415-885-3701
                                e-mail: cancerresource@ucsfmedctr.org
                                           www.cancer.ucsf.edu/crc/
The Cancer Resource Center supports wellness and the healing process by providing patients and their loved ones with information emotional support and community resources. The CRC maintains a multimedia library provides access to specialized health databases and offers research assistance. We host diverse support

groups and classes and direct people to other community resources. All CRC programs are free.
Frank Mccorm PhD, Director

2208 Jonsson Comprehensive Cancer Center University of California At Los Angeles
University of California At Los Angeles
8-684 Factor Building 310-825-5268
Los Angeles, CA 90095-1781 888-662-8252
Fax: 310-206-5553
e-mail: jcccinfo@mednet.ucla.edu
www.cancer.ucla.edu
UCLA's Jonsson Comprehensive Cancer Center (JCCC) has established an international reputation for developing new cancer therapies providing the best in experimental treatments and expertly guiding and training the next generation of medical researchers.
Judith Gasson, Director
James Economou, Executive Director

2209 Pediatric Cancer Research Laboratory Children's Hospital of Orange County
Children's Hospital of Orange County
1201 W.LA Veta Ave 714-997-3000
Orange, CA 92868-3874 Fax: 714-532-8380
www.choc.org
CHOC is the first hospital devoted exclusively to caring for children in Orange County.
Dr Mitchell Cairo, Director

2210 Rebecca and John Moores UCSD Cancer Center
3855 Health Sciences Drive 585-534-7600
La Jolla, CA 92093-0658 Fax: 858-534-7628
e-mail: dedavis@ucsd.edu
www.cancer.ucsd.edu
One of the just 39 centers in the US to hold a National Cancer Institute designation as a Comprehensive Cancer Center. As such it ranks among the top centers in the nation conducting basic and clinical cancer research providing advanced patient care and serving the community through outreach and education programs.
John Alksne, Professor Surgery
Michael Andre, Adjunct Professor Radiology

2211 Salk Institute Cancer Center
Salk Institute for Biological Studies
PO Box 85800 858-453-4100
San Diego, CA 92186-5800 Fax: 858-453-8534
e-mail: communications@salk.edu
www.salk.edu
The Cancer Center was established in 1970. It is one of only eight basic research cancer centers in the country designated by the National Cancer Institute. The center includes 22 faculty members 150 postdoctoral researchers 45 graduate students and 80 research assistants. It comprises about half of the research at the Salk Institute.
Walter Eckhart, Professor and Laboratory Head
William R Brody, President

2212 Santa Barbara Breast Cancer Institute
5333 Hollister Avenue 805-964-8883
Santa Barbara, CA 93111-2341
Otto Sartorius, Director

2213 Stanford University: Beckman Center for Molecular and Genetic Medicine
School of Medicine, Department of Biochemistry
291 Campus Drive Rm LK3C02 650-723-3622
Stanford, CA 94305-5101 Fax: 650-724-9733
cmgm.stanford.edu
Dr Paul Berg, Emeritus Professor Biochemistry
Philip A Pizzo MD, Dean

2214 USC/Norris Comprehensive Cancer Center
1441 Eastlake Avenue
Los Angeles, CA 90033-1048 323-865-3000
uscnorriscancer.usc.edu
Major regional and national resource for cancer research treatment prevention and education.
Peter A Jones, Director
Nikias C.L Max, President

2215 University of California Berkeley Cancer Research Laboratory
449 Life Science Addition 510-642-4711
Berkeley, CA 94720-2751 Fax: 510-642-5741
e-mail: crl@berkeley.edu
www.crl.berkeley.edu/?q=crl
Basic research with a special emphasis on mammary cancer and tumor immunotherapy.
Astar Winoto, Director
Judith Yee, Manager

2216 University of California: Los Angeles Bone Marrow Transplantation Program
200 UCLA Medical Plaza
Los Angeles, CA 90024 310-206-6889
www.healthcare.ucla.edu/transplant
Treatment of leukemia and anemia.
David W Golde MD, Director
Gabriel Danovitch, M.D., Medical Director, Proffessor of Medicine

2217 AMC Cancer Research Center
1600 Pierce Street 303-233-6501
Denver, CO 80214 800-321-1557
Fax: 303-239-3400
e-mail: contactus@amc.org
www.amc.org
Offers research activities publications meetings educational activities public services testing services community-based cancer control programs and knowledge of cancer mortality rates.
Alice Norton, Executive Director
Gail Eckhardt, Clinical Science

2218 Colorado Cancer Research Program
2253 S Oneida Street 303-777-2663
Denver, CO 80224 888-785-6789
Fax: 303-777-2642
e-mail: ccrp@co-cancerresearch.org
www.co-cancerresearch.org
A nonprofit community-based cancer program established to provide community hospitals and physicians access to a wide range of cancer research trials in order to provide their patients with greater options for the treatment control and prevention.
Jane Hajovsky, Executive Director
Eduardo Pajon, Principal Investigator

2219 University of Colorado Cancer Center
13001 E 17th Place 303-724-3155
Aurora, CO 80045 800-473-2288
Fax: 303-724-3162
e-mail: CancerCenter.Webmaster@uchsc.edu
www.uccc.info
UCCC consortium is the hub for cancer research in Colorado. With eight programs 17 shared core resources and nearly 400 members from three universities and six institutions UCCC is responsible for the majority of cancer research in the Rocky Mountain region.
Dan Theodorescu MD PhD, Director
Laurie Gasper MD, Associate Director for Clinical Research

2220 Yale University Comprehensive Cancer Center
333 Cedar Street 203-785-4095
New Haven, CT 06520-8028 866-925-3226
Fax: 203-785-4116
www.yalecancercenter.org
A National Cancer Institute designated comprehensive cancer center for over 30 years Yale Cancer Center is one of only 40 Centers in the nation and the only comprehensive center in Southern New England.
Thomas Lynch, Director
Kevin Vest, PT, MBA, FACHE, Deputy Director

District of Columbia

2221 Georgetown University: Vincent T Lombardi Cancer Research Center
3800 Reservoir Road NW
Washington, DC 20057   202-444-4000
www.lombardi.georgetown.edu
Established in 1970 the Lombardi Comprehensive Cancer Center is named for the legendary Green Bay Packers and Washington Redskins coach Vince Lombardi who was treated for cancer at Georgetown University Hospital.
Louis M Weiner, Director
Peter G Shields, Deputy Director

2222 Howard University Cancer Center
2041 Georgia Avenue NW   202-806-7697
Washington, DC 20060-0001   Fax: 202-462-8928
e-mail: ladams-campbell@howard.edu
www.cancer.howard.edu
Reduce the burden of cancer through research education and service with emphasis on the unique ethnic and cultural aspects of minority and underserved populations.
Lucile Adams-Campbel, Director
Wayne A I Frederick, Interim Director

2223 Melanoma Research Foundation
1411 K Street NW   202-347-9675
Washington, DC 20005   800-673-1290
Fax: 202-347-9678
e-mail: info@melanoma.org
www.melanoma.org
Founded in October 1996 by melanoma patients and their families to support research which will lead to cure for melanoma. Strictly a volunteer organization - not one person will receive compensation for his or her efforts.
Steve Silverstein, President & CEO
william G Reilly, President/Owner

Florida

2224 Rambaugh-Goodwin Institute for Cancer Research
1850 NW 69th Avenue   954-587-9020
Plantation, FL 33313   Fax: 954-587-6378
e-mail: info@rgicr.org
www.rgicr.org
RGI is committed to rapidly developing anti-cancer therapies in conjunction with industrial and academic partners using efficient models of cancer growth and metastasis with the aim of moving novel compounds to market in the shortest time possible.
Claire Thuning-Robin, Director

2225 UM/Sylvester Comprehensive Cancer Center
1475 NW 12th Avenue   305-243-1000
Miami, FL 33136   800-545-2292
www.sylvester.org
UMHC offers an outpatient clinic a 40-bed inpatient unit a comprehensive treatment unit the Mohs surgery center/dermatology clinic the Rosenfield GI Center a cardiology lab and clinic a radiology/imaging suite an interventional radiology clinic the Spine Institute clinics on-site laboratory and pharmacy the Courtelis Center for Psychosocial Oncology the Jill Selevan Chapel a cafeteria as well as administrative offices.
Joan Scheiner, Chair
Jayne S. Malfitano, Vice Chair

Georgia

2226 Emory University: Georgia Center for Cancer Statistics
Rollins School of Public Health
201 Dowman Drive   404-727-6123
Atlanta, GA 30322   Fax: 404-727-7261
e-mail: gccs@sph.emory.edu
www.sph.emory.edu/gccs
Serves as a cancer registry for five counties of metropolitan Atlanta and ten rural counties of central Georgia.
James W Wagner, President

2227 Emory University: Winship Cancer Institute
1365-C Clifton Road NE   404-778-1900
Atlanta, GA 30322   888-946-7447
www.winshipcancer.emory.edu
A clinical cancer center coordinating basic and clinical cancer research.
Walter Currans, Executive Director
Fadlo Khuri MD, Deputy Directory for Basic Research

Hawaii

2228 Pacific Health Research Institute
3375 Koapaka Street   808-524-4411
Honolulu, HI 96819   Fax: 808-524-5559
e-mail: info@phrei.org
www.phrihawaii.org
Located in Honolulu Hawaii Pacific Health Research Institute (PHRI) is the largest independent biomedical research institute in the state. Since its founding on 1960 as an independent not for profit 501(c)(3) research institute PHRI today has become a leader in biomedical research in the Pacific. Indeed its researchers are performing complex investigations aimed at conquering some of the most debilitating and lethal diseases that afflict humankind.
Vicki L Shambaugh, MA, MPH, Director
Helen Petrovitch, Executive Director

2229 University of Hawaii: Cancer Research Center
1236 Lauhala Street   808-586-2985
Honolulu, HI 96813   Fax: 808-586-2982
e-mail: cvogel@crch.hawaii.edu
www.crch.org
The mission of the Cancer Research Center of Hawaii is to reduce the burden of cancer through research education and service with an emphasis on the unique ethnic culture and environmental characteristics of Hawaii and the Pacific.
Carl-Wilhelm Vogel, Professor (Researcher)
Michele Carbone, Interim Cancer Center Director

Illinois

2230 Cancer and Leukemia Group B
230 W Monroe   773-702-9171
Chicago, IL 60606   Fax: 312-345-0117
e-mail: marciak@uchicago.edu
www.calgb.org
Integral unit of the Institute specializing in leukemia research and prevention.
Marcia Kelly, Administrative Coordinator
Michael Kelly, Director Protocol Operations

2231 Kellogg Cancer Care Center Evanston Hospital
Evanston Hospital
2650 Ridge Avenue   847-570-2000
Evanston, IL 60201   888-364-6400
www.enh.org
Integral unit of the Evanston Hospital this center researches treatment and diagnosis of cancer including phase 1 and phase 2 studies.
Mark R Neaman, President, CEO
Jeffery H Hillebrand, COO

2232 Leukemia Research Foundation
3520 Lake Avenue   847-424-0600
Wilmette, IL 60091-1064   888-558-5385
Fax: 847-424-0606
e-mail: info@lrfmail.org
www.leukemia-research.org
To conquer leukemia lymphoma and myelodysplastic syndromes by funding research into their causes and cures and to enrich the quality of life of those touched by these diseases.
Kevin Radelet, Executive Director
Cindy Kane, Senior Director of Development

2233 Oncology Hematology Associates of Central Illinois
8940 N Wood Sage Road   309-243-3000
Peoria, IL 61615-7828   866-662-6564
www.illinoiscancercare.com
Research into cancer treatments.
Robert Cooper, Director
Paul A S Fishkin, Hematology Internal Medicine Medical O

2234 Robert H Lurie Comprehensive Cancer Center of Northwestern University
Galter Pavilion 675 N Street Clair   312-695-0990
Chicago, IL 60611   866-587-4322
                                        Fax: 312-695-1352
                              e-mail: cancer@northwestern.edu
                                    www.lurie.northwestern.edu
Lurie Cancer Center is a founding member of the National Comprehensive Cancer Network an exclusive alliance of 21 of the nation's leading cancer centers.
Steven T Rosen, Director
Leonidas Platanias, Deputy Director

2235 University of Chicago Cancer Research Center
5841 S Maryland Avenue   773-702-6180
Chicago, IL 60637   877-824-0600
                          e-mail: cancerresources@uccrc.org
                                        www.cancer.uchicago.edu
The University of Chicago Cancer Research Center (UCCRC) employs a wealth of intellectual technological and financial resources to pursue a comprehensive collaborative research program involving more than 200 renowned scientists and clinicians.
Mary Ellen Connellan, Executive Director
Justin Ullman, President

2236 University of Chicago: Clinical Nutrition Research Unit
5841 S Maryland Avenue   773-702-6180
Chicago, IL 60637-1463   877-824-0600
                        e-mail: feedback@bsd.uchicago.edu
                                            www.uchicago.edu
Provide superior healthcare in a compassionate manner ever mindful of each patient's dignity and individuality.
Michael M Le Beau PhD, Director
James L Madara, CEO

Indiana

2237 Mary Margaret Walther Program Walther Cancer Institute
Walther Cancer Institute
9292 N Meridian Street   317-708-6101
Indianapolis, IN 46260   Fax: 317-708-6102
                                    e-mail: info@walther.org
                                            www.walther.org
Focuses research on all types of cancer studies.
Leonard J Betley, Chairman
James E Ruckle, President/CEO

Iowa

2238 Iowa Oncology Research Association
300 E Locust   515-244-7586
Des Moines, IA 50309   888-244-6061
                                        Fax: 515-244-3037
                                   e-mail: sherrijr@iora.org
                                                www.iora.org
Clinical cancer studies and research.
Sherri Rickabaugh, Administrator
Becky Berrett, Research Assistants

2239 University of Iowa: Holden Comprehensive Cancer Center
UI Hospitals and Clinics
University of Iowa   319-353-8620
Iowa City, IA 52242-1002   800-777-8442
                                        Fax: 319-353-8988
                        e-mail: cancer-center@uiowa.edu
                          www.uihealthcare.com/depts/cancercenter
The Holden Cancer Center promotes interactive high-quality cancer research high-quality health care related to the prevention detection and treatment of cancer and educates cancer professionals and the citizens of Iowa about cancer.
Jean E Robillard, Vice President for Medical Affairs
Kenneth P Kates, CEO

Kansas

2240 Kansas State University: Terry C Johnson Center for Basic Cancer Research
Center for Basic Cancer Research

1 Chalmers Hall   785-532-6705
Manhattan, KS 66506   Fax: 785-532-6707
                                  e-mail: marcia@k-state.edu
                                www.k-state.edu/cancer.center
The mission of the Terry C. Johnson Center for Basic Cancer Research is to further the understanding of cancers by funding basic cancer research and supporting higher education training and public outreach.
Rob Denell, Director
S Keith Chapes, Associate Director

Kentucky

2241 Henry Vogt Cancer Research Institute James Graham Brown Cancer Center
James Graham Brown Cancer Center
2301 S 3rd Street   502-852-5555
Louisville, KY 40208   800-334-8635
                                      e-mail: info@ulh.org
                                www.louisville.edu/hsc/centers
The overall goal of the scientists in the Henry Vogt Cancer Research Institute is to study mechanisms relevant to tumor cell biology at the basic and translational level in order to provide insights that will contribute to the ultimate prevention and cure of malignant diseases.
Donald M Miller, Director
John W Eaton, Deputy Director

2242 Kentucky Cancer Program
2365 Harrodsburg Road   859-219-0772
Lexington, KY 40504-3381   Fax: 859-219-0548
                                   e-mail: dka@kcp.uky.edu
                                            www.kcp.uky.edu
The KCP provides a variety of cancer programs and services to health professionals the public patients and survivors.
Debra Armstong, Director
Diane Frasure, Administrative Associate

2243 University of Kentucky: Children Cancer Study Group
Markey Cancer Center
800 Rose Street   859-257-4500
Lexington, KY 40536-93   800-333-8874
                                        Fax: 859-323-2074
                                www.ukhealthcare.uky.edu/markey/
Kentucky Children's Hospital is the only children's hospital in the region. Patients range in age from infants through adolescents and have a variety of illness and injuries.
Michael Karpf, Executive Vice President for Health Affa
Frank Butler, VP for Medical Center Operations

2244 University of Kentucky: Lucille Parker Markey Cancer Center
800 Rose Street   859-247-4500
Lexington, KY 40536   800-333-8874
                                        Fax: 859-323-2074
                                www.ukhealthcare.uky.edu/markey/
The Markey Cancer Center mission is to eliminate the morbidity and mortality of cancer through a comprehensive program of research education clinical care and community outreach.
Alfred M Cohen MD FACS, Director
Michael Karpf, Executive Vice President for Health Affa

Louisiana

2245 Baton Rouge Regional Tumor Registry Mary Bird Perkins Cancer Center
Mary Bird Perkins Cancer Center
4950 Essen Lane   225-767-0847
Baton Rouge, LA 70809   Fax: 225-215-1215
                                            www.marybird.org
The Louisiana Tumor Registry is composed of a central office and regional registries that collect and process cancer incidence data from the state's eight established geographic regions. These eight geographic areas are based on Louisiana's historic health districts.
Todd D Stevens, President, CEO
J Gerald Jolly, Chairman

2246 Tulane University Pulmonary Diseases Critical Care and Enviromental Medicine
School of Medicine

1430 Tulane Avenue
New Orleans, LA 70112
504-988-5187
800-588-5300
e-mail: medsch@tulane.edu
www.som.tulane.edu/pulmdis/facilities
Provides state-of-the-art care to patients and teaching to trainees through several areas of academic excellence that include: Interstitial Lung Diseases; Asthma; Cystic Fibrosis; Sleep Disorders; Interventional Pulmonology; Lung Cancer; Smoking Cessation; Critical Care; and Environmental Medicine.
Lee Hamm, MD, Senior Vice President and Dean
Roy Weiner, Associate Dean for Clinical Research

Maryland

2247 Frederick Cancer Research Center
PO Box B
Frederick, MD 21702-1201
301-846-1000
Fax: 301-846-1108
web.ncifcrf.gov
Direct research into the causes treatment and prevention of cancer AIDS and related diseases.
Craig W Reynolds, Associate Director
Jo Anne Barb, Secretary

2248 Johns Hopkins University: Sydney Kimmel Comprehensive Cancer Center
The Harry and Jeanette Weinberg Buidling
401 N Broadway
Baltimore, MD 21231-0005
410-955-5222
www.hopkinskimmelcancercenter.org
Johns Hopkins Kimmel Cancer Center has active programs in clinical research laboratory research education community outreach and prevention and control.
Ronald J Danielles, President
Edward Miller MD, Dean of Medical Faculty, CEO

2249 National Foundation for Cancer Research National Foundation for Cancer Research
National Foundation for Cancer Research
4600 E W Highway
Bethesda, MD 20814-3206
301-654-1250
800-321-2873
Fax: 301-654-5824
e-mail: info@nfcr.org
www.nfcr.org
NFCR promotes and facilitates collaboration among scientists to accelerate the pace of discovery from bench to bedside. NFCR is committed to Research for a Cure - cures for all types of cancers.
Franklin C Salisbury Jr, President
Sujuan BA, Phd., COO

2250 Warren Grant Magnuson Clinical Center
National Institute of Health
9000 Rockville Pike
Bethesda, MD 20892
301-496-4000
800-411-1222
Fax: 301-480-9793
TTY: 866-411-1010
e-mail: prpl@mail.cc.nih.gov
www.clinicalcenter.nih.gov/index.html
Established in 1953 as the research hospital of the National Institutes of Health. Designed so that patient care facilities are close to research laboratories so new findings of basic and clinical scientists can be quickly applied to the treatment of patients. Upon referral by physicians, patients are admitted to NIH clinical studies.
John Gallin, Clinical Center Director
David Henderson, Deputy Director for Clinical Care

Massachusetts

2251 Boston University Cancer Research Center
820 Harrison Avenue
Boston, MA 02118
617-638-8265
Fax: 617-638-6518
e-mail: sfenness@bu.edu
www.bumc.bu.edu/clinicaltrials
The Office of Clinical Research (OCR) was established on July 1 1998 to serve as the central focus for clinical research support conduct and training at Boston University Medical Center.
Douglas V Faller, Director
Salli Fennessey, Manager

2252 Dana-Farber Institute: Department of Biostatistics and Computational Biology
450 Brookline Avenue
Boston, MA 02115-5450
617-632-3000
Fax: 617-632-2444
e-mail: biostatistics@jimmy.harvard.edu
www.dana-farber.org
Integral unit of the Institute organized into laboratories of biostatistics computing and epidemiology.
Marvin Zelen, Researcher
Edward J Benz, President, CEO

2253 David H. Koch Institute for Integrative Ca ncer Research
MIT Center for Cancer
Koch Institute at MIT 76-158
Cambridge, MA 02142
617-253-6403
Fax: 617-324-2238
e-mail: cancer@mit.edu
www.ki.mit.edu
The mission of MIT Cancer Center is to apply tools of basic science and technology to determine how cancer is caused progresses and responds to treatment. Through this effort they have developed an increasingly complete understanding of the nature of cancer cells which has led directly to improved treatments for the disease.
Dr Tyler Jacks, Director
Dr Jaqueline Lees, Associate Director

Michigan

2254 Gershenson Radiation Oncology Center Barbara Ann Karmanos Cancer Institute
Barbara Ann Karmanos Cancer Institute
4100 John Road
Detroit, MI 48201
313-745-9191
800-527-6266
Fax: 313-745-2314
e-mail: info@karmanos.org
www.karmanos.org
Radiation therapy and cancer treatment and research.
Gerold Bepler, President

2255 Meyer L Prentis Comprehensive Cancer Center of Metropolitan Detroit
Barbara Ann Karmanos Cancer Institute
4100 John Road
Detroit, MI 48201
313-745-9191
800-527-6266
Fax: 313-745-2314
e-mail: info@karmanos.org
www.karmanos.org

Gerald Bepler, President

2256 Meyer L Prentis Comprehensive Cancer Cente Barbara Ann Karmanos Cancer Institute
4100 John Road
Detroit, MI 48201
313-745-9191
800-527-6266
Fax: 313-745-2314
e-mail: info@karmanos.org
www.karmanos.org

Gerald Bepler, President

2257 University of Michigan: Cancer Center Cancer Research Committee
Cancer Research Committee
1500 E Medical Center Drive
Ann Arbor, MI 48109-094
734-764-0039
800-865-1125
Fax: 734-936-9582
www.cancer.med.umich.edu
The U-M Comprehensive Cancer Center provides its patients diagnostic treatment and support services in a collaborative environment focused on excellence in patient care.
Eric R Fearon, Associate Director for Science
Max S Wicha, Director

2258 Wayne State University Center for Molecular Medicine and Genetics
Wayne State University School of Medicine
3127 Scott Hall
Detroit, MI 48201
313-577-5323
Fax: 313-577-5218
e-mail: sshaw@wayne.edu
www.genetics.wayne.edu

Research focusing on human conditions such as cancer and neuromuscular disorders.
Lawrence I Grossman, Professor/Director
Jeffrey A Loeb, Associate Director

Minnesota

2259 Mayo Comprehensive Cancer Center
200 First Street SW
Rochester, MN 55905-0001
507-284-2511
Fax: 507-284-0161
TTY: 507-284-9786
www.mayo.edu
Scientists and physician investigators conduct wide-ranging research to improve patient care while training the next generation of medical scholars.
Denis Cortese, President/Chief Executive Officer
Robert A Rizza, Director

2260 University of Minnesota Masonic Cancer Center
Division of Oncology
420 Delaware Street SE
Minneapolis, MN 55455
612-624-8484
800-226-2376
Fax: 612-626-3069
e-mail: ccinfo@umn.edu
www.cancer.umn.edu
The Masonic Cancer Center fosters this mission by creating a collaborative research environment focused on the causes prevention detection and treatment of cancer; applying that knowledge to improve quality of life for patients and survivors; and sharing its discoveries with other scientists students professionals and the community.
Brian Steeves, Deputy Director
Ann D Cieslak, Executive Director

Missouri

2261 Cancer Research Center
3501 Berrywood Drive
Columbia, MO 65201
573-875-2255
Fax: 873-443-1202
www.cancerresearchcenter.org
Not only does the Cancer Research Center offer research they also offer community outreach programs to educate church groups civic clubs and other organizations about their research and cancer prevention.
Dr. Abe Eisenstark, Research Director
Jack Bozarth, Director

Nebraska

2262 Lincoln Cancer Center
4600 Valley Road
Lincoln, NE 68510-4844
402-483-2827
Fax: 402-483-4184
Barb Morton, Director

2263 University of Nebraska at Omaha Eppley Institute for Research in Cancer
University of Nebraska
985950 Nebraska Medical Center
Omaha, NE 68198-5950
402-559-4090
e-mail: hmmaurer@unmc.edu
www.unmc.edu/eppley
To improve the health of Nebraska through premier educational programs innovative research the highest quality patient care and outreach to underserved populations.
Harold M Maurer, Chancellor
Thomas H Rosenquist, Vice Chancellor

New Hampshire

2264 Norris Cotton Cancer Center Dartmouth-Hitchcock Medical Center
Dartmouth-Hitchcock Medical Center
One Medical Center Drive
Lebanon, NH 03756
603-653-9000
800-639-6918
Fax: 603-653-9003
e-mail: cancercenter@dartmouth.edu
www.cancer.dartmouth.edu

The Cancer Center provides a positive environment for treatment cure and recovery for patients with all forms of cancer.
Mark Israel MD, Director
Burton L Eisenberg, Deputy Director

New Mexico

2265 University of New Mexico: Cancer Research and Treatment Center
1201 Camino de Salud NE
Albuquerque, NM 87131-5001
505-272-4946
800-432-6806
Fax: 505-925-0100
www.cancer.unm.edu
One of the nation's 60 premier National Cancer Institute (NCI)-Designated Cancer Centers and we have been named one of America's Best Cancer Hospitals by U.S. News & World Report. UNM Cancer Center provides cancer diagnosis and treatment to over 40% of the adults and virtually all of the children diagnosed with cancer each year in New Mexico.
Cheryl Willman, Director/CEO
John A Trotter, Deputy EVP for Health Sciences

2266 University of New Mexico: Center for Non-Invasive Diagnosis
Mind Imaging Center/University of New Mexico
1101 Yale Boulevard NE
Albuquerque, NM 87131-0001
505-277-0111
Fax: 505-272-4056
www.hsc.unm.edu
Cardiology and cancer research.
David Lepre, Executive Director

New York

2267 Ackerman Institute for the Family
149 E 78th Street
New York, NY 10075
212-879-4900
Fax: 212-744-0206
e-mail: ackerman@ackerman.org
www.ackerman.org
Independent nonprofit research organization specializing in family therapy teaching and clinical services.
Lois Braverman, President/CEO
Evan Imber-B PhD, Director

2268 Albany Medical College Joint Center for Cancer and Blood Disorders
43 New Scotland Avenue
Albany, NY 12208
518-262-3125
877-AMC-8008
Fax: 518-262-3165
TTY: 518-262-1180
www.amc.edu
Offers research in the fields of cancer and blood disorders focusing on radiotherapy pathology and surgery.
Herbert Abbott, General Pediatric
Kevin Costello, Internal Medicine

2269 Albert Einstein Cancer Center Albert Einstein College of Medicine
Albert Einstein College of Medicine
1300 Morris Park Avenue
Bronx, NY 10461
718-430-2302
Fax: 718-430-2000
e-mail: aecc@aecom.yu.edu
www.einstein.yu.edu/centers/cancer/
The goal of AECC is to foster basic clinical population-based and translational research that addresses all aspects of the cancer problem.
Allen M Spiegel MD, Dean
David Goldman, Director

2270 Association for Research of Childhood Cancer
PO Box 251
Buffalo, NY 14225-0251
716-681-4433
e-mail: president@arocc.org
www.arocc.org
The Association was chartered by New York State in that year as a not-for-profit corporation whose primary purpose was to fund the major pediatric research centers in Western New York.
Larry Lorenz, Vice President
Anne O'Donnel, President

2271 Bassett Research Institute
One Atwell Road
Cooperstown, NY 13326   607-547-3456
                                     800-227-7388
e-mail: research.institute@bassett.edu
www.bassett.org
Research institute committed to seeking new information and new
strategies for preventing detecting and treating disease.
William F Streck MD, President/CEO

2272 Cancer Institute of Brooklyn
927 49th Street   718-972-5816
Brooklyn, NY 11219-2923   Fax: 718-972-8693
Jo-Ann Hertz, Executive Director

2273 Cancer Research Institute: New York
One Exchange Plaza 55 Broadway   212-688-7515
New York, NY 10006   800-992-2623
                                     Fax: 212-832-9376
e-mail: info@cancerresearch.org
www.cancerresearch.org
The Cancer Research Institute is the world's only non-profit organization dedicated exclusively to the support and coordination of
laboratory and clinical efforts that will lead to the immunological
treatment control and prevention of cancer.
Jill O'Donnel-Tormey, Executive Director
Leslie Anson, Assistant to the Executive Director

2274 Columbia University Comprehensive Cancer Center
630 W 168th Street   212-305-4186
New York, NY 10032   Fax: 212-305-6889
/www.cumc.columbia.edu/
Lee Goldman, President
Anne L Taylor, Vice Dean

**2275 Medical Foundation of Buffalo Hauptman-Woodward Medical
Research Insti**
Hauptman-Woodward Medical Research Institute
700 Ellicott Street   716-898-8600
Buffalo, NY 14203-1102   Fax: 716-898-8660
www.hwi.buffalo.edu
Nonprofit organization devoted to cancer research.
Herbert A Hauptman PhD, President/Nobel Laureate
Eaton E Lattman, Executive Director & CEO

2276 Memorial Sloan-Kettering Cancer Center
1275 York Avenue   212-639-2000
New York, NY 10065   888-675-7722
e-mail: publicaffairs@mskcc.org
www.mskcc.org
Sloan-Kettering Institute has endeavored to lead the way in basic
science research oftentimes translating those advances into clinical treatments.
Harold Varmus, President, CEO
Paul A Marks, President Emeritus

**2277 New York University Cancer Institute New York University
Medical Center**
New York University Medical Center
530 First Avenue   212-263-7300
New York, NY 10016   888-769-8633
                                     Fax: 212-263-0715
www.nyucancerinstitute.org
The mission of the NYU Cancer Institute is to decrease and elimi-
nate cancer as a significant health problem throughout New York
the national and the world by developing and maintaining excel-
lent programs in patient care research education and prevention.
William Carroll, Director
Lauren E Hackett, Executive Director of Administration

2278 Roswell Park Cancer Institute National Cancer Institute
Elm & Carlton Streets   716-845-2300
Buffalo, NY 14263   877-275-7724
e-mail: askrpci@roswellpark.org
www.roswellpark.org
Roswell Park Cancer Institute has made fundamental contributions to reducing the cancer burden and has successfully maintained an exemplary leadership role in setting the national
standards for cancer care research and education.
Donald L Trump MD, Director
Ann Gioia, Director

2279 State University of New York Health Science Center At Brooklyn
450 Clarkson Avenue
Brooklyn, NY 11203   718-270-1000
www.downstate.edu
Downstate includes Colleges of Medicine Nursing and Health Related Professions and a School of Graduate Studies as well as its
own teaching hospital an M.P.H. Program and extensive research
facilities.
John C LaRosa, President
John B Clark, Interim Chancellor

2280 University of Rochester: James P Wilmot Cancer Center
601 Elmwood Avenue   585-275-5823
Rochester, NY 14642   866-494-5668
                                     Fax: 585-276-0158
www.urmc.rochester.edu
To use education science and technology to improve health transforming the patient experience with fresh ideas and approaches
steeped in disciplined science and delivered by health care professionals who innovate take intelligent risks and care about the lives
they touch.
Jonathan W. Friedberg M.D., Director
Gregory Connolly, M.D., Hematology Oncology

North Carolina

**2281 Cancer Center of Wake Forest University at Bowman Gray
School of Medicine**
Wake Forest University School Of Medicine
Medical Center Boulevard   336-716-2011
Winston-Salem, NC 27157   800-446-2255
                                     Fax: 336-716-9593
e-mail: medadmit@wfubmc.edu
www1.wfubmc.edu/cancer
Provide a superb education as well as personal support. Beyond the
academic experiences offered at our medical school we encourage
the development of our students as caring physicians dedicated to
providing the very best care professionally and personally to all
patients.
William B Applegate M D M P, Dean
John D McConnell, CEO

2282 Duke Comprehensive Cancer Center
2424 Erwin Road   919-684-3377
Durham, NC 27705   888-ASK-DUKE
                                     Fax: 919-684-5653
www.cancer.duke.edu
One of only 39 centers in the country designated by the National
Cancer Institute (NCI) as a 'comprehensive cancer center ' Duke
combines cutting-edge research with compassionate care. Our
team of nationally recognized physicians and staff treat nearly 6
000 new patients per year giving them the extensive experience
that yields better results. In fact U.S. News & World Report rates
Duke #7 in the nation for cancer care and best in the Southeast.
H Kim Lyerly, Director
Anthony Means, Deputy Director

**2283 University of North Carolina UNC Lineberger Comprehensive
Cancer Center**
School of Medicine
450 est Dr   919-966-3036
Chapel Hill, NC 27514   866-869-1856
                                     Fax: 919-966-3015
e-mail: lccc@med.unc.edu
www.unclineberger.org
The Center provides multidisciplinary programs for most cancers
giving patients the benefit of many medical specialists in one place
often in one visit.
H Shelton Earp, Director
Michael O'Malley, Associate Director

Ohio

2284 Case Western Reserve University: Ireland Cancer Center
University Hospitals of Cleveland
11100 Euclid Avenue   216-844-1529
Cleveland, OH 44106   888-844-8447
www.uhhospitals.org/irelandcancer
Thomas F Senty, CEO

2285 Children's Hospital Research Foundation
700 Childrens Drive   614-722-2000
Columbus, OH 43205-2696   614-792-8401
Fax: 61 -35 -079
e-mail: CommunityLink@NationwideChildrens.org
www.nationwidechildrens.org
Offers research activities into Reye's Syndrome genetics and children's cancer chemotherapy.
Richard McClead, Medical Director
Richard J Brilli, Chief Medical Officer

2286 Medical College of Toledo: Cancer Research Division
Department of Pathology
3000 Arlington Avenue   419-383-4000
Toledo, OH 43614-2595   800-321-8383
Fax: 419-383-6130
e-mail: utmc.webmaster@utoledo.edu
www.utmc.utoledo.edu
Researches into all aspects of cancer.
Jill Zyrek-Betts, Assistant Professor

2287 Ohio State University Comprehensive Cancer Center
Arthur G James Cancer Hospital
300 W 10th Avenue   614-293-7521
Columbus, OH 43210-1240   e-mail: michael.caligiuri@osumc.edu
www.osucc.osu.edu
A national and international leader in research, which translates to high-quality patient care and educational programs for residents of Ohio and beyond.
Michael A Caligiuri M D, Director
John C Byrd, Associate Director

2288 Ohio State University General Clinical Research Center
The Ohio State University   614-293-8750
Columbus, OH 43210   Fax: 614-293-3796
e-mail: william.malarkey@osumc.edu
www.crc.osu.edu
Provides facilities and financial support for inpatient and outpatient cancer research.
William Malaykey, Program Director
David Phillips, Administrative Director

2289 The Cancer Prevention Institute
23 Jasper St   937-227-9400
Dayton, OH 45409   877-274-4543
Fax: 937-297-6970
e-mail: info@pch-dayton.org
www.premiercommunityhealth.org
Nonprofit organization focusing research activities primarily on cancer prevention anti-cancer drugs early diagnosis of cancer and bone marrow toxicity. previously known as the Hipple Cancer Research Center.
Stephen McHugh, Treasurer
Diane Ewing, Chair

Oklahoma

2290 Natalie Warren Bryant Cancer Center St. Francis Hospital
St. Francis Hospital
6600 S Yale Avenue   918-488-6688
Tulsa, OK 74136   e-mail: webadministrator@saintfrancis.com
www.saintfrancis.com/locations/nwbcc
Jake Henry Jr, President/Chief Executive Officer
Barry Steichen, Executive Vice President/Chief Administr

2291 Oklahoma Medical Research Foundation Immunobiolgy & Cancer Research
Oklahoma Medical Research Foundation
825 North East 13th Street   405-271-6673
Oklahoma City, OK 73104-5005 800-522-0211
Fax: 405-271-7016
e-mail: OMRF-President@omrf.org
www.omrf.org
Dr. Stephen Prescott, President

2292 Samuel Roberts Noble Foundation Biomedical Division
Samuel Roberts Noble Foundation
2510 Sam Noble Parkway   580-223-5810
Ardmore, OK 73401   Fax: 580-224-6217
www.noble.org

One of the largest international offshore drilling contractors in the world.
Michael A Cawley, CEO/President
Bill Goddard, Trustee

Pennsylvania

2293 Abramson Cancer Center of the University of Pennsylvania
3535 Market Street
Philadelphia, PA 19104-3309   800-789-PENN
Fax: 215-349-5445
e-mail: craig@mail.med.upenn.edu
www.penncancer.com
National leader in cancer research patient care and education.
Douglas L Fraker MD, Deputy Director
Caryn Lerman, Interim Director

2294 Allegheny Singer Research Institute West Penn Allegheny Health System
West Penn Allegheny Health System
4800 Friendship Avenue   412-362-8677
Pittsburgh, PA 15224   877-284-2000
Fax: 412-359-8610
e-mail: tchakurd@wpahs.org
www.wpahs.org
Christopher Olivia MD, President, CEO

2295 Eastern Cooperative Oncology Group
1818 Market Street   215-789-3645
Philadelphia, PA 19103   800-4CA-NCER
Fax: 267-256-5291
www.ecog.dfci.harvard.edu
Studies into cancer including biological response modifiers and cancer studies.

2296 Fox Chase Cancer Center
333 Cottman Avenue   215-728-6900
Philadelphia, PA 19111-2497 888-369-2427
www.fccc.edu
Linda Fliescher MPH PhD, Assistant Vice President for Communicati
Theresa Berger MBE, Project Manager

2297 Temple University FELS Institute for Cancer Research
School of Medicine
3500 N Broad Street   215-707-7000
Philadelphia, PA 19140   Fax: 215-707-7000
www.temple.edu/medicine
Policies and programs are oriented toward research and training in cancer-related basic biological and biochemical sciences with progressive extension into the areas of molecular developmental and chemical biology to advance knowledge of the etiology and pathogenesis of cancer. A major goal of the Institute is to utilize the advances made in basic science programs to develop novel targeted therapies for the treatment of cancer.
John M Daly MD, Dean
Diane Omdal, Director, Research Administration

2298 University of Pittsburgh Cancer Institute
5150 Centre Avenue   412-647-2811
Pittsburgh, PA 15232   e-mail: PCI-INFO@upmc.edu
www.upci.upmc.edu
Since 1985 the UPCI has been committed to improving the understanding of how cancer develops; to characterizing new lifesaving approaches for cancer prevention detection diagnosis and treatment; and to educating future generations of scientists and clinicians.
Nancy E Davidson MD, Committee Chair
Adam Brufsky MD PhD, Associate Director

Rhode Island

2299 Brown University Division of Biology and Medicine
BioMed Research Admin, Brown Medical School
The Warren Alpert Medical School of   401-863-3330
Providence, RI 02912-0001   Fax: 401-863-2660
www.biomed.brown.edu

Interdisciplinary studies in biological and medical sciences including studies in health care problems and fields of research such as cancer and diabetes.
John Perry, Senior Associate Dean
Edward J Wing, Medicine / Biological Sciences

2300 Roger Williams Clinical Cancer Research Center
Roger Williams General Hospital
825 Chalkstone Avenue
Providence, RI 02908   401-456-2000
                                   www.rwmc.com

Kenneth Belcher, President
Sheri L. Smith, Ph.D., Chair

South Carolina

2301 Children's Center for Cancer and Blood Disorders
University of South Carolina School of Medicine
7 Richland Medical Park
Columbia, SC 29203   803-434-7000
                                   www.palmettohealth.org
Joint clinical and basic research of juvenile cancer and blood disorders.
Charles D Beaman Jr, CEO

Tennessee

2302 St. Jude Children's Research Hospital
262 Danny Thomas Place   901-495-3300
Memphis, TN 38105   Fax: 901-495-4011
                                   e-mail: donors@stjude.com
                                   www.stjude.org
One of the world's premier pediatric cancer research centers.
Harvey J Cohen, Chair
William Evan PharmD, Director/CEO

2303 University of Tennessee Memphis: Cancer Center
66 N. Pauline St   901-448-5150
Memphis, TN 38163-0001   Fax: 901-528-5033
Alvin M Mauer MD, Director

Texas

2304 Baylor University Bone Marrow Transplantation Research Center
Baylor Research Institute
3500 Gaston Avenue   214-820-2687
Dallas, TX 75246   800-422-9567
                                   www.baylorhealth.com
Offers bone marrow transplantation research in leukemia studies.
John B McWhorter, President
Irving D Prengler, VP Medical Staff Affairs

2305 Cancer Therapy and Research Center
7979 Wurzbach Road   210-450-1000
San Antonio, TX 78229   800-340-2872
                                   www.ctrc.net
The mission of the Cancer Therapy & Research Center is to conquer cancer through research prevention and treatment.
Ian M Thompson MD, Director

2306 San Antonio Cancer Institute
7703 Floyd Curl Drive   210-567-7000
San Antonio, TX 78229-3900   Fax: 210-567-2709
                                   www.uthscsa.edu/
Dr Tyler J Curiel, Director
William L Henrich MD MACP, President

2307 Southwest Foundation for Biomedical Research
PO Box 760549
San Antonio, TX 78245-0549   210-258-9400
                                   www.sfbr.org
Advancing the health of our global community through innovative biomedical research.
John R Hurd, Chairman
Lewis J Moorman III, Vice-Chairman

2308 University of Texas: MD Anderson Cancer Center
1515 Holcombe Boulevard   713-792-2121
Houston, TX 77030-4009   800-392-1611
                                   www.mdanderson.org
To eliminate cancer in Texas the nation and the world through outstanding programs that integrate patient care research and prevention and through education for undergraduate and graduate students trainees professionals employees and the public.
John Mendelsohn, President -Executive Committee
Raymond DuBois, Executive Vice President

2309 University of Texas: Medical Branch at Galveston Cancer Center
301 University Boulevard   409-772-1011
Galveston, TX 77555   Fax: 409-747-1938
                                   TTY: 409-772-4200
                                   e-mail: public.affairs@utmb.edu
                                   www.utmb.edu
The mission of The University of Texas Medical Branch at Galveston is to provide scholarly teaching innovative scientific investigation and state-of-the-art patient care in a learning environment to better the health of society.
B Mark Evers, Director
David L Calender, President

Utah

2310 Brigham Young University Cancer Research Center
181 Benson Science Building   801-422-3913
Provo, UT 84602   e-mail: cancer_research@byu.edu
                                   www.cancerresearch.byu.edu
Provide a rigorous research training program for students.
Daniel L Simmons, Director
Cecil O. Samuelson, President

2311 Huntsman Cancer Institute University of Utah School of Medicine
University of Utah School of Medicine
2000 Circle of Hope   801-585-0303
Salt Lake City, UT 84112   877-585-0303
                                   Fax: 801-585-5886
                                   e-mail: public.affairs@hci.utah.edu
                                   www.huntsmancancer.org
Understand cancer from its beginnings to use that knowledge in the creation and improvement of cancer treatments to relieve the suffering of cancer patients and to provide education about cancer risk prevention and care.
Mary C Beckerle, Executive Director
Wallace Akerley, Senior Director of Clinical Research

Vermont

2312 University of Vermont Cancer Center University of Vermont
University of Vermont
E-213 Given Buildinge   802-656-4414
Burlington, VT 05405   877-540-4673
                                   Fax: 802-656-8788
                                   e-mail: info@vermontcancer.org
                                   www.vermontcancer.org
Richard Branda, Interim Director
Marianne Baggs, Assistant to the Director

Virginia

2313 Cancer Research Foundation of America
1600 Duke Street   703-836-4412
Alexandria, VA 22314-3421   800-227-2732
                                   Fax: 703-836-4413
                                   e-mail: mmcleod@crfa.org
                                   www.preventcancer.org
Prevention and early detection of cancer through research education and community outreach to all populations including children and the underserved.
Carolyn R Aldige, President and Founder
Marcia Myers Carlucci, Chairman

2314 Virginia Commonwealth University: Massey Cancer Center
401 College Street   804-828-0450
Richmond, VA 23298-5017   877-4MA-SSEY
                                                     Fax: 804-828-8453
                                              e-mail: massey@vcu.edu
                                                     www.massey.vcu.edu
The mission of the University of Central Arkansas is to maintain
the highest academic quality and to ensure that its programs remain
current and responsive to the diverse needs of those it serves.
Gordon D Ginder MD, Director
Steven Grant MD, Associate Director

Washington

2315 Fred Hutchinson Cancer Research Center
1100 Fairview Avenue N   206-288-7222
Seattle, WA 98109-1024   800-804-8824
                                                     Fax: 206-288-1025
                                              e-mail: hutchdoc@fhcrc.org
                                                     www.fhcrc.org
At Fred Hutchinson Cancer Research Center our interdisciplinary
teams of world-renowned scientists and humanitarians work together to prevent diagnose and treat cancer HIV/AIDS and other
diseases.
Lee Hartwell, Director/President
Mark Groudine, Executive Vice President and Deputy Dire

West Virginia

2316 West Virginia University: Mary Babb Randolph Cancer Center
Mary Babb Randolph Cancer Center Clinic
One Medical Center Drive   304-293-4500
Morgantown, WV 26506   877-427-2894
                                                     Fax: 304-598-4553
                                              www.wvucancer.org/pages/
Premier cancer facility with a national reputation of excellence in
cancer treatment prevention and research.
Augusto Ochoa, Director
Lori K Acciavatti, Professional Technologists

Wisconsin

2317 University of Wisconsin Paul P Carbone Comprehensive Cancer Center
600 Highland Avenue   608-263-6400
Madison, WI 53792-6164   800-622-8942
                                                     Fax: 608-263-8613
                                              e-mail: gxw@medicine.wisc.edu
                                                     www.cancer.wisc.edu
The University of Wisconsin Paul P. Carbone Comprehensive Cancer Center is the only comprehensive cancer center in Wisconsin as
designated by the National Cancer Institute. An integral part of the
UW School of Medicine and public Health this cancer center unites
more than 250 physicians and scientists who work together in
translating discoveries from research laboratories into new
treatments that benefit cancer patients.
George Wildi MD, Director
Kelly Sitkin, Development Director

Support Groups & Hotlines

2318 American Cancer Society: San Jose Prostate Cancer Support Group
3369 Union Avenue
San Jose, CA 95124-2033   408-559-8553
                                                     www.cancer.org

2319 American Foundation for Urologic Disease: Us Too Line
1128 N Charles Street   301-727-2908
Baltimore, MD 21201-5506   800-828-7866
                                              e-mail: admin@afud.org
                                                     www.afud.org
Provides information and referrals for family members, victims
and other individuals concerned with prostate cancer.

2320 American Institute for Cancer Research
1759 R Street NW   202-328-7744
Washington, DC 20009   800-843-8114
                                                     Fax: 202-328-7226
                                              e-mail: aicrweb@aicr.org
                                                     www.aicr.org
Melvin Huston, Chairman
Lawrence Pratt, Vice-Chairman

2321 Cancer Information Service
National Cancer Institute
1100 Fairview Avenue North   206-667-4675
Seattle, WA 98109-1024   800-422-6237
                                                     Fax: 206-667-7792
                                                     TTY: 800-332-8615
                                                     www.cancer.gov
Provides the latest and most accurate cancer information to patients, their families, the public, and health professionals. Also
provides personalized responses to specific questions about cancer and assistance to smokers who want to quit.
Nancy Zbaren, Program Director

2322 Cancer Support Community
3276 Mc Nutt Avenue   925-933-0107
San Francisco, CA 94597-1909   Fax: 925-933-0249
                                              www.cancersupportcommunity.net
Offers understanding, support and guidance to people with cancer
and those who care about them.
James Bouquin, President & Executive Director
Margaret Stauffer, Vice President & Program Director

2323 Cancervive
11636 Chayote Street   310-203-9232
Los Angeles, CA 90049   800-486-2873
                                                     Fax: 310-471-4618
                                              e-mail: cancervivr@aol.com
                                                     www.cancervive.org
Dedicated to providing support, public education and advocacy to
those who have experienced this disease. The mission of
Cancervive is to assist survivors to reclaim their lives after cancer.
Susan Nessim Keeney, Founder/President

2324 Center for Cancer Survival
104 W Anapamu Street   805-962-6221
Santa Barbara, CA 93101-3126
Nonprofit, nonmedical outreach education program teaching specific emotional, mental and spiritual skills for survival on their
journey of recovery from cancer.
Richard Sheldon, Founder

2325 Collaborative Medicine Center
10 Willow Street   415-383-3197
Mill Valley, CA 94941-2895
Not specifically a cancer treatment center but works with cancer
patients by using a variety of supportive modalities. The emphasis
at the center is on helping people learn to support and activate their
own healing processes.
Martin L Rossman MD

2326 Commonwealth Cancer Help Program
451 Mesa Road   415-868-0970
Bolinas, CA 94924   Fax: 415-868-2230
                                              e-mail: commonweal@commonweal.org
                                              www.commonweal.org/programs/cancer-help/
An educational program designed to help participants reduce the
stress of cancer, explore health habits, be with others experiencing
the same difficulties and consider information on established and
complementary therapeutic options.
Michael Lerner, President
Susan Braun, Executive Director

2327 Corporate Angel Network
Westchester County Airport
One Loop Road   914-328-1313
White Plains, NY 10604-1215   866-328-1313
                                                     Fax: 914-328-3938
                                              e-mail: info@corpangelnetwork.org
                                                     www.corpangelnetwork.org
To ease the emotional stress, physical discomfort and financial
burden of travel for cancer patients by arranging free flights to

treatment cetners, using the empty seats on corporate aircraft flying on routine business.
Peter H. Fleiss, Executive Director
Randall Greene, President & CEO

2328 Exceptional Cancer Patients/ECaP
532 Jackson Park Drive 814-337-8192
Meadville, CT 16335 Fax: 814-337-0699
e-mail: info@ecap-online.org, info@mind-body.org
www.ecap-online.org/home.htm
The mission of EcaP/Exceptional Cancer Patients is to provide exceptional resources, comprehensive professional training programs and extraordinary interdisciplinary retreats that help people facing the challenges of cancer and other chronic illnesses discover their inner healing resources.
Bernie Siegal MD, Founder
Barry Bittman MD, Chief Executive Officer

2329 Gilda's Club: Grand Rapids
1806 Bridge Street NW 616-453-8300
Grand Rapids, MI 49504 Fax: 616-453-8355
e-mail: info@gildasclubgr.org
www.gildasclubgr.org
A free cancer support community of children, adults, families and friends.
Leann Arkema, President/CEO
Davis Sesbastian, Chair

2330 Gilda's Club: New York City
502 Eigth Avenue 718-788-1600
Brooklyn, NY 11215 Fax: 718-788-0322
e-mail: info@gildasclubnyc.org
www.gildasclubnyc.org
Creates welcoming communities of free support for everyone living with cancer - men, women, teens and children - along with their families and friends. The innovative program is an essential complement to medical care, providing networking and support groups, workshops, lectures and social activities, all free of charge.
Robert Easton, Chairman of the Board
Lily Safani, CEO

2331 Gilda's Club: Quad Cities
1234 E River Drive 319-326-7504
Davenport, IA 52803 877-926-7504
Fax: 563-323-1658
e-mail: qc@gildasclubqc.org
www.gildasclubqc.org
A cancer support community providing people living with cancer, and all who touch their lives, access to other people going through the same experience.
Claudia Robinson, CEO
Melissa Wright, Program Director

2332 Gilda's Club: South Florida
119 Rose Drive 954-763-6776
Fort Lauderdale, FL 33316 Fax: 954-763-6761
e-mail: info@gildasclubsouthflorida.org
www.gildasclubsouthflorida.org
A free cancer support community for women, men, children, and teens with all types of cancer and their families and friends. Offer networking groups, lectures, workshops, specialized children's and teen programs, and social events in a nonresidential, non-medical, home-like setting.
Shelley Goren, CEO
Sara Howley Callari, Chair

2333 I Can Cope
American Cancer Society
1599 Clifton Road NE 404-320-3333
Atlanta, GA 30329-4250 800-227-2345
www.cancer.org
An educational program for people facing cancer, either personally, or as a friend or family caregiver. Helps dispel cancer myths by presenting straightforward facts and answers to your cancer-related questions

2334 International Association of Cancer Victors and Friends
7740 W Manchester Avenue 310-822-5032
Playa del Rey, CA 90293-8449 Fax: 310-822-4193
e-mail: IACUF@Inetworld.net
Offers reports and information on alternative therapies and recent cancer studies.
Ann Cinquina

2335 JamesCare For Life Support Groups & Services
James Cancer Hospital & Solove Research Institute
300 W 10th Avenue 614-293-5066
Columbus, OH 43210 800-293-5066
Fax: 614-293-2565
e-mail: jamesline@osumc.edu
www.cancer.osu.edu
JamesCare for Life Cancer Support Groups and Services provides a wide range of resources and services to assist patients and families on their journey. This group offers support for patients and families to share experiences, express concerns, and learn more about the impact of cancer and available treatments.
Michael A Caligiuri, CEO
Jeff Walker, Senior Executive Director

2336 Look Good... Feel Better
American Cancer Society
1599 Clifton Road NE 404-320-3333
Atlanta, GA 30329-4250 800-227-2345
www.lookgoodfeelbetter.org
A community-based, free, national service. Teaches female cancer patients beauty tips to look better and feel good about how they look during chemotherapy and radiation treatments

2337 Lung Cancer Alliance Support Group
888 16th Street NW 202-463-2080
Washington, DC 20006 800-298-2436
e-mail: kay@lungcanceralliance.org
www.lungcanceralliance.org
Dedicated solely to support and advocacy for all those living with or at risk for lung cancer.
T.Joseph Lopez, Chairman
Cheryl Healton, President & CEO

2338 National Foundation for Cancer Research Hotline
4600 E W Highway 301-654-1250
Bethesda, MD 20814 800-321-2873
Fax: 301-654-5824
e-mail: info@nfcr.org
www.nfcr.org
To support cancer research and public education relating to prevention, earlier diagnosis, better treatments and ultimately, a cure for cancer. Promotes and facilitates collaboration among scientists to accelerate the pace of discovery from bench to bedside.
Silas Deane, VP Marketing/Communications

2339 National Health Information Center
PO Box 1133 310-565-4167
Washington, DC 20013-1133 800-336-4797
Fax: 301-984-4256
e-mail: info@nhic.org
www.health.gov/nhic
A health information referral service sponsored by the Office of Disease Prevention and Health Promotion. Puts health professionals and consumers who have health questions in touch with those organizations that are best able to provide answers.
Ellen Langhans, Chairwoman
Linda Harris, Lead, Health Communication and e-health

2340 National Hospice Helpline
1731 King Street 703-837-1500
Alexandria, VA 22314 800- 64- 646
Fax: 703-837-1233
e-mail: nhcpo_info@nhpco.org
www.nhpco.org
Offers more information on hospice in general and offers referrals to a hospice program in your area.
Ronald Fried, Chair
Linda Rock, Vice Chair

2341 PDQ
National Cancer Institute

6116 Executive Boulevard   301-402-5874
Bethesda, MD 20892-8322   800-422-6237
  www.cancer.gov
An NCI database that contains the latest information about cancer treatment, screening, prevention, genetics, supportive care, and complementary and alternative medicine, plus clinical trials.
Mark Greene MD, Editor-in-Chief

2342   **Reach to Recovery**
American Cancer Society
1599 Clifton Road NE   404-320-3333
Atlanta, GA 30329-4250   800-227-2345
  www.cancer.org
Provides support for people recentlry diagnosed with breast cancer; people facing a possible diagnosis of breast cancer; those interested in or who have undergone a lumpectomy or mastectomy; those considering breast reconstruction; those who have lymphedema; those who are undergoing or who have completed treatment such as chemotherapy and radiation therapy; people facing breast cancer recurrence or metastasis

2343   **United Ostomy Associations of America Advocacy Hotline**
PO Box 512
Northfield, MN 55057-0512   800-826-0826
  e-mail: info@uoaa.org
  www.ostomy.org
A national network for bowel and urinary diversion support groups in the United States. The goal is to provide a nonprofit association that will serve to unify and strengthen its member support groups, which are organized for the benefit of people who have, or will have intestinal or urinary diversions and their caregivers.
Dave Rudzin, President

2344   **Wainwright House Cancer Support Programs**
260 Stuyvesant Avenue   914-967-6080
Rye, NY 10580-3115
Weeklong residential retreats offered four times a year to cancer patients. Retreats are devoted to cancer patient education, health promotion and stress management.
Richard Grossman, Program Director

2345   **Women's Suffrage for Prostate Cancer Awareness**
743 Caribou Court
Sunnyvale, CA 94087-4229   800-776-2262
  e-mail: info@pcawomen.org
  www.pcawomen.org
Women have banded together here to help people cope with the effects of prostate cancer on their lives and educate others about it. Members understand problems of patients and families and are here to support and educate.
Judith P. Barnhard, CPA, Chairman
May Barnhard, PC, Chairman

Books

2346   **3rd Opinion: International Directory to Complementary Therapy Centers**
Avery Publishing Group
120 Old Broadway   516-741-2155
New Hyde Park, NY 11040-5000
Discusses over 300 alternative treatment cancer centers, educational centers, support groups and other research services.

2347   **A Breast Cancer Journey: Your Personal Guidebook**
American Cancer Society
1599 Clifton Road NE   404-320-3333
Atlanta, GA 30329-4250   800-227-2345
Helps women steer through the maze of information, empowering them to take control of their disease, treatment choices, health care team and life. Guidebook format encourages the reader to organize her information in a logical, easily accessible manner, record personal feelings and concerns and understand the details of practical matters such as paperwork and insurance, legal and sexual issues, side effects of treatment, and helping the entire family with support.
440 pages paperback
ISBN: 0-944235-20-4

2348   **American Cancer Society Cancer Book**
Doubleday & Company
666 5th Avenue
New York, NY 10103-0001   212-765-6500
  www.penguinrandomhouse.com
Publishes 135 cancer organizations, centers, support services and various programs.

2349   **American Cancer Society's Guide to Complementary/Alternative Cancer Methods**
American Cancer Society
1599 Clifton Road NE   404-320-3333
Atlanta, GA 30329-4250   800-227-2345
Helps the public, the consumer and patients and their families understand what works, what's dangerous, and how best to evaluate the hundreds of claims that can be found on the internet and in the popular press. Each entry is researched and based on scientific evidence. Possible problems or complications are identified and clearly highlighted for easy reference. Covers a broad range, including herbs, vitamins, minerals, diet, manual healing and biological methods. Clear, understandable language.
464 pages hardcover
ISBN: 0-944235-20-4

2350   **American Cancer Society's Guide to Pain Control**
American Cancer Society
1599 Clifton Road NE   404-320-3333
Atlanta, GA 30329-4250   800-227-2345
Provides a wealth of information, including talking to your health care team about pain, understanding what pain is and where it comes from, current drug and non-drug treatments and dealing with the financial burden of pain treatment. Includes information on how to record, chart and rate pain, guidelines for pain management, a comprehensive list of medications and other methods of pain relief and an informative resource guide.
400 pages paperback
ISBN: 0-944235-20-4

2351   **American Cancer Society's Healthy Eating Cookbook: A Celebration of Food...**
American Cancer Society
1599 Clifton Road NE   404-320-3333
Atlanta, GA 30329-4250   800-227-2345
More than 200 pages of irresistable recipes that turn healthy eating into a celebration of good food. Features photos and recipes from a host of the American Cancer Society's celebrity friends and fans. Includes hundreds of recipes, celebrity photos and essays, a handy Smart Substitution reference section and numerous tips for healthy cooking, including smart shopping, using leftovers and eating out.
216 pages hardcover
ISBN: 0-944235-20-4

2352   **Bowel Cancer**
Oxford University Press
2001 Evans Road   800-445-9714
Cary, NC 27513-2010   800-451-7556
  Fax: 919-677-1303
  e-mail: custserv.us@oup.com
  www.global.oup.com
Offers information and public awareness on the disease of bowel cancer.
152 pages

2353   **Breast Cancer**
Branden Publishing Company
Branden Books   617-734-2045
Wellesley, MA 02482   Fax: 617-734-2046
  www.branden.com
Paperback
ISBN: 0-828319-49-9

2354   **Cancer Dictionary**
Facts on File
11 Penn Plaza   212-967-8800
New York, NY 10001   800-322-8755
  Fax: 800-678-3633
352 pages Paperback

2355   **Cancer Facts and Figures**
American Cancer Society

1599 Clifton Road NE 404-320-3333
Atlanta, GA 30329-4250 800-227-2345
Publishes over 57 treatment centers.

2356 Cancer Rates and Risks
National Cancer Institute
Building 31
Bethesda, MD 20892-0001 800-422-6237
This book is a compact guide to statistics, risk factors, and risks for major cancer sites.
136 pages

2357 Cancer Sourcebook
Karen Bellenir, author
Omnigraphics
155 W. Congress 313-961-1340
Detroit, MI 48226-4105 313-961-1383
Fax: 800-875-1340
e-mail: contact@omnigraphics.com
www.omnigraphics.com
Offers basic information on cancer types, symptoms, diagnostic methods, and treatments. Includes statistics on cancer occurrences worldwide and the risks associated with known carcinogens and activities.
2003 1119 pages
ISBN: 0-780806-33-6

2358 Cancer Therapy: Ind. Consumer's Guide to Non-Toxic Treatment & Prevention
Ralph W. Moss, author
Equinox Press
Cancer Decisions
Lemont, PA 16851 814-238-3367
800-980-1234
Fax: 814-238-3367
www.cancerdecisions.com
A must for cancer patients and their families who want: Practical information on the most promising non-toxic treatments; Scientific evidence in readable language; Well-documented resource lists and medical references.
523 pages
ISBN: 1-881025-06-3
Ralph Moss, Medical Writer

2359 Cancer in the Family: Helping Children Cope with a Parent's Illness
American Cancer Society
1599 Clifton Road NE 404-320-3333
Atlanta, GA 30329-4250 800-227-2345
A diagnosis of cancer changes a family forever. Ordinary responsibilities become more demanding, and parents sometimes need assistance in balancing all of their children's needs. This book outlines steps to take to help children understand what happens when a parent has been diagnosed with cancer. Offers suggestions for talking to children, helping them cope, answering difficult questions, managing role changes and disruptions in routines, recognizing signs that your child needs help.
272 pages paperback
ISBN: 0-944235-20-4

2360 Caregiving: A Step-By-Step Resource for Caring for the Person w/Cancer at Home
American Cancer Society
1599 Clifton Road NE 404-320-3333
Atlanta, GA 30329-4250 800-227-2345
This practical guide offers manageable solutions to the myriad conditions and situations the caregiver may face, from physical to emotional conditions and dealing with health care providers and insurance carriers, to taking care of his or her own needs as well as those of the patient. East to use, this handy reference offers thorough, concise check-lists, questions to ask, signs and symptoms to note, and where to turn for more help.
336 pages paperback
ISBN: 0-944235-20-4

2361 Celebrate! Healthy Entertaining for Any Occasion
American Cancer Society
1599 Clifton Road NE 404-320-3333
Atlanta, GA 30329-4250 800-227-2345
You can celebrate in style without taking a break from healthy eating or delicious food. This book combines 20 festive, fun theme menus with easy recipes that don't sacrifice taste. Each menu offers a combination of approximately 8 manageable recipes, including appetizers, main dishes, side dishes, desserts and even beverages. Activities and decorating ideas in each section help make entertaining a breeze.
272 pages paperback
ISBN: 0-944235-20-4

2362 Choices: Realistic Alternatives in Cancer Treatment
Harper Collins
Avenue of the Americas
New York, NY 10019 800-331-3761
Fax: 800-822-4090
www.naturalpedia.com
Covers a wide gamut of information that includes treatment centers, associations, research groups, and other facilities that are equipped to assist cancer patients and their families.

2363 Colorectal Cancer: A Compassionate Resource for Patients and Their Families
American Cancer Society
5900 Wilshire Boulevard 323-634-0080
Los Angles, CA 90036-4250 800-227-2345
www.oreilly.com
The information in this article is meant to educate and should not be used as an alternative for professional medical care.
290 pages paperback
ISBN: 0-944235-20-4

2364 Consumer's Guide to Cancer Drugs
American Cancer Society
1599 Clifton Road NE 404-320-3333
Atlanta, GA 30329-4250 800-227-2345
Created for patients, cancer survivors and caregivers. Provides detailed information for the more than 200 medicines used to treat cancer or the symptoms of cancer. Drugs are listed alphabetically by generic name and described in depth. Detailed descriptions include common side effects, precautions and other important facts. All generic and trade names are listed in the index for easy cross-reference. Easy-to-understand language.
448 pages paperback
ISBN: 0-944235-20-4

2365 Coping: A Young Woman's Guide to Breast Cancer Prevention
Rosen Publishing Group
29 E 21st Street 212-777-3017
New York, NY 10010 800-237-9932
Fax: 888-436-4643
e-mail: customerservice@rosenpub.com
www.rosenpublishing.com
Breast cancer research has revealed the genetic predisposition of some cancers. This guide explains the nature of cancer, the risk of cancer and the ways to reduce that risk, especially for young women with a family history of breast cancer.

ISBN: 0-825929-67-1

2366 Everyone's Guide to Cancer Therapy
Andrews McMeel Publishing, LLC
c/o Simon & Schuster
Riverside, NJ 08075 800-851-8923
Fax: 816-581-7486
e-mail: order-desk@Distican.com
www.andrewsmcmeel.com
How cancer is diagnosed, treated, and managed day to day.
2002 960 pages Paperback
ISBN: 0-740718-56-8

2367 Health Consequences of Smoking: Cancer & Chronic Lung Disease in the Workplace
DIANE Publishing Company
330 Pusey Ave 610-461-6200
Darby, PA 19023 800-782-3833
Fax: 610-461-6130
e-mail: dianepublishing@gmail.com
www.dianepublishing.net
Examines the relationship between cigarette smoking and occupational exposures. Establishes that in order to protect the workers fully, forces of labor, management, insurers and government must become as engaged in attempts to reduce the prevalence of ciga-

rette smoking as they are in occupational exposure. Tables and figure. Extensive bibliography, index.
542 pages Paperback
ISBN: 0-788123-11-4
Herman Baron, Publisher

2368 Healthy and Hearty Diabetic Cooking
Diabetes Self-Management Books
PO Box 11477
Des Moines, IA 50381-0001   800-664-9269
James Hazlett, Editor

2369 Home Care Guide for Cancer
John's Hopkins University Press
2715 N Charles Street   410-516-6900
Baltimore, MD 21218-4319   800-537-5487
                                  Fax: 410-516-6998
                                  www.press.jhu.edu
This easy to use workbook was designed for home caregivers, patients, support groups and education programs; it features easy to read type and index for quick reference and advice on twenty common cancer caregiving problems.
1996 260 pages Paperback
ISBN: 0-943126-30-4
Peter Houts, Editor

2370 I Choose to Fight: Tom Harper's Courageous Victory Over Cancer
Prentice Hall
15 Columbus Circle
New York, NY 10023-7707   212-373-8000
                                  www.prenhall.com
A semi, auto-biographical account of Tom Harper's ordeal with testicular cancer, an afflication in young men.

2371 Informed Decisions: The Complete Book of Cancer Diagnosis, Treatment and Recovery
American Cancer Society
1599 Clifton Road NE   404-320-3333
Atlanta, GA 30329-4250   800-227-2345
Offers the latest information on every aspect of cancer, from detection to recovery. Covers everything from cancer causes and risk, screening and diagnostic tests, and treatment strategies to coping tips and questions to ask your doctor. Includes tips on how to effectively deal with the system and get the most advanced care in the country. Helps cancer patients and families make the right kinds of decisions- decisions that suit your particular needs and desires, and help you feel in control.
690 pages hardcover
ISBN: 0-944235-20-4

2372 Love Knot
Jones & Bartlett Publishers
40 Tall Pine Drive   978-443-5000
Sudbury, MA 01776   800-832-0034
                                  Fax: 978-443-8000
                                  e-mail: info@jblearning.com
                                  www.jblearning.com
It is a world-leading provider of instructional, assessment, and learning-performance management solutions for the secondary, post-secondary, and professional markets
232 pages Paperback
ISBN: 0-763714-12-7
Joy Stark, Associate Marketing Manager

2373 My Prostate and Me: Dealing with Prostate Cancer
Addison Books
2719 Houston Avenue
Houston, TX 77009-7607   800-829-9653

2374 National Cancer Institute Fact Book
National Cancer Institute
Building 31
Bethesda, MD 20892-0001   800-422-6237
This book presents general information about the National Cancer Institute including budget data, grants and contracts and historical information.

2375 No Less a Woman
Firestone Touchstone Paperbacks/Simon & Schuster
200 Old Tappan Road
Old Tappan, NJ 07675-7005   800-999-5479
Offers intimate interviews that explore the major issues of coping and surviving breast cancer, from diagnosis and treatment to physical and psychological recovery. In their own words, ten women describe how they successfully adjusted to the changes in their bodies and their feelings about themselves.
288 pages
ISBN: 0-671868-99-3

2376 Organizing and Maintaining Support Groups for Parents
Candlelighters' Childhood Cancer Foundation
7910 Woodmont Avenue   301-657-8401
Bethesda, MD 20814-3015   800-366-2223
Benefits of self-help support groups, activities, referral systems and parent/professional relations.

2377 Prostate Cancer: A Survivor's Guide
Don Kaltenbach and Tim Richards, author
Dattoli Cancer Foundation
2803 Fruitville Road   941-365-5599
Sarasota, FL 24237   800-915-1001
                                  Fax: 941-366-3786
                                  e-mail: info@dattolifoundation.org
                                  www.dattolifoundation.org
Written with the aid of leading prostate cancer specialists, this book clearly explains tests, the latest statistics and how to interpret them.
updated 2003 256 pages
ISBN: 0-964008-89-0

2378 Prostate Cancer: What Every Man and His Family Needs to Know
American Cancer Society
1599 Clifton Road NE   404-320-3333
Atlanta, GA 30329-4250   800-227-2345
Written by a team of internationally known and respected medical experts, this newly revised edition explains everything a man needs to know about prostate cancer, the most common form of cancer (excluding skin cancer) among American men.
322 pages paperback
ISBN: 0-944235-20-4

2379 Prostate Health Workbook
Newton Malerman, author
Hunter House Publishing
424 Church Street   615-255-2665
Nashville, TE 37219   800-266-5592
                                  Fax: 615-255-5081
                                  e-mail: ordering@hunterhouse.com
                                  www.turnerpublishing.com
A practical guide for the prostate cancer patients.
2002 160 pages Paperback
Newton Malerman, Author

2380 Singing from the Soul
Bone Marrow Foundation
515 Madison Avenue   212-838-3029
New York, NY 10022-5102   800-365-1336
                                  Fax: 212-223-0081
                                  e-mail: THEBMF@BoneMarrow.org
                                  www.bonemarrow.org
Jose Carreras' autobiography describes in eloquent detail his bone marrow transplant experience.

2381 Teratologies: A Cultural Study of Cancer
Routledge
8th Floor, 711 3rd Avenue   212-216-7800
New York, NY 10017   Fax: 212-564-7854
                                  e-mail: orders@taylorandfrancis.com
                                  www.routledge.com
A distinctively feminist look at how cancer is perceived, experienced and theorized in contemporary society. Beginning with powerful personal accounts of her own illness, as well as self-help manuals and patients' personal stories, Jackie Stacey explores changing beliefs about the causes and treatments of cancer in both biomedecine and its increasingly popular alternative counterparts.
304 pages
Jackie Stacey, Author

2382 The Mountain You've Climbed: A Parent's Guide to Childhood Cancer Survivorship
500 North Broadway 314-241-1600
Saint Louis, MO 63101 Fax: 314-241-1996
e-mail: krudd@children-cancer.org
www.nationalchildrenscancersociety.org
This guide is designed to answer parent's questions regarding childhood cancer, address issues related to diagnosis and offer suggestions on how to integrate the cancer experience into all areas of the family's life. It addresses issues beginning from the time of diagnosis through the completion of treatment and beyond.
Mark Slocomb, Chairman
Mark Stolze, President/CEO

2383 Understanding Breast Cancer Genetics
Barbara T Zimmerman, PhD, author
University Press of Mississippi
3825 Ridgewood Road 601-432-6205
Jackson, MS 39211-6492 Fax: 601-432-6217
e-mail: kburgess@ihl.state.ms.us
www.upress.state.ms.us
Clinical explanations for the genetic causes of the disease women most greatly fear.
2004 128 pages Paperback
ISBN: 1-578065-79-8
Barbara T. Zimmerman, Ph.D., Author

2384 Understanding Cancer Therapies
Helen S L Chan, MD, author
University Press of Mississippi
3825 Ridgewood Road 601-432-6205
Jackson, MS 39211-6492 Fax: 601-432-6217
e-mail: kburgess@ihl.state.ms.us
www.upress.state.ms.us
A practical and hopeful guide to the many treatments available.
2006 144 pages Paperback
ISBN: 1-578066-89-1
Helen S. L. Chan, M.D., Author

2385 Understanding Colon Cancer
A Richard Adrouny, MD; FACP, author
University Press of Mississippi
3825 Ridgewood Road 601-432-6205
Jackson, MS 39211-6492 Fax: 601-432-6217
e-mail: kburgess@ihl.state.ms.us
www.upress.state.ms.us
For the general reader a concise manual of facts, warnings, prevention, treatments, and forecasts.
2002 168 pages Paperback
ISBN: 1-578062-03-9
A. Richard Adrouny, M.D., F.A.C.P., Author

2386 When a Parent Has Cancer: A Guide to Caring for Your Children
Harper Collins
10 E 53rd Street
New York, NY 10022 212-207-7000
www.harpercollins.com

ISBN: 0-060187-09-3
Wendy S. Harpham M.D., Author

2387 Women and Cancer: A Compassionate Reource for Patients and Their Families
American Cancer Society
1599 Clifton Road NE 404-320-3333
Atlanta, GA 30329-4250 800-227-2345
Concise, thorough and up-to-date, this book provides women who have been diagnosed with cancer information about the four most common cancers of the reproductive system- breast, cervical, endometrial and ovarian cancer. Each chapter describes how each organ is structured and how it functions, and the risks and benefits of new drug therapies, radiation and chemotherapy, and surgical procedures. Includes patient stories and addresses the full range of issues faced by patients and their families.
290 pages paperback
ISBN: 0-944235-20-4

2388 Young People with Cancer: A Handbook for Parents
Barry Leonard, author
DIANE Publishing Company
330 Pusey Avenue 610-461-6200
Darby, PA 19023 800-782-3833
Fax: 610-461-6130
e-mail: dianepublishing@gmail.com
www.dianepublishing.net
Gives you information on all stages of your child's cancer. It tells you what to expect and suggests ways to prepare for different situations.
109 pages Paperback
ISBN: 0-756736-59-5
Herman Baron, Publisher

Children's Books

2389 Cancer
Franklin Watts Grolier
90 Old Sherman Turnpike 203-797-3500
Danbury, CT 06816-0001 800-621-1115
Fax: 203-797-3197
www.auth.grolier.com
Discusses causes such as chemicals, viruses, radiation and oncogenes, as well as diagnosis, types of cancers, immune defenses and common treatments.
96 pages Grades 7-12
ISBN: 0-531108-03-1

2390 Cancer: Overview Series
Lucent Books
Thomson Gale
Farmington Hills, MI 48331-9187 800-877-4253
Fax: 800-363-4253
e-mail: gale.customerservice@thomson.com
www.gale.com/lucent
Questions are answered for young adults on the issues of cancer prevention and treatment.
1999 112 pages
ISBN: 1-560063-63-7

2391 Help Yourself: Tips for Teenagers with Cancer
National Cancer Institute
Building 31
Bethesda, MD 20892-0001 800-422-6237
This magazine-style booklet is designed to provide information and support adolescents with cancer.
37 pages

2392 Hospital Days: Treatment Ways
National Cancer Institute
Building 31
Bethesda, MD 20892-0001 800-422-6237
Coloring book helping to orient children with cancer to hospital and treatment procedures.
26 pages

2393 Kathy's Hats: A Story of Hope
Trudy Krisher, author
Albert Whitman & Company
250 South Northwest Hgwy 847-232-2800
Suite 320ÿ, IL 60068-2723 800-255-7675
Fax: 847-581-0039
e-mail: mail@awhitmanco.com
www.albertwhitman.com
When Kathy turns nine she learns she has cancer. When she loses her hair due to the chemotherapy, she feels ugly and awkward. This is a matter-of-fact book about a tough time and subject, and its calm and respectable treatment well serves a story that is indeed one of hope.
32 pages Hardcover
ISBN: 0-807541-16-6

2394 Kemo Shark
Kidscope
2045 Peachtree Roadÿÿ
Atlanta, GA 30309-1107 404-233-0001
www.kidscope.org

Color comic book designed to help children with the psychological and physiological changes in a family where a parent has cancer and chemotherapy.

2395 Kid's 1st Cookbook: Delicious-Nutritious Treats to Make Yourself
American Cancer Society
1599 Clifton Road NE 404-320-3333
Atlanta, GA 30329-4250 800-227-2345
Do creepy spiders, sloppy dogs and tornado swirls sound edible to you? They will to kids. Inside this beautifully illustrated hardcover edition are activities, colorful recipes and cooking tips that will turn meal preparation into exciting family fun. Kids of all ages can take charge, don a chef's hat and create delicious and nutricious snacks and dishes for every meal.
96 pages hardcover
ISBN: 0-944235-20-4

2396 Living with Cancer
Franklin Watts Grolier
90 Old Sherman Turnpike 203-797-3500
Danbury, CT 06816-0001 800-621-1115
Fax: 203-797-3197
www.auth.grolier.com
Shows how persons with cancer can overcome their illness and lead productive lives.
32 pages Grades 5-7
ISBN: 0-531108-59-7

2397 My Book for Kids with Cancer
Waterfront Books
98 Brookes Avenue
Burlington, VT 05401-3326 800-639-6063
www.waterfrontbooks.com/
Frustrated because he couldn't find any books about kids who survived cancer, Jason decided to write his own.
32 pages

2398 Our Mom Has Cancer
American Cancer Society
1599 Clifton Road NE 404-320-3333
Atlanta, GA 30329-4250 800-227-2345
When Abigail and Adrienne's mom told them she had cancer, they were afraid. But when the girls couldn't find any books that explained what might happen to their mother and what they might expect, they wrote one themselves. The girls, ages 9 and 11, tell readers that when their mother was tired during treatment, friends and family pitched in to help cook and to push her in her wheelchair. When chemotherapy made their mom's hair fall out, they threw a hat party for her.
32 pages hardcover
ISBN: 0-944235-20-4

2399 Sammie's New Mask: A Coloring Book for Friends of Children with Cancer
500 North Broadway 314-241-1600
Saint Louis, MO 63101 Fax: 314-241-1996
e-mail: krudd@children-cancer.org
www.thenccs.org
Sammie's New Mask is about a young girl named Sammie and her friend, Jack, who has cancer. This story addresses Sammie's concerns and common misconceptions about cancer. This coloring book is designed for children in kindergarten through third grade.
K-3rd Grade
Mark Slocomb, Chairman
Mark Stolze, President/CEO

2400 Sammy's Mommy Has Cancer: For Children Who Have a Loved One with Cancer
Sherry Kohlenberg, author
Magination Press (American Psychological Assoc.)
750 First Street NE 202-336-5510
Washington, DC 20002-4242 800-374-2721
Fax: 202-336-5502
TDD: 202-336-6123
e-mail: magination@apa.org
www.apamaginationpress.apa.org
Sherry Kohlenberg wrote this book after she was diagnosed with breast cancer for her son. It is a warm, sensitive, straightforward story that will help young children understand and accept the changes in their lives when a parent is diagnosed with a life threatening illness. Parents will welcome this valuable aid in explaining the illness to their children. Both the story and the introduction offer useful suggestions for involving children in the jiys and sorrows of good and bad days.
1993 32 pages Softcover
ISBN: 0-945354-55-X

2401 Silver Kiss
Delacorte
568 Broadway
New York, NY 10012-4039 212-354-6500
www.foursquare.com
This moving tale describes the feelings of Zoe as her mother dies of cancer and her family attempts to shield her from seeing the slow decline in her mother.
Grades 8-12

2402 Silver Linings: Living with Cancer
Vantage Press
516 W 34th Street 212-736-1767
New York, NY 10001-1395 Fax: 212-736-2273
Highly personal journey of one woman's battle with breast cancer for over thirty-five years. From operations, radiation treatments, and hormone therapy and her faith and hope while induring them.

ISBN: 0-533113-52-0

2403 The Mountain You've Climbed: A Young Adult Guide to Childhood Cancer Survivorship
500 North Broadway 314-241-1600
Saint Louis, MO 63101 Fax: 314-241-1996
e-mail: krudd@children-cancer.org
www.thenccs.org
This guide is designed to answer questions and address issues related to cancer survivorship for people ages 15 to 24. As survivorship rates continue to increase, the knowledge regarding late-effects also continues to increase. This survivorship guide will answer questions as well as address healthy living styles for your future.
Ages 15-24
Mark Slocomb, Chairman
Mark Stolze, President/CEO

2404 They Never Want to Tell You: Children Talk About Cancer
Harvard University Press
79 Garden Street 617-495-2600
Cambridge, MA 02138 800-448-2242
Fax: 617-495-5898
www.hup.harvard.edu
A comprehensive book that focuses on eight children who share their various experiences with cancer.
Grades 7-12
ISBN: 0-674883-70-5

2405 Waiting for Johnny Miracle
Harper & Row
10 E 53rd Street 212-207-7000
New York, NY 10022-5299
This powerful book focuses on Becky, a 17-year-old girl who must face the fear of cancer after being diagnosed with a malignant tumor. This book brings up the painful issues that come with the pain, treatment and death of cancer.
Grades 8-12

2406 Why God Gave Me Pain
Loyola University Press
3441 N Ashland Avenue 773-281-1818
Chicago, IL 60657-1355
Using a girl's diary entries, this book expounds on the side effects of cancer as well as the psychological ramifications of the debilitating disease.

Magazines

2407 American Journal of Clinical Oncology: Cancer Clinical Trials
Raven Press

1185 Ave of the Americas
New York, NY 10036-2601

212-930-9500
800-777-2295
www.lib.stu.edu.cn

Offers outstanding coverage of ongoing research in cancer treatment. This journal is the primary source for timely updates covering all aspects of cancer management.
BiMonthly
ISBN: 0-277373-2 -
Luther W Brady, Editor

2408   Cancer Detection and Prevention Journal
Elsevier
Journals Cust Ser Dept.
Orlando, FL 32887-4800

877-839-7126
Fax: 407-363-1354
e-mail: usjcs@elsevier.com
www.elsevier.com

A peer-refereed journal devoted to cancer prevention by predictive and preventitive oncology. It is uniquely focused on advances in genetics, molecular medicine and biotechnologies that have an impact on clinical oncology modalities.
2002-present

2409   Cancer Nursing: An International Journal for Cancer Care
Lippincott Williams & Wilkins
Wolters Kluwer Health
Riverwoods, IL 60015-1600

847-580-5000
800-638-3030
Fax: 301-223-2400
e-mail: orders@lww.com
www.lww.com

Addresses the whole spectrum of problems arising in the care and support of cancer patients- prevention and early detection, geriatric and pediatric cancer nursing, medical and surgical oncology, ambulatory care, nutritional support, psychosocial aspects of cancer, patient responces to all treatment modalities, and specific nursing interventions.
BiMonthly
ISBN: 0-162220-X -

2410   Diseases of the Colon and Rectum
American Society of Colon and Rectal Surgeons
85 W Algonquin Road
Arlington Heights, IL 60005

847-290-9184
Fax: 847-290-9203
e-mail: ascrs@fascrs.org
www.fascrs.org

Diseases of the Colon and Rectum (DCR) is the official journal of the American Society of Colon and Rectal Surgeons and is mailed to all members on a mothly basis as a member benefit. Non-member subscribers have access to the online version of DCR.
journal

2411   Pancreas
Raven Press
1185 Ave of the Americas
New York, NY 10036-2601

212-930-9500
800-777-2295

Provides a central forum for communication of original works involving both basic and clinical research on the exocrine and endocrine pancreas and their consequences in the disease state.
8x Year
ISBN: 0-885317-7 -
Vay Liang W Go, Editor

2412   Practice Parameters
American Society of Colon and Rectal Surgeons
85 W Algonquin Road
Arlington Heights, IL 60005

847-290-9184
Fax: 847-290-9203
e-mail: ascrs@fascrs.org
www.fascrs.org

Parameters that have been published in the scientific journal Diseases of the Colon and Rectum, along with other scientific journals. They can be found on the website under Professionals.

2413   Roswellness Magazine
Roswell Park Cancer Institute
Elm & Carlton Streets
Buffalo, NY 14263

716-845-2300
877-275-7724
e-mail: askrpci@roswellpark.org
www.roswellpark.org

A consumer magazine promoting good health habits, cancer prevention and early detection, and the services of Roswell Park Cancer Institute.
2x/year
Donald L Trump MD, FACP, President/CEO
Candace Johnson PhD, Deputy Director

2414   Skin Cancer Foundation Journal
Skin Cancer Foundation
149 Madison Avenue
New York, NY 10016-8728

212-725-5176
800-754-6490
Fax: 212-725-5751
e-mail: info@skincancer.org
www.skincancer.org

A collection of articles by physicians, scientists and lay writers on the subject.

Newsletters

2415   Candlelighters' Quarterly
Childhood Cancer Foundation
7910 Woodmont Avenue
Bethesda, MD 20814

301-657-8401
800-366-2223

Artlices on living with and treating pediatric/adolescent cancer, written by and for parents and professionals in the field. Includes reviews, resources, pen pal column, and more.

2416   Candlelighters' Youth Newsletter
Childhood Cancer Foundation
7910 Woodmont Avenue
Bethesda, MD 20814-3015

301-657-8401
800-366-2223

Offers information to teenagers and young adults on cancer issues, medical information, camps and programs.
Quarterly

2417   Exceptional Cancer Patients/ECaP Newsletter
Exceptional Cancer Patients/ECaP
532 Jackson Park Drive
Meadville, CT 16335

814-337-8192
Fax: 814-337-0699
e-mail: info@ecap-online.org, info@mind-body.org
www.ecap-online.org/home.htm

E-newsletter with inspirational articles
2x/year
Bernie Siegal MD, Founder
Barry Bittman MD, Chief Executive Officer

2418   Melanoma Newsletter
Skin Cancer Foundation
149 Madison Avenue
New York, NY 10016-8728

212-725-5176
800-754-6490
Fax: 212-725-5751
e-mail: info@skincancer.org
www.skincancer.org

For medical investigators and practitioners.

2419   Nutrition Action Healthletter
Center for Science in the Public Interest
One Rideau St
Ottawa, OT 20009-5736

613-244-7337
Fax: 613-244-1559
e-mail: cspi@cspinet.org
www.cspinet.org

The nation's leading consumer group concerned with food and nutrition issues. Focuses on diseases that result from consuming too many calories, too much fat, sodium and sugar such as cancer and heart disease.
16 pages 10 per year
Stephen Schmidt, Editor

2420   Oncology Times: The News Center for the Cancer Care Team
Lippincott Williams & Wilkins
Wolters Kluwer Health
Riverwoods, IL 60015-1600

847-580-5000
800-638-3030
Fax: 301-223-2400
e-mail: orders@lww.com
www.lww.com

Reports on breaking clinical news in oncology, radiology, surgery, chemotherapy, and biological and gene therapy, as well as the pro-

fessional, political, reimbursement, and practice management issues that affect those treating cancer patients.
2x Monthly

2421 Options: New Directions in the War on Cancer
People Against Cancer
604 E Street   515-972-4444
Otho, IA 50569-0010   Fax: 515-972-4415
e-mail: info@peopleagainstcancer.com
www.peopleagainstcancer.com
Published by People Against Cancer.
8 pages
Frank Wiewel, Executive Director

2422 Phoenix: Newsletter
Candlelighters' Childhood Cancer Foundation
7910 Woodmont Avenue   301-657-8401
Bethesda, MD 20814-3015   800-366-2223
For adult survivors of childhood cancer.

2423 Sun and Skin News
Skin Cancer Foundation
149 Madison Avenue   212-725-5176
New York, NY 10016-8728   800-754-6490
Fax: 212-725-5751
e-mail: info@skincancer.org
www.skincancer.org
Deals with skin cancer and related subjects in nontechnical terms.

2424 Support for People with Oral and Head and Neck Cancer
PO Box 53   516-759-5333
Locust Valley, NY 11560-0053   800-377-0928
Fax: 516-671-8794
e-mail: info@spohnc.org
www.spohnc.org
This a patient run support program. Other services include patient networking oportunities, a national newsletter, a resource library and insurance information and assistance.
Nancy E Leupold, President/Founder

2425 The Phoenix
United Ostomy Associations of America, Inc.
The Phoenix Magazine   949-600-7296
Mission Viejo, CA 92690   800-826-0826
e-mail: publisher@uoaa.org
www.uoaa.org
The Phoenix magazine is the official publication of the United Ostomy Associations of America, Inc. and is published four times a year- December, March, June, and September.
Quarterly

2426 Voice of Hope
National Children's Cancer Society
500 North Broadway   314-241-1600
Saint Louis, MO 63101   Fax: 314-241-1996
e-mail: krudd@children-cancer.org
www.thenccs.org
It educates donors on how their support is furthering the N.C.C.S. mission, and acknowledges supporters. Distributed to donors of the N.C.C.S.
3x/year
Mark Slocomb, Chairman
Mark Stolze, President/CEO

Pamphlets

2427 Advanced Cancer: Living Each Day
National Cancer Institute
Building 31
Bethesda, MD 20892-0001   800-422-6237
Booklet delving into all aspects of everyday living with cancer. Offers information on coping, how children react, facing the unknown, living wills, additional resources and making treatment decisions.
30 pages

2428 After Breast Cancer: A Guide to Followup Care
National Cancer Institute
Building 31
Bethesda, MD 20892-0001   800-422-6237
Explains the importance of checking for possible signs of recurring cancer by receiving regular mammograms, getting breast exams from a doctor, and continuing monthly breast self-exams.
15 pages

2429 Basic Family Library
Candlelighters' Childhood Cancer Foundation
7910 Woodmont Avenue   301-657-8401
Bethesda, MD 20814-3015   800-366-2223
A bibliography of materials on childhood cancers, medical support, death and bereavement and materials for children.

2430 Brachytherapy and IMRT
Michael Dattoli, Jennifer Cash, and Don Kaltenbach, author
Dattoli Cancer Foundation
2803 Fruitville Road   941-365-5599
Sarasota, FL 34237   800-915-1001
Fax: 941-366-3786
e-mail: info@dattolifoundation.org
www.dattolifoundation.org
A primer on seed implants and Intensity Modulated Radiation Therapy (IMRT). This booklet provides a comprehensive overview of prostate cancer treatment protocols that utilize brachytherapy and IMRT either with or without hormonal therapy.
50 pages Booklet

2431 Breast Biopsy: What You Should Know
National Cancer Institute
Building 31   301-496-4000
Bethesda, MD 20892-0001
Offers information on what happens before, during and after a breast biopsy.

2432 Breast Cancer: Understanding Treatment Options
National Cancer Institute
Building 31
Bethesda, MD 20892-0001   800-422-6237
Summarizes the biopsy procedure and examines the pros and cons of various types of breast surgery. It discusses lumpectomy and radiation therapy as primary treatment.
19 pages

2433 Breast Exams: What You Should Know
National Cancer Institute
Building 31
Bethesda, MD 20892-0001   800-422-6237
Provides answers to questions about breast cancer and breast screening methods.
10 pages

2434 Camps for Children with Cancer and their Siblings
Candlelighters' Childhood Cancer Foundation
7910 Woodmont Avenue   301-657-8401
Bethesda, MD 20814-3015   800-366-2223
A listing by state of day and overnight camp programs, children served and programs.

2435 Cancer Tests You Should Know About: A Guide for People 65 and Over
National Cancer Institute
Building 31
Bethesda, MD 20892-0001   800-422-6237
Describes the cancer tests important for people age 65 and older. Informs men and women of the exams they should be requesting when they schedule checkups with their doctors.
14 pages

2436 Cancer of the Bladder: Research Report
National Cancer Institute
Building 31
Bethesda, MD 20892-0001   800-422-6237
Offers information on the types of bladder cancer, mortality rates, diagnosis, symptoms, therapies, rehabilitation, clinical trials, and selected references.

2437 Cancer of the Colon and Rectum: Research Report
National Cancer Institute
Building 31
Bethesda, MD 20892-0001   800-422-6237

Informative pamphlet offering factual statistics on causes and prevention, detection, diagnosis, staging, treatment, followup, clinical trials and selected references.

2438 Cancer of the Ovary: Research Report
National Cancer Institute
Building 31
Bethesda, MD 20892-0001
800-422-6237

2439 Cancer of the Pancreas: Research Report
National Cancer Institute
Building 31
Bethesda, MD 20892-0001
800-422-6237
Offers information on the various types of pancreatic cancer, treatments, surgical procedures, chemotherapy, biological therapy, hormone therapy, clinical trials and selected references.

2440 Cancer of the Uterus: Endometrial Cancer
National Cancer Institute
Building 31
Bethesda, MD 20892-0001
800-422-6237
Offers information on the description and function of the uterus, incidence and mortality, possible causes and prevention, detection, diagnosis, staging, treatment, clinical trials and selected references.

2441 Cancer of the Uterus: Research Report
National Cancer Institute
Building 31
Bethesda, MD 20892-0001
800-422-6237

2442 Candlelighters Guide to Bone Marrow Transplants in Children
Candlelighters' Childhood Cancer Foundation
7910 Woodmont Avenue
301-657-8401
Bethesda, MD 20814-3015
800-366-2223
For parents who are contemplating a BMT or harvest for their child or whose child is undergoing the procedure.

2443 Chemotherapy and You: A Guide to Self-Help During Treatment
National Cancer Institute
Building 31
Bethesda, MD 20892-0001
800-422-6237
Explains chemotherapy and addresses problems and concerns of patients undergoing this treatment.

2444 Chew or Snuff is Real Bad Stuff
National Cancer Institute
Building 31
301-435-3848
Bethesda, MD 20892-2580
800-422-6237
www.nci.nih.gov
Designed for young adults, this brochure describes the health and social effects of using smokeless tobacco products.

2445 Clearing the Air: A Guide to Quitting Smoking
National Cancer Institute
Building 31
Bethesda, MD 20892-0001
800-422-6237
Offers hints on quitting smoking and cancer prevention.
24 pages

2446 Cutaneous Melanoma of the Head and Neck
American Academy of Otolaryngology
1650 Diagonal Road
703-836-4444
Alexandria, VA 22314-3357
Fax: 703-683-5100
www.entnet.org
Self-instruction package.
Paperback
ISBN: 1-567720-22-6

2447 Diet, Nutrition and Cancer Prevention: The Good News
National Cancer Institute
Building 31
Bethesda, MD 20892-0001
800-422-6237
Provides an overview of dietary guidelines that may assist individuals in reducing their risks for some cancers.
16 pages

2448 Diet, Nutrition and Cancer Prevention: A Guide to Food Choices
National Cancer Institute
Building 31
Bethesda, MD 20892-0001
800-422-6237

Describes what is known about diet, nutrition and cancer prevention. Provides information about foods that contain components like fiber, fat and vitamins that may affect a person's risk of getting certain cancers.

2449 Dilemmas of Providing Help in a Crisis: The Role of Friends & Parents
Candlelighters' Childhood Cancer Foundation
7910 Woodmont Avenue
301-657-8401
Bethesda, MD 20814-3015
800-366-2223

2450 Do the Right Thing: Get a Mammogram
National Cancer Institute
Building 31
Bethesda, MD 20892-0001
800-422-6237
Targets black women age 40 and older. Describes the importance of regular mammograms in the early detection of breast cancer.

2451 Eating Hints: Recipes and Tips for Better Nutrition During Cancer Treatment
National Cancer Institute
Building 31
Bethesda, MD 20892-0001
800-422-6237
Provides recipes that help patients meet their needs for good nutrition during treatment.

2452 Facing Forward: A Guide for Cancer Survivors
National Cancer Institute
Building 31
Bethesda, MD 20892-0001
800-422-6237
Presents a concise overview of important survivor issues, including ongoing health needs, psychosocial concerns, insurance and employment.
43 pages

2453 Facts About Lung Cancer
American Lung Association
1740 Broadway
New York, NY 10019-4315
212-315-8700
www.librarylovers.org.au

2454 Facts About Radon
American Lung Association
1740 Broadway
New York, NY 10019-4315
212-315-8700
www.librarylovers.org.au

2455 Help, Hope, Believe
National Children's Cancer Society
500 North Broadway
314-241-1600
Saint Louis, MO 63101
Fax: 314-241-1996
e-mail: krudd@children-cancer.org
www.thenccs.org
N.C.C.S. Informational Brochure
3x/year
Mark Slocomb, Chairman
Mark Stolze, President/CEO

2456 Helping Children Cope While a Sibling Undergoes Bone Marrow Transplant
Bone Marrow Foundation
515 Madison Avenue
212-838-3029
New York, NY 10022-5102
Fax: 212-223-0081
e-mail: THEBMF@BoneMarrow.org
www.bonemarrow.org
Discusses the wide array of emotions felt by the entire family as a child receives a bone marrow transplant.

2457 If You've Thought About Breast Cancer
Rose Kushner Breast Cancer Advisory Center
PO Box 224
Kensington, MD 20895-0224
Fax: 301-897-3444

2458 Immune System: How it Works
National Cancer Institute
Building 31
Bethesda, MD 20892-0001
800-422-6237
Written for the high school level, this booklet explains the human immune system for the general public. It describes the sophistica-

tion of the body's immune responses, the impact of immune disorders and the relation of the immune system to cancer therapies.
28 pages

2459 Informed Consent: Does the Current Process Reflect Current Treatments
Candlelighters' Childhood Cancer Foundation
7910 Woodmont Avenue   301-657-8401
Bethesda, MD 20814-3015   800-366-2223

2460 Insurance Articles
Candlelighters' Childhood Cancer Foundation
7910 Woodmont Avenue   301-657-8401
Bethesda, MD 20814-3015   800-366-2223
Includes: Tips on securing health insurance for childhood cancer survivors and patients, Stay a step ahead of you insuruer, and others.

2461 Interpreting Your PSA and Related Prostate Cancer Blood Tests
Michael Dattoli, Jennifer Cash, and Don Kaltenbach, author
Dattoli Cancer Foundation
2803 Fruitville Road   941-365-5599
Sarasota, FL 34237   800-915-1001
                                    Fax: 941-366-3786
                        e-mail: info@dattolifoundation.org
                               www.dattolifoundation.org
Provides a comprehensive overview of the PSA (prostate specific antigen) blood test and other related lab tests including the PSA velocity, free and bound PSA, and the PAP (prostatic Acid Phosphatase) blood test.
2006 50 pages Booklet

2462 Leading Self-Help Groups: Report on Workshop for Leaders of Groups
Candlelighters' Childhood Cancer Foundation
7910 Woodmont Avenue   301-657-8401
Bethesda, MD 20814-3015   800-366-2223

2463 Letter to a Friend Whose Child is Newly Diagnosed with Cancer
Candlelighters' Childhood Cancer Foundation
7910 Woodmont Avenue   301-657-8401
Bethesda, MD 20814-3015   800-366-2223

2464 Managing Your Child's Eating Problems During Cancer Treatment
National Cancer Institute
Building 31
Bethesda, MD 20892-0001   800-422-6237
Contains information about the importance of nutrition, side effects of cancer and its treatment.
32 pages

2465 Mastectomy: A Treatment for Breast Cancer
National Cancer Institute
Building 31
Bethesda, MD 20892-0001   800-422-6237
Presents information about the different types of breast surgery, explains what to expect at the hospital and during the recovery period.
25 pages

2466 Melanoma: Research Report
National Cancer Institute
Building 31
Bethesda, MD 20892-0001   800-422-6237
Offers information on types of skin cancer, detection, diagnosis, staging, treatment, clinical trials, selected references and additional information for patients with skin cancer.

2467 Nutrition for Patients Receiving Chemotherapy/Radiation Treatment
National Cancer Institute
Building 31
Bethesda, MD 20892-0001   800-422-6237
Describes the importance of maintaining nutritional intake while receiving chemotherapy and radiation.

2468 Once a Year for a Lifetime
National Cancer Institute
Building 31
Bethesda, MD 20892-0001   800-422-6237
Targets all women age 40 and older describing the importance of regular mammograms in the early detection of breast cancer.

2469 Oral Cancers: Research Report
National Cancer Institute
Building 31
Bethesda, MD 20892-0001   800-422-6237
Describes types of oral cancer, causes and risk factors, symptoms, prevention, detection, diagnosis, treatment, staging, methods of treatments, followup care, clinical trials and selected references for more information.

2470 Pap Test: It Can Save Your Life
National Cancer Institute
Building 31
Bethesda, MD 20892-0001   800-422-6237
Easy-to-read pamphlet tells women of the importance of getting a Pap test, how often to get it done and where to go to get it.

2471 Preparing your Child for a Bone Marrow Transplant
Bone Marrow Foundation
515 Madison Avenue   212-838-3029
New York, NY 10022-5102   Fax: 212-223-0081
                        e-mail: THEBMF@BoneMarrow.org
                                  www.bonemarrow.org
Discusses the wide array of emotions felt by the entire family as a child receives a bone marrow transplant.

2472 Questions and Answers About Breast Lumps
National Cancer Institute
Building 31
Bethesda, MD 20892-0001   800-422-6237
Describes some of the most common noncancerous breast lumps and what can be done about them.
22 pages

2473 Questions and Answers About Choosing a Mammography Facility
National Cancer Institute
Building 31
Bethesda, MD 20892-0001   800-422-6237
Lists questions to ask in selecting a quality mammography facility.

2474 Questions and Answers About DES Exposure During Pregnancy and Before Birth
National Cancer Institute
Building 31
Bethesda, MD 20892-0001   800-422-6237

2475 Questions and Answers About Metastatic Cancer
National Cancer Institute
Building 31
Bethesda, MD 20892-0001   800-422-6237
Presents information on detection, treatment methods and common areas of reoccurrence.

2476 Questions and Answers About Pain Control
National Cancer Institute
Building 31
Bethesda, MD 20892-0001   800-422-6237
Discusses pain control using both medical and nonmedical methods.

2477 Radiation Therapy and You: A Guide To Self-Help During Treatment
National Cancer Institute
Building 31
Bethesda, MD 20892-0001   800-422-6237
Explains radiation therapy and addresses concerns of patients receiving radiation treatment.

2478 Recurrence: What Do I Do Now?
Dattoli Cancer Foundation
2803 Fruitville Road   941-365-5599
Sarasota, FL 34237   800-915-1001
                                    Fax: 941-366-3786
                        e-mail: info@dattolifoundation.org
                               www.dattolifoundation.org

This booklet offers comprehensive information on the issues surrounding ruccurence: detection, risk categories, treatment options including radiation, brachytherapy, and hormone therapy.
58 pages Booklet

2479 Research Report: Adult Kidney Cancer and Wilms' Tumor
National Cancer Institute
Building 31
Bethesda, MD 20892-0001   800-422-6237

2480 Skin Cancers, Basal Cell and Squamous Cell Carcinomas: Research Report
National Cancer Institute
Building 31
Bethesda, MD 20892-0001   800-422-6237
Offers information on types of skin cancer, incidence and mortality, risk factors, prevention, symptoms, detection, diagnosis, staging, treatment, followup care and clinical trials.

2481 Students with Cancer: A Resource for the Educator
National Cancer Institute
Building 31
Bethesda, MD 20892-0001   800-422-6237
Designed for teachers who have students with cancer in their classrooms or schools.
22 pages

2482 Sunlight, Ultraviolet Radiation and the Skin
National Cancer Institute
Building 31
Bethesda, MD 20892-0001   800-422-6237

2483 Support Systems for Parents of Children with Cancer
Candlelighters' Childhood Cancer Foundation
7910 Woodmont Avenue   301-657-8401
Bethesda, MD 20814-3015   800-366-2223

2484 Taking Time: Support for People with Cancer & People Who Care for Them
National Cancer Institute
Building 31
Bethesda, MD 20892-0001   800-422-6237
Discusses the emotional sides of cancer. how to deal with the disease and learn to talk with friends, family members and others about cancer.

2485 Talking with Your Child About Cancer
National Cancer Institute
Building 31
Bethesda, MD 20892-0001   800-422-6237
Designed for the parent whose child has been diagnosed with cancer.
16 pages

2486 Testicular Cancer: Research Report
National Cancer Institute
Building 31
Bethesda, MD 20892-0001   800-422-6237

2487 Testicular Self-Examination
National Cancer Institute
Building 31
Bethesda, MD 20892-0001   800-422-6237
Contains information about risks and symptoms of testicular cancer and provides instructions on how to perform testicular self-examination.

2488 What You Need to Know About Bladder Cancer
National Cancer Institute
Building 31   301-496-4000
Bethesda, MD 20892-0001
Offers information on the history, symptoms, diagnosis, treatment, followup care, support groups, medical terms and resources for more information.

2489 What You Need to Know About Cancer
National Cancer Institute
Building 31
Bethesda, MD 20892-0001   800-422-6237
Offers information on signs and symptoms, diagnosis, treatment, early detection and advances in medical technology.

2490 What You Need to Know About Cancer of The Colon and Rectum
National Cancer Institute
Building 31
Bethesda, MD 20892-0001   800-422-6237
Offers information on symptoms, diagnosis, treatments, and support for cancer patients.

2491 What You Need to Know About Cervical Cancer
National Cancer Institute
Building 31
Bethesda, MD 20892-0001   800-422-6237
Areas covered include early detection, symptoms, treatments, diagnosis, followup care, support, medical terms and resources.

2492 What You Need to Know About Esophagal Cancer
National Cancer Institute
Building 31
Bethesda, MD 20892-0001   800-422-6237
Offers information on symptoms, causes, preventions, diagnosis, support, medical terms and available resources.

2493 What You Need to Know About Kidney Cancer
National Cancer Institute
Building 31
Bethesda, MD 20892-0001   800-422-6237
Offers factual information on diagnosis, symptoms, prevention, treatment and referral sources.

2494 What You Need to Know About Larynx Cancer
National Cancer Institute
Building 31
Bethesda, MD 20892-0001   800-422-6237
Offers information on what cancer is, symptoms, diagnosis, treatment options, side effects of medication, rehabilitation, learning to speak again, living with cancer, causes and preventions, medical terms and resources.

2495 What You Need to Know About Lung Cancer
National Cancer Institute
Building 31
Bethesda, MD 20892-0001   800-422-6237
Offers information on types of lung cancer, symptoms, diagnosis, treatments, support, medical terms and resources.

2496 What You Need to Know About Oral Cancers
National Cancer Institute
Building 31
Bethesda, MD 20892-0001   800-422-6237
Offers information on symptoms, diagnosis, treatments, rehabilitation, followup care, support, medical terms and resources for cancer patients.

2497 What You Need to Know About Ovarian Cancer
National Cancer Institute
Building 31
Bethesda, MD 20892-0001   800-422-6237
Early detection, symptoms, diagnosis, treatments, medical terms and resources for further information.

2498 What You Need to Know About Pancreatic Cancer
National Cancer Institute
Building 31
Bethesda, MD 20892-0001   800-422-6237
Offers information on symptoms, diagnosis, treatment, support, medical terms and resources.

2499 What You Need to Know About Prostate Cancer
National Cancer Institute
Building 31
Bethesda, MD 20892-0001   800-422-6237
Offers information on symptoms, diagnosis, treatment options, side effects of medications, followup care, living with cancer and support resources for patients.

2500 What You Need to Know About Skin Cancer
National Cancer Institute
Building 31
Bethesda, MD 20892-0001   800-422-6237

Offers information on types of skin cancer, symptoms, causes, prevention, treatment planning, treating skin cancer, research and medical terms.

2501 What You Need to Know About Testicular Cancer
National Cancer Institute
Building 31
Bethesda, MD 20892-0001   800-422-6237
Offers information on the symptoms, diagnosing of testicular cancer, side effects of treatments, followup care, support for patients, cancer research, medical terms and resources.

2502 What You Need to Know About Uterine Cancer
National Cancer Institute
Building 31
Bethesda, MD 20892-0001   800-422-6237
Offers information on symptoms, diagnosing cancer of the uterus, treatments, followup care, support for patients, medical terms and resources.

2503 What You Need to Know About...
National Cancer Institute
Building 31
Bethesda, MD 20892-0001   800-422-6237
This is a series of booklets, broken down in this directory. Each provides information about a specific type of cancer. These booklets discuss emotional issues, treatment, diagnosis, symptoms and questions to ask the doctor about cancer.

2504 What are Clinical Trials All About?
National Cancer Institute
Building 31
Bethesda, MD 20892-0001   800-422-6237
Explains clinical trials (studies of new cancer treatments) to help patients decide if they want to take part in a trial.

2505 When Cancer Recurs: Meeting the Challenge Again
National Cancer Institute
Building 31
Bethesda, MD 20892-0001   800-422-6237
Offers information on why cancer can recur, where cancers can recur, diagnosing recurrent cancer, treatment methods and resources that offer more help.

2506 When Someone in Your Family Has Cancer
National Cancer Institute
Building 31
Bethesda, MD 20892-0001   800-422-6237
Written for young people whose parent or sibling has cancer.
28 pages

2507 Who is This Person Who Helped Save My Life
Bone Marrow Foundation
515 Madison Avenue   212-838-3029
New York, NY 10022-5102   Fax: 212-223-0081
e-mail: THEBMF@BoneMarrow.org
www.bonemarrow.org
Discusses the wide range of emotions for a patient in the process of searching for and identifying a donor.

2508 Why Do You Smoke?
National Cancer Institute
Building 31
Bethesda, MD 20892-0001   800-422-6237
Contains a self-test to determine why people smoke and suggest alternatives that can help them stop and prevent cancer.

2509 Wish Fulfillment Organizations
Candlelighters' Childhood Cancer Foundation
7910 Woodmont Avenue   301-657-8401
Bethesda, MD 20814-3015   800-366-2223
A list of groups granting wishes of children with life-threatening, chronic or terminal illnesses, with criteria and contacts.

2510 Young People with Cancer: A Handbook for Parents
National Cancer Institute
Building 31
Bethesda, MD 20892-0001   800-422-6237

Discusses the most common types of childhood cancer, treatments, and side effects and issues that may arise when a child is diagnosed with cancer.
86 pages

Audio & Video

2511 Beyond the Loss of the Breast
Fanlight Productions
4196 Washington Street   617-469-4999
Boston, MA 02131-1731   800-937-4113
Fax: 617-469-3379
e-mail: fanlight@fanlight.com
www.fanlight.com
This video addresses breast cancer throught the personal narratives and poetry of two women living with recurrent breast cancer and the film maker, whose mother died from metastatic disease.
1994 25 Minutes
ISBN: 1-572951-68-0

2512 Living with Ovarian Cancer
National Ovarian Cancer Coalition
2501 Oak Lawn Avenue   561-393-0005
Dallas, TX 5219   888-682-7426
Fax: 561-393-7275
e-mail: nocc@ovarian.org
www.ovarian.org
Videotape for women who have been recently diagnosed with ovarian cancer. Created to orient and inform patients and their families; describes the experiences of individuals intimately connected with the disease.
Suzy Lockwood-Rayermann RN, Chair
Julene Fabrizio, President

2513 Not Just a Cancer Patient
Fanlight Productions
4196 Washington Street   617-469-4999
Boston, MA 02131-1731   800-937-4113
Fax: 617-469-3379
e-mail: fanlight@fanlight.com
www.fanlight.com
Focuses on several articulate teenagers who are undergoing cancer treatment to help caregivers understand the needs and feelings of this population.
1991 23 Minutes
ISBN: 1-572950-86-2

2514 Skin Cancer: Preventable and Curable
Skin Cancer Foundation
149 Madison Avenue   212-725-5176
New York, NY 10016-8728   800-754-6490
Fax: 212-725-5751
e-mail: info@skincancer.org
www.skincancer.org

Web Sites

2515 American Academy of Dermatology
www.aad.org
An organization of doctors who specialize in diagnosing and treating skin problems.

2516 American Cancer Society
www.cancer.org
Provides free printed materials, offers a range of services to patients and their families.

2517 American Lung Association
www.lung.org
A voluntary organization interested in the prevention and control of lung disease.

2518 American Prostate Society
www.ameripros.org
Organization dedicated exclusively to using existing medical capabilities to reduce death due to prostate cancer and to reduce unnecessary or ineffective prostate surgery.

2519 American Society of Colon and Rectal Surgeons

www.fascrs.org

Represents more than 1000 board certified colon and rectal surgeons and other surgeons dedicated to advancing and promoting the science and practice of the treatment of patients with diseases and disorders affecting the colon, rectum and anus.

2520 Association for the Cure of Cancer of the Prostate

www.capcure.org

2521 Bone Marrow Foundation

www.bonemarrow.org

The Bone Marrow Foundation offers financial assistance and free support services to bone marrow/stem cell transplant patients and their families. The foundation relies 100% on private donations to provide these vital services.

2522 Healing Well

www.healingwell.com

An online health resource guide to medical news, chat, information and articles, newsgroups and message boards, books, disease-related web sites, medical directories, and more for patients, friends, and family coping with disabling diseases, disorders, or chronic illnesses.

2523 Health Finder

www.healthfinder.gov

Searchable, carefully developed web site offering information on over 1000 topics. Developed by the US Department of Health and Human Services, the site can be used in both English and Spanish.

2524 Healthlink USA

www.healthlinkusa.com

Health information concerning treatment, cures, prevention, diagnosis, risk factors, research, support groups, email lists, personal stories and much more. Updated regularly.

2525 Helios Health

www.helioshealth.com

Online resource for your health information. Detailed information about specific health topics, access to expert advice from our Medical Advisory Board, and up-to-date health news.

2526 International Association of Eating Disorders Professionals

www.iaedp.com

Supplies printed information and sponsors meetings and other activities. Publishes a directory of speech instructors and maintains a list of sources for supplies for laryngectomee.

2527 Leukemia and Lymphoma Society

www.leukemia.org

A national voluntary health agency dedicated to curing leukemia, lymphoma, Hodgkin's disease and myeloma and to improving the quality of life of patients and their families.

2528 MedicineNet

www.medicinenet.com

An online resource for consumers providing easy-to-read, authoritative medical and health information.

2529 Medscape

www.medscape.com

Medscape offers specialists, primary care physicians, and other health professionals the Web's most robust and integrated medical information and educational tools.

2530 National Alliance of Breast Cancer Organizations

www.nabco.org

A network of breast cancer organizations that provides information, assistance and referral to anyone with questions about breast cancer and acts as a voice for the interests and concerns of breast cancer survivors and women at risk.

2531 National Ovarian Cancer Coalition

www.ovarian.org

Our mission is to raise awareness about ovarian cancer and to promote education about the disease.

2532 Support for People with Oral and Head and Neck Cancer

www.spohnc.org

Nonprofit organization founded in 1991 to address the broad emotional, physical and humanistic needs of oral and head and neck cancer patients.

2533 United Ostomy Association

www.uoa.org

A national network for bowel and urinary diversion support groups in the United States. Its goal is to provide a nonprofit association that will serve to unify and strengthen its member support groups, which are organized for the benefit of people who have, or will have intestinal or urinary diversions and their caregivers.

2534 WebMD

www.webmd.com

Provides credible information, supportive communities, and in-depth reference material about health subjects. A source for original and timely health information as well as material from well known content providers.

2535 Webhelp

www.webhelp.com

Provides links to information, including research, treatment, prevention, support, and more.

Description

2536 Carpal Tunnel Syndrome

Carpal Tunnel Syndrome, CTS, is a painful, often debilitating condition caused by compression of the median nerve as it passes through the wrist (carpal tunnel) to the hand. CTS most commonly occurs in women aged 30 to 50 years. The incidence is highest among keyboard users, secretaries, musicians, assembly-line workers, and others who engage in repetitive handwork.

An initial indication of CTS is a feeling that the hand is asleep. Typically, the patient wakes at night with numbness and tingling of the affected hand. The most serious functional problem occurs when it becomes difficult or impossible to move the thumb into a grasping position with the other fingers. In advanced cases, pain associated with CTS may radiate up the arm to the shoulder. While job-related movement is the most common cause of CTS, people with underlying conditions, such as diabetes, gout, rheumatoid arthritis, obesity and pregnancy, are more prone to experience symptoms. Although less common, the onset of CTS can stem from trauma, such as a blow to the hand or wrist.

Diagnosis involves the Phalen Test, in which the hands are placed together, back to back and the wrist is flexed. This maneuver generally produces tingling of the hand in a patient with CTS. Diagnosis is confirmed by testing how quickly an impulse is transmitted along the median nerve.

The condition can most often be successfully treated based on an understanding of workplace movement issues — ergonomics. keyboard users, and those engaged in similar activities, should adjust their seats and backrests to assure that their arms are positioned comfortably during work sessions. For mild cases of CTS, a lightweight brace, especially worn at night, can decrease symptoms by holding the wrist stable. Marked improvement may arise from wearing a brace for a week or two. However, in many cases, it is recommended that the sufferer cease working until symptoms have improved. Exercises and deep-tissue massage can strengthen the wrist and hand.

Over-the-counter anti-inflammatory medications, such as ibuprofen and aspirin, can also reduce symptoms of mild Carpal Tunnel Syndrome. In more acute conditions, cortisone injections may be administered. When symptoms are severe and persistent, surgery may be required to reduce pressure on the nerves. The most common surgery is an open incision technique called open carpal tunnel release, which usually improves the condition dramatically. A newer and less invasive procedure is endoscopic carpal tunnel release, which uses a smaller incision and visualizes the operative field using a fiber optic camera.

National Agencies & Associations

2537 American Academy of Orthopaedic Surgeons
6300 N River Road
Rosemont, IL 60018-4262

847-823-7186
800-346-2267
Fax: 847-823-8125
e-mail: custserv@aaos.org
www7.aaos.org

The American Academy of Orthopaedic Surgeons provides education and practice management services for orthopaedic surgeons and allied health professionals. The Academy also serves as an advocate for improved patient care and to inform the public.
Joshua J Jacobs, President
Andrew N Pollak, Treasurer

2538 American Chronic Pain Association
PO Box 850
Rocklin, CA 95677

800-533-3231
Fax: 916-632-3208
e-mail: ACPA@pacbell.net
www.theacpa.org

ACPA mission is to facilitate peer support and education for individuals with chronic pain and their families so that these individuals may live more fully in spite of their pain and to raise awareness among the health care community and policy makers.
Penny Cowan, Executive Director
Mary Jane Bentÿ, Development and Distance Education at th

2539 American Society for Surgery of the Hand
822 W. Washington Boulevard
Chicago, IL 60607

312-880-1900
Fax: 847-384-1435
e-mail: info@assh.org
www.assh.org

The mission of the ASSH is to advance the science and practice of hand and upper extremity surgery through education research and advocacy on behalf of patients and practitioners.
Mark C Anderson CAE, Executive VP, CEO
W. P. Andre Lee, President

2540 Arthritis Trust of America
7376 Walker Road
Fairview, TN 37602-8141

615-799-1002
e-mail: admin@arthritistrust.org
www.arthritistrust.org

The Arthritis Trust of America provides information about auto-immune or collagen tissue diseases such as Rheumatoid Arthritis and related diseases. They provide publications and physician referrals and when funds are available they fund research.
Perry A Chapdelaine BA MA, Executive Director
Cheryl Jacobsen, President

2541 National Institute of Arthritis and Musculoskeletal and Skin Disease (NIAMS)
1 AMS Circle
Bethesda, MD 20892-3675

301-495-4484
888-226-4267
Fax: 301-718-6366
TTY: 301-565-2966
e-mail: niamsinfo@mail.nih.gov
www.niams.nih.gov

The NIAMS Information Clearinghouse provides information about various forms of arthritis and rheumatic disease and bone, muscle, and skin diseases. It distributes patient and professional education materials and refers people to other sources of information.
Stephen I Katz MD, PhD, Director/Chairman
Lynda F Bonewald Ph.D, Lefkowitz Professor

Research Centers

2542 Center for Neurology & Stroke Baptist Hospital Office
Baptist Hospital Office
333 West Thomas Road
Phoenix, AZ 85015

602-335-0300
Fax: 602-249-3118
e-mail: info@cnsaz.com
www.cnsaz.com

Providing comprehensive testing and consulting for neurological disorders.

2543 Michigan Hand Center
1111 Leffingwell Avenue NE
Grand Rapids, MI 49525
616-459-7101
800-582-7244
Fax: 616-957-0444
e-mail: info@michiganhandcenter.com
www.oamichigan.com

Janid Pike, Director
Samuel Agnew, MD,FACS

2544 National Institute of Arthritis & Musculoskeletal Skin Diseases
National Institutes of Health
I AMS Circle
Bethesda, MD 20892-3675
301-495-4484
Fax: 301-718-6366
TTY: 301-565-2966
e-mail: niamsinfo@mail.nih.gov
www.niams.nih.gov

Support Groups & Hotlines

2545 National Health Information Center
PO Box 1133
Washington, DC 20013-1133
310-565-4167
800-336-4797
Fax: 301-984-4256
e-mail: info@nhic.org
www.health.gov/nhic

A health information referral service sponsored by the Office of Disease Prevention and Health Promotion. Puts health professionals and consumers who have health questions in touch with those organizations that are best able to provide answers.
Ellen Langhans, Chairwoman
Linda Harris, Lead, Health Communication and e-health

Books

2546 Occupational Therapy Practice Guidelines for Adults with Carpal Tunnel Syndrome
American Occupational Therapy Association
4720 Montgomery Lane
Bethesda, MD 20814-1220
301-652-6611
Fax: 240-762-5150
TDD: 800-377-8555
www.aota.org

13 pages Paperback
ISBN: 1-569001-47-2

2547 Pain Free Typing Techniques: Simple Solutions to Prevent Strain Injury
Howard Richman, author

Sound Feelings Publishing
18375 Ventura Boulevard
Tarzana, CA 91356
818-757-0600
e-mail: information@soundfeelings.com
www.soundfeelings.com

This 12 page booklet provides drug-free treatments and suggestions for repetitive motion disorder and cumulative trauma disorders. Unconventional concepts for increasing human performance are revealed, which help prevent computer-related illnesses including hand pain, wrist pain, and other keyboard ergonomics. Most repetitive motion disorders and overuse injuries can be improved by correcting certain angles and positions.
1999 12 pages Booklet
ISBN: 1-882060-80-6

Pamphlets

2548 Carpal Tunnel Syndrome
Arthritis Foundation
535 Connecticut Avenue
Norwalk, CT 06854-0669
203-828-0349
800-283-7800
Fax: 404-872-0457
e-mail: jmitchell@belvoir.com
www.harvardhealthcontent.com

Offers an introduction to Carpal Tunnel, causes, symptoms, diagnosis and resources.

Web Sites

2549 Avoiding Carpal Tunnel Syndrome
www.indiana.edu/~ucsstaff/cts.html
A guide for computer keyboard users, by Mark Sheehan, reprinted from the University Computing Times.

2550 CTD Resource Network
www.ctdrn.org
This is an organization providing educational material and charitable assistance related to the prevention and treatment of cumulative trauma disorders, also known as repetitive strain injuries.

2551 Carpal Tunnel Syndrome Home Page
www.ctsplace.com
Information about carpal tunnel syndrome (CTS) and how to prevent it.

2552 Computer-Related Repetitive Strain Injury
rsi.unl.edu
Contains advice on proper posture and equipment from Paul Marxhausen, an engineering electronics technician.

2553 Health Finder
www.healthfinder.gov
Searchable, carefully developed web site offering information on over 1000 topics. Developed by the US Department of Health and Human Services, the site can be used in both English and Spanish.

2554 MedicineNet
www.medicinenet.com
An online resource for consumers providing easy-to-read, authoritative medical and health information.

2555 Neurology Channel
www.healthcommunities.com
Find clearly explained, medically accurate information regarding conditions, including an overview, symptoms, causes, diagnostic procedures and treatment options. On this site it is possible to ask questions and get information from a neurologist and connect to people who have similar health interests.

2556 RSI Resources
www.geocities.com/HotSprings/1702
Information on carpal tunnel and other repetitive strain injuries.

Description

2557 **Celiac Disease**

Celiac disease, also called celiac sprue, is a chronic disease in which the small bowel cannot absorb most nutrients. This inability, called malabsorption, is caused by inflammation of the bowel triggered by a sensitivity to gluten, a cereal protein found in wheat and rye, and less so in barley and oats.

The disease may appear when a child is first given wheat products, generally in the second year of life. Some cases, however, do not appear until a person is in their twenties, or later, with women showing symptoms 10 to 15 years earlier than men. Affected children will fail to grow normally. Adults may lose weight despite a voracious appetite. There is no typical presentation of celiac disease. However, painful abdominal distention and passage of large, loose stools are common; iron deficiency anemia and vitamin deficiencies may appear.

Family incidence is a valuable clue. Celiac disease is more common in people with Type I diabetes and certain forms of thyroid and skin disease. Blood tests are helpful in making the diagnosis, but the most definitive test is examination of a small sample of the inflamed bowel.

Withdrawal of dietary gluten is the treatment for celiac disease; eating even small amounts of gluten-containing foods can prevent remission and cause relapse. Vitamins and minerals may also have to be supplemented. See also *Gastrointestinal Disorders* and *Crohn's Disease*.

National Agencies & Associations

2558 **American Celiac Society**
PO Box 23455   504-737-3293
New Orleans, LA 70183   Fax: 973-669-8808
e-mail: americanceliacsociety@yahoo.com
www.americanceliacsociety.org
Nonprofit tax exempt organization that supports efforts in education research and mutual support. Helps to set up support groups sponsors conferences seek funding for education and research identify ingredients in foods and educate the public.
Annette Bentley, President
James Bentley, Vice-President

2559 **Canadian Celiac Association**
5025 Orbitor Drive Building 1   905-507-6208
Mississauga, ON, L4W 4-4Y5   800-363-7296
Fax: 905-507-4673
e-mail: info@celiac.ca
www.celiac.ca

A national organization dedicated to providing services and support to persons with celiac disease and dermatitis herpetiformis through programs of awareness, advocacy, education and research.
Anne Wraggett, President
Bill Shank, Executive Vice President

2560 **Celiac Sprue Association: USA**
PO Box 31700   402-558-0600
Omaha, NE 68131-700   877-CSA-4CSA
Fax: 402-643-4108
e-mail: celiacs@csaceliacs.org
www.csaceliacs.org
Member based nonprofit support organization dedicated to helping individuals with celiac disease and dermatitis herpetiformis

worldwide through education information and research. Includes over 150 support contacts nationwide and Cel-Kids Network.
Mary Schluckebier, Executive Director
Diane Craig, President

2561 **Gluten Intolerance Group: GIG**
31214 124th Avenue SE   253-833-6655
Auburn, WA 98092-3667   Fax: 253-833-6675
e-mail: info@gluten.net
www.gluten.net
Provides instructional and general information materials as well as counseling and access to gluten-free products and ingredients to persons with celiac sprue and their families, operates telephone information and referral service and conducts educational seminars.
Cynthia Kupp RDCD, Executive Director

Support Groups & Hotlines

2562 **American Celiac Society Hotline**
Dietary Support Coalition
PO BOX 23455   504-737-3293
New Orleans, LA 70183
Provides practical assistance to members and individuals with celiac disease and information about the disease to the public.
Annette Bentley, President
James Bentley, Vice President

2563 **Celiac Disease Foundation**
20350 Ventura Boulevard   818-716-1513
Woodlands Hills, CA 91364-1838   Fax: 818-267-5577
e-mail: cdf@celiac.org
www.celiac.org/
Provides services and support to persons with celiac disease and dermatitis herpetiformis, through programs of awareness, education, advocacy and research; telephone information and referral services; medical advisory board annual educational conference and quarterly newsletters.
Marcia Riches, President
Richard Tasoff, Vice-President

2564 **National Health Information Center**
PO Box 1133   310-565-4167
Washington, DC 20013   800-336-4797
Fax: 301-984-4256
e-mail: info@nhic.org
www.health.gov/nhic
Offers a nationwide information referral service, produces directories and resource guides.
Ellen Langhans, Chairwoman
Linda Harris, Lead, Health Communication and e-health

Books

2565 **CSA/USA Cookbook Series**
Celiac Sprue Association/USA
PO Box 31700   402-558-0600
Omaha, NE 68131   877-272-4272
Fax: 402-643-4108
e-mail: celiacs@csaceliacs.org
www.csaceliacs.org
Three cookbooks compiled from CSA members' contributions. Each contains a section of cooking hints, information on adapting recipes and a variety of special topics related to cooking gluten-free.
34 pages Annual
Mary Schluckebier, Executive Director

2566 **Cooperative Gluten-Free Commercial Products Listing**
Celiac Sprue Association/USA
PO Box 31700   402-558-0600
Omaha, NE 68131   877-272-4272
Fax: 402-643-4108
e-mail: celiacs@csaceliacs.org
www.csaceliacs.org
Listing of gluten-free products compiled from written documentation recieved by the Celiac Sprue Association from manufacturers and distributors. Also includes vendor information for companies

specializing in gluten-free products and phone numbers of companies.
2006 Annual
Mary Schluckebier, Executive Director

2567 Diets to Help Gluten and Wheat Allergy
HarperCollins Canada Limited/Order Department
1995 Markham Road
Scarborough, M1B-5M8   800-387-0117
Fax: 800-668-5788
This book offers sound and practical advice on gluten allergy wheat sensitivity and Celiac disease.
96 pages
ISBN: 0-722529-10-4

2568 Gluten Intolerance
American Dietetic Association
1120 Connecticut Ave NW   202-775-8277
Washington, DC 20036   800-877-1600
www.eatright.org
Resource and recipe book.

2569 The Gluten-Free Gourmet
Bette Hagman, author
Gluten Intolerance Group: GIG
31214 124th Avenue SE   253-833-6655
Auburn, WA 98092-3667   Fax: 253-833-6675
e-mail: customerservice@gluten.org
www.gluten.net
225 recipes.
272 pages
ISBN: 0-805064-84-2
Cynthia Kupper RDCD, Executive Director

Newsletters

2570 GIG Quarterly Magazine
Gluten Intolerance Group: GIG
31214 124th Avenue SE   253-833-6655
Auburn, WA 98092-3667   Fax: 253-833-6675
e-mail: customerservice@gluten.org
www.gluten.net
Member magazine. Offers updated medical and technological information for patients with celiac disease, their families and healthcare professionals.
Quarterly
Cynthia Kupper RDCD, Executive Director

2571 Lifeline
Celiac Sprue Association/USA
PO Box 31700   402-558-0600
Omaha, NE 68131   877-272-4272
Fax: 402-643-4108
e-mail: celiacs@csaceliacs.org
www.csaceliacs.org
Quarterly newsletter for members; contains up-to-date research information, personal stories from celiacs, cooking tips, recipes and contact information for support chapters and resource units.
Mary Schluckebier, Executive Director

2572 Whooo's Report
American Celiac Society
PO Box 23455   504-737-3293
New Orleans, LA 70183   e-mail: amerceliacsoc@netscape.net
Provides practical assistance to members and individuals with celiac disease and information about the disease to the public.

Pamphlets

2573 Celiac Disease
Gluten Intolerance Group: GIG
31214 124th Avenue SE   253-833-6655
Auburn, WA 98092-3667   Fax: 253-833-6675
e-mail: customerservice@gluten.org
www.gluten.net
Offers facts and statistics on celiac disease.
Cynthia Kupper RDCD, Executive Director

2574 Celiac Disease: A Hidden Epidemic
Peter Greene, MD, author
Harper Collins Publishers
10 East 53rd Street
New York, NY 10022   212-207-7000
www.harpercollins.com
An inside-out examination and explanation of Celiac Disease.
2006 352 pages
ISBN: 0-060766-93-X
Peter H.R. Green M.D., Author
Rory Jones, Author

2575 Dermatitis Herpetiformis
Gluten Intolerance Group: GIG
31214 124th Avenue SE   253-833-6655
Auburn, WA 98092-3667   Fax: 253-833-6675
e-mail: customerservice@gluten.org
www.gluten.net
Offers facts and statistics on dermatitis herpetformis.
Cynthia Kupper RDCD, Executive Director

2576 Grains and Flours
Celiac Sprue Association/USA
PO Box 31700   402-558-0600
Omaha, NE 68131   877-272-4272
Fax: 402-643-4108
e-mail: celiacs@csaceliacs.org
www.csaceliacs.org
A variety of different gluten-free flour mixtures, to experiment with and discover your favorite!
Mary Schluckebier, Executive Director

2577 Guide to Gluten-Free Diets
American Allergy Association
PO Box 7273   650-322-1663
Menlo Park, CA 94026-7273
Offers information on safe substitutes for baking and cooking. Differentiates celiac disease from wheat allergy. Sources of gluten in diet with warnings on when to check with the manufacturer.

2578 Patient Packet
Celiac Sprue Association/USA
PO Box 31700   402-558-0600
Omaha, NE 68131   877-272-4272
Fax: 402-643-4108
e-mail: celiacs@csaceliacs.org
www.csaceliacs.org
A basic information packet for the newly-diagnosed celiac. Provided free of charge to individuals, physicians, dietitians, and family members.
Mary Schluckebier, Executive Director

2579 Quick Start Diet Guide
Gluten Intolerance Group: GIG
31214 124th Avenue SE   253-833-6655
Auburn, WA 98092-3667   Fax: 253-833-6675
e-mail: customerservice@gluten.org
www.gluten.net
Packet available to download on website.
Cynthia Kupper RDCD, Executive Director

Audio & Video

2580 CD-A NIH Consensus Conference
Celiac Sprue Association/USA
PO Box 31700   402-558-0600
Omaha, NE 68131   877-272-4272
Fax: 402-643-4108
e-mail: celiacs@csaceliacs.org
www.csaceliacs.org
Celiac Disease - A NIH Consensus Conference - Reaching Out to Improve the Health of Millions.
Mary Schluckebier, Executive Director

Web Sites

2581   Celiac Disease & Gluten-Free Diet Online Resource Center

www.celiac.com

Internet based support organization that provides important resources and information for people on gluten-free diets due to celiac disease, gluten intolerance or wheat allergy.

2582   Celiac Disease Foundation

www.celiac.org/

Provides services and support to persons with celiac disease and dermatitus herpetiformis, through programs of awareness, education, advocacy and research; telephone information and referral services; medical advisory board; and special educational seminars and quarterly meetings.

2583   Celiac Sprue Association: USA

www.csaceliacs.org

Member based, nonprofit support organization dedicated to helping individuals with celiac disease and dermatitis herpetiformis worldwide through education, information and research. Includes over 90 support chapters, 50 resource units, and Cel-Kids Network. Sponsors an annual conference, publishes educational materials, conducts a summer youth camp and provides phone and on-line counseling.

2584   Gluten Intolerance Group: GIG

www.gluten.org

Provides instructional and general information materials, as well as counseling and access to gluten-free products and ingredients to persons with celiac sprue and their families, operates telephone information and referral service, conducts educational seminars for health professionals, conducts and supports research, offers leadership and assistance to contacts and provides for a gluten-free kids camp.

2585   Healing Well

www.healingwell.com

An online health resource guide to medical news, chat, information and articles, newsgroups and message boards, books, disease-related web sites, medical directories, and more for patients, friends, and family coping with disabling diseases, disorders, or chronic illnesses.

2586   Health Finder

www.healthfinder.gov

Searchable, carefully developed web site offering information on over 1000 topics. Developed by the US Department of Health and Human Services, the site can be used in both English and Spanish.

2587   Healthlink USA

www.healthlinkusa.com

Health information concerning treatment, cures, prevention, diagnosis, risk factors, research, support groups, email lists, personal stories and much more. Updated regularly.

2588   Helios Health

www.helioshealth.com

Online resource for your health information. Detailed information about specific health topics, access to expert advice from our Medical Advisory Board, and up-to-date health news.

2589   MedicineNet

www.medicinenet.com

An online resource for consumers providing easy-to-read, authoritative medical and health information.

2590   Medscape

www.medscape.com

Medscape offers specialists, primary care physicians, and other health professionals the Web's most robust and integrated medical information and educational tools.

2591   WebMD

www.webmd.com

Provides credible information, supportive communities, and in-depth reference material about health subjects. A source for original and timely health information as well as material from well known content providers.

Description

2592 ## Cerebral Palsy

Cerebral palsy, CP, applies to disorders of voluntary movement resulting from damage to areas in the brain. CP can be caused by birth trauma, insufficient oxygen supplied to the infant at or before birth, premature birth or a severe systemic disease, such as meningitis, during early infancy. However, the exact cause is often difficult to establish.

Children with cerebral palsy may not be identified until they reach 1-2 years of age and may show only lagging motor development. Therefore, children known to be at risk should be followed closely. Increased spastic movements are the most common symptoms, but children may also show weakness, poor sense of balance, involuntary movements and abnormal walking. In more severe cases, difficulty in speaking and mental retardation may also be present.

Since there is no known cure for cerebral palsy, the goal of treatment is to develop maximal independence. Therapy may include physical and occupational rehabilitation, the use of leg braces, speech training and special orthopedic surgery. Parents need assistance and guidance in understanding their child's status and potential.

National Agencies & Associations

2593 **American Academy for Cerebral Palsy and Developmental Medicine**
555 E Wells St.
Milwaukee, WI 53202
414-918-3014
Fax: 414-276-2146
e-mail: info@aacpdm.org
www.aacpdm.org
A multidisciplinary scientific society devoted to the study of cerebral palsy and other childhood onset disabilities, promoting professional education for the treatment and management of these conditions and to improving the quality of life for people with the condition.
1550 members
Maureen O'Donnel, President
Scott Hoffinger, Treasurer

2594 **Canadian Cerebral Palsy Sports Association**
720 Belfast Rd
Ottawa, Ontario, K1G 0-5K9
613-748-1430
866-247-9934
Fax: 613-748-1355
e-mail: info@ccpsa.ca
www.ccpsa.ca
Is an athlete focused national organization administering and governing sport opportunities targeted to athletes with CP and related disabilities.
Sandy Hermiston, President
Marie Dannhaeuser, Executive Director

2595 **Easter Seals**
233 S Wacker Drive
Chicago, IL 60606
312-726-6200
800-221-6827
Fax: 312-726-1494
TTY: 312-726-4258
e-mail: info@easter-seals.org
www.easter-seals.org
Provides services to children and adults with disabilities as well as support to their families.
Stephen F Rossman, Chairman

2596 **Independent Living Research Utilization Project**
2323 S Shepherd
Houston, TX 77019
713-520-0232
Fax: 713-520-5785
TTY: 713-520-0232
e-mail: ilru@ilru.org
www.ilru.org
A national center for information training research and technical assistance in independent living. Goal is to expand the body of knowledge in independent living and to improve utilization of results of research programs and demonstration projects.
Lex Frieden, Director
Linda CoVan, Grant Coordinator

2597 **National Rehabilitation Information Center**
8201 Corporate Drive
Landover, MD 20785
301-459-5900
800-346-2742
Fax: 301-459-4263
TTY: 301-459-5984
e-mail: narincinfo@heitechservices.com
www.naric.com/
One of the three components of the office of Special Education and Rehabilitative Services. Operates in concert with the Rehabilitation Services Administration and the Office of Special Education Programs.
Mark Odum, Director
Jessica H. Chaiken, Media and Information Services Manager

2598 **United Cerebral Palsy Associations**
1660 L Street NW
Washington, DC 20036
202-776-0406
800-872-5827
Fax: 202-776-0414
TTY: 202-973-7197
e-mail: info@ucp.org
www.ucp.org
A network of approximately 119 state and local voluntary agencies which provide services conduct public and professional education programs and support research in cerebral palsy.
Stephen Bennett, President, CEO
Michael E Hill, Senior Vice President

State Agencies & Associations

Alabama

2599 **United Cerebral Palsy of Alabama**
301 EA Darden Drive
Anniston, AL 36202
256-237-8203
Fax: 256-235-2388
e-mail: executivedirector@ecaucp.org
www.ecaucp.org
United Cerebral Palsy provides information, advocacy, referral services for persons with disabilities and/or their families. UCP also operates an equipment loan program, conducts parent workshops, disseminates written literature on topics of interest.
Linda Johns, Executive Director
Shannon Priddy, Development Director

2600 **United Cerebral Palsy of East Central Alabama**
301 EA Darden Drive
Anniston, AL 36202
256-237-8203
Fax: 256-235-2388
e-mail: executivedirector@ecaucp.org
www.ecaucp.org
United Cerebral Palsy provides information, advocacy, referral services for persons with disabilities and/or their families. UCP also operates an equipment loan program, conducts parent workshops, disseminates written literature on topics of interest to people with disabilities.
Donald Turner, Chairman of the Board
John Rogers, Treasurer

2601 **United Cerebral Palsy of Greater Birmingha m**
120 Oslo Circle
Birmingham, AL 35211
205-944-3900
800-654-4483
Fax: 205-944-3990
e-mail: gedwards@ucpbham.com
www.ucpbham.com
United Cerebral Palsy provides information, advocacy, referral services for persons with disabilities and/or their families. UCP also operates an equipment loan program, conducts parent work-

shops, disseminates written literature on topics of interest to people with disabilities.
Gary Edwards, Executive Director
Jennifer H Ellison, Chief Development Officer

2602   United Cerebral Palsy of Huntsville & Tennessee Valley
2075 Max Luther Drive   256-852-5600
Huntsville, AL 35810   Fax: 256-852-6722
e-mail: tracyc@ucphuntsville.org
www.ucp.org
United Cerebral Palsy provides information, advocacy, referral services for persons with disabilities and/or their families. UCP also operates an equipment loan program, conducts parent workshops, disseminates written literature on topics of interest.
Cheryl Smith, Executive Director
Tim Reeves, President

2603   United Cerebral Palsy of Mobile
3058 Dauphin Square Connector   251-479-4900
Mobile, AL 36607   Fax: 251-479-4998
e-mail: info@ucpmobile.org
www.ucp.org
United Cerebral Palsy provides information, advocacy, referral services for persons with disabilities and/or their families. UCP also operates an equipment loan program, conducts parent workshops, disseminates written literature on topics of interest.
Glenn Harger, President/CEO
Susan Watson, VP/COO

2604   United Cerebral Palsy of Northwest Alabama
4212 Jackson Highway   256-381-4310
Sheffield, AL 35660   Fax: 256-381-4378
e-mail: alison@ucpshoals.org
www.ucpshoals.org
United Cerebral Palsy provides information, advocacy, referral services for persons with disabilities and/or their families. UCP also operates an equipment loan program, conducts parent workshops, disseminates written literature on topics of interest.
Alison Isbell, Director
Linda Williamson, Development Director/WEE-CARE Director

2605   United Cerebral Palsy of West Alabama
1100 UCP Parkway   205-345-3031
Northport, AL 35476   Fax: 205-345-3035
e-mail: lisasucp@comcast.net
www.ucpa.org
United Cerebral Palsy provides information, advocacy, referral services for persons with disabilities and/or their families. UCP also operates an equipment loan program, conducts parent workshops, disseminates written literature on topics of interest.
Lisa D Skelton, Executive Director
Brenda Ewart, Development Director

Alaska

2606   United Cerebral Palsy of Alaska/PARENTS
4743 E Northern Lights Boulevard   907-337-7678
Anchorage, AK 99508   800-478-7678
Fax: 907-337-7671
TTY: 907-337-7629
e-mail: parents@parentsinc.org
www.ucpa.org
Provides information, advocacy, referral services for persons with disabilities and/or their families. UCP also operates an equipment loan program, conducts parent workshops, disseminates written literature on topics of interest to people with disabilities.

Arizona

2607   United Cerebral Palsy of Central Arizona
1802 Parkside Lane   602-943-5472
Phoenix, AZ 85027   Fax: 602-943-4936
e-mail: info@ucpofaz.org
www.ucpa.org
United Cerebral Palsy provides information, advocacy, referral services for persons with disabilities and/or their families. UCP also operates an equipment loan program, conducts parent workshops, disseminates written literature on topics of interest.
Dan Rossi, Executive Director
Perry Bramlett, Chief Human Resources Officer

2608   United Cerebral Palsy of Southern Arizona
635 N Craycroft Road   520-795-3108
Tucson, AZ 85711   Fax: 520-795-3196
e-mail: staff@ucpsa.org
www.ucpsa.org
United Cerebral Palsy provides information, advocacy, referral services for persons with disabilities and/or their families. UCP also operates an equipment loan program, conducts parent workshops, disseminates written literature on topics of interest.
Cindy Mars, Executive Director
Gary Bahman, Finance Director

Arkansas

2609   United Cerebral Palsy of Central Arkansas
9720 N Rodney Parham Road   501-224-6067
Little Rock, AR 72227   Fax: 501-227-5591
e-mail: general@ucpcark.org
www.ucpark.org
United Cerebral Palsy provides information, advocacy, referral services for persons with disabilities and/or their families. UCP also operates an equipment loan program, conducts parent workshops, disseminates written literature on topics of interest.
Woody Connette, Chair
Ian Ridlon, Vice-Chairman

California

2610   United Cerebral Palsy of Central California
4224 North Cedar Avenue   559-221-8272
Fresno, CA 93726-3700   Fax: 559-221-9347
e-mail: info@ccucp.org
www.ccucp.org/
United Cerebral Palsy provides information, advocacy, referral services for persons with disabilities and/or their families. UCP also operates an equipment loan program, conducts parent workshops, disseminates written literature on topics of interest to people with disabilities.
Mark Lanier, Presdient
Carol Klonnger, Vice-President

2611   United Cerebral Palsy of Greater Sacramento o
191 Lathrop Way   916-565-7700
Sacramento, CA 95815   Fax: 916-565-7773
e-mail: ucp@ucpsacto.org
www.ucpsacto.org
UCP provides programs and services for people with all types of developmental disabilities. These services include: day programs for adults, an in-home respite service, transportation, independent living services, information and referral services.
Doug Bergman, President/CEO
Tanya Hartle, COO

2612   United Cerebral Palsy of Los Angeles & Ventura Counties
6430 Independence Avenue   818-782-2211
Woodland Hills, CA 91367   Fax: 818-909-9106
e-mail: mail@ucpla.com
www.ucpla.org
United Cerebral Palsy provides information, advocacy, referral services for persons with disabilities and/or their families. UCP also operates an equipment loan program, conducts parent workshops, disseminates written literature on topics of interest to people with disabilities.
Ronald S Cohen, Chief Executive Officer
Clark Jensen, Chief Operating Officer

2613   United Cerebral Palsy of Orange County
980 Roosevelt   949-333-6400
Irvine, CA 92602   Fax: 949-333-6400
e-mail: info@ucp-oc.org
www.ucp-oc.org
United Cerebral Palsy provides information, advocacy, referral services for persons with disabilities and/or their families. UCP also operates an equipment loan program, conducts parent workshops, disseminates written literature on topics of interest.
Paul Pulver, Executive Director¯
Lauren Mille Beeler, Director of Therapy Services

2614   United Cerebral Palsy of San Diego County
8525 Gibbs Drive   858-571-7803
San Diego, CA 92123   Fax: 858-571-0919
e-mail: ucp@ucpsd.org
www.ucpa.org
United Cerebral Palsy provides information, advocacy, referral
services for persons with disabilities and/or their families. UCP
also operates an equipment loan program, conducts parent workshops, disseminates written literature on topics of interest.
David Carucci, Executive Director
Mary Krieger, Associate Executive Director

2615   United Cerebral Palsy of San Joaquin, Calaveras & Amador
Counties
333 W Benjamin Holt Drive   209-956-0290
Stockton, CA 95207   Fax: 209-956-0294
e-mail: slarson@ucpsj.org
www.ucp.org
United Cerebral Palsy provides information, advocacy, referral
services for persons with disabilities and/or their families. UCP
also operates an equipment loan program, conducts parent workshops, disseminates written literature on topics of interest to
people with disabilities.
Leslie Heier, Interim Executive Director
Theresa Galano-Burke, Executive Assistant

2616   United Cerebral Palsy of San Luis Obispo
3620 Sacramento Drive   805-543-2039
San Luis Obispo, CA 93401   877-UCP-CAR1
Fax: 805-543-2045
e-mail: shaftmt@aol.com
www.ucp-slo.org
United Cerebral Palsy provides information, advocacy, referral
services for persons with disabilities and/or their families. UCP
also operates an equipment loan program, conducts parent workshops, disseminates written literature on topics of interest to
people with disabilities.
Mark Shaffer, UCP Executive Director
Karl Winkler, UCP Administrative Assistant

2617   United Cerebral Palsy of Santa Barbara County
6430 Independence Avenue   818-782-2211
Woodland Hills, CA 91367   888-733-4227
Fax: 818-909-9106
e-mail: mail@ucpla.org
www.ucpla.org
United Cerebral Palsy provides information, advocacy, referral
services for persons with disabilities and/or their families. UCP
also operates an equipment loan program, conducts parent workshops, disseminates written literature on topics of interest.
Ellen Kessler, Chairperson
Nick Roxborough, President

2618   United Cerebral Palsy of Santa Clara & San Mateo Counties
512 E Maude Avenue   650-917-6900
Sunnyvale, CA 94085-4431   Fax: 650-948-8503
e-mail: info@ucpscsm.org
www.ucpscsm.org/
United Cerebral Palsy provides information, advocacy, referral
services for persons with disabilities and/or their families. UCP
also operates an equipment loan program, conducts parent workshops, disseminates written literature on topics of interest.
Stephen Bennett, President/CEO National Office (DC)
Armetta Parker, Marketing/Communications Director (DC)

2619   United Cerebral Palsy of Stanislaus County
1213 13th Street   209-577-2122
Modesto, CA 95353   Fax: 209-577-2392
e-mail: rlonczak@ucpstan.org
www.ucpstan.org
United Cerebral Palsy provides information, advocacy, referral
services for persons with disabilities and/or their families. UCP
also operates an equipment loan program, conducts parent workshops, disseminates written literature on topics of interest to
people with disabilities.
Robert S Lonczak, Executive Director
Jeanette Jones, Program~Coordinator

2620   United Cerebral Palsy of the Golden Gate
1970 Broadway   510-832-7430
Oakland, CA 94612   Fax: 510-839-1329
e-mail: info@ucpgg.org
www.ucp.org
United Cerebral Palsy provides information, advocacy, referral
services for persons with disabilities and/or their families. UCP
also operates an equipment loan program, conducts parent workshops, disseminates written literature on topics of interest.
Karen Glatze, Administrator
Dori Maxon, SNAP Program Director

2621   United Cerebral Palsy of the Inland Empire
35-325 Date Palm Drive   760-321-8184
Cathedral City, CA 92234   877-512-2224
Fax: 760-321-8284
e-mail: info@ucpie.org
www.ucp.org
United Cerebral Palsy provides information, advocacy, referral
services for persons with disabilities and/or their families. UCP
conducts parent workshops, disseminates written literature on topics of interest to people with disabilities.
Roger M Alexander, Chair
Micki James, Vice Chair

2622   United Cerebral Palsy of the North Bay
3835 Cypress Drive   707-766-9990
Petaluma, CA 94954   800-872-5827
Fax: 202-776-0414
e-mail: info@ucpnb.org
www.ucp.org
United Cerebral Palsy's mission is to advance the independence,
productivity and full citizenship of people with disabilities
through an affiliate network.
Margaret Farman, Executive Director
Ron Hamilton, Chief of Operations

Colorado

2623   United Cerebral Palsy of Colorado
801 Yosemite Street   303-691-9339
Denver, CO 80230-5708   866-701-2277
Fax: 303-691-0846
www.cpco.org
United Cerebral Palsy provides information, advocacy, referral
services for persons with disabilities and/or their families. UCP
also operates an equipment loan program, conducts parent workshops, disseminates written literature on topics of interest.
Jim Reuter, Chairman of the Board
Judith I Ham, President/CEO

Connecticut

2624   United Cerebral Palsy of Eastern Connecticut
42 Norwich Road   860-447-3800
Quaker Hill, CT 06375   Fax: 860-443-8272
e-mail: email@ucpect.org
www.ucp.org
United Cerebral Palsy provides information, advocacy, referral
services for persons with disabilities and/or their families. UCP
also operates an equipment loan program, conducts parent workshops, disseminates written literature on topics of interest to
people with disabilities.
Margaret Morrison, Executive Director
Patricia Mansfield, Executive Director

2625   United Cerebral Palsy of Greater Hartford
80 Whitney Street   860-236-6201
Hartford, CT 06105   Fax: 860-218-2454
e-mail: jmcmahon@sunrisegroup.org
www.ucphartford.org
United Cerebral Palsy provides information, advocacy, referral
services for persons with disabilities and/or their families. UCP
also operates an equipment loan program, conducts parent workshops, disseminates written literature on topics of interest to
people with disabilities.
Pam Reid, Regional Administrator
Sean Thompson, In-Home Support Coordinator

2626   United Cerebral Palsy of Southern Connecticut
94-96 South Turnpike Road   203-269-3511
Wallingford, CT 06492   Fax: 203-269-7411
                    e-mail: ucpasouthernct@yahoo.com
                                         www.ucpa.org
United Cerebral Palsy provides information, advocacy, referral services for persons with disabilities and/or their families. UCP also operates an equipment loan program, conducts parent workshops, disseminates written literature on topics of interest to people with disabilities.

Delaware

2627   United Cerebral Palsy of Delaware
700 A River Road   302-764-2400
Wilmington, DE 19809-2746   Fax: 302-764-8713
                    e-mail: wmccool@ucpde.org
                    www.ucp.org/ucp_local.cfm/52
United Cerebral Palsy provides information, advocacy, referral services for persons with disabilities and/or their families. UCP also operates an equipment loan program, conducts parent workshops, disseminates written literature on topics of interest.
Michelle Welch, President
D Bruce McClenathan, Vice President

District of Columbia

2628   United Cerebral Palsy of Washington DC
1818 New York Avenue   202-526-0146
Washington, DC 20002   Fax: 202-526-0519
                    e-mail: dcarter@ucpdc.org
                                         www.ucpdc.org
United Cerebral Palsy provides information, advocacy, referral services for persons with disabilities and/or their families. UCP also operates an equipment loan program, conducts parent workshops, disseminates written literature on topics of interest.
Mark A Simione, Board President
Roderick Johnson, Board Secretary

2629   United Cerebral Palsy of Washington DC & Northern Virginia
1818 New York Avenue NE   202-526-0146
Washington, DC 20002   Fax: 202-526-0519
                    e-mail: webmaster@ucpdcnova.org
                                         www.ucpdc.org
United Cerebral Palsy provides information, advocacy, referral services for persons with disabilities and/or their families. UCP also operates an equipment loan program, conducts parent workshops, disseminates written literature on topics of interest to people with disabilities.
Mark Simione, President
George Connors, 1st Vice President

Florida

2630   United Cerebral Palsy of Central Florida
3305 S Orange Avenue   407-852-3300
Orlando, FL 32806   Fax: 407-852-3301
                    e-mail: mbetts@ucpcdc.org
                                         www.ucpcfl.org
United Cerebral Palsy provides information, advocacy, referral services for persons with disabilities and/or their families. UCP also operates an equipment loan program, conducts parent workshops, disseminates written literature on topics of interest.
Ilene E Wilkins, President & Chief Executive Officer
Jill Wisth, Chief Financial Officer

2631   United Cerebral Palsy of East Central Florida
1100 Jimmy Ann Drive   386-274-6474
Daytona Beach, FL 32117   Fax: 386-274-6532
                    e-mail: info@ucpecf.org
                                         www.ucp.org

Barry Pollack, President/CEO
Kelly Johanessen, VP of Operations

2632   United Cerebral Palsy of Florida
1830 Buford Court   850-922-5630
Tallahassee, FL 32308   Fax: 850-922-1258
                    e-mail: gloriawe@earthlink.net
                                         www.ucp.org

United Cerebral Palsy provides information, advocacy, referral services for persons with disabilities and/or their families. UCP also operates an equipment loan program, conducts parent workshops, disseminates written literature on topics of interest.

2633   United Cerebral Palsy of North Florida: Tender Loving Care
1241 NE Avenue   850-769-7960
Panama City, FL 32401   Fax: 850-769-1060
                    e-mail: kimberly.mcmanus@comcast.net
                                         www.ucp.org
United Cerebral Palsy provides information, advocacy, referral services for persons with disabilities and/or their families. UCP also operates an equipment loan program, conducts parent workshops, disseminates written literature on topics of interest to people with disabilities.

2634   United Cerebral Palsy of Northeast Florida
3311 Beach Boulevard   904-396-1462
Jacksonville, FL 32207   Fax: 904-396-1199
                    e-mail: cpnefagency@hotmail.com

2635   United Cerebral Palsy of Northwest Florida
2912 North East Street   850-432-1596
Pensacola, FL 32501-1324   Fax: 850-432-1930
                    e-mail: information@ucpnwfl.org
                                         www.ucpnwfl.org/
The number one service provider in Northwest Florida for individuals with cerebral palsy and other developmental disabilities, UCP provides information ,advocacy and referral services for persons with disabilities and/or their families. Additionally, UCP offers individuals assistance with daily living skills training, computer training, basic education, speech, physical and occupational therapy, residential, supported living and finding long-term employment.
Brain Bell, Chair
Michelle Fielder, Vice-Chairman

2636   United Cerebral Palsy of Sarasota-Manatee
1090 S Tamiami Trail   941-957-3599
Sarasota, FL 34236   Fax: 947-957-3499
                    e-mail: ucpwendy@aol.com
                                         www.ucpsarasota.org
United Cerebral Palsy provides information, advocacy, referral services for persons with disabilities and/or their families. UCP also operates an equipment loan program, conducts parent workshops, disseminates written literature on topics of interest.
Barnett A Greenberg, Chairperson
Mark Famiglio, President

2637   United Cerebral Palsy of South Florida
2700 W 81st Street   305-325-1080
Hialeah, FL 33016   Fax: 305-325-1313
                    e-mail: info@ucpsouthflorida.org
                                         www.ucp.org
United Cerebral Palsy provides information, advocacy, referral services for persons with disabilities and/or their families. UCP also operates an equipment loan program, conducts parent workshops, disseminates written literature on topics of interest.
Joseph Aniello, President & CEO
Linda Gluck, Vice President & CFO

2638   United Cerebral Palsy of Tallahassee
1830 Buford Court   850-878-2141
Tallahassee, FL 32308   Fax: 850-922-1258
                    e-mail: gloriawe@earthlink.net
                                         www.ucp.org
United Cerebral Palsy provides information, advocacy, referral services for persons with disabilities and/or their families. UCP also operates an equipment loan program, conducts parent workshops, disseminates written literature on topics of interest.

2639   United Cerebral Palsy of Tampa Bay
2215 E Henry Avenue   813-239-1179
Tampa, FL 33610   800-749-5155
                                         Fax: 813-237-3091
                    e-mail: kryals@advanceability.org
                                         www.ucptampa.org
United Cerebral Palsy provides information, advocacy, referral services for persons with disabilities and/or their families. UCP also operates an equipment loan program, conducts parent work-

shops, disseminates written literature on topics of interest to people with disabilities.
Jim King, Executive Director
Dawn Gosselin, Executive Development Assistant / Events

Georgia

2640 United Cerebral Palsy of Georgia
3300 NE Expressway
Atlanta, GA 30341
770-676-2000
Fax: 770-455-8040
e-mail: info@ucpga.org
www.ucp.org
United Cerebral Palsy provides information, advocacy, referral services for persons with disabilities and/or their families. UCP also operates an equipment loan program, conducts parent workshops, disseminates written literature on topics of interest to people with disabilities.
Diane Wilush, Executive Director
Kevin Walton, Associate Executive Director

Hawaii

2641 United Cerebral Palsy of Hawaii
414 Kuwili Street
Honolulu, HI 96817-5050
808-532-6744
800-606-5654
Fax: 808-532-6747
e-mail: ucpa@diverseabilities.org
www.ucpahi.org
United Cerebral Palsy provides information, advocacy, referral services for persons with disabilities and/or their families. UCP also operates an equipment loan program, conducts parent workshops, disseminates written literature on topics of interest.
Jerry Pupillo, President
Stephen Hink, 1st Vice President

Idaho

2642 United Cerebral Palsy of Idaho
5420 W Franklin Road
Boise, ID 83705
208-377-8070
888-289-3281
Fax: 208-322-7133
e-mail: info@ucpidaho.org
www.ucp.org
United Cerebral Palsy provides information, advocacy and referral services for persons with disabilities and/or their families.
Kim Kane, Executive Director
Kathy Griffin, Program Director

Illinois

2643 United Cerebral Palsy Land of Lincoln
101 N 16th Street
Springfield, IL 67203
217-525-6522
Fax: 217-525-9017
e-mail: info@ucpll.org
www.ucp.org
United Cerebral Palsy provides information, advocacy, referral services for persons with disabilities and/or their families. UCP also operates an equipment loan program, conducts parent workshops, disseminates written literature on topics of interest.
Brenda L Yarnell, President/CEO
Kathy Leuelling, Chief Operating Officer

2644 United Cerebral Palsy of East Central Illinois
1023 N Water
Decatur, IL 62523
217-428-5033
Fax: 217-428-5094
ww.ucpa.org
United Cerebral Palsy provides information, advocacy, referral services for persons with disabilities and/or their families. UCP also operates an equipment loan program, conducts parent workshops, disseminates written literature on topics of interest.
Woody Connette, Chair

2645 United Cerebral Palsy of Greater Chicago
547 W Jackson
Chicago, IL 60661
312-765-0419
Fax: 312-765-0503
TTY: 312-368-0179
e-mail: pdulle@ucpnet.org
www.ucpnet.org

United Cerebral Palsy provides information, advocacy, referral services for persons with disabilities and/or their families. UCP also operates an equipment loan program, conducts parent workshops, disseminates written literature on topics of interest to people with disabilities.
Paul J Dulle, President/CEO
Peggy Childs, Executive Vice President

2646 United Cerebral Palsy of Illinois
310 E Adams
Springfield, IL 62701
877-550-8274
877-550-8274
Fax: 217-528-9739
TTY: 877-550-8274
e-mail: cpil@sbcglobal.net
www.ucpillinois.org
United Cerebral Palsy provides information, advocacy, referral services for persons with disabilities and/or their families. UCP also operates an equipment loan program, conducts parent workshops, disseminates written literature on topics of interest to people with disabilities.
Don Moss, Executive Director
Alice Foss, Associate Director

2647 United Cerebral Palsy of Southern Illinois
9 Cusumano Professional Plaza Drive
Mount Vernon, IL 62864
618-244-2505
Fax: 618-244-3568
e-mail: ucpsi@onemain.com
www.ucpa.org
United Cerebral Palsy provides information, advocacy, referral services for persons with disabilities and/or their families. UCP also operates an equipment loan program, conducts parent workshops, disseminates written literature on topics of interest to people with disabilities.

2648 United Cerebral Palsy of Will County
311 S Reed Street
Joliet, IL 60436
815-744-3500
Fax: 815-744-3504
e-mail: ucpwill@ucpwill.org
www.ucp.org
United Cerebral Palsy provides information, advocacy, referral services for persons with disabilities and/or their families. UCP also operates an equipment loan program, conducts parent workshops, disseminates written literature on topics of interest to people with disabilities.
Samuel Mancuso, President & Chief Executive Officer
Stephanie Bergner, Family Support/Respite Administrator

2649 United Cerebral Palsy of the Blackhawk Region
7399 Forest Hills Road
Rockford, IL 61111
815-636-7132
Fax: 815-282-8835
e-mail: ucpbr@aol.com
www.ucpa.org
United Cerebral Palsy provides information, advocacy, referral services for persons with disabilities and/or their families. UCP also operates an equipment loan program, conducts parent workshops, disseminates written literature on topics of interest to people with disabilities.

2650 United Cerebral Palsy: Eastern Seals
230 W Monroe Street
Chicago, IL 60606
312-726-6200
800-221-6827
Fax: 312-726-1494
www.stsweb.indstate.edu
United Cerebral Palsy provides information, advocacy, referral services for persons with disabilities and/or their families. UCP also operates an equipment loan program, conducts parent workshops, disseminates written literature on topics of interest.
John Rogers, IT consultant
Tyler Howe, Project Manager

Indiana

2651 United Cerebral Palsy Association of Indiana
1915 West 18th Street
Indianapolis, IN 46202-1016
317-632-3561
Fax: 317-632-3338
e-mail: donnar@ucpaindy.org
www.ucpa.org
United Cerebral Palsy provides information, advocacy, referral services for persons with Cerebral Palsy and/or their families. UCP also provides funding for equipment and operates an equipment

loan program, disseminates written literature on topics of interest to people with disabilities.
Donna L Roberts, Executive Director

2652 United Cerebral Palsy Associations
6100 N Keystone Avenue   317-632-3561
Indianapolis, IN 46220   Fax: 317-632-3338
e-mail: donnar@ucpaindy.org
www.ucpaindy.org
United Cerebral Palsy provides information, advocacy, referral services for persons with Cerebral Palsy and/or their families. UCP also provides funding for equipment and operates an equipment loan program, disseminates written literature on topics of interest.
Donna L Roberts, Executive Director
Beth Allison, Case Manager

2653 United Cerebral Palsy of the Wabash Valley
621 Poplar Street   812-232-6305
Terre Haute, IN 47807   Fax: 812-234-3683
e-mail: ucp.wv@verizon.net
www.ucpwv.org
United Cerebral Palsy provides information, advocacy, referral services for persons with disabilities and/or their families. UCP also operates an equipment loan program, conducts parent workshops, disseminates written literature on topics of interest to people with disabilities.
Jacquie Denehie, Executive Director
Brain Garcia, President

Kansas

2654 United Cerebral Palsy of Kansas
5111 E 21st Street   316-688-1888
Wichita, KS 67208   Fax: 316-688-5687
e-mail: davej@cprf.org
www.ucp.org
United Cerebral Palsy provides information, advocacy, referral services for persons with disabilities and/or their families. UCP also operates an equipment loan program, conducts parent workshops, disseminates written literature on topics of interest.
Dave Jones, Executive Director
Amelia Ornelas, Office Manager

Louisiana

2655 United Cerebral Palsy of Baton Rouge McMains Children's Developmental Center
1805 College Drive   225-923-3420
Baton Rouge, LA 70808   Fax: 225-922-9316
e-mail: jketcham@mcmainscdc.org
www.mcmainscdc.org
United Cerebral Palsy provides information, advocacy, referral services for persons with disabilities and/or their families. UCP also operates an equipment loan program, conducts parent workshops, disseminates written literature on topics of interest.
Janet Ketcham, Director
Norman Landry, President

2656 United Cerebral Palsy of Greater New Orleans
1000 Leonidas St & Leake Avenue   504-865-0003
New Orleans, LA 70118   Fax: 504-865-0300
e-mail: info@ucpgno.com
www.ucpgno.org
United Cerebral Palsy provides information, advocacy, referral services for persons with disabilities and/or their families. UCP also operates an equipment loan program, conducts parent workshops, disseminates written literature on topics of interest to people with disabilities.
Tommy Freel, Chair
Joanne Rinardo, Treasurer

Maine

2657 United Cerebral Palsy of Northeastern Maine
700 Mount Hope Avenue   207-941-2952
Bangor, ME 04401   877-603-0030
Fax: 207-941-2955
e-mail: office@ucpofmaine.org
www.ucp.org

United Cerebral Palsy provides information, advocacy, referral services for persons with disabilities and/or their families. UCP also operates an equipment loan program, conducts parent workshops, disseminates written literature on topics of interest to people with disabilities.
Bobbi-Jo Yeager, Executive Director
Tricia Kail, Director of Services

Maryland

2658 United Cerebral Palsy of Central Maryland
1700 Reistertown Road   410-484-4540
Baltimore, MD 21208-2935   Fax: 410-484-1807
TTY: 800-451-2452
e-mail: info@ucp-cm.org
www.ucp.org
United Cerebral Palsy provides information, advocacy, referral services for persons with disabilities and/or their families. UCP also operates an equipment loan program, conducts parent workshops, disseminates written literature on topics of interest.
Diane Coughlin, President and CEO
Judy Cox, Assistant to the President

2659 United Cerebral Palsy of Prince Georges & Montgomery Counties
4409 Forbes Boulevard   301-459-0566
Lanham, MD 20706   Fax: 301-459-7691
TTY: 301-459-7691
TDD: 301-262-4982
e-mail: ucppgmc@aol.com
www.ucppgmc.org
Provides information, advocacy, referral services for persons with disabilities and/or their families. UCP also operates an equipment loan program, conducts parent workshops, disseminates written literature on topics of interest to people with disabilities.
Charles McNelly, Executive Director
Diane Dekoladenu, Program Director

2660 United Cerebral Palsy of Southern Maryland
221 Chinquapin Round Road   410-280-2003
Annapolis, MD 21401   Fax: 410-269-5757
e-mail: ucpinfo@ucpsm.org
www.ucpsm.org
United Cerebral Palsy provides information, advocacy, referral services for persons with disabilities and/or their families. UCP also operates an equipment loan program, conducts parent workshops, disseminates written literature on topics of interest to people with disabilities.

Massachusetts

2661 United Cerebral Palsy of Berkshire County
208 W Street   413-442-1562
Pittsfield, MA 01201   Fax: 413-499-4077
e-mail: info@ucpberkshire.org
www.ucp.org
United Cerebral Palsy provides information, advocacy, referral services for persons with disabilities and/or their families. UCP also operates an equipment loan program, conducts parent workshops, disseminates written literature on topics of interest to people with disabilities.
Christine Singer, Executive Director
Joni Thomas, Director of Development

2662 United Cerebral Palsy of MetroBoston
71 Arsenal Street   617-926-5480
Watertown, MA 02472   Fax: 617-926-3059
e-mail: ucpboston@ucpboston.org
www.ucp.org
United Cerebral Palsy provides information, advocacy, referral services for persons with disabilities and/or their families. UCP also operates an equipment loan program, conducts parent workshops, disseminates written literature on topics of interest.
Todd Kates, Executive Director
Roberta Jaro, Associate Executive Director

Michigan

2663 United Cerebral Palsy of Metropolitan Detroit
23077 Greenfield   248-557-5070
Southfield, MI 48075   Fax: 248-557-0224
e-mail: main@ucpdetroit.org
www.ucp.org
United Cerebral Palsy provides information, advocacy, referral services for persons with disabilities and/or their families. UCP also operates an equipment loan program, conducts parent workshops, disseminates written literature on topics of interest.
Leslynn Angel, President & CEO
Latoya Jones, Chief Financial Officer

2664 United Cerebral Palsy of Michigan
4970 Northwind Drive   517-203-1200
E Lansing, MI 48823   800-828-2714
Fax: 517-203-1203
e-mail: ucp@ucpmichigan.org
www.ucp.org
United Cerebral Palsy provides information, advocacy, referral services for persons with disabilities and/or their families. UCP also operates an equipment loan program, conducts parent workshops, disseminates written literature on topics of interest.
Linda Potter, Executive Director
Linda Carey, Office Manager

Minnesota

2665 United Cerebral Palsy of Central Minnesota
510 25th Avenue North   320-253-0765
St. Cloud, MN 56303-3255   Fax: 320-253-6753
e-mail: info@ucpcentralmn.org
www.ucpcentralmn.org
Provides information, advocacy, referral services for persons with disabilities and/or their families. UCP conducts parent workshops, disseminates free newsletter. Computers go round recycles quality used computers to persons with disabilities. UCP awards scholarship for post secondary education.
Shelly Gaetz, President
Sue Schlosser, Vice-President

2666 United Cerebral Palsy of Minnesota
1821 University Avenue W   651-646-7588
St Paul, MN 55104-2892   877-528-5678
Fax: 651-646-3045
e-mail: ucpmnStacey@hotmail.com
www.ucp.org
United Cerebral Palsy provides information, advocacy, referral services for persons with disabilities and/or their families. UCP also operates an equipment loan program, conducts parent workshops, disseminates written literature on topics of interest.
Stacey Vogele, Executive Director
Ramsey Lee, Events Coordinator

Missouri

2667 United Cerebral Palsy of Greater Kansas City
1044 Main Street   816-531-4454
Kansas City, MO 64105   Fax: 816-531-3383
e-mail: bscott@ucpkc.org
www.ucp.org
Provides information, advocacy, referral services for persons with disabilities and/or their families. UCP also operates residential programs and care management for seniors.
Bruce A Scott, President & CEO
Sam T Switzer, Senior Vice President & CFO

2668 United Cerebral Palsy of Greater St. Louis
13975 Mancester Rd   636-227-6030
Manchester, MO 63011-3999   Fax: 636-779-2270
e-mail: forkoshr@ucpstl.org
www.ucpheartland.org/
United Cerebral Palsy provides information, advocacy, referral services for persons with disabilities and/or their families. UCP also operates an equipment loan program, conducts parent workshops, disseminates written literature on topics of interest to people with disabilities.
Woody Connette, Chair
Lan Ridlon, Vice Chair

2669 United Cerebral Palsy of Northwest Missouri
3303 Frederick Avenue   816-364-3836
St. Joseph, MO 64506   Fax: 816-390-8546
e-mail: ucp@ucpnwmo.org
www.ucpa.org
United Cerebral Palsy provides information, advocacy, referral services for persons with disabilities and/or their families. UCP also operates an equipment loan program, conducts parent workshops, disseminates written literature on topics of interest to people with disabilities.
Jared Bronner, President
Shawn Drew, Vice-President

Nebraska

2670 United Cerebral Palsy of Nebraska
920 S 107th Avenue   402-502-3572
Omaha, NE 68114   800-729-2556
Fax: 402-502-6791
e-mail: jennyh@ucpnebraska.org
www.ucp.org
United Cerebral Palsy provides information, advocacy, referral services for persons with disabilities and/or their families. UCP also operates an equipment loan program, conducts parent workshops, disseminates written literature on topics of interest.
Carol Hahn, Executive Director
Anne Brodin, Financial & Services Director

Nevada

2671 United Cerebral Palsy of Northern Nevada
4068 S McCarran Boulevard   775-331-3323
Reno, NV 89502-7532   Fax: 775-331-7913
e-mail: upcnn@ucpnn.org
www.ucpnv.org
United Cerebral Palsy provides information, advocacy, referral services for persons with disabilities and/or their families. UCP also provides employment and supported living services and disseminates written literature on topics of interest.
E. Sue Saunders, Chairperson
Julie Ann Utley, Vice Chairperson

New Jersey

2672 United Cerebral Palsy of Hudson County
721 Broadway   201-436-2200
Bayonne, NJ 07002   Fax: 201-436-6642
e-mail: kkearney@ucpofhudsoncounty.org
www.ucp.org
United Cerebral Palsy provides information, advocacy, referral services for persons with disabilities and/or their families. UCP also operates an equipment loan program, conducts parent workshops, disseminates written literature on topics of interest to people with disabilities.
Nick Starita, Executive Director
Keith J Kearney, Associate Executive Director

2673 United Cerebral Palsy of Morris-Somerset
245 Main Street   908-879-2243
Chester, NJ 07930   Fax: 908-879-8363
e-mail: info@ucpnj.org
www.ucpa.org
United Cerebral Palsy provides information, advocacy, referral services for persons with disabilities and/or their families. UCP also operates an equipment loan program, conducts parent workshops, disseminates written literature on topics of interest.

2674 United Cerebral Palsy of New Jersey
1005 Whitehead Road Extension   609-392-4004
Ewing, NJ 08638   888-322-1918
Fax: 609-882-4054
TTY: 609-882-0620
e-mail: info@cpofnj.org
www.cpofnj.org
United Cerebral Palsy provides information, advocacy, referral services for persons with disabilities and/or their families. UCP

also operates an equipment loan program, conducts parent workshops, disseminates written literature on topics of interest.
Mathew Jacobs, President
Warren Kelemen, Vice-President

New York

2675   Center for the Disabled
314 S Manning Boulevard   518-437-5700
Albany, NY 12208   e-mail: bulgaro@cftd.org
          www.cfdsny.org
United Cerebral Palsy provides information, advocacy, referral services for persons with disabilities and/or their families. UCP also operates an equipment loan program, conducts parent workshops, disseminates written literature on topics of interest to people with disabilities.
Alan Krafchin, CEO/President
Patrick J Rielly, Chief Operating Officer

2676   Cerebral Palsy Associations of New York State
90 State Street   518-436-0178
Albany, NY 12207   Fax: 518-436-8619
          e-mail: AffiliateServices@cpofnys.org
          www.cpofnys.org
Provides information, advocacy, referral services for persons with disabilities and/or their families. CP also operates an equipment loan program, conducts parent workshops and disseminates written literature on topics of interest to people with disabilities.
Michael Alvaro, Executive Vice President
Susan Constantino, President & CEO

2677   Niagara Cerebral Palsy
9812 Lockport Road   716-297-0798
Niagara Falls, NY 14304   Fax: 716-297-0998
          e-mail: info@niagaracp.org
          www.ucpaofniagara.com
Provides educational, residential, vocational and recreational programs.

2678   Prospect Child And Family Center
133 Aviation Road   518-798-0170
Queensbury, NY 12804   Fax: 518-798-0533
          e-mail: pcfccent@prospectcenter.com
          www.prospectcenter.com

Gary Edie, President
Eli Socolof, Vice-President

2679   United Cerebral Palsy of Chemung County
1118 Charles Street   607-734-7107
Elmira, NY 14901   Fax: 607-734-7334
          www.chemungcp.com
United Cerebral Palsy provides information, advocacy, referral services for persons with disabilities and/or their families. UCP also operates an equipment loan program, conducts parent workshops, disseminates written literature on topics of interest to people with disabilities.
Mark Peters, Executive Director
Leisa Alger, Associate Executive Director

2680   United Cerebral Palsy of Fulton & Montgomery Counties
67 Division Street   518-842-3511
Amsterdam, NY 12010   Fax: 518-843-6042
          www.ucpa.org
United Cerebral Palsy provides information, advocacy, referral services for persons with disabilities and/or their families. UCP also operates an equipment loan program, conducts parent workshops, disseminates written literature on topics of interest to people with disabilities.

2681   United Cerebral Palsy of Greater Suffolk
250 Marcus Boulevard   631-232-0011
Hauppauge, NY 11788   Fax: 631-232-4422
          e-mail: info@ucp-suffolk.org
          www.ucp-suffolk.org
United Cerebral Palsy provides information, advocacy, referral services for persons with disabilities and/or their families. UCP also operates an equipment loan program, conducts parent workshops, disseminates written literature on topics of interest.
Stephen H Friedman, President & CEO
James Monnier, Board of Directors

2682   United Cerebral Palsy of Nassau County
380 Washington Avenue   516-378-2000
Roosevelt, NY 11575   Fax: 516-868-4089
          e-mail: info@ucpn.org
          www.ucpn.org
United Cerebral Palsy provides information, advocacy, referral services for persons with disabilities and/or their families. UCP also operates an equipment loan program, conducts parent workshops, disseminates written literature on topics of interest to people with disabilities.
Robert Masterson, President
Thomas Connolly, Executive Vice President

2683   United Cerebral Palsy of New York City
80 Maiden Lane   212-683-6700
New York, NY 10038-4811   800-GIV-EUCP
          Fax: 212-685-8394
          e-mail: info@ucpnyc.org
          www.ucpnyc.org
United Cerebral Palsy provides information, advocacy, referral services for persons with disabilities and/or their families. UCP also operates an equipment loan program, conducts parent workshops, disseminates written literature on topics of interest.
Edward R. Matthews, Chief Executive Officer
Gary Geresi, President

2684   United Cerebral Palsy of Putnam & Southern Dutchess Counties
40 John Barrett Road   845-878-9078
Patterson, NY 12563   Fax: 845-878-3203
          e-mail: hvcs@aol.com
          www.ucpa.org
United Cerebral Palsy provides information, advocacy, referral services for persons with disabilities and/or their families. UCP also operates an equipment loan program, conducts parent workshops, disseminates written literature on topics of interest to people with disabilities.

2685   United Cerebral Palsy of Queens: Queens Centers for Progress
81-15 164th Street   718-380-3000
Jamaica, NY 11432   Fax: 718-380-0483
          TTY: 718-969-0270
          e-mail: info@queenscp.org
          www.queenscp.org
Provides information advocacy and referral services for persons with disabilities and/or their families. Offers an equipment loan program parent workshops and written literature on topics of interest to people with disabilities.
George Wildi Berger, President
Joseph A Cristiano, Vice-President

2686   United Cerebral Palsy of Westchester County
1186 King Street   914-937-3800
Rye Brook, NY 10573   Fax: 914-937-0967
          www.cpwestchester.org
United Cerebral Palsy provides information advocacy referral services for persons with disabilities and/or their families. UCP also operates an equipment loan program conducts parent workshops disseminates written literature on topics of interest to people with disabilities.
Richard Osterer, President
Richard Eising, Executive Vice President

2687   United Cerebral Palsy of Western New York
7 Community Drive   716-894-0130
Buffalo, NY 14225   Fax: 716-894-8257
          e-mail: ucpawny1@aol.com
          www.ucpa.org
United Cerebral Palsy provides information advocacy referral services for persons with disabilities and/or their families. UCP also operates an equipment loan program conducts parent workshops disseminates written literature on topics of interest to people with disabilities.

2688   United Cerebral Palsy of the North Country
4 Commerce Lane   315-379-9667
Canton, NY 13617   Fax: 315-379-9388
          e-mail: ucpa@imcnet.net
          www.cpnorthcountry.org/
United Cerebral Palsy provides information advocacy referral services for persons with disabilities and/or their families. UCP also

operates an equipment loan program conducts parent workshops disseminates written literature on topics of interest to people with disabilities.

North Carolina

2689 Easter Seals UCP North Carolina & Virginia
2315 Myron Drive 919-783-8898
Raleigh, NC 27607 800-662-7119
Fax: 919-782-5486
e-mail: QM@nc.eastersealsucp.com
www.nc.easterseals.com
A lifelong partner to families managing disabilities and mental health challenges. Serves more than 20,000 individuals and their families annually through an array of services. Enhances the quality of life for individuals and maximizes their potential for engaging in their communities.
Connie L Cochran, President/CEO

Ohio

2690 United Cerebral Palsy of Central Ohio
440 Industrial Mile Road 614-279-0109
Columbus, OH 43228-2411 Fax: 914-279-2527
e-mail: tfitch@ucpofcentralohio.org
www.ucpofcentralohio.org
United Cerebral Palsy provides information advocacy referral services for persons with disabilities and/or their families. UCP also operates an equipment loan program conducts parent workshops disseminates written literature on topics of interest to people with disabilities.
Charles Dyas, President/Executive Committee Chair
Diane Dierna, Vice-President

2691 United Cerebral Palsy of Cincinnati
3601 Victory Parkway 513-221-4606
Cincinnati, OH 45229 Fax: 513-872-5262
e-mail: sschiller@ucp-cincinnati.org
www.ucp-cincinnati.org
United Cerebral Palsy provides information advocacy referral services for persons with disabilities and/or their families. UCP also operates an equipment loan program conducts parent workshops disseminates written literature on topics of interest to people with disabilities.
Susan Schiller, Executive Director, Development Director

2692 United Cerebral Palsy of Greater Cleveland
10011 Euclid Avenue 216-791-8363
Cleveland, OH 44106 Fax: 216-721-3372
e-mail: sdean@ucpcleveland.org
www.ucpcleveland.org/
United Cerebral Palsy provides information, advocacy, referral services for persons with disabilities and/or their families. UCP also operates an equipment loan program, conducts parent workshops, disseminates written literature on topics of interest to people with disabilities.
Mathew Cox, Chair
Sean Wenger, Vice-Chairman

2693 United Cerebral Palsy of Greater Dane
10011 Euclid Avenue 216-791-8363
Cleveland, OH 44106 Fax: 216-721-3372
e-mail: sdean@ucpcleveland.org
www.ucpcleveland.org
United Cerebral Palsy provides information advocacy referral services for persons with disabilities and/or their families. UCP also operates an equipment loan program conducts parent workshops disseminates written literature on topics of interest to people with disabilities.
Robert J Darden, President
Douglas A Neary, Vice President

Oklahoma

2694 United Cerebral Palsy of Oklahoma
10400 Greenbriar Place 405-759-3562
Oklahoma City, OK 73159 Fax: 405-917-7082
e-mail: info@ucpok.org
www.ucpok.org

United Cerebral Palsy provides information advocacy referral services for persons with disabilities and/or their families. UCP also operates an equipment loan program conducts parent workshops disseminates written literature on topics of interest to people with disabilities.

Oregon

2695 United Cerebral Palsy of Oregon & SW Washington
11731 NE Glenn Widing Drive 503-777-4166
Portland, OR 97220 800-473-4581
Fax: 503-771-8048
e-mail: ucpa@ucpaorwa.org
www.ucp.org
United Cerebral Palsy provides information advocacy referral services for persons with disabilities and/or their families. UCP also operates an equipment loan program conducts parent workshops disseminates written literature on topics of interest to people with disabilities.
Bud Thoune, Executive Director
Doug Taylor, Development and Marketing Director

Pennsylvania

2696 United Cerebral Palsy Central PA
44 S 38th Street 717-975-0611
Camp Hill, PA 17011 Fax: 717-975-0839
e-mail: kidscenter@ucpcentralpa.org
www.ucp.org
United Cerebral Palsy provides information advocacy referral services for persons with disabilities and/or their families. UCP also operates an equipment loan program conducts parent workshops disseminates written literature on topics of interest to people with disabilities.
Jeffrey W Cooper, President/CEO
Jennifer Brubaker~, Director of Administrative Services

2697 United Cerebral Palsy of Beaver, Butler & Lawrence Counties
101 Hindman Lane 724-482-4765
Butler, PA 16001 Fax: 724-283-5945
www.ucpa.org
United Cerebral Palsy provides information, advocacy, referral services for persons with disabilities and/or their families. UCP also operates an equipment loan program, conducts parent workshops, disseminates written literature on topics of interest to people with disabilities.

2698 United Cerebral Palsy of Northwestern Pennsylvania
3745 W 12th Street 814-836-9113
Erie, PA 16505 Fax: 814-833-3919
e-mail: leaton@mecaup.com
www.ucpa.org
United Cerebral Palsy provides information advocacy referral services for persons with disabilities and/or their families. UCP also operates a wheelchair ramp building program, conducts parent workshops and offers adaptive recreation activities.
Laura Eaton, Executive Director

2699 United Cerebral Palsy of Pennsylvania
908 N Second Street 717-441-6044
Harrisburg, PA 17102 866-761-6129
Fax: 717-236-2046
e-mail: kimberlycossar@wannarassoc.com
www.ucp.org
United Cerebral Palsy provides information advocacy referral services for persons with disabilities and/or their families. UCP also operates an equipment loan program conducts parent workshops disseminates written literature on topics of interest to people with disabilities.
Joan Martin, Executive Director
Vini Portzline, Policy Information Exchange

2700 United Cerebral Palsy of Philadelphia Vicinity
102 E Mermaid Lane 215-242-4200
Philadelphia, PA 19118 Fax: 215-247-4229
TTY: 215-248-7620
e-mail: ucpkravitz@aol.com
www.ucpphila.org
United Cerebral Palsy provides information advocacy referral services for persons with disabilities and/or their families. UCP also

operates an equipment loan program conducts parent workshops disseminates written literature on topics of interest to people with disabilities.
Gary J Weyhmuller, President
David J Barnhart, Vice President

2701 United Cerebral Palsy of Pittsburgh
4638 Centre Avenue   412-683-7100
Pittsburgh, PA 15213   Fax: 412-683-4160
                              e-mail: info@ucppittsburgh.org
                                                    www.ucp.org
United Cerebral Palsy provides information advocacy referral services for persons with disabilities and/or their families. UCP also operates an equipment loan program conducts parent workshops disseminates written literature on topics of interest to people with disabilities
Al Condeluci, CEO
Joyce Redmerski, Chief Financial Officer

2702 United Cerebral Palsy of South Central Pennsylvania
788 Cherry Tree Court   717-632-5552
Hanover, PA 17331   800-333-3873
                                        Fax: 717-632-2315
                        e-mail: phoughton@ucpsouthcentral.org
                                                    www.ucp.org
Provides early intervention, in home personal care and community integration services for children and adults with disabilities in York, Adams and Franklin counties.
Paulette Houghton, Executive Director
William Long, Director of Operations

2703 United Cerebral Palsy of Southern Alleghenies Region
119 Jari Drive   814-262-9600
Johnstown, PA 15904   877-371-1110
                                        Fax: 814-262-9650
                                    e-mail: info@ucpsar.org
                                                  www.alucp.org
United Cerebral Palsy provides information, advocacy, referral services for persons with disabilities and/or their families. UCP also operates an equipment loan program, conducts parent workshops, disseminates written literature on topics of interest.
Marie Polinsky, CEO
Mark Malzi, CFO

2704 United Cerebral Palsy of Southwestern Pennsylvania
190 N Main Street   724-229-0851
Washington, PA 15301   Fax: 724-229-9252
                                    e-mail: info@ucpswpa.org
                                                    www.ucp.org
United Cerebral Palsy provides information, advocacy, referral services for persons with disabilities and/or their families. UCP also operates an equipment loan program, conducts parent workshops, disseminates written literature on topics of interest.

2705 United Cerebral Palsy of Western Pennsylvania
2904 Seminary Drive   724-832-8272
Greensburg, PA 15601   Fax: 724-837-8278
                            e-mail: ucp@ucpofwesternpa.org
                                                  www.ucpa.org
United Cerebral Palsy provides information, advocacy, referral services for persons with disabilities and/or their families. UCP also operates an equipment loan program, conducts parent workshops, disseminates written literature on topics of interest.

Rhode Island

2706 United Cerebral Palsy of Rhode Island
200 Main Street   401-728-1800
Pawtucket, RI 02860   Fax: 401-728-0182
                                      e-mail: info@ucpri.org
                                                  www.ucpri.org
United Cerebral Palsy provides information, advocacy, referral services for persons with disabilities and/or their families. UCP also operates an equipment loan program, conducts parent workshops, disseminates written literature on topics of interest to people with disabilities.
Peter Quattromani, Executive Director & CEO
Karl Provost, CFO

Tennessee

2707 United Cerebral Palsy of Middle Tennessee
1200 9th Avenue N   615-242-4091
Nashville, TN 37208   Fax: 615-242-3582
                            e-mail: request@ucpnashville.org
                                              www.ucpmidtn.org/
United Cerebral Palsy provides information, referral services for persons with disabilities and/or their families. UCP also operates an equipment loan program, conducts parent workshops, disseminates written literature on topics of interest to people with disabilities.
Deana Claiborne, Executive Director
Diane Dietrich, Director of Development

2708 United Cerebral Palsy of the Mid-South
3239 players club Parkway   901-761-4277
Memphis, TN 38125   Fax: 901-761-7876
                                  e-mail: ucp@ucpmemphis.org
                                              www.ucpmemphis.org
United Cerebral Palsy provides information, advocacy, referral services for persons with disabilities and/or their families. UCP also operates an equipment loan program, conducts parent workshops, disseminates written literature on topics of interest to people with disabilities.
Michael Nolen, Chief Executive Officer
Kelly Burrow, Executive Vice-President of Development

Texas

2709 United Cerebral Palsy of Greater Houston
4500 Bissonet   713-838-9050
Bellaire, TX 77401   Fax: 713-838-9098
                                  e-mail: ucp@ucphouston.org
                                                  www.ucpa.org
United Cerebral Palsy provides information, advocacy, referral services for persons with disabilities and/or their families. UCP also operates an equipment loan program, conducts parent workshops, disseminates written literature on topics of interest to people with disabilities.

2710 United Cerebral Palsy of Metropolitan Dallas
8802 Harry Hines Boulevard   214-247-4505
Dallas, TX 75235   800-999-1898
                                        Fax: 214-351-2610
                            e-mail: billknudsen@ucpdallas
                                                www.ucpdallas.org
United Cerebral Palsy provides information, advocacy, referral services for persons with disabilities and/or their families. UCP also operates an equipment loan program, conducts parent workshops, disseminates written literature on topics of interest to people with disabilities.
Bill Knudsen, President / Chief Executive Officer
Becky Adams, Chief Operations Officer

2711 United Cerebral Palsy of Tarrant County
1555 Merrimac Circle   817-332-7171
Fort Worth, TX 76107   Fax: 817-332-7601
                                      e-mail: info@ucptc.org
                                                  www.ucpa.org
United Cerebral Palsy provides information, advocacy, referral services for persons with disabilities and/or their families. UCP also operates an equipment loan program, conducts parent workshops, disseminates written literature on topics of interest to people with disabilities.

2712 United Cerebral Palsy of Texas
1016 La Posada Drive   512-472-8696
Austin, TX 78752   800-798-1492
                                        Fax: 512-472-8026
                                    e-mail: info@ucptexas.org
                                                  www.ucpa.org
United Cerebral Palsy provides information, advocacy, referral services for persons with disabilities and/or their families. UCP also operates an equipment loan program, conducts parent workshops, disseminates written literature on topics of interest.

2713 United Cerebral Palsy of Utah
PO Box 65219
S Salt Lake, UT 84165
801-266-1805
Fax: 801-266-2404
e-mail: shellyp@ucputah.org
www.ucpa.org
United Cerebral Palsy provides information, advocacy, referral
services for persons with disabilities and/or their families. UCP
also operates an equipment loan program, conducts parent workshops, disseminates written literature on topics of interest.

2714 Cerebral Palsy of Virginia
5825 Arrowhead Drive
Virginia Beach, VA 23462
757-497-7474
Fax: 757-497-0868
e-mail: kap@cerebralpalsyofvirginia.org
www.cerebralpalsyofvirginia.org
Cerebral Palsy provides information, advocacy, referral services
for persons with disabilities and/or their families. Cerebral Palsy
also operates an equipment loan program, summer computer camp,
art works job training program and much more.
Kathy Prendergast, Executive Director
Michelle Majority, Associate Executive Director

2715 United Cerebral Palsy of Pierce County
6315 S 19th Street
Tacoma, WA 98466-6217
253-565-1463
Fax: 253-565-1463
e-mail: info@ucp-sps.org
www.ucpa.org
United Cerebral Palsy provides information, advocacy, referral
services for persons with disabilities and/or their families. UCP
also operates an equipment loan program, conducts parent workshops, disseminates written literature on topics of interest to
people with disabilities.

2716 United Cerebral Palsy of Greater Dane County
2801 Coho Street
Madison, WI 53713
608-273-4434
Fax: 608-273-3426
e-mail: ucpgdc@ucpdane.org
www.ucpdane.org
Provides information, advocacy, referral services for persons with
disabilities and/or their families. UCP also conducts parent workshops and disseminates written literature on topics of interest to
people with disabilities.
Wade Harrison, President
Rich Cooper, Vice-President

2717 United Cerebral Palsy of North Central Wisconsin
108 Scott Street
Wausau, WI 54401
715-842-8700
800-472-4408
www.ucpa.org
United Cerebral Palsy provides information, advocacy, referral
services for persons with disabilities and/or their families. UCP
also operates an equipment loan program, conducts parent workshops, disseminates written literature on topics of interest to
people with disabilities.

2718 United Cerebral Palsy of Southeastern Wisconsin
7519 W Oklahoma Avenue
Milwaukee, WI 53219
414-329-4500
888-482-7739
Fax: 414-329-4510
TTY: 414-329-4511
e-mail: info@ucpsew.org
www.ucpsew.org/
United Cerebral Palsy provides information, advocacy, referral
services for persons with disabilities and/or their families. UCP
also operates an equipment loan program, conducts parent workshops, disseminates written literature on topics of interest to
people with disabilities.
Scott Andreson, Presdient
Emmett Prosser, Secretary

2719 United Cerebral Palsy of Wisconsin
206 Water Street
Eau Claire, WI 54703
715-832-1782
Fax: 715-832-8203
e-mail: ucp1ruth@sbcglobal net
www.ucpwcw.org/
United Cerebral Palsy provides information, advocacy, referral
services for persons with disabilities and/or their families. UCP
also operates an equipment loan program, conducts parent workshops, disseminates written literature on topics of interest to
people with disabilities.
Connie Werlein, President
Randi Johnson, Vice-President

Research Centers

**2720 Orthopaedic Biomechanics Laboratory Shriners Hospital for
Crippled Children**
Shriners Hospital for Crippled Children
2181 Westlawn Building
Iowa City, IA 52242-1100
319-335-7529
Fax: 319-335-7530
Offers research and studies into cerebral palsy.
Stephen R Skinner, Clinical Director

Support Groups & Hotlines

2721 Family Support Network
215 Centennial Mall S
Lincoln, NE 68508-1813
402-477-2992
800-245-6081

2722 National Health Information Center
PO Box 1133
Washington, DC 20013-1133
310-565-4167
800-336-4797
Fax: 301-984-4256
e-mail: info@nhic.org
www.health.gov/nhic
A health information referral service sponsored by the Office of
Disease Prevention and Health Promotion. Puts health profession-
als and consumers who have health questions in touch with those
organizations that are best able to provide answers.
Ellen Langhans, Chairwoman
Linda Harris, Lead, Health Communication and e-health

Books

2723 An Introduction to Your Child Who Has Cerebral Palsy
Medic Publishing Company
PO Box 89
Redmond, WA 98073-0089
425-881-2883
Information and answers to questions for parents of children with
cerebral palsy.

2724 Children with Cerebral Palsy
Woodbine House
6510 Bells Mill Road
Bethesda, MD 20817-1636
301-897-3570
800-843-7323
Fax: 301-897-5838
e-mail: info@woodbinehouse.com
www.woodbinehouse.com
Explains what Cerebral Palsy is, and discusses its diagnosis and
treatment. Also offers information and advice concerning daily
care, early intervention, therapy, educational options and family
life.
432 pages Paperback
ISBN: 0-933149-15-8

2725 Discovery Book
United Cerebral Palsy Association
1660 L Street NW
Washington, DC 20036-5602
202-776-0406
800-872-5827
Fax: 202-776-0414
ucpnatl@ucpa.org

2726 Individuals with Cerebral Palsy
Mainstream
1030 5th Street NW
Washington, DC 20001-2504
202-898-1400
e-mail: info@mainstreaminc.org
www.mainstreaminc.org

Mainstreaming individuals with cerebral palsy into the workplace.
12 pages

2727 **Occupational Therapy Practice Guidelines for Adults with Cerebral Palsy**
American Occupational Therapy Association
4720 Montgomery Lane
Bethesda, MD 20814-1220
301-652-6611
Fax: 240-762-5150
TDD: 800-377-8555
www.aota.org

15 pages
ISBN: 1-569001-59-6

Children's Books

2728 **Can't You Be Still?**
Gemma B Publishing
776 Corydon Avenue
Winnipeg, MB, R3M 0Y1,
204-452-7566
Fax: 204-475-9903
e-mail: gempub@mts.net
www.gemmab.mb.ca
On Ann's first day at school, the other students are both fascinated and horrified by her cerebral palsy. She wins them over by helping them jump into the water and swim. Available in Braille.
24 pages Paperback
ISBN: 0-969647-70-0
Sarah Yates, President

2729 **Cerebral Palsy**
Franklin Watts Grolier
90 Old Sherman Tpke
Danbury, CT 06816-0001
203-797-3500
800-621-1115
Fax: 203-797-3197
www.auth.grolier.com
A look at the causes, detection, prevention, effects and treatment of Cerebral Palsy.
112 pages Grades 7-12
ISBN: 0-531125-29-7

2730 **Here's What I Mean To Say**
Gemma B Publishing
776 Corydon Avenue
Winnipeg, MB, R3M 0Y1,
204-452-7566
Fax: 204-475-9903
e-mail: gempub@mts.net
www.gemmab.mb.ca
In this books Ann's battle to read is assisted by an angel, who helps her read the directions in Jay's computer game. Is the angel read or is this the magic of reading? Available in Braille.
32 pages Paperback
ISBN: 0-969647-72-7
Sarah Yates, President

2731 **Mine for Keeps**
Little, Brown & Company
34 Beacon Street
Boston, MA 02108-1415
617-227-0730
800-343-9204
Sarah Jean Copeland was born with cerebral palsy. At four years of age she was placed in a school for handicapped children but made such good progress that she could return home. Coming home for Sarah meant a new school, and new adjustments to her parents, two sisters, and her brother. At first Sarah was scared and didn't think she could do all the things she needed to do, but she soon learned her fears were not well-founded.
186 pages Hardcover

2732 **My Brother Matthew**
Woodbine House
6510 Bells Mill Road
Bethesda, MD 20817-1636
800-843-7323
www.woodbinehouse.com
A book written from the point of view of the brother of Matthew, a boy with multiple disabilities, David describes the incidents characterizing how life in his family changes.
28 pages Grades K-5

2733 **Nobody Knows!**
Gemma B Publishing
776 Corydon Avenue
Winnipeg, MB, R3M 0Y1,
204-452-7566
Fax: 204-475-9903
e-mail: gempub@mts.net
www.gemmab.mb.ca
An adventure during which a frustrated Ann goes out to find someone who understand what she wants. She meets a turtle and an alligator, who like her don't use words to communicate. Available in Braille.
24 pages Paperback
ISBN: 0-969647-71-9
Sarah Yates, President

Newsletters

2734 **Family Support Bulletin**
United Cerebral Palsy Associations
1660 L Street NW
Washington, DC 20036-1202
202-842-1266
800-872-5827

Pamphlets

2735 **Cerebral Palsy: Facts & Figures**
United Cerebral Palsy Associations
1825 K Street NW
Washington, DC 20006
202-776-0406
800-872-5827
Fax: 202-776-0414
www.ucp.org
Offers information on what cerebral palsy is, the effects, causes, types, and prevention.

Audio & Video

2736 **A Day At A Time**
Filmakers Library
3212 Duke Street
Alexandria, VA 22314-1798
212-808-4980
Fax: 212-808-4983
e-mail: sales@alexanderstreet.com
www.academicvideostore.com
The story of twin girls with Cerebral Palsy, whose family is determined that they have every opportunity to participate in and lead normal lives. Winner of a number of awards. DVD or VHS $195, Classroom Rental $75
VHS or DVD
Sue Oscar, Co-President

Web Sites

2737 **American Academy for Cerebral Palsy and Developmental Medicine**
AACPDM.org
A multidisciplinary scientific society devoted to the study of cerebral palsy and other childhood onset disabilities, to promoting professional education for the treatment and management of these conditions, and to improving the quality of life for people with these disabilities.

2738 **Healing Well**
www.healingwell.com
An online health resource guide to medical news, chat, information and articles, newsgroups and message boards, books, disease-related web sites, medical directories, and more for patients, friends, and family coping with disabling diseases, disorders, or chronic illnesses.

2739 **Health Finder**
www.healthfinder.gov
Searchable, carefully developed web site offering information on over 1000 topics. Developed by the US Department of Health and Human Services, the site can be used in both English and Spanish.

2740 **Healthlink USA**
www.healthlinkusa.com
Health information concerning treatment, cures, prevention, diagnosis, risk factors, research, support groups, email lists, personal stories and much more. Updated regularly.

2741 Helios Health

www.helioshealth.com

Online resource for your health information. Detailed information about specific health topics, access to expert advice from our Medical Advisory Board, and up-to-date health news.

2742 MedicineNet

www.medicinenet.com

An online resource for consumers providing easy-to-read, authoritative medical and health information.

2743 Medscape

www.medscape.com

Medscape offers specialists, primary care physicians, and other health professionals the Web's most robust and integrated medical information and educational tools.

2744 National Institute of Neurological Disorders and Stroke

www.ninds.nih.gov

The mission of NINDS is to reduce the burden of neurological disease - a burden borne by every age group, by every segment of society, by people all over the world.

2745 National Rehabilitation Information Center

www.naric.com/

The National Rehabilitation Information Center (NARIC) is the library of the National Institute on Disability, Independent Living, and Rehabilitation Research (NIDILRR.).

2746 Neurology Channel

www.healthcommunities.com

Find clearly explained, medically accurate information regarding conditions, including an overview, symptoms, causes, diagnostic procedures and treatment options. On this site it is possible to ask questions and get information from a neurologist and connect to people who have similar health interests.

2747 United Cerebral Palsy Associations

ucp.org

United Cerebral Palsy (UCP) educates, advocates and provides support services to ensure a life without limits for people with a spectrum of disabilities.

2748 WebMD

www.webmd.com

Provides credible information, supportive communities, and in-depth reference material about health subjects. A source for original and timely health information as well as material from well known content providers.

Description

2749 Chronic Fatigue Syndrome

Chronic Fatigue Syndrome, CFS, is an illness characterized by longstanding fatigue that impairs daily functioning. It may be accompanied by sore throat, swollen glands, muscle and joint pain, headaches, sleeplessness, and impaired memory or concentration. Profound or life-altering fatigue—the disease's hallmark—usually comes on suddenly and persists for at least six months, and often for years.

The cause of CFS is controversial. One theory is that a chronic viral infection is involved. Allergic reactions have also been proposed, and various immunologic abnormalities have been reported. Another theory involves proposed disturbances in the hormonal (endocrine) system. Psychological factors may be the cause, although CFS is distinct from typical depression or anxiety. Because the cause is unknown, there is no single test or group of tests that can diagnose CFS. Therefore, the goal in evaluating an individual with presumed CFS is to exclude other treatable illnesses.

Given the difficulty in proving a diagnosis or understanding the cause of CFS, it is not surprising that many treatments have been offered for it. Antidepressants appear to be the most successful treatment studied so far; as many as 80 percent of patients report benefit. Other therapies, including nutritional supplements, hormones, antiviral drugs and steroids have been mostly disappointing.

Patients with CFS need emotional support from physicians and family, due to the debilitating nature of the disease. Individual and group therapy may help some individuals. See also *Fibromyalgia*.

National Agencies & Associations

2750 American Academy of Sleep Medicine
2510 North Frontage Road   630-737-9700
Darien, IL 60561   Fax: 630-737-9790
www.aasmnet.org
A unique multi-disciplinary organization for both individual members and center members. The individual member branch includes clinicians involved in the diagnosis and treatment of patients with disorders of sleep and alertness.
Amy Aronsky, Director
M Safwan Badr, President

2751 International Association for Chronic Fatigue
27 N Wacker Drive   847-258-7248
Chicago, IL 60606   Fax: 847-579-0975
e-mail: Admin@iacfsme.org
www.IACFS.net
A nonprofit organization of research scientists, physicians, licensed medical healthcare professionals and other individuals and institutions interested in promoting the stimulation, coordination and exchange of ideas for CFS research and patient care.
Newsletter
Fred Friedberg, President
Staci R Stevens, Vice President

2752 National Chronic Fatigue Syndrome and Fibromyalgia Association
PO Box 18426   816-737-1343
Kansas City, MO 64133-8426   Fax: 816-524-6782
e-mail: information@ncfsfa.org
www.ncfsfa.org
Compiles and provides peer reviewed, scientifically accurate educational materials to inform the public, health professionals, patients and their families about the nature and impact of chronic fatigue syndrome, fibromyalgia and related disorders. Offers a support group.
Orvalene Prewitt, President

2753 National Institute of Allergy and Infectious Diseases
Office of Communications
6610 Rockledge Drive   301-402-1663
Bethesda, MD 20892-6612   866-284-4107
Fax: 301-402-1020
TDD: 800-877-8339
e-mail: af10r@nih.gov
www.niaid.nih.gov
Offers information and educational materials on Chronic Fatigue Syndrome and other disorders.
Anthony S Fauci, MD, Director

2754 Option Institute
2080 South Undermountain Road   413-229-2100
Sheffield, MA 01257   800-714-2779
Fax: 413-229-8931
e-mail: participantsupport@option.org
www.option.org
Self-defeating beliefs, along with attitudes and judgments, can lead to a host of physical and psychological challenges, including Chronic Fatigue Syndrome. The Option Institute offers programs designed to help you gain new perspectives on the attitudes and judgments that may be affecting your life, especially those regarding and surrounding Chronic Fatigue Syndrome.
Barry Kaufman, Co-Founder
Samahria Ltye Kaufman, Co-Founder

Foundations

2755 National CFIDS Foundation
103 Aletha Road   781-449-3535
Needham, MA 02492   Fax: 781-449-8606
e-mail: info@ncf-net.org
www.ncf-net.org
The goals of the Foundation are to help fund medical research to find a cause, expedite treatments and eventually a cure for this devastating disease. The NCF also strives to provide information, education, and support to those people who have CFIDS (also known as chronic fatigue syndrome (CFS), myalgic encephalomyelitis (ME) and many other names)— as well as related illnesses such as Gulf War Illness (GWI) and Multiple Chemical Sensitivities (MCS). Provides guides, articles, and newsletters.
Gail Kansky, President
Prof. Alan Cocchetto, Medical Advisor

Support Groups & Hotlines

2756 Centers for Disease Control and Prevention
1600 Clifton Road
Atlanta, GA 30333   800-232-4636
TTY: 888-232-6348
e-mail: cdcinfo@cdc.gov
www.cdc.gov
Collaborating to create the expertise, information, and tools that people and their communities need to protect their health - through health promotion, prevention of disease, injury and disability, and preparedness for new health threats.
Thomas R Frieden MD MPH, Director

2757 Chronic Fatigue Syndrome & Fibromyalgia Support
7250 Clearvista Dr   317-252-9223
Indianapolis, IN 46256
Offers emotional support, education and information about CFS and FMS through statewide monthly meetings and a quarterly

newsletter. Provides 24-hour hotline and physician/attorney referrals. Financial assistance for members. Support group meets twice a month at Community Hospital North Professional Building and at other locations throughout Indiana.

2758 National Chronic Fatigue Syndrome and Fibromyalgia Association
PO Box 18426
816-737-1343
Kansas City, MO 64133
Fax: 816-524-6782
e-mail: information@ncfsfa.org
www.ncfsfa.org
To educate and inform the public about the nature and impact of Chronic Fatigue Syndrome and Fibromyalgia and related disorders.
Orvalene Prewitt, President

2759 National Health Information Center
PO Box 1133
310-565-4167
Washington, DC 20013-1133
800-336-4797
Fax: 301-984-4256
e-mail: info@nhic.org
www.health.gov/nhic
A health information referral service sponsored by the Office of Disease Prevention and Health Promotion. Puts health professionals and consumers who have health questions in touch with those organizations that are best able to provide answers.
Ellen Langhans, Chairwoman
Linda Harris, Lead, Health Communication and e-health

Books

2760 CFIDS in Children Packet
CFIDS Association of America
PO Box 220398
Charlotte, NC 28222-0398
800-442-3437
This packet contains articles about CFIDS and children.
60 pages

2761 CFS Cookbook
CFIDS Association of America
PO Box 220398
Charlotte, NC 28222-0398
800-442-3437
Gourmet recipes designed to combat the monotony associated with CFIDS, allergy and immune-compromised diets.
218 pages

2762 Chronic Fatigue Syndrome Cookbook: Delicious & Wellness-Enhancing Recipes
DIANE Publishing Company
330 Pusey Avenue
610-461-6200
Darby, PA 19023
800-782-3833
Fax: 610-461-6130
e-mail: dianepublishing@gmail.com
www.dianepublishing.net
These recipes help combat the boredom of the CFS diet usually recommended and still satisfy all of your nutritional requirements as a CFS sufferer. In addition, the book includes a comprehensive look at the do's and don't's of a CFS diet, quick recipes for those days when you are too tired to cook and an insightful medical introduction.
218 pages Hardcover
ISBN: 0-756753-28-7
Herman Baron, Publisher

2763 Chronic Fatigue Syndrome and the Yeast Connection
CFIDS Association of America
PO Box 220398
Charlotte, NC 28222-0398
800-442-3437
Dr. Crook explains the possible role of multiple entities, including yeast overgrowth, allergies and chemical sensitivities, in CFS and how each contributes to immune dysregulation.
386 pages

2764 Chronic Fatigue Syndrome: Information for Physicians
Barry Leonard, author
DIANE Publishing Company

330 Pusey Avenue
610-461-6200
Darby, PA 19023
800-782-3833
Fax: 610-461-6130
e-mail: dianepublishing@gmail.com
www.dianepublishing.net
Includes a historical perspective on chronic fatigue syndrome; epidemiology; clinical picture; evaluation of patients; patient management; etiologic theories; public health service resources; fact sheet; resources for patients, overview of the CFS research program; NIAID and NIAID/Johns Hopkins hospital study, which seeks volunteers, management strategies for CFS; the relationship between nuerally mediatec hypotension and CFS and fibromyalgia and CFS; solving diagnostic and therapeutic dilemmas.
60 pages Paperback
ISBN: 0-788143-78-6
Herman Baron, Publisher

2765 Chronic Fatigue Syndrome: The Limbic Hypothesis
CFIDS Association of America
PO Box 220398
Charlotte, NC 28222-0398
800-442-3437
A detailed thesis proposing CFS as a limbic system encephalopathy in the context of a dysregulated neuroimmune system.
259 pages

2766 Chronic Fatigue: Your Complete Exercise Guide
Human Kinetics Press
1607 N Market Street
217-351-5076
Champaign, IL 61820-5076
800-747-4457
Fax: 217-351-1549
e-mail: info@hkusa.com
www.humankinetics.com
1993 144 pages Paperback
ISBN: 0-873223-93-4
Steve Ruhlig, Marketing Director

2767 Coping With CFS
CFIDS Association of America
PO Box 220398
704-365-2343
Charlotte, NC 28222-0398
800-442-3437
Fax: 704-365-9755
e-mail: info@cfids.org
www.cfids.org
Offers practical, established coping strategies for living better with CFIDS. Based on Dr. Friedberg's experiences as a person with CFIDS and a counselor to PWCs.
176 pages
Jon Sterling, Chairman
Kim Kenny, President/CEO

2768 Disability and Chronic Fatigue Syndrome
The Haworth Press
10 Alice Street
607-722-5857
Binghamton, NY 13904-1580
800-429-6784
Fax: 800-895-0582
e-mail: getinfo@haworthpressinc.com
www.impresaitalia.info
Discusses the difficult subject of how to diagnose disability in chronic fatigue syndrome patients, how to determine the severity of a patient's disability, and how new disability guidelines would make more chronic fatigue patients eligible to apply for disability benefits.
121 pages Paperback
ISBN: 0-789005-01-8
Bill Cohen, Publisher
Sandy Jones, VP Marketing

2769 Doctor's Guide to Chronic Fatigue Syndrome
CFIDS Association of America
PO Box 220398
Charlotte, NC 28222-0398
800-442-3437
Written by one of the world's leading experts on CFIDS.
275 pages

2770 Fifty Things You Should Know About the Chronic Fatigue Syndrome Epidemic
St. Martin's Press

175 5th Avenue
New York, NY 10010-7848

212-674-5151
800-221-7945
Fax: 212-420-9314

1993
ISBN: 0-312950-43-8

2771 Hope and Help for Chronic Fatigue Syndrome
CFIDS Association of America
PO Box 220398
Charlotte, NC 28222-0398

704-365-2343
800-442-3437
Fax: 704-365-9755
e-mail: info@cfids.org
www.cfids.org

Insight into the experience of having CFIDS, the physical and emotional impact, difficulty in obtaining a diagnosis, available methods of treatment and key strategies for regaining control over your life.
216 pages
Jon Sterling, Chairman
Kim Kenny, President/CEO

2772 International Classification of Sleep Disorders
American Academy of Sleep Medicine
2510 North Frontage Road
Darien, IL 60561

630-737-9700
Fax: 630-737-9790
e-mail: cme@aasmnet.org
www.aasmnet.org

A comprehensive manual for physicians and other healthcare professionals containing information on 84 sleep disorders. The extensive text describes the diagnostic features of each disorder and includes specific diagnostic and severity criteria for each disorder.
396 pages Paperback

2773 Living with CFS: A Personal Story of the Struggle for Recovery
CFIDS Association of America
PO Box 220398
Charlotte, NC 28222-0398

800-442-3437

Describes the pain associated with the author's loss of livelihood, impaired physical and mental functioning and the strain on his marriage and friendships, while maintaining hope for recovery.
224 pages
ISBN: 1-560250-75-5

2774 Living with ME
CFIDS Association of America
PO Box 220398
Charlotte, NC 28222-0398

800-442-3437
Fax: 704-365-9755

The author describes M.E. (mylagic encephalomyelitis - the British term for chronic fatigue syndrome), and discusses practical methods for coping and comments on various treatments.

2775 Music Appreciation
CFIDS Association of America
PO Box 220398
Charlotte, NC 28222-0398

800-442-3437

A full-length collection of poems by Skloot who has been disabled by CFIDS since 1988.
105 pages

2776 Night-Side: CFS and the Illness Experience
CFIDS Association of America
PO Box 220398
Charlotte, NC 28222-0398

704-365-2343
800-442-3437
Fax: 704-365-9755
e-mail: info@cfids.org
www.cfids.org

An honest and ultimately hopeful exploration of what it means to have your life shattered by disease.
190 pages
Jon Sterling, Chairman
Kim Kenny, President/CEO

2777 Recovering From the Chronic Fatigue Syndrome: A Guide to Self-Empowerment
Berkley Books
200 Madison Avenue
New York, NY 10016-3903

212-951-8800
www.penguinputnam.com

This book teaches persons with CFIDS to take control of their illness and to help themselves find the road to recovery.
1993 224 pages Paperback
ISBN: 0-399518-07-0

2778 Running on Empty
CFIDS Association of America
PO Box 220398
Charlotte, NC 28222-0398

704-365-2343
800-442-3437
Fax: 704-365-9755
e-mail: info@cfids.org
www.cfids.org

Landmark guide to CFIDS has just been revised and re-released. A must read for the newly disgnosed.
315 pages
Jon Sterling, Chairman
Kim Kenny, President/CEO

2779 Self-Caring Fatigue
Rodale Press
604 East Stree
Otho, IA 50569-0099

715-191-0217
515-972-4444
Fax: 515-972-4415
e-mail: info@peopleagainstcancer.com
www.rodale.com

A step-by-step plan to uncover and eliminate the causes of chronic fatigue.
1993 320 pages
ISBN: 0-875961-61-4

2780 Solving the Puzzle of CFS
2730 Wilshire Boulevard
Santa Monica, CA 90403-4724

310-453-4424
Fax: 310-966-9196

Magazines

2781 CFIDS Chronicle
CFIDS Association of America
PO Box 220398
Charlotte, NC 28222-0398

704-362-2343
800-442-3437
Fax: 704-365-9755

The largest and most comprehensive periodical specifically pertaining to chronic fatigue syndrome information in the world.

2782 Feel Good Catalog
2895 W Oxford Avenue
Englewood, CO 80110-4370

303-790-1045
800-997-6789

Variety of items to ease pain.

2783 Journal SLEEP
American Academy of Sleep Medicine
One Westbrook Corp Center
Westchester, IL 60154

708-492-0930
Fax: 708-492-0943
www.journalslep.org

Publishes articles ranging from clinical investigations of sleep/wake disorders and medical problems during sleep, to investigations of the basic physiological and biochemical events and anatomical structures involved in normal and abnormal sleep. Includes psychological and psycho-physiological research, as well as research in relevant areas of circadian and biological rhythms.
10x Year
ISBN: 0-161810-5 -

2784 Journal of the Chronic Fatigue Syndrome
Haworth Medical Press
10 Alice Street
Binghamton, NY 13904-1503

607-722-5857
800-429-6784
Fax: 607-722-0012
www.impresaitalia.info

Peer reviewed medical journal containing CFIDS scientific abstract information. Appropriate for patients as well as medical professionals.
Quarterly
Nancy Klimas MD, Founding Co-Editor

Newsletters

2785   Health Points
TyH Publications
17007 E Colony Drive
Fountain Hills, AZ 85268   800-801-1406
                            e-mail: editor@e-tyh.com
National newsletter with articles on complementary therapy, latest
nutrition news, disability issues and much more. Focus is on
fibromyalgia, chronic fatigue, arthritis and chronic pain.
Quarterly

2786   Heart of America News
National Chronic Fatigue Syndrome & Fibromyalgia
PO Box 18426
Kansas City, MO 64133-8426   660-313-2000
Offers scientifically accurate information, medical updates, infor-
mational references, articles on coping and living with Chronic Fa-
tigue Syndrome and more, based on peer-reviewed materials.
Quarterly

2787   National Forum
103 Aletha Road   781-449-3535
Needham, MA 02492   Fax: 781-449-8606
                              e-mail: info@ncf-net.org
                                    www.ncf-net.org
The Forum's focus: CFIDS/ME, FMS, GWI, MCS and related ill-
nesses.
Gail Kansky, President

2788   Syndrome Sentinel
Massachusetts CFIDS Association
808 Main Street
Waltham, MA 02451-8533   781-893-4415
                                    www2.shore.net
This quarterly newsletter contains articles written by health-care
professionals working with these conditions. Contributors include
traditional and alternative experts, as well as personal stories from
people with these chronic syndromes and their significant others.

2789   The National Forum
The National CFIDS Foundation
103 Aletha Road   781-449-3535
Needham, MA 02492   Fax: 781-449-8606
                              e-mail: info@ncf-net.org
                                    www.ncf-net.org
Offers the latest information on CFIDS treatments being tried
throughout the United States.

Pamphlets

2790   Americans with Disabilities Act: CFS and Employment
National Chronic Fatigue Syndrome & Fibromyalgia
PO Box 18426
Kansas City, MO 64133-8426   660-313-2000

2791   CFIDS Membership Packet
CFIDS Association of America
PO Box 220398
Charlotte, NC 28222-0398   800-442-3437
                                    Fax: 704-365-9755
Offers pamphlets, brochures, information on local support groups
for members.

2792   CFIDS in Children
CFIDS Association of America
PO Box 220398
Charlotte, NC 28222-0398   800-442-3437
Describes the special difficulties faced by children with CFIDS.

2793   CFS in the Workplace
National Chronic Fatigue Syndrome & Fibromyalgia
PO Box 18426
Kansas City, MO 64133   660-313-2000

2794   Chronic Fatigue Syndrome & School Success
National Chronic Fatigue Syndrome & Fibromyalgia
PO Box 18426
Kansas City, MO 64133-8426   660-313-2000

2795   Chronic Fatigue Syndrome in Children
National Chronic Fatigue Syndrome & Fibromyalgia
PO Box 18426   660-313-2000
Kansas City, MO 64133

2796   Chronic Fatigue Syndrome in Men
National Chronic Fatigue Syndrome & Fibromyalgia
PO Box 18426   660-313-2000
Kansas City, MO 64133-8426

2797   Chronic Fatigue Syndrome: A Pamphlet for Physicians
National Institute of Allergy & Infectious Disease
5601 Fishers Lane   301-402-1663
Bethesda, MD 20892-2520   Fax: 301-402-0120
                           e-mail: niaidnews@niaid.nih.gov
                                     www.niaid.nih.gov
Offers information on epidemiology, clinical procedures, evaluations, patient management, neuropsychologic features and
etiologic theories.

2798   Chronic Fatigue Syndrome: The Thief of Vitality
National Chronic Fatigue Syndrome & Fibromyalgia
PO Box 18426   660-313-2000
Kansas City, MO 64133-8426

2799   Coping Skills
National Chronic Fatigue Syndrome & Fibromyalgia
PO Box 18426   660-313-2000
Kansas City, MO 64133-8426

2800   Disability Packet
CFIDS Association of America
PO Box 220398
Charlotte, NC 28222-0398   800-442-3437
Includes nine Chronicle articles about disability benefits and how
persons with CFIDS can secure Social Security Disability Insur-
ance benefits.
42 pages

2801   Facts About Chronic Fatigue Syndrome
Centers for Disease Control & Prevention
Division of Viral Dis   404-639-3311
Atlanta, GA 30333

2802   Fibromyalgia
National Chronic Fatigue Syndrome & Fibromyalgia
PO Box 18426   660-313-2000
Kansas City, MO 64133-8426

2803   March is Chronic Fatigue Syndrome Awareness Month Tips
National Chronic Fatigue Syndrome & Fibromyalgia
PO Box 18426   660-313-2000
Kansas City, MO 64133

2804   Neuropsychological Rehabilitation Suggestions/Techniques
National Chronic Fatigue Syndrome & Fibromyalgia
PO Box 18426   660-313-2000
Kansas City, MO 64133-8426

2805   School's Guide for Students with CFS
National Chronic Fatigue Syndrome & Fibromyalgia
PO Box 18426   660-313-2000
Kansas City, MO 64133-8426

2806   Social Security Disability Benefits Information
National Chronic Fatigue Syndrome & Fibromyalgia
PO Box 18426   660-313-2000
Kansas City, MO 64133-8426

2807   Suicide is Not an Option
National Chronic Fatigue Syndrome
PO Box 18426   660-313-2000
Kansas City, MO 64133-8426

2808   Understanding CFIDS
CFIDS Association of America
PO Box 220398
Charlotte, NC 28222-0398   800-442-3437
Provides an extensive overview of CFIDS and answers the most
commonly asked questions about the disease.

2809   Understanding the Emotions Surrounding CFS
National Chronic Fatigue Syndrome & Fibromyalgia

PO Box 18426   660-313-2000
Kansas City, MO 64133-8426

Audio & Video

2810 Behavioral and Circadian Sleep Problems of Infancy and Childhood
American Academy of Sleep Medicine
2510 North Frontage Road   630-737-9700
Darien, IL 60561   Fax: 708-492-0943
                                        e-mail: cme@aasmnet.org
                                              www.aasmnet.org
Addresses the problems of sleep disorders in children and outlines the types of disturbances, both of a medical and behavioral nature, that are commonly identified.
66 slides

2811 CFS and Self-Esteem
CFIDS Association of America
PO Box 220398
Charlotte, NC 28222-0398   800-442-3437
Addresses the sources of low self-esteem in persons with CFIDS and offers reassurance and practical techniques for increasing self-confidence.
Audiotape

2812 CFS: Addressing the Realities of a Chronic Illness
National Chronic Fatigue Syndrome & Fibromyalgia
PO Box 18426   660-313-2000
Kansas City, MO 64133-8426
This video offers reliable information featuring patients and a medical professional.

2813 CFS: Unraveling the Mystery
CFIDS Association of America
PO Box 220398
Charlotte, NC 28222-0398   800-442-3437
An excellent videotape for convincing skeptics that CFIDS is a real disease.
Videotape

2814 Chronic Fatigue Syndrome: For Those Who Care
CFIDS Association of America
PO Box 220398
Charlotte, NC 28222-0398   800-442-3437
An audiotape designed for friends and family of persons with CFIDS.
Audiotape

2815 Chronic Fatigue Syndrome: Information, Relaxation/Healing Exercise
CFIDS Association of America
PO Box 220398
Charlotte, NC 28222-0398   800-442-3437
Includes a comprehensive overview of CFS and relaxation/healing and imagery/stress reduction exercises for persons with CFIDS.
Audiotape

2816 Fibromyalgia
National Chronic Fatigue Syndrome & Fibromyalgia
PO Box 18426   660-313-2000
Kansas City, MO 64133
Videotape

2817 HHS Satelite Video on Chronic Fatigue Syndrome and Fibromyalgia Association
National Chronic Fatigue Syndrome and Fibromyalgia
PO Box 18426   660-313-2000
Kansas City, MO 64133-8426

2818 Living Hell: The Real World of Chronic Fatigue Syndrome
CFIDS Association of America
PO Box 220398
Charlotte, NC 28222-0398   800-442-3437
An emotional exposure of the tragedy of CFIDS.
Videotape

2819 Neurocognitive Aspects of CFS
CFIDS Association of America

PO Box 220398
Charlotte, NC 28222-0398   800-442-3437
A description of CFIDS-associated neurocognitive deficits and strategies for coping with them and the embarrassment and frustration they cause.
Audiotape

Web Sites

2820 American Association for Chronic Fatigue Syndrome
                                              www.aacfs.org
A non profit organization of research scientists, physicians, licensed medical healthcare professionals, and other indviduals and institutions interested in promoting the stimulation, coordination, and exchange of ideas for CFS research and patient care.

2821 CFIDS Association of America
                                              solvecfs.org
An organization focused on myalgic encephalomyelitis (ME) and Chronic Fatigue Syndrome (CFS) since being founded in 1987.

2822 Centers for Disease Control and Prevention
                                              www.cdc.gov
CDC works 24/7 to protect America from health, safety and security threats, both foreign and in the U.S. Whether diseases start at home or abroad, are chronic or acute, curable or preventable, human error or deliberate attack, CDC fights disease and supports communities and citizens to do the same.

2823 Healing Well
                                              www.healingwell.com
An online health resource guide to medical news, chat, information and articles, newsgroups and message boards, books, disease-related web sites, medical directories, and more for patients, friends, and family coping with disabling diseases, disorders, or chronic illnesses.

2824 Health Finder
                                              www.healthfinder.gov
Searchable, carefully developed web site offering information on over 1000 topics. Developed by the US Department of Health and Human Services, the site can be used in both English and Spanish.

2825 Healthlink USA
                                              www.healthlinkusa.com
Health information concerning treatment, cures, prevention, diagnosis, risk factors, research, support groups, email lists, personal stories and much more. Updated regularly.

2826 Helios Health
                                              www.helioshealth.com
Online resource for your health information. Detailed information about specific health topics, access to expert advice from our Medical Advisory Board, and up-to-date health news.

2827 Journal of Chronic Fatigue Syndrome
                                              www.cfs-news.org/jcfs.htm
Offers multidisciplinary original research, practical clinical management, case reports, and literature reviews to keep the entire health care delivery team well informed.

2828 MedicineNet
                                              www.medicinenet.com
An online resource for consumers providing easy-to-read, authoritative medical and health information.

2829 Medscape
                                              www.medscape.com
Medscape offers specialists, primary care physicians, and other health professionals the Web's most robust and integrated medical information and educational tools.

2830 Option Institute
                                              www.option.org/cfs.shtml
Self-defeating beliefs, along with attitudes and judgments, can lead to a host of physical and psychological challenges, including Chronic Fatigue Syndrome. The Option Institute offers programs designed to help you gain new perspectives on the attitudes and judgments that may be affecting your life, especially those regarding and surrounding Chronic Fatigue Syndrome.

2831 **Sleepnet**

www.sleepnet.com

Links all the sleep information located on the internet. Provides a place for everyone to read and post questions, or responses.

2832 **WebMD**

www.webmd.com

Provides credible information, supportive communities, and in-depth reference material about health subjects. A source for original and timely health information as well as material from well known content providers.

Description

2833 **Chronic Pain**

Chronic pain is defined as pain persisting for more than one month after resolution of an acute injury or pain that persists or recurs for more than three months. The pain may begin for unknown reasons, or may begin with some injury or illness but persist long after the triggering event is gone. Human pain has physiological causes but also has psychological components differing for each person. Many Americans suffer from chronic pain. The annual cost, including treatment and lost work days, now hovers around $100 billion in the US.

Doctors and patients have tried almost every conceivable type of therapy for chronic pain. Drug treatments include narcotics (codeine and morphine), non-narcotic painkillers such as acetaminophen, and nonsteroidal anti-inflammatory drugs such as ibuprofen. Use of antidepressants, either alone or in conjunction with pain medications, can be beneficial. Doctors may inject drugs to block the nerves that carry the pain signal, or may even cut the nerve. Physical measures include heat or cold application, application of electrical stimuli (TENS), stretching, and general conditioning exercises. Psychological treatment includes psychotherapy, meditation, hypnosis and biofeedback-relaxation. Because of the complexity of chronic pain and its treatment, some doctors have begun to specialize in management of pain, and have organized multidisciplinary pain clinics which offer expertise from anesthesiology, rheumatology, neurosurgery, psychology and physical therapy.

A realistic goal of therapy is to improve one's daily functioning; for instance, being able to return to work or pleasurable activities. Those able to achieve this status will often state that the pain is still there but that it does not bother them like it once did. Whatever the stage of one's condition, peer support is important, and is available from local in-person support groups or from Internet chat rooms and bulletin boards.

National Agencies & Associations

2834 **American Chronic Pain Association**
PO Box 850
Rocklin, CA 95677   800-533-3231
                          Fax: 916-632-3208
                e-mail: ACPA@pacbell.net
                      www.theacpa.org
ACPA mission is to facilitate peer support and education for individuals with chronic pain and their families so that these individuals may live more fully in spite of their pain; and to raise awareness among the health care community and policy makers.
Penny Cowan, Executive Director

2835 **American Osteopathic Association**
142 E. Ontario St.   312-202-8000
Chicago, IL 60611   800-621-1773
                          Fax: 312-202-8200
                e-mail: info@osteopathic.org
                      www.osteopathic.org
Serving as the professional family for more than 110,000 osteopathic physicians (DOs) and osteopathic medical students, the American Osteopathic Association (AOA) promotes public health and encourages scientific research.
Robert S. Juhasz, DO, President
Adrienne White-Faines, Executive Director

2836 **American Pain Society**
4700 W Lake Avenue   847-375-4715
Glenview, IL 60025   866-574-2654
                          Fax: 847-375-6479
                e-mail: info@americanpainsociety.org
                      www.americanpainsociety.org
A multidisciplinary organization of basic and clinical scientists practicing clinicians policy analysts and others. Mission is to advance pain-related research education treatment and professional practice.
Catherine H Underwood, Executive Director
Seddon R Savage MD, MS, President

2837 **American Physical Therapy Association**
1111 North Fairfax Street   703-684-2782
Alexandria, VA 22314   800-999-2782
                          Fax: 703-684-7343
                          TDD: 703-683-6748
                e-mail: memberservices@apta.org
                      www.apta.org
The American Physical Therapy Association (APTA) is an individual membership professional organization representing more than 90,000 member physical therapists (PTs), physical therapist assistants (PTAs), and students of physical therapy.
Paul Rockar, Jr, PT, DPT, MS, President
J. Michael Bowers, Chief Executive Officer

2838 **International Association for the Study of Pain**
111 Queen Anne Avenue N   206-283-0311
Seattle, WA 98109-4955   Fax: 206-283-9403
                e-mail: iaspdesk@iasp-pain.org
                      www.iasp-pain.org
The International Association for the Study of Pain is the leading professional forum for science practice and education in the field of pain.
Eija Anneli Kalso MD, President
Judith A Paice PhD, RN, President Elect

2839 **International Pelvic Pain Society Women's Medical Plaza**
Women's Medical Plaza
1100 E Woodfield Road   847-517-8712
Schaumburg, IL 60173   800-624-9676
                          Fax: 847-517-7229
                e-mail: info@pelvicpain.org
                      www.pelvicpain.org
Short range goal is to recruit organize and educate health care professionals actively involved with the treatment of patients who have chronic pelvic pain.
Fred Marion Howard, Chairman of the Board
Richard P Marvel MD, President

2840 **National Association of Myofascial Trigger Point Therapists**
                e-mail: president@namtpt.org
                      www.myofascialtherapy.org
The NAMTPT is a professional organization dedicated increasing the public awareness of and access to myofascial pain treatment.
Mary Biancalana, President
Julie Zuleger, Vice President

2841 **National Fibromyalgia & Chronic Pain Association**
31 Federal Avenue   801-200-3627
Logan, UT 84321   e-mail: info@fmcpaware.org
                      www.fmcpaware.org
Jan Chambers, president and founder of the NFMCPA, a 501(c) nonprofit organization, recognized the need for an organization to bring together advocacy, research and education for the fibromyalgia (FM) and overlapping conditions.
Janet Favero Chambers, President

2842 Reflex Sympathetic Dystrophy Syndrome Association (RSDSA)
PO Box 502   203-877-3790
Milford, CT 06460   877-662-7737
Fax: 203-882-8362
e-mail: info@rsds.org
www.rsds.org
Nonprofit professional and consumer organization founded to support research into the cause, treatment and cure of reflex sympathetic dystrophy syndrome. RSDSA also organizes support groups, promote awareness among health professionals and develop educational programs.
Paul R Charlesworth, President
James E Tyrrell Jr, Chairman of the Board

Support Groups & Hotlines

2843 National Health Information Center
PO Box 1133   310-565-4167
Washington, DC 20013-1133   800-336-4797
Fax: 301-984-4256
e-mail: info@nhic.org
www.health.gov/nhic
A health information referral service sponsored by the Office of Disease Prevention and Health Promotion. Puts health professionals and consumers who have health questions in touch with those organizations that are best able to provide answers.
Ellen Langhans, Chairwoman
Linda Harris, Lead, Health Communication and e-health

Books

2844 ACPA Facilitator Guide & Materials
American Chronic Pain Association
PO Box 850   916-632-0922
Rocklin, CA 95677   800-533-3231
Fax: 916-632-3208
e-mail: acpa@theacpa.org
www.theacpa.org
This guide will help you and others in your community organize an ACPA chapter. The manual contains how-to information on organizing an ACPA chapter, sharing responsibility for the group with others, finding a meeting place, conducting the first meeting, and generating public interest in your area. You must be an ACPA member to purchase this manual.
Penny Cowan, Executive Director

2845 ACPA Family Manual
Penny Cowan, author
American Chronic Pain Association
PO Box 850   916-632-0922
Rocklin, CA 95677   800-533-3231
Fax: 916-632-3208
e-mail: acpa@theacpa.org
www.theacpa.org
A manual designed with the needs of those who live with a person who has chronic pain.
149 pages
ISBN: 0-967387-82-5
Penny Cowan, Executive Director

2846 ACPA Journal Reflections of You
American Chronic Pain Association
PO Box 850   916-632-0922
Rocklin, CA 95677   800-533-3231
Fax: 916-632-3208
e-mail: acpa@theacpa.org
www.theacpa.org
A daily meditation and personal journal book which provides positive and motivating thoughts to stimulate your thinking and challenge you to personal growth. Your daily entries in the journal will help track your progress and show when you have reached your personal goal.
Penny Cowan, Executive Director

2847 ACSM's Exercise Management for Persons with Chronic Disease & Disabilities
Human Kinetics Press

1607 N Market Street   800-747-4457
Champaign, IL 61820-5076   800-747-4457
Fax: 217-351-1549
e-mail: info@hkusa.com
www.humankinetics.com
1993 384 pages Hardcover
ISBN: 0-736038-72-8
Steve Ruhlig, Marketing Director

2848 Essential Guide to Chronic Illness: The Active Patient's Handbook
James W Long, author
DIANE Publishing Company
330 Pusey Avenue   610-461-6200
Darby, PA 19023   800-782-3833
Fax: 610-461-6130
e-mail: dianepublishing@gmail.com
www.dianepublishing.net
A comprehensive guide to dealing with nearly 50 chronic illness and conditions from acne to Zollinger-Ellison syndrome, including diabetes, menopause, migraines, rheumatoid arthritis and psoriasis.
625 pages Paperback
ISBN: 0-788169-03-3
Herman Baron, Publisher

2849 From Patient to Person: First Steps
American Chronic Pain Association
PO Box 850   916-632-0922
Rocklin, CA 95677   800-533-3231
Fax: 916-632-3208
e-mail: acpa@theacpa.org
www.theacpa.org
A workbook designed to help anyone who has a chronic pain problem to gain a better understanding of how one can begin to cope with all the problems that their pain creates.

ISBN: 0-967387-80-9
Penny Cowan, Executive Director

2850 Occupational Therapy Practice Guidelines for Adults with Low Back Pain
American Occupational Therapy Association
4720 Montgomery Lane   301-652-6611
Bethesda, MD 20814-1220   Fax: 240-762-5150
TDD: 800-377-8555
www.aota.org
15 pages
ISBN: 1-569001-49-9

2851 Occupational Therapy Practice Guidelines for Adults with Hip Fracture/Replacement
American Occupational Therapy Association
4720 Montgomery Lane   301-652-6611
Bethesda, MD 20814-1220   Fax: 240-762-5150
TDD: 800-377-8555
www.aota.org
10 pages
ISBN: 1-569001-48-0

2852 Staying Well: Advanced Pain Management for ACPA Members
American Chronic Pain Association
PO Box 850   916-632-0922
Rocklin, CA 95677   800-533-3231
Fax: 916-632-3208
e-mail: acpa@theacpa.org
www.theacpa.org
This workbook is designed for those who have a working knowledge of the basics of pain management. This workbook provides additional skills necessary to continue to move forward in the journey to wellness.

ISBN: 0-969387-81-7
Penny Cowan, Executive Director

2853 Understanding Chronic Pain
Angela Koestler, PhD; Ann Myers, MD, author
University Press of Mississippi

3825 Ridgewood Road
Jackson, MS 39211-6492

601-432-6205
Fax: 601-432-6217
e-mail: kburgess@ihl.state.ms.us
www.upress.state.ms.us

A handbook for people coping with chronic pain and suffering and for those who seek to understand and support them.
2002 184 pages Paperback
ISBN: 1-578064-40-6
Kathy Burgess, Advertising/Marketing Services Manager

2854 **Your Pain is Real: Free Yourself from Chronic Pain, Breakthrough Med. Trtmnt.**
DIANE Publishing Company
330 Pusey Avenue
Darby, PA 19023

610-461-6200
800-782-3833
Fax: 610-461-6130
e-mail: dianepublishing@gmail.com
www.dianepublishing.net

A complete, authoritative and hopeful book on the subject of chronic pain relief. Offers revolutionary ways to relieve all types and degrees of painful conditions. Also offers breakthrough medical treatments, clear guidelines for seeking expert care and the latest scientific findings on pain management.
252 pages Hardcover
ISBN: 0-756753-70-8
Herman Baron, Publisher

Newsletters

2855 **American Chronic Pain Association**
PO Box 850
Rocklin, CA 95677-0850

916-632-0922
800-533-3231
Fax: 916-632-3208
e-mail: acpa@theacpa.org
www.theacpa.org

A nonprofit organization with over 400 chapters in the US, Canada, Australia, New Zealand and Russia. The purpose of this organization is to provide a support system for those suffering chronic pain through group activities.
Quart w/ mbrshp
Penny Cowan, Executive Founder & Director

2856 **Health Points**
TyH Publications
17007 E Colony Drive
Fountain Hills, AZ 85268

800-801-1406
e-mail: editor@e-tyh.com

National newsletter with articles on complementary therapy, latest nutrition news, disability issues and much more. Focus is on fibromyalgia, chronic fatigue, arthritis and chronic pain.
Quarterly

Audio & Video

2857 **ACPA Relaxation Tapes**
American Chronic Pain Association
PO Box 850
Rocklin, CA 95677

916-632-0922
800-533-3231
Fax: 916-632-3208
e-mail: acpa@theacpa.org
www.theacpa.org

Audio tapes offering information on pain relief, breath relaxation and autogenic relaxation. These tapes are designed to help persons regain control of their bodies through exercises in relaxation techniques. $10.00-$25.00.
Audio Tapes
Penny Cowan, Executive Director

2858 **ACPA Video: 10 Steps from Patient to Person**
American Chronic Pain Association
PO Box 850
Rocklin, CA 95677

916-632-0922
800-533-3231
Fax: 916-632-3208
e-mail: acpa@theacpa.org
www.theacpa.org

The video, featuring Penny Cowan, founder of the ACPA, discussed the value of a multidisciplinary pain management program and what is necessary to maintain wellness long term.
Penny Cowan, Executive Director

2859 **Affirmation Tape**
American Chronic Pain Association
PO Box 850
Rocklin, CA 95677

916-632-0922
800-533-3231
Fax: 916-632-3208
e-mail: acpa@theacpa.org
www.theacpa.org

Designed to help you focus on positive things about yourself and builds self-esteem.
Penny Cowan, Executive Director

2860 **Relaxation Tape**
American Chronic Pain Association
PO Box 850
Rocklin, CA 95677

916-632-0922
800-533-3231
Fax: 916-632-3208
e-mail: acpa@theacpa.org
www.theacpa.org

Tape one includes pain relief and breath relaxation. Tape two includes general relaxation and autogenic relaxation.
Penny Cowan, Executive Director

Web Sites

2861 **American Chronic Pain Association**

www.theacpa.org
Facilitating peer support and education for individuals with chronic pain and their families so that these individuals may live more fully in spite of their pain.

2862 **American Pain Society**

ampainsoc.org
Multidisciplinary organization of basic and clinical scientists, practicing clinicians, policy analysts, and others.

2863 **Discovery Health**

www.discoverylife.com
A source of information on various health topics, including chronic pain and its symptoms and treatments.

2864 **Healing Well**

www.healingwell.com
An online health resource guide to medical news, chat, information and articles, newsgroups and message boards, books, disease-related web sites, medical directories, and more for patients, friends, and family coping with disabling diseases, disorders, or chronic illnesses.

2865 **Health Finder**

www.healthfinder.gov
Searchable, carefully developed web site offering information on over 1000 topics. Developed by the US Department of Health and Human Services, the site can be used in both English and Spanish.

2866 **Healthlink USA**

www.healthlinkusa.com
Health information concerning treatment, cures, prevention, diagnosis, risk factors, research, support groups, email lists, personal stories and much more. Updated regularly.

2867 **Helios Health**

www.helioshealth.com
Online resource for your health information. Detailed information about specific health topics, access to expert advice from our Medical Advisory Board, and up-to-date health news.

2868 **International Pelvic Pain Society**

www.pelvicpain.org/
Short range goal is to recruit, organizae, and educate health care professionals actively invlved with the treatment of patients who have chronic opelvic pain. It also aims to bring hope to men and women who suffer from chronic pelvic pain by significantly raising public awareness and impacting individual lives.

2869 MedicineNet

www.medicinenet.com

An online resource for consumers providing easy-to-read, authoritative medical and health information.

2870 Medscape

www.medscape.com

Medscape offers specialists, primary care physicians, and other health professionals the Web's most robust and integrated medical information and educational tools.

2871 WebMD

www.webmd.com

Provides credible information, supportive communities, and in-depth reference material about health subjects. A source for original and timely health information as well as material from well known content providers.

Description

2872 ## Congenital Heart Disease

Congenital Heart Disease (CHD) represents the most common group of congenital (present from birth) anomalies. CHD can be thought of as a group of disorders that result from the abnormal formation of the heart in utero. The heart develops between the 2nd and 6th week of gestation, and may be affected by genetic mutation, maternal systemic medications or toxins (e.g. alcohol abuse). The incidence of CHD in the population is about 8 cases in 1,000 live births, or just under 1%. About half of these cardiac defects are considered to be minor and can be followed clinically while the other half fall into the categories of major CHD. This latter group often requires surgery early in life to either completely repair the heart defect or in some cases, to redirect blood through the cardiovascular system to palliate the structural abnormality.

CHD can be divided into three major categories: left to right shunting lesions, left heart obstructive lesions and those that lead to marked cyanosis (decreased oxygen delivery to the organs and tissues), the so called cyanotic heart diseases.

The left to right shunting lesions are the most common of the three groups and include the ventricular septal defect (VSD), the atrial septal defect (ASD), the atrioventricular septal defect (also referred to as the AV canal), and the patent ductus arteriosus. In all of these left to right shunting lesions, there is a progressive increase in the amount of blood sent from the left side of the heartacross the given defect (hole) into the right side that delivers blood to the lungs. There is as a result, too much blood entering the pulmonary circuit and this can lead to problems with breathing and feeding for infants in the first few months of life.

The more common left heart obstructive diseases include aortic stenosis, coarctation of the aorta and the hypoplastic left heart syndrome. Each of these can lead to a marked reduction in the amount of blood flow that is able to leave the left side of the heart and can be delivered to the organs and tissues. This leads to marked abnormalities in the way the organs and tissues function and can cause serious and emergent problems for infants in the first week or two of life.

Cyanotic heart disease are those cardiac malformations that lead to a bluish discoloration of the baby as there is insufficient oxygenated blood that is delivered to the body with or without inadequate blood delivered to the lungs to pick up oxygen. The more common disorders in this group are tetralogy of Fallot, Transposition of the great arteries, tricuspid atresia and truncus arteriosus.

With the remarkable advances in neonatal cardiac surgery and interventional cardiac catheterization, almost all of the cardiac malformations can be aggressively addressed with excellent results, even in the youngest and smallest of patients. Overall, survival from all cardiac surgeries in children with CHD is greater than 95%, and even for the most complex of CHD it is approaching 90%. These children often require long-term follow-up from a pediatric cardiologist, but the vast majority lead healthy active lives. See also *Birth Defects*.

National Agencies & Associations

2873 **Adult Congenital Heart Association**
6757 Greene Street
Philadelphia, PA 19119-3508
215-849-1260
888-921-ACHA
Fax: 215-849-1261
e-mail: Info@achaheart.org
www.achaheart.org
The Adult Congenital Heart Association (ACHA) is a nonprofit organization which seeks to improve the quality of life and extend the lives of adults with congenital heart defects through education, outreach, advocacy and promotion of research.
Amy Verstappen, President
Tim Clair, Chief Operating Officerÿ

2874 **Congenital Heart Information Network**
101 N Washington Avenue
Margate City, NJ 08402-1195
609-822-1572
Fax: 609-822-1574
e-mail: mb@tchin.org
www.tchin.org
C.H.I.N. is a national organization that provides reliable information support services, financial assistance and resources to families of children with congenital heart defects and acquired heart disease and adults with congenital heart defects.
Mona Barmash, President

2875 **Kids with Heart National Association for Children's Heart Disorders**
1578 Careful Drive
Green Bay, WI 54307-2504
920-498-0058
800-538-5390
e-mail: michelle@kidswithheart.org
www.kidswithheart.org
Kids with Heart is a nonprofit organization founded in 1985 dedicated to providing support for families affected by congenital heart defects through surgical care packages.
Michelle Rin BA, President
Dean Rintamaki, Vice President

2876 **Schneeweiss Adult Congenital Heart Disease Center**
New York Presbyterian Hospital
161 Fort Washington Avenue
New York, NY 10032
212-305-6936
Fax: 212-305-0490
www.congenitalheart.hs.columbia.edu
We provide such diagnostic services such as echocardiography cardiac MRI and cardiac catheterization. Highly specialized care is provided by a team of physicians specifically interested in the problems of adults with congenital heart disease.
Marlon S Rosenbaum MD, Director
Jonathan Ginns, Adult Congenital Heart Disease

Web Sites

2877 **Heartpoint**
www.heartpoint.com
Heartpoint provides information about specific heart defects.

2878 **MedicineNet**
www.medicinenet.com
An online resource for consumers providing easy-to-read, authoritative medical and health information.

2879 **Medline Plus**
www.nlm.nih.gov/medlineplus
This website includes information about congenital heart disease and includes links regarding support and treatment.

2880 **Yale: Congenital Heart Disease**
www.yale.edu/imaging/chd

This web site provides in-depth information regarding various types of heart conditions.

Description

2881 Cooley's Anemia (Thalassemia)

Cooley's anemia, or beta-Thalassemia major, is an inherited disorder characterized by abnormal production of hemoglobin in the red blood cells. There are two forms of beta-Thalassemia: beta-Thalassemia minor, in which the person has no symptoms, and beta-Thalassemia major, or Cooley's anemia, which is a severe, debilitating disease. Although a baby who has Cooley's anemia appears normal at birth, growth rates are impaired, and puberty may be significantly delayed or absent. Without therapy, there is a general decline. The skin becomes pale or jaundiced, facial bones become more prominent and pronounced, and the spleen becomes enlarged.

While there is no cure for Cooley's anemia, there are treatments such as blood transfusions, which can reduce some symptoms of the disease. However, children with Cooley's anemia should receive as few transfusions as possible because of the danger of iron overload from the "heme" portion of hemoglobin. Chelation, or binding, of the excess iron associated with multiple, repetitive transfusions is important, and is accomplished with deferoxamine. Removal of the spleen may reduce transfusion requirements.

Because there is no cure for beta-Thalassemia major, genetic screening of at-risk populations is very important, notably for persons of Mediterranean, African and Southeast Asian ancestry. Prenatal diagnosis can also be performed.

National Agencies & Associations

2882 American Hellenic Educational Progressive Association
1909 Q Street NW
Washington, DC 20009
202-232-6300
Fax: 202-232-2140
e-mail: ahepa@ahepa.org
www.ahepa.org
The mission of the AHEPA Family is to promote Hellenism Education Philanthropy Civic Responsibility and Family and Individual Excellence.
Basil N Mossaidis, Executive Director

2883 American Society of Hematology
2021 L Street NW
Washington, DC 20036
202-776-0544
866-828-1231
Fax: 202-776-0545
www.hematology.org
A professional society serving both clinicians and scientists around the world who are working to conquer blood diseases.
Martha Liggett, Esq., Executive Director
LaFaundra Neville-Ingram, CAP, Executive Assistant

2884 Fanconi Anemia Research Foundation
1801 Willamette Street
Eugene, OR 97401
541-687-4658
888-326-2664
Fax: 541-687-0548
e-mail: info@fanconi.org
www.fanconi.org
Funds research and provides education and support services worldwide to families affected with Fanconi anemia a rare genetic aplastic anemia that leads to bone marrow failure acute myelogenous leukemia and squamous cell carcinomas.

2885 National Association of Special Education Teachers
1250 Connecticut Ave, NW
Washington, DC 20036
800-754-4421
Fax: 800-754-4421
e-mail: contactus@naset.org
www.naset.org
The National Association of Special Education Teachers (NASET) is a national membership organization dedicated to rendering all possible support and assistance to those preparing for or teaching in the field of special education.
Dr. Roger Pierangelo, Co-Executive Director
Dr. George Giuliani, Co-Executive Director

State Agencies & Associations

California

2886 Cooley's Anemia Foundation (CAF): California
2629 Foothill Boulevard
La Crescenta, CA 91214
800-601-2821
Fax: 212-279-5999
e-mail: info@cooleysanemia.org
www.cooleysanemia.org
The Cooley's Anemia Foundation (CAF) is dedicated to serving people afflicted with various forms of thalassemia, most notably the major form of this genetic blood disease, Cooley's anemia/thalassemia major. CAF's mission is advancing the treatment and curing the disease.
Christine Giannamore, Coordinator
Gina Cioffi Esq, National Office Executive Director

Illinois

2887 Cooley's Anemia Foundation (CAF): Illinois Oakbrook Towers
Oakbrook Towers
40 N Tower Road
Altbrook, IL 62503
847-602-2616
800-522-7222
Fax: 212-279-5999
e-mail: info@cooleysanemia.org
www.cooleysanemia.org
The Cooley's Anemia Foundation (CAF) is dedicated to serving people afflicted with various forms of thalassemia most notably the major form of this genetic blood disease Cooley's anemia/thalassemia major. CAF's mission is advancing the treatment and curing the disease.
Bruce Rod, President Illinois Office
Gina Cioffi, National Office Executive Director

Maryland

2888 Cooley's Anemia Foundation (CAF): Capital Area
15321 Peach Orchard Avenue
Silver Spring, MD 20905
301-989-8947
800-522-7222
Fax: 212-279-5999
e-mail: info@cooleysanemia.org
www.cooleysanemia.org
The Cooley's Anemia Foundation (CAF) is dedicated to serving people afflicted with various forms of thalassemia most notably the major form of this genetic blood disease Cooley's anemia/thalassemia major. CAF's mission is advancing the treatment and curing the disease.
Carl C Vitaliti, President Capital Area Office
Gina Cioffi Esq, National Office Executive Director

Massachusetts

2889 Cooley's Anemia Foundation (CAF): Massachusetts Chapter
44 Joseph Road
Newton, MA 02460-1122
617-332-5952
800-522-7222
Fax: 212-279-5999
e-mail: info@cooleysanemia.org
www.cooleysanemia.org
The Cooley's Anemia Foundation (CAF) is dedicated to serving people afflicted with various forms of thalassemia most notably the major form of this genetic blood disease Cooley's ane-

mia/thalassemia major. CAF's mission is advancing the treatment and curing the disease.

Rudi Viscomi, President Massachusetts Office
Gina Cioffi, National Office Executive Director

New Jersey

2890   Cooley's Anemia Foundation (CAF): New Jersey Chapter
29 Alyson Place   732-688-2279
Bloomfield, NJ 07003   800-522-7222
                                          Fax: 212-279-5999
e-mail: info@cooleysanemia.org
www.cooleysanemia.org

The Cooley's Anemia Foundation (CAF) is dedicated to serving people afflicted with various forms of thalassemia most notably the major form of this genetic blood disease Cooley's anemia/thalassemia major. CAF's mission is advancing the treatment and curing the disease.

Christine Somma, President New Jersey Office
Gina Cioffi, National Office Executive Director

New York

2891   Cooley's Anemia Foundation (CAF): Rochester
                                               585-482-5587
                                               800-522-7222
                                          Fax: 212-279-5999
e-mail: info@cooleysanemia.org
www.cooleysanemia.org

The Cooley's Anemia Foundation (CAF) is dedicated to serving people afflicted with various forms of thalassemia most notably the major form of this genetic blood disease Cooley's anemia/thalassemia major. CAF's mission is advancing the treatment and curing the disease.

Shirley Cammilleri, President Rochester Office
Gina Cioffi Esq, National Office Executive Director

2892   Cooley's Anemia Foundation (CAF): Buffalo
135 Wellington Road   716-834-8903
Buffalo, NY 14216   800-522-7222
                                          Fax: 212-279-5999
e-mail: info@cooleysanemia.org
www.cooleysanemia.org

The Cooley's Anemia Foundation (CAF) is dedicated to serving people afflicted with various forms of thalassemia most notably the major form of this genetic blood disease Cooley's anemia/thalassemia major. CAF's mission is advancing the treatment and curing the disease.

Dennis Locurto, President Buffalo Office
Gina Cioffi Esq, National Office Executive Director

2893   Cooley's Anemia Foundation (CAF): Long Island
111 Cherry Valley Avenue   516-358-9100
Garden City, NY 11530   800-522-7222
                                          Fax: 516-358-9101
e-mail: info@cooleysanemia.org
www.cooleysanemia.org

The Cooley's Anemia Foundation (CAF) is dedicated to serving people afflicted with various forms of thalassemia most notably the major form of this genetic blood disease Cooley's anemia/thalassemia major. CAF's mission is advancing the treatment and curing the disease.

Thomas Rotolo, President Long Island Office
Janice Cenzoprano, Vice President Long Island Office

2894   Cooley's Anemia Foundation (CAF): Queens
157-26 9th Avenue   718-746-7677
Beachurst, NY 11357   800-522-7222
                                          Fax: 718-746-7678
e-mail: info@cooleysanemia.org
www.cooleysanemia.org

The Cooley's Anemia Foundation (CAF) is dedicated to serving people afflicted with various forms of thalassemia most notably the major form of this genetic blood disease Cooley's anemia/thalassemia major. CAF's mission is advancing the treatment and curing the disease.

Paul Tucci, President Queen Office
Abbey Chakalis, Events Manager

2895   Cooley's Anemia Foundation (CAF): Staten Island
16B Dreyer Avenue   718-761-5380
Staten Island, NY 10314   800-522-7222
                                          Fax: 718-761-5381
e-mail: info@cooleysanemia.org
www.cooleysanemia.org

The Cooley's Anemia Foundation (CAF) is dedicated to serving people afflicted with various forms of thalassemia most notably the major form of this genetic blood disease Cooley's anemia/thalassemia major. CAF's mission is advancing the treatment and curing the disease.

Gina Cioffi Esq, National Office Executive Director
Craig Butler, National Office Communications Director

2896   Cooley's Anemia Foundation (CAF): Suffolk Chapter Office
740 Smithtown Bypass   631-863-0532
Smithtown, NY 11787   800-522-7222
                                          Fax: 631-863-0535
e-mail: info@cooleysanemia.org
www.cooleysanemia.org

The Cooley's Anemia Foundation (CAF) is dedicated to serving people afflicted with various forms of thalassemia most notably the major form of this genetic blood disease Cooley's anemia/thalassemia major. CAF's mission is advancing the treatment and curing the disease.

Gina Cioffi Esq, National Office Executive Director
Craig Butler, National Office Communications Director

2897   Cooley's Anemia Foundation (CAF): Westches ter/Rockland Chapter
3 Samuel Purdy Lane   914-232-1808
Katonah, NY 10536   800-522-7222
                                          Fax: 212-279-5999
e-mail: info@cooleysanemia.org
www.cooleysanemia.org

The Cooley's Anemia Foundation (CAF) is dedicated to serving people afflicted with various forms of thalassemia most notably the major form of this genetic blood disease Cooley's anemia/thalassemia major. CAF's mission is advancing the treatment and curing the disease.

Peter Chieco, President Westchester/Rockland Office
Janet Manning, Executive Director

Texas

2898   Cooley's Anemia Foundation (CAF): Texas
4504 Astor Road   214-324-6147
Mesquite, TX 75150-2320   800-522-7222
                                          Fax: 214-324-0612
e-mail: info@cooleysanemia.org
www.cooleysanemia.org

The Cooley's Anemia Foundation (CAF) is dedicated to serving people afflicted with various forms of thalassemia most notably the major form of this genetic blood disease Cooley's anemia/thalassemia major.

Mateen Shah, President
Gina Cioffi Esq, National Office Executive Director

Foundations

2899   Cooleys Anemia Foundation
330 Seventh Avenue
New York, NY 10001   800-522-7222
                                          Fax: 212-279-5999
e-mail: info@cooleysanemia.org
www.cooleysanemia.org

Our mission is advancing the treatment and cure for this fatal blood disease, enhancing the quality of life of patients and educating the medical profession, trait carriers and the public about Cooley's anemia/thalassemia major.

Gina Cioffi, Esq, National Executive Director
Craig Butler, Communications Director

Support Groups & Hotlines

2900 **National Health Information Center**
PO Box 1133
Washington, DC 20013

310-565-4167
800-336-4797
Fax: 301-984-4256
e-mail: info@nhic.org
www.health.gov/nhic

A health information referral service sponsored by the Office of Disease Prevention and Health Promotion. Puts health professionals and consumers who have health questions in touch with those organizations that are best able to provide answers.
Ellen Langhans, Chairwoman
Linda Harris, Lead, Health Communication and e-health

Books

2901 **Genes, Blood & Courage**
129-09 26th Avenue
Flushing, NY 11354

212-598-0911
800-522-7222
www.cooleysanemia.org

2902 **What is Cooley's Anemia**
330 Seventh Ave
New York, NY 10001

212-279-8090
800-522-7222
Fax: 718-321-3340
e-mail: info@cooleysanemia.org
www.cooleysanemia.org

Patient and family handbook.
Jayne Restivo, National Executive Director

2903 **What is Thalassemia?**
Cooley's Anemia Foundation
330 Seventh Ave
New York, NY 10001

212-279-8090
800-522-7222
Fax: 718-321-3340
e-mail: info@cooleysanemia.org
www.cooleysanemia.org

A guide to help thalassemics and their parents understand thalassemia, the reasons for treatment and the hope for the future.
Jayne Restivo, National Executive Director

Children's Books

2904 **Coloring Book on Thalassemia**
330 Seventh Ave
New York, NY 10001

212-279-8090
800-522-7222
Fax: 718-321-3340
e-mail: info@cooleysanemia.org
www.cooleysanemia.org

Available in English, Italian, Greek and Chinese.
Jayne Restivo, National Executive Director

Magazines

2905 **AHEPAN Magazine**
American Hellenic Educational Progressive Assn
1909 Q Street NW
Washington, DC 20009

202-232-6300
Fax: 202-232-2140
e-mail: ahepa@ahepa.org
www.ahepa.org

This magazine includes all of the AHEPA organizations.
Quarterly
Basil N Mossaidis, Executive Director

Newsletters

2906 **Lifeline**
Cooley's Anemia Foundation
330 Seventh Ave
New York, NY 10001

212-279-8090
800-522-7222
Fax: 718-321-3340
e-mail: info@cooleysanemia.org
www.cooleysanemia.org

A newsletter published by Cooley's Anemia Foundation.
Jayne Restivo, National Executive Director

Pamphlets

2907 **Desferal Q&A**
330 Seventh Ave
New York, NY 10001

212-279-8090
800-522-7222
Fax: 718-321-3340
e-mail: info@cooleysanemia.org
www.cooleysanemia.org

Guideline for home infusion.
Jayne Restivo, National Executive Director

2908 **What is Thalassemia Trait?**
Cooley's Anemia Foundation
330 Seventh Ave
New York, NY 10001

212-279-8090
800-522-7222
Fax: 718-321-3340
e-mail: info@cooleysanemia.org
www.cooleysanemia.org

This booklet offers information on the thalassemia trait.
1995
Jayne Restivo, National Executive Director

Audio & Video

2909 **TAG Annual Patient/Family Conference Video**
Cooley's Anemia Foundation
Thalassemia Action Group
New York, NY 10001

800-522-7222
Fax: 212-279-5999
e-mail: TAG@cooleysanemia.org
www.cooleysanemia.org/

Video from the Thalassemia Action Group/TAG Annual Patient/Family Conference held in March of each year.
Gina Cioffi Esq, National Executive Director
Craig Butler, Communications Director

2910 **To Live**
Cooley's Anemia Foundation
330 Seventh Avenue
New York, NY 10001

800-522-7222
Fax: 212-279-5999
e-mail: info@cooleysanemia.org
www.cooleysanemia.org/

An informative and educational video from Cooley's Anemia Foundation.
Gina Cioffi Esq, National Executive Director
Craig Butler, Communications Director

2911 **You're Not Alone**
Cooley's Anemia Foundation
330 Seventh Avenue
New York, NY 10001

212-279-8090
800-522-7222
Fax: 718-321-3340
e-mail: info@cooleysanemia.org
www.cooleysanemia.org

An informative and educational video from Cooley's Anemia Foundation.
Gina Cioffi Esq, National Executive Director
Craig Butler, Communications Director

Web Sites

2912 **Healing Well**

www.healingwell.com

An online health resource guide to medical news, chat, information and articles, newsgroups and message boards, books, disease-related web sites, medical directories, and more for patients, friends, and family coping with disabling diseases, disorders, or chronic illnesses.

2913 **Health Finder**

www.healthfinder.gov

Searchable, carefully developed web site offering information on over 1000 topics. Developed by the US Department of Health and Human Services, the site can be used in both English and Spanish.

2914 Healthlink USA

www.healthlinkusa.com

Health information concerning treatment, cures, prevention, diagnosis, risk factors, research, support groups, email lists, personal stories and much more. Updated regularly.

2915 Helios Health

www.helioshealth.com

Online resource for your health information. Detailed information about specific health topics, access to expert advice from our Medical Advisory Board, and up-to-date health news.

2916 MedicineNet

www.medicinenet.com

An online resource for consumers providing easy-to-read, authoritative medical and health information.

2917 Medscape

www.medscape.com

Medscape offers specialists, primary care physicians, and other health professionals the Web's most robust and integrated medical information and educational tools.

2918 WebMD

www.webmd.com

Provides credible information, supportive communities, and in-depth reference material about health subjects. A source for original and timely health information as well as material from well known content providers.

Description

2919 Crohn's Disease

Crohn's disease is a chronic inflammation in the lining of the digestive tract, generally in the small bowel or part of the colon. The cause is unknown, although the disease is more common in some families and racial groups. Although not a proven cause, periods of emotional stress have been linked with flare-ups of the disease. Onset is typically before age 30, with the peak incidence between 14 and 24 years.

Common symptoms include diarrhea, weight loss, fever, abdominal pain and loss of appetite. If the disease is extensive it may cause deficiencies of essential vitamins and other nutrients. Sometimes inflammation occurs outside the gut, attacking the eyes, joints or skin. Local complications include bowel perforation with formation of abscesses or fistulas which drain out to the skin. Established chronic Crohn's disease is characterized by lifelong exacerbations. These patients carry an increased risk of cancer of the small bowel and colon/rectum.

Therapy depends on the location of the disease and on its severity. Although no specific therapy is known, drug treatment can range from simple anti-diarrheal medications to anti-inflammatory drugs and immunosuppressives. Surgery may be necessary to treat complications. In all cases, careful attention should be paid to the patient's nutritional status and psychological well-being. See also *Gastrointestinal Disorders* and *Celiac Disease*.

National Agencies & Associations

2920 CCFA Camps Across America Crohn's & Colitis Foundation of America

Crohn's & Colitis Foundation of America
386 Park Avenue S
New York, NY 10016
212-685-3440
800-932-2423
Fax: 212-779-4098
e-mail: info@ccfa.org
www.ccfa.org

A chance for children with Crhon's disease or ulcerative colitis to have a camping experience. Because CCFA camps are offered by chapters across the country every camp has its own flavor and style. Activities, as well as the length of stay may vary from child to child.
Richard Geswell, President

2921 Crohn's & Colitis Foundation of America

386 Park Avenue S
New York, NY 10016
212-685-3440
800-932-2423
Fax: 212-779-4098
e-mail: info@ccfa.org
www.ccfa.org

CCFA's mission is to cure and prevent Crohn's disease and ulcerative colitis through research and to improve the quality of life of children and adults affected by this disease through education and support. The foundation offers patient and professional support.
Richard Geswell, President

2922 Ileitis and Colitis Educational Foundation

Central DuPage Hospital
25 N Winfield Road
Winfield, IL 60190
630-933-1600
Fax: 630-933-1300
TTY: 630-933-4833
e-mail: cdh_information@cdh.org
www.cdh.org

Offers support groups fund-raising activities educational materials and public awareness campaigns pertaining to these disorders.
Luke McGuinness, President, CEO
Richard A Mark, Vice Chair

2923 International Foundation for Functional Gastrointestinal Disorders (IFFGD)

PO Box 170864
Milwaukee, WI 53217-8076
414-964-1799
888-964-2001
Fax: 414-964-7176
e-mail: iffgd@iffgd.org
www.iffgd.org

Nonprofit education, support and research organization devoted to increasing awareness and understanding of functional gastrointestinal disorders, including irritable bowel syndrome (IBS), constipation, diarrhea, pain, and incontinence. Mission is to inform, assist and support people affected by these disorders.
Nancy J Norton, President

2924 National Institute of Diabetes, Digestive & Kidney Diseases

National Institute of Health
1 Information Way
Bethesda, MD 20892-3560
800-860-8747
Fax: 703-738-4929
TTY: 866-569-1162
e-mail: ndic@info.niddk.nih.gov
www.diabetes.niddk.nih.gov

Conducts and supports research on many of the most serious diseases affecting public health. The Institute supports much of the clinical research on the diseases of internal medicine and related subspecialty fields as well as many basic science disciplines.
Dr. Griffin Rodgers, Acting Director

2925 Pediatric Crohn's and Colitis Association

PO Box 188
Newton, MA 02468
617-489-5854
e-mail: questions@pcca.hypermart.net
www.pcca.hypermart.net

Focuses on all aspects of pediatric and adolescent Crohn's disease and ulcerative colitis, including medical, nutritional, psychological and social factors. Activities include information sharing, educational forums, newsletters and hospital outreach programs.

2926 Reach Out for Youth with Ileitis and Colitis

PO Box 857
Melville, NY 11747
631-293-3102
TTY: 631-293-3103
e-mail: info@reachoutforyouth.org
www.reachoutforyouth.org

Provides educational seminars and individual and group support to patients and their families. Fundraising efforts support the center's programs, clinical and laboratory research, and purchase of state-of-the-art equipment.
Susan Spellman, Founder and Executive Director

2927 United Ostomy Association

PO Box 512
Northfield, MN 55057
800-826-0826
Fax: 507-645-5168
e-mail: info@uoa.org
www.uoa.org

A national network for bowel and urinary diversion support groups in the United States. Its goal is to provide a nonprofit association that will serve to unify and strengthen its member support groups, which are organized for the benefit of people who have, or will have intestinal or urinary diversions and their caregivers.
David Rudzin, President
Daine Miterko, UOAA Advocacy Chair

2928 World Ostomy and Continence Nurses Society

15000 Commerce Parkway
Mt Laurel, NJ 08054
888-224-9626
Fax: 856-439-0525
e-mail: wocn_info@wocn.org
www.wocn.org

Membership comprises nurses that specialize in enterostomal therapy.
Phyllis Kupsick, MSN, FNP-BC, CW, President
Carolyn Watts, MSN, RN, CWON, President-Elect

State Agencies & Associations

Alabama

2929 CCFA Alabama Chapter
244 Goodwin Crest Drive
Birmingham, AL 35259

205-941-9900
800-249-1993
Fax: 205-941-1411
e-mail: ptalty@ccfa.org OR info@ccfa.org
www.ccfa.org/chapters/alabama/

Crohn's and Colitis Foundation of America is a non-profit, volunteer-driven organization dedicated to finding the cure for Crohn's disease and ulcerative colitis.
Pat Talty, Executive Director

Arizona

2930 CCFA Southwest Chapter: Arizona
8098 Via de Negocio
Scottsdale, AZ 85258

480-246-3676
877-259-2104
Fax: 480-246-3679
e-mail: southwest@ccfa.org
www.ccfa.org/chapters/southwest/

Crohn's and Colitis Foundation of America is a non-profit volunteer-driven organization dedicated to finding the cure for Crohn's disease and ulcerative colitis.
Kathie Gadberry, Executive Director
Bernadette Sewer, Development Coordinator

California

2931 CCFA California: Greater Los Angeles Chapter
1640 S Sepulveda Boulevard
Los Angeles, CA 90025

310-478-4500
866-831-9157
Fax: 310-478-4546
e-mail: losangeles@ccfa.org
www.ccfa.org/chapters/losangeles/

Crohn's and Colitis Foundation of America is a non-profit volunteer-driven organization dedicated to finding the cure for Crohn's disease and ulcerative colitis.
Iyad Zabaneh, Development Coordinator
Kerri Yoder, Education Manager

Colorado

2932 CCFA Rocky Mountain Chapter
1777 S Bellaire Street
Denver, CO 80222

303-639-9163
866-768-2232
Fax: 303-568-0424
e-mail: rockymountain@ccfa.org
www.ccfa.org/chapters/rockymountain/

Crohn's and Colitis Foundation of America is a non-profit volunteer-driven organization dedicated to finding the cure for Crohn's disease and ulcerative colitis.
Nancy Freimuth, Walk Manager
Mackenzie Lyle, Interim Executive Director

Connecticut

2933 CCFA Central Connecticut Chapter
P O Box 275
Branford, CT 06405

203-208-3130
e-mail: mgrande@ccfa.org
www.ccfa.org/chapters/centralct/

Crohn's and Colitis Foundation of America is a non-profit volunteer-driven organization dedicated to finding the cure for Crohn's disease and ulcerative colitis.
Sally Connolly, Board President

2934 CCFA Northern Connecticut Affiliate Chapter
PO Box 370614
W Hartford, CT 06137-0614

212-679-1570
800-932-2423
Fax: 212-679-3567
e-mail: info@ccfa.org
www.ccfa.org/chapters/northernct/

Crohn's and Colitis Foundation of America is a non-profit volunteer-driven organization dedicated to finding the cure for Crohn's disease and ulcerative colitis.
Marilyn Hagg Blohm, Executive Director National Headquarters
Jeff Neale, Public Relations National Headquarters

Florida

2935 CCFA Florida Chapter
2250 N Druid Hills Road
Boca Raton, FL 30329-2391

404-982-0616
877-664-2929
Fax: 404-982-0656
e-mail: kkeohane@ccfa.org
www.ccfa.org/chapters/florida/

Crohn's and Colitis Foundation of America is a non-profit volunteer-driven organization dedicated to finding the cure for Crohn's disease and ulcerative colitis.
Deborah Barnard, Development Manager
Lacy Woods, Administrator

Georgia

2936 CCFA Georgia Chapter
2250 N Druid Hills Road
Atlanta, GA 30329

404-982-0616
800-472-6795
Fax: 404-982-0656
e-mail: georgia@ccfa.org
www.ccfa.org/chapters/georgia/

Crohn's and Colitis Foundation of America is a non-profit volunteer-driven organization dedicated to finding the cure for Crohn's disease and ulcerative colitis.
Marcia Greenburg, Executive Director
Karen Rittenbaum, Development Director

Illinois

2937 CCFA Illinois: Carol Fisher Chapter
2250 E Devon Avenue
Des Plaines, IL 60018

847-827-0404
800-886-6664
Fax: 847-827-6563
e-mail: Illinois@ccfa.org
www.ccfa.org/chapters/illinois/

Crohn's and Colitis Foundation of America is a non-profit volunteer-driven organization dedicated to finding the cure for Crohn's disease and ulcerative colitis.
Marianne Floriano, Executive Director
Kristina Sickles, Development Coordinator

Indiana

2938 CCFA Indiana Chapter
931 E 86th Street
Indianapolis, IN 46240

317-259-8071
800-332-6029
Fax: 317-259-8091
e-mail: indiana@ccfa.org
www.ccfa.org/chapters/indiana/

Crohn's and Colitis Foundation of America is a non-profit volunteer-driven organization dedicated to finding the cure for Crohn's disease and ulcerative colitis.
Scott Baumruck, Development Director
Dawn Drinkut, Development Assistant

Iowa

2939 CCFA Iowa Chapter
PO Box 1184
Johnston, IA 50131-0016

515-664-8961
Fax: 319-277-6293
e-mail: iowa@ccfa.org
www.ccfa.org/chapters/iowa/

Crohn's and Colitis Foundation of America is a non-profit volunteer-driven organization dedicated to finding the cure for Crohn's disease and ulcerative colitis.
Tony Kline, Chapter President
Abbie Hansen, Vice President Communications

Kansas

2940 CCFA Mid-America Chapter: Kansas
1034 S Brentwood
St Louis, MO 63117

314-863-4747
800-783-8006
Fax: 314-863-4749
e-mail: sskodak@ccfa.org
www.ccfa.org/chapters/midamerica/

Crohn's and Colitis Foundation of America is a non-profit volunteer-driven organization dedicated to finding the cure for Crohn's disease and ulcerative colitis.
Steve Skodak, Executive Director
Andi Harrington, Development Manager

Louisiana

2941 CCFA Louisiana Chapter
7611 Maple Street
New Orleans, LA 70118
504-861-3433
866-382-2232
Fax: 504-861-3466
e-mail: lams@ccfa.org
www.ccfa.org/chapters/louisiana
Crohn's and Colitis Foundation of America is a non-profit volunteer-driven organization dedicated to finding the cure for Crohn's disease and ulcerative colitis.
David Lee Thomas, Development Director
Gail C Smith, Development Assistant

Maryland

2942 CCFA Maryland Chapter
10400 Little Patuxent Parkway
Columbia, MD 21044
443-276-0861
800-618-5583
Fax: 443-276-0865
e-mail: maryland@ccfa.org
www.ccfa.org/chapters/md-southde
Crohn's and Colitis Foundation of America is a non-profit volunteer-driven organization dedicated to finding the cure for Crohn's disease and ulcerative colitis.
Robert J Milanchus, Regional Executive Director
Mary Glagola, President

Massachusetts

2943 CCFA New England Chapter: Massachusetts
280 Hillside Avenue
Needham, MA 02494
781-449-0324
800-314-3459
Fax: 781-449-0325
e-mail: ne@ccfa.org
www.ccfa.org/chapters/ne
Crohn's and Colitis Foundation of America is a non-profit volunteer-driven organization dedicated to finding the cure for Crohn's disease and ulcerative colitis.
Jess Adani, Development Manager
Kristin Patmos, Education Manager

Michigan

2944 CCFA Michigan Chapter: Farmington Hills
31313 N Western Highway
Farmington Hills, MI 78334
248-737-0900
Fax: 248-737-0904
e-mail: michigan@ccfa.org
www.ccfa.org/chapters/michigan
Crohn's and Colitis Foundation of America is a non-profit volunteer-driven organization dedicated to finding the cure for Crohn's disease and ulcerative colitis.
Bernard L Riker, Executive Director
Gilda Hauser, Development Manager

Minnesota

2945 CCFA Minnesota Chapter
1885 University Avenue W
Saint Paul, MN 55104
651-917-2424
888-422-3266
Fax: 651-917-2425
e-mail: Minnesota@ccfa.org
www.ccfa.org/chapters/minnesota
Crohn's and Colitis Foundation of America is a non-profit volunteer-driven organization dedicated to finding the cure for Crohn's disease and ulcerative colitis.
Maggie Brown, Take Steps Manager
Ruby Lanoux, Development Manager

Missouri

2946 CCFA Mid-America Chapter: Missouri
1034 S Brentwood
Saint Louis, MO 63117
314-863-4747
800-783-8006
Fax: 314-863-4749
e-mail: info@ccfa.org
www.ccfa.org/chapters/midamerica
Crohn's and Colitis Foundation of America is a non-profit volunteer-driven organization dedicated to finding the cure for Crohn's disease and ulcerative colitis.
Steve Skodak, Executive Director
Andi Harrington, Development Manager

New Jersey

2947 CCFA New Jersey Chapter
45 Wilson Avenue
Manalapan, NJ 07726
732-786-9960
Fax: 732-786-9964
e-mail: newjersey@ccfa.org
www.ccfa.org/chapters/newjersey
Crohn's and Colitis Foundation of America is a non-profit volunteer-driven organization dedicated to finding the cure for Crohn's disease and ulcerative colitis.
Rosemarie Golombos, Executive Director
Barbara Fedorchak, Chapter Development Manager

New York

2948 CCFA Greater New York Chapter: National Headquarters
386 Park Avenue S
New York, NY 10016-8804
800-932-2423
800-932-2423
Fax: 212-679-3567
e-mail: info@ccfa.org
www.ccfa.org
Crohn's and Colitis Foundation of America is a non-profit volunteer-driven organization dedicated to finding the cure for Crohn's disease and ulcerative colitis.
Marilyn Hagg Blohm, Executive Director
Jeff Neale, Public Relations/Media Director

2949 CCFA Long Island Chapter
585 Stewart Avenue
Garden City, NY 11530
516-222-5530
Fax: 516-222-5535
e-mail: longisland@ccfa.org
www.ccfa.org/chapters/longisland
Crohn's and Colitis Foundation of America is a non-profit volunteer-driven organization dedicated to finding the cure for Crohn's disease and ulcerative colitis.
Marilyn Hagg Blohm, Executive Director National Office
Jeff Neale, Public Relations/Media National Office

2950 CCFA Rochester/Southern Tier Chapter
2117 Buffalo Road
Rochester, NY 14624
585-617-4771
800-932-2423
e-mail: rochester@ccfa.org
www.ccfa.org/chapters/rochester
Crohn's and Colitis Foundation of America is a non-profit volunteer-driven organization dedicated to finding the cure for Crohn's disease and ulcerative colitis.
Marilyn Hagg Blohm, Executive Director National Headquarters
Jeff Neale, Public Relations

2951 CCFA Upstate/Northeastern New York Chapter
4 Normanskill Boulevard
Delmar, NY 12054
518-439-0252
e-mail: upstateny@ccfa.org
www.ccfa.org/chapters/upstateny
Crohn's and Colitis Foundation of America is a non-profit volunteer-driven organization dedicated to finding the cure for Crohn's disease and ulcerative colitis.
Linda Winston, Chapter President
Peter Purcel MD, Medical Advisory Chair

2952 CCFA Western New York Chapter
2714 Sheridan Drive
Tonawanda, NY 14150-0224
716-833-2870
800-932-2423
e-mail: jpetri@ccfa.org
www.ccfa.org/chapters/westernny

Crohn's and Colitis Foundation of America is a non-profit volunteer-driven organization dedicated to finding the cure for Crohn's disease and ulcerative colitis.
Marilyn Hagg Blohm, Executive Director National Headquarters
Jeff Neale, Public Relations

North Carolina

2953 CCFA Carolinas Chapter
2901 N Davidson Street
Charlotte, NC 28205
704-332-1611
877-332-1611
Fax: 704-332-1612
e-mail: carolinas@ccfa.org
www.ccfa.org/chapters/carolinas
Crohn's and Colitis Foundation of America is a non-profit volunteer-driven organization dedicated to finding the cure for Crohn's disease and ulcerative colitis.
Angela Parks, Development Director
Julie Perkins, Special Events/Development Manager

2954 CCFA South Carolina Chapter
2901 N Davidson Street
Charlotte, NC 28205
704-332-1611
877-632-1611
Fax: 704-332-1612
e-mail: carolinas@ccfa.org
www.ccfa.org/chapters/carolinas
Crohn's and Colitis Foundation of America is a non-profit volunteer-driven organization dedicated to finding the cure for Crohn's disease and ulcerative colitis.
Angela Parks, Development Manager
Tewanna Sanders, Education & Support Manager

Ohio

2955 CCFA Central Ohio Chapter
5008 Pine Creek Drive
Westerville, OH 43081
614-865-1933
800-625-5977
Fax: 614-865-1934
e-mail: centralohio@ccfa.org
www.ccfa.org/chapters/centralohio
Crohn's and Colitis Foundation of America is a non-profit volunteer-driven organization dedicated to finding the cure for Crohn's disease and ulcerative colitis.
Janelle Gasaway, Take Steps Manager
Kelly Bush, Development Coordinator

2956 CCFA Northeast Ohio Chapter
23775 Commerce Park Road
Beachwood, OH 44122
216-831-2692
866-345-2232
Fax: 216-831-2792
e-mail: neohio@ccfa.org
www.ccfa.org/chapters/neohio
Crohn's and Colitis Foundation of America is a non-profit volunteer-driven organization dedicated to finding the cure for Crohn's disease and ulcerative colitis.
Kristin Knipp, Development Coordinator
Patty Kaplan, Development Manager NE Ohio Chapter

2957 CCFA Southwest Ohio Chapter
8 Triangle Park Drive
Cincinnati, OH 45246
513-772-3550
877-283-7513
Fax: 513-772-7599
e-mail: SWOhio@ccfa.org
www.ccfa.org/chapters/swohio
Crohn's and Colitis Foundation of America is a non-profit volunteer-driven organization dedicated to finding the cure for Crohn's disease and ulcerative colitis.
Rachel Spradlin, Take Steps Manager
Jenny Southers, Development Manager SE Ohio Chapter

Oklahoma

2958 CCFA Oklahoma Chapter
4504 E 67th Street
Tulsa, OK 74136
918-523-8540
800-658-1533
Fax: 918-523-8560
e-mail: jsummers@ccfa.org
www.ccfa.org/chapters/oklahoma

Crohn's and Colitis Foundation of America is a non-profit volunteer-driven organization dedicated to finding the cure for Crohn's disease and ulcerative colitis.
Judy Summers, Regional Executive Director
Christopher Woods, President

Pennsylvania

2959 CCFA Philadelphia/Delaware Valley Chapter
367 E Street Road
Trevose, PA 19053
215-396-9100
888-340-4744
Fax: 215-396-1170
e-mail: Philadelphia@ccfa.org
www.ccfa.org/chapters/philadelphia
Crohn's and Colitis Foundation of America is a non-profit volunteer-driven organization dedicated to finding the cure for Crohn's disease and ulcerative colitis.
Barbara Berman, Executive Director
Suzanne Rhodeside, Development Director

2960 CCFA Western Pennsylvania/West Virginia Chapter
300 Penn Center Boulevard
Pittsburgh, PA 15235
412-823-8272
877-823-8272
Fax: 412-823-8276
e-mail: wpawv@ccfa.org
www.ccfa.org/chapters/wpawv
Crohn's and Colitis Foundation of America is a non-profit volunteer-driven organization dedicated to finding the cure for Crohn's disease and ulcerative colitis.
10-12 pages
Jamie Rhoades, Development Manager
Susan Kukic, Executive Director

Tennessee

2961 CCFA Tennessee Chapter
95 White Bridge Road
Nashville, TN 37205
615-356-0444
866-814-2232
Fax: 615-356-0445
e-mail: tennessee@ccfa.org
www.ccfa.org/chapters/tennessee
Crohn's and Colitis Foundation of America is a non-profit volunteer-driven organization dedicated to finding the cure for Crohn's disease and ulcerative colitis.
Michelle J Chianese, Education & Support Manager
Nicole Boisvert, Walk Manager

Texas

2962 CCFA Houston Gulf Coast/South Texas Chapter
5120 Woodway
Houston, TX 77056
713-572-2232
800-785-2232
Fax: 713-572-2433
e-mail: infohouston@ccfa.org
www.ccfa.org/chapters/houston
Crohn's and Colitis Foundation of America is a non-profit volunteer-driven organization dedicated to finding the cure for Crohn's disease and ulcerative colitis.
Brandy Bendele, Walk Manager
Erin Fagan, Development Manager

2963 CCFA North Texas Chapter
12801 N Central Expressway
Dallas, TX 75243
972-386-0607
Fax: 972-386-0509
e-mail: ntexas@ccfa.org
www.ccfa.org/chapters/ntexas
Crohn's and Colitis Foundation of America is a non-profit volunteer-driven organization dedicated to finding the cure for Crohn's disease and ulcerative colitis.
Rachel Wallace, Development Manager
Sharon Seagraves, Executive Director

Virginia

2964 CCFA Greater Washington DC/Virginia Chapter
4085 Chain Bridge Road   703-865-6130
Fairfax, VA 22314   877-807-5271
                                    Fax: 703-865-8873
                    e-mail: washingtondc@ccfa.org
                    www.ccfa.org/chapters/washingtondc
Crohn's and Colitis Foundation of America is a non-profit volunteer-driven organization dedicated to finding the cure for Crohn's disease and ulcerative colitis.
Eileen Pugh, Executive Director
Stephanie Campbell, Development Coordinator

Washington

2965 CCFA Washington State Chapter
9 Lake Bellevue Drive   425-451-8455
Bellevue, WA 98005   877-703-6900
                                    Fax: 425-451-1708
                    e-mail: northwest@ccfa.org
                    www.ccfa.org/chapters/northwest
Crohn's and Colitis Foundation of America is a non-profit volunteer-driven organization dedicated to finding the cure for Crohn's disease and ulcerative colitis.
Linda Huse, Executive Director
Jennifer Simmons, Development Manager

Wisconsin

2966 CCFA Wisconsin Chapter
1126 S 70th Street   414-475-5520
W Allis, WI 53214   877-586-5588
                                    Fax: 414-475-5502
                    e-mail: wisconsin@ccfa.org
                    www.ccfa.org/chapters/wisconsin
Crohn's and Colitis Foundation of America is a non-profit volunteer-driven organization dedicated to finding the cure for Crohn's disease and ulcerative colitis.
Jan Lenz, Executive Director
Nadine Davis, Development Coordinator

Libraries & Resource Centers

2967 National Digestive Diseases Information Clearinghouse
2 Information Way
Bethesda, MD 20892-3570   800-891-5389
                                    Fax: 703-738-4929
                                    TTY: 866-569-1162
                    e-mail: nddic@info.niddk.nih.gov
                    www.digestive.niddk.nih.gov
Established to increase knowledge and understanding about digestive diseases among people with these conditions and their families, health care professionals, and the general public. To carry out this mission, NDDIC works closely with a coordinating panel of representatives from Federal agencies, voluntary organizations on the national level, and professional groups to identify and respond to informational needs about digestive diseases.
Kathy Kranzfelder, Director

Research Centers

2968 Hahnemann University, Krancer Center for Inflammatory Bowel Disease Research
230 N Broad St   215-762-7000
Philadelphia, PA 19102   Fax: 215-762-8109
                    www.hahnemannhospital.com
Research into the causes and treatments of ulcerative colitis and Crohn's disease.
Dr. Harris Clearfield, Director

Support Groups & Hotlines

2969 Crohn's & Colitis Foundation of America Hotline
Crohn's & Colitis Foundation of America

386 Park Avenue S
New York, NY 10016   800-932-2423
                    e-mail: info@ccfa.org
                    www.ccfa.org
Our mission is to cure and prevent Crohn's disease and ulcerative colitis through research and to improve the quality of life of children and adults affected by these digestive disease through education and support. Known collectively as inflammatory bowel disease (IBD), these painful chronic illnesses affect up to one million Americans, including approximately 100,000 children under the age of 18.
Maura Breen, Chairman
Paul Salerno, Treasurer

2970 National Health Information Center
PO Box 1133   310-565-4167
Washington, DC 20013   800-336-4797
                                    Fax: 301-984-4256
                    e-mail: info@nhic.org
                    www.health.gov/nhic
A health information referral service sponsored by the Office of Disease Prevention and Health Promotion. NHIC puts health professionals and consumers who have health questions in touch with those organizations that are best able to provide answers.

Books

2971 Crohn's Disease and Ulcerative Colitis Fact Book
Crohn's & Colitis Foundation of America
386 Park Avenue S   212-685-3440
New York, NY 10016-8804   800-932-2423
                                    Fax: 212-779-4098
                    e-mail: info@ccfa.org
                    www.ccfa.org
Written in layman's language, this first complete guide is helpful in understanding and coping with inflammatory bowel diseases.

2972 Managing Your Child's Crohn's Disease or Ulcerative Colitis
Crohn's & Colitis Foundation of America
386 Park Avenue S   212-685-3440
New York, NY 10016-8804   800-932-2423
                                    Fax: 212-779-4098
                    e-mail: info@ccfa.org
                    www.ccfa.org
Full-length book on Crohn's disease and ulcerative colitis, specifically targeted for parents of children and teenagers; includes topics on cause and diagnosis, treatment, surgery, hospitalization, diet and nutrition, school and social issues and resources for the patient.
$16.95 Members

2973 Ostomy Book: Living Comfortably with Colostomies, Ileostomies and Urostomies
Barbara Dorr Mullen and Kerry Anne McGinn, author
Bull Publishing Company
PO Box 1377thur Boulevard
Boulder, CO 80306   800-676-2855
                                    Fax: 303-545-6354
                    www.bullpub.com
This book provides complete information on everything from details of surgery to the management of the appliances. Just as importantly, it is a beautifully told story of the entire expereince from diagnosis through rehabilitation to looking forward to a full and happy life.

ISBN: 0-923521-12-7

2974 People...Not Patients: Source Book for Living with Bowel Disease
Chron's & Colitis Foundation of America
386 Park Avenue S   212-685-3440
New York, NY 10016-8804   800-932-2423
                                    Fax: 212-779-4098
                    e-mail: info@ccfa.org
                    www.ccfa.org
Contains the essential information you need to help you cope with Chron's disease and ulcerative colitis after you leave the doctor's office.

2975 Treating IBD
Crohn's & Colitis Foundation of America
386 Park Avenue S   212-685-3440
New York, NY 10016-8804   800-932-2423
                                Fax: 212-779-4098
                              e-mail: info@ccfa.org
                                      www.ccfa.org
Patient's guide to the medical and surgical management of Inflammatory Bowel Disease, this book gives information on treating crohn's disease and ulcerative colitis, including drug therapies, advances in nutritional care, and recently developed surgical alternatives.

2976 Understanding Crohn Disease and Ulcerative Colitis
Jon Zonderman, Ronald S Vender, MD, author
University Press of Mississippi
3825 Ridgewood Road   601-432-6205
Jackson, MS 39211-6492   Fax: 601-432-6217
                     e-mail: kburgess@ihl.state.ms.us
                              www.upress.state.ms.us
For patients and caregivers an overview of the nature and treatments of inflammatory bowel disease.
2000 128 pages Paperback
ISBN: 1-578062-03-9
Kathy Burgess, Advertising/Marketing Services Manager

Magazines

2977 Colon and Rectal Surgery
International Academy of Proctology
PO Box 1716   765-342-3686
Martinsville, IN 46151   Fax: 765-342-4173
Information for professionals involved with colon and rectal surgery.
George Donnally MD

2978 Digestive Health Matters
Intl. Foundation for Gastrointestinal Disorders
PO Box 170864   414-964-1799
Milwaukee, WI 53217-0864   888-964-2001
                                Fax: 414-964-7176
                              e-mail: iffgd@iffgd.org
                                      www.iffgd.org
Quarterly journal focuses on upper and lower gastrointestinal disorders in adults and children. Educational pamphlets and factsheets are available. Patient and professional membership.

2979 Foundation Focus
Crohn's & Colitis Foundation of America
386 Park Avenue S   212-685-3440
New York, NY 10016-8804   800-932-2423
                                Fax: 212-779-4098
                              e-mail: info@ccfa.org
                                      www.ccfa.org
Magazine for CCFA supporters.

2980 Phoenix Magazine
United Ostomy Association of America
PO Box 512
Northfield, MN 55057   800-826-0826
                                Fax: 507-645-5168
                              e-mail: info@uoaa.org
                                      www.ostomy.org
America's leading ostomy patient magazine providing colostomy, ileostomy, urostomy and continent diversion information, management techniques, new products and much more.
Quarterly
David Rudzin, President

Newsletters

2981 Crohn's Disease, Ulcerative Colitis, and School
Pediatric Crohn's & Colitis Association
PO Box 188   617-489-5854
Newton, MA 02468   e-mail: questions@pcca.hypermart.net
                              pcca.hypermart.net

Information on Crohn's Disease and Ulcerative Colitis, including medical, nutritional, psychological and social factors.

2982 IBD File
Crohn's & Colitis Foundation of America
386 Park Avenue S   212-685-3440
New York, NY 10016-8804   800-932-2423
                                Fax: 212-779-4098
                              e-mail: info@ccfa.org
                                      www.ccfa.org
Offers updated information and the latest medical news about Crohn's Disease and Colitis.

2983 Inflammatory Bowel Disease
Gastro-Intestinal Research Foundation
70 E Lake Street   312-332-1350
Chicago, IL 60601   Fax: 312-332-4757
                              e-mail: info@girf.org
                     www.giresearchfoundation.org
Newsletter and patient pamphlet.

2984 Inner Circle
Reach Out for Youth with Ileitis and Colitis
84 Northgate Circle   516-293-3102
Melville, NY 11747   Fax: 516-293-3103
                              www.rightdiagnosis.com
Provides information to patients with ileitis and colitis and their families.

2985 Inside Story
Reach Out for Youth with Ileitis and Colitis
84 Northgate Circle   516-293-3102
Melville, NY 11747   Fax: 516-293-3103
                              www.rightdiagnosis.com
Provides information to patients with ileitis and colitis and their families.

Pamphlets

2986 ABC's of Pediatric Inflammatory Bowel Disease
Pediatric Crohn's & Colitis Association
PO Box 188   617-489-5854
Newton, MA 02468   e-mail: questions@pcca.hypermart.net
                              pcca.hypermart.net
Information on Pediatric Inflammatory Disease, including medical, nutritional, psychological and social factors.

2987 CCFA: A Case for Support
Crohn's & Colitis Foundation of America
386 Park Avenue S   212-685-3440
New York, NY 10016-8804   800-932-2423
                                Fax: 212-779-4098
                              e-mail: info@ccfa.org
                                      www.ccfa.org
Reviews the work of the Crohn's and Colitis Foundation of America, sponsors a nationally recognized research program, which seeks to improve treatment and ultimately find the cure for inflammatory bowel disease.

2988 Coping with Crohn's and Colitis is Tough
Crohn's & Colitis Foundation of America
386 Park Avenue S   212-685-3440
New York, NY 10016-8804   800-932-2423
                                Fax: 212-779-4098
                              e-mail: info@ccfa.org
                                      www.ccfa.org
Offers information on the Crohn's and Colitis Association. Also offers factual information and statistics on the diseases.

2989 Crohn's Disease
NDDIC
2 Information Way   301-496-3583
Bethesda, MD 20892-0001   800-891-5389
                                Fax: 301-907-8906
                     e-mail: nddic@info.niddlc.nin.gov
                                 www.niddk.nih.gov

October 1992

2990 Guide for Children and Teenagers to Crohn's Disease/Ulcerative Colitis
Crohn's & Colitis Foundation of America
386 Park Avenue S   212-685-3440
New York, NY 10016-8804   800-932-2423
                                Fax: 212-779-4098
                                e-mail: info@ccfa.org
                                      www.ccfa.org
Offers important information on these illnesses to children and teens.

2991 Ileostomy Guide
United Ostomy Associations of America, Inc.
PO Box 66
Fairview, TN 37062-0066   800-826-0826
                                e-mail: info@uoaa.org
                                      www.uoaa.org
Written for persons who have recently had an ileostomy, this guidebook covers a spectrum of topics including basic facts about ileostomies, information for patients, helpful ideas and practical tips.
28 pages

2992 Questions & Answers About Diet and Nutrition
Crohn's & Colitis Foundation of America
386 Park Avenue S   212-685-3440
New York, NY 10016-8804   800-932-2423
                                Fax: 212-779-4098
                                e-mail: info@ccfa.org
                                      www.ccfa.org
Raises important facts about how diet and nutrition affect persons with Crohn's Disease.

2993 Questions and Answers About Complications
Crohn's & Colitis Foundation of America
386 Park Avenue S   212-685-3440
New York, NY 10016-8804   800-932-2423
                                Fax: 212-779-4098
                                e-mail: info@ccfa.org
                                      www.ccfa.org
Medical facts and complications from surgery.

2994 Questions and Answers About Crohn's Disease & Ulcerative Colitis
Crohn's & Colitis Foundation of America
386 Park Avenue S   212-685-3440
New York, NY 10016-8804   800-932-2423
                                Fax: 212-779-4098
                                e-mail: info@ccfa.org
                                      www.ccfa.org
Offers information on the illness and answers the most frequently asked questions about Crohn's Disease. Also includes a glossary of IBD terms.

2995 Questions and Answers About Emotional Factors in Ileitis and Colitis
Crohn's & Colitis Foundation of America
386 Park Avenue S   212-685-3440
New York, NY 10016-8804   800-932-2423
                                Fax: 212-779-4098
                                e-mail: info@ccfa.org
                                      www.ccfa.org
Answers some of the most commonly asked questions about ileitis and colitis and the role of emotional factors in their cause and course.

2996 Questions and Answers About Pregnancy in Ileitis and Colitis
Crohn's & Colitis Foundation of America
386 Park Avenue S   212-685-3440
New York, NY 10016-8804   800-932-2423
                                Fax: 212-779-4098
                                e-mail: info@ccfa.org
                                      www.ccfa.org
Answers questions about inflammatory bowel disease concerning conception, pregnancy, delivery and nursing.

2997 Questions and Answers About Surgery
Crohn's & Colitis Foundation of America

386 Park Avenue S   212-685-3440
New York, NY 10016-8804   800-343-3637
                                Fax: 212-779-4098
                                e-mail: info@ccfa.org
                                      www.ccfa.org
Answers questions and offers basic facts about surgery for persons suffering from Crohn's Disease and Ulcerative Colitis.

2998 Teacher's Guide to Crohn's Disease and Ulcerative Colitis
Crohn's & Colitis Foundation of America
386 Park Avenue S   212-685-3440
New York, NY 10016-8804   800-932-2423
                                Fax: 212-779-4098
                                e-mail: info@ccfa.org
                                      www.ccfa.org
The purpose of this brochure is to increase the support and encouragement given to young people with Crohn's disease and ulcerative colitis by teachers who understand their illness.

2999 Crohn's Disease, Ulcerative Colitis and Your Child
Crohn's & Colitis Foundation of America
386 Park Avenue S   212-685-3440
New York, NY 10016-8804   800-932-2423
                                Fax: 212-779-4098
                                e-mail: info@ccfa.org
                                      www.ccfa.org
Answers questions about IBD in children, providing information on early signs, growth and developments, treatments and special problems in school.

Web Sites

3000 Crohn's & Colitis Foundation of America
                                      www.ccfa.org
The Crohn's & Colitis Foundation of America (CCFA) is a non-profit, volunteer-driven organization dedicated to finding the cures for Crohn's Disease and ulcerative colitis. It was founded in 1967 by Irwin M. and Suzanne Rosenthal, William D. and Shelby Modell, and Henry D. Janowitz, M.D. Since there founding over four decades ago, CCFA has remained at the forefront of research in Crohn's disease and ulcerative colitis.

3001 Healing Well
                                  www.healingwell.com
An online health resource guide to medical news, chat, information and articles, newsgroups and message boards, books, disease-related web sites, medical directories, and more for patients, friends, and family coping with disabling diseases, disorders, or chronic illnesses.

3002 Health Finder
                                  www.healthfinder.gov
Searchable, carefully developed web site offering information on over 1000 topics. Developed by the US Department of Health and Human Services, the site can be used in both English and Spanish.

3003 Healthlink USA
                                  www.healthlinkusa.com
Health information concerning treatment, cures, prevention, diagnosis, risk factors, research, support groups, email lists, personal stories and much more. Updated regularly.

3004 MedicineNet
                                  www.medicinenet.com
An online resource for consumers providing easy-to-read, authoritative medical and health information.

3005 Medscape
                                  www.medscape.com
Medscape offers specialists, primary care physicians, and other health professionals the Web's most robust and integrated medical information and educational tools.

3006 National Digestive Diseases Information Clearinghouse
                                  www.niddk.nih.gov
Offers various educational information, resources and reprints focusing on Colitis, Ulcerative Colitis and Crohn's disease.

3007 Pediatric Crohn's and Colitis Association
                                  pcca.hypermart.net

Focuses on all aspects of pediatric and adolescent Crohn's disease and ulcerative colitis, including medical, nutritional, psychological and social factors. Activities include information sharing, educational forums, newsletters and hospital outreach programs, as well as support of research.

3008   United Ostomy Association

www.uoa.org

A national network for bowel and urinary diversion support groups in the United States. Its goal is to provide a nonprofit association that will serve to unify and strengthen its member support groups, which are organized for the benefit of people who have, or will have intestinal or urinary diversions and their caregivers.

3009   WebMD

www.webmd.com

Provides credible information, supportive communities, and in-depth reference material about health subjects. A source for original and timely health information as well as material from well known content providers.

Description

3010 Cystic Fibrosis

Cystic fibrosis, CF, is an inherited disease of the exocrine (mucus-producing) glands, primarily affecting the gastrointestinal and respiratory tracts. The mucus that is secreted by persons with the disease is especially thick, thus blocking, rather than lubricating, passageways in the lungs and digestive tract. CF is the most common life-shortening genetic disease in the white population, occurring in 1 in 3,000 live births in the United States, but it occurs in people of all ethnic and racial backgrounds.

In the newborn with CF, thick fecal material may cause partial obstruction of the intestine, which then may contort and rupture. Later in life, blockage of secretions from the pancreas results in frequent, foul-smelling, fatty stools, distention of the abdomen and slowed growth. Damage to the lung occurs as thick mucus secretions plug airways. Fifty percent of all patients develop breathing problems marked by a chronic cough, wheezing and repeated lung infections.

The course of CF is usually determined by the degree to which the lungs are affected, and varies greatly from patient to patient. The prognosis is poor, but advances in therapy have helped many survive well into adulthood. Treatment usually includes aggressive use of antibiotics and other drugs to prevent lung complications, physical therapy, adequate nutrition and psychosocial support.

The first CF gene therapy research began in 1993, and scientists have identified mutations in a CF regulator genethat cause cells to produce abnormally thick mucus. Gene therapy to replace the defective gene with a functional copy is currently under study. Genetic screening is now available.

National Agencies & Associations

3011 Childhood Liver Disease Research Network
340 E. Huron Street
Ann Arbor, MI 48104   e-mail: Briaa.Robinson@arborresearch.org
childrennetwork.org
The Childhood Liver Disease Research Network (ChiLDReN) is a collaborative team of doctors, nurses, research coordinators, medical facilities and patient support organizations.
Briaa Robinson, Project Assistant

3012 Cystic Fibrosis Worldwide
50 Elm Street
Southbridge, MA 01550   508-764-2730
Fax: 508-765-8883
e-mail: information@cfww.org
www.cfww.org
IACFA is a non profit organization headquartered in Zurich Switzerland. The purpose and direction of the organization is to assist in improving the quality of life by identifying common problems and attempting to define possible solutions.
Christine Noke, Executive Director
Mitch Messer, President

Foundations

3013 Cystic Fibrosis Foundation
6931 Arlington Road   301-951-4422
Bethesda, MD 20814   800-344-4823
Fax: 301-951-6378
e-mail: info@cff.org
www.cff.org
The mission of the Cystic Fibrosis Foundation is to assure the development of the means to cure and control cystic fibrosis and to improve the quality of life for those with the disease.
Catherine C. McLoud, Chairman
Robert J Beall, Ph.D., President/CEO

Libraries & Resource Centers

3014 Children's Hospital of Orange County
455 S Main Street   714-997-3000
Orange, CA 92868-3874   e-mail: mail@choc.org
www.choc.org
Our mission is to nuture, advance and protect the health and well-being of children.
Kimberly C Cripe, President/CEO

Research Centers

Arizona

3015 Cystic Fibrosis Center: Phoenix Childrens Hospital
1919 E Thomas Road   602-546-1000
Phoenix, AZ 85016   888-908-5437
Fax: 602-460-23
www.phoenixchildrens.com
Robert Meyer, President and Chief Executive Officer
Bruce Morgenstern, Medical Staff President

Arkansas

3016 Arkansas Cystic Fibrosis Center Arkansas Children's Hospital
Arkansas Children's Hospital
1 Children's Way   501-364-1100
Little Rock, AR 72202   Fax: 501-364-3930
TTY: 501-364-1184
e-mail: pedspulmonary@uams.edu
www.arpediatrics.org
Provide high-quality specialized care to patients from comprehensive diagnosis to ongoing treatment.
John L Carroll, Division Chief
Dennis E Schellhase, Director

California

3017 Children's Hospital of Los Angeles
4650 Sunset Boulevard   323-660-2450
Los Angeles, CA 90027   e-mail: webmaster@chla.usc.edu
www.childrenshospitalalla.org
Provides the highest quality healthcare for children who are the sickest and most seriously injured in our region and beyond.
Richard D Cordova, President/CEO
Rodney B Hanners, Senior Vice President & Chief Operating

3018 Childrens Hospital at Oakland
747 52nd Street
Oakland, CA 94609   510-428-3000
www.childrenshospitaloakland.org
The mission of Children's Hospital Oakland is to ensure the delivery of the highest quality pediatric care for all children through regional primary and subspecialty networks; a strong education and teaching program a diverse workforce state of the art research programs and facilities; and nationally recognized child advocacy efforts.
Bertram Lubin, President and Chief Executive Officer
Kathleen Hogue Gonzalez, Vice President, Research Administration

3019 Cystic Fibrosis Center: Cedars-Sinai Medical Center
Cedars-Sinai Medical Center

8700 Beverly Boulevard
Los Angeles, CA 90048

310-423-3277
800-233-2771
Fax: 310-423-4131
www.cedars-sinai.edu

3020 Cystic Fibrosis Center: University of California at San Francisco
400 Parnassus Avenue
San Francisco, CA 94122-0106

415-353-2961
Fax: 415-476-9278
e-mail: ucsf.org?
pulmonary.ucsf.edu

Provides comprehensive evaluation as well as inpatient and outpatient care for patients with cystic fibrosis.
Mary Ellen Kleinhenz, Adult CF Director
Dennis Niels MD, Pediatric CF Director

3021 Cystic Fibrosis Research
2672 Bayshore Parkway
Mountain View, CA 94043

650-404-9975
Fax: 650-404-9981
e-mail: cfri@cfri.org
www.cfri.org

Cystic Fibrosis Research exists to fund research to provide educational and personal support and spread awareness of Cystic Fibrosis a life threatening genetic disease.
Carroll Jenkins, Executive Director
David Soohoo, Director of Programs

3022 Memorial Miller Children's Hospital Cystic Fibrosis Center
2801 Atlantic Avenue
Long Beach, CA 90806

562-933-2000
Fax: 562-933-8501
e-mail: enussbaum@memorialcare.org
www.memorialcare.org/miller

provides a multidisciplinary approach to asthma cystic fibrosis sleep disorders and the entire spectrum of chronic and acute lung and airway disorders in children.
Eliezer Nuss, Medical Director
Barry Arbuckle, President

3023 Stanford CF Center Packard Children's Hospital At Stanford
Packard Children's Hospital At Stanford
725 Welch Road
Palo Alto, CA 94304-1601

650-497-8000
e-mail: jkirby@leland.stanford.edu
cfcenter.stanford.edu

Colleen Dunn, Administrator
Cassie Everson, Research Coordinator

Colorado

3024 Denver Childrens Hospital
1830 Franklin Street
Denver, CO 80218

72 -77 -136
800-624-6553
Fax: 303-832-9245
TTY: 720-777-9390
www.thechildrenshospital.org

Frank Accurs, Director
Jim Schmerling, President, CEO

Connecticut

3025 University of Connecticut Health Center
263 Farmington Avenue
Farmington, CT 06030-0001

860-679-2000
TTY: 860-679-2242
TDD: 860-679-2242
e-mail: president@uconn.edu
www.uchc.edu

Philip E Austin, President
Cato T Laurencin, Vice President for Health Affairs

3026 Yale University Cystic Fibrosis Research Center
Yale Pediatrics
333 Cedar Street
New Haven, CT 06510

203-432-4771
e-mail: sheila.rivera@yale.edu
www.yalepediatrics.org

One of only two in the state of Connecticut the CF Center in the Children's Hospital at the Yale-New Haven Hospital offers a multidisciplinary team approach to provide the most comprehensive state of the art care of CF patients.
Marie Egan, Director
Richard C Levin, President

District of Columbia

3027 Metropolitan DC Cystic Fibrosis Center Children s Hospital National Medical Cen
Children s Hospital National Medical Center
111 Michigan Avenue NW
Washington, DC 20010-2970

202-476-5000
TTY: 800-855-1155
e-mail: tbear@cnmc.org
www.childrensnational.org

An active clinical and basic science research program that exists within the center.
Roberta Alessi, Senior Vice President
Mark Batshaw, Executive Vice President and Chief Acade

Florida

3028 Cystic Fibrosis Center: All Children's Hospital
Department of Pulmonology
501 6th Street S
Saint Petersburg, FL 33701

727-898-7451
800-456-4543
Fax: 727-767-4218
www.allkids.org

Anthony D Kriseman, Pulmonology
Joseph (Jay) Fleece III, Chair

3029 Miami Childrens Hospital Division of Pulmonology
3100 SW 62nd Avenue
Miami, FL 33155-3309

305-666-6511
800-432-6837
Fax: 305-663-8417
e-mail: info@mch.com
www.mch.com

Division evaluates and treats many respiratory disorders including asthma chronic lung disease cystic fibrosis pneumonia and tuberculosis. The Division is strongly committed to a multidisciplinary medical approach to these complex disorders.
Moises Simps, Director
M Narendra Kini, President, CEO

3030 Nemours Childrens Clinic
807 Childrens Way
Jacksonville, FL 32207

904-390-3600
Fax: 904-390-3699
www.nemours.org

Nemours Children's Clinic is one integrated multispecialty group practice with locations in four states seeing patients from across the US and the world.
David J Bailey, President, CEO
Robert Bridges, Executive Vice-President

Georgia

3031 Department of Pediatrics Medical College of Georgia
1120 15th Street
Augusta, GA 30912

706-721-3466
Fax: 706-721-7311
e-mail: pwalling@ georgiahealth.edu
www.mcg.edu/pediatrics

Dr William Kanto Jr, Chairperson Pediatrics

3032 Emory University: Cystic Fibrosis Center
201 Dowman Drive
Atlanta, GA 30322-1028

404-727-6123
Fax: 404-727-4828
e-mail: lwolfen@emory.edu
www.emory.edu

Lindy Wolfen MD, Director
Jim Wagner, President

Illinois

3033 Comer Children's Hospital at the University of Chicago
5841 S Maryland Avenue
Chicago, IL 60637

773-702-1000
888-824-0200
www.uchospitals.edu

3034 Comer Children's Hospital at the Universit
5721 S Maryland Avenue
Chicago, IL 60637

773-702-1000
888-824-0200
www.uchicagokidshospital.org

To provide superior healthcare in a compassionate manner ever mindful of each patient's dignity and individuality.

3035 Cystic Fibrosis Center: Childrens Memorial Hospital
2300 Childrens Plaza   773-880-4000
Chicago, IL 60614-3363   800-543-7362
e-mail: cf@childrensmemorial.org
www.childrensmemorial.org
The Cystic Fibrosis Center at Children's Memorial Hospital has
been a CFF-accredited CF care center since 1963. It is committed
to providing exemplary care to each patient and family focused on
individualized preventative care active management of lung health
and nutrition and patient family education.
Susanna McCo, Director
Patrick M Magoon, President, CEO

**3036 Cystic Fibrosis Center: Park Ridge Lutheran General Children's
Hospital**
Lutheran General Children's Hospital
1775 Dempster Street   847-723-154
Park Ridge, IL 60068   Fax: 847-696-3041
www.advocatehealth.com/lgch
James H Skogsbergh, President, CEO

3037 Loyola University Medical Center: Department of Pediatrics
2160 S 1st Avenue   708-327-9120
Maywood, IL 60153   888-584-7888
www.loyolamedicine.org
Vicki Keough, Dean and Professor

3038 Saint Francis Medical Center Peoria Pulmonary Association
530 NE Glen Oak Avenue
Peoria, IL 61637   309-655-2000
www.osfsaintfrancis.org
Dr. Denise Mammolito, President

Indiana

3039 The Riley Cystic Fibrosis Center
1701 North Senate Boulevard   317-962-2000
Indianapolis, IN 46202   800-248-1199
www.rileychildrenshospital.com
The Riley Cystic Fibrosis Center is the only Cystic Fibrosis Foundation accredited Cystic Fibrosis Center in the state. The Center
provides state-of-the-art CF care at Riley and across the state.
Daniel Fink, President, CEO

Iowa

3040 Blank Childrens Hospital Pediatric Pulmonology Clinic
Children's Health Center
1212 Pleasant Street
Des Moines, IA 50309   515-241-6548
www.blankchildrens.org
David Starke, President, CEO
Ken Cheyne, Medical Director

**3041 Pediatric Allergy & Pulmonary Division University of Iowa
Healthcare**
University of Iowa Healthcare
200 Hawkins Drive   319-356-2296
Iowa City, IA 52242   e-mail: allerpulm@uiowa.edu
www.uihealthcare.com/depts/med/pediatric
The Division of Allergy and Pulmonology offers evaluation and
management of allergic disorders in children with too many infections and acute and chronic breathing disorders of childhood and
adolescence.
Jody Kurtt RN, Director

Kansas

3042 Kansas University Medical Center: Cystic Fibrosis Center
3901 Rainbow Boulevard   913-588-5000
Kansas City, KS 66160   800-332-4199
TDD: 913-588-7963
e-mail: gperry@kumc.edu
www2.kumc.edu
Barbara F Atkinson, Executive Vice Chancellor

**3043 St. Joseph Medical Center Cystic Fibrosis Care and Teaching
Center**
929 N. St. Francis   316-268-5000
Wichita, KS 67214   Fax: 316-583-90
e-mail: contact@viachristi.org
www.viachristi.org
Kay Glasner, Director
Maria Loving, Public Relations Specialist

Kentucky

3044 Kentucky University: Cystic Fibrosis Center
800 Rose Street   859-257-1000
Lexington, KY 40536-0298   800-333-8874
Fax: 859-257-7706
www.ukhealthcare.uky.edu
The cystic fibrosis team works with more than 175 patients and is
dedicated to working with the most advanced therapies to improve
the life of every patient.
Jamshed F Kanga, Director
Dr. Michael Karpf, Executive Vice President

3045 Kosair Childrens Cystic Fibrosis Center
Suite 201
Louisville, KY 40202-2021   502-629-6000
www.nortonhealthcare.com
The Cystic Fibrosis Center is one of 120 centers in the United
States accredited by the National Cystic Fibrosis Foundation. Spe-
cialists provide diagnosis and multidisciplinary care for cystic fi-
brosis patients of all ages. Professional education and training is
also provided.
Nemie Eid, Medical Director
Stephen A Williams, President, CEO

Louisiana

3046 Ernest N Morial Asthma, Allergy & Respiratory Disease Center
Louisiana State University School of Medicine
1901 Perdido Street   504-568-4634
New Orleans, LA 70112-3932   888-695-8647
Fax: 504-568-4295
e-mail: dthoma2@lsumc.edu
www.lsuhsc.edu
Warren R Summer, Director
Larry H. Hollierÿ, President and Chief Operating Officer

Maine

3047 Central Maine Cystic Fibrosis Center
300 Main Street   207-795-0111
Lewiston, ME 04240-7027   Fax: 207-795-2303
www.cmhc.org
Ralph V Harder, Director
Peter Chkale, Chief Executive Officer

3048 Maine Medical Center: Cystic Fibrosis Clinical Center
22 Bramhall Street   207-662-0111
Portland, ME 04102-3175   877-339-3107
Fax: 207-775-6024
TTY: 207-662-4900
www.mmc.org
Richard W Peterson, President, CEO

3049 Maine Medical Center: Cystic Fibrosis Clin
22 Bramhall Street   207-662-0111
Portland, ME 04102-3175   877-339-3107
Fax: 207-775-6024
TTY: 207-662-4900
www.mmc.org
Richard W Peterson, President, CEO

Maryland

3050 Cystic Fibrosis Center: National Institute of Health NIDDK
Building 31 Room 9A06
Bethesda, MD 20892-2560   301-496-3583
www2.niddk.nih.gov
Dr Griffin Rodgers, Acting Director

3051 **Cystic Fibrosis Foundation**
6931 Arlington Road
Bethesda, MD 20814   301-951-4422
     800-344-4823
     Fax: 301-951-6378
     e-mail: info@cff.org
     www.cff.org
The mission of the Cystic Fibrosis Foundation a nonprofit donor-supported organization is to assure the development of the means to cure and control cystic fibrosis and to improve the quality of life for those with the disease.
Robert J Beall, President and CEO

Massachusetts

3052 **Baystate Medical Center Wesson Memorial Unit**
Wesson Memorial Unit
759 Chestnut Street
Springfield, MA 01199   413-794-0000
     e-mail: Marian.Panto@bhs.org
     www.baystatehealth.com
BMC serves as a regional resource for specialty medical care and research while providing comprehensive primary medical services to the community.
Mark R Tolosky, President & Chief Executive Officer
Paula S Dennison, Senior Vice President Human Resources

3053 **Childrens Hospital Medical Center Cystic Fibrosis Center**
300 Longwood Avenue
Boston, MA 02115   617-355-6000
     Fax: 617-730-0373
     TTY: 617-730-0152
     www.childrenshospital.org
The Cystic Fibrosis Center at Children's Hospital Boston is one of the oldest and largest cystic fibrosis centers in the United States and was founded by Dr. Harry Schwachman one of the earliest physician investigators to help characterize the disorder.
Terry Spence, Director
Sandra Fenwick, President, CEO

3054 **Cystic Firbrosis Center: Tufts New England Medical Center**
Pediatric Pulmonology and Allergy Department
800 Washington Street
Boston, MA 02111   617-636-5000
     www.nemc.org
We strive to heal to comfort to teach to learn and to seek the knowledge to promote health and prevent disease.
Ellen Zane, President and Chief Executive Officer
Margaret Vosburgh, Chief Operating Officer

3055 **Massachusetts General Hospital**
55 Fruit Street
Boston, MA 02114-2622   617-726-2000
     Fax: 617-726-6989
     TTY: 617-724-8800
     TDD: 617-724-8800
     www.massgeneral.org
Peter L Slavin, President
David Torchi, Chairman and Chief Executive Officer

3056 **University of Massachusetts Memorial Medical Center**
55 Lake Avenue N
Worcester, MA 01655   508-334-1000
     www.umassmemorial.org
UMass Memorial Medical Center is the region's trusted academic medical center committed to improving the health of the people of Central New England through excellence in clinical care service teaching and research.
Walter Ettinger, President
George Brenckle, Senior Vice President and Chief Informat

Michigan

3057 **East Lansing Cystic Fibrosis Center Michigan State University**
Michigan State University
1200 E Michigan Avenue
Lansing, MI 48912   517-364-5440
     Fax: 517-364-5413
     phd.msu.edu
Eliane F Eakin, Director
H Dele Davies, Department Chair

3058 **Kalamazoo Center for Medical Studies Michigan State University**
Michigan State University

1000 Oakland Drive
Kalamazoo, MI 49008-1202   269-337-4400
     800-275-5267
     Fax: 269-337-4234
     e-mail: programs@kcms.msu.edu
     www.med.wmich.edu
John M. Dunn, Chairman of the Board
Paul A. Spaude, President & CEO

3059 **University of Michigan: Cystic Fibrosis Center**
A Alfred Taubman Health Care Center
1500 E Medical Center Drive
Ann Arbor, MI 48109-0318   734-936-4000
     Fax: 734-936-7635
     TTY: 800-649-3777
     TDD: 800-649-3777
     www.med.umich.edu
Samya Z Nasr, Director
Douglas L Strong, CEO

Minnesota

3060 **University of Minnesota: Cystic Fibrosis Center**
University of Minnesota Hospital
420 Delaware Street SE
Minneapolis, MN 55455   612-624-0962
     800-688-5252
     Fax: 612-624-0696
     e-mail: cfcenter@umn.edu
     www.med.umn.edu/peds/cfcenter/home.html
The mission was to develop approaches to understanding and treating the complications of CF.
Warren E Regelmann, Co-Director
Jordan M Dunitz, Co-Director

Mississippi

3061 **University of Mississippi Medical Center**
2500 N State Street
Jackson, MS 39216-4500   601-984-5046
     Fax: 601-984-1973
     www.umc.edu
Suzanne Mill, Director
Daniel W Jones, Chancellor

Missouri

3062 **Children's Mercy Hospital Children's Mercy Hospitals & Clinics**
Children's Mercy Hospitals & Clinics
2401 Gilham Road
Kansas City, MO 64108   816-234-3000
     866-512-2168
     Fax: 816-842-6107
     TTY: 816-234-3816
     e-mail: webmaster@cmh.edu
     www.childrensmercy.org
Children's Mercy Hospital provides the highest level of medical care technology services equipment and facilities in promoting the health and well-being of children in the region from birth through adolescence.
Randall L O'Donnell PhD, President/CEO
V Fred Burry, Executive Medical Director/Executive Vic

3063 **University of Missouri Columbia Cystic Fibrosis Center**
University of Missouri/Dept of Child Health
One Hospital Drive N712
Columbia, MO 65212-1   573-882-6882
     Fax: 573-821-54
     e-mail: clarksonb@health.missouri.edu
     www.ch.missouri.edu/cysticfibrosis.htm
Peter Konig, Director
Melissa Lawson, Division Director

3064 **Washington University: Cystic Fibrosis Center**
St. Louis Children's Hospital
660 S Euclid Avenue
Saint Louis, MO 63110   314-454-2694
     888-678-4357
     Fax: 314-454-2515
     www.medschool.wustl.edu/
Dedicated to the treatment of patients with cystic fibrosis (CF) for more than 4 decades. The Cystic Fibrosis Clinical Center and affiliated programs has developed into a premier clinical and research program.
Thomas Ferko, Director

Nebraska

3065 University of Nebraska Medical Center Cystic Fibrosis Center
The Nebraska Medical Center 402-552-2000
Omaha, NE 68198-5190 800-922-0000
Fax: 402-559-7062
e-mail: necfcntr@unmc.edu
www.unmc.edu

Harold M Maurer, Chancellor
Hari Bandla, Associate Professor

Nevada

3066 Children's Lung Specialists
3838 Meadow Lane 702-598-4411
Las Vegas, NV 89107 Fax: 702-598-1988
e-mail: cls@childrens-lung-specialists.com
www.childrens-lung-specialists.com
The certified Cystic Fibrosis Center of Southern Nevada.
Ruben MD, Director/President/Owner
Craig Nakamu, Assistant Director

New Hampshire

3067 New Hampshire Cystic Fibrosis Care Teaching and Research Center
DarthmouthHitchcock Medical Center
One Medical Center Drive 603-650-5000
Lebanon, NH 03756 Fax: 603-500-07
TTY: 603-650-8034
www.dhmc.org

William Boyl, Director
Dennis Stoke, Director

New Jersey

3068 Monmouth Medical Center: Cystic Fibrosis & Pediatric Pulmonary Center
Monmouth Medical Center
95 Old Short Hills Road 732-222-5200
West Orange, NJ 7052 888-724-7123
Fax: 908-222-4472
e-mail: info@sbhcs.com
www.sbhcs.com

Peri Kamalakar, Director of Pediatric Hematology/Oncolog

3069 Monmouth Medical Center: Cystic Fibrosis & Monmouth Medical Center
368 Lakehurst Road 732-222-5200
Toms River, NJ 08755 888-724-7123
Fax: 908-222-4472
e-mail: info@sbhcs.com
www.sbhcs.com

Peri Kamalakar, Director of Pediatric Hematology/Oncolog

3070 New Jersey Medical School
185 S Orange Avenue 973-972-4595
Newark, NJ 07101-1709 Fax: 973-972-5965
e-mail: webnjms@umdnj.edu
njms.umdnj.edu
The mission of New Jersey Medical School is to educate students physicians and scientists to meet society's current and future healthcare needs through patient-centered education; pioneering research; innovative clinical rehabilitative and preventive care; and collaborative community outreach.
Maria L. Soto-Greene, MD, Vice Dean
Robert L Johnson MD, Dean

New York

3071 Albany Medical College Pediatric Pulmonary & Cystic Fibrosis Center
Department of Pediatrics
43 New Scotland Avenue 518-262-3125
Albany, NY 12208 877-262-8008
Fax: 518-262-6884
www.amc.edu

Scott Scroed, Division Chief

3072 Armond V Mascia Cystic Fibrosis Center NY Medical College
Division of Pediatrics Pulmonology
New York Medical College 914-594-4000
Valhalla, NY 10595 Fax: 914-594-4336
e-mail: pedpulm@nymc.edu
www.nycmc.edu
Provides comprehensive inpatient and outpatient consultation and management for children suffering from a broad variety of respiratory problems. They are the only accredited Cystic Fibrosis center in the Hudson Valley. The center is dedicated to teaching research and patient care.
Allen Dozer, Chief
Karl P Alder MD, President, CEO

3073 CF & Pediatric Pulmonary Care Center
Mount Sinai Hospital
One Gustave L Levy Place 212-241-6500
New York, NY 10029-6574 800-637-4624
Fax: 212-876-3255
www.mountsinai.org
Center staff perform outpatient and inpatient consultations with an integrated multidisciplinary team of professionals who are dedicated specifically to the practice of Pediatric Pulmonary Medicine.
Dennis S Charney, Dean, Executive Vice President

3074 Childrens Lung and Cystic Fibrosis Center
Women and Children's Hospital of Buffalo
140 Hodge Avenue 716-878-7000
Buffalo, NY 14222-2099 Fax: 716-888-3945
e-mail: AMTaylor@kaleidahealth.org
www.wchob.org
Services for infants children and teenagers with cystic fibrosis and other chronic respiratory conditions.
Annise Taylor, Manager
Cheryl Klass, President

3075 Cystic Fibrosis Center St. Vincent's Hospital & Medical Center
St. Vincent's Hospital & Medical Center of NY
36 7th Avenue 212-604-8895
New York, NY 10011-6600 Fax: 212-604-3899
www.svcmc.org

Maria Berdel, Co-Director
Patricia Wal MD, Co-Director

3076 Pulomonolgy Morgan Stanley Children's Hospital
Morgan Stanley Children's Hospital
3959 Broadway 212-305-5437
New York, NY 10032-3702 877-NYP-WELL
www.childrensnyp.org

Meyer Kattan, Director

3077 State University of NY Hospital: Upstate Medical Center
750 E Adams Street 315-464-5540
Syracuse, NY 13210-1834 877-464-5540
TDD: 315-464-5769
www.upstate.edu/uh

Stephen R Goodman, Vice President
David R. Smith, President

North Carolina

3078 UNC Cystic Fibrosis Center Department of Pediatrics
Department of Pediatrics
7011 Thurston-Bowles Building 919-966-1077
Chapel Hill, NC 27599-7248 Fax: 919-966-7524
www.med.unc.edu/cystfib/CFcent.htm
A large multidisciplinary group focused on the pathogenesis and other lung diseases.
Richard C Boucher, Director
Margaret Lei, Director

3079 Western Michigan University School of Medi cine
350 Hanes House 919-684-3364
Durham, NC 27710 888-275-3853
Fax: 919-684-2292
www.pulmonary.duke.edu
Provides primary and consultative care for patients with various lung diseases on an inpatient and outpatient basis.
Monica Kraft, Division Chief
Gina Brewer, Administrative Assistant

North Dakota

3080   St. Alexius Medical Heart and Lung Clinic
900 E Broadway Avenue   701-530-7000
Bismarck, ND 58501   877-530-5550
                                     Fax: 701-530-8984
                                     TTY: 701-530-5555
                                     TDD: 701-530-5555
                                     www.st.alexius.org
Specializes in services such as cardiac consultation cardiac surgery cardiac catheterization electrophysiology angioplasty intracoronary stents rotoblade asthma emphysema cystic fibrosis chronic lung disease. lung cancer allergy and anesthesia.
John Castleberry, Chair
Sr. Nancy Miller, OSB, President

Ohio

3081   Case Western Reserve University: Cystic Fibrosis Center
10900 Euclid Avenue   216-368-2000
Cleveland, OH 44106-2624   Fax: 216-844-5916
                                     e-mail: Mds11@case.edu
                                     www.case.edu

Barbara Snyder, President

3082   Columbus Children's Hospital: Cystic Fibrosis Center
700 Childrens Drive   614-722-2000
Columbus, OH 43205-0296   Fax: 614-722-4755
                                     www.nationwidechildrens.org

Dr Steve Allen, CEO
Elizabeth D Allen, Physician

3083   Lewis H Walker MD: Cystic Fibrosis Center
Children's Hospital Medical Center of Akron
One Perkins Square   330-543-1000
Akron, OH 44308-1062   800-262-0333
                                     TTY: 330-543-8080
                                     www.akronchildrens.org/respiratory
One of six CF centers in the state of Ohio providing comprehensive care for patients who suffer from this disease. The center which is part of the Robert T. Stone Respiratory Center actively participates in clinical trials to research new drug therapies to manage cystic fibrosis.
Nathan Krayn, Director Cystic Fibrosis Center
William H Considine, President, CEO

3084   Pediatric Pulmonary Center The Children's Medical Center of Dayton
The Children's Medical Center of Dayton
1 Children's Plaza   937-641-3000
Dayton, OH 45404-1815   800-228-4055
                                     Fax: 937-641-4500
                                     www.childrensdayton.org
David Kinsaul, President, CEO
Robert Fink, Medical Director

3085   University of Cincinnati College of Medicine Division of Pediatrics
Children s Hospital Medical Center
3333 Burnet Avenue   513-636-4200
Cincinnati, OH 45229-3039   800-344-2462
                                     Fax: 513-636-0345
                                     TTY: 513-636-4900
                                     e-mail: thomas.boat@cchmc.org
                                     www.cincinnatichildrens.org
The University of Cincinnati Department of Pediatrics consists entirely of staff members from Cincinnati Children's Hospital Medical Center one of the nation's leading pediatric research and teaching institutions.
Michael Fisher, President, CEO
Thomas F Boat, Professor of Pediatrics

Oklahoma

3086   University of Oklahoma: Cystic Fibrosis Center
Department of Pediatrics

940 NE 13th Street   405-271-4401
Oklahoma City, OK 73104   Fax: 405-271-8710
                                     e-mail: brenda-freese@ouhsc.edu
                                     www.oumedicine.com
James A Royall, Professor/Chief Pediatric Pulmonology
Terrence L Stull MD, Chairman

Oregon

3087   Oregon Health & Science University
3181 SW Sam Jackson Park Road   503-494-8311
Portland, OR 97239-3098   e-mail: contactus@ohsuhealth.com
                                     www.ohsuhealth.com
Oregon Health & Science University is a leading health and research university that strives for excellence in patient care education research and community service.
Joseph Rober, President
Steven D Stadum, Executive Vice President

Pennsylvania

3088   Cystic Fibrosis Center: Polyclinic Medical Center
Polyclinic Medical Center
PO Box 8700   717-231-8900
Harrisburg, PA 17105-8700   800-334-1007
                                     Fax: 717-782-4679
                                     www.pinnaclehealth.org

Muttiah Gane, Director
Michael A Young, FACHE, President/CEO

3089   Pediatric Pulmonary and Cystic Fibrosis Center
St. Christopher's Hospital for Children
3601 A Street   215-427-5000
Philadelphia, PA 19134   888-STC-RIS
                                     Fax: 215-427-5555
                                     www.stchristophershospital.com
A team of pediatric pulmonary medicine experts treats children with a wide range of acute and chronic lung diseases such as cystic fibrosis bronchopulmonary dysplasia apnea respiratory infections bronchiolitis congenital malformations including chest wall deformities and pneumonia.
Laurie Varlo, Director

3090   University of Pennsylvania: Penn Lung Center
Hospital of The University of Pennsylvania
3 Ravdin Suite F   215-662-4000
Philadelphia, PA 19104   800-789-7366
                                     www.pennhealth.com
Penn Lung Center of the University of Pennsylvania Health System is a multidisciplinary resource for consultation second opinion diagnosis and ongoing treatment of patients with lung disease.
Leslie A Litzky, Associate Professor of Pathology and Lab
Maryl Kreide, Assistant Professor of Medicine

3091   University of Pittsburgh Cystic Fibrosis Center: Children's Hospital
Department of Cell Biology And Physiology
S362 BST   412-648-9362
Pittsburgh, PA 15261   Fax: 412-648-8330
                                     e-mail: cdpweb@pitt.edu
                                     www.cbp.pitt.edu/centers/cfrc.html
The primary goal of the Center is to focus the attention of new and established investigators on multidisciplinary approaches designed to improve the understanding and treatment of cystic fibrosis (CF).
Raymond A Frizzell, Director
Carol A Bertrand, Research Assistant Professor

Rhode Island

3092   Rhode Island Hospital: Cystic Fibrosis Center
Department of Pediatrics
593 Eddy Street   401-444-4000
Providence, RI 02903   Fax: 401-444-2168
                                     e-mail: mschechter@lifespan.org
                                     www.lifespan.org

Michael S Schechter, Director
George A Vecchione, President, CEO

South Carolina

3093 Medical University of South Carolina: Cystic Fibrosis Center
171 Ashley Avenue 803-792-1414
Charleston, SC 29403 800-424-6872
Fax: 843-876-1435
www.musc.edu/cfcenter
The objectives of the Cystic Fibrosis Center at MUSC are to offer unsurpassed care to patients with cystic fibrosis to teach medical students house staff medical care providers and general public about cystic fibrosis and to learn about cystic fibrosis through clinical and laboratory research.
Isabel Virella-Lowell, MD, Director
W Stuart Smith, Vice President, Executive Director

Tennessee

3094 Memphis Cystic Fibrosis Center LeBonheur Children's Medical Center
LeBonheur Children's Medical Center
848 Adams Ave 901-287-5437
Memphis, TN 38103 e-mail: info@lebonheur.org
www.lebonheur.org
Meri Armour, President, CEO

3095 Vanderbilt Children's Hospital
2200 Childrens Way 615-936-1000
Nashville, TN 37232 866-936-7811
www.vanderbiltchildrens.com
Children's Hospital provides top-level care while including the family as an essential element of a child's treatment plan.
Luke Gregory, Chief Executive Officer
Jonathan Gitlin, Vice Chancellor

Texas

3096 Cook Children's Medical Center: Cystic Fibrosis Clinic
4214 Andrews Highway
Midland, TX 79701 432-570-5693
www.cookchildrens.org
James C Cunningham MD, Director
Paula Webb, Vice President of Nursing Services

3097 Cystic Fibrosis Care and Teaching Center Children's Medical Center
Children's Medical Center
1935 Medical District Dr 214-456-7000
Dallas, TX 75235 Fax: 214-456-2563
www.childrens.com
The Dallas Cystic Fibrosis Care and Teaching Center manages the outpatient and inpatient care of approximately 400 infants children adolescents and adults.
Claude Prest MD, Director
Brenda Urbanczyk, Practice Administrator

3098 Cystic Fibrosis-Lung Disease Center: Santa Rosa Children's Hospital
CHRISTUS Center for Children and Families
333 N Santa Rosa 210-704-2011
San Antonio, TX 78207 Fax: 210-704-2651
www.santarosahealth.org
Serving more than 150 000 children each year CSRCH is a 200-plus bed facility and is the only academic Children's hospital in San Antonio partnering with The University of Texas Health Science Center at San Antonio while collaborating with private pediatricians to provide comprehensive pediatric services at one location since 1959.
Donna Beth Willey-Courand MD, Director
Patrick Carrier, President, CEO

3099 Texas Childrens Cystic Fibrosis Care Center
Texas Children's Clinical Care Center
6701 Fannin Street 832-824-1000
Houston, TX 77030 800-364-5437
Fax: 832-825-3072
e-mail: pulmonarymedicine@texaschildrenshospital
www.texaschildrenshospital.org

Provides comprehensive clinical services to help patients families and referring physicians deal with the many problems cystic fibrosis causes.
Mark A. Wallace, President and Chief Executive Officer
Dr. Mark Kline, Physician-in-Chief

3100 Tri-Services Military Cystic Fibrosis Center
Brooke Army Medical Center/Pediatrics Department
3851 Roger Brooke Drive 210-916-3400
Fort Sam Houston, TX 78234-6320 Fax: 210-916-3076
e-mail: ted.cieslak@cen.amedd.army.mil
www.bamc.amedd.army.mil
COL Ted Cieslak, Chief of Pediatrics
Joseph Caravalho, Commanding Officer

Utah

3101 University of Utah Intermountain Cystic Fibrosis Center
University Hospital & Clinics
50 N. Medical Drive 801-581-2121
Salt Lake City, UT 84132 800-824-2073
Fax: 801-585-5350
e-mail: judy.carle@hsc.utah.edu
www.med.utah.edu
Barbara A Chatfield MD, Director Pediatric Program
Loris Betz, Senior VP, Executive Dean

Vermont

3102 Medical Center Hospital of Vermont Cystic Fibrosis Center
Cystic Fibrosis Center
111 Colchester Avenue 802-847-0000
Burlington, VT 05401-7152 800-358-1144
Fax: 802-555-2323
www.fahc.org
Tom Lahiri MD, Director
Melinda L Estes, President, CEO

Virginia

3103 Eastern Virginia Medical School Children's Hospital of The King's Daught
Children's Hospital of The King's Daughters
601 Children's Lane 757-668-7000
Norfolk, VA 23507 e-mail: healthinfo@chkd.org
www.chkd.org
Provider of quality children's health services
James D. Dahling, President and Chief Executive Officer
Kathy Abshire, Vice President, Finance

3104 University of Virginia School of Medicine Cystic Fibrosis Center
Department of Pediatrics
PO Box 800793 434-924-2250
Charlottesville, VA 22908 800-251-3627
Fax: 434-243-6618
www.healthsystem.virginia.edu
Comprehensive care for children and adults with cystic fibrosis.
Steven T DeKosky MD, Vice President, Dean
Sharon L Hostler, Senior Associate Dean

Washington

3105 University of Washington: Cystic Fibrosis Center
University of Washington Medical Center/Adult Prog
1959 NE Pacific Street 206-598-6116
Seattle, WA 98195 Fax: 206-598-4610
www.washington.edu
UW Medicine works to improve the health of the public by advancing medical knowledge
Ronald Gibson, Center Director
Ronald Gibson, Professor and Center Director

West Virginia

3106 West Virginia University Cystic Fibrosis Center
Pediatrics Department

PO Box 9214
Morgantown, WV 26506-9214
304-293-1201
Fax: 304-293-1216
e-mail: kmoffett@hsc.wvu.edu
www.hsc.wvu.edu

The Hospital providing the full range of services including allergy/immunology cardiology child development critical care cystic fibrosis endocrinology adolescent medicine gastroenterology genetics and metabolic disease hematology/oncology neonatology nephrology neurology and apnea evaluation. Services provided by faculty with joint appointments include ophthalmology urology orthopedics psychiatry surgery and cardiothoracic surgery.
Kathryn S Moffett MD, Director
Giovanni Piedimonte, Chair

Wisconsin

3107 Medical College of Wisconsin: Cystic Fibrosis Clinic
Children's Hospital of Wisconsin
PO Box 1997
Milwaukee, WI 53201-1997
414-266-2000
877-266-8989
www.chw.org

Children's Hospital and Health System is an independent health care system dedicated solely to the health and well-being of children.
Robert Kliegman MD, Executive VP
Peter J Bartz, Cardiology Pediatric

3108 University of Wisconsin-Madison: Cystic Fibrosis/Pulmonary Center
Clinical Science Center
600 Highland Avenue
Madison, WI 53792
608-263-6400
800-323-8942
www.uwhealth.org

UW Health represents the academic medical care providers of the University of Wisconsin-Madison and its affiliated organizations.
Michael J Rock, Faculty
Prasad S Dalvie, Radiology

Support Groups & Hotlines

3109 National Health Information Center
PO Box 1133
Washington, DC 20013-1133
310-565-4167
800-336-4797
Fax: 301-984-4256
e-mail: info@nhic.org
www.health.gov/nhic

A health information referral service sponsored by the Office of Disease Prevention and Health Promotion. Puts health professionals and consumers who have health questions in touch with those organizations that are best able to provide answers.

Books

3110 Cystic Fibrosis: A Guide for Patient and Family
Raven Press
1185 Ave of the Americas
New York, NY 10036-2601
212-930-9500
800-777-2295
253 pages Softcover
ISBN: 0-397516-53-3

3111 Understanding Cystic Fibrosis
Karen Hopkin, PhD, author
University Press of Mississippi
3825 Ridgewood Road
Jackson, MS 39211-6492
601-432-6205
Fax: 601-432-6217
e-mail: kburgess@ihl.state.ms.us
www.upress.state.ms.us

A useful guide for families and patients.
1998 128 pages Paperback
ISBN: 0-878059-67-9
Kathy Burgess, Advertising/Marketing Services Manager

Children's Books

3112 Give Me One Wish
Norton Publishers

500 5th Avenue
New York, NY 10110-0002
212-354-5500
800-233-4830
www.scholastic.com/

This book reads like a novel because it re-enacts the author's daughter's bout with cystic fibrosis.
Grades 10-12

3113 Robyn's Book: A True Diary
Scholastic
730 Broadway
New York, NY 10003-9511
212-505-3000
800-325-6149

This book chronicles the life of the author and her battle with cystic fibrosis.
Grades 7-12

3114 Toothpick
Holiday
40 E 49th Street
New York, NY 10017-1105
212-688-0085

This book uses relationships between two different teenagers to parallel the life of a person with cystic fibrosis.
Grades 6-9

Newsletters

3115 Better Breathing Bulletin
American Lung Association of Connecticut
45 Ash Street
East Hartford, CT 06108-3294
860-289-5401
800-586-4872
Fax: 860-289-5405
www.alact.org

This newsletter is aimed at persons with chronic lung problems.
John E Zinn, President/CEO

3116 Commitment
Cystic Fibrosis Foundation
6931 Arlington Road
Bethesda, MD 20814-5231
301-951-4422
800-344-4823
Fax: 301-951-6378
e-mail: info@cff.org
www.cff.org

Offers general information on cystic fibrosis, fund-raising features, public policy and news from across the nation on cystic fibrosis.

Pamphlets

3117 Consumer Fact Sheet
Cystic Fibrosis Foundation
6931 Arlington Road
Bethesda, MD 20814-5231
301-951-4422
800-344-4823
Fax: 301-951-6378
e-mail: info@cff.org
www.cff.org

Offers a brief introduction to cystic fibrosis, symptoms, causes, treatments and offers illustrations pertaining to drainage positions.

3118 Cystic Fibrosis: A Guide for Parents
American Lung Association
1740 Broadway
New York, NY 10019-4315
212-315-8700

Comprehensive booklet covering topics such as treatment, social aspects, inheritance, genetics and outlook for the future.
24 pages

3119 For Adults with Cystic Fibrosis: Facts on Reproduction
National Maternal and Child Health Clearinghouse
2070 Chain Bridge Road
Vienna, VA 22182-2588
703-442-9051
888-275-4772
Fax: 703-821-2098
e-mail: ask@hrsa.gov
www.ask.hrsa.gov

The purpose of this booklet is to review the reproductive issues that are unique to individuals with cystic fibrosis.

3120 Foundation Facts
Cystic Fibrosis Foundation

6931 Arlington Road
Bethesda, MD 20814-5231

301-951-4422
800-344-4823
Fax: 301-951-6378
e-mail: info@cff.org
www.cff.org

Offers information on the fund-raising and grants offered and supported by the foundation.

3121 Here's Everything You'll Need to Save Money with the CFF Health Services
CFF Home Health & Pharmacy Services
6931 Arlington Road
Bethesda, MD 20814-5223

800-342-6967
Fax: 800-233-3504

Offers information on the Cystic Fibrosis Foundation's home health services.

3122 Home Line
Cystic Fibrosis Foundation
6931 Arlington Road
Bethesda, MD 20814-5231

301-951-4422
800-344-4823
Fax: 301-951-6378
e-mail: info@cff.org
www.cff.org

Offers information on services and programs offered by the foundation.

Audio & Video

3123 Alex: The Life of a Child
Cystic Fibrosis Foundation
6931 Arlington Road
Bethesda, MD 20814

301-951-4422
800-344-4823
Fax: 301-951-6378
e-mail: info@cff.org
www.cff.org

The story of Alexandra Deford, a young girl who lost her battle with CF at the age of 8, has touched the hearts of millions and has helped to put a face to this disease. Alex's courage and strength is a true inspiration, and in the decades since her death, much progress has been made in the fight against CF. VHS only.
1986 1 Hr 35 Minutes
Robert J Beall, PhD, President/CEO

3124 Embers of the Fire
Mary Kondrat, author
Fanlight Productions
4196 Washington Street
Boston, MA 02131-1731

617-469-4999
800-937-4113
Fax: 617-469-3379
e-mail: fanlight@fanlight.com
www.fanlight.com

Offers a straight forward explanation of the disease with a primary focus on the stories of several courageous young people with cystic fibrosis during a week at summer camp. Addresses their fears of rejection, isolation and death while demonstrating the ways they have learned to lead fulfilling lives.
1992 28 Minutes
ISBN: 1-572950-98-6

3125 Expanding the Horizon of Hope: 50 Years of Progress
Cystic Fibrosis Foundation
6931 Arlington Road
Bethesda, MD 20814

301-951-4422
800-344-4823
Fax: 301-951-6378
e-mail: info@cff.org
www.cff.org

This film highlights the progress that has been made in CF research and care over the past 50 years, as well as the challenges that still lie ahead. It pays tribute to all who are involved in the CF effort—from researchers and clinicians, to patients and their families, to volunteers, donors and staff. DVD only.
2005 60 Minutes
Robert J Beall, PhD, President/CEO

3126 Faces of Cystic Fibrosis
Cystic Fibrosis Foundation

6931 Arlington Road
Bethesda, MD 20814

301-951-4422
800-344-4823
Fax: 301-951-6378
e-mail: info@cff.org
www.cff.org

Through the words of people with CF and their family members, hear the story of how the fight against CF has evolved into a story of hope and optimism that was never possible before...and how none of this would be possible without the dedication and efforts of volunteers. Available in VHS/DVD.
2001 11 Minutes
Robert J Beall, PhD, President/CEO

3127 Information About the Sweat Test
Cystic Fibrosis Foundation
6931 Arlington Road
Bethesda, MD 20814

301-951-4422
800-344-4823
Fax: 301-951-6378
e-mail: info@cff.org
www.cff.org

See and hear some basic information about the sweat test, the standard diagnostic test for CF. It is intended to help families better understand the sweat testing procedure and what to expect when the test is conducted. VHS only.
3.47 Minutes
Robert J Beall, PhD, President/CEO

Web Sites

3128 Healing Well
www.healingwell.com
An online health resource guide to medical news, chat, information and articles, newsgroups and message boards, books, disease-related web sites, medical directories, and more for patients, friends, and family coping with disabling diseases, disorders, or chronic illnesses.

3129 Health Finder
www.healthfinder.gov
Searchable, carefully developed web site offering information on over 1000 topics. Developed by the US Department of Health and Human Services, the site can be used in both English and Spanish.

3130 Healthlink USA
www.healthlinkusa.com
Health information concerning treatment, cures, prevention, diagnosis, risk factors, research, support groups, email lists, personal stories and much more. Updated regularly.

3131 Helios Health
www.helioshealth.com
Online resource for your health information. Detailed information about specific health topics, access to expert advice from our Medical Advisory Board, and up-to-date health news.

3132 MedicineNet
www.medicinenet.com
An online resource for consumers providing easy-to-read, authoritative medical and health information.

3133 Medscape
www.medscape.com
Medscape offers specialists, primary care physicians, and other health professionals the Web's most robust and integrated medical information and educational tools.

3134 WebMD
www.webmd.com
Provides credible information, supportive communities, and in-depth reference material about health subjects. A source for original and timely health information as well as material from well known content providers.

Description

3135 Diabetes Mellitus

Diabetes mellitus is a condition in which the body lacks enough insulin to control its own blood glucose (sugar) level. Ordinarily, the pancreas releases enough of this hormone to let the body's cells absorb and metabolize glucose. In Type I diabetes (formerly called juvenile-onset diabetes and affecting 10 percent of diabetic patients), the pancreas simply stops producing insulin. In Type II, commonly affecting overweight individuals older than 40, the pancreas might release normal, reduced, or even elevated levels of insulin, but the body's cells are resistant to the insulin's action. In either case, blood glucose levels rise (hyperglycemia) until the kidney starts to dump sugar into the urine. The patient may experience excessive thirst and urination, hunger, weakness and weight loss. In extreme cases, when there is either insufficient insulin or the body undergoes stress, or strenuous exercise, some components of the blood become seriously altered and the patient may lapse into a coma. Long-term complications include an increased risk of coronary heart disease and other vascular diseases, such as stroke, vision loss and kidney failure.

Type I appears to be caused by a genetic predisposition that may express itself after an acute insult, often a viral infection. Genetic factors are important in Type II diabetes which runs strongly in families. It is much more common in obese people, as well as among African-Americans, Hispanics and Native Americans.

Prevention ofacute and long-term complications requires careful management including maintaining the proper diet and exercise, blood glucose monitoring and medications. Thorough education of the patient and relevant family members is absolutely critical.

Some individuals with Type II diabetes can control their disease through diet, exercise and weight loss alone. Some will have to take oral medication that helps the pancreas make more insulin or makes the body more sensitive to insulin. Some Type II diabetics, and all Type I diabetics, need to take insulin. Research has shown that tight control of diabetes through frequent blood testing and proper adjustment of the dosage of insulin is most beneficial. Insulin is generally given in multiple injections throughout the day, with preparations varying by length of effectiveness. Closest control of glucose levels is achieved by giving insulin through a continuously-connected insulin pump. Pancreas transplantation is considered only for patients who also need some other organ, generally a kidney.

National Agencies & Associations

3136 American Association of Diabetes Educators
200 W Madison Street
Chicago, IL 60606
800-338-3633
e-mail: aade@aadenet.org
www.aadenet.org

An independent multidisciplinary organization of health professionals involved in teaching persons with diabetes. The mission is to enhance the competence of health professionals who teach persons with diabetes and advance the specialty practice of diabetes.
Donna Tomky, President
Tami Ross, VP

3137 American Diabetes Association
1701 N Beauregard Street
Alexandria, VA 22311
804-225-8038
888-342-2383
Fax: 804-225-8211
e-mail: askada@diabetes.org
www.diabetes.org

The nation's leading voluntary organization concerned with diabetes and its complications. The mission of the organization is to prevent and cure diabetes and to improve the lives of persons with diabetes. Offers a network of offices nationwide.
Julie Heverly, Area Director
Larry Hausner, CEO

3138 Diabetes Exercise and Sports Association
310 West Liberty
Louisville, KY 40202
502-581-0207
800-898-4322
Fax: 502-581-0206
e-mail: desa@diabetes-exercise.org
www.diabetes-exercise.org

Exists to enhance the quality of life for people with diabetes through exercise and physical fitness.
Paula Harper, Founder
Guy Hornsby, Chair

3139 Juvenile Diabetes Foundation: International
26 Broadway
New York, NY 10004
800-533-2873
Fax: 212-785-9595
e-mail: info@jdrf.org
www.jdf.org

Focuses energies on fund-raising, referrals, educational materials and information pertaining to juvenile diabetes.
Jeffery Brewer, President

3140 National Certification Board for Diabetes Educators
330 E Algonquin Road
Arlington Heights, IL 60005
847-228-9795
877-239-3233
Fax: 847-228-8469
e-mail: info@ncbde.org
www.ncbde.org

The Board for Diabetes Educators is dedicated to promoting excellence in the field of diabetes education through the development maintenance and protection of the certified Diabetes Educator credential and the certification process.
Samuel Abbate, Chair
Lance Hoxie, Chief Executive Officer

3141 National Diabetes Action Network for the Blind
National Federation of the Blind
200 East Wells Street
Baltimore, MD 21230
410-659-9314
Fax: 410-685-5653
e-mail: nfb@nfb.org
www.nfb.org

Leading support and information organization of persons losing vision due to diabetes. Provides personal contact and resource information with other blind diabetics about non-visual techniques of independently managing diabetes and monitoring glucose levels.
Marc Maurer, President
Fredric Schroeder, First Vice President

3142 National Institute of Diabetes, Digestive & Kidney Diseases
National Institutes of Health
1 Information Way
Bethesda, MD 20892-2560
800-860-8747
Fax: 703-738-4929
TTY: 866-569-1162
e-mail: ndic@info.niddk.nih.gov
www.diabetes.niddk.nih.gov

Conducts and supports research on many of the most serious diseases affecting public health. The Institute supports much of the clinical research on the diseases of internal medicine and related subspecialty fields as well as many basic science disciplines.
Dr. Griffin Rodgers, Acting Director

State Agencies & Associations

Alabama

3143 American Diabetes Association: Alabama
3918 Montclair Road   205-870-5172
Birmingham, AL 35213   888-DIA-BETE
                                  Fax: 205-879-2903
                        e-mail: acasey@diabetes.org
                                   www.diabetes.org

Aimee Casey, Executive Director
Stephanie Willis, Director

3144 Juvenile Diabetes Research Foundation: Birmingham
14 Office Park Circle   205-871-0333
Birmingham, AL 35223   Fax: 205-871-0355
                         e-mail: alabama@jdf.org
                              www.jdrf.org/alabama

Karin Scott, Executive Director
Sarah Hendren, Special Events Manager

Alaska

3145 American Diabetes Association: Alaska
801 W Fireweed Lane   907-272-1424
Anchorage, AK 99503   888-DIA-BETE
                                  Fax: 907-272-1428
                      e-mail: mcassano@diabetes.org
                                   www.diabetes.org

Michelle Cassano, Executive Director
Phoebe O'Connell, Manager

Arizona

3146 American Diabetes Association: Arizona
8125 N 23rd Avenue   602-861-4731
Phoenix, AZ 85021   Fax: 602-995-1344
                                   www.diabetes.org

Edyth Haro, Manager
Lynda Brown, Special Events Manager

3147 American Diabetes Association: Arizona, Border Area
333 W Ft Lowell Rd   520-795-3711
Tucson, AZ 85705   888-DIA-BETE
                                  Fax: 520-795-1179
                       e-mail: fgomez@diabetes.org
                                   www.diabetes.org

Fred Gomez, Executive Director
Heidi Goldsmith, Manager

3148 American Diabetes Association: Atlanta Met
8125 N 23rd Avenue   602-861-4731
Phoenix, AZ 85021   Fax: 602-995-1344
                       e-mail: kbisko@diabetes.org
                                   www.diabetes.org

Karen Bisko, Executive Director
Suzanne Miller, Director

3149 American Diabetes Association: Northern Arizona
5333 N 7th Street   602-861-4731
Phoenix, AZ 85014   Fax: 602-995-1344
                      e-mail: llandon@diabetes.org
                                   www.diabetes.org

Laura Landon, Executive Director
Suzanne Miller, Programs Director

3150 Juvenile Diabetes Research Foundation: Phoenix Chapter
4343 E Camelback Road   602-224-1800
Phoenix, AZ 85018   Fax: 602-224-1801
                   e-mail: desertsouthwest@jdrf.org
                              www.jdrf.org/arizona

Marci Zimmerman, Executive Director
Valerie Jones, Associate Executive Director

Arkansas

3151 American Diabetes Association: Arkansas
320 Executive Court   501-221-7444
Little Rock, AR 72205   888-DIA-BETE
                                  Fax: 501-221-3138
                       e-mail: rselig@diabetes.org
                                   www.diabetes.org

Rick Selig, Director
Charlotte Williams, Associate Manager

3152 Juvenile Diabetes Research Foundation: Northwest Arkansas Branch
4241 Gabel Dr   479-443-9190
Fayetteville, AR 72703   Fax: 479-443-2692
                       e-mail: nwarkansas@jdrf.org
                                   www.nwark.jdrf.org

Deb Euculano, Special Events Manager

California

3153 American Diabetes Association: California
2720 Gateway Oaks Drive   916-924-3232
Sacramento, CA 95833   888-DIA-BETE
                                  Fax: 916-924-0529
                      e-mail: AskADA@diabetes.org
                                   www.diabetes.org/

The American Diabetes Association is a nonprofit health organization providing diabetes research, information and advocacy. Founded in 1940, the American Diabetes Association conducts programs in all 50 states and the District of Columbia.
Michael D Farley CFRE, Chief Community Relations Officer
Richard Kahn PhD, Chief Scientific/Medical Officer

3154 Diabetes Society of Santa Clara Valley
4040 Moorpark Avenue   408-241-1922
San Jose, CA 95117   888-DIA-BETE
                                  Fax: 408-241-1972
                  e-mail: Info@thediabetessociety.org
                                   www.diabetes.org

The Diabetes Society is dedicated to providing education and information to those who have diabetes educating the general public about the seriousness of this disease, and supporting research aimed at preventing complications and finding a cure.
Douglas Metz DPM/MPH, Executive Director
Thomas Smith, Program/Camp Director

3155 Juvenile Diabetes Research Foundation: Bakersfield Chapter
712 19th Street   661-636-1305
Bakersfield, CA 93301   Fax: 661-636-1307
                     e-mail: Bakersfield@jdrf.org
                              www.jdrf-bakersfield.org

The Juvenile Diabetes Research Foundation International (JDRF) is a charitable funder and advocate of type 1 (juvenile) diabetes research worldwide. The mission of JDRF is to find a cure for diabetes and its complications through the support of research.
Allison Perkins Thomas, Bakersfield Branch Manager
Arnold Donald, President/CEO Corporate Office (NY)

3156 Juvenile Diabetes Research Foundation: Inl and Empire Chapter
1001 East Cooley Drive   909-424-0100
Colton, CA 92324   Fax: 909-424-0044
                    e-mail: inlandempire@jdrf.org
                              www.inlandempire.jdrf.org

The Juvenile Diabetes Research Foundation International (JDRF) is a charitable funder and advocate of type 1 (juvenile) diabetes research worldwide. The mission of JDRF is to find a cure for diabetes and its complications through the support of research.
Jamie Brunelle, Board of Directors
Evelyn Edinin, Board of Directors

3157 Juvenile Diabetes Research Foundation: Los Angeles Chapter
800 West Sixth Street   213-233-9901
Los Angeles, CA 90017   Fax: 213-622-6276
                      e-mail: losangeles@jdrf.org
                              www.jdrf.org/losangeles

The Juvenile Diabetes Research Foundation International (JDRF) is a charitable funder and advocate of type 1 (juvenile) diabetes re-

search worldwide. The mission of JDRF is to find a cure for diabetes and its complications through the support of research.
Mark Rieck, Executive Director
Dennis Ellman Esq, Board of Directors President

3158 Juvenile Diabetes Research Foundation: Nor thern California Inland Chapter
1329 Howe Avenue
Sacramento, CA 95825
916-920-0790
Fax: 916-920-0367
e-mail: northernca@jdrf.org
www.jdrf.org/norcal
The Juvenile Diabetes Research Foundation International (JDRF) is a charitable funder and advocate of type 1 (juvenile) diabetes research worldwide. The mission of JDRF is to find a cure for diabetes and its complications through the support of research.
Victoria Webster, Executive Director
Molly Atkinson, Special Events Coordinator

3159 Juvenile Diabetes Research Foundation: Ora nge County Chapter
17992 Mitchell South
Irvine, CA 92614
949-553-0363
Fax: 949-553-8813
e-mail: orangecounty@jdrf.org
www.jdrfoc.org
The Juvenile Diabetes Research Foundation International (JDRF) is a charitable funder and advocate of type 1 (juvenile) diabetes research worldwide. The mission of JDRF is to find a cure for diabetes and its complications through the support of research.
Louise Cummings, Executive Director
John Giovannone, President

3160 Juvenile Diabetes Research Foundation: San Diego Chapter
5677 Oberlin Drive
San Diego, CA 92121
858-597-0240
Fax: 858-597-2072
e-mail: sandiego@jdrf.org
www.jdrf-sandiego-news.org
The Juvenile Diabetes Research Foundation International (JDRF) is a charitable funder and advocate of type 1 (juvenile) diabetes research worldwide. The mission of JDRF is to find a cure for diabetes and its complications through the support of research.
Linda Riley, Executive Director
Katherine Griswold, Special Events Manager

Colorado

3161 American Diabetes Association: Denver
2480 W 26th Avenue
Denver, CO 80211
720-855-1102
Fax: 720-855-1302
e-mail: AskADA@diabetes.org
www.diabetes.org/
The American Diabetes Association is a nonprofit health organization providing diabetes research, information and advocacy. Founded in 1940 the American Diabetes Association conducts programs in all 50 states and the District of Columbia.
Michael D Farley CFRE, Chief Community Relations Officer
Richard Kahn, Chief Scientific/Medical Officer

3162 Juvenile Diabetes Research Foundation: Colorado Springs Chapter
3710 Sinton Road
Colorado Springs, CO 80907
719-633-8110
Fax: 719-633-8155
e-mail: lpage@jdrf.org
www.jdrfcoloradosprings.org
The Juvenile Diabetes Research Foundation International (JDRF) is a charitable funder and advocate of type 1 (juvenile) diabetes research worldwide. The mission of JDRF is to find a cure for diabetes and its complications through the support of research.
Lynn Page, Branch Manager
Andi Chernushin, President

3163 Juvenile Diabetes Research Foundation: Roc ky Mountain Chapter
5613 DTC Parkway
Greenwood Village, CO 80111
303-779-0525
Fax: 303-720-1630
e-mail: RockyMountain@jdrf.org
www.jdrf.org/rockymountain
The Juvenile Diabetes Research Foundation International (JDRF) is a charitable funder and advocate of type 1 (juvenile) diabetes re-

search worldwide. The mission of JDRF is to find a cure for diabetes and its complications through the support of research.
James Buckles, Executive Director
Nancy L Walters, Special Events Director

Connecticut

3164 American Diabetes Association: Connecticut
306 Industrial Park Road
Middletown, CT 06457
203-639-0385
888-DIA-BETE
Fax: 860-632-5098
e-mail: AskADA@diabetes.org
www.diabetes.org
The American Diabetes Association is a nonprofit health organization providing diabetes research, information and advocacy. Founded in 1940 the American Diabetes Association conducts programs in all 50 states and the District of Columbia.
Michael D Farley CRFE, Chief Community Relations Officer
Richard Kahn, Chief Scientific/Medical Officer

3165 Juvenile Diabetes Research Foundation: Greater New Haven Chapter
2969 Whitney Avenue
Hamden, CT 06518
203-248-1880
Fax: 203-248-1820
e-mail: newhaven@jdf.org
www.jdrf.org/greaternewhaven
The Juvenile Diabetes Research Foundation International (JDRF) is a charitable funder and advocate of type 1 (juvenile) diabetes research worldwide. The mission of JDRF is to find a cure for diabetes and its complications through the support of research.
Mary K Kessler, Executive Director
Will Martinez, Board of Directors President

3166 Juvenile Diabetes Research Foundation: Fai rfield County Chapter
200 Connecticut Avenue
Norwalk, CT 06854
203-854-0658
Fax: 203-854-0798
e-mail: fairfield@jdrf.org
www.jdrf.org/fairfieldcounty
The Juvenile Diabetes Research Foundation International (JDRF) is a charitable funder and advocate of type 1 (juvenile) diabetes research worldwide. The mission of JDRF is to find a cure for diabetes and its complications through the support of research.
Barbara Rose, Executive Director
Michelle Tighe, Special Events Coordinator

3167 Juvenile Diabetes Research Foundation: Nor th Central CT and Western MA
18 North Main Street
West Hartford, CT 06107
860-561-1153
Fax: 860-561-3440
e-mail: northcentralct@jdrf.org
www.jdrf.org/index.cfm?page_id=100619
The Juvenile Diabetes Research Foundation International (JDRF) is a charitable funder and advocate of type 1 (juvenile) diabetes research worldwide. The mission of JDRF is to find a cure for diabetes and its complications through the support of research.
Mary Ann Slomski, Executive Director
Ellen Kellie, Special Events Coordinator

Delaware

3168 American Diabetes Association: Delaware
100 W 10th Street
Wilmington, DE 19801
302-656-0030
888-342-2383
Fax: 302-656-7331
e-mail: AskADA@diabetes.org
www.diabetes.org
The American Diabetes Association is a nonprofit health organization providing diabetes research, information and advocacy. Founded in 1940 the American Diabetes Association conducts programs in all 50 states and the District of Columbia.
Michael D Farley CFRE, Chief Community Relations Officer
Richard Kahn, Chief Scientific/Medical Officer

3169 Juvenile Diabetes Research Foundation: Del aware
100 West 10th Street
Wilmington, DE 19801
302-888-1117
Fax: 302-888-1878
e-mail: delaware@jdrf.org
www.jdrf.org/delaware

The Juvenile Diabetes Research Foundation International (JDRF) is a charitable funder and advocate of type 1 (juvenile) diabetes research worldwide. The mission of JDRF is to find a cure for diabetes and its complications through the support of research.
Ellen Rubesin, Executive Director
Stephanie Bucksner, Special Events Coordinator

District of Columbia

3170 American Diabetes Association: District of Columbia
1025 Connecticut Avenue NW   202-331-8303
Washington, DC 20036   888-342-2383
                                    Fax: 202-331-1402
                        e-mail: AskADA@diabetes.org
                                    www.diabetes.org
The American Diabetes Association is a nonprofit health organization providing diabetes research, information and advocacy. Founded in 1940 the American Diabetes Association conducts programs in all 50 states and the District of Columbia.
Michael D Farley CFRE, Chief Community Relations Officer
Richard Kahn, Chief Scientific/Medical Officer

3171 Juvenile Diabetes Research Foundation: Cap itol Chapter
1400 K Street NW   202-371-0044
Washington, DC 20005   Fax: 202-371-0046
                          e-mail: capitol@jdrf.org
                               www.jdrfcapitol.org
The Juvenile Diabetes Research Foundation International (JDRF) is a charitable funder and advocate of type 1 (juvenile) diabetes research worldwide. The mission of JDRF is to find a cure for diabetes and its complications through the support of research.
Pam Gatz, Executive Director
Carrie Hamilton, Special Events Director

Florida

3172 American Diabetes Association: Northeast F lorida/Southeast Georgia
8384 Baymeadows Road   904-730-7200
Jacksonville, FL 32256   888-342-2383
                                    Fax: 940-730-7933
                        e-mail: AskADA@diabetes.org
                                    www.diabetes.org
The American Diabetes Association is a nonprofit health organization providing diabetes research, information and advocacy. Founded in 1940 the American Diabetes Association conducts programs in all 50 states and the District of Columbia.
Sheri Criswell, Executive Director
Richard Kahn, Chief Scientific/Medical Officer

3173 American Diabetes Association: Seattle
1101 N Lake Destiny Road   407-660-1926
Maitland, FL 32751   Fax: 407-660-1080
                        e-mail: AskADA@diabetes.org
                                    www.diabetes.org
The American Diabetes Association is a nonprofit health organization providing diabetes research, information and advocacy. Founded in 1940 the American Diabetes Association conducts programs in all 50 states and the District of Columbia.
Pauline Lowe, Executive Director
Richard Kahn, Chief Scientific/Medical Officer

3174 American Diabetes Association: South Coast Regional/Central Florida
1101 North Lake Destiny Road   407-660-1926
Maitland, FL 32751   888-342-2383
                                    Fax: 407-660-1080
                        e-mail: AskADA@diabetes.org
                                    www.diabetes.org
The American Diabetes Association is a nonprofit health organization providing diabetes research, information and advocacy. Founded in 1940, the American Diabetes Association conducts programs in all 50 states and the District of Columbia, reaching hundreds of communities.
Michael D Farley CFRE, Chief Community Relations Officer
Richard Kahn, Chief Scientific/Medical Officer

3175 Juvenile Diabetes Research Foundation: Cen tral Florida Chapter
279 Douglas Avenue   407-774-2166
Altamonte Springs, FL 32714   Fax: 407-774-2168
                      e-mail: centralflorida@jdrf.org
                            www.jdrf.org/centralflorida
The Juvenile Diabetes Research Foundation International (JDRF) is a charitable funder and advocate of type 1 (juvenile) diabetes research worldwide. The mission of JDRF is to find a cure for diabetes and its complications through the support of research.
Kendra Presley, Special Events Manager
Gwen Bell, Office Manager

3176 Juvenile Diabetes Research Foundation: Flo rida Sun Coast Chapter
3333 Clark Road   941-929-0621
Sarasota, FL 34231   Fax: 941-929-0602
                     e-mail: floridasuncoast@jdrf.org
                                www.jdrf.org/index.cfm
The Juvenile Diabetes Research Foundation International (JDRF) is a charitable funder and advocate of type 1 (juvenile) diabetes research worldwide. The mission of JDRF is to find a cure for diabetes and its complications through the support of research.
Sara Rankin, Executive Director
Jeannie Kawcak, Special Events Coordinator

3177 Juvenile Diabetes Research Foundation: Gre ater Palm Beach County Chapter
1450 Centrepark Boulevard   561-686-7701
West Palm Beach, FL 33401   Fax: 561-686-7702
                  e-mail: greaterpalmbeach@jdrf.org
                         www.jdrf.org/greaterpalmbeach
The Juvenile Diabetes Research Foundation International (JDRF) is a charitable funder and advocate of type 1 (juvenile) diabetes research worldwide. The mission of JDRF is to find a cure for diabetes and its complications through the support of research.
Lora Hazelwood, Executive Director
Esther Swann, Special Events Coordinator

3178 Juvenile Diabetes Research Foundation: Nor th Florida Chapter
8400 Baymeadows Way   904-739-2101
Jacksonville, FL 32256   Fax: 904-739-2693
                       e-mail: northflorida@jdrf.org
                             www.jdrf.org/northflorida
The Juvenile Diabetes Research Foundation International (JDRF) is a charitable funder and advocate of type 1 (juvenile) diabetes research worldwide. The mission of JDRF is to find a cure for diabetes and its complications through the support of research.
Brooks Biagini, Executive Director
Wendy Smit, Special Events Assistant

3179 Juvenile Diabetes Research Foundation: Sou th Florida Chapter
3411 NW 9th Avenue   954-565-4775
Fort Lauderdale, FL 33309   Fax: 954-565-4767
                       e-mail: southflorida@jdrf.org
                 www.jdrf.org/chapters/FL/South-Florida
The Juvenile Diabetes Research Foundation International (JDRF) is a charitable funder and advocate of type 1 (juvenile) diabetes research worldwide. The mission of JDRF is to find a cure for diabetes and its complications through the support of research.
Ingrid Velarde, Special Events Coordinator
Katelyn Tolzien, Special Events Coordinator

3180 Juvenile Diabetes Research Foundation: Tam pa Bay Chapter
5959 Central Avenue   727-344-2873
Saint Petersburg, FL 33710   Fax: 727-384-9009
                          e-mail: tampabay@jdrf.org
                                        www.jdf.org
The Juvenile Diabetes Research Foundation International (JDRF) is a charitable funder and advocate of type 1 (juvenile) diabetes research worldwide. The mission of JDRF is to find a cure for diabetes and its complications through the support of research.
Arnold Donald, President/CEO Corporate Office
Robin Harding, EVP Development & COO

Georgia

3181 American Diabetes Association: Atlanta Met ro
17 Executive Park 404-320-7100
Atlanta, GA 30329 888-342-2383
Fax: 404-320-0025
e-mail: AskADA@diabetes.org
www.diabetes.org
The American Diabetes Association is a nonprofit health organization providing diabetes research, information and advocacy. Founded in 1940 the American Diabetes Association conducts programs in all 50 states and the District of Columbia, reaching hundreds of communities
Michael Gault, Senior Executive Director
Richard Kahn, Chief Scientific/Medical Officer

3182 American Diabetes Association: Savannah
5105 Paulsen Street 912-353-8110
Savannah, GA 31405 888-343-2383
Fax: 912-353-9114
e-mail: AskADA@diabetes.org
www.diabetes.org
The American Diabetes Association is a nonprofit health organization providing diabetes research, information and advocacy. Founded in 1940 the American Diabetes Association conducts programs in all 50 states and the District of Columbia.
Maria Center, Director
Richard Kahn, Chief Scientific/Medical Officer

3183 Juvenile Diabetes Research Foundation: Geo rgia Chapter
400 Perimeter Center Terrace 404-420-5990
Atlanta, GA 30346 Fax: 404-420-5995
e-mail: georgia@jdrf.org
www.jdrfgeorgia.org/
The Juvenile Diabetes Research Foundation International (JDRF) is a charitable funder and advocate of type 1 (juvenile) diabetes research worldwide. The mission of JDRF is to find a cure for diabetes and its complications through the support of research.
Rob Shaw, Executive Director
Scott Whiteside, EVP/General Manager

Hawaii

3184 American Diabetes Association: Hawaii
1500 S Beretania Street 808-947-5979
Honolulu, HI 96826 888-342-2383
Fax: 808-947-5978
e-mail: AskADA@diabetes.org
www.diabetes.org
The American Diabetes Association is a nonprofit health organization providing diabetes research, information and advocacy. Founded in 1940 the American Diabetes Association conducts programs in all 50 states and the District of Columbia.
Majken Mechling, Executive Director
Richard Kahn, Chief Scientific/Medical Officer

3185 Juvenile Diabetes Research Foundation: Haw aii Chapter
1019 Waimanu Street 808-988-1000
Honolulu, HI 96814 Fax: 808-597-8758
e-mail: hawaii@jdrf.org
www.jdf.org
The Juvenile Diabetes Research Foundation International (JDRF) is a charitable funder and advocate of type 1 (juvenile) diabetes research worldwide. The mission of JDRF is to find a cure for diabetes and its complications through the support of research.
Arnold Donald, President/CEO Corporate
Robin Harding, EVP/Develpment & COO Corporate

Illinois

3186 American Diabetes Association: Greater Ill inois
2580 Federal Drive 217-875-9011
Decatur, IL 62526 888-342-2383
Fax: 217-875-6849
e-mail: AskADA@diabetes.org
www.diabetes.org
The American Diabetes Association is a nonprofit health organization providing diabetes research, information and advocacy. Founded in 1940 the American Diabetes Association conducts programs in all 50 states and the District of Columbia, reaching hundreds of communities.
Donna Scott, Executive Director
Richard Kahn, Chief Scientific/Medical Officer

3187 American Diabetes Association: Northern Il linois
30 North Michigan Avenue 312-346-1805
Chicago, IL 60602 888-343-2383
Fax: 312-346-5342
e-mail: AskADA@diabetes.org
www.diabetes.org
The American Diabetes Association is a nonprofit health organization providing diabetes research, information and advocacy. Founded in 1940, the American Diabetes Association conducts programs in all 50 states and the District of Columbia, reaching hundreds of communities.
Michael D Farley CFRE (Corporate), Chief Community Relations Officer
Richard Kahn, Chief Scientific/Medical Officer

3188 Juvenile Diabetes Research Foundation: Gre ater Chicago Chapter
500 North Dearborn Street 312-670-0313
Chicago, IL 60610 Fax: 312-670-0250
e-mail: illinois@jdrf.org
www.jdrfillinois.org
The Juvenile Diabetes Research Foundation International (JDRF) is a charitable funder and advocate of type 1 (juvenile) diabetes research worldwide. The mission of JDRF is to find a cure for diabetes and its complications through the support of research.
Amy Franze, Executive Director
Janine Tobola, Director Office Operations

Indiana

3189 American Diabetes Association: Northern In diana/Northern Ohio
6415 Castleway W Drive 317-352-9226
Indianapolis, IN 46250 888-342-2383
Fax: 317-594-0748
e-mail: AskADA@diabetes.org
www.diabetes.org
The American Diabetes Association is a nonprofit health organization providing diabetes research, information and advocacy. Founded in 1940 the American Diabetes Association conducts programs in all 50 states and the District of Columbia.
Jennifer Pferrer, Executive Director
Richard Kahn, Chief Scientific/Medical Officer

3190 Diabetes Youth Foundation of Indiana
7311 Tousley Drive 317-750-9310
Indianapolis, IN 46256-9212 Fax: 317-243-4418
e-mail: dyfjulie@yahoo.com
www.dyfofindiana.org
This nonprofit group whose mission is to improve the lives of children with diabetes and their families.
Julie Shutt, Executive Director
Rick Crosslin, Camp Director

3191 Juvenile Diabetes Research Foundation: Ind iana State Chapter
8465 Keystone Crossing 317-202-0352
Indianapolis, IN 46240 Fax: 317-202-0357
e-mail: indianastate@jdrf.org
www.jdrf.org/indiana
The Juvenile Diabetes Research Foundation International (JDRF) is a charitable funder and advocate of type 1 (juvenile) diabetes research worldwide. The mission of JDRF is to find a cure for diabetes and its complications through the support of research.
Henry Rodriguez MD, Chapter President

3192 Juvenile Diabetes Research Foundation: Nor thern Indiana Chapter
2004 Ironwood Circle 574-273-1810
South Bend, IN 46635 Fax: 574-273-1870
e-mail: northernindiana@jdrf.org
www.jdrf.org
The Juvenile Diabetes Research Foundation International (JDRF) is a charitable funder and advocate of type 1 (juvenile) diabetes re-

search worldwide. The mission of JDRF is to find a cure for diabetes and its complications through the support of research.
Arnold Donald, President/CEO Corporate
Robin Harding, EVP/Development & COO Corporate

Iowa

3193 American Diabetes Association: Cedar Rapid s District
St Luke's Resource Center 319-247-5124
Cedar Rapids, IA 52406 888-342-2383
Fax: 319-247-5125
e-mail: AskADA@diabetes.org
www.diabetes.org
The American Diabetes Association is a nonprofit health organization providing diabetes research, information and advocacy. Founded in 1940 the American Diabetes Association conducts programs in all 50 states and the District of Columbia.
Jennifer Petsche, Manager
Richard Kahn, Chief Scientific/Medical Officer

3194 Juvenile Diabetes Research Foundation: Eas tern Iowa Chapter
701 10th Street SE 319-393-3850
Cedar Rapids, IA 52403 Fax: 319-393-3852
e-mail: easterniowa@jdrf.org
www.jdrf.org/easterniowa
The Juvenile Diabetes Research Foundation International (JDRF) is a charitable funder and advocate of type 1 (juvenile) diabetes research worldwide. The mission of JDRF is to find a cure for diabetes and its complications through the support of research.
Ann Elise Walsh, Special Events Manager
Mary Henry, Special Events Coordinator

3195 Juvenile Diabetes Research Foundation: Gre ater Iowa Chapter
5444 NW 96th Street 515-986-1512
Johnston, IA 50131 Fax: 515-986-1513
e-mail: greateriowa@jdif.org
www.jdrf.org/greateriowa
The Juvenile Diabetes Research Foundation International (JDRF) is a charitable funder and advocate of type 1 (juvenile) diabetes research worldwide. The mission of JDRF is to find a cure for diabetes and its complications through the support of research.
Jean Howieson, Special Events Director
Judy Greaves, Office Administrator

Kansas

3196 American Diabetes Association: Kansas
837 S Hillside 316-684-6091
Wichita, KS 67211 888-342-2383
Fax: 316-684-5675
e-mail: AskADA@diabetes.org
www.diabetes.org
The American Diabetes Association is a nonprofit health organization providing diabetes research, information and advocacy. Founded in 1940 the American Diabetes Association conducts programs in all 50 states and the District of Columbia.
Sarah Beth Webb, Director
Richard Kahn, Chief Scientific/Medical Officer

Kentucky

3197 American Diabetes Association: Kentucky
161 St Matthews Avenue 502-452-6072
Louisville, KY 40207 888-342-2383
Fax: 502-893-2698
e-mail: AskADA@diabetes.org
www.diabetes.org
The American Diabetes Association is a nonprofit health organization providing diabetes research, information and advocacy. Founded in 1940 the American Diabetes Association conducts programs in all 50 states and the District of Columbia.
Samantha Carroll, Associate Director
Richard Kahn, Chief Scientific/Medical Officer

3198 Juvenile Diabetes Research Foundation: Kentuckiana Chapter
133 Evergreen Road 502-485-9397
Louisville, KY 40243 866-485-9397
Fax: 502-485-9591
e-mail: kentuckiana@jdrf.org
www.jdf.org/chapters/ky/kentuckiana

The Juvenile Diabetes Research Foundation International (JDRF) is a charitable funder and advocate of type 1 (juvenile) diabetes research worldwide. The mission of JDRF is to find a cure for diabetes and its complications through the support of research.
Twynette S Davidson, Executive Director
Joe Salvagne, Chapter President

Louisiana

3199 American Diabetes Association: Louisana
2644 S Sherwood Forest Boulevard 225-216-3980
Baton Rouge, LA 70816 888-342-2383
Fax: 225-295-7005
e-mail: AskADA@diabetes.org
www.diabetes.org

Paige Grogan, Associate Manager
Lori Koonce, Associate Manager

3200 Juvenile Diabetes Research Foundation: Bat on Rouge Chapter
9457 Brookline Avenue 225-932-9511
Baton Rouge, LA 70809 Fax: 225-932-9514
e-mail: batonrouge@jdrf.org
www.jdrf.org/batonrouge

Kristy Andries, President/Development Chair
Danielle Graham, Special Events Assistant

3201 Juvenile Diabetes Research Foundation: Lou isiana Chapter
2201 Veterans Memorial Bouelvard 504-828-2873
Metairie, LA 70002 Fax: 504-828-4922
e-mail: louisiana@jdrf.org
www.jdrf.org/louisiana

Sam Robinson, President Board of Directors
Becky Spinnato, Vice President Fundraising

3202 Juvenile Diabetes Research Foundation: Shr eveport Chapter
2001 East 70th Street 318-798-1195
Shreveport, LA 71105 Fax: 318-798-1194
e-mail: jburns@jdrf.org
www.jdrf.org/shreveport

Jeff Knutson, President Board of Directors
Craig Floyd, Vice President Fundraising

Maine

3203 American Diabetes Association: Maine
80 Elm Street 207-774-7717
Portland, ME 04101 888-342-2383
Fax: 207-774-7714
e-mail: AskADA@diabetes.org
www.diabetes.org

Emily Silevinac, Associate Manager
Ryan Williams, Associate Manager

3204 Juvenile Diabetes Research Foundation: New England/Maine Chapter
33 Silver Street 207-761-0133
Portland, ME 04101 Fax: 207-761-1687
e-mail: maine@jdrf.org OR eburgo@jdrf.org
www.jdrf.org/maine
Heidi Daniels, New England Chapter Executive Director
Emily Hampton Burgo, Branch Manager

Maryland

3205 American Diabetes Association: Maryland
800 Wyman Park Drive 410-265-0075
Baltimore, MD 21211 888-342-2383
Fax: 410-235-4048
e-mail: AskADA@diabetes.org
www.diabetes.org

Kathy Rogers, Executive Director
Dotty Raynor, Director

3206 Juvenile Diabetes Research Foundation: Mar yland Chapter
200 East Joppa Road 410-823-0073
Towson, MD 21286 Fax: 410-823-0416
e-mail: maryland@jdrf.com
www.jdrf.org/maryland/
Rebecca Maude, Executive Director
Dotty Raynor, Outreach Manager

Massachusetts

3207 American Diabetes Association: Boston
330 Congress Street
Boston, MA 02210

617-482-4580
888-342-2383
Fax: 617-482-1824
e-mail: AskADA@diabetes.org
www.diabetes.org

Christopher Boynton, Executive Director
Lori Glowacki, Director of Special Events

3208 Juvenile Diabetes Research Foundation: New England/Bay State Chapter
20 Walnut Street
Wellesley, MA 02481

781-431-0700
Fax: 781-431-8836
e-mail: baystate@jdrf.org
www.jdrf.org/baystate

Heidi Daniels, New England Chapter Executive Director
Virginia Irving, Associate Executive Director

Michigan

3209 American Diabetes Association: Michigan
3940 Broadmoor Avenue SE
Grand Rapids, MI 49512

616-458-9341
888-342-2383
Fax: 616-575-9930
e-mail: AskADA@diabetes.org
www.diabetes.org

Darla Hill, Coordinator
Sharice Purman, Director

3210 Juvenile Diabetes Research Foundation: Metropolitan Detroit/SE Michigan
24359 Northwestern Highway
Southfield, MI 48075-2020

248-355-1133
Fax: 248-355-1188
e-mail: metrodetroit@jdrf.org
www.jdrfdetroit.org

Rita L Combest, Development Director
Susan Kossik, Development Manager

3211 Juvenile Diabetes Research Foundation: Wes t Michigan Chapter
5075 Cascade Road SE
Grand Rapids, MI 49546

616-957-1838
Fax: 616-957-1169
e-mail: westmichigan@jrdf.org
www.jdrf.org/westmichigan

Annette Guilfoyle, Executive Director
Maxine Gray, Special Events Coordinator

Minnesota

3212 American Diabetes Association: Minnesota
Parkdale Center
Saint Louis Park, MN 55416

763-593-5333
888-342-2383
Fax: 952-582-9000
e-mail: AskADA@diabetes.org
www.diabetes.org

Jenni Hargraves, Executive Director
Becky Barnett, Associate Manager

3213 Juvenile Diabetes Research Foundation: Min nesota Chapter
2626 East 82nd Street
Bloomington, MN 55425

952-851-0770
800-663-1860
Fax: 952-851-0766
e-mail: minnesota@jdrf.org
www.jdrf.org/minnesota

Jackie Casey, Executive Director
Angie McCarthy, Special Events Manager

Mississippi

3214 American Diabetes Association: Mississippi
16 Northtown Drive
Jackson, MS 39211

601-932-1118
888-342-2383
Fax: 601-932-1988
e-mail: AskADA@diabetes.org
www.diabetes.org

The nation's leading voluntary health organization providing diabetes research, information and advocacy. Our mission is to pre-vent and cure diabetes and to improve the lives of all people affected by diabetes.
Mary D Fortune, Executive Vice President
Stephanie J Coghlan MBA, Senior Regional Director

Missouri

3215 American Diabetes Association: Missouri
1944-A Sunshine
Springfield, MO 65804

417-890-8400
888-342-2383
Fax: 417-890-8484
e-mail: AskADA@diabetes.org
www.diabetes.org

Renee Paulsell, Executive Director
Jennifer Cotner-Jone, Associate Director

3216 Juvenile Diabetes Research Foundation: St. Louis Chapter
225 S Meramec Avenue
Clayton, MO 63105

314-726-6778
Fax: 314-726-6778
e-mail: metrostlouis@jdrf.org
www.jdrfstl.org

M Marie Davis, Executive Director
William Schmitt, Corporate Development

Montana

3217 American Diabetes Association: Montana
3203 3rd Avenue N
Billings, MT 59101

406-256-0616
888-342-2383
Fax: 406-896-0289
e-mail: AskADA@diabetes.org
www.diabetes.org

Karen Talmadge, Chair
Laurelean Gaines, President

Nebraska

3218 American Diabetes Association: Nebraska
14216 Dayton Circle
Omaha, NE 68137

402-571-1101
888-342-2383
Fax: 402-572-8141
e-mail: AskADA@diabetes.org
www.diabetes.org

Shawn Murphy, Executive Director
Kortney Krill, Associate Manager

3219 Juvenile Diabetes Research Foundation: Lin coln Chapter
1540 S 70th Street
Lincoln, NE 68506

402-484-8300
Fax: 402-484-8302
e-mail: lincoln@jdrf.org
www.jdrf.org/lincoln

Deb Gokie, Executive Director
Maggie Pavelka, Special Events Assistant

3220 Juvenile Diabetes Research Foundation: Oma ha Council Bluffs Chapter
9202 W Dodge Road
Omaha, NE 68114

402-397-2873
Fax: 402-572-3343
e-mail: omaha@jdrf.org
www.jdrf.org/omaha

Shawn Reynolds, Executive Director
Melissa Shapiro, Special Events Coordinator

Nevada

3221 American Diabetes Association: Nevada
2785 E Desert Inn Road
Las Vegas, NV 89121

702-369-9995
888-342-2383
Fax: 702-369-3717
e-mail: AskADA@diabetes.org
www.diabetes.org

Mary Stokes, Manager
Carly Rohrer, Associate Manager

3222 Juvenile Diabetes Research Foundation: Nevada Chapter
5542 S Fort Apache Road   702-732-4795
Las Vegas, NV 89148   Fax: 702-732-1635
                                          e-mail: nevada@jdf.org
                                          www.jdrf.org/nevada

Stuart Mason, Nevada Chapter Co-Founder
Flora Mason, Nevada Chapter Co-Founder

3223 Juvenile Diabetes Research Foundation: Nor thern Nevada Branch
5335 Kietzke Lane   775-786-1881
Reno, NV 89511   Fax: 775-827-0131
                                          e-mail: northernnevada@jdrf.org
                                          www.jdrf.org/northernnevada

Molly Dillon, Branch Manager
Arnie Pitts, Board of Directors President

New Hampshire

3224 American Diabetes Association: New Hampshire
249 Canal Street   603-627-9579
Manchester, NH 03101   888-342-2383
                                          Fax: 603-669-1477
                                          www.diabetes.org

3225 Juvenile Diabetes Research Foundation: New England/New Hampshire Chapter
2 Wellman Avenue   603-595-2595
Nashua, NH 03064   Fax: 603-595-2073
                                          e-mail: newhampshire@jdrf.org
                                          www.jdrf.org/newhampshire

Brooke Edwards, Special Events Coordinator
Heidi Daniels, New England Chapter Executive Director

New Jersey

3226 American Diabetes Association: New Jersey
CentrePoint II Suite 103   732-469-7979
Bridgewater, NJ 08807   888-342-2383
                                          Fax: 732-469-4887
                                          e-mail: AskADA@diabetes.org
                                          www.diabetes.org

James Roberts, Executive Director
Pamela Hooper, Director

3227 Juvenile Diabetes Research Foundation: South Jersey Chapter
1415 Route 70 E   856-429-1101
Cherry Hill, NJ 08034   Fax: 856-429-1105
                                          e-mail: southjersey@jdrf.org
                                          www.jdrf.org/southjersey

Stephen Blocher, Executive Director
Robin Berger, Special Events Coordinator

3228 Juvenile Diabetes Research Foundation: Cen tral Jersey Chapter
740 Broad Street   732-219-6654
Shrewsbury, NJ 07702   Fax: 732-219-8722
                                          e-mail: centraljersey@jdrf.org
                                          www.jdrf.org/chapters/NJ/Central-Jersey

Lori McLane, Executive Director
Beckie Burlew, Special Events Coordinator

3229 Juvenile Diabetes Research Foundation: Mid -Jersey Chapter
28 Kennedy Boulevard   732-296-7171
East Brunswick, NJ 08816   Fax: 732-296-1433
                                          e-mail: midjersey@jdrf.org
                                          www.jdrf.org/NJ/Mid-Jersey

Elizabeth Giardina Preston, Chapter Executive Director
Sandra Hilsenrath, Special Events Coordinator

3230 Juvenile Diabetes Research Foundation: Roc kland County/Northern New Jersey
560 Sylvan Avenue   201-568-4838
Englewood Cliffs, NJ 07632   Fax: 201-568-5360
                                          e-mail: rockland@jdrf.org
                                          www.jdrf.org/northernnj

Douglas Rouse, Executive Director
Allison Hartstone, Special Events Coordinator

New Mexico

3231 American Diabetes Association: New Mexico
2625 Pennsylvania NE   505-266-5716
Albuquerque, NM 87110   888-342-2383
                                          Fax: 505-268-4533
                                          e-mail: AskADA@diabetes.org
                                          www.diabetes.org

Betsey Robinson, Associate Director
Lisa Johnson, Manager

3232 Juvenile Diabetes Research Foundation: Albuquerque
2501 San Pedro NE   505-255-4005
Albuquerque, NM 87110   Fax: 505-260-1430
                                          e-mail: newmexico@jdrf.org
                                          www.jdrf.org/newmexico

Joann Perrine, Branch Manager
Elizabeth Romero, Fundraising Assistant

New York

3233 American Diabetes Association: New York
Pine W Plaza Building 2   518-218-1755
Albany, NY 12205   888-342-2383
                                          Fax: 518-218-0114
                                          e-mail: AskADA@diabetes.org
                                          www.diabetes.org

Amy R Young, District Director
Karen Dooley, Associate Manager

3234 Juvenile Diabetes Research Foundation
Executive Office/Corporate Headquarters
120 Wall Street   212-725-4925
New York, NY 10005-4001   800-533-2873
                                          Fax: 212-785-9595
                                          e-mail: info@jdrf.org
                                          www.jdrf.org/

Allan J Lewis, President/Chief Executive Officer
Amy C Franze, EVP Development

3235 Juvenile Diabetes Research Foundation: Long Island/South Shore Chapter
532 Broadhollow Road   631-414-1126
Melville, NY 11747   Fax: 631-414-1133
                                          e-mail: longisland@jdrf.org
                                          www.jdrf.org/longisland

Barbara Rogus, Executive Director
Christina Colandro, Special Events Manager

3236 Juvenile Diabetes Research Foundation: Buf falo/Western New York Chapter
331 Alberta Drive   716-833-2873
Buffalo, NY 14226   Fax: 716-833-0199
                                          e-mail: westernny@jdrf.org
                                          www.jdrf.org/westernny

Karen Swierski, Executive Director
Jennifer Hickok, Special Events Manager

3237 Juvenile Diabetes Research Foundation: Hud son Valley Chapter
Hollowbrook Office Park   845-297-8600
Wappinger Falls, NY 12590   Fax: 845-297-7887
                                          e-mail: hudsonvalley@jdrf.org
                                          www.letscurediabetes.com

Charlie Lawrence, Branch Manager
Linda Delia, Events Assistant

3238 Juvenile Diabetes Research Foundation: New York Chapter
432 Park Avenue S   212-689-2860
New York, NY 10016   Fax: 212-689-4038
                                          e-mail: newyorkchapter@jdrf.org
                                          www.nyc.jdrf.org

Mania Boyder, New York City Chapter Executive Director

3239 Juvenile Diabetes Research Foundation: Nor theastern New York
6 Greenwood Drive   518-477-2873
East Greenbush, NY 12061   Fax: 518-477-7004
                                          e-mail: northeastny@jdrf.org
                                          www.jdrf.org/NortheasternNY

Bev Kennedy, Executive Director
Darlene Robbiano, Special Events Manager

3240 Juvenile Diabetes Research Foundation: Roc hester Branch/Western New York Chapter
1200-A Scottsville Road
Rochester, NY 14624   585-546-1390
                                  Fax: 585-546-1404
                       e-mail: rochester@jdrf.org
                             www.jdrf.org/rochester

Mary Anne Fox, Executive Director
Lisa Swindon, Senior Development Coordinator

3241 Juvenile Diabetes Research Foundation: Wes tchester County Chapter
30 Glenn Street   914-686-7700
White Plains, NY 10603   Fax: 914-686-7701
                       e-mail: westchester@jdrf.org
                             www.jdrf.org/westchester

Katherine Cintron, Executive Director
Dejan Popovich, Special Events Coordinator

North Carolina

3242 American Diabetes Association: North Carolina
222 South Church Street   704-373-9111
Charlotte, NC 28202   888-342-2383
                                  Fax: 704-373-9113
                                     www.diabetes.org

Dianne Roth, Executive Director

3243 Juvenile Diabetes Research Foundation: Triangle/Eastern North Carolina Chapter
2210 Millbrook Road   919-431-8330
Raleigh, NC 27604   Fax: 919-431-8373
                          e-mail: triangle@jdrf.org
                               www.jdrftriangle.org

Jim Burson, Chapter President
Courtney Davies, Executive Director

3244 Juvenile Diabetes Research Foundation: Cha rlotte Chapter
205 Regency Executive Park Drive   704-561-0828
Charlotte, NC 28217   Fax: 704-561-9920
                         e-mail: charlotte@jdrf.org
                                  www.gwc.jdrf.org

Brenning Johnston, Volunteer Coordinator

3245 Juvenile Diabetes Research Foundation: Pie dmont Triad Chapter
1401-B Old Mill Circle   336-768-1027
Winston-Salem, NC 27103   Fax: 336-768-1029
                          e-mail: piedmont@jdrf.org
                                  www.jdrf.org/triad

Brad Calloway, President Board of Directors
Tom Brinkley, VP Fundraising & Development

North Dakota

3246 American Diabetes Association: Nashville
1323 23rd Street S   701-234-0123
Fargo, ND 58103   Fax: 701-235-3080
                       e-mail: AskADA@diabetes.org
                                     www.diabetes.org

Stephanie Chimeziri, Associate Director

3247 American Diabetes Association: North Dakota
1323 23rd Street South   701-234-0123
Fargo, ND 58103   888-342-2383
                                  Fax: 701-235-3080
                                     www.diabetes.org

Ohio

3248 American Diabetes Association: Ohio
4500 Rockside Road   216-328-9989
Independence, OH 44131   888-342-2383
                                  Fax: 216-328-0007
                       e-mail: AskADA@diabetes.org
                                     www.diabetes.org

Jill Pupa, Executive Director
Patti Clair, Associate Director

3249 Juvenile Diabetes Research Foundation/JDRF
1293-H Lyons Road   937-439-2873
Dayton, OH 45458   Fax: 937-439-4086
                            e-mail: dayton@jdrf.org
                                www.jdrf.org/dayton

Karen Myers, Executive Director
Vicky Williams, Office Manager

3250 Juvenile Diabetes Research Foundation: Mid-Ohio Chapter
1550 Old Henderson Rd   614-464-2873
Columbus, OH 43220   Fax: 614-464-2877
                           e-mail: midohio@jdrf.org
                               www.jdrf.org/midohio

Staci Perkins, Executive Director
Roberta Smedes, Office Manager

3251 Juvenile Diabetes Research Foundation: Akr on/Canton Chapter
5000 Rockside Road
Canton, OH 44131   888-718-3061
                                  Fax: 216-328-8340
                          e-mail: jcallahan@jdrf.org
                  www.jdrf.org/chapters/OH/Northeast-Ohio

Laura E Maciag, Executive Director
Danielle Thompson, Special Events Manager

3252 Juvenile Diabetes Research Foundation: Gre ater Cincinnati Chapter
8041 Hosbrook Road   513-793-3223
Cincinnati, OH 45236-3830   Fax: 513-936-5333
                         e-mail: cincinnati@jdrf.org
                              www.jdrf.org/cincinnati

Bill Rice, Executive Director
Bethe Ferguson, Special Events Coordinator

3253 Juvenile Diabetes Research Foundation: Tol edo/Northwest Ohio Chapter
3450 W Central Avenue   419-873-1377
Toledo, OH 43606   800-533-2873
                                  Fax: 419-720-6339
                      e-mail: northwestohio@jdrf.org
                            www.jdrf.org/northwestohio

Megan Meyer, Executive Director
Marna Cousino, Special Events Coordinator

Oklahoma

3254 American Diabetes Association: Oklahoma
3000 United Founders Boulevard   405-840-3881
Oklahoma City, OK 73112   888-342-2383
                                  Fax: 405-840-3899
                       e-mail: AskADA@diabetes.org
                                     www.diabetes.org

Diane Sarantakos, Executive Director
Andrea Barnett, Associate Manager

3255 Juvenile Diabetes Research Foundation: Cen tral Oklahoma Chapter
2601 NW Expressway   405-810-0070
Oklahoma City, OK 73112   888-533-9255
                                  Fax: 405-810-0078
                          e-mail: oklahoma@jdrf.org
                               www.jdrf.org/centralok

Renee MacDonald, Executive Director
Shannon Scott, Special Events Coordinator

3256 Juvenile Diabetes Research Foundation: Tul sa Green County Chapter
4606 E 67th Street   918-481-5807
Tulsa, OK 74136   Fax: 918-481-5823
                             e-mail: tulsa@jdrf.org
                             www.jdrf.org/tulsa-green

Brandi Sullivan, Executive Director
Angela Peterson, Special Events Coordinator

Oregon

3257 American Diabetes Association: Oregon
2350 Oakmont Way 541-343-0735
Eugene, OR 97401 888-342-2383
Fax: 541-342-1491
e-mail: AskADA@diabetes.org
www.diabetes.org

Cynthia Benton, Associate Director

3258 Juvenile Diabetes Research Foundation: Ore gon/SW Washington Chapter
7460 SW Hunziker Street 503-643-1995
Portland, OR 97223 866-598-9074
Fax: 503-598-9087
e-mail: oregon-washington@jdrf.org
www.jdrf.org/oregon

Ashleigh Farleigh, Special Events Manager
Debbie Secor, Special Events Assistant

Pennsylvania

3259 American Diabetes Association: Pennsylvania
3544 Progress Avenue 717-657-4310
Harrisburg, PA 17110 888-342-2383
Fax: 717-657-4320
www.diabetes.org

3260 American Diabetes Association: Western Pennsylvania
300 Penn Center Boulevard 412-824-1181
Pittsburgh, PA 15235 888-342-2383
Fax: 412-824-2191
e-mail: AskADA@diabetes.org
www.diabetes.org

Terri Seidman, Area Manager
Steven Shivak, Executive Director

3261 Juvenile Diabetes Research Foundation: Central Pennsylvania Chapter
119 Aster Drive 717-901-6489
Harrisburg, PA 17112 Fax: 717-901-6573
e-mail: centralpa@jdrf.org
www.jdrf.org/centralpa

Susan Harral, Executive Director
Kate Severs, Special Events Assistant

3262 Juvenile Diabetes Research Foundation: Ber ks County Chapter
619 Wellington Avenue 610-775-4169
West Lawn, PA 19609
Tammy A. Edwards, Contact

3263 Juvenile Diabetes Research Foundation: Nor thwestern Pennsylvania Chapter
1700 Peach St 814-452-0635
Erie, PA 16501 Fax: 814-452-0645
e-mail: northwestpa@jdrf.org
www.jdrf.org/northwestpa

Douglas K White, Executive Director
Amy Bement, Special Events Assistant

3264 Juvenile Diabetes Research Foundation: Phi ladelphia Chapter
225 City Line Avenue 610-664-9255
Bala Cynwyd, PA 19004 Fax: 610-664-9585
e-mail: philadelphia@jdrf.org
www.jdrf.org/philadelphia

Ellen Rubesin, Executive Director
Kathy Farren, Special Events Director

3265 Juvenile Diabetes Research Foundation: Wes tern Pennsylvania
960 Penn Avenue 412-471-1414
Pittsburgh, PA 15222 888-528-8788
Fax: 412-471-1417
e-mail: westernpa@jdrf.org
www.jdrf.org/westernpa

David R Donahue, Executive Director
Kimberly A McElroy, Office Manager

Rhode Island

3266 American Diabetes Association: Rhode Island
146 Clifford St 401-351-0498
Providence, RI 02903 888-342-2383
Fax: 401-351-1674
www.jdf.org

South Carolina

3267 American Diabetes Association: South Carolina
2711 Middleburg Drive 803-799-4246
Columbia, SC 29204 888-342-2383
Fax: 803-799-5792
www.diabetes.org

3268 Juvenile Diabetes Research Foundation: Palmetto Chapter
810 Dutch Square Blvd 803-782-1477
Columbia, SC 29210 Fax: 803-782-8975
e-mail: palmetto@jdrf.org
www.jdrfpalmetto.org/about.aspx

Michael Slapnik, President
Dana Bruce, Executive Director

3269 Juvenile Diabetes Research Foundation: Low Country Chapter
520 Folly Road 843-345-0369
Charleston, SC 29412 Fax: 843-406-7957
e-mail: dmenefee@jdrf.org
www.jdrf.org/lowcountry
Pam Nestor McAdams, Events/Walk Director South Coastal Chptr

South Dakota

3270 Juvenile Diabetes Research Foundation: Sio ux Falls Chapter
PO Box 88540 605-338-2295
Sioux Falls, SD 57109-8540

Tennessee

3271 American Diabetes Association: Nashville
4205 Hillsboro Road 615-298-3066
Nashville, TN 37215 888-342-2383
Fax: 615-292-5357
e-mail: AskADA@diabetes.org
www.diabetes.org

Glenda Berry, Executive Director
Harlyn Hardin, Director of Programs

3272 American Diabetes Association: Tennessee
5583 Murray Road 901-682-8232
Memphis, TN 38119 888-342-2383
Fax: 901-682-8170
e-mail: AskADA@diabetes.org
www.diabetes.org

John Carroll, Director
Daniele Cain, Coordinator

3273 Juvenile Diabetes Research Foundation: East Tennessee Chapter
355 Trane Lane 865-544-0768
Knoxville, TN 37919 Fax: 865-544-4312
e-mail: EastTennessee@jdrf.org
www.easttennessee.jdrf.org

3274 Juvenile Diabetes Research Foundation: Mid dle Tennessee Chapter
105 Westpark Drive 615-383-6781
Nashville, TN 37027 Fax: 615-383-4284
e-mail: MidTennessee@jrdf.org
www.midtennessee.jdrf.org

Joe Bide, Vice President

Texas

3275 American Diabetes Association: Texas
4150 International Plaza 817-332-7110
Fort Worth, TX 76109 888-342-2383
Fax: 817-732-6244
www.diabetes.org

3276 Juvenile Diabetes Research Foundation: South Central Texas Chapter
8700 Crownhill Boulevrad
San Antonio, TX 78209
210-822-5336
Fax: 210-822-1443
e-mail: scentraltexas@jdrf.org
www.sctx-jdrf.org

Doug Koskie, President
Brigitte West, Secretaryÿ

3277 Juvenile Diabetes Research Foundation: Dal las Chapter
9400 North Central Expressway
Dallas, TX 75231-5063
214-373-9808
Fax: 214-373-6337
e-mail: dallas@jrdf.org
www.jdrfdallas.org

Dave Johnson, President
Michael Keith, Treasurer

3278 Juvenile Diabetes Research Foundation: Gre ater Fort Worth/ Arlington Chapter
3840 Hulen Street
Fort Worth, TX 76107-2127
817-332-2601
Fax: 817-332-5641
e-mail: grfortworth@jdrf.org
www.jdf.org

3279 Juvenile Diabetes Research Foundation: Hou ston/Gulf Coast Chapter
2425 Fountain View
Houston, TX 77057
713-334-4400
Fax: 713-334-4040
e-mail: houston@jdrf.org
www.jdf.org

3280 Juvenile Diabetes Research Foundation: Wes t Texas Chapter
Clay Desta Towers, 10 Desta Drive
Midland, TX 79705
432-570-5643
Fax: 432-682-0765
e-mail: westtexas@jdrf.org
www.jdf.org

Utah

3281 American Diabetes Association: Utah
1245 E Brickyard Road
Salt Lake City, UT 84106
801-363-3024
888-342-2383
Fax: 801-363-3031
www.diabetes.org

Vermont

3282 American Diabetes Association: Vermont
1 Kennedy Drive
S Burlington, VT 05403
802-654-7716
888-342-2383
Fax: 802-658-9145
www.diabetes.org

Virginia

3283 American Diabetes Association: Richmond
4335 Cox Road
Glen Allen, VA 23060
804-225-8038
888-342-2383
Fax: 804-270-4742
www.diabetes.org

3284 American Diabetes Association: Virginia
870 Greenbrier Circle
Chesapeake, VA 23320
757-424-6662
888-342-2383
Fax: 757-420-0490
www.diabetes.org

3285 Juvenile Diabetes Research Foundation: Gre ater Blue Ridge Chapter
3959 Electric Road
Roanoke, VA 24018
540-772-1975
888-849-0510
Fax: 540-772-6672
e-mail: greaterblueridge@jdrf.org
www.jdrfgreaterblueridge.org

Mary Lou Bruce, Board President
Annette Kirby, Secretary

Washington

3286 American Diabetes Association: Seattle
Metropolitan Park E
Seattle, WA 98101
206-282-4616
888-342-2383
Fax: 206-903-8107
www.diabetes.org

Linda Henderson, Executive Director
Sarah Popelka, Director

3287 American Diabetes Association: Washington
1200 Sixth Avenue
Spokane, WA 99204
509-624-7478
888-342-2383
Fax: 509-624-7212
www.diabetes.org

3288 Juvenile Diabetes Research Foundation: Seattle Guild
1215 Fourth Avenue
Seattle, WA 98161-1101
206-343-0873
Fax: 206-343-7015
e-mail: terickson@jdrf.org
www.jdrfnorthwest.org

Nadie Heichel, Executive Director
Becky Baumgardner, Office Manager

3289 Juvenile Diabetes Research Foundation: Sea ttle Chapter
1333 N Northlake Way
Seattle, WA 98103-8900
206-545-1510
Fax: 206-545-1511
www.jdf.org

3290 Juvenile Diabetes Research Foundation: Spo kane County Area Chapter
9 South Washington
Spokane, WA 99201
509-459-6307
Fax: 509-459-6392
e-mail: inlandnw@jdrf.org
http://www.jdrf.org/index.cfm

Kay C Dightman, Contact

West Virginia

3291 American Diabetes Association: West Virginia
PO Box 238
Hurricane, WV 25526
304-768-2596
888-342-2383
Fax: 304-562-1887
e-mail: rahearn@diabetes.org
diabetes.org

Karen Talmadge, Chair
Lurelean Gaines, President

3292 Juvenile Diabetes Research Foundation: Hun tington Chapter
PO Box 2903
Huntington, WV 25728
304-525-4533

Wisconsin

3293 American Diabetes Association: Wisconsin
1701 North Beauregard Street Alexan
Monona, WI 53713
608-222-7785
888-342-2383
Fax: 608-222-7795
e-mail: bfolco@diabetes.org
www.diabetes.org

Barb Folco, Manager
Jay Kemp, Coordinator

3294 Juvenile Diabetes Research Foundation: Southeastern Chapter
3333 North Mayfair Road
Wauwatosa, WI 53222
414-453-4673
Fax: 414-453-4919
e-mail: southeastwi@jdrf.org
www.sewi.jdrf.org/

3295 Juvenile Diabetes Research Foundation: Gre ater Madison Chapter
434 S. Yellowstone Drive
Madison, WI 53719
608-833-2873
Fax: 608-833-9214
e-mail: westernwi@jdrf.org
www.jdrfwesternwisconsin.org/

Douglas Berry, President
Aaron Weinbe Swenson, Treasurer

3296 Juvenile Diabetes Research Foundation: Nor theast Wisconsin Chapter
1800 Appleton Road 920-997-0038
Menasha, WI 54952-0101 Fax: 920-997-0039
e-mail: northeastwi@jdrf.org
www.jdrf.org
Julie Kersten, Executive Director
Dana Paschen, Special Events Coordinator

Libraries & Resource Centers

3297 Diabetes Control Program
California Department of Health Services
PO Box 997413 916-552-9888
Sacramento, CA 95899-7413 Fax: 916-552-9988
http://www.caldiabetes.org/
Our mission is to prevent diabetes and its complications in California's diverse communities.
Susan Lopez-Payan, Interim Chief

3298 Division of Diabetes Translation
National Center for Chronic Disease Prevention
1600 Clifton Rd 800-232-4636
Atlantia, GA 30333-3717 Fax: 770-488-5966
TTY: 888-232-6348
e-mail: cdcinfo@cdc.gov
www.cdc.gov/diabetes
The Division of Diabetes Translation's (DDT) goal is to reduce the burden of diabetes in the United States. The division works to achieve this goal by combining support for public health-oriented diabetes prevention and control programs (DPCPs) and translating diabetes research findings into widespread clinical and public health practice.

3299 Health Science Library
Marshall University
1600 Medical Center Drive
Huntington, WV 25701 304-691-1700
www.musom.marshall.edu/library
The Health Sciences Library's primary mission is serving the informational needs of the students, faculty, and staff at Marshall University and the Cabell-Huntington Hospital. The Library also plays an important role in providing information services to hospitals and healthcare professionals in the Huntington and the Tri-State area.
Edward Dzierzak, Director

3300 Joslin Center at University of Maryland Medicine
22 S Greene Street
Baltimore, MD 21201 800-492-5538
TDD: 800735225800
e-mail: joslin@umms001.ab.umd.edu
www.umm.edu/joslindiabetes
The Joslin Center at University of Maryland Medicine meets the highest standards of care for people with diabetes. Its programs reflect a philosophy which have been the hallmark of Joslin's care — a comprehensive team approach to diabetes treatment with programs designed to help children and adults with diabetes take charge of their own health and well-being.
Thomas W Donner, MD, Director

3301 Naomi Berrie Diabetes Center at Columbia University Medical Center
Russ Berrie Medical Science Pavillion
1150 St. Nicholas Avenue 212-851-5494
New York, NY 10032 Fax: 212-851-5459
e-mail: diabetes@columbia.edu
nbdiabetes.org
The special focus of the Naomi Berrie Diabetes Center is on families — a concept that differentiates it from almost every other diabetes treatment facility in America. People with diabetes are strongly encouraged to involve their entire families in the treatment process.
Robin Goland, MD, Co-Director
Rudolph Liebel, Co-Director

3302 National Diabetes Information Clearinghous e
One Information Way
Bethesda, MD 20892-3560 800-860-8747
Fax: 703-738-4929
TTY: 866-8569-116
e-mail: ndic@info.niddk.nih.gov
diabetes.niddk.nih.gov
To serve as a diabetes informational, educational, and referral resource for health professionals and the public. NDIC is a service of the NIDDK.

3303 Schulze Diabetes Institute
University of Minnesota
420 Delaware Street SE 612-626-3016
Minneapolis, MN 55455 e-mail: diitinfo@umn.edu
www.med.umn.edu
Formerly the Diabetes Institute for Immunology and Transplantation
David Sutherland MD, PhD, Director
Bernard Hering, Director

3304 Tallahassee Memorial Diabetes Center
Tallahassee Memorial Health Care
1300 Miccosukee Road 850-431-5404
Tallahassee, FL 32308 800-662-4278
Fax: 850-431-6325
www.tmh.org/diabetes
TMH provides comprehensive, patient-centered services to both children and adults. The Diabetes Center uses a team approach that involves the patient, physicians, nurse educators, registered dietitians with access to a diabetes counselor and registered pharmacists and social worker.
Richard M Bergenstal, MD, Medical Director

Research Centers

3305 Barbara Davis Center for Childhood Diabetes
13001 E 17th Place 303-724-2323
Aurora, CO 80045-6511 Fax: 303-724-6839
e-mail: george.eisenbarth@uchsc.edu
www.uchsc.edu/misc/diabetes
Research and educational organization.
Marian Rewers, Clinical Director
George S Eisenbarth, Executive Director

3306 Baylor College of Medicine: Children's General Clinical Research Center
One Baylor Plaza 713-798-4780
Houston, TX 77030 Fax: 713-790-1345
e-mail: pedi-webmaster@bcm.edu
www.bcm.edu/pediatrics
Offers research into juvenile aspects of immunology and infectious diseases including diabetes research activities.
Lisa Bomgaars, Medical Director
Mark A Ward, Director

3307 Benaroya Research Institute Virginia Mason Medical Center
Virginia Mason Medical Center
1201 9th Avenue 206-583-6525
Seattle, WA 98101-2795 Fax: 206-223-7543
e-mail: info@benaroyaresearch.org
www.benaroyaresearch.org
Immunology and diabetes research.
Robert B Lemon, Chair
Gerald Nepom, Director

3308 Diabetes Education and Research Center The Franklin House
The Franklin House
PO Box 897 215-829-3426
Philadelphia, PA 19105 Fax: 215-829-5807
e-mail: webmaster@dibeteseducationandresearchcen
www.diabeteseducationandresearchcenter.o
Is a non-profit organization serving the needs of people living in Philadelphia PA and surrounding communities. The goal of the Foundation is to improve the health of people with diabetes.

3309 Diabetes Research and Training Center: University of Alabama at Birmingham
Department of Medicine

1530 3rd Avenue S
Birmingham, AL 35294-1150
205-934-4011
Fax: 205-934-4389
TTY: 205-934-4642
www.main.uab.edu

The DRTC works to develop and evaluate new models of diabetes care and to facilitate translational diabetes research.
Dr Carol Garrison, President
William Ferniany, CEO

3310 Division on Endocrinology Northwestern University Feinberg School
Northwestern University Feinberg School of Medicin
251 East Huron Street
Chicago, IL 60611
312-926-6895
Fax: 312-503-7757
e-mail: help@medicine.northwestern.edu
www.medicine.northwestern.edu

Nonprofit organization focusing research activities on endocrinology metabolism nutrition and specializing in diabetes.
Joe Bass, MD, PhD, Chief of the Division of Endocrinology
Grazia Aleppo, MD, Director, Endocrinology Clinical Practic

3311 Endocrinology Research Laboratory Cabrini Medical Center
Cabrini Medical Center
227 E 19th Street
New York, NY 10003-7457
212-222-7464
e-mail: info@cabrininty.org
www.cabrininy.org

Focuses on the effects of insulin and insulin-like growth factors on human body functions.
Dr Leonid Poretsky, Director

3312 Indiana University: Area Health Education Center
714 N Senate Avenue
Indianapolis, IN 46202
317-278-8893
Fax: 317-278-0392
e-mail: ahec@iupui.edu
www.ahec.iupui.edu

A collaborative statewide system for community-based primary health care professions education that fosters the continuing improvement of health care services for all citizens in Indiana.
Richard D Kiovsky, MD, Director
Jonathan C Barclay, Associate Director

3313 Indiana University: Center for Diabetes Research
340 West 10th Street
Indianapolis, IN 46202-3082
317-274-8157
Fax: 317-274-1437
e-mail: rconsidi@iupui.edu
www.medicine.iu.edu

Our goal is to promote the training of scientists whose research will develop new understandings of the basis of the disease and its complications and to cultivate basic science research that can speed the discovery of more effective therapies.
Robert Considine, Associate Professor of Medicine
D Craig Brater MD, Dean

3314 Indiana University: Pharmacology Research Laboratory
Division of Clinical Pharmacology
1001 W 10th Street
Indianapolis, IN 46202
317-630-8795
Fax: 317-630-8185
e-mail: tamllewi@iupui.edu
www.medicine.iupui.edu/clinpharm

We will train highly skilled compassionate and altruistic professionals both generalists and specialists to be future leaders in medical practice academia and industry.
David A Flockhart, Division Director
John T Callaghan, Associate Professor of Medicine

3315 International Diabetes Center at Nicollet
3800 Park Nicollet Boulevard
Saint Louis Park, MN 55416-2533
952-993-3393
888-825-6315
Fax: 952-993-1302
e-mail: idcdiabetes@parknicollet.com
www.parknicollet.com/diabetes

Research center which improves the quality of life of individuals with diabetes and those at risk of developing diabetes by undertaking clinical care education research and outreach activities that stimulate and support health.
Richard Berg MD, Executive Director

3316 Joslin Diabetes Center
One Joslin Place
Boston, MA 02215-5306
617-732-2400
800-567-5461
Fax: 617-322-40
e-mail: diabetes@joslin.harvard.edu
www.joslin.org

An internationally recognized leader in diabetes and endocrine disease treatment research and patient and professional education affiliated with Harvard Medical School. In addition to its headquarters in Boston's Longwood Medical area Joslin has affiliated treatment centers across the nation. Established in 1898.
John L Brooks, Chairman of the Board
Martin J Abrahamson, Senior VP, Medical Director

3317 Metabolic Research Institute
1515 N Flagler Drive
West Palm Beach, FL 33401
561-802-3060
Fax: 561-802-3260
e-mail: moreinformation@metabolic-institute.com
www.metabolic-institute.com

The Metabolic Research Institute specializes in clinical studies involving endocrinology disorders complications of endocrinology disorders metabolic problems and selected renal disease.
William A Kaye, Co-Director
Barry Horowitz, Co-Director

3318 Sansum Diabetes Research Institute
2219 Bath Street
Santa Barbara, CA 93105-4321
805-682-7638
Fax: 805-682-3332
e-mail: info@sansum.org
www.sansum.org

A research institute devoted to the prevention treatment and cure of diabetes.
Lois Jovanovich, CEO & Chief Scientific Officer
Wendy Bevier, Associate Investigator

3319 University of Chicago: Comprehensive Diabetes Center
5841 S Maryland Avenue
Chicago, IL 60637
773-702-2371
800-989-6740
e-mail: diabetes@uchospitals.edu
www.kovlerdiabetescenter.org

The University of Chicago Kovler Diabetes Center offers a unique fully comprehensive approach to diagnosing and treating diabetes. Focuses on children adolescents and adults with diabetes as well as individuals at the highest risk for serious complications.
Louis H Philipson, Medical Director
Christopher Rhodes, Kovler Diabetes Center Pediatric Program

3320 University of Colorado: General Clinical Research Center, Pediatric
13001 E 17th Place
Aurora, CO 80045
720-777-2957
Fax: 72 -77 -727
e-mail: CTRCAdmin@tchden.org
www.uchsc.edu/pedsgcrc

Focuses on developmental studies and diabetes research.
Ronald J Sokol, Program Director
Philip S Zeitler, Associate Program Director

3321 University of Iowa: Diabetes Research Center
Department of Internal Medicine
200 Hawkins Drive
Iowa City, IA 52242
319-353-7842
www.int-med.uiowa.edu

The Diabetes Research Center combines the talents of experienced clinical investigators molecular biologists and vascular physiologists in an integrated multidisciplinary approach toward the study and treatment of abnormalities of vascular reactivity which characterize diabetes mellitus.
Ken Kates, Chief Executive Officer
John Swenning, Associate Director

3322 University of Kansas Cray Diabtetes Center
3901 Rainbow Boulevard
Kansas City, KS 66160-7376
913-588-5000
Fax: 913-588-4023
TTY: 913-588-7963
e-mail: geaks@kumc.edu
www.kumc.edu

The KU Medical Center is a complex institution whose basic functions include research education patient care and community service involving multiple constituencies at state and national levels.
Barbara Atkinson, Executive Vice Chancellor

3323 **University of Massachusetts: Diabetes and Endocrinology Research Center**
55 Lake Avenue N
Worcester, MA 01655   508-856-8989
e-mail: evelyn.vignola@umassmed.edu
www.umassmed.edu
UMMS has exploded onto the national scene as a major center for research, and in the past four decades, UMMS researchers have made pivotal advances in HIV, cancer, diabetes, infectious disease and in understanding the molecular basis of disease.
Micheal F Collins MD, Senior VP
Michael P Czech, Professor and Chair

3324 **University of Miami: Diabetes Research Institute**
200 S Park Road
Hollywood, FL 33021   954-964-4040
800-321-3437
Fax: 954-964-7036
e-mail: info@drif.org
www.diabetesresearch.org
The Diabetes Research Institute (DRI) is an innovator in many fields of diabetes research but one of its primary strengths lies in islet cell transplantation, a cellular therapy that restores insulin production to normalize blood sugar control.
Thomas D Stern, Chairman
Camillo Ricordi, DRI Scientific Director

3325 **University of New Mexico General Clinical Research Center**
University of New Mexico Hospital
The University of New Mexico
Albuquerque, NM 87131-2240   505-277-0111
Fax: 505-272-0266
e-mail: mburge@salud.unm.edu
hsc.unm.edu/som/gcrc
Diabetes research.
Steve McKernan, CEO
Richard Larson, Vice President for Research

3326 **University of Pennsylvania Diabetes and Endocrinology Research Center**
700 Clinical Research Building (CRB   215-898-4365
Philadelphia, PA 19104   Fax: 215-898-5408
e-mail: gburgese@mail.med.upenn.edu
www.med.upenn.edu/idom/derc
The Penn Diabetes and Endocrinology Research Center (DERC) participates in the nationwide inter-disciplinary program established over two decades ago by the NIDDK to foster research and training in the areas of diabetes and related endocrine and metabolic disorders.
Mitchell A Lazar, Director
Morris J Birnbaum, Co Director

3327 **University of Pittsburgh: Department of Molecular Genetics and Biochemistry**
200 Lothrop Street
Pittsburgh, PA 15261   412-648-9570
Fax: 412-624-8997
e-mail: info@mmg.pitt.edu
www.mgb.pitt.edu
MMG students and fellows routinely publish their research in outstanding journals, present their science at international conferences and go on to achieve positions at prestigious laboratories and institutions.
J Richard Chaillet, Associate Professor
Bruce A McClane, Professor

3328 **University of Tennessee: General Clinical Research Center**
1265 Union Avenue
Memphis, TN 38104   901-516-2212
Fax: 901-516-7013
e-mail: bsalpert@utmem.edu
www.utmem.edu/crc
Congress directed the National Institutes of Health to establish clinical research centers throughout the United States to launch an all-out attack on human diseases.
Bruce S Alpert MD, Program Director
Teresa Carr, Research Nurses

3329 **University of Texas General Clinical Research Center**
7400 Merton Minter Boulevard
San Antonio, TX 78229   409-772-1950
Fax: 409-772-8097
e-mail: public.affairs@utmb.edu
www.utmb.edu/gcrc

Focuses on diabetes and infectious disease research.
Michael Lich MD, Program Director
Garland D Anderson, Principal Investigator

3330 **University of Washington Diabetes: Endocrinology Research Center**
DVA Puget Sound Health Care System
1660 S Columbian Way
Seattle, WA 98108   206-616-4860
Fax: 206-764-2693
e-mail: derc@u.washington.edu
www.depts.washington.edu/diabetes
The primary purpose of the DERC is to facilitate and enhance the diabetes-related research of approximately 100 Affiliate Investigators at the University of Washington
Jerry P Palmer MD, Director
David E Cummings, Deputy Director

3331 **Vanderbilt University Diabetes Center**
1211 Medical Center Drive
Nashville, TN 37232   615-322-5000
e-mail: dc.brown@vanderbilt.edu
www.mc.vanderbilt.edu/diabetes/vdc
The Vanderbilt Diabetes Center provides complete care for children and adults with diabetes under one roof
Joe C Davis, Chair in Biomedical Sciences
Alvin C Powers, Director Vanderbilt Diabetes Center

3332 **Veterans Affairs Medical Center: Research Service**
500 Foothill Drive
Salt Lake City, UT 84148   801-582-1565
Fax: 801-584-1289
www.va.gov
Diabetes and cancer research.
James Floyd, Director
Byron Bair, Director

3333 **Warren Grant Magnuson Clinical Center**
National Institute of Health
9000 Rockville Pike
Bethesda, MD 20892   301-496-4000
800-411-1222
Fax: 301-480-9793
TTY: 866-411-1010
e-mail: prpl@mail.cc.nih.gov
clinicalcenter.nih.gov
Established in 1953 as the research hospital of the National Institutes of Health. Designed so that patient care facilities are close to research laboratories so new findings of basic and clinical scientists can be quickly applied to the treatment of patients. Upon referral by physicians, patients are admitted to NIH clinical studies.
John Gallin, Director
David Henderson, Deputy Director for Clinical Care

3334 **Washington University: Diabetes Research and Training Center**
School of Medicine
660 S Euclid Avenue
Saint Louis, MO 63110   314-362-0558
Fax: 314-747-2692
e-mail: apermutt@wustl.edu
drtc.im.wustl.edu
DRTC investigators were involved in conducting 60 investigator-initiated diabetes-related clinical research protocols on the WU GCRC
Jean Schaffer MD, Professor of Medicine
Kristin E Mondy, Medicine/Infectious Diseases

Support Groups & Hotlines

3335 **American Diabetes Association National Center**
1701 N Beauregard Street
Alexandria, VA 22311   800-342-2383
Fax: 703-549-6995
e-mail: askada@diabetes.org
www.diabetes.org
To prevent and cure diabetes and to improve the lives of all people affected by diabetes.
John W Griffin Jr, Chair of the Board
Larry Hausner, CEO

3336 Diabetes Society
1165 Lincoln Avenue
San Jose, CA 95125
408-287-3785
Fax: 408-287-2701
e-mail: ckassouf@diabetessociety.org
www.diabetessociety.org
The Diabetes Society was organized in 1963 as the result of efforts by a group of mothers of children with diabetes. Today, the Diabetes Society offers its services to the estimated 140,000 people with diabetes in the Santa Clara Valley.
Greg Price, Board President
Carol Kassouf, CEO

3337 Juvenile Diabetes International Hotline
Juvenile Diabetes Research Foundation Int'l
26 Broadway
New York, NY 10004
800-533-2873
Fax: 212-785-9595
e-mail: info@jdrf.org
www.jdf.org
The leading charitable funder and advocate of type 1 (juvenile) diabetes research worldwide.
Robert Wood Johnson IV, Chairman
Jeffrey Brewer, President/CEO

3338 National Health Information Center
PO Box 1133
Washington, DC 20013
310-565-4167
800-336-4797
Fax: 301-984-4256
e-mail: info@nhic.org
www.health.gov/nhic
A health information referral service sponsored by the Office of Disease Prevention and Health Promotion. Puts health professionals and consumers who have health questions in touch with those organizations that are best able to provide answers.

Books

3339 101 Tips for Improving Your Blood Sugar
American Diabetes Association
1701 North Beauregard Str
Alexandria, VA 22311-3447
800-342-2383
Fax: 703-549-6995
www.diabetes.org
Tips for 101 common situations and questions to reduce the risk of complications from blood sugar at the wrong level.
122 pages

3340 Balance Your Act: A Book for Adults with Diabetes
Pritchett & Hull
3440 Oakcliff Road
Atlanta, GA 30340-3079
800-774-1124
1993 96 pages Paperback
ISBN: 0-939838-14-1

3341 Buyer's Guide
American Diabetes Association
1701 North Beauregard Str
Alexandria, VA 22311-3447
800-342-2383
Fax: 703-549-6995
www.diabetes.org
A catalog listing all manufacturers of insulin, syringes, pumps, test strips, monitors and more.

3342 Caring for the Diabetic Soul
American Diabetes Association
1701 North Beauregard Str
Alexandria, VA 22311-3447
800-342-2383
Fax: 703-549-6995
www.diabetes.org
Restoring emotional balance for yourself and your family.
213 pages

3343 Clinical Practice Recommendations
American Diabetes Association
1701 North Beauregard Str
Alexandria, VA 22311-3447
800-342-2383
Fax: 703-549-6995
www.diabetes.org

Features all current position and consensus statements of the American Diabetes Association.

3344 Complete Weight Loss Workbook
American Diabetes Association
1701 North Beauregard Str
Alexandria, VA 22311-3447
800-342-2383
Fax: 703-549-6995
www.diabetes.org
A unique, brisk, practical workbook that offers a series of fresh, memorable tests, checklists, worksheets, mini-cases, calculation exercises, mental reminders, and other practical aids to losing weight and staying fit for good.
252 pages

3345 Computer Planned Menus for Health Professionals
American Diabetes Association
1701 North Beauregard Str
Alexandria, VA 22311-3447
800-342-2383
Fax: 703-549-6995
www.diabetes.org
Input a patient's dietary prescription, food preferences, and budget, and the program produces individualized menus. Professional version includes license to distribute these customized menus.

3346 Control Diabetes the Easy Way
Random House Trade Books
400 Hahn Road
Westminster, MD 21157-4663
800-733-3000
Fax: 800-659-2436

ISBN: 0-679778-03-9

3347 Convenience Food Facts
American Diabetes Association
1701 North Beauregard Str
Alexandria, VA 22311-3447
800-342-2383
Fax: 703-549-6995
www.diabetes.org
Helps to serve appetizing convenience foods low in sodium, cholesterol, and fat.
459 pages Softcover

3348 Cooking a la Heart
American Diabetes Association
1701 North Beauregard Str
Alexandria, VA 22311-3447
800-342-2383
Fax: 703-549-6995
www.diabetes.org
Recipes that include a complete nutrient profile with diabetic exchanges.

3349 Diabetes & Pregnancy: What to Expect
American Diabetes Association
1701 North Beauregard Str
Alexandria, VA 22311-3447
800-342-2383
Fax: 703-549-6995
www.diabetes.org
Information concerning an unborn baby's development, tests to expect, labor and delivery, birth control, and more.

3350 Diabetes A to Z
American Diabetes Association
1701 North Beauregard Str
Alexandria, VA 22311-3447
800-342-2383
Fax: 703-549-6995
www.diabetes.org
Dictionary-style guidebook discussing basic terms and issues concerning diabetes. Third edition.
202 pages

3351 Diabetes Care Made Easy
Chronimed Publishing
PO Box 59032
Minneapolis, MN 55459-0032
612-513-6475
800-848-2793
Fax: 612-443-2806
Written and designed for both adults and for children with limited reading skills, this easy-to-read book explains how to exercise and

eat for better health, prevent foot problems, test blood sugar, cope with emotions, take insulin, and more. Also available in Spanish.
180 pages Paperback
ISBN: 1-885115-31-8

3352   Diabetes Education Goals
American Diabetes Association
1701 North Beauregard Str
Alexandria, VA 22311-3447   800-342-2383
                                      Fax: 703-549-6995
                                      www.diabetes.org
Features advice on how to assess, plan, and evaluate patient education and counseling programs. Covers both short-term and in-depth goals. Focuses on the education process and assessing the unique needs of each patient.
64 pages Softcover

3353   Diabetes Low-Fat & No-Fat Meals in Minutes
John Wiley and Sons, Inc.
Cust Ser-Consumer Accts
Indianapolis, IN 46256   877-762-2974
                                      Fax: 800-597-3299
                                      e-mail: consumers@wiley.com
                                      www.wiley.com
Includes more than 250 recipes, 60 days of diabetic menus, and 16 pages of full-color photographs. Each recipe features a complete nutrition analysis, including diabetic exchanges.
1998 352 pages
ISBN: 1-565610-84-9

3354   Diabetes Medical Nutrition Therapy
American Diabetes Association
1701 North Beauregard Str
Alexandria, VA 22311-3447   800-342-2383
                                      Fax: 703-549-6995
                                      www.diabetes.org
A professional guide to management and nutrition education resources. Provides in-depth coverage of nutrition assessment, goal setting, intervention, and outcome evaluation. Information is provided on specific resources and case studies are cited for practical examples.
Softcover

3355   Diabetes Mellitus: A Practical Handbook
Bull Publishing Company
PO Box 1377
Boulder, CO 80306   800-676-2855
                                      Fax: 303-545-6354
                                      www.bullpub.com
This helpful and user friendly practical guide addresses the everyday concerns of all diabetics.
2002 Paperback
ISBN: 0-923521-72-0

3356   Diabetes Self-Management
RA Rapaport Publishing
150 W 22nd Street   212-989-0200
New York, NY 10011-2421   800-234-0923
                                      Fax: 212-989-4786
                                      e-mail: editor@diabetes-self-mgmt.com
                                      www.diabetesselfmanagement.com
Publishes practical, how to information, focusing on the day-to-day and long term aspects of diabetes in a positive and upbeat style. Gives subscribers up-to-date news, facts and advice to help them maintain their wellness and make informed decisions regarding their health.
Ingird Strauch, Executive
Richard A. Rapaport, Publisher

3357   Diabetes Sourcebook
Dawn D Matthews, author
Omnigraphics
155 W. Congress   313-961-1340
Detroit, MI 48226-4105   313-961-1383
                                      Fax: 800-875-1340
                                      e-mail: contact@omnigraphics.com
                                      www.omnigraphics.com
This Sourcebook contains information for people seeking to understand the risk factors, complications, and management of the different types of diabetes. It includes information about testing,

diagnosis, medications, and other topics related to living with diabetes.
2003 622 pages
ISBN: 0-780806-29-8

3358   Diabetes Teaching Guide for People Who Use Insulin
Joslin Diabetes Center
1 Joslin Place   617-732-2400
Boston, MA 02215-5306   Fax: 617-732-2562
                                      e-mail: diabetes@joslin.harvard.edu
                                      www.joslin.org
Discusses the causes of diabetes, the role of diet and exercise, meal planning and complications. Also provide information on drawing blood, mixing and injecting insulin.

3359   Diabetes Youth Curriculum: A Toolbox for Educators
Chronimed Publishing
PO Box 59032   612-513-6475
Minneapolis, MN 55459-0032   800-848-2793
                                      Fax: 612-443-2806
Program consisting of two volumes: the Curriculum and the Resource and Activities Guide (listed separately). Divided into sections dealing with general development concepts and specific guidelines for ages 6 to 8, 9 to 11, and 12 to 16.
136 pages Paperback
ISBN: 0-937721-49-2

3360   Diabetes: A Guide to Living Well
American Diabetes Association
1701 North Beauregard Str
Alexandria, NY 22311   800-342-2383
                                      Fax: 703-549-6995
                                      e-mail: ADAorders@pbd.com
                                      www.diabetes.org
Offers a guide to helping the person with diabetes design a program of individualized self-care and gain the willingness to follow it. Also tells how to deal with diet, exercise, stress, emotions, negative beliefs, and self-image.
242 pages Paperback
ISBN: 1-580402-09-7

3361   Diabetes: Your Complete Exercise Guide
Human Kinetics Publishers
PO Box 5076   217-351-1549
Champaign, IL 61825-5076   800-747-4457
                                      Fax: 217-351-5076
Part of the Cooper Clinic and Research Institute Fitness Series providing exercise rehabilitation for persons with diabetes.
144 pages Paperback
ISBN: 0-873224-27-2

3362   Diabetes: Your Questions Answered
Paul Drury and Wendy Gatling, author
Elsevier
Book Cust Ser Dept
St. Louis, MO 63146   800-545-2522
                                      Fax: 800-535-9935
                                      e-mail: usbkinfo@elsevier.com
                                      www.elsevier.com
This new volume in the popular Your Questions Answered series uses a question-and-answer format to provide easy access to hands-on guidance on the management of diabetes. Its succinct, practical coverage explores the latest evidence-based practice guilines and their interpretation. Case vignettes illustrate the clinical relevance of the material.
2004 380 pages Softcover
ISBN: 0-443073-89-9

3363   Diabetic Gourmet
Diabetes Self-Management Books
PO Box 10676
Des Moines, IA 50336-0676   800-664-9269

3364   Diabetic's Guide to Health and Fitness
Human Kinetics Publishers
PO Box 5076   217-351-1549
Champaign, IL 61825-5076   800-747-4457
                                      Fax: 217-351-5076
272 pages Paperback
ISBN: 0-880113-47-2

3365 Direct and Indirect Costs of Diabetes in the US
American Diabetes Association
1701 North Beauregard Str
Alexandria, VA 22311-3447   800-342-2383
                                  Fax: 703-549-6995
                                  www.diabetes.org
Examines the specific costs of diabetes, as well as all the costs of
health care for people with diabetes and compares those costs with
the total cost of health care for the US population without diabetes.
32 pages Softcover

3366 Dr. Bernstein's Diabetes Solution
Richard K Bernstein, MD, author
Little, Brown and Company
Haworth Public School   201-384-5526
New York, NY 07641   800-759-0190
                                  Fax: 201-384-8619
                        e-mail: publicity@littlebrown.com
                        www.hachettebookgroupusa.com
A complete guide to achieving normal blood sugars with strong
emphasis on diet and up-to-date information on products, insulins,
and oral agents.
512 pages Hardcover
ISBN: 0-316099-06-6

3367 Easy & Elegant Entrees
American Diabetes Association
1701 North Beauregard Str
Alexandria, VA 22311-3447   800-342-2383
                                  Fax: 703-549-6995
                                  www.diabetes.org
Recipes that are low in fat and calories.

3368 Exchanges for All Occasions
American Diabetes Association
1701 North Beauregard Str
Alexandria, VA 22311-3447   800-342-2383
                                  Fax: 703-549-6995
                                  www.diabetes.org
Meal planning suggestions for traveling, entertaining, camping,
dining out, and more.

3369 Family Cookbook: Volumes I-IV
American Diabetes Association
1701 North Beauregard Str
Alexandria, VA 22311-3447   800-342-2383
                                  Fax: 703-549-6995
                                  www.diabetes.org
Unforgettable recipes for the whole family. Great for diabetics.

3370 Fitness Book: For People with Diabetes
American Diabetes Association
1701 North Beauregard Str
Alexandria, VA 22311-3447   800-342-2383
                                  Fax: 703-549-6995
                                  www.diabetes.org
Advice on learning to exercise to lose weight, exercise safely, increase your competitive edge, get your mind and body ready to exercise, and more.
149 pages

3371 Great Starts & Fine Finishes
American Diabetes Association
1701 North Beauregard Str
Alexandria, VA 22311-3447   800-342-2383
                                  Fax: 703-549-6995
                                  www.diabetes.org
Healthy select cookbook offering great meals in minutes.

3372 Healthy Eater's Guide to Family & Chain Restaurants
American Diabetes Association
1701 North Beauregard Str
Alexandria, VA 22311-3447   800-342-2383
                                  Fax: 703-549-6995
                                  www.diabetes.org
Advice on safe choices from fast-food menus, complete with nutri-
tion values and exchanges.

3373 Healthy Homestyle Cookbook
American Diabetes Association

1701 North Beauregard Str
Alexandria, VA 22311-3447   800-342-2383
                                  Fax: 703-549-6995
                                  www.diabetes.org
Lay-flat binding for hands-free reference.
181 pages

3374 How to Cook for People with Diabetes
American Diabetes Association
1701 North Beauregard Str
Alexandria, VA 22311-3447   800-342-2383
                                  Fax: 703-549-6995
                                  www.diabetes.org
One hundred and fifty recipes featuring unusual techniques.
205 pages

3375 If Your Child Has Diabetes: An Answer Book for Parents
Putnam Publishing Group
200 Madison Avenue   212-951-8400
New York, NY 10016-3903
Provides information and recommendations for parents of children
with diabetes on subjects such as school, recreation, medical and
life insurance and employment as well as general information
about diabetes.

3376 Intensified Insulin Management for You
Chronimed Publishing
PO Box 59032   612-513-6475
Minneapolis, MN 55459-0032   800-848-2793
                                  Fax: 612-443-2806
Manual helping those with diabetes to understand and use an intensified insulin regimen under the guidance of their health care provider. A personalized program for advanced diabetes self-care that
focuses on emotional and intellectual goals as well as on how diet
and exercise fit into an intensified regimen.
85 pages Paperback
ISBN: 0-937721-84-0

3377 Intensive Diabetes Management
American Diabetes Association
1701 North Beauregard Str
Alexandria, VA 22311-3447   800-342-2383
                                  Fax: 703-549-6995
                                  www.diabetes.org
Delivers practical advice on how to help your patients achieve
better glucose control through intensified management.
128 pages Softcover

3378 Learning to Live Well with Diabetes
Chronimed Publishing
PO Box 59032   612-513-6475
Minneapolis, MN 55459-0032   800-848-2793
                                  Fax: 612-443-2806
Updated and revised edition reflects the latest medical advances,
technologies, and research. In straight-forward language, it ex-
plains how to take charge of your diabetes and live an active,
healthy life.
525 pages Paperback
ISBN: 0-937721-79-4

3379 Life with Diabetes: A Series of Teaching Outlines
American Diabetes Association
1701 North Beauregard Str
Alexandria, VA 22311-3447   800-342-2383
                                  Fax: 703-549-6995
                                  www.diabetes.org
Presents a comprehensive curriculum for diabetes education. Each
outline includes a statement of purpose, prerequisites for attending
the session, materials needed for teaching the session, recommended teaching method, a content outline, instructor notes, an
evaluation and documentation plan, and suggested readings
related to each topic.

3380 Managing Type II Diabetes
Chronimed Publishing
PO Box 59032   612-513-6475
Minneapolis, MN 55459-0032   800-848-2793
                                  Fax: 612-443-2806
Revised and updated guide for people with Type II diabetes. Offers
the latest medical advances and practical advice. Includes tips on

dealing with emotions, finding motivation to manage diabetes, preventing and treating complications, monitoring blood glucose, and more.
192 pages Paperback
ISBN: 1-885115-26-1

3381 Managing Your Gestational Diabetes
Chronimed Publishing
PO Box 59032   612-513-6475
Minneapolis, MN 55459-0032   800-848-2793
                                                        Fax: 612-443-2806
Gives answers to questions on weight gain, injecting insulin, and preventing complications.
128 pages Paperback
ISBN: 1-565610-52-0

3382 Manual of Pediatric Nutrition
B.C Decker, Inc.
50 King Street E, Floor 2   905-522-7017
Ontario, Canada L8N 3K7,   800-568-7281
                                                        Fax: 905-522-7839
                                              e-mail: info@bcdecker.com
                                                        www.bcdecker.com
A comprehensive guide that provides an overview of nutritional care for both healthy and ill pediatric patients.
2005 500 pages
ISBN: 1-550093-08-8

3383 Maximizing the Role of Nutrition in Diabetes Management
American Diabetes Association
1701 North Beauregard Str
Alexandria, VA 22311-3447   800-342-2383
                                                        Fax: 703-549-6995
                                                        www.diabetes.org
Integrates medical, nutritional, and behavioral sciences and recognizes the importance of each in total diabetes care.
64 pages Softcover

3384 Medical Management of Pregnancy Complicated by Diabetes
American Diabetes Association
1701 North Beauregard Str
Alexandria, VA 22311-3447   800-342-2383
                                                        Fax: 703-549-6995
                                                        www.diabetes.org
Information on every aspect of pregnancy and diabetes, providing precise protocols for treatment. Techniques for managing blood glucose levels from the time of conception through every stage of pregnancy.
136 pages Softcover

3385 Medical Management of Type I Diabetes
American Diabetes Association
1701 North Beauregard Str
Alexandria, VA 22311-3447   800-342-2383
                                                        Fax: 703-549-6995
                                                        www.diabetes.org
Instruction on all issues impacting patients with Type 1 diabetes, including: blood glucose regulation, nutrition, exercise, blood pressure, blood lipid levels, and other key elements.
176 pages Softcover

3386 Medical Management of Type II Diabetes
American Diabetes Association
1701 North Beauregard Str
Alexandria, VA 22311-3447   800-342-2383
                                                        Fax: 703-549-6995
                                                        www.diabetes.org
Complete overview of Type II diabetes, including diagnosis and classification, pathogenesis, and prevention/treatment of complications.
112 pages Softcover

3387 Month of Meals Set of 5
American Diabetes Association
1701 North Beauregard Str
Alexandria, VA 22311-3447   800-342-2383
                                                        Fax: 703-549-6995
                                                        www.diabetes.org

Each planner offers twenty-eight day's worth of tasty selections including a holiday planner, ethnic meals, fast foods, meat and potatoes, and vegetarian dishes. Available individually.
5 planners

3388 Outsmarting Diabetes
Richard S Beaser, author
John Wiley and Sons, Inc.
Cust Ser-Consumer Accts
Indianapolis, IN 46256   877-762-2974
                                                        Fax: 800-597-3299
                                            e-mail: consumers@wiley.com
                                                        www.wiley.com
Shows how intensive control can dramatically reduce the effects of insulin-dependent diabetes and the risk of long-term complications.
256 pages Paperback
ISBN: 0-471346-94-4

3389 Pumping Insulin
John Walsh PA, CDE and Ruth Roberts, MA, author
Torrey Pines Publishing
The Diabetes Mall   619-497-0900
San Diego, CA 92103   800-988-4772
                                                        Fax: 619-497-0900
                                                        www.diabetesnet.com
Features information for achieving excellent blood sugar control, correcting pump problems quickly, and lowering risks for complications.
322 pages Paperback
John Walsh,PA,CDE, Author
Ruth Roberts MA, Author

3390 Quick and Easy Meals and Menus
Diabetes Self-Management Books
PO Box 11066
Des Moines, IA 50380-0001   800-664-9269

3391 Quick and Healthy Recipes & Ideas
American Diabetes Association
1701 North Beauregard Str
Alexandria, VA 22311-3447   800-342-2383
                                                        Fax: 703-549-6995
                                                        www.diabetes.org
More than 190 recipes with complete nutrition information for each.

3392 Quick and Hearty Main Dishes
American Diabetes Association
1701 North Beauregard Str
Alexandria, VA 22311-3447   800-342-2383
                                                        Fax: 703-549-6995
                                                        www.diabetes.org
Offers recipes for main courses.

3393 Raising a Child with Diabetes: A Guide for Parents
American Diabetes Association
1701 North Beauregard Str
Alexandria, VA 22311-3447   800-342-2383
                                                        Fax: 703-549-6995
                                                        www.diabetes.org
You'll learn how to help your child adjust to insulin to allow for favorite foods, have a busy schedule and still feel healthy and strong, negotiate the twists and turns of being different, and much more.

3394 Real Life Parenting of Kids with Diabetes
Virginia Nasmyth Loy, author
McGraw-Hill Companies
Returns Department
Dubuque, IA 52002   877-833-5524
                                                        Fax: 609-308-4484
                             e-mail: pbg.ecommerce_custserv@mcgraw-hill.com
                                                        www.mcgraw-hill.com
Virginia Loy had engineered successful management of her two sons' diabetes for 12 years at the time of publication. She is offering her organized, experienced, and practical advice to parents, for helping children to cope with and manage their diabetes from elementary school through college.
2001 188 pages Paperback
ISBN: 1-580400-83-3

3395 Resource and Activities Guide
Chronimed Publishing
PO Box 59032
Minneapolis, MN 55459-0032
612-513-6475
800-848-2793
Fax: 612-443-2806

For use with the Diabetes Youth Curriculum. Contains 300 educational activities that correspond with the text in the Curriculum and can easily be removed for photocopying.
260 pages Loose Leaf
ISBN: 0-937721-50-6

3396 Right from the Start
American Diabetes Association
1701 North Beauregard Str
Alexandria, VA 22311-3447
800-342-2383
Fax: 703-549-6995
www.diabetes.org

Addresses issues such as: learning to take charge, coping, changing one's eating habits, getting fit, self-testing, family issues, preventive care, finances, as well as resources to turn to for further information and support. Available for both Type 1 and Type 2.
Pkg. of 25

3397 Savory Soups and Salads
American Diabetes Association
1701 North Beauregard Str
Alexandria, VA 22311-3447
800-342-2383
Fax: 703-549-6995
www.diabetes.org

Offers exciting recipes for quick and healthy side dishes.

3398 Simple and Tasty Side Dishes
American Diabetes Association
1701 North Beauregard Str
Alexandria, VA 22311-3447
800-342-2383
Fax: 703-549-6995
www.diabetes.org

Healthy recipes for the diabetic.

3399 Special Celebrations and Parties Cookbook
American Diabetes Association
1701 North Beauregard Str
Alexandria, VA 22311-3447
800-342-2383
Fax: 703-549-6995
www.diabetes.org

Offers a list of more than 150 holiday recipes.

3400 Take-Charge Guide to Type I Diabetes
American Diabetes Association
1701 North Beauregard Str
Alexandria, VA 22311-3447
800-342-2383
Fax: 703-549-6995
www.diabetes.org

Offers answers to the most important questions regarding Type 1 diabetes.

3401 Therapy for Diabetes Mellitus and Related Disorders
American Diabetes Association
1701 North Beauregard Str
Alexandria, VA 22311-3447
800-342-2383
Fax: 703-549-6995
www.diabetes.org

Guides through the treatment of specific problems of persons with diabetes. Represents the views and experience of leading clinicians in a concise, practical approach to treatment.
384 pages

3402 Type 2 Diabetes: Your Healthy Living Guide
American Diabetes Association
1701 North Beauregard Str
Alexandria, VA 22311-3447
800-342-2383
Fax: 703-549-6995
www.diabetes.org

A thorough guide to staying healthy with Type 2. Includes everything from choosing a health care team and eating and exercising properly to self-monitoring, insulin, dealing with complications, and keep mentally fit.
180 pages

3403 Using Insulin
Torrey Pines Press

The Diabetes Mall
San Diego, CA 92103
619-497-0900
800-988-4772
Fax: 619-497-0900
www.diabetesnet.com

How to take charge of your blood sugars in diabetes. Information on feeling better, improving your health, and achieving peace of mind.
316 pages Paperback
John Walsh,PA,CDE, Author
Ruth Roberts MA, Author

3404 Voice of the Diabetic
200 East Wells Street
Columbia, MO 65201
573-875-8911
e-mail: epc@roudley.com
www.nfb.org

Personal stories and practical guidelines by blind diabetics and medical professionals, medical news, resource column and a recipe corner.

3405 Weight Management for Type II Diabetes
John Wiley and Sons, Inc.
Cust Ser-Consumer Accts
Indianapolis, IN 46256
877-762-2974
Fax: 800-597-3299
e-mail: consumers@wiley.com
www.wiley.com

An interactive, personalized guide that helps you manage your weight and your diabetes by making gradual lifestyle changes. Details how to set reasonable goals, keep pace with an exercise program, design your own meal plan, manage stress, and more.
1997 224 pages Paperback
ISBN: 0-471347-50-7

3406 When Diabetes Complicates Your Life
Chronimed Publishing
PO Box 59032
Minneapolis, MN 55459-0032
612-513-6475
800-848-2793
Fax: 612-443-2806

Directly addresses the subject of diabetic complications. This revised edition includes chapters on nerves and circulation, kidneys, and eyes. Enhancements to the new edition include a chapter on vitamins, herbs, and supplements, and reference to the latest research.
Feb 1998 208 pages Paperback
ISBN: 1-565611-27-6

Children's Books

3407 Diabetes
Franklin Watts Grolier
90 Old Sherman Turnpike
Danbury, CT 06816-0001
203-797-3500
800-621-1115
Fax: 203-797-3197
www.auth.grolier.com

Looks at the differences between juvenile and adult-onset diabetes, discusses the history of the disease, causes, complications and treatments.
128 pages Grades 7-12
ISBN: 0-531108-82-1

3408 Dinosaur Tamer
American Diabetes Association
1701 North Beauregard Str
Alexandria, VA 22311-3447
800-342-2383
Fax: 703-549-6995
www.diabetes.org

Twenty-five fictional stories that will entertain, enlighten, and ease your child's frustrations about having diabetes. Each tale evaporates the fear of insulin shots, blood tests, going to diabetes camp, and more.
Ages 8-12

3409 Even Little Kids Get Diabetes
Connie Pirner, author
Albert Whitman & Company

250 South Northwest Hgwy
Suite 320ÿ, IL 60068-2723

847-232-2800
800-255-7675
Fax: 847-581-0039
e-mail: mail@awhitmanco.com
www.albertwhitmanco.com

A preschooler tells how it was discovered when she was only two, that she has this common disease and describes her daily treatment and the precautions her family must observe.
24 pages Hardcover
ISBN: 0-807521-58-8
Alison Acheson, Author
Mike Allegra, Author

3410 Everyone Likes to Eat
John Wiley and Sons, Inc.
Customer Service-Consumer Accounts
Indianapolis, IN 46256

877-762-2974
Fax: 800-597-3299
e-mail: consumers@wiley.com
www.wiley.com

Revised and up-to-date second edition. How children can eat most of the foods they enjoy and still take care of their diabetes. Intended for elementary-school-age children, this guide is filled with activities, puzzles, and problem-solving exercises.
128 pages Paperback
ISBN: 0-471346-82-1

3411 Grilled Cheese
American Diabetes Association
1701 North Beauregard Str
Alexandria, VA 22311-3447

800-342-2383
Fax: 703-549-6995
www.diabetes.org

Story designed to ease children's fears and frustrations of having diabetes.

3412 Kiss the Candy Days Good-bye
Delacorte Press
1540 Broadway
New York, NY 10036-4039

212-354-6500

This book focuses on Jimmy who is surprised to learn he has diabetes after seeming so healthy and fit. The story contains information on symptoms and the dangers of untreated diabetes.
Grades 6-8

3413 Living with Diabetes
Franklin Watts Grolier
90 Old Sherman Turnpike
Danbury, CT 06816-0001

203-797-3500
800-621-1115
Fax: 203-797-3197
www.auth.grolier.com

Shows how persons with diabetes can control their illness and lead productive lives.
32 pages Grades 5-7
ISBN: 0-531108-44-9

3414 Shira: A Legacy of Courage
Doubleday
666 5th Avenue
New York, NY 10103-0001

212-354-6500

A biographical account of Shira Putter's fight with a rare form of diabetes. Using the victim's diary, this book is both powerful and poignant, as well as an educational resource for all people struggling with diabetes.
Grades 4-9

3415 Sun, the Rain and the Insulin
American Diabetes Association
1701 North Beauregard Str
Alexandria, VA 22311-3447

800-342-2383
Fax: 703-549-6995
www.diabetes.org

Author chronicles a week at a summer diabetes camp, using her expertise and experience to capture the journey and the fight to cope that all people go through when diabetes hits the family.

Magazines

3416 Countdown
Juvenile Diabetes Foundation International
432 Park Avenue S
New York, NY 10016-8013

212-889-7575
Fax: 212-725-7259

Offers the latest news and information in diabetes research and treatment to everyone from an international arena of diabetes investigators to parents of small children with diabetes, from physicians to school teachers, from pharmacists to corporate executives.
Sandy Dylak, Editor

3417 Diabetes
American Diabetes Association
1701 North Beauregard Str
Alexandria, VA 22311-3447

800-342-2383
Fax: 703-549-6995
www.diabetes.org

A peer-reviewed journal focusing on laboratory research.
Monthly

3418 Diabetes Care
American Diabetes Association
1701 North Beauregard Str
Alexandria, VA 22311-3447

800-342-2383
Fax: 703-549-6995
www.diabetes.org

A peer-reviewed journal emphasizing reviews, commentaries and original research on topics of interest to clinicians.
Monthly

3419 Diabetes Forecast
American Diabetes Association
1701 North Beauregard Str
Alexandria, VA 22311-3447

800-342-2383
Fax: 703-549-6995
www.diabetes.org

The monthly lifestyle magazine for people with diabetes, featuring complete, in-depth coverage of all aspects of living with diabetes.
Monthly

3420 Diabetes Spectrum: From Research to Practice
American Diabetes Association
1701 N Beauregard Street
Alexandria, VA 22311

800-342-2383
Fax: 703-549-6995
www.diabetes.org

A journal translating research into practice and focusing on diabetes education and counseling.
Quarterly

3421 Joslin Magazine
Joslin Diabetes Center
1 Joslin Place
Boston, MA 02215-5306

617-732-2400
Fax: 617-732-2562
e-mail: diabetes@joslin.harvard.edu
www.joslin.org

3422 Voice of the Diabetic
Ed Bryant, author
National Federation of the Blind
200 East Wells Street
Baltimore, MD 21230-4998

410-659-9314
Fax: 410-685-5653
e-mail: subscribe@diabetes.nfb.org
www.nfb.org

The leading publication in the diabetes field. Each issue addresses the problems and concerns of diabetes, with a special emphasis for those who have lost vision due to diabetes. Available in print and on cassette.
28 pages Quarterly
Eileen Ley, Director of Publishing
Elizabeth Lunt, Editor

Newsletters

3423 Clinical Diabetes
American Diabetes Association

1701 North Beauregard Str
Alexandria, VA 22311-3447   800-342-2383
                                   Fax: 703-549-6995
                                   www.diabetes.org
A bimonthly newsletter providing practical treatment information
for primary care physicians.
BiMonthly

3424 Diabetes Advisor
American Diabetes Association
1701 N Beauregard Street   703-549-1500
Alexandria, VA 22311   800-342-2383
                                  Fax: 703-549-6995
                                  e-mail: askada@diabetes.org
                                  www.diabetes.org
Offers informative articles and research in the area of diabetes for
professionals and patients. Offers facts and research on diagnosis,
symptoms, technology and the newest devices for persons with di-
abetes, as well as referral and hotline numbers.
Bi-Monthly
John G Graham IV, CEO

3425 Diabetes Dateline
National Diabetes Information Clearinghouse
1 Information Way   301-496-3583
Bethesda, MD 20205   800-860-8747
                                  Fax: 301-907-8906
                                  e-mail: ndic@info.niddck.nih.gov
                                  www.niddk.nih.gov
BiAnnually

3426 Diabetes Educator
American Association of Diabetes Educators
444 N Michigan Avenue   312-644-2233
Chicago, IL 60611-3959   Fax: 312-644-4411
                                  www.aadenet.org
Offers information to health professionals working with persons
with diabetes.
James J Balija, Executive Director

3427 Kid's Corner
American Diabetes Association
1701 North Beauregard Str
Alexandria, VA 22311-3447   800-342-2383
                                   Fax: 703-549-6995
                                   www.diabetes.org
A mini-magazine for kids that offers word searches, puzzles and
jokes - plus an encouraging story in each issue about kids with diabetes.
8 pages Quarterly

Pamphlets

3428 Dental Tips for Diabetics
National Diabetes Information Clearinghouse
1 Information Way   301-496-3583
Bethesda, MD 20892-0001   800-860-8747
                                  Fax: 301-907-8906
                                  e-mail: ndic@info.niddk.nih.gov
                                  www.niddk.nih.gov
Discusses the relationship between diabetes and periodontal disease. Describes the symptoms of periodontal problems and preventive measures.

3429 Diabetes Dateline
National Diabetes Information Clearinghouse
1 Information Way
Bethesda, MD 20892-0001   800-860-8747
                                  Fax: 301-634-0716
                                  TTY: 866-569-1162
                                  e-mail: ndic@info.niddk.nih.gov
                                  www.diabetes.niddk.nih.gov
This bulletin features news about current issues in diabetes research and control, special events, patient and professional meeting, and new publications available from NDIC and other
organizations.
Quarterly

3430 Diabetes and Brief Illness
Chronimed Publishing
PO Box 59032   612-513-6475
Minneapolis, MN 55459-0032   800-848-2793
                                  Fax: 612-443-2806
This booklet gives self-care instructions and eating suggestions to
prevent development of ketoacidosis during brief illness that dis-
rupts normal eating.
12 pages Pack of 10

3431 Diabetes and Exercise
Chronimed Publishing
PO Box 59032   612-513-6475
Minneapolis, MN 55459-0032   800-848-2793
                                  Fax: 612-443-2806
Exercise and weight loss tips and precautions for those with both
insulin and non-insulin-dependent diabetes.
36 pages Pack of 10

3432 Diabetes in Pregnancy
March of Dimes
1275 Mamaroneck Avenue   914-997-4488
White Plains, NY 10605   Fax: 212-254-3518
                                  e-mail: NY639@marchofdimes.com
                                  www.marchofdimes.com
Fact Sheets: one or two page review written for the general public.

3433 Diabetic Foot Care
American Diabetes Association
1701 North Beauregard Str
Alexandria, VA 22311-3447   800-342-2383
                                   Fax: 703-549-6995
                                   www.diabetes.org
Booklet discussing early detection and prompt treatment of diabetic foot problems.
12 pages

3434 Gestational Diabetes: What To Expect
American Diabetes Association
7 Washington Square   518-218-1755
Albany, NY 22311   800-342-2383
                                  Fax: 703-549-6995
                                  e-mail: ADAorders@pbd.com
                                  www.diabetes.org
A complete comprehensive guide for women with gestational diabetes. Explains the stages in your baby's development, the types of
prenatal testing you may recieve, and what to expect during labor,
delivery, and beyond.
100 pages
ISBN: 1-580402-33-X

3435 Healthy Eating
Chronimed Publishing
PO Box 59032   612-513-6475
Minneapolis, MN 55459-0032   800-848-2793
                                  Fax: 612-443-2806
Offers simple guidelines for choosing healthful foods, lowering
fat intake, and timing meals and snacks. Available in Spanish.
Pack of 10

3436 Healthy Food Choices
American Diabetes Association
1701 North Beauregard Str
Alexandria, VA 22311-3447   800-342-2383
                                   Fax: 703-549-6995
                                   www.diabetes.org
Pamphlet containing the basics of good nutrition.

3437 Hypoglycemia The Other Sugar Disease
Anita Flegg, author
Book Coach Press
3-390 MacKay Street   613-746-3334
Ontario, Canada K1M 2C4,   e-mail: info@bookcoachpress.com
                                  www4.bookcoachpress.com
This book is filled with dozens of real-life practical tips and will
give you the tools to feel better and take control of your life.

3438 Insulin-Dependent Diabetes
National Diabetes Information Clearinghouse

1 Information Way
Bethesda, MD 20892-0001 800-860-8747
Fax: 301-634-0716
TTY: 866-569-1162
e-mail: ndic@info.niddk.nih.gov
www.diabetes.niddk.nih.gov
Explains diabetes and how it develops and describes the differences between the two major forms of diabetes, insulin-dependent and noninsulin-dependent.

3439 Low Blood Sugar
Chronimed Publishing
PO Box 59032 612-513-6475
Minneapolis, MN 55459-0032 800-848-2793
Fax: 612-443-2806

Pack of 10

3440 Noninsulin-Dependent Diabetes
National Diabetes Information Clearinghouse
1 Information Way
Bethesda, MD 20892-0001 800-860-8747
Fax: 301-634-0716
TTY: 866-569-1162
e-mail: ndic@info.niddk.nih.gov
www.diabetes.niddk.nih.gov
Describes the symptoms and diagnosis of noninsulin-dependent diabetes; diabetes management, including diet, oral drugs, and insulin; glucose monitoring; and complications.
1992 35 pages

3441 Recognizing and Treating Low Blood Sugar (Hypoglycemia)
Chronimed Publishing
PO Box 59032 612-513-6475
Minneapolis, MN 55459-0032 800-848-2793
Fax: 612-443-2806
The causes, symptoms, and treatment of low blood sugar are clearly presented in this booklet, including guidelines for using glucagon.
12 pages Pack of 10

3442 Taking Care of Gestational Diabetes
International Diabetes Center at Park Nicollet
3800 Park Nicollet Blvd 952-993-3874
Minneapolis, MN 55416-2699 888-637-2675
Fax: 952-993-0501
e-mail: idccustsvc@parknicollet.com
www.idcpublishing.com
Available in Spanish. Empowering women to make healthy choices for a healthy pregnancy, a healthy baby, and a healthy lifestyle. This book covers food planning, testing, targets, medications and more.
242 pages

3443 Understanding Gestational Diabetes
National Diabetes Information Clearinghouse
1 Information Way
Bethesda, MD 20892-0001 800-860-8747
Fax: 301-634-0716
TTY: 866-569-1162
e-mail: ndic@info.niddk.nih.gov
www.diabetes.niddk.nih.gov
A guide for women who develop diabetes during pregnancy. It discusses symptoms and diagnosis of gestational diabetes, risk factors, tests during pregnancy and daily management including the use of insulin and blood gluclose monitoring.
44 pages

Audio & Video

3444 ADA Clinical Education Series on CD-Rom
American Diabetes Association
1701 North Beauregard Str
Alexandria, VA 22311-3447 800-342-2383
Fax: 703-549-6995
www.diabetes.org
Features complete texts of Medical Management of Type 1 Diabetes, Medical Management of Type 2 Diabetes, Therapy for Diabetes Mellitus and Related Disorders, 2nd Ed., and Medical Management of Pregnancy Complicated by Diabetes, 2nd Ed.
CD-Rom

3445 Black Experience
American Diabetes Association
1701 North Beauregard Str 203-639-0385
Alexandria, CT 22311-7137 800-342-2383
Fax: 703-549-6995
www.diabetes.org
Designed to increase awareness of diabetes in the black community.
L Butcher, District Director

3446 Diabetes & Exercise Video
American Diabetes Association
1701 North Beauregard Str
Alexandria, VA 22311-3447 800-342-2383
Fax: 703-549-6995
www.diabetes.org
A video offering information on how to maintain good health and exercise in controlling diabetes.

3447 Label Reading and Shopping
American Diabetes Association/Conn. Affiliate
1701 North Beauregard Str 203-639-0385
Alexandria, CT 22311-7137 800-342-2383
Fax: 703-549-6995
www.diabetes.org
Provides practical information on how to shop and what to look for on labels.
Videotape

3448 Living Well with Diabetes
American Diabetes Association/Conn. Affiliate
1701 North Beauregard Str 203-639-0385
Alexandria, CT 22311-7137 800-342-2383
Fax: 703-549-6995
www.diabetes.org
Presents two patient role models who are successfully following a treatment plan for noninsulin dependent diabetes.
Videotape

3449 On Top of My Game: Living with Diabetes
American Diabetes Association/Conn. Affiliate
1701 North Beauregard Str 203-639-0385
Alexandria, CT 22311-7137 800-342-2383
Fax: 703-549-6995
www.diabetes.org
Six patients and their families share their day-to-day frustrations and successes in managing diabetes.
Videotape

3450 Physicians Guide to Type I Diabetes
American Diabetes Association/Conn. Affiliate
1701 North Beauregard Str 203-639-0385
Alexandria, CT 22311-7137 800-342-2383
Fax: 703-549-6995
www.diabetes.org
Principles of good care in the diagnosis and management of Type I.
Videotape

3451 Survival Skills for Diabetic Children
Ajn Company
20 West 44th Street 212-686-7220
New York, NY 10036-2961 800-226-6256
Fax: 212-686-7232
www.chamber.nyc
How to provide insulin-dependent children with education, supervision, and support.
1988 28 minutes

3452 Understanding Diabetes: A User's Guide to Novolin
American Diabetes Association/Conn. Affiliate
1701 North Beauregard Str 203-639-0385
Alexandria, CT 22311 800-342-2383
Fax: 703-549-6995
www.diabetes.org

Basic information about diabetes and the role insulin plays in blood glucose control.
Videotape

original and timely health information as well as material from well known content providers.

Web Sites

3453 American Association of Diabetes Educators

www.aabenet.org

The mission is to enhance the competence of health professionals who teach persons with diabetes, advance the specialty practice of diabetes education, and to improve the quality of diabetes education and care for all those affected by diabetes.

3454 American Diabetes Association

www.diabetes.org

Offers a network of 52 affiliates with over 55,000 volunteers, including a professional membership of more than 10,000 physicians, social workers, nutritionists, educators and nurses.

3455 Diabetes Dictionary

diabetes.niddk.nih.gov

A publication of National Diabetes Information Clearinghouse. The Clearinghouse provides information about diabetes to people with diabetes and to their families, health care professionals, and the public. The NDIC answers inquiries, develops and distributes publications, and works closely with professional and patient organizations and Government agencies to coordinate resources about diabetes.

3456 Diabetes Exercise and Sports Association

www.diabetes-exercise.org

Exists to enhance the quality of life for people with diabetes through exercise and physical fitness.

3457 Healing Well

www.healingwell.com

An online health resource guide to medical news, chat, information and articles, newsgroups and message boards, books, disease-related web sites, medical directories, and more for patients, friends, and family coping with disabling diseases, disorders, or chronic illnesses.

3458 Health Finder

www.healthfinder.gov

Searchable, carefully developed web site offering information on over 1000 topics. Developed by the US Department of Health and Human Services, the site can be used in both English and Spanish.

3459 Healthlink USA

www.healthlinkusa.com

Health information concerning treatment, cures, prevention, diagnosis, risk factors, research, support groups, email lists, personal stories and much more. Updated regularly.

3460 Helios Health

www.helioshealth.com

Online resource for your health information. Detailed information about specific health topics, access to expert advice from our Medical Advisory Board, and up-to-date health news.

3461 MedicineNet

www.medicinenet.com

An online resource for consumers providing easy-to-read, authoritative medical and health information.

3462 Medscape

www.medscape.com

Medscape offers specialists, primary care physicians, and other health professionals the Web's most robust and integrated medical information and educational tools.

3463 National Diabetes Information Clearinghous e

www.niddk.nih.gov

Offers various materials, resources, books, pamphlets and more for persons and families in the area of diabetes.

3464 WebMD

www.webmd.com

Provides credible information, supportive communities, and in-depth reference material about health subjects. A source for

Description

3465 Down Syndrome

Down syndrome is a collection of inherited abnormalities caused by an extra chromosome. Instead of having the normal number of chromosomes (46), children with Down syndrome have an extra chromosome 21. (Because there are three copies of chromosome 21 instead of the normal two, Down syndrome is often called trisomy 21). This chromosomal abnormality results in altered growth and development. Approximately 4,000 children are born with Down syndrome every year in the United States. The overall incidence is about 1 in every 700 live births, but there is a marked variability depending on maternal age. In the early childbearing years, the incidence is about 1/2000 live births; for mothers over 40, it rises to at least 1/100 if not more frequent with advancing age.

Down syndrome is associated with a wide variety of clinical signs, although most individuals do not possess all of them. Common findings include decreased muscle tone, slanting eyes with folds of skin in the inside corners, white spots appearing in the irises of the eyes, and single creases across the palms of one or both hands. Physically, children with Down syndrome have broad feet with short toes, short ears and necks, small heads and small oral cavities. Mental development in the child with Down syndrome is impaired; the mean IQ is approximately 50. Hearing and speech abilities may also be hampered. However, many children with Down syndrome can reach surprisingly high levels of achievement. Congenital heart disease is found in nearly half of patients, and there is an increased susceptibility to acute leukemia. Today, most patients survive well into adulthood, although problems such as Alzheimer's Disease and psychiatric illness may increase with age.

It is essential that parents enroll their children with Down syndrome in an infant development program. These programs advise parents on how to help a child with Down syndrome in language, cognitive, social and motor skills.

National Agencies & Associations

3466 ARC The ARC of the United States
The ARC of the United States
1660 L Street NW
Washington, DC 20036   301-565-3842
800-433-5255
Fax: 301-565-3843
e-mail: info@thearc.org
www.thearc.org
Works to include all children and adults with cognitive intellectual and developmental disabilities in every community.
Mohan Mehra, President
Nancy Webster, Vice President

3467 Aleh Foundation Aleh Institustions USA
Aleh Institustions USA
5317 13th Avenue
Brooklyn, NY 11219   718-851-4596
800-317-2534
Fax: 718-851-4597
e-mail: shlomo@alehfoundation.com
www.alehfoundation.org

Founded in 1983, the Aleh Rehabilitation Center has served as a residential facility to close to 200 children with multiple, physical and mental disabilities. These children and their families benefit from a wide range of services in a caring, supportive atmosphere.
Rabbi Shlomo Braun, Founder & Director

3468 Canadian Down Syndrome Society
5005 Dalhousie Drive NW
Calgary Alberta, T3N-5R8   403-270-8500
800-883-5608
Fax: 403-270-8291
e-mail: info@cdss.ca
www.cdss.ca
Resource linking parents and professionals through advocacy education and providing information.
Krista J Flint, Executive Director

3469 National Association for Down Syndrome
PO Box 206
Wilmette, IL 60091   630-325-9112
e-mail: info@nads.org
www.nads.org
A non-for-profit organization founded in Chicago in 1961 by parents of children with Down syndrome who felt a need to create a better environment and bring about understanding and acceptance of people with Down syndrome.
Jackie Rotondi, President
Diane Urhausen, Executive Director

3470 National Dissemination Center for Children with Disabilities
1825 Connecticut Avenue NW
Washington, DC 20009   202-884-8200
800-695-0285
Fax: 202-884-8441
TTY: 202-884-8200
e-mail: nichcy@aed.org
www.nichcy.org
Publishes free, fact filled newsletters. Arranges workshops. Advises parents on the laws entitling children with disabilities to special education and other services.
Dr Suzanne Ripley, Contact

3471 National Down Syndrome Congress
1370 Center Drive
Atlanta, GA 30338   770-604-9500
800-232-6372
Fax: 770-604-9898
e-mail: info@ndsccenter.org
www.NDSCcenter.org
The mission of the NDSC is to provide information, advocacy, and support concerning all aspects of life for individuals with Down Syndrome.
Brooks Robertson, President
Sue Joe, Resources Specialist

3472 National Down Syndrome Society
666 Broadway
New York, NY 10012   212-460-9330
800-221-4602
Fax: 212-979-2873
e-mail: info@ndss.org
www.ndss.org
NDSS supports researchers seeking the causes of and answers to many of the medical genetic behavioral and learning problems associated with Down syndrome. Also sponsors symposia and conferences for parents and professionals provides advocacy.
Jon Colman, President
Betsy Goodwin, Founder

3473 National Early Childhood Technical Assistance System
University of North Carolina, Chapel Hill
Campus Box 8040 UNC-CH
Chapel Hill, NC 27599-0001   919-962-2001
Fax: 919-966-7463
e-mail: nectac@unc.edu
www.nectac.org
Assists states and other entities in developing comprehensive services for children with special needs through the age of eight and their families.
Lynne Kahn, Director & Principal Investigator
Joan Danaher, Associate Director Information Resources

State Agencies & Associations

California

3474 Down Syndrome Association of Los Angeles
16461 Sherman Way
Van Nuys, CA 91406

818-786-0001
Fax: 818-786-0004
e-mail: info@dsala.org
www.dsala.org

Offers information on Down syndrome, counseling, resources, facts, laws and other forms of information.
Gail Williamson, Executive Director
Sandra Baker, Office Administrator/Spanish Coordinator

Colorado

3475 Mile High Down Syndrome Association
2121 S Oneida Street
Denver, CO 80224

303-797-1699
Fax: 303-756-6144
e-mail: info@mhdsa.org
www.mhdsa.org

Mac Macsovits, Executive Director
Melissa Davis, Volunteer Coordinator

Connecticut

3476 Connecticut Down Syndrome Congress
263 Farmington Avenue
Farmington, CT 06030-0485

205-351-1157
888-486-8537
e-mail: manager@ctdownsyndrome.org
www.ctdownsyndrome.org

Sheryl Knapp, Secretary
Walter Glomb, President

District of Columbia

3477 Administration for Children and Families
370 L'Enfant Promenade
Washington, DC 20447

www.acf.hhs.gov

The Administration for Children & Families (ACF) is a division of the U.S. Department of Health & Human Services (HHS). ACF promotes the economic and social well-being of families, children, individuals and communities.
Mark Greenberg, Acting Assistant Secretary
Jeff Hild, Chief of Staff

3478 National Institute for Occupational Safety and Health
395 E Street, SW
Washington, DC 20201

202-245-0625
800-232-4636
Fax: 513-533-8347
TTY: 888-232-6348
www.cdc.gov/niosh/

The National Institute for Occupational Safety and Health (NIOSH) is the U.S. federal agency that conducts research and makes recommendations to prevent worker injury and illness.
John Howard, MD, Director
Frank Hearl, PE, Chief of Staff

Florida

3479 Gold Coast Down Syndrome Organization
2255 Glades Road
Boca Raton, FL 33431

561-912-1231
Fax: 561-912-1232
e-mail: gcdso@bellsouth.net
www.goldcoastdownsyndrome.org

Gold Coast Down syndrome Organization is a private nonprofit corporation dedicated to making the future brighter for people with Down syndrome in Palm Beach County, Florida.
Sue Killan, President
Tina Trujillo, Secretary

3480 Goodwill Industries-Suncoast
Goodwill Industries-Suncoast
10596 Gandy Boulevard
St. Petersburg, FL 33702

727-523-1512
888-279-1988
Fax: 727-577-2749
e-mail: gw.marketing@goodwill-suncoast.rog
www.goodwill-suncoast.org

A nonprofit community based organization whose purpose is to improve the quality of life for people who are disabled, disadvantaged and/or aged. This mission is accomplished through a staff of over 1,200 employees providing independent living skills, affordable housing, career assessment and planning, job skills, training, placement, and job retention assistance with useful employment. Annually, Goodwill Industries-Suncoast serves over 30,000 people in Citrus, Hernando, Levy, Marion and more.
Martin W Gladysz, Chair
R Lee Waits, President/CEO

Georgia

3481 Division of Adolescent and School Health
4770 Buford Hwy, NE
Atlanta, GA 30341

800-232-4636
TTY: 888-232-6348
www.cdc.gov/HealthyYouth

CDC promotes the health and well-being of children and adolescents to enable them to become healthy and productive adults.

3482 Down Syndrome Association of Atlanta
2221 Peachtree Rd
Atlanta, GA 30309

404-320-3233
Fax: 404-228-7475
e-mail: contactus@AtlantaDSAA.org
www.dsaatl.org

Hawaii

3483 Hawaii Down Syndrome Congress
419 Keoniana Street
Honolulu, HI 96815

808-949-1999
e-mail: Conkay@AOL.com
www.downscity.com

Constance K Smith, President

Indiana

3484 Indiana Down Syndrome Foundation
2625 N. Meridian Street #49
Indianapolis, IN 46208

317-925-7617
888-989-9255
Fax: 317-925-7619
e-mail: info@dsindiana.org
www.indianadsf.org

Lisa Tokarz-Guiterre, Executive Director
Jeff Huffman, President

Maryland

3485 Agency for Healthcare Research and Quality
540 Gaither Road
Rockville, MD 20850

301-427-1364
www.ahrq.gov/index.html

The Agency for Healthcare Research and Quality's (AHRQ) mission is to produce evidence to make health care safer, higher quality, more accessible, equitable, and affordable, and to work within the U.S. Department of Health and Human Services and with other partners to make sure that the evidence is understood and used.
Richard G. Kronick, PhD, Director, Director
Sharon B. Arnold, PhD, Deputy Director

3486 Centers for Medicare and Medicaid Services
7500 Security Boulevard
Baltimore, MD 21244

410-786-3000
877-267-2323
TTY: 866-226-1819
e-mail: Mandy.Cohen@cms.hhs.gov
www.cms.gov

US federal agency which administers Medicare, Medicaid, and the State Children's Health Insurance Program.
Dr. Mandy Cohen, M.D., MPH, Chief of Staff
Timothy P. Love, Chief Operating Officer

3487 National Human Genome Research Institute
Building 31, Room 4B09
Bethesda, MD 20892

301-402-0911
Fax: 301-402-2218
www.genome.gov

The National Human Genome Research Institute began as the National Center for Human Genome Research (NCHGR), which was established in 1989 to carry out the role of the National Institutes

of Health (NIH) in the International Human Genome Project (HGP).
Eric D. Green, M.D., Ph.D., Director
Lawrence Brody, Ph.D., Director, Division of Genomics & Society

3488 National Institute of General Medical Sciences
45 Center Drive MSC 6200   301-496-7301
Bethesda, MD 20892   e-mail: info@nigms.nih.gov
www.nigms.nih.gov
The National Institute of General Medical Sciences (NIGMS) supports basic research that increases understanding of biological processes and lays the foundation for advances in disease diagnosis, treatment and prevention.
Jon R. Lorsch, Ph.D., Director
Judith H. Greenberg, Ph.D., Deputy Director

3489 National Institute on Drug Abuse
6001 Executive Boulevard   301-443-1124
Bethesda, MD 20892   e-mail: dd279k@nih.gov
www.drugabuse.gov
NIDA's mission is to lead the Nation in bringing the power of science to bear on drug abuse and addiction.
Nora D. Volkow, M.D., Director
David Daubert, Acting Associate Director for Management

3490 U.S. Food and Drug Administration
10903 New Hampshire Ave   301-796-8240
Silver Spring, MD 20993   888-463-6332
www.fda.gov
FDA is responsible for protecting the public health by assuring the safety, efficacy and security of human and veterinary drugs, biological products, medical devices, our nation's food supply, cosmetics, and products that emit radiation.
Stephen Ostroff, M.D., Acting Commissioner
James Tyler, Chief Financial Officer

Massachusetts

3491 Massachusetts Down Syndrome Congress
20 Burlington Mall Road   781-221-0024
Melrose, MA 02176   800-664-MDSC
Fax: 781-221-0011
e-mail: mdsc@mdsc.org
www.mdsc.org
Maureen Gallagher, Executive Director
Sarah Cullen, Outreach Coordinator

Minnesota

3492 Down Syndrome Association of Minnesota
656 Transfer Road   651-603-0720
St Paul, MN 55114   800-511-3696
Fax: 651-603-0726
e-mail: dsamn@dsamn.org
www.dsamn.org
A non-profit organization dedicated to ensuring that all individuals with Down syndrome and their families receive the support necessary to participate in, contribute to and achieve the fulfillment of life in their community.
Craig Parker, President
Kathleen Forney, Executive Director

New York

3493 Association for Children with Down Syndrome
4 Fern Place   516-933-4700
Plainview, NY 11803   Fax: 516-933-9524
e-mail: msmith@acds.org
www.acds.org
Nonprofit educational program that combines national information and research dissemination with direct services at the local level. Services include early intervention, pre-school, recreation programs and residential homes.
Michael M Smith, Executive Director
Cecilia Barry, Principal

North Carolina

3494 National Institute of Environmental Health Sciences
111 T.W. Alexander Drive   919-541-4580
Research Triangle Park, NC 27709   e-mail: carroll1@niehs.nih.gov
www.niehs.nih.gov
The mission of the NIEHS is to discover how the environment affects people in order to promote healthier lives.
Linda S. Birnbaum, Ph.D., Director
Richard Woychik, Ph.D., Deputy Director

Ohio

3495 Down Syndrome Association of Greater Cinci nnati
644 Linn Street   513-761-5400
Cincinnati, OH 45203-1734   Fax: 513-761-5401
e-mail: dsagc@dsagc.com
www.dsagc.com
The mission of the Down Syndrome Association of Greater Cincinnati is to provide information resources and support to individuals with Down syndrome, their families, and their communities.
Janet Gora, Executive Director
Nora Lindsay Quinn, Event Coordinator

Tennessee

3496 Down Syndrome Association of Middle Tennessee
111 N Wilson Boulevard   615-386-9002
Nashville, TN 37205-2411   Fax: 615-386-9754
e-mail: dsamt@bellsouth.net
www.dsamt.org
A nonprofit organization of families whose mission is to enhance the quality of life for all individuals with Down Syndrome by providing information and support to families professionals and the community.
Sheila Moore, Executive Director
Erin Kice, Program Coordinator

Texas

3497 Down Syndrome Guild of Dallas
701 N Central Expressway   214-267-1374
Richardson, TX 75080-1174   Fax: 972-234-2510
www.downsyndromedallas.org
Kelly Drablos, President
Tamara White, Secretary

3498 Texas Association on Mental Retardation
TAMR Headquarters   512-349-7470
Austin, TX 78755   Fax: 512-349-2117
e-mail: pat.holder@tamr-web.com
www.tamr-web.com
An organization made up of professionals, parents, consumers and advocates. Our goal is to create an accessible system of services and resources which support personal choice and promotes lives of dignity and self-determination.
Pat Holder

Virginia

3499 Down Syndrome Association of Hampton Roads
The Endependence Center   757-466-3696
Norfolk, VA 23502   e-mail: DSAHR@verizon.net
www.dsahr.org
The Down Syndrome Association of Hampton Roads is a not-for-profit organization serving the needs of individuals with Down Syndrome and their families. The association is supported by a board of directors, an advisory board and dedicated volunteers.
Andrea Anderson, President
Florence Thacker, Secretary

3500   Down Syndrome Association of Wisconsin
3211 South Lake Drive
Milwaukee, WI 53235
414-327-3729
866-327-3729
Fax: 414-327-1329
e-mail: info@dsaw.org
www.dsaw.org

An organization created by families for families of individuals and for individuals with Down Syndrome. Our primary mission is to provide each person with Down Syndrome the support needed to achieve personal goals and develop self-esteem.
Tom Oday, President
Nicole Cook, Treasurer

Libraries & Resource Centers

3501   Adult Down Syndrome Center of Lutheran General Hospital
1999 Dempster Street
Park Ridge, IL 60068
847-318-2303
www.advocatehealthc.com

The Adult Down Syndrome Center is a comprehensive medical resource providing multidisciplinary medical and psychosocial care for adults with Down syndrome, with an emphasis on health promotion.
Brian Chicoine MD, Medical Director

3502   Ann Whitehill Down Syndrome Program
Riley Hospital for Children
702 Barnhill Drive
Indianapolis, IN 46202
800-248-1199
www.iuhealth.org

Brings together specialists from many areas to address the medical and psychosocial needs of children with Down Syndrome. We also refer the family to local resources for therapy and developmental programs.
Evans Parker, President
William Cast, CEO

3503   Blick Clinic for Developmental Disabilities
640 W Market Street
Akron, OH 44303-1465
330-762-5425
Fax: 330-762-4019
e-mail: blickclinic@blickclinic.com
www.blickclinic.com

Blick Clinic is a private, non-profit outpatient clinic which began by a group of parents of children with developmental disabilities and a few volunteer professionals. Together, they developed the Clinic into a single, comprehensive source of diagnostic, evaluation, treatment, and support group services to persons with developmental disabilities.

3504   Center for Disabilities and Development
University of Iowa Hospitals and Clinics
100 Hawkins Drive
Iowa City, IA 52242-1011
319-353-6900
877-686-0031
Fax: 319-356-8284
TTY: 877-686-0032
e-mail: CDD-Webmaster@uiowa.edu
www.healthcare.uiowa.edu/cdd

Provides comprehensive health care and services to people with disabilities of all ages and their families through a combination of outpatient, impatient, and community based programs. UHS provides information, evaluation, treatment recommendations, and training related to aging and disabilities. UHS provides both preservice and inservice training programs for service providers and others who provide services to individuals with disabilities.

3505   Children's Hospital of Philadelphia
34th St & Civic Center Boulevard
Philadelphia, PA 19104-4399
215-590-1000
www.chop.edu

The oldest hospital dedicated exclusively to pediatrics, strives to be the world leader in the advancement of healthcare for children by integrating excellent patient care, innovative research and quality professional education into all of its programs.

3506   Children's Neurodevelopment Center
Hasbro Children's Hospital
167 Point Street
Providence, RI 02903
401-444-3500
www.lifespan.org/

The Children's Neurodevelopment Center (CNDC) at Hasbro Children's Hospital provides evaluation and treatment of children with neurological, genetic, developmental, metabolic and behavioral disorders.
Timothy J. Babineau, President and Chief Executive Officer
Kenneth E. Arnold, Senior Vice President and General Counse

3507   Dartmouth-Hitchcock Medical Center - Genetics and Development
One Medical Center Drive
Lebanon, NH 03756-0001
603-653-1400
Fax: 603-653-3585
www.employees.dartmouth-hitchcock.org

Dartmouth-Hitchcock Clinic is committed to a regional, integrated, comprehensive healthcare system, which can evolve under physician leadership, lay administrative support and public trustee guidance. DHC and its partnering DHMC organizations are recognized as leaders in using scientific methods to improve health care delivery.
Carol B Andrew EdD, MS
Mary Beth Dinulos, MD

3508   Developmental Evaluation Clinic
Westchester Institute for Human Development
Cedarwood Hall
Valhalla, NY 10595-1681
914-493-8150
e-mail: wihd@wihd.org
www.wihd.org

WIHD envisions a future where all people, including children and adults living with disabilities, fully participate in society, live healthy and productive lives, and have access to culturally appropriate services and supports, emerging technologies, competent professionals, caring families, caregivers, and communities.

3509   Developmental Medicine Center (DMC)
Children's Hospital Boston
300 Longwood Avenue
Boston, MA 02115
617-355-6000
Fax: 617-730-0373
TTY: 617-730-0152
www.childrenshospital.org

Provides developmental evaluation and treatment services for children aged birth to adolescence with a wide range of developmental, behavioral and learning difficulties
Leonard A Rappaport MD, MS, Program Director
Sandra Fenwick, President, CEO

3510   Down Syndrome Center of Western Pennsylvania
One Children's Hospital Drive
Pittsburgh, PA 15224-2524
412-692-5325
Fax: 412-692-5723
www.chp.edu

The Down Syndrome Center of Western Pennsylvania has a lending library of books, videos, audio cassettes and periodicals; provides current information about Down syndrome to families and professionals; maintains a file of articles on issues relating to Down Syndrome and publishes a quarterly newsletter in conjunction with the Down Syndrome Group of Western Pennsylvania.
Dr William Cohen, MD, Director

3511   Down Syndrome Clinic of Houston
6701 Fannin Street, 16th Floor
Dallas, TX 75235-7701
832-822-3478
Fax: 832-825-3399
e-mail: downsyndrome@texaschildrenshospital.org
www.texaschildreshospital.org

The mission of the Down Syndrome Clinic of Houston is to help individuals with Down syndrome reach his or her fullest potential. We accomplish our goal by offering a clinic where children receive complete evaluations by a multidisciplinary team. Families will obtain needed strategies for management of common concerns.
Nirupama Madduri, MD, Chief of Service
Jennifer Chung, Clinic Coordinator

3512   Dr. Gertrude A Barber National Institute
136 E Avenue
Erie, PA 16507-1899
814-453-7661
Fax: 814-455-1132
e-mail: BNIerie@barberinstitute.org
www.barberinstitute.org

We believe that all persons have the capacity for growth and fulfillment, and to that end they must be afforded every opportunity to at-

tain the greatest use of thier potential within themselves and their community.
John Barber, JD, President/CEO
Maureen Barber-Carey, EdD, Executive Vice President

3513 Jane and Richard Thomas Center for Down Syndrome
Cincinnati Center for Developmental Disorders
3333 Burnet Avenue   513-636-4200
Cincinnati, OH 45229-3039   800-344-2462
Fax: 513-636-0527
TTY: 513-636-4900
www.cincinnatichildrens.org
The Jane and Richard Thomas Center for Down Syndrome conducts research and offers interdisciplinary evaluations and intervention for infants, children, adolescents and young adults with Down syndrome. By providing a range of comprehensive services within one center, families can now spend less time pursuing services through multiple agencies and professionals.
David J Schonfeld MD, Division Head
Michael Fisher, President and CEO

3514 Kennedy Krieger Institute
707 N Broadway   443-923-9200
Baltimore, MD 21205-1888   800-873-3377
Fax: 410-550-9292
e-mail: info@kennedykrieger.org
www.kennedykrieger.org
Kennedy Krieger Institute is an internationally recognized facility located in Baltimore, Maryland dedicated to improving the lives of children and adolescents with pediatric developmental disabilities through patient care, special education, research, and professional training. Our clinical programs offer an interdisciplinary approach in treatment tailored to the individual needs of each child.
Gary W Goldstein, President

3515 LaRabida Children's Hospital: Developmental Disabilities & Delays
6501 South Promontory Drive   773-363-6700
Chicago, IL 60649   e-mail: info@larabida.org
www.larabida.org
La Rabida Children's Hospital is dedicated to excellence in caring for children with chronic illness, disabilities, or who have been abused, allowing them to achieve their fullest potential through expertise and innovation within the health care and academic communities.
Paula Kienberger Jaudes, MD, President/CEO

3516 Marcus Institute for Development and Learning
1920 Briarcliff Road   404-727-9450
Atlanta, GA 30329   Fax: 404-727-9598
e-mail: Marcus_Info@MarcusInstitute.org
www.marcus.org
Our mission is to provide information, services and programs to people with developmental disabilities and their families, as well as those who live and work with them. We offer integrated state-of-the-art clinical, behavioral, educational and family support services through a single organization to reduce the stress and aggravation for families who may have a child with mild to severe disabilities.
Charles M Shaffer, Jr, President/CEO
Dr Claire Coles, Director Fetal Alcohol Center

3517 MeritCare Children's Hospital Down Syndrome Outpatient Service
Coordinated Treatment Center
736 Broadway   701-234-6600
Fargo, ND 58122-4420   800-828-2901
Fax: 701-234-6965
www.meritcare.com
MeritCare Children's Hospital offers a multidisciplinary outpatient service to help accommodate the special medical developmental, behavioral, family and community needs of patients with Down Syndrome.

3518 Mt. Washington Pediatric Clinic
1708 W Rogers Avenue   410-578-8600
Baltimore, MD 21209-4596   Fax: 410-466-1715
www.mwph.org

The primary purpose of the Mt. Washington Pediatric Hospital and its affiliates is to sponsor and promote the provision of the highest quality pediatric health care services in a nurturing environment.
Sheldon J Stein, President/CEO
Robert H Imhoff, III, VP Development

3519 Santa Rosa Medical Center
PO Box 7330   210-228-2386
San Antonio, TX 78207-0330   www.srmcfl.com
Philip Wright, CEO

3520 UCSF Children's Hospital Health Library
505 Parnassus Avenue
San Francisco, CA 94143   415-476-1000
www.ucsfhealth.org
This Health Library is an online resource to supplement information your doctors, nurses and pharmacists may provide. Our library includes a medical dictionary and an online calendar of our health events. We have news about our research advances and treatments, patient education materials and listings of other helpful Web sites.
Mark Laret, CEO

3521 University of Maryland: Department of Pediatrics
22 South Greene Street   410-328-8667
Baltimore, MD 21201   Fax: 410-328-3981
http://www.umm.edu/pediatrics/
Recognized throughout Maryland and the mid-Atlantic region as a valuable resource for critically and chronically ill children, the University of Maryland Hospital for Children combines state-of-the-art medicine with family-centered care.

3522 University of Washington: Experimental Education Unit
Box 357925   206-543-4011
Seattle, WA 98195-7925   Fax: 206-543-8480
www.eeuweb.org
The Experimental Education Unit (EEU) is a state-certified special education school that serves children from birth to age 7 with diverse abilities. Faculty at the EEU conduct research projects, and provide training opportunties to undergraduate and graduate students, educators, and other professionals.
Rick Neel, Director

Research Centers

3523 Institute for Basic Research in Developmental Disabilities
44 Holland Avenue   718-494-0600
Albany, NY 12229-0001   866-946-9733
Fax: 718-494-0833
TTY: 866-933-4889
www.omr.state.ny.us
Conducts research into neurodegenerative diseases Alzheimer's disease developmental disabilities fragile X syndrome Down's Syndrome autism epilepsy and basic science issues underlying all developmental disabilities.
W Ted Brown, Director
Raju K Pullarkat, Chair Developmental Biochemistry

3524 Kennedy Krieger Institute - Down Syndrome
10 Center Drive   301-496-4000
Bethesda, MD 20892   888-554-2080
Fax: 443-923-9138
TTY: 443-923-2645
e-mail: webmaster@kennedykrieger.org
clinicalcenter.nih.gov
Dedicated to improving the lives of children and adolescents with pediatric developmental disabilities through patient care special education research and professional training.
John Gallin, Director
Char Koller, Research

3525 National Institute of Child Health and Human Development
PO Box 3006
Rockville, MD 20847   800-370-2943
Fax: 301-984-1473
TTY: 888-320-6942
e-mail: NICHDInformationResourceCenter@mail.nih.
www.nichd.nih.gov
Duane Alexander MD, Director

Support Groups & Hotlines

3526 Down Syndrome Association of Greater Cinci nnati
644 Linn Street 513-761-5400
Cincinnati, OH 45203-1734 Fax: 513-761-5401
e-mail: janet@dsagc.com
www.dsagc.com

Janet Gora, Executive Director
Collette Maddy, Office Coordinator

3527 National Down Syndrome Congress
1370 Center Drive 770-604-9500
Atlanta, GA 30338 800-232-6372
Fax: 770-604-9898
e-mail: info@ndsccenter.org
www.ndsccenter.org

Provides information, advocacy and support concerning all aspects of life for individuals with Down syndrome.
David Tolleson, Executive Director
Jim Faber, President

3528 National Down Syndrome Society Hotline
666 Broadway 212-460-9330
New York, NY 10012 800-221-4602
Fax: 212-979-2873
e-mail: info@ndss.org
www.ndss.org

NDSS supports researchers seeking the causes of and answers to many of the medical, genetic, behavioral and learning problems associated with Down syndrome; sponsors symposia and conferences for parents and professionals; performs advocacy; provides information and refferal through a toll-free number; and develops and disseminates educational materials.
Jon Colman, President
Patricia Baker, Program Manager

3529 Parents of Children with Down Syndrome
Arc of Montgomery County
11600 Nebel Street 301-984-5777
Rockville, MD 20852-2538 Fax: 301-816-2429
TTY: 301-881-1548
e-mail: asachs@arcmontmd.org
www.arcmontmd.org/

Activities include formal and informal meetings, parent-to-parent support, contacting new parents of down syndrome children to offer support and information on community resources, providing information on doctors, hospitals and professionals.
Petere Holden, Executive Director
John Slavcoff, President of the Board

Books

3530 ACDS Infant, Toddler & Pre-school Curriculum for Children
Association for Children with Down Syndrome
4 Fern Place 516-933-4700
Plainview, NY 11803 Fax: 516-933-9524
e-mail: msmith@acds.org
www.acds.org

This curriculum is user friendly for parents, educators, related service professionals and other caregivers. It provides checklists and teaching strategies to facilitate aquisition of skills in cognition, self-help, socialization, speech and language, gross and fine motor skills plus much more.
Michael M. Smith, Executive Director

3531 Babies with Down Syndrome
Woodbine House
6510 Bells Mill Road 301-897-3570
Bethesda, MD 20817-1636 800-843-7323
www.telebyte.com

Praised as the finest book ever written for new parents, this book covers everything they need to know about rearing these beautiful and special children in a loving environment.
237 pages Paperback
ISBN: 0-933149-02-6

3532 Bethy and the Mouse: God's Gifts in Special Packages
Faith and Life Press

718 Main Street 316-283-5100
Newton, KS 67114-0344
A father's account of his special children, Bethy with Down Syndrome and The Mouse who has been born with microcephaley. A tender story of a father's love.
164 pages Paperback
ISBN: 0-873031-11-3

3533 Breast Feeding the Baby with Down Syndrome
LaLeche League International
35 E. Wacker Drive 312-646-6260
Chicago, IL 60601-4048 Fax: 312-644-8557
e-mail: llli@llli.org
www.llli.org

16 pages Pamphlet

3534 Cara: Growing with a Retarded Child
Temple University Press
1852 North 10th Street 215-926-2140
Philadelphia, PA 19122 800-621-2736
www.temple.edu/tempress

The author offers information and experiences on raising her daughter, Cara, who has Down syndrome.

3535 Communication Skills in Children with Down Syndrome
Woodbine House
6510 Bells Mill Road
Bethesda, MD 20817 800-843-7323
www.woodbinehouse.com

Offers parents a chance to learn what to expect as communication skills progress from infancy through early teenage years. Discussions are included on speech and language therapy, hearing problems, school performance and intelligibility issues.
150 pages Paperback
ISBN: 0-933149-53-0

3536 Current Approaches to Down's Syndrome
Greenwood Publishing Group, Inc/Praeger Publishers
P.O. Box 1911 805-968-1911
Santa Barbara, CA 93117-6926 800-368-6868
Fax: 866-270-3856
e-mail: CustomerService@abc-clio.com
www.greenwood.com

An exploration of current initiatives relating to Down syndrome in the medical, educational and social fields.
447 pages
ISBN: 0-275902-12-9
Vince Burns, VP
Brian Stratford, Editor

3537 Differences in Common: Straight Talk on Mental Retardation/Down Syndrome
Woodbine House
22 Corporate Woods Blvd 518-738-0020
Albany, NY 12211 800-843-7323
e-mail: info@dsahrc.org
www.dsahrc.org

A collection of essays by the mother of an adult son who has Down syndrome. Focuses on mainstreaming, terminology, parent groups and advocacy.
M Trainer, Editor

3538 Down Syndrome: A Review of Current Knowledge
Jean-Adolphe Rondal, Juan Perera, and Lynn Nadek, author
John Wiley and Sons, Inc.
111 River Street 201-748-6000
Hoboken, NJ 07030 877-762-2974
Fax: 201-748-6088
e-mail: info@wiley.com
www.wiley.com

1999 350 pages Hardcover
Stephen M. Smith, President and CEO
John Kritzmacher, EVP, CFO

3539 Down Syndrome: An Update and Review for Primary Care Physicians
Dartmouth-Hitchcock Medical Center
22 Corporate Woods Blvd 518-738-0020
Albany, NY 12211-0001 e-mail: info@dsahrc.org
www.dsahrc.org

An excellent medical review of Down syndrome intended for physicians.
WC Cooley, Editor

3540 Down Syndrome: The Facts
Oxford University Press
2001 Evans Road   212-726-6000
Cary, NC 27513-2010   800-451-7556
                                        Fax: 919-677-1303
                                        www.oup-usa.org
A book for parents who have a child with Down syndrome written by a pediatrician who works with Down syndrome children.
M Selikowitz, Editor

3541 From 17 Months to 17 Years...A Look at Down Syndrome
Bonnie Lavender
22 Corporate Woods Blvd   518-738-0020
Albany, NY 12211   e-mail: info@dsahrc.org
                                         www.dsahrc.org
Includes profiles of six families who have children with Down syndrome. Offers photographs and accompanying text that detail each family's experiences with Down syndrome.
B Lavender, Editor
GJ Lega, Editor

3542 Medical and Surgical Care for Children with Down Syndrome
Woodbine House
6510 Bells Mill Road
Bethesda, MD 20817-1636   800-843-7323
                                         www.woodbinehouse.com
Provides detailed and easy-to-understand information for parents on a wide range of medical conditions and treatments including: heart disease, recurrent infections, thyroid problems, eye problems, skin conditions, ear, nose and throat problems, orthopedic conditions, leukemia, facial and dental concerns and neurological problems.
320 pages Paperback
ISBN: 0-933149-54-9

3543 Parent's Guide to Down Syndrome: Toward a Brighter Future
Siegfried M Pueschel, MD, PhD, JD, MPH, author
Brookes Publishing Company
Cust Ser Department
Baltimore, MD 21285-0624   800-638-3775
                                        Fax: 410-337-8539
                           e-mail: custserv@brookespublishing.com
                                        www.brookespublishing.com
A comprehensive reference book especially for new parents but useful and informative to seasoned parents as well. Range of topics include a history of Down syndrome, physical characterisitcs, developmental expectations, early intervention, feeding the young child and the school years.
2001 338 pages Paperback
ISBN: 1-557664-52-8

3544 Parents of Children with Down Syndrome
11600 Nebel Street   301-984-5792
Rockville, MD 20852-2538   Fax: 301-816-2429
Activities include formal and informal meetings, parent-to-parent support, contacting new parents of down syndrome children to offer support and information on community resources, providing information on doctors, hospitals and professionals.

3545 Paul
Miriam Perrone
440 Park Avenue   912-638-8551
Saint Simons Island, GA 31522-4357
How a determined mother carved a semi-independent life for her now-grown Down's syndrome child.

3546 Show Me No Mercy
Cokesbury
Nashville of This young adult man with Down syndrome relates the experience of This 37 Years to be reunited with his son after a family tragedy separates them.
R Perske, Editor

3547 Since Owen
Johns Hopkins University Press

2715 N Charles Street   410-516-6900
Baltimore, MD 21218-2105   Fax: 410-516-6968
                                          www.press.jhu.edu
A well written book displaying understanding from a veteran parent communicating with other parents of children with disabilities.
466 pages
Kathleen Keane, Director
Erik A. Smist, Director, Finance and Administration

3548 Teaching the Infant with Down Syndrome: A Guide for Parents & Professionals
Pro-Ed, Inc.
8700 Shoal Creek Blvd   512-451-3246
Austin, TX 78757-6897   800-897-3202
                                        Fax: 512-451-8542
                                        e-mail: info@proedinc.com
                                        www.proedinc.com
A manual providing teaching ideas and activities that can be used to assist an infant's development.
MJ Hanson, Editor

3549 To Give an Edge: A Guide for New Parents of Children with Down's Syndrome
Viking Press
7000 Washington Avenue S   612-941-8780
Eden Prairie, MN 55344-3580
A guide for new parents designed to provide information about the disorder and how other parents of children with Down syndrome have coped.
JE Rynders, Editor
JM Horrobin, Editor

3550 Understanding Down's Syndrome An Introduction for Parents
Brookline Books
8 Trumbull Rd   413-584-0184
Northampton, MA 01060   Fax: 617-734-3952
                                    e-mail: brbooks@yahoo.com
                                    www.brooklinebooks.com
The author provides answers and explanations to the countless questions directed to him during his twenty years' involvement with Down syndrome individuals and their families.
Softcover
ISBN: 1-571290-09-5

Children's Books

3551 Our Brother Has Down's Syndrome: An Introduction for Children
Firefly Books
50 Staples Avenue   416-499-8412
Richmond Hill,   416-499-8313
                                    e-mail: info@fireflybooks.com
                                    www.fireflybooks.com
Two young sisters tell about their little brother with Down syndrome in this color picture book.
21 pages
S Cairo, Editor

3552 Secret Place of the Stairs
Harper & Row
10 E 53rd Street   212-207-7000
New York, NY 10022-5299
A story that weaves many themes, including the institutionalizing of the protagonist's sister, her parents' divorce and her own expectations.
Grades 7-10

3553 We Can Do It!
Macmillan
175 Fifth Avenue
New York, NY 10010-6221   646-307-5151
                                        www.macmillan.com
A colorful book of photographs that show the daily activities of young children with different developmental delays, including Down syndrome.
L Dwight, Editor

Magazines

3554   Down Syndrome, Papers and Abstracts for Professionals
666 Broadway   301-963-1857
New York, NY 10012
e-mail: info@ndss.org
www.ndss.org
Quarterly review of research literature pertaining to Down syndrome.
Sara Weir, President
Robert P. Taishoff, Chairman

3555   Exceptional Parent Magazine
6 Pickwick Lane   617-730-5800
Woodcliff Lake, NJ 07677-5071   Fax: 201-746-0179
www.eparent.com
A publication dealing with many issues affecting exceptional children and their families.
Monthly
Joseph M. Valenzano, Jr., President, CEO
Rick Rader, Editor-in-Chief

Newsletters

3556   Down Syndrome News
National Down Syndrome Congress
30 Mansell Court   770-604-9500
Roswell, GA 30076-1655   800-232-6372
Fax: 770-604-9898
e-mail: NDSC.center@aol.com
www.ndsccenter.org
Contains book reviews, articles and items of interest to those touched by Down syndrome.
10x Annually
Marilyn Tolbert, President
Bret Bowerman, 1st Vice President

3557   Down Syndrome Today
Down Syndrome Today Publications
666 Broadway   516-654-3242
New York, NY 10012-0212   800-221-4602
www.ndss.org
Offers information, articles, resources and materials for the parent and professional working and nurturing patients and persons with Downs syndrome.
Sara Weir, President
Robert P. Taishoff, Chairman

3558   National Down Syndrome Society Update
666 Broadway   212-460-9330
New York, NY 10012-2317   800-221-4602
Fax: 212-979-2873
www.ndss.org
Offers information on the activities of the society, new breakthroughs in medical technology, articles offering state of the art information to families and individuals with Down syndrome, and answers to questions about the illness.
12 pages Quarterly
Sara Weir, President
Robert P. Taishoff, Chairman

3559   On the Up with Down Syndrome
Carole Shafer, author
Down Syndrome Association of Wisconsin
9401 West Beloit Road   414-327-3729
Milwaukee, WI 53227   866-327-3729
Fax: 414-327-1329
e-mail: thomtalent@aol.com
www.dsaw.org
Offers the exchange of ideas and experiences. Free to our members. Membership is $20.00/year.
Quarterly
Ron Irwin, Board President
Robbin Lyons, Newsletter Contact

Pamphlets

3560   Alzheimer's Disease and Down Syndrome
National Down Syndrome Society
666 Broadway   212-460-9330
New York, NY 10012-2317   800-221-4602
www.ndss.org
1995
Sara Weir, President
Robert P. Taishoff, Chairman

3561   Down Syndrome
March of Dimes
1275 Mamaroneck Avenue   914-997-4488
White Plains, NY 10605   Fax: 212-254-3518
e-mail: NY639@marchofdimes.com
www.marchofdimes.com

3562   Heart and Down Syndrome
National Down Syndrome Society
666 Broadway   212-460-9330
New York, NY 10012-2317   800-221-4602
www.ndss.org
1995
Sara Weir, President
Robert P. Taishoff, Chairman

3563   Life Planning and Down Syndrome
National Down Syndrome Society
666 Broadway   212-460-9330
New York, NY 10012-2317   800-221-4602
www.ndss.org
Sara Weir, President
Robert P. Taishoff, Chairman

3564   Neurology of Down Syndrome
National Down Syndrome Society
666 Broadway   212-460-9330
New York, NY 10012-2317   800-221-4602
www.ndss.org
1995
Sara Weir, President
Robert P. Taishoff, Chairman

3565   New Parents
Association for Children with Down Syndrome
4 Fern Place   516-933-4700
Plainview, NY 11803   Fax: 516-933-9524
e-mail: msmith@acds.org
www.acds.org
Bibliography compiled for parents who have just given birth to a child with Down syndrome. Free upon reciept of a stamped, self-addressed envelope.
Michael Smith, Executive Director

3566   Sexuality in Down Syndrome
National Down Syndrome Society
666 Broadway   212-460-9330
New York, NY 10012-2317   800-221-4602
www.ndss.org
1995
Sara Weir, President
Robert P. Taishoff, Chairman

3567   Speech and Language in Children and Adolescents with Down Syndrome
National Down Syndrome Society
666 Broadway   212-460-9330
New York, NY 10012-2317   800-221-4602
www.ndss.org
1995
Sara Weir, President
Robert P. Taishoff, Chairman

Audio & Video

3568   Adaptation to the Initial Crisis
Lawren Productions

100 Brook Hill Drive
West Nyack, NY 10994-1556
845-353-7500
800-872-7423
Fax: 845-353-4141
e-mail: online@cambridge.org
www.cambridge.org/us
A family learns to adapt to the birth of a child with a handicap.

3569 Bernardsville Beginnings
National Down Syndrome Society
666 Broadway
New York, NY 10012-2317
212-460-9330
800-221-4602
Fax: 212-979-2873
www.ndss.org
Follows Alison through her first full year in a first grade inclusion program. Step-by-step account of teaching staff preparation, classroom experiences, a portrayal of one girl's successful adjustment, and a whole class matured by the experience.
23 minutes
Sara Weir, President
Robert P. Taishoff, Chairman

3570 Bittersweet Waltz
National Down Syndrome Society
666 Broadway
New York, NY 10012-2317
212-460-9330
800-221-4602
Fax: 212-979-2873
e-mail: info@ndss.org
www.ndss.org
Experience of Alec and his first year included in a regular fifth grade class. From a point of view of a parent, a child, and the school administration.
18 minutes
Sara Weir, President
Robert P. Taishoff, Chairman

3571 Colin and Ricky
Lawren Productions
930 Pitner Avenue
Evanston, IL 60202-1556
847-328-6700
800-421-2363
A young boy comes to deal with his disappointment surrounding the birth of his baby brother with Down syndrome.

3572 Congratulations: An Introduction to Down Syndrome for Parents/Family/Friends
New Challenges
96 Ogden Avenue
White Plains, NY 10605
914-287-0723
Film for parents which addresses some of the most commonly asked questions about raising a child with Down syndrome.

3573 Daddy's Girl
Carle Media
110 W Main Street
Urbana, IL 61801-2715
217-384-4838
A film starring a twelve-year-old actress with Down syndrome, dealing with her divorced father's inability to accept the fact that his daughter has Down syndrome.
Carolyn Baxley

3574 Down Syndrome: See the Potential
Down Syndrome Association of Charlotte
666 Broadway
New York, NY 10012
800-221-4602
www.ndss.org
Video highlighting the capability of children with Down syndrome.
Sara Weir, President
Robert P. Taishoff, Chairman

3575 Gifts of Love
National Down Syndrome Society
666 Broadway
New York, NY 10012-2317
212-460-9330
800-221-4602
Fax: 212-979-2873
www.ndss.org
Four families of children with Down syndrome talk about their feelings and experiences with their children, particularly during

the first six years. All the children live at home and attend programs in their communities.
25 minutes
Sara Weir, President
Robert P. Taishoff, Chairman

3576 Infant Motor Development: A Look at the Phases
Communication Skill Builders/Therapy Skill Builder
3830 E Bellevue
Tucson, AZ 85733
520-323-7500
A video depicting development in and activities for infants birth through 12 months.

3577 New Expectations
Lawren Productions
930 Pitner Avenue
Evanston, IL 60202-1556
800-421-2363
Focuses on the emotional and technical aspects of Down syndrome. Highlights four persons at various life stages from infancy to adulthood in the areas of education and employment.

3578 New Set of Fears, a New Set of Hopes
Meyer Children's Rehabilitation Institute
Resource Center
Omaha, NE 68131
402-559-7467
800-232-6372
Explores the way a family adjusts as they go through the life cycle with their child who has Down syndrome.

3579 Opportunities to Grow
National Down Syndrome Society
666 Broadway
New York, NY 10012-2317
212-460-9330
800-221-4602
Fax: 212-979-2873
e-mail: info@ndss.org
www.ndss.org
Sequel to Gifts of Love video shows how people with Down syndrome, ages 6 to 26, participate equally in all phases of community life. Vignettes of 15 young men and women illustrate how inclusion, education, computer facilitation, socialization programs, and employment training help them to fulfill their potential.
25 minutes
Sara Weir, President
Robert P. Taishoff, Chairman

3580 Stepping Stones
AIT
PO Box A
Bloomington, IN 47402-0120
800-457-4509
Series of video programs on teaching basic skills to at-risk, special needs and normally developed children.

3581 Thanks Mom and Dad: Profiles of Patrick
University of Washington
CDMRC Mail Stop WJ-10
Seattle, WA 98195-0001
206-543-4011
800-232-6372
Documentary on the life of Patrick, a young man with Down syndrome from birth through his graduation from high school.

3582 You Don't Outgrow Down Syndrome
National Association for Down Syndrome
1460 Renaissance Drive
Park Ridge, IL 60068-4542
630-325-9112
847-376-8908
e-mail: info@nads.org
www.nads.org
Winner of the second annual International Rehabilitation Film Festival.
Steve Connors, President
Sarah Alzamora, First Vice President

Web Sites

3583 Aleh Foundation
www.aleh.org
ALEH is Israel's largest and most advanced network of residential facilities for children with severe disabilities.

3584 Down Syndrome
www.downsyn.com

A resource for new paretns of children with Down syndrome. Provides a personnel perspective from parents who also have children with Down syndrome.

3585 Healing Well

www.healingwell.com

An online health resource guide to medical news, chat, information and articles, newsgroups and message boards, books, disease-related web sites, medical directories, and more for patients, friends, and family coping with disabling diseases, disorders, or chronic illnesses.

3586 Health Finder

www.healthfinder.gov

Searchable, carefully developed web site offering information on over 1000 topics. Developed by the US Department of Health and Human Services, the site can be used in both English and Spanish.

3587 Healthlink USA

www.healthlinkusa.com

Health information concerning treatment, cures, prevention, diagnosis, risk factors, research, support groups, email lists, personal stories and much more. Updated regularly.

3588 Helios Health

www.helioshealth.com

Online resource for your health information. Detailed information about specific health topics, access to expert advice from our Medical Advisory Board, and up-to-date health news.

3589 MedicineNet

www.medicinenet.com

An online resource for consumers providing easy-to-read, authoritative medical and health information.

3590 Medscape

www.medscape.com

Medscape offers specialists, primary care physicians, and other health professionals the Web's most robust and integrated medical information and educational tools.

3591 National Down Syndrome Society

www.ndss.org

NDSS works to obtain a better understanding of Down syndrome, the potential of people with Down syndrome, to support research about the condition, and to provide information and referral services for families and professionals.

3592 WebMD

www.webmd.com

Provides credible information, supportive communities, and in-depth reference material about health subjects. A source for original and timely health information as well as material from well known content providers.

Description

3593 # Eating Disorders (Anorexia Nervosa, Bulimia)

Anorexia nervosa and bulimia nervosa are eating disorders characterized by a disturbed sense of body image and an irrational fear of obesity. They are manifested by abnormal patterns relating to food and by self-induced, marked weight loss.

Anorexia is a psychiatric disorder in which dieting and a desire for thinness leads to excessive weight loss. About 95 percent of persons with this disorder are female, although males can be affected. The onset usually occurs during adolescence and some sufferers are in their 60s. Anorexia nervosa is characterized by self-starvation, food preoccupation and rituals, compulsive exercising, and often a resulting absence of menstrual cycles. The cause is unknown, although social factors appear to play an important role, including advertisements that equate thinness with desirability. Denial is a prominent feature, and sufferers usually resist treatment.

Bulimia is characterized by recurring episodes of binge eating followed by efforts to avoid weight gain, such as purging through self-induced vomiting or abuse of laxatives and/or diuretics (water pills). Unlike patients with anorexia, those with bulimia usually have normal weight. Binges are often triggered by psychological stress and carried out in secret. Warning signs of bulimia include eating uncontrollably, frequent use of the bathroom, erosion of dental enamel of the front teeth (from vomiting), and painless swollen salivary glands. Bulimia may coexist with anorexia.

Anorexia nervosa is associated with a 10 percent death rate, generally from a sudden disturbance of heart rhythm. Fortunately, most sufferers will eventually return to a normal or near-normal body weight, although many continue to struggle with body image and unhealthy eating patterns. Treatment for both illnesses is similar, beginning with the need to restore body weight. Initial treatment may require hospitalization for physical stabilization. Long-term psychological treatment and behavior modification is often necessary and focuses on behavioral and emotional growth for both the individual with the eating disorder and their family. See also *Obesity.*

National Agencies & Associations

3594 **Academy for Eating Disorders**
111 Deer Lake Road
Deerfield, IL 60015-1577
847-498-4274
Fax: 847-480-9282
e-mail: info@aedweb.org
www.aedweb.org
AED is an association of multidisciplinary professionals promoting effective treatment, developing prevention initiatives, advocating for the field, stimulating research and sponsoring an annual conference.
Pamela K. Keel, PhD, FAED, President
Carla Slawson, MBA, Executive Director

3595 **American Dietetic Association**
120 S Riverside Plaza
Chicago, IL 60606-6995
312-899-0040
800-877-1600
e-mail: media@eatright.org
www.eatright.org
ADA offers nutrition information consumer tips nutrition fact sheets consumer frequently asked questions and referrals to registered dieticians.
Patricia M Babjak, Chief Executive Officer
Judith C Rodriguez, President

3596 **Anna Westin Foundation**
PO Box 268
Chaska, MN 55318
952-361-3051
e-mail: kitty@annawestinfoundation.org
www.annawestinfoundation.org
The Anna Westin Foundation is dedicated to the prevention and treatment of eating disorders. They are committed to preventing the tragic loss of life to anorexia nervosa and bulimia and to raising public awareness of those dangerous illnesses.
Kitty Westin, President

3597 **Anorexia Nervosa & Bulimia Association**
1500 Ouellette Avenue
Windsor, N8X 1-1C0
519-969-0227
e-mail: info@bana.ca
www.bana.ca
Facilitate advocate and coordinate support for any individual directly or indirectly affected by eating disorders and to raise public awareness through improved communication and the provision of education within our community.
Steven Richards, President
Sarah Woodruff, Vice-President

3598 **Dads and Daughters**
34 E Superior Street
Duluth, MN 55802
218-772-3942
888-824-DADS
Fax: 218-728-0314
e-mail: info@dadsanddaughters.org
www.thedadman.com
Provides tools to strengthen father-daughter relationships and transform pervasive cultural messages that value daughters more for how they look than who they are.
Gregg Rutter, Development Director
David Sadker, Author ofyTeachers

3599 **Eating Disorders Action Group**
6156 Quinpool Road
Halifax Nova Scotia, B3L 1-3Z9
902-443-9944
e-mail: reception@edag.ca
www.edag.ca
A community based charitable organization dedicated to promoting healthy body image and self esteem and to supporting individuals who experience disordered eating.

3600 **Eating Disorders Anonymous**
PO Box 55876
Phoenix, AZ 85078-5876
www.4eda.org
EDA provides information about local support group meetings.

3601 **Eating Disorders Coalition for Research, Policy and Action**
720 7th Street NW
Washington, DC 20001-4303
202-543-9570
Fax: 202-543-9570
e-mail: manager@eatingdisorderscoalition.org
www.eatingdisorderscoalition.org
Advocates at the federal level on behalf of people with eating disorders their families and professionals working with these populations. Promotes federal support for improved access to care.
David Jaffe, Executive Director
Jeanine Cogan, Policy Director

3602 **Healthy Weight Network**
402 S 14th Street
Hettinger, ND 58639
701-567-2646
Fax: 701-567-2602
e-mail: hwj@healthyweight.net
www.healthyweight.net
Promotes information and resources pertaining to the Health at Any Size paradigm.
Frances M Berg MS, Founder/Editor

3603 International Association of Eating Disorders Professionals
PO Box 1295
Pekin, IL 61555-1295
309-346-3341
800-800-8126
Fax: 309-346-2874
e-mail: iaedpmembers@earthlink.net
www.iaedp.com
IAEDP Offers professional counseling and assistance to the medical community, courts, law enforcement officials and social welfare agencies.
Mary Bellofatto, President
Emmett R Bishop, Immediate Past President

3604 Jessie's Hope Society
11739 23rd Street
Maple Ridge, V2X-5X8
604-466-4877
877-288-0877
Fax: 604-466-4897
e-mail: info@jessieshope.org
www.jessieshope.org
Promote positive body image by fostering in youth within communities and across cultures throughout British Columbia.
Connie Coniglio, Chair
Mimi Hudson, Secretary

3605 National Association of Anorexia Nervosa and Associated Disorders
750 E Diehl Road
Naperville, IL 60563
630-577-1330
Fax: 847-433-4632
e-mail: anadhelp@anad.org
www.anad.org
Works to prevent eating disorders and provides numerous programs — all free — to help victims and families including hotlines, support groups, referrals, information packets and newsletters. Educational/prevention programs include presentations and early detection.
Vivian Hanse Meehan, Founder/President
Laura Discipio, Executive Director

3606 National Eating Disorder Information Centre
ES 7-421, 200 Elizabeth Street
Toronto, Ontario, M5G-2C4
416-340-4156
866-633-4220
Fax: 416-340-4736
e-mail: nedic@uhn.on.ca
www.nedic.ca
Promotes healthy lifestyles, including both healty eating and appropriate, enjoyable exercise.
Merryl Bear MEd, Director
Jessica Rust, Administrative Coordinator

3607 National Eating Disorders Association
603 Stewart Street
Seattle, WA 98101
206-382-3587
800-931-2237
Fax: 206-829-8501
e-mail: info@NationalEatingDisorders.org
www.nationaleatingdisorders.org
Our mission is to eliminate eating disorders and body dissatisfaction through prevention efforts education referral and support services advocacy training and research.
Lynn S Grefe MA, Chief Executive Officer
Molly Bauthues, Communications Manager

3608 National Eating Disorders Screening Program
One Washington Street
Wellesley Hills, MA 02481
781-239-0071
Fax: 781-431-7447
e-mail: smhinfo@mentalhealthscreening.org
www.mentalhealthscreening.org
Offers eating disorders screening.
Douglas G Jacobs MD, President/Medical Director

3609 National Women's Health Information Center
8270 Willow Oaks Corporate Drive
Fairfax, VA 22031
800-994-9662
Fax: 703-560-6598
TTY: 888-220-5446
TDD: 888-220-5446
e-mail: Wanda.jones@hhs.gov
www.4woman.gov
Government agency with free health information for women.
Wanda K Jones PhD, Deputy Assistant Secretary for Health
Frances E Ashe-Goins, Deputy Director

3610 Weight-Control Information Network National Institutes of Health
National Institutes of Health
1 WIN Way
Bethesda, MD 20892-3665
202-828-1025
877-946-4627
Fax: 202-828-1028
e-mail: win@info.niddk.nih.gov
www.win.niddk.nih.gov/index.htm
Information on obesity weight-control and nutrition.
BiAnnual

State Agencies & Associations

Connecticut

3611 Renfrew Center of Connecticut
1445 E. Putnam Avenue
Wilton, CT 06897
800-736-3739
Fax: 203-563-9936
e-mail: foundation@renfrew.org
www.renfrewcenter.com

District of Columbia

3612 Administration for Children and Families
370 L'Enfant Promenade
Washington, DC 20447
www.acf.hhs.gov
The Administration for Children & Families (ACF) is a division of the U.S. Department of Health & Human Services (HHS). ACF promotes the economic and social well-being of families, children, individuals and communities.
Mark Greenberg, Acting Assistant Secretary
Jeff Hild, Chief of Staff

3613 National Institute for Occupational Safety and Health
395 E Street, SW
Washington, DC 20201
202-245-0625
800-232-4636
Fax: 513-533-8347
TTY: 888-232-6348
www.cdc.gov/niosh/
The National Institute for Occupational Safety and Health (NIOSH) is the U.S. federal agency that conducts research and makes recommendations to prevent worker injury and illness.
John Howard, MD, Director
Frank Hearl, PE, Chief of Staff

Florida

3614 Renfrew Center of Miami
151 Majorca Avenue
Coral Gables, FL 33134
800-REN-FREW
Fax: 305-445-2729
e-mail: info@renfrewcenter.com
www.renfrewcenter.com

3615 Renfrew Center of South Florida
7700 Renfrew Lane
Coconut Creek, FL 33073
800-736-3739
Fax: 954-698-9007
e-mail: info@renfrewcenter.com
www.renfrewcenter.com

Georgia

3616 Division of Adolescent and School Health
4770 Buford Hwy, NE
Atlanta, GA 30341
800-232-4636
TTY: 888-232-6348
www.cdc.gov/HealthyYouth
CDC promotes the health and well-being of children and adolescents to enable them to become healthy and productive adults.

Maryland

3617 Agency for Healthcare Research and Quality
540 Gaither Road
Rockville, MD 20850
301-427-1364
www.ahrq.gov/index.html

The Agency for Healthcare Research and Quality's (AHRQ) mission is to produce evidence to make health care safer, higher quality, more accessible, equitable, and affordable, and to work within the U.S. Department of Health and Human Services and with other partners to make sure that the evidence is understood and used.
Richard G. Kronick, PhD, Director, Director
Sharon B. Arnold, PhD, Deputy Director

3618 Centers for Medicare and Medicaid Services
7500 Security Boulevard
Baltimore, MD 21244
410-786-3000
877-267-2323
TTY: 866-226-1819
e-mail: Mandy.Cohen@cms.hhs.gov
www.cms.gov
US federal agency which administers Medicare, Medicaid, and the State Children's Health Insurance Program.
Dr. Mandy Cohen, M.D., MPH, Chief of Staff
Timothy P. Love, Chief Operating Officer

3619 National Center for Complementary and Integrative Health
9000 Rockville Pike
Bethesda, MD 20892
888-644-6226
TTY: 866-464-3615
e-mail: nccih-info@mail.nih.gov
nccih.nih.gov
The National Center for Complementary and Integrative Health (NCCIH) is the Federal Government's lead agency for scientific research on the diverse medical and health care systems, practices, and products that are not generally considered part of conventional medicine.
Josephine P. Briggs, M.D., Director
David Shurtleff, Ph.D., Deputy Director

3620 National Human Genome Research Institute
Building 31, Room 4B09
Bethesda, MD 20892
301-402-0911
Fax: 301-402-2218
www.genome.gov
The National Human Genome Research Institute began as the National Center for Human Genome Research (NCHGR), which was established in 1989 to carry out the role of the National Institutes of Health (NIH) in the International Human Genome Project (HGP).
Eric D. Green, M.D., Ph.D., Director
Lawrence Brody, Ph.D., Director, Division of Genomics & Society

3621 St. Joseph's Medical Center
7601 Osler Drive
Towson, MD 21204
410-337-1000
www.stjosephtowson.com

John Tolmie, President/CEO

3622 U.S. Food and Drug Administration
10903 New Hampshire Ave
Silver Spring, MD 20993
301-796-8240
888-463-6332
www.fda.gov
FDA is responsible for protecting the public health by assuring the safety, efficacy and security of human and veterinary drugs, biological products, medical devices, our nation's food supply, cosmetics, and products that emit radiation.
Stephen Ostroff, M.D., Acting Commissioner
James Tyler, Chief Financial Officer

Massachusetts

3623 Massachusetts Eating Disorder Association
92 Pearl Street
Newton, MA 02458
617-558-1881
866-343-MEDA
Fax: 617-558-1771
e-mail: info@medainc.com
www.medainc.org
A nonprofit organization dedicated to the treatment and prevention of eating disorders. MEDA provides help line resource and referral, assessments, client consultations, individual therapy, support groups and an intensive evening treatment program.
100+ Members
Rebecca Manley, Founder
Beth Mayer, CEO

New Jersey

3624 American Anorexia Bulimia Association: New Jersey Chapter
10 Station Place
Metuchen, NJ 08840
609-252-0202
Fax: 609-688-1544
e-mail: njaaba@NJAABA.org
www.njaaba.org

3625 Renfrew Center of Northern New Jersey
174 Union Street
Ridgewood, NJ 07450
800-736-3739
Fax: 201-652-6253
e-mail: info@renfrewcenter.org
www.renfrewcenter.com

New York

3626 Renfrew Center of New York
11 E 36th Street
New York, NY 10016
800-736-3739
Fax: 212-686-1865
e-mail: info@renfrewcenter.org
www.renfrewcenter.com

3627 Westchester Task Force on Eating Disorders/American Anorexia Bulimia
3 Mount Joy Avenue
Scarsdale, NY 10583-2632
914-472-3701

North Carolina

3628 National Institute of Environmental Health Sciences
111 T.W. Alexander Drive
Research Triangle Park, NC 27709
919-541-4580
e-mail: carroll1@niehs.nih.gov
www.niehs.nih.gov
The mission of the NIEHS is to discover how the environment affects people in order to promote healthier lives.
Linda S. Birnbaum, Ph.D., Director
Richard Woychik, Ph.D., Deputy Director

Pennsylvania

3629 American Anorexia Bulimia Association of Philadelphia
PO Box 1287
Langhorne, PA 19047
215-221-1864
Fax: 215-702-8944
www.aabaphila.org

3630 Pennsylvania Educational Network for Eating Disorders
4801 McKnight Road
Pittsburgh, PA 15237
412-215-7967
www.pened.org
PENED is a nonprofit organization providing education, support, and referral information to the general and professional public.
Anita Sincro Maier, Therapist
Ralph F. Wilps, Therapist

3631 Renfrew Center of Bryn Mawr
735 Old Lancaster Road
Bryn Mawr, PA 19010
800-736-3739
Fax: 610-527-9361
e-mail: info@renfrewcenter.org
www.renfrewcenter.com

3632 Renfrew Center of Philadelphia
475 Spring Lane
Philadelphia, PA 19128
800-REN-FREW
Fax: 215-482-7390
e-mail: info@renfrew.org
www.renfrewcenter.com

Research Centers

3633 Academy for Eating Disorders
111 Deer Lake Road
Deerfield, IL 60015-1577
847-498-4274
Fax: 847-480-9282
e-mail: info@aedweb.org
www.aedweb.org

Disseminate knowledge regarding eating disorders to members of the Academy other professionals and the general public
Debra Katzman, President
Susie Orbach, Board of Advisor

3634   Center for the Study of Anorexia and Bulimia
1841 Broadway at 60th Street   212-333-3444
New York, NY 10023   Fax: 212-333-5444
www.icpnyc.org
The Institute is composed of a group of 150 professionally trained licensed psychotherapists who offer a full range of psychotherapeutic services including individual and group psychotherapy and psychoanalysis in addition to more specialized treatment services.
Jim M Pollack CSW, Executive Director/Director of Treatment
Ron Taffel, Chair

3635   Division of Digestive & Liver Diseases of Cloumbia University
630 W 168th Street   212-305-5960
New York, NY 10032-3784   Fax: 212-305-8466
e-mail: hjw14@columbia.edu
www.cumc.columbia.edu
The Division's faculty members are devoted to research and the clinical care of patients with gastrointestinal, liver and nutritional disorders. The Division is also responsible for the Gastroenterology Training Program at the medical center and for teaching medical students, interns, residents, fellows and attending physicians aspects of gastrointestinal and liver diseases.
Howard J Worman MD, Division Director
Karen Wisdom, Director

3636   Harris Center for Education and Advocacy in Eating Disorders
2 Longfellow Place   617-726-8470
Boston, MA 02114   Fax: 617-726-1595
e-mail: dherzog@partners.org
www.harriscentermgh.org
Conducts research provides a newsletter and information.
David B Herzog MD, Director
David B Herzog, Director

Support Groups & Hotlines

3637   AABA Support Group
Chippenham Medical Center
7101 Jahnke Rd.   804-320-3911
Richmond, VA 23225
Elliot Spanier, Contact

3638   About Kids GI Disorders
IFFGD
PO Box 170864   414-964-1799
Milwaukee, WI 53217-8076   888-964-2001
Fax: 414-964-7176
e-mail: iffgd@iffgd.org
www.aboutkidsgi.org
About Kids is the pediatric branch of the International Foundation for Functional Gastrointestinal Disorders (IFFGD), a registered nonprofit education and research organization founded in 1991. Their mission is to inform, assist, and support those affected by gastrointestinal (GI) disorders, addressing issues of digestive health in children through support of education and research. IFFGD promotes awareness among the public, health care providers, researchers, and regulators.
Nancy J Norton, President/Founder

3639   Association of Gastrointestinal Motility D isorders
AGMD International Corporate Headquarters
12 Roberts Drive   781-275-1300
Bedford, MA 01730   Fax: 781-275-1304
e-mail: digestive.motility@gmail.com
www.agmd-gimotility.org
A non-profit international organization which serves as an integral educational resource concerning digestive motility diseases and disorders. Also functions as an important information base for members of the medical and scientific communities. Also provides a forum for patients suffering from digestive motility diseases and disorders as well as their families and members of the medical, scientific, and nutritional communities.
Mary Angela DeGrazia-DiTucci, President/Patient/Founder

3640   Coconut Creek Eating Disorders Support Group
Renfrew Center
7700 NW 48th Avenue   954-698-9222
Coconut Creek, FL 33073-3508   877-367-3383
Fax: 954-698-9007
www.renfrew.org
Samuel Menagad, Director

3641   Eating Disorder Resource Center
330 W 58th Street   212-989-3987
New York, NY 10019   e-mail: info@edrcnyc.org
www.edrcnyc.org
A specialized treatment program for women and men who were suffering from bulimia. Now EDRC treats eating disorders of all kinds, offering individual, group, family and couples treatment for those challenged by bulimia, binge eating disorder, anorexia and other kinds of body dysmorphia.
Judith Brisman, Director & Founder
Senna Lauer, Marketing Assistant

3642   Eating Disorders Association of New Jersey
10 Station Place
Metuchen, NJ 08840   800-522-2230
Fax: 732-906-9307
e-mail: info@edanj.org
www.edanj.org
A non-profit state organization whose mission is to provide supportive services and resources to indivudals affected by eating disorders, including family members and friends.

3643   First Presbyterian Church in the City of New York Support Groups
First Presbyterian Church in the City of New York
12 West 12th Street   212-675-6150
New York, NY 10011   e-mail: fpcnyc@fpcnyc.org
www.fpcnyc.org
The First Presbyterian Church in the City of New York provides numerous programs and supports groups for both adults and children including an educational program for autistic children.
Jon M Walton, Senior Pastor
Sarah Segal Mccaslin, Associate Pastor

3644   Holliswood Hospital Psychiatric Care, Serv ices and Self-Help/Support Groups
87-37 Palermo Street   718-776-8181
Holliswood, NY 11423   800-486-3005
Fax: 718-776-8572
e-mail: HolliswoodInfo@libertymgt.com
www.holliswoodhospital.com/
The Holliswood Hospital, a 110-bed private psychiatric hospital located in a quiet residential Queens community, is a leader in providing quality, acute inpatient mental health care for adult, adolescent, geriatric and dually diagnosed patients. Holliswood Hospital treats patients with a broad range of psychiatric disorders. Additionally, specialized services are available for patients with psychiatric diagnoses compounded by chemical dependency, or a history of physical or sexual abuse.
Susan Clayton, Support Group Coordinator
Angela Hurtado, Support Group Coordinator

3645   National Health Information Center
PO Box 1133   310-565-4167
Washington, DC 20013   800-336-4797
Fax: 301-984-4256
e-mail: info@nhic.org
www.health.gov/nhic
A health information referral service sponsored by the Office of Disease Prevention and Health Promotion. Puts health professionals and condumers who have health questions in touch with those organizations that are best able to provide answers.

3646   Pediatric/Adolescent Gastroesophageal Reflux Association
PO Box 7728   301-601-9541
Silver Spring, MD 20901   888-887-7729
e-mail: gergroup@aol.com
www.reflux.org
Provides information and support to parents, patients and doctors about Gastroesophageal Reflux.
Beth Anderson, Director

3647 Richmond Support Group
Warwick Medical & Professional Ctr
Richmond, VA
804-320-7881

Books

3648 Anorexia Nervosa & Recovery: A Hunger for Meaning
The Haworth Press
One Haworth Center
Holland, MI 49423
616-393-3000
800-344-2600
e-mail: getinfo@haworth.com
www.haworth.com

1993 146 pages Paperback
ISBN: 0-918393-95-7

3649 Bearly Any Fat Cookbook
Obesity Foundation
8757 Georgia Avenue
Silver Spring, MD 20910-2202
301-563-6526
301-563-6595
e-mail: editor@obesity.org
www.obesity.org
Perfect cookbook to assist anyone in a weight reduction program.
Francesca M. Dea, Executive Director
Kathie Cleary, Senior Director, Finance

3650 Body Betrayed
American Psychiatric Press
1400 K Street NW
Washington, DC 20005-2403
202-682-6268
Fax: 202-789-2648
A book concentrating on women, eating disorders and treatments.
440 pages Hardcover
ISBN: 0-880485-22-1

3651 Bulimia: A Guide to Recovery
Gurze Books
PO Box 2238
Carlsbad, CA 92018-9883
800-756-7533
Fax: 760-434-5476
e-mail: gzcatl@aol.com
www.bulimia.com
This intimate guidebook offers a complete understanding of bulimia and a plan for recovery. It includes a two-week program to stop bingeing, things-to-do instead of bingeing, a two-week guide for support groups, specific advice for loved ones and Eating Without Fear, Hall's story of self-cure which has inspired thousands of other bulimics.
280 pages Paperback
ISBN: 0-936077-31-X

3652 Conversations with Anorexics
Jason Aronson
P.O. Box 15556
Amsterdam, NL -7100
800-782-0015
Fax: 201-840-7242
e-mail: mail@aronson.com
www.aronson.com
A Compassionate and Hopeful Journey through the Therapeutic Process.
238 pages
ISBN: 1-568212-61-5
Robert D. Aronson, Director
Lisa Rooimans, Assistant

3653 Coping with Eating Disorders
Rosen Publishing Group
29 E 21st Street
New York, NY 10010
212-777-3017
800-237-9932
Fax: 888-436-4643
e-mail: customerservice@rosenpub.com
www.rosenpublishing.com
This book offers practical suggestions on coping with eating disorders.
ISBN: 0-823929-74-4
Barbara Moe, Author

3654 Cult of Thinness
Oxford University Press

2001 Evans Road
Cary, NC 27513-2010
212-726-6000
800-451-7556
Fax: 919-677-1303
www.oup-usa.org
1996 256 pages
ISBN: 0-195082-41-9

3655 Deadly Diet: Recovering from Anorexia & Bulimia
New Harbinger Publications
5674 Shattuck Avenue
Oakland, CA 94609-1662
800-748-6273
Fax: 510-652-5472
e-mail: customerservice@newharbinger.com
www.newharbinger.com
1993 265 pages Paperback
ISBN: 1-879237-42-3

3656 Eating Diorders Resource Catalogue
Gurze Books
PO Box 2238
Carlsbad, CA 92018-9883
800-756-7533
Fax: 760-434-5476
www.bulimia.com
This catalogue of resources contains over 140 books, videos and audiotapes, lists of national organizations and treatment facilities and basic facts about eating disorders. It is widely distributed by individuals who are suffering, their loved ones, the health care professionals who treat them and educators who are working towards prevention.
24 pages Annual

3657 Eating Disorder Sourcebook
Gurze Books
PO Box 2238
Carlsbad, CA 92018-2238
800-756-7533
Fax: 760-434-5476
e-mail: gzcatl@aol.com
www.bulimia.com
An ideal book for someone with a loved one who has an eating disorder but who knows little about this subject, this new release presents a clear overview of basic issues.
222 pages Paperback

3658 Eating Disorders Resource Catalogue
Gurze Books
PO Box 2238
Carlsbad, CA 92018-9883
800-756-7533
Fax: 760-434-5476
www.bulimia.com
This catalogue of resources contains over 140 books, videos and audiotapes, lists of national organizations and treatment facilities and basic facts about eating disorders. It is widely distributed by individuals who are suffering, their loved ones, the health care professionals who treat them and educators who are working towards prevention.
28 pages Annual

3659 Eating Disorders-Overview Series
Lucent Books
Thomson Gale
Farmington Hills, MI 48331-9187
800-877-4253
Fax: 800-414-5043
e-mail: gale.customerservice@thomson.com
www.gale.com/lucent
This book examines how eating disorders can be identified, who is affected by them, and how they can be treated.
2001
ISBN: 1-560066-59-8

3660 Eating Disorders: When Food Turns Against You
Franklin Watts Grolier
90 Old Sherman Tpke
Danbury, CT 06816-0001
203-797-3500
Fax: 203-797-3197
www.grolier.com
1993 96 pages
ISBN: 0-531111-75-0

3661 Emotional Eating: A Practical Guide to Taking Control
Free Press

1230 Ave of the Americas
New York, NY 10020

800-223-7445
Fax: 800-943-9831
e-mail: info@simonsays.com
www.simonsays.com

1003 200 pages
ISBN: 0-029002-15-0

3662 Encyclopedia of Obesity and Eating Disorders
Facts on File
132 West 31st Street   212-967-8800
New York, NY 10001   800-322-8755
                               Fax: 800-678-3633
e-mail: custserv@factsonfile.com
www.infobasepublishing.com
From abdominoplasty to Zung Rating Scale, this volume defines and explains these disorders, along with medical and other problems associated with them.
272 pages Hardcover

3663 Endorphins: Eating Disorders & Other Addictive Behavior
WW Norton & Company
500 5th Avenue   212-354-5500
New York, NY 10110-0054   800-233-4830
                               Fax: 212-869-0856
www.wwnorton.com

1993 320 pages
ISBN: 0-393701-56-5

3664 Etiology and Treatment of Bulimia Nervosa
Jason Aronson
P.O.Box 15556
Amsterdam, NB 1001-7100   800-782-0015
                               Fax: 201-767-1576
www.aronson.com

352 pages Softcover
ISBN: 1-568213-39-5

3665 Evaluation and Management of Eating Disorders
Human Kinetics Publishers
8600 Rockville Pike   217-351-1549
Bethesda, MD 20894-5076   800-747-4457
                               Fax: 217-351-5076
www.ncbi.nlm.nih.gov

368 pages Cloth
ISBN: 0-873229-11-8

3666 Fear of Being Fat
Jason Aronson
P.O.Box 15556
Amsterdam, NB 1001-7100   800-782-0015
                               Fax: 201-840-7242
www.aronson.com

366 pages
ISBN: 0-876688-99-7

3667 Getting Better Bit(e) by Bit(e)
Gurze Books
PO Box 2238
Carlsbad, CA 92018-2238   800-756-7533
                               Fax: 760-434-5476
e-mail: gzcatl@aol.com
www.bulimia.com
This practical book on recovery from bulimia and binge eating is packed with lists, exercises, case studies, discussions, insights and specific things to do. This book also addresses the day-to-day problems faced by eating disorder sufferers and concentrates on key behavior changes necessary for progress.
143 pages Paperback

3668 Going Backwards
Scholastic
730 Broadway   212-505-3000
New York, NY 10003-9511   800-325-6149
www.thesaurus.com
A story that weaves the themes of acceptance, death, mortality and family loyalty to present a controversial plot.
Grades 7-10
Michele Turner, CEO
Jim Conning, SVP of Engineering

3669 Golden Cage: The Enigma of Anorexia Nervosa
Gurze Books
PO Box 2283
Carlsbad, CA 92018-2283   800-756-7533
                               Fax: 760-434-5476
e-mail: gzcatl@aol.com
www.bulimia.com

3670 Group Psychotherapy for Eating Disorders
American Psychiatric Press
PO Box 1295   202-682-6268
Pekin, IL 61555-2403   800-800-8126
                               Fax: 202-789-2648
e-mail: info@eatingdisordersreview.com
eatingdisordersreview.com
The first book to fully explore the use of group therapy in the treatment of eating disorders.
353 pages Hardcover
ISBN: 0-880484-19-5

3671 Helping Athletes with Eating Disorders
Human Kinetics Publishers
165 West 46th Street   212-575-6200
New York, NY 10036-5076   800-931-2237
                               Fax: 212-575-1650
https://www.nationaleatingdisorders.org
Gives readers the information they need to identify and address major eating disorders such as: anorexia, bulimia nervosa, and eating disorders not otherwise specified.
208 pages Cloth
ISBN: 0-873223-83-7
Ric Clark, Chair
Mary Curran, Vice-Chair

3672 Hope and Recovery: A Mother-Daughter Story About Anorexia Nervosa & Bulimia
Franklin Watts Grolier
65 West 36th St.
New York, NY 10018-0001   800-621-1115
                               Fax: 800-374-4329
www.kirkusreviews.com/
Mother and daughter tell a story of a young woman's recovery from the horror of an eating disorder. This compelling account shows how anorexia and bulimia can affect an entire family.
192 pages
ISBN: 0-531111-40-7
Herb Simon, Chairman
Marc Winkelman, President and Publisher

3673 Hungry Self: Women, Eating and Identity
Gurze Books
PO Box 2283
Carlsbad, CA 92018-2283   800-756-7533
                               Fax: 760-434-5476
e-mail: gzcatl@aol.com
www.bulimia.com

3674 Insights in the Dynamic Psychotherapy of Anorexia and Bulimia
Jason Aronson
P.O.Box 15556   646-415-2561
Amsterdam, NB 1001-1523   800-782-0015
                               Fax: 201-840-7242
www.aronson.com

320 pages Hardcover
ISBN: 0-876685-68-8
Robert D. Aronson, Director
Lisa Rooimans, Assistant

3675 It's Not Your Fault
Gurze Books
PO Box 2238
Carlsbad, CA 92018-2238   800-756-5476
                               Fax: 760-434-5476
e-mail: gzcatl@aol.com
www.bulimia.com
In this comprehensive, medically sound guide to overcoming eating disorders, Dr. Marx defines the warnings signs of eating disorders, explores causes, at risk populations, the role of drug therapy and advises patients and families where and how they can find help.

3676   Making Peace with Food
Gurze Books
PO Box 2238
Carlsbad, CA 92018-2238   800-756-7533
                                    Fax: 760-434-5476
                              e-mail: gzcatl@aol.com
                                    www.bulimia.com
This unique, full sized workbook is designed to help anyone who
experienced compulsive eating, yo-yo dieting, food and body anxiety, or associated eating disorders. Filled with ideas, workbook
pages, exercises and resources, Kano's book is an excellent aid to
clarifying and overcoming your personal diet/weight struggle.
224 pages Paperback

3677   Meals Without Squeals Sense
Bull Publishing
PO Box 1377   303-545-6350
Boulder, CO 80306   800-676-2855
                                    Fax: 303-545-6354
                                    www.bullpub.com
Straight forward information on childrens growth accompanies
age specific, child tested recipes. Explained is how common feed-
ing problems can be solved and show ways to offer children posi-
tive experiences with food.
2006 288 pages
ISBN: 1-933503-00-4
Emily Sewell, CFO
Claire Cameron, Director of Marketing

3678   My Name is Caroline
Doubleday
666 Fifth Avenue   212-354-6500
New York, NY 10103
A poignant tale of one woman's battle with bulimia throughout her
life as a successful student, athlete, scholar and musician.
Grades 10-12

3679   Obesity: Theory and Therapy
Raven Press
8600 Rockville Pike   212-930-9500
Bethesda, MD 20894-2601   800-777-2295
                                    www.ncbi.nlm.nih.gov
A classic reference for clinicians dealing with obesity, this volume
provides the most up-to-date research, preclinical and clinical
information.
500 pages
ISBN: 0-881678-84-8

3680   Practice Guidelines for Eating Disorders
American Psychiatric Press
1000 Wilson Boulevard   202-682-6268
Arlington, VA 22209-2403   Fax: 202-789-2648
                         e-mail: psychiatryonline@psych.org
                                    psychiatryonline.org
Designed for health care professionals, this guideline includes information on all aspects of anorexia nervosa and bulimia nervosa,
including self-induced vomiting, use of laxatives and vigorous exercise to prevent weight gain.
38 pages Paperback
ISBN: 0-890423-00-8

**3681   Psychodynamic Technique in the Treatment of the Eating
Disorders**
Jason Aronson
P.O.Box 15556   646-415-2561
Amsterdam, NB 1001-7100   800-782-0015
                                    Fax: 201-840-7242
                              e-mail: mail@aronson.com
                                    www.aronson.com

440 pages Hardcover
ISBN: 0-876686-22-6
Robert D. Aronson, Director
Lisa Rooimans, Assistant

3682   Self-Starvation
Jason Aronson

P.O.Box 15556   646-415-2561
Amsterdam, NB 1001-7100   800-782-0015
                                    Fax: 201-840-7242
                              e-mail: mail@aronson.com
                                    www.aronson.com
312 pages Softcover
ISBN: 1-568218-22-2
Robert D. Aronson, Director
Lisa Rooimans, Assistant

3683   Starving to Death in a Sea of Objects
Jason Aronson
P.O.Box 15556   646-415-2561
Amsterdam, NB 1001-7100   800-782-0015
                                    Fax: 201-840-7242
                              e-mail: mail@aronson.com
                                    www.aronson.com
How emancipation becomes security for anorexics.
464 pages Softcover
ISBN: 0-876684-35-5
Robert D. Aronson, Director
Lisa Rooimans, Assistant

3684   Surviving an Eating Disorder: Perspectives & Strategies
Gurze Books
PO Box 2238
Carlsbad, CA 92018-2238   800-756-7533
                                    Fax: 760-434-5476
                              e-mail: gzcatl@aol.com
                                    www.bulimia.com
Parents, spouses and friends of individuals with food problems
will find practical guidelines in this book for helping themselves
and their loved ones.
222 pages Paperback

3685   Treating Bulimia: A Psychoeducational Approach
American Anorexia/Bulimia Association
165 W 46th Street   212-575-6200
New York, NY 10036-2501   e-mail: amanbu@aol.com
                                    lifestream.aol.com

3686   When Food is Love
Gurze Books
PO Box 2238   760-434-7533
Carlsbad, CA 92018-2238   800-756-7533
                                    Fax: 760-434-5467
                              e-mail: gzcatl@aol.com
                                    www.gurze.com
Drawing on her own personal experience, Roth explores similarities between eating and loving such as fantasizing, wanting the for-
bidden, creating drama, control issues, and the experience of
relationship.
205 pages Paperback

3687   Withering Child
University of Georgia Press
320 South Jackson Street
Athens, GA 30602   404-542-2830
                                        800-266-5842
                                    Fax: 706-542-2558
                         e-mail: books@ugapress.uga.edu
                                    www.uga.edu/ugapress

1993 288 pages
ISBN: 0-820315-60-5
Lisa Bayer, Director
Chantel Dunham, Director of Development

Children's Books

3688   Billy's Story
Metro Intergroup of Overeaters Anonymous
117 W 26th Street
New York, NY 10001   212-206-8621
                                    www.billysstory.com

3689   I Was a Fifteen-Year-Old Blimp
Harper & Row
10 E 53rd Street   212-207-7000
New York, NY 10022-5299

This story focuses on Gabby, a teenage girl who overhears others discuss her weight and takes radical steps to become popular.
Grades 6-9

Magazines

3690 BASH Magazine
Bulimia Anorexia Self-Help/Behavior Adaptation
PO Box 39903
Saint Louis, MO 63139-8903   800-762-3334
A journal of eating and mood disorders.
Monthly

Newsletters

3691 AABA Newsletter
American Anorexic and Bulemic Association
905 S. Fillmore   806-345-6300
Amarillo, TX 79105-2501   Fax: 806-345-6363
                                          e-mail: firm@bf-law.com
                                               www.bf-law.com
This newsletter is published three times a year and is mailed to the members of the AABA. The AABA is a tax-exempt, nonprofit organization with a membership of professionals, sufferers of eating disorders, and their family and friends.

3692 Eating Disorders Review
Gurze Books
PO Box 2238
Carlsbad, CA 92018-9883   800-756-7533
                                          Fax: 760-434-5476
                                          e-mail: gzcatl@aol.com
                                               www.bulimia.com
Presents current clinical information for the professional treating eating disorders. Features summeries of relevant research from journals and unpublished studies, abstracts, nutritional notes, questions and answers, book reviews and reproducible client handouts.
8 pages BiMonthly
Joel Yager MD, Editor-in-Chief
Liegh Cohn, Publisher

3693 National Association of Anorexia Nervosa and Associated Disorders Newsletter
750 E Diehl Road   630-577-1330
Naperville, IL 60563   Fax: 847-433-4632
                                          e-mail: anadhelp@anad.org
                                               www.anad.org
2 pages Quarterly
Vivian Hansen Meehan, President
Dawn Ries, Administrator

3694 WIN Notes
Weight-control Information Network
1 WIN Way   202-828-1025
Bethesda, MD 20892-3665   877-946-4627
                                          Fax: 202-828-1028
                                  e-mail: win@mathewsgroup.com
                              www.niddk.nih.gov/health/nutrit/win.htm
Addresses the health information needs of individuals with weight-control problems. Available on the WIN web site.
BiAnnual
Griffin P. Rodgers, Director

3695 Working Together
Anorexia Nervosa and Associated Disorders
PO Box 7   847-831-3438
Highland Park, IL 60035-0007   Fax: 847-433-4632
                                               www.thesaurus.com
Designed for individuals, families, group leaders and professionals concerned with eating disorders. Provides updates on treatments, resources, conferences, programs, articles by therapists, recovered victims, group members and leaders.
Quarterly
Michele Turner, CEO
Jim Conning, SVP of Engineering

Pamphlets

3696 Applying New Attitudes & Directions
Anorexia Nervosa and Associated Disorders
PO Box 7   847-831-3438
Highland Park, IL 60035-0007   Fax: 847-433-4632
                                          e-mail: anad20@aol.com
Self-help booklet offering an eight-step program to recovery with suggestions, information and recovery stories.
Dawn Ries, Administrator

Audio & Video

3697 Bulimia: A Guide to Recovery
Gurze Books
PO Box 2238
Carlsbad, CA 92018-2238   800-756-7533
                                          Fax: 760-434-5476
                                          e-mail: gzcatl@aol.com
                                               www.bulimia.com
This newly rediscovered tape is an inspirational talk by Lindsey Hall on the relationship between bulimia, self-esteem and love. This was one of Lindsey's last public appearances, where she addressed a 1991 eating disorers conference in Colorado Springs.
Audio tape

Web Sites

3698 Anorexia Nervosa & Related Eating Disorders
                                               www.anred.com
A nonprofit organization that provides information about anorexia nervosa, bulimia nervosa, binge eating disorder, and other less-well-known food and weight disorders.

3699 GERD Information Resource Center
                                               www.gerd.com
A resource center with educational resources on Gastroesophageal Reflux Disease (GERD).

3700 Gastroenterology Therapy Online
                                          www.gastrotherapy.com
An informational website with resources for many kinds of diseases.

3701 Healing Well
                                          www.healingwell.com
An online health resource guide to medical news, chat, information and articles, newsgroups and message boards, books, disease-related web sites, medical directories, and more for patients, friends, and family coping with disabling diseases, disorders, or chronic illnesses.

3702 Health Finder
                                          www.healthfinder.gov
Searchable, carefully developed web site offering information on over 1000 topics. Developed by the US Department of Health and Human Services, the site can be used in both English and Spanish.

3703 Healthlink USA
                                          www.healthlinkusa.com
Health information concerning treatment, cures, prevention, diagnosis, risk factors, research, support groups, email lists, personal stories and much more. Updated regularly.

3704 Helios Health
                                          www.helioshealth.com
Online resource for your health information. Detailed information about specific health topics, access to expert advice from our Medical Advisory Board, and up-to-date health news.

3705 MedicineNet
                                          www.medicinenet.com
An online resource for consumers providing easy-to-read, authoritative medical and health information.

3706 Medscape
                                          www.medscape.com

Medscape offers specialists, primary care physicians, and other health professionals the Web's most robust and integrated medical information and educational tools.

3707   National Association for Anorexia Nervosa and Associated Disorders

www.anad.org

ANAD provides educational/prevention programs include presentations and early detection packets for schools and community groups, sponsoring local and national training conferences for health professionals, and working with electronic and print media. Undertakes and encourages research, fights insurance discrimination.

3708   National Eating Disorders Association

www.NationalEatingDisorders.org

National nonprofit organization dedicated to increasing the awareness and prevention of eating disorders.

3709   WebMD

www.webmd.com

Provides credible information, supportive communities, and in-depth reference material about health subjects. A source for original and timely health information as well as material from well known content providers.

3710   Weight-control Information Network

www.niddk.nih.gov

The Weight-control Information Network (WIN) was established in 1994 to provide the general public, health professionals, and the media with up-to-date, science-based information on obesity, weight control, physical activity, and related nutritional issues. WIN provides tip sheets, fact sheets, and brochures for a range of audiences. Some of WIN's content is available in Spanish.

Description

3711 Endometriosis

Endometriosis is a hormonal condition in which the tissue that normally lines the inside of the uterus (endometrium) is also found outside the uterus, generally on the outer surface of pelvic organs. These cells respond to the woman's hormonal cycles, and swell and bleed at the time of menses. This causes pain, generally worse with each period, pelvic masses and alterations of the menstrual cycle. The pain may be aggravated by intercourse or defecation. Although the reported incidence varies, endometriosis is commonly found in 10 to 15 percent of women between the ages of 25 and 44 years. It is estimated that 25 to 50 percent of infertile women have this disorder.

Treatment depends on the severity of the symptoms and the age and reproductive wishes of the patient. The pain associated with mild cases may be treated with non-steroidal anti-inflammatory drugs. More severe cases may respond to suppression of ovarian function. Laparoscopic surgery may destroy some of the collection of tissue, and is often used in hopes of improving fertility. Hysterectomy (removal of the uterus) is used for intractable cases, especially in women who do not desire future pregnancy.

National Agencies & Associations

3712 American Association of Gynecologic Laproscopists
6757 Katella Avenue
Cypress, CA 90630-4505
714-503-6200
800-554-2245
Fax: 714-503-6201
e-mail: lmichels@aagl.org
www.aagl.com

Our global commitment to women's healthcare is embodied in our continuing medical education of physicians and professionals to further promote the well documented high standards of minimally invasive gynecologic surgery.
Linda Michels, Executive Director
Franklin D Loffer, EVP/Medical Director

3713 American Society for Reproductive Medicine
1209 Montgomery Highway
Birmingham, AL 35216-2809
205-978-5000
Fax: 205-978-5005
e-mail: asrm@asrm.com
www.asrm.com

A private, nonprofit medical organization devoted to advancing the knowledge, understanding and expertise in all phases of reproductive medicine and biology. Offers patient education brochures, recommended readings and support. Publishes professional journal and consumer publications.
Robert W Rebar, MD, Executive Director
Andrew LaBarbera, Scientific Director

3714 Endometriosis Association
630 Ibis Drive
Delray Beach, FL 33444
561-274-7442
800-239-7280
Fax: 561-274-0931
e-mail: exec-comm@endocenter.org
www.endocenter.org

Nonprofit international organization dedicated to helping women and girls suffering from endometriosis. Services include chapter and support groups, crisis/counseling assistance, education of the public and medical community materials including books and videos.
Ann Koerner, Operations Manager

3715 Endometriosis Association International
8585 N 76th Place
Milwaukee, WI 53223
414-355-2200
800-992-3636
Fax: 414-355-6065
www.endometriosisassn.org

Offers a 24 hour crisis call hotline, support groups, education in the form of literature including fact sheets, brochures, newsletters, articles educational videos, books and research.
Mary Lou Ballweg, President/Executive Director
Carolyn Keith, Co-Founder

3716 Hysterectomy Educational Resources & Services (HERS) Foundation
422 Bryn Mawr Avenue
Bala Cynwyd, PA 19004
610-667-7757
888-750-4377
Fax: 610-677-8096
e-mail: hersfdn@earthlink.net
www.hersfoundation.com

A nonprofit foundation which provides information about the alternatives to hysterectomy, the risks of the alternatives, and the consequences of the surgery. HERS provides telephone counseling by appointment for a fee of $5.00 per quarter hour. The fee can be waived if necessary. HERS also provides copies of a medical journals, a quarterly newsletter, and a free lending library of books, videos and audio tapes.

3717 International Pelvic Pain Society Women's Medical Plaza
Women's Medical Plaza
1100 E Woodfield Road
Schaumburg, IL 60173
847-517-8712
800-624-9676
Fax: 847-517-7229
e-mail: info@pelvicpain.org
www.pelvicpain.org

Short range goal is to recruit organize and educate health care professionals actively involved with the treatment of patients who have chronic pelvic pain.
Fred Marion Howard, Chairman of the Board
Howard Taylo Sharp, President

3718 National Women's Health Network
1413 K Street
Washington, DC 20005
202-682-2640
Fax: 202-682-2648
e-mail: nwhn@nwhn.org
www.womenshealthnetwork.org

Nonprofit organization that does not accept financial support from pharmaceutical or tobacco companies or medical device manufacturers. Advocates for national policies that protect and promote all women's health and provides evidence-based independent information.
Bindiya Patel, Chairperson
Malika Redmond, Action Vice Chair

Foundations

3719 Fertility Research Foundation
877 Park Avenue
New York, NY 10021
212-744-5500
888-439-2999
Fax: 212-744-6536
e-mail: info@frfbaby.com
www.frfbaby.com

Offers information on treatment and the latest research on male and female infertility.
Masood Khatamee MD, Executive Director

Libraries & Resource Centers

3720 National Womens Health Resource Center
157 Broad Street
Red Bank, NJ 07701
877-986-9472
Fax: 732-249-4671
e-mail: info@healthywomen.org
www.healthywomen.org

The not-for-profit National Women's Health Resource Center (NWHRC) is the leading independent health information source for women. NWHRC develops and distributes up-to-date and objective women's health information based on the latest advances in medical research and practice.

Elizabeth Battaglino Cahill, Executive Vice President
Amber McCracken, Director Communications

Research Centers

3721   Dartmouth Medical School: Microbiology Department
Department of Microbiology & Immunology
1 Rope Ferry Road   603-650-1200
Hanover, NH 03755-1404   877-DMS-1797
                                     Fax: 603-650-1202
                        e-mail: microbiology@dartmouth.edu
                                    www.dms.dartmouth.edu
Dartmouth Medical School is a beacon of discovery and learning stimulating inquiry and harnessing ingenuity for new solutions and better health
Ann Hill, Administrative Assistant
Gregory J MacDonald, Assistant Professor of Medicine

3722   Endometriosis Association Research Program : Vanderbuilt University
1211 Medical Center Drive   615-322-5000
Nashville, TN 37232   Fax: 615-343-8881
                                    www.mc.vanderbilt.edu
Heather Arnold, Senior Secretary

3723   Endometriosis Reseach Center and Women's Hospital
The Endometriosis Research Center
630 Ibis Drive   561-274-7442
Delray Beach, FL 33444   800-239-7280
                                     Fax: 561-274-0931
                                       www.endocenter.org
A nonprofit organization dedicated to establishing a center to conduct research and provide women education and treatment.
Ann Koerner, Operations Manager

3724   University of Tennessee: Division of Reproductive Endocrinology
956 Court Avenue
Memphis, TN 38163   901-528-5859
                        www.utmem.edu/obgyn/reproductive.htm
Studies into endometriosis.
Dr. Jon Buster, Chief
Kennard Brown, Executive Vice Chancellor & Chief Operat

Support Groups & Hotlines

3725   National Health Information Center
PO Box 1133   310-565-4167
Washington, DC 20013   800-336-4797
                                     Fax: 301-984-4256
                                    e-mail: info@nhic.org
                                      www.health.gov/nhic
A helath information referral service sponsored by the Office of Disease Prevention and Health Promotion. Puts health professionals and consumers who have health questions in touch with those organizations that are best able to provide answers.

3726   RESOLVE Helpline
1760 Old Meadow Road   703-556-7172
McLean, VA 22102   Fax: 703-506-3266
                                         www.resolve.org
A nationwide network mandated to promote reproductive health and to ensure equal access to all family building options for men and women experienceing infertility or other reproductive disorders.
Barbara Collura, President/ CEO
Margaret Cha Berardelli, Director

Books

3727   Alternatives for Women with Endometriosis Guide by Women for Women
Third Side Press

3 Marina Road   773-271-3029
Yarmouth, MA 04096-1863   Fax: 773-271-0459
                                   e-mail: thirdside@aol.com
                                    www.womentowomen.com
174 pages
ISBN: 1-879427-12-5

3728   Coping with Endometriosis
Avery Putnam Penguin
375 Hudson Street   212-366-2000
New York, NY 10014   800-847-5515
                                     Fax: 800-775-4829
                        e-mail: online@penguinputnam.com
                                    www.penguinputnam.com
Educates readers about the disease, focusing on the particular psychological and emotional concerns that those suffering from endometriosis may have.
322 pages
ISBN: 1-583330-74-7

3729   Endometriosis Sourcebook
Endometriosis Association
8585 N 76th Place   414-355-2200
Milwaukee, WI 53223   800-992-3636
                                     Fax: 414-355-6065
                        e-mail: endo@endometriosisassn.org
                                   www.EndometriosisAssn.org
Comprehensive, authorative and up-to-date resource that includes information about treatment options, strategies for coping with the disease and its effects on you and those around you.
473 pages Paperback
ISBN: 0-809232-63-4
Mary Lou Ballweg, Founder/Executive Director

3730   Endometriosis and Infertility and Traditio nal Chinese Medicine
Blue Poppy Press
1990 57th Court N.   303-447-8372
Boulder, CO 80301   800-487-9296
                                     Fax: 303-245-8362
                        e-mail: honora@bluepoppy.com
                                   www.bluepoppy.com/press
An easy to understand guide to Chinese medicine as it relates to endometriosis and infertility.
105 pages Paperback
ISBN: 0-936185-14-7
Honora Wolfe, Marketing Director

3731   Endometriosis: A Key to Healing through Nutrition
Endometriosis Association
8585 N 76th Place   414-355-2200
Milwaukee, WI 53223   800-992-3636
                                     Fax: 414-355-6065
                        e-mail: endo@endometriosisassn.org
                                   www.endometriosisassn.org
An excellent resource tool to help patients begin making changes in their diets.
Mary Lou Ballweg, Founder/Executive Director

3732   Endometriosis: A Natural Approach
Ulysses Press
PO Box 3440   510-601-8301
Berkeley, CA 94703   800-377-2542
                                     Fax: 510-601-8307
                        e-mail: ulysses@ulyssespress.com
                                      www.ulyssespress.com
This is a solid resource, written in a clear, basic tone, for anyone who needs information about the widespread disease known as endometriosis. Chapters cover all aspects of endometriosis, from what it is and what causes it, to diagnosis, natural therapies, and conventional treatments.
120 pages
ISBN: 1-569750-88-2
Ray Riegert, Publisher
Leslie Henriques, Co-Publisher

3733   Endometriosis: Advanced Management and Surgical Techniques
Springer Verlag

175 5th Avenue
New York, NY 10010

212-460-1500
800-777-4643
Fax: 212-473-6272
e-mail: service@springer-ny.com
www.springer-ny.com

This book provides a practical, clinical, and thorough examination of both the medical and surgical treatment of this disease.
Derk Haank, CEO
Martin Mos, COO

3734   Endometriosis: Complete Reference for Taking Charge of Your Health
Contemporary Books/McGraw-Hill Companies
8585 N. 76th Place
Milwaukee, WI 53223

414-355-2200
Fax: 414-355-6065
www.endometriosisassn.org

An authoritative guide on endometriosis, including its prevention and relationship with other diseases. Special sections are dedicated to endo and menopause, endo and teenagers, endo and nutrition, endo and cancer as well as endo and environmental toxins.

Newsletters

3735   Endometriosis Association Newsletter
Endometriosis Association
8585 N 76th Place
Milwaukee, WI 53223

414-355-2200
800-992-3636
Fax: 414-355-6065
e-mail: endo@EndometriosisAssn.org
www.EndometriosisAssn.org

Contains research updates and latest health news that affects women and girls with endometriosis. Regular features such as crisis call helpers, news and announcements, and request for contact provide networking and support assistance.
10 pages Bi-Monthly
Mary Lou Ballweg, Executive Director

Pamphlets

3736   Infertility: Causes and Treatment
American College/Obstetricians and Gynecologists
409 12th Street SW
Washington, DC 20024

202-638-5577
800-673-8444
Fax: 304-728-2171
www.acog.com

To obtain a free copy of this publication, please send a self-addressed stamped #10 envelope and request by title.

Audio & Video

3737   Monroe Institute Surgical Support Tapes
Endometriosis Association
8585 N 76th Place
Milwaukee, WI 53223-2633

414-355-2200
800-992-3636
Fax: 414-355-6065
e-mail: endo@endometriosisassn.org
www.EndometriosisAssn.org

Anxiety is normal for women before surgery, so women with endometriosis will be happy to hear this wonderful series of audiotapes specifically developed for relaxation.
Audiotape
Mary Lou Ballweg, Founder/Executive Director

Web Sites

3738   American Society for Reproductive Medicine
www.asrm.com
Devoted to advancing the knowledge, understanding and expertise in all phases of reproductive medicine and biology. Offers patient education brochures, recommended readings and support.

3739   Endometriosis Association
www.EndometriosisAssn.org
Nonprofit organization dedicated to helping women and girls suffering from endometriosis. Services include chapter and support groups, crisis/counseling assistance, education of the public and the medical community. Materials, including books, video/audiotapes, CDs, newsletters and articles mostly based on data from the Association's research registries and its extensive research program, including a flagship scientific team at Vanderbuilt University School of Medicine.

3740   Endometriosis Research Center
www.endocenter.org
Maintain and offer a vast database of unbased and fact-based materials on every aspect of Endometriosis to practitioners, researchers, patients and all those interested in the disease.

3741   Endometriosis Support Group
www.geocities.com/HotSprings/5422
Online support group and question forum for endometriosis.

3742   Healing Well
www.healingwell.com
An online health resource guide to medical news, chat, information and articles, newsgroups and message boards, books, disease-related web sites, medical directories, and more for patients, friends, and family coping with disabling diseases, disorders, or chronic illnesses.

3743   Health Finder
www.healthfinder.gov
Searchable, carefully developed web site offering information on over 1000 topics. Developed by the US Department of Health and Human Services, the site can be used in both English and Spanish.

3744   Healthlink USA
www.healthlinkusa.com
Health information concerning treatment, cures, prevention, diagnosis, risk factors, research, support groups, email lists, personal stories and much more. Updated regularly.

3745   Helios Health
www.helioshealth.com
Online resource for your health information. Detailed information about specific health topics, access to expert advice from our Medical Advisory Board, and up-to-date health news.

3746   International Pelvic Pain Society
www.pelvicpain.org/
Short range goal is to recruit, organize, and educate health care professionals actively involved with the treatment of patients who have chronic pelvic pain. They also work to bring hope to men and women who suffer from chronic pelvic pain by significantly raising public awareness and impacting individual lives.

3747   MedicineNet
www.medicinenet.com
An online resource for consumers providing easy-to-read, authoritative medical and health information.

3748   Medscape
www.medscape.com
Medscape offers specialists, primary care physicians, and other health professionals the Web's most robust and integrated medical information and educational tools.

3749   Universe of Women's Health
www.obgyn.net
A comprehensive website dedicated to women's health.

3750   WebMD
www.webmd.com
Provides credible information, supportive communities, and in-depth reference material about health subjects. A source for original and timely health information as well as material from well known content providers.

Description

3751 Fabry Disease

Fabry disease is an inherited fat storage disorder caused by deficiency of an enzyme involved in the biodegradation of lipids (fats). As abnormal storage of the fatty compound increases with time, blood vessels become narrowed, leading to decreased blood flow. The problem occurs in all blood vessels in the body, but affects in particular the skin, kidneys, heart, brain and nerves.

In children, Fabry begins with pain and burning sensations in hands and feet that is worse with exercise and hot weather. Other symptoms include a dark red rash around the waist, decreased ability to perspire and cloudiness of the cornea, which usually does not affect vision.

As those with Fabry's grow older, they may have impaired circulation, leading to early heart attacks and strokes. As kidneys become more involved, many patients require kidney transplants or dialysis. Gastrointestinal symptoms include frequent bowel movements shortly after eating. Patients with Fabry disease usually survive into adulthood but have a reduced life expectancy.

Currently, there is no cure for Fabry disease and treatment typically deals with controlling its symptoms. Pain in hands and feet respond to several medications. Gastrointestinal hyperactivity may be controlled by taking a nutritional supplement. Enzyme replacement therapy was given a dramatic boost in 2003 when the FDA approved a new synthetic enzyme. It is given intravenously and reduces lipid (fat) accumulation in many types of cells.

National Agencies & Associations

3752 Association for Neuro-Metabolic Disorders

3901 Rainbow Boulevard
Kansas City, KS 66160

913-588-5000
800-334-7980
TTY: 913-588-7963
e-mail: VOLK4OLKS@aol.com
www.kumc.edu

Serves as an advocate organization for families of patients with neuro-methabolic disorders such as phenylketonuria, maple syrup urine disease, galactosemia and biotinidase. Provides educational information for parents and children and provides networking.
Barbara F Atkinson MD, Executive Vice Chancellor

3753 Genetic and Rare Diseases Information Center

Genetic and Rare Diseases Informati
Gaithesburg, MD 20898-8126

301-251-4925
888-205-2311
Fax: 301-251-4911
TTY: 888-205-3223
e-mail: GARDinfo@nih.gov
www.rarediseases.info.nih.gov/GARD

Provides free and immediate access to accurate, reliable information about genetic and rare diseases. Also provides assistance to patients and families, health professionals and other interested parties.
Stephen C. Groft, Director
P.J. Brooks, Health Scientist Administrator

3754 International Center for Fabry Disease Mt. Sinai School of Medicine

Mt. Sinai School of Medicine
One Gustave L Levy Place
New York, NY 10029

212-241-6500
866-322-7963
e-mail: fabry.disease@mssm.edu
www.mssm.edu

Clinical research center attended by a staff of physicians and nurses specially trained to understand and meet the needs of individuals with Fabry disease. Services offered to both men and women of all ages include diagnosis, evaluation and treatment consultation.
Robert J Desnick PhD MD, Professor and Chair
Dennis Charney, Executive VP

3755 National Institute of Neurological Disorders and Stroke (NINDS)

NIH Neurological Institute
Bethesda, MD 20824

301-496-5751
800-352-9424
Fax: 301-496-0296
TTY: 301-468-5981
www.ninds.nih.gov

The mission of NINDS is to reduce the burden of neurological disease - a burden borne by every age group, by every segment of society, by people all over the world.
Story C Landis PhD, Director
Walter J Koroshetz, Deputy Director

3756 National Organization for Rare Disorders (NORD)

55 Kenosia Avenue
Danbury, CT 06813-1968

203-744-0100
800-999-6673
Fax: 203-798-2291
TDD: 203-797-9590
e-mail: orphan@rarediseases.org
www.rarediseases.org

The National Organization for Rare Disorders(NORD), a 501(c)3 organization, is a unique federation of voluntary health organizations dedicated to helping people with rare orphan diseases and assisting the organizations that serve them. NORD is committed to the identification, treatment, and cure of rare disorders through programs of education, advocacy, research, and service.
Frank Sasinowski, Chair
Carolyn Asbury, Vice Chair

3757 National Tay-Sachs and Allied Disease Association

2001 Beacon Street
Brighton, MA 02135

800-906-8723
800-906-8723
Fax: 617-277-0134
e-mail: info@ntsad.org
www.ntsad.org

A mutual support group coordinated by staff and volunteers who are parents of affected children of affected adults. One of several programs supported and sponsored by the association.
Bradley L Campbell, President
Stewart Altman, Vice President

Research Centers

3758 Lysosomal Disease Center at the University of Pittsburgh

E1650 Biomedical Science Tower
Pittsburgh, PA 15261

800-334-7980
pitt.edu

Offers diagnosis management treatment and genetic counseling for people with or at risk for lysosomal storage disease and their families.
John A Barrenger MD PhD, Director
Erin O'Rourk, Manager

3759 National Gaucher Disease Foundation

2227 Idlewood Road
Tucker, GA 30084

770-934-2910
800-504-3189
Fax: 770-934-2911
e-mail: rhonda@gaucherdisease.org
www.gaucherdisease.org

Provides information and assistance for those affected by Gaucher disease.
Rhonda P Buyers, CEO/Executive Director
Barbara Lichtenstein, Programs Director National Gaucher Care

Support Groups & Hotlines

3760 Fabry Support & Information Group
108 NE 2nd Street Suite C
Concordia, MO 64020
660-463-1355
Fax: 660-463-1356
e-mail: info@fabry.org
www.fabry.org
To raise awareness of Fabry disease and its symptoms. The website provides mutual self-help by linking patients and family members/caregivers. In this way they can support and encourage one another.
J Johnson, Founder

Web Sites

3761 A World of Genetic Societies
www.faseb.org/genetics
FASEB's Mission is to advance health and welfare by promoting progress and education in biological and biomedical sciences through service to member societies and collaborative advocacy.

3762 Alliance of Genetic Support Groups
www.geneticalliance.org
Genetic Alliance is a nonprofit health advocacy organizations. Its network includes more than 1,200 disease-specific advocacy organizations, as well as thousands of universities, private companies, government agencies, and public policy organizations. The network is a dynamic and growing open space for shared resources, creative tools, and innovative programs.

3763 Fabry Support & Information Group
www.fabry.org
Fabry Support & Information Group (FSIG) is a 501(c)(3) nonprofit organization. There mission is to raise awareness of Fabry disease and its symptoms. The FSIG website provides mutual self-help by linking patients and family members/caregivers. In this way they can support and encourage one another. An increased understanding of Fabry disease and emotional support may alleviate some of the burden associated with this rare disorder.

3764 Gene Clinics
www.genetests.org
GeneTests is a medical genetics information resource developed for physicians, genetic counselors, other healthcare providers and researchers.

3765 International Center for Fabry Disease
www.mountsinaifpa.org
The International Center for Fabry Disease at Icahn School of Medicine is dedicated to the diagnosis and treatment of Fabry disease. There comprehensive clinical and research program offers diagnostic testing, complete evaluations, consultations, and treatment, as well as counseling for couples at risk to have children with Fabry disease.

3766 International Storage Disease Collaborative
www.pediatrics.med.umn/edu/isdcsg/
This study group focuses on stem cell and bone marrow transplantation. Has discussion page/general information.

3767 MedicineNet
www.medicinenet.com
An online resource for consumers providing easy-to-read, authoritative medical and health information.

3768 Morbus Fabry
home.t-online.de
Fabry information and links to other sites.

3769 NIH's National Institute of Neurological Disorders & Strokes
www.ninds.nih.gov
The mission of NINDS is to seek fundamental knowledge about the brain and nervous system and to use that knowledge to reduce the burden of neurological disease.

3770 National Organization for Rare Disorders (NORD)
www.rarediseases.org
The NORD is a unique federation of voluntary health organizations dedicated to helping people with rare orphan diseases and assisting the organization that serve them.

3771 National Society of Genetic Counselors
nsgc.org
The National Society of Genetic Counselors (NSGC) promotes the professional interests of genetic counselors and provides a network for professional communication. Local and national continuing education opportunities and the discussion of all issues relevant to human genetics and the genetic counseling profession are an integral part of membership in NSGC.

3772 OMIM: Fabry Disease
omim.org/entry/301500
Description of disease and links to research papers written.

3773 Pediatric Database: Fabry Disease
www.icondata.com
Description of disease.

3774 Support-Group.Com: Fabry Disease
www.support-group.com
Fabry Disease discussion forum.

Description

3775 Fibromyalgia Syndrome

Fibromyalgia syndrome, FMS, also called fibrositis or fibromyositis, is a condition of widespread muscular pain and fatigue. It strikes mostly women between the ages of 20 and 50, and may affect as many as one in 20 adult females. The pain ranges from mild discomfort to complete disability and may vary from day to day. Physical over-exertion, changes in weather, drafty environments, stress, depression, and hormonal changes can all contribute to flare-ups in FMS symptoms.

In addition to widespread pain, FMS also causes a decreased sense of energy, disturbances of sleep, and varying degrees of anxiety and depression. Other medical conditions sometimes associated with fibromyalgia include tension headaches, migraine, irritable bowel syndrome, premenstrual tension syndrome, chronic fatigue syndrome, cold intolerance, and restless leg syndrome.

A physician's diagnosis of FMS is usually based on the following criteria: widespread musculoskeletal pain; tenderness at 11 or more of 18 specific tender points, which are exquisitely more tender than adjacent sites; and scans of the brain. Fibromyalgia may remit spontaneously with decreased stress but can recur at frequent intervals or become chronic.

There is currently no commonly accepted cure for this condition. Aspirin and other drugs used to treat musculoskeletal pain partially improve symptoms. Antidepressant drugs, taken in low doses, have been shown to provide restorative sleep. Patients may also benefit from regular aerobic exercises, local applications of heat, gentle massage and reduced stress in their lives. See also *Chronic Fatigue Syndrome*.

National Agencies & Associations

3776 American Fibromyalgia Syndrome Association
6380 East Tanque Verde 520-733-1570
Tucson, AZ 85715 Fax: 520-290-5550
e-mail: kthorson@afsafund.org
www.afsafund.org
Nonprofit organization whose primary mission is to seed research in FMS and CFS. We acknowledge that patient and physician education, public awareness and advocacy are all important ingredients in aiding the lives of people with FMS and CFS.
Kristen Thorson, President
Steve Thorson, VP

3777 FM-CFS Canada
99 Fifth Avenue
Ottawa, Ontario, K1S-5P5 www.fm-cfs.ca
Dedicated to advancing Fibromyalgia (FM) and Chronic Fatigue Syndrome (CFS) education, research and treatment.
Graham Mayes, President/Director
Ed Napke, VP/Director

3778 National Chronic Fatigue Syndrome and Fibromyalgia Association
PO Box 18426 816-737-1343
Kansas City, MO 64133 Fax: 816-524-6782
e-mail: information@ncfsfa.org
www.ncfsfa.org

Offering a support group, medical and patient information plus research.
Orvalene Prewitt, President

3779 National Chronic Fatigue Syndrome and Fibr
PO Box 18426 816-737-1343
Kansas City, MO 64133 Fax: 816-524-6782
e-mail: information@ncfsfa.org
www.ncfsfa.org
Offering a support group medical and patient information plus research.
Orvalene Prewitt, President

3780 National Fibromyalgia Association
2121 S Towne Centre Place 714-921-0150
Anaheim, CA 92806 Fax: 714-921-6920
e-mail: kfox@fmaware.org
www.fmaware.org
Develops and extends programs dedicated to improving the quality of life for people with Fibromyalgia by increasing the awareness of the public media government and medical communities. Supports an ongoing media presence and assist local support groups.
Lynne Matallana, Founder/President
Rae Marie Gleason, Executive Director

3781 National Fibromyalgia Partnership (NFP)
PO Box 160
Linden, VA 22642 866-725-4404
Fax: 866-666-2727
e-mail: mail@fmpartnership.org
www.fmpartnership.org
The NFP is a 501(c)(3) non-profit, membership organization which publishes medically accurate information on Fibromyalgia to patients, health care professionals and the public. Information and resources not listed in this volume are available in print and/or on the NFP Web site. It also provides support and start-up information to support groups.
Tamara K Liller, President & Director of Publications
Jacqueline M Yencha, Vice-President, Asst Dir of Publications

3782 National Hemophilia Foundation/Hemophilia and AIDS/HIV Network (HANDI)
116 W 32nd Street 212-328-3700
New York, NY 10001 Fax: 212-328-3777
www.hemophilia.org
Dedicated to the treatment and the cure of hemophilia AIDS and other blood related disorders. This foundation wished to improve the quality of life of all those affected through promotion and support of research education and other services.
Val Bias, CEO
Neil Frick, Vice President

3783 National ME/FM Action Network
National ME/FM Action Network 613-829-6667
Suite 512, K2H8V- 8V7 Fax: 613-829-8518
www.mefmaction.net
A non-profit organization dedicated to advancing the recognition and understanding of Myalgic Encephalomyelitis/Chronic Fatigue Syndrome (ME/CFS) and Fibromyalgia Syndrome (FMS) through education, advocacy, support, and research.
Lydia E. Neilson, Founder and Chief Executive Officer
Margaret Parlor, President

3784 Option Institute
2080 S Undermountain Road 413-229-2100
Sheffield, MA 01257 800-714-2779
Fax: 413-229-8931
e-mail: participantsupport@option.org
www.option.org
Self-defeating beliefs along with attitudes and judgments can lead to a host of physical and psychological challenges, including Fibromyalgia. The Option Institute offers programs designed to help you gain new perspectives on the attitudes and judgments that can hamper progress.
Barry Kaufman, Co-Founder
Samahria Lyt Kaufman, Co-Founder

Libraries & Resource Centers

3785 Fibromyalgia Resources Group
103 Sherwood Hill Road
Brewster, NY 10509
845-278-5944
Fax: 845-278-2641
e-mail: kindness@fibrobetsy.com
Personalized patient service searches and distributes information on patient recommended, fibromyalgia literate doctors world wide. Information packet is included with each doctor list emailed. Doctor recommendations are welcome.
Betsy Jacobson, President

Support Groups & Hotlines

3786 Fibromyalgia Network
PO Box 31750
Tucson, AZ 85751-1750
520-290-5508
800-853-2929
Fax: 520-290-5550
e-mail: inquiry@fmnetnews.com
www.fmnetnews.com
Provides individuals with ad-free, patient-focused information that can be use today.

3787 National Chronic Fatigue Syndrome and Fibromyalgia Association Support Group
PO Box 18426
Kansas City, MO 64133
816-737-1343
Fax: 816-524-6782
e-mail: information@ncfsfa.org
www.ncfsfa.org
To educate and inform the public about the nature and impact of Chronic Fatigue Syndrome and Fibromyalgia and related disorders.
Orvalene Prewitt, President

3788 National Health Information Center
PO Box 1133
Washington, DC 20013
310-565-4167
800-336-4797
Fax: 301-984-4256
e-mail: info@nhic.org
www.health.gov/nhic
A health information referral service sponsored by the Office of Disease Prevention and Health Promotion. Puts health professionals and consumers who have health questions in touch with those organizations that are best able to provide answers.

3789 Rocky Mountain CFIDS/FMS Association
7020 E Girard Avenue
Denver, CO 80224
303-423-7367
e-mail: link@rmcfa.org
www.rmcfa.org
An educational resource for patients, medical professionals and those affected by these diseases.
Tim Smith, President
Mike Munoz, Executive Director

Books

3790 All About Fibromyalgia
Oxford University Press
198 Madison Avenue
New York, NY 10016-4314
212-726-6033
800-451-7556
Fax: 212-726-6447
www.oup-usa.org

ISBN: 0-195147-53-7

3791 Delicate Balance: Living Successfully with Chronic Illness
Perseus Books Group
5500 Central Avenue
Boulder, CO 80301
800-386-5656
Fax: 303-449-3356
e-mail: info@perseuspublishing.com
www.perseuspublishing.com
Up to date and practical advice and inspiration for the millions of Americans who struggle daily against chronic illness. From locating a suitable healthcare provider and making sense of the powerful emotions that accompany chronic illness, to seeking accomodations from the Americans with Disabilities Act, this book is helpful and hopeful.
312 pages
ISBN: 0-738203-23-8

3792 Fibromyalgia
NAMSIC/National Institutes of Health
1 AMS Circle
Bethesda, MD 20892-0001
301-495-4484
877-226-4267
Fax: 301-718-6366
TTY: 301-565-2966
e-mail: niamsinfo@mail.nih.gov
www.nih.gov/niams

3793 Fibromyalgia & Other Central Pain Syndromes
Daniel Wallace, Daniel Clauw, author
Lippincott Williams & Wilkins
16522 Hunters Green Pkwy
Hagerstown, MD 21740-2116
301-223-2300
800-638-3030
Fax: 301-223-2400
e-mail: orders@lww.com
www.lww.com
Devoted to fibromyalgia and other centrally mediated chronic pain syndromes. Leading experts examine the latest research findings on these syndromes and present evidence-based reviews of current controversies.
2005
ISBN: 0-781752-61-2

3794 Fibromyalgia Guidelines: The Concensus Diagnosis & Treatment Protocols
FM-CFS Canada
16522 Hunters Green Pkwy
Hagerstown, MD 21740-5P5
301-223-2300
800-638-3030
Fax: 301-223-2400
e-mail: orders@lww.com
www.lww.com
This entire special issue of the Journal of Musculoskeletal Pain [JMP] is devoted to presentation of what will likely to be called the Canadian Consensus Document on Fibromyalgia Syndrome (FMS). The document encompasses a very broad scope, involving a clinical case definition, diagnosis, and management of FMS.
130 pages

3795 Fibromyalgia Relief Book: 213 Ideas for Improving Your Quality of Life
Walker & Company
435 Hudson Street
New York, NY 10014
212-727-8300
Fax: 212-727-0984
e-mail: orders@walkerbooks.com
www.walkerbooks.com

208 pages Paperback
ISBN: 0-802775-53-5
Josh Wood, Sales Director

3796 Fibromyalgia Supporter
Anadem Publishing Company
3620 N High Street
Columbus, OH 43214
800-633-0055
Fax: 614-262-6630
e-mail: anadem@anadem.com
www.anadem.com

3797 Fibromyalgia Survivor
Anadem Publishing Company
3620 N High Street
Columbus, OH 43214
800-633-0055
Fax: 614-262-6630
e-mail: anadem@anadem.com
www.anadem.com

ISBN: 0-964689-12-X

3798 Fibromyalgia Syndrome and Chronic Fatigue Syndrome in Young People
Fibromyalgia Network
PO Box 31750
Tucson, AZ 85751-1750
800-853-2929
Fax: 520-290-5550
www.fmnetnews.com

Guide for parents.
Kristin Thorson, Editor

3799 Fibromyalgia and Chronic Myofascial Pain Syndrome: a Survivor Manual
New Harbinger Publishers
5674 Shattuck Avenue
Oakland, CA 94609
800-748-6273
Fax: 510-652-5472
e-mail: customerservice@newharbinger.com
www.newharbinger.com
Written from the perspective of myofacial pain syndrome.
432 pages

3800 Fibromyalgia, Managing the Pain
Anadem Publishing Company
3620 N High Street
Columbus, OH 43214-3611
800-633-0055
Fax: 614-262-6630
e-mail: anadem@anadem.com
www.anadem.com
Comprehensive guide to the syndrome, including chapters on diagnosis, medication, physical medicine treatments, occupational adjustments, advice on flare ups and some medical and legal aspects of FMS.

3801 Inside Fibromyalgia
Anadem Publishing Company
3620 N High Street
Columbus, OH 43214
614-262-2539
800-633-0055
Fax: 614-262-6630
e-mail: anadem@anadem.com
www.anadem.com
Written by a physician who has fibromyalgia. From the newest medications to alternative therapies and everything in between, Dr. Pellegrino helps you develop a plan for healing today and tomorrow.
Paperback
ISBN: 1-890018-36-8

3802 Laugh at Your Muscles
Anadem Publishing Company
3620 N High Street
Columbus, OH 43214-3611
800-633-0055
Fax: 614-262-6630
e-mail: anadem@anadem.com
www.anadem.com

3803 Taking Charge of Fibromyalgia
FMS Educational Systems
P O Box 500
Salem, OR 97308
503-315-7257
Fax: 503-315-7205
e-mail: nfra@firstpac.com
www.nfra.net
Written by three professionals who have fibromyalgia and who often update the book.

3804 Taking Control of TMJ: Your Total Wellness Program
Robert O Uppgaard, DDS, author
New Harbinger Publications
5674 Shattuck Avenue
Oakland, CA 94609
800-748-6273
Fax: 510-652-5472
e-mail: customerservice@newharbinger.com
www.newharbinger.com
Six-step wellness program helps readers understand what TMJ is and provides exercises to improve jaw functioning, relieve pain and deal with trigger points, eliminate harmful habits, deal with contributing stress, and evaluate and improve your diet and exercise habits. Additional chapters cover the connection between TMJ, whiplash, and fibromyalgia.
2004 200 pages Paperback
ISBN: 1-572241-26-8

3805 Understanding Post-Traumatic Fibromyalgia
Anadem Publishing Company

3620 N High Street
Columbus, OH 43214-3611
800-633-0055
Fax: 614-262-6630
e-mail: anadem@anadem.com
www.anadem.com
Anyone with post-traumatic fibromyalgia will benefit from reading this book focusing exclusively on this condition.

Magazines

3806 FM Monograph
National Fibromyalgia Partnership
140 Zinn Way
Linden, VA 22642
866-725-4404
Fax: 866-666-2727
e-mail: mail@fmpartnership.org
www.fmpartnership.org
Publishes a print quarterly (available online and in booklet form in English, Spanish, and French) which provides information on fibromyalgia symptoms, diagnosis, treatment, and research. Comprehensive resource packets and reprints are also available on a variety of subjects. Technical support is provided to fibromyalgia support organizations worldwide.
Quarterly
Tamara Liller, President

3807 Fibromyalgia AWARE
National Fibromyalgia Association
1000 Bristol Street N.
Newport Beach, CA 92660
714-921-0150
Fax: 714-921-6920
e-mail: nfa@FMaware.org
www.FMaware.org
Official publication of the National Fibromyalgia Association. Available to members and contributors.

3808 Fibromyalgia Frontiers
National Fibromyalgia Partnership (NFP)
PO Box 160
Linden, VA 22642
866-725-4404
Fax: 866-666-2727
e-mail: mail@fmpartnership.org
www.fmpartnership.org
Publishes a print quarterly (available online and in booklet form in English, Spanish, and French) which provides information on fibromyalgia symptoms, diagnosis, treatment, and research. Comprehensive resource packets and reprints are also available on a variety of subjects. Technical support is provided to fibromyalgia support organizations worldwide. Included with membership into NFP.
Quarterly
Tamara Liller, President

3809 Journal of Musculoskeletal Pain
Haworth Medical Press
10 Alice Street
Binghamton, NY 13904-1503
607-722-5857
800-429-6784
Fax: 607-722-0012
e-mail: getinfo@haworthpress.com
www.haworthpress.com
Peer reviewed medical journal containing FMS scientific abstract information. Appropriate for medical professionals as well as amateur.
Quarterly

Newsletters

3810 Fibromyalgia Clinic Kentfield Rehabilitation Newsletter
Fibromyalgia Clinic
25 Sir Francis Drake Blvd
Santa Ana, CA 92799
714-230-3150
Fax: 714-850-0153
www.dynamicchiropractic.com

3811 Florida Fibromyalgia News
FMS Association of Florida
P.O. Box 100221
Gainesville, FL 32610-4848 e-mail: painresearch@medicine.ufl.edu
rheum.med.ufl.edu
Quarterly newsletter.

3812 Health Points
TyH Publications
17007 E Colony Drive
Fountain Hills, AZ 85268
800-801-1406
e-mail: editor@e-tyh.com
www.healthpts.com
National newsletter with articles on complementary therapy, latest nutrition news, disability issues and much more. Focus is on fibromyalgia, chronic fatigue, arthritis and chronic pain.
Quarterly
J. Mark Lambright, President & CEO
Don Springer, Chief Operating Officer

3813 Healthwatch
CFIDS and Fibromyalgia Health Resource
2040 Alameda Padre Serra
Santa Barbara, CA 93103
800-366-6056
Fax: 805-963-4515
e-mail: cutomerservice@prohealthinc.com
www.prohealth.com
Healthwatch serves fibromyalgia and chronic fatigue syndrome sufferers by focusing on reporting the latest news in research and treatment, making hard-to-find nutritional supplements available at low prices, and raising needed funds for medical research.

3814 Journal of Musculoskeletal Medicine
Cliggott Publishing Company
27 Warren Street
Hackensack, NJ 07601-6074
201-487-9655
Fax: 201-487-9656
e-mail: wspc@wspc.com
www.worldscientific.com
This journal provides a unique and efficient monthly update on the management of musculoskeletal disorders. Offers articles regarding orthopedics, rheumatology, sports medicine, etc.

3815 To Your Health and Healthpoints
To Your Health
12005 Saguaro Blvd
Fountain Hills, AZ 85268
480-837-7590
800-801-1406
Fax: 480-837-1875
www.e-tyh.com
Resource catalogue and newspaper for FMS, CFIDS, arthritis, and chronic pain. Features vitamins and health products developed specifically for FMS and CFIDS making hard-to-find, recommended nutritional supplements available to fibromyalgia and chronic fatigue syndrome sufferers at a manufacturer-direct low price.

Audio & Video

3816 Audio Cassette Program on Fibromyalgia
Arthritis Foundation/Research Cassettes
111 E Wacker Drive
Chicago, IL 60601-3713
312-616-3470
Covers treatment and research taped during a patient education forum.

3817 Fibromyalgia Interval Training
Arthritis Foundation Distribution Center
235 East 42nd Street
New York, NY 10017-6996
800-879-3477
Fax: 770-442-9742
www.arthritis.com
Designed for people with fibromyalgia, the video features warm water exercises in shallow and deep water, including warmup, stretching, upper and lower body exercises, aerobics, strengthing, cool-down and relaxation. Designed to help you manage the pain, stiffness and fatigue of fibromyalgia.

3818 Fibromyalgia Stretch Video & Strength and Toning Video
Oregon Fibromyalgia Foundation
1221 SW Yamhill
Portland, OR 97205
503-228-3217
www.myalgia.com
These videos offer comprehensive stretching and strength and toning regimens developed by exercise physiologist Sharon Clark PhD, FNP, specifically for people with FMS. Fibromyalgia patients are shown demonstrating these unique stretching and strength and toning programs. Prices are per video and do not include shipping and handling.

3819 Fibromyalgia: Face to Face
Ontario Fibromyalgia Association
250 Cloor Street E
Toronto, Ontario, M4W
416-979-7228
A 14 minute insight into living with FMS from people, including children, who are coping with this syndrome.

3820 Improving Muscle Tone and Strength
Oregon Fibromyalgia Foundation
235 Berry Road
Hartford, ME 04220
207-224-7471
www.atabendintheroad.com
A video developed by exercise physiologist Sharon Clark, PhD, RN, specifically for people with fibromyalgia.

Web Sites

3821 American Fibromyalgia Research Association
www.afsafund.org
Charitable organization whose primary mission is to seed research in FMS and CFS. We acknowledge that patient and physician education, public awareness and advocacy are all important ingredients in aiding the lives of people with FMS and CFS.

3822 FM/CFS Canada
www.fm-cfs.ca
Dedicated to advancing Fibromyalgia (FM) and Chronic Fatigue Syndrome (CFS) education, research and treatment.

3823 Healing Well
www.healingwell.com
An online health resource guide to medical news, chat, information and articles, newsgroups and message boards, books, disease-related web sites, medical directories, and more for patients, friends, and family coping with disabling diseases, disorders, or chronic illnesses.

3824 Health Finder
www.healthfinder.gov
Searchable, carefully developed web site offering information on over 1000 topics. Developed by the US Department of Health and Human Services, the site can be used in both English and Spanish.

3825 Healthlink USA
www.healthlinkusa.com
Health information concerning treatment, cures, prevention, diagnosis, risk factors, research, support groups, email lists, personal stories and much more. Updated regularly.

3826 Helios Health
www.helioshealth.com
Online resource for your health information. Detailed information about specific health topics, access to expert advice from our Medical Advisory Board, and up-to-date health news.

3827 MedicineNet
www.medicinenet.com
An online resource for consumers providing easy-to-read, authoritative medical and health information.

3828 Medscape
www.medscape.com
Medscape offers specialists, primary care physicians, and other health professionals the Web's most robust and integrated medical information and educational tools.

3829 My Fibromyalgia & Chronic Fatigue Syndrome
www.fms-help.com
A compassionate, Christian-based site for people with Fibromyalgia (FMS), Chronic Fatigue & Immune Dysfunction Syndrome (CFIDS) and Myalgic Encephalomyelitis (M.E.)

3830 National Fibromyalgia Association
www.fmaware.org
Information for fibromyalgia patients and the general public.

3831   National Fibromyalgia Partnership (NFP)
PO Box 160
Linden, VA 22642   866-725-4404
                                              Fax: 866-666-2727
                           e-mail: mail@fmpartnership.org
                                   www.fmpartnership.org

The NFP is a 501(c)(3) non-profit, membership organization which publishes medically accurate information on fibromyalgia to patients, health care professionals and the public. Information and resources not listed in this volume are available in print and/or on the NFP website. It also provides support and start-up informaiton to support groups. Additional website: www.frontiersnews.org

Tamara K Liller, President & Director of Publications
Jacqueline M Yencha, Vice-President, Asst Dir of Publications

3832   Neurology Channel
                                   www.healthcommunities.com

Find clearly explained, medically accurate information regarding conditions, including an overview, symptoms, causes, diagnostic procedures and treatment options. On this site it is possible to ask questions and get information from a neurologist and connect to people who have similar health interests.

3833   Option Institute
Option Institute
                                   www.option.org/fibromyalgia.html

Self-defeating beliefs, along with attitudes and judgments, can lead to a host of physical and psychological challenges, including Fibromyalgia. The Option Institute offers programs designed to help you gain new perspectives on the attitudes and judgments that may be affecting your life, especially those regarding and surrounding Fibromyalgia.

3834   WebMD
                                           www.webmd.com

Provides credible information, supportive communities, and in-depth reference material about health subjects. A source for original and timely health information as well as material from well known content providers.

Description

3835 Gastrointestinal Disorders

The digestive tract is responsible for taking food into the body, processing it into simple chemicals that can be absorbed to nourish the body, and expelling the remainder.

Motility disorders of the gastrointestinal (GI) tract are conditions in which there is a failure of normal top-to-bottom movement of gastric contents. In reflux, the food content moves from the stomach back into the esophagus, irritating that organ and causing heartburn, the most common symptom. This is known as GERD, or gastro-esophageal reflux disease, and sometimes causes choking or coughing. Complications include inflammation and even ulceration of the esophagus. It is a problem in infants, but also occurs in adults especially with advancing age. Occasionally, an ulcer may develop in a segment of the GI tract, typically in the stomach or duodenum. An infectious agent, H. pylori, plays a central role in peptic ulcer disease. In achalasia, the normal movement of food down the GI tract by peristalsis is disrupted, and contents of the esophagus are unable to move into the stomach. As a result, the person chokes on food or liquid. Chest pain and coughing at night may also occur.

Other motility disorders reflect the bowel's inability to move its contents forward properly. Children may be born with Hirschprung's disease in which peristalsis is absent or abnormal in the large bowel, resulting in partial or complete obstruction. The most common motility disorder in adults is called irritable bowel syndrome; also known as functional bowel or spastic colitis, it causes variable degrees of abdominal pain and bloating, diarrhea and/or constipation.

Outpouchings in the walls of the lower GI tract, called diverticula, sometimes trap nutrient waste, and may become infected, bleed, and rupture. Finally, the digestive tract may fail in its primary task of absorbing nutrients, known as malabsorption syndromes. Rarely it will absorb too much of something. In hemochromatosis, for instance, the bowel takes in too much iron from the diet, and the excess is stored in and damages the liver, pancreas, heart, and gonads. More commonly, the body absorbs too little nutrient rather than too much. For instance, celiac disease, or sprue, is a disorder caused by intolerance to gluten, a cereal protein in wheat rye, barley, and oats. Lactose intolerance is an inability to digest a carbohydrate in dairy products. Treatment for malabsorption syndromes includes dietary modifications and, in more serious cases, supplementation with intravenous feedings known as parenteral nutrition.

National Agencies & Associations

3836 American College of Gastroenterology
PO Box 342260
Bethesda, MD 20827-2260

301-263-9000
www.acg.gi.org

ACG serves clinical and scientific information needs of member physicians and surgeons who specialize in digestive and related disorders. Emphasis is on scholarly practice, teaching and research.
Delbert H Chumley MD, President
Edgar Achkar, Director

3837 American Dietetic Association
120 S Riverside Plaza
Chicago, IL 60606-6995

312-899-0040
800-877-1600
e-mail: media@eatright.org
www.eatright.org

ADA serves the public through the promotion of optimal nutrition health and well-being.
Patricia M Babjak, Chief Executive Officer
Judith Rodriguez, President

3838 American Gastroenterological Association National Office
National Office
4930 Del Ray Avenue
Bethesda, MD 20814

301-654-2055
Fax: 301-654-5920
e-mail: member@gastro.org
www.gastro.org

AGA fosters the development and application of the science of gastroenterology by providing leadership and aid including patient care, research, teaching, continuing education, scientific communication and matters of national health policy.
Ian L Taylor MD, President
Loren Lane, Vice President

3839 American Hemochromatosis Society
4044 W Lake Mary Boulevard
Lake Mary, FL 32746-2012

407-829-4488
888-655-4766
Fax: 407-333-1284
e-mail: mail@americanhs.org
www.americanhs.org

Educates the public, the medical community and the media by distributing the most current information available on hereditary hemochromatosis (HH) including DNA screening for HH and pediatric HH; also facilitates patient empowerment through an online network.
Sandra Thomas, President/Founder

3840 American Motility Society
45685 Harmony Lane
Belleville, MI 48111

734-699-1130
Fax: 734-699-1136
e-mail: admin@motilitysociety.org
www.motilitysociety.org

Promotes research and sponsors professional education seminars about gastrointestinal motility topics including disorders of esophageal, gastric, small intestinal, and colonic function; and sponsors biennial meetings (even years), syposia and courses.
Michael Cami MD, President
Lori Ennis, Executive Director

3841 American Pancreatic Association
PO Box 14906
Minneapolis, MN 55414

612-626-9797
Fax: 612-625-7700
e-mail: apa@umn.edu
www.american-pancreatic-association.org

Provides forum for presentation of scientific research related to the pancreas.
Martin Freeman, President
Ashok Saluja, Secretary-Treasurer

3842 American Pseudo-Obstruction and Hirschsprung's Disease Society
1825 Connecticut Avenue NW
Washington, DC 20009

202-884-8200
800-695-0285
Fax: 202-884-8441
TTY: 202-884-8200
e-mail: nichcy@aed.org
www.nichcy.org

Promotes public awareness of gastrointestinal motility disorders in particular intestinal pseudo-obstruction and Hirschsprung's disease; provides education and support to individuals and families of children who have been diagnosed with these disorders.

3843   American Society for Gastrointestinal Endoscopy
1520 Kensington Road   630-573-0600
Oak Brook, IL 60523   800-353-2743
                                          Fax: 630-573-0691
                                      e-mail: info@asge.org
                                               www.asge.org
ASGE provides information training and practice guidelines about
gastrointestinal endoscopic techniques.
M Brian Fennerty, President
Gregory G Ginsberg, President-Elect

3844   American Society for Parenteral and Enteral Nutrition (ASPEN)
8630 Fenton Street   301-587-6315
Silver Spring, MD 20910-3805   Fax: 301-587-2365
                                    e-mail: aspen@nutr.org
                                        www.nutritioncare.org
Offers information and continuing medical education to professionals involved in the care of parenterally and enterally fed patients. Membership includes complimentary subscriptions to two
peer reviewed journals.
Charles Ston Vanway, President
Tom Jaksic, Vice President

3845   American Society of Adults with Pseudo-Obstruction
International Corporate Headquarters
19 Carrol Road   781-935-9776
Woburn, MA 01801-6161   Fax: 781-933-4151
ASAP educates the general public and medical community about
chronic intestinal pseudo-obstruction (CIP) and other related digestive motility disorders; serves as an integral source of information for patients of all ages with CIP and related disorders.

3846   Center for Digestive Disorders: Central
25 N Winfield Road   630-933-1600
Winfield, IL 60190   877-933-4234
                                          Fax: 630-933-1300
                                          TTY: 630-933-4833
                              e-mail: cdh_information@cdh.org
                                               www.cdh.org
Multifaceted program to meet the needs of people who suffer from
gastrointestinal problems; offers literature, videotapes and educational meetings and, if medical care is needed, appropriate
referrals are made.
Luke McGuinness, President/CEO
Jim Spear, Executive Vice President/CFO

3847   Cyclic Vomiting Syndrome Association
10520 W Bluemound Road   414-342-7880
Milwaukee, WI 53226   Fax: 414-342-8980
                                   e-mail: cvsa@cvsaonline.org
                                               www.cvsaonline.org
CVSA provides opportunities for patients, families and professionals to offer and receive support and share knowledge about cyclic vomiting syndrome; actively promotes and facilitates medical
research about nausea and vomiting.
Kathleen Adams, President, Co Founder
Jennifer Dhuse, Secretary

3848   Digestive Disease National Coalition
507 Capitol Court NE   202-544-7497
Washington, DC 20002   Fax: 202-546-7105
                                   e-mail: ddnc@hmcw.org
                                               www.ddnc.org
Informs the public and the health care community about digestive
disorders; seeks Federal funding for research education and training; and represents members' interests regarding Federal and State
legislation that affects digestive diseases research.
Linda Aukett, Chairperson
James DeGerome, President

3849   International Academy of Proctology
2209 John R Wooden Drive   765-342-3686
Martinsville, IN 46151   Fax: 765-342-4173
Encourages study of diseases of the colon and accessory organs of
digestion and conducts seminars.

3850   International Foundation for Functional Gastrointestinal Disorders
700 W.Viginia St   414-964-1799
Milwaukee, WI 53204-8076   888-964-2001
                                          Fax: 414-964-7176
                                    e-mail: iffgd@iffgd.org
                                               www.iffgd.org
IFFGD is a nonprofit education support and research organization
devoted to increasing awareness and understanding of functional
gastrointestinal disorders, including irritable bowel syndrome
(IBS), constipation, diarrhea, pain, and incontinence.
Nancy J Norton, President

3851   Iron Overload Diseases Association
525 Mayflower Road   561-586-8246
W Palm Beach, FL 33405   866-768-8629
                                          Fax: 561-842-9881
                                  e-mail: iod@ironoverload.org
                                               www.ironoverload.org
Conducts professional education symposiums and exhibits at medical meetings; serves and counsels hemochromatosis patients and
families; offers doctor referrals; promotes patient advocacy concerning insurance, Medicare, blood banks, and the FDA.
Roberta Crawford, Founder/President

3852   National Digestive Diseases Information Clearinghouse
Two Information Way
Bethesda, MD 20892-3570   800-891-5389
                                          Fax: 703-738-4929
                                          TTY: 866-569-1162
                            e-mail: nddic@info.niddk.nih.gov
                                               www.digestive.niddk.nih.gov
Offers various educational information, public resources and re-
prints, public awareness materials and more on digestive
disorders.
Griffin P Rodgers MD MACP, Director

3853   North American Society for Pediatric Gastroenterology and Nutrition
PO Box 6   215-233-0808
Flourtown, PA 19031   Fax: 215-233-3918
                                 e-mail: naspghan@naspghan.org
                                               www.naspghan.org
Promotes research and provides a forum for professionals in the ar-
eas of pediatric GI liver disease, gastroenterology, and nutrition.
Associated with fellow organizations in Europe and Australia
(ESPGAN, AUSPGAN).
Margaret K Stallings, Executive Director
Philip M Sherman, President

3854   Pediatric Adolescent Gastroesophageal Reflux Association
PO Box 7728   301-601-9541
Silver Spring, MD 20907   888-887-7729
                                  e-mail: gergroup@aol.com
                                               www.reflux.org
PAGER's mission is to: (1) gather and disseminate information on
pediatric gastroesophageal reflux (GER) and related disorders; (2)
provide educational and emotional support to patients with GER,
their families, and professionals; (3) promote awareness of GER
within both the medical community and the general public; and (4)
promote research into the causes, treatments and eventual cure for
pediatric GER.
Beth Anderson, Director

3855   Society for Surgery of the Alimentary Tract
900 Cummings Center   978-927-8330
Beverly, MA 01915   Fax: 978-524-8890
                                               www.ssat.com
SSAT provides a forum for exchange of information among physi-
cians specializing in alimentary tract surgery.
David W Rattner, President
David M Mahvi, President-Elect

3856   Society of American Gastrointestinal Endoscopic Surgeons
11300 W Olympic Boulevard   310-437-0544
Los Angeles, CA 90064   Fax: 310-437-0585
                                               www.sages.org

SAGES encourages study and practice of gastrointestinal endoscopy laparoscopy and minimal access surgery.

Jo Buyske, President
Steven D Schwaitzberg, President-Elect

3857   Society of Gastroenterology Nurses and Associates
401 N Michigan Avenue   312-321-5165
Chicago, IL 60611-4267   800-245-7462
                                       Fax: 312-673-6694
                             e-mail: sgna@smithbucklin.com
                                          www.sgna.org
SGNA provides members with continuing education opportunities practice and training guidelines and information about trends and development in the field of gastroenterology.

Peggy Gauthier, President
Leslie Stewart, President-Elect

3858   United Ostomy Association
PO Box 512
Northfield, MN 55057   800-826-0826
                                       Fax: 507-645-5168
                                     e-mail: info@uoaa.org
                                          www.uoaa.org
A national network for bowel and urinary diversion support groups in the United States. Its goal is to provide a nonprofit association that will serve to unify and strengthen its member support groups, which are organized for the benefit of people who have, or will have intestinal or urinary diversions and their caregivers.

Dave Rudzin, President
Diane Miterko, Chair

Foundations

3859   American Porphyria Foundation
4900 Woodway   713-266-9617
Houston, TX 77056   866-APF-3635
                                       Fax: 713-840-9552
                              e-mail: porphyrus@aol.com
                                   www.porphyriafoundation.com
The APF is dedicated to improving the health and well-being of individuals and families affected by porphyria. Our mission is to enhance public awareness about porphyria, develop educational programs and distributing educational material for patients and physicians and support research to improve treatment and ultimately lead to a cure.

Desiree H Lyon, Executive Director
James Young, Chairman

3860   Gastro-Intestinal Research Foundation
70 East Lake Street   312-332-1350
Chicago, IL 60601-5907   Fax: 312-332-4757
                                     e-mail: girf@girf.org
                                          www.girf.org
Provides funds for equipment, laboratories and the support of investigators and young physicians in the University of Chicago Gastroenterology Section, a group of full-time dedicated doctors who seek solutions to all kinds of gastrointestinal illnesses, affecting the esophagus, the stomach, the small intestine, the large intestine, the liver, the gallbladder, and the pancreas.

Jennifer Hanauer, Director
Stephen Wright, GIRF Staff

3861   Oley Foundation
43 New Scotland Ave   518-262-5079
Albany, NY 12208-3478   800-776-6539
                                       Fax: 518-262-5528
                                          www.oley.org
Promotes and advocates education and research in home parenteral and enteral nutrition; provides support and networking to patients through information clearinghouse and regional volunteer networks; sponsors meetings and conferences, including annual patient/clinician conference; maintains speakers bureau.

Joan Bishop, Executive Director
Cathy Harrington, Administrative Assistant

Research Centers

3862   Baylor College of Medicine: General Clinical Research Center for Adults
One Baylor Plaza   713-798-4951
Houston, TX 77030   e-mail: dbier@bcm.edu
                                  www.bcm.edu/pediatrics
Endocrinology, genetics and gastroenterology research.

Dennis M Bier MD, Program Director
Paul Klotman, President

3863   Digestive Disorders Associates Ridgely Oaks Professional Center
Ridgely Oaks Professional Center
621 Ridgely Avenue   41 -22 -488
Annapolis, MD 21401   800-273-0505
                                       Fax: 410-224-6971
                                       TTY: 800-735-2258
                                          www.dda.net
Specialize in the diagnosis and treatment of diseases of the entire digestive system including esophagus stomach small and large intestine colon liver pancreas and gall bladder.

Michael S Epstein, Founder
Charles E King, Doctor

3864   Gastrointestinal Research Foundation
70 E Lake Street   312-332-1350
Chicago, IL 60601-5915   Fax: 312-332-4757
                                     e-mail: info@girf.org
                                          www.girf.org
Founded to help combat gastrointestinal diseases. Raises funds to support research at the Center for study of the Digestive Diseases at the University of Chicago Medical Center and to support advanced training for scientists. Sponsors educational activities for the public.

Martin N Sandler, Co-Founder
Steven R Davidson, Co-Chairman

3865   University of California: Davis Gastroenterology & Nutrition Center
Pediatric GI Medical Center
4900 Broadway
Sacramento, CA 95820-2214   ÿ91- 73- 904
                                    www.ucdmc.ucdavis.edu
Research into gastrointestinal mobility and electro-physiology nutrition support and references for the public and patient evaluations.

Bonnie Hyatt, Assistant Director
Jenny Carrick, Senior Director of Communications and Ma

3866   University of California: Los Angeles Center for Ulcer Research
LA Medical Center
Building 115 Room 117   310-312-9284
Los Angeles, CA 90073   Fax: 310-268-4963
                             e-mail: cureadmn@mednet.ucla.edu
                                    www.cure.med.ucla.edu
Offers basic and clinical research related to peptic ulcer disease including causes checks and balances and stress-ulcer relationships.

Enrique Rozengurt, Director
Emeran Mayer, Co-Director

3867   University of Michigan Michigan Gastrointestinal Peptide Research Ctr.
U-M Health System
1500 E Medical Center Drive
Ann Arbor, MI 48109   734-936-4000
                                       Fax: 734-763-2535
                              e-mail: GutPeptide@umich.edu
                                  www.med.umich.edu/mgpc
Research into gastroenterology including chemistry of gut hormones is studied.

Chung Owyang MD, Director
Juanita Merc MD PhD, Associate Director

3868   University of Pennsylvania: Harrison Department of Surgical Research
3400 Spruce Street   215-662-4000
Philadelphia, PA 19104   800-789-PENN
                                       Fax: 215-615-0471
                            e-mail: julie.koehler@uphs.upenn.edu
                              www.uphs.upenn.edu/surgery/res/harrisonr

Offers research and studies on surgical transplantations gastrointestinal physiology.
Julie Hagan Koehler MBA, Business Director
Georgina Suarez, Administrative Assistant

Support Groups & Hotlines

3869 National Health Information Center
PO Box 1133
Washington, DC 20013
310-565-4167
800-336-4797
Fax: 301-984-4256
e-mail: info@nhic.org
www.health.gov/nhic
A health information referral service sponsored by the Office of Disease Prevention and Health Promotion. Puts health professionals and consumers who have health questions in touch with those organizations that are best able to provide answers.

3870 Pull-thru Network
2312 Savoy Street
Hoover, AL 35226-1528
205-978-2930
e-mail: ptnmail@charter.net
www.pullthrough.org
Dedicated to the needs of those born wutith anorectal malformation or colon disease and any of the associated diagnoses.

Magazines

3871 ASAP Forum
ASAP International Corporate Headquarters
19 Carroll Road
Woburn, MA 01801
781-935-9776
Fax: 781-933-4151
e-mail: asapgi@sprynet.com
Educates the general public and medical community about chronic intestinal pseudo-obstruction (CIP) and other related digestive motility disorders; serves as an integral source of information for patients of all ages with CIP and related disorders, their families, and members of the medical community.

3872 American Journal of Gastroenterology
American College of Gastroenterology
6400 Goldsboro Rd
Bethesda, MD 20817-1656
301-263-9000
Fax: 703-931-4520
www.acg.gi.org
Serves clinical and scientific information needs of member physicians and surgeons, who specialize in digestive and related disorders. Emphasis is on scholarly practice, teaching, and research.
Thomas F Fise, Executive Director

3873 American Journal of Gastrointestinal Surgery
Society for Surgery of the Alimentary Tract
500 Cummings Center
Beverly, MA 01915
978-927-8330
Fax: 978-524-8890
e-mail: ssat@prri.com
www.ssat.com
Provides information for physicians specializing in gastrointestinal surgery.
Robin S. McLeod, Chair
Fabrizio Michelassi, President

3874 Clinical Perspectives in Gastroenterology
American Gastroenterological Association
4930 Del Ray Avenue
Bethesda, MD 20814
301-654-2055
Fax: 301-654-5920
e-mail: member@gastro.org
www.gastro.org
Focuses on research, medical and professional developments in the science of gastroenterology.
John I. Allen, President
Michael Camilleri, President-Elect

3875 Digestive Health Matters
Intl. Foundation for Gastrointestinal Disorders
700 W. Virginia St.
Milwaukee, WI 53204-0864
414-964-1799
888-964-2001
Fax: 414-964-7176
e-mail: iffgd@iffgd.org
www.iffgd.org

Quarterly journal focuses on upper and lower gastrointestinal disorders in adults and children. Educational pamphlets and factsheets are available. Patient and professional membership.
Nancy Norton, President
William Norton, VP

3876 Gastroenterology
American Gastroenterological Association
4930 Del Ray Avenue
Bethesda, MD 20814-3002
301-654-2055
Fax: 301-654-5920
e-mail: member@gastro.org
www.gastro.org
Focuses on research, medical and professional developments in the science of gastroenterology.
John I. Allen, President
Michael Camilleri, President-Elect

3877 Gastroenterology Nursing
Society of Gastroenterology Nurses and Associates
330 N. Wabash Ave.
Chicago, IL 60611
312-321-5165
800-245-7462
Fax: 312-673-6694
e-mail: sgna@sba.com
www.sgna.org
Provides members with information about trends and development in the field of gastroenterology nursing.
Colleen Keith, President
Lisa Fonkalsrud, President-Elect

3878 Gastrointestinal Endoscopy
American Society for Gastrointestinal Endoscopy
3300 Woodcreek Dr.
Downers Grove, IL 60515
630-573-0600
866-353-2743
Fax: 630-963-8332
e-mail: info@asge.org
www.asge.org
Provides information, training, and practice guidelines about gastrointestinal endoscopic techniques.
Adjournia Jones, Manager of Operations
Angela Saylor, Accounting Assistant Manager

3879 Journal of Parenteral and Enteral Nutrition
ASPEN
8630 Fenton Street
Silver Spring, MD 20910-3805
301-587-6315
Fax: 301-587-2365
e-mail: aspen@nutr.org
www.nutritioncare.org
Offers information to professionals involved in the care of parenterally and enterally fed patients.
100 pages BiMonthly
Adrian Nickel, Director Communications/Marketing

3880 Journal of Pediatric Gastroenterology and Nutrition
N American Society for Pediatric Gastroenterology
6900 Grove Road
Thorofare, NJ 08086
609-848-1000
Fax: 609-848-5274
www.jpgn.org/
Provides information for professionals in the areas of pediatric GI liver disease, gastroenterology, and nutrition.

3881 Journal of the American Dietetic Association
American Dietetic Association
120 South Riverside Plaza
Chicago, IL 60606-6995
312-899-0040
800-877-1600
Fax: 312-899-1979
www.eatright.org
Professional journal of the ADA.

3882 Nutrition in Clinical Practice
ASPEN
8630 Fenton Street
Silver Spring, MD 20910-3805
301-587-6315
Fax: 301-587-2365
e-mail: aspen@nutr.org
www.nutritioncare.org
Offers information to professionals involved in the care of parenterally and enterally fed patients.
100 pages BiMonthly
Adrian Nickel, Director Communications/Marketing

3883 Pancreas
American Pancreatic Association

3 Bethesda Metro Center
Bethesda, MD 20814-6904

301-961-1508
866-726-2737
Fax: 301-657-9776
e-mail: info@pancreasfoundation.org
pancreasfoundation.org

Provides information on scientific research related to the pancreas.
Joseph M. Titlebaum, Chair
Jessica Kruse, Secretary

3884 Phoenix Magazine
United Ostomy Association of America
PO Box 512
Northfield, MN 55057

800-826-0826
Fax: 507-645-5168
e-mail: info@uoaa.org
www.uoa.org

America's leading ostomy patient magazine providing colostomy, ileostomy, urostomy and continent diversion information, management techniques, new products and much more.
Quarterly
David Rudzin, President

Newsletters

3885 ADA Courier
American Dietetic Association
120 South Riverside Plaza
Chicago, IL 60606-6995

312-899-0040
800-877-1600
Fax: 312-899-1979
www.eatright.org

Information for the public on the promotion of optimal nutrition, health, and well-being.
Sonja L. Connor, President
Evelyn F. Crayton, President-Elect

3886 APF Newsletter
4900 Woodway
Houston, TX 77056

713-266-9617
Fax: 713-840-9552
e-mail: porphyrus@aol.com
www.porphyriafoundation.com

Provides updates on treatment and research, as well as informative articles on patients and specialists who treat porphyria. It's mailed to all Sponsors of the APF.
Desiree H Lyon, Executive Director
James V. Young, Chairman

3887 ASAP Capsule
ASAP International Corporate Headquarters
19 Carroll Road
Woburn, MA 01801

781-935-9776
Fax: 781-933-4151
e-mail: asapgi@sprynet.com

Professional membership newsletter for ASAP, an organization which educates the general public and medical community about chronic intestinal pseudo-obstruction (CIP) and other related digestive motility disorders; serves as an integral source of information for patients of all ages with CIP and related disorders, their families, and members of the medical community.

3888 ASAP Digest
ASAP International Corporate Headquarters
19 Carroll Road
Woburn, MA 01801

781-935-9776
Fax: 781-933-4151
e-mail: asapgi@sprynet.com

General membership newsletter for ASAP. Educates the general public and medical community about chronic intestinal pseudo-obstruction (CIP) and other related digestive motility disorders; serves as an integral source of information for patients of all ages with CIP and related disorders, their families, and members of the medical community.

3889 Clinical Updates
American Society for Gastrointestinal Endoscopy
3300 Woodcreek Dr.
Downers Grove, IL 60515

630-573-0600
Fax: 630-963-8332
e-mail: info@asge.org
www.asge.org

Provides information, training, and practice guidelines about gastrointestinal endoscopic techniques.
Quarterly
Colleen M. Schmitt, President
Douglas O. Faigel, President-elect

3890 Code V
Cyclic Vomiting Syndrome Association (CVSA)
13180 Caroline Court
Elm Grove, WI 53122-1732

614-837-2586
Fax: 614-837-6543
e-mail: drwaites@infinet.com
www.beaker.iupui.edu/cvsa

Newsletter for members of the CVSA.

3891 Hemochromatosis Awareness
Hemochromatosis Foundation
PO Box 8569
Albany, NY 12208

518-489-0972
Fax: 518-489-0227
www.hemochromatosis.org

Provides information to the public, families, professionals and government agencies about hereditary hemochromatosis (HH); conducts and raises funds for research; encourages early screening for HH; holds symposiums and meetings; and offers genetic counseling along with support for patients, families, and professionals.
Margit Krikker MD, Medical Director

3892 Ironic Blood
Iron Overload Diseases Association
433 Westward Drive
Taylors, SC 29687-5123

561-840-8512
Fax: 561-842-9881
e-mail: info@irondisorders.org
www.irondisorders.org

Information for hemochromatosis patients and families.

3893 Lifeline Letter
Oley Foundation
Albany Medical Center
Albany, NY 12208-3478

518-262-5079
800-776-6539
Fax: 518-262-5528
e-mail: bishopj@mail.amc.edu
www.oley.org

Information on home parenteral and enteral nutrition for patients and the public.
16 pages Bi-Monthly
Joan Bishop, Executive Director

3894 Ostomy Quarterly
United Ostomy Association
P.O. Box 512
Northfield, MN 55057

800-826-0826
e-mail: info@uoa.org
www.uoa.org

First person stories, ostomy management advice from an ET and MD, organization news and ostomy product information.
72 pages Quarterly
Susan Burns, President
Jim Murray, 1st Vice President

3895 Pull-thru Network News
Pull-thru Network
4 Woody Lane
Westport, CT 06880

203-221-7530
e-mail: Pullthrunw@aol.com
members.aol.com/pullthrunw/Pullthru.html

Provides information to patients and families of children who have had or will have pull-through surgery to correct an imperforate anus or associated malformation, Hirschsprung's disease, or other fecal incontinence problems.

3896 SGNA News
Society of Gastroenterology Nurses and Associates
330 N. Wabash Ave.
Chicago, IL 60611

312-321-5165
800-245-7462
Fax: 312-321-5165
e-mail: sgna@sba.com
www.sgna.org

Provides members with information about trends and development in the field of gastroenterology.

3897 WIN Notes
Weight-control Information Network

1 WIN Way 301-496-3583
Bethesda, MD 20892-3665 877-946-4627
Fax: 202-828-1028
e-mail: win@mathewsgroup.com
www.niddk.nih.gov/health/nutrit/win.htm
Addresses the health information needs of individuals with weight-control problems. Available on the WIN web site.
BiAnnual

Pamphlets

3898 Acute Intermittent Porphyria
American Prophyria Foundation
PO Box 22712
Houston, TX 77227 713-266-9617
www.enterprise.net
An informational brochure published by the American Porphyria Foundation.

3899 Common Questions About Porphyria
American Prophyria Foundation
PO Box 22712
Houston, TX 77227 713-266-9617
www.enterprise.net
An informational brochure published by the American Porphyria Foundation.

3900 Diet and Nutrition in Porphyria
American Prophyria Foundation
PO Box 22712
Houston, TX 77227 713-266-9617
www.enterprise.net
An informational brochure published by the American Porphyria Foundation.

3901 Drugs and Porphyria
American Prophyria Foundation
PO Box 22712
Houston, TX 77227 713-266-9617
www.enterprise.net
An informational brochure published by the American Porphyria Foundation.

3902 Erythropoietic Protoporphyria
American Prophyria Foundation
PO Box 22712
Houston, TX 77227 713-266-9617
www.enterprise.net
An informational brochure published by the American Porphyria Foundation.

3903 Hematin
American Prophyria Foundation
PO Box 22712
Houston, TX 77227 713-266-9617
www.enterprise.net
An informational brochure published by the American Porphyria Foundation.

3904 Iron Overload Alert
Iron Overload Diseases Association
433 Westward Drive 561-840-8512
Taylors, SC 29687-5123 Fax: 561-842-9881
e-mail: info@irondisorders.org
www.irondisorders.org
Information for hemochromatosis patients and families.

3905 Issues in Women's Gastrointestinal Health
Gastro-Intestinal Research Foundation
70 E Lake Street 312-332-1350
Chicago, IL 60601 Fax: 312-332-4757
e-mail: info@girf.org
www.girf.org
Patient education pamphlet.
Howard Grill, President

3906 Porphyria Cutanea Tarda
American Prophyria Foundation

PO Box 22712
Houston, TX 77227 713-266-9617
www.enterprise.net
An informational brochure published by the American Porphyria Foundation.

Audio & Video

3907 A Day in the Life of a Child
Albany Medical Center 518-262-5079
Albany, NY 12208-3478 800-776-6539
Fax: 518-262-5528
www.oley.org
In this video you are welcomed into the household of the Miller family. The Millers have three children, one of whom is tube fed. Jessica has been dependent on tube-feedings since birth, and her family is prepared to show you just what that means. They share tips for keeping a sterile environment in a house with three children, and tips for helping Jessica fit in with her peers.
Joan Bishop, Executive Director

3908 Cleveland Clinic Teaching Conference
Hemochromatosis Foundation
PO Box 8569 518-489-0972
Albany, NY 12208 Fax: 518-489-0227
www.hemochromatosis.org
Provides information to the public, families, and professionals about hereditary hemochromatosis.

3909 Family Teaching Conference
Hemochromatosis Foundation
PO Box 8569 518-489-0972
Albany, NY 12208 Fax: 518-489-0227
www.hemochromatosis.org
Provides information to the public, families, and professionals about hereditary hemochromatosis.

3910 Life with Mic-Key
Albany Medical Center 518-262-5079
Albany, NY 12208-3478 800-776-6539
Fax: 518-262-5528
www.oley.org
Serves as an informative and introductory guide for adapting to life with a Mic-key low profile feeding tube. Low profile means that the Mic-key tube lies very close to the patient's body and does not stick out. It's slim design allows more air to circulate around the stoma site and makes it easy to care for. The Mic-key tube uses a balloon to hold it in place and comes with several important accessories, including two types of extensions sets and an anti-reflux valve.
10 Minutes
Joan Bishop, Executive Director

3911 Mealtime Notions - The 'Get Permission' Approach to Mealtimes and Oral Motor
Marsha Dunn Klein, MED, OTR/L, author
Albany Medical Center 518-262-5079
Albany, NY 12208-3478 800-776-6539
Fax: 518-262-5528
www.oley.org
This video explores the development of trusting feeding relationships, understanding the child's pace, and strategies for increasing permissive behavior. Tools discussed in this video include an introduction to the sensory continuum, a description of the around the bowl technique, and tips for removing the stress from your child's mealtime.
10 Minutes
Joan Bishop, Executive Director

Web Sites

3912 American College of Gastroenterology (ACG)
www.acg.gi.org
Serves clinical and scientific information needs of member physicians and surgeons, who specialize in digestive and related disorders. Emphasis is on scholarly practice, teaching, and research.

3913 American Gastroenterological Association (AGA)

www.gastro.org

Fosters the development and application of the science of gastroenterology by providing leadership and aid, including patient care, research, teaching, continuing education, scientific communication, and matters of national health policy pertaining to gastroenterology.

3914 American Hemochromatosis Society

www.americanhs.org

Educates the public, the medical community, and the media by distributing the most current information available on hereditary hemochromatosis (HH), including DNA screening for HH and pediatric HH; also facilitates patient empowerment through an online network.

3915 American Porphyria Foundation

PO Box 22712
Houston, TX 77227

713-266-9617
Fax: 713-840-9552
e-mail: porphyrus@aol.com
www.porphyriafoundation.com

Advances awareness, research, and treatment of the porphyrias; provides self-help services for members; and provides referrals to porphyria treatment specialists.

Karl E Anderson, MD, Chairman

3916 American Pseudo-Obstruction and Hirschsprung's Disease Society

Promotes public awareness of gastrointestinal motility disorders, in particular intestinal pseudo-obstruction and Hirschsprung's Disease; provides education and support to individuals and families of children who have been diagnosed with these disorders through parent-to-parent contact, publications, and educational symposia; and encourages and supports medical research in the area of gastrointestinal motility disorders.

3917 American Society for Gastrointestinal Endoscopy

www.asge.org

ASGE provides information, training, and practice guidelines about gastrointestinal endoscopic techniques.

3918 American Society of Abdominal Surgeons

www.abdominalsurg.org

ASAS sponsors extensive continuing education program for physicians in the field of abdominal surgery and maintains library.

3919 Background on Functional Gastrointestinal Disorders

www.med.unc.edu

Statistical background information on gastrointestinal disorders.

3920 Children's Motility Disorder Foundation

www.motility.org

CMDF works to increase awareness of pediatric motility disorders in the general public and among the physicians most likely to encounter children suffering from these conditions, such as pediatricians and family practice doctors. Supports medical research regarding the causes, treatment, and potentially life-threatening disorders.

3921 Cyclic Vomiting Syndrome Association

www.cvsaonline.org/

CVSA provides opportunities for patients, families, and professionals to offer and receive support and share knowledge about cyclic vomiting syndrome; actively promotes and facilitates medical research about nausea and vomiting; increases worldwide public and professional awareness; and serves as a resource center for information.

3922 Gastrointestinal Research Foundation

www.girf.org

Founded to help combat gastrointestinal diseases. Raises funds to support research at the Center for the study of the Digestive Diseases at the University of Chicago Medical Center and to support advanced training for scientists. Sponsors educational activities for the public.

3923 Healing Well

www.healingwell.com

An online health resource guide to medical news, chat, information and articles, newsgroups and message boards, books, disease-related web sites, medical directories, and more for patients, friends, and family coping with disabling diseases, disorders, or chronic illnesses.

3924 Health Finder

www.healthfinder.gov

Searchable, carefully developed web site offering information on over 1000 topics. Developed by the US Department of Health and Human Services, the site can be used in both English and Spanish.

3925 Healthlink USA

www.healthlinkusa.com

Health information concerning treatment, cures, prevention, diagnosis, risk factors, research, support groups, email lists, personal stories and much more. Updated regularly.

3926 Helios Health

www.helioshealth.com

Online resource for your health information. Detailed information about specific health topics, access to expert advice from our Medical Advisory Board, and up-to-date health news.

3927 Hemochromatosis Foundation

www.hemochromatosis.org

Provides information to the public, families, and professionals about hereditary hemochromatosis (HH); conducts and raises funds for research; encourages early screening for HH; holds symposiums and meetings; and offers genetic counseling along with support for patients, families, and professionals.

3928 International Foundation for Functional Gastrointestinal Disorders

www.iffgd.org

IFFGD is a nonprofit education, support and research organization devoted to increasing awareness and understanding of functional gastrointestinal disorders, including irritable bowel syndrome (IBS), constipation, diarrhea, pain, and incontinence. Mission is to inform, assist and support people affected by these disorders.

3929 MedicineNet

www.medicinenet.com

An online resource for consumers providing easy-to-read, authoritative medical and health information.

3930 Medscape

www.medscape.com

Medscape offers specialists, primary care physicians, and other health professionals the Web's most robust and integrated medical information and educational tools.

3931 National Digestive Diseases Information Clearinghouse

www.niddk.nih.gov

Offers various educational information, public resources and reprints, public awareness materials and more on digestive disorders.

3932 North American Society for Pediatric Gastroenterology and Nutrition

www.naspghan.org

NASPGHAN strives to improve the care of infants, children and adolescents with digestive disorders by promoting advances in clinical care, research and education.

3933 Nutrition in Clinical Practice

www.nutritioncare.org

NCP is indexed by PubMed (MEDLINE), Cumulative Index to Nursing and Allied Health Literature, International Nursing Index, International Pharmaceutical Index, Reference Update, Silver Platter, TOXLINE and UMI.

3934 Oley Foundation

www.oley.org

Enriches the lives of those requiring home IV & tube feeding through education, outreach, & networking.

3935 Pediatric Adolescent Gastroesophageal Assn

www.reflux.org

Discussions led by local experts, family medical histories and check swabs, supervised nap room and separate activity room for kids, trained babysitters available.

3936 Pediatric/Adolescent Gastroesophageal Reflux Association

www.reflux.org

PAGER gathers and disseminates information on pediatric gastroesophageal reflux and related disorders; provides support and education to patients, their families, and the public; promotes the general welfare of patients, their families, and the public; promotes the general welfare of patients with gastroesophageal reflux and their families; and promotes public awareness of the condition.

3937   Pull-thru Network

www.pullthrunetwork.org

Pull-thru Network (PTN) was founded in 1988 and has grown to be one of the largest organizations in the world dedicated to the needs of those born with an anorectal malformation or colon disease and any of the associated diagnoses

3938   Society for Surgery of the Alimentary Tract

www.ssat.com

SSAT provides a forum for exchange of information among physicians specializing in alimentary tract surgery.

3939   Society of American Gastrointestinal Endoscopic Surgeons

www.sages.org

SAGES encourages study and practice of gastrointestinal endoscopy, laparoscopy, and minimal acces surgery.

3940   WebMD

www.webmd.com

Provides credible information, supportive communities, and in-depth reference material about health subjects. A source for original and timely health information as well as material from well known content providers.

Description

3941 Gaucher's Disease

Gaucher's disease is an inherited disorder of metabolism of fats. These metabolic products can not be broken down properly because of a deficiency of an enzyme called glucocerebroside. Symptoms can include fatigue, anemia, bleeding problems (such as nosebleeds and easy bruising), enlargement of the spleen and/or liver, bone pain, easily fractured bones and brown pigmentation of the skin. The degree of symptoms and complications vary by age of onset and the degree of involvement of the disorder's clinical forms. Diagnosis is based on finding Gaucher's typical cells in the bone marrow.

The treatment for Gaucher's disease is enzyme replacement, called Cerezyme, administered intravenously. Removal of the spleen and blood transfusions may be necessary. Current research is aimed at genetic therapy.

National Agencies & Associations

3942 National Foundation for Jewish Genetic Diseases
One Gustave L Levy Place 212-241-6500
New York, NY 10029-6574 Fax: 212-241-6947
www.mssm.edu/jewish_genetics
This foundation was created to raise funds for and to inform the public about genetic diseases which afflict descendants of eastern and central European Jews. It sponsors medical symposia from time to time.
R J Desnick PhD MD, Center Director
Dennis S Charney, Executive VP

3943 National Gaucher Foundation
2227 Idlewood Road
Tucker, GA 33008
800-504-3189
Fax: 770-934-2911
e-mail: ngf@gaucherdisease.org
www.gaucherdisease.org
National foundation providing information and assistance for those affected by Gaucher disease as well as education and outreach to increase public awareness.
Robin A Ely MD, President/Medical Director
Rhonda P Buyers, CEO/Executive Director

3944 National Organization for Rare Disorders (NORD)
55 Kenosia Avenue 203-744-0100
Danbury, CT 06813-1968 800-999-6673
Fax: 203-798-2291
TDD: 203-797-9590
e-mail: orphan@rarediseases.org
www.rarediseases.org
The NORD is a unique federation of voluntary health organizations dedicated to helping people with rare orphan diseases and assisting the organizations that serve them.
Frank Sasinowski, Chair
Carolyn Asbury, Vice Chair

Research Centers

3945 Children's Gaucher Research Fund
8110 Warren Court 916-797-3700
Granite Bay, CA 95746-2123 Fax: 916-797-3707
e-mail: research@childrensgaucher.org
www.childrensgaucher.org
A nonprofit organization that raises funds to coordinate support research to find a cure for Type 2 and Type 3 Gaucher Disease.
Roscoe Brady, Scientific Advisory Board
Gregory Grabowski, Scientific Advisory Board

3946 Comprehensive Gaucher Treatment Center at Tower Hermatology Oncology
9090 Wilshire Boulevard 310-888-8680
Beverly Hills, CA 90211 888-248-4456
Fax: 310-285-7298
e-mail: info@gaucherwest.com
www.gaucherwest.com
The Comprehensive Gaucher Treatment Center at Tower Hermatology Oncology under the direction of Dr. Barry Rosenbloom provides clinical evaluations for the diagnosis and treatment of patient's with Gaucher disease. We provide a multi-disciplinary program that includes Hermatology Genetics Orthopedics and Radiology. To ensure continuity of care we provide assistance to other physicians regarding testing diagnosis evaluation and management of the Gaucher patient.
Barry Rosenbloom, Director
Cheryl Elzinga, Gaucher Coordinator

3947 LAC/USC Imaging Science Center
1975 Zonal Avenue 323-442-1900
Los Angeles, CA 90089-9034 Fax: 323-442-2722
e-mail: nestrada@usc.edu
www.usc.edu/schools/medicine
Provides a Gaucher Disease radiology consultant: Michael R Terk MD.and Muskuloskeletal Imaging.
Coreen Rodgers, COO
Sherri Sammon, Associate Director

Support Groups & Hotlines

3948 Brave Kids
151 Sawgrass Corners Drive 904-280-1895
Ponte Vedra Beach, FL 32082 800-568-1008
Fax: 904-280-1897
e-mail: info@bravekids.org
www.bravekids.org
An organization that offers support for parents and children suffering from serious health problems.
Kristen Fitzgerald, Founder

3949 National Health Information Center
PO Box 1133 310-565-4167
Washington, DC 20013 800-336-4797
Fax: 301-984-4256
e-mail: info@nhic.org
www.health.gov/nhic
Offers a nationwide information referral service, produces directories and resource guides.

Newsletters

3950 Gaucher Disease Newsletter
National Gaucher Foundation
61 General Early Drive 301-816-1515
Harpers Ferry, WV 25425-3151 800-504-3189
Fax: 770-934-2911
e-mail: rhonda@gaucherdisease.org
www.gaucherdisease.org
Offers information on the latest research, treatments and technology for persons affected by Gaucher Disease. Also includes legislative and medical information.
Quarterly
Brian E. Berman, President
Michael David Epstein, Chairman/Secretary

Pamphlets

3951 Gaucher Disease Fact Sheet
National Gaucher Foundation
61 General Early Drive 301-816-1515
Harpers Ferry, WV 25425-3151 800-504-3189
Fax: 770-934-2911
e-mail: rhonda@gaucherdisease.org
www.gaucherdisease.org

Offers information on what Gaucher Disease is, the symptoms, risks, treatments and the workings of the National Gaucher Foundation.
Brian E. Berman, President
Michael David Epstein, Chairman/Secretary

3952 Living with Gaucher Disease
National Gaucher Foundation
61 General Early Drive   301-816-1515
Harpers Ferry, WV 25425-3151   800-504-3189
                                          Fax: 770-934-2911
                     e-mail: rhonda@gaucherdisease.org
                                  www.gaucherdisease.org
A guide for parents, families and relatives that teach them how to deal with and cope with a diagnosis of Gaucher Disease.
24 pages
Brian E. Berman, President
Michael David Epstein, Chairman/Secretary

Audio & Video

3953 Pain & Hope
National Gaucher Foundation
61 General Early Drive   301-816-1515
Harpers Ferry, WV 25425-3151   800-504-3189
                                          Fax: 770-934-2911
                     e-mail: rhonda@gaucherdisease.org
                                  www.gaucherdisease.org
A patient and family perspective on Gaucher Disease.
Brian E. Berman, President
Michael David Epstein, Chairman/Secretary

Web Sites

3954 Gaucher Disease Homepage
                              www.gaucherdisease.org
Information on Gaucher disease, including symptoms, treatment, prevalence, resources, support, and news.

3955 Healing Well
                              www.healingwell.com
An online health resource guide to medical news, chat, information and articles, newsgroups and message boards, books, disease-related web sites, medical directories, and more for patients, friends, and family coping with disabling diseases, disorders, or chronic illnesses.

3956 Health Finder
                              www.healthfinder.gov
Searchable, carefully developed web site offering information on over 1000 topics. Developed by the US Department of Health and Human Services, the site can be used in both English and Spanish.

3957 Healthlink USA
                              www.healthlinkusa.com
Health information concerning treatment, cures, prevention, diagnosis, risk factors, research, support groups, email lists, personal stories and much more. Updated regularly.

3958 Helios Health
                              www.helioshealth.com
Online resource for your health information. Detailed information about specific health topics, access to expert advice from our Medical Advisory Board, and up-to-date health news.

3959 MedicineNet
                              www.medicinenet.com
An online resource for consumers providing easy-to-read, authoritative medical and health information.

3960 Medscape
                              www.medscape.com
Medscape offers specialists, primary care physicians, and other health professionals the Web's most robust and integrated medical information and educational tools.

3961 WebMD
                              www.webmd.com

Provides credible information, supportive communities, and in-depth reference material about health subjects. A source for original and timely health information as well as material from well known content providers.

Description

3962 Growth Disorders

There are many conditions that make a child grow more slowly than average. Any sort of severe chronic illness, especially one involving the digestive system, may cause this. Certain genetic conditions such as Turner syndrome, a sex chromosome abnormality or achondroplasia (skeletal maldevelopment) will predictably limit growth and eventual adult height. Endocrine, or hormonal, causes of short stature include underactivity of the thyroid gland (hypothyroidism) or pituitary gland, where growth hormone (GH) is normally formed. Finally, there are many cases where the child's height is significantly below that of peers, yet none of these conditions is present. This may reflect two parents who are themselves quite short, or may be completely unexplained.

If slow growth is related to low levels of GH, therapy with synthetic GH is extremely effective. Regular injections will be necessary for a prolonged period until an acceptable height is reached.

Regardless of the underlying cause, a child whose disorder is recognized at birth or who is not growing as quickly as the rest of his or her peers should receive a complete evaluation by a pediatric endocrinologist or other growth specialist.

National Agencies & Associations

3963 Dwarf Athletic Association of America
708 Gravenstein Highway N
Sebastopol, CA 95472
972-317-8299
888-598-3222
Fax: 972-966-0184
e-mail: daaa@flash.net
www.daaa.org

Develops, promotes and provides quality amateur level athletic opportunities for dwarf athletes in the US. Our mission is to encourage people with dwarfism to participate in sports regardless of their level of skill.
Amy B Andrews, Board President
Mike Cekanor, Board VP

3964 Genetic Alliance
4301 Connecticut Avenue NW
Washington, DC 20008
202-966-5557
Fax: 202-966-8553
e-mail: info@geneticalliance.org
www.geneticalliance.org

Improves health through the authentic engagement of communities and individuals. The goal is to build capacity within the genetics community. Transform health through genetics, and promote an environment of opennes cetnered on the health of individuals, families and communities.
Sharon F Terry MA, President/CEO
Greg Biggers, Entrepreneur-In-Residence

3965 Little People of America
250 El Camino Real
Tustin, CA 92780
714-368-3689
888-LPA-2001
Fax: 714-368-3367
e-mail: info@lpaonline.org
www.lpaonline.org

Focuses research, support and information on persons who are short in stature.
Lois Gerage-Lamb, President
Bill Bradford, Senior VP

3966 Little People's Research Fund (LPRF)
616 Old Edmondson Avenue
Catonsville, MD 21228
410-747-1100
800-232-LPRF
Fax: 410-747-1374
e-mail: lprf@lprf.org
www.lprf.org

LPRF supports research into the disabling conditions of skeletal dysplasia (dwarfism), promotes patient care and education of the medical community as well as the general public. It assists families by sponsoring clinics in various states.
Steven E Kopits MD, Medical Advisor

3967 National Institute of Child Health and Human Development
PO Box 3006
Rockville, MD 20847
800-370-2943
Fax: 866-760-5947
TTY: 888-320-6942
e-mail: NICHDInformationResourceCenter@mail.nih.
www.nichd.nih.gov

Duane Alexander MD, Director

Foundations

3968 Human Growth Foundation
997 Glen Cove Avenue
Glen Head, NY 11545
516-671-4041
800-451-6434
Fax: 516-671-4055
e-mail: hgf1@hgfound.org
www.hgfound.org

Our mission is to help children, and adults with disorders of growth and growth hormone through research, education, support, and advocacy. The Foundation is dedicated to helping medical science to better understand the process of growth. It is composed of concerned parents and friends of children, and adults, with growth problems; and, interested health professionals.
Patricia D Costa, Executive Director
Pisit Pitukcheewanont, President

3969 MAGIC Foundation for Children's Growth
6645 West North Avenue
Oak Park, IL 60302
708-383-0808
800-362-4423
Fax: 708-383-0899
e-mail: dianne@magicfoundation.org
www.magicfoundation.org

Provides support services for the families of children afflicted with a wide variety of chronic and/or critical disorders, syndromes and that affect a child's growth.
Dianne Tamburrino, Executive Director
Susan Smith, Director Medical Education

3970 March of Dimes Birth Defects Foundation
1275 Mamaroneck Avenue
White Plains, NY 10605
914-997-4488
www.marchofdimes.com

Our mission is to improve the health of babies by preventing birth defects, premature birth, and infant mortality.

Research Centers

3971 Case Western Reserve University: Bolton Brush Growth Study Center
2123 Abington Road
Cleveland, OH 44106-4905
216-368-4649
Fax: 216-368-3204
e-mail: mgh4@po.cwru.edu
dental.cwru.edu/bolton-brush

Investigations and research into the growth and development of the human body. Extensive collection of longitudinal human growth data.
Mark G Hans, Director
Aaron Weinbe, Associate Professor and Chairman

3972 International Skeletal Dysplasia Registry Medical Genetics Institute
Medical Genetics Institute
8700 Beverly Boulevard
Los Angeles, CA 90048
310-423-3277
800-233-2771
Fax: 310-423-0462
www.csmc.edu

Provides patient services for skeletal dysplasia patients particularly research in dwarfism.
David L Rimoin MD PhD, Director
Xiao-Ning Chen, Research Scientist

3973   New Jersey Institute of Technology Center for Biomedical Engineering
University Heights   973-596-8449
Newark, NJ 07102-1982   Fax: 973-596-6056
e-mail: william.c.hunter@njit.edu
www.njit.edu

Offers research into facial and bone disorders.
Robert A Altenkirch, President
Joel Bloom, Vice President

3974   WM Krogman Center for Research in Child Growth and Development
3101 Walnut Street   215-898-1470
Philadelphia, PA 19104-6003   e-mail: mannj@upenn.edu
www.upenn.edu

Focuses research and studies on growth disorders and birth defects.
Amy Gutmann, President

Support Groups & Hotlines

3975   National Health Information Center
PO Box 1133   310-565-4167
Washington, DC 20013   800-336-4797
Fax: 301-984-4256
e-mail: info@nhic.org
www.health.gov/nhic

Offers a nationwide information referral service, produces directories and resource guides.

Books

3976   Growing Children: A Parent's Guide
Human Growth Foundation
997 Glen Cove Avenue   516-671-4041
Glen Head, NY 11545   800-451-6434
Fax: 516-671-4055
e-mail: hgf1@hgfound.org
www.hgfound.org

Offers parents information on the normal pattern of their child's growth, growth charts, recognition of growth problems, evaluation of growth problems and resources for more information.
Pisit Pitukcheewanont, President
Emily L. Germain-Lee, Vice President

3977   Short and OK
Human Growth Foundation
997 Glen Cove Avenue   516-671-4041
Glen Head, NY 11545   800-451-6434
Fax: 516-671-4055
e-mail: hgf1@hgfound.org
www.hgfound.org

Guide for parents of short children offering information on behavior issues, medical issues and psychological warning signs.
54 pages
Pisit Pitukcheewanont, President
Emily L. Germain-Lee, Vice President

Pamphlets

3978   Achondroplasia
Human Growth Foundation
997 Glen Cove Avenue   516-671-4041
Glen Head, NY 11545   800-451-6434
Fax: 516-671-4055
e-mail: hgf1@hgfound.org
www.hgfound.org

Signs, causes and prevention of achondroplasia.
Pisit Pitukcheewanont, President
Emily L. Germain-Lee, Vice President

3979   Growth Hormone Testing
Human Growth Foundation
997 Glen Cove Avenue   516-671-4041
Glen Head, NY 11545   800-451-6434
Fax: 516-671-4055
e-mail: hgf1@hgfound.org
www.hgfound.org

What to expect during the testing period.
Pisit Pitukcheewanont, President
Emily L. Germain-Lee, Vice President

3980   Intrauterine Growth Retardation
Human Growth Foundation
997 Glen Cove Avenue   516-671-4041
Glen Head, NY 11545   800-451-6434
Fax: 516-671-4055
e-mail: hgf1@hgfound.org
www.hgfound.org

Explains some of the reasons for an infant's failure to grow normally in intrauterine life.
Pisit Pitukcheewanont, President
Emily L. Germain-Lee, Vice President

3981   Most Frequently Asked Questions with Growth Hormone Deficiency
Human Growth Foundation
997 Glen Cove Avenue   516-671-4041
Glen Head, NY 11545   800-451-6434
Fax: 516-671-4055
e-mail: hgf1@hgfound.org
www.hgfound.org

Provides a brief overview for parents about Growth Hormone Deficiency.
Pisit Pitukcheewanont, President
Emily L. Germain-Lee, Vice President

3982   Septo-Optic Dysplasia
Human Growth Foundation
997 Glen Cove Avenue   516-671-4041
Glen Head, NY 11545   800-451-6434
Fax: 516-671-4055
e-mail: hgf1@hgfound.org
www.hgfound.org

Also known as DeMorsier Syndrome. Describes the disease and the different treatments that can lead to the significant improvement in the quality of life.
Pisit Pitukcheewanont, President
Emily L. Germain-Lee, Vice President

Web Sites

3983   Alliance of Genetic Support Groups
www.geneticalliance.org
Genetic Alliance is a nonprofit health advocacy organization. Its network includes more than 1,200 disease-specific advocacy organizations, as well as thousands of universities, private companies, government agencies, and public policy organizations. The network is a dynamic and growing open space for shared resources, creative tools, and innovative programs.

3984   Atomz
www.pediatricservices.com
Provides resources to help all families obtain the information they need for the development of their children. Pediatric Services offers bilingual services - English and Espanol.

3985   Healing Well
www.healingwell.com
An online health resource guide to medical news, chat, information and articles, newsgroups and message boards, books, disease-related web sites, medical directories, and more for patients, friends, and family coping with disabling diseases, disorders, or chronic illnesses.

3986   Health Finder
www.healthfinder.gov
Searchable, carefully developed web site offering information on over 1000 topics. Developed by the US Department of Health and Human Services, the site can be used in both English and Spanish.

3987 Healthlink USA

www.healthlinkusa.com

Health information concerning treatment, cures, prevention, diagnosis, risk factors, research, support groups, email lists, personal stories and much more. Updated regularly.

3988 Helios Health

www.helioshealth.com

Online resource for your health information. Detailed information about specific health topics, access to expert advice from our Medical Advisory Board, and up-to-date health news.

3989 Human Growth Foundation

www.HGFound.org

Organization committed to expanding and accelerating research into growth hormone deficiency. Provides education and support to those affected by growth disorders and their families and fosters the exchange of information with the medical community.

3990 MedicineNet

www.medicinenet.com

An online resource for consumers providing easy-to-read, authoritative medical and health information.

3991 Medscape

www.medscape.com

Medscape offers specialists, primary care physicians, and other health professionals the Web's most robust and integrated medical information and educational tools.

3992 OHSU Homepage Search

www.ohsu.edu

A search which provides several links for information on growth disorders.

3993 WebMD

www.webmd.com

Provides credible information, supportive communities, and in-depth reference material about health subjects. A source for original and timely health information as well as material from well known content providers.

Description

3994 Head Injuries

Head Injuries, or Traumatic Brain Injuries, cover a range of severity. Currently, there are 5.3 million Americans living with a disability because of a head or brain injury. Concussion, the most common injury, is the momentary loss of consciousness. It usually resolves without any major complications. Damage can result from penetration of the skull or from acceleration/deceleration of the brain that occurs in severe automobile accidents. Injuries can include brain bruising and bleeding into the brain, resulting in swelling that can be life threatening because the skull, as a rigid structure, cannot expand.

Postconcussion syndrome commonly follows a mild injury and can include temporary headaches, dizziness, mild mental slowing and sleepiness. A moderate head or brain injury results in loss of consciousness usually lasting from minutes to a few hours, followed by a few days or weeks of confusion. Loss of consciousness for greater than two minutes implies a worse outcome. Cognitive and psychological impairments lasting many months or even permanently are usual consequences of moderate injury. A severe injury almost always results in prolonged unconsciousness or coma lasting days to weeks or longer. People who sustain a severe head or brain injury often have brain contusions, hematomas (a collection of blood) and/or damage to the nerve fibers or axons. Many people who sustain a severe brain injury make significant improvements in the first year or two. After that improvement tends to slow down, but may continue for years. Some physical and/or cognitive impairments are permanent. See also *Brain Tumors*.

National Agencies & Associations

3995 American Brain Tumor Association
2720 River Road
Des Plaines, IL 60018-4117
847-827-9910
800-886-2282
Fax: 847-827-9918
e-mail: info@abta.org
www.abta.org

Services includes over 40 publications which address brain tumors their treatment and coping with the disease. Materials address brain tumors in all age groups. Provide free social service consultations and a mentorship program for new brain tumor support groups.
Elizabeth M Wilson, Executive Director
Geri Jo Duda, Patient Services

3996 Brain Injury Association
1608 Spring Hill Road
Vienna, VA 22182
703-761-0750
800-444-6443
Fax: 703-761-0755
e-mail: info@biausa.org
www.biausa.org

The BIA's mission is to create a better future through brain injury prevention research education and advocacy. Offers information on state and national offices treatment and rehabilitation conferences prevention financial development and more.
Susan H Connors, President/CEO
Mary S Reitter, EVP/COO

3997 Dynamic Rehab
1800 W Big Beaver Road
Troy, MI 48084
281-485-4144
888-DYN-MIC
Fax: 281-485-4196
e-mail: dynmaicrehab@sbcglobal.net
www.dynamicrehab.net

Primary focus is the production and distribution of motivational videotapes and workshops.
Greta Ludwig PT, Owner/Physical Therapist
Teresa Turner, Owner/Physical Therapist

3998 FASST, Friends & Survivors Standing Together
21100 W. Capitol Drive
Pewaukee, WI 53072
Fax: 262-790-9670

Nonprofit organization supporting brain injured people and their caregivers. Information, support groups and more.

3999 Family Caregiver Alliance/National Center on Caregiving
180 Montgomery Street
San Francisco, CA 94104
415-434-3388
800-445-8106
Fax: 415-434-3508
e-mail: info@caregiver.org
www.caregiver.org

Caregiver information and assistance via phone or e-mail; fact sheets and publications describing and documenting caregiver needs and services.
Kathleen Kelly, Executive Director
Ping Hao, President

4000 International Brain Injury Association
5909 Ashby Manor Place
Alexandria, VA 22313
703-960-0027
Fax: 703-960-6603
e-mail: chaynes@hdipub.com
www.internationalbrain.org

Provides scientific and medical leadership worldwide in the field of brain injury.
Nathan Zasler, Chairman
Margaret Roberts, Executive Director/Administration

4001 National Health Information Center
PO Box 1133
Washington, DC 20013
301-565-4167
800-336-4797
Fax: 301-984-4256
e-mail: info@nhic.org
www.health.gov/nhic

Offers a nationwide information referral service, produces directories and resource guides.

4002 Rainbow House
4149 W 26th Street
Chicago, IL 60623
773-521-1815
www.rainbow-house.org

Rainbow House is a Chicago-based nonprofit organization whose mission is to end domestic violence. Rainbow House has offered domestic violence prevention programs support and outreach services and resources to survivors across the City of Chicago.
Angel Beltran, Chair
Rosy Mares, Vice Chair

4003 TPN: The Perspective Network
PO Box 121012
W Melbourne, FL 32912-1012
770-844-6898
Fax: 770-844-6898
e-mail: TPN@tbi.org
www.tbi.org

The Perspective Network provides forums and resources for persons with families, caregivers, friends and the professionals who serve them. Their goals are to promote a sense of community and to increase public awareness of brain injury.

State Agencies & Associations

Alabama

4004 Alabama Head Injury Foundation
3100 Lorna Road
Hoover, AL 35216
205-823-3818
800-433-8002
Fax: 205-823-4544
e-mail: ahif1@bellsouth.net
http://www.ahif.org

Services provided to Alabamians with traumatic brain injury or spinal cord injury include information, housing, respite care, recreation programs, resource coordination.
Keith Belt, President
Charles D Priest, Executive Director

Arizona

4005 Brain Injury Association of Arizona
5025 E Washington Street
Phoenix, AZ 85034
602-508-8024
888-500-9165
Fax: 602-508-8285
e-mail: info@biaaz.org
www.biaaz.org
Information and resources for brain injury survivors and their families. Support group listings available. Educational training, conference for families and survivors, neuro-specific resources and helpline.
Lisa Counters, President
Rebecca Armendariz, VicePresident

Arkansas

4006 Brain Injury Association of Arkansas
PO Box 26236
Little Rock, AR 72221-6236
501-374-3585
800-444-6443
Fax: 501-918-6595
e-mail: info@brainassociation.org
www.brainassociation.org

Dana Austen, President
Kortney Coats, Vice President

Colorado

4007 Brain Injury Association of Colorado
4200 W Conejos Place
Denver, CO 80204
303-355-9969
800-955-2443
Fax: 303-355-9968
e-mail: informationreferral@biacolorado.org
www.biacolorado.org
William Levis, President
Gavin Attwood, Executive Director

Connecticut

4008 Brain Injury Association of Connecticut
200 Day Hill Road
Windsor, CT 06095
86 - 2 - 02
800-278-8242
Fax: 86 - 2 - 05
e-mail: general@biact.org
www.biact.org
500 Members
Paul A Slager, President
Julie Peters, Executive Director

Delaware

4009 Brain Injury Association of Delaware
840 Walker Road
Dover, DE 19904
302-346-2083
800-411-0505
Fax: 888-258-3694
e-mail: biadresourcecenter@cavtel.net
www.biausa.org/Delaware
Devon Dorman, President
Esther Curtis, Executive Director

Florida

4010 Brain Injury Association of Florida
1637 Metropolitan Boulevard
Tallahassee, FL 32308
850-410-0103
800-992-3442
Fax: 850-410-0105
e-mail: biaftalla@biaf.org
www.biaf.org
Valerie E Breen, President/CEO

4011 Choices for Work Program Goodwill Industries-Suncoast
Goodwill Industries-Suncoast
10596 Gandy Boulevard
St Petersburg, FL 33702
727-523-1512
888-279-1988
Fax: 727-563-9300
TTY: 727-579-1068
e-mail: gw.marketing@goodwill-suncoast.com
www.goodwill-suncoast.org
A nonprofit community based organization whose purpose is to improve the quality of life for people who are disabled, disadvantaged and/or aged. This mission is accomplished through a staff of over 1,200 employees providing independent living skills, affordable housing, career assessment and job skills training and opportunities.
Deborah A. Passerini, President
Oscar J. Horton, Chair

4012 Pensacola Brain Injury TBI/ABI Support Group
TBI/ABI Support Group
2001 N E Street
Pensacola, FL 32507
850-457-2870
e-mail: hens8250@bellsouth.net
pensacolabrainnetwork.com/sys-tmpl/door
Survivors and caregivers oriented association. Publishes monthly magazine.
Peggy Henshall, Support Group Coordinator

Hawaii

4013 Brain Injury Association of Hawaii
420 Kuwili Street
Honolulu, HI 96817-1474
808-791-6942
Fax: 808-454-1975
e-mail: biahi@hawaiiantel.net
www.biausa.org/Hawaii

Ian Mattoch, President
Mary Wilson, Executive Director

Idaho

4014 Brain Injury Association of Idaho
PO Box 414
Boise, ID 83701-0414
208-342-0999
888-374-3447
Fax: 208-333-0026
e-mail: info@biaid.org
www.biaid.org

Michelle Featherston, President

Illinois

4015 Brain Injury Association of Illinois
PO Box 64420
Chicago, IL 60664-0420
312-726-5699
800-699-6443
Fax: 312-630-4011
e-mail: info@biail.org
www.biail.org
Philicia L Deckard, Executive Director
Irene Pedersen, Founder

Indiana

4016 Brain Injury Association of Indiana
9531 Valparaiso Court
Indianapolis, IN 46268
317-356-7722
866-854-4246
Fax: 31 - 8 - 17
e-mail: info@biai.org
www.biausa.org/Indiana

Anna Garrett, Executive Director
Laura C Trexler, TBI Grant Program Director

Iowa

4017 Brain Injury Association of Iowa
7025 Hickman Road
Urbandale, IA 50322
319-466-7455
800-444-6443
Fax: 800-381-0812
e-mail: info@biaia.org
www.biaia.org

Geoffrey Lauer, Executive Director

Kansas

4018 Brain Injury Association of Kansas and Greater Kansas City
6405 Metcalf Avenue
Overland Park, KS 66202

913-754-8883
800-444-6443
Fax: 816-842-1531
e-mail: info@biaks.org
www.biaks.org

Rob Flores, President
Betsy Johnson, Executive Director

Kentucky

4019 Brain Injury Association of Kentucky
7410 New Lagrange Roadd
Louisville, KY 40222

502-493-0609
800-592-1117
Fax: 502-426-2993
www.biak.us

Chell Austin, Executive Director
Wes Wilkinson, Development Director

Maine

4020 Brain Injury Association of Maine
13 Washington Street
Waterville, ME 04901

207-861-9900
800-275-1233
Fax: 207-861-4617
e-mail: info@biame.org
www.biame.org

Mary Lombardo, President
Leslie DuVall, Director of Operations

Maryland

4021 Brain Injury Association of Maryland
2200 Kernan Drive
Baltimore, MD 21207

410-448-2924
800-221-6443
Fax: 410-448-3541
e-mail: info@biamd.org
www.biamd.org

Patricia Janus, President
Diane Tripplet, Executive Director

Massachusetts

4022 Brain Injury Association of Massachusetts
30 Lyman Street
Westborough, MA 01581

508-475-0032
800-242-0030
Fax: 508-475-0400
e-mail: biama@biama.org
www.biama.org

Shahriar Khaksari, President
Arlene Korab, Executive Director

Michigan

4023 Brain Injury Association of Michigan
7305 Grand River
Brighton, MI 48114-2334

810-229-5880
800-444-6443
Fax: 810-229-8947
e-mail: info@biami.org
www.biami.org

Our mission is to enhance the lives of those affected by brain injury through education, advocacy, research and local support groups and to reduce the incidence of brain injury through prevention.
Katie Knight, Program Coordinator
Michael F Dabbs, President

Minnesota

4024 Brain Injury Association of Minnesota
34 13th Avenue NE
Minneapolis, MN 55413

612-378-2742
800-669-6442
Fax: 612-378-2789
e-mail: info@braininjurymn.org
www.braininjurymn.org

20-24 pages
Andrew Kiragu, Board Chairman

Mississippi

4025 Brain Injury Association of Mississippi
2727 Old Canton
Jackson, MS 39296-5912

601-981-1021
800-444-6443
Fax: 601-981-1039
e-mail: info@msbia.org
www.msbia.org

Howard T Katz, Chairman
Lee Jenkins, Executive Director

Missouri

4026 Brain Injury Association of Missouri
10270 Page Avenue
Saint Louis, MO 63132-1322

314-426-4024
800-444-6443
Fax: 314-426-3290
e-mail: info@biamo.org
www.biamo.org

Information and referral services and support groups through the state of Missouri.
John Bennett, President of the Board
Terrie Price, VP

Montana

4027 Brain Injury Association of Montana
1280 S 3rd W
Missoula, MT 59801

406-541-6442
800-241-6442
Fax: 406-541-4360
e-mail: biam@biamt.org
www.biamt.org

Bobbi Perkins, President
Kristen Morgan, Program Director

New Hampshire

4028 Brain Injury Association of New Hampshire
109 N State Street
Concord, NH 03301

603-225-8400
800-773-8400
Fax: 603-228-6749
e-mail: mail@bianh.org
www.bianh.org

Brant Elkind, President
Steven Wade, Executive Director

New Jersey

4029 Brain Injury Association of New Jersey
825 Georges Road
N Brunswick, NJ 08902

732-745-0200
800-669-4323
Fax: 732-745-0211
e-mail: info@bianj.org
www.bianj.org

Barbara Parker, President

New Mexico

4030 Brain Injury Association of New Mexico
3234 Candelaria NE
Albuquerque, NM 87107

505-292-7414
88 - 2 - 74
Fax: 505-271-8983
e-mail: info@braininjurynm.org
www.braininjurynm.org

John Tiwald, Board President
Mark Pedrotty, VP

New York

4031 Brain Injury Association of New York State
10 Colvin Avenue
Albany, NY 12206-1242

518-459-7911
800-228-8201
Fax: 518-482-5285
e-mail: info@bianys.org
www.bianys.org

Marie Cavallo, President
Judith Avner, Executive Director

4032 RRTC on Community Integration of Persons with TBI
2323 S Shepherd   713-630-0526
Houston, TX 77019   800-732-8124
                                          Fax: 713-630-0529
e-mail: terri.hudler-hull@memorialhermann.org
www.tbicommunity.org

Karen A Hart PhD, Director Of Training
Sunil Kothari, Medical Director

North Carolina

4033 Brain Injury Association of North Carolina
2113 Cameron Street   919-833-9634
Raleigh, NC 27605   800-377-1464
                                          Fax: 919-833-5415
e-mail: bianc@bianc.net
www.tbicommunity.org

Cindy Boyd, Board Chairman
Sandra Farmer, President

Ohio

4034 Brain Injury Association of Ohio
855 Grand View Avenue   614-481-7100
Columbus, OH 43215-1123   866-644-6242
                                          Fax: 614-481-7103
e-mail: help@biaoh.org
www.biaoh.org

Jon Fishpaw, President
Suzanne Minnich, Executive Director

Oklahoma

4035 Brain Injury Association of Oklahoma
PO Box 88   580-233-4363
Hillsdale, OK 73743-0088   800-444-6443
                                          Fax: 580-233-4546
e-mail: brainhelp@braininjuryoklahoma.org`
www.braininjuryoklahoma.org

Tracy Grammer, President
Gary Clarke, Chairman

Oregon

4036 Brain Injury Association of Oregon
PO Box 549   503-740-3155
Molalla, OR 97038   800-544-5243
                                          Fax: 503-961-8730
e-mail: info@biaoregon.org
www.biaoregon.org

Tootie Smith, President
Sherry Stock, Executive Director

Pennsylvania

4037 Brain Injury Association of Pennsylvania
950 Walnut Bottom Road   717-657-3601
Carlisle, PA 17015   866-635-7097
                                          Fax: 717-692-5567
e-mail: info@biapa.org
www.biapa.org

Drew Nagele, Chairman of Board Development Committee
Stewart L Cohen, Chairman

Rhode Island

4038 Brain Injury Association of Rhode Island
935 Park Avenue   401-461-6599
Cranston, RI 02910-2743   Fax: 401-461-6561
e-mail: braininjuryctr@biaofri.org
www.biaofri.org

Michael Baker, Co-President
Colleen McCarthy, Co-President

South Carolina

4039 Brain Injury Association of South Carolina
800 Dutch Square Boulevard   803-731-9823
Columbia, SC 29210   877-TBI-FACT
                                          Fax: 803-731-4804
e-mail: scbraininjury@bellsouth.net
www.biausa.org/sc

Elaine Phillips, President
Joyce Davis, Executive Director

Tennessee

4040 Brain Injury Association of Tennessee
955 Woodland St   615-248-5878
Nashville, TN 37206   877-757-2428
                                          Fax: 615-383-1176
e-mail: biaoftn@yahoo.com
www.biaoftn.org

Guynn Edwards, President
Pam Bryan, Executive Director

Texas

4041 Brain Injury Association of Texas
316 W 12th Street   512-326-1212
Austin, TX 78701   800-392-0040
                                          Fax: 512-478-3370
e-mail: info@biatx.org
www.biatx.org

Jane Boutte, President

Utah

4042 Brain Injury Association of Utah
1800 S W Temple   801-484-2240
Salt Lake City, UT 84115   800-281-8442
                                          Fax: 801-484-5932
e-mail: biau@sisna.com
www.biau.org

Teresa Such-Niebar, President
Ron S Roskos, Executive Director

Vermont

4043 Brain Injury Association of Vermont
92 S Main Street   802-244-6850
Waterbury, VT 05676   877-856-1772
                                          Fax: 802-244-4005
e-mail: support1@biavt.org
www.biavt.org

Marsha Bancroft, President
Trevor Squirrell, Executive Director

Virginia

4044 Brain Injury Association of America's National Family Helpline
1608 Spring Hill Road   703-761-0750
Vienna, VA 22182   800-444-6443
                                          Fax: 703-761-0755
e-mail: FamilyHelpline@biausa.org
www.biausa.org

Greg Oshanick, Chairman
Susan Conners, President and CEO

4045 Brain Injury Association of Virginia
1506 Willow Lawn Drive   804-355-5748
Richmond, VA 23230   800-444-6443
                                          Fax: 804-355-6381
e-mail: info@biav.net
www.biav.net

Anne McDonnell, Executive Director
Lynette Scott, Program Director

Washington

4046 Brain Injury Association of Washington
800 Jefferson Street   206-388-0900
Seattle, WA 98104   800-523-5438
                                        Fax: 206-388-0901
                                        e-mail: info@biawa.org
                                        www.biawa.org

Richard Adler, President
Gene van den Bosch, Executive Director

West Virginia

4047 Brain Injury Association of West Virginia
PO Box 574   304-766-4892
Institute, WV 25112-0574   800-356-6443
                                        Fax: 304-766-4940
                                        e-mail: mdavis@brainman.com
                                        www.biausa.org/WVirginia

Michael W Davis, Board of Director
Linda Arthur, Board of Director

Wisconsin

4048 Brain Injury Association of Wisconsin
21100 W Capitol Drive   262-790-9660
Pewaukee, WI 53072   800-882-9282
                                        Fax: 262-790-9670
                                        e-mail: admin@execpc.com
                                        www.biaw.org

Advocacy, education, prevention, information, resources, and support groups in regards to traumatic brain injury.
David Voss, President
Mark Warhus, Executive Director

Wyoming

4049 Brain Injury Association of Wyoming
111 W 2nd Street   307-473-1767
Casper, WY 82601   800-643-6457
                                        Fax: 307-237-5222
                                        e-mail: biaw@tribcsp.com
                                        www.biausa.org/Wyoming

Larry Plemmons, President
Jack Nokes, Director

Foundations

4050 Brain Trauma Foundation
708 Third Avenue   212-772-0608
New York, NY 10017-4201   Fax: 212-772-2035
                                        e-mail: info@braintrauma.org
                                        www.braintrauma.org

Our goal at the Brain Trauma Foundation is to improve the outcome of TBI patients through Guideline development, clinical research, professional education, and quality improvement programs.
Quarterly
Jamshid Ghajar, MD, President
Pamela Drexel, Executive Director

Research Centers

4051 Brady Institute Jamaica Hospital Medical Center
Jamaica Hospital Medical Center
8900 Van Wyck Expressway   718-206-6000
Jamaica, NY 11418-2897   Fax: 718-206-6559
                                        www.jamaicahospital.org

The James and Sarah Brady Institute for Traumatic Brain Injury.
David P Rosen, President & CEO
Neil Foster Phillips, Chairman

4052 Dana Alliance for Brain Initiatives
745 Fifth Avenue   212-223-4040
New York, NY 10151   Fax: 212-317-8721
                                        e-mail: danainfo@dana.org
                                        www.dana.org

A non-profit organization of more than 250 neuroscientists which was formed to help provide information about the personal and public benefits of brain research.
Jane Nevins, Vice President
Edward F Rover, President

4053 Institute for Rehabilitation and Research
1333 Moursund Street   713-799-5000
Houston, TX 77030   800-447-3422
                                        Fax: 713-874-1798
                                        e-mail: tirr.referrals@memorialhermann.org
                                        www.tirr.org

Carl Josehart, CEO
Gerard F. Francisco, Chief Medical Officer

4054 New York University Medical Center Head Trauma Program
Reet   212-998-9819
New York, NY 10010-4020   Fax: 212-340-7158
Research pertaining to young adults suffering from head injuries.
Dr Yehuda Ben-Yishay, Coordinator

4055 Ohio State University Laboratory of Psychobiology
1835 Neil Avenue   614-292-8185
Columbus, OH 43210-1222   Fax: 614-292-4537
                                        www.psy.ohio-state.edu/labs
Studies done on recovery of function after brain damage.
Laura Peterson, Lab Coordinator
James Walton, Research Associate

4056 Rehabilitation Institute of Michigan
261 Mack Avenue   313-745-1203
Detroit, MI 48201   Fax: 313-745-2376
                                        www.rimrehab.org
Physical medicine and rehabilitation medicine.
William H Restum PhD, President
Horacio Varg Jr, Interim Executive Director

4057 Thomas Jefferson University Ischemia-Shock Research Center
1020 Locust Street   215-503-4400
Philadelphia, PA 19107-6731   Fax: 215-503-9920
                                        e-mail: jgsbs-info@jefferson.edu
                                        www.jefferson.edu
Promotes research into head injuries and clinical studies.

4058 Thomas Jefferson University Ischemia-Shock
1020 Walnut Street   215-955-6000
Philadelphia, PA 19107   Fax: 215-923-7932
                                        www.jefferson.edu
Promotes research into head injuries and clinical studies.

4059 Tulane University: US-Japan Biomedical Research Laboratories
1430 Tulane Avenue   504-988-5187
New Orleans, LA 70112   Fax: 504-394-7169
                                        e-mail: medsch@tulane.edu
                                        www.tulane.edu/som/
Focuses research efforts on neuroendocrinology and neurosciences.
Benjamin P Sachs, MB, BS, Senior Vice President, Dean
Mary Brown, MBA, Vice President

4060 UCLA Neuropsychiatric Institute
760 Westwood Plaza   310-825-2631
Los Angeles, CA 90095   800-825-9989
                                        Fax: 310-825-9179
                                        e-mail: pwhybrow@mednet.ucla.edu
                                        www.semel.ucla.edu
Devote to teach research and patient care in psychiatry neuroscience and related fields.
Peter Whybrow, Director

4061 University of California: Irvine Brain Imaging Center
101 The City Drive S   949-824-7872
Irvine, CA 92697-3960   Fax: 949-824-7873
                                        e-mail: BIC@msx.hsis.uci.edu
                                        www.bic.uci.edu
Offers PET scan analysis of brain functions focusing on brain damage brain tumors and head injuries.
Steven L Small, PhD, MD, Director
David B Keator, MCS, Technical Director

4062 University of California: San Francisco Laboratory for Neurotrauma
1001 Potrero Avenue
San Francisco, CA 94110-3518
415-206-8313
www.ucsf.edu

Research done into traumatic brain and head injuries.
Lawrence H Pitts MD

4063 University of Memphis: Department of Psych ology
Memphis State University
202 Psychology Building
901-678-2000
Memphis, TN 38152
Fax: 901-678-2579
e-mail: psycadvise@memphis.edu
www.memphis.edu/psychology/

Evaluation and development of assessment and treatment procedures for neurologically impaired persons.
Guy Mittleman, Professor Director of CAPR
Frank Andrasik, Professor, Chair

4064 Virginia Commonwealth University: Rehab Research and Training Center
1314 W Main Street
804-828-1851
Richmond, VA 23284-2011
Fax: 804-828-2193
TTY: 804-828-2494
www.vcu.edu/rrtcweb/

Focuses research on traumatic brain and head injuries.
Paul Wehman, Director
Jeanne Dalton, Public Relations Assistant Specialist

4065 Wayne State University: Gurdjian-Lissner Biomechanics Laboratory
Department of Neurological Surgery
4160 John R Street
313-831-0777
Detroit, MI 48201
877-486-7978
Fax: 313-966-0368
e-mail: neurosurgery@med.wayne.edu
www.neurosurgery.med.wayne.edu

Head and neck injury research.
Murali Guthikonda, MD, FACS, Professor (Clinician-Educator) and Chair
Patti Bekowies, MBA, Chief Administrative Officer

Support Groups & Hotlines

Alabama

4066 Alabama Head Injury Foundation Helpline
3100 Lorna Road
205-823-3818
Hoover, AL 35216-5451
800-433-8002
Fax: 205-823-4544
e-mail: ahif1@bellsouth.net
www.ahif.org/

The Alabama Head Injury Foundation (AHIF) was founded by professionals and families in 1983 to increase public awareness of Traumatic Brain Injury (TBI) and to stimulate the development of supportive services. AHIF provides accessible resources, services and programs that meet the unique needs of individuals with traumatic brain injury (TBI) as well as spinal cord injury (SCI) in certain programs.
Charles D Priest, Executive Director
Janet Massey, Executive Assistant

Arizona

4067 Brain Injury Association of Arizona
5025 E Washington Street
602-508-8024
Phoenix, AZ 85034
888-500-9165
Fax: 602-508-8285
e-mail: info@biaaz.org
www.biaaz.org

Information and resources for brain injury survivors and their families. Support group listings available. Educational training, conference for families and survivors, neuro-specific resources and helpline.
Kim Halloran, Executive Director
Jeanne Andersen, Information & Referral Manager

Arkansas

4068 Brain Injury Association of Arkansas Helpl ine
PO Box 26236
501-374-3585
Little Rock, AR 72221-6236
866-610-4841
Fax: 501-918-6595
e-mail: info@brainassociation.org
www.bia-ar.org

Founded in 1980, the Brain Injury Association of America (BIAA) is a national organization serving and representing individuals, families and professionals who are touched by a life-altering, often devastating, traumatic brain injury (TBI). BIAA provides information, education and support through its network of chartered state affiliates, local chapters and support groups across the country to assist the 5.3 million Americans currently living with traumatic brain injury and their families.
Dana Austen, President Arkansas State Office
Kortney E Gold, Vice President

California

4069 Brain Injury Association of California Hel pline
3501 Mall View Road
661-872-4903
Bakersfield, CA 93306
Fax: 661-873-2508
e-mail: calbiainfo@yahoo.com
www.biacal.org/

Founded in 1980, the Brain Injury Association of America (BIAA) is a national organization serving and representing individuals, families and professionals who are touched by a life-altering, often devastating, traumatic brain injury (TBI). BIAA provides information, education and support through its network of chartered state affiliates, local chapters and support groups across the country to assist the 5.3 million Americans currently living with traumatic brain injury and their families.
Paula Daoutis, Administrative Director
Ursula Pesta, Project Coordinator

4070 Jodi House
625 Chapala St.
805-563-2882
Santa Barbara, CA 93101
Fax: 805-563-3982
e-mail: info@jodihouse.org
www.jodihouse.org

Jodi House is a community-based, post-rehabilitation day program that provides opportunities for social interaction, life skill training, recreation, and support for adults living with acquired brain injury (i.e. from head trauma, tumor, and stroke) and their families.
Gayle Cummings, Co-President
Timothy Morton-Smith, Co-President/Vice President of Finance

Colorado

4071 Brain Injury Association of Colorado Helpline
1385 South Colorado Boulevard
303-355-9969
Denver, CO 80222
800-955-2443
Fax: 303-355-9968
e-mail: biacolo@aol.com
www.BIAColorado.org

Dannis Schanel, LCSW, CBIST, President
Gavin Attwood, Exececutive Director

Connecticut

4072 Brain Injury Association of Connecticut Helpline
200 Day Hill Road
860-219-0291
Windsor, CT 06095-1304
800-278-8242
Fax: 860-219-0568
e-mail: general@biact.org
www.biact.homestead.com/

Supports persons with brain injuries and their families by promoting services to facilitate full inclusion within their local community and to increase awareness and understanding of brain injury and its prevention through community education.
500 Members
Paul A. Slager, Esq., President
Dr. Johnny Magwood, BSME, MBA, DBA, Vice President

Delaware

4073 Brain Injury Association of Delaware Helpl ine
32 West Loockerman Street   302-346-2083
Dover, DE 19904   800-411-0505
                                          Fax: 302-678-3183
                   e-mail: biadresourcecenter@cavdel.net
                                          www.biaofde.org//
Founded in 1980, the Brain Injury Association of America (BIAA) is a national organization serving and representing individuals, families and professionals who are touched by a life-altering, often devastating, traumatic brain injury (TBI). BIAA provides information, education and support through its network of chartered state affiliates, local chapters and support groups across the country to assist the 5.3 million Americans currently living with traumatic brain injury and their families.
Elizabeth Furber, President Delaware State Office
Timothy J Walker, Vice President

Florida

4074 Brain Injury Association of Florida
1637 Metropolitan Blvd   850-410-0103
Tallahassee, FL 32308   800-992-3442
                                          Fax: 850-410-0105
                                       e-mail: admin@biaf.org
                                              www.biaf.org

Gary Clarke, Chairman
Valerie Breen, President/CEO

Hawaii

4075 Brain Injury Association of Hawaii
420 Kuwili Street   808-436-8977
Honolulu, HI 96817   e-mail: biahi@hawaiiantel.net
                                        www.biausa.org/Hawaii
Dedicated to serving those affected by brain injury throughgh advocacy, prevention, and support
Mary Wilson, Executive Director
Ian Mattoch, President

Illinois

4076 American Brain Tumor Association Patient Line
8550 W. Bryn Mawr Ave   773-577-8750
Chicago, IL 60631-4117   800-886-2282
                                          Fax: 773-577-8738
                                       e-mail: info@abta.org
                                              www.abta.org

Offers emergency support, information and referrals for patients and their families.
Ronald Petrocelli, MD, Chair
Elizabeth M Wilson, President, CEO

4077 Brain Injury Association of Illinois Helpline
PO Box 64420   312-726-5699
Chicago, IL 60664-420   800-699-6443
                                          Fax: 312-630-4011
                                       e-mail: info@biail.org
                                              www.biail.org
Works with all people with brain inquiries and their families with professionals who serve them. Provides camp oppurtunities, support groups, educational seminars, information and referrals and a quarterly newsletter.
Irene Pedersen, Founder
Philicia L Deckard, Executive Director

Indiana

4078 Brain Injury Association of Indiana Helpli ne
9531 Valparaiso Court   317-356-7722
Indianapolis, IN 46268   866-854-4246
                                          Fax: 317-802-1768
                                       e-mail: info@biai.org
                                              www.biai.org
Founded in 1980, the Brain Injury Association of America (BIAA) is a national organization serving and representing individuals, families and professionals who are touched by a life-altering, often devastating, traumatic brain injury (TBI). BIAA provides informa-

tion, education and support through its network of chartered state affiliates, local chapters and support groups across the country to assist the 5.3 million Americans currently living with traumatic brain injury and their families.
Nancy Ritter, Chairperson
Anna Garrett, Executive Director

Iowa

4079 Brain Injury Alliance of Iowa Helpline
Brain Injury Association of America
7025 Hickman Road   319-272-2312
Urbandale, IA 50322   855-444-6443
                                          Fax: 319-272-2109
                                       e-mail: info@biaia.org
                                              www.biaia.org
Geoffrey Lauer, Executive Director
Natasha Retz, Director of Programs and Services

Kansas

4080 Brain Injury Association of Kansas and Greater Kansas City Helpline
6701 W. 64th Street   913-754-8883
Overland Park, KS 66202   800-783-1356
                                          Fax: 816-842-1531
                                  e-mail: rabramowitz@biaks.org
                                              www.biaks.org

Whitney Sunderland, President
Robin Abramowitz, Executive Director

Kentucky

4081 Brain Injury Alliance of Kentucky
7321 New LaGrange Road   502-493-0609
Louisville, KY 40222   800-592-1117
                                          Fax: 502-426-2993
                                  e-mail: chell.austin@biak.us
                                              www.biak.us
Founded in 1980, the Brain Injury Association of America (BIAA) is a national organization serving and representing individuals, families and professionals who are touched by a life-altering, often devastating, traumatic brain injury (TBI). BIAA provides information, education and support through its network of chartered state affiliates, local chapters and support groups across the country to assist the 5.3 million Americans currently living with traumatic brain injury and their families.
Andrew Horne, President Kentucky State Office
Chell Austin, Executive Director

Louisiana

4082 Brain Injury Association of Louisiana Help line
c/o National Headquarters Office
8325 Oak Street   504-982-0685
New Orleans, LA 70118   800-444-6443
                                          Fax: 703-761-0755
                                       e-mail: info@biala.org
                                              www.biala.org/
Founded in 1980, the Brain Injury Association of America (BIAA) is a national organization serving and representing individuals, families and professionals who are touched by a life-altering, often devastating, traumatic brain injury (TBI). BIAA provides information, education and support through its network of chartered state affiliates, local chapters and support groups across the country to assist the 5.3 million Americans currently living with traumatic brain injury and their families.
Janet Clark, Chairman
Tommy Lotz, Executive Director

Maryland

4083 Brain Injury Association of Maryland Helpl ine
Kernan Hospital
2200 Kernan Drive   410-448-2924
Baltimore, MD 21207   800-221-6443
                                          Fax: 410-448-3541
                                       e-mail: info@biamd.org
                                              www.biamd.org

Founded in 1980, the Brain Injury Association of America (BIAA) is a national organization serving and representing individuals, families and professionals who are touched by a life-altering, often devastating, traumatic brain injury (TBI). BIAA provides information, education and support through its network of chartered state affiliates, local chapters and support groups across the country to assist the 5.3 million Americans currently living with traumatic brain injury and their families.
Mark Huslage, President Maryland State Office
Bryan Thomas Pugh, Executive Director

Massachusetts

4084 Brain Injury Association of Massachusetts Helpline
30 Lyman Street · · · · · · · · · · · · · · · 508-475-0032
Westborough, MA 01581 · · · · · · · · · 800-242-0030
Fax: 508-475-0400
TTY: 508-948-0593
e-mail: biama@biama.org
www.biama.org
Founded in 1980, the Brain Injury Association of America (BIAA) is a national organization serving and representing individuals, families and professionals who are touched by a life-altering, often devastating, traumatic brain injury (TBI). BIAA provides information, education and support through its network of chartered state affiliates, local chapters and support groups across the country to assist the 5.3 million Americans currently living with traumatic brain injury and their families.
Teresa Hayes, President Massachusetts State Office
Mathew Martino, Executive Board

4085 VALT Support Group (Vital Active Life After Trauma)
53 Linden Street · · · · · · · · · · · · · · · 617-277-6327
Brookline, MA 02149

Michigan

4086 Brain Injury Association of Michigan Helpline
7305 Grand River · · · · · · · · · · · · · · · 810-229-5880
Brighton, MI 48114-2334 · · · · · · · · · 800-444-6443
Fax: 810-229-8947
e-mail: info@biami.org
www.biami.org
Deborah Newton, Chair
Michael F Dabbs, President

Minnesota

4087 Brain Injury Alliance of Minnesota
34 13th Avenue North East · · · · · · · · 612-378-2742
Minneapolis, MN 55413 · · · · · · · · · · 800-669-6442
Fax: 612-378-2789
e-mail: info@braininjurymn.org
www.braininjurymn.org
Tom Gode, Executive Director

Mississippi

4088 Brain Injury Association of Mississippi Helpline
2727 Old Canton Road · · · · · · · · · · · · 601-981-1021
Jackson, MS 39216-5912 · · · · · · · · · · 800-444-6443
Fax: 601-981-1039
e-mail: ljenkins@msbia.org
www.msbia.org/
Howard T Katz, MD, Chair
Lee Jenkins, Executive Director

Missouri

4089 Brain Injury Association of Missouri Helpline
2265 Schuetz Road · · · · · · · · · · · · · · 314-426-4024
St Louis, MO 63146-1322 · · · · · · · · · 800-444-6443
Fax: 314-426-3290
e-mail: info@biamo.org
www.biamo.org
Information and referral services and support groups throughout the state of Missouri.
Eric Hart, Psy.D, Board President
Stephanie Cooper, Executive Director

Montana

4090 Brain Injury Alliance of Montana
1280 South 3rd Street West · · · · · · · · 406-541-6442
Missoula, MT 59801 · · · · · · · · · · · · · 800-241-6442
Fax: 406-243-2349
e-mail: kristen@biamt.org
www.biamt.org
Kristen Morgan, MSW, Program Director
Molly Walsh, Outreach Coordinator

New Hampshire

4091 Brain Injury Association of New Hampshire
Brain Injury Association of America
109 N State Street · · · · · · · · · · · · · · · 603-225-8400
Concord, NH 03301-4447 · · · · · · · · · 800-773-8400
Fax: 603-228-6749
e-mail: mail@bianh.org
www.bianh.org
Laura Flashman, PhD, President
Steven D Wade, Executive Director

New Jersey

4092 Brain Injury Alliance of New Jersey
Brain Injury Association of America
825 Georges Road · · · · · · · · · · · · · · · 732-745-0200
North Brunswick, NJ 08902 · · · · · · · · 800-669-4323
Fax: 732-745-0211
e-mail: info@bianj.org
www.bianj.org
Edward Kim, MD, MBA, Chairperson
Barbara Geiger-Parker, President/CEO

New Mexico

4093 Brain Injury Alliance of New Mexico
3232 Candelaria NE · · · · · · · · · · · · · · 505-292-7414
Albuquerque, NM 87107 · · · · · · · · · · 888-292-7415
Fax: 505-271-8983
e-mail: braininjurynm@msn.com
www.braininjurynm.org
Founded in 1980, the Brain Injury Association of America (BIAA) is a national organization serving and representing individuals, families and professionals who are touched by a life-altering, often devastating, traumatic brain injury (TBI). BIAA provides information, education and support through its network of chartered state affiliates, local chapters and support groups across the country to assist the 5.3 million Americans currently living with traumatic brain injury and their families.
John Tiwald, Board President New Mexico State Office
Mark Pedrotty, PhD, Vice President

New York

4094 Brain Injury Association of New York State Helpline
10 Colvin Avenue · · · · · · · · · · · · · · · 518-459-7911
Albany, NY 12206-1242 · · · · · · · · · · 800-228-8201
Fax: 518-482-5285
e-mail: info@bianys.org
www.bianys.org
Marie Cavallo, Ph.D, President
Judith Avner, Executive Director

4095 Cafe Plus
216 W Manlius Street · · · · · · · · · · · · 315-446-3124
East Syracuse, NY 13057 · · e-mail: cafeplus@dreamscape.com
www.dreamscape.com/cafeplus
For people who have survived a head-injury or some type of head trauma.
David Listowski, Manager

4096 Hy Feinstein Clubhouse
Long Island Head Injury Association
300 Kennedy Drive · · · · · · · · · · · · · · 631-543-2245
Hauppauge, NY 11788 · · · · · · · · Fax: 631-543-2261
e-mail: lgiordano@headinjuryassoc.org
www.headinjuryassociation.org/feinstein.

The LIHIA provides a place for people with head injury to participate in meaningful work, to have the opportunity to meet and build friendships and ultimately seek employment within the community.
Stuart Gleiber, President
Leonard Feinstein, Vice President

North Carolina

4097 Brain Injury Association of North Carolina Helpline
2113 Cameron Street
Raleigh, NC 27605
919-833-9634
800-377-1464
Fax: 919-833-5415
e-mail: bianc@bianc.net
www.bianc.net/

Susan Baker, Director of Finance
Cindy Boyd, Fundraising Chair

North Dakota

4098 Brain Injury Association of North Dakota
1225 South 12th Street
Bismarck, ND 58504
877-525-2724
Fax: 701-845-1175
e-mail: braininjurynd@gmail.co
www.braininjurynd.com/
Founded in 1980, the Brain Injury Association of America (BIAA) is a national organization serving and representing individuals, families and professionals who are touched by a life-altering, often devastating, traumatic brain injury (TBI). BIAA provides information, education and support through its network of chartered state affiliates, local chapters and support groups across the country to assist the 5.3 million Americans currently living with traumatic brain injury and their families.
April Fairfield, Executive Director
Rebecca Quinn, Eastern Region Contact

Ohio

4099 Brain Injury Association of Ohio
855 Grandview Avenue
Columbus, OH 43215-1000
614-481-7100
800-444-6443
Fax: 614-481-7103
e-mail: help@biaoh.org
www.biaoh.org

Stephanie Ramsey, President
Jon Fishpaw, First Vice President

Oklahoma

4100 Brain Injury Association of Oklahoma Helpl ine
3015 E. Skelly Dr.
Tulsa, OK 74105-0088
918-789-0406
800-765-6809
Fax: 918-712-9019
e-mail: braininjuryoklahoma@gmail.com
www.braininjuryoklahoma.org
Founded in 1980, the Brain Injury Association of America (BIAA) is a national organization serving and representing individuals, families and professionals who are touched by a life-altering, often devastating, traumatic brain injury (TBI). BIAA provides information, education and support through its network of chartered state affiliates, local chapters and support groups across the country to assist the 5.3 million Americans currently living with traumatic brain injury and their families.
Adam Sherman, PhD, President Oklahoma State Office
Mary Dobbs, Vice-President

Oregon

4101 Brain Injury Alliance of Oregon
Brain Injury Association of America
2145 NW Overton Street
Portland, OR 97210
503-413-7707
800-544-5243
Fax: 503-413-6849
e-mail: biaor@biaoregon.org
www.biaoregon.org

Non-profit providing information and referral, support groups, prevention, education, training, and advocacy for those with brain injury, families, and professionals.
Ralph Wiser, President
Chuck McGilvrary, Vice-President

Rhode Island

4102 Brain Injury Association of Rhode Island H elpline
935 Park Avenue
Cranston, RI 02910-2743
401-461-6599
Fax: 401-461-6561
e-mail: braininjuryctr@biaofri.org
www.biausa.org/RI/
Founded in 1980, the Brain Injury Association of America (BIAA) is a national organization serving and representing individuals, families and professionals who are touched by a life-altering, often devastating, traumatic brain injury (TBI). BIAA provides information, education and support through its network of chartered state affiliates, local chapters and support groups across the country to assist the 5.3 million Americans currently living with traumatic brain injury and their families.
Michael L. Baker, Co-President
Sharon Brinkworth, Executive Director

Tennessee

4103 Brain Injury Association of Tennessee Help line
955 Woodland Street
Nashville, TN 37206
615-248-2541
800-444-6443
Fax: 615-383-1176
e-mail: biaoftn@yahoo.com
www.braininjurytn.org/
Founded in 1980, the Brain Injury Association of America (BIAA) is a national organization serving and representing individuals, families and professionals who are touched by a life-altering, often devastating, traumatic brain injury (TBI). BIAA provides information, education and support through its network of chartered state affiliates, local chapters and support groups across the country to assist the 5.3 million Americans currently living with traumatic brain injury and their families.
Guynn Edwards, President Tennessee State Office
Pam Bryan, Executive Director

Utah

4104 Brain Injury Alliance of Utah
Brain Injury Association of America
5280 Commerce Dr.
Murray, UT 84107
801-716-4993
800-281-8442
Fax: 801-716-4995
e-mail: info@biau.org
www.biau.org/

Antonietta Anna Russo, Ph.D., President
Ron S Roskos, Executive Director

Vermont

4105 Brain Injury Association of Vermont Helpli ne
92 South Main Street
Waterbury, VT 05676
802-244-6850
877-856-1772
Fax: 802-244-4005
e-mail: support1@biavt.org
www.biavt.org
Founded in 1980, the Brain Injury Association of America (BIAA) is a national organization serving and representing individuals, families and professionals who are touched by a life-altering, often devastating, traumatic brain injury (TBI). BIAA provides information, education and support through its network of chartered state affiliates, local chapters and support groups across the country to assist the 5.3 million Americans currently living with traumatic brain injury and their families.
Marsha Bancroft, President Vermont State Office
Trevor Squirrell, Executive Director

Virginia

4106 Brain Injury Association of Virginia Helpline
1506 Willow Lawn Dr
Richmond, VA 23230-5018
804-355-5748
800-444-6443
Fax: 804-355-6381
e-mail: info@biav.net
www.biav.net

Nonprofit organization providing information and resources related to brain injury to individuals with brain injuries, their families and professionals who deal with brain injury.
Kimberly Moore, President
Anne McDonnell, Executive Director

Washington

4107 Brain Injury Association of Washington Hel pline
P.O. Box 3044
Seattle, WA 98114
206-467-4800
877-982-4292
Fax: 206-467-4808
e-mail: info@braininjurywa.org
www.braininjurywa.org/

Founded in 1980, the Brain Injury Association of America (BIAA) is a national organization serving and representing individuals, families and professionals who are touched by a life-altering, often devastating, traumatic brain injury (TBI). BIAA provides information, education and support through its network of chartered state affiliates, local chapters and support groups across the country to assist the 5.3 million Americans currently living with traumatic brain injury and their families.
Mark T Long, President Washington State Office
Deborah Crawley, Executive Director

4108 Brain Injury Resource Center
Brain Injury Resource Center
PO Box 84151
Seattle, WA 98124-5451
206-621-8558
Fax: 206-329-4355
e-mail: brain@headinjury.com
www.headinjury.com

Disseminates head injury information and provides referrals to facilitate adjustment to life following head injury. Organizes seminars for professionals, head injury survivors, and their families.
Constance Miller MA, Founder/President
B Parker Lindner MPA, Communications Specialist

West Virginia

4109 Brain Injury Association of West Virginia Helpline
Brain Injury Association of America
PO Box 574
Institute, WV 25112-574
304-400-4506
800-356-6443
Fax: 304-766-4940
e-mail: mdavis@brainman.com

Michael W Davis, President

Wisconsin

4110 Brain Injury Alliance of Wisconsin
21100 W. Capitol Dr.
Brookfield, WI 53072
262-790-9660
800-882-9282
Fax: 262-790-9670
e-mail: admin@execpc.com
www.biaw.org

Founded in 1980, the Brain Injury Association of America (BIAA) is a national organization serving and representing individuals, families and professionals who are touched by a life-altering, often devastating, traumatic brain injury (TBI). BIAA provides information, education and support through its network of chartered state affiliates, local chapters and support groups across the country to assist the 5.3 million Americans currently living with traumatic brain injury and their families.
Audrey Nelson, President Wisconsin State Office
Lori Schultz, Executive Director

Wyoming

4111 Brain Injury Alliance of Wyoming
111 West 2nd Street
Casper, WY 82601
307-473-1767
800-643-6457
Fax: 307-237-5222
e-mail: director@wybia.org
www.wybia.org/

Dorothy Cronin, Director

Books

4112 An Educational Challenge: Meeting the Needs of Students with Brain Injury
Brain Injury Association
2775 South Quincy Street
Arlington, VA 22206
703-998-2020
800-444-6443
Fax: 703-236-6001
e-mail: info@brainline.org
www.brainline.org

Noel Gunther, Executive Director
Christian Lindstrom, Director

4113 Brain Injury Glossary
HDI Publishers
5215 Ashe Rd.
Bakersfield, CA 93313
661-872-3408
800-922-4994
Fax: 661-872-5150
e-mail: spersel@neuroskills.com
www.neuroskills.com

Contains glossary and descriptions of health care providers.
Mark J. Ashley, President and CEO

4114 Brainlash
Demos Medical Publishing
11 West 42nd Street
New York, NY 10036
212-683-0072
Fax: 212-683-0118
e-mail: support@demosmedical.com
www.demosmedpub.com

Maximize your recovery from mild brain injury.
376 pages
ISBN: 1-888799-37-4
Dr. Diana M Schneider

4115 Coming Home: A Discharge Manual for Families of Persons with a Brain Injury
HDI Publishers
5215 Ashe Rd.
Bakersfield, CA 93313
661-872-3408
800-922-4994
Fax: 661-872-5150
e-mail: spersel@neuroskills.com
www.neuroskills.com

Mark J. Ashley, President and CEO

4116 Communication Disorders Following Traumatic Brain Injury
Pro-Ed, Inc.
8700 Shoal Creek Blvd
Austin, TX 78757-6897
512-451-3246
800-897-3202
Fax: 800-397-7633
e-mail: info@proedinc.com
www.proedinc.com

For graduates and professionals, this text takes a holistic approach toward treating the client with traumatic brain injury.
439 pages Paperback
ISBN: 0-890792-95-X
Lindy Jordaan, Marketing Coordinator

4117 Dano Cerebral: Guia Para Familias y Cuidadores
Brain Injury Association/HDI Publishers/Catalogue
PO Box 131401
Houston, TX 77219
800-321-7037
Fax: 713-526-7787

This book, written in Spanish, is a thorough, well-researched guide for people with brain injury, their families and caregivers. Up-to-date information covers such topics as Intensive Care- admittance and discharge; Mechanics of brain injury; Coma; Consequences of brain injury; Mental and Emotional symptoms among many others.
158 pages 1994

4118   From the Ashes
Phoenix Project
PO Box 84151
Seattle, WA 98124-5451   206-621-8558
                               e-mail: brain@headinjury.com
                                     www. headinjury.com
A self-help book that addresses the trauma that comes with a head
injury and introduces methods of building a fulfilling and produc-
tive life.
108 pages

4119   Handbook of Head Truma: Acute Care to Recovery
Plenum Publishing Corporation
233 Spring Street   212-620-8000
New York, NY 10013-1522   800-221-9369
                                    Fax: 212-463-0742
                               e-mail: books@plenum.com
                                     journals.lww.com

466 pages
ISBN: 0-306439-47-6
Nathan R. Selden, President
Zoher Ghogawala, VP

4120   Head Injury and the Family: A Life and Living Perspective
St. Lucie Press
100 E Linton Boulevard   407-274-9906
Delary Beach, FL 33483   Fax: 407-274-9927
One of the best books written in this area. Easy to read, written with
family, caregivers and patients in mind. Includes exercises and vignettes.

4121   Integrating Community Resources
HDI Publishers
540 Gaither Road   301-427-1104
Rockville, MD 20850   800-321-7037
                                    Fax: 713-956-2288
                                         www.ahrq.gov

4122   Living with Brain Injury: A Guide for Families
Brain Injury Association/HDI Publishers/Catalogue
PO Box 131401   512-785-4469
Houston, TX 77219   800-321-7037
                                    Fax: 713-526-7787
                          e-mail: rusty@sheltoninteractive.com
                                  www.richardsenelick.com
This book will help readers- families, persons with brain injury
and professionals alike- through this uncharted territory. topics include: How brain injury is caused and how it can be treated: Physical, cognitive and behavioral symptoms; Questions family
members commonly ask.
145 pages 1998
Richard C. Senelick, Author

4123   National Directory of Brain Injury Rehabilitatiom
Brain Injury Association
2775 South Quincy Street   703-998-2020
Arlington, VA 22206   800-444-6443
                                    Fax: 703-236-6001
                               e-mail: info@brainline.org
                                     www.brainline.org
Desk reference for professionals listing brain injury rehabilitation
programs and individual service providers nationwide.
Noel Gunther, Executive Director
Christian Lindstrom, Director

4124   National Directory of Head Injury Rehabilitation Services
Brain Injury Association
2775 South Quincy Street   703-998-2020
Arlington, VA 22206   800-444-6443
                                    Fax: 703-236-6001
                               e-mail: info@brainline.org
                                     www.brainline.org

Noel Gunther, Executive Director
Christian Lindstrom, Director

4125   Planning for the Future
Brain Injury Association

2775 South Quincy Street   703-998-2020
Arlington, VA 22206   800-444-6443
                                    Fax: 703-236-6001
                               e-mail: info@brainline.org
                                     www.brainline.org
This book provides a meaningful life for a child with a disability
after your death.
Noel Gunther, Executive Director
Christian Lindstrom, Director

4126   Recovery from Brain Damage in the Elderly
Aspen Publishers
8600 Rockville Pike
Bethesda, MD 20894-0990   800-638-8437
                                    www.ncbi.nlm.nih.gov
Recovery and rehabilitation techniques in the area of brain damage
in the elderly.

4127   Sexuality and the Person with Traumatic Brain Injury
Brain Injury Association
1000 Thomas Jefferson   202-403-5600
Washington, DC 20007   800-444-6443
                                    Fax: 703-236-6001
                                    TTY: 877-334-3499
                               e-mail: msktc@air.org
                                       www.msktc.org

**4128   Stress Management Following Head Injury: Strategies for
Families and Caregivers**
Brain Injury Association
2775 South Quincy Street   703-998-2020
Arlington, VA 22206   800-444-6443
                                    Fax: 703-236-6001
                               e-mail: info@brainline.org
                                     www.brainline.org

Noel Gunther, Executive Director
Christian Lindstrom, Director

4129   TBI Tool Kit
HDI Publishers
2775 South Quincy Street   703-998-2020
Arlington, VA 22206   800-321-7037
                                    Fax: 713-956-2288
                               e-mail: info@brainline.org
                                     www.brainline.org

Noel Gunther, Executive Director
Christian Lindstrom, Director

**4130   Traumatic Brain Injury Rehabilitation: Brain Injury Consortium
Monograph Series**
St. Lucie Press
250 Greenwich St.   212-772-0608
New York, NY 10007   Fax: 407-274-9927
                                    www.braintrauma.org
Assistive technology, under the Americans with Disabilities Act,
is that designed for and used by individuals with the intent of elimi-
nating, ameliorating, or compensating for functional limitations.
Coverage includes impaired functions that limit vocational out-
come, behavior concerns in the workplace, maximizing a client's
residual knowledge skills, use of computers and adapting work
environments.
Jamshid Ghajar, President
Alan Quasha, Chairman

4131   Traumatic Head Injury: Cause, Consequence and Challenge
Brain Injury Association/HDI Publishers/Catalogue
785 Market St.
San Francisco, CA 94103   800-445-8106
                                    Fax: 713-526-7787
                                    https://caregiver.org
A resource book on traumatic brain injury which translates technical medical information on brain injury into simple, easy-to-understand language for persons with brain injury and their families.
Covered topics: a general overview of brain injury; similarities
and differences among people with brain injury; types and consequences of brain injury; recovery and rehabilitation; accepting and
coping with change.
60 pages 1993
Ping Hao, President
Jacquelyn Kung, VP

4132 **Why Did it Happen on a School Day: My Family's Experience with Brain Injury**
Brain Injury Association
2775 South Quincy Street
Arlington, VA 22206
703-998-2020
800-444-6443
Fax: 703-236-6001
www.brainline.org

Noel Gunther, Executive Director
Christian Lindstrom, Director

4133 **Working After Brain Injury**
HDI Publishers
2775 South Quincy Street
Arlington, VA 22206
703-998-2020
800-321-7037
Fax: 713-956-2288
www.brainline.org

Noel Gunther, Executive Director
Christian Lindstrom, Director

Magazines

4134 **Journal of Head Trauma Rehabilitation**
Aspen Publishers
2001 Market Street
Philadelphia, PA 19103-3129
215-521-8300
800-638-8437
www.lww.com
Scholarly journal designed to provide information on clinical management and rehabilitation of the head-injured for the practicing professional.

Jennifer E. Brogan, Vice President
Kivmars Bowling, Senior Publisher

4135 **Mouth Magazine**
PO Box 558
Topeka, KS 66601-0558
785-272-2578
Fax: 785-272-7348
www.mouthmag.org

Bi-monthly magazine with subscription.
Lucy Gwin, Editor-designer
Cal Grandy, General Officer

Newsletters

4136 **BIAW News**
Brain Injury Association of Wisconsin
N63 W23583 Main Street
Sussex, WI 53089
262-790-9660
800-882-9282
Fax: 262-790-9670
e-mail: admin@biaw.org
www.biaw.org

David Voss, President
Mark Warhus, Executive Director

4137 **Brain Injury Source**
Brain Injury Association
1608 Spring Hill Road
Vienna, VA 22182
703-761-0750
800-444-6443
Fax: 703-761-0755
e-mail: BIAV@visi.net
www.biausa.org

Written for and by professionals in the field. Blends professionally written articles on information and research in brain injury with a user friendly format that incorporates graphics and charts to effectively deliver the messages. Full color.
50+ pages Quarterly

4138 **Brain Waves**
Brain Injury Association of Florida
1637 Metropolitan Blvd
Tallahassee, FL 32308
850-410-0103
800-992-3442
Fax: 850-410-0105
e-mail: admin@biaf.org
www.biaf.org

Each issue highlights a topic related to TBI and TBI resources.
Bi-Annually
Valerie E Breen, President/CEO

4139 **Brainstorm**
Brain Injury Association of Arizona
5025 E. Washington Street
Phoenix, AZ 85034
602-508-8024
888-500-9165
Fax: 602-323-9165
e-mail: info@biaaz.org
www.biaaz.org
A newsletter serving persons with brain injury, their families and professionals.
8 pages Quarterly
Robert Djergaian, Board President
Tom Nielsen, Vice President

4140 **TBI Challenge!**
Brain Injury Association of America
1608 Spring Hill Road
Vienna, VA 22182-3010
703-761-0750
800-444-6443
Fax: 703-761-0755
www.biausa.org
Exclusively for and about persons with brain injury. Provides information to individuals with brain injury and their families. Professionals will benefit from the perspectives provided in Kid's Corner, Relatively Speaking, Ask the Lawyer, Information and Resources and Ask the Doctor.
bimonthly

Pamphlets

4141 **A Survey of Accredited and Other Rehabilitation Facilities**
Brain Injury Association
6951 East Southpoint Road
Tucson, AZ 85756
703-236-6000
800-444-6443
Fax: 520-318-1129
www.carf.org
Education, training and cognitive rehabilitation in barin injury programs.
Herb Zaretsky, Board Chair

4142 **About Head Injuries**
Channing L Bete Company
P.O.BOX 84151
Seattle, WA 98124
206-621-8558
800-628-7733
www.headinjury.com
Covers basic information including identifying the members of the treatment team and how to take care of yourself as a caregiver.

4143 **Adolescents with Closed Head Injuries: A Report of Initial Cognitive Deficits**
Brain Injury Association
P.O.BOX 84151
Seattle, WA 98124
206-621-8558
800-444-6443
Fax: 703-236-6001
www.headinjury.com

4144 **Basic Questions About Head Injury & Disability**
Brain Injury Association
P.O.BOX 84151
Seattle, WA 98124
206-621-8558
800-444-6443
Fax: 703-236-6001
www.headinjury.com

4145 **Behavioral and Psychosocial Sequelae of Pediatric Head Injury**
Brain Injury Association
P.O.BOX 84151
Seattle, WA 98124
206-621-8558
800-444-6443
Fax: 703-236-6001
www.headinjury.com

4146 **Brain Damage is a Family Affair**
Brain Injury Association
P.O.BOX 84151
Seattle, WA 98124
206-621-8558
800-444-6443
Fax: 703-236-6001
www.headinjury.com

4147 **Brain Injuries: A Guide for Families & Caretakers**
Brain Injury Association

P.O.BOX 84151
Seattle, WA 98124

206-621-8558
800-444-6443
Fax: 703-236-6001
www.headinjury.com

4148   Brain Injury: A Home Based Cognitive Rehabilitation Program
HDI Publishers
2775 South Quincy Street
Arlington, VA 22206

703-998-2020
800-321-7037
Fax: 713-956-2288
e-mail: info@brainline.org
www.brainline.org

4149   Catastrophic Injury Cases: The Relationship of Traumatic Brain Injury
Brain Injury Association
P.O.BOX 84151
Seattle, WA 98124

206-621-8558
800-444-6443
Fax: 703-236-6001
www.headinjury.com

4150   Children with Disabilities: Understanding Sibling Issues
Brain Injury Association
P.O.BOX 84151
Seattle, WA 98124

206-621-8558
800-444-6443
Fax: 703-236-6001
www.headinjury.com

4151   Counseling Head Injured Patients: Guidelines for Community Health Workers
Brain Injury Association
P.O.BOX 84151
Seattle, WA 98124

206-621-8558
800-444-6443
Fax: 703-236-6001
www.headinjury.com

4152   Education Concerns for the Traumatically Head Injured Student
Brain Injury Association
P.O.BOX 84151
Seattle, WA 98124

206-621-8558
800-444-6443
Fax: 703-236-6001
www.headinjury.com

4153   From One Family Member to Another
Brain Injury Association
P.O.BOX 84151
Seattle, WA 98124

206-621-8558
800-444-6443
Fax: 703-236-6001
www.headinjury.com

A mother tells the story of her son's injury and recovery. Gives suggestions for structuring the home environment.

4154   Guide to Selecting and Monitoring Head Injury Rehabilitation Services
Brain Injury Association
P.O.BOX 84151
Seattle, WA 98124

206-621-8558
800-444-6443
Fax: 703-236-6001
www.headinjury.com

4155   Head Injury Survivor on Campus: Issues & Resources
Brain Injury Association
P.O.BOX 84151
Seattle, WA 98124

206-621-8558
800-444-6443
Fax: 703-236-6001
www.headinjury.com

4156   Head Injury: A Booklet for Families
Brain Injury Association
P.O.BOX 84151
Seattle, WA 98124

206-621-8558
800-444-6443
Fax: 703-236-6001
www.headinjury.com

4157   Head Injury: A Guide for Families
HDI Publishers
P.O.BOX 84151
Seattle, WA 98124

206-621-8558
800-321-7037
Fax: 713-956-2288
www.headinjury.com

Structured by problem with examples and practical coping strategies.

4158   Hearing Loss Following Head Injury
Brain Injury Association
P.O.BOX 84151
Seattle, WA 98124

206-621-8558
800-444-6443
Fax: 703-236-6001
www.headinjury.com

4159   Hiring Persons with a Brain Injury: What to Expect
HDI Publishers
P.O.BOX 84151
Seattle, WA 98124

206-621-8558
800-321-7037
Fax: 713-956-2288
www.headinjury.com

4160   Individual Psychotherapy with the Brain Injured Adult
Brain Injury Association
P.O.BOX 84151
Seattle, WA 98124

206-621-8558
800-444-6443
Fax: 703-236-6001
www.headinjury.com

Review of literature on substance abuse and head injury. Includes statistics, and treatment options, strategies and extensive bibliography.

4161   Information General Sobre: Lesion Cerebral
Brain Injury Association
P.O.BOX 84151
Seattle, WA 98124

206-621-8558
800-444-6443
Fax: 703-236-6001
www.headinjury.com

4162   Introductory Information for Families
Brain Injury Association
P.O.BOX 84151
Seattle, WA 98124

206-621-8558
800-444-6443
Fax: 703-236-6001
www.headinjury.com

A collection of readings on basic information about TBI and a guide for selecting rehabilitation facilities.

4163   Know Your Brain
Nat'l Institute of Neurological Disorders & Stroke
PO Box 5801
Bethesda, MD 20824

301-496-5751
800-352-9424
Fax: 301-402-2186
www.ninds.nih.gov

Basic information about the brain, neuroscience research, and disorders of the brain.

4164   Legal and Financial Issues for Families
Brain Injury Association
P.O.BOX 84151
Seattle, WA 98124

206-621-8558
800-444-6443
Fax: 703-236-6001
www.headinjury.com

Packet designed for families that explores some of the legal and financial issues faced after TBI.

4165   Life After Brain Injury: Who am I
HDI Publishers
2775 South Quincy Street
Arlington, VA 22206

703-998-2020
800-321-7037
Fax: 713-956-2288
e-mail: info@brainline.org
www.brainline.org

A well-structured book. Dicusses specific problems areas. Includes good examples and gives lists of practical coping strategies.

4166   Mild Brain Injury: Damage and Outcome
Brain Injury Association
P.O.BOX 84151
Seattle, WA 98124

206-621-8558
800-444-6443
Fax: 703-236-6001
www.headinjury.com

4167   Neuropsychology of Attention and Memory
Brain Injury Association
P.O.BOX 84151
Seattle, WA 98124

206-621-8558
800-444-6443
Fax: 703-236-6001
www.headinjury.com

4168 Persisting Problems After Mild Head Injury: A Review of the Syndrome
Brain Injury Association
P.O.BOX 84151
Seattle, WA 98124
206-621-8558
800-444-6443
Fax: 703-236-6001
www.headinjury.com

4169 Post-Traumatic Headaches: Subtypes & Behavioral Treatments
Brain Injury Association
P.O.BOX 84151
Seattle, WA 98124
206-621-8558
800-444-6443
Fax: 703-236-6001
www.headinjury.com

4170 Recovery and Cognitive Retraining After Craniocerebral Trauma
Brain Injury Association
P.O.BOX 84151
Seattle, WA 98124
206-621-8558
800-444-6443
Fax: 703-236-6001
www.headinjury.com

4171 Relationships Between Personality Disorders
Brain Injury Association
P.O.BOX 84151
Seattle, WA 98124
206-621-8558
800-444-6443
Fax: 703-236-6001
www.headinjury.com
Social Disturbances and physical disability following TBI.

4172 Resources List of Organizations
Brain Injury Association
P.O.BOX 84151
Seattle, WA 98124
206-621-8558
800-444-6443
Fax: 703-236-6001
www.headinjury.com

4173 Severe Brain Injury
Brain Injury Association
P.O.BOX 84151
Seattle, WA 98124
206-621-8558
800-444-6443
Fax: 703-236-6001
www.headinjury.com
This pamphlet is in hand out format and would be appropriate for use in clinic or hospital setting.

4174 Spouses of Persons Who Are Brain Injured: Overlooked Victims
Brain Injury Association
P.O.BOX 84151
Seattle, WA 98124
206-621-8558
800-444-6443
Fax: 703-236-6001
www.headinjury.com

4175 Stress Management Following Head Injury: Strategies for Families & Caregivers
Brain Injury Association
P.O.BOX 84151
Seattle, WA 98124
206-621-8558
800-444-6443
Fax: 703-236-6001
www.headinjury.com

4176 Subarachnoid Hemorrhage & Aneurysm
University Hospital & Clinics
269 Hanover Street
Hanover, MA 02339
781-826-5556
888-272-4602
Fax: 781-826-5566
e-mail: debra@bafound.org
www.bafound.org
This pamphlet includes easy to read, general information plus a glossary and schematic diagrams. This pamphlet would be most appropriate for use with recently head injured patients.
Christine Buckley, Executive Director??
Debra Coulter?, Director of Information Technology

4177 Substance Abuse Task Force White Paper
Brain Injury Association
P.O.BOX 84151
Seattle, WA 98124
206-621-8558
800-444-6443
Fax: 703-236-6001
www.headinjury.com

Review of literature on substance abuse and head injury. Includes statistics, and treatment options, strategies and extensive bibliography.

4178 Susan's Dad: A Child's Story of Head Injury
Brain Injury Association
P.O.BOX 84151
Seattle, WA 98124
206-621-8558
800-444-6443
Fax: 703-236-6001
www.headinjury.com

4179 Teaching Persons with A Brain Injury: What to Expect
HDI Publishers
1608 Spring Hill Road
Vienna, VA 22182
703-761-0750
800-444-6443
Fax: 703-761-0755
www.biausa.org
Daniel S. Chamberlain, Chairman
Susan H. Connors, President and CEO

4180 Unseen Injury: Minor Head Injury
Brain Injury Association
P.O.BOX 84151
Seattle, WA 98124
206-621-8558
800-444-6443
Fax: 703-236-6001
www.headinjury.com

4181 What is Anoxic Brain Injury
Brain Injury Association
P.O.BOX 84151
Seattle, WA 98124
206-621-8558
800-444-6443
Fax: 703-236-6001
www.headinjury.com

4182 When Your Child Goes to School After an Injury
Brain Injury Association
P.O.BOX 84151
Seattle, WA 98124
206-621-8558
800-444-6443
Fax: 703-236-6001
www.headinjury.com

4183 When Your Child is Seriously Injured: The Emotional Impact on Families
Brain Injury Association
P.O.BOX 84151
Seattle, WA 98124
206-621-8558
800-444-6443
Fax: 703-236-6001
www.headinjury.com

4184 Working After A Head Injury
HDI Publishers
1608 Spring Hill Road
Vienna, VA 22182
703-761-0750
800-444-6443
Fax: 703-761-0755
www.biausa.org
Daniel S. Chamberlain, Chairman
Susan H. Connors, President and CEO

Audio & Video

4185 A Fate Better than Death
Brain Injury Association
P.O.BOX 84151
Seattle, WA 98124
206-621-8558
800-444-6443
Fax: 703-236-6001
www.headinjury.com
Video features 4 young adults with traumatic brain injury. Focuses on support groups.

4186 Neuropsychological Assessment: What it Does & Does Not Do
Brain Injury Association
P.O.BOX 84151
Seattle, WA 98124
206-621-8558
800-444-6443
Fax: 703-236-6001
www.headinjury.com
This pamphlet is in hand out format and would be appropriate for use in clinic or hospital setting.

4187 Peter Wegner Is Alive and Well and Living in Providence
Filmakers Library

3212 Duke Street   212-808-4980
Alexandria, VA 22314-1798   Fax: 212-808-4983
                           e-mail: sales@alexanderstreet.com
                                      www.filmakers.com

Peter Wegner was a professor at Brown University when he recveived an award in London and was hit by a bus there. The film follows the challenges and decisions faced by his family, in dealing with the serious brain injuries sustained. Comatose, brain surgery, how can a person decide the right path for their loved one? Winner of American Psychology Award. DVD or VHS $195, Classroom Rental $55
VHS or DVD
Sue Oscar, Co-President

4188   Unseen Injury: Minor Head Injury
Brain Injury Association
P.O.BOX 84151   206-621-8558
Seattle, WA 98124   800-444-6443
                                    Fax: 703-236-6001
                                    www.headinjury.com
Designed specifically for viewing by family members.

4189   Surviving Coma: The Journey Back
Brain Injury Association
P.O.BOX 84151   206-621-8558
Seattle, WA 98124   800-444-6443
                                    Fax: 703-236-6001
                                    www.headinjury.com
21 minutes

Web Sites

4190   Agency for Healthcare: Research Facility
                                      www.ahcpr.gov
The Agency for Healthcare Research and Quality's (AHRQ) mission is to produce evidence to make health care safer, higher quality, more accessible, equitable, and affordable, and to work within the U.S. Department of Health and Human Services and with other partners to make sure that the evidence is understood and used.

4191   American Brain Tumor Association
                                        www.abta.org
Provides comprehensive resources that support the complex needs of brain tumor patients and caregivers, as well as the critical funding of research in the pursuit of breakthroughs in brain tumor diagnosis, treatment and care.

4192   Brain Injury Association
                                       www.biausa.org
Seeking to improve the quality of life for people with brain injuries and their families through information and resource referral, legislative advocacy, prevention awareness, and professional education. BIA's mission is to create a better future through brain injury prevention, research, education and advocacy.

4193   Brain Research Institute: Medicine School University of California, Los Angeles
                                      www.bri.ucla.edu
The UCLA Brain Research Institute (BRI) is a catalyst for education, outreach, and research collaborations among current and future scientists, engineers and clinicians who seek to understand the healthy and diseased brain.

4194   Headinjury.Com
                                    www.headinjury.com
Maintained by the Head Injury Hotline, a non-profit clearinghouse founded and operated by head injury activist. The primary goal are to empower through education, resources and support. The basic premise is that the medical system is deeply flawed and that the brain injury rehab industry is no exception. The site integrates resources from diverse organizations including support groups, rehabilitation and research sites.

4195   Healing Well
                                    www.healingwell.com
An online health resource guide to medical news, chat, information and articles, newsgroups and message boards, books, disease-related web sites, medical directories, and more for patients, friends, and family coping with disabling diseases, disorders, or chronic illnesses.

4196   Health Finder
                                    www.healthfinder.gov
Searchable, carefully developed web site offering information on over 1000 topics. Developed by the US Department of Health and Human Services, the site can be used in both English and Spanish.

4197   Healthlink USA
                                    www.healthlinkusa.com
Health information concerning treatment, cures, prevention, diagnosis, risk factors, research, support groups, email lists, personal stories and much more. Updated regularly.

4198   Helios Health
                                     www.helioshealth.com
Online resource for your health information. Detailed information about specific health topics, access to expert advice from our Medical Advisory Board, and up-to-date health news.

4199   MedicineNet
                                      www.medicinenet.com
An online resource for consumers providing easy-to-read, authoritative medical and health information.

4200   Medscape
                                       www.medscape.com
Medscape offers specialists, primary care physicians, and other health professionals the Web's most robust and integrated medical information and educational tools.

4201   Neurology Channel
                                  www.healthcommunities.com
Find clearly explained, medically accurate information regarding conditions, including an overview, symptoms, causes, diagnostic procedures and treatment options. On this site it is possible to ask questions and get information from a neurologist and connect to people who have similar health interests.

4202   Road Less Traveled
                                       www.lesstravel.org
Dedicated to survivors and families of victims of Traumatic Brain Injury.

4203   TBI Help
                                        www.tbihelp.com
Information concerning head injury.

4204   Traumatic Brain Injury
                                  www.traumaticbraininjury.com
Internet resource for education, advocacy, research and support for brain injury survivors, their families, and medical and rehabilitation professionals.

Description

4205 Hearing Impairment

Approximately 21 million Americans have some degree of hearing impairment or Deafness. This common problem affects people of all ages, and the loss can range from mild to severe.

Hearing loss is divided into four categories: conductive, sensorineural, mixed and central. Conductive hearing loss is caused by a defect in the external ear canal or middle ear, and can be helped by hearing aids, medical treatment or surgery. Sensorineural hearing loss results from damage to the inner ear and to the primary nerve that transmits sound waves to the brain. Mixed hearing loss is a combination of conductive and sensorineural defects. Central hearing loss results from impairment of brain function.

Hearing loss may be present at birth or begin later in life. Causes include infections (such as meningitis), injury, prolonged noise exposure, hereditary diseases and side effects of certain drugs. Amplification of sound with hearing aids helps almost all persons with mild-to-severe conductive or sensorineural hearing loss. Profoundly deaf persons who cannot be helped by hearing aids may benefit from a cochlear implant, a specialized device inserted into the inner ear. Children with hearing impairments may have slow or inaccurate speech development, or problems with concentration. Early diagnosis usually helps children improve their auditory ability, through the use of hearing aids, educational programs and speech therapy. Hearing loss in adults, if moderate or severe, is usually obvious to the patient family members. In young children, however, the problem is easily overlooked and the opportunity for early intervention can be lost.

National Agencies & Associations

4206 ABLEDATA
8630 Fenton Street
Silver Spring, MD 20910
301-608-8998
800-227-0216
Fax: 301-608-8958
TTY: 301-608-8912
e-mail: abledata@macrointernational.com
www.abledata.com
An information and referral service that uses computer listings and a large file system to answer requests related to assistive devices. Houses a large file system library and contacts with other sources which enables them to answer just about any question.
Katherine Belknap, Project Director
Steve Lowe, Associate Project Manager/Webmaster

4207 ADARA
PO Box 480
Myersville, MD 21773
501-224-6678
Fax: 501-868-8812
TTY: 501-868-8850
e-mail: adaraorg@comcast.net
www.adara.org
Professional networking for excellence in service delivery with individuals who are deaf or hard of hearing. A partnership of national organizations, local affiliates, professional sections and individual members working together to support social services.
Barry Critchfield, President
Michelle Niehaus, President-Elect

4208 Academy of Doctors of Audiology
3493 Lansdowne Dr.
Lexington, KY 40517
866-493-5544
Fax: 859-271-0607
www.audiologist.org
Encourages audiology training programs to include pertinent aspects of hearing aid dispensing in their curriculum.
Nancy N Green, President
Brian Urban, President-Elect

4209 Academy of Rehabilitative Audiology
PO Box 952
DeSoto, TX 75123
e-mail: ara@audrehab.org
www.audrehab.org
Provides professional education research and interest in programs for hearing handicapped persons.
Kathleen Cienkowski, Ph.D., President
Linda Thibodeau, Ph.D., President-Elect

4210 American Academy of Audiology
11480 Commerce Park Drive
Reston, VA 20191
703-790-8466
800-222-2336
Fax: 703-790-8631
e-mail: infoaud@audiology.org
www.audiology.org
A professional organization of individuals dedicated to providing high quality hearing care to the public. Provides professional development education and research and provides increased public awareness of hearing disorders and audiologic services.
Bettie Borton, President
Erin Miller, President-Elect

4211 American Academy of Otolaryngology: Head
1650 Diagonal Road
Alexandria, VA 22314-3357
703-836-4444
Fax: 703-684-4288
TTY: 703-519-1585
e-mail: executiveservices@entnet.org
www.entnet.org
The missions of the AAO-HNS and its foundation are to advance the art and science of otolaryngology-head and neck surgery through state-of-the-art education, research and learning; and to unite, serve and represent the interests of its members and their families.
James L. Netterville, President
Richard W. Waguespack, President-Elect

4212 American Association of the Deaf-Blind
PO Box 2831
Kensington, MD 20891-3803
301-495-4403
Fax: 301-495-4404
TTY: 301-495-4402
e-mail: AADB-Info@aadb.org
www.aadb.org
Promotes better opportunities and services for deaf-blind people. The mission of this organization is to assure that a comprehensive, coordinated system of services is accessible to all deaf-blind people, enabling them to achieve their maximum potential.
600 Members
Jill Gaus, President
Lynn Jansen, Vice President

4213 American Auditory Society
PO Box 779
Pennsville, NJ 08070
877-746-8315
Fax: 650-763-9185
e-mail: amaudsoc@comcast.net
www.amauditorysoc.org
Publishes Ear & Hearing and The Bulletin of the American Auditory Society.
Linda Hood, PhD, President
Darla M. Eastlack, Executive Director

4214 American Hearing Research Foundation
310 W. Lake Street
Elmhurst, IL 60126-4539
630-617-5079
Fax: 630-563-9181
e-mail: sparmet@american-hearing.org
www.american-hearing.org
Supports medical research and education into the causes prevention and cures of deafness, hearing losses and balance disorders.

Also keeps physicians and the public informed of the latest developments in hearing research and education.

Richard G. Muench, Chairman
Alan G. Micco, President

4215 American Society for Deaf Children
800 Florida Avenue NE, #2047   202-644-9204
Washington, DC 20002-3695   800-942-2732
                                             Fax: 410-795-0965
                                             TTY: 717-334-8808
                                 e-mail: asdc@deafchildren.org
                                         www.deafchildren.org

A nonprofit parent-helping-parent organization promoting a positive attitude toward signing and deaf culture. Also provides support encouragement and current information about deafness to families with deaf and hard of hearing children.

Beth S Benedict PhD, President
Joseph Finnegan, VP

4216 American Speech-Language-Hearing Association
2200 Research Boulevard   301-296-5700
Rockville, MD 20850   800-638-8255
                                             Fax: 301-296-8580
                                             TTY: 301-296-5650
                                  e-mail: actioncenter@asha.org
                                                  www.asha.org

A professional and scientific organization for speech-language pathologists and audiologists concerned with communication disorders. Provides informational materials and a toll-free HELPLINE number for consumers to inquire about speech, language or hearing disorders.

Patricia A. Prelock, PhD, President
Elizabeth S. McCrea, PhD, President -Elect

4217 American Tinnitus Association
522 SW Fifth Avenue   503-248-9985
Portland, OR 97204-0005   800-634-8978
                                             Fax: 503-248-0024
                                       e-mail: tinnitus@ata.org
                                                   www.ata.org

Provides information about tinnitus and referrals to local contacts/support groups nationwide. Also provides a bibliography service, funds scientific research related to tinnitus and offers workshops to professionals. Works to promote public education.

Thomas J. Lobl, PhD, Chair
Melanie F. West, Vice-Chair

4218 Association of Late-Deafened Adults
8038 Macintosh Lane   815-332-1515
Rockford, IL 61107   866-402-2532
                                             Fax: 877-907-1738
                                             TTY: 815-332-1515
                                        e-mail: info@alda.org
                                                  www.alda.org

Serves as a resource and information center for late-deafened adults and works to increase public awareness of the special needs of late-deafened adults.

Mary Lou Mistretta, President
Dave Litman, President-Elect

4219 Auditory-Verbal International
1390 Chain Bridge Road   703-739-1049
McLean, VA 22101   Fax: 703-739-0395
                                             TTY: 703-739-0874
                                    e-mail: audiverb@aol.com
                                        www.auditory-verbal.org

Dedicated to helping children who have hearing losses learn to listen and speak. Promotes the Auditory-Verbal Therapy approach which is based on the belief that the overwhelming majority of these children can hear and talk by using their residual hearing ability.

Chellie Lisenby, Executive Director
Steven R Rech, President

4220 Better Hearing Institute
1444 I Street NW   202-449-1100
Washington, DC 20005   800-327-9355
                                             Fax: 202-216-9646
                                             TTY: 703-642-0580
                                   e-mail: mail@betterhearing.org
                                            www.betterhearing.org

A nonprofit educational organization that implements national public information programs on hearing loss and available medical, surgical, hearing aid and rehabilitation assistance for millions with uncorrected hearing problems.

Sergei Kochk PhD, Executive Director
Renee La Mura, Administrative Director

4221 CAPCOM
6707 Old Dominion Drive   202-363-0535
McLean, VA 22101   800-241-2232
                                             TTY: 703-749-1876

Conducts research on the special needs of the hearing impaired including senior citizens. Presents workshops on law and the deaf and on promoting productive working relationships for the hearing impaired employees of agencies and corporations.

4222 Canine Assistance for the Disabled CADI
CADI
3958 Union Road   314-892-2554
Saint Louis, MO 63125   e-mail: supportdogs@MSN.com

The mission of Support Dogs Inc. is to give people with disabilities greater independence and improve lives through the help of a support or touch dog and promote canines as partners through abilities education.

4223 Center on Employment: Rochester Institute of Technology
National Technical Institute for the Deaf
52 Lomb Memorial Drive   585-475-6400
Rochester, NY 14623-5604   Fax: 585-475-7570
                                             TTY: 585-475-6400
                                       e-mail: ntidcoe@rit.edu
                                            www.ntid.rit.edu/nce

Operated by the National Technical Institute for the Deaf at Rochester Institute of Technology, the NTIC Center on employment was established to promote successful employment of RIT's deaf students and graduates.

John Macko, Director
Lorie Fidurko, Office Assistant

4224 Cochlear Implant Association
5335 Wisconsin Avenue NW   202-895-2781
Washington, DC 20015-2052   Fax: 202-895-2782
                                e-mail: pwms.cici@worldnet.att.net

Provides information and support to implant users and their families, professionals and the general public.

John McCelland, President
Lorie Singer, VP

4225 Convention of American Instructors of the Deaf
PO Box 377   817-354-8414
Bedford, TX 76095-0377   TTY: 817-354-8414
                                      e-mail: caid@swbell.net
                                                  www.caid.org

An organization that promotes professional development communication and information among educators of deaf individuals and other interested people.

Keith Mousley, President
Larry Quinsland, Ph.D, Vice-President

4226 Council on Education of the Deaf College of Education
College of Education
343 A Erickson Hall   330-672-0735
East Lansing, MI 48824-0001   Fax: 330-672-2498
                                             TTY: 330-672-2396
                                     e-mail: catalyst@kent.edu
                            www.deafed.net/PageText.asp?hdnPageId=58

Offers information and referral services to the hearing impaired.

Dr Karen Dilka, Executive Director
Dr Carmel Collum Yarger, President

4227 Deaf Artists of America
302 Goodman Street N
Rochester, NY 14607-1148
Fax: 716-244-3690
TTY: 315-224-3460
www.deafed.net/publisheddocs/sub/ivc39.h
Organized to bring support and recognition to deaf and hard of hearing artists. The goals are to publish information about deaf artists, provide cultural and educational opportunities, exhibit and market deaf artists' work and collect and disseminate information.
Tom Willard, Executive Director

4228 Deaf REACH
3521 12th Street NE
Washington, DC 20017
202-832-6681
Fax: 202-832-8454
TTY: 202-832-6681
e-mail: lweinstock@deaf-reach.org
www.deaf-reach.org
Offers group homes for mentally ill adults, day programs for the developmentally disabled deaf, referrals case management and housing placement. Serves adults with disabilities, specifically deaf and/or low-income.
Annette Reichman, President
Jon Tomar, VP

4229 Deafness Research Foundation
641 Lexington Avenue
New York, NY 10022
212-328-9480
866-454-3924
Fax: 212-328-9484
TTY: 888-435-6104
e-mail: info@drf.org
www.drf.org
The nation's largest voluntary health organization entirely committed to public awareness and support for basic and clinical research into deafness and hearing disabilities. Sponsors a broad program of innovative research and education.
Elizabeth Thorp, President, CEO
Clifford Tallman, Principal

4230 Deafness and Communicative Disorders Branch
Department of Education
400 Maryland Ave., SW
Washington, DC 20202-2736
202-205-8730
800-872-5327
Fax: 800-437-0833
TTY: 202-205-8352
e-mail: annette.reichman@ed.gov
www.ed.gov/offices/OSERS/RSA.html
Promotes improved and expanded rehabilitation services for deaf and hard of hearing people and individuals with speech or language impairments.
Annette Reichman, Branch Chief

4231 Dogs for the Deaf
10175 Wheeler Road
Central Point, OR 97502
541-826-9220
800-990-3647
Fax: 541-826-6696
TTY: 541-826-9220
TDD: 541-826-9220
e-mail: info@dogsforthedeaf.org
www.dogsforthedeaf.org
Trains ear dogs to alert deaf persons to certain sounds. Dogs are chosen from pet adoption shelters and assigned on the basis of a prioritized waiting list. Four to five months of training teaches them to alert their masters to a number of sounds.
Robin Dickson, President/CEO
Vaughn Maurice, General Manager

4232 EAR Foundation
1817 Patterson Street
Nashville, TN 37203
615-627-2724
800-545-4327
Fax: 615-627-2728
TTY: 615-627-2724
TDD: 615-627-2724
e-mail: info@earfoundation.org
www.earfoundation.org
A national non-profit organization committed to the goal of better hearing and balance through public and professional education programs including The Meniere's Network and the Young Ears program. The Meniere's Network is a national network of patient outreach.
Amy Nielsen, Associate Director

4233 Hands Organization: Advocacy Network for the Deaf and Hearing Impaired
Advocacy Network For The Deaf And Hearing Impaired
PO Box 17755
Chicago, IL 60617-0755
773-978-8552
TTY: 773-978-8552
Advocacy for the deaf and hearing impaired; information and referrals educational events sign language summer youth camps and newsletters.

4234 Hear Now: Starkey Hearin Foundation
The Starkey Hearing Foundation
6700 Washington Avenue S
Eden Prairie, MN 55344
866-354-3254
Fax: 952-828-6900
e-mail: info@StarkeyFoundation.org
www.sotheworldmayhear.org
Committed to making technology accessible to deaf and hard of hearing individuals throughout the United States. Also raises funds to provide hearing aids, cochlear implants and related services to children and adults who have hearing losses.
Richard Brown, President
Brady Forseth, Executive Director

4235 Hearing Education and Awareness for Rocker s
1405 Lyon Street
San Francisco, CA 94115
415-409-3277
Fax: 415-552-4296
TTY: 415-476-7600
e-mail: hear@hearnet.com
www.hearnet.com
Educates the public about the real dangers of hearing loss resulting from repeated exposure to excessive noise levels.
Kathy Peck, Executive Director
John Doyle, Secretary

4236 Hearing Loss Association of America
7910 Woodmont Avenue
Bethesda, MD 20814-3079
301-657-2248
Fax: 301-913-9413
TTY: 301-657-2248
e-mail: info@hearingloss.org
www.hearingloss.org
Promotes awareness and information about hearing loss communication assistive devices and alternative communication skills through publications exhibits and presentations.
Diana D. Bender, Ph.D, President
Anna Gilmore Hall, Executive Director

4237 Helen Keller National Center for Deaf/Blind Youth and Adults
141 Middle Neck Road
Sands Point, NY 11050-1299
516-944-8900
Fax: 516-944-7302
TTY: 516-944-8637
e-mail: hkncinfo@hknc.org
www.hknc.org
The national center and its 10 regional offices providing diagnostic evaluations comprehensive vocational and personal adjustment training and job preparation and placement for people who are deaf/blind from every state and territory.

4238 House Ear Institute
2100 W 3rd Street
Los Angeles, CA 90057
213-483-4431
800-388-8612
Fax: 213-483-8789
TTY: 213-484-2642
TDD: 213-484-2642
e-mail: info@hei.org
www.hei.org
A national non-profit otologic research and educational institute that provides information on hearing and balance disorders.
John W House MD, President
James D Boswell, CEO

4239 International Hearing Dog
5901 E 89th Avenue
Henderson, CO 80640
303-287-3277
Fax: 303-287-3425
TTY: 303-287-3277
TDD: 303-287-3277
e-mail: info@hearingdog.org
www.ihdi.org

Trains dogs to hear for deaf persons - telephones, doorbells, babies etc.
Samuel Cheris, Chairman
Valerie Foss-Brugger, President/ Executive Director

4240 International Hearing Society
16880 Middlebelt Road   734-522-7200
Livonia, MI 48154   800-521-5247
                                          Fax: 734-522-0200
                              e-mail: tom.higgins8@verizon.net
                                            www.ihsinfo.org
A nonprofit professional association which represents Hearing Instrument Specialists in the United States, Canada and several other countries. The society is recognized for promoting and maintaining the highest possible standards for its members.
Thomas Higgins, President
Kathleen Mennillo, Executive Director

4241 John Tracy Clinic
806 W Adams Boulevard   213-748-5481
Los Angeles, CA 90007-2505   800-522-4582
                                          Fax: 213-749-1651
                                          TTY: 213-747-2924
                                                www.jtc.org/
An educational facility for preschool age children who have hearing losses and their families. In addition to on-site services worldwide correspondence courses in English and Spanish are offered to parents whose children are of preschool age and are hard of hearing.
Michael D. Barker, Chair
J. Gaston Kent, President and Chief Executive Officer

4242 Listening and Spoken Language Knowledge Ce nter
3417 Volta Place NW   202-337-5220
Washington, DC 20007   Fax: 202-337-8314
                                          TTY: 202-337-5221
                                  e-mail: info@agbell.org
                     www.listeningandspokenlanguage.org/
The world's oldest and largest membership organization promoting the use of spoken language by children and adults who are hearing impaired. Members include parents of children with hearing loss, adults who are deaf or hard of hearing and educators.
Lyn Robertson, Ph.D., President
Alexander T Graham, Executive Director/CEO

4243 National Association of the Deaf
8630 Fenton Street   301-587-1788
Silver Spring, MD 20910-4500   Fax: 301-587-1791
                                   e-mail: nad.info@nad.org
                                                www.nad.org
The nation's largest constituency organization safeguarding the accessibility and civil rights of 28 million deaf and hard of hearing Americans in education, employment, health care and telecommunications. A private, nonprofit organization.
Christopher Wagner, President
Howard A Rosenblum, CEO

4244 National Captioning Institute
3725 Concorde Parkway   703-917-7600
Chantilly, VA 20151   Fax: 703-917-9853
                                          TTY: 703-917-7600
                             e-mail: jagudelo@ncicap.org
                                             www.ncicap.org
Advocates captioned television for people who want to see, as well as hear, the dialogue of a television program. It not only enables deaf and hard-of-hearing people to understand all of a program's content but it is also beneficial for new Americans learning English.
Gene Chao, President, CEO
Drake Smith, Chief Technology Officer

4245 National Center for Voice and Speech: Univ ersity of Iowa
The University Of Iowa
250 Hawkins Drive   319-335-6600
Iowa City, IA 52242   Fax: 319-335-6603
                               e-mail: ingo-titze@uiowa.edu
                                              www.ncvs.org
This is a consortium of institutions focusing on voice and speech disorders. The members of this consortium are the University of Iowa, the Denver Center for Performing Arts, the University of Wisconsin-Madison and the University of Utah.
Ingo Titze PhD, Executive Director
Eric Hunter, Deputy Executive Director

4246 National Consortium on Deaf-Blindness
Teaching Research
345 N Monmouth Avenue
Monmouth, OR 97361   800-438-9376
                                          Fax: 503-838-8150
                                          TTY: 800-854-7013
                                e-mail: info@nationaldb.org
                                          www.nationaldb.org
Collects organizes and disseminates information related to children and youth who are deaf-blind and connects consumers of deaf-blind information to sources of information about deaf-blindness assistive technology and deaf-blind people.
John Reiman
Kathy McNulty

4247 National Dissemination Center for Children
1825 Connecticut Avenue NW   202-884-8200
Washington, DC 20009   800-695-0285
                                          Fax: 202-884-8441
                                          TTY: 202-884-8200
                                e-mail: nichcy@fhi360.org
                                             www.nichcy.org
Publishes free fact filled newsletters. Arranges workshops. Advises parents on the laws entitling children with disabilities to special education and other services.
Bruce Ramirez, Executive Director
John Westbrook, Director

4248 National Family Association for Deaf-Blind
141 Middle Neck Road
Sands Point, NY 11050   800-225-0411
                                          Fax: 516-883-9060
                                e-mail: NFADB@aol.com
                                              www.nfadb.org
NFADB advocates for all persons who are deaf-blind of any chronological age and cognitive ability, supports national policy to benefit people who are deaf-blind, encourages the founding and strengthening of family organizations in each state and shares information.
Susan Green, President
Cynthia Jackson-Glenn, Treasurer

4249 National Institute on Deafness and other Communication Disorders
National Institutes Of Heath
31 Center Drive   301-496-7243
Bethesda, MD 20892-2320   800-241-1044
                                          Fax: 301-402-0018
                                          TTY: 800-241-1055
                            e-mail: nidcdinfo@nidcd.nih.gov
                                          www.nidcd.nih.gov
A national resources center for information about hearing, balance, smell, taste, voice, speech and language.
Dr. James F Battey, Jr., M.D., Ph.D, Director
Marin Allen PhD, Chief Office of Health Communication

4250 National Organization for Hearing Research
P.O. Box 421   610-649-6114
Narberth, PA 19072   Fax: 610-668-1428
                                          TTY: 610-664-3135
                             e-mail: info@nohrfoundation.org
                                          www.nohrfoundation.org
This organization is a nonprofit private foundation seeking to fund exceptional researchers with $5 000 seed money grants.

4251 Rainbow Alliance of the Deaf
309 Millside Drive
Columbus, OH 43230   e-mail: president@rad.org
                                                www.rad.org
A national organization serving the deaf gay and lesbian community. Represents approximately 24 chapters throughout the United States Canada and Europe.
Larry Pike, President
Steven Schumacher, Secretary

4252 Registry of Interpreters for the Deaf
333 Commerce Street
Alexandria, VA 22314
703-838-0030
Fax: 703-838-0454
TTY: 703-838-0459
e-mail: ridinfo@rid.org
www.RID.org
A membership organization with almost 4 000 members including professional interpreters and translators persons with deafness or hearing impairments and professionals in related fields.
Brenda Walker Prudhom, President/Board of Directors
Shane H. Feldman, Executive Director

4253 Society of Hearing Impaired Physicians
1999 Mowry Avenue
Fremont, CA 94538-1622
510-797-2939
Fax: 510-797-0168
e-mail: fphship@aol.com
This Society aids and assists physicians medical students and prospective medical students whose hearing impairment may necessitate different tools and/or approaches to medical practice and training.

4254 Telecommunications for the Deaf
8630 Fenton Street
Silver Spring, MD 20910
301-589-3786
Fax: 301-589-3797
TTY: 301-589-3006
e-mail: info@tdi-online.org
www.tdi-online.org
A nonprofit consumer advocacy organization promoting full visual and other access to information and telecommunications for people who are deaf, hard of hearing, deaf-blind and speech impaired.
Claude Stout, Executive Director
Scott Recht, Business Manager

4255 Tripod
1727 W Burbank Boulevard
Burbank, CA 91506
818-972-2080
Fax: 818-972-2090
TTY: 818-972-2080
e-mail: info@tripod.org
www.tripod.org
TRIPOD is a nonprofit organization dedicated to providing support and services for deaf and hard of hearing children and their families. TRIPOD offers model local educational programs, Montessori, bilingual parent, infant, toddler and preschool programs.

4256 USA Deaf Sports Federation
PO Box 910338
Lexington, KY 40591-0338
605-367-5760
Fax: 605-782-8441
TTY: 605-367-5761
e-mail: HomeOffice@usdeafsports.org
www.usdeafsports.org
A governing body for all deaf sports and recreation in the United States.
Jack C. Lamberton, President
Chris Kaftan, Secretary

State Agencies & Associations

Alabama

4257 Alabama Institute for Deaf and Blind
205 East South Street
Talladega, AL 35160
256-761-3200
Fax: 256-761-3344
TTY: 256-761-3200
e-mail: mascia.john@aidb.state.al.us
www.aidb.org
Dr. John Mascia, President
Dr. Frieda Meacham, Vice President, Instructional Programs

Arizona

4258 Arizona Association of the Deaf
5025 N Central Avenue
Phoenix, AZ 85012
e-mail: tposedly@aol.com
www.azadinc.org
This organization shall be organized and operated exclusively to promote the welfare of deaf and hard of hearing residents of the state of Arizona in education, economic, security, social equality, and just rights and privileges as citizens.
Tom Buell, President
Joy Saunders, Vice President

Arkansas

4259 Arkansas Association of the Deaf
26 Corporate Hill Drive
Little Rock, AR 72205
e-mail: hdketchum@aol.com
www.arkad.org
The mission of the Arkansas Association of the Deaf is to promote the educational, economic, and social welfare of Arkansans who are deaf or hard of hearing.
Holly Ketchum, President
Billie Jordan, 1st Vice President

District of Columbia

4260 Administration for Children and Families
370 L'Enfant Promenade
Washington, DC 20447
www.acf.hhs.gov
The Administration for Children & Families (ACF) is a division of the U.S. Department of Health & Human Services (HHS). ACF promotes the economic and social well-being of families, children, individuals and communities.
Mark Greenberg, Acting Assistant Secretary
Jeff Hild, Chief of Staff

4261 Shiloh Senior Center for the Hearing Impaired
913 P Street NW
Washington, DC 20001
202-232-1425
TTY: 202-667-9779
Senior programs, sponsored by the DC Office on Aging in co-ordination with grantee: Shiloh Baptist Church serving the entire Metro Washington area's deaf and hard-of-hearing senior citizens.

Florida

4262 Florida Association of the Deaf
7852 Mansfield Hollow Rd.
Delray Beach, FL 33446
e-mail: junc@fadcentral.org
www.fadcentral.org
The mission of the Florida Association of the Deaf is to promote, protect, and preserve the rights and quality of life of Deaf and hard of hearing individuals in the state of Florida.
June McMahon, President
Lissette Molina, Vice President

Georgia

4263 Agency for Toxic Substances and Disease Registry
4770 Buford Hwy NE
Atlanta, GA 30341
800-232-4636
TTY: 888-232-6348
www.atsdr.cdc.gov
The Agency for Toxic Substances and Disease Registry (ATSDR), based in Atlanta, Georgia, is a federal public health agency of the U.S. Department of Health and Human Services. ATSDR serves the public by using the best science, taking responsive public health actions, and providing trusted health information to prevent harmful exposures and diseases related to toxic substances.
Patrick Breysse, PhD, CIH, Director
Donna Knutson, PhD, Acting Deputy Director

4264 Georgia Association of the Deaf
PO Box 615
Hiram, GA 30141-1616
e-mail: turqcat9992000@yahoo.com
www.gadeaf.org
Julie Burton, President
Russell Fleming, Vice President

Illinois

4265 Illinois Association of the Deaf
PO Box 1275
Oak Park, IL 60304
773-237-1877
Fax: 847-740-2319
TTY: 847-740-2319
e-mail: botz@iadeaf.org
www.iadeaf.org

The Illinois Association of the Deaf is a non-profit, political, educational, social economic, welfare of the deaf, and cultural organization made up of deaf, hard of hearing, and hearing members.
Angela Botz, President
Crystal Kelley Schwartz, Vice-President

Kansas

4266 Kansas Association of the Deaf
PO Box 10085   785-273-0612
Olathe, KS 66051   Fax: 785-273-9063
e-mail: president@deafkansas.org
www.deafkansas.org
The mission of the Kansas Association of the Deaf a state-wide, non-profit organization is to assure that an extensive, organized system of services is accessible to all deaf or hard of hearing people in Kansas.
Ann Cooper, President
Pam Siebert, Vice-President

Kentucky

4267 Kentucky Association of the Deaf
1707 Richmond Drive
Louisville, KY 40205-1407
Fax: 606-272-7747
TTY: 606-223-3999
e-mail: president@kydeaf.org
www.kydeaf.org
The mission of the Kentucky Association of the Deaf is to advocate for the deaf and hard of hearing in Kentucky by promoting equality, accessibility, and quality of life through employment, services, education and welfare.
Sharon White, President
Arlen Finke, Vice-President

Louisiana

4268 Louisiana Association of the Deaf
3112 Valley Creek Drive
Baton Rouge, LA 70808   225-341-6406
Fax: 225-923-1235
TTY: 225 923-1266
e-mail: info@lad1908.org
www.lad1908.org

Lou Cannon, President
Cindy Robillard, VP

Maryland

4269 Agency for Healthcare Research and Quality
540 Gaither Road
Rockville, MD 20850   301-427-1364
www.ahrq.gov/index.html
The Agency for Healthcare Research and Quality's (AHRQ) mission is to produce evidence to make health care safer, higher quality, more accessible, equitable, and affordable, and to work within the U.S. Department of Health and Human Services and with other partners to make sure that the evidence is understood and used.
Richard G. Kronick, PhD, Director, Director
Sharon B. Arnold, PhD, Deputy Director

4270 Centers for Medicare and Medicaid Services
7500 Security Boulevard   410-786-3000
Baltimore, MD 21244   877-267-2323
TTY: 866-226-1819
e-mail: Mandy.Cohen@cms.hhs.gov
www.cms.gov
US federal agency which administers Medicare, Medicaid, and the State Children's Health Insurance Program.
Dr. Mandy Cohen, M.D., MPH, Chief of Staff
Timothy P. Love, Chief Operating Officer

4271 National Human Genome Research Institute
Building 31, Room 4B09   301-402-0911
Bethesda, MD 20892   Fax: 301-402-2218
www.genome.gov
The National Human Genome Research Institute began as the National Center for Human Genome Research (NCHGR), which was established in 1989 to carry out the role of the National Institutes

of Health (NIH) in the International Human Genome Project (HGP).
Eric D. Green, M.D., Ph.D., Director
Lawrence Brody, Ph.D., Director, Division of Genomics & Society

4272 National Institute of Biomedical Imaging and Bioengineering
9000 Rockville Pike   301-496-8859
Bethesda, MD 20892   e-mail: info@nibib.nih.gov
www.nibib.nih.gov
The mission of the National Institute of Biomedical Imaging and Bioengineering (NIBIB) is to improve health by leading the development and accelerating the application of biomedical technologies.
Roderic I. Pettigrew, Ph.D., M.D., Director
Marcella Canada, Administrative Officer

4273 U.S. Food and Drug Administration
10903 New Hampshire Ave   301-796-8240
Silver Spring, MD 20993   888-463-6332
www.fda.gov
FDA is responsible for protecting the public health by assuring the safety, efficacy and security of human and veterinary drugs, biological products, medical devices, our nation's food supply, cosmetics, and products that emit radiation.
Stephen Ostroff, M.D., Acting Commissioner
James Tyler, Chief Financial Officer

Massachusetts

4274 Massachusetts State Association of the Deaf
PO Box 276   781-388-9114
Reading, MA 01867   Fax: 781-388-9015
TTY: 781-388-9115
e-mail: MSADeaf@aol.com
www.msad.org
The Massachusetts State Association of the Deaf is a statewide nonprofit organization serving the estimated 350 000 deaf and hard of hearing Massachusetts citizens and their families.
Justine Barros, President
Michelle Donatello, Vice President

Michigan

4275 Michigan Deaf Association
6093 133rd Ave
Saugatuck, MI 49453   Fax: 586-775-0906
e-mail: info@mideaf.org
www.mideaf.org
MDA is a non-profit, tax exempt organization with a mission to help improve the lives of Deaf and Hard of Heating citizens of Michigan. MDA is affiliated with he National Association of the Deaf whose mission is to promote, protect, and preserve the rights of the deaf and hearing impaired communities.
Scot A Pott, President
Kat Vogtmann, 1st Vice-President

New York

4276 Center for Hearing and Communication
50 Broadway   917-305-7700
New York, NY 10004   Fax: 917-305-7888
TTY: 917-305-7999
e-mail: inf@lhh.org
www.chchearing.org
A private not-for-profit rehabilitation agency for infants, children and adults who are hard of hearing and deaf. The League's mission is to improve the quality of life for people with all degrees of hearing loss.
Laurie Hanin, Executive Director
Ellen Lafargue, Director Audiology

North Carolina

4277 National Institute of Environmental Health Sciences
111 T.W. Alexander Drive   919-541-4580
Research Triangle Park, NC 27709 e-mail: carroll1@niehs.nih.gov
www.niehs.nih.gov

The mission of the NIEHS is to discover how the environment affects people in order to promote healthier lives.
Linda S. Birnbaum, Ph.D., Director
Richard Woychik, Ph.D., Deputy Director

4278 North Carolina Association of the Deaf
1200 Revolution Mill Drive
Greensboro, NC 27405   919-773-2974
                                        Fax: 919-834-0127
                        e-mail: NCAD2011@gmail.com
                                        www.ncadeaf.org
Christina Bryant, Chairperson

North Dakota

4279 North Dakota Association of the Deaf
1115 11th Avenue North
Fargo, ND 58102
                        e-mail: rolewitz @ hotmail.com
                                        www.nddeaf.org
The North Dakota Association of the Deaf is actively involved in issues affecting Deaf citizens in North Dakota.
Michele Rolewitz, President
Cody Duncan, Vice President

Oklahoma

4280 Oklahoma Association of the Deaf
2737 Sunnybrook Lane
Enid, OK 73703
                        e-mail: Mlznull@aol.com
                                        www.ok-oad.org
The purpose of Oklahoma Association of the Deaf is to promote the interests of the deaf and to advance the social, educational, cultural and economic well-being of the deaf.
Lynn Null, President
Ka Ann Varner, Vice President

Oregon

4281 Oregon Association of the Deaf
999 Locust Street NE
Salem, OR 97301
                        e-mail: contact@deaforegon.com
                                        www.deaforegon.com
The Oregon Association of the Deaf is a non-profit organization working toward a better life for the deaf. Their mission is to create an opportunity for the Deaf of Oregon to join together in planning, devising, conducting and participating in activities.
Daniel Sloan, Committee
Wendy Stanley, Committee

Rhode Island

4282 Rhode Island Association of the Deaf
PO Box 40853
Providence, RI 02940
                        e-mail: riadsec@gmail.com
                                        www.riadeaf.blogspot.in/
Heather Niedbala, Vice-President
Neil Leahey, Treasurer

Texas

4283 Texas Association of the Deaf
PO Box 1982
Manchaca, TX 78652-3570
                        e-mail: steve@deaftexas.org
                                        www.deaftexas.org
Texas Association of the Deaf is an organization for persons who are deaf or hard of hearing. It is a membership organization to provide information and education including surveys and studies to bring the viewpoint on various issues affecting the lives of the deaf and hearing impaired.
Steve C Baldwin, President
Chris Kearney, VP

Virginia

4284 National Science Foundation
4201 Wilson Blvd
Arlington, VA 22230   703-292-5111
                                        TDD: 703-292-5090
                        e-mail: info@nsf.gov
                                        www.nsf.gov

NSF is the only federal agency whose mission includes support for all fields of fundamental science and engineering, except for medical sciences.
France A. Cordova, Director
Richard O. Buckius, Chief Operating Officer

4285 Virginia Association of the Deaf
5251 College Drive
Dublin, VA 24084   757-587-9555
                                        Fax: 757-461-5376
                                        TTY: 757-461-7527
                        e-mail: vadpresident007@yahoo.com
                                        www.vad.org
LaDonna Larsen, President
Chuck Kelley, VP

Wisconsin

4286 Wisconsin Association of the Deaf
PO Box 114
Delavan, WI 53115-4230   608-825-9791
                                        TTY: 414-607-3297
                        e-mail: wisdeaf@gmail.com
                                        www.wisdeaf.org/
The mission of the Wisconsin Association of the Deaf is to ensure that a comprehensive and coordinated system of resources is accessible to Wisconsin people who are deaf or hard of hearing, enabling them to achieve their maximum potential.
Jenny Buechner-Madison, President
Steph Buell, Vice President

Wyoming

4287 Deaf Association of Wyoming
PO Box 20107
Cheyenne, WY 82003   307-635-1125
                        e-mail: president@dawyoming.org
                                        www.dawyoming.org
The Deaf Association of Wyoming is a state non-profit organizations; which is associated with the Association of the Deaf. Membership is open to all deaf persons, parents of deaf children, interpreters, professionals who work with deaf and all interested parties.
Heather Parsons, President
Bill Bitner, VP

Libraries & Resource Centers

4288 Captioned Films/Videos
National Association of the Deaf
8630 Fenton Street
Silver Spring, MD 20910-4500   301-587-1788
                                        Fax: 301-587-1791
                                        TTY: 301-587-1789
                                        www.nad.org
The mission of the National Association of the Deaf is to promote,protect,and preserve the rights and quality of life of eaf and hard of hearing individuals in the United States of America.
Jason Stark, Director-Described and Captioned Media P

4289 Captioned Media Program
National Association of the Deaf
8630 Fenton Street
Silver Spring, MD 20910-4500   301-587-1788
                                        Fax: 301-587-1791
                                        TTY: 301-587-1789
                                        www.nad.org
Free loans of educational and entertainment captioned films and videos for deaf and hard of hearing people.
Jason Stark, Director

4290 Friends of Libraries for Deaf Action USA
2930 Craiglawn Road
Silver Spring, MD 20904-1816   202-727-2255
                                        Fax: 301-572-5168
                                        TTY: 301-572-5168
                        e-mail: folda86@aol.com
                                        www.folda.net/
Library services for people with disabilities.
Alice L Hagemeyer, President
Merrie A Davidson, Associate

4291 Library Services to the Deaf Community
District of Columbia Public Library

901 G Street NW
Washington, DC 20001
202-727-2145
TTY: 202-727-2255
e-mail: library_deaf_dc@yahoo.com
www.dclibrary.org

Assures that the deaf community is aware of existing library and information services by the District of Columbia Public Library; promotes public awareness about the deaf community, deaf history and culture, American Sign Language, and assistive technology for people with hearing loss.

John W Hill Jr, President
Bonnie R Cohen, VP

4292 Listening and Spoken Knowledge Center
3417 Volta Place NW
Washington, DC 20007-2737
202-337-5220
Fax: 202-337-8314
TTY: 202-337-5221
e-mail: info@agbell.org
www.listeningandspokenlanguage.org/

Contains one of the world's largest historical collections of publications, documents and information on deafness. In addition to the main collection, which includes books, periodicals and indexed clipping files dating from the turn of the century, the library also houses a significant archival collection dealing with the history of deafness since the 16th century.

Lyn Robertson, Ph.D., President
Alexander T Graham, Executive Director/CEO

4293 Wallace Memorial Library
Rochester Institute of Technology
90 Lomb Memorial Drive
Rochester, NY 14623
585-475-2562
www.rit.edu/alumni/benefits/library.php

Information on physical disabilities and deafness.
Chandra McKenzie, Assistant Provost/Director

Research Centers

4294 Boys Town National Research Hospital
555 N 30th Street
Omaha, NE 68131
402-498-6511
800-320-1171
Fax: 402-498-6331
TTY: 800 320-1171
www.boystownhospital.org

An internationally recognized center for state-of-the-art research diagnosis treatment of patients with ear diseases hearing and balance disorders cleft lip and palate and speech/language problems. Also includes programs such as Parent/Child Workshops Center for Childhood Deafness Register for Heredity Hearing Loss Center for Hearing research Center for Abused Handicapped and summer programs for gifted deaf teens and college students.

John K Arch, Executive VP
Edward M. Kolb, Medical Director

4295 Center for Hearing Loss in Children Boystown National Research Hospital
Boystown National Research Hospital
555 N 30th Street
Omaha, NE 68131-2136
402-498-6511
800-282-6657
Fax: 402-498-6331
TTY: 800 320-1171
e-mail: chilic@boystown.org
www.boystownhospital.org

The Center for Hearing Loss in Children unites professionals from a variety of disciplines to focus on research training information dissemination and continuing education in the area of childhood deafness.

John K Arch, Executive VP
Edward M. Kolb, Medical Director

4296 Central Institute for the Deaf
825 S Taylor Avenue
Saint Louis, MO 63110-1502
314-977-0132
877-444-4574
Fax: 314-977-0023
TTY: 314-977-0037
e-mail: rfeder@cid.edu
www.cid.edu

Central Institute for the Deaf is a private nonprofit auditory-oral school for children who have hearing impairments. We teach children with hearing loss birth-12 to listen talk and succeed in the mainstream.

Ned Lemkemeier, President
Robin M Feder, Executive Director

4297 City University of New York Center for Research in Speech and Hearing
365 Fifth Avenue
New York, NY 10016-4309
212-817-7000
877-428-6942
Fax: 212-817-1537
e-mail: strangepin@aol.com
www.gc.cuny.edu

Programmable research of digital and auditory hearing aids and sensory aids for the speech and hearing impaired person.

Dr. William Kelly, President
Marilyn Marzolf, Chief of Staff

4298 Civitan International Research Center
1530 3rd Avenue S
Birmingham, AL 35294-0001
205-934-8900
800-UAB-CIRC
Fax: 205-975-6330
www.circ.uab.edu

Studies of deaf children.
Dr Harald Sontheimer, Director
Dr Alan Percy, Medical Director

4299 Cleveland Hearing and Speech Center
11635 Euclid Avenue
Cleveland, OH 44106-4319
216-231-0787
Fax: 216-231-2135
TTY: 216-231-5266
e-mail: jkeatley@chsc.org
www.chsc.org

Offers research and studies into speech language and hearing disorders.

David J Abood, President
Bernard P Henri PhD, Executive Director

4300 David T Siegel Institute for Communicative Disorders
Humana Hospital-Michael Reese
3033 S Cottage Grove Avenue
Chicago, IL 60616-3346
773-791-2900
Fax: 773-791-4014

Conducts behavioral research on language development and sign language for the deaf.
Edward Applebaum, Chief Service

4301 Eaton-Peabody Laboratory of Auditory Physiology
Massachusetts Eye & Ear Institute
243 Charles Street
Boston, MA 02114-3002
617-573-3745
Fax: 617-720-4408
e-mail: eplweb@mit.edu
research.meei.harvard.edu/EPL

Auditory system and auditory information processing including ear-brain interactions in normal and pathologic hearing.

John Fernandez, President, CEO
Thane Benson, Consultant

4302 Gallaudet University: Center for Auditory and Speech Sciences
800 Florida Avenue NE
Washington, DC 20002-3660
202-651-5000
866-637-0102
Fax: 202-651-5295
TTY: 202-651-5005
e-mail: publicrelations@gallaudet.edu
www.gallaudet.edu

Develops new hearing tests that use speech sounds to measure hearing loss.

Dr T Alan Hurwitz, President
Deborah DeStefano, Special Assistant to the President

4303 Hear Center
301 E Del Mar Boulevard
Pasadena, CA 91101
626-796-2016
Fax: 626-796-2320
e-mail: info@hearcenter.org
www.hearcenter.org

Auditory and verbal program designed to help hearing impaired children infants and adults lead normal and productive lives. Seeks to develop auditory techniques to aid people who have communication problems due to deafness.

Ellen Simon, Executive Director
Deborah Lorino, Office Manager

4304 Houston Ear Research Foundation
7737 SW Freeway   713-771-9966
Houston, TX 77074-1867   800-843-0807
                                    Fax: 713-771-0546
                                    TTY: 800-843-0807
                          e-mail: info@houstoncochlear.org
                                 www.houstoncochlear.org
Aims to improve health care and education for deaf and hearing-impaired children.
Jan Gilden, Clinical Audiologist
Mary Lynn McDonald

4305 Loyola University of Children: Parmly Hearing Institute
1032 W Sheridan Road   773-274-3000
Chicago, IL 60660   Fax: 773-508-2719
                               e-mail: webmaster@luc.edu
                                            www.luc.edu
Engage in the comparative study of sensory systems including hearing vision speech perception vestibular function and the special senses of the lateral-line organ and electroreception in fish.
Richard Fay, PhD, Director
Dr William Yost, Professor of Psychology

4306 Northern Illinois University Research and Training Center
1425 W Lincoln Highway   815-753-1000
DeKalb, IL 60115-2825   800-892-3050
                                    Fax: 815-753-6520
                               e-mail: helpdesk@niu.edu
                                            www.niu.edu
Conducts research resource development and training/technical assistance projects geared toward enhancing the employment independent living and quality of life outcomes for traditionally underserved people who are deaf.
Douglas D Baker, President

4307 Ohio State University Otological Research Laboratories
410 W 10th Avenue   614-293-8103
Columbus, OH 43210   800-293-5123
                                    Fax: 614-293-5506
                        e-mail: OSUCareConnection@osumc.edu
                                 www.medicalcenter.osu.edu
Clinical and basic research in otology.
Larry Anstine, CEO
Peter Geier, Chief Operating Officer

4308 Ohio University Therapy Associates: Hearing, Speech and Language Clinic
W218 Grover Center   740-593-1000
Athens, OH 45701   Fax: 740-593-0287
                               e-mail: webteam@ohio.edu
                               www.ohio.edu/hearingspeech
Focuses on hearing and speech impairments.
Brooke Hallowell, Director
Davida Parsons, Clinical Director

4309 Oregon Health Sciences University Oregon Hearing Research Center Tinnitus Clinic
3181 S W Sam Jackson Park Road   503-494-7954
Portland, OR 97239-3098   Fax: 503-945-5656
                                    TTY: 503-494-0910
                                    e-mail: ohrc@ohsu.edu
                          www.ohsu.edu/xd/health/services/ent/serv
The first medical clinic in the world established exclusively for the treatment of chronic tinnitus. During the last 25 years we have successfully treated more than 7 000 patients with severe tinnitus. The Clinic also treats patients with hyperacusis (hypersensitivity to sounds).
William Martin PhD, Director
Baker Yong-Bing Shi, MD, PhD, Assistant Professor

4310 Regional Resource Center on Deafness Western Oregon State College
Western Oregon State College
345 N Monmouth Avenue   503-838-8444
Monmouth, OR 97361   877-877-1593
                                    TTY: 503-838-8000
                                 e-mail: rrcd@wou.edu
                          www.wou.edu/education/sped/rrcd.php
Improve the employment and independent living status of deaf and hard-of-hearing people by increasing the number of rehabilitation professionals and their community partners nationwide who have the necessary knowledge and communication skills to serve this population.
Cheryl Davis, Director
Konnie Sayers, Administrative Assistant

4311 Rehabilitation Engineering on Hearing Enha ncement
Lexington Center
800 Florida Avenue NE   202-651-5335
Washington, DC 20002   Fax: 202-651-5324
                                    TTY: 202-651-5335
                          e-mail: info@hearingresearch.org
                                 www.hearingresearch.org
A federally funded center that conducts research into hearing aid technology and alternate technologies.
Matthew H Bakke Ph D, Director
James J Mahshie PhD, Director

4312 Research and Training Center for Persons Who are Deaf or Hard of Hearing
University of Arkansas
26 Corporate Hill Drive   501-686-9691
Little Rock, AR 72205-3822   Fax: 501-686-9698
                                    TTY: 501-686-9691
                               e-mail: dwatson@uark.edu
                                 www.uark.edu/depts/rehabres
Rehabilitation of deaf and hearing impaired individuals.
Douglas Watson, Director
Glenn B Anderson, Professor Director of Training

4313 Rochester Institute of Technology: Nationa l Technical Institute for the Deaf
Lyndon Baines Johnson Building
52 Lomb Memorial Drive   585-475-6400
Rochester, NY 14623   Fax: 585-475-5978
                                    TTY: 585-475-6400
                          e-mail: gbuckley@ntid.rit.edu
                                 www.ntid.rit.edu
Provides technical and professional education and training for deaf students.
Dr Gerard Buckley, President

4314 Scottish Rite Center for Childhood Language Disorders
2800 - 16th Street NW   202-232-8155
Washington, DC 20009-3602   Fax: 202-483-8169
                                            dcsr.org
Association offering speech-language evaluations and treatment hearing screening and consultation and referrals to children ages birth to 18 years with hearing or speech disorders.
Dr Tommie L Robinson, Director

4315 Speech Simulation Research Foundation
PO Box 824   757-442-2755
Nassawadox, VA 23413-0824
Focuses on hearing and speech disorders.
Monte Penney, Director

4316 State University College at Fredonia Youngerman Clinic
W123 Thompson Hall   716-673-3203
Fredonia, NY 14063   Fax: 716-673-3332
                          e-mail: melissa.sidor@fredonia.edu
                                 www.fredonia.edu
Studies communication disorders including hearing and speech.
Melissa Sidor, Director

4317 State University College at Plattsburgh Auditory Research Laboratory
101 Broad Street
Plattsburgh, NY 12901-2170   518-564-2000
                                 www.plattsburgh.edu
Dr John Ettling, President
Anne Hansen, Vice-President

4318 Syracuse University Institute for Sensory Research
Syracuse University
621 Skytop Road   315-443-4164
Syracuse, NY 13244-1   Fax: 315-443-1184
                               e-mail: rlsmith@syr.edu
                                    www.isr.syr.edu

Sensory processing and hearing disorders.
Robert L Smith, Director

4319   Temple University Speech and Hearing Science Laboratories
1801 N Broad Street   215-204-7000
Philadelphia, PA 19122   e-mail: president@temple.edu
                                                    www.temple.edu

Speech and hearing studies.
Neil D Theobald, President
Kevin G Clark, Senior Advisor to the President/Interim

4320   Temple University: Section of Auditory Research
1801 N Broad Street   215-204-7000
Philadelphia, PA 19122   Fax: 215-707-6417
                                 e-mail: president@temple.edu
                                                    www.temple.edu

Neil D Theobald, President
Kevin G Clark, Senior Advisor to the President/Interim

4321   The University of Memphis: School of Commu nication Sciences and Disorders
Memphis State University
101 Wilder Tower   901-678-2111
Memphis, TN 38152-3520   800-669-2678
                                             Fax: 901-251-82
                             e-mail: recruitment@memphis.edu
                                           www.memphis.edu/ausp

Offers research into hearing loss and deafness as well as speech impairments.
Shirley C Raines, President
Walt Manning, Associate Director

4322   Trace Center University of Wisconsin: Madison
University of Wisconsin: Madison
1550 Engineering Drive   608-262-6966
Madison, WI 53706-2274   Fax: 608-262-8848
                                            TTY: 608-263-5408
                                 e-mail: info@trace.wisc.edu
                                                    trace.wisc.edu

Research and development center working with communication control and computer access technologies for people with disabilities.
Gregg C Vanderheiden, Center Director
Julie Gamradt, Communication Director

4323   University of Alabama Speech and Hearing Center
5721 USA Drive N   251-445-9378
Mobile, AL 36688-2   Fax: 251- 44- 937
                       e-mail: sh-cntr@jaguar1.usouthal.edu
                        www.southalabama.edu/alliedhealth/speech

Providing undergraduate master's and doctoral programs that challenge the student to achieve the highest standards of academic learning scientific inquiry and clinical excellence.
Robert E Moore, Chair
Elizabeth M Adams, Assistant Professor of Audiology

4324   University of Chicago: Temporal Bone Laboratory for Ear Research
5841 S Maryland Avenue   773-702-1000
Chicago, IL 60637-1463   888-824-0200
                                            Fax: 773-702-6809
                                                    www.uchospitals.edu
Focuses on hearing impairments and deafness research.
Dr Raul Hinojasa, Director

4325   University of Maine: Communication Science s & Disorders
5724 Dunn Hall   207-581-2006
Orono, ME 04469-5724   Fax: 207-581-2060
                          e-mail: Luanne.Wasson@umit.maine.edu
                                                    www.umaine.edu/comscidis
Speech disorders of adults and children including hearing impairments and deafness.
Judy Stickles, Clinic Director
Amy Engler Booth, Audiologist

4326   University of Michigan Communicative Disorders Clinic
412 Maynard Street   734-764-1817
Ann Arbor, MI 48109-2054   Fax: 734-764-7084
                               e-mail: kkellogg@chartermi.net
                                                    www.umich.edu/comdis

Focuses on communicative disorders including hearing impairments and speech disorders.
Mary Sue Coleman, President
Joerg Lahann, Assistant Professor of Biomedical Engine

4327   University of Michigan: Kresge Hearing Research Institute
1150 W Medical Center Drive   734-764-8111
Ann Arbor, MI 48109-0500   Fax: 734-764-0014
                                            TTY: 734-764-8110
                                  e-mail: josef@umich.edu
                                                    www.khri.med.umich.edu
Focuses on hearing and auditory disorders.
Josef M Miller, Director
Sue Kelch, Research Administrator

4328   University of Nebraska: Lincoln
1400 R Street   402-472-7211
Lincoln, NE 68588   Fax: 402-472-7697
                                 e-mail: jbernthal1@unl.edu
                                                    www.unl.edu
Focuses on hearing impairments and deaf research.
Harvey Perlman, Chancellor
Marjorie Kostelnik, Dean Education Human Science

4329   University of North Carolina at Chapel Hill Division of Speech & Hearing
321 S. Columbia Street   919-966-1007
Chapel Hill, NC 27599-1   Fax: 919-966-0100
                                 e-mail: idiana@med.unc.edu
                                                    www.med.unc.edu/ahs/sphs

The Division of Speech and Hearing Sciences prepares clinical practitioners in speech-language pathology and audiology to be scholars teachers and researchers in both the theoretical and applied aspects of human communication sciences and disorders.
Jackson Roush, PhD, Director
Lee McLean, PhD, Professor and Associate Dean

4330   University of Oklahoma: Health Sciences Ce nter
University of Oklahoma
1100 N Lindsey   405-271-4000
Oklahoma City, OK 73104   Fax: 405-713-60
                                                    www.ouhsc.edu

Dr. Dewayne Andrews, Senior Vice President and Provost
Kenneth D Rowe, Vice President for Administration and Fi

4331   University of Texas at Dallas Callier Center for Communication Disorders
1966 Inwood Road   214-905-3000
Dallas, TX 75235-7205   Fax: 214-905-3022
                                            TDD: 214-905-3012
                          e-mail: roeser@callier.utdallas.edu
                                                    www.callier.utdallas.edu

Focuses on communication and behavioral disorders including hearing impairments and deafness research.
Tom Campbell, Executive Director
Phillip L Wilson, Head of Audiology

4332   University of Washington Department of Speech & Hearing Sciences
1417 NE 42nd Street   206-685-7400
Seattle, WA 98105-6246   Fax: 206-543-1093
                          e-mail: sphscadv@u.washington.edu
                                    www.depts.washington.edu/sphsc/
Communication sciences and disorders.
Joan Hanson, Clinic Manager
Mary Wood, Assistant to the Chair

4333   Yeshiva University: Institute of Communication Disorders
Montefiore Medical Center
500 West 185th Street   212-960-5400
New York, NY 10033   Fax: 718-515-8235
                               e-mail: mfried@montefiore.org
                                                    www.yu.edu
Studies on communicative disorders including speech and hearing.
Richard M Joel, President
Josh Joseph, VP, Chief of Staff

Support Groups & Hotlines

4334 Aurora of Central New York
518 James Street
Syracuse, NY 13203-2282
315-422-7263
Fax: 315-422-4792
TTY: 315-422-9746
TDD: 315-422-9746
e-mail: auroracny@auroraofcny.org
Professional counseling services helps to assist individuals and their families deal with the trauma of hearing or vision loss.
Debra Chaken, Executive Director

4335 Beginnings for Parents of Children Who are Deaf or Hard of Hearing
302 Jefferson Street
Raleigh, NC 27605
919-715-4092
800-541-4327
Fax: 919-715-4093
TTY: 919-715-4092
e-mail: raleigh@ncbegin.org
www.ncbegin.org/
Beginnings provides support to parents of deaf and hard-of-hearing children in an unbiased, family-centered atmosphere. In addition, Beginnings also offers impartial information on communication options, placement and educational programs, and workshops for professional personnel who work with deaf and hard-of-hearing children. Advocacy and support for young people from birth to age 21 is available.
Jim Johnson, President
Dr Joni Y Alberg, Executive Director

4336 Children of Deaf Adults
PO Box 30715
Santa Barbara, CA 93130-0715
805-682-0997
www.coda-international.org
Promotes family awareness and individual growth in hearing children of deaf parents.
Carmel Batson, President
Millie Brother, Founder

4337 Children's Rights Program
Alexander Graham Bell Association
3417 Volta Place NW
Washington, DC 20007
202-337-5220
866-337-5220
Fax: 202-337-8314
e-mail: info@agbell.org
www.agbell.org
Actively advocates for the legal rights of children with hearing impairments and for legislation to upgrade the delivery of services to children and adults who are hearing impaired.
Gerri A Hanna, Director Advocacy/Policy

4338 Dial-a-Hearing Screening Test
PO Box 1880
Media, PA 19063
610-544-7700
800-222-3277
Fax: 610-543-2802
e-mail: dahst@aol.com
Hearing help information center. Provides local phone number for Dial-a-Hearing Screening Test and hearing information.
George Biddle, Executive Director

4339 International Hearing Society
International Hearing Society (IHS)
16880 Middlebelt Road
Livonia, MI 48154
734-522-7200
800-521-5247
Fax: 734-522-0200
e-mail: chelms@ihsinfo.org
http://ihsinfo.org/IhsV2/Home/Index.cfm
Hearing Aid Helpline, a service of International Hearing Society (IHS), provides a referral service for locating qualified hearing healthcare professionals. IHS is a professional association representing Hearing Instrument Specialists worldwide engaged in the practice of testing human hearing, selecting, fitting and dispensing of hearing instruments. Founded in 1951, the Society conducts programs in competency accreditation, education, training promoting specialty-level certification.
Thomas Higgins, President
Todd Beyer, Secretary

4340 John Tracy Clinic on Deafness
806 W Adams Boulevard
Los Angeles, CA 90007-2599
213-748-5481
800-522-4582
Fax: 213-749-1651
www.jtc.org
Hotline.
Michael D Barker, Chair
J.Gaston Kent, President & CEO

4341 National Health Information Center
PO Box 1133
Washington, DC 20013
310-565-4167
800-336-4797
Fax: 301-984-4256
e-mail: info@nhic.org
www.health.gov/nhic
Offers a nationwide information referral service, produces directories and resource guides.

4342 Project Eyes and Ears
1844 T Street SE
Washington, DC 20020-4635
202-889-7045
Fax: 202-889-6312
Disseminates information about resources to families and service providers, provides transition services for pre-kindergarten children who are deaf-blind and integrates children into normalized settings.
Janice Wellborn

Books

4343 A Child with Hearing Loss in Your Classroom? Don't Panic!
Alexander Graham Bell Association
3417 Volta Place NW
Washington, DC 20007-2737
202-337-5220
Fax: 202-337-8314
TTY: 202-337-5220
e-mail: info@agbell.org
www.listeningandspokenlanguage.org
Designed for mainstream teachers, this booklet discusses educational needs for students with hearing impairments. It especially focuses on students' language skills and their abilities to follow directions, learn new concepts, and comprehend reading. Candid advice about getting support from professionals, implementing and mantaining an IEP, improving classroom acoustic environments and using the PATERR approach.
1993 25 pages

4344 A New Civil Right: Telecommunications Equality for Deaf and Hard of Hearing
Karen Peltz Strauss, author
Hearing Loss Association of America
7910 Woodmont Avenue
Bethesda, MD 20814-3079
301-657-2248
Fax: 301-913-9413
TTY: 301-657-2249
e-mail: info@hearingloss.org
www.hearingloss.org
This book provides a compelling picture of the challenges and the realization that FCC regulation is required for people with hearing loss to receive the functional equivalence of what everyone else takes for granted.
2006 Hardcover
Anna Gilmore Hall, Executive Director
Lise Hamlin, Director of Public Policy

4345 A Quiet World: Living with Hearing Loss
David G Myers, author
Hearing Loss Association of America
7910 Woodmont Avenue
Bethesda, MD 20814-3079
301-657-2248
Fax: 301-913-9413
TTY: 301-657-2249
e-mail: info@hearingloss.org
www.hearigloss.org
A social psychologist, teacher, and author. The Author's gradual hearing loss caused serious trouble in his career and in his relationships with loved ones as he approached 50. He tells the story of his journey from denial to acceptance to an exploration of the technologies that offer help.
2000 Hardcover
Anna Gilmore Hall, Executive Director
Lise Hamlin, Director of Public Policy

4346   ASL PAH! Deaf Students' Essays About their Language
Sign Media
4020 Blackburn Lane   301-421-0268
Burtonsville, MD 20866-1167   800-475-4756
                                        Fax: 301-421-0270
                                        TTY: 301-421-4460
                              e-mail: info@signmedia.com
                                        www.signmedia.com
Tape/text combination featuring student essays on the role of ASL in their lives. The tape offers additional insights from the student authors. The text is not a transcript of the tape.
1979 Paperback/Video
ISBN: 0-932130-14-3
Barabara Olmert, Director Marketing

4347   ASL in Schools: Policies and Curriculum
Gallaudet University
800 Florida Avenue, NE   773-568-1550
Washington, DC 20002-3819   800-621-2736
                                        Fax: 800-621-8476
                                        TTY: 888-630-9347
                          e-mail: gupress@gallaudet.edu
                                      gupress.gallaudet.edu
Conference participants questioned experts on bilingual education for deaf students and discussed policy issues faced by educators across the United States.
139 pages

4348   Academic Acceptance of ASL
Gallaudet University
800 Florida Avenue, NE   773-568-1550
Washington, DC 20002-3819   800-621-2736
                                        Fax: 800-621-8476
                                        TTY: 888-630-9347
                          e-mail: gupress@gallaudet.edu
                                      gupress.gallaudet.edu
This monograph presents a dozen articles that demonstrate clearly and convincingly that the study of ASL affords the same educational values and the same intellectual rewards as the study of any other foreign language.
196 pages

4349   Access for All: Integrating Deaf, Hard of Hearing and Hearing Preschoolers
Gallaudet University
800 Florida Avenue, NE   773-568-1550
Washington, DC 20002-3819   800-621-2736
                                        Fax: 800-621-8476
                                        TTY: 888-630-9347
                          e-mail: gupress@gallaudet.edu
                                      gupress.gallaudet.edu
Describes a model program for integrating the Deaf and hard of hearing children in early education.
150 pages Book & Video

4350   American Deaf Culture
Gallaudet University
800 Florida Avenue, NE   773-568-1550
Washington, DC 20002-3819   800-621-2736
                                        Fax: 800-621-8476
                                        TTY: 888-630-9347
                          e-mail: gupress@gallaudet.edu
                                      gupress.gallaudet.edu
This book presents a collection of classic articles which have been selected to provide a variety of perspectives on language and culture of deaf people in America.
132 pages

4351   American Deaf Culture: An Anthology
Sign Media
4020 Blackburn Lane   301-421-0268
Burtonsville, MD 20866-1167   800-475-4756
                                        Fax: 301-421-0270
                                        TTY: 301-421-4460
                              e-mail: info@signmedia.com
                                        www.signmedia.com

Features deaf and hearing authors offering their experience and perspectives on cultural values, ASL, social interaction in the Deaf community, education, folklore and more.
Paperback
ISBN: 0-932130-09-7
Barbara Olmert, Director Marketing
Sherman Wilcox, Editor

4352   American Sign Language: A Beginning Course
National Association of the Deaf
8630 Fenton Street   301-587-1788
Silver Spring, MD 20910-4500   Fax: 301-587-1791
                                        TTY: 301-587-1789
                              e-mail: nad.info@nad.org
                                                nad.org
An interactive approach to teaching and learning American Sign Language, with 700 sign illustrations, each accompanied by an object drawing.
199 pages Paperback
ISBN: 0-913072-64-8
Christopher Wagner, President
Melissa S. Draganac-Hawk, Vice-President

4353   An Invisible Condition: The Human Side of Hearing Loss
SHHH Publications
7910 Woodmont Avenue   301-657-2248
Bethesda, MD 20814-3572   Fax: 301-913-9413
                                        www.hearingloss.org
Offers editorials from the SHHH Journal that have shaped the past decade of self help with their focus on the plight and hopes and the aspirations of hard of hearing people everywhere.
Rocky Stone, Author

4354   Angels and Outcasts: An Anthology of Deaf Characters in Literature
Gallaudet University
800 Florida Avenue, NE   773-568-1550
Washington, DC 20002-3819   800-621-2736
                                        Fax: 800-621-8476
                                        TTY: 888-630-9347
                          e-mail: gupress@gallaudet.edu
                                      gupress.gallaudet.edu
Collection of writings by and about deaf people revealing attitudes and prejudices common to western cultures.
375 pages
Trent Batson, Co-Editor
Eugene Bergman, Co-Editor

4355   Approaching Equality
TJ Publishers
817 Silver Spring Avenue   301-585-4440
Silver Spring, MD 20910-4617   800-999-1168
                                        Fax: 301-585-5930
                                        TTY: 301-585-4441
                              e-mail: tjpubinc@aol.com
Written by the former chair of the Commission on the Education of the deaf, this book reviews the dramatic developments in the education of deaf children.
112 pages Softcover
ISBN: 0-932666-39-6
Angela K Thames, President
Jerald A Murphy, VP

4356   Assessment & Management of Mainstreamed Hearing-Impaired Children
Pro-Ed, Inc.
8700 Shoal Creek Blvd   512-451-3246
Austin, TX 78757-6897   800-897-3202
                                        Fax: 800-397-7633
                              e-mail: info@proedin.com
                                        www.proedinc.com
The theoretical and practical considerations of developing appropriate programming for hearing-impaired children who are being educated in mainstream educational settings are presented in this book.
415 pages Hardcover
ISBN: 0-890794-58-8
Linda Jordan, Marketing Coordinator

4357 Assessment of Hearing Impaired People
Gallaudet University
800 Florida Avenue, NE   773-568-1550
Washington, DC 20002-3819   800-621-2736
                                     Fax: 800-621-8476
                                     TTY: 888-630-9347
                           e-mail: gupress@gallaudet.edu
                                     gupress.gallaudet.edu
This is a comprehensive review of 62 tests used by educational institutions, rehabilitation agencies, and mental health centers.
128 pages Softcover

4358 At Home Among Strangers
Gallaudet University
800 Florida Avenue, NE   773-568-1550
Washington, DC 20002-3819   800-621-2736
                                     Fax: 800-621-8476
                                     TTY: 888-630-9347
                           e-mail: gupress@gallaudet.edu
                                     gupress.gallaudet.edu
Details the history and culture of the deaf community.
336 pages
Jerome D. Schein, Author

4359 Basic Course in Manual Communication
National Association of the Deaf
8630 Fenton Street   301-587-1788
Silver Spring, MD 20910-4500   Fax: 301-587-1791
                                     TTY: 301-587-1789
                             e-mail: nad.info@nad.org
                                     nad.org
Over 700 signs are grouped according to shape, location, and movement. Also includes dialogues for practice.
158 pages Paperback
Christopher Wagner, President
Melissa S. Draganac-Hawk, Vice-President

4360 Basic Sign Communication: Student Materials
National Association of the Deaf
8630 Fenton Street   301-587-1788
Silver Spring, MD 20910-4500   Fax: 301-587-1791
                                     TTY: 301-587-1789
                             e-mail: nad.info@nad.org
                                     nad.org
Includes study and reference materials for all three levels of Basic Sign Communication.
232 pages Paperback
ISBN: 0-913072-56-7
Christopher Wagner, President
Melissa S. Draganac-Hawk, Vice-President

4361 Basic Sign Communication: Vocabulary
National Association of the Deaf
8630 Fenton Street   301-587-1788
Silver Spring, MD 20910-4500   Fax: 301-587-1791
                                     TTY: 301-587-1789
                             e-mail: nad.info@nad.org
                                     nad.org
Features sections on Sign Vocabulary, Numbers, and Classifiers. Contains 1000 illustrated signs, organized alphabetically by gloss for quick reference.
162 pages Paperback
ISBN: 0-913072-55-9
Christopher Wagner, President
Melissa S. Draganac-Hawk, Vice-President

4362 Basic Vocabulary and Language Thesaurus for Hearing Impaired Children
Alexander Graham Bell Association
3417 Volta Place NW   202-337-5220
Washington, DC 20007-2737   Fax: 202-337-8314
                                     TTY: 202-337-5220
                              e-mail: info@agbell.org
                           www.listeningandspokenlanguage.org
This simple thesaurus lists spontaneous vocabulary used by normally hearing children and lets patients and teachers check so that children with hearing losses have mastered these words.
1977 76 pages

4363 Basic Vocabulary: American Sign Language for Parents and Children
TJ Publishers
817 Silver Spring Avenue   301-585-4440
Silver Spring, MD 20910-4617   800-999-1168
                                     Fax: 301-585-5930
                                     TTY: 301-585-4441
                              e-mail: tjpubinc@aol.com
Carefully selected words and signs include those families use every day. Alphabetically organized vocabulary incorporates developmental lists helpful to both deaf and hearing children and over 1,000 clear sign language illustrations.
240 pages Softcover
ISBN: 0-932666-00-0
Angela K Thames, President
Jerald A Murphy, VP

4364 Being in Touch
Gallaudet University
800 Florida Avenue, NE   773-568-1550
Washington, DC 20002-3819   800-621-2736
                                     Fax: 800-621-8476
                                     TTY: 888-630-9347
                           e-mail: gupress@gallaudet.edu
                                     gupress.gallaudet.edu
Provides information on hearing and vision loss.
80 pages

4365 Best Practices in Educational Interpreting
Sign Enhancers
4450 La Crosse Ave   503-304-4501
San Diego, CA 92117-2941   800-767-4461
                                     Fax: 503-304-1063
                                     TTY: 503-304-4501
                       e-mail: SignEnhancers@iCloud.com
                                     www.signenhancers.com
Specific recommendations of best practices for working in preschool through graduate school. Case studies focus on real-life situations with suggested solutions and questions for further thought.
269 pages
ISBN: 0-205263-11-9

4366 Between Friends
Beltone Electronics Corporation
2601 Patriot Blvd.   847-832-3300
Glenview, IL 60026-6772   800-235-8663
                                     www.beltone.com
For hearing aid wearers: quizzes, jokes, health, recipes and financial items.
6 pages
Renee Rockoff, Editor

4367 Black and Deaf in America
TJ Publishers
817 Silver Spring Avenue   301-585-4440
Silver Spring, MD 20910-4617   800-999-1168
                                     Fax: 301-585-5930
                                     TTY: 301-585-4441
                              e-mail: tjpubinc@aol.com
An in depth look at some of the problems of the black deaf community, including undereducation and underemployment. This book includes an important chapter on signs used in the black community and presents interviews with prominent Black deaf individuals who share their joys, fears and hope for the future.
91 pages Softcover
ISBN: 0-932666-18-3
Angela K Thames, President
Jerald A Murphy, VP

4368 Blueprint for Conversational Competence
Alexander Graham Bell Association
3417 Volta Place NW   202-337-5220
Washington, DC 20007-2737   Fax: 202-337-8314
                                     TTY: 202-337-5220
                              e-mail: info@agbell.org
                           www.listeningandspokenlanguage.org
A book that develops conversational skills in children with hearing impairments.
175 pages

4369 **Book of Name Signs**
Gallaudet University
800 Florida Avenue, NE
Washington, DC 20002-3819
773-568-1550
800-621-2736
Fax: 800-621-8476
TTY: 888-630-9347
e-mail: gupress@gallaudet.edu
gupress.gallaudet.edu
This text discusses the rules for ASL name sign formulation and their appropriate uses and presents a list of over 400 name signs.
112 pages

4370 **Broken Ears: Wounded Hearts**
Gallaudet University
800 Florida Avenue, NE
Washington, DC 20002-3819
773-568-1550
800-621-2736
Fax: 800-621-8476
TTY: 888-630-9347
e-mail: gupress@gallaudet.edu
gupress.gallaudet.edu
An intimate journey into the lives of a deaf, multihandicapped child and her young hearing parents.
186 pages Hardcover

4371 **CUED Speech Resource Book for Parents of Deaf Children**
Alexander Graham Bell Association
3417 Volta Place NW
Washington, DC 20007-2737
202-337-5220
Fax: 202-337-8314
TTY: 202-337-5220
e-mail: info@agbell.org
www.listeningandspokenlanguage.org
A comprehensive book describing cued speech, getting started, your child's rights in and out of school and families expectations with special attention on siblings and peer relationships.
832 pages Hardcover

4372 **Can't Your Child Hear?**
Gallaudet University
800 Florida Avenue, NE
Washington, DC 20002-3819
773-568-1550
800-621-2736
Fax: 800-621-8476
TTY: 888-630-9347
e-mail: gupress@gallaudet.edu
gupress.gallaudet.edu
Is deafness a difference to be accepted or a defect to be corrected? This comprehensive reference will help parents, as well as educators and other professionals, recognize their options in understanding and handling a child who is deaf.
340 pages Softcover

4373 **Chelsea: The Story of a Signal Dog**
Gallaudet University
800 Florida Avenue, NE
Washington, DC 20002-3819
773-568-1550
800-621-2736
Fax: 800-621-8476
TTY: 888-630-9347
e-mail: gupress@gallaudet.edu
gupress.gallaudet.edu
A story of a young deaf couple and their dog who acts as their ears.
169 pages

4374 **Choices in Deafness**
Woodbine House
6510 Bells Mill Road
Bethesda, MD 20817-1636
800-843-7323
e-mail: info@woodbinehouse.com
www.woodbinehouse.com
Serving as an invaluable guide to the world of deaf education, this expanded edition covers a wide variety of communication options for children with hearing impairments. By providing medical, audiological, and educational information. It also contains numerous case studies. This indispensible book is an outstanding resource for parents.
1996 212 pages
ISBN: 0-933149-09-3
Sue Schwartz, Ph.D., Author/ Editor

4375 **Chuck Baird**
Gallaudet University

800 Florida Avenue, NE
Washington, DC 20002-3819
773-568-1550
800-621-2736
Fax: 800-621-8476
TTY: 888-630-9347
e-mail: gupress@gallaudet.edu
gupress.gallaudet.edu
Contains 35 full-color plates of the artwork of the deaf artist.
55 pages

4376 **Classroom Notetaker**
Alexander Graham Bell Association
3417 Volta Place NW
Washington, DC 20007-2737
202-337-5220
Fax: 202-337-8314
TTY: 202-337-5220
e-mail: info@agbell.org
www.listeningandspokenlanguage.org
This detailed manual for instructors, administrators and staff note takers promotes classroom notetaking within long-term educational programs as vital for students who are deaf and hard of hearing from elementary school to college. This book will help readers to sell a notetaking program to schools and will give a good foundation for designing and implementing a notetaking program in a school or college.
1996 150 pages

4377 **Closer Look: The English Program at the Model Secondary School for the Deaf**
Gallaudet University
800 Florida Avenue, NE
Washington, DC 20002
773-568-1550
800-621-2736
Fax: 800-621-8476
TTY: 888-630-9347
e-mail: gupress@gallaudet.edu
gupress.gallaudet.edu
Program highlighting student-centered activities using carefully selected novels and literature texts to enhance students' reading comprehension and writing abilities through interaction with real literature.
67 pages

4378 **Cochlear Implant Auditory Training Guidebook**
Alexander Graham Bell Association
3417 Volta Place NW
Washington, DC 20007-2737
202-337-5220
Fax: 202-337-8314
TTY: 202-337-5220
e-mail: info@agbell.org
www.listeningandspokenlanguage.org
This guidebook full of reproducible masters was designed for parents and professionals working with children ages four and up who have cochlear implants. It includes an easy to follow hierarchy for listening goals and a quick placement test to help you find where to start.
236 pages

4379 **Cochlear Implantation for Infants and Children**
Alexander Graham Bell Association
3417 Volta Place NW
Washington, DC 20007-2737
202-337-5220
Fax: 202-337-8314
TTY: 202-337-5220
e-mail: info@agbell.org
www.listeningandspokenlanguage.org
This comprehensive text presents the surgical, medical, audiological speech and language and habilitation aspects of cochlear implants in infants and children.
1997 263 pages

4380 **Cognition, Education and Deafness**
Gallaudet University
800 Florida Avenue, NE
Washington, DC 20002-3819
773-568-1550
800-621-2736
Fax: 800-621-8476
TTY: 888-630-9347
e-mail: gupress@gallaudet.edu
gupress.gallaudet.edu
The work of 54 authors is gathered in this definitive collection of current research on deafness and cognition. The articles are grouped into seven sections: cognition, problem solving, thinking processes, language development, reading methodologies, measurement of potential and intervention programs.
260 pages Hardcover

4381 Communicate with Me: Conversation Skills for Deaf Students
Gallaudet University
800 Florida Avenue, NE   773-568-1550
Washington, DC 20002-3819   800-621-2736
                                          Fax: 800-621-8476
                                          TTY: 888-630-9347
                              e-mail: gupress@gallaudet.edu
                                      gupress.gallaudet.edu
Students learn how to begin and end conversations, choose appropriate topics and maintain subjects.
160 pages

4382 Communication Access for Persons with Hearing Loss
Mark Ross, author
Hearing Loss Association of America
7910 Woodmont Avenue   301-657-2248
Bethesda, MD 20814-3079   Fax: 301-913-9413
                                          TTY: 301-657-2249
                              e-mail: info@hearingloss.org
                                      www.hearingloss.org
Communication access for persons with hearing loss covers both visual and hearing techniques devoted to persons with hearingloss, ranging from mild to profound.
Anna Gilmore Hall, Executive Director
Lise Hamlin, Director of Public Policy

4383 Communication Issues Among Deaf People
Gallaudet University
800 Florida Avenue, NE   773-568-1550
Washington, DC 20002-3819   800-621-2736
                                          Fax: 800-621-8476
                                          TTY: 888-630-9347
                              e-mail: gupress@gallaudet.edu
                                      gupress.gallaudet.edu
Monograph discussing important aspects of communication including total communication and the value of ASL.
138 pages

4384 Communication Issues Among Deaf People: Eyes, Hands and Voices
National Association of the Deaf
8630 Fenton Street   301-587-1788
Silver Spring, MD 20910-4500   Fax: 301-587-1791
                                          TTY: 301-587-1789
                              e-mail: nad.info@nad.org
                                      nad.org
Includes over thirty relevant articles reflecting a wide range of perceptions and attitutes on communication among deaf people.
145 pages
Christopher Wagner, President
Melissa S. Draganac-Hawk, Vice-President

4385 Communication Rules for Hard of Hearing People
Hearing Loss Association of America
7910 Woodmont Avenue   301-657-2248
Bethesda, MD 20814-3079   Fax: 301-913-9413
                                          TTY: 301-657-2249
                              e-mail: info@hearingloss.org
                                      www.hearingloss.org
To open the world of communication to people with hearing loss through education, information, support and advocacy.
Anna Gilmore Hall, Executive Director
Lise Hamlin, Director of Public Policy

4386 Communication and Adult Hearing Loss
Alexander Graham Bell Association
3417 Volta Place NW   202-337-5220
Washington, DC 20007-2737   Fax: 202-337-8314
                                          TTY: 202-337-5220
                              e-mail: info@agbell.org
                              www.listeningandspokenlanguage.org
This informative book was written for anyone who wants to communicate more effectively with a person with adult hearing loss.
1993 136 pages

4387 Comprehensive Signed English Dictionary
Harris Communications
6541 City W Parkway   612-906-1180
Eden Prairie, MN 55344-3248   Fax: 612-946-0924
                                      gupress.gallaudet.edu

Complete dictionary offers 3100 signs, including signs reflecting contemporary vocabulary.
457 pages
Harry Bornstein, Co-Editor
Karen L. Saulnier, Co-Editor

4388 Consumer Handbook on Dizziness and Vertigo
Dennis Poe, MD, author
Hearing Loss Association of Amercia
7910 Woodmont Avenue   301-657-2248
Bethesda, MD 20814-3079   Fax: 301-913-9413
                                          TTY: 301-657-2249
                              e-mail: info@hearingloss.org
                                      www.hearingloss.org
Learn the differences between dizziness and vertigo.
Hardcover
ISBN: 0-966182-64-2
Anna Gilmore Hall
Lise Hamlin, Director of Public Policy

4389 Conversational Sign Language II: An Intermdiate Advanced Manual
Harris Communications
6541 City W Parkway   612-906-1180
Eden Prairie, MN 55344-3248   Fax: 612-946-0924
                                      gupress.gallaudet.edu
This book presents English words and their American Sign Language equivalents.
218 pages
William J. Madsen, Author

4390 Dancing Without Music
Gallaudet University
800 Florida Avenue, NE   773-568-1550
Washington, DC 20002-3819   800-621-2736
                                          Fax: 800-621-8476
                                          TTY: 888-630-9347
                              e-mail: gupress@gallaudet.edu
                                      gupress.gallaudet.edu
Investigates being deaf and its social ramifications.
320 pages
Beryl Lieff Benderly, Author

4391 Deaf Children in Public Schools Placement, Context, and Consequences
Gallaudet University
800 Florida Avenue, NE   773-568-1550
Washington, DC 20002-3819   800-621-2736
                                          Fax: 800-621-8476
                                          TTY: 888-630-9347
                              e-mail: gupress@gallaudet.edu
                                      gupress.gallaudet.edu
Assesses the progress of three second-grade deaf students to demonstrate the importance of placement, context, and language in their development.
August 1997 250 pages
ISBN: 1-563680-62-9
Claire L. Ramsey, Author

4392 Deaf Culture, Our Way
Gallaudet University
800 Florida Avenue, NE   773-568-1550
Washington, DC 20002-3819   800-621-2736
                                          Fax: 800-621-8476
                                          TTY: 888-630-9347
                              e-mail: gupress@gallaudet.edu
                                      gupress.gallaudet.edu
A revised edition of Silence is Golden, Sometimes, this new edition contains sections on Classic Humor, Bathroom Tales, Classic Hazards and New Technology.
115 pages

4393 Deaf Empowerment, Emergence, Struggle and Rhetoric
Gallaudet University
800 Florida Avenue, NE   773-568-1550
Washington, DC 20002-3819   800-621-2736
                                          Fax: 800-621-8476
                                          TTY: 888-630-9347
                              e-mail: gupress@gallaudet.edu
                                      gupress.gallaudet.edu

Examines the rhetorical foundation that motivated Deaf people to work for social change during the past two centuries. Assesses the goal of a multicultural society and offers suggestions for community building through a new humanitarianism.
July 1997 192 pages Hardcover
ISBN: 1-563680-61-0

4394   Deaf Heritage: A Narrative History of Deaf America
National Association of the Deaf
8630 Fenton Street   301-587-1788
Silver Spring, MD 20910-4500   Fax: 301-587-1791
                                                   TTY: 301-587-1789
                                         e-mail: nad.info@nad.org
                                                            nad.org
In-depth history of Deaf America contains pictures, vignettes, and biographical profiles.
483 pages Paperback
Christopher Wagner, President
Melissa S. Draganac-Hawk, Vice-President

4395   Deaf Heritage: Student Text and Workbook
National Association of the Deaf
8630 Fenton Street   301-587-1788
Silver Spring, MD 20910-4500   Fax: 301-587-1791
                                                   TTY: 301-587-1789
                                         e-mail: nad.info@nad.org
                                                            nad.org
Each chapter is followed by a vocabulary section and workbook activities including questions and follow-up activities for students.
115 pages Paperback
Christopher Wagner, President
Melissa S. Draganac-Hawk, Vice-President

4396   Deaf History Unveiled: Interpretations from the New Scholarship
Gallaudet University
800 Florida Avenue, NE   773-568-1550
Washington, DC 20002-3819   800-621-2736
                                                   Fax: 800-621-8476
                                                   TTY: 888-630-9347
                                         e-mail: gupress@gallaudet.edu
                                                    gupress.gallaudet.edu
Essays written by internationally renowned deaf studies scholars.
316 pages
John Vickrey Van Cleve, Editor

4397   Deaf Like Me
Gallaudet University
800 Florida Avenue, NE   773-568-1550
Washington, DC 20002-3819   800-621-2736
                                                   Fax: 800-621-8476
                                                   TTY: 888-630-9347
                                         e-mail: gupress@gallaudet.edu
                                                    gupress.gallaudet.edu
Written by the uncle and father of a deaf girl, this is an account of parents coming to terms with deafness.
292 pages
Thomas S. Spradley, Co-Author
James P. Spradley, Co-Author

4398   Deaf President Now! The 1988 Revolution at Gallaudet University
Gallaudet University
800 Florida Avenue, NE   773-568-1550
Washington, DC 20002-3819   800-621-2736
                                                   Fax: 800-621-8476
                                                   TTY: 888-630-9347
                                         e-mail: gupress@gallaudet.edu
                                                    gupress.gallaudet.edu
This book chronicles the events leading up to the revolution in which deaf people won social change for themselves and all disabled people.
240 pages
John B. Christiansen, Co-Author
Sharon N. Barnartt, Co-Author

4399   Deaf Sport: The Impact of Sports Within the Deaf Community
Gallaudet University

800 Florida Avenue, NE   773-568-1550
Washington, DC 20002-3819   800-621-2736
                                                   Fax: 800-621-8476
                                                   TTY: 888-630-9347
                                         e-mail: gupress@gallaudet.edu
                                                    gupress.gallaudet.edu
Describes the full ramifications of athletics for deaf people.
224 pages
David A. Stewart, Author

4400   Deaf Students and the School-to-Work Transition
Gallaudet University
800 Florida Avenue, NE   773-568-1550
Washington, DC 20002-3819   800-621-2736
                                                   Fax: 800-621-8476
                                                   TTY: 888-630-9347
                                         e-mail: gupress@gallaudet.edu
                                                    gupress.gallaudet.edu
Studies severely and profoundly hearing impaired students as they leave high school and enter the work force.
278 pages

4401   Deaf Studies Curriculum Guide
Gallaudet University
800 Florida Avenue, NE   773-568-1550
Washington, DC 20002-3819   800-621-2736
                                                   Fax: 800-621-8476
                                                   TTY: 888-630-9347
                                         e-mail: gupress@gallaudet.edu
                                                    gupress.gallaudet.edu
Designed to help students explore the history, language and culture of deaf people.
250 pages

4402   Deaf Women: A Parade Through the Decades
Gallaudet University
800 Florida Avenue, NE   773-568-1550
Washington, DC 20002-3819   800-621-2736
                                                   Fax: 800-621-8476
                                                   TTY: 888-630-9347
                                         e-mail: gupress@gallaudet.edu
                                                    gupress.gallaudet.edu
A compilation of information, history, anecdotes and research that showcases many deaf women from all walks of American life.
192 pages

4403   Deaf and Hard of Hearing Individuals
Mainstream
1030 5th Street NW   202-898-1400
Washington, DC 20001-2504
Mainstreaming deaf individuals into the workplace.
12 pages

4404   Deaf in America: Voices from a Culture
Gallaudet University
800 Florida Avenue, NE   773-568-1550
Washington, DC 20002-3819   800-621-2736
                                                   Fax: 800-621-8476
                                                   TTY: 888-630-9347
                                         e-mail: gupress@gallaudet.edu
                                                    gupress.gallaudet.edu
Written by authors who are themselves deaf.
134 pages

4405   Deafness and Child Development
Gallaudet University
800 Florida Avenue, NE   773-568-1550
Washington, DC 20002-3819   800-621-2736
                                                   Fax: 800-621-8476
                                                   TTY: 888-630-9347
                                         e-mail: gupress@gallaudet.edu
                                                    gupress.gallaudet.edu
Provides rational, informed and balanced approaches to the effects of deafness in child development.
236 pages

4406   Deafness: 1993-2013
National Association of the Deaf

8630 Fenton Street
Silver Spring, MD 20910

301-587-1788
Fax: 301-587-1791
TTY: 301-587-1789
e-mail: nad.info@nad.org
nad.org

Over 30 articles cover such topics as magnet schools, deaf identity, technology, multicultural education, communication, leadership, and sign language research.
Paperback
Christopher Wagner, President
Melissa S. Draganac-Hawk, Vice-President

4407 Deafness: A Personal Account
Faber & Faber
19 Union Square W
New York, NY 10003-3304

781-721-1427
e-mail: contact@faber.co.uk
www.faber.co.uk

Poet, critic and translator David Wright's enduring memoir (now with a substantial new introduction by the author) describes with humor and insight his early life, his development as a poet, and little-known history of deaf education.
202 pages

4408 Deafness: An Autobiography
Gallaudet University
800 Florida Avenue, NE
Washington, DC 20002-3819

773-568-1550
800-621-2736
Fax: 800-621-8476
TTY: 888-630-9347
e-mail: gupress@gallaudet.edu
gupress.gallaudet.edu

This book is intended to explore the author's own experiences with deafness, and satisfy the curiosity about the condition of deaf people.
238 pages

4409 Deafness: Historical Perspectives
National Association of the Deaf
8630 Fenton Street
Silver Spring, MD 20910

301-587-1788
Fax: 301-587-1791
TTY: 301-587-1789
e-mail: nad.info@nad.org
nad.org

Focuses on the history of deaf people. Topics cover a spectrum from a history of deaf theaters, to a genealogy of our first deaf families, to a conversation with a ghost.
Paperback
Christopher Wagner, President
Melissa S. Draganac-Hawk, Vice-President

4410 Deafness: Life and Culture II
National Association of the Deaf
8630 Fenton Street
Silver Spring, MD 20910

301-587-1788
Fax: 301-587-1791
TTY: 301-587-1789
e-mail: nad.info@nad.org
nad.org

Continues to explore the variety and diversity of the deaf experience.
133 pages Paperback
ISBN: 0-913072-79-6
Christopher Wagner, President
Melissa S. Draganac-Hawk, Vice-President

4411 Directory of Auditory-Oral Programs
Alexander Graham Bell Association
3417 Volta Place NW
Washington, DC 20007-2737

202-337-5220
Fax: 202-337-8314
TTY: 202-337-5220
e-mail: info@agbell.org
www.listeningandspokenlanguage.org

This directory lists auditory/oral programs in public and private schools, auditory-oral programs in speech and hearing centers and therapists who offer private tutoring and auditory-oral therapy.
67 pages

4412 Discovering Sign Language
Gallaudet University

800 Florida Avenue, NE
Washington, DC 20002-3819

773-568-1550
800-621-2736
Fax: 800-621-8476
TTY: 888-630-9347
e-mail: gupress@gallaudet.edu
gupress.gallaudet.edu

Here is a book of information about deaf people and sign communication.
104 pages Softcover

4413 Douglas Tilden, the Man and His Legacy
Gallaudet University
800 Florida Avenue, NE
Washington, DC 20002-3819

773-568-1550
800-621-2736
Fax: 800-621-8476
TTY: 888-630-9347
e-mail: gupress@gallaudet.edu
gupress.gallaudet.edu

A beautiful tribute to the Deaf sculptor, Douglas Tilden.
216 pages

4414 Ear Book
Gallaudet University
800 Florida Avenue, NE
Washington, DC 20002-3819

773-568-1550
800-621-2736
Fax: 800-621-8476
TTY: 888-630-9347
e-mail: gupress@gallaudet.edu
gupress.gallaudet.edu

A how-to book on obtaining and using an otoscope, recognizing and managing common ear disorders, when to call the doctor and when your child needs ear tubes.
136 pages Softcover

4415 Ear Gear: A Student Workbook on Hearing and Hearing Aids
Gallaudet University
800 Florida Avenue, NE
Washington, DC 20002-3819

773-568-1550
800-621-2736
Fax: 800-621-8476
TTY: 888-630-9347
e-mail: gupress@gallaudet.edu
gupress.gallaudet.edu

Attractive workbook designed to teach elementary-age children about hearing loss and the use of hearing aids.
75 pages

4416 Educating Deaf Children Bilingually
Gallaudet University
800 Florida Avenue, NE
Washington, DC 20002-3819

773-568-1550
800-621-2736
Fax: 800-621-8476
TTY: 888-630-9347
e-mail: gupress@gallaudet.edu
gupress.gallaudet.edu

Discusses perspectives and practices of educating deaf children with goals of age-level achievement.
120 pages

4417 Educating the Deaf: Psychology, Principles and Practices
Gallaudet University
800 Florida Avenue, NE
Washington, DC 20002-3819

773-568-1550
800-621-2736
Fax: 800-621-8476
TTY: 888-630-9347
e-mail: gupress@gallaudet.edu
gupress.gallaudet.edu

Offers extensive coverage of the background and history of the education of the deaf, as well as specific information on working with multihandicapped students.
383 pages

4418 Education and Deafness
Longman Publishing Group
95 Church Street
White Plains, NY 10601-1515

914-993-5000

This comprehensive introduction to educating students with hearing impairments provides extensive coverage of the interrelated issues that affect the teaching of these students. It concentrates on the severely to profoundly hearing impaired but includes an entire

chapter devoted to students whose impairments are less severe (hard-of-hearing students).
320 pages Paperback
ISBN: 0-801300-26-6

4419 Educational and Development Aspects of Deafness
Gallaudet University
800 Florida Avenue, NE   773-568-1550
Washington, DC 20002-3819   800-621-2736
                                    Fax: 800-621-8476
                                    TTY: 888-630-9347
                          e-mail: gupress@gallaudet.edu
                                  gupress.gallaudet.edu
Book detailing the ongoing revolution in the education of deaf children.
415 pages
Donald F. Moores, Co-Editor
Kathryn P. Meadow-Orlans, Co-Editor

4420 Empowerment and Black Deaf Persons
Gallaudet University
800 Florida Avenue, NE   773-568-1550
Washington, DC 20002-3819   800-621-2736
                                    Fax: 800-621-8476
                                    TTY: 888-630-9347
                          e-mail: gupress@gallaudet.edu
                                  gupress.gallaudet.edu
Conference proceedings focusing on the guidance and training of African American deaf individuals.
175 pages

4421 Encyclopedia of Deafness and Hearing Disorders
Facts on File
11 Penn Plaza   212-967-8800
New York, NY 10001   800-322-8755
                                    Fax: 800-678-3633
A comprehensive guide to all aspects of hearing impairments.

4422 Eye-Centered: A Study of Spirituality of Deaf People
NCOD
814 Thayer Avenue   301-587-7992
Silver Spring, MD 20910-4500
The findings of the five-year De Sales Project conducted by The National Catholic Office for the Deaf.

4423 FM Auditory Trainers: A Winning Choice for Students, Teachers and Parents
Alexander Graham Bell Association
3417 Volta Place NW   202-337-5220
Washington, DC 20007-2737   Fax: 202-337-8314
                                    TTY: 202-337-5220
                            e-mail: info@agbell.org
                      www.listeningandspokenlanguage.org
A practical guide to the selection and use of FM trainers in class or at home.
67 pages

4424 For Teachers of the Hearing Impaired
Gallaudet University
800 Florida Avenue, NE   773-568-1550
Washington, DC 20002-3819   800-621-2736
                                    Fax: 800-621-8476
                                    TTY: 888-630-9347
                          e-mail: gupress@gallaudet.edu
                                  gupress.gallaudet.edu
Contains practical articles by and for teachers of hearing impaired children.

4425 Foundations of Spoken Language for Hearing Impaired Children
Alexander Graham Bell Association
3417 Volta Place NW   202-337-5220
Washington, DC 20007-2737   Fax: 202-337-8314
                                    TTY: 202-337-5220
                            e-mail: info@agbell.org
                      www.listeningandspokenlanguage.org
This guide traces the individual progress of a child's speech development.
1978 87 pages

4426 Free Hand: Education of the Deaf
TJ Publishers
817 Silver Spring Avenue   301-585-4440
Silver Spring, MD 20910-4617   800-999-1168
                                    Fax: 301-585-5930
                                    TTY: 301-585-4441
                            e-mail: tjpubinc@aol.com
Based on the proceedings of a 1990 symposium on the educational uses of ASL, A Free Hand presents papers by prominent educators, researchers and linguists in the changing role of American sign language in the classroom.
204 pages Softcover
ISBN: 0-932666-40-X
Angela K Thames, President
Jerald A Murphy, VP

4427 GA and SK Etiquette
Gallaudet University
800 Florida Avenue, NE   773-568-1550
Washington, DC 20002-3819   800-621-2736
                                    Fax: 800-621-8476
                                    TTY: 888-630-9347
                          e-mail: gupress@gallaudet.edu
                                  gupress.gallaudet.edu
This booklet presents guidelines for proper usage of the TDD.
53 pages

4428 Gallaudet Encyclopedia of Deaf People and Deafness
Gallaudet University
800 Florida Avenue, NE   773-568-1550
Washington, DC 20002-3819   800-621-2736
                                    Fax: 800-621-8476
                                    TTY: 888-630-9347
                          e-mail: gupress@gallaudet.edu
                                  gupress.gallaudet.edu
Three-volume set of research and information on deaf people and deafness.
1400 pages
John V. Van Cleve, Editor

4429 Growing Together: Information for Parents of Deaf & Hard of Hearing Children
Gallaudet University
800 Florida Avenue, NE   773-568-1550
Washington, DC 20002-3819   800-621-2736
                                    Fax: 800-621-8476
                                    TTY: 888-630-9347
                          e-mail: gupress@gallaudet.edu
                                  gupress.gallaudet.edu
This publication answers questions often asked by parents of children with a hearing loss.
92 pages

4430 Handtalk Zoo
Macmillan Publishing Company
6535 Nova Drive   954-530-8746
Davie, FL 33317-6221   800-257-5755
                                    Fax: 954-530-6247
                            e-mail: post@mcp.com
                                    www.mcp.com
Wonderful photographs are used to show children at the zoo communicating with sign language.
28 pages Hardcover
ISBN: 0-027008-01-0

4431 Hearing Aid Handbook
Gallaudet University
800 Florida Avenue, NE   773-568-1550
Washington, DC 20002-3819   800-621-2736
                                    Fax: 800-621-8476
                                    TTY: 888-630-9347
                          e-mail: gupress@gallaudet.edu
                                  gupress.gallaudet.edu
A complete guide for wearers and clinicians for the use and maintenance of hearing aids.
172 pages Paperback
Donna S. Wayner, Author

4432 Hearing Impaired Children and Youth and Developmental Disabilities
Gallaudet University
800 Florida Avenue, NE
Washington, DC 20002-3819
773-568-1550
800-621-2736
Fax: 800-621-8476
TTY: 888-630-9347
e-mail: gupress@gallaudet.edu
gupress.gallaudet.edu
Offers insights from 24 experts to help clarify relationships between hearing impairments and developmental difficulties.
416 pages

4433 Hearing Loss Help
Impact Publications
9104 Manassas Drive
Manassas Park, VA 20111-5211
703-361-7300
Fax: 703-335-9469
e-mail: query2@impactpublications.com
www.impactpublications.com
Self-help guide provides factual information on how we hear, and on the causes and symptoms of hearing loss. Gives practical information on ways to improve everyday communication and create better listening conditions, and covers assistive listening devices.

4434 Hearing Loss and Hearing Aids: A Bridge to Healing
Richard Carmen, author
Hearing Loss Association of America
7910 Woodmont Avenue
Bethesda, MD 20814-3079
301-657-2248
Fax: 301-913-9413
TTY: 301-657-2249
e-mail: info@hearingloss.org
www.hearingloss.org
The Consumer Handbook on hearing loss and hearing aids.
Softcover
ISBN: 0-966182-61-8
Anna Gilmore Hall, Executive Director
Lise Hamlin, Director of Public Policy

4435 Hispanic Deaf
Gallaudet University
800 Florida Avenue, NE
Washington, DC 20002-3819
773-568-1550
800-621-2736
Fax: 800-621-8476
TTY: 888-630-9347
e-mail: gupress@gallaudet.edu
gupress.gallaudet.edu
Hispanic students now make up the largest minority in education for deaf students. This timely collection includes articles by many of the professionals most closely involved with the education of this very special population.
213 pages Hardcover

4436 History of Special Education: From Isolation to Integration
Gallaudet University
800 Florida Avenue, NE
Washington, DC 20002-3819
773-568-1550
800-621-2736
Fax: 800-621-8476
TTY: 888-630-9347
e-mail: gupress@gallaudet.edu
gupress.gallaudet.edu
Comprehensive volume examining the facts and events that shaped this field in Western Europe, United States and Canada.
464 pages
Margret A. Winzer, Author

4437 Hollywood Speaks
Gallaudet University
800 Florida Avenue, NE
Washington, DC 20002-3819
773-568-1550
800-621-2736
Fax: 800-621-8476
TTY: 888-630-9347
e-mail: gupress@gallaudet.edu
gupress.gallaudet.edu
How deafness has been treated in movies and how it provides yet another window onto social history in addition to a fresh angle from which to view Hollywood.
167 pages Hardcover

4438 Hometown Heroes: Successful Deaf Youth in America
Gallaudet University
800 Florida Avenue, NE
Washington, DC 20002-3819
773-568-1550
800-621-2736
Fax: 800-621-8476
TTY: 888-630-9347
e-mail: gupress@gallaudet.edu
gupress.gallaudet.edu
A lively book showcasing more than 40 deaf and hard-of-hearing teenagers in the United States.
108 pages

4439 How Hearing Impacts Relationships
Richard Carmen, author
Hearing Loss Association of America
7910 Woodmont Avenue
Bethesda, MD 20814-3079
301-657-2248
Fax: 301-913-9413
TTY: 301-657-2249
e-mail: info@hearingloss.org
www.hearingloss.org
At last families of loved ones with untreated hearing loss can know they are not alone and what options are available.
Softcover
ISBN: 0-966182-63-4
Anna Gilmore Hall, Executive Director
Lise Hamlin, Director of Public Policy

4440 How the Student with Hearing Loss Can Succeed in College
Alexander Graham Bell Association
3417 Volta Place NW
Washington, DC 20007-2737
202-337-5220
Fax: 202-337-8314
TTY: 202-337-5220
e-mail: info@agbell.org
www.listeningandspokenlanguage.org
This revised book details how students who are deaf or hard of hearing and professionals must work together for students in college to be successful.
1996 304 pages

4441 How to Survive a Hearing Loss
Gallaudet University
800 Florida Avenue, NE
Washington, DC 20002-3819
773-568-1550
800-621-2736
Fax: 800-621-8476
TTY: 888-630-9347
e-mail: gupress@gallaudet.edu
gupress.gallaudet.edu
This book presents the results of the author's intensive research about hearing and the ear.
241 pages
Charlotte Himber, Author

4442 Hug Just Isn't Enough
Gallaudet University
800 Florida Avenue, NE
Washington, DC 20002-3819
773-568-1550
800-621-2736
Fax: 800-621-8476
TTY: 888-630-9347
e-mail: gupress@gallaudet.edu
gupress.gallaudet.edu
Photos of deaf children and excerpts from interviews with parents of deaf youngsters.

4443 I Didn't Hear the Dragon Roar
Gallaudet University
800 Florida Avenue, NE
Washington, DC 20002-3819
773-568-1550
800-621-2736
Fax: 800-621-8476
TTY: 888-630-9347
e-mail: gupress@gallaudet.edu
gupress.gallaudet.edu
The remarkable true story of a deaf woman's journey from Hong Kong to Katmandu.
251 pages

4444 IDEA Advocacy for Children Who are Deaf or Hard of Hearing
Alexander Graham Bell Association
3417 Volta Place NW
Washington, DC 20007-2737
202-337-5220
Fax: 202-337-8314
TTY: 202-337-5220
e-mail: info@agbell.org
www.listeningandspokenlanguage.org

This book offers up to date information about the 1997 Individuals with Disabilities Education Act which affects children who are deaf or hard of hearing.
1997 96 pages

4445   Implications and Complications for Deaf Students of Full Inclusion Movement
Gallaudet University
800 Florida Avenue, NE   773-568-1550
Washington, DC 20002-3819   800-621-2736
                                            Fax: 800-621-8476
                                            TTY: 888-630-9347
                                   e-mail: gupress@gallaudet.edu
                                            gupress.gallaudet.edu
A collection of papers discussing the full inclusion movement.
80 pages

4446   In Silence: Growing Up Hearing in a Deaf World
Gallaudet University
800 Florida Avenue, NE   773-568-1550
Washington, DC 20002-3819   800-621-2736
                                            Fax: 800-621-8476
                                            TTY: 888-630-9347
                                   e-mail: gupress@gallaudet.edu
                                            gupress.gallaudet.edu
Author's story of growing up as a hearing child of deaf parents.
335 pages
Ruth Sidransky, Author

4447   In This Sign
Gallaudet University
800 Florida Avenue, NE   773-568-1550
Washington, DC 20002-3819   800-621-2736
                                            Fax: 800-621-8476
                                            TTY: 888-630-9347
                                   e-mail: gupress@gallaudet.edu
                                            gupress.gallaudet.edu
A modern classic following a family of deaf parents and their hearing impaired child through several decades of growth and pain, tragedy and triumph.
275 pages

4448   Inclusion?
Gallaudet University
800 Florida Avenue, NE   773-568-1550
Washington, DC 20002-3819   800-621-2736
                                            Fax: 800-621-8476
                                            TTY: 888-630-9347
                                   e-mail: gupress@gallaudet.edu
                                            gupress.gallaudet.edu
This book defines quality education for deaf and hard of hearing students.
213 pages

4449   International Directory of Periodicals Related to Deafness
Gallaudet University
800 Florida Avenue, NE   773-568-1550
Washington, DC 20002-3819   800-621-2736
                                            Fax: 800-621-8476
                                            TTY: 888-630-9347
                                   e-mail: gupress@gallaudet.edu
                                            gupress.gallaudet.edu
Offers information on more than 500 magazines and journals related to deafness.
150 pages

4450   International Telephone Directory for TDD Users
Gallaudet University
800 Florida Avenue, NE   773-568-1550
Washington, DC 20002-3819   800-621-2736
                                            Fax: 800-621-8476
                                            TTY: 888-630-9347
                                   e-mail: gupress@gallaudet.edu
                                            gupress.gallaudet.edu
Offers 12,000 TDD members and organizations serving deaf people.
190 pages

4451   Introduction to Communication
Gallaudet University

800 Florida Avenue, NE   773-568-1550
Washington, DC 20002-3819   800-621-2736
                                            Fax: 800-621-8476
                                            TTY: 888-630-9347
                                   e-mail: gupress@gallaudet.edu
                                            gupress.gallaudet.edu
Curriculum materials exploring the areas of sound, hearing and interpersonal communication.
100 pages

4452   Invisible Condition: The Human Side of Hearing Loss
Howard E Stone, author
Hearing Loss Association of America
7910 Woodmont Avenue   301-657-2248
Bethesda, MD 20814-3079   Fax: 301-913-9413
                                            TTY: 301-657-2249
                                     e-mail: info@hearingloss.org
                                            www.hearingloss.org
A collection of 14 years of editorials by the author from the SHHH Journal. An inspiration book that transcends hearing loss.
1993
Anna Gilmore Hall, Executive Director
Howard E. Stone, Author

4453   Its Your Turn Now: Using Dialogue Journals with Deaf Students
Gallaudet University
800 Florida Avenue, NE   773-568-1550
Washington, DC 20002-3819   800-621-2736
                                            Fax: 800-621-8476
                                            TTY: 888-630-9347
                                   e-mail: gupress@gallaudet.edu
                                            gupress.gallaudet.edu
Based on years of experience, this book reviews teachers' questions and answers.
130 pages

4454   Journey Into the Deaf World
DawnSignPress
6130 Nancy Ridge Drive   858-625-0600
San Diego, CA 92121-3223   800-549-5350
                                            Fax: 858-625-2336
                                            TTY: 858-625-0600
                                 e-mail: comments@dawnsign.com
                                            www.dawnsign.com
Provides explanation about the nature and meaning of the deaf world. Comprehensive work discusses latest findings and theories for deaf studies students and professionals working with deaf people.
528 pages Paperback
ISBN: 0-915035-63-4
Harlan Lane, Co-Author
Robert Hoffmeister, Co-Author

4455   Journey Out of Silence
Dora Tinglestad Weber, author
Hearing Loss Association of America
7910 Woodmont Avenue   301-657-2248
Bethesda, MD 20814-3079   Fax: 301-913-9413
                                            TTY: 301-657-2249
                                     e-mail: info@hearingloss.org
                                            www.hearingloss.org
Dora Weber, who made a long and arduous journey out of silence, shares her experiences in an effort to encourage those who are hearing impaired and to increase the sensitivity of those who are not.
Softcover
ISBN: 1-890676-30-6
Anna Gilmore Hall, Executive Director
Lise Hamlin, Director of Public Policy

4456   Joy of Signing
Gospel Publishing House
1445 N Boonville Avenue   417-831-8000
Springfield, MO 65802-1894   800-641-4310
                                            Fax: 417-862-5881
                               e-mail: CustSrvOrders@ag.org
                                            gospelpublishing.com

Illustrated sign language text with descriptions of the origin of selected signs and examples of how each is used. Second edition.
352 pages
Lottie L. Riekehof, Author

4457 Kaleidoscope of Deaf America
Harris Communications
8630 Fenton Street · 301-587-1788
Silver Spring, MD 20910-3248 · Fax: 301-587-1791
TTY: 301-587-1789
nad.org

Puts you in touch with the trends, the events and the thinking that is shaping your future.
79 pages

4458 Kendall Demonstration Elementary School Curriculum Guides
Gallaudet University
800 Florida Avenue, NE · 773-568-1550
Washington, DC 20002-3819 · 800-621-2736
Fax: 800-621-8476
TTY: 888-630-9347
e-mail: gupress@gallaudet.edu
gupress.gallaudet.edu

These guides provide detailed information to help teachers organize curriculum, structure classes and develop individualized education programs.
18 months+

4459 Kid-Friendly Parenting with Deaf and Hard of Hearing Children
Gallaudet University
800 Florida Avenue, NE · 773-568-1550
Washington, DC 20002-3819 · 800-621-2736
Fax: 800-621-8476
TTY: 888-630-9347
e-mail: gupress@gallaudet.edu
gupress.gallaudet.edu

A step-by-step guide offering parents hundreds of ideas and play activities for children ages 3 to 12.
336 pages
Daria Medwid, Co-Author
Denise Chapman Weston, Co-Author

4460 Learning to Hear Again
Alexander Graham Bell Association
3417 Volta Place NW · 202-337-5220
Washington, DC 20007-2737 · Fax: 202-337-8314
TTY: 202-337-5220
e-mail: info@agbell.org
www.listeningandspokenlanguage.org

This audiologic rehabilitation curriculum guide is designed to help audiologists and speech language pathologist provide rehabilitation and education for adults with hearing losses. The authors are practicing audiologists and have used these methods successfully in individual and group sessions. This comprehensive manual comprises lesson plans, activities and materials ready to be duplicated and distributed to clients.
1996 224 pages

4461 Learning to See: American Sign Language as a Second Language
Gallaudet University
800 Florida Avenue, NE · 773-568-1550
Washington, DC 20002-3819 · 800-621-2736
Fax: 800-621-8476
TTY: 888-630-9347
e-mail: gupress@gallaudet.edu
gupress.gallaudet.edu

Provides a comprehensive introduction to the history and structure of ASL to the deaf community.
134 pages

4462 Least Restrictive Environment: The Paradox of Inclusion
LRP Publications
P.O. Box 24668
West Palm Beach, FL 33416-0980 · 800-341-7874
Fax: 561-622-2423
e-mail: custserv@lrp.com
www.lrp.com

Analyzes relevant federal law and the inclusion reform movement, and discusses the premise that an effort to force one generic place-ment on all children will create more problems than thought imaginable.
Paperback

4463 Legal Rights for the Deaf and Hard of Hearing
Hearing Loss Association of America
7910 Woodmont Avenue · 301-657-2248
Bethesda, MD 20814-3079 · Fax: 301-913-9413
TTY: 301-657-2249
e-mail: info@hearingloss.org
www.hearingloss.org

A comprehensive analysis of recent laws passed to protect the rights of and guarantee equal access for people with hearing loss. The book explains in layman's terminology how legislation affects individuals with disabilities in everyday life.
2002 Softcover
Anna Gilmore Hall, Executive Director
Lise Hamlin, Director of Public Policy

4464 Legal Rights of Hearing-Impaired People
Gallaudet University
800 Florida Avenue, NE · 773-568-1550
Washington, DC 20002-3819 · 800-621-2736
Fax: 800-621-8476
TTY: 888-630-9347
e-mail: gupress@gallaudet.edu
gupress.gallaudet.edu

Includes updated interpretations of legislation affecting hearing-impaired people, including chapters dealing with the ADA.
297 pages

4465 Lessons in Laughter: The Autobiography of a Deaf Actor
Gallaudet University
800 Florida Avenue, NE · 773-568-1550
Washington, DC 20002-3819 · 800-621-2736
Fax: 800-621-8476
TTY: 888-630-9347
e-mail: gupress@gallaudet.edu
gupress.gallaudet.edu

Born deaf of deaf parents, Bernard Bragg dreamed of using sign language to act. This book recounts how he starred in his own television show.
237 pages

4466 Let's Learn About Deafness
Gallaudet University
800 Florida Avenue, NE · 773-568-1550
Washington, DC 20002-3819 · 800-621-2736
Fax: 800-621-8476
TTY: 888-630-9347
e-mail: gupress@gallaudet.edu
gupress.gallaudet.edu

Hands-on school classroom activities for the deaf student.
82 pages

4467 Listen to Me: Auditory Exercises for Adults
Alexander Graham Bell Association
3417 Volta Place NW · 202-337-5220
Washington, DC 20007-2737 · Fax: 202-337-8314
TTY: 202-337-5220
e-mail: info@agbell.org
www.listeningandspokenlanguage.org

Helps hard of hearing teenagers and adults to listen, lip read, pick up clues from conversations and remember what they have heard.
65 pages

4468 Listen with the Heart: Relationships and Hearing Loss
Hearing Loss Association of America
7910 Woodmont Avenue · 301-657-2248
Bethesda, MD 20814-3079 · Fax: 301-913-9413
TTY: 301-657-2249
e-mail: info@hearingloss.org
www.hearingloss.org

Written for family and friends as well as professionals. It is an excellent text for college and graduate level courses in psychology, mental health counseling, speech and hearing, special education, and deaf education.
Anna Gilmore Hall, Executive Director
Michael A. Harvey, Author

4469 Listening
National Catholic Office for the Deaf
7201 Buchnan Street   301-577-1684
Landover Hills, MD 20784-4500   e-mail: Info@ncod.org
                                                www.ncod.org
Published as a pastoral service for the hearing impaired.

4470 Listening & Talking
Alexander Graham Bell Association
3417 Volta Place NW   202-337-5220
Washington, DC 20007-2737   Fax: 202-337-8314
                                                TTY: 202-337-5220
                                       e-mail: info@agbell.org
                        www.listeningandspokenlanguage.org
This guide promotes spoken language in young hearing-impaired
children.
191 pages

**4471 Listening to Learn: A Handbook for Parents with
Hearing-Impaired Children**
Alexander Graham Bell Association
3417 Volta Place NW   202-337-5220
Washington, DC 20007-2737   Fax: 202-337-8314
                                                TTY: 202-337-5220
                                       e-mail: info@agbell.org
                        www.listeningandspokenlanguage.org
Developed by teachers, this handbook provides parents with the
essential steps necessary to develop effective spoken communication with their children.
98 pages

4472 Listening: Ways of Hearing in a Silent World
Hannah Merker, author
Hearing Loss Association of America
7910 Woodmont Avenue   301-657-2248
Bethesda, MD 20814-3079   Fax: 301-913-9413
                                                TTY: 301-657-2249
                                  e-mail: info@hearingloss.org
                                          www.hearingloss.org
This book is about one woman's evocative account of her percep-
tions and rememberance of sound.
1999
Anna Gilmore Hall, Executive Director
Lise Hamlin, Director of Public Policy

4473 Literature Journal
Gallaudet University
800 Florida Avenue, NE   773-568-1550
Washington, DC 20002-3819   800-621-2736
                                                Fax: 800-621-8476
                                                TTY: 888-630-9347
                               e-mail: gupress@gallaudet.edu
                                          gupress.gallaudet.edu
This book includes extensive examples of student and teacher entries taken from actual journals of deaf high school students.
44 pages

4474 Living with Hearing Loss
Marcia B Dugan, author
Hearing Loss Association of America
7910 Woodmont Avenue   301-657-2248
Bethesda, MD 20814-3079   Fax: 301-913-9413
                                                TTY: 301-657-2249
                                  e-mail: info@hearingloss.org
                                          www.hearingloss.org
Living with Hearing Loss takes the reader from A to Z on the kinds
and causes of hearing loss and its common early signs. Topics In-
clude: Seeking Professional Evaluations, Hearing Aids, Assistive
Technology, Speechreading, Communication Tips, Cochlear Im-
plants, Dealing with Tinnitus, and resources.
2003
ISBN: 1-563681-34-0
Anna Gilmore Hall, Executive Director
Lise Hamlin, Director of Public Policy

**4475 Looking Back: A Reader on the History of Deaf Communities &
Sign Language**
Gallaudet University

800 Florida Avenue, NE   773-568-1550
Washington, DC 20002-3819   800-621-2736
                                                Fax: 800-621-2736
                                                TTY: 888-630-9347
                               e-mail: gupress@gallaudet.edu
                                          gupress.gallaudet.edu
Renowned researchers from around the world present provocative
findings in six areas relating to the deaf culture.
558 pages

4476 Loss for Words
Gallaudet University
800 Florida Avenue, NE   773-568-1550
Washington, DC 20002-3819   800-621-2736
                                                Fax: 800-621-8476
                                                TTY: 888-630-9347
                               e-mail: gupress@gallaudet.edu
                                          gupress.gallaudet.edu
The author's touching story of her life as an interpreter for her parents, head of her household by the age of eight and a teacher and
helper to both of her deaf parents.
208 pages

4477 Mainstreaming Deaf and Hard of Hearing Students
Gallaudet University
800 Florida Avenue NE   773-568-1550
Washington, DC 20002-3695   800-621-2736
                                                Fax: 800-621-8476
                                                TTY: 888-630-9347
                               e-mail: gupress@gallaudet.edu
                                          gupress.gallaudet.edu
Gallaudet University is the world leader in liberal education and
career development for deaf and hard-of-hearing undergraduate
students.
40 pages

4478 Man Without Words
Gallaudet University
800 Florida Avenue, NE   773-568-1550
Washington, DC 20002-3819   800-621-2736
                                                Fax: 800-621-8476
                                                TTY: 888-630-9347
                               e-mail: gupress@gallaudet.edu
                                          gupress.gallaudet.edu
Author relates her experiences teaching sign language to a 27 year
old deaf Mexican man who had no education and no language.
203 pages

4479 Martimer
APSEA-RCHI
Box 308   902-667-3808
Amherst, NS, B4H 3Z6,   Fax: 902-667-0893
Periodical describing programs and services provided by the
APSEA Resource Center for the Hearing Impaired.
Phyllis Cameron, Editor

4480 Mask of Benevolence: Disabling the Deaf Community
Gallaudet University
800 Florida Avenue, NE   773-568-1550
Washington, DC 20002-3819   800-621-2736
                                                Fax: 800-621-8476
                                                TTY: 888-630-9347
                               e-mail: gupress@gallaudet.edu
                                          gupress.gallaudet.edu
Written by a doctor who does not view deafness as a handicap but
rather a different state of hearing.
310 pages

4481 Meeting Halfway in ASL
MSM Productions
1095 Meigs Street   716-442-6370
Rochester, NY 14620-3380   Fax: 716-442-6371
                                                TTY: 716-442-6370
                               e-mail: Books@deaflife.com
                                          www.deaflife.com

Illustrated photographic sign-language book containing 1,300 photos.

ISBN: 0-963401-67-
Bernard Bragg, Co-Author
Jack R. Olson, Co-Author

4482 Meeting the Challenge: Hearing-Impaired Professionals in the Workplace
Gallaudet University
800 Florida Avenue, NE   773-568-1550
Washington, DC 20002-3819   800-621-2736
                                      Fax: 800-621-8476
                                      TTY: 888-630-9347
                       e-mail: gupress@gallaudet.edu
                                   gupress.gallaudet.edu
Provides information on communication methods, educational backgrounds and job search tactics used by more than 1500 participants and their current employment conditions.
236 pages

4483 Mental Health Services for Deaf People
Gallaudet University
800 Florida Avenue, NE   773-568-1550
Washington, DC 20002-3819   800-621-2736
                                      Fax: 800-621-8476
                                      TTY: 888-630-9347
                       e-mail: gupress@gallaudet.edu
                                   gupress.gallaudet.edu
Contains information on over 350 mental health programs and services for deaf people across the United States.
210 pages

4484 Missing Words: The Family Handbook on Adult Hearing Loss
Gallaudet University
800 Florida Avenue, NE   773-568-1550
Washington, DC 20002-3819   800-621-2736
                                      Fax: 800-621-8476
                                      TTY: 888-630-9347
                       e-mail: gupress@gallaudet.edu
                                   gupress.gallaudet.edu
Written by a mother who lost her hearing and her daughter, learning to cope.
304 pages

4485 Mother Father Deaf: Living Between Sound and Silence
Harvard University Press
79 Garden Street   617-495-2600
Cambridge, MA 02138-1423   800-448-2242
                                      Fax: 617-495-5898
                      e-mail: contact_hup@harvard.edu
                                      www.hup.harvard.edu
Based on interviews with 150 adult hearing children of deaf parents who chart the sometimes difficult middle ground between spoken and signed language.
Paul Preston, Author

4486 Moving Toward the Standards
Gallaudet University
800 Florida Avenue, NE   773-568-1550
Washington, DC 20002-3819   800-621-2736
                                      Fax: 800-621-8476
                                      TTY: 888-630-9347
                       e-mail: gupress@gallaudet.edu
                                   gupress.gallaudet.edu
A national action plan for mathematics education reform for the deaf.
55 pages

4487 Music in Motion
Modern Signs Press
PO Box 1181   562-596-8548
Los Alamitos, CA 90720-1181   800-572-7332
                                      Fax: 562-795-6614
                                      TTY: 562-493-4168
              e-mail: modsigns@modernsignspress.com
                                   www.modernsignspress.com

Includes guitar notes and glossary of sign descriptions for 325-word vocabulary.
109 pages
ISBN: 0-916708-07-1

4488 NAD Deaf Awareness Kit
National Association of the Deaf
8630 Fenton Street   301-587-1788
Silver Spring, MD 20910   Fax: 301-587-1791
                                      TTY: 301-587-1789
                             e-mail: nad.info@nad.org
                                              nad.org
Includes information that can be used both during Deaf Awareness Week and year-round to recognize the accomplishments and heritage of the deaf community.
Christopher Wagner, President
Melissa S. Draganac-Hawk, Vice-President

4489 Never the Twain Shall Meet: The Communications Debate
Gallaudet University
800 Florida Avenue, NE   773-568-1550
Washington, DC 20002-3819   800-621-2736
                                      Fax: 800-621-8476
                                      TTY: 888-630-9347
                       e-mail: gupress@gallaudet.edu
                                   gupress.gallaudet.edu
Should sign language be used in the education of Deaf children or should they be forced to deal with a hearing, speaking world on its own terms?.
129 pages

4490 Next Step
Gallaudet University
800 Florida Avenue, NE   773-568-1550
Washington, DC 20002-3819   800-621-2736
                                      Fax: 800-621-8476
                                      TTY: 888-630-9347
                       e-mail: gupress@gallaudet.edu
                                   gupress.gallaudet.edu
A national conference focusing on issues related to substance abuse in the deaf and hard of hearing population.
209 pages

4491 No Sound
Harris Communications
6541 City W Parkway   612-906-1180
Eden Prairie, MN 55344-3248   Fax: 612-946-0924
A moving, highly informative autobiography of Julius Wiggins, founder and president of the newspaper Silent News. Second edition.
211 pages

4492 No Walls of Stone: An Anthology of Literature by Deaf Writers
Gallaudet University
800 Florida Avenue, NE   773-568-1550
Washington, DC 20002-3819   800-621-2736
                                      Fax: 800-621-8476
                                      TTY: 888-630-9347
                       e-mail: gupress@gallaudet.edu
                                   gupress.gallaudet.edu
Short fiction, essays, verse and drama written by the deaf and hard of hearing writer.
240 pages
Jill Jepson, Editor

4493 None So Deaf
Gallaudet University
800 Florida Avenue, NE   773-568-1550
Washington, DC 20002-3819   800-621-2736
                                      Fax: 800-621-8476
                                      TTY: 888-630-9347
                       e-mail: gupress@gallaudet.edu
                                   gupress.gallaudet.edu
A student history of education of deaf people and the development of sign language.
51 pages Paperback

4494 Odyssey of Hearing Loss: Tales of Triumph
Michael A Harvey, PhD, author
Hearing Loss Association of America

7910 Woodmont Avenue
Bethesda, MD 20814-3079

301-657-2248
Fax: 301-913-9413
TTY: 301-657-2249
e-mail: info@hearingloss.org
www.hearingloss.org

A glimpse into the lives of 10 people; each showing how sharing insights about hearing loss helps people on the road to healing and a life well examined.

Anna Gilmore Hall, Executive Director
Michael A. Harvey, Author

4495   Okada Hearing Ear Guide
RR 1 Box 640F
Fontana, WI 53125-9714

414-275-5226

Trains dogs to aid hearing-impaired persons.

4496   On My Own
Gallaudet University
800 Florida Avenue, NE
Washington, DC 20002-3819

773-568-1550
800-621-2736
Fax: 800-621-8476
TTY: 888-630-9347
e-mail: gupress@gallaudet.edu
gupress.gallaudet.edu

Book examining doorbell devices, alarm clocks, telephone amplifiers and other assistive devices for the deaf.
50 pages Teacher's Guide

4497   Oral Interpreting Selections from Papers from Kirsten Gonzales
Alexander Graham Bell Association
3417 Volta Place NW
Washington, DC 20007-2737

202-337-5220
Fax: 202-337-8314
TTY: 202-337-5220
e-mail: info@agbell.org
www.listeningandspokenlanguage.org

These six easy to read articles discuss speech reading and oral interpreting. The articles answer questions that are frequently asked by professionals and the general public.
30 pages

4498   Other Side of Silence
Gallaudet University
800 Florida Avenue, NE
Washington, DC 20002-3819

773-568-1550
800-621-2736
Fax: 800-621-8476
TTY: 888-630-9347
e-mail: gupress@gallaudet.edu
gupress.gallaudet.edu

Explores the deaf community through interviews from across the country.
256 pages

4499   Our Forgotten Children
Alexander Graham Bell Association
3417 Volta Place NW
Washington, DC 20007-2737

202-337-5220
Fax: 202-337-8314
TTY: 202-337-5220
e-mail: info@agbell.org
www.listeningandspokenlanguage.org

This simple book describes characteristics of hard-of-hearing children in the school and discusses their educational requirements, psychological and social needs and amplification options.
68 pages

4500   Our Forgotten Children: Hard of Hearing Pupils in the Schools
Julia M Davis, PhD, author
Hearing Loss Association of America
7910 Woodmont Avenue
Bethesda, MD 20814-3079

301-657-2248
Fax: 301-913-9413
TTY: 301-657-2249
e-mail: info@hearingloss.org
www.hearingloss.org

Important resource about the educational environment.
2001
Anna Gilmore Hall, Executive Director
Lise Hamlin, Director of Public Policy

4501   Outsiders in a Hearing World
Gallaudet University

800 Florida Avenue, NE
Washington, DC 20002-3819

773-568-1550
800-621-2736
Fax: 800-621-2736
TTY: 888-630-9347
e-mail: gupress@gallaudet.edu
gupress.gallaudet.edu

The author gives a sociologist's view of what it is like to be deaf.
240 pages

4502   Parents and Teachers: Partners in Language Development
Alexander Graham Bell Association
3417 Volta Place NW
Washington, DC 20007-2737

202-337-5220
Fax: 202-337-8314
TTY: 202-337-5220
e-mail: info@agbell.org
www.listeningandspokenlanguage.org

Outlines the essential role of the teacher and parent in the development of language in the school aged child with hearing impairment.
386 pages

4503   Perigee Visual Dictionary of Signing
Harris Communications
6541 City W Parkway
Eden Prairie, MN 55344-3248

612-906-1180
Fax: 612-946-0924

An A-to-Z guide to American Sign Language vocabulary.
450 pages

4504   Perspectives Folio: Mainstreaming
Gallaudet University
800 Florida Avenue, NE
Washington, DC 20002-3819

773-568-1550
800-621-2736
Fax: 800-621-8476
TTY: 888-630-9347
e-mail: gupress@gallaudet.edu
gupress.gallaudet.edu

Presents 14 articles from Perspectives magazine that offer practical, experience-based advice on mainstreaming for parents and students themselves.
39 pages

4505   Perspectives on Deafness
National Association of the Deaf
8630 Fenton Street
Silver Spring, MD 20910

301-587-1788
Fax: 301-587-1791
TTY: 301-587-1789
e-mail: nad.info@nad.org
nad.org

Focuses on the many perspectives which constitute diversity within the deaf community.
Paperback
Christopher Wagner, President
Melissa S. Draganac-Hawk, Vice-President

4506   Place of Their Own: Creating the Deaf Community in America
Gallaudet University Press
800 Florida Avenue, NE
Washington, DC 20002-3819

773-568-1550
800-621-2736
Fax: 800-621-8476
TTY: 888-630-9347
e-mail: gupress@gallaudet.edu
gupress.gallaudet.edu

Traces the history of deaf people and views deafness not from the perspective of a pathology, but of culture, not as a disease or disability to overcome or be cured, but as the distinguishing characteristic of a distinct community of individuals whose history and achievement are worthy of study.

4507   Politics of Deafness
Gallaudet University
800 Florida Avenue, NE
Washington, DC 20002

773-568-1550
800-621-2736
Fax: 800-621-8476
TTY: 888-630-9347
e-mail: gupress@gallaudet.edu
gupress.gallaudet.edu

Embarks upon a postmodern examination of the search for identity in deafness and its relationship to the prevalent Hearing culture that has marginalized Deaf people.
June 1997 304 pages Softcover
ISBN: 1-563680-58-0
Owen Wrigley, Author

4508 Possible Dream: Mainstream Experiences of Hearing-Impaired Students

Alexander Graham Bell Association
3417 Volta Place NW
Washington, DC 20007-2737

202-337-5220
Fax: 202-337-8314
TTY: 202-337-5220
e-mail: info@agbell.org
www.listeningandspokenlanguage.org

This collection highlights the experiences of auditory-oral children who are Bell Association financial aid winners and their families.
66 pages
Mildred L Oberkotter, Editor

4509 Post Milan

Gallaudet University
800 Florida Avenue, NE
Washington, DC 20002-3819

773-568-1550
800-621-2736
Fax: 800-621-8476
TTY: 888-630-9347
TDD: 800-621-8476
e-mail: gupress@gallaudet.edu
gupress.gallaudet.edu

Timely issues covering trends in ASL and ASL/English literacy.
323 pages

4510 PreReading Strategies

Gallaudet University
800 Florida Avenue, NE
Washington, DC 20002-3819

773-568-1550
800-621-2736
Fax: 800-621-8476
TTY: 888-630-9347
e-mail: gupress@gallaudet.edu
gupress.gallaudet.edu

Here is a wealth of good advice for preparing students to understand what they read, building comprehension and enjoyment.
65 pages

4511 Psychoeducational Assessment of Hearing-Impaired Students

Pro-Ed, Inc.
8700 Shoal Creek Blvd
Austin, TX 78757-6897

512-451-3246
800-897-3202
Fax: 512-451-8542
e-mail: info@proedinc.com
www.proedinc.com

This book includes a comprehensive presentation of issues and procedures related to the assessment of hearing-impaired students.
251 pages Paperback
ISBN: 0-890794-55-3
Lindy Jordaan, Marketing Coordinator

4512 Reading and Deafness

Pro-Ed, Inc.
8700 Shoal Creek Blvd
Austin, TX 78757-6897

512-451-3246
800-897-3202
Fax: 800-397-7633
e-mail: info@proedinc.com
www.proedinc.com

Three areas are looked at in this book: deaf children's prereading development of real-world knowledge; cognitive abilities and linguistic skills.
422 pages Hardcover
ISBN: 0-887441-07-6
Lindy Jordaan, Marketing Coordinator

4513 Rebuilt: My Journey Back to the Hearing World
Michael Chorost, author

Hearing Loss Association of America
7910 Woodmont Avenue
Bethesda, MD 20814-3079

301-657-2248
Fax: 301-913-9413
TTY: 301-657-2249
e-mail: info@hearingloss.org
www.hearingloss.org

Brimming with insight and written with charm and self-deprecating humor, Rebuilt unveils, in personal terms, the astounding possibilities of a new technological age.
240 pages Paperback
ISBN: 0-618717-60-9
Anna Gilmore Hall, Executive Director
Lise Hamlin, Director of Public Policy

4514 Say That Again, Please

Gallaudet University
800 Florida Avenue, NE
Washington, DC 20002-3819

773-568-1550
800-621-2736
Fax: 800-621-8476
TTY: 888-630-9347
e-mail: gupress@gallaudet.edu
gupress.gallaudet.edu

This book serves to enlighten those who are interested.
370 pages

4515 Schedules of Development for Hearing Impaired Infants and their Parents

Alexander Graham Bell Association
3417 Volta Place NW
Washington, DC 20007-2737

202-337-5220
Fax: 202-337-8314
TTY: 202-337-5220
e-mail: info@agbell.org
www.listeningandspokenlanguage.org

Written for parents and teachers, this assessment record of verbal learning will help to evaluate each child's language development.
1977 14 pages

4516 Science of Sound

Gallaudet University
800 Florida Avenue, NE
Washington, DC 20002-3819

773-568-1550
800-621-2736
Fax: 800-621-8476
TTY: 888-630-9347
e-mail: gupress@gallaudet.edu
gupress.gallaudet.edu

This exciting book is carefully designed to help hearing-impaired students understand, use and enjoy the principles of sound.
32 pages

4517 Seeds of Disquiet: One Deaf Woman's Experience

Gallaudet University
800 Florida Avenue, NE
Washington, DC 20002-3819

773-568-1550
800-621-2736
Fax: 800-621-8476
TTY: 888-630-9347
e-mail: gupress@gallaudet.edu
gupress.gallaudet.edu

This book relates to the story of how Cheryl Heppner reacted to two severe losses in her hearing.
192 pages

4518 Seeing Voices: A Journey Into the World of the Deaf

Gallaudet University
800 Florida Avenue, NE
Washington, DC 20002-3819

773-568-1550
800-621-2736
Fax: 800-621-8476
TTY: 888-630-9347
e-mail: gupress@gallaudet.edu
gupress.gallaudet.edu

Dr. Sacks takes us into the world of deaf people.
180 pages

4519 Sign Communication: A Family Affair

Gallaudet University
800 Florida Avenue, NE
Washington, DC 20002-3819

773-568-1550
800-621-2736
Fax: 800-621-8476
TTY: 888-630-9347
e-mail: gupress@gallaudet.edu
gupress.gallaudet.edu

Book designed to help hearing parents communicate effectively with their deaf children on issues of good health and personal growth.
132 pages

4520 Sign Language Feelings
Gallaudet University
800 Florida Avenue, NE   773-568-1550
Washington, DC 20002-3819   800-621-2736
Fax: 800-621-8476
TTY: 888-630-9347
e-mail: gupress@gallaudet.edu
gupress.gallaudet.edu
Worksheets teach signs for happy, sad and all of the feelings in between.

4521 Sign Language Interpreters and Interpreting
Gallaudet University
800 Florida Avenue, NE   773-568-1550
Washington, DC 20002-3819   800-621-2736
Fax: 800-621-8476
TTY: 888-630-9347
e-mail: gupress@gallaudet.edu
gupress.gallaudet.edu
This monograph presents articles about personal characteristics and abilities of interpreters, the effects of lag time on interpreter errors, and the interpretation of register.
161 pages

4522 Sign Language Made Simple
Gospel Publishing House
1445 N Boonville Avenue   417-862-2781
Springfield, MO 65802-1894   800-641-4310
Fax: 417-862-7566
e-mail: CustSrvOrders@ag.org
gospelpublishing.com
Illustrated sign language text with descriptions of the origin of selected signs and examples of how each is used. Second edition.
240 pages
Edgar D. Lawrence, Author

4523 Sign Language Talk
Franklin Watts Grolier
557 Broadway   573-632-1632
New York, NY 10012-0001   800-724-6527
Fax: 203-797-3197
www.grolier.com
Using 300 easy-to-follow illustrations, this book introduces the structure of sign language, shows how sentences are formed and how signed conversations differ from spoken ones.
96 pages
ISBN: 0-531105-97-0

4524 Sign Language and the Deaf Community: Essays in Honor of William Stokoe
National Association of the Deaf
8630 Fenton Street   301-587-1788
Silver Spring, MD 20910   Fax: 301-587-1791
TTY: 301-587-1789
e-mail: nad.info@nad.org
nad.org
Collection of essays, written by professionals in the field of sign language research and usage, describing how information has dramatically altered society's understanding of deaf people and their culture.
267 pages Paperback
Christopher Wagner, President
Melissa S. Draganac-Hawk, Vice-President

4525 Signed English Starter
Harris Communications
6541 City W Parkway   612-906-1108
Eden Prairie, MN 55344-3248   Fax: 612-946-0924
gupress.gallaudet.edu
The first book to use when learning Signed English.
208 pages
Harry Bornstein, Co-Author
Karen L. Saulnier, Co-Author

4526 Signing Exact English
Modern Signs Press

PO Box 1181   562-596-8548
Los Alamitos, CA 90720-1181   800-572-7332
Fax: 562-795-6614
TTY: 562-493-4168
e-mail: modsigns@modernsignspress.com
www.modernsignspress.com
A reference manual containing manual signs representing nearly 4,000 words, plus signs for letters, numbers, prefixes and suffixes.
1993 479 pages Softcover
ISBN: 0-196708-23-3

4527 Signing Illustrated
Gallaudet University
800 Florida Avenue, NE   773-568-1550
Washington, DC 20002-3819   800-621-2736
Fax: 800-621-8476
TTY: 888-630-9347
e-mail: gupress@gallaudet.edu
gupress.gallaudet.edu
A guide presenting illustrations of over 1,350 signs.
85 pages

4528 Signing Naturally: Teacher's Curriculum Guide-Level 1
DawnSignPress
6130 Nancy Ridge Drive   619-625-0600
San Diego, CA 92121-3223   800-549-5350
Fax: 619-625-2336
e-mail: DawnSign@aol.com
www.dawnsign.com
Guide and video.
336 pages 22 minutes
ISBN: 0-915035-07-3

4529 Signs Everywhere
Modern Signs Press
PO Box 1181   562-596-8548
Los Alamitos, CA 90720-1181   800-572-7332
Fax: 562-795-6614
TTY: 562-493-4168
e-mail: modsigns@modernsignspress.com
www.modernsignspress.com
Includes signs for cities, towns and states through United States, Canada and Mexico. Drawings and descriptions of the signs accompany maps showing locations of states and cities.
280 pages
ISBN: 0-916708-05-5

4530 Signs for Computing Terminology
National Association of the Deaf
8630 Fenton Street   301-587-1788
Silver Spring, MD 20910-4500   Fax: 301-587-1791
TTY: 301-587-1789
e-mail: nad.info@nad.org
nad.org
Contains over 600 computer related sign illustrations used by deaf and hearing computer specialists.
182 pages Paperback
ISBN: 0-913072-63-X
Christopher Wagner, President
Melissa S. Draganac-Hawk, Vice-President

4531 Silent Alarm: On the Edge with a Deaf EMT
Gallaudet University
800 Florida Avenue, NE   773-568-1550
Washington, DC 20002-3819   800-621-2736
Fax: 800-621-8476
TTY: 888-630-9347
e-mail: gupress@gallaudet.edu
gupress.gallaudet.edu
Silent Alarm tells the gripping story of survival and the good that the author did as a topnotch EMT.
160 pages
Steven L. Schrader, Author

4532 Silent Garden: Raising Your Deaf Child
Gallaudet University

800 Florida Avenue, NE
Washington, DC 20002

773-568-1550
800-621-2736
Fax: 800-621-8476
TTY: 888-630-9347
e-mail: gupress@gallaudet.edu
gupress.gallaudet.edu

Provides parents with a firm foundation for making the difficult decisions necessary for their deaf child's future. Includes information on critical concerns, communication, technological alternative, and reassurance through case studies and interviews.
304 pages Softcover
ISBN: 1-563680-58-0

4533   Simultaneous Communication, ASL and Other Communication Modes
Gallaudet University
800 Florida Avenue, NE
Washington, DC 20002-3819

773-568-1550
800-621-2736
Fax: 800-621-8476
TTY: 888-630-9347
e-mail: gupress@gallaudet.edu
gupress.gallaudet.edu

This monograph presents four major articles that examine issues surrounding communications in an educational environment.
236 pages

4534   Sing Praise
Sunday School Board of the Southern Baptists
127 9th Avenue N
Nashville, TN 37234-0001   800-458-2772
For use by interpreters to the deaf.

4535   Sociolinguistics in Deaf Communities
Gallaudet University
800 Florida Avenue, NE
Washington, DC 20002-3819

773-568-1550
800-621-2736
Fax: 800-621-8476
TTY: 888-630-9347
e-mail: gupress@gallaudet.edu
gupress.gallaudet.edu

The first volume in a series offering assessments and up-to-date information on sign language linguistics.
280 pages
Ceil Lucas, Editor

4536   Software to Go
Gallaudet University
800 Florida Avenue, NE
Washington, DC 20002-3819

773-568-1550
800-621-2736
Fax: 800-621-8476
TTY: 888-630-9347
e-mail: gupress@gallaudet.edu
gupress.gallaudet.edu

Lists and describes commercial software that may be borrowed by educators of hearing impaired students.
100 pages

4537   Sound and Sign, Childhood Deafness and Mental Health
Gallaudet University
800 Florida Avenue, NE
Washington, DC 20002-3819

773-568-1550
800-621-2736
Fax: 800-621-8476
TTY: 888-630-9347
e-mail: gupress@gallaudet.edu
gupress.gallaudet.edu

Presents research to support beliefs that deaf children should be educated using a combination manual and oral communication in residual hearing and speech.
265 pages

4538   Speak to Me
Gallaudet University
800 Florida Avenue, NE
Washington, DC 20002-3819

773-568-1550
800-621-2736
Fax: 800-621-8476
TTY: 888-630-9347
e-mail: gupress@gallaudet.edu
gupress.gallaudet.edu

A story of a single mother confronted with the deafness of her son.
160 pages
Marcia Calhoun Forecki, Author

4539   Speech and the Hearing-Impaired Child
Alexander Graham Bell Association
3417 Volta Place NW
Washington, DC 20007-2737

202-337-5220
Fax: 202-337-8314
TTY: 202-337-5220
e-mail: info@agbell.org
www.listeningandspokenlanguage.org

Provides a systematic approach to the teaching of speech and a challenge to all involved in the development of spoken language skills in hearing-impaired children.
402 pages

4540   Speechreading in Context
Gallaudet University
800 Florida Avenue, NE
Washington, DC 20002-3819

773-568-1550
800-621-2736
Fax: 800-621-8476
TTY: 888-630-9347
e-mail: gupress@gallaudet.edu
gupress.gallaudet.edu

This useful guide for teachers and therapists approaches speechreading instruction with the help of context cues.
32 pages

4541   Speechreading: A Way to Improve Understand ing
Harriet Kaplan, author
Hearing Loss Association of America
7910 Woodmont Avenue
Bethesda, MD 20814

301-657-2248
Fax: 301-913-9413
TTY: 3016572249
e-mail: info@hearingloss.org
www.hearingloss.org

Discusses the nature and process of speechreading, its benefits, and its limitations. This useful book clarifies commonly-held misconceptions about speechreading. The beginning chapters address difficult communication situations and problems related to the speaker, the speechreader, and the environment It then offers strategies to manage them.
160 pages Paperback
Anna Gilmore Hall, Executive Director
Lise Hamlin, Director of Public Policy

4542   Study of American Deaf Folklore
Gallaudet University
800 Florida Avenue, NE
Washington, DC 20002-3819

773-568-1550
800-621-2736
Fax: 800-621-8476
TTY: 888-630-9347
e-mail: gupress@gallaudet.edu
gupress.gallaudet.edu

Presents a discussion of the different functions that folklore serves in the community.
156 pages

4543   Substance Abuse and Recovery: Empowerment of Deaf Persons
Gallaudet University
800 Florida Avenue, NE
Washington, DC 20002-3819

773-568-1550
800-621-2736
Fax: 800-621-8476
TTY: 888-630-9347
e-mail: gupress@gallaudet.edu
gupress.gallaudet.edu

Professionals in the field of substance abuse and deafness present their views on abuse.
217 pages

4544   Talk with Me
Alexander Graham Bell Association
3417 Volta Place NW
Washington, DC 20007-2737

202-337-5220
Fax: 202-337-8314
TTY: 202-337-5220
e-mail: info@agbell.org
www.listeningandspokenlanguage.org

Written by a clinical psychologist and mother, this book educates parents and professionals about crucial early decisions that affect

the speech, language, auditory, social and emotional development of children with hearing impairments.
222 pages

4545 Teaching English to the Deaf as a Second Language
Depart. of English, Gallaudet University
800 Florida Avenue NE   773-568-1550
Washington, DC 20002   800-621-2736
                               Fax: 800-621-8476
                               TTY: 888-630-9347
                               e-mail: gupress@gallaudet.edu
                               gupress.gallaudet.edu
Publishes articles of practical interest to classroom teachers of hearing impaired and second language students.

Kendall Green

4546 There's a Hearing Impaired Child in my Class
Gallaudet University
800 Florida Avenue, NE   773-568-1550
Washington, DC 20002-3819   800-621-2736
                               Fax: 800-621-8476
                               TTY: 888-630-9347
                               e-mail: gupress@gallaudet.edu
                               gupress.gallaudet.edu
This complete package provides basic facts about deafness, practical strategies for teaching hearing impaired children, and the question-and-answer information for all students.
44 pages

4547 Thirteen Keys to A Successful High School Experience
Alexander Graham Bell Association
3417 Volta Place NW   202-337-5220
Washington, DC 20007-2737   Fax: 202-337-8314
                               TTY: 202-337-5220
                               e-mail: info@agbell.org
                               www.listeningandspokenlanguage.org
In this booklet, three students who have profound hearing losses share their mainstream education experiences. This booklet is great for teachers of any age child and many of the suggestions to make mainstreaming easier are practical and easy to implement.
1996 28 pages

4548 Toward Effective Public School Programs for Deaf Students
Thomas N. Kluwin, Donald F. Moores, Gonter Gaustad, author
Teachers College Press
1234 Amsterdam Avenue   212-678-3929
New York, NY 10027   Fax: 212-678-4149
                               e-mail: tcpress@tc.columbia.edu
                               www.teacherscollegepress.com
Examining various options for providing effective education-including the highly controversial practice of mainstreaming-the editors base their study on one of the largest and longest-running studies ever of public school programs for the deaf.
272 pages
ISBN: 0-807731-59-5
Martha Gonter Gaustad, Editors

4549 Understanding Deafness Socially
Gallaudet University
800 Florida Avenue, NE   773-568-1550
Washington, DC 20002-3819   800-621-2736
                               Fax: 800-621-8476
                               TTY: 888-630-9347
                               e-mail: gupress@gallaudet.edu
                               gupress.gallaudet.edu
Articles on the social dynamics of deafness.
196 pages

4550 Understanding Ear Infections
Alexander Graham Bell Association
3417 Volta Place NW   202-337-5220
Washington, DC 20007-2737   Fax: 202-337-8314
                               TTY: 202-337-5220
                               e-mail: info@agbell.org
                               www.listeningandspokenlanguage.org
Based on medical research, this clinical aid for medical and hearing professionals explains ear infections and their complications to patients and their families. Sturdily designed of cardboard and

spiral-bound, each page has photos and diagrams that explain each topic and answer commonly asked questions about ear infections.
1993 27 pages

4551 Viewpoints on Deafness
National Association of the Deaf
8630 Fenton Street   301-587-1788
Silver Spring, MD 20910   Fax: 301-587-1791
                               TTY: 301-587-1789
                               e-mail: nad.info@nad.org
                               nad.org
Monograph presents a collection of viewpoints on deafness.
157 pages Paperback
Christopher Wagner, President
Melissa S. Draganac-Hawk, Vice-President

4552 Visible Speech
SRC Software Research Corporation
Box 4277, Station A   250-727-3744
Victoria, BC, V8X 3X8,
Computerized speech culture, analysis and computer-based speech training.
6 pages
AE Wright, Publisher

4553 Voyage to an Island
Gallaudet University
800 Florida Avenue, NE   773-568-1550
Washington, DC 20002-3819   800-621-2736
                               Fax: 800-621-8476
                               TTY: 888-630-9347
                               e-mail: gupress@gallaudet.edu
                               gupress.gallaudet.edu
This book recounts the story of how the author, a deaf woman from Finland, adjusts to moving to the exotic island of St. Lucia.
248 pages
Raija Nieminen, Author

4554 Week the World Heard Gallaudet
Gallaudet University
800 Florida Avenue, NE   773-568-1550
Washington, DC 20002-3819   800-621-2736
                               Fax: 800-621-8476
                               TTY: 888-630-9347
                               e-mail: gupress@gallaudet.edu
                               gupress.gallaudet.edu
This book gives the readers a day-by-day description of the Deaf President Now movement as it unfolded from March 6 to 13, 1988.
176 pages Paperback

4555 What is an Audiogram?
Gallaudet University
800 Florida Avenue, NE   773-568-1550
Washington, DC 20002-3819   800-621-2736
                               Fax: 800-621-8476
                               TTY: 888-630-9347
                               e-mail: gupress@gallaudet.edu
                               gupress.gallaudet.edu
Here's a cheery friend to solve the mysteries of the audiogram.
16 pages

4556 What's that Pig Outdoors? A Memoir of Deafness
Henry Kisor, author
Pengiuin Group
1325 South Oak Street   217-333-0950
Champaign, IL 61820-3657   800-526-0275
                               Fax: 217-244-8082
                               e-mail: uipress@uillinois.edu
                               www.press.uillinois.edu
Life of a journalist who is deaf and lives in a hearing world lipreading. Discusses some of the technical advances which help the deaf.
288 pages Hardcover
ISBN: 0-140148-99-2
Henry Kisor, Author

4557 When Your Child is Deaf: A Guide for Parents
Alexander Graham Bell Association

3417 Volta Place NW
Washington, DC 20007-2737

202-337-5220
Fax: 202-337-8314
TTY: 202-337-5220
e-mail: info@agbell.org
www.listeningandspokenlanguage.org

This book gives encouragement and advice to parents on their essential roles in teaching speech to their child.
182 pages

4558   When the Mind Hears
Gallaudet University
800 Florida Avenue, NE
Washington, DC 20002-3819

773-568-1550
800-621-2736
Fax: 800-621-8476
TTY: 888-630-9347
e-mail: gupress@gallaudet.edu
gupress.gallaudet.edu

Told largely from the vantage point of Laurent Clerc.
460 pages

4559   Who Speaks for the Deaf Community?
National Association of the Deaf
8630 Fenton Street
Silver Spring, MD 20910

301-587-1788
Fax: 301-587-1791
TTY: 301-587-1789
e-mail: nad.info@nad.org
nad.org

Paperback
Christopher Wagner, President
Melissa S. Draganac-Hawk, Vice-President

4560   Wired for Sound
Gallaudet University
800 Florida Avenue, NE
Washington, DC 20002-3819

773-568-1550
800-621-2736
Fax: 800-621-8476
TTY: 888-630-9347
e-mail: gupress@gallaudet.edu
gupress.gallaudet.edu

Secondary school edition of Ear Gear, this attractive workbook is designed to give older students an in-depth understanding of hearing and hearing aids.
156 pages
Carole Bugosh Simko, Author

4561   Working with Deaf People: Accessibility and Accommodation in the Workplace
2600 S 1st Street
Springfield, IL 62704-4730

217-789-8980
Fax: 217-789-9130
e-mail: books@ccthomas.com
www.ccthomas.com

Reveals the kinds of patterns of work adjustment problems that can surface among deaf employees, including the points of view of both supervisors an deaf people.
250 pages Paperback
ISBN: 0-398061-26-2
Charles C Thomas, Publisher

4562   Working with Deaf Persons in Sunday School
Sunday School Board of the Southern Baptists
127 9th Avenue N
Nashville, TN 37234-0001

800-458-2772

Provides guidance for organizing and conducting Sunday School classes/departments for deaf children, youth and adults.

4563   Writer's Workshop
Gallaudet University
800 Florida Avenue, NE
Washington, DC 20002-3819

773-568-1550
800-621-2736
Fax: 800-621-8476
TTY: 888-630-9347
e-mail: gupress@gallaudet.edu
gupress.gallaudet.edu

Offers suggestions to teachers who are interested in turning the classroom into an environment where students learn to express themselves in writing.
95 pages

4564   You Just Don't Understand
Deborah Tannen, author
Hearing Loss Association of America
7910 Woodmont Avenue
Bethesda, MD 20814-3079

301-657-2248
Fax: 301-913-9413
TTY: 301-657-2249
e-mail: info@hearingloss.org
www.hearingloss.org

Studded with lively and entertaining examples of real conversations, this book gives you the tools to understand what went wrong — and to find a common language in which to strengthen relationships at work and at home. A classic in the field of interpersonal relations, this book will change forever the way you approach conversations.
Softcover
ISBN: 0-060959-62-2
Anna Gilmore Hall, Executive Director
Lise Hamlin, Director of Public Policy

4565   You and Your Deaf Child
Gallaudet University
800 Florida Avenue, NE
Washington, DC 20002-3819

773-568-1550
800-621-2736
Fax: 800-621-8476
TTY: 888-630-9347
e-mail: gupress@gallaudet.edu
gupress.gallaudet.edu

This guide for parents explores how families interact to deal with the special impact of a child who is hearing impaired.
1997 224 pages 2nd edition
John W. Adams, Author

Children's Books

4566   ABC's of Finger Spelling
Modern Signs Press
PO Box 1181
Los Alamitos, CA 90720-1181

562-596-8548
800-572-7332
Fax: 562-795-6614
TTY: 562-493-4168
e-mail: modsigns@modernsignspress.com
www.modernsignspress.com

Helps teach upper and lower case letters of the alphabet. Includes printed letters and easy-to-follow drawings of the hand shapes.
60 pages
ISBN: 0-916708-13-6

4567   Alphabet of Animal Signs
Garlic Press
899 South College Mall Rd
Bloomington, IN 47401-5337

541-345-0063
800-789-0554
Fax: 800-789-5576
e-mail: kadler@ipgbook.com
www.garlicpress.com

Presents animal illustrations and associated signs for each letter of the alphabet.
16 pages Paperback
ISBN: 0-931993-65-2
Stan Collins, Author

4568   Animal Signs: A First Book of Sign Language
Gallaudet University
800 Florida Avenue, NE
Washington, DC 20002-3819

773-568-1550
800-621-2736
Fax: 800-621-8476
TTY: 888-630-9347
e-mail: gupress@gallaudet.edu
gupress.gallaudet.edu

Full-color photos of animals and their signs.
16 pages Ages 1-4
Debbie Slier, Author

4569   Another Handful of Stories
Gallaudet University

800 Florida Avenue, NE
Washington, DC 20002-3819
773-568-1550
800-621-2736
Fax: 800-621-8476
TTY: 888-630-9347
e-mail: gupress@gallaudet.edu
gupress.gallaudet.edu

Second book contains a series of 37 stories told by deaf individuals.
124 pages

4570 At Grandma's House
Modern Signs Press
PO Box 1181
Los Alamitos, CA 90720-1181
562-596-8548
800-572-7332
Fax: 562-795-6614
TTY: 562-493-4168
e-mail: modsigns@modernsignspress.com
www.modernsignspress.com

Pictures, signs and printed words tell the tale of April, a cuddly little rabbit who loves to play with her beloved Grandma.
28 pages

4571 Be Happy, Not Sad
Modern Signs Press
PO Box 1181
Los Alamitos, CA 90720
562-596-8548
800-572-7332
Fax: 562-795-6614
TTY: 562-493-4168
e-mail: modsigns@modernsignspress.com
www.modernsignspress.com

These books help children understand hard to explain emotions through signing. Includes Be Happy Not Sad coloring workbook.
2 Book Set

4572 Belonging
Gallaudet University
800 Florida Avenue, NE
Washington, DC 20002-3819
773-568-1550
800-621-2736
Fax: 800-621-8476
TTY: 888-630-9347
e-mail: gupress@gallaudet.edu
gupress.gallaudet.edu

Gustie Blaine loses her hearing after an illness and must now learn to accept her loss and understand the changes it brings.
176 pages
Virginia M. Scott, Author

4573 Chris Gets Ear Tubes
Gallaudet University
800 Florida Avenue, NE
Washington, DC 20002-3819
773-568-1550
800-621-2736
Fax: 800-621-8476
TTY: 888-630-9347
e-mail: gupress@gallaudet.edu
gupress.gallaudet.edu

A helpful book for parents and children to share concerning ear tubes and hospitals.
44 pages

4574 Clerc: The Story of His Early Years
Gallaudet University
800 Florida Avenue, NE
Washington, DC 20002-3819
773-568-1550
800-621-2736
Fax: 800-621-8476
TTY: 888-630-9347
e-mail: gupress@gallaudet.edu
gupress.gallaudet.edu

A novel by Laurent Clerc, a deaf teacher who helped Gallaudet establish schools to educate deaf Americans.
208 pages

4575 Come Sign with Us: Sign Language Activities for Children
Gallaudet University
800 Florida Avenue, NE
Washington, DC 20002-3819
773-568-1550
800-621-2736
Fax: 800-621-8476
TTY: 888-630-9347
e-mail: gupress@gallaudet.edu
gupress.gallaudet.edu

Revised version, offering more follow-up activities, including many in context, to teach children sign language. Features more than 300 line drawings of both adults and children signing familiar words, phrases, and sentences using ASL. Shows how to form each sign exactly and also presents the origins of ASL, facts about deafness, and the deaf community.
160 pages Softcover
ISBN: 1-563680-51-3
Jan C. Hafer, Co-Author
Robert M. Wilson, Co-Author

4576 Day We Met Cindy
Gallaudet University
800 Florida Avenue, NE
Washington, DC 20002-3819
773-568-1550
800-621-2736
Fax: 800-621-8476
TTY: 888-630-9347
e-mail: gupress@gallaudet.edu
gupress.gallaudet.edu

A picture storybook telling the story of Cindy, the hearing impaired aunt of one of the students of a first grade class.
32 pages
Anne Marie Starowitz, Author

4577 Finger Alphabet
Gallaudet University
800 Florida Avenue, NE
Washington, DC 20002-3819
773-568-1550
800-621-2736
Fax: 800-621-8476
TTY: 888-630-9347
e-mail: gupress@gallaudet.edu
gupress.gallaudet.edu

Includes activities for improving fingerspelling.
30 pages

4578 Flying Fingers Club
Gallaudet University
800 Florida Avenue, NE
Washington, DC 20002-3819
773-568-1550
800-621-2736
Fax: 800-621-8476
TTY: 888-630-9347
e-mail: gupress@gallaudet.edu
gupress.gallaudet.edu

Three young friends, one deaf and two hearing find they can communicate secretly in sign language.
104 pages

4579 Gift of the Girl Who Couldn't Hear
Alexander Graham Bell Association
3417 Volta Place NW
Washington, DC 20007-2737
202-337-5220
Fax: 202-337-8314
TTY: 202-337-5220
e-mail: info@agbell.org
www.listeningandspokenlanguage.org

This fictional novel for middle school readers introduces Eliza, a gifted singer and Lucy, her best friend who has been deaf since birth.
79 pages

4580 Goldilocks and the Three Bears
Gallaudet University
800 Florida Avenue, NE
Washington, DC 20002-3819
773-568-1550
800-621-2736
Fax: 800-621-8476
TTY: 888-630-9347
e-mail: gupress@gallaudet.edu
gupress.gallaudet.edu

Offers children ages 3-8 the classic story with new words and matching signs in Signed English.
48 pages Casebound
ISBN: 1-563680-57-2
Harry Bornstein, Co-Author
Karen L. Saulnier, Co-Author

4581 Grandfather Moose
Modern Signs Press

PO Box 1181
Los Alamitos, CA 90720-1181

562-596-8548
800-572-7332
Fax: 562-795-6614
TTY: 562-493-4168
e-mail: modsigns@modernsignspress.com
www.modernsignspress.com

Offers exciting and beautifully illustrated rhymes, games and chants in sign language.
32 pages

4582 Handful of Stories
Gallaudet University
800 Florida Avenue, NE
Washington, DC 20002-3819

773-568-1550
800-621-2736
Fax: 800-621-8476
TTY: 888-630-9347
e-mail: gupress@gallaudet.edu
gupress.gallaudet.edu

Sometimes incredible, moving and amusing, these stories are based on the personal experiences of deaf storytellers.
118 pages

4583 Handmade Alphabet
Gallaudet University
800 Florida Avenue, NE
Washington, DC 20002-3819

773-568-1550
800-621-2736
Fax: 800-621-8476
TTY: 888-630-9347
e-mail: gupress@gallaudet.edu
gupress.gallaudet.edu

This book presents 26 beautiful color drawings showing a hand forming a letter of the manual alphabet.
26 pages

4584 Hasta Luego, San Diego
Gallaudet University
800 Florida Avenue, NE
Washington, DC 20002-3819

773-568-1550
800-621-2736
Fax: 800-621-8476
TTY: 888-630-9347
e-mail: gupress@gallaudet.edu
gupress.gallaudet.edu

A Flying Fingers Club mystery.
104 pages
Jean F. Andrews, Author

4585 Hearing Loss
Franklin Watts Grolier
557 Broadway
New York, NY 10012-0001

203-797-3500
800-724-6527
Fax: 203-797-3197
www.grolier.com

Offers a concise explanation of how and why hearing losses occur, how the ear works and how to protect your hearing.
144 pages Grades 7-12
ISBN: 0-531125-19-0

4586 I Have a Sister, My Sister is Deaf
TJ Publishers
817 Silver Spring Avenue
Silver Spring, MD 20910-4617

301-585-4440
800-999-1168
Fax: 301-585-5930
TTY: 301-585-4441
e-mail: tjpubinc@aol.com

An emphatic, affirmative look at the relationship between siblings, as a young deaf child is affectionately described by her older sister. This Coretta Scott King honor award winner helps young children develop an understanding that deaf children share the same interests as hearing children.
1977 32 pages Softcover
ISBN: 0-064430-59-6
Angela K Thames, President
Jerald A Murphy, VP

4587 I Was So Mad!
Modern Signs Press

PO Box 1181
Los Alamitos, CA 90720-1181

562-596-8548
800-572-7332
Fax: 562-795-6614
TTY: 562-493-4168
e-mail: modsigns@modernsignspress.com
www.modernsignspress.com

Includes manual alphabet and glossary of signs.
40 pages
ISBN: 0-916708-16-0

4588 In Our House
Modern Signs Press
PO Box 1181
Los Alamitos, CA 90720-1181

562-596-8548
800-572-7332
Fax: 562-795-6614
TTY: 562-493-4168
e-mail: modsigns@modernsignspress.com
www.modernsignspress.com

This colorful picturebook tells the story of Joy and Jason helping Mom and Dad around the house. Has a 140-word vocabulary listed in an alphabetical glossary.
32 pages
ISBN: 0-191670-81-1

4589 Invisible Inc #4
Alexander Graham Bell Association
3417 Volta Place NW
Washington, DC 20007-2737

202-337-5220
Fax: 202-337-8314
TTY: 202-337-5220
e-mail: info@agbell.org
www.listeningandspokenlanguage.org

The intrepid trio accept an invitation to doom as they solve the mystery behind their school's haunted computer.
1996 42 pages

4590 King Midas With Selected Sentences in ASL
Gallaudet University
800 Florida Avenue, NE
Washington, DC 20002-3819

773-568-1550
800-621-2736
Fax: 800-621-8476
TTY: 888-630-9347
e-mail: gupress@gallaudet.edu
gupress.gallaudet.edu

Fairytale retold with full color illustrations and American Sign Language sentences.
72 pages Casebound
ISBN: 0-930323-75-0

4591 Learning to Sign in my Neighborhood
Gallaudet University
800 Florida Avenue, NE
Washington, DC 20002-3819

773-568-1550
800-621-2736
Fax: 800-621-8476
TTY: 888-630-9347
e-mail: gupress@gallaudet.edu
gupress.gallaudet.edu

Here are signs to learn and pictures to color, all in one friendly book.
32 pages

4592 Little Green Monsters
Modern Signs Press
PO Box 1181
Los Alamitos, CA 90720-1181

562-596-8548
800-572-7332
Fax: 562-795-6614
TTY: 310-493-4168
e-mail: modsigns@modernsignspress.com
www.modernsignspress.com

Forty-five word vocabulary in signs and printed words introduces concept of directionality. Includes manual alphabet and glossary of signs.
36 pages

4593 Little Red Riding Hood
Gallaudet University

800 Florida Avenue, NE
Washington, DC 20002-3819

773-568-1550
800-621-2736
Fax: 800-621-8476
TTY: 888-630-9347
e-mail: gupress@gallaudet.edu
gupress.gallaudet.edu

A beloved folktale that is told in American Sign Language format.
48 pages
Harry Bornstein, Co-Author
Karen L. Saulnier, Co-Author

4594   Living with Deafness
Franklin Watts Grolier
557 Broadway
New York, NY 10012-0001

203-797-3500
800-724-6527
Fax: 203-797-3197
www.grolier.com

Shows how deaf persons can overcome their disability and live happy, productive lives.
32 pages Grades 5-7
ISBN: 0-531108-42-2

4595   Mandy
Gallaudet University
800 Florida Avenue, NE
Washington, DC 20002-3819

773-568-1550
800-621-2736
Fax: 800-621-8476
TTY: 888-630-9347
e-mail: gupress@gallaudet.edu
gupress.gallaudet.edu

A beautiful story about a young deaf girl's relationship with her grandmother.
32 pages

4596   Matthew Pinkowski's Special Summer
Gallaudet University
800 Florida Avenue, NE
Washington, DC 20002-3819

773-568-1550
800-621-2736
Fax: 800-621-8476
TTY: 888-630-9347
e-mail: gupress@gallaudet.edu
gupress.gallaudet.edu

Matthew begins his special summer by moving to Minnesota, where he meets some special friends.
150 pages

4597   Messy Monsters, Jungle Joggers and Bubble Baths
Alexander Graham Bell Association
3417 Volta Place NW
Washington, DC 20007-2737

202-337-5220
Fax: 202-337-8314
TTY: 202-337-5220
e-mail: info@agbell.org
www.listeningandspokenlanguage.org

This child's work book is filled with poems, stories and delightful drawings that make speaking lip reading and using residual hearing fun for the elementary school aged child.
97 pages

4598   Mother Goose in Sign
Garlic Press
899 South College Mall Rd
Bloomington, IN 47401-5337

541-345-0063
800-789-0554
Fax: 800-789-5576
e-mail: orders@ipgbook.com
www.garlicpress.com

Fully illustrated Mother Goose nursery rhymes in sign language.
16 pages Paperback
ISBN: 0-931993-66-0
SH Collins, Contact

4599   My ABC Signs of Animal Friends
DawnSignPress
6130 Nancy Ridge Drive
San Diego, CA 92121-3223

619-625-0600
800-549-5350
Fax: 619-625-2336
e-mail: DawnSign@aol.com
www.dawnsign.com

Sign language primer for both hearing and deaf children from birth to age five.
32 pages
ISBN: 0-915035-31-6

4600   My First Book of Sign
Gallaudet University
800 Florida Avenue, NE
Washington, DC 20002-3819

773-568-1550
800-621-2736
Fax: 800-621-8476
TTY: 888-630-9347
e-mail: gupress@gallaudet.edu
gupress.gallaudet.edu

This book makes signing fun for children from three to eight.
76 pages

4601   My Signing Book of Numbers
Gallaudet University
800 Florida Avenue, NE
Washington, DC 20002-3819

773-568-1550
800-621-2736
Fax: 800-621-8476
TTY: 888-630-9347
e-mail: gupress@gallaudet.edu
gupress.gallaudet.edu

Picture book helps children learn their numbers in sign language.
56 pages

4602   Nick's Mission
Alexander Graham Bell Association
3417 Volta Place NW
Washington, DC 20007-2737

202-337-5220
Fax: 202-337-8314
TTY: 202-337-5220
e-mail: info@agbell.org
www.listeningandspokenlanguage.org

Twelve-year-old Nick plans to spend his summer vacation at the lake, snorkeling and playing with Wags, his dog, not at speech therapy as his mother has planned. But the summer will embroil Nick and Wags in an exciting mystery that includes kidnapping, smuggling, stolen macaws and maybe even speech therapy.
1996 148 pages

4603   Now I Understand
Gallaudet University
800 Florida Avenue, NE
Washington, DC 20002-3819

773-568-1550
800-621-2736
Fax: 800-621-8476
TTY: 888-630-9347
e-mail: gupress@gallaudet.edu
gupress.gallaudet.edu

Explores what happens when a hard-of-hearing boy is mainstreamed.
56 pages

4604   Number and Letter Games
Gallaudet University
800 Florida Avenue, NE
Washington, DC 20002-3819

773-568-1550
800-621-2736
Fax: 800-621-8476
TTY: 888-630-9347
e-mail: gupress@gallaudet.edu
gupress.gallaudet.edu

A fascinating way to learning sign language with games, riddles and map skills for children and adults.
30 pages

4605   Nursery Rhymes from Mother Goose
Gallaudet University
800 Florida Avenue, NE
Washington, DC 20002-3819

773-568-1550
800-621-2736
Fax: 800-621-8476
TTY: 888-630-9347
e-mail: gupress@gallaudet.edu
gupress.gallaudet.edu

The complete nursery rhyme is presented in Signed English.
64 pages

4606   Popsicles are Cold
Modern Signs Press

PO Box 1181
Los Alamitos, CA 90720-1181

562-596-8548
800-572-7332
Fax: 562-795-6614
TTY: 562-493-4168
e-mail: modsigns@modernsignspress.com
www.modernsignspress.com

Colorful pictures and rhyming words highlight this storybook with a 33-word vocabulary in signs and printed words.
32 pages

4607 **Season of Change**
Gallaudet University
800 Florida Avenue, NE
Washington, DC 20002-3819

773-568-1550
800-621-2736
Fax: 800-621-8476
TTY: 888-630-9347
e-mail: gupress@gallaudet.edu
gupress.gallaudet.edu

A cheerful teenager tired of having people treat her as a problem just because she does not hear very well.
108 pages
Lois L. Hodge, Author

4608 **Secret Signing: A Sign Language Activity Book**
Gallaudet University
800 Florida Avenue, NE
Washington, DC 20002-3819

773-568-1550
800-621-2736
Fax: 800-621-8476
TTY: 888-630-9347
e-mail: gupress@gallaudet.edu
gupress.gallaudet.edu

Children will enjoy this activity book with signs.
64 pages Level K-1

4609 **Secret in the Dorm Attic**
Gallaudet University
800 Florida Avenue, NE
Washington, DC 20002-3819

773-568-1550
800-621-2736
Fax: 800-621-8476
TTY: 888-630-9347
e-mail: gupress@gallaudet.edu
gupress.gallaudet.edu

Susan, Donald and Matt are back, as the Flying Fingers Club solving yet another mystery.
104 pages

4610 **Sesame Street Sign Language ABC**
Gallaudet University
800 Florida Avenue, NE
Washington, DC 20002-3819

773-568-1550
800-621-2736
Fax: 800-621-8476
TTY: 888-630-9347
e-mail: gupress@gallaudet.edu
gupress.gallaudet.edu

Muppets learn words and letters signed by Linda Bove.
30 pages

4611 **Sesame Street Sign Language Fun**
Gallaudet University
800 Florida Avenue, NE
Washington, DC 20002-3819

773-568-1550
800-621-2736
Fax: 800-621-8476
TTY: 888-630-9347
e-mail: gupress@gallaudet.edu
gupress.gallaudet.edu

This book uses the Muppets to explain concepts such as opposites, words and feelings.
62 pages

4612 **Sign Numbers**
Modern Signs Press
PO Box 1181
Los Alamitos, CA 90720-1181

562-596-8548
800-572-7332
Fax: 562-795-6614
TTY: 562-493-4168
e-mail: modsigns@modernsignspress.com
www.modernsignspress.com

A manual teaching sign language and written numbers that includes printed numbers and easy-to-follow drawings of the number hand shapes.
60 pages

4613 **Sign-Me-Fine**
Gallaudet University
800 Florida Avenue, NE
Washington, DC 20002-3819

773-568-1550
800-621-2736
Fax: 800-621-8476
TTY: 888-630-9347
e-mail: gupress@gallaudet.edu
gupress.gallaudet.edu

Written for young adults, this book introduces American Sign Language and how it differs from English.
120 pages
Laura Greene, Co-Author
Eva Barash Dicker, Co-Author

4614 **Signed Language Coloring Books**
Gallaudet University
800 Florida Avenue, NE
Washington, DC 20002-3819

773-568-1550
800-621-2736
Fax: 800-621-8476
TTY: 888-630-9347
e-mail: gupress@gallaudet.edu
gupress.gallaudet.edu

Six coloring books made up of easy-to-color pictures that include the printed, signed and fingerspelled words for each image.
16 pages

4615 **Signing for Kids**
Gallaudet University
800 Florida Avenue, NE
Washington, DC 20002-3819

773-568-1550
800-621-2736
Fax: 800-621-8476
TTY: 888-630-9347
e-mail: gupress@gallaudet.edu
gupress.gallaudet.edu

Contains 17 chapters dealing with special areas of interest to children like pets, family, friends and people.
142 pages

4616 **Signs for Me: Basic Vocabulary for Children, Parents and Teachers**
DawnSignPress
6130 Nancy Ridge Drive
San Diego, CA 92121-3223

619-625-0600
800-549-5350
Fax: 619-625-2336
e-mail: DawnSign@aol.com
www.dawnsign.com

ASL/English vocabulary primer filled with all the basics for preschoolers. The focus is on learning ASL signs and English words for better language development. Illustrates the meaning of the sign, the sign itself, and the English word in bold print.
112 pages
ISBN: 0-915035-27-8

4617 **Silent Dances**
Gallaudet University
800 Florida Avenue, NE
Washington, DC 20002-3819

773-568-1550
800-621-2736
Fax: 800-621-8476
TTY: 888-630-9347
e-mail: gupress@gallaudet.edu
gupress.gallaudet.edu

Space adventure story featuring a deaf graduate of Gallaudet University.
275 pages

4618 **Silent Garden: Raising Your Deaf Child**
Alexander Graham Bell Association
3417 Volta Place NW
Washington, DC 20007-2737

202-337-5220
Fax: 202-337-8314
TTY: 202-337-5220
e-mail: info@agbell.org
www.listeningandspokenlanguage.org

This book provides parents of deaf children with crucial information on the possibilities afforded their children. Ogden, deaf since birth and a professor of deaf studies offers parents the foundation

for making the difficult decisions necessary to start their children on the road to realizing their full potential.
1996 313 pages

4619 Silent Observer
Gallaudet University
800 Florida Avenue, NE
Washington, DC 20002-3819
773-568-1550
800-621-2736
Fax: 800-621-8476
TTY: 888-630-9347
e-mail: gupress@gallaudet.edu
gupress.gallaudet.edu

Lovely illustrations tell the story of an affectionate memoir of childhood presented through the eyes of a deaf girl.
48 pages
Christy MacKinnon, Writer and Illustrator

4620 Simple Signs
Gallaudet University
800 Florida Avenue, NE
Washington, DC 20002-3819
773-568-1550
800-621-2736
Fax: 800-621-8476
TTY: 888-630-9347
e-mail: gupress@gallaudet.edu
gupress.gallaudet.edu

Charming, full-color pictures and hints introducing ASL to children.
32 pages

4621 Sleeping Beauty
Gallaudet University
800 Florida Avenue, NE
Washington, DC 20002-3819
773-568-1550
800-621-2736
Fax: 800-621-8476
TTY: 888-630-9347
e-mail: gupress@gallaudet.edu
gupress.gallaudet.edu

Classic story with full-color illustrations and line drawings of more than 30 sentences rendered in ASL, offering new dimensions of imagination while also strengthening young readers' language skills.
64 pages
ISBN: 0-930323-97-1

4622 Songs in Sign
Gallaudet University
800 Florida Avenue, NE
Washington, DC 20002-3819
773-568-1550
800-621-2736
Fax: 800-621-8476
TTY: 888-630-9347
e-mail: gupress@gallaudet.edu
gupress.gallaudet.edu

Fully illustrated sign English.
30 pages

4623 Very Special Sister
Gallaudet University
800 Florida Avenue, NE
Washington, DC 20002-3819
773-568-1550
800-621-2736
Fax: 800-621-8476
TTY: 888-630-9347
e-mail: gupress@gallaudet.edu
gupress.gallaudet.edu

Tells the story of Laura who is deaf and her delight at the fact that she will soon have a brother.
36 pages
Dorothy Hoffman Levi, Author

4624 Where Is Spot?
Gallaudet University
800 Florida Avenue, NE
Washington, DC 20002-3819
773-568-1550
800-621-2736
Fax: 800-621-8476
TTY: 888-630-9347
e-mail: gupress@gallaudet.edu
gupress.gallaudet.edu

A Signed English edition of a childhood favorite.
20 pages

4625 Word Signs: A First Book of Sign Language
Gallaudet University
800 Florida Avenue, NE
Washington, DC 20002-3819
773-568-1550
800-621-2736
Fax: 800-621-8476
TTY: 888-630-9347
e-mail: gupress@gallaudet.edu
gupress.gallaudet.edu

Full-color photos of basic words and their signs.
16 pages Ages 1-4
Debbie Slier, Author

Magazines

4626 American Annals of the Deaf
Convention of American Instructors of the Deaf
800 Florida Avenue NE
Washington, DC 20002-3660
773-568-1550
800-621-2736
Fax: 800-621-8476
TTY: 888-630-9347
e-mail: gupress@gallaudet.edu
gupress.gallaudet.edu

Scholarly journal at the forefront of research related to the education of deaf people. Annual reference Issue identifies programs and services for deaf people nationwide.
64 pages 5x Year
Donald Moores, Editor
Mary E Carew, Managing Editor

4627 American Journal of Audiology
American Speech-Language-Hearing Association
2200 Research Boulevard
Rockville, MD 20850-3226
301-897-5700
800-498-2071
e-mail: actioncenter@asha.org
www.asha.org

AJA is a twice-yearly journal of clinical practice for audiologists and hearing researchers.
Russell L Malone PhD, Editor

4628 American Journal of Speech-Language Pathology
American Speech-Language-Hearing Association
10801 Rockville Pike
Rockville, MD 20852-3226
301-897-5700
800-638-8255
Fax: 301-296-8580
TTY: 301-296-5650
ajslp.pubs.asha.org

AJSLP reports peer-reviewed, primary research findings (basic and applied) concerning an array of clinically oriented topics transcending all aspects of clinical practice in speech-language pathology.
Russell L Malone PhD, Editor

4629 Audiology Today
11480 Commerce Park Drive
Reston, VA 20191-2019
703-790-8466
800-222-2336
Fax: 703-476-5157
e-mail: infoaud@audiology.org
www.audiology.org

AT is the American Academy of Audiology's award-winning magazine of, by, and for audiologists.
David Fabry, PhD, Content Editor
Amy Miedema, CAE, Executive Editor

4630 Auricle
Auditory-Verbal International
2121 Eisenhower Avenue
Alexandria, VA 22314-4688
703-739-1049
Fax: 703-739-0395
TTY: 703-739-0874
e-mail: audiverb@aol.com
www.auditory-verbal.org

To provide the choice of listening and speaking as the way of life for children and adults who are deaf on hard of hearing.
Magazine
Sara Lake, Executive Director/CEO/Publisher
Mary Benson, Executive Assistant

4631 Deaf Life
MSM Productions

1095 Meigs Street
Rochester, NY 14620-3380
716-442-6370
Fax: 585-442-6371
www.deaflife.com

This magazine focuses on profiles, news, controversial issues, cultural topics and more relating to the Deaf community.
50 pages Monthly
Matthew Moore, Publisher

4632 Deaf Sports Review
American Athletic Association of the Deaf
PO Box 910338
Lexington, KY 40591-1737
801-393-8710
Fax: 801-393-2263
TTY: 801-393-7916
e-mail: HomeOffice@usdeafsports.org
www.usdeafsports.org

A magazine that describes deaf athletes and past and upcoming events.
Quarterly
Shirley Platt, Editor

4633 Deaf USA
Eye Festival Communications
6917B Woodley Avenue
Van Nuys, CA 91406-4844
818-902-9800
Fax: 818-902-9840

Provides news coverage on all activities and issues of interest to deaf and hard of hearing readers as well as professionals and associates within this specialized market.
Monthly
David Rosenbaum, Editor

4634 Deaf-Blind American
American Association of the Deaf-Blind
PO Box 8064
Silver Spring, MD 20907-4500
301-563-9064
800-735-2258
Fax: 301-588-8705
TTY: 301-588-6545
e-mail: aadb-info@aadb.org
www.aadb.org

A journal of the American Association of the Deaf-Blind with articles on new technology, legislation news affecting deaf-blind Americans, success stories on deaf-blind, conference news, and many other topics of interest to deaf-blind people.
4x Year
Jamie McNamara, Editor

4635 Hearing Health
363 Seventh Avenue
New York, NY 10001
212-257-6140
866-454-3924
e-mail: info@hhf.org
hearinghealthfoundation.org

A publication for deaf and hard-of-hearing people, as well as hearing health care professionals, libraries, agencies, schools and organizations.
BiMonthly
Paula Bartone-Bonillas, Editor

4636 Journal of AAA
American Academy of Audiology
1735 N Lynn Street
Arlington, VA 22209-2019
703-524-1923
800-222-2336
Fax: 703-524-2303

James Jerger, Editor

4637 Journal of Speech-Language-Hearing Research
American Speech-Language-Hearing Association
10801 Rockville Pike
Rockville, MD 20852-3226
301-897-5700
800-638-8255
Fax: 301-296-8580
TTY: 301-296-5650
ajslp.pubs.asha.org

The bimonthly Journal of Speech, Language, and Hearing Research (JSHLR)-an online-only, international, peer-reviewed scholarly journal-has been published continuously since 1936.
Russell L Malone PhD, Editor

4638 Language, Speech and Hearing Services in the Schools
American Speech-Language-Hearing Association

10801 Rockville Pike
Rockville, MD 20852
301-897-5700
800-638-8255
Fax: 301-296-8580
TTY: 301-296-5650
ajslp.pubs.asha.org

Professional journal for clinicians, audiologists and speech-language pathologists.

Russell L Malone PhD, Editor

4639 NADmag
National Association of the Deaf
8630 Fenton Street
Silver Spring, MD 20910
301-587-1788
Fax: 301-587-1791
TTY: 301-587-1789
e-mail: nad.info@nad.org
nad.org

Each NADmag focuses on a specific theme, such as technology and telecommunications, human services, deaf culture, education, and interpreting.
32 pages Bi-Monthly
Christopher Wagner, President
Melissa S. Draganac-Hawk, Vice-President

4640 Perspectives in Education and Deafness
Gallaudet University
800 Florida Avenue, NE
Washington, DC 20002-3819
773-568-1550
800-621-2736
Fax: 800-621-8476
TTY: 888-630-9347
e-mail: gupress@gallaudet.edu
gupress.gallaudet.edu

A practical, reader-friendly magazine, offering help and advice in and beyond the classroom, tuned to the needs of today's students, teachers, and families.
5x Annually
Mary Abrams Perica, Editor

4641 SHHH Journal
Self Help For Hard of Hearing People
7910 Woodmont Avenue
Bethesda, MD 20814-3079
301-657-2248
Fax: 301-913-9413
TTY: 301-657-2249
www.hearingloss.org

An educational journal about hearing loss for hard-of-hearing people.
BiMonthly
Barbara G Harris, Editor

4642 Silent News
1425 Jefferson Road
Rochester, NY 14623-3139
716-272-4900
Fax: 716-272-4904
TTY: 716-272-4900

Covers news and events of interest to deaf and hard-of-hearing people all over the world.
Monthly
Tom Willard, Editor

4643 Silent News Job Bulletin
1425 Jefferson Road
Rochester, NY 14623-3139
716-272-4900
Fax: 716-272-4904
TTY: 716-272-4900

Lists current job openings and career opportunities working with deaf and hard-of-hearing people.
BiAnnually

4644 Tinnitus Today
American Tinnitus Association
PO Box 5
Portland, OR 97207-0005
503-248-9985
800-634-8978
Fax: 503-248-0024
e-mail: tinnitus@ata.org
www.ata.org

A quarterly magazine published by the American Tinnitus Association.
28 pages Quarterly
ISBN: 1-530656-9 -
Cara James, Executive Director
Paul Morris, Development Director

4645   USA Deaf Sports Federation
3607 Washington Boulevard
Ogden, UT 84403-1737

801-393-8710
Fax: 801-393-2263
TTY: 801-393-7916
e-mail: homeoffice@usadsf.org
www.usadsf.org

A glossy magazine called Deaf Sports Review featuring articles on all deaf sports and recreation.
Dr. Bobbie Beth Scoggins, President
Valerie Kinney, Administrative Assistant

4646   Volta Review
Alexander Graham Bell Association
3417 Volta Place NW
Washington, DC 20007-2737

202-337-5220
Fax: 202-337-8314
TTY: 202-337-5220
e-mail: info@agbell.org
www.listeningandspokenlanguage.org

A professionally reviewed journal highlighting research and studies in the field of deafness.
5x Year
Michelle Vanderhoff, Managing Editor

4647   Volta Voices
Alexander Graham Bell Association
3417 Volta Place NW
Washington, DC 20007-2737

202-337-5220
Fax: 202-337-8314
TTY: 202-337-5220
e-mail: info@agbell.org
www.listeningandspokenlanguage.org

A magazine highlighting inspirational stories from parents of children who are deaf, legislative news, technology update and stories pertaining to speech, speech reading, and the use of residual hearing.
BiMonthly
Michelle Vanderhoff, Managing Editor

4648   World Around You
Gallaudet University
800 Florida Avenue, NE
Washington, DC 20002-3819

773-568-1550
800-621-2736
Fax: 800-621-8476
TTY: 888-630-9347
e-mail: gupress@gallaudet.edu
gupress.gallaudet.edu

A current events magazine directed at keeping junior high and high school deaf and hard-of-hearing students informed about deaf people and the deaf community.
5x Year
Cathryn Carroll, Editor

Newsletters

4649   AAAD Bulletin
American Athletic Association of the Deaf
3607 Washington Boulevard
Ogden, UT 84403-1737

801-393-8710
Fax: 801-393-2263
TTY: 801-393-7916

A newsletter describing deaf athletes and upcoming events.
Quarterly
Shirley Platt, Editor

4650   ADARA Updated
ADARA
PO Box 251554
Little Rock, AR 72225-1554

501-868-8850
Fax: 501-868-8812

Updates readers on events, resources, legislation, information of national interest, conferences, workshops and employment opportunities. Information from and about local chapters, special interest sections, and national organizations is included in this publication.
Quarterly
Nanncy Long PhD, Editor

4651   ALDA News
Association of Late-Deafened Adults

8038 Macintosh Lane
Rockford, IL 61107

815-332-1515
Fax: 877-907-1738
TTY: 815-332-1515
e-mail: info@alda.org
www.alda.org

Marilyn Howe, Publisher

4652   Adult Bible Lessons for the Deaf
Sunday School Board of the Southern Baptists
127 9th Avenue N
Nashville, TN 37234-0001

800-458-2772

Bible study quarterly that relates to the needs of deaf and hearing impaired persons.
Quarterly

4653   Audiology Express
American Academy of Audiology
1735 N Lynn Street
Arlington, VA 22209-2019

703-524-1923
800-222-2336
Fax: 703-524-2303

4654   Better Hearing News
Better Hearing Institute
5021B Backlick Road
Annandale, VA 22003-6043

703-642-0580
800-327-9355
Fax: 703-750-9302

Quarterly
Jerry J Rizzo, Executive Director

4655   Canine Listener
Dogs for the Deaf
10175 Wheeler Road
Central Point, OR 97502

541-826-9220
800-990-3647
Fax: 541-826-6696
TTY: 541-826-9220
TDD: 541-826-9220
e-mail: info@dogsforthedeaf.org
www.dogsforthedeaf.org

Offers information on various dogs for the deaf that are available, hotlines, support groups and articles on the newest technology for the hard of hearing person.
Quarterly
Robin Dickson, President/CEO

4656   Caption Center News
Caption Center
125 Western Avenue
Boston, MA 02134-1008

617-429-9225
Fax: 617-562-0590

Reports developments in closed captioning for persons with hearing impairments.

4657   Deaf Artists of America
302 Goodman Street N
Rochester, NY 14607-1148

716-244-3460
Fax: 716-244-3690
TTY: 716-244-3460

Tom Willard, Editor

4658   Deaf Episcopalian
Episcopal Conference of the Deaf
PO Box 27459
Philadelphia, PA 19118-0459

215-247-1059
e-mail: Bmose@aol.com
www.ecdeaf.org

Preston H. Colangelo Dn., Contact

4659   Deaf Work
Baptist Sunday School Board
127 9th Avenue N
Nashville, TN 37234-0002

615-251-2000

Offers information for religious workers and church educators who teach the handicapped.

4660   Deafpride Advocate
Deafpride
1350 Potomac Avenue SE
Washington, DC 20003-4412

202-675-6700

4661   Endeavor
American Society for Deaf Children

800 Florida Avenue, NE
Washington, DC 20002-1373

717-334-7922
800-942-2732
Fax: 410-795-0965
TTY: 717-334-7922
e-mail: asdc1@aol.com
www.deafchildren.org

Newsletter for parents of deaf children.
36 pages Quarterly
Tami Hossler, Editor

4662 Frat
National Fraternal Society of the Deaf
1300 W NW Highway
Mt Prospect, IL 60056-2217

847-392-9282
Fax: 847-392-9298
TTY: 708-392-1409

Offers fraternal insurance information and news about members.
BiMonthly
Wayne D Shook, Editor

4663 GA-SK Newsletter
Telecommunications for the Deaf
8630 Fenton Street
Silver Spring, MD 20910-3822

301-589-3786
Fax: 301-589-3797
TTY: 301-589-3006

A newsletter focusing on issues for the deaf and hearing impaired person.
Quarterly
Barry Solomon, Editor
Alfred Sonnenstrahl, Manager

4664 Gallaudet Today
Galladet University
800 Florida Avenue, NE
Washington, DC 20002

202-651-5000
Fax: 212-599-0039
e-mail: president@gallaudet.edu
www.gallaudet.edu

A university publication with both general and special issues on deafness-related topics.
Quarterly
Vickie Walter, Editor

4665 Hear
Deafness Research Foundation
15 W 39th Street
New York, NY 10018-3806

212-768-1181

Offers information on the Foundation's activities and events, technical updates on assistive devices, legislative and medical information on the latest breakthroughs and laws for the hearing impaired, book reviews and resources.
Monte H Jacoby, Executive Director

4666 NTID Focus
National Technical Institute for the Deaf
52 Lomb Memorial Drive
Rochester, NY 14623-5604

716-475-6906
Fax: 716-475-5623
TTY: 716-475-6906
e-mail: ntidmc@rit.edu
www.rit.edu/ntid

A college publication featuring news and stories about NTID programs and community members.
TriAnnual
Kathryn Shwartz, Editor

4667 Newsletter of American Hearing Research
American Hearing Research Foundation
275 N. York Street
Elmhurst, IL 60126-4539

630-617-5079
Fax: 630-563-9181
e-mail: blederer@american-hearing.org
www.american-hearing.org

Concerned with hearing research and education.
6-8 pages 3 per year
William L Lederer, Executive Director
Sharon Parmet, Development/Communications Associate

4668 Newsline
Sertoma Foundation
1912 E Meyer Boulevard
Kansas City, MO 64132-1141

816-333-8300
Fax: 816-333-4320
e-mail: infosertoma@sertomahq.org
www.sertoma.org

Reports on activities of the Sertoma Foundation in the field of speech and hearing impairments.

4669 Otoscope
EAR Foundation
1817 Patterson Street
Nashville, TN 37203

615-329-7807
800-545-4327
Fax: 615-329-7935
TTY: 615-329-7849
e-mail: ear@earfoundation.org
www.earfoundation.org

8-14 pages Quarterly
Amy Nielsen, Director Educational Programs

4670 Research at Gallaudet
Gallaudet University
800 Florida Avenue, NE
Washington, DC 20002-3819

773-568-1550
800-621-2736
Fax: 800-621-8476
TTY: 888-630-9347
e-mail: gupress@gallaudet.edu
gupress.gallaudet.edu

Newsletter reporting research and activities of the Institute.

4671 Speech and Deafness Newsletter
Hearing, Speech
1620 18th Avenue
Seattle, WA 98122-2798

206-323-5770

Agency newsletter for membership and community.
8 pages
Patty Tumberg, Editor

4672 Tech Talk
Caption Center
125 Western Avenue
Boston, MA 02134-1008

617-492-9225
Fax: 617-562-0590

4673 USA Deaf Sports Federation
PO Box 910338
Lexington, KY 40591-1737

801-393-8710
Fax: 801-393-2263
TTY: 801-393-7916
e-mail: HomeOffice@usdeafsports.org
www.usdeafsports.org

A matte newsletter called USADSF Bulletin featuring articles on all deaf sports and recreation.
Jack C. Lamberton?, President
Jeffrey L.? Salit, Vice President

Pamphlets

4674 25 Ways to Promote Spoken Language in Your Child with a Hearing Loss
Alexander Graham Bell Association
3417 Volta Place NW
Washington, DC 20007-2737

202-337-5220
Fax: 202-337-8314
TTY: 202-337-5220
e-mail: info@agbell.org
www.listeningandspokenlanguage.org

This pamphlet teaches twenty-five golden rules about preparing your child to listen and to speak.
1995 62 pages

4675 Aging and Hearing Loss: Some Commonly Asked Questions
National Information Center on Deafness
800 Florida Avenue NE
Washington, DC 20002-3660

773-568-1550
800-621-2736
Fax: 800-621-8476
TTY: 888-630-9347
e-mail: gupress@gallaudet.edu
gupress.gallaudet.edu

Discusses the hearing evaulation, tests used to determine type and extent of hearing loss and what an audiogram tells us.

4676 Alerting and Communication Devices for Deaf and Hard of Hearing People
National Information Center on Deafness

800 Florida Avenue NE
Washington, DC 20002

773-568-1550
800-621-2736
Fax: 800-621-8476
TTY: 888-630-9347
e-mail: gupress@gallaudet.edu
gupress.gallaudet.edu

Describes general communication in everyday life.
Loraine DiPietro, M.A., Co-Author
Pettyt Williams, Ph.D., Co-Author

4677 Alexander Graham Bell's Life
Alexander Graham Bell Association
3417 Volta Place NW
Washington, DC 20007-2737

202-337-5220
Fax: 202-337-8314
TTY: 202-337-5220
e-mail: info@agbell.org
www.listeningandspokenlanguage.org

This pamphlet highlights Alexander Gram Bell's professional and personal involvement with deafness as a teacher of the deaf; a friend of many notable persons, including Helen Keller; a scientist interested in acoustics; the inventor of the telephone; and the founder of the Bell Association.
1996

4678 All About the New Generation of Hearing Aids
National Information Center on Deafness
800 Florida Avenue NE
Washington, DC 20002-3660

773-568-1550
800-621-2736
Fax: 800-621-8476
TTY: 888-630-9347
e-mail: gupress@gallaudet.edu
gupress.gallaudet.edu

Explains the terms digital hearing aid, and digitally controlled hearing aid.

4679 Assistive Devices Demonstration Centers
National Information Center on Deafness
800 Florida Avenue NE
Washington, DC 20002-3660

773-568-1550
800-621-2736
Fax: 800-621-8476
TTY: 888-630-9347
e-mail: gupress@gallaudet.edu
gupress.gallaudet.edu

A resource list identifying demonstration centers across the United States.

4680 Books for Parents of Deaf and Hard of Hearing Children
National Information Center on Deafness
800 Florida Avenue NE
Washington, DC 20002

773-568-1550
800-621-2736
Fax: 800-621-8476
TTY: 888-630-9347
e-mail: gupress@gallaudet.edu
gupress.gallaudet.edu

Identifies books written for parents and everday experiences of deaf and hard of hearing children.

4681 Care of the Ears and Hearing for Health
American Hearing Research Foundation
275 N. York Street
Elmhurst, IL 60126-4539

630-617-5079
Fax: 630-563-9181
e-mail: blederer@american-hearing.org
www.american-hearing.org

Offers information on ear infections relating to chronic progressive deafness.
William L Lederer, Executive Director
Sharon Parmet, Development/Communications Associate

4682 Consumer's Guide to Hearing Aids
Hearing Loss Association of America
7910 Woodmont Avenue
Bethesda, MD 20814-3079

301-657-2248
Fax: 301-913-9413
TTY: 301-657-2249
e-mail: info@hearingloss.org
www.hearingloss.org

Color booklet illustrating the different styles of hearing aids and comparing different models and features. Illustrates the technology pyramid and hearing aid pricing.
2006 24 pages
Anna Gilmore Hall, Executive Director
Lise Hamlin, Director of Public Policy

4683 Deaf Culture Videotapes
National Information Center on Deafness
800 Florida Avenue NE
Washington, DC 20002-3660

773-568-1550
800-621-2736
Fax: 800-621-8476
TTY: 888-630-9347
e-mail: gupress@gallaudet.edu
gupress.gallaudet.edu

This list identifies deaf culture and deaf history videotapes available from the Historic Film Collection of the National Association of the Deaf.

4684 Deaf Culture: Suggested Readings
National Information Center on Deafness
800 Florida Avenue NE
Washington, DC 20002-3660

773-568-1550
800-621-2736
Fax: 800-621-8476
TTY: 888-630-9347
e-mail: gupress@gallaudet.edu
gupress.gallaudet.edu

A selected reading list providing annotations for 62 books highlighting the community, and history of deaf people.

4685 Deafness: A Fact Sheet
National Information Center on Deafness
800 Florida Avenue NE
Washington, DC 20002-3660

773-568-1550
800-621-2736
Fax: 800-621-8476
TTY: 888-630-9347
e-mail: gupress@gallaudet.edu
gupress.gallaudet.edu

4686 Developing Cognition in Young Children Who are Deaf
Hope
343 A Erickson Hall
East Lansing, MI 48824-4648

435-752-9533
Fax: 435-752-9533
e-mail: catalyst@kent.edu
www.deafed.net

Presents interesting, updated information on the importance of early cognition development in young children who are deaf. Contains many ideas for ways to promote early thinking skills, especially those that promote and enhance early communication and language development.

4687 Ear and Hearing
National Information Center on Deafness
800 Florida Avenue NE
Washington, DC 20002-3660

773-568-1550
800-621-2736
Fax: 800-621-8476
TTY: 888-630-9347
e-mail: gupress@gallaudet.edu
gupress.gallaudet.edu

An illustrated publication of the ear and what can go wrong with it.

4688 Educating Deaf Children: An Introduction
National Information Center on Deafness
800 Florida Avenue NE
Washington, DC 20002-3660

773-568-1550
800-621-2736
Fax: 800-621-8476
TTY: 888-630-9347
e-mail: gupress@gallaudet.edu
gupress.gallaudet.edu

Describes the different settings in which deaf children are currently educated.

4689 Facts About Hearing Aids
Alexander Graham Bell Association
3417 Volta Place NW
Washington, DC 20007-2737

202-337-5220
Fax: 202-337-8314
TTY: 202-337-5220
e-mail: info@agbell.org
www.listeningandspokenlanguage.org

This brochure describes defferent types of hearing aids, factors to consider when choosing a hearing aid, the best way to go about purchasing a hearing aid. It also addresses cost and provides information on hearing conservation.

4690   Facts and Fancies About Hearing Aids
American Hearing Research Foundation
275 N. York Street
Elmhurst, IL 60126-4539
630-617-5079
Fax: 630-563-9181
e-mail: blederer@american-hearing.org
www.american-hearing.org
Offers information on types of hearing aids and hearing aid evaluations.
William L Lederer, Executive Director
Sharon Parmet, Development/Communications Associate

4691   Genetics and Deafness
National Information Center on Deafness
800 Florida Avenue NE
Washington, DC 20002-3660
773-568-1550
800-621-2736
Fax: 800-621-8476
TTY: 888-630-9347
e-mail: gupress@gallaudet.edu
gupress.gallaudet.edu
Written for deaf people and their families who wish to learn more about the relationship between heredity and deafness.

4692   Hearing Loss: Information for Professionals in the Aging Network
National Information Center on Deafness
800 Florida Avenue NE
Washington, DC 20002-3660
773-568-1550
800-621-2736
Fax: 800-621-8476
TTY: 888-630-9347
e-mail: gupress@gallaudet.edu
gupress.gallaudet.edu
Introduces professionals in the aging network to the realities of hearing loss.

4693   How Does Your Child Hear and Talk?
American Speech-Language-Hearing Association
2200 Research Boulevard
Rockville, MD 20850-3226
301-296-5700
800-638-8255
Fax: 301-296-8580
TTY: 301-296-5650
e-mail: nsslha@asha.org
www.asha.org
Offers a chart to parents on children's growth pertaining to their hearing and speech.

4694   Late-Deafened Adults: A Selected Annotated Bibliography
National Information Center on Deafness
800 Florida Avenue NE
Washington, DC 20002-3660
773-568-1550
800-621-2736
Fax: 800-621-8476
TTY: 888-630-9347
e-mail: gupress@gallaudet.edu
gupress.gallaudet.edu
A selected reading list of books and articles for late-deafened people and their families.

4695   Leading National Publications of and for Deaf People
National Information Center on Deafness
800 Florida Avenue NE
Washington, DC 20002
773-568-1550
800-621-2736
Fax: 800-621-8476
TTY: 888-630-9347
e-mail: gupress@gallaudet.edu
gupress.gallaudet.edu
Identifies publications with national circulations to deaf audiences.

4696   Making New Friends
National Information Center on Deafness
800 Florida Avenue NE
Washington, DC 20002-3660
773-568-1550
800-621-2736
Fax: 800-621-8476
TTY: 888-630-9347
e-mail: gupress@gallaudet.edu
gupress.gallaudet.edu
Identifies resources that offer opportunities for deaf people.

4697   Meniere's Disease: Hearing Loss & Inner Ear Blood Flow
Self Help for Hard of H
7910 Woodmont Avenue
Bethesda, MD 20814-3079
301-657-2248
Fax: 301-913-9413
TTY: 301-657-2249
e-mail: national@shhh.org
www.hearingloss.org
Includes a personal narrative.

4698   National Information Center on Deafness Brochure
National Information Center on Deafness
800 Florida Avenue NE
Washington, DC 20002
773-568-1550
800-621-2736
Fax: 800-621-8476
TTY: 888-630-9347
e-mail: gupress@gallaudet.edu
gupress.gallaudet.edu
A description of services offered by NICD.

4699   Noise Can Be Harmful to Your Health
Deafness Research Foundation
15 W 39th Street
New York, NY 10018-3806
212-768-1181
Offers information, including a chart of noise levels, low to harmful, and the effects these noise levels have on your hearing.

4700   Otitis Media
Deafness Research Foundation
15 W 39th Street
New York, NY 10018-3806
212-768-1181
Offers information on Otitis Media, prevention, causes, treatments and symptoms.

4701   Perspectives Folio: Parent-Child
Gallaudet University
800 Florida Avenue, NE
Washington, DC 20002-3819
773-568-1550
800-621-2736
Fax: 800-621-8476
TTY: 888-630-9347
e-mail: gupress@gallaudet.edu
gupress.gallaudet.edu
Seven articles emphasizing family communication while providing important information for parents about deafness and the deaf culture.
29 pages

4702   Publications from the National Information Center on Deafness
National Information Center on Deafness
800 Florida Avenue NE
Washington, DC 20002-3660
773-568-1550
800-621-2736
Fax: 800-621-8476
TTY: 888-630-9347
e-mail: gupress@gallaudet.edu
gupress.gallaudet.edu
Order form and explanations of NICD publications.

4703   Questions and Answers About Employment of Deaf People
National Information Center on Deafness
800 Florida Avenue NE
Washington, DC 20002-3660
773-568-1550
800-621-2736
Fax: 800-621-8476
TTY: 888-630-9347
e-mail: gupress@gallaudet.edu
gupress.gallaudet.edu

4704   Questions and Answers on Hearing Loss
Self Help for Hard of H
7910 Woodmont Avenue
Bethesda, MD 20814-3079
301-657-2248
Fax: 301-913-9413
TTY: 301-657-2249
e-mail: national@shhh.org
www.hearingloss.org

4705   So You Have Had an Ear Operation...What Next?
American Hearing Research Foundation
275 N. York Street
Elmhurst, IL 60126-4539
630-617-5079
Fax: 630-563-9181
e-mail: blederer@american-hearing.org
www.american-hearing.org

Offers information on ear infections and surgery.
William L Lederer, Executive Director
Sharon Parmet, Development/Communications Associate

4706 Statewide Services for Deaf and Hard of Hearing People
National Information Center on Deafness
800 Florida Avenue NE
Washington, DC 20002

773-568-1550
800-621-2736
Fax: 800-621-8476
TTY: 888-630-9347
e-mail: gupress@gallaudet.edu
gupress.gallaudet.edu

A resource list of states that have established commissions and other offices to serve deaf people.

4707 Travel Resources for Deaf and Hard of Hearing People
National Information Center on Deafness
800 Florida Avenue NE
Washington, DC 20002

773-568-1550
800-621-2736
Fax: 800-621-8476
TTY: 888-630-9347
e-mail: gupress@gallaudet.edu
gupress.gallaudet.edu

A publication list of travel industry resources for deaf and hard of hearing people.

4708 What are TTY's? TDDs? TTs?
National Information Center on Deafness
800 Florida Avenue NE
Washington, DC 20002-3660

773-568-1550
800-621-2736
Fax: 800-621-8476
TTY: 888-630-9347
e-mail: gupress@gallaudet.edu
gupress.gallaudet.edu

Discusses text telephones used by deaf people.

4709 World of Sound
International Hearing Society
16880 Middlebelt Road
Livonia, MI 48154-3367

313-478-2610
Fax: 313-478-4520

The purpose of this booklet is to provide basic information for those with questions about hearing loss, hearing aids and Hearing Instrument Specialists.

4710 You Don't Have to Hate Meetings: Try Computer-Assisted Notetaking Instead
Self Help for Hard of H
7910 Woodmont Avenue
Bethesda, MD 20814-3079

301-657-2248
Fax: 301-913-9413
TTY: 301-657-2249
e-mail: national@shhh.org
www.hearingloss.org

Audio & Video

4711 ASL Poetry: Selected Works of Clayton Valli
DawnSignPress
6130 Nancy Ridge Drive
San Diego, CA 92121-3223

858-625-0600
800-549-5350
Fax: 858-625-2336
TTY: 858-625-0600
e-mail: comments@dawnsign.com
www.dawnsign.com

Twenty one original Valli poems recited by a diversity of native signers. Guided experience through the richness of poetry in another language.
105 minutes
ISBN: 0-915035-23-5
Clayton Valli, Director

4712 Basic Course in American Sign Language Vid eotape Package
TJ Publishers
2544 Tarpley Road
Carrollton, TX 75006

972-416-0800
800-999-1168
Fax: 972-416-0944
e-mail: customerservice@tjpublishers.com
www.tjpublishers.com/index.html

The A Basic Course in American Sign Language Vocabulary Videotape features four Deaf models signing each vocabulary word

contained in all 22 lessons of the text plus the alphabet and numbers. The tape has captions and voice which can be turned off to sharpen visual acuity. It is ideal for classroom reinforcement and independent home study.
Angela K Thames, President
Jerald A Murphy, VP

4713 Beginning Reading and Sign Language Video
TJ Publishers
2544 Tarpley Road
Carrollton, TX 75006

972-416-0800
800-999-1168
Fax: 972-416-0944
e-mail: customerservice@tjpublishers.com
www.tjpublishers.com/index.html

Learning sign improves reading, motor skills and visual perception and increases language acquisition abilities. For kids from 2 to 12, this video picture book features deaf actress Susan Bressler signing over a hundred words at the zoo, at home and around the community.
Video
Angela K Thames, President
Jerald A Murphy, VP

4714 Come Sign With Us
Gallaudet University
800 Florida Avenue, NE
Washington, DC 20002-3819

773-568-1550
800-621-2736
Fax: 800-621-8476
TTY: 888-630-9347
e-mail: gupress@gallaudet.edu
gupress.gallaudet.edu

Lessons including fingerspelling and signing are overviewed.
90 minutes
ISBN: 1-563680-50-5
Jan C. Hafer, Co-Author
Robert M. Wilson, Co-Author

4715 Deaf Children Signers
Harris Communications
15155 Technology Drive
Eden Prairie, MN 55344

952-906-1180
800-825-6758
Fax: 952-906-1099
TTY: 800-825-9187
e-mail: info@harriscomm.com
www.harriscomm.com

This 5-part collection of children signers is great for children, teachers, parents and interpreters.
Robert Harris Ph.D, Founder/President/CEO

4716 Deaf Culture Autobiographies
Harris Communications
15155 Technology Drive
Eden Prairie, MN 55344

952-906-1180
800-825-6758
Fax: 952-906-1099
TTY: 800-825-9187
e-mail: info@harriscomm.com
www.harriscomm.com

Inspiring videotapes offer encouragement and enlightenment to the hearing impaired. Total of eight videotapes.
Robert Harris Ph.D, Founder/President/CEO

4717 Deaf Culture Series
Harris Communications
15155 Technology Drive
Eden Prairie, MN 55344

952-906-1180
800-825-6758
Fax: 952-906-1099
TTY: 800-825-9187
e-mail: info@harriscomm.com
www.harriscomm.com

Each video in this 5-part series features a variety of Deaf talent. It is an excellent resource for Deaf studies programs, Interpreter Preparation programs and Sign Language programs.
Robert Harris Ph.D, Founder/President/CEO

4718 Deaf Mosaic Series
Harris Communications

15155 Technology Drive
Eden Prairie, MN 55344

952-906-1180
800-825-6758
Fax: 952-906-1099
TTY: 800-825-9187
e-mail: info@harriscomm.com
www.harriscomm.com

A national magazine show produced monthly by Gallaudet University, this show has been awarded nine Emmys. As the only nation-wide program about the Deaf community, these videotapes are the best of the best from the shows programs.
Robert Harris Ph.D, Founder/President/CEO

4719 Diagnosis and Treatment of Unilateral Hearing Loss
American Academy of Otolaryngology
1650 Diagonal Road
Alexandria, VA 22314-3357

703-836-4444
Fax: 703-683-5100
www.entnet.org

This CD-ROM focuses on evaluation and treatment of unilateral hearing loss arising from skull base lesion.

4720 Do You Hear That?
Alexander Graham Bell Association
3417 Volta Place NW
Washington, DC 20007-2737

202-337-5220
Fax: 202-337-8314
TTY: 202-337-5220
e-mail: info@agbell.org
www.listeningandspokenlanguage.org

This video documents auditory-verbal therapy as it is practiced at North York General Hospital in Toronto, Canada.
1992 35 minutes

4721 Fantastic Series
Gallaudet University Bookstore
800 Florida Avenue NE
Washington, DC 20002-3660

773-568-1550
800-621-2736
Fax: 800-621-8476
TTY: 888-630-9347
e-mail: gupress@gallaudet.edu
gupress.gallaudet.edu

Tapes designed to encourage both deaf and hearing children to use their imaginations.
Ages 6-10

4722 Fingers that Tickle and Delight
National Association of the Deaf
8630 Fenton Street
Silver Spring, MD 20910

301-587-1788
Fax: 301-587-1791
TTY: 301-587-1789
e-mail: nad.info@nad.org
nad.org

One's woman's experiences from childhood, school, marriage, her career as a teacher and interpreter trainer, and her life as an entertainer. Closed captioned.
13+ 32 minutes
Christopher Wagner, President
Melissa S. Draganac-Hawk, Vice-President

4723 Fingerspelling and Numbers Software
American Sign Language (ASL) Productions
c/o Harris Communications
Eden Prairie, MN 55344

952-906-1180
800-767-4461
Fax: 952-906-1099
TTY: 800-767-4461
e-mail: ASLProductions@harriscomm.com
www.americansignlanguageproductions.com

Fingerspelling practice partner that allows you to control the speed and vocabulary level. Requires Windows 3.1 or greater.
Robert Harris Ph.D, Founder/President-Harris Communications
Jenna Cassell, Founder ASL Productions

4724 Getting in Touch
Research Press
2612 N Mattis Avenue
Champaign, IL 61822-1053

217-352-3273
800-519-2707
Fax: 217-352-1221
e-mail: rp@researchpress.com
www.researchpress.com

Shows how to create an individualized communications system based on the abilities and needs of the child. Illustrates seven basic communication procedures that involve the use of touch cues and object cues.

4725 Gospel of Luke
Gallaudet University Bookstore
800 Florida Avenue NE
Washington, DC 20002-3660

773-568-1550
800-621-2736
Fax: 800-621-8476
TTY: 888-630-9347
e-mail: gupress@gallaudet.edu
gupress.gallaudet.edu

A set of five videotapes of the Gospel of Luke told in ASL.
Set of five

4726 Granny Good's Sign of Christmas
Gallaudet University Bookstore
800 Florida Avenue NE
Washington, DC 20002-3660

773-568-1550
800-621-2736
Fax: 800-621-8476
TTY: 888-630-9347
e-mail: gupress@gallaudet.edu
gupress.gallaudet.edu

Twas The Night Before Christmas told in American Sign Language.

4727 Hearing Loss and Rehabilitation
American Academy of Otolaryngology
1650 Diagonal Road
Alexandria, VA 22314-3357

703-836-4444
Fax: 703-683-5100
www.entnet.org

Slides

4728 I Can Hear!
Alexander Graham Bell Association
3417 Volta Place NW
Washington, DC 20007-2737

202-337-5220
Fax: 202-337-8314
TTY: 202-337-5220
e-mail: info@agbell.org
www.listeningandspokenlanguage.org

This inspirational video describes the auditory-verbal approach for developing speech and language for hearing impaired children and adults.
1992 23 minutes

4729 I Can Hear!: II
Alexander Graham Bell Association
3417 Volta Place NW
Washington, DC 20007-2737

202-337-5220
Fax: 202-337-8314
TTY: 202-337-5220
e-mail: info@agbell.org
www.listeningandspokenlanguage.org

An exciting videotape that gives more examples of auditory-verbal therapy and a variety of kids who have been taught to speak using this method.
1996 19 minute video

4730 I See What You Say: Self Help Lip Reading Program
Alexander Graham Bell Association
3417 Volta Place NW
Washington, DC 20007-2737

202-337-5220
Fax: 202-337-8314
TTY: 202-337-5220
e-mail: info@agbell.org
www.listeningandspokenlanguage.org

Easy to follow videotape and manual for consumers teaches visual recognition of speech sounds in single words and phrases.
1995 54 minutes

4731 Interpreters in Public Schools Kit
Sign Media
4020 Blackburn Lane
Burtonsville, MD 20866-1167

301-421-0268
800-475-4756
Fax: 301-421-0270
TTY: 301-421-4460
e-mail: info@signmedia.com
www.signmedia.com

Videotapes individually specialized for administrators, classroom teachers and for interpreters. Provides practical insights to some of

the most crucial issues and problems facing mainstreamed programs. Contains reproducible printed material.
Three videos
Barbara Olmert, Director Marketing

4732 Interview with Kirsten Gonzales
Alexander Graham Bell Association
3417 Volta Place NW
Washington, DC 20007-2737
202-337-5220
Fax: 202-337-8314
TTY: 202-337-5220
e-mail: info@agbell.org
www.listeningandspokenlanguage.org
Interviews a longtime user and trainer of oral interpreters who offers techniques in articulation and natural gestures.
20 minutes

4733 It's Not Just Hearing AIDS: Deaf People and the Epidemic
National Association of the Deaf
8630 Fenton Street
Silver Spring, MD 20910
301-587-1788
Fax: 301-587-1791
TTY: 301-587-1789
e-mail: nad.info@nad.org
nad.org
Straightforward and factual information on how AIDS is transmitted, who gets AIDS, procedures for an HIV test, and an interview with a person who actually has the AIDS virus.
9 - 13+ Video
Christopher Wagner, President
Melissa S. Draganac-Hawk, Vice-President

4734 Joy of Signing
Gallaudet University Bookstore
800 Florida Avenue NE
Washington, DC 20002-3660
773-568-1550
800-621-2736
Fax: 800-621-8476
TTY: 888-630-9347
e-mail: gupress@gallaudet.edu
gupress.gallaudet.edu
Three tapes full of useful information to help increase skill and comfort with sign.
1 Videotape

4735 King Midas
Gallaudet University
800 Florida Avenue, NE
Washington, DC 20002-3819
773-568-1550
800-621-2736
Fax: 800-621-8476
TTY: 888-630-9347
e-mail: gupress@gallaudet.edu
gupress.gallaudet.edu
Now the tale of King Midas and his golden touch is charmingly retold with full-color illustrations, and key sentences shown in American Sign Language (ASL).
30 minutes
ISBN: 0-930323-71-8
Robert Newby, Author

4736 King Midas Videotape
Gallaudet University Bookstore
800 Florida Avenue NE
Washington, DC 20002-3660
773-568-1550
800-621-2736
Fax: 800-621-8476
TTY: 888-630-9347
e-mail: gupress@gallaudet.edu
gupress.gallaudet.edu
Story of King Midas told in American Sign Language.
Robert Newby, Author

4737 Learning to Communicate: The First Three Years Videotape
Alexander Graham Bell Association
3417 Volta Place NW
Washington, DC 20007-2737
202-337-5220
Fax: 202-337-8314
TTY: 202-337-5220
e-mail: info@agbell.org
www.listeningandspokenlanguage.org
This video shows normal communication development in young children under three years of age. It discusses factors which can affect speech and language development, including anatomy and environment. Closed captioned.
11 minutes

4738 Let's Be Friends
Britannica Film Company
345 4th Street
San Francisco, CA 94107-1206
415-597-5555
The teacher left the room and asked Shelly, a hearing impaired child to be the mother. Margaret, an emotionally disturbed child, became frightened and verbally attacked Shelly. The teacher worked to get them to become friends and understand each other's problems.
Films

4739 Once Upon a Time - Children's Classics Ret old in American Sign Language
Harris Communications
15155 Technology Drive
Eden Prairie, MN 55344
952-906-1180
800-825-6758
Fax: 952-906-1099
TTY: 800-825-9187
e-mail: info@harriscomm.com
www.harriscomm.com
Children's classics come alive on videotapes.
Robert Harris Ph.D, Founder/President/CEO

4740 Parent Sign Video Series
TJ Publishers
2544 Tarpley Road
Carrollton, TX 75006
972-416-0800
800-999-1168
Fax: 972-416-0944
e-mail: customerservice@tjpublishers.com
www.tjpublishers.com/index.html
Ten instructional videotapes specifically designed for parents of deaf children, present frequently used vocabulary and phrases. The tapes are perfect for home use and as a compliment to sign language and educational programs. Deaf and hearing parents, each having a deaf and a hearing child, reflect common communication needs of all families.
Video
Angela K Thames, President
Jerald A Murphy, VP

4741 People vs. Noise
Better Hearing Institute
1444 I Street, NW
Washington, DC 20005-6043
202-449-1100
Fax: 202-216-9646
e-mail: mail@betterhearing.org
www.betterhearing.org

4742 Read My Lips
Alexander Graham Bell Association
3417 Volta Place NW
Washington, DC 20007-2737
202-337-5220
Fax: 202-337-8314
TTY: 202-337-5220
e-mail: info@agbell.org
www.listeningandspokenlanguage.org
A six videotape series that takes adults from lip reading to basic words to complex phrases and sentences in a variety of real life situations.

4743 See What I'm Saying
Thomas Kaufman, author
Fanlight Productions
32 Court Street
Brooklyn, NY 11201-1731
718-488-8900
800-876-1710
Fax: 718-488-8642
e-mail: rentals@icarusfilms.com
www.fanlight.com
Follows Patricia, a deaf child from a hearing, Spanish speaking family, through her first year of elementary school. Illustrates how the acquisition of communication skills enhances a child's self-esteem, confidence and family relationships. Open captioned.
1992 31 Minutes
ISBN: 1-572950-90-0

4744 Seeing and Hearing Speech: Lessons in Lipreading and Listening
Hearing Loss Association of America
7910 Woodmont Avenue
Bethesda, MD 20814-3079
301-657-2248
Fax: 301-913-9413
TTY: 301-657-2249
e-mail: info@hearingloss.org
www.hearingloss.org

This CD-Rom helps people with hearing loss learn to combine what they see with what they hear to understand speech better in difficult situations. This interactive CD-ROM contains carefully planned lessons to improve speech understanding through lipreading.
CD-ROM
Anna Gilmore Hall, Executive Director
Lise Hamlin, Director of Public Policy

4745   Show & Tell: Explaining Hearing Loss to Teachers
Alexander Graham Bell Association
3417 Volta Place NW   202-337-5220
Washington, DC 20007-2737   Fax: 202-337-8314
                                                  TTY: 202-337-5220
                                  e-mail: info@agbell.org
                        www.listeningandspokenlanguage.org
This video introduces mainstreamed teachers to the challenges that hearing impairments impose on normal communication.
20 minutes

4746   Show 'N' Tell Stories
Modern Signs Press
PO Box 1181   562-596-8548
Los Alamitos, CA 90720-1181   800-572-7332
                                                  Fax: 562-795-6614
                                                  TTY: 562-493-4168
                        e-mail: modsigns@modernsignspress.com
                               www.modernsignspress.com
A bilingual storytelling series for Deaf children and their families, featuring both Signing Exact English (SEE) and American Sign Language (ASL).
Videotape

4747   Sign-Me-A-Story
DawnSignPress
6130 Nancy Ridge Drive   858-768-0428
San Diego, CA 92121-3223   800-549-5350
                                                  Fax: 858-625-2336
                                                  TTY: 858-625-0600
                                  e-mail: info@dawnsign.com
                                        www.dawnsign.com/
Linda Bove, the deaf actress from Sesame Street, introduces children to American Sign Language. Teaches simple signs and then acts out fairy tales. Stories are voiced and closed captioned, accessible to all.
30 minutes
ISBN: 0-394892-32-1
Joe Dannis, Founder/Publisher/President

4748   Sleeping Beauty Videotape
Gallaudet University Bookstore
800 Florida Avenue NE   773-568-1550
Washington, DC 20002-3660   800-621-2736
                                                  Fax: 800-621-8476
                                                  TTY: 888-630-9347
                                  e-mail: gupress@gallaudet.edu
                                        gupress.gallaudet.edu
Presents the entire story of Sleeping Beauty told in American Sign Language.

4749   Sleeping Beauty: With Selected Sentences in ASL
Gallaudet University
800 Florida Avenue, NE   773-568-1550
Washington, DC 20002-3819   800-621-2736
                                                  Fax: 800-621-8476
                                                  TTY: 888-630-9347
                                  e-mail: gupress@gallaudet.edu
                                        gupress.gallaudet.edu
Features the full story in ASL and includes vocabulary and sentence structure focusing on adjectives, with a voice-over throughout.
30 minutes
ISBN: 0-930323-98-X

4750   Sound Hearing
Hearing Loss Association of America

7910 Woodmont Avenue   301-657-2248
Bethesda, MD 20814-3079   Fax: 301-913-9413
                                                  TTY: 301-657-2249
                                  e-mail: info@hearingloss.org
                                        www.hearingloss.org
Provides listening samples to illustrate sound, hearing, and hearing loss. Listeners will hear as people who have hearing loss might, listening to music, a story, etc.
CD-ROM, 26 mins
Anna Gilmore Hall, Executive Director
Lise Hamlin, Director of Public Policy

4751   Telecoil: Plugging Into Sound
Hearing Loss Association of America
7910 Woodmont Avenue   301-657-2248
Bethesda, MD 20814-3079   Fax: 301-913-9413
                                                  TTY: 301-657-2249
                                  e-mail: info@hearingloss.org
                                        www.hearingloss.org
In The Telecoil: Plugging Into Sound, members of SHHH give accounts of their experiences with using the telecoil, describing how the telecoil makes a noticeable difference in their social and professional lives.
Open Captioned
Anna Gilmore Hall, Executive Director
Lise Hamlin, Director of Public Policy

4752   Telecoil: Plugging into Sound
7910 Woodmont Avenue   301-657-2248
Bethesda, MD 20814-3079   Fax: 301-913-9413
                                                  TTY: 301-657-2249
                                  e-mail: national@shhh.org
                                        www.hearingloss.org
Guide for consumers concerning why they should include a telecoil in their hearing aid. SHHH members are featured, talking about their experiences. Includes 50 brochures. Open-captioned.
1996 10 minutes

4753   Telling Stories
Harris Communications
15155 Technology Drive   952-906-1180
Eden Prairie, MN 55344   800-825-6758
                                                  Fax: 952-906-1099
                                                  TTY: 800-825-9187
                                  e-mail: info@harriscomm.com
                                        www.harriscomm.com
This international, award winning play, now on video, uses the symbols and myths drawn from the struggles between the world of the deaf and the world of the hearing.
Robert Harris Ph.D, Founder/President/CEO

4754   Treasure
Gallaudet University Bookstore
800 Florida Avenue NE   773-568-1550
Washington, DC 20002-3660   800-621-2736
                                                  Fax: 800-621-8476
                                                  TTY: 888-630-9347
                                  e-mail: gupress@gallaudet.edu
                                        gupress.gallaudet.edu
Ella Mae Lentz, a well-known deaf poet, signs some of her poems.

4755   Unheard Voices
Hearing Loss Association of America
7910 Woodmont Avenue   301-657-2248
Bethesda, MD 20814-3079   Fax: 301-913-9413
                                                  TTY: 301-657-2249
                                  e-mail: info@hearingloss.org
                                        www.hearingloss.org
Unheard Voices is a candid and compassionate portrayal of people coping with the life-changing impact of hearing loss. Open-captioned.
23 minutes
Anna Gilmore Hall, Executive Director
Barbara Kelley, Deputy Executive Director

Web Sites

4756   Alexander Graham Bell Association
                        www.listeningandspokenlanguage.org

They helps families, health care providers and education professionals understand childhood hearing loss and the importance of early diagnosis and intervention. Through advocacy, education, research and financial aid, AG Bell helps to ensure that every child and adult with hearing loss has the opportunity to listen, talk and thrive in mainstream society.

4757   American Academy of Audiology

www.audiology.org

Provides professional development, education and research and provides increased public awareness of hearing disorders and audiologic services.

4758   American Academy of Otolaryngology

www.entnet.org

Advance the art and science of otalaryngology-head and neck surgury through state-of-the-art education, research, and learning; and to unite, serve, and represent the interests of its members and their patients to the public.

4759   American Society for Deaf Children

www.deafchildren.org

Provides support, encouragement, and current information about deafness to families with deaf and hard of hearing children.

4760   American Tinnitus Association

www.ata.org

Provides information about tinnitus and referrals to local contacts/support groups nationwide.

4761   Auditory-Verbal International

www.auditory-verbal.org

Promotes the Auditory-Verbal Therapy approach, which is based on the belief that the overwhelming majority of these children can hear and talk by using their residual hearing and hearing aids.

4762   Better Hearing Institute

www.betterhearing.org

Information programs on hearing loss and available medical, surgical, hearing aid, and rehabilitation assistance for millions with uncorrected hearing problems.

4763   Council on Education of the Deaf

www.deafed.net

Offers information and referral services to the hearing impaired.

4764   Deafness Research Foundation

hearinghealthfoundation.org

4765   EAR Foundation

www.earfoundation.org

Provides the general public support services promoting the integration of the hearing and balance impaired into mainstream society and to educate young people and adults about hearing preservation and early detection of hearing loss, enabling them to prevent at an early age hearing and balance disorders.
Molli C. Conti, Executive Director

4766   Healing Well

www.healingwell.com

An online health resource guide to medical news, chat, information and articles, newsgroups and message boards, books, disease-related web sites, medical directories, and more for patients, friends, and family coping with disabling diseases, disorders, or chronic illnesses.

4767   Health Finder

www.healthfinder.gov

Searchable, carefully developed web site offering information on over 1000 topics. Developed by the US Department of Health and Human Services, the site can be used in both English and Spanish.
Rick Smith, President & CEO
Rebecca Frank, Chief Development Officer

4768   Healthlink USA

www.healthlinkusa.com

Health information concerning treatment, cures, prevention, diagnosis, risk factors, research, support groups, email lists, personal stories and much more. Updated regularly.

4769   Hear Now

www.starkeyhearingfoundation.org

Hear Now is the application-based program of Starkey Hearing Foundation that provides assistance to low-income Americans. Each person they help is fit with new, top-of-the-line digital hearing aids that are customized to their hearing loss.
Molli C. Conti, Executive Director

4770   Hearing Education and Awareness for Rocker

www.hearnet.com

Educates the public about the real dangers of hearing loss resulting from repeated exposure to excessive noise levels.

4771   Helios Health

www.helioshealth.com

Online resource for your health information. Detailed information about specific health topics, access to expert advice from our Medical Advisory Board, and up-to-date health news.

4772   House Ear Institute

houseclinic.com

A national non-profit otologic research and educational institute that provides information on hearing and balance disorders.

4773   John Tracy Clinic

www.jtc.org

An educational facility for preschool age children who have hearing losses and their families. In addition to on-site services, worldwide correspondence courses in English and Spanish are offered to parents whose children are of preschool age and are hard of hearing, deaf, or deaf-blind.

4774   MedicineNet

www.medicinenet.com

An online resource for consumers providing easy-to-read, authoritative medical and health information.

4775   Medscape

www.medscape.com

Medscape offers specialists, primary care physicians, and other health professionals the Web's most robust and integrated medical information and educational tools.

4776   National Association of the Deaf

www.nad.org

Focus on advocacy, captioned media, deafness-related information/publications, legal assistance and more.

4777   National Captioning Institute

ncicap.org

Advocates captioned television for people who want to see, as well as hear, the dialogue of a television program. It not only enables deaf and hard-of-hearing people to understand all of a program's content, but it is also beneficial for new Americans learning English as a second language, as well as children learning to read.

4778   National Information Center on Deafness

www.gallaudet.edu

Provides information or referrals on questions about deafness, including general information, education, research, legislation, assistive devices and more. Offers a bibliography of readings available on 30 topics relating to deafness.

4779   National Information Clearinghouse on Children Who are Deaf-Blind

nationaldb.org

Collects, organizes and disseminates information related to children and youth who are deaf-blind and connects consumers of deaf-blind information to sources of information about deaf-blindness, assistive technology and deaf-blind people.

4780   National Institute on Deafness and Other Communication Disorders

www.nih.gov/nidcd

A national resources center for information about hearing, balance, smell, taste, voice, speech and language.

4781   Registry of Interpreters for the Deaf

www.RID.org

Professional interpreters and translators, persons with deafness or hearing impairments and professionals in related fields.

4782   Self-Help for Hard of Hearing People

www.hearingloss.org

Promotes awareness and information about hearing loss, communication, assistive devices, and alternative communication skills through publications, exhibits and presentations.

4783 USA Deaf Sports Federation

www.usdeafsports.org

Website published by a governing body for all deaf sports and recreation in the United States.

Marybeth Leamyini, Communications Director

4784 WebMD

www.webmd.com

Provides credible information, supportive communities, and in-depth reference material about health subjects. A source for original and timely health information as well as material from well known content providers.

Description

4785 ## Heart Disease

There is a wide range of heart (cardiac) diseases that can be divided into several major categories: heart failure; problems in electrical conduction; heart rate and rhythm; and malfunction of the heart valves. Coronary disease relates to the arteries that supply oxygen to the heart muscle itself.

Heart failure is the general inability of the heart to function effectively as the pumping mechanism to distribute oxygenated blood and nutrients to the cells and tissues. As the heart's pumping action declines, blood does not get distributed properly and normal circulation gets disrupted. As a result, the fluid accumulates, or backs up, causing swelling (edema) in the body, often noticeable in the ankles, as well as within the lungs (pulmonary edema) causing difficulty in breathing. Numerous mechanisms are responsible for heart failure so treatment is aimed at the underlying causes, improving heart contractibility (and thus pump efficiency), and removal of excess fluid through the kidneys.

Problems in the electrical conduction that makes the heart contract result in irregular heart rate and rhythm, either slower, faster, or, in life-threatening situations, absence of heart beat or ineffective heart contractions. Specific medications and procedures are used in treatment, again depending on the underlying problem.

New diagnostic (angiography) and therapeutic catheter techniques have been developed to accurately identify the rhythm problem, and in some cases, cure it bydelivering radio frequency energy to the abnormal pathway.

Malfunctions of heart valves are also common, but surgical advances enable successful repair and replacement of defective or diseased valves.

The arteries that directly supply the heart (known as coronary arteries) can also be affected by disease processes. Deposits or fatty plaques may cause narrowing of the arteries, or the arteries can become blocked by a clot that originated somewhere else in the body. Either way, the heart may be deprived of oxygenated blood and the particular muscle that is fed by the artery is injured or dies. Angina is chest pain produced when the heart is not receiving enough oxygen but no direct damage occurs. A heart attack (or myocardial infarction) occurs when the heart is deprived of its blood for a significant amount of time. The outcome of a heart attack depends on the amount of damage sustained by the affected heart muscle and the speed with which treatment is started. Immediate medical intervention has a marked effect on long-term prognosis. Administration of agents that dissolve the clot (blood thinners, antithrombotics) significantly reduce heart attack deaths when given within 6 hours of the onset of chest pain. Catheter interventions (angioplasty) can include balloons and metallic stents that are placed in coronary arteries to push obstructions against the arterial walls thereby re-opening the vessel. The most recent advance is a stent that is coated with a drug that is coated to prevent reformation of the clot.

The symptoms of heart disease are varied, but may include chest pain, difficulty breathing, fatigue, palpitations, dizziness and fainting. See also *Congenital Heart Disease*.

National Agencies & Associations

4786 **American Heart Association**
7272 Greenville Avenue
Dallas, TX 75231   800-242-8721
www.americanheart.org
Supports research education and community service programs with the objective of reducing premature death and disability from cardiovascular diseases and stroke; coordinates the efforts of health professionals and other engaged in the fight against heart disease.
Nancy Brown, CEO

4787 **Canadian Adult Congenital Heart Network**
2233 Argentia Road   905-826-6665
Mississauga, L5N 2-2L2   e-mail: erwin.oechslin@cachnet.org
www.cachnet.org
Was created to pool the knowledge and experience of congenital heart disease professionals in Canada to help strengthen their skills and knowledge of the discipline, and to create a community of individuals committed to caring for adults with congenital heart disease and their families.
Dr Erwin Oechslin, President
Dr Ariane Marelli, Vice-President

4788 **Children's Heart Society**
PO BOX 52088   780-454-7665
Edmonton, AB T6G 2-2T5   888-247-9404
Fax: 780-454-7665
e-mail: childrensheart@shaw.ca
www.childrensheart.org
Supports families of children with acquired and congenital heart disease.
Shannon Moroz, President
Tina Krieger, Vice-President

4789 **National Heart, Lung and Blood Institute**
National Institutes of Health
PO BOX 30105   301-592-8573
Bethesda, MD 20824   Fax: 301-592-8563
TTY: 240-629-3255
e-mail: NHLBIinfo@nhlbi.nih.gov
www.nhlbi.nih.gov
Primary responsibility of this organization is the scientific investigation of heart, blood vessel, lung and blood disorders. Oversees research, demonstration, prevention, education, control and training activities in these fields and emphasizes the prevention and control of heart diseases.
Gary H Gibbons, Director
Susan B Shurin, Deputy Director

4790 **Pulmonary Hypertension Association**
801 Roeder Road   301-565-3004
Silver Spring, MD 20910   800-748-7274
Fax: 301-565-3994
e-mail: pha@PHAssociation.org
www.PHAssociation.org
A nonprofit organization for pulmonary hypertension patients, families, caregivers and PH-treating medical professionals. The mission of the Pulmonary Hypertension Association (PHA) is to find ways to prevent and cure pulmonary hypertension, and to provide hope for the pulmonary hypertension community through support, education, advocacy and awareness.
Vallerie McLaughlin, MD, Chair
Rino Aldrighetti, President

Research Centers

4791 Arizona Heart Institute
2632 N 20th Street
Phoenix, AZ 85006-1300
602-266-2200
800-345-4278
Fax: 602-604-5047
e-mail: information@azheart.com
www.azheart.com
Edward Diethrich, Medical Director and Founder

4792 Baylor College of Medicine: Debakey Heart Center
Texas Medical Center
1 Baylor Plaza
Houston, TX 77030-3411
713-798-4710
Fax: 713-798-3692
e-mail: president@bcm.edu
www.bcm.tmc.edu
Research activities have an emphasis on therapeutic intervention and prevention of heart disease.
James T Hackett, Chair
Paul Klotman MD, President

4793 Bees-Stealy Research Foundation
2001 4th Avenue
San Diego, CA 92101-2303
619-235-8744
Fax: 619-234-8190
Basic cardiac research.
HD Peabody Jr, Director

4794 Bockus Research Institute Graduate Hospital
Graduate Hospital
415 S 19th Street
Philadelphia, PA 19146-1464
215-893-2000
Offers research in cardiovascular diseases with emphasis on muscle tissue studies.
Dr Robert Cox, Director

4795 Boston University, Whitaker Cardiovascular Institute
715 Albany Street
Boston, MA 02118
617-638-4887
Fax: 617-638-4066
www.bumc.bu.edu
Offers basic and clinical care research relating to cardiovascular diseases.
Gary J Balady MD, Clinical Investigator

4796 Cardiovascular Research and Training Center University of Alabama
THT Room 311
Birmingham, AL 35294-6
205-934-3624
Fax: 205-345-96
Robert C Bueourge, Director

4797 Children's Heart Institute of Texas
PO Box 3966
Corpus Christi, TX 78463-3966
512-887-4505
Fax: 512-887-0539
Offers research and statistical information on pediatric cardiology.
Laura Berlanga, Director

4798 Cleveland Clinic Lerner Research Institute
9500 Euclid Avenue
Cleveland, OH 44195
216-444-3900
Fax: 216-444-3279
e-mail: dicorlp@ccf.org
www.lerner.ccf.org
Research institute focusing on diseases of the cardiovascular system.
Paul E DiCorleto PhD, Institute Chairman
Guy M Chisolm, III, PhD, Institute Vice-Chair

4799 Columbia University Irving Center for Clinical Research Adult Unit
Presbyterian Hospital
116 Street and Broadway
New York, NY 10027
212-854-1754
Fax: 212-053-13
e-mail: askcuit@columbia.edu
www.columbia.edu
Research center focusing on pulmonary diseases.
Lee C Bollinger, President
John H Coatsworth, Provost

4800 Congenital Heart Disease Anomalies Support, Education & Resources CHASER
2112 N Wilkins Road
Swanton, OH 43558-9445
419-825-5575
Fax: 419-825-2880
e-mail: myer106w@wonder.em.cdc.gov
www.csun.edu
An organization established to meet the emotional and educational needs of parents and professionals who deal with congenital heart disease in children. Offers resource materials and support for parent to parent networking.

4801 Creighton University Cardiac Center
3006 Webster Street
Omaha, NE 68131-2137
402-280-4566
800-237-7828
Fax: 402-280-4938
thecardiaccenter.creighton.edu
Research into the clinical aspects of cardiology and heart disease.
Tami Ward, Nurse Practitioner
Kimberly Harm, Nurse Practitioner

4802 Duke University Pediatric Cardiac Catheterization Laboratory
T901/Children's Health Center
Durham, NC 27705-0001
919-681-4080
Fax: 919-681-2714
e-mail: john.rhodes@duke.edu
pediatrics.duke.edu
Research into pediatric cardiology.
Joseph St Geme, III, MD, Chair
Kay Marshall, Chief Administrator

4803 Florida Heart Research Institute
4770 Biscayne Boulevard
Miami, FL 33137
305-674-3020
Fax: 305-535-3642
e-mail: pak@floridaheart.org
www.miamiheartresearch.org
General cardiovascular research.
Kathleen T DuCasse, Chief Executive Officer

4804 Framingham Heart Study
73 Mount Wayte Avenue
Framingham, MA 01702-5828
508-935-3418
Fax: 508-626-1262
e-mail: LLehmann1@partners.org
www.framinghamheartstudy.org
Lisa Soleymani Lehmann, M.D.,, Chair

4805 General Clinical Research Center at Beth Israel Hospital
330 Brookline Avenue
Boston, MA 02215-5400
617-667-7000
800-667-5356
TDD: 800-439-0183
www.bidmc.org
Studies into cardiology pulmonary disorders and heart disease.
Stephen B Kay, Chair
Kevin Tabb, MD, President & Chief Executive Officer

4806 General Clinical Research Center: University of California at LA
Center for Health Sciences
10833 Le Conte Avenue
Los Angeles, CA 90095
310-825-7177
Fax: 310-206-5012
e-mail: lshakerirwin@mednet.ucla.edu.
www.gcrc.medsch.ucla.edu
Cardiovascular and heart disease disorders and illness research.
Isidro Salus MD, Program Director
Gerald Levey, Principal Investigator

4807 Hahnemann University Likoff Cardiovascular Institute
Broad & Vine Streets
Philadelpia, PA 19102
215-854-8100
Diseases of the heart and vessels.
William S Frankl MD, Director

4808 Harvard Throndike Laboratory Harvard Medical Center
Harvard Medical Center
330 Brookline Avenue
Boston, MA 02215-5400
617-735-3020
Fax: 617-735-4833
Dr James Morgan, Director

4809 Heart Disease Research Foundation
50 Court Street
Brooklyn, NY 11201-4801
718-649-6210
Robert A Teters, Director

4810 Heart Research Foundation of Sacramento
1007 39th Street
Sacramento, CA 95816-5502
916-456-3365
e-mail: rjfrink@pol.net
www.hrfsac.org

Dr Frink, Founder/Principal Investigator

4811 Hope Heart Institute
1380 112th Ave. NE
Bellvue, WA 98004
425-456-8700
Fax: 425-456-8701
e-mail: info@hopeheart.org
www.hopeheart.org

Heart and blood vessel research.
Dr Lester R Sauvage MD, Founder
Cherie Skager, Interim Executive Director

4812 John L McClellan Memorial Veterans' Hospital Research Office
4300 W 7th Street
Little Rock, AR 72205-5446
501-257-1000
Fax: 501-671-2510
www2.va.gov

Karl David Straub MD, Chief Staff

4813 Krannert Institute of Cardiology
1801 N Senate Boulevard
Indianapolis, IN 46202-4832
317-962-0500
800-843-2786
Fax: 317-962-0501
medicine.iupui.edu/krannert
The cardiovascular program at the Indiana University School of Medicine is recognized throughout the world for its commitment to excellence in patient care research and education. While we're known for our experience and ability to take care of the most complex cardiovascular problems we are equally focused on prevention and early detection.
Peng-Sheng Chen, MD, Division Director
Eric Williams, MD, Associate Dean

4814 Loyola University of Chicago Cardiac Transplant Program
2160 S 1st Avenue
Maywood, IL 60153-3304
708-216-9000
888-584-7888
Fax: 708-216-4918
www.loyolamedicine.org/
Loyola University Health System is committed to excellence in patient care and the education of health professionals. They believe that our Catholic heritage and Jesuit traditions of ethical behavior academic distinction and scientific research lead to new knowledge and advance our healing mission in the communities we serve.
Larry M Goldberg, President & CEO
Wendy S Leutgens, Senior Vice President and COO

4815 Medstar Georgetown University Hospital Facility
3800 Reservoir Road NW
Washington, DC 20007-2195
202-444-2000
www.georgetownuniversityhospital.org
Studies of medical sciences with particular emphasis on heart disease.
Dr Richard Goldberg, President

4816 Mount Sinai Medical Center
4300 Alton Road
Miami Beach, FL 33140-2997
305-674-2121
Fax: 305-743-09
www.msmc.com

General cardiovascular research.
Steven D Sonenreich, President & Chief Executive Officer

4817 Oklahoma Medical Research Foundation: Cardiovascular Research Program
825 NE 13th Street
Oklahoma City, OK 73104-5097
405-271-6673
800-522-0211
Fax: 405-271-3980
e-mail: contact@omrf.org
www.omrf.ouhsc.edu
The Cardiovascular Biology Research Program investigates fundamental mechanisms involved in blood coagulation inflammation and atherogenesis with special emphasis on the regulation of theses processes.
Dr Stephen M Prescott, President
Mike D Morgan, Executive Vice President & COO

4818 Pennsylvania State University Artificial Heart Research Project
Milton S Hershey Medical Center
500 University Drive
Hershey, PA 17033-2391
717-531-8407
Fax: 717-531-5011
www.psu.edu

William S Pierce MD, Director

4819 Preventive Medicine Research Institute
900 Bridgeway
Sausalito, CA 94965-2158
415-332-2525
Fax: 415-325-30
e-mail: Tandis@pmri.org
www.pmri.org
Nonprofit organization focusing on prevention and treatment of heart disease through modification of diet exercise and relaxation techniques.
Dean Ornish, MD, Founder & President
Anne Ornish, Vice President, Director of Program Deve

4820 Purdue University William A Hillenbrand Biomedical Engineering Center
AA Potter Engineering Center
206 S. Martin Jischke Drive
W Lafayette, IN 47907-2032
765-494-2995
877-598-4233
Fax: 765-494-6628
e-mail: WeldonBME@purdue.edu
engineering.purdue.edu/BME
Cardiology and heart disease research.
Brian J Knoy, Director of Development
Kathryn Copper, Secretary

4821 Rockefeller University Laboratory of Cardiac Physiology
1230 York Avenue
New York, NY 10065
212-327-8000
Fax: 212-327-7974
e-mail: pubinfo@rockefeller.edu
www.rockefeller.edu
Causes of cardiac arrhythmias and prevention of heart disease.
David Rockefeller, Honorary Chair
Russell L Carson, Chair

4822 San Francisco Heart & Vascular Institute
1900 Sullivan Avenue
Daly City, CA 94015-2200
650-991-6712
800-82H-EART
Fax: 650-755-7315
e-mail: webmaster@sfhi.com
www.sfhi.com
At Seton Medical Center we are committed to providing a full range of high quality services and state-of-the-art cardiovascular treatments for our patients. Our medical nursing and social services staff provide quality care and compassion as a coordinated team focusing on the medical emotional and spiritual needs of patients and their families.
Colman J Ryan, MD, Executive Medical Director
Michael Girolami, MD, Chief of Cardiology

4823 Specialized Center of Research in Ischemic Heart Disease
1802 6th Avenue South
Birmingham, AL 35294-0001
205-934-4011
800-822-8816
www.health.uab.edu

Coronary artery disease.
Will Ferniany, CEO
Becky Armstrong, Program Manager

4824 Texas Heart Institute St Lukes Episcopal Hospital
St Lukes Episcopal Hospital
6770 Bertner Avenue
Houston, TX 77030-0345
832-355-4011
800-292-2221
Fax: 713-791-3089
e-mail: mmattsson@heart.thi.tmc.edu
www.texasheartinstitute.org

Denton A Cooley MD, President Emeritus
James T Willerson MD, President, Medical Director

4825 University of Alabama at Birmingham: Congenital Heart Disease Center
1720 2nd Avenue South
Birmingham, AL 35294
205-934-4011
Fax: 205-934-7514
TDD: 205-934-4642
www.uab.edu

Ray L Watts, MD, President
Linda Lucas, PhD, Provost

4826 University of California San Diego General Clinical Research Center
UCSD Medical Center
200 W Arbor Drive
San Diego, CA 92103-1910
619-543-3102
858-657-7000
Fax: 619-435-36
www.health.ucsd.edu
General clinical research.
Paul Viviano, Chief Executive Officer and Associate Vi
Margarita Baggett, Interim Chief Operating Officer and Chie

4827 University of California: Cardiovascular Research Laboratory
Center for Health Sciences
UCLA Medical Center
Los Angeles, CA 90024
310-825-6824
Fax: 310-206-5777
Cellular and subcellular cardiac conditions.
Dr Glenn Langer, Director

4828 University of Cincinnati Department of Pathology & Laboratory Medicine
234 Goodman Street
Cincinnati, OH 45219-0529
513-584-7284
Fax: 513-584-3892
e-mail: pathology@uc.edu
pathology.uc.edu

Fred V Lucas, MD, Chair of Pathology
James Hill, Business Manager

4829 University of Iowa: Iowa Cardiovascular Center
College of Medicine
200 Hawkins Drive
Iowa City, IA 52242
319-335-8588
Fax: 319-335-6969
www.int-med.uiowa.edu
The purpose is to coordinate the cardiovascular programs of the College into a more cohesive unit to permit us to 1) utilize our cardiovascular resources optimally 2) intensify expand and integrate basic and clinical research programs in areas related to cardiovascular research and 3) evaluate the role of new measures for prevention diagnosis and treatment of cardiovascular disease.
Barry London, MD, PhD, Director Cardiovascular Medicine

4830 University of Michigan Pulmonary and Critical Care Division
University Hospital
1500 E Medical Center Drive
Ann Arbor, MI 48109
734-647-9342
888-287-1084
Fax: 734-763-4585
www2.med.umich.edu/healthcenters/clinic_
Kevin Michael Chan, MD, Division Director

4831 University of Michigan: Cardiovascular Med icine
325 Briarwood Circle
Ann Arbor, MI 48108-0001
734-647-9000
Fax: 734-936-0133
www2.med.umich.edu/departments/cvc/servi
Focuses on the diagnosis, treatment and prevention of cardiovascular and heart diseases.
Kim Allen Eagle, MD, Division Director

4832 University of Missouri Columbia Division of Cardiothoracic Surgery
School of Medicine
Columbia, MO 65212
573-882-2121
Fax: 573-884-0437
e-mail: AldenM@missouri.edu
www.missouri.edu
Cardiac surgery research.
Mike Alden, Director
Brian Foster, Provost

4833 University of Pennsylvania Muscle Institut e
School of Medicine
700A Clinical Research Building
Philadelphia, PA 19104-2646
215-573-9758
Fax: 215-898-2653
e-mail: mafoster@mail.med.upenn.edu
www.med.upenn.edu/pmi/
Studies in tissue science.
E. Michael Ostap, PhD, Director

4834 University of Pittsburgh: Human Energy Research Laboratory
4200 Fifth Avenue
Pittsburgh, PA 15260-0001
412-624-4141
www.pitt.edu

Focuses on exercise and cardiac rehabilitation.
Mark A Nordenberg, Chancellor
Patricia E Beeson, Provost and Senior Vice Chancellor

4835 University of Rochester: Clinical Research Center
601 Elmwood Avenue
Rochester, NY 14642-0001
585-275-2907
Fax: 585-256-3805
e-mail: germaine_reinhardt@urmc.rochester.edu
www.urmc.rochester.edu/crc/
Studies of normal tissue functions pertaining to heart diseases.
Thomas A Pearson, MD, MPH, PhD, Director, Principal Investigator
Giovanni Schifitto , MD, Program Director

4836 University of Southern California: Coronary Care Research
1200 N State Street
Los Angeles, CA 90033-1029
213-226-7242
Dr. L Julian Haywood, Director

4837 University of Tennessee: Division of Cardiovascular Diseases
920 Madison Avenue
Memphis, TN 38163-0001
901-448-5750
Fax: 901-448-8084
www.utmem.edu\cardiology
Cardiovascular system disorders including heart disease prevention and treatment.
Karl T Weber MD, Director

4838 University of Texas Southwestern Medical Center at Dallas
University of Texas
5323 Harry Hines Boulevard
Dallas, TX 75390-7208
214-648-3111
Fax: 214-483-11
www.utsouthwestern.edu
Cardiology department research.
Daniel K Podolsky, MD, President
J. Gregory Fitz, MD, Executive Vice President

4839 University of Utah: Artificial Heart Research Laboratory
50 North Medical Drive
Salt Lake City, UT 84132-1414
801-581-2121
Fax: 801-581-4044
healthsciences.utah.edu
Cardiac and blood vessel research.
Allen Stephens, Associate Director

4840 University of Utah: Cardiovascular Genetic Research Clinic
420 Chipeta Way
Salt Lake City, UT 84132-0001
801-581-3888
Fax: 801-581-6862
www.medicine.utah.edu/internalmedicine/c
Cardiovascular genetics research.
Dr Roger Williams, Founder

4841 Urban Cardiology Research Center
2300 Garrison Boulevard
Baltimore, MD 21216-2308
410-945-8600
Causes diagnosis and treatment of cardiovascular diseases.
Arthur White MD, Director

4842 Warren Grant Magnuson Clinical Center
National Institute of Health
10 Center Drive MSC 1078
Bethesda, MD 20892
301-496-3311
800-411-1222
Fax: 301-496-2390
TTY: 866-411-1010
e-mail: mmichael@cc.nih.gov
www.dnrc.nih.gov/reports/programs/ncc.as
Established in 1953 as the research hospital of the National Institutes of Health. Designed so that patient care facilities are close to research laboratories so new findings of basic and clinical scientists can be quickly applied to the treatment of patients. Upon referral by physicians, patients are admitted to NIH clinical studies.
Madeline Michael, Chief, Clinical Nutrition Services

4843 Yeshiva University General Clinical Research Center
500 West 185th Street
New York, NY 10033
212-960-5400
www.yu.edu
Cardiovascular research.
Dr Henry Kressel, Chairman
Richard M Joel, President

Support Groups & Hotlines

4844 American Autoimmune Related Diseases Association
22100 Gratiot Avenue   586-776-3900
East Detroit, MI 48021   800-598-4668
                                          Fax: 586-776-3903
                                    e-mail: aarda@aarda.org
                                              www.aarda.org
Awareness, education, referrals for patients with any type of auto-immune disease.
Stanley M Finger, PhD, Chairman of the Board
Virginia T Ladd, President & Executive Director

4845 Mended Hearts
8150 N. Central Expressway   214-206-9259
Dallas, TX 75206   888-432-7899
                                          Fax: 214-295-9552
                                e-mail: info@mendedhearts.org
                                          www.mendedhearts.org
Mutual support for persons who have heart disease, their families, friends, and other interested persons.
Gordon Littlefield, President of the Board
Donnette Smith, Executive Vice President

4846 Mitral Valve Prolapse Program of Cincinnati Support Group
10525 Montgomery Road   513-745-9911
Cincinnati, OH 45242   e-mail: kscordo@wright.edu
                                        www.nursing.wright.edu
Brings together persons frightened by their symptoms in order to learn to better cope with MVP. Fosters use of non-drug therapies. Supervised exercise sessions, diagnostic evaluations and specialized testing. Information and referrals, conferences, literature, group meetings, MVP Hot Line, and assistance in starting groups.

4847 National Health Information Center
PO Box 1133   310-565-4167
Washington, DC 20013   800-336-4797
                                          Fax: 301-984-4256
                                      e-mail: info@nhic.org
                                          www.health.gov/nhic
Offers a nationwide information referral service, produces directories and resource guides.

4848 National Society for MVP and Dysautonomia
880 Montclair Road   205-595-8229
Birmingham, AL 35213   866-595-8229
                                          Fax: 205-595-8222
                        e-mail: nancysawyermd@bellsouth.net
Assists individuals suffering from mitral valve prolapse syndrome and dysautonomia to find support and understanding. Education on symptoms and treatment. Other areas of focus are Fibromyalgia and Sjogren's Syndrome.
Nancy Sawyer, MD

4849 Pulmonary Hypertension Association
801 Roeder Road   301-565-3004
Silver Spring, MD 20910   800-748-7274
                                          Fax: 301-565-3994
                            e-mail: PHCR@PHAssociation.org
                                          www.phassociation.org
A nonprofit organization funded and for pulmonary hypertension patients. Our mission is to seek a cure, provide hope, support, education and to promote awareness and advocate for the PH community.
Vallerie McLaughlin, MD, Chair
Rev. Steve White, PhD, Chair-Elect

4850 Society of Mitral Valve Prolapse Syndrome
PO Box 431   630-250-9327
Itasca, IL 60143-0431   Fax: 630-773-0478
                                e-mail: bonnie0107@aol.com
                                www.mitralvalveprolapse.com/
Provides support and education to patients, families and friends about mitral valve prolapse syndrome.
Jim Durante, Co-Founder
Bonnie Durante, Co-Founder

Books

4851 Advances in Cardiac and Pulmonary Rehabilitation
Haworth Press
10 Alice Street   607-722-5857
Binghamton, NY 13904-1580   800-429-6784
                                          Fax: 607-722-0012
                                          www.haworthpress.com
Enhance your rehabilitation program with this authoritative volume.
74 pages Hardcover
ISBN: 0-866569-86-0

4852 Congenital Heart Disease
Northwestern University Press
625 Colfax Street   847-491-5313
Evanston, IL 60208-4210   800-621-2736
                                          www.nupress.nwu.edu

1993 300 pages
ISBN: 1-880416-82-4
Dory Kranz, Executive Director
Pip Marks, Director Outreach Services

4853 Dr. Dean Ornish's Program for Reversing Heart Disease
Random House Trade Books
400 Hahn Road
Westminster, MD 21157-4663   800-733-3000
                                          Fax: 800-659-2436
                                          deanornish.com/books

ISBN: 0-804110-38-7
Andrea Liptak, Founder

4854 Expert Guide to Beating Heart Disease: What You Absolutely Must Know
Dr. Harlan M. Krumholz, author
HarperCollins
195 Broadway   212-207-7000
New York, NY 10007-5299   e-mail: orders@harpercollins.com
                                          www.harpercollins.com
Translates key medical data into clear guidelines capturing the highest treatment standards for heart disease. Profiles care alternatices from supplements to stress reduction as well as treatments on the horizon.
2005 288 pages
ISBN: 0-060578-34-3
Brian Murray, President and CEO
Michael Morrison, President and Publisher

4855 Heart Disease
Franklin Watts Grolier
90 Old Sherman Turnpike   203-797-3500
Danbury, CT 06816-0001   800-621-1115
                                          Fax: 203-797-3197
                                              www.grolier.com
Using diagrams, this book discusses strokes and other blood vessel disorders, as well as their treatment and prevention.
112 pages Grades 7-12
ISBN: 0-531108-84-8
Debbie Fields, Executive Director

4856 Heart of a Child: What Families Need to Know About Heart Disorders
Johnss Hopkins University Press
2715 N Charles Street   410-935-6900
Baltimore, MD 21218-4319   800-537-5487
                                          Fax: 410-516-6968
                                              www.press.jhu.edu

1993 352 pages Paperback
ISBN: 0-801866-36-7
Doris Farrelly, Contact

4857 Living with Heart Disease
Franklin Watts Grolier
90 Old Sherman Turnpike   203-797-3500
Danbury, CT 06816-0001   800-621-1115
                                          Fax: 203-797-3197
                                              www.grolier.com

Shows how persons with heart disease can overcome their illness and lead productive lives.
32 pages Grades 5-7
ISBN: 0-531108-45-7
Dory Kranz, Executive Director
Pip Marks, Director Outreach Services

4858 Mitral Valve Prolapse Syndrome/Dysautonomia Survival Guide
Society of Mitral Valve Prolapse Syndrome
PO Box 431   630-250-9327
Itasca, IL 60143-0431   Fax: 630-773-0478
e-mail: bonnie0107@aol.com
www.mitralvalveprolapse.com
Provides support and education to patients, families and friends about mitral valve prolapse syndrome.
175 pages
ISBN: 1-572243-03-1

4859 What Every Woman Must Know About Heart Disease
Warner Books
1271 Ave of the Americas   212-484-2900
New York, NY 10020-1300   Fax: 818-507-5596
e-mail: nylandimmunojobs@boxter.com
www.twbookmark.com

1996
ISBN: 0-446519-86-3

4860 Women Take Heart
Putnam Publishing Group
1380 112th Ave NE   425-456-8700
Bellevue, WA 98004-3903   Fax: 425-456-8701
www.hopeheart.org

1993 224 pages
ISBN: 0-399138-88-9
Cherie Skager, Executive Director
Carol Coughlin, Manager of Development Operations

4861 Women and Heart Disease
Random House Trade Books
400 Hahn Road   301-592-8573
Bethesda, MD 20824-4663   800-733-3000
Fax: 800-659-2436
www.nhlbi.nih.gov

ISBN: 0-345386-20-5
Kathleen B. O'Sullivan, Executive Officer
Ariel Herman, Deputy Executive Officer

Children's Books

4862 Village by the Sea
Franklin Watts Grolier
90 Old Sherman Turnpike   203-797-3500
Danbury, CT 06816-0001   Fax: 203-797-3197
www.grolier.com
This story focuses on the relationship between Emma and her father as he prepares to undergo bypass surgery.
Grades 5-8

Newsletters

4863 American Heart Association News
American Heart Association
7272 Greenville Avenue   214-706-1162
Dallas, TX 75231-5129   800-242-8721
Fax: 214-696-5211
www.heart.org
News reports and journal reports on the latest information concerning heart disease.

4864 And the Beat Goes On
Society of Mitral Valve Prolapse Syndrome
PO Box 431   630-250-9327
Itasca, IL 60143-0431   Fax: 630-773-0478
e-mail: bonnie0107@aol.com
www.mitralvalveprolapse.com

Bi-monthly newsletter. Provides support and education to patients, families and friends about mitral valve prolapse syndrome.
6 pages

4865 Heartstyle
American Heart Association
7272 Greenville Avenue   214-706-1162
Dallas, TX 75231-5129   800-242-8721
Fax: 214-696-5211
www.heart.org
Reports on heart and blood vessel diseases and stroke.
Quarterly

4866 MVPS & Anxiety
Society of Mitral Valve Prolapse Syndrome
PO Box 431   630-250-9327
Itasca, IL 60143-0431   Fax: 630-773-0478
e-mail: bonnie0107@aol.com
www.mitralvalveprolapse.com

6 pages

Pamphlets

4867 About High Blood Pressure
American Heart Association
7272 Greenville Avenue   214-706-1162
Dallas, TX 75231-5129   800-242-8721
Fax: 214-696-5211
www.heart.org
Offers information on what blood pressure is, risk factors and at risk persons.

4868 American Heart Association Diet
American Heart Association
7272 Greenville Avenue   214-706-1162
Dallas, TX 75231-5129   800-242-8721
Fax: 214-696-5211
www.heart.org
An eating plan for healthy americans.

4869 Cholesterol and Your Heart
American Heart Association
7272 Greenville Avenue   214-706-1162
Dallas, TX 75231-5129   800-242-8721
Fax: 214-696-5211
www.heart.org
Offers information on lowering blood cholesterol levels.

4870 Congenital Heart Defects
March of Dimes
1275 Mamaroneck Avenue   914-997-4488
White Plains, NY 10605   Fax: 212-254-3518
e-mail: NY639@marchofdimes.com
www.marchofdimes.com

4871 E is for Exercise
American Heart Association
7272 Greenville Avenue   214-706-1162
Dallas, TX 75231-5129   800-242-8721
Fax: 214-696-5211
www.heart.org
Offers information on what kinds of exercise are the best and how to exercise properly.

4872 Easy Food Tips for Heart Healthy Eating
American Heart Association
7272 Greenville Avenue   214-706-1162
Dallas, TX 75231-5129   800-242-8721
Fax: 214-696-5211
www.heart.org
Offers food selection hints for fat-controlled meals.

4873 Eat Well, But Wisely
American Heart Association
7272 Greenville Avenue   214-706-1162
Dallas, TX 75231-5129   800-242-8721
Fax: 214-696-5211
www.heart.org
Offers information on good nutrition to reduce the risks of heat attacks.

4874 Exercise and Your Heart
American Heart Association
7272 Greenville Avenue
Dallas, TX 75231-5129
214-706-1162
800-242-8721
Fax: 214-696-5211
www.heart.org

Offers information on how to get enough exercise from daily activities, what the benefits of exercise are and what the risks of exercising are.

4875 Heart Defects
Association of Birth Defect Children
7272 Greenville Avenue
Dallas, TX 75231-5603
800-242-8721
www.heart.org

Informational sheet on the causes, symptoms and statistics of heart defects and heart disease in children.

4876 How to Have Your Cake and Eat It Too
American Heart Association
7272 Greenville Avenue
Dallas, TX 75231-5129
214-706-1162
800-242-8721
Fax: 214-696-5211
www.heart.org

A guide to low-fat, low-cholesterol eating.

Web Sites

4877 American Heart Association
www.americanheart.org

Supports research, education and community service programs with the objective of reducing premature death and disability from cardiovascular diseases and stroke; coordinates the efforts of health professionals, and other engaged in the fight against heart and circulatory disease.

4878 Healing Well
www.healingwell.com

An online health resource guide to medical news, chat, information and articles, newsgroups and message boards, books, disease-related web sites, medical directories, and more for patients, friends, and family coping with disabling diseases, disorders, or chronic illnesses.

4879 Health Finder
www.healthfinder.gov

Searchable, carefully developed web site offering information on over 1000 topics. Developed by the US Department of Health and Human Services, the site can be used in both English and Spanish.

4880 Healthlink USA
www.healthlinkusa.com

Health information concerning treatment, cures, prevention, diagnosis, risk factors, research, support groups, email lists, personal stories and much more. Updated regularly.

4881 Helios Health
www.helioshealth.com

Online resource for your health information. Detailed information about specific health topics, access to expert advice from our Medical Advisory Board, and up-to-date health news.

4882 MedicineNet
www.medicinenet.com

An online resource for consumers providing easy-to-read, authoritative medical and health information.

4883 Medscape
www.medscape.com

Medscape offers specialists, primary care physicians, and other health professionals the Web's most robust and integrated medical information and educational tools.

4884 National Heart, Lung and Blood Institute
www.nhlbi.nih.gov

Primary responsibility of this organization is the scientific investigation of heart, blood vessel, lung and blood disorders. Oversees research, demonstration, prevention, education, control and training activities in these fields and emphasizes the prevention and control of heart diseases.

4885 WebMD
www.webmd.com

Provides credible information, supportive communities, and in-depth reference material about health subjects. A source for original and timely health information as well as material from well known content providers.

Description

4886 Hemophilia

Hemophilia is a genetic disorder that disrupts the body's normal blood clotting function because there is a deficiency of specific proteins known as clotting factors—specifically, factor VIII and factor IX. About 20,000 Americans are affected with the disorder and, currently, there is no cure.

Hemophilia is linked to the X-chromosome because that is where both factor genes are located. As a result, hemophilia affects males almost exclusively, with females being carriers, whose sons have a 50 percent chance of having the disorder.

Hemophiliacs, like anyone else, will bleed if injured, but they will bleed longer and more profusely. They may also bleed in response to injuries that are inconsequential in other people. For instance, normal daily activities may cause bleeding within a joint, leading to severe pain and swelling, and over time destroying the joint.

The severity of hemophilia varies dramatically depending on the factor VIII and IX levels, thus, affecting a person's prognosis and need for therapy. Treatment is with transfusions of the appropriate factor, and usually has to be repeated frequently. Most hemophiliacs treated with plasma concentrate in the early 1980s are infected with HIV contracted from contaminated blood and transfusions. HIV is now responsible for over half of deaths among hemophiliacs.

Most hemophiliacs are now treated at comprehensive hemophilia centers, which offer not just factor replacement but multispecialty expertise, sophisticated laboratory testing, physical therapy and psychological support. New techniques allow for identification of carrier females in these families. This is important for genetic counseling and family planning.

National Agencies & Associations

4887 American Red Cross Blood Services

2025 E Street, NW
Washington, DC 20006
202-303-5214
800-733-2767
e-mail: lkeefe@arlingtonredcross.org
www.redcross.org

Distributes a wide variety of plasma therapeutics to benefit people with hemophilia A and B, immune disorders and hypoalbuminemia.
Bonnie McElveen Hunter, Chairman of the Board
Gail J McGovern, President & CEO

4888 Baxter Hyland Division

One Baxter Parkway
Deerfield, IL 60015-1900
224-948-2000
800-422-9837
Fax: 800-568-5020
www.baxter.com

Government affairs office that monitors and selectively lobbies on issues relating to Medicare Medicaid Orphan Drugs and other subjects relating to hemophilia.
Robert L Parkinson, Jr, Chairman of the Board & CEO
David P Scharf, Corporate Vice President and General Cou

4889 Canadian Hemophilia Society

400-1255 University Street
Montreal, Quebec, H3B3B-3B6
514-848-0503
800-668-2686
Fax: 514-848-9661
e-mail: chs@hemophilia.ca
www.hemophilia.ca

Strives to improve the health and quality of life for all people with inherited bleeding disorders and to find a cure.
Craig Upshaw, President
David Page, National Executive Director

4890 Hemophilia Health Services

201 Great Circle Road
Nashville, TN 37228
615-352-2500
866-712-5200
Fax: 800-330-0756
e-mail: info@hemophiliahealth.com
www.hemophiliahealth.com

Largest homecare company devoted solely to serving people with bleeding disorders.
Ken Trader, VP of Sales and Marketing

4891 National Hemophilia Foundation

116 W 32nd Street
New York, NY 10001
212-328-3700
800-424-2634
Fax: 212-328-3777
e-mail: info@hemophilia.org
www.hemophilia.org

Dedicated to the treatment and the cure of hemophilia, related bleeding disorders and complications of those disorders or their treatment, including HIV infection, as well as improving the quality of life of all those affected.
Jorge de la Riva, Chair
Val Bias, Chief Executive Officer

4892 World Federation of Hemophilia

1425, boul. Ren,-L,vesque
Montreal, H3G1T-1T7
514-875-7944
Fax: 514-875-8916
e-mail: wfh@wfh.org
www.wfh.org

An international not-for-profit organization to improving the lives of people with hemophilia and related bleeding disorders.
John E Bournas, CEO/Executive Director
Elizabeth Myles, Chief Operating Officer

State Agencies & Associations

Alabama

4893 Hemophilia and Bleeding Disorders of Alaba ma, Inc.

151 Market Place
Montgomery, AL 36117-1640
334-277-9446
855-469-4232
Fax: 334-272-9167
www.hbda.us/

Brian Ward, Chairman
Vicki Jackson, Executive Director

Arkansas

4894 Hemophilia Foundation of Arkansas

351 Valley Oak Lane
Austin, AR 72007
501-941-3109
888-941-4366
e-mail: angieclark1315@sbcglobal.net
www.hemophilia.org

Angie Clark, President
John Little, VP

California

4895 Central California Chapter of the National Hemophilia Foundation

PO Box 163689
Sacramento, CA 95816
916-448-0370
Fax: 916-489-1569
e-mail: cchfsac@yahoo.com
www.cchfsac.org

A very small and family-oriented chapter. Offers an active youth group, an annual summer camp, a men's and women's group and

various family activities for persons living in the central California valley from its center in Sacramento to the borders of Nevada.
Sean Hubbert, President
Tracey Huntington, Vice-President

4896   Hemophilia Association of San Diego County
3550 Camino Del Rio North
San Diego, CA 92108
619-325-3570
Fax: 619-325-4350
e-mail: info@hasdc.org
www.hasdc.org
Provides summer camp programs for young persons with hemophilia, sponsors educational programs for the general public, sponsors support groups for parents to help them deal with hemophilia, monitors legislation pertaining to hemophilia and related conditions.
Mike Brown, Board President
Melissa Pregill, Executive Director

4897   Hemophilia Foundation of Northern California
6400 Hollis Street
Emeryville, CA 94608-3024
510-658-3324
Fax: 510-658-3384
e-mail: merlin.wedepohl@hemofoundation.org
www.hemofoundation.org
A volunteer, nonprofit organization serving the needs of people with hemophilia and other related bleeding disorders in 35 counties in Northern California. Provides hemophilia literature, scholarships, youth programs and annual summer camps.
Merlin Wedepohl, Executive Director
Nancy Trunzo, Office Manager and Walk Manager

4898   Hemophilia Foundation of Southern California
6720 Melrose Avenue
Hollywood, CA 90038
323-525-0440
800-371-4123
Fax: 323-525-0445
e-mail: hfsc@hemosocal.org
www.hemosocal.org

Tamara Kato, President
Linda Corrente, Executive Director

Colorado

4899   Colorado Chapter National Hemophilila Foun dation
2465 Sheridan Blvd
Edgewater, CO 80214
720-626-1263
88 - 7 - 02
e-mail: info@cohemo.org
www.cohemo.org

Amy Board, Executive Director

Florida

4900   Florida Hemophilia Association
915 Middle River Drive
Ft Lauderdale, FL 33304
813-367-0050
888-880-8330
Fax: 813-367-0051
e-mail: dadamkin@floridahemophilia.org
www.floridahemophilia.org

Barbie Arrebola, President
Debbi Adamkin, Executive Director

Georgia

4901   Hemophilia Foundation of Georgia
8800 Roswelll Road
Atlanta, GA 30350
770-518-8272
Fax: 770-518-3310
e-mail: mail@hog.org
www.hog.org
Established to help Georgia residents with hemophilia lead normal and productive lives. Because this organization is comprised of patients, their friends and families, it is especially motivated to provide the best in personalized and comprehensive services.
Patricia Dominic, CEO
Andrew Maurer, Chief Governance Officer

Hawaii

4902   Hemophilia Foundation of Hawaii Kapiolani Medical Center
Kapiolani Medical Center

45-1031B. Wailele Road
Kaneohe, HI 96744
808-782-5506
Fax: 808-638-2910
e-mail: hawaiihemophiliafoundation@hotmail.com
www.hawaiihemo.org/
Cinda Hueu, President
Jennifer Chun, Executive Director

Idaho

4903   Hemophilia Foundation of Idaho
4696 Overland Road
Boise, ID 83705-1622
208-344-4476
866-453-4476
Fax: 208-344-4476
e-mail: tmagrini@hemophilia.org
www.idahoblood.org/
Shane Bell, President
Taryn Magrini, Executive Director

Illinois

4904   Hemophilia Foundation of Illinois
332 S. Michigan Avenue
Chicago, IL 60604
312-427-1495
Fax: 312-427-1602
e-mail: brobinson.hfi@mindspring.com
www.hemophiliaillinois.org
Serves as an information source referral service and advocate for persons with hemophilia and their families. The mission of this chapter is to provide counseling, educational information and support services to persons affected by hemophilia and related disorders.
Mike Toohey, President
Robert P Robinson, Executive Director

Indiana

4905   Hemophilia Foundation of Indiana
5172 E 65th Street
Indianapolis, IN 46220
317-570-0039
800-241-2873
Fax: 317-570-0058
e-mail: cfeay@hoii.org
www.hemophiliaofindiana.org
Scott Ehnes, Executive Director
Briana Vieke, Program Director

Kentucky

4906   Kentucky Hemophilia Foundation
1850 Taylor Avenue
Louisville, KY 40213
502-456-3233
800-582-2873
Fax: 502-456-3234
e-mail: info@kyhemo.org
www.kyhemo.org
Assists individuals with hemophilia and related inherited bleeding disorders through education, advocacy and support services. Services include quarterly newsletter, post secondary education scholarship, summer camp for children, seminars and support functions.
Quarterly
Eric Marcum, President
Ursela Lacer, Executive Director

Louisiana

4907   Louisiana Chapter of the National Hemophilia Foundation
3636 S Sherwood Forest
Baton Rouge, LA 70816-2285
225-291-1675
800-749-1680
Fax: 225-291-1679
e-mail: contact@lahemo.org
www.lahemo.org/
Lori Keels, Executive Director
Edgar Guedry, President

Maryland

4908 Hemophilia Foundation of Maryland
13 Class Court
Parkville, MD 21234-2602
410-661-2307
800-964-3131
Fax: 410-661-2308
e-mail: Miller8043@comcast.net
www.hfmonline.org

The Hemophilia foundation of Maryland is a private not for profit organization which devotes its efforts to improving the quality of life for persons affected with bleeding disorders and their complications.
Harvey Gates, President
Emma Miller-Clark, Executive Director

Massachusetts

4909 New England Hemophilia Association
347 Washington Street
Dedham, MA 02026
781-326-7645
Fax: 781-329-5122
e-mail: info@newenglandhemophilia.org
www.newenglandhemophilia.org

New England Hemophilia Association is dedicated to improving the quality of life for persons with bleeding disorders (hemophilia, von Willebrands, and other factor deficiencies) and their families through education, support and advocacy.
Patrick Mancini, President
Kevin R Sorge, Executive Director

Michigan

4910 Hemophilia Foundation of Michigan
1921 W Michigan Avenue
Ypsilanti, MI 48197
734-544-0015
800-482-3041
Fax: 734-544-0095
e-mail: hfm@hfmich.org
www.hfmich.org

Coordinates funding, professional education, and networking, with Hemophilia Treatment Centers in Michigan, Indiana, and Ohio. Provides educational services, including workshops, meetings, symposiums, and numerous publications.
Carrie Reaume, Executive Director
Suzanne Kapica, Regional Coordinator

Minnesota

4911 Hemophilia Foundation of Minnesota and the Dakotas
750 S Plaza Drive
Mendota Heights, MN 55120
651-406-8655
Fax: 651-406-8656
e-mail: hemophiliafound@visi.com
www.hfmd.org

A nonprofit organization established to be a leader and a catalyst within the community to enable and inspire members to impact their own lives, with the ultimate aim of cures for both hemophilia and HIV/AIDS.
John Schulte, President/Board of Directors
James Paist, Executive Director

Mississippi

4912 Mississippi Hemophilia Foundation
PO Box 13608
Jackson, MS 39236
601-957-2706
e-mail: haleyjones80@yahoo.com
www.mshemophilia.com/

Haley Jones, President
Leslee Loden, Vice-President

Missouri

4913 Gateway Hemophilia Association
14248 F Manchester Road
Manchester, MO 63011
314-482-5973
877-623-8300
Fax: 314-729-7033
e-mail: NicFahey@gatewayhemophilia.org
www.gatewayhemophilia.org

Nic Fahey, President
Bridget Tyrey, Executive Director

Nebraska

4914 Nebraska Chapter of the National Hemophilia Foundation
215 Centennial Mall S
Lincoln, NE 68508
402-742-5663
Fax: 402-742-5677
e-mail: office@nebraskanhf.org
www.nebraskanhf.org

The mission of this chapter is to provide support, education, communication and advocacy for men, women and children challenged by Hemophilia. Services provided include a toll free telephone hotline for persons seeking information on HIV and hemophilia.
Jason Everts, President
Kristi Harvey-Simi, Executive Director

Nevada

4915 Hemophilia Foundation of Nevada
7473 W. Lake Mead Blvd.
Las Vegas, NV 89128
702-564-4368
Fax: 702-446-8134
e-mail: Info@hfnv.org
www.hfnv.org

Dennis Flynn, President Executive Committee
Kelli Walters, Executive Director

New Mexico

4916 Hemophilia Foundation of New Mexico
PO Box 51494
Albuquerque, NM 87181
505-341-9321
866-341-9321
Fax: 505-292-5818
e-mail: sangredeoro@comcast.net
www.hemophilia.org

Lori Long, President
Loretta Cordova, Executive Director

New York

4917 Hemophilia Center of Western New York
936 Delaware Ave
Buffalo, NY 14209
716-896-2470
866-434-6551
Fax: 716-218-4010
e-mail: info@hemophiliawny.com
www.hemophiliawny.com

Robert Long, Chairman
Thomas Long, President

4918 National Hemophilia Foundation: Mary M. Gooley Hemophilia Center
1415 Portland Avenue
Rochester, NY 14621
585-922-5700
Fax: 585-922-5775
e-mail: robert.fox@rochestergeneral.org
www.hemocenter.org

Robert Fox, CEO/ President
Linda Magliocco, Senior Vice President

North Carolina

4919 Hemophilia Foundation of North Carolina
260 Town Hall Dr.
Morrisville, NC 27560
919-319-0014
800-990-5557
Fax: 919-319-0016
e-mail: info@hemophilia-nc.org
www.hemophilia-nc.org

A nonprofit organization that serves as an information source for the hemophilia community of North Carolina. Supply the most up-to-date information concerning hemophilia and hemophilia related HIV/AIDS.
Steven Peretti, PhD, President
Leonard Poe, Vice President & Advocacy Chair

Ohio

4920 Central Ohio Chapter of the National Hemophilia Foundation
200 E. Campus View Blvd
Columbus, OH 43235-0345
614-985-3752
800-847-0345
Fax: 614-985-3601
e-mail: ralexander@hemophilia.org
www.nhfcentralohio.org

Jeff Stewart, President
Rob Alexander, Executive Director

4921 Northern Ohio Chapter of the National Hemophilia Foundation
One Independence Place
5000 Rockside Road
Independence, OH 44131
216-834-0051
800-554-HEMO
Fax: 216-834-0055
e-mail: jtooley@nohf.org
www.nohf.org

Marlene Piatak, President
Janet Tooley, Executive Director

4922 Northwest Ohio Hemophilia Association
2121 Hughes Drive
Toledo, OH 43606
419-291-5882
Fax: 419-479-3269
e-mail: carla@nwohemophilia.org
www.nwohemophilia.org/

Jim Knepp, President
Carla Wells, Executive Director

4923 Southwestern Ohio Chapter of the National Hemophilia Foundation
3131 S Dixie Drive
Moraine, OH 45439
937-298-8000
Fax: 937-298-8080
e-mail: info@swohiohemophilia.org
www.swohiohemophilia.org

This chapter serves persons with hemophilia and blood clotting disorders in an 11 county area. It is dedicated to offering people with hemophilia and related blood disorders and their families educational opportunities about the diseases.
Dena Shepard, President
John Gale, Executive Director

Oklahoma

4924 Oklahoma Chapter of the National Hemophilia Foundation
720 W. Wilshire Blvd
Oklahoma City, OK 73116
405-463-6634
800-735-3855
e-mail: tayers@okhemophilia.org
www.okhemophilia.org

Tom Ayers, President
Bob Goodley, Executive Director

Oregon

4925 Hemophilia Foundation of Oregon
10940 SW Barnes Rd #129
Portland, OR 97225
503-297-7207
Fax: 503-297-0127
e-mail: info@hemophiliaoregon.org
www.hemophiliaoregon.org/

Jeremy Swanlund, President
Marita Postma, Executive Director

Pennsylvania

4926 Delaware Valley Chapter of the National Hemophilia Foundation
14 E. 6th Street
Lansdale, PA 19446
215-393-3611
Fax: 215-393-9419
e-mail: hemophilia@navpoint.com
www.hemophiliasupport.org

Thomas Galvin, President
William Widerman, Vice-President

4927 Western Pennsylvania Chapter of the National Hemophilia Foundation
20411 Rt. 19
Cranberry Township, PA 16066
724-741-6160
800-824-0016
Fax: 724-741-6167
e-mail: info@westpennhemophilia.org
www.westpennhemophilia.org

Brings together and serves as a focal point for those segments of the community most concerned with hemophilia. They include medical and social service providers, people with hemophilia and their families educators and the general public.
Scott E Miller, President
Nathan Rost, Vice-President

Rhode Island

4928 Rhode Island Hemophilia Foundation
347 Washington Street
Dedham, MA 02026
781-326-7645
Fax: 781-329-5122
e-mail: info@newenglandhemophilia.org
www.newenglandhemophilia.org

Patrick Mancini, President
Kevin R Sorge, Executive Director

South Carolina

4929 Hemophilia Association of South Carolina
PO Box 3874
Sumter, SC 29151
864-350-9941
888-829-4849
e-mail: information@hemophiliaofsouthcarolina.ne
www.hemophiliaofsouthcarolina.net/

Sue Martin, President

Tennessee

4930 Tennessee Hemophilia & Bleeding Disorder Foundation
1819 Ward Drive
Murfreesboro, TN 37129-5281
615-900-1486
888-703-3269
Fax: 615-900-1487
e-mail: mary@thbdf.org
www.thbdf.org

Offers a hemophilia clinic, social workers and consultants, a state hemophilia program, blood donor programs, counseling programs, genetic counseling, literature and resources, summer camp, grants, and more for the hemophilia and HIV/AIDS community.
Kent Russ, President
Mary Hord, Executive Director

Texas

4931 Lone Star Chapter of the National Hemophilia Foundation
10500 NW Freeway
Houston, TX 77092
713-686-6100
888-LSC-NHF1
Fax: 832-383-4601
e-mail: Debbiedelariva@yahoo.com
www.lonestarhemophilia.org

Nick Zasowski, President

4932 Texas Central Chapter of the National Hemophilia Foundation
12700 Hillcrest Road
Dallas, TX 75230
972-386-3865
Fax: 214-654-9954
e-mail: mail@texcen.org
www.texcen.org

A group of volunteers seeking solutions to the various aspects of the hemophilia problem. Supports blood drives sponsors a summer camp for hemophiliac children, conducts educational member meetings, arranges for genetic counseling and sponsors group support meetings.
Shannon Brush, President
Brendan Hayes, Executive Director

Utah

4933 Utah Chapter of the National Hemophilia Foundation
772 E 3300 S
Salt Lake City, UT 84106
801-484-0325
877-463-6893
Fax: 801-746-2488
www.hemophiliautah.org

Offers educational information, pamphlets, fundraising events and more for persons and families affected by hemophilia.
Reg Ecker, President
Scott Muir, Executive Director

Virginia

4934 Hemophilia Association of the Capital Area
10560 Main Street
Fairfax, VA 22030-1504
703-352-7641
Fax: 540-427-6589
e-mail: admin@HACAcares.org
www.hacacares.org
A nonprofit organization serving persons with bleeding disorders and their families in northern Virginia Washington DC and Montgomery and Prince George's Counties in Maryland. This chapter's mission is to improve the quality of life for persons with hemophilia.
Miriam Goldstein, President
Karen Krzmarzick, Executive Director

4935 United Virginia Chapter of the National Hemophilia Foundation
PO Box 188
Midlothian, VA 23113-8824
804-748-7896
800-266-8438
Fax: 800-266-8438
e-mail: info@vahemophilia.org
www.vahemophilia.org

Kelly Waters, Executive Director
Heather Conner, Administrative Assistant

Washington

4936 Bleeding Disorder Foundation of Washington
9639 Firdale Avenue
Edmonds, WA 98020
206-533-1660
Fax: 206-533-1686
e-mail: general@bdfwa.org
www.bdfwa.org

Caprice Sauter, President
Stephanie Simpson, Executive Director

4937 Inland Empire Bleeding Disorders
1010 Riverside Drive
W Richland, WA 99353
509-967-7417
866-710-4323
e-mail: iebd4u@verizon.net
www.hemophilia.org

Debbie Campeau, President
Jill McCary, President

Wisconsin

4938 Great Lakes Hemophilia Foundation
638 N 18th Street
Milwaukee, WI 53233
414-257-0200
888-797-GLHF
Fax: 414-257-1225
e-mail: info@glhf.org
www.glhf.org
The only Wisconsin organization that addresses the physical, emotional social and financial needs of individuals affected by hemophilia. This chapter supports high-quality cost-effective programs for patient care, education, research and public awareness.
Bill Finn, President
Danielle Leitner Baxter, Executive Director

Foundations

4939 National Hemophilia Foundation
116 West 32nd Street
New York, NY 10001
212-328-3700
800-424-2634
Fax: 212-328-3777
e-mail: info@hemophilia.org
www.hemophilia.org
The National Hemophilia Foundation is dedicated to finding better treatments and cures for bleeding and clotting disorders and to preventing the complications of these disorders through education, advocacy and research.
Jorge de la Riva, Chair
Val Bias, Chief Executive Officer

Research Centers

4940 Albany Medican Center
43 New Scotland Avenue
Albany, NY 12208-3479
518-262-3125
800-773-7080
Fax: 518-262-6320
e-mail: albanyhtc@mail.amc.edu
www.amc.edu
Providing excellence in medical education biomedical research and patient care.
Joanne Faunce, President

4941 Albert Einstein Medical Center Hemophilia Program
5501 Old York Road
Philadelphia, PA 19141
215-456-7890
Fax: 215-456-6179
www.einstein.edu
With humanity humility and honor to heal by providing exceptionally intelligent and responsive healthcare and education for as many as we can reach
Barry R Freedman, CEO/ President
John Finger, Chief Administrative Officer

4942 American Red Cross Hemophilia Center
2025 E Street, NW
Washington, DC 20006-0905
202-303-5214
800-733-2767
Fax: 608-233-8318
www.redcross.org

Greg Mandell, CEO
Sandra Fenwick, President

4943 Boston Hemophilia Center Fegan 5 Children's Hospital
Fegan 5 Children's Hospital
300 Longwood Avenue
Boston, MA 02115
617-355-6000
800-355-7944
Fax: 617-730-0152
TTY: 617-730-0152
www.childrenshospital.org
The program offers comprehensive care to people with hemophilia and their families. Our services range from medical treatment counseling and support to discounts on clotting-factor replacement and other products that people with hemophilia require.
Dr James Mandell, CEO
Sandra Fenwick, President

4944 Bowman Grey School of Medicine: Hemophilia Diagnostic Center
Wake Forest University
Department of Pediatrics
Winston Salem, NC 27157-0001
919-716-4324
Fax: 910-716-7100
Christine A MD, Director
Michael Fisher, CEO

4945 Children's Hospital Hemophilia Treatment Center
3333 Burnet Avenue
Cincinnati, OH 45229
513-636-4200
800-344-2462
Fax: 513-636-5599
TTY: 513-636-4900
www.cincinnatichildrens.org
Cincinnati Children's will improve child health and transform delivery of care through fully integrated globally recognized research education and innovation.
Ralph Gruppo Cohen MD, Medical Director

4946 Childrens Hospital of Philadelphia Hemophilia Program
Division of Hematology
34th Street and Civic Center Boulev
Philadelphia, PA 19104
215-590-3437
800-879-2467
Fax: 215-903-92
www.chop.edu
The Children's Hospital of Philadelphia the oldest hospital in the United States dedicated exclusively to pediatrics strives to be the world leader in the advancement of healthcare for children by integrating excellent patient care innovative research and quality professional education into all of its programs.
Leslie J Raffini, Physician
Char Witmer, Physician

4947 Christus Santa Rosa Health System
Children's Hospital

333 N Santa Rosa Street
San Antonio, TX 78207-3108
210-704-2011
877-ALL-KIDZ
Fax: 210-704-2396
www.christussantarosa.org
Patrick Carrier, Presidnet, CEO

4948   Comprehensive Hemophilia Diagnostic and Treatment Center
University of North Carolina
101 Manning Drive
Chapel Hill, NC 27514
919-966-4131
Fax: 919-966-3036
e-mail: lccc@med.unc.edu
www.unchealthcare.org
Multidisciplinary clinics are dedicated to patients with hemophilia (through the Comprehensive Hemophilia Diagnostic and Treatment Center) sickle cell disease brain tumors late effects of anticancer therapy as well as general hematology/oncology.
William RN

4949   Comprehensive Pediatric Hemophilia Center University of South Florida
University of South Florida
450 W Drive
Tampa, FL 33612-4742
813-974-2201
Sara Griggs Kirschke

4950   Eastern Michigan Hemophilia Center St. Joseph Hospital
St. Joseph Hospital
302 Kensington Avenue
Flint, MI 48503-2044
810-762-8656
Leslie RN

4951   Eau Claire Hemophilia Center
900 W Clairemont Avenue
Eau Claire, WI 54701
715-839-4418
Fax: 715-833-4976
Vicky Anders RN, Program Manager

4952   Fairview-University Hemophilia & Thrombosis Center
Harvard Street at E River Road
Minneapolis, MN 55455
612-626-6455
800-688-5252
Fax: 612-625-4955
Serves over 700 adults and children in Minnesota with inherited bleeding disorders. Offers access to current technologies and treatments. Special programs include patient support group family retreats and camps.
Linda Swanso Macfarlane, Director

4953   Great Plains Regional Hemophilia Center University of Iowa Hospitals
University of Iowa Hospitals
200 Howkins Drive
Iowa City, IA 52242
319-384-8442
800-777-8442
Fax: 319-567-59
www.uiowa.edu

Donald E Fahner MD

4954   Greater Grand Rapids Pediatric Hemophilia Program
DeVos at Spectrum Health Systems
100 Michigan NE
Grand Rapids, MI 49503
616-391-2033
James B Trujillo, Financial Administer
W Hoots, Medical Director

4955   Gulf States Hemophilia Diagnostic and Treatment Center
University of Texas Health Science Center Houston
6655 Travis Street
Houston, TX 77030-3005
713-500-8360
800-464-1440
Fax: 713-500-8364
www.livingwithhaemophilia.com
Marisela Thompson, Chief Executive Officer
Joan Curran, Chief Government Relations and External

4956   Gundersen Clinic Comprehensive Hemophilia Treatment Center
Gundersen Clinic
1900 S Avenue
LaCrosse, WI 54601
608-782-7300
800-362-9567
Fax: 608-775-6692
e-mail: info@GundLuth.org
www.gundersenhealth.org/
Jeffrey E Thompson, Chief Executive Officer
Julio Bird, Executive Vice President

4957   Hematology Treatment Center of the Great Lakes Hemophilia Foundation
638 North 18th Street
Milwaukee, WI 53233-2178
414-257-0200
888-797-GLHF
Fax: 414-257-1225
e-mail: info@glhf.org
www.glhf.org
Bill Finn, President
Danielle Leitner Baxter, Executive Director

4958   Hemophilia Association of the Huntington Area
Marshall University School of Medicine
1600 Medical Center Drive
Huntington, WV 25703-1518
304-691-1384
877-691-1600
Fax: 304-691-1375
McKowen, Dean, Vice President
Andrew Tendleton, Medical Director

4959   Hemophilia Center of Central Pennsylvania Penn State Milton S Hershey Medical Cent
Penn State Milton S Hershey Medical Center
500 University Drive
Hershey, PA 17033
717-531-8521
800-243-1455
Fax: 717-310-4021
TTY: 717-531-4395
www.pennstatehershey.org/
Harold L Paz, Chief Executive Officer
Alan L Brechbill, Executive Director

4960   Hemophilia Center of Rhode Island Rhode Island Hospital
Rhode Island Hospital
593 Eddy Street
Providence, RI 02903
401-444-5184
Fax: 401-444-5017
www.rirad.org
Brian Stainken, President
Terrance Healey, Vice-President

4961   Hemophilia Center of West Virginia University Health Sciences Center
University Health Sciences Center
Medical Center Drive
Morgantown, WV 26506
304-293-4229
Fax: 304-293-3793
John S Holmberg, Executive Director
Thomas Long, President

4962   Hemophilia Center of Western New York Erie County Medical Center
Erie County Medical Center
936 Delaware Ave
Buffalo, NY 14209-3021
716-896-2470
866-434-6551
Fax: 716-218-4010
www.hemophiliawny.com
The center provides a variety of services to the hemophilia and HIV/AIDS community. Included among these services are diagnostics registration outpatient treatment home care programs home visits school visits dental services and counseling services. Offers an adult unit and a pediatric unit.
Robert Long, Chairman
Thomas Long, President

4963   Hemophilia Center of the Huntington Hospital
100 W California Boulevard
Pasadena, CA 91105-3023
626-397-5000
www.huntingtonhospital.com
At Huntington our mission is to excel at the delivery of health care to our community.
Stephen Ralph, President and Chief Executive Officer
Jim Noble, Executive Vice President, COO and CFO

4964   Hemophilia Clinic: Childrens' Rehabilitation Service
1870 Pleasant Avenue
Mobile, AL 36617
334-479-8617
800-879-8163
Fax: 334-450-5037
e-mail: djackson@rehab.state.al.us
www.hemophilia.org
Dianna Jackson

4965   Hemophilia Treatment Center at Children's National Medical Center
Department of Hematology/Oncology

111 Michigan Avenue NW
Washington, DC 20010

202-884-3622
Fax: 202-884-2976
www.livingwithhaemophilia.com

Gordon L Cowen, President

4966 Los Angeles Orthopaedic Hospital
2400 S Flower Street
Los Angeles, CA 90007-2629

213-742-1000
Fax: 213-742-1103
e-mail: info@laoh.ucla.edu
www.orthohospital.org

Anthony A Scaduto, M.D, Presidnent, CEO

4967 Louisiana Comprehensive Hemophilia Care Center
1430 Tulane Avenue
New Orleans, LA 70112-2699

504-988-5433
Fax: 504-883-08
e-mail: cleissi@tulane.edu
tulane.edu

Cindy Leissinger, MD, Chief

4968 Maine Hemophilia Treatment Center
19 Bramhall Street
Portland, ME 04102

207-885-7683
Fax: 207-885-7565

Nancy Roy Langstraat, Director

4969 Mayo Comprehensive Hemophilia Center Mayo Clinic
Mayo Clinic
200 1st Street SW
Rochester, MN 55905

507-284-2511
800-660-4582
Fax: 507-284-8286
www.mayoclinic.org/hemophilia/

A World Federation of Hemophilia-designated International Hemophilia Training Center provides multidisciplinary assessment and care of persons with bleeding disorders. Offers consultation with hemotologists specializing in the care of pediatric and adult patients a special consultation laboratory testing center and more.
Harlan ARNP

4970 Miami Comprehensive Hemophilia Center Jackson Medical Towers
Jackson Medical Towers
1500 NW
Miami, FL 33136-3609

305-243-4791
Fax: 305-324-9785

Susan Schmal MD, Head Physician

4971 Michigan State University Hemophilia Comprehensive Care Clinic
Michigan State University
2900 Hannah Boulevard
E Lansing, MI 48823

517-353-9385
800-759-5595
Fax: 517-353-9421

John Penner Gioia RN

4972 Missouri Illinois Regional Hemophilia Comprehensive Treatment Center
3635 Vista Avenue & Grand Boulevard
Saint Louis, MO 63104-1003

314-268-5275
Fax: 314-268-5104

Kathleen P Crist MD, Vice President

4973 Mountain State Regional Hemophilia Center
University of Arizona Health Sciences Center
1501 N Campbell Avenue
Tucson, AZ 85724-0001

520-626-1197
Fax: 520-626-1460
e-mail: phanthourath@ahsc.arizona.edu
www.ahsc.arizona.edu

Anoma Phanthourath, Deputy & Chief of Staff

4974 Nadeene Brunini Comprehensive Hemophilia Care Center
St Michael s Medical Center
197 Route 18 South
East Brunswick, NJ 08816-2011

732-249-6000
Fax: 732-249-7999
e-mail: hemnj@comcast.net
www.hanj.org

Hemophilia and other bleeding disorder treatment center.
Louis

4975 North Dakota Comprehensive Hemophilia Center
Roger Maris Cancer Center
820 4th Street N
Fargo, ND 58122-0001

701-234-7544
800-437-4010
Fax: 701-234-7592

A treatment center for diseases of hemotosis and thrombosis which includes a clinical research program in bleeding disorders. Hemotologists are available for consultation 24 hours a day.

4976 North Dakota Hemostasis and Thrombosis Treatment Center
Roger Maris Cancer Center
820 4th Street N
Fargo, ND 58122-0001

701-234-7544
800-437-4010
Fax: 701-234-7577
www.meritcare.com

A treatment center for diseases of hemotosis and thrombosis which includes a clinical research program in bleeding disorders. Hemotologists are available for consultation 24 hours a day.
Dr Nathan Podolsky MD, President

4977 North Texas Comprehensive Pediatric Hemophilia Center
1935 Motor Street
Dallas, TX 75235-7701

214-456-2382
Fax: 214-456-6133
www.hemophiliaregion6.org

Andrea Johns Steele, President
Ann Gilbert, Director

4978 Northwest Ohio Hemophilia Treatment Center
The Toledo Hospital
2142 N Cove Boulevard
Toledo, OH 43606-3895

419-471-2291
Fax: 412-916-01
www.toledochildrens.org

4979 Oklahoma Comprehensive Hemophilia Diagnostic Treatment Center
940 NE 13th Street
Oklahoma City, OK 73126-0307

405-271-3661
800-688-5288
Fax: 405-271-3756

Beverly Stev Kasper, Hematology
Richard W Cook, Chairman, CEO

4980 Puget Sound Blood Center
921 Terry Avenue
Seattle, WA 98104-1256

206-292-6500
800-398-7888
e-mail: schedule@psbc.org
www.psbc.org

Dr. James P AuBuchon, President, CEO
David C Fennell, Chief Operating Officer and Chief Inform

4981 Regional Hemophilia Treatment Center Children's Hospital of Michigan
Children's Hospital of Michigan
1921 W. Michigan Avenue
Ypsilanti, MI 48197-2196

734-544-0015
800-482-3041
Fax: 734-544-0095
www.hfmich.org

Carrie Reaume, Executive Director
Suzanne Kapica, Regional Coordinator

4982 Richland Memorial Comprehensive Pediatric Hemophilia Center
Children's Hospital for Cancer & Blood Disorders
7 Richland Medical Park Drive
Columbia, SC 29203

803-434-3533
Fax: 803-434-4598

Daniel Fink, Chief Executive Officer & President

4983 Riley Hemophilia & Hemophilia Center Riley Hospital for Children
Riley Hospital for Children
705 Riley Hospital Drive
Indianapolis, IN 46202-5200

317-944-5000
800-248-1199
Fax: 317-278-0616
e-mail: mheiny@iupui.edu
rileychildrenshospital.com

Jeff Sperring, MD, Presindent, CEO
Paul R Haut, MD, Chief Medical Officer

4984 SouthWestern Medical Center
University of Texas Southwestern Medical Center
5323 Harry Hines Boulevard
Dallas, TX 75390-7208

214-648-3111
www.utsouthwestern.edu

Daniel K Podolsky, MD, President
J. Gregory Fitz, MD, Executive Vice-President

4985 Southern Tier Hemophilia Center United Health Services-Wilson Hospital
United Health Services-Wilson Hospital
33-57 Harrison Street   607-763-6436
Johnson City, NY 13790   Fax: 607-763-5514
Doris Michal RN

4986 St. Joseph's Hemophilia Center
2927 N 7th Avenue   602-406-3770
Phoenix, AZ 85013-4102
Rachel Stuar MD, Director

4987 Ted R Montoya Hemophilia Program University of New Mexico
University of New Mexico
Albuquerque, NM 87131-0001   505-277-0111
                               800-225-5866
                               Fax: 505-272-6845
                               www.unm.edu

Prasad Mathe Barchi, President

4988 Tennessee Hemophilia and Bleeding Disorder Foundation
1819 Ward Drive   615-900-1486
Murfreesboro, TN 37129   888-703-3269
                               Fax: 615-900-1487
                               e-mail: mary@thbdf.org
                               www.thbdf.org

Kent Russ, President
Mary Hord, Executive Director

4989 The Vanderbilt Hemostasis Clinic
2200 Children's Way   615-936-1765
Nashville, TN 37232-9830   866-372-5663
                               Fax: 615-936-8400
                               www.mc.vanderbilt.edu/vhtc
The mission of the Vanderbilt Hemostasis-Thrombosis Clinic is to provide the highest quality compassionate care for individuals with inherited disorders of bleeding or clotting. The team emphasizes the empowerment of patients in their own care while also providing opportunities to participate in scientific advances in the diagnosis and treatment of bleeding and clotting disorders.
Anne T Neff, Director of Hemostasis Clinic
Mary G Hudson, Nurse Coordinator

4990 Thomas Jefferson University: Cardenza Foundation for Hematologic Research
1020 Walnut Street   215-955-6000
Philadelphia, PA 19107-5005   Fax: 215-955-2342
                               www.jefferson.edu

Robert L Abildgaard MD

4991 Tufts Medical Center
Tufts New England Medical Center
800 Washington Street   617-636-5000
Boston, MA 02111-1526   Fax: 617-636-7738
                               e-mail: webinfo@tuftsmedicalcenter.org
                               www.tuftsmedicalcenter.org
Comprehensive care for pediatric and young adult individuals with bleeding and prothrombotic disorders.
Eric Beyer, President and Chief Executive Officer
Michael Wagner, Chief Medical Officer

4992 UCD Northern Central California Hemophilia Program
PO Box 163689   916-448-0370
Sacramento, CA 95816-2208   Fax: 916-489-1569
                               e-mail: cchfsac@yahoo.com
                               www.cchfsac.org
An all-volunteer nonprofit organization dedicated to helping people with bleeding disorders.
Sean Hubbert, President
Tracey Huntington, Vice President

4993 UCSD Comprehensive Hemophilia Treatment Center
9500 Gilman Drive   619-471-0336
La Jolla, CA 92093   Fax: 858-822-6444
                               e-mail: kdherbst@ucsd.edu
                               hem-onc.ucsd.edu
Sanford J Shattil, M.D., Professor of Medicine
Edward Ball, MD, Professor of Medicine

4994 University Medical Center Hemophilia Program
1800 W Charleston Boulevard
Las Vegas, NV 89102-2329   702-383-2000
                               www.umcsn.com
Lawrence Weekly, Chair
Chris Giunchigliani, Vice Chair

4995 University Treatment Center of University Hospitals of Cleveland
11100 Euclid Avenue   216-844-8447
Cleveland, OH 44106   888-844-8447
                               Fax: 216-844-5431
                               www.uhhospitals.org
Thomas F Zenty III, CEO

4996 University of Cincinnati Adult Hemophilia Treatment Program
231 Bethesda Avenue   513-558-4233
Cincinnati, OH 45267-0001   Fax: 513-558-3878
Kathleen E Coleman, President

4997 University of Michigan Hemophilia Center
1500 E Medical Center Drive   734-764-1817
Ann Arbor, MI 48109   Fax: 734-635-15
                               www.umich.edu

Mary Sue Hord, Executive Director

4998 Vermont Regional Hemophilia Center
108 Cherry Street   802-863-7200
Burlington, VT 05402   800-464-4343
                               Fax: 802-865-7754
                               e-mail: vtadap@vdh.state.vt.us
                               healthvermont.gov
Provides care to persons with types of bleeding disorders. We see people from Vermont and upstate New York.
Miriam Huste Kinsaul, President, CEO
Emmett Broxson, Director Hemothology

4999 West Central Ohio Hemophilia Center Childens Medical Center
Childens Medical Center
1 Childrens Plaza   937-641-3000
Dayton, OH 45404-1815   800-228-4055
                               Fax: 937-641-5878
                               www.childrensdayton.org
The center provides complete care for individuals and families with hemophilia and related bleeding disorders. Some of the services offered include a comprehensive clinic emergency treatment network consultations diagnostic coagulation laboratory home infusion programs HIV/AIDS education and counseling and more.
Elizabeth H Ey, Chair
Deborah Feldman, President/ CEO

Support Groups & Hotlines

5000 National Health Information Center
PO Box 1133   310-565-4167
Washington, DC 20013   800-336-4797
                               Fax: 301-984-4256
                               e-mail: info@nhic.org
                               www.health.gov/nhic
Offers a nationwide information referral service, produces directories and resource guides.

Books

5001 Avoiding Indecision and Hesitation with Hemophilia-Related Emergencies
American Health Consultants
7 Penn Plaza   212-328-3700
New York, NY 10001   800-688-2421
                               Fax: 212-328-3777
                               http://www.hemophilia.org
Provides detailed information necessary for physicians, and ED staff to deal effectively and expeditiously with hemophilia emergencies.
12 pages
Neil Frick, VP for Research
John Indence, VP for Marketing & Communications

5002 Federal Medicaid Drug Program
1730 E Street NW
Washington, DC 20006-5300   202-628-9292
Discusses changes in government reimbursement and its effect on plasma derived products distributed by the American Red Cross. Includes law information, individual state billing procedures and Medicaid program coverage for the hemophilia community.

5003 Guide to Insurance Coverage for People with Hemophilia
Armour Pharmaceutical Company
820 First Street NE   202-675-6984
Washington, DC 20002-3930   800-230-9797
                                  Fax: 972-616-6211
                                  www.hemophiliafed.org
An educational guide designed to assist with health insurance concerns.
Tracy Cleghorn, President
Scott Boling, Co-Vice President

5004 Hemophilia Camp Directory
National Hemophilia Foundation
116 W 32nd Street   212-219-8180
New York, NY 10001-3212   800-424-2634
                                  Fax: 212-328-3777
                                  www.hemophilia.org
Lists camps in the United States for children with hemophilia and other coagulation disorders.
16 pages

5005 Procedure Coding for Hemophilia Treatment
Armour Pharmaceutical Company
820 First Street NE   202-675-6984
Washington, DC 20002-3930   800-230-9797
                                  Fax: 972-616-6211
                                  www.hemophiliafed.org
Educational guide designed to facilitate the appropriate use of CPT codes for the hemophilia community.
Tracy Cleghorn, President
Scott Boling, Co-Vice President

Children's Books

5006 Adventures of Maxx
Nova Factor
1620 Century Centery Pkwy   901-348-8129
Memphis, TN 38137   800-424-2634
                                  Fax: 901-385-3778
                                  legendofmaxx.com
An activity book for children with hemophilia, this publication is intended to be both educational and entertaining.
15 pages

5007 Children's Hemophilia Book
Porton Products Limited
37-39 West Main St.   978-352-7657
Georgetown, MA 01833-2006   Fax: 978-352-6254
                                  e-mail: info@kelleycom.com
                                  www.kelleycom.com
Coloring book that discusses what hemophilia is, bleeding episodes and treatment from a child's point of view.
25 pages

5008 Harold Talks About How He Inherited Hemophilia
Kentucky Hemophilia Foundation
1850 Taylor Avenue   502-456-3233
Louisville, KY 40213-1571   800-582-2873
                                  Fax: 502-634-9995
                                  e-mail: info@kyhemo.org
                                  www.kyhemo.org
Children's brochure explaining hemophilia causes, symptoms and living a regular life.

5009 Harold's Secret: A Boy with Hemophilia
Bayer
400 Morgan Lane   203-937-2765
West Haven, CT 06516-4175
A comic book for youngsters pertaining to children with hemophilia and understanding of the illness among school friends.
16 pages

5010 Understanding Hemophilia: A Young Person's Guide
Armour Pharmaceuticals Company
820 First Street NE   202-675-6984
Washington, DC 20002-3930   800-230-9797
                                  Fax: 972-616-6211
                                  www.hemophiliafed.org
This publication is designed for young persons with hemophilia. Presented in very basic and accessible language, this text with colored illustrations points out what hemophilia is, how to cope and more.
91 pages

Magazines

5011 HEMALOG
Maleria Medica
101 W 23rd Street   212-725-5151
New York, NY 10011-2490   Fax: 212-725-2794
                                  e-mail: hemalog@hotmail.com
                                  www.humalog.com
The purpose of Hemalog is to serve as a national forum for the hemophilia community, providing current news, information, opinion and contact with others in the community. The material contained in this journal reflects the experience and opinion of a wide range of people connected with hemophilia and encourages story and art contributions.
36 pages Quarterly

5012 HemAware
National Hemophilia Foundation
7 Penn Plaza   212-328-3700
New York, NY 10001-3212   800-424-2634
                                  Fax: 212-328-3777
                                  www.hemophilia.org
NHF magazine that offers treatment news about bleeding disorders and provides comprehensive articles on the latest developments in treatment and research as well as highlighting new programs and new resources in the field.
Bi-Monthly
Neil Frick, VP for Research
John Indence, VP for Marketing & Communications

5013 Human Factor
Hemophilia Health Services
410 West Lowe   641-472-4480
Fairfield, IA 52556-4206   800-800-6606
                                  Fax: 641-472-5412
                                  e-mail: hfi@humanfactors.com
                                  www.humanfactors.com
This journal is provided as a free service for the purpose of informing, educating and empowering the hemophilia community.
Quarterly
Eric Schaffer, CEO
Jay More, Global President

Newsletters

5014 Artery
Hemophilia Foundation of Michigan
1921 W. Michigan Avenue   734-544-0015
Ypsilanti, MI 48197-2973   800-482-3041
                                  Fax: 734-544-0095
                                  www.hfmich.org
Offers information on the chapter's activities and events, support groups and hotlines, technical and medical updates pertaining to the hemophilia and HIV/AIDS community.
Quarterly

5015 Big Red Factor
National Hemophilia Foundation: Nebraska
215 Centennial Mall South   402-742-5663
Lincoln, NE 68508   Fax: 402-742-5677
                                  e-mail: office@nebraskanhf.org
                                  www.nebraskanhf.org/chapter/
Chapter newsletter offering legislative and medical updates, technology, resources, assistive devices and more for persons affected by hemophilia and other blood disorders.

5016 Bloodlines
Hemophilia Association of San Diego County
3550 Camino del Rio North
San Diego, CA 92108   619-325-3570
                    Fax: 619-325-4350
                    e-mail: info@hasdc.org
                    www.hasdc.org
Updates membership on the newest techniques and technologies on the treatment of hemophilia.
Quarterly

5017 Concentrate
Hemophilia of North Carolina
2 Centerview Drive   919-852-4788
Greensboro, NC 27407-3708
Offers information on summer camps, resources, book reviews, parent information and articles pertaining to hemophilia.
Monthly

5018 Factor Nine News
Coalition for Hemophilia B
225 W 34th Street   212-628-3445
New York, NY 10122
                    Fax: 212-554-6906
                    e-mail: cfb@web-depot.com
                    www.boygenius.com/cfb
Offers information on FDA approvals, annual meetings and the latest in technology and information regarding hemophilia.

5019 Hemophilia NewsBriefs
Great Lakes Hemophilia Foundation
638 North 18th Street   414-257-0200
Milwaukee, WI 53233
                    Fax: 414-257-1225
                    e-mail: info@glhf.org
                    www.glhf.org

Bill Finn, President
Jeff Koopmeiners, Vice President

5020 Infusion
Kentuckian Hemophilia Foundation
982 Eastern Parkway   510-634-8161
Louisville, KY 40217-1571   800-582-CURE
                    Fax: 510-568-6111
                    e-mail: officeinfo@HFNonline.org
                    www.hfnconline.org
Offers information on summer camps, association activities and events, national projects touching on hemophilia and HIV related disorders and articles on the newest breakthroughs and technology for fighting bleeding disorders.
Quarterly

5021 Initiatives
Quantum Health Resources
790 The City Drive S   714-750-1610
Orange, CA 92868-4941
Aimed at keeping patients and other interested individuals informed on important economic trends, legislation and medical issues.
Quarterly

5022 Linking Factor
National Hemophila Foundation: Utah Chapter
340 E 400 S
Salt Lake City, UT 84111-2909   800-800-6606
A newsletter offering chapter association news and information.
BiMonthly

5023 New England Hemophilia Association Newsletter
347 Washington St.   781-326-7645
Dedham, MA 02026-4558   800-228-6342
                    Fax: 781-329-5122
                    e-mail: info@newenglandhemophilia.org
                    www.newenglandhemophilia.org
New England Hemophilia Association is dedicated to improving the quality of life for persons with bleeding disorders (hemophilia, von Williebrands, and other factor deficiencies) and their families through education, support and advocacy. NEHA is a chapter of the National Hemophilia Foundation.
Quarterly
Patrick Mancini, President
William McCartney, Treasurer

5024 TN Hemo & Bleeding Disorders Foundation Newsletter
TN Hemo & Bleedin Disorders Foundation
1819 Ward Drive   615-220-4868
Murfreesboro, TN 37129-5281   888-703-3269
                    Fax: 615-220-4889
                    e-mail: mary@thbdf.org
                    www.thbdf.org
3x/year
Suzie Harlan, President
Chris Cassada, Vice President

5025 Ways & Means
Quantum Health Resources
790 The City Drive S   714-750-1610
Orange, CA 92868-4941
Features pertinent health care information for hemophilia patients and their families.
Quarterly

5026 Infusion
Northern California Chapter of the NHF
7700 Edgewater Drive
Oakland, CA 94621-3023   650-568-NCHF
                    www.infusion.com
Informs members of medical, dental and orthopedic treatment advances and the latest research in the field. Helps to keep people with hemophilia and their families aware of relevant local and national meetings and includes important updates regarding research and treatment.
BiMonthly
Alim Somani, President
John Michell, Chief Operating Officer

Pamphlets

5027 Anyone Can Have a Bleeding Problem
Hemophilia Foundation of Michigan
411 Huronview Boulevard   734-761-2535
Ann Arbor, MI 48103-2973   800-482-3041
Offers information on Hemophilia and Von Willebrand's Disease. How persons can get it, prevention and causes of the illnesses.

5028 Article Reprint Exchange
HANDI-The National Hemophilia Foundation
7 Penn Plaza   212-328-3700
New York, NY 10001-3212   800-424-2634
                    Fax: 212-328-3777
                    www.hemophilia.org
Offers various reprinted articles concerning hemophilia and the newest medical technology.
Neil Frick, VP for Research
John Indence, VP for Marketing & Communications

5029 Basics of HIV Disease: Questions and Answers
National Hemophilia Foundation
7 Penn Plaza   212-328-3700
New York, NY 10001-3212   800-424-2634
                    Fax: 212-328-3777
                    www.hemophilia.org
This publication contains basic information about hemophilia and HIV disease.
1992 28 pages
Neil Frick, VP for Research
John Indence, VP for Marketing & Communications

5030 Clotting Agents Are Lifesavers
Hemophilia Foundation of Michigan
411 Huronview Boulevard   734-761-2535
Ann Arbor, MI 48103-2973
Offers information on what hemophilia is, treatments, occurances, heredity, Von Willebrand's Disease, patient services and direct services for hemophiliacs and HIV/AIDS patients.

5031 Comprehensive Care
National Hemophilia Foundation
7 Penn Plaza   212-328-3700
New York, NY 10001-3212   800-424-2634
                    Fax: 212-328-3777
                    www.hemophilia.org

Discusses the nature of comprehensive care and its functions and defines the care team. Also touches upon essential resources, HIV, and the benefits of comprehensive care.
1991 12 pages
Neil Frick, VP for Research
John Indence, VP for Marketing & Communications

5032   Comprehensive Services for Persons with Hemophilia
Hemophilia Foundation of Minnesota/Dakotas
7 Penn Plaza   212-328-3700
New York, NY 10001-3712   Fax: 212-328-3777
                                                      www.hemophilia.org
Offers information on what hemophilia is and information and resources for persons with hemophilia and other bleeding disorders.
Neil Frick, VP for Research
John Indence, VP for Marketing & Communications

5033   Consumer Bill of Rights and Responsibilities for Healthcare Service
National Hemophilia Foundation
7 Penn Plaza   212-328-3700
New York, NY 10001-3212   800-424-2634
                                              Fax: 212-328-3777
                                                      www.hemophilia.org
Serves as a set of goals for both the provider and consumer in seeking, providing, and receiving high quality health care within a setting of honesty and respect.
1994
Neil Frick, VP for Research
John Indence, VP for Marketing & Communications

5034   Countdown to a Cure
Louisiana Hemophilia Foundation
3636 S Sherwood Forest   225-291-1675
Baton Rouge, LA 70816-2285   Fax: 225-291-1679
                              e-mail: lahemophilia@hipoint.net
                              www.louisianahemophilia.org/
Offers information on chapter resources and services for hemophiliacs and their families. Offers information and services to families/patients affected by bleeding disorders.

5035   Fight Hemophilia with Facts Not Fiction
Great Lakes Hemophilia Foundation
638 North 18th Street   414-257-0200
Milwaukee, WI 53233   Fax: 414-257-1225
                                                      www.glhf.org
Offers information on what hemophilia is, research information and treatments.

5036   Get Real and Be Safe!
National Hemophilia Foundation
7 Penn Plaza   212-328-3700
New York, NY 10001-3212   800-424-2634
                                              Fax: 212-328-3777
                                                      www.hemophilia.org
Comic book style, this pamphlet offers information to young adults on the hazards and precautions of sex. Offers an Ask The Doctor question and answer section to books and resources for young adults on safer sex and HIV/AIDS.
1991 14 pages
Neil Frick, VP for Research
John Indence, VP for Marketing & Communications

5037   Guidelines for Finding Childcare
National Hemophilia Foundation
7 Penn Plaza   212-328-3700
New York, NY 10001-3212   800-424-2634
                                              Fax: 212-328-3777
                                                      www.hemophilia.org
Information for parents on how to hire a good babysitter, information on daycare centers, how to tell daycare staff about hemophilia, cooperative childcare and suggested reading for parents.
1987 10 pages
Neil Frick, VP for Research
John Indence, VP for Marketing & Communications

5038   HIV Disease in People with Hemophilia: Your Questions Answered
National Hemophilia Foundation

7 Penn Plaza   212-328-3700
New York, NY 10001-3212   800-424-2634
                                              Fax: 212-328-3777
                                                      www.hemophilia.org
Discusses hemophilia and HIV disease, AIDS, management of HIV disease, risks to sexual partners, and issues for children with hemophilia.
1991 48 pages
Neil Frick, VP for Research
John Indence, VP for Marketing & Communications

5039   HIV Infection and Hemophilia
Hemophilia Foundation of Illinois
7 Penn Plaza   212-328-3700
New York, NY 10001-4434   800-424-2634
                                              Fax: 212-328-3777
                                                      www.hemophilia.org
Offers information on HIV/AIDS relating to persons with hemophilia.
Neil Frick, VP for Research
John Indence, VP for Marketing & Communications

5040   Hemophilia: Current Medical Management
National Hemophilia Foundation
7 Penn Plaza   212-328-3700
New York, NY 10001-3212   800-424-2634
                                              Fax: 212-328-3777
                                                      www.hemophilia.org
Provides an overview of all aspects of hemophilia treatment, including prophylaxis, home therapy, inhibitors, orthopedic solutions, surgery, and dental care.
1994 30 pages
Neil Frick, VP for Research
John Indence, VP for Marketing & Communications

5041   How to Control Bleeds: Inspired by Vince, an 8-year-old Boy with Hemophilia
Bayer
400 Morgan Lane   203-937-2765
West Haven, CT 06516-4175
An educational comic book story by Vince about hemophilia and treatment for bleeds.
26 pages

5042   Living with HIV: Talking with Your Child
Bobbie Steinhart, author
National Hemophilia Foundation
7 Penn Plaza   212-328-3700
New York, NY 10001-3212   800-424-2634
                                              Fax: 212-328-3777
                                                      www.hemophilia.org
A pamphlet directed at caregivers of young children living with hemophilia and HIV disease.
1990 8 pages
Neil Frick, VP for Research
John Indence, VP for Marketing & Communications

5043   Mild Hemophilia
National Hemophilia Foundation
7 Penn Plaza   212-328-3700
New York, NY 10001-3212   800-424-2634
                                              Fax: 212-328-3777
                                                      www.hemophilia.org
Defines mild hemophilia and details its discovery, diagnosis, inheritance, symptoms, treatment, and activity limitations.
1994 25 pages
Neil Frick, VP for Research
John Indence, VP for Marketing & Communications

5044   Participating in a Clinical Trial: Your Life, Your Choice
National Hemophilia Foundation
7 Penn Plaza   212-328-3700
New York, NY 10001-3212   800-424-2634
                                              Fax: 212-328-3777
                                                      www.hemophilia.org
This brochure explains what clinical trials are and what they are like for patients, describes what kinds of HIV therapies are being tested in clinical trials, and lists questions to ask before joining a

trial. This publication is ideal for patients, their families, and/or healthcare personnel who counsel HIV-positive patients.
1994 6 pages
Neil Frick, VP for Research
John Indence, VP for Marketing & Communications

5045 Physical Therapy in Hemophilia
Nationa Hemophilia Foundation
7 Penn Plaza   212-328-3700
New York, NY 10001-3832   800-424-2634
                                                              Fax: 212-328-3777
                                                              www.hemophilia.org
Targeted at physical therapy students or new therapists at comprehensive hemophilia care clinics. Also provides basic treatment care information for persons with hemophilia and their families.
1986 13 pages
Neil Frick, VP for Research
John Indence, VP for Marketing & Communications

5046 Simple & Complex: A Hemophilia Primer
Western Pennsylvania Chapter of the NHF
8326 Naab Rd   412-685-2231
Indianapolis, IN 46260-1531   Fax: 412-683-2568
                                                              www.ihtc.org
Offers information on what hemophilia is, explains AIDS and HIV infection, offers information on the treatments for hemophilia and what hemophilia care costs.
Ike G. Batalis, President and CEO
Phillip E. Himelstein, Founder

5047 Student with Hemophilia: A Resource for the Educator
National Hemophilia Foundation
7 Penn Plaza   212-328-3700
New York, NY 10001-3212   800-424-2634
                                                              Fax: 212-328-3777
                                                              www.hemophilia.org
Written for teachers, nurses, and other school personnel, this booklet aims to dispel the myths and fears surrounding hemophilia.
1995 16 pages
Neil Frick, VP for Research
John Indence, VP for Marketing & Communications

5048 Treatment of Hemophilia: Current Orthopedic Management
Marvin Gilbert, Jerome Wiedel, author
National Hemophilia Foundation
7 Penn Plaza   212-328-3700
New York, NY 10001-3212   800-424-2634
                                                              Fax: 212-328-3777
                                                              www.hemophilia.org
Covers a wide range of orthopedic treatment issues, including hemophilic arthropathy, clinical considerations, diagnostic imaging, surgical and nonsurgical treatments, hemophilic synovitis, soft-tissue bleeding, the hemophilia pseudotumor, fracture care, other musculoskelatal problems, and HIV infections.
1995 25 pages
Neil Frick, VP for Research
John Indence, VP for Marketing & Communications

5049 Understanding Hepatitis
Leonard Seeff, Maribel Johnson, author
National Hemophilia Foundation
7 Penn Plaza   212-328-3700
New York, NY 10001-3212   800-424-2634
                                                              Fax: 212-328-3777
                                                              www.hemophilia.org
Provides comprehensive information about viral hepatitis for people with bleeding disorders, their caregivers, and families. Discusses the different hepatitis viruses, viral transmissions, how the liver is affected by hepatitis, blood product concerns, prevention, diagnosis, treatment, and psychosocial issues.
1997 24 pages
Neil Frick, VP for Research
John Indence, VP for Marketing & Communications

5050 Von Willebrand Disease: A Guide for Patients and Families
Hemophilia Health Services
6820 Charlotte Pike
Nashville, TN 37209-4206   800-800-6606

Offers information on this disease, explains the causes, treatments, prevention and offers resources and books.

5051 What Is Hemophilia?
Hemophilia Foundation of Georgia
8800 Roswell Road   770-518-8272
Atlanta, GA 30328-1689   800-866-4366
                                                              Fax: 770-518-3310
                                                              e-mail: hog@america.net
                                                              www.hog.org
Offers information on what hemophilia is, common factors in hemophilia, the cost and treatments offered to hemophiliacs and more.
Dan Maddock, Chief Governance Officer
Amy Greene, Secretary

5052 What Women Should Know About HIV Infection AIDS and Hemophilia
Hemophilia Foundation of Illinois
7 Penn Plaza   212-328-3700
New York, NY 10001-4434   800-424-2634
                                                              Fax: 212-328-3777
                                                              www.hemophilia.org
For spouses/partners of men with hemophilia and women with bleeding disorders. Provides information about HIV/AIDS and how it affects women in the hemophilia community.
25 pages
Neil Frick, VP for Research
John Indence, VP for Marketing & Communications

5053 What You Should Know About Hemophilia
National Hemophilia Foundation
7 Penn Plaza   212-328-3700
New York, NY 10001-3212   800-424-2634
                                                              Fax: 212-328-3777
                                                              www.hemophilia.org
Defines hemophilia, explains its effects, and provides a historical overview of treatment and treatment complications.
1991 13 pages
Neil Frick, VP for Research
John Indence, VP for Marketing & Communications

5054 Who Will Tell Them of Your Special Needs?
MedicAlert
2323 Colorado Avenue
Turlock, CA 95382-2018   800-432-5378
Offers information on MedicAlert bracelets, personal identification medical information needed for treatment in case of emergency.

Audio & Video

5055 Song of Superman
National Hemophilia Foundation
7 Penn Plaza   212-328-3700
New York, NY 10001-3212   800-424-2634
                                                              Fax: 212-328-3777
                                                              www.hemophilia.org
Designed to help young people with bleeding disorders come to terms with their HIV status, sexuality, and living with HIV. The video explores issues of disclosure in relationships and safer sex through dramatic scenes and frank testimonials by young people living with hemophilia and/or HIV. The companion workbook contains group exercises that follow each of the main topics of the video and serve as a bridge to discussion.
1993 49 pages
Neil Frick, VP for Research
John Indence, VP for Marketing & Communications

5056 Treat Yourself to a Brighter Future - It's Time to Hit the Freedom Trail
c/o Hemophilia Association of the Capital Area
10560 Main Street   703-352-7641
Fairfax, VA 22030-7182   Fax: 540-427-6589
                                                              e-mail: admin@HACAcares.org
                                                              www.hacacares.org/ed_publist.html
A booklet and videotape published by the American Red Cross providing a list of required supplies and equipment for self-infusion concentrates for persons with hemophilia A. It is an instructional

piece for home self-infusion and concise text and illustrations depict seven steps for self-infusion.

20 pages Video & Booklet
Steve Long, President
Eboni Morris, Vice President

Web Sites

5057   American Red Cross Blood Services

www.redcross.org/services/biomed
Distributes a wide variety of plasma therapeutics to benefit people with hemophilia A and B, immune disorders and hypoalbuminemia.

5058   Healing Well

www.healingwell.com
An online health resource guide to medical news, chat, information and articles, newsgroups and message boards, books, disease-related web sites, medical directories, and more for patients, friends, and family coping with disabling diseases, disorders, or chronic illnesses.

5059   Health Finder

www.healthfinder.gov
Searchable, carefully developed web site offering information on over 1000 topics. Developed by the US Department of Health and Human Services, the site can be used in both English and Spanish.

5060   Healthlink USA

www.healthlinkusa.com
Health information concerning treatment, cures, prevention, diagnosis, risk factors, research, support groups, email lists, personal stories and much more. Updated regularly.

5061   Helios Health

www.helioshealth.com
Online resource for your health information. Detailed information about specific health topics, access to expert advice from our Medical Advisory Board, and up-to-date health news.

5062   MedicineNet

www.medicinenet.com
An online resource for consumers providing easy-to-read, authoritative medical and health information.

5063   Medscape

www.medscape.com
Medscape offers specialists, primary care physicians, and other health professionals the Web's most robust and integrated medical information and educational tools.

5064   National Hemophilia Foundation

www.hemophilia.org
Information on the treatment and the cure of hemophilia, related bleeding disorders and complications of those disorders or their treatment, including HIV infection, as well as improving the quality of life of all those affected.

5065   WebMD

www.webmd.com
Provides credible information, supportive communities, and in-depth reference material about health subjects. A source for original and timely health information as well as material from well known content providers.

Description

5066 Hepatitis

Hepatitis, or inflammation of the liver, has multiple causes and several stages. Hepatitis is usually caused by viruses or by excess alcohol consumption. Less common causes include prescription medications, accidental poisoning, and auto-immune diseases in which the body attacks its own liver.

The severity of the disease is highly variable. At an early stage, hepatitis may cause no symptoms, vague mild symptoms, or overwhelming disease. Early symptoms include vague abdominal pain, jaundice, fever, loss of appetite and nausea. If the disease becomes chronic, it may lead to irreversible scarring, or cirrhosis, which causes weakness, fatigue and weight loss. Late stage disease includes fluid accumulation in the abdominal cavity, gastrointestinal bleeding and mental changes. Abdominal pain and liver enlargement are generally present. Advanced cirrhosis is a risk factor for cancer of the liver.

There are four major kinds of viral hepatitis. Type A is very common world-wide, is spread by contaminated food and water, and generally causes a mild to moderately severe illness that runs its course over several weeks and disappears without further damage. Type B is also very common, and is spread by bodily fluids, generally through blood transfusion, sexual intercourse, sharing of needles or contaminated items like shaving razors and tattoo needles. The disease may resolve without further consequences, but frequently becomes chronic and may lead to cirrhosis as well as chronic infections. Hepatitis C is also spread through blood transfusion and needle sharing. Although it is not usually severe at onset, it can lead to the same serious consequences as type B. Finally, there is a type D, which is spread by blood products, and only infects people who already have Type B. Type D is associated with a more severe course.

Prevention of any of these forms of viral hepatitis depends on avoiding the usual routes of transmission. In addition, there is an effective vaccine available for hepatitis B. Close family contacts of persons with this disease should receive the vaccine if they have not yet received it as part of routine childhood immunization.

Treatment of hepatitis is largely supportive, but antiviral drugs and interferon are used in certain stages of Type B and Type C infection. End-stage or overwhelming infection may necessitate liver transplantation. See also *Liver Disease*.

National Agencies & Associations

5067   American Hepatitis Association
133 E 58th Street
New York, NY 10022   212-753-8068

Conducts educational and prevention programs concerning hepatitis provides screening and vaccines and offers support groups for individuals with hepatitis.
Gerberding, MD, Director

5068   Centers for Disease Control and Prevention Hepatitis Branch
1600 Clifton Road   404-639-2709
Atlanta, GA 30333   800-232-4636
TTY: 888-232-6348
www.cdc.gov/ncidod/diseases/hepatitis
Monitors the rates of viral hepatitis in the United States; provides epidemiologic assistance for outbreaks of viral hepatitis; coordinates and implements epidemiologic studies to define the risk factors for acute and chronic viral hepatitis; provides viral hepatitis reference/diagnostic services; serves as the World Health Organization Collaborating Center for Reference and Research on Viral Hepatitis.
Julie Louise Foy, Contact
Judy Greenspan, Contact

5069   HIV/Hepatitis C in Prison (HIP) Committee
California Prison Focus   510-665-1935
San Francisco, CA 94103   e-mail: contact@prisons.org
www.prisons.org/hivin
The HIV/HCV in Prison Committee of California Prison Focus works on behalf of prisoners to fight for consistent access to quality medical care including access of all new HIV and hepatitis C medications, diagnostic testing and combination therapies.
Michelle Wexler MD, Executive Director
Diane C Peterson, Associate Director for Immunization

5070   Hepatitis Foundation International
504 Blick Drive   301-879-6891
Silver Spring, MD 20904-2901   800-891-0707
Fax: 301-879-6890
e-mail: info@hepatitisfoundation.org
www.hepfi.org
Grassroots support network for persons with viral hepatitis. Provides education about the prevention diagnosis and treatment of viral hepatitis as well as phone network support and various literature.
Thelma King Thiel, CEO
Theodore Karrison, Vice-Chairman

5071   Immunization Action Coalition
1573 Selby Avenue   651-647-9009
Saint Paul, MN 55104   Fax: 651-647-9131
e-mail: admin@immunize.org
www.immunize.org
The mission of the Immunization Action Coalition is to boost immunization rates and prevent disease. The coalition promotes physician, community and family awareness of and responsibility for appropriate immunization of all children and adults against all diseases.
Deborah L Wexler, MD, Executive Director
Litjen Tan, MS, PhD, Chief Strategy Officer

5072   Inter-Provincial Roof Consultants, Ltd.
5828 176th Street   604-576-5740
Surrey, V3S 4-6J9   800-616-2437
Fax: 604-576-5790
e-mail: inbox@iprc.ca
www.iprc.ca
Through partnerships and collaboration, will work to reduce the incidence of new HIV/AIDS/HEP C and other blood borne pathogens and to improve the quality of life for those infected and affected.
Sean M Lang, President/Owner/Chief Consultant/Spec Wr
Mike Kosman, Consultant/Spec Writer/Roof Observer

5073   National Hepatitis C Coalition
PO Box 5058   951-766-8238
Hemet, CA 92544   e-mail: mail@nationalhepatitis-c.org
www.nationalhepatitis-c.org
The National Hepatitis C Coalition is a 501(c)(3) tax exempt organization that relies on private donations from good folks like you in order to continue helping others with hepatitis C.
Patty Krueger, Co-Founder

Foundations

5074 Hepatitis B Foundation
3805 Old Easton Road
Doylestown, PA 18902
215-489-4900
Fax: 215-489-4313
e-mail: info@hepb.org
www.hepb.org

We are dedicated to finding a cure and improving the quality of life for those affected by hepatitis B worldwide. Our commitment includes funding focused research, promoting disease awareness, supporting immunization and treatment initiatives, and serving as the primary source of information for patients and their families, the medical and scientific community, and the general public.

Joel Rosen, Chairman, Esq
Timothy M Block, PhD, President

Libraries & Resource Centers

5075 Hepatitis Education Project
911 Western Avenue
Seattle, WA 98104
206-732-0311
Fax: 206-732-0312
e-mail: hep@scn.org
www.hepeducation.org

The mission of the Hepatitis Education Project is to help raise awareness among patients, medical personnel and the public of the facts concerning hepatitis patients and the resources available to help those who live with the disease.

Steve Graham, President
Michael Ninburg, Executive Director

Support Groups & Hotlines

5076 Christ Hospital Hepatitis C Support Group
Christ Hospital
176 Palisade Avenue
Jersey City, NJ 07306
201-795-1230
e-mail: dkatz65717@aol.com

For anyone interested in becoming advocates for increasing awareness of this illness.

Graham, President
Michael Ninburg, Executive Director

5077 Hepatitis Education Project
911 Western Avenue
Seattle, WA 98104
206-732-0311
e-mail: hepinfo@hepeducation.org
www.hepeducation.org

Helps raise awareness among patients, medical personeel and the public of the facts concerning hepatitis patients and the resources available to help those who live with the disease

Steve Graham, President
Michael Ninburg, Executive Director

5078 National Health Information Center
PO Box 1133
Washington, DC 20013
310-565-4167
800-336-4797
Fax: 301-984-4256
e-mail: info@nhic.org
www.health.gov/nhic

Offers a nationwide information referral service, produces directories and resource guides.

Borden, NE Regional Contact

Books

5079 Hepatitis B Prevention: A Resource Guide
National Digestive Diseases Info. Clearinghouse
2 Information Way
Bethesda, MD 20824
301-496-3583
800-891-5389
Fax: 301-907-8906
e-mail: nddic@info.niddk.uih.goc
www.niddk.nih.gov

Designed to assist health care and other professionals who work in planning or administering hepatitis B prevention programs.
252 pages

5080 Understanding Hepatitis
James L Achord, MD, author
University Press of Mississippi
3825 Ridgewood Road
Jackson, MS 39211-6492
601-432-6205
Fax: 601-432-6217
e-mail: kburgess@ihl.state.ms.us
www.upress.state.ms.us

For general readers a comprehensive discussion of the causes and of the treatments of hepatitis.
2002 152 pages Paperback
ISBN: 1-578064-36-8

5081 Viral Hepatitis: Scientific Basis and Clinical Management
Churchill Livingstone
PO Box 3188
Secaucus, NJ 07096-3188
201-319-9800
800-553-5426
Fax: 201-319-9659
www.harcourt-international.com/cl/

1997 800 pages Hardcover
ISBN: 0-443057-97-4

Magazines

5082 Hepatitis Magazine
Quality Publishing Services
523 N Sam Houston Pkwy E
Houston, TX 77060
281-272-2744
800-310-7047
Fax: 281-847-5440
e-mail: info@hepatitismag.com
www.hepatitismag.com

Magazine for those with hepatitis. Price listed is for a one year subscription.
Quarterly

Newsletters

5083 American Liver Foundation: Progress Newsletter
39 Broadway
New York, NY 10006-4826
212-668-1000
800-465-4837
Fax: 212-483-8179
e-mail: info@liverfoundation.org
www.liverfoundation.org

The American Liver Foundation is the nation's leading nonprofit organization promoting liver health and disease prevention. ALF provides research education and sdvocacy for those affected by liver-related diseases, including hepatitis
8 pages 2 per year

5084 B Connected
3805 Old Easton Road
Doylestown, PA 18902
215-489-4900
Fax: 215-489-4313
e-mail: info@hepb.org
www.hepb.org

Features practical health tips, frequently asked questions, and other useful information for patients and families to live well with chronic hepatitis B. Available in both print and online versions.
3x/year
Joel Rosen, Chairman
Timothy M. Block, President

5085 B-Informed Newsletter
Hepatitis B Foundation
3805 Old Easton Road
Doylestown, PA 18902
215-489-4900
Fax: 215-489-4313
e-mail: info@hepb.org
www.hepb.org

Includes a Drug Watch of approved and experimental therapies for Hepatitis B, reasearch updates, Foundation news and events, and feature articles on special topics. Available in print and online.
Joel Rosen, Chairman
Timothy M. Block, President

5086 Hepatitis Alert
Hepatitis Foundation International (HFI)

8121 Georgia Avenue
Silver Spring, MD 20910-1423
301-565-9410
800-891-0707
Fax: 973-875-5044
e-mail: hfi@intac.com
www.hepfi.org

Provides information for the public, patients, educators, and medical professionals about the diagnosis, treatment, and prevention of viral hepatitis.
Karen Wirth, Chair
Dane R. Christiansen, Vice Chair

5087 Hepatitis B Coalition News
Hepatitis B Coalition
2550 University Ave W
Saint Paul, MN 55114-6328
651-647-9009
Fax: 651-647-9131
e-mail: admin@inmunize.org
www.immunize.org

Newsletter with brochures, articles, videotapes, audio-cassette tapes and manuals for different ethnic populations.
Deborah L. Wexler, MD, Executive Director
Litjen Tan, MS, PhD, Chief Strategy Officer

5088 NEEDLE TIPS & the Hepatitis B Coalition News
Hepatitis B Coalition
2550 University Ave W
St. Paul, MN 55114-6328
651-647-9009
Fax: 651-647-9131
e-mail: admin@immunize.org
www.immunize.org

Information on immunization for health professionals.
28 pages 2x Year
Deborah L. Wexler, MD, Executive Director
Litjen Tan, MS, PhD, Chief Strategy Officer

5089 VACCINATE ADULTS! Coalition News
Hepatitis B Coalition
2550 University Ave W
St. Paul, MN 55114-6328
651-647-9009
Fax: 651-647-9131
e-mail: admin@immunize.org
www.immunize.org

Information on immunization: adult medicine specialist.
12 pages 2x Year
Deborah L. Wexler, MD, Executive Director
Litjen Tan, MS, PhD, Chief Strategy Officer

Pamphlets

5090 Advice to Parents of Children with HBV
Hepatitis B Foundation
3805 Old Easton Road
Doylestown, PA 18902
215-489-4900
Fax: 215-489-4313
e-mail: info@hepb.org
www.hepb.org

Provides information to people affected by hepatitis B and their loved ones. Current HBV research, telephone numbers, and a medical glossary.
Joel Rosen, Chairman
Timothy M. Block, President

5091 Caring for Your Liver
Hepatitis Foundation International (HFI)
8121 Georgia Avenue
Silver Spring, MD 20910-1423
301-565-9410
800-891-0707
Fax: 973-875-5044
e-mail: hfi@intac.com
www.hepfi.org

Information for the person with hepatitis.
Karen Wirth, Chair
Dane R. Christiansen, Vice Chair

5092 Caution! Treating Children with Acetaminophen
Hepatitis Foundation International (HFI)
8121 Georgia Avenue
Silver Spring, MD 20910-1423
301-565-9410
800-891-0707
Fax: 973-875-5044
e-mail: hfi@intac.com
www.hepfi.org

Information on hepatitis.
Karen Wirth, Chair
Dane R. Christiansen, Vice Chair

5093 Chronic Viral Hepatitis Backgrounder
Schering Corporation
2000 Galloping Hill Road
Kenilworth, NJ 07033
908-298-4000
www.sch-plough.com

Offers information and statistics on viral hepatitis.

5094 Cirrhosis: Many Causes
American Liver Foundation
39 Broadway
New York, NY 10066-1000
212-668-1000
800-223-0179
Fax: 212-483-8179
e-mail: info@liverfoundation.org
www.liverfoundation.org

Gives basic facts about cirrhosis including causes, signs, symptoms and treatments.
David Ticker, Chief Financial Officer
Lynn Seim, Chief Operating Officer

5095 Diagnosis and Treatment
Hepatitis Foundation International (HFI)
8121 Georgia Avenue
Silver Spring, MD 20910-1423
301-565-9410
800-891-0707
Fax: 973-875-5044
e-mail: hfi@intac.com
www.hepfi.org

Information for the person with hepatitis.
Karen Wirth, Chair
Dane R. Christiansen, Vice Chair

5096 Health Insurance
Hepatitis Foundation International (HFI)
8121 Georgia Avenue
Silver Spring, MD 20910-1423
301-565-9410
800-891-0707
Fax: 973-875-5044
e-mail: hfi@intac.com
www.hepfi.org

Information on hepatitis and health insurance.
Karen Wirth, Chair
Dane R. Christiansen, Vice Chair

5097 Helpful Tips for Carriers of HBV
Hepatitis Foundation International (HFI)
8121 Georgia Avenue
Silver Spring, MD 20910-1423
301-565-9410
800-891-0707
Fax: 973-875-5044
e-mail: hfi@intac.com
www.hepfi.org

Information for people with Hepatitis B.
Karen Wirth, Chair
Dane R. Christiansen, Vice Chair

5098 Hepatitis
National Institute of Allergy & Infectious Disease
5601 Fishers Lane
Bethesda, MD 20892-0001
301-402-1663
Fax: 301-402-0120
e-mail: niaidnews@niaid.nih.gov
www.niaid.nih.gov/default.htm

A pamphlet discussing the cause, symptoms, transmission, diagnosis, tests, prevention and the latest research on Hepatitis.

5099 Hepatitis A and B Vaccination
Hepatitis Foundation International (HFI)
8121 Georgia Avenue
Silver Spring, MD 20910-1423
301-565-9410
800-891-0707
Fax: 973-875-5044
e-mail: hfi@intac.com
www.hepfi.org

Information on hepatitis vaccination.
Karen Wirth, Chair
Dane R. Christiansen, Vice Chair

5100 Hepatitis A, B & C
Hepatitis Foundation International (HFI)
8121 Georgia Avenue
Silver Spring, MD 20910-1423
301-565-9410
800-891-0707
Fax: 973-875-5044
e-mail: hfi@intac.com
www.hepfi.org

Information for the person with hepatitis.
Karen Wirth, Chair
Dane R. Christiansen, Vice Chair

5101 Hepatitis A, B & C: Liver Disease You Should Know About
American Liver Foundation
1425 Pompton Avenue
Cedar Grove, NJ 07009
800-465-4837
Fax: 973-256-3214
e-mail: info@liverfoundation.org
www.liverfoundation.org
Explains viral hepatitis, transmission, symptoms, testing and acute chronic hepatitis.

5102 Hepatitis B Prevention
National Center For Infectious Diseases
Hepatitis Branch
Atlanta, GA 30333
404-332-4555
Explains what hepatitis B is, what behaviors are risky and how to protect oneself against it.

5103 Hepatitis Fact Sheet
www.cdc.gov/ncidod/diseases/hepatitis/c
Offers information on the causes, symptoms, prevention and treatments for hepatitis.

5104 How Many Times a Day Do You Risk Being Infected with Hepatitis B?
American Liver Foundation
1425 Pompton Avenue
Cedar Grove, NJ 07009
800-465-4837
Fax: 973-256-3214
e-mail: info@liverfoundation.org
www.liverfoundation.org
A flyer emphasizing the importance of vaccination against hepatitis B.

5105 Is Your Liver Giving You the Silent Treatment?
Hepatitis Foundation International (HFI)
8121 Georgia Avenue
Silver Spring, MD 20910-1423
301-565-9410
800-891-0707
Fax: 973-875-5044
e-mail: hfi@intac.com
www.hepfi.org
Provides information for patients with hepatitis.
Karen Wirth, Chair
Dane R. Christiansen, Vice Chair

5106 Living with Hepatitis C: Self Help Tips
Hepatitis Foundation International (HFI)
8121 Georgia Avenue
Silver Spring, MD 20910-1423
301-565-9410
800-891-0707
Fax: 973-875-5044
e-mail: hfi@intac.com
www.hepfi.org
Information for people with Hepatitis C.
Karen Wirth, Chair
Dane R. Christiansen, Vice Chair

5107 Protect Yourself and Those You Love Against HBV
Hepatitis B Foundation
3805 Old Easton Road
Doylestown, PA 18902
215-489-4900
Fax: 215-489-4313
e-mail: info@hepb.org
www.hepb.org
Provides information to people affected by hepatitis B and their loved ones.
Joel Rosen, Chairman
Timothy M. Block, President

5108 Q and A: Hepatitis B Prevention
SmithKline Beecham Pharmaceuticals
1 Franklin Plaza
Philadelphia, PA 19102-1282
215-751-4000
Informational booklet written for healthcare personnel by the manufacturer of Engerix-B vaccine, reviews hepatitis B prevention.

5109 Someone You Know Has Hepatitis B
Hepatitis B Foundation

3805 Old Easton Road
Doylestown, PA 18902
215-489-4900
Fax: 215-489-4313
e-mail: info@hepb.org
www.hepb.org
Provides information to people affected by hepatitis B and their loved ones.
Joel Rosen, Chairman
Timothy M. Block, President

5110 Tips on Coping with Chronic Hepatitis
Hepatitis Foundation International (HFI)
8121 Georgia Avenue
Silver Spring, MD 20910-1423
301-565-9410
800-891-0707
Fax: 973-875-5044
e-mail: hfi@intac.com
www.hepfi.org

Information for people with hepatitis.
Karen Wirth, Chair
Dane R. Christiansen, Vice Chair

5111 Viral Hepatitis: Everybody's Problem?
American Liver Foundation
39 Broadwa
New York, NY 10006-1000
212-668-1000
800-223-0179
Fax: 212-483-8179
e-mail: info@liverfoundation.org
www.liverfoundation.org
Covering a broad range of topics including: a definition of the disease, descriptions of types of infections, transmission, symptoms, treatment options and prevention of hepatitis.
David Ticker, Chief Financial Officer
Lynn Seim, Chief Operating Officer

5112 What Health Care Workers Should Know About Hepatitis B
Channing L Bete Company
2550 University Ave W
St. Paul, MN 55114
651-647-9009
800-628-7733
Fax: 651-647-9131
www.immunize.org
Presents information in easy-to-read, simple English for health care workers about hepatitis B.
15 pages
Deborah L. Wexler, MD, Executive Director
Litjen Tan, MS, PhD, Chief Strategy Officer

Audio & Video

5113 Hepatitis B Video
Hepatitis B Foundation
3805 Old Easton Road
Doylestown, PA 18902
215-489-4900
Fax: 215-489-4313
e-mail: info@hepb.org
www.hepb.org
Provides information to people affected by hepatitis B and their loved ones.
Joel Rosen, Chairman
Timothy M. Block, President

5114 Hepatitis C: A Viral Mystery
Terry Strauss, Stephen Steady, author
Fanlight Productions
4196 Washington Street
Boston, MA 02131-1731
617-469-4999
800-937-4113
Fax: 617-469-3379
e-mail: fanlight@fanlight.com
www.fanlight.com
This timely video is about living with a serious, chronic illness. In addition to discussing the medical treatments available, the video also explores alternatives which appear to help some people.
2000 30 Minutes
ISBN: 1-572953-08-X

Web Sites

5115 HIV/Hepatitis C in Prison (HIP) Committee
www.prisons.org/hivin.htm

Fighting for consistent access to quality medical care including access to all new HIV and Hepatitis C medications, diagnostic testing and combination therapies.

5116   Healing Well

www.healingwell.com

An online health resource guide to medical news, chat, information and articles, newsgroups and message boards, books, disease-related web sites, medical directories, and more for patients, friends, and family coping with disabling diseases, disorders, or chronic illnesses.

5117   Health Finder

www.healthfinder.gov

Searchable, carefully developed web site offering information on over 1000 topics. Developed by the US Department of Health and Human Services, the site can be used in both English and Spanish.

5118   Healthlink USA

www.healthlinkusa.com

Health information concerning treatment, cures, prevention, diagnosis, risk factors, research, support groups, email lists, personal stories and much more. Updated regularly.

5119   Healthy Lives

www.healthylives.com/hepatitis

5120   Helios Health

www.helioshealth.com

Online resource for your health information. Detailed information about specific health topics, access to expert advice from our Medical Advisory Board, and up-to-date health news.

5121   Hepatitis B Coalition

www.immunize.org

The Immunization Action Coalition (IAC) works to increase immunization rates and prevent disease by creating and distributing educational materials for health professionals and the public that enhance the delivery of safe and effective immunization services.

5122   Hepatitis Information Network

www.hepnet.com

5123   MedicineNet

www.medicinenet.com

An online resource for consumers providing easy-to-read, authoritative medical and health information.

5124   Medscape

www.medscape.com

Medscape offers specialists, primary care physicians, and other health professionals the Web's most robust and integrated medical information and educational tools.

5125   WebMD

www.webmd.com

Provides credible information, supportive communities, and in-depth reference material about health subjects. A source for original and timely health information as well as material from well known content providers.

Description

5126 Hydrocephalus

The normal brain and spinal cord are surrounded with a watery substance called cerebro-spinal fluid, CSF, which collects within the brain in several larger pools called ventricles, connected to one another through tiny channels. The CSF is formed in some of these ventricles, circulates widely and is eventually reabsorbed. If CFS production exceeds reabsorption, or if the fluid is blocked from circulating and it may build up pressure that expands the ventricles and presses on the normal brain tissue, causing hydrocephalus, or water on the brain.

Hydrocephalus can cause change in behavior, headache, visual loss, vomiting and weakness. Hydrocephalus may be congenital, that is, present from birth. If it occurs in a child whose skull bones have not yet fused together, it may cause the head to enlarge.

In adults whose brains are encased in the rigid skull, there is no room to expand and pressure builds up in the brain. Excess CSF may be in response to infection such as meningitis or to blockage of CSF movement by tumor. Treatment and outlook depend on the underlying cause. Medical therapy may cause limited temporary improvement. Surgical treatment may be able to correct the underlying cause. If it cannot, the surgeon may still give substantial relief by placing a shunt which allows extra CSF to drain from the ventricles to some other part of the body.

National Agencies & Associations

5127 Association of Hydrocephalus Education Advocacy & Discussion (AHEAD)
1730 Autumn Leaf Lane
Huntingdon Valley, PA 19006-1515   215-355-4728
Organized by young adults with hydrocephalus for the purpose of providing telephone support nationwide.
Lane Fischetti, Founder
Jamie Fischetti, Secretary

5128 Guardians of Hydrocephalus Research Foundation
2618 Avenue Z   718-743-4473
Brooklyn, NY 11235-2023   Fax: 718-743-1171
e-mail: ghrf2618@aol.com
www.ghrforg.org
Non-profit organization made up of concerned parents and dedicated volunteers. The goal is to wipe out this top ranking birth defect.
Michael Kranz, Director of Research
Pip Marks, Director of Support & Education

5129 Hydrocephalus Association Hydrocephalus Association
Hydrocephalus Association
4340 East West Highway   301-202-3811
Bethesda, MD 20814   888-598-3789
Fax: 301-202-3813
e-mail: info@hydroassoc.org
www.hydroassoc.org
The association provides support education and advocacy for families and professionals. The goal is to insure that families and individuals dealing with the complexities of hydrocephalus receive personal support, comprehensive educational materials and outreach.
Barrett O'Connor, Chair
Dawn Mancuso, Chief Executive Officer

5130 Hydrocephalus Foundation
910 Rear Broadway   781-942-1161
Saugus, MA 01906   e-mail: HyFII@netscape.net
www.hydrocephalus.org
Dedicated to providing support educational resources and networking opportunities to patients and families affected by hydrocephalus. The Foundation also promotes related research and facilitates the training of healthcare professionals to improve patient care.
Greg A Tocco, Founder & Executive Director
Michael Tocco R.Ph., M.Ed., President

5131 National Hydrocephalus Foundation
12413 Centralia Road   562-924-6666
Lakewood, CA 90715   888-857-3434
Fax: 562-924-6666
e-mail: debbifields@nhfonline.org
www.nhfonline.org
The foundation is a national organization with almost 30 years of history. We provide information and education along with peer-to-peer support a physician referral sheet along with patient and family comments and several different types of help sheets.
Michael Fields, President
Debbi Fields, Executive Director

5132 Spina Bifida & Hydrocephalus Association of Nova Scotia
15 Laura Drive   902-679-1124
Nova Scotia, B3G 1-1B6   800-304-0450
Fax: 902-679-1433
e-mail: info@sbhans.ca
www.sbhans.ca
It is a non-profit, registered charitable organization affiliated with the Spina Bifida and Hydrocephalus Association of Canada, and currently has one chapter in Cape Breton.

5133 Spina Bifida & Hydrocephalus Association o f Ontario
555 Richmond Street West   416-214-1056
Toronto, Ontario, M5V 3-3B1   800-387-1575
Fax: 416-214-1446
e-mail: provincial@sbhao.on.ca
www.sbhao.on.ca/
It is a non-profit registered charitable organization affiliated with the Spina Bifida and Hydrocephalus Association of Canada and currently has one chapter in Cape Breton.
Marc Garson, Chair
Joan Booth, Executive Director

5134 The Kidney Foundation of Canada
300-5165 Sherbrooke Street W   514-369-4806
Montreal, QC H4A 1-1T6   800-361-7494
Fax: 514-369-2472
e-mail: info@kidney.ca
www.kidney.ca
A national volunteer organization committed to reducing the burden of kidney disease through: funding and stimulating innovative research; providing education and support; promoting access to high quality healthcare; and increasing public awareness and commitment to advancing kidney health and organ donation.
Dr Julian Midgley, President
Andrew MacRitchie, Treasurer

5135 World Hypertension League
Medical University of Ohio   419-383-5270
Toledo, OH 43614-5809   Fax: 419-383-3120
e-mail: gmonhollen@meduohio.edu
hsc.utoledo.edu
Devoted to the advancement of hypertension prevention and control through joint efforts of all national leagues and societies.
Lloyd A Gross, Chairman
Raymond Moser, Vice Chairman

State Agencies & Associations

Maryland

5136 Hydrocephalus Association
4340 East West Highway   301-202-3811
Bethesda, MD 20814   888-598-3789
                                     Fax: 301-202-3813
                              e-mail: info@hydroassoc.org
                                     www.hydroassoc.org
Founded in 1976 this group was formed as a group of concerned families and patients with hydrocephalus to share information and experiences in dealing with this disease locally and nationwide.
Barrett O'Connor, Chair
Dawn Mancuso, Chief Executive Officer

Michigan

5137 Hydrocephalus Support Group of Michigan Children's Hospital of Michigan
Children's Hospital of Michigan
3901 Beaubien   313-745-5437
Detroit, MI 48201   Fax: 313-993-8744
Founded in 1992 this group provides information to families and gives them support.
Mary Smellie

Pennsylvania

5138 Hydrocephalus Association of Philadelphia
PO Box 2099   610-497-0375
Boothwyn, PA 19061-8099   Fax: 610-497-2836
Founded in 1992 the Association provides support information advocacy and telephone support to families in Pennsylvania New Jersey and Delaware.
Halmi, Director

Rhode Island

5139 Hydrocephalus Association of Rhode Island
PO Box 343   401-723-6065
Valley Falls, RI 02864-0343
Founded in 1993 the mission of this Association is to provide information support and advocacy for individuals with hydrocephalus and for friends and family members.
Gabriella Pike, President

Texas

5140 Hydrocephalus Association of North Texas
PO Box 670552
Dallas, TX 74637-0552   214-528-2877
                        http://nhfonline.org/treatment.php?id=or
Founded in 1987 the mission is to provide information and support to parents of children with hydrocephalus in the state of Texas and neighboring states.
Beverly Pozzi

Washington

5141 Children's Hydrocephalus Support Group
PO Box 1611   425-482-0479
Woodinville, WA 98072   e-mail: lpoliski@hydrosupport.org
                                     www.hydrosupport.org
Founded in 1993 the group of Seattle provides support to individuals with hydrocephalus.
Lori Poliski, Co-Founder
Paul Gross, Co-Founder

Support Groups & Hotlines

5142 Hydrocephalus Parents Support Group
1325 Louis Street   908-722-4691
Manville, NJ 08835
Founded in 1993, the group provides support for parents of children with hydrocephalus.
Andrea

5143 National Health Information Center
PO Box 1133   310-565-4167
Washington, DC 20013   800-336-4797
                                     Fax: 301-984-4256
                                   e-mail: info@nhic.org
                                     www.health.gov/nhic
Offers a nationwide information referral service, produces directories and resource guides.
Sansone, Executive Director
Mary Trifault, Executive Associate

Books

5144 Hydrocephalus: A Guide for Patients, Families, and Friends
O'Reilly and Associates
1005 Gravenstein Hwy N   707-827-7019
Sebastopol, CA 95472   800-889-8969
                                     Fax: 707-824-8268
                               e-mail: order@oreilly.com
                                     www.oreilly.com
Hydrocephalus: A Guide for Patients, Families, and Friends provides individuals and families with the guidance, information and support needed to make the right decisions at the right time.
350 pages Paperback
ISBN: 1-565924-10-X

5145 Spina Bifida Association of America: Insights into Spina Bifida
Spina Bifida Association of America
1600 Wilson Blvd.   202-944-3285
Arlington, VA 22209-4226   800-621-3141
                                     Fax: 202-944-3295
                                  e-mail: sbaa@sbaa.org
                                     www.sbaa.org
News on medical, legislative and education topics relevant to individuals with spina bifida.
bi-monthly
Megan Sorensen, Chair
Wilson Neyland, Chair-Elect

Children's Books

5146 Loving Ben
Delacorte
1540 Broadway   212-354-6500
New York, NY 10036-4039
This is a moving story of a sister who cares for her baby brother and tries to help him learn despite his birth defects and deteriorating health.
Grades 7-10

Newsletters

5147 Alliance of Genetic Support Groups
4301 Connecticut Ave NW   202-966-5557
Washington, DC 20008   800-336-4363
                                     Fax: 202-966-8553
                            e-mail: info@geneticalliance.org
                                     www.geneticalliance.org
A coalition of voluntary genetic support groups, consumers and professionals addressing the needs of individuals and families affected by genetic disorders from a national perspective.
Sharon Terry, President and CEO
Natasha Bonomme, Vice President of Strategic Development

5148 Hydrocephalus Association Newsletter
Hydrocephalus Association
4340 East West Highway   301-202-3811
Bethesda, MD 20814-2912   888-598-3789
                                     Fax: 301-202-3813
                              e-mail: info@hydroassoc.org
                                     www.hydroassoc.org
Offers information on association news, conference articles, meetings, support and educational groups.
12 pages Quarterly
Aseem Chandra, Chair
Craig Brown, Senior Vice Chair

5149 Hydrocephalus Parents Support Group Newsletter
PO Box 1611
Woodinville, WA 98072   425-482-0479
                     e-mail: lpoliski@hydrosupport.org
                     www.hydrosupport.org
Founded in 1993, the group provides support for parents of children with hydrocephalus.

5150 Hydrocephalus Support Group Newsletter
PO Box 1611
Woodinville, WA 98072-4236   425-482-0479
                     Fax: 314-995-4108
                     e-mail: lpoliski@hydrosupport.org
                     www.hydrosupport.org
Founded in 1986, this group provides information, education and support to anyone dealing with hydrocephalus.

5151 National Hydrocephalus Foundation Newsletter
12413 Centrailia Road   562-924-6666
Lakewood, CA 90715-1623   888-857-3434
                     Fax: 562-924-6666
                     e-mail: info@nhfonline.org
                     www.nhfonline.org
Founded in 1979, the foundation is a national organization whose purpose is to provide information and education, along with peer support newsletter quarterly. Group meeting quarterly in Long Beach, CA. $35 a year.
Quarterly
Debbi Fields, Executive Director

5152 New York University Medical Center Auxiliary of Tisch Hospital
560 1st Avenue
New York, NY 10016   212-263-5040
                     www.nyukidshealth.org
Conducts national symposiums on hydrocephalus.

Pamphlets

5153 About Hydrocephalus: A Book for Families
Hydrocephalus Association
4340 East West Highway   301-202-3811
Bethesda, MD 20814-2912   888-598-3789
                     Fax: 301-202-3813
                     e-mail: info@hydroassoc.org
                     www.hydroassoc.org
A booklet in either English or Spanish, detailing all aspects of hydrocephalus from diagnosis and treatment to complications and follow-up care.
36 pages Paperback
Aseem Chandra, Chair
Craig Brown, Senior Vice Chair

5154 About Normal Pressure Hydrocephalus: A Book for Adults & Their Families
Hydrocephalus Association
870 Market Street   415-732-7040
San Francisco, CA 94102-2912   888-598-3789
                     Fax: 415-732-7044
                     e-mail: info@hydroassoc.org
                     www.hydroassoc.org
Booklet discusses the diagnosis and treatment of adult-onset normal pressure hydrocephalus.
24 pages Paperback
Dory Kranz, Executive Director
Pip Marks, Director Outreach Services

5155 Directory of Neurosurgeons Who Treat Adults
Hydrocephalus Association
870 Market Street   415-732-7040
San Francisco, CA 94102-2912   888-598-3789
                     Fax: 415-732-7044
                     e-mail: info@hydroassoc.org
                     www.hydroassoc.org
Names and addresses of neurosurgeons who treat adult-onset normal pressure hydrocephalus and adult-acquired hydrocephalus, listed alphabetically and geographically.
Dory Kranz, Executive Director
Pip Marks, Director Outreach Services

5156 Directory of Pediatric Neurosurgeons
Hydrocephalus Association
870 Market Street   415-732-7040
San Francisco, CA 94102-2912   888-598-3789
                     Fax: 415-732-7044
                     e-mail: info@hydroassoc.org
                     www.hydroassoc.org
Names and addresses of more than 200 neurosurgeons who specialize in pediatrics, listed alphabetically and geographically.
Dory Kranz, Executive Director
Pip Marks, Director Outreach Services

5157 Endoscopic Third Ventriculotomy
Hydrocephalus Association
870 Market Street   415-732-7040
San Francisco, CA 94102-2912   888-598-3789
                     Fax: 415-732-7044
                     e-mail: info@hydroassoc.org
                     www.hydroassoc.org
Series includes information on primary care, learning disabilities, eye problems, social skills development, headaches, endoscopic third ventriculostomy, shunts and more.
Dory Kranz, Executive Director
Pip Marks, Director Outreach Services

5158 Eye Problems Associated with Hydrocephalus in Children
Hydrocephalus Association
870 Market Street   415-732-7040
San Francisco, CA 94102-2912   888-598-3789
                     Fax: 415-732-7044
                     e-mail: info@hydroassoc.org
                     www.hydroassoc.org
Series includes information on primary care, learning disabilities, eye problems, social skills development, headaches, endoscopic third ventriculostomy, shunts and more.
Dory Kranz, Executive Director
Pip Marks, Director Outreach Services

5159 Fact Sheet: Hydrocephalus
Hydrocephalus Association
870 Market Street   415-732-7040
San Francisco, CA 94102-2912   888-598-3789
                     Fax: 415-732-7044
                     e-mail: info@hydroassoc.org
                     www.hydroassoc.org
Available in Spanish.
Dory Kranz, Executive Director
Pip Marks, Director Outreach Services

5160 Headaches and Hydrocephalus
Hydrocephalus Association
870 Market Street   415-732-7040
San Francisco, CA 94102-2912   888-598-3789
                     Fax: 415-732-7044
                     e-mail: info@hydroassoc.org
                     www.hydroassoc.org
Series includes information on primary care, learning disabilities, eye problems, social skills development, headaches, endoscopic third ventriculostomy, shunts and more.
Dory Kranz, Executive Director
Pip Marks, Director Outreach Services

5161 Hospitalization Tips
Hydrocephalus Association
870 Market Street   415-732-7040
San Francisco, CA 94102-2912   888-598-3789
                     Fax: 415-732-7044
                     e-mail: info@hydroassoc.org
                     www.hydroassoc.org
1997
Dory Kranz, Executive Director
Pip Marks, Director Outreach Services

5162 How to Be an Assertive Parent on the Treatment Team
Hydrocephalus Association
870 Market Street   415-732-7040
San Francisco, CA 94102-2912   888-598-3789
                     Fax: 415-732-7044
                     e-mail: info@hydroassoc.org
                     www.hydroassoc.org
Dory Kranz, Executive Director
Pip Marks, Director Outreach Services

5163 ID Card for Third Ventriculostomy Patients
Hydrocephalus Association
870 Market Street   415-732-7040
San Francisco, CA 94102-2912   888-598-3789
                                  Fax: 415-732-7044
                   e-mail: info@hydroassoc.org
                               www.hydroassoc.org

Dory Kranz, Executive Director
Pip Marks, Director Outreach Services

5164 LINK Directory Information
Hydrocephalus Association
870 Market Street   415-732-7040
San Francisco, CA 94102-2912   888-598-3789
                                  Fax: 415-732-7044
                   e-mail: info@hydroassoc.org
                               www.hydroassoc.org

A nationwide network of individuals listed in directory format giving members direct access to others in similar circumstances.
Dory Kranz, Executive Director
Pip Marks, Director Outreach Services

5165 Learning Disabilities in Children with Hydrocephalus
Hydrocephalus Association
870 Market Street   415-732-7040
San Francisco, CA 94102-2912   888-598-3789
                                  Fax: 415-732-7044
                   e-mail: info@hydroassoc.org
                               www.hydroassoc.org

Available in Spanish.
Dory Kranz, Executive Director
Pip Marks, Director Outreach Services

5166 Nonverbal Learning Disorder Syndrome
Hydrocephalus Association
870 Market Street   415-732-7040
San Francisco, CA 94102-2912   888-598-3789
                                  Fax: 415-732-7044
                   e-mail: info@hydroassoc.org
                               www.hydroassoc.org

1998
Dory Kranz, Executive Director
Pip Marks, Director Outreach Services

5167 Prenatal Hydrocephalus: A Book for Parents
Hydrocephalus Association
870 Market Street   415-732-7040
San Francisco, CA 94102-2912   888-598-3789
                                  Fax: 415-732-7044
                   e-mail: info@hydroassoc.org
                               www.hydroassoc.org

Dory Kranz, Executive Director
Pip Marks, Director Outreach Services

5168 Resource Guide
Hydrocephalus Association
870 Market Street   415-732-7040
San Francisco, CA 94102-2912   888-598-3789
                                  Fax: 415-732-7044
                               www.hydroassoc.org

A comprehensive listing of 450 articles on all aspects of hydrocephalus. Articles may be ordered from the association for a small fee.
Dory Kranz, Executive Director
Pip Marks, Director Outreach Services

5169 Resource Guide: Normal Pressure Hydrocephalus/Adult Onset
Hydrocephalus Association
870 Market Street   415-732-7040
San Francisco, CA 94102-2912   888-598-3789
                                  Fax: 415-732-7044
                   e-mail: info@hydroassoc.org
                               www.hydroassoc.org

Dory Kranz, Executive Director
Pip Marks, Director Outreach Services

5170 Social Skills Development in Children with Hydrocephalus
Hydrocephalus Association

870 Market Street   415-732-7040
San Francisco, CA 94102-2912   888-598-3789
                                  Fax: 415-732-7044
                   e-mail: info@hydroassoc.org
                               www.hydroassoc.org

Dory Kranz, Executive Director
Pip Marks, Director Outreach Services

5171 Survival Skills for the Family Unit
Hydrocephalus Association
870 Market Street   415-732-7040
San Francisco, CA 94102-2912   888-598-3789
                                  Fax: 415-732-7044
                   e-mail: info@hydroassoc.org
                               www.hydroassoc.org

Dory Kranz, Executive Director
Pip Marks, Director Outreach Services

5172 Understanding Your Child's Education Needs/Individualized Education Program
Hydrocephalus Association
870 Market Street   415-732-7040
San Francisco, CA 94102-2912   888-598-3789
                                  Fax: 415-732-7044
                   e-mail: info@hydroassoc.org
                               www.hydroassoc.org

Dory Kranz, Executive Director
Pip Marks, Director Outreach Services

Audio & Video

5173 Hydrocephalus: A Neglected Disease
Guardians of Hydrocephalus Research Foundation
2640 East 28 Street   718-743-9650
Brooklyn, NY 11235-2023   Fax: 718-743-9650
                   e-mail: GHRF2618@aol.com
                               www.homestead.com

The Guardians of Hydrocephalus Research Foundation (GHRF) is a non-profit group dedicated to research into the cause and treatment of hydrocephalus
Marie Fischetti, Founder

Web Sites

5174 Healing Well
                               www.healingwell.com
An online health resource guide to medical news, chat, information and articles, newsgroups and message boards, books, disease-related web sites, medical directories, and more for patients, friends, and family coping with disabling diseases, disorders, or chronic illnesses.

5175 Health Finder
                               www.healthfinder.gov
Searchable, carefully developed web site offering information on over 1000 topics. Developed by the US Department of Health and Human Services, the site can be used in both English and Spanish.

5176 Healthlink USA
                               www.healthlinkusa.com
Health information concerning treatment, cures, prevention, diagnosis, risk factors, research, support groups, email lists, personal stories and much more. Updated regularly.

5177 Helios Health
                               www.helioshealth.com
Online resource for your health information. Detailed information about specific health topics, access to expert advice from our Medical Advisory Board, and up-to-date health news.

5178 Hydrocephalus Association
                               www.hydroassoc.org
Provides support, education and advocacy for families and professionals. The goal is to insure that families and individuals dealing with the complexities of hydrocephalus receive personal support, comprehensive educational materials and on-going medical care.

5179 Hydrocephalus Center

www.patientcenters.com/hydrocephalus

An online reference that was created especially as a resource for those with hydrocephalus and their families.

5180 MedicineNet

www.medicinenet.com

An online resource for consumers providing easy-to-read, authoritative medical and health information.

5181 Medscape

www.medscape.com

Medscape offers specialists, primary care physicians, and other health professionals the Web's most robust and integrated medical information and educational tools.

5182 Neurology Channel

www.healthcommunities.com

Find clearly explained, medically accurate information regarding conditions, including an overview, symptoms, causes, diagnostic procedures and treatment options. On this site it is possible to ask questions and get information from a neurologist and connect to people who have similar health interests.

5183 WebMD

www.webmd.com

Provides credible information, supportive communities, and in-depth reference material about health subjects. A source for original and timely health information as well as material from well known content providers.

Description

5184 Hypertension

Hypertension is an abnormal elevation of blood pressure. Blood pressure is noted as a top number (systolic) over a bottom number (diastolic) with a reading of 120/80 being recognized as normal. Hypertension is defined as a systolic pressure greater than 140 and/or a diastolic pressure greater than 90. It is a common disorder that affects about 20 percent of the population. Primary, or essential, hypertension is the most common form, and it has no known cause. It is more prevalent in African-Americans, males, and those with a family history of high blood pressure. Other risk factors include obesity, diabetes, high levels of fat and cholesterol, smoking, sedentary lifestyle and psychological stress. It is a significant risk factor for coronary heart disease, heart failure, stroke, and kidney failure.

Patients with hypertension generally have no symptoms. Diagnosis is made by simple measurement with a blood pressure cuff. Several measurements are necessary at different times to establish the diagnosis.

Treatment of hypertension is done in a step-wise fashion beginning with lifestyle modifications (weight reduction, regular exercise, smoking cessation, a low salt, fat and cholesterol diet and improved stress reduction.) If medications are necessary, doctors can choose from a wide variety of effective and usually well-tolerated drugs. Therapy generally must be lifelong.

Occasionally the blood pressure may be refractory, or difficult to control with medicines. In this instance, screening is needed for unusual causes of hypertension, such as renovascular disease (narrowing of the arteries feeding the kidneys), hyperaldosteronism (a tumor or overgrowth of the adrenal gland which secretes hormones that raise the blood pressure), or aortic coarctation (a congenital malformation of the major blood vessels near the heart.) If no specifically treatable cause is identified, the patient will require combination therapy with high doses of drugs. Given a commitment to doing so, it is almost always possible to control the pressure.

National Agencies & Associations

5185 American Society of Hypertension
45 Main Street   212-696-9099
Brooklyn, NY 11201   Fax: 347-916-0267
e-mail: ash@ash-us.org
www.ash-us.org
To organize and conduct educational seminars, materials and products in all aspects of hypertension and other cardiovascular diseases.
William B White, President
Torry Mark Sansone, Executive Director

5186 National Heart, Lung & Blood Institute
PO Box 30105   301-592-8573
Bethesda, MD 20824-0105   Fax: 301-592-8563
TTY: 240-629-3255
e-mail: nhlbiinfo@nhlbi.nih.gov
www.nhlbi.nih.gov

Primary responsibility of this organization is the scientific investigation of heart, blood vessel, lung and blood disorders. Oversee research, demonstration, prevention, education and training activities in these fields and emphasizes the control of stroke.
Gary H Gibbons, MD, Director

5187 National Hypertension Association
324 E 39th Street   212-889-3557
New York, NY 10016   Fax: 212-447-7032
e-mail: nathypertension@aol.com
www.nathypertension.org
Conducts research on the cause of hypertension through basic laboratory and clinical studies sponsors seminars and symposia to keep the medical profession and public abreast of services and advances in the treatment of hypertension.
William M Manger, MD, PhD, Chairman

5188 National Stroke Association
9707 E Easter Lane   303-649-9299
Centennial, CO 80112-3747   800-787-6537
Fax: 303-649-1328
e-mail: Info@stroke.org
www.stroke.org
A national organization whose sole purpose is to reduce the incidence and impact of stroke through prevention treatment rehabilitation and research and support for stroke survivors and their families. NSA produces a variety of education materials and other support services.
Michael D Walker, MD, Chairman
James Baranski, CEO

5189 Pulmonary Hypertension Association
801 Roeder Road   301-565-3004
Silver Spring, MD 20910   800-748-7274
Fax: 301-565-3994
e-mail: pha@PHAssociation.org
www.PHAssociation.org
A nonprofit organization for pulmonary hypertension patients families caregivers and PH-treating medical professionals. The mission of the Pulmonary Hypertension Association (PHA) is to find ways to prevent and cure pulmonary hypertension.
Vallerie McLaughlin, MD, Chair
Rino Aldrighetti, President & CEO

5190 Sentry Health Monitors
200 East Randolph   877-446-3743
Chicago, IL 60601   Fax: 301-476-9388
e-mail: lcreasman@sentryhealthmonitors.com
www.lifeclinic.com
The lifeclinic.com web site was developed to provide an in-depth resource for information about prevalent, long-term health conditions and an online service to track your health over time. It also provides the information, resources and tools that can help patients and their families.
Leslie Creasman, Manager of Customer Service

Research Centers

5191 Creighton University Midwest Hypertension Research Center
601 N 30th Street   402-280-4507
Omaha, NE 68131-2137   Fax: 402-280-4101
Dr William PhD, Director

5192 Hahnemann University: Division of Surgical Research
230 N Broad Street   215-762-7000
Philadelphia, PA 19102   866-884-4HUH
Fax: 215-762-8109
www.hahnemannhospital.com
Studies hypertension and management of stress ulcers.
Teuro Matsum Carretero, Division Head
William H Beierwaltes, Scientist

5193 Henry Ford Hospital: Hypertension and Vascular Research Division
2799 W Grand Boulevard   313-972-1693
Detroit, MI 48202-2689   Fax: 313-876-1479
e-mail: ocarret1@hfhs.org
www.hypertensionresearch.org

Basic biomedical research seeks to understand: The role of vaso-constrictors and vasodilators (angiotensin II bradykinin nitric oxide natriuretic peptides) in the regulation of blood pressure development of hypertension and development of target organ damage (myocardial infarction heart failure vascular injury and renal disease); The generation of reactive oxygen species by blood vessels and kidney cells and how this contributes to target organ damage; and The mechanisms by which therape
William H Beierwaltes, Ph.D., Faculty
Oscar A Carretero, Faculty

5194 Indiana University: Hypertension Research Center
425 University Boulevard 317-274-4591
Indianapolis, IN 46202-0001 800-274-4862
Fax: 317-278-0673
www.indiana.edu/medical
The mission of the Center is to conduct research in the causes diagnosis treatment and prevention of high blood pressure and its complications.
Dr Myron Rom MPH, Director
Eric Schips, Divisional Administrator

5195 New York University General Clinical Research Center
NYU Medical Center
550 First Avenue 212-263-7300
New York, NY 10016 Fax: 212-263-8501
www.med.nyu.edu
Focuses in the areas of hypertension and studies into endocrinology.
Robert I Grossman, MD, Dean & CEO
Steven B Abramson, MD, Senior Vice President and Vice Dean for

5196 University of Michigan: Division of Hypertension
1500 E Medical Center 734-615-0863
Ann Arbor, MI 48109 855-855-0863
www.med.umich.edu
Excellence in medical education patient care and research.
Douglas L Stoulil, Study Coordinator

5197 University of Minnesota: Hypertensive Research Group
611 Beacon Street SE 612-624-1438
Minneapolis, MN 55455
Research pertaining to hypertension and stress disorders.
Jack Massry, Head

5198 University of Southern California: Division of Nephrology
2025 Zonal Avenue 323-442-5100
Los Angeles, CA 90033-1034 Fax: 213-226-3958
www.usc.edu/health/internal/divisions/ne
Research into hypertension and sleep disorders.
Gbemisola A Adeseun, MD, MPH, Faculty
Vito M Campese, MD, Faculty

5199 University of Virginia: Hypertension and Atherosclerosis Unit
Medical Center 804-924-8470
Charlottesville, VA 22908-0001 Fax: 804-924-2581
Dr Carlos DVM, Director

5200 Wake Forest University: Arteriosclerosis Research Center
Department of Comparative Medicine
300 S Hawthorne Road 336-764-3600
Winston-Salem, NC 27103-2732 Fax: 336-764-5818
Hypertension research.
Thomas Clark

Support Groups & Hotlines

5201 National Health Information Center
PO Box 1133 310-565-4167
Washington, DC 20013 800-336-4797
Fax: 301-984-4256
e-mail: info@nhic.org
www.health.gov/nhic
Offers a nationwide information referral service, produces directories and resource guides.

Books

5202 Courage: Poems & Positive Thoughts for Stroke Survivors
National Stroke Association
9707 E Easter Lane 303-649-9299
Centennial, CO 80112-3747 800-787-6537
Fax: 303-649-1328
e-mail: info@stroke.org
www.stroke.org
Words of inspiration from survivors and caregivers.
83 pages
Colette Lafosse, Director Rehabilitation/Recovery Program

5203 Discovery Circles
National Stroke Association
9707 E Easter Lane 303-649-9299
Centennial, CO 80112-3747 800-787-6537
Fax: 303-649-1328
e-mail: info@stroke.org
www.stroke.org
NSA's guide to organizing and facilitating stroke support groups. This detailed manual describes the support group structure and the facilitator's role.
213 pages
Dave Egger, Publisher
Nancy Coulter, Editor

5204 Magic of Humor in Caregiving
National Stroke Association
9707 E Easter Lane 303-649-9299
Centennial, CO 80112-3747 800-787-6537
Fax: 303-649-1328
e-mail: info@stroke.org
www.stroke.org
A dynamic researching tool focusing on the necessity of humor in daily caregiving interaction.
Colette Lafosse, Director Rehabilitation/Recovery Program
James R. Sherman, Author

5205 Management of Hypertension
EMIS Medical Publishers
Durant, OK 74702-1607 580-924-0643
800-225-0694
Fax: 580-924-9414

ISBN: 0-929240-62-6
Kenneth H. Coope, Publisher

5206 November Days
National Stroke Association
9707 E Easter Lane 303-649-9299
Centennial, CO 80112-3747 800-787-6537
Fax: 303-649-1328
e-mail: info@stroke.org
www.stroke.org
A caregiver's story of her struggle with a loved one's stroke.
225 pages

5207 Ted's Stroke: The Caregiver's Story
National Stroke Association
9707 E Easter Lane 303-649-9299
Centennial, CO 80112-3747 800-787-6537
Fax: 303-649-1328
e-mail: info@stroke.org
www.stroke.org
Personal experiences, guidance and tips for caregivers.
175 pages
ISBN: 0-962487-61-9
Seven Locks, Publisher

5208 Women in Your Life: Protect Yourself, Protect Your Family
National Stroke Association
9707 E Easter Lane 303-649-9299
Centennial, CO 80112-3747 800-787-6537
Fax: 303-649-1328
e-mail: info@stroke.org
www.stroke.org
Valuable information about the unique toll stroke takes on women.
Colette Lafosse, Director Rehabilitation/Recovery Program

Magazines

5209 American Journal of Hypertension
American Society of Hypertension
45 Main Street   212-696-9099
New York, NY 11201   Fax: 347-916-0267
                                   e-mail: ash@ash-us.org
                                   www.ash-us.org

5210 Ethnicity & Disease
International Society on Hypertension in Blacks
2045 Manchester Street NE   404-875-6263
Atlanta, GA 30324-4110   Fax: 404-875-6334
                                   e-mail: member@ishib.org
                                   www.ishib.org
International journal on ethnic minority population differences in diease patterns. Provides a comprehensive source of information on the causal relationships in the etiology of common illnesses through the study of ethnic patterns of disease.
Quarterly
John Willey, Publisher
Melanie T Cockfield, Director Administration

5211 Ethnicity Disease
International Society on Hypertension in Blacks
2045 Manchester Street NE   404-875-6263
Atlanta, GA 30324-4110   Fax: 404-875-6334
                                   e-mail: member@ishib.org
                                   www.ishib.org
Determined to accomplish the overall mission to improving the health and life expectancy of ethnic minority populations around the world. Publishes a quarterly journal and holds an annual conference.
150 pages Quarterly
Christopher T Fitzpatrick, CEO
Melanie T Cockfield, Director Administration

5212 Magazine of the National Institute of Hypertension Studies
13217 Livernois Avenue   313-931-3427
Detroit, MI 48238-3162
Association news.

Newsletters

5213 News Report
National Hypertension Association
324 E 30th Street   212-889-3557
New York, NY 10016-8329   Fax: 212-447-7032
                                   e-mail: nathypertension@aol.com
                                   www.nathypertension.org
Offers information and medical updates regarding hypertension. Recent book publication: 100 Questions and Answers about Hypertension by WM Manger, MD, PhD, and RW Gifford, Jr, MT available throught National Hypertension Association.
W.M. Manger MD, PhD, Chairman

Pamphlets

5214 African-Americans and Stroke
National Stroke Association
9707 E Easter Lane   303-649-9299
Centennial, CO 80112-3747   800-787-6537
                                   Fax: 303-649-1328
                                   e-mail: info@stroke.org
                                   www.stroke.org
Colette Lafosse, Director Rehabilitation/Recovery Program

5215 Aneurysm Answers
National Stroke Association
9707 E Easter Lane   303-649-9299
Centennial, CO 80112-3747   800-787-6537
                                   Fax: 303-649-1328
                                   e-mail: info@stroke.org
                                   www.stroke.org
Colette Lafosse, Director Rehabilitation/Recovery Program

5216 Check Your Pulse, America: Atrial Fibrillation
National Stroke Association
9707 E Easter Lane   303-649-9299
Centennial, CO 80112-3747   800-787-6537
                                   Fax: 303-649-1328
                                   e-mail: info@stroke.org
                                   www.stroke.org
Colette Lafosse, Director Rehabilitation/Recovery Program

5217 Cholesterol and Stroke
National Stroke Association
9707 E Easter Lane   303-649-9299
Centennial, CO 80112-3747   800-787-6537
                                   Fax: 303-649-1328
                                   e-mail: info@stroke.org
                                   www.stroke.org
Colette Lafosse, Director Rehabilitation/Recovery Program

5218 High Blood Pressure and Stroke
National Stroke Association
9707 E Easter Lane   303-649-9299
Centennial, CO 80112-3747   800-787-6537
                                   Fax: 303-649-1328
                                   e-mail: info@stroke.org
                                   www.stroke.org
Colette Lafosse, Director Rehabilitation/Recovery Program

5219 Mobility: Issues Facing Stroke Survivors and Their Families
National Stroke Association
9707 E Easter Lane   303-649-9299
Centennial, CO 80112-3747   800-787-6537
                                   Fax: 303-649-1328
                                   e-mail: info@stroke.org
                                   www.stroke.org
Colette Lafosse, Director Rehabilitation/Recovery Program

5220 Recurrent Stroke
National Stroke Association
9707 E Easter Lane   303-649-9299
Centennial, CO 80112-3747   800-787-6537
                                   Fax: 303-649-1328
                                   e-mail: info@stroke.org
                                   www.stroke.org
Colette Lafosse, Director Rehabilitation/Recovery Program

5221 Smoking Cessation: Be Smoke Free in 3 Minutes
National Stroke Association
9707 E Easter Lane   303-649-9299
Centennial, CO 80112-3747   800-787-6537
                                   Fax: 303-649-1328
                                   e-mail: info@stroke.org
                                   www.stroke.org
Colette Lafosse, Director Rehabilitation/Recovery Program

5222 Transient Ischemic Attack
National Stroke Association
9707 E Easter Lane   303-649-9299
Centennial, CO 80112-3747   800-787-6537
                                   Fax: 303-649-1328
                                   e-mail: info@stroke.org
                                   www.stroke.org
Seemant Chaturvedi MD, Author
Steven R. Levine MD, Author

Audio & Video

5223 Stroke: Touching the Soul of Your Family
National Stroke Association
9707 E Easter Lane   303-649-9299
Centennial, CO 80112-3747   800-787-6537
                                   Fax: 303-649-1328
                                   e-mail: info@stroke.org
                                   www.stroke.org
Fifteen minute video chronicling three stroke survivors and their courageous struggle to overcome daily challenges and educate others about stroke.
Colette Lafosse, Director Rehabilitation/Recovery Program

Web Sites

5224 American Society of Hypertension

www.ash-us.org

To organize and conduct educational seminars, materials, and products in all aspects of hypertension and other cardiovascular diseases.

5225 Healing Well

www.healingwell.com

An online health resource guide to medical news, chat, information and articles, newsgroups and message boards, books, disease-related web sites, medical directories, and more for patients, friends, and family coping with disabling diseases, disorders, or chronic illnesses.

5226 Health Finder

www.healthfinder.gov

Searchable, carefully developed web site offering information on over 1000 topics. Developed by the US Department of Health and Human Services, the site can be used in both English and Spanish.

5227 Healthlink USA

www.healthlinkusa.com

Links to websites which may include treatment, cures, diagnosis, prevention, support groups, email lists, messageboards, personal stories, risk factors, statistics, research and more.

5228 Helios Health

www.helioshealth.com

Online resource for your health information. Detailed information about specific health topics, access to expert advice from our Medical Advisory Board, and up-to-date health news.

5229 Hypertension: Journal of the American Heart Association

hyper.ahajournals.org

Lists current issues of journals about hypertension and the American Heart Association.

5230 Inter-American Society of Hypertension

www.iashonline.org

Website hosted by IASH, a non-profit professional organization devoted to the understanding, prevention and control of hypertension and vascular diseases in the American population. Members from 20 different countries in the Americas as well as Europe, Australia and Asia. Stimulates research and the exchange of ideas in hypertension and vascular diseases amoung physicians and scientists. Promotes the detection, control and prevention of hypertension and other cardiovascular risk factors.

5231 Lifeclinic.Com

www.lifeclinic.com

Online information about blood pressure, hypertension, diabetes, cholesterol, stroke, heart failure and more. Maintains current, up-to-date and accurate information for patients to help them manage their conditions better and to improve communications between them and their doctors.

5232 Mayo Clinic Health Oasis

www.mayohealth.org

Mission is to empower people to manage their health, by providing useful and up-to-date information and tools that reflect the expertise and standard of excellence of the Mayo Clinic.

5233 MedicineNet

www.medicinenet.com

An online resource for consumers providing easy-to-read, authoritative medical and health information.

5234 Medscape

www.medscape.com

Medscape offers specialists, primary care physicians, and other health professionals the Web's most robust and integrated medical information and educational tools.

5235 National Heart, Lung & Blood Institute

www.nhlbi.nih.gov

Information on the scientific investigation of heart, blood vessel, lung and blood disorders. Oversee research, demonstration, prevention, education and training activities in these fields and emphasizes the control of stroke.

5236 WebMD

www.webmd.com

Provides credible information, supportive communities, and in-depth reference material about health subjects. A source for original and timely health information as well as material from well known content providers.

Description

5237 Impotence

Impotence, also called erectile dysfunction (ED), is defined as the inability of a male to achieve and maintain an erection of sufficient quality to allow sexual intercourse. ED is very common, affecting millions of American males. Although it may occur at any age, it becomes dramatically more common with advancing age. Impotence may be caused by diabetes, circulatory disturbance, genital injury, hormonal disorders, medication side effects, depression, surgery (for instance, prostate removal) and many less well-characterized physical and psychological states. Impotence may be situational, that is, involving place, time, partner and degree of self-esteem.

Few cases of impotence are completely cured, but several kinds of effective treatment exist, including correction, if possible, of underlying causes. Oral medications that increase blood flow to the penis have been effective in many instances. Psychological factors that accompany ED should be considered in every case, including behavioral therapy and counseling, as needed.

National Agencies & Associations

5238 American Urological Association American Foundation for Urologic Disease
American Foundation for Urologic Disease
1000 Corporate Boulevard
Linthicum, MD 21090
410-689-3700
866-746-4282
Fax: 410-689-3800
e-mail: aua@AUAnet.org
www.auafoundation.org
The American Foundation for Urologic Disease Inc. is a charitable organization established to raise funds for research lay education and patient advocacy for the prevention detection management and cure of urologic disease.
Pramod C Sogani, MD, FACS, FRCS c, President
Gopal H Badlani, MD, Secretary

5239 Impotence Institute of America
119 S Ruth Street
Maryville, TN 37803
865-379-2154
800-669-1603
e-mail: iwatenn@aol.com
A non-profit organization dedicated to education about impotence. The IIA is a division of the Impotence World Association. Provides information on the causes, impact and treatments on this topic. Also publishes a quarterly newsletter on impotence topics.

5240 Impotence Resource Center of the Geddings Osbon Sr Foundation
PO Box 1593
Augusta, GA 30903
800-433-4215
Fax: 706-821-2782
e-mail: impotence@afud.org
www.impotence.org
Offers a free medical discussion where the consumer can obtain accurate unblessed information in a confidential understanding and thoughtful manner.
Rodgers, Director

5241 National Kidney and Urologic Diseases Information Clearinghouse
31 Center Drive MSC 2560
Bethesda, MD 20892-2560
301-496-3583
800-891-5390
Fax: 301-907-8906
e-mail: nkudic@info.niddk.nih.gov
www.niddk.nih.gov

Provides information about diseases of the kidneys and urologic system to people with such afflictions and to their families, health care professionals and the public. Answers inquiries; develops, reviews and distributes publications.
Dr Griffin P Rodgers, Director
Camille M Hoover, Executive Officer

Research Centers

5242 Central New York Male Sexual Dysfunction Center
357 Genesee Street
Oneida, NY 13421
315-363-8862
888-269-6732
Fax: 315-363-5477
www.cnymsdc.com
Burman, Director

5243 Male Sexual Dysfunction Clinic
3401 N Central Avenue
Chicago, IL 60634
800-788-2873
800-788-2873
Fax: 847-231-4130
e-mail: info@msdclinic.com
www.msdclinic.com
Helping men overcome male sexual dysfunctions such as impotence since 1981.
Sheldon O MD, Director

5244 New York Male Reproductive Center: Sexual Dysfunction Unit
161 Fort Washington Avenue
New York, NY 10032
212-305-0123
Fax: 212-305-0126
e-mail: rshabsigh@urology.columbia.edu
The New York Male Reproductive Center at Columbia-Presbyterian Medical Center offers state-of-the-art diagnosis and treatment for impotence. Treatments include surgical and non-surgical procedures.
Ridwan Shabs

Support Groups & Hotlines

5245 Impotence Information Center
PO Box 9
Minneapolis, MN 55440
800-843-4315
MacKenzie, Founder

5246 Impotents Anonymous
8630 Fenton Street
Silver Spring, MD 20910-3803
301-588-5777
Serves as an educational organization providing concerned individuals with information regarding impotence.
Bruce

5247 National Health Information Center
PO Box 1133
Washington, DC 20013
310-565-4167
800-336-4797
Fax: 301-984-4256
e-mail: info@nhic.org
www.health.gov/nhic

Offers a nationwide information referral service, produces directories and resource guides.
MPA, Executive Director
John M Barry MD, President

Books

5248 Impotence: How to Overcome It
HealthProInk Publishing
562 Wind Drift Lane
Spring Lake, MI 49456-2168
313-355-3686
Priyantha Hettiarachchi, Author

5249 It's Not All in Your Head
Impotence Institute of America
8201 Corporate Drive
Landover, MD 20785-2230
301-577-0650
A couple's guide to overcoming impotence.
Gordon J. G. Asmundson PhD, Author
Steven Taylor PhD, Author

Newsletters

5250 Impotence Worldwide
8201 Corporate Drive
Landover, MD 20785-2230   301-577-0650
Provides information from professionals and lay persons concerning impotence plus manufactured product information.
Monthly

5251 Your Sexuality & Health
Impotence Resource Center
333 City Boulevard West,   714-456-2951
Orange, CA 92868-1593   800-433-4215
                                       Fax: 714-456-7263
e-mail: nfo@centerforreconstructiveurology.org
www.centerforreconstructiveurology.org
Quarterly newsletter that features articles by medical experts and highlights current research and tidbits of healthy living advice.
Quarterly

Pamphlets

5252 Answers to the Most Asked Questions About Impotence
Impotence World Services
8201 Corporate Drive   301-577-0650
Landover, MD 20785-2230

5253 Impotence Causes and Treatments
American Medical Systems
10700 Bren Road E   952-933-4666
Minnetonka, MN 55343   800-843-4315
                                       Fax: 952-930-6157
www.visitams.com
Offers information on what impotence is, physical and emotional causes, treatments, questions and answers.

5254 Male Treatment Guide
Impotence Resource Center
333 City Boulevard West,   714-456-2951
Orange, CA 92868-1593   800-433-4215
                                       Fax: 714-456-7263
e-mail: nfo@centerforreconstructiveurology.org
www.centerforreconstructiveurology.org
Explains impotence - what it is, what causes it and how it is treated.
Free

5255 Woman's Perspective
Impotence Resource Center
334 City Boulevard West,   714-456-2952
Orange, CA 92869-1593   800-433-4215
                                       Fax: 714-456-7264
e-mail: nfo@centerforreconstructiveurology.org
www.centerforreconstructiveurology.org
Talking with your partner about impotence and choosing a treatment together.
Free

Audio & Video

5256 Impotence Treatment Options
Impotence Resource Center
335 City Boulevard West,   714-456-2953
Orange, CA 92870-1593   800-433-4215
                                       Fax: 714-456-7265
e-mail: nfo@centerforreconstructiveurology.org
www.centerforreconstructiveurology.org
Actual taping of a men's sexual health seminar - presented by Gary Leach, MD.

5257 Male Treatment Guide
Impotence Resource Center
336 City Boulevard West,   714-456-2954
Orange, CA 92871-1593   800-433-4215
                                       Fax: 714-456-7266
e-mail: nfo@centerforreconstructiveurology.org
www.centerforreconstructiveurology.org

Explains impotence - what it is, what causes it and how it is treated.
Audio Tape

5258 Medical Management of Impotence
Impotence Resource Center
337 City Boulevard West,   714-456-2955
Orange, CA 92872-1593   800-433-4215
                                       Fax: 714-456-7267
e-mail: nfo@centerforreconstructiveurology.org
www.centerforreconstructiveurology.org

5259 Woman's Perspective
Impotence Resource Center
338 City Boulevard West,   714-456-2956
Orange, CA 92873-1593   800-433-4215
                                       Fax: 714-456-7268
e-mail: nfo@centerforreconstructiveurology.org
www.centerforreconstructiveurology.org
Talking with your partner about impotence and choosing a treatment together.
Audio Tape

Web Sites

5260 American Foundation for Urologic Disease

e-mail: nfo@centerforreconstructiveurology.org
www.urologyhealth.org
The Urology Care Foundation is committed to promoting urology research and education. They work with researchers, healthcare professionals, patients and caregivers to improve patients' lives.

5261 Family Meds

www.familymeds.com
At Familymeds.com VIPPS certified online pharmacy, they process all of our prescriptions through a fully U.S. and Connecticut licensed and accredited pharmacy based in Farmington, CT.

5262 Healing Well

www.healingwell.com
An online health resource guide to medical news, chat, information and articles, newsgroups and message boards, books, disease-related web sites, medical directories, and more for patients, friends, and family coping with disabling diseases, disorders, or chronic illnesses.

5263 Health Finder

www.healthfinder.gov
Searchable, carefully developed web site offering information on over 1000 topics. Developed by the US Department of Health and Human Services, the site can be used in both English and Spanish.

5264 Healthlink USA

www.healthlinkusa.com
Health information concerning treatment, cures, prevention, diagnosis, risk factors, research, support groups, email lists, personal stories and much more. Updated regularly.

5265 Helios Health

www.helioshealth.com
Online resource for your health information. Detailed information about specific health topics, access to expert advice from our Medical Advisory Board, and up-to-date health news.

5266 Impotence Resource Center of the Geddings Osbon Sr Foundation

www.centerforreconstructiveurology.org
A regional, national, and international tertiary referral center dedicated to the treatment of disorders of the male urethra and external genitalia. In addition to patient care, there mission includes clinical and laboratory research and teaching.

5267 Impotence Specialists.com

www.impotencespecialists.com
Offers information on physicians in your area, treatment options, online resources and more. A guide to the nation's impotence specialists.

5268 Impotence World Association

www.impotence.com

Informs and educates the public on the subject of impotence and its causes and treatments. Serving the impotence industry since 1983 by bringing total care to the treatment of impotence.

5269   MedicineNet

www.medicinenet.com

An online resource for consumers providing easy-to-read, authoritative medical and health information.

5270   Medscape

www.medscape.com

Medscape offers specialists, primary care physicians, and other health professionals the Web's most robust and integrated medical information and educational tools.

5271   WebMD

www.webmd.com

Provides credible information, supportive communities, and in-depth reference material about health subjects. A source for original and timely health information as well as material from well known content providers.

Description

5272 Incontinence

Urinary incontinence is the involuntary leakage of urine, whether during waking or sleeping hours. One common type is urge incontinence, resulting from involuntary bladder contractions. The person feels a sudden urge to urinate, so intense that it may not be controlled long enough to reach the toilet. Common causes of urge incontinence are urinary tract infections, spinal cord injury, and kidney stones. Stress incontinence is the instantaneous leakage of urine without bladder contractions. It manifests as loss of urine during stress events, such as coughing, sneezing, laughing, or lifting. This may occur in women due to weak bladder tone from multiple pregnancies. In men, stress incontinence can occur after prostate removal or trauma to the bladder. Overflow incontinence, in which the bladder cannot control urine output, can be caused by nerve injury, alcoholism, and some diseases. Symptoms include urgency, and having to urinate more often (frequency) and at night (nocturia).

Treatment of incontinence focuses on therapy for the underlying causes. Infections are treated with the appropriate antibiotics. Stress incontinence in women can be treated with exercises to strengthen the bladder muscles. Other therapies include biofeedback and electrical stimulation. Severe cases may require surgical repair. Urinary incontinence remains largely a neglected problem, despite the fact that it can often be successfully treated.

National Agencies & Associations

5273 International Foundation for Functional Gastrointestinal Disorders (IFFGD)

700 W. Virginia Street
Milwaukee, WI 53204-8076

414-964-1799
888-964-2001
Fax: 414-964-7176
e-mail: iffgd@iffgd.org
www.iffgd.org

Nonprofit education, support and research organization devoted to increasing awareness and understanding of functional gastrointestinal disorders including irritable bowel syndrome (IBS), constipation, diarrhea, pain and incontinence.
Nancy J Norton, Co-Founder & President
William Norton, Co-Founder

5274 Intestinal Disease Foundation

100 W Station Square Drive
Pittsburgh, PA 15219-1122

412-261-5888
877-587-9606
Fax: 412-471-2722
www.intestinalfoundation.org

Provides one-on-one telephone support, educational programs and materials and self-help groups for people with irritable bowel syndrome (IBS), diverticular disease, inflammatory bowel diseases and short bowel syndrome; sponsors educational seminars; provides educational materials.
Harriet Gibb Deng, Chairperson
Nancy Muller, Executive Director

5275 National Association for Continence

PO Box 1019
Charleston, SC 29402-1019

843-377-0900
800-BLA-DDER
Fax: 843-377-0905
e-mail: memberservices@nafc.org
www.nafc.org

Founded as Help for Incontinent People, NAFC is the foremost consumer advocacy organization dedicated to helping people who struggle with incontinence and related voiding dysfunction. Its mission is focused on public education, awareness and collaboration.
Donna Browdie, Chair
James Firman EdD, President/CEO

5276 National Council on Aging

1901 L Street NW
Washington, DC 20036

202-479-1200
800-677-1116
Fax: 202-479-0735
TTY: 202-479-6674
TDD: 202-479-6674
e-mail: info@ncoa.org
www.ncoa.org

Organizations and professionals promoting the dignity self-determination and well-being of older persons.
Richard Gartley, President/Founder
Elizabeth LaGro, Vice President, Communications & Educati

5277 Simon Foundation for Continence

PO Box 815
Wilmette, IL 60091

847-864-3913
800-237-4666
Fax: 847-864-9758
e-mail: info@simonfoundation.org
www.simonfoundation.org

Seeks to bring the topic of incontinence out of the closet and remove the associated stigma; provides educational materials to patients their families and the health care professionals who provide patient care.
Cheryle

5278 Urology Care Foundation

1000 Corporate Boulevard
Linthicum, MD 21090

410-689-3700
800-828-7866
Fax: 410-689-3998
e-mail: info@urologycarefoundation.org
www.urologyhealth.org

A charitable organization whose mission is the prevention and cure of urologic diseases through the expansion of research education and public awareness.
Sandra Vasso Norton, President

Support Groups & Hotlines

5279 Greater New York Pull-Thru Network

62 Edgewood Avenue
Wyckoff, NJ 07481

201-891-5977

National support network providing emotional support and information to patients and families of children who have had or will have a pull-thru type surgery to correct an imperforate anus or associated malformation, Hirschsprung's or other fecal incontinence problems. Support group meetings held quarterly.

5280 National Health Information Center

PO Box 1133
Washington, DC 20013

301-565-4167
800-336-4797
Fax: 301-984-4256
e-mail: info@nhic.org
www.health.gov/nhic

Offers a nationwide information referral service, produces directories and resource guides.
Gartley, Founder/President
Elizabeth LaGro, Vice President, Communications & Educati

5281 Simon Foundation Helpline for Incontinence Information

Simon Foundation for Continence
PO Box 815
Wilmette, IL 60091

847-864-3913
800-237-4666
Fax: 847-864-9758
e-mail: info@simonfoundation.org
www.simonfoundation.org

Offers information and help to persons with incontinence problems and professionals who work with them.
Cheryle Brown MD, Director

5282 University of California at San Francisco Women's Continence Center
2356 Sutter Street
San Francisco, CA 94115
415-885-7788
877-366-8532
coe.ucsf.edu/wcc
Offers a comprehensive array of clinical services for women with incontinence, urethal or bladder dysfuntion and pelvic support problems.
Jeanette S Vecchiarello, President/Board of Directors
Doni DeBolt, Executive Director

Books

5283 Managing Incontinence: a Guide to Living with Loss of Bladder Control
Simon Foundation for Incontinence
PO Box 815
Wilmette, IL 60091
847-864-3913
800-237-4666
Fax: 847-864-9768
e-mail: simoninfo@simonfoundation.org
www.simonfoundation.org
Seeks to bring the topic of incontinence out of the closet and remove the associated stigma; provides information to patients, their families and the health care professionals who provide patient care.
Quarterly
Cheryle B Gartley, President
Cheryle Gartley, Author

5284 Pocket Guide for Continence Care
National Association for Continence
PO Box 1019
Charleston, SC 29402
843-377-0900
800-252-3337
Fax: 843-377-0905
e-mail: memberservices@nafc.org
www.nafc.org
Condensed version of the Blueprint for Continence Care, this guide is designed for a first line supervisor or any health care professional in any eldercare environment to help address any issues related to bladder health. The guide is perfect for a quick referral because it can actually fit in the healthcare professional's pocket.
Nancy Muller, Executive Director
Caryn Antos, Publicity/Publications Associate

5285 Resource Guide: Products and Services for Incontinence
National Association for Continence
PO Box 1019
Charleston, SC 29402
843-377-0900
800-252-3337
Fax: 843-377-0905
e-mail: memberservices@nafc.org
www.nafc.org
Complete directory of products and services available. Categories include disposable products, reusable products, skin care products, deodorizing products, pelvic organ support devices, medications to treat incontinence and others. Also includes a listing of distributors and mail/phone order companies.
Nancy Muller, Executive Director
Caryn Antos, Publicity/Publications Associate

5286 Your Personal Guide to Bladder Health
National Association for Continence
PO Box 1019
Charleston, SC 29402
843-377-0900
800-252-3337
Fax: 843-377-0905
e-mail: memberservices@nafc.org
www.nafc.org
Designed for residents of assisted living environments, other older individuals living independently and their involved family members. It encompasses a wide variety of informative topics, including diet and daily habits, pelvic muscle exercises odor control and more.
48 pages
Nancy Muller, Executive Director
Caryn Antos, Publicity/Publications Associate

Magazines

5287 Digestive Health Matters
Intl. Foundation for Gastrointestinal Disorders
PO Box 170864
Milwaukee, WI 53217-0864
414-964-1799
888-964-2001
Fax: 414-964-7176
e-mail: iffgd@iffgd.org
www.iffgd.org
Quarterly journal focuses on upper and lower gastrointestinal disorders in adults and children. Educational pamphlets and factsheets are available. Patient and professional membership.

Newsletters

5288 Discoveries
National Association for Continence
PO Box 1019
Charleston, SC 29402
843-377-0900
800-252-3337
Fax: 843-377-0905
e-mail: memberservices@nafc.org
www.nafc.org
Compendium comprised of the most recently released incontinence products and newly approved protocol. Includes editorial sections, authored by leading clinicians and researchers, describing new product technology and research in other medical advances related to continence care.
32 pages BiAnnual
Nancy Muller, Executive Director
Caryn Antos, Publicity/Publications Associate

5289 Informer
Simon Foundation for Incontinence
PO Box 815
Wilmette, IL 60091
847-864-3913
800-237-4666
Fax: 847-864-9768
e-mail: simoninfo@simonfoundation.org
www.simonfoundation.org
Seeks to bring the topic of incontinence out of the closet and remove the associated stigma; provides information to patients, their families, and the health care professionals who provide patient care.
Quarterly
Cheryle B Gartley, President
Bret Easton Ellis, Author

5290 Intestinal Fortitude
Intestinal Disease Foundation
One Station Square
Pittsburgh, PA 15219
412-261-5888
Fax: 412-471-2722
www.intestinalfoundation.org
Newsletter, brochures and books for Intestinal Disease Foundation members.
Dwight Franklin, Author

5291 Participate
IFFGD
PO Box 17864
Milwaukee, WI 53217-0864
414-964-1799
888-964-2001
Fax: 414-964-7176
e-mail: iffgd@iffgd.org
www.aboutincontinence.org
Provides information for people affected by the various forms of functional bowel disorders, including irritable bowel syndrome, constipation, diarrhea, pain and incontinence.
Quarterly

5292 Pull-Thru Network News
Greater New York Pull-Thru Network
62 Edgewood Avenue
Wyckoff, NJ 07481-3456
201-891-5977
www.pullthrough.org
Quarterly newsletter for patients and families who have had or will have a pull-thru type surgery to correct an imperforate anus or associated malformation, Hirschsprung's or other fecal incontinence problem.

5293 Quality Care
National Association for Continence
PO Box 1019   843-377-0900
Charleston, SC 29402   800-252-3337
                                          Fax: 843-377-0905
                            e-mail: memberservices@nafc.org
                                              www.nafc.org

Quarterly newsletter addressing causes, symptoms, management and treatment options for incontinence and related disorders.
Quarterly
Nancy Muller, Executive Director
Caryn Antos, Publicity/Publications Associate

Pamphlets

5294 Bladder Control for Women
National Kidney and Urologic Diseases Information
3 Information Way
Bethesda, MD 20892-3580   800-891-5390
                                          Fax: 301-907-8906
                          e-mail: nkudic@info.nidkk.nih.gov
                                       www.kidney.niddk.nih.gov
Comprehensive introduction to the causes, symptoms, and treatments for bladder control problems in women.

5295 Exercising Your Pelvic Muscles
National Kidney and Urologic Diseases Information
3 Information Way
Bethesda, MD 20892-3580   800-891-5390
                                          Fax: 301-907-8906
                          e-mail: nkudic@info.nidkk.nih.gov
                                       www.kidney.niddk.nih.gov
A description of exercises for the pelvic floor muscles, called Kegel exercises, and how they can help to restore or maintain bladder control.

5296 Menopause and Bladder Control
National Kidney and Urologic Diseases Information
3 Information Way
Bethesda, MD 20892-3580   800-891-5390
                                          Fax: 301-907-8906
                          e-mail: nkudic@info.nidkk.nih.gov
                                       www.kidney.niddk.nih.gov
An introduction to the changes to your body that occur during menopause, how these changes can result in loss of bladder control, and how your health care team can help you restore or maintain bladder control.

5297 NAFC Fact Sheets
National Association for Continence
PO Box 1019   843-377-0900
Charleston, SC 29402   800-252-3337
                                          Fax: 843-377-0905
                            e-mail: memberservices@nafc.org
                                              www.nafc.org
Offering helpful tips and information on a variety of topics, the sheets provide consumers and professionals with the necessary information on managing incontinence. Some titles include medications, diet and daily habits, odor control, prostatectomy and many more.
Nancy Muller, Executive Director
Caryn Antos, Publicity/Publications Associate

5298 Pregnancy, Childbirth, and Bladder Control
National Kidney and Urologic Diseases Information
3 Information Way
Bethesda, MD 20892-3580   800-891-5390
                                          Fax: 301-907-8906
                          e-mail: nkudic@info.nidkk.nih.gov
                                       www.kidney.niddk.nih.gov
A look at the effects that pregnancy and childbearing can have on bladder control and ways you can counter those effects.

5299 Talking to Your Health Care Team About Bladder Control
National Kidney and Urologic Diseases Information

3 Information Way
Bethesda, MD 20892-3580   800-891-5390
                                          Fax: 301-907-8906
                          e-mail: nkudic@info.nidkk.nih.gov
                                       www.kidney.niddk.nih.gov
Tips for giving your health care provider the information needed to diagnose and treat your bladder control problem. Includes a questionnaire for you to fill out and take to your first appointment.

5300 Urinary Incontinence in Women
National Kidney and Urologic Diseases Information
3 Information Way
Bethesda, MD 20892-3580   800-891-5390
                                          Fax: 301-907-8906
                          e-mail: nkudic@info.nidkk.nih.gov
                                       www.kidney.niddk.nih.gov
An overview of the types, diagnosis, and treatment of urinary incontinence in women.

5301 What Your Female Patients Want to Know About Bladder Control
National Kidney and Urologic Diseases Information
3 Information Way
Bethesda, MD 20892-3580   800-891-5390
                                          Fax: 301-907-8906
                          e-mail: nkudic@info.nidkk.nih.gov
                                       www.kidney.niddk.nih.gov
Fact sheet with tips for health care providers on raising the issue of incontinence with female patients who may be reluctant to talk about their problem.

5302 Your Body's Design for Bladder Control
National Kidney and Urologic Diseases Information
3 Information Way
Bethesda, MD 20892-3580   800-891-5390
                                          Fax: 301-907-8906
                          e-mail: nkudic@info.nidkk.nih.gov
                                       www.kidney.niddk.nih.gov
An introduction to the female urinary system. Includes diagrams of the bladder and pelvic floor muscles.

5303 Your Daily Bladder Diary
National Kidney and Urologic Diseases Information
3 Information Way
Bethesda, MD 20892-3580   800-891-5390
                                          Fax: 301-907-8906
                          e-mail: nkudic@info.nidkk.nih.gov
                                       www.kidney.niddk.nih.gov
An easy-to-use form for patients to note liquid intake, trips to the bathroom, urine leaks, and other details that may help explain your incontinence.

5304 Your Medicines and Bladder Control
National Kidney and Urologic Diseases Information
3 Information Way
Bethesda, MD 20892-3580   800-891-5390
                                          Fax: 301-907-8906
                          e-mail: nkudic@info.nidkk.nih.gov
                                       www.kidney.niddk.nih.gov
Booklet describing the effects that your medications could have on bladder control, with a recommendation for discussing all your medicines with your doctor.

Audio & Video

5305 Solution Starts with You
Simon Foundation for Continence
PO Box 815   847-864-3913
Wilmette, IL 60091   800-237-4666
                                          Fax: 847-864-9758
                       e-mail: cbgartley@simonfoundation.org
                                      www.simonfoundation.org
Seeks to bring the topic of incontinence out of the closet and remove the associated stigma; provides information to patients, their families, and the health care professionals who provide patient care.
Quarterly
Cheryle Gartley, Founder/President
Jasmine Schmidt, Director of Education

Web Sites

5306   American Foundation for Urologic Disease

www.urologyhealth.org
The Urology Care Foundation is committed to promoting urology research and education. They work with researchers, healthcare professionals, patients and caregivers to improve patients' lives.

5307   Healing Well

www.healingwell.com
An online health resource guide to medical news, chat, information and articles, newsgroups and message boards, books, disease-related web sites, medical directories, and more for patients, friends, and family coping with disabling diseases, disorders, or chronic illnesses.

5308   Health Finder

www.healthfinder.gov
Searchable, carefully developed web site offering information on over 1000 topics. Developed by the US Department of Health and Human Services, the site can be used in both English and Spanish.

5309   Healthlink USA

www.healthlinkusa.com
Health information concerning treatment, cures, prevention, diagnosis, risk factors, research, support groups, email lists, personal stories and much more. Updated regularly.

5310   Helios Health

www.helioshealth.com
Online resource for your health information. Detailed information about specific health topics, access to expert advice from our Medical Advisory Board, and up-to-date health news.

5311   MedicineNet

www.medicinenet.com
An online resource for consumers providing easy-to-read, authoritative medical and health information.

5312   Medscape

www.medscape.com
Medscape offers specialists, primary care physicians, and other health professionals the Web's most robust and integrated medical information and educational tools.

5313   National Association for Continence

www.nafc.org
Interactive website packed with useful information about diagnosis, treatment options and management solutions for incontinence. The site currentlyfeatures a specialist search engine of healthcare providers who have recieved specific training in the diagnosis and treatment of incontinence to assist consumers in locating a specialist in their area. Other features include archived Quality Care articles, a message board, online database of active support groups and much more.

5314   Simon Foundation for Continence

www.simonfoundation.org
Seeks to bring the topic of incontinence out of the closet and remove the associated stigma; provides educational materials to patients, their families, and the health care professionals who provide patient care.

5315   WebMD

www.webmd.com
Provides credible information, supportive communities, and in-depth reference material about health subjects. A source for original and timely health information as well as material from well known content providers.

Description

5316 Infertility

Infertility is defined as the failure to achieve conception by couples who have not used contraception for at least one year, and affects 1 in 5 couples in the United States.

Female causes of infertility include dysfunction of the ovaries (20 percent of couples), blockage of the tubes connecting the ovaries to the uterus (30 percent), and abnormal secretions (5 percent). Infertility in males is mostly related to sperm disorders (35 percent of couples), either insufficient production of sperm, ineffective sperm, or defective delivery of sperm. Unidentified factors account for the remaining 10 percent of couples.

A variety of tests are needed to determine the exact cause of infertility and then identify the appropriate treatment options. Failure to conceive can be both an emotional and financial burden on couples. Counseling and psychological support are important parts of treatment.

National Agencies & Associations

5317 Adopt-A-Special-Kid America
8201 Edgewater Drive
Oakland, CA 94621
510-553-1748
888-680-7349
Fax: 510-553-1747
e-mail: info@aask.org
www.aask.org/
Adopt-A-Special-Kid provides information on adoption of children with special needs.
Roberto Hribek, Chair
Ken Mosesian, Executive Director

5318 American Fertility Association
315 Madison Avenue
New York, NY 10017-0004
888-917-3777
Fax: 718-601-7722
e-mail: info@theafa.org
www.theafa.org
Purpose is to educate the public about reproductive disease and support families during struggles with infertility and adoption. Exists to serve the unique needs of men and women confronting infertility issues.
Don Giudice, MD, PhD, President
Robert W Rebar MD, Executive Director

5319 American Society for Reproductive Medicine
1209 Montgomery Highway
Birmingham, AL 35216-2809
205-978-5000
Fax: 205-978-5005
e-mail: asrm@asrm.org
www.asrm.com
Purpose is to educate the public about reproductive disease and support families during struggles with infertility and adoption. Exists to serve the unique needs of men and women confronting infertility issues.
Linda C. Coffey, President

5320 Hysterectomy Educational Resources & Services (HERS) Foundation
422 Bryn Mawr Avenue
Bala Cynwyd, PA 19004
610-667-7757
888-750-4377
Fax: 610-677-8096
e-mail: HERS@hersfoundation.org
www.hersfoundation.com
A nonprofit foundation which provides information about the alternatives to hysterectomy the risks of the alternatives and the consequences of the surgery. HERS provides telephone counseling by appointment.
Nora W Berger, MD, Member of Advisory Board
Geoffrey Sher, MD, Member of Advisory Board

5321 International Council on Infertility Information Dissemination
PO Box 6836
Arlington, VA 22206
703-379-9178
Fax: 703-379-1593
e-mail: INCIIDinfo@inciid.org
www.inciid.org
Provides information on infertility pregnancy loss adoption high risk pregnancy and parenting after the above.
Gary S Collura, President/CEO
Margaret Chandler Berardelli, Director, Development

5322 RESOLVE: The National Infertility Association
1760 Old Meadow Road
McLean, VA 22102
703-556-7172
Fax: 703-506-3266
e-mail: info@resolve.org
www.resolve.org
A nationwide nonprofit consumer organization serving the unique needs of those striving to build a family. Provides compassionate and informed help to people who are experiencing the infertility crisis and strives to increase the visibility of infertility in the community.
Barbara Collura, Executive Director
Dawn Gannon, Professional Outreach Manager

State Agencies & Associations

Alabama

5323 RESOLVE of Alabama
1760 Old Meadow Road
McLean, VA 22102
703-556-7172
888-473-3062
Fax: 703-506-3266
e-mail: info@southeast.resolve.org
www.southeast.resolve.org/
Barbara Nelson, President
Denny Ceizyk, VP

Arizona

5324 RESOLVE of Valley of the Sun
PO Box 36252
Phoenix, AZ 85067-6252
602-995-3933
e-mail: resolveaz@hotmail.com
www.resolveaz.org
Tina Collura, President/CEO
Margaret Chandler Berardelli, Director, Development

Arkansas

5325 RESOLVE Affiliate of Northwest Arkansas
2230 Country Way
Fayetteville, AR 72703-4215
501-521-3763
888-895-6055
e-mail: info@southcentral.resolve.org
www.southcentral.resolve.org/
Barbara Waldron, CA/San Diego Chair

California

5326 RESOLVE of Greater Los Angeles
PO Box 12529
Newport Beach, CA 92658
310-326-2630
877-203-7771
e-mail: info@southwest.resolve.org
www.southwest.resolve.org
Mari Waldron, CA/San Diego Chair

5327 RESOLVE of Greater San Diego
PO Box 12529
Newport Beach, CA 92658-7385
310-326-2630
877-203-7771
e-mail: info@southwest.resolve.org
www.southwest.resolve.org
Mari Munoz, Northern California Coordinator

5328 RESOLVE of Northern California
312 Sutter Street
San Francisco, CA 94108
415-788-6772
888-591-6663
Fax: 415-788-6774
e-mail: info@northpacific.resolve.org
www.northpacific.resolve.org/
Volunteer-based organization that provides infertility education adoption information advocacy and support.
Tracie Fletcher, Local Area Affiliate Chair

Colorado

5329 RESOLVE of Colorado
PO Box 260725
Littleton, CO 80163-0725
303-469-5261
888-592-4449
e-mail: info@mountain.resolve.org
www.mountain.resolve.org/
Jennifer Malave, Support Services
Maryann Post, Helpline Coordinator

Connecticut

5330 RESOLVE of Fairfield County
PO Box 930
S Norwalk, CT 06856-0930
914-686-1490
888-765-2810
Fax: 203-255-2561
e-mail: info@northeast.resolve.org
northeast.resolve.org
Anne Odeen-Lodato,, Chair
Erin Lasker, Executive Director

5331 RESOLVE of Greater Hartford
PO Box 290964
Wethersfield, CT 06129
781-890-2225
e-mail: admin@resolvenewengland.org
www.resolvenewengland.org/
Pam Bare, Regional Chair
Cindy Peterson, Volunteer Coordinator

District of Columbia

5332 RESOLVE of the Washington Metro Area
PO Box 3423
Merrifield, VA 22116-3423
202-362-5555
888-583-4441
e-mail: info@midatlantic.resolve.org
www.res.pub30.convio.net/Regions/mid-atl
Cindy Gedaro, Florida, Orlando Coordinator

Florida

5333 RESOLVE Affiliate of Central Florida
1050 W Morse Boulevard
Winter Park, FL 32789
407-637-0142
888-473-3062
e-mail: resolveofcentralflorida@gmail.com
www.southeast.resolve.org/
Susanna Witt, Florida, Tampa Coordinator
Kathy Fountain, Florida, Tampa Coordinator

5334 RESOLVE of North Florida
1929 Logging Lane
Jacksonville, FL 32221-2071
904-737-0140
888-473-3062
e-mail: Nicole@theadoptionconsultancy.com
www.southeast.resolve.org/
Nicole Linder, Cooordinator

5335 RESOLVE of South Florida
3342 SW 51 Street
Ft Lauderdale, FL 33312
954-749-9500
888-473-3062
e-mail: resolvesf@yahoo.com
www.southeast.resolve.org/
Elise Badey, Coordinator
Renee Whitley, Advocacy Chair

Georgia

5336 RESOLVE of Georgia
3904 N Druid Hills Road
Decatur, GA 30333
404-233-8443
888-473-3062
e-mail: Katie9924@hotmail.com
southeast.resolve.org
Kate Collura, President/CEO
Margaret Chandler Berardelli, Director, Development

Hawaii

5337 RESOLVE of Hawaii
PO Box 29193
Honolulu, HI 96820
808-528-8559
888-591-6663
e-mail: info@resolveofhawaii.org
www.res.pub30.convio.net/Regions/north-p
Barbara Collura, President/CEO
Margaret Chandler Berardelli, Director, Development

Illinois

5338 RESOLVE of Illinois
PO Box 56
Hinsdale, IL 60521
773-743-1623
888-255-1399
e-mail: info@greatlakes.resolve.org
www.res.pub30.convio.net/Regions/great-l
Barbara Collura, President/CEO
Margaret Chandler Berardelli, Director, Development

Indiana

5339 RESOLVE of Indiana
5155 Sandy Court
Pittsboro, IN 46167-9129
317-329-9519
888-255-1399
e-mail: info@greatlakes.resolve.org
www.res.pub30.convio.net/Regions/great-l
Barbara Collura, President/CEO
Margaret Chandler Berardelli, Director, Development

Iowa

5340 RESOLVE Affiliate of Iowa
1348 Atlantic
Dunuque, IA 52001
319-557-2763
888-959-0333
e-mail: info@midwest.resolve.org
www.res.pub30.convio.net/Regions/midwest
Barbara Verhiley, Kentucky State Coordinator

Kentucky

5341 RESOLVE of Kentucky
851 Van Dyke Mill Road
Taylorsville, KY 40071-9502
502-834-7568
888-255-1399
e-mail: kentucky@greatlakes.resolve.org
www.res.pub30.convio.net/Regions/great-l
Stephanie Collura, President/CEO
Margaret Chandler Berardelli, Director, Development

Louisiana

5342 RESOLVE of Louisiana
PO Box 55693
Metairie, LA 70055-5693
504-454-6987
888-895-6055
e-mail: info@southcentral.resolve.org
www.res.pub30.convio.net/Regions/south-c
Barbara Bare, Regional Chair
Cindy Peterson, Volunteer Coordinator

Massachusetts

5343 RESOLVE of the Bay State
395 Totten Pond Road
Waltham, MA 02451-1553
781-890-2225
Fax: 781-890-2249
e-mail: admin@resolvenewengland.org
www.resolvenewengland.org/
Information on the Massachusetts chapter of a national, nonprofit consumer based infertility support organization. Information and a

variety of services to answer your questions about infertility, treatments, coping techniques and insurance issues.
1,000 Homes
Pam Rollinger, Detroit, MI Area Coordinator

Michigan

5344 RESOLVE of Michigan
3601 W Thirteen Mile Road   586-412-8712
Royal Oak, MI 48068-9998   888-255-1399
e-mail: info@greatlakes.resolve.org
www.res.pub30.convio.net/Regions/great-l
Kathy Collura, President/CEO
Margaret Chandler Berardelli, Director, Development

Minnesota

5345 RESOLVE of Minnesota
1161 E Wayzata Boulevard   651-659-0333
Wayzata, MN 55391   888-959-0333
e-mail: info@midwest.resolve.org
www.res.pub30.convio.net/Regions/midwest
Barbara Myrick, Missouri Local Area Coordinator

Missouri

5346 RESOLVE of St. Louis, Missouri
PO Box 411072   314-567-8788
Saint Louis, MO 63141-3072   888-959-0333
e-mail: MMyrickResolveMissouri@Yahoo.com
www.res.pub30.convio.net/Regions/midwest
Melissa Isaacson, Nevada Chair

Nevada

5347 RESOLVE of Nevada
Barbara Greenspun Women's Care Center
8280 W Warm Springs Road   702-616-4900
Las Vegas, NV 89074   877-203-7771
e-mail: rpbooklover@cox.net
www.res.pub30.convio.net/Regions/southwe
Robyn Odeen-Lodato, Chair
Erin Lasker, Executive Director

New Hampshire

5348 RESOLVE of New Hampshire
131 Daniel Webster Highway   781-890-2225
Nashua, NH 03060-5224   e-mail: admin@resolvenewengland.org
www.resolvenewengland.org/
Pam Griffiths, New Jersey Coordinator

New Jersey

5349 RESOLVE of New Jersey
1830 Front Street   908-322-9180
Scotch Plains, NJ 07076-0335   888-RNJ-2810
e-mail: griffithskm@yahoo.com
www.res.pub30.convio.net/Regions/northea
Kim Rodriguez, New Mexico State Coordinator

New Mexico

5350 RESOLVE of New Mexico
PO Box 93386   505-291-5066
Albuquerque, NM 87199   888-895-6055
e-mail: nmresolve@yahoo.com
www.res.pub30.convio.net/Regions/south-c
Rachel Soto-Lugo, President Advocacy Chair
April R Simanoff, VP Outreach Coordinator

New York

5351 RESOLVE of Long Island
PO Box 303   631-385-5026
Long Island, NY 11714   e-mail: racchair@northeast.resolve.org
www.northeast.resolve.org
Arelys Malave, Support Services
Maryann Post, Helpline Coordinator

5352 RESOLVE of New York City
178 Columbus Avenue   212-799-7400
New York, NY 10023   888-765-2810
e-mail: info@northeast.resolve.org
www.res.pub30.convio.net/Regions/northea
Anne Malave, Support Services
Maryann Post, Helpline Coordinator

5353 RESOLVE of the Capital District
PO Box 14591   518-242-3848
Albany, NY 12212-4591   888-765-2810
e-mail: info@northeast.resolve.org
www.res.pub30.convio.net/Regions/northea
Anne Pell, North Carolina Coordinator

North Carolina

5354 RESOLVE of North Carolina
101 Gettysburg Drive   919-380-8497
Cary, NC 27513   888-473-3062
e-mail: resolvenc@gmail.com
www.southeast.resolve.org/
Terry Collura, President/CEO
Margaret Chandler Berardelli, Director, Development

Ohio

5355 RESOLVE of Ohio
3000 NW Boulevard   614-340-0905
Columbus, OH 43221   888-255-1399
Fax: 614-340-0916
e-mail: info@greatlakes.resolve.org
www.res.pub30.convio.net/Regions/great-l
Barbara Zornes, Oklahoma State Coordinator

Oklahoma

5356 RESOLVE of Oklahoma
PO Box 18151   405-949-8857
Oklahoma City, OK 73154-0151   888-895-6055
e-mail: christina-zornes@ouhsc.edu
www.res.pub30.convio.net/Regions/south-c
Christy Collura, President/CEO
Margaret Chandler Berardelli, Director, Development

Oregon

5357 RESOLVE of Oregon
PO Box 175   503-762-0449
Scappoose, OR 97056   888-591-6663
e-mail: resolve_oregon@yahoo.com
www.res.pub30.convio.net/Regions/north-p
Barbara Fries, Philadelphia Coordinator

Pennsylvania

5358 RESOLVE of Philadelphia
PO Box 2456   215-849-3920
Southeastern, PA 19399-2456   888-765-2810
e-mail: phillyresolve@gmail.com
www.res.pub30.convio.net/Regions/northea
Katie Collura, President/CEO
Margaret Chandler Berardelli, Director, Development

5359 RESOLVE of Pittsburgh
PO Box 11203   703-861-2910
Pittsburgh, PA 15238-0203   888-255-1399
e-mail: info@greatlakes.resolve.org
www.res.pub30.convio.net/Regions/great-l
Barbara

5360 RESOLVE of Southcentral Pennsylvania
PO Box 402   717-234-8583
Camp Hill, PA 17001-0402
Odeen-Lodato,, Chair
Erin Lasker, Executive Director

Rhode Island

5361 RESOLVE of the Ocean State
PO Box 28201   781-890-2225
Providence, RI 02908-0201 e-mail: admin@resolvenewengland.org
www.resolvenewengland.org/
Pam Collura, President/CEO
Margaret Chandler Berardelli, Director, Development

South Carolina

5362 RESOLVE of South Carolina
204 Fernbrook Circle   864-542-9092
Spartanburg, SC 29307-2966   888-473-3062
e-mail: info@southeast.resolve.org
www.southeast.resolve.org/
Barbara Myers, Tennessee Coordinator

Tennessee

5363 RESOLVE of Tennessee
4770 Riverdale Road   615-244-5582
Memphis, TN 38141-8529   888-473-3062
e-mail: resolvetn@gmail.com
www.southeast.resolve.org/
Jessica Collura, President/CEO
Margaret Chandler Berardelli, Director, Development

Texas

5364 RESOLVE of Central Texas
PO Box 49783   512-453-2171
Austin, TX 78765   888-895-6055
e-mail: info@southcentral.resolve.org
www.res.pub30.convio.net/Regions/south-c
Barbara Collura, President/CEO
Margaret Chandler Berardelli, Director, Development

5365 RESOLVE of Dallas/Fort Worth
434 N Manus Drive
Dallas, TX 77244   888-895-6055
e-mail: info@southcentral.resolve.org
www.res.pub30.convio.net/Regions/south-c
Barbara Collura, President/CEO
Margaret Chandler Berardelli, Director, Development

5366 RESOLVE of Houston
PO Box 441212   713-975-5324
Houston, TX 77244-1212   888-895-6055
e-mail: info@southcentral.resolve.org
www.res.pub30.convio.net/Regions/south-c
Barbara Collura, President/CEO
Margaret Chandler Berardelli, Director, Development

5367 RESOLVE of South Texas
PO Box 782061   210-967-6771
San Antonio, TX 78278   888-895-6055
e-mail: info@southcentral.resolve.org
www.res.pub30.convio.net/Regions/south-c
Barbara Barron, Salt Lake City Coordinator

Utah

5368 RESOLVE of Utah
PO Box 57531   801-483-4024
Salt Lake City, UT 84157-0531   888-592-4449
e-mail: resolveutah@gmail.com
www.res.pub30.convio.net/Regions/mountai
Jennifer Odeen-Lodato,, Chair
Erin Lasker, Executive Director

Vermont

5369 RESOLVE of Vermont
PO Box 1094   781-890-2225
Williston, VT 05495-1094 e-mail: admin@resolvenewengland.org
www.resolvenewengland.org/
Pam Guthrie, Chair
Carol Knoph, Chair

Wisconsin

5370 RESOLVE of Wisconsin
PO Box 13842   262-521-4590
Wauwatosa, WI 53213-0842   888-255-1399
e-mail: info@greatlakes.resolve.org
www.res.pub30.convio.net/Regions/great-l
Barbara Jansen, Executive Director
Asgerally T Fazleabas, President

5371 Society for the Study of Reproduction
1619 Monroe Street   608-256-2777
Madison, WI 53711-2063   Fax: 608-256-4610
e-mail: ssr@ssr.org
www.ssr.org
International scientific society promotes the study of reproductive
biology by fostering interdisciplinary communication within the
science by holding conferences and by publishing meritorious
studies.
2,400 members
Susan S Suarez, President
Judith Jansen, Executive Director

Foundations

5372 Fertility Research Foundation
877 Park Avenue   212-744-5500
New York, NY 10021   888-439-2999
Fax: 212-744-6536
e-mail: info@frfbaby.com
www.frfbaby.com
Offers information on treatment and the latest research on male
and female infertility.
Masood Khatamee MD, Executive Director

Libraries & Resource Centers

5373 National Women's Health Resource Center
157 Broad Street
Red Bank, NJ 07701   877-986-9472
Fax: 732-530-3347
e-mail: info@healthywomen.org
www.healthywomen.org
NWHRC provides the most current women's health care information through website articles, online mini-courses, a monthly electronic newsletter, and periodic news releases.
Eve Dryer, Chair
Elizabeth Battaglino, Chief Executive Officer

Research Centers

5374 California Center for Population Research
759 Chestnut Street
Springfield, MA 01199-1001   413-784-5252
www.tufts.edu
Dr Donald Higby, Director

5375 Fertility Clinic at the Shepherd Spinal Center
Shepherd Spinal Center
2020 Peachtree Road NW
Atlanta, GA 30309-1465   404-352-2020
www.shepherd.org
This clinic makes it possible for paralyzed men to father children.
Gary Ulicny, Chief Executive Officer

5376 Fertility and Women's Health Care Center
130 Maple Street   413-781-8220
Springfield, MA 01103-2202   Fax: 413-732-9088
Conducts basic and clinical studies of male and female infertility.
Ronald K Burke MD, Head

5377 Melpomene Institute for Women's Health Research
550 Rice Street   651-789-0140
Saint Paul, MN 55103   Fax: 651-292-9417
e-mail: shawne@melpomene.org
www.melpomene.org

Focuses on women's health including fertility issues.
Judy Mahle Lutter, President

5378 University of California: UCLA Population Research Center
4284 Public Affairs Building 310-206-7566
Los Angeles, CA 90095-2006 Fax: 310-825-8762
e-mail: stats@ccpr.ucla.edu
www.ccpr.ucla.edu
Clinical investigations of overpopulation and infertility.
Judith A Seltzer, Director
Jennie Brand, Associate Director

5379 University of Michigan Reproductive Sciences Program
1500 East Medical Center Drive 734-764-8123
Ann Arbor, MI 48109 Fax: 734-763-5992
e-mail: juckno@umich.edu
www.med.umich.edu/OBGYN/research/rsp/
Research done into reproductive medicine and infertility treatments.
Timothy R. B Johnson, Chair
Janet Hall, Clinical Department Administrator

5380 Vanderbilt University: Center for Fertility and Reproductive Research
Nashville, TN 37232-0001 615-322-6576
Fax: 615-343-4902
Reproductive biology and fertility research.

5381 Wayne State University: University Women's Care
26400 W 12 Mile Road 248-352-8200
Southfield, MI 48034 Fax: 248-356-8224
wayne.edu
Reproductive endocrine infertility and gynecologic surgery research. The research spans the woman's life cycle. Research projects include: endometriosis polycystic ovary syndrome sexual dysfunction fibroids and menopause. Additional studies pertaining to women's health and male infertility.
Elizabeth Pu MD, Associate Professor
Nancy Angel RN, Research Nurse Coordinator

Support Groups & Hotlines

5382 National Health Information Center
PO Box 1133 301-565-4167
Washington, DC 20013 800-336-4797
Fax: 301-984-4256
e-mail: info@nhic.org
www.health.gov/nhic
Offers a nationwide information referral service, produces directories and resource guides.

5383 National Infertility Network Exchange
PO Box 204 516-794-5772
East Meadow, NY 11554 Fax: 516-794-0008
e-mail: info@nine-infertility.org
www.nine-infertility.org/
The National Infertility Network Exchange (NINE) is a national, notfor profit organization for persons and couples with impaired fertility. NINE supportes the decision of legal and medical means to build families as well as the decision to remain childfree.

Books

5384 Adopt the Baby You Want
Simon & Schuster
1230 Ave of the Americas 212-698-7000
New York, NY 10020-1586 800-223-2348
A how-to adoption book written by an attorney specializing in all areas of adoption.
272 pages
Susan Shultz, Author
Michael R. Sullivan, Author

5385 Adopting After Infertility: The Decision, the Commitment, the Experience
American Society for Reproductive Medicine

1209 Montgomery Highway 205-978-5000
Birmingham, AL 35216-2809 Fax: 205-978-5018
e-mail: asrm@asrm.com
www.asrm.com
Emphasizes the importance of communication between partners and offers several guidelines for maintaining a healthy relationship during such a stressful process.
318 pages

5386 Adoption Directory
American Society for Reproductive Medicine
1209 Montgomery Highway 205-978-5000
Birmingham, AL 35216-2809 Fax: 205-978-5018
e-mail: asrm@asrm.com
www.asrm.com
An extensive reference text covering such specifics as state statutes, adoption agencies, exchanges and agencies.
515 pages

5387 Adoption Fact Book
American Society for Reproductive Medicine
1209 Montgomery Highway 205-978-5000
Birmingham, AL 35216-2809 Fax: 205-978-5018
e-mail: asrm@asrm.com
www.asrm.com
A comprehensive source of statistics, regulations and facts on adoption.
277 pages

5388 Adoption Resource Book
Harper Collins
10 E 53rd Street 212-207-7000
New York, NY 10022-5299 800-242-7737
Explores and describes all types and styles of adoption and provides excellent resources for each path taken.
421 pages Third edition
Lois Gilman, Author

5389 Baby of Your Own: New Ways to Overcome Infertility
Taylor Publishing Company
1550 W Mockingbird Lane 214-637-2800
Dallas, TX 75235-5007
Provides current information regarding the psychological aspects of infertility.
244 pages

5390 Conquering Infertility: A Guide for Couples
Prentice Hall Press
15 Columbus Circle 212-373-8000
New York, NY 10023-7707
Covers various aspects of infertility.

5391 Consumer's Guide to Insurance
American Society for Reproductive Medicine
1209 Montgomery Highway 205-978-5000
Birmingham, AL 35216-2809 Fax: 205-978-5018
e-mail: asrm@asrm.com
www.asrm.com
A how-to book for infertile couples who are experiencing difficulty with insurance reimbursement.
106 pages

5392 Consumer's Legal Guide to Today's Health Care
American Society for Reproductive Medicine
1209 Montgomery Highway 205-978-5000
Birmingham, AL 35216-2809 Fax: 205-978-5018
e-mail: asrm@asrm.com
www.asrm.com
Provides accurate and up-to-date information concerning patient rights and medical care.
384 pages
Stephen L. Isaacs, Author

5393 Designs on Life
American Society for Reproductive Medicine
1209 Montgomery Highway 205-978-5000
Birmingham, AL 35216-2809 Fax: 205-978-5018
e-mail: asrm@asrm.com
www.asrm.com

Provides real life stories regarding assisted reproductive technology.
276 pages

5394 Family Bonds: Adoption and the Politics of Parenting
American Society for Reproductive Medicine
1209 Montgomery Highway   205-978-5000
Birmingham, AL 35216-2809   Fax: 205-978-5050
                    www.lawdigitalcommons.bc.edu
A well organized book is written for people struggling with some of the issues encountered in their journey through infertility and ultimately adoption.
1993 273 pages
Elizabeth Bartholet, Author

5395 Fertility and Pregnancy Guide for DES Daughters and Sons
American Society for Reproductive Medicine
1209 Montgomery Highway   205-978-5000
Birmingham, AL 35216-2809   Fax: 205-978-5018
                    e-mail: asrm@asrm.com
                    www.asrm.com
Guide offering information related to the reproductive potential of individuals who have been exposed to DES in utero.
48 pages

5396 For Want of a Child: A Psychologist and His Wife Explore Infertility
Continuum Publishing Corporation
370 Lexington Avenue   212-532-3650
New York, NY 10017-6503
A psychologist and his wife go through the emotional effects and challenges of infertility.

5397 Getting Pregnant When You Thought You Couldn't
Warner Books
1271 Ave of the Americas
New York, NY 10020   www.twbookmark.com
A concise guide to understanding infertility that covers issues from diagnosis to treatment and is useful for couples at any stage of infertility treatment.
1993 512 pages
Helane S. Rosenberg, Author

5398 Guide for the Childless Couple
American Society for Reproductive Medicine
1209 Montgomery Highway   205-978-5000
Birmingham, AL 35216-2809   Fax: 205-978-5018
                    e-mail: asrm@asrm.com
                    www.asrm.com
A short text which focuses on the emotional aspects of infertility, including its effects on marriage and self-esteem.
201 pages

5399 Guide to In Vitro Fertilization & Other Assisted Reproduction Methods
Pharos Books
200 Park Avenue   212-692-3700
New York, NY 10166-0005   800-221-4816
This book discusses assisted reproductive technologies from a laboratory and a patient's perspective.

5400 Having Your Baby By Donor Insemination
Houghton Mifflin Company
222 Berkeley Street
Boston, MA 02116   617-351-5000
                    www.hmco.com
A resource guide to donor insemination which discusses the experience, traditions and techniques of donor insemination, sperm freezing, and known vs. anonymous donors.
352 pages

5401 Healing the Infertile Family
University of California Press
1445 Lower Ferry Road   205-978-5000
Ewing, NJ 08618   800-777-4726
                    Fax: 800-999-1958
        e-mail: orders@cpfs.pupress.princeton.edu

This well-written book is dedicated to the psychological concerns of the infertile couple.
335 pages
ISBN: 0-520211-80-4

5402 Hormones
American Society for Reproductive Medicine
1209 Montgomery Highway   205-978-5000
Birmingham, AL 35216-2809   Fax: 205-978-5018
                    e-mail: asrm@asrm.com
                    www.asrm.com
Highly recommended text for patients who are suffering from reproductive disorders.
216 pages

5403 How Can I Help?: A Handbook for Practical Suggestions for Infertility
American Society for Reproductive Medicine
1209 Montgomery Highway   205-978-5000
Birmingham, AL 35216-2809   Fax: 205-978-5018
                    e-mail: asrm@asrm.com
                    www.asrm.com
Designed to provide greater understanding of the infertility experience.
18 pages

5404 How to Be a Successful Fertility Patient
American Society for Reproductive Medicine
1209 Montgomery Highway   205-978-5000
Birmingham, AL 35216-2809   Fax: 205-978-5018
                    e-mail: asrm@asrm.com
                    www.asrm.com
Offers extensive interviews with dozens of male and female infertility patients.
1993 447 pages
Peggy Robin, Author

5405 In Pursuit of Fertility
American Society for Reproductive Medicine
1209 Montgomery Highway   205-978-5000
Birmingham, AL 35216-2809   Fax: 205-978-5018
                    e-mail: asrm@asrm.com
                    www.asrm.com
A comprehensive text which can be used as a tool for couples who want to achieve an understanding of their problem as well as treatment options.
348 pages
Robert R. Franklin, Author

5406 In Vitro Fertilization
Facts on File
11 Penn Plaza   212-967-8800
New York, NY 10001   800-322-8755
                    Fax: 800-678-3633
The A.R.T. of making babies. (Assisted Reproductive Technology) A complete and caring overview of the options available to infertile couples.
208 pages Hardcover
ISBN: 0-816032-69-6

5407 Infertility Book: A Comprehensive Medical & Emotional Guide
American Society for Reproductive Medicine
1209 Montgomery Highway   205-978-5000
Birmingham, AL 35216-2809   Fax: 205-978-5018
                    e-mail: asrm@asrm.com
                    www.asrm.com
Enables the infertile couple to learn how to take control and educate themselves about the trials and tribulations of infertility treatment.
420 pages Softcover
Robert D. Nachtigall, Author
Carla Harkness, Author

5408 Infertility: A Comprehensive Text
Appleton & Lange
11 W 19th Street   203-838-4400
New York, NY 10011-4209   800-423-1359
A medical reference book.

5409 Issues in Reproductive Management
Thieme Med Publishers
381 Park Avenue S   212-683-5088
New York, NY 10016-8806   Fax: 212-779-9020
1993
ISBN: 0-865775-05-2

5410 Lethal Secrets: The Psychology of Donor Insemination
Warner Books
1271 Ave of the Americas
New York, NY 10020   www.twbookmark.com
An interview of a cross-section of people who participated in do-
nor insemination.
1993 277 pages
ISBN: 1-567430-20-1

5411 Lifeline: The Action Guide to Adoption Search
American Society for Reproductive Medicine
1209 Montgomery Highway   205-978-5000
Birmingham, AL 35216-2809   Fax: 205-978-5018
                                e-mail: asrm@asrm.com
                                          www.asrm.com
A very interesting text describing how an adoptee or adoptive par-
ent may track down birth parents.
384 pages
Virgil L. Klunder, Author

5412 Long-Awaited Stork: A Guide to Parenting After Infertility
Jossey-Bass
350 Sansome Street   415-433-1740
San Francisco, CA 94104   Fax: 415-433-0499
                                e-mail: webperson@jbp.com
                                          www.josseybass.com
An excellent resource for couples who are moving from being pa-
tients to being parents.
300 pages
ISBN: 0-787940-53-4
Ellen Sarasohn Glazer, Author

5413 Love Cycles: The Science of Intimacy
Random House
1540 Broadway   212-782-9000
New York, NY 10036   Fax: 212-302-7985
                                   www.athenainstitute.com
Book providing patients with refreshing, scientific concepts of
rhythms and relationships between the sexes.
330 pages
Winifred B. Cutler, Author

5414 Loving Journeys Guide to Adoption
American Society for Reproductive Medicine
1209 Montgomery Highway   205-978-5000
Birmingham, AL 35216-2809   Fax: 205-978-5018
                                e-mail: asrm@asrm.com
                                          www.asrm.com
Describes the basic prerequisits agencies and social workers expectations of prospective adoptive parents. Part two offers a directory of state-by-state listings of public and private adoption
agencies and adoption attorneys.
394 pages
Elaine L. Walker, Author

5415 Male Body
Firestone Touchstone Paperbacks/Simon & Schuster
200 Old Tappan Road
Old Tappan, NJ 07675-7005   800-999-5479
An informative and reassuring reference written to meet increasing interest in male health issues. This book discusses varied aspects of health such as infections and injuries, vasectomies, the
emotional aspects of sexual difficulties and preventive measures
that can be taken against AIDS and other sexually transmitted
diseases.
208 pages
ISBN: 0-671864-26-2

5416 Men, Women and Infertility
American Society for Reproductive Medicine

1209 Montgomery Highway   205-978-5000
Birmingham, AL 35216-2809   Fax: 205-978-5018
                                e-mail: asrm@asrm.com
                                          www.asrm.com
A helpful book offering suggestions for a positive self-image and
high self-esteem through the trauma of infertility.
1993 256 pages
Aline P. Zoldbrod, Author

5417 Miscarriage Women: Sharing from the Heart
American Society for Reproductive Medicine
1209 Montgomery Highway   205-978-5000
Birmingham, AL 35216-2809   Fax: 205-978-5018
                                e-mail: asrm@asrm.com
                                          www.asrm.com
A well organized book offering help and information to benefit pa-
tients who have experienced pregnancy loss as well as profession-
als working with these couples.
1993 258 pages
Shelly Marks, Author
Marie Allen, Author

5418 Missed Conceptions: Overcoming Infertility
McGraw-Hill
1221 Ave of the Americas   212-512-2000
New York, NY 10020
Book about infertility and the emotional agony that goes along
with it. Addresses all aspects surrounding infertility care and offers in-depth discussions of the many fertility options now
available.
377 pages

5419 Motherhood: A Feminist Perspective
American Society for Reproductive Medicine
1209 Montgomery Highway   205-978-5000
Birmingham, AL 35216-2809   Fax: 205-978-5018
                                e-mail: asrm@asrm.com
                                          www.asrm.com
A compilation of papers from conference proceedings designed to
define motherhood. Offers information on infertility, emotional
and financial difficulties and daily living.
234 pages

**5420 Mothers of Thyme: Customs and Rituals of Infertility and
Miscarriage**
Lida Rose Press
PO Box 15076
Ann Arbor, MI 48106
An interesting book that offers details on rituals and misconcep-
tions concerning infertility and miscarriage.
128 pages
ISBN: 0-962595-75-6

5421 Never to Be a Mother
Harper Collins Publishers
10 E 53rd Street   212-207-7000
New York, NY 10022-5299   800-242-7737
Offers childless women a plan for confronting their grief, anger
and guilt, as well as offering alternative ways to mother and live.

5422 No-Hysterectomy Option
American Society for Reproductive Medicine
1209 Montgomery Highway   205-978-5000
Birmingham, AL 35216-2809   Fax: 205-978-5018
                                e-mail: asrm@asrm.com
                                          www.asrm.com
An excellent reference for women faced with decisions regarding
hysterectomy.
265 pages
Herbert A. Goldfarb, Author

5423 One Women's Passionate Quest to Complete Her Family
Viking Penguin
375 Hudson Street   212-366-2000
New York, NY 10014-3658
The author presents a highly emotional account of the years of an-
guish, disappointment, and finally the joy she achieved in trying to
complete her family.

5424 Overcoming Infertility
Doubleday
666 5th Avenue
New York, NY 10103-0001
212-765-6500
800-223-6834
Paints a clear picture of the medical and emotional aspects of infertility.

5425 Preventing Miscarriage: The Good News
American Society for Reproductive Medicine
1209 Montgomery Highway
Birmingham, AL 35216-2809
205-978-5000
Fax: 205-978-5018
e-mail: asrm@asrm.com
www.asrm.com
Provides information on possible causes of miscarriages with information on infections, abnormalities and more.
240 pages Softcover
Jonathan Scher, Author
Carol Dix, Author

5426 Reproductive Hazards in the Workplace: Mending Jobs, Managing Pregnancies
Regina H Kenen, PhD, author
Haworth Press
10 Alice Street
Binghamton, NY 13904-1580
607-722-5857
800-429-6784
Fax: 607-722-0012
www.haworthpress.com
Offers information on the history and present of potential reproductive hazards. Includes pregnancy hazard hotlines, specific contact points where women can get information on working environments and more.
286 pages Hardcover
ISBN: 1-560241-54-3

5427 Resolving Infertility
RESOLVE: National Infertility Association
1310 Broadway
Somerville, MA 02144-1779
617-623-1156
888-623-0744
Fax: 617-623-0252
e-mail: info@resolve.org
www.resolve.org
Understanding the options and choosing solutions when you want to have a baby is a definitive resource to help you sort out the options and negative through the experience with confidence. This book tells you everything you need to know about infertility treatment and exploring other family building options.
370 pages
ISBN: 0-062735-22-5
Bonny Gilbert, Executive Director
Diane Aronson, Author

5428 Science and Babies: Private Decisions, Public Dilemmas
American Society for Reproductive Medicine
1209 Montgomery Highway
Birmingham, AL 35216-2809
205-978-5000
Fax: 205-978-5018
e-mail: asrm@asrm.com
www.asrm.com
Offers a superb summary of key reproductive issues ranging from conception to contraception.
250 pages

5429 Silent Sorrow
Delta-Dell Publishers
666 5th Avenue
New York, NY 10103-0001
212-765-6500
800-223-6834
A book dealing with the emotional and psychological aspects of losing a child.

5430 Surrogate Motherhood: The Legal and Human Issues
Harvard University Press
79 Garden Street
Cambridge, MA 02138-1423
617-495-2600
A discussion of the psychological, legal and policy questions raised by surrogacy.

5431 Surviving Infertility
Tapestry Books
PO Box 359
Ringoes, NJ 08551-0359
908-806-6695
800-765-2367
Fax: 732-288-2999

A valuable source of support and practical advice for coping with the many intense feelings associated with being infertile.
389 pages

5432 Surviving Pregnancy Loss: A Complete Sourcebook for Women & Their Families
American Society for Reproductive Medicine
1209 Montgomery Highway
Birmingham, AL 35216-2809
205-978-5000
Fax: 205-978-5018
e-mail: asrm@asrm.com
www.asrm.com
Contains practical approaches to coping with the emotional and psychological problems associated with pregnancy loss.
298 pages
Bonnie Gradstein, Author
Rochelle Friedman, Author

5433 Sweet Grapes: How to Stop Being Infertile and Living Again
American Society for Reproductive Medicine
1209 Montgomery Highway
Birmingham, AL 35216-2809
205-978-5000
Fax: 205-978-5018
e-mail: asrm@asrm.com
www.asrm.com
Recommended for couples nearing the end of their options or for those who are unsure if they wish to pursue infertility therapy.
Michael Carter, Author
Jean W. Carter, Author

5434 To Love a Child
Addison Wesley Publishing
PO Box 165
Clifton Park, MA 12065
518-859-4424
800-447-2226
e-mail: directoratTLC@aol.com
www.toloveachild.net
A thoughtful and informative overview of alternatives to bio/genetic parenting.

5435 Understanding and Infertility
Tapestry Books
PO Box 359
Ringoes, NJ 08551-0359
908-806-6695
800-765-2367
Fax: 732-288-2999
Provides specific advice to the family on how to be supportive of members and/or friends who suffer from infertility.
28 pages

5436 WHO Laboratory Manual
American Society for Reproductive Medicine
1209 Montgomery Highway
Birmingham, AL 35216-2809
205-978-5000
Fax: 205-978-5018
e-mail: asrm@asrm.com
www.asrm.com

Third edition

5437 Waiting: A Diary of Loss and Hope in Pregnancy
American Society for Reproductive Medicine
1209 Montgomery Highway
Birmingham, AL 35216-2809
205-978-5000
Fax: 205-978-5018
e-mail: asrm@asrm.com
www.asrm.com
Provides clear insight into coping with the trials and tribulations of infertility.
121 pages

5438 Without Child
American Society for Reproductive Medicine
1209 Montgomery Highway
Birmingham, AL 35216-2809
205-978-5000
Fax: 205-978-5018
e-mail: asrm@asrm.com
www.asrm.com
Covers topics including the doctor-patient relationship, religion and infertility, living child-free and the adoption process for persons without children investigating their options.
226 pages

5439 Women Without Children
Pharos Books
200 Park Avenue
New York, NY 10166-0005
212-692-3700
800-221-4816
Offers women without children support through their struggle and decision making.

Children's Books

5440 Mommy, Did I Grow in Your Tummy? Where Some Babies Come From
American Society for Reproductive Medicine
1209 Montgomery Highway   205-978-5000
Birmingham, AL 35216-2809   Fax: 205-978-5018
e-mail: asrm@asrm.com
www.asrm.com

Illustrated book that helps parents explain the different ways children can come into the world, including IVF, surrogacy, game donation and adoption.
28 pages Ages 4-8
Kathy Clo, Author
Elaine R. Gordon, Author

Magazines

5441 American Society for Reproductive Medicine: Clinic Specific Annual Report
1209 Montgomery Highway   205-978-5000
Birmingham, AL 35216-2809   Fax: 205-978-5018
e-mail: asrm@asrm.com
www.asrm.com
Gives the success rates of treatment for fertility centers around the country.

5442 Biology of Reproduction
1603 Monroe Street   608-256-2777
Madison, WI 53711-2021   Fax: 608-256-4610
e-mail: bor@ssr.org
www.biolreprod.org
A monthly, peer-reviewed journal.
250 pages Monthly

5443 Family Building Magazine
RESOLVE: National Infertility Association
1310 Broadway   617-623-1156
Somerville, MA 02144-1779   888-623-0744
Fax: 617-623-0252
e-mail: info@resolve.org
www.resolve.org
Offers various information on the newest technology and advances in infertility treatments, support groups, helplines, centers and in depth articles written by professionals in the field.
15-18 pages Quarterly
Bonny Gilbert, Executive Director

5444 Infertility and Adoption
RESOLVE: National Infertility Association
1310 Broadway   617-623-1156
Somerville, MA 02144-1779   888-623-0744
Fax: 617-623-0252
e-mail: info@resolve.org
www.resolve.org
Published by RESOLVE: The National Infertility Association.
Bonny Gilbert, Executive Director
Roy Sokol, Author

5445 Journal of Occupational & Environmental Medicine
Williams & Wilkins
351 W Camden Street   301-528-4000
Baltimore, MD 21201-7912   800-638-0672

Newsletters

5446 Hers Newsletter
Hysterectomy Educational Resources & Services
422 Bryn Mawr Avenue   610-667-7757
Bala Cynwyd, PA 19004-2708   800-777-4377
Fax: 610-667-8096
e-mail: hersfdn@aol.com
www.hersfoundation.com
Offers information and support for women who have had or are going through hysterectomies.
Quarterly
Nora W Coffey, President

5447 RESOLVE of the Bay State
PO Box 541553   781-647-1614
Waltham, MA 02454-1553   Fax: 781-899-7207
e-mail: admin@resolveofthebaystate.org
www.resolveofthebaystate.org
Information on the Massachusetts chapter of a national, nonprofit, consumer based infertility support organization. Information on a variety of services to answer your questions about infertility, treatments, coping techniques, insurance issues and family building options.

Pamphlets

5448 ART-Assisted Reproductive Technologies
Serono Symposia USA
100 Longwater Circle
Norwell, MA 02061-1616   800-283-8088

5449 Abnormal Uterine Bleeding
American Society for Reproductive Medicine
1209 Montgomery Highway   205-978-5000
Birmingham, AL 35216-2809   Fax: 205-978-5018
e-mail: asrm@asrm.com
www.asrm.com

1996
Malcolm G. Munro, Author

5450 Adoption
American Society for Reproductive Medicine
1209 Montgomery Highway   205-978-5000
Birmingham, AL 35216-2809   Fax: 205-978-5018
e-mail: asrm@asrm.com
www.asrm.com

1990

5451 Affording Your Infertility
Serono Symposia USA
100 Longwater Circle
Norwell, MA 02061-1616   800-283-8088

5452 Age and Fertility
American Society for Reproductive Medicine
1209 Montgomery Highway   205-978-5000
Birmingham, AL 35216-2809   Fax: 205-978-5018
e-mail: asrm@asrm.com
www.asrm.com

1996

5453 Bibliography
RESOLVE: National Infertility Association
1310 Broadway   617-623-1156
Somerville, MA 02144-1779   888-623-0744
Fax: 617-623-0252
e-mail: info@resolve.org
www.resolve.org
Annotated guide to books and articles on medical and emotional aspects of infertility.
Bonny Gilbert, Executive Director

5454 Birth Defects of the Female Reproductive System
American Society for Reproductive Medicine
1209 Montgomery Highway   205-978-5000
Birmingham, AL 35216-2809   Fax: 205-978-5018
e-mail: asrm@asrm.com
www.asrm.com

1993

5455 Coping with the Holidays
RESOLVE
1310 Broadway   781-643-0744
Somerville, MA 02144-1779

5456 Donor Insemination
American Society for Reproductive Medicine

1209 Montgomery Highway   205-978-5000
Birmingham, AL 35216-2809   Fax: 205-978-5018
                                       e-mail: asrm@asrm.com
                                       www.asrm.com
1995
Christopher L. R. Barratt, Author
Ian Douglas Cooke, Author

5457   Early Menopause (Premature Ovarian Failure)
American Society for Reproductive Medicine
1209 Montgomery Highway   205-978-5000
Birmingham, AL 35216-2809   Fax: 205-978-5018
                                       e-mail: asrm@asrm.com
                                       www.asrm.com
1996

5458   Ectopic Pregnancy
American Society for Reproductive Medicine
1209 Montgomery Highway   205-978-5000
Birmingham, AL 35216-2809   Fax: 205-978-5018
                                       e-mail: asrm@asrm.com
                                       www.asrm.com
1996
Isabel Stabile, Author

5459   Emotional Aspects of Infertility
RESOLVE: National Infertility Association
1310 Broadway   617-623-1156
Somerville, MA 02144-1779   888-623-0744
                                       Fax: 617-623-0252
                                       e-mail: info@resolve.org
                                       www.resolve.org
Published by RESOLVE: The National Infertility Association.
Bonny Gilbert, Executive Director

5460   Ending Infertility Treatment
RESOLVE: National Infertility Association
1310 Broadway   617-623-1156
Somerville, MA 02144-1779   888-623-0744
                                       Fax: 617-623-0252
                                       e-mail: info@resolve.org
                                       www.resolve.org
Published by RESOLVE: The National Infertility Association.
Bonny Gilbert, Executive Director

5461   Endometriosis
American Society for Reproductive Medicine
1209 Montgomery Highway   205-978-5000
Birmingham, AL 35216-2809   Fax: 205-978-5018
                                       e-mail: asrm@asrm.com
                                       www.asrm.com
Available in Spanish.
1994
Michael Vernon, Author
Dian Shepperson Mills, Author

5462   Environmental Toxins and Fertility
RESOLVE: National Infertility Association
1310 Broadway   617-623-1156
Somerville, MA 02144-1779   888-623-0744
                                       Fax: 617-623-0252
                                       e-mail: info@resolve.org
                                       www.resolve.org
Published by the National Infertility Association (RESOLVE).
Bonny Gilbert, Executive Director

5463   Fertility After Cancer Treatment
American Society for Reproductive Medicine
1209 Montgomery Highway   205-978-5000
Birmingham, AL 35216-2809   Fax: 205-978-5018
                                       e-mail: asrm@asrm.com
                                       www.asrm.com
1995

5464   Getting Started: How Do I Know If I'm Infertile?
RESOLVE
1310 Broadway   781-643-0744
Somerville, MA 02144-1779

5465   Hirsutism and Polycystic Ovarian Syndrome
American Society for Reproductive Medicine

1209 Montgomery Highway   205-978-5000
Birmingham, AL 35216-2809   Fax: 205-978-5018
                                       e-mail: asrm@asrm.com
                                       www.asrm.com
1995

5466   Husband Insemination
American Society for Reproductive Medicine
1209 Montgomery Highway   205-978-5000
Birmingham, AL 35216-2809   Fax: 205-978-5018
                                       e-mail: asrm@asrm.com
                                       www.asrm.com
1995

5467   IVF & GIFT: A Guide to Assisted Reproductive Technologies
American Society for Reproductive Medicine
1209 Montgomery Highway   205-978-5000
Birmingham, AL 35216-2809   Fax: 205-978-5018
                                       e-mail: asrm@asrm.com
                                       www.asrm.com
Available in Spanish.
1995

5468   If You are Having Trouble Conceiving
American Society for Reproductive Medicine
1209 Montgomery Highway   205-978-5000
Birmingham, AL 35216-2809   Fax: 205-978-5018
                                       e-mail: asrm@asrm.com
                                       www.asrm.com

5469   Infertility Insurance
Serono Symposia USA
100 Longwater Circle
Norwell, MA 02061-1616   800-283-8088

5470   Infertility: An Overview
American Society for Reproductive Medicine
1209 Montgomery Highway   205-978-5000
Birmingham, AL 35216-2809   Fax: 205-978-5018
                                       e-mail: asrm@asrm.com
                                       www.asrm.com
Available in Spanish.
1994

5471   Infertility: Causes and Treatment
American College/Obstetricians and Gynecologists
409 12th Street SW
Washington, DC 20024   www.acog.com
To obtain a free copy of this publication, please send a self-ad-
dressed stamped #10 envelope and request by title. (#AP002)
Nicole Ellisson, Author

5472   Infertility: Coping and Decision Making
American Society for Reproductive Medicine
1209 Montgomery Highway   205-978-5000
Birmingham, AL 35216-2809   Fax: 205-978-5018
                                       e-mail: asrm@asrm.com
                                       www.asrm.com
1995

5473   Infertility: The Emotional Roller Coaster
Serono Symposia USA
100 Longwater Circle
Norwell, MA 02061-1616   800-283-8088

5474   Insights Into Infertility
Serono Symposia USA
100 Longwater Circle
Norwell, MA 02061-1616   800-283-8088

5475   Introduction to Infertility: The First Steps
RESOLVE: National Infertility Association
1310 Broadway   617-623-1156
Somerville, MA 02144-1779   888-623-0744
                                       Fax: 617-623-0252
                                       e-mail: info@resolve.org
                                       www.resolve.org
Published by RESOLVE: The National Infertility Association.
Bonny Gilbert, Executive Director

5476 Laparoscopy and Hysteroscopy
American Society for Reproductive Medicine
1209 Montgomery Highway   205-978-5000
Birmingham, AL 35216-2809   Fax: 205-978-5018
e-mail: asrm@asrm.com
www.asrm.com

1995

5477 Male Infertility
Serono Symposia USA
100 Longwater Circle
Norwell, MA 02061-1616   800-283-8088

5478 Male Infertility and Vasectomy Reversal
American Society for Reproductive Medicine
1209 Montgomery Highway   205-978-5000
Birmingham, AL 35216-2809   Fax: 205-978-5018
e-mail: asrm@asrm.com
www.asrm.com

1995

5479 Managing Family & Friends
RESOLVE
1310 Broadway   781-643-0744
Somerville, MA 02144-1779

5480 Miscarriage
American Society for Reproductive Medicine
1209 Montgomery Highway   205-978-5000
Birmingham, AL 35216-2809   Fax: 205-978-5018
e-mail: asrm@asrm.com
www.asrm.com

1995

5481 Myths & Facts
RESOLVE
1310 Broadway   781-643-0744
Somerville, MA 02144-1779

5482 Ovulation Detection
American Society for Reproductive Medicine
1209 Montgomery Highway   205-978-5000
Birmingham, AL 35216-2809   Fax: 205-978-5018
e-mail: asrm@asrm.com
www.asrm.com

1995

5483 Ovulation Drugs
American Society for Reproductive Medicine
1209 Montgomery Highway   205-978-5000
Birmingham, AL 35216-2809   Fax: 205-978-5018
e-mail: asrm@asrm.com
www.asrm.com

1995

5484 Patient Information Series Publications
American Society for Reproductive Medicine
1209 Montgomery Highway   205-978-5000
Birmingham, AL 35216-2809   Fax: 205-978-5018
e-mail: asrm@asrm.com
www.asrm.com
Offers a set of 20 various brochures ranging from artificial insemination to male infertility problems.

5485 Pelvic Pain
American Society for Reproductive Medicine
1209 Montgomery Highway   205-978-5000
Birmingham, AL 35216-2809   Fax: 205-978-5018
e-mail: asrm@asrm.com
www.asrm.com

1997

5486 Pregnancy After Infertility
American Society for Reproductive Medicine
1209 Montgomery Highway   205-978-5000
Birmingham, AL 35216-2809   Fax: 205-978-5018
e-mail: asrm@asrm.com
www.asrm.com

1997

5487 Premenstrual Syndrome (PMS)
American Society for Reproductive Medicine
1209 Montgomery Highway   205-978-5000
Birmingham, AL 35216-2809   Fax: 205-978-5018
e-mail: asrm@asrm.com
www.asrm.com

1997
Syndrome Sullivan, Author
Ronald V. Norris, Author

5488 Third Party Reproduction (Donor Eggs, Donor Sperm, Donor Embryos, & Surrogacy)
American Society for Reproductive Medicine
1209 Montgomery Highway   205-978-5000
Birmingham, AL 35216-2809   Fax: 205-978-5018
e-mail: asrm@asrm.com
www.asrm.com

1996

5489 Tubal Factor Infertility
American Society for Reproductive Medicine
1209 Montgomery Highway   205-978-5000
Birmingham, AL 35216-2809   Fax: 205-978-5018
e-mail: asrm@asrm.com
www.asrm.com

1995

5490 Understanding: A Guide to Impaired Fertility for Family and Friends
American Society for Reproductive Medicine
1209 Montgomery Highway   205-978-5000
Birmingham, AL 35216-2809   Fax: 205-978-5018
e-mail: asrm@asrm.com
www.asrm.com
A pamphlet designed for families of patients with infertility and for distribution to individuals who may want to become involved in the counseling and support of these couples.
28 pages
Patricia I. Johnston, Author

5491 Unexplained Infertility
American Society for Reproductive Medicine
1209 Montgomery Highway   205-978-5000
Birmingham, AL 35216-2809   Fax: 205-978-5018
e-mail: asrm@asrm.com
www.asrm.com

1997

5492 Uterine Fibroids
American Society for Reproductive Medicine
1209 Montgomery Highway   205-978-5000
Birmingham, AL 35216-2809   Fax: 205-978-5018
e-mail: asrm@asrm.com
www.asrm.com

1997
Togas Tulandi, Author

Audio & Video

5493 Candid Talk About Loss in Adoption
Mary Martin Mason
4505 York Avenue S   612-922-1136
Minneapolis, MN 55410-1422
Discusses losses incurred by the adopted persons and adoptive persons issues for children adopted into different race families.
Videotape

5494 Coping with Infertility
Distributed By UC Video
425 Ontario Street SE   612-627-4444
Minneapolis, MN 55414-3002
Features five couples talking about their infertility experiences.
Odessa Flores

5495 Infertility: Exploring the Male Factor
American Society for Reproductive Medicine
1209 Montgomery Highway   205-978-5000
Birmingham, AL 35216-2809   Fax: 205-978-5018
e-mail: asrm@asrm.com
www.asrm.com

A well-orchestrated video discussing male factor infertility, including the infertility workup, physical exam, semen analysis, and surgical options available.
1993 47 minutes

5496 One, Two, Three, Zero: Infertility
Filmmaker's Library
133 E 58th Street   212-355-6545
New York, NY 10022-1236
Videotape

5497 Six Phases of Infertility Treatment: Medical & Emotional Aspects
RESOLVE of Maryland
PO Box 19049   410-243-0235
Baltimore, MD 21284-9049
Gives an overview of infertility treatment, addressing the medical and emotional aspects.
Videotape

5498 So You're Going to Adopt
Mary Martin Mason
4505 York Avenue S   612-922-1136
Minneapolis, MN 55410-1422
This video prepares adoptive parents for pre and post adoption issues.
Videotape

Web Sites

5499 Adopt-A-Special-Kid America
www.adoptaspecialkid.org
Adopt-A-Special-Kid provides information on adoption of children with special needs.

5500 American Society for Reproductive Medicine
www.asrm.com
Devoted to advancing the knowledge, understanding and expertise in all phases of reproductive medicine and biology. Offers patient education brochures, recommended readings and support.

5501 Center for Disease Control
www.cdc.gov
Reproductive health information source. Also a resource for the Society of Reproductive Technology. Invitro fertilization data reports and men's reproductive health. Interesting well balanced site.

5502 Fertilethoughts.com
www.fertilethoughts.com
A support sytem concerned with helping reach a goal of finding the perfect doctor, the diagnosis, as well as the treatment.

5503 Healing Well
www.healingwell.com
An online health resource guide to medical news, chat, information and articles, newsgroups and message boards, books, disease-related web sites, medical directories, and more for patients, friends, and family coping with disabling diseases, disorders, or chronic illnesses.

5504 Health Finder
www.healthfinder.gov
Searchable, carefully developed web site offering information on over 1000 topics. Developed by the US Department of Health and Human Services, the site can be used in both English and Spanish.

5505 Healthlink USA
www.healthlinkusa.com
Health information concerning treatment, cures, prevention, diagnosis, risk factors, research, support groups, email lists, personal stories and much more. Updated regularly.

5506 Helios Health
www.helioshealth.com
Online resource for your health information. Detailed information about specific health topics, access to expert advice from our Medical Advisory Board, and up-to-date health news.

5507 Infertility Books
www.infertilitybooks.com

Nonprofit site includes book titles regarding infertility and a short explanation of each book and how to get it.

5508 International Council on Infertility Information Dissemination
www.inciid.org
A nonprofit organization that helps individuals and couples explore their family-building options.

5509 Internet Health Resources
www.ihr.com/infertility
This web site provides extensive information about IVF, ICSI, infertility clinics, donor egg and surrogacy services, sperm banks, pharmacies, infertility books and videotapes, sperm testing, infertility newsgroups and support organizations, and drugs and medications.

5510 Ivf.com
www.ivf.com
Goal is to provide the latest women's healthcare innovations to address infertility, polycystic ovaries, endometriosis, and pelvic pain treatment.

5511 MedicineNet
www.medicinenet.com
An online resource for consumers providing easy-to-read, authoritative medical and health information.

5512 Medscape
www.medscape.com
Medscape offers specialists, primary care physicians, and other health professionals the Web's most robust and integrated medical information and educational tools.

5513 National Institutes of Health
www.medlineplus.gov
Information regarding all aspects of infertility. Some of the topics include: Latest news, overview of anatomy and physiology, clinical trails, diagnoses and symptoms, treatment, genetics, plus lots of links to other sites. Type infertility into the search engine.

5514 RESOLVE
www.resolve.org
Provides help to people who are experiencing the infertility crisis and strives to increase the visibility of infertility issues via concerted advocacy and public education.

5515 Uterine Artery Embolization
www.uterlinearteryembolization.com
Provides information on Uterine Artery Embolization, or Uterine Fibroid Embolization as an alternative to hysterectomy or myomectomy as a treatment for uterine fibroids.

5516 WebMD
www.webmd.com
Provides credible information, supportive communities, and in-depth reference material about health subjects. A source for original and timely health information as well as material from well known content providers.

Description

5517 Kidney Disease

The diseases that affect the kidney can be divided into diseases of the kidney itself, such as nephritis, polycystic kidney disease, kidney infections and stones, and diseases of other body systems that cause damage to the kidneys, such as diabetes, high blood pressure and lupus. In either instance, disruption of kidney function results in failure to remove excess fluids and wastes from the blood. This may lead to end stage kidney, or renal, failure.

Symptoms of kidney disease and their severity, depend on the underlying cause. If there is damage or disease in the urinary tract, there can be pain when urinating, blood in the urine, or changes in frequency and urgency of urination. If excess fluid cannot be removed, there may be swelling around the eyes and ankles. When the kidney is damaged directly, back or flank tenderness may be present. In many cases, kidney disease causes no symptoms until the advanced stages, although it may be detected much earlier through tests of blood or urine.

Treatment is directed to the cause, and may include antibiotics for infections, removal of kidney stones by surgery or ultrasound waves, management of the systemic disease such as diabetes, dietary modification, especially of salt and protein intake, and close monitoring and correction of fluids and electrolytes. Treatment may also include control of high blood pressure, which can be caused by kidney disease and further damage the kidney. The most severe cases of kidney failure require either dialysis, in which the blood's toxins are mechanically filtered and removed, or a kidney transplant.

National Agencies & Associations

5518 Alabama Kidney Foundation
31 Center Drive MSC 2560
Bethesda, MD 20892-3580

301-496-6325
800-891-5390
Fax: 301-480-3510
e-mail: starr@mail.nih.gov
www.niddk.nih.gov

Strives to increase knowledge and understanding about diseases of the kidneys and urologic system among people with these conditions their families health care professionals and the general public.
Dr Robert Star, Director

5519 American Association of Kidney Patients
2701 N Rocky Point Drive
Tampa, FL 33607-1796

813-636-8100
800-749-2257
Fax: 813-636-8122
e-mail: info@aakp.org
www.aakp.org

Serves the needs and interests of all kidney patients and their families. Founded in 1969 by kidney patients, for kidney patients, the purpose of this association is to help patients and their families cope with the emotional, physical and social impact of kidney disease.
Sam Pederson, President
Paul T Conway, Vice-President

5520 National Diabetes Information Clearinghous e
11921 Rockville Pike
Rockville, MD 20852

301-881-3052
800-638-8299
Fax: 301-881-0898
e-mail: patientservice@kidneyfund.org
www.akfinc.org

A nonprofit national health organization providing direct financial assistance to thousands of Americans who suffer from kidney disease.
John P Butler, Chair
LaVarne A Burton, President/ CEO

5521 National Institute of Diabetes & Digestive & Kidney Diseases
National Institutes of Health
1 Information Way
Bethesda, MD 20892-2560

301-496-4000
800-860-8747
Fax: 703-738-4929
TTY: 866-569-1162
e-mail: ndic@info.niddk.nih.gov
www.diabetes.niddk.nih.gov

Conducts and supports research on many of the most serious diseases affecting public health. The Institute supports much of the clinical research on the diseases of internal medicine and related subspecialty fields as well as many basic science disciplines.
Dr Griffin Rodgers, Acting Director

5522 National Kidney Foundation
30 E 33rd Street
New York, NY 10016

212-889-2210
800-622-9010
Fax: 212-689-9261
e-mail: info@kidney.org
www.kidney.org

A major voluntary health organization dedicated to preventing kidney and urinary tract diseases improving the health and well-being of individuals and families affected by these diseases and increasing the availability of all organs for transplantation.
Bruce Skyer, Chief Executive Officer
Joseph Vassalotti, MD, Chief Medical Officer

State Agencies & Associations

Alabama

5523 Alabama Chapter of the American Association of Kidney Patients
PO BOX 12505
Birmingham, AL 35202-2238

205-934-2111
800-750-3331
Fax: 205-975-6682
e-mail: jack@alkidney.org
www.alkidney.org

Gwen Deierhoi, President
E.W. Jackson III, Executive Director

Arizona

5524 Arizona Kidney Foundation
4203 E Indian School Road
Phoenix, AZ 85018

602-840-1644
Fax: 602-840-2360
www.azkidney.org

Leonard J McDonald, Chair
Jeffrey D Neff, Chief Executive Officer

5525 Central Arizona Chapter of the American Association of Kidney Patients
4401 W Hatcher Road
Glendale, AZ 85302-3821

602-939-7248

Dale A Ester, President

Arkansas

5526 National Kidney Foundation of Arkansas
1818 N Taylor Street
Little Rock, AR 72207

501-664-4343
800-622-9010
Fax: 816-221-7984
e-mail: nkfar@kidney.org
www.kidney.org

Nonprofit health organization. Our mission is to prevent kidney and urinary tract disease improve the health and well being of indi-

viduals and families affected by these diseases and increase the availability of all organs for transplantation.
R D Todd Baur, Member of the Board of Directors
Derek E Bruce, Member of the Board of Directors

California

5527 Harbor-South Bay Orange County Chapter of the American Assoc. of Kidney Patients
PO Box 8 714-527-8009
Seal Beach, CA 90740 e-mail: delrita@aol.com
www.aakp.org

Rita McQuire, President

5528 Los Angeles Chapter of the American Association of Kidney Patients
9854 National Boulevard 310-364-1807
Los Angeles, CA 90034 e-mail: aakpla@yahoo.com
www.aakp.org

Robin Siegal, President

5529 National Kidney Foundation of Northern California
131 Steuart Street 415-543-3303
San Francisco, CA 94105 888-427-5653
Fax: 415-543-3331
e-mail: infopacific@kidney.org
www.kidney.org/site/503/index.cfm
Work with kidney patients both pre ESRD dialysis and transplant. Financial assistance educational workshops scholarships children's and family camps transplant games information and referral.
Brad J Small, Division President
Connie M Nieri, Division Director of Finance/Operations

5530 National Kidney Foundation of Southern California
15490 Ventura Boulevard 818-783-8153
Sherman Oaks, CA 91403 800-747-5527
Fax: 818-783-8160
e-mail: nkfsca@kidney.org
www.kidney.org

Pier Merone, Division President
Natalie Kanooni, Division Program Manager

5531 Redding Chapter of the American Association of Kidney Patients
790 Pioneer Drive 530-241-6451
Redding, CA 96001-0258 e-mail: teamward@c-zone.net
www.aakp.org

5532 Sacramento Valley Chapter of the American Association of Kidney Patients
565 Morrison Avenue 916-924-1996
Sacramento, CA 95838

Colorado

5533 Colorado Chapter of the American Association of Kidney Patients
PO Box 8442 303-758-8610
Denver, CO 80201

5534 National Kidney Foundation of Colorado: Idaho, Montana, and Wyoming
650 South Cherry Street 720-748-9991
Denver, CO 80246 800-596-7943
Fax: 720-748-1273
e-mail: nkfcmw@kidney.org
www.kidney.org/site/505/

Brandi Krause, State Director
Stacey Lux, Development Director

5535 Western Slope Chapter of the American Association of Kidney Patients
1539 Ptarmigan Ridge 970-244-9196
Grand Junction, CO 81056
Vicki Hathaway, CEO
Donna Sciacca, Director of Patient Programs/Services

Connecticut

5536 National Kidney Foundation of Connecticut
1463 Highland Avenue 203-439-7912
Cheshire, CT 06410 800-441-1280
Fax: 203-439-7934
e-mail: nkfct@kidney.org
www.kidney.org/site/102/index.cfm

Marcia Hilditch, Program Manager
Deb Ramada, Development Coordinator

District of Columbia

5537 Georgetown University Center for Hypertension and Renal Disease Research
3800 Reservoir Road NW 202-687-9183
Washington, DC 20007 Fax: 202-687-7893
e-mail: wilcoxch@qunet.georgetown.edu
www.georgetown.edu/research/hrdrc
International institute for basic and clinical investigation education and clinical practice in hypertension and renal disease.
Christopher Englert, Jr. CAE, President/CEO

5538 National Kidney Foundation of the National Capital Area
5335 Wisconsin Avenue NW 202-244-7900
Washington, DC 20015-2030 Fax: 202-244-7405
e-mail: infowdc@kidney.org
www.kidney.org/site/203/index.cfm

Pamela D Gatz, Division President
Sherrita Lancaster, Division Office Manager

Florida

5539 American Association of Kidney Patients
2701 N Rocky Point Drive 813-636-8100
Tampa, FL 33607 800-749-2257
Fax: 813-636-8122
e-mail: info@aakp.org
www.aakp.org

Sam Pederson, President
Paul T Conway, Vice-President

5540 Kidney Association of South Florida
6801 Lake Worth Road 561-434-4559
Lake Worth, FL 33467 e-mail: jansym@bellsouth.net
www.aakp.org

Jan Symonette, President

5541 National Kidney Foundation of Florida
1040 Woodcock Road 407-894-7325
Orlando, FL 32803 800-927-9659
Fax: 407-895-0051
e-mail: nkf@kidneyfla.org
www.kidney.org/site/204/index.cfm

Andrew Helfan, President
Stephanie Hutchinson, CEO

5542 South Florida Chapter of the American Association of Kidney Patients
5217 Northlake Boulevard 561-471-2588
Palm Beach Gardens, FL 33418 e-mail: diazgray@aol.com
www.aakp.org

Robert Kirby, President

5543 Sunshine Chapter of the American Association of Kidney Patients
PO Box 4716 305-821-4827
Hialeah, FL 33014-0716
Elaine Printup

Georgia

5544 Atlanta Georgia Chapter of the American Association of Kidney Patients
6409 Lakeview Drive 404-932-1100
Buford, GA 30518
Pamela Sachs, Division President
Tracy Jenny, Division Program Director

5545 National Kidney Foundation of Georgia
2951 Flowers Road S
Atlanta, GA 30341
770-452-1539
800-633-2339
Fax: 770-452-7564
e-mail: nkfga@kidney.org
www.kidney.org
Barbara McDowell, President

5546 Rome Georgia Chapter of the American Association of Kidney Patients
118 Woodcrest Drive
Rome, GA 30161
706-232-8989
Hazel Hayashida, Chief Executive Officer
Diana Pinard, Director of Organization Planning

Hawaii

5547 National Kidney Foundation of Hawaii
1314 S King Street
Honolulu, HI 96814
808-593-1515
800-488-2277
Fax: 808-589-5993
e-mail: Glen@kidneyhi.org
www.kidneyhi.org
Hawaii's leading voluntary health agency to the education prevention and treatment of kidney and urinary tract diseases and increase the availability of all organs for transplantation in Hawaii.
Aileen Utterdyke, President
Glen Hayashida, CEO

Idaho

5548 National Kidney Foundation of Colorado, Idaho, Montana, and Wyoming
650 South Cherry Street
Denver, CO 80246
720-748-9991
800-596-7943
Fax: 720-748-1273
e-mail: nkfcmw@kidney.org
www.kidney.org/site/505/
Brandi Krause, State Director
Stacey Lux, Development Director

Illinois

5549 Chicagoland Chapter of the American Association of Kidney Patients
70 Lincoln Oaks Drive
Chicago, IL 60514
708-325-3475
Gloria Lang, Chief Executive Officer
Kate Grubbs O'Connor, Chief Operating Officer

5550 National Kidney Foundation of Illinois
215 W Illinois
Chicago, IL 60654
312-321-1500
Fax: 312-321-1505
e-mail: kidney@nkfi.org
www.nkfi.org
Mark L Schwartz, President
Kate Grubbs O'Connor, Chief Executive Officer

Indiana

5551 National Kidney Foundation of Indiana
911 E 86th Street
Indianapolis, IN 46240-1840
317-722-5640
800-382-9971
Fax: 317-722-5650
e-mail: nkfi@kidneyindiana.org
www.kidney.org/site/303/index.cfm
The mission of the NKFI is to prevent kidney and urinary tract disease improve the health and well-being of individuals and family affected by these disease and increase the availability of all organs for transplantation.
Margie Evans Fort, Chief Executive Officer
Heather Gallagher, Communications Director

Iowa

5552 Iowa Chapter of the Association of Kidney Patients
2203 75th Place
Davenport, IA 52806-1107
319-391-1194
Dave Hagarty, Executive Director
Lori Donald, Accounting Coordinator

Kansas

5553 National Kidney Foundation of Kansas and Western Missouri
6405 Metcalf Avenue
Overland Park, KS 66202
913-262-1551
800-596-7943
Fax: 913-722-4841
e-mail: nkfkswmo@kidney.org
www.kidney.org/site/305/index.cfm
Sherri Denny, Regional Administrative Assistant
Alexandra Wilson, Special Events Manager

Kentucky

5554 National Kidney Foundation of Kentucky
250 E Liberty Street
Louisville, KY 40202
502-585-5433
800-737-5433
Fax: 502-585-1445
e-mail: infonkfk@kidney.org
www.nkfk.org
April Enix, Director of Development
Nital Desai, Community Outreach Manager

Louisiana

5555 Bayou Area Chapter of the American Association of Kidney Patients
PO Box 400
Lockport, LA 70374
504-532-3542
Louisiana Kranze, Chief Executive Officer
Tracey Eldridge, Director of Special Events

5556 National Kidney Foundation of Louisiana
8200 Hampson Street
New Orleans, LA 70118
504-861-4500
800-462-3694
Fax: 504-861-1976
e-mail: info@kidneyla.org
www.kidneyla.org
Shawn Donelon, Chairman
Torie Kranze, Chief Executive Officer

Maine

5557 National Kidney Foundation of Maine
85 Astor Avenue
Norwood, ME 02062
781-278-0222
800-542-4001
Fax: 781-278-0333
e-mail: nkfofmrnv@kidneyhealth.org
www.kidney.org/site/105/index.cfm
Andrea Savisky RN CNN, Division Program Director
Mark Daley, Division Donor Records Director/User Ser

Maryland

5558 National Kidney Foundation of Maryland
Heaver Plaza, 1301 York Road
Lutherville, MD 21093-2136
410-494-8545
800-671-5369
Fax: 410-494-8549
e-mail: cshafer@kidneymd.org
www.kidneymd.org
Also covers the Harrisburg area of Pennsylvania and portions of Virginia and West Virginia.
Cassie Shafer, President/CEO
Christie Vera, Vice President of Development and Market

Massachusetts

5559 National Kidney Foundation of MA/RI/NH/VT
85 Astor Avenue   781-278-0222
Norwood, MA 02062   800-542-4001
                                              Fax: 781-278-0333
                    e-mail: nkfofmrnv@kidneyhealth.org
                        www.kidney.org/site/105/index.cfm
Andrea Savisky RN CNN, Division Program Director
Mark Daley, Division Donor Records Director/User Ser

Michigan

5560 Michigan Kidney Foundation
1169 Oak Valley Drive   734-222-9800
Ann Arbor, MI 48108   800-482-1455
                                              Fax: 734-222-9801
                              e-mail: info@nkfm.org
                                      www.nkfm.org

Andrew Boschma, Chairman
Daniel M Carney, President/CEO

Minnesota

5561 National Kidney Foundation of Minnesota
1970 Oakcrest Avenue   651-636-7300
Saint Paul, MN 55113   800-596-7943
                                              Fax: 651-636-9700
                            e-mail: jille@kidney.org
                     www.kidney.org/site/313/index.cfm
Also covers North Dakota and South Dakota.
Jill Evenocheck, Division President
Amy Busack, Regional Vice-President

Mississippi

5562 National Kidney Foundation of Mississippi
3000 Old Canton Road   601-981-3611
Jackson, MS 39216   800-232-1592
                                              Fax: 601-981-3612
                          e-mail: gail@kidneyms.org
                                   www.kidneyms.org

Paul Howell, President
Lee Parrott, Vice President

Missouri

5563 National Kidney Foundation of Eastern Missouri and Metro East
1001 Craig Road   314-961-2828
Creve Coeur, MO 63146   800-489-9585
                                              Fax: 314-961-0888
                          e-mail: nkfemo@kidney.org
                     www.kidney.org/site/308/index.cfm

Chad Iseman, State Director
Alayna Tatum, Special Events Manager

Montana

5564 National Kidney Foundation of Colorado/Idaho/Montana/Wyoming
650 South Cherry Street   720-748-9991
Denver, CO 80246   800-596-7943
                                              Fax: 720-748-1273
                          e-mail: nkfcmw@kidney.org
                              www.kidney.org/site/505/

Brandi Krause, State Director
Stacey Lux, Development Director

Nebraska

5565 Nebraska Kidney Association
11725 Arbor Street   402-932-7200
Omaha, NE 68144-2116   800-642-1255
                                              Fax: 402-933-0087
                       e-mail: nkfnoffice@kidneyne.org
                                   www.kidneyne.org
Improve the lives of all Nebraskans through advocacy, education,
early disease detection and patient services.

New Hampshire

5566 National Kidney Foundation of MA/RI/NH/VT
85 Astor Avenue   781-278-0222
Norwood, MA 02062   800-542-4001
                                              Fax: 781-278-0333
                    e-mail: nkfofmrnv@kidneyhealth.org
                        www.kidney.org/site/105/index.cfm
Andrea Savisky RN CNN, Division Program Director
Mark Daley, Division Donor Records Director/User Ser

New Jersey

5567 Garrett Mountain Chapter of the American Association of Kidney Patients
PO Box 8496   973-523-3959
Haledon, NJ 07538
Hurwitz, President

5568 Meadowlands Chapter of the American Association of Kidney Patients
PO Box 3032   201-471-5674
Clifton, NJ 07012-3032
Howard

5569 Northern New Jersey Chapter of the American Association of Kidney Patients
1095 Stone Street   732-382-1092
Rahway, NJ 07065-1913
Burnett

New Mexico

5570 National Kidney Foundation of New Mexico
3167 San Mateo Boulevard NE   505-830-3542
Albuquerque, NM 87110   800-282-0190
                                              Fax: 816-221-7984
                          e-mail: nkfnm@kidney.org
                                      www.kidney.org

Connie Giarrusso, President
Shirley Baer, Executive Director

New York

5571 Kidney & Urology Foundation of America
2 West 47th Street   212-629-9770
New York, NY 10036   800-633-6628
                                              Fax: 212-629-5652
                      e-mail: info@kidneyurology.org
                                www.kidneyurology.org
Sam Giarrusso, President
Kerri Shapiro, Director of Operations/Administration

5572 Long Island Chapter of the American Association of Kidney Patients
2 Maplewood Avenue   516-756-9126
Farmingdale, NY 11735
Margie Ng Makhuli, Chief Executive Officer
Laura Squadrito, Director of Programs and Services

5573 National Kidney Foundation of Central New York
731 James Street   315-476-0311
Syracuse, NY 13203   877-8KI-DNEY
                                              Fax: 315-476-3707
                         e-mail: info@cnykidney.org
                       www.kidney.org/site/110/index.cfm
Nannette Carbone, Chief Executive Officer
Susan Burns, Director of Administration

5574 National Kidney Foundation of Northeast New York
1971 Western Avenue   518-458-9697
Albany, NY 12203   800-622-9010
                                              Fax: 518-458-9690
                          e-mail: info@nkfneny.org
                www.kidney.org/about/local_info.cfm?sear
Carol MS Ed CFRE, Executive Director
Mary Jones, Division Development Director

5575 National Kidney Foundation of Western New York
310 Packetts Landing
Fairport, NY 14450
585-598-3963
800-724-9421
Fax: 585-598-3966
e-mail: infoupny@kidney.org
www.kidney.org/site/109/index.cfm
Nonprofit health organization.
Joanne Spink, Division President
Megan Alchowiak, Community Outreach Manager

5576 New York Chapter of the American Association of Kidney Patients
450 Clarkson Avenue
Brooklyn, NY 11203
718-270-1548
e-mail: linda.cohen@downstate.edu
www.aakp.org
Linda Welch, Kidney Early Evaluation Program Contact

North Carolina

5577 National Kidney Foundation of North Carolina
5950 Fairview Road
Charlotte, NC 28210
704-552-1351
800-356-5362
Fax: 704-552-7870
www.nkfnc.org
Kenya Welch, Kidney Early Evaluation Program Contact

Ohio

5578 Miami Valley Ohio Chapter of the American Association of Kidney Patients
4511 W State Route
W Milton, OH 45383
513-698-5847
Bob B Gold, Division President
Danielle Estep, Division Program Director

5579 National Kidney Foundation of Ohio
2800 Corporate Exchange Drive
Columbus, OH 43231-2804
614-882-6184
800-242-2133
Fax: 614-882-6564
e-mail: nkfoh@kidney.org
www.nkfofohio.org
Patti V.B. Gold, Division President
Danielle Estep, Division Program Director

Oklahoma

5580 American Association of Kidney Patients: Tulsa Chapter
911 North Woodland Drive
Sand Springs, OK 74063
918-241-3969
800-749-2257
e-mail: jasonmikles@hotmail.com
Jason Tallent, CEO

5581 National Kidney Foundation of Oklahoma
10600 S Pennsylvania Avenue
Oklahoma City, OK 73170
816-221-9559
800-622-9010
Fax: 816-221-7984
e-mail: nkfok@kidney.org
www.kidney.org/about/local_info.cfm?sear
Jeff Baumgardner, CEO
Glenda McClure, Operations Manager

Pennsylvania

5582 Lehigh Valley Chapter of the American Association of Kidney Patients
1242 N 19th Street
Allentown, PA 18104-3058
610-776-1091
e-mail: info@aakp.org
www.aakp.org
Jill Spink, Division President
Mary Reilly, Development Director

5583 National Kidney Foundation of Delaware Valley
111 S Independence Mall E
Philadelphia, PA 19106
215-923-8611
800-697-7007
Fax: 215-923-2199
e-mail: nkfdv@kidney.org
www.kidney.org/site/112/index.cfm
Also covers Delaware and Southern New Jersey.
Joseph Mullen, Chairman
Joanne Spink, Division President

5584 National Kidney Foundation of Western Pennsylvania
3109 Forbes Avenue
Pittsburgh, PA 15213
412-261-4115
800-261-4115
Fax: 412-261-1405
e-mail: info@kidneyall.org
www.kidney.org/site/113/index.cfm
Also covers Northern West Virginia.
James Sullivan, Chairman
David Vanella, Vice Chairman

Rhode Island

5585 National Kidney Foundation of MA/RI/NH/VT
85 Astor Avenue
Norwood, MA 02062
781-278-0222
800-542-4001
Fax: 781-278-0333
e-mail: nkfofmrnv@kidneyhealth.org
www.kidney.org/site/105/index.cfm
Andrea Savisky RN CNN, Division Program Director
Mark Daley, Division Donor Records Director/User Ser

South Carolina

5586 National Kidney Foundation of South Carolina
508 Hampton Street
Columbia, SC 29201
803-798-3870
800-488-2277
Fax: 803-799-3871
e-mail: karen.bailey@kidney.org
www.kidney.org/site/209/index.cfm
Beth Irick, Division President
Karen Bailey, Division Senior Administrative Assistant

South Dakota

5587 National Kidney Foundation Serving Minneso ta, Dakotas & Iowa Division Office
1970 Oakcrest Avenue
Saint Paul, MN 55113
651-636-7300
800-596-7943
Fax: 651-636-9700
e-mail: jille@kidney.org
www.kidney.org/site/313/index.cfm
Jill Evenocheck, Division President
Amy Busack, Regional Vice President

Tennessee

5588 National Kidney Foundation of East Tennessee
5201 Kingston Pike
Knoxville, TN 37919-1523
865-688-5481
800-242-2133
Fax: 865-688-5495
e-mail: nkfetn@kidney.org
www.kidney.org/about/local_info.cfm?sear
The National Kidney Foundation of East Tennessee works to prevent kidney and urinary tract diseases improve the health and well-being of individuals and family members affected by these diseases and increase the availability of all organs for transplantation.
Helen

5589 National Kidney Foundation of West Tennessee
857 Mount Moriah Road
Memphis, TN 38117
901-683-6185
800-273-3869
Fax: 901-683-6189
e-mail: info@nkfwtn.org
www.kidney.org/about/local_info.cfm?sear
Bruce Skyer, Chief Executive Officer
Joseph Vassalotti, MD, Chief Medical Officer

5590 National Kidney Foundation of West Texas
5429 Lyndon B Johnson Fwy
Dallas, TX 75240
214-351-2393
877-543-6397
Fax: 214-351-3797
e-mail: texasinfo@kidney.org
www.kidney.org/site/406/index.cfm
Marrie Collins, President
Mark Edwards, Division Program Director

5591 Tennessee Kidney Foundation
95 White Bridge Road   615-383-3887
Nashville, TN 37205-2613   800-380-3887
Fax: 615-383-2647
e-mail: info@tennesseekidneyfoundation.org
www.tennesseekidneyfoundation.org
Ron Carter, President
Bob Horton, First Vice President

Texas

5592 American Association of Kidney Patients: Piney Woods Chapter
PO Box 1012   903-537-7031
Mount Vernon, TX 75457   800-749-2257
e-mail: edwinhargraves@webtv.net
Edwin Wager, President

5593 Lone Star Chapter of the American Association of Kidney Patients
10042 Sugarloaf Drive
San Antonio, TX 78245   210-523-1605
www.aakp.org
Robert Eaton, CEO
Cameron Hernholm, Director of Development

5594 National Kidney Foundation of North Texas
5429 Lyndon B Johnson Freeway   214-351-2393
Dallas, TX 75240   877-543-6397
Fax: 214-351-3797
e-mail: texasinfo@kidney.org
www.kidney.org/site/406/index.cfm
Public and professional education about kidney and urinary tract diseases. Peer mentoring medical emergency identification jewelry kidney early evaluation program Camp Reynal transplant games.
Marrie Collins, President
Mark Edwards, Division Program Director

5595 National Kidney Foundation of Southeast Texas
5429 Lyndon B Johnson Freeway   214-351-2393
Dallas, TX 75240   877-543-6397
Fax: 214-351-3797
e-mail: texasinfo@kidney.org
www.kidney.org/site/406/index.cfm
Provides services for people who suffer with kidney and urinary tract diseases.
Marrie Collins, President
Mark Edwards, Division Program Director

5596 National Kidney Foundation of Texas
5429 Lyndon B Johnson Fwy   214-351-2393
Dallas, TX 75240   877-543-6397
Fax: 214-351-3797
e-mail: texasinfo@kidney.org
www.kidney.org/site/406/index.cfm
Marie Collins, Division President
Mark Edwards, Divisional Program Director

5597 National Kidney Foundation of the Texas Coastal Bend
PO Box 9172   361-884-5892
Corpus Christi, TX 78469   Fax: 361-884-2332
e-mail: info@coastalbendkidneyfoundation.org
www.coastalbendkidneyfoundation.org
Bess Stone, President
Becky Gardner, Executive Director

Utah

5598 National Kidney Foundation of Utah
3707 N Canyon Road   801-226-5111
Provo, UT 84604-4585   800-869-5277
Fax: 801-226-8278
e-mail: NKFU@KidneyUT.org
www.kidneyut.org
Serving kidney dialysis and transplant patients through out Utah providing patient service and support programs medical research and public and patient education regarding kidney disease and its treatment and prevention and the promotion of organ donations.
E.J. Garn, Chairman
Deen Vetterli, Chief Executive Officer

Vermont

5599 National Kidney Foundation of MA/RI/NH/VT
85 Astor Avenue   781-278-0222
Norwood, MA 02062   800-542-4001
Fax: 781-278-0333
e-mail: nkfofmrnv@kidneyhealth.org
www.kidney.org/site/105/index.cfm
Andrea Savisky RN CNN, Division Program Director
Mark Daley, Division Donor Records Director/User Ser

Virginia

5600 National Kidney Foundation of Virginia
1622 East Parham Road   804-288-8342
Richmond, VA 23228   800-543-6398
Fax: 804-282-7835
e-mail: eleanor.myers@kidney.org
www.kidney.org/site/203/index.cfm
An affiliate of the National Kidney Foundation it serves kidney patients and their families in Virginia and portions of West Virginia. Mission includes professional and public education prevention and working to increase the availability of all organs for donation.
Eleanor Myers, Regional Program Director
Liz King, Community Outreach Manager

Wisconsin

5601 National Kidney Foundation of Wisconsin
16655 W Bluemound Road   262-821-0705
Brookfield, WI 53005-5935   800-543-6393
Fax: 262-821-5641
e-mail: nkfw@kidneywi.org
www.kidneywi.org
Offers prevention detection and education programs for those at risk for kidney disease. The National Kidney Foundation of Wisconsin is making life's better through its programs and services. Brochures are offered at no charge.
Mary Braband, Chair
Cindy Huber, Chief Executive Officer

Wyoming

5602 National Kidney Foundation of Colorado/Idaho/Montana/Wyoming
650 South Cherry Street   720-748-9991
Denver, CO 80246   800-596-7943
Fax: 720-748-1273
e-mail: nkfcmw@kidney.org
www.kidney.org/site/505/
Brandi Krause, State Director
Stacey Lux, Development Director

Research Centers

5603 Kidney Disease Institute
Wadsworth Center for Laboratories and Research
Empire State Plaza   518-474-7354
Albany, NY 12237   Fax: 518-737-71
e-mail: dohweb@health.state.ny.us
www.nyhealth.gov
An information and referral organization for polycystic kidney disease autoimmune kidney disease and transplantation.
Andrew M Cuomo, Governor
Nirav R Shah, Commissioner

5604 Lovelace Medical Foundation
2425 Ridgecrest Drive SE   505-348-9400
Albuquerque, NM 87108-5127   Fax: 505-348-8567
e-mail: info@lrri.org
www.lrri.org
Jackie Lovelace Johnson, Director
Frank Bond, Director

5605 Lovelace Respiratory Research Institute
615 S Preston Street   502-852-7350
Louisville, KY 40202-0001   Fax: 502-852-7643
e-mail: cbrown@kdp.louisville.edu
kdpnet.kdp.louisville.edu

Educates residents and patients regarding kidney diseases and offers a dialysis clinic for people afflicted with kidney disease.
George R Ottensmeyer, President

5606 Nevada Kidney Disease & Hypertension Cente rs
210 S Desplaines Street 312-654-2720
Chicago, IL 60661 Fax: 312-654-0118
e-mail: charlotte.chapple@ainmd.com
www.ainmd.com/
A medical group practicing nephrology in the Chicago metropolitan area and it suburbs. Includes 21 nephrologists with expertise in many areas in the field of nephrology including hypertension chronic and acute renal failure hemodialysis and peritoneal dialysis glomerulonephritis acid base disturbances fluid and electrolytes management. Provides personal high quality care to patients with kidney diseases.
Eduardo Kantor MD, Founder

5607 PKD Foundation Polycystic Kidney Disease Foundation
Polycystic Kidney Disease Foundation
9221 Ward Parkway 816-931-2600
Kansas City, MO 64114-3367 800-PKD-CURE
Fax: 816-931-8655
e-mail: pkdcure@pkdcure.org
www.pkdcure.org
The foundation exists to win the war with PKD. Their mission is to promote research into the treatment and cure of polycystic kidney disease by raising financial support for peer approved biomedical research projects and fostering public awareness among medical professionals patients and the general public.
Frank Condella, Jr, Chair
Michelle Davis, Interim CEO and Chief Development Office

5608 University of Kansas Kidney and Urology Research Center
3901 Rainbow Boulevard 913-588-5000
Kansas City, KS 66160 Fax: 913-588-3995
TTY: 913-588-7963
www.kumc.edu
Jared J Brosius, Chief
Joseph Messana, Professor/ Service Chief

5609 University of Michigan Nephrology Division
University of Michigan Health System
1500 E Medical Center Drive 734-936-5645
Ann Arbor, MI 48109 Fax: 734-763-4151
www.med.umich.edu/intmed/nephrology
Focuses on kidney research.
Eric Mullen, Division Administrator
Susan Geisser, Financial Consultant

5610 University of Rochester: Nephrology Research Program
601 Elmwood Avenue 585-275-3660
Rochester, NY 14642-0001 Fax: 716-442-9201
www.urmc.rochester.edu
Focuses on kidney disorders.
David A Bushinsky, MD, Division Chief

5611 Warren Grant Magnuson Clinical Center
National Institute of Health
10 Center Drive MSC 1078 301-496-3311
Bethesda, MD 20892 800-411-1222
Fax: 301-496-2390
TTY: 866-411-1010
e-mail: mmichael@cc.nih.gov
www.dnrc.nih.gov/reports/programs/ncc.as
Established in 1953 as the research hospital of the National Institutes of Health. Designed so that patient care facilities are close to research laboratories so new findings of basic and clinical scientists can be quickly applied to the treatment of patients. Upon referral by physicians, patients are admitted to NIH clinical studies.
John Slatopolsky, Director

5612 Washington University Chromalloy American Kidney Center
One Barnes-Jewish Hospital Plaza 314-362-7209
Saint Louis, MO 63110-1036 Fax: 314-747-3743
renal.wustl.edu
Offers a dialysis unit for people afflicted with kidney disease.
Dr Eduardo Lanning RN/JD, President Board of Directors
Sean Tully, Vice President Board of Directors

Support Groups & Hotlines

5613 Kidneeds
Greater Cedar Rapids Community Foundation
200 First Street Southwest 319-366-2862
Cedar Rapids, IA 52404 Fax: 319-386-0431
e-mail: kidneedsmpgn@yahoo.com
www.medicine.uiowa.edu/kidneeds/
Primary mission of kidneeds is to fund research on membranoproliferative giomerulonephritis type 2 (MPON type 2, aka, dense deposit disease). Phone support and annual newsletter availiable. No computerized version availiable. No mailing list availble.
Lynne

5614 National Health Information Center
PO Box 1133 310-565-4167
Washington, DC 20013 800-336-4797
Fax: 301-984-4256
e-mail: info@nhic.org
www.health.gov/nhic
Offers a nationwide information referral service, produces directories and resource guides.
Cathcart, Executive Director

Books

5615 Family and ADPKD: A Guide for Children and Parents
Polycystic Kidney Disease Foundation
9221 Ward Parkway 816-931-2600
Kansas City, MO 64114 800-753-2873
Fax: 816-931-8655
e-mail: pkdcure@pkdcure.org
www.pkdcure.org
This book focuses on the questions most commonly asked by children and parents about ADPKD. It is divided into two sections: one for children and one for parents.
48 pages
ISBN: 0-961456-75-2
Dave Switzer, National Director, Educational Programs
Arlene B. Chapman, Author

5616 Kidney Beginnings: A Patient's Guide to Li ving with Reduced Kidney Function
American Association of Kidney Patients
3505 E Frantage Road 813-636-8100
Tampa, FL 33607 800-749-2257
Fax: 813-636-8122
e-mail: info@aakp.org
www.aakp.org
Provides patients with the information they need to take control of their healthcare and do what is necessary to preserve and protect their kidney function. The book addresses concerns of those at risk for kidney disease and their family members; featuring information about the workings of the kidneys, common medications, hypertention, testing, and answers to health, diet and lifestyle questions.
62 pages
Kim Buettner, Executive Director

5617 Kidney Cooking
National Kidney Foundation of Georgia
1639 Tullie Circle NE
Atlanta, GA 30329-2304 404-248-1315
A unique cookbook with over one hundred recipes that have been analyzed for sodium, potassium and protein content.

5618 Nutrition & the Kidney
Little Brown & Company
34 Beacon Street 617-227-0730
Boston, MA 02108-1415 Fax: 617-227-4633
1993 480 pages
ISBN: 0-316575-00-3

5619 PKD Patient's Manual
Polycystic Kidney Disease Foundation

9221 Ward Parkway
Kansas City, MO 64114

816-931-2600
800-753-2873
Fax: 816-931-8655
e-mail: pkdcure@pkdcure.org
www.pkdcure.org

Covers everything from cysts to how persons can be active if they have ARPKD.

Dave Switzer, National Director, Educational Programs

5620   Q&A on PKD
Polycystic Kidney Disease Foundation
9221 Ward Parkway
Kansas City, MO 64114

816-931-2600
800-753-2873
Fax: 816-931-8655
e-mail: pkdcure@pkdcure.org
www.pkdcure.org

A goldmine of information for the PKD patient and physician. Includes 88 pages of PKD questions and answers by the scientific advisers of the PKR Foundation.

88 pages Paperback
ISBN: 0-961456-72-8
Dave Switzer, National Director, Educational Programs

5621   Real Lifestyles Manual
R&D Laboratories
4204 Glencoe Avenue
Marina Del Rey, CA 90292-5612

800-338-9066

A complete renal guide including diets for hemodialysis and CAPD patients. Delicious menus, ADA exchange lists, gourmet recipes with nutritional analysis for renal patients and exercises.

5622   Your Child, Your Family & ARPKD
Polycystic Kidney Disease Foundation
9221 Ward Parkway
Kansas City, MO 64114

816-931-2600
800-753-2873
Fax: 816-931-8655
e-mail: pkdcure@pkdcure.org
www.pkdcure.org

This second edition book focuses on the questions most commonly asked about ARPKD in order to help families understand more about the disease.

Dave Switzer, National Director, Educational Programs

5623   Your Child, Your Family and Autosomal Recessive Polycystic Kidney Disease
Polycystic Kidney Disease Foundation
9221 Ward Parkway
Kansas City, MO 64114

816-931-2600
800-753-2873
Fax: 816-931-8655
e-mail: pkdcure@pkdcure.org
www.pkdcure.org

This secong edition book focuses on the questions most commonly asked about autosomal recessive PKD in order to help families understand more about the disease.

26 pages Paperback
Dave Switzer, National Director, Educational Programs

Magazines

5624   Kindey Beginnings: The Magazine
American Association of Kidney Patients
3505 E Frantage Road
Tampa, FL 33607

813-636-8100
800-749-2257
Fax: 813-636-8122
e-mail: info@aakp.org
www.aakp.org

This quarterly member magazine provides articles, news items and information of interest to those at risk or recently diagnosed with kidney disease, their famliy, and healthcare professionals.

Kmi Buettner, Executive Director

5625   aakpRENALIFE
American Association of Kidney Patients
35052 E Frantage Road
Tampa, FL 33607

813-636-8100
800-749-2257
Fax: 813-636-8122
e-mail: info@aakp.org
www.aakp.org

The official publication for AAKP members, offering articles, news and health care information for kidney patients,and health care professionals.

BiMonthly
Kim Buettner, Executive Director

Newsletters

5626   Family Focus
National Kidney Foundation
30 E 33rd Street
New York, NY 10016-5337

212-889-2210
800-622-9010
Fax: 212-689-9261
www.kidney.org

A patient and family newspaper targeted toward dialysis populations.

Quarterly

5627   PKD Progress
PKD Foundation
4901 Main Street
Kansas City, MO 64112-2634

816-931-2600
800-753-2873
Fax: 816-931-8655
e-mail: pkdcure@pkdcure.org
www.pkdcure.org

Offers information and updated medical news for persons and professionals with an interest in kidney disorders.

Monthly
Dave Switzer, Marketing/Public Relations Director

5628   Renal Recipes Quarterly
R&D Laboratories
4204 Glencoe Avenue
Marina Del Rey, CA 90292-5612

800-338-9066

Features timely holiday and ethnic food menus and recipes, shopping and food tips, analysis of nutrients and calculation of food exchanges.

Quarterly

5629   Transplant Chronicles
National Kidney Foundation
30 E 33rd Street
New York, NY 10016

212-889-2210
800-622-9010
Fax: 212-689-9261
www.kidney.org

A patient and family newsletter targeted towards transplant recipients.

Quarterly

Pamphlets

5630   About Kidney Stones
National Kidney Foundation
30 E 33rd Street
New York, NY 10016

212-889-2210
800-622-9010
Fax: 212-689-9261
www.kidney.org

Discusses causes, treatment and prevention of kidney stones.

5631   Advance Directives: A Guide for Patients and Their Families
National Kidney Foundation
30 E 33rd Street
New York, NY 10016-5337

212-889-2210
800-622-9010
Fax: 212-689-9261
www.kidney.org

Everyone has the right to make an advance directive, which is a legal document stating how you want decisions made concerning your medical care when your no longer able to make them yourself. This booklet describes the different types of advance directives and the medical decisions they cover.

12 pages Package

5632   American Kidney Fund Helps When Nobody Else Will
American Kidney Fund

6110 Executive Boulevard
Rockville, MD 20852-3915

301-881-3052
800-638-8299
Fax: 301-881-0898
e-mail: helpline@AFINC.org
www.kidneyfund.org

Focuses on the services and programs offered by the American Kidney Fund.

5633 At Home with AAKP
American Association of Kidney Patients
3505 E Frantage Road
Tampa, FL 33607

813-636-8100
800-749-2257
Fax: 813-636-8122
e-mail: info@aakp.org
www.aakp.org

A free publication, this was developed to address the growing need for information about home dialysis treatment options.
Kim Buettner, Executive Director

5634 Children and Kidney Disease
American Kidney Fund
6110 Executive Boulevard
Rockville, MD 20852-3915

301-881-3052
800-638-8299
Fax: 301-881-0898
www.arbon.com/kidney/

5635 Choosing a Treatment for Kidney Failure
National Kidney Foundation
30 E 33rd Street
New York, NY 10016

212-889-2210
800-622-9010
Fax: 212-689-9261
www.kidney.org

Introduces treatment options for kidney failure and explains the pros and cons of each.
16 pages

5636 Diabetes and Kidney Disease
National Kidney Foundation
30 E 33rd Street
New York, NY 10016-5337

212-889-2210
800-622-9010
Fax: 212-689-9261
www.kidney.org

Explains the connection between diabetes and kidney disease covering prevention, recognition and treatments.
12 pages Pkg. of 100
Edgar V. Lerma, Author
Vecihi Batuman, Author

5637 Dialysis Patient: An Informative Guide for the Dentist
American Kidney Fund
6110 Executive Boulevard
Rockville, MD 20852-3915

301-881-3052
800-638-8299
Fax: 301-881-0898
www.arbon.com/kidney/

5638 Diet Guide for the CAPD Patient
American Kidney Fund
6110 Executive Boulevard
Rockville, MD 20852-3915

301-881-3052
800-638-8299
Fax: 301-881-0898
www.arbon.com/kidney/

5639 Diet Guide for the Hemodialysis Patient
American Kidney Fund
6110 Executive Boulevard
Rockville, MD 20852-3915

301-881-3052
800-638-8299
Fax: 301-881-0898
www.arbon.com/kidney/

5640 Facts About Kidney Diseases and Their Treatment
American Kidney Fund
6110 Executive Boulevard
Rockville, MD 20852-3915

301-881-3052
800-638-8299
Fax: 301-881-0898
www.arbon.com/kidney/

Offers information about what kidneys are and their functions, diagnosis and treatment of kidney disease.

5641 Facts About Kidney Stones
American Kidney Fund

6110 Executive Boulevard
Rockville, MD 20852-3915

301-881-3052
800-638-8299
Fax: 301-881-0898
www.arbon.com/kidney/

5642 Glomerulonephritis
National Kidney Foundation
30 E 33rd Street
New York, NY 10016-5337

212-889-2210
800-622-9010
Fax: 212-689-9261
www.kidney.org

Defines the types of Glomerulonephritis, signs, causes and symptoms.
8 pages Pkg. of 100
Graeme Catto, Author

5643 Hemodialysis
National Kidney Foundation
30 E 33rd Street
New York, NY 10016

212-889-2210
800-622-9010
Fax: 212-689-9261
www.kidney.org

Introduces and explains the hemodialysis treatment process.
12 pages Pkg. of 100
C. Ronco, Author
M.H. Rosner, Author

5644 High Blood Pressure and Your Kidneys
National Kidney Foundation
30 E 33rd Street
New York, NY 10016-5337

212-889-2210
800-622-9010
Fax: 212-689-9261
www.kidney.org

Offers a description of hypertension, including symptoms, detection, causes and effects. Also available in Spanish.
8 pages Pkg. of 100
Dr.Randall Hammett, Author

5645 High Blood Pressure and its Effects on the Kidneys
American Kidney Fund
6110 Executive Boulevard
Rockville, MD 20852

301-881-3052
800-638-8299
Fax: 301-881-0898
www.arbon.com/kidney/

5646 Kid
American Kidney Fund
6110 Executive Boulevard
Rockville, MD 20852-3915

301-881-3052
800-638-8299
Fax: 301-881-0898
www.arbon.com/kidney/

5647 Kidney Disease: A Guide for Patients and Their Families
American Kidney Fund
6110 Executive Boulevard
Rockville, MD 20852

301-881-3052
800-638-8299
Fax: 301-881-0898
www.arbon.com/kidney/

Offers information on how the kidneys work, symptoms of kidney disease, kidney failure and treatment alternatives.

5648 Kidney Transplant: A New Lease on Life
National Kidney Foundation
30 E 33rd Street
New York, NY 10016

212-889-2210
800-622-9010
Fax: 212-689-9261
www.kidney.org

A brochure that answers common questions about transplants, such as patient expectations, drug therapy, complications including rejection and recovery.
10 pages Pkg. of 100

5649 Kidneys for Kids
American Kidney Fund
6110 Executive Boulevard
Rockville, MD 20852-3915

301-881-3052
800-638-8299
Fax: 301-881-0898
www.arbon.com/kidney/

5650 Nutrition and Changing Kidney Function
National Kidney Foundation

30 E 33rd Street
New York, NY 10016-5337

212-889-2210
800-622-9010
Fax: 212-689-9261
www.kidney.org

Explains how to slow the progression of kidney disease by controlling the intake of vitamins, minerals, fluids, calories and proteins.
12 pages Pkg. of 100

5651 Organ Donor Program
National Kidney Foundation
30 E 33rd Street
New York, NY 10016-5337

212-889-2210
800-622-9010
Fax: 212-689-9261
www.kidney.org

A comprehensive description of the organ donor program that explains organ and tissue donation, brain death, routine inquiry and becoming an organ donor.
12 pages Pkg. of 100

5652 Peritoneal Dialysis
National Kidney Foundation
30 E 33rd Street
New York, NY 10016

212-889-2210
800-622-9010
Fax: 212-689-9261
www.kidney.org

Introduces and explains the peritoneal dialysis treatment process
8 pages
K.D. Nolph, Author

5653 Understanding Nephrotic Syndrome
American Kidney Fund
6110 Executive Boulevard
Rockville, MD 20852-3915

301-881-3052
800-638-8299
Fax: 301-881-0898
www.arbon.com/kidney/

5654 Urinary Tract Infections
National Kidney Foundation
30 E 33rd Street
New York, NY 10016-5337

212-889-2210
800-622-9010
Fax: 212-689-9261
www.kidney.org

Defines urinary tract infections, its symptoms, causes and treatments.
10 pages Pkg. of 100

5655 Warning Signs of Kidney Disease
National Kidney Foundation
30 E 33rd Street
New York, NY 10016-5337

212-889-2210
800-622-9010
Fax: 212-689-9261
www.kidney.org

A one-panel leaflet that numbers and lists the six early warning signs of kidney disease.
Pkg. of 100

5656 Winning the Fight Against Silent Killers
National Kidney Foundation
30 E 33rd Street
New York, NY 10016-5337

212-889-2210
800-622-9010
Fax: 212-689-9261
www.kidney.org

Written for the African-American community, this brochure discusses the increased risk of high blood pressure and diabetes in this population.
12 pages Pkg. of 100

5657 Your Kidneys: Master Chemists of the Body
National Kidney Foundation
30 E 33rd Street
New York, NY 10016-5337

212-889-2210
800-622-9010
Fax: 212-689-9261
www.kidney.org

Offers an overview of kidneys and urinary system, describing the kidneys' filtering system, hereditary, congenital and acquired kidney diseases.
12 pages Pkg. of 100

Audio & Video

5658 It's Just Part of My Life
National Kidney Foundation
30 E 33rd Street
New York, NY 10016-5337

212-889-2210
800-622-9010
Fax: 212-689-9261
www.kidney.org

A 15-minute program for adolescent dialysis patients and their families.

5659 People Like Us
National Kidney Foundation
30 E 33rd Street
New York, NY 10016-5337

212-889-2210
800-622-9010
Fax: 212-689-9261
www.kidney.org

A seven-part video series targeted toward the newly-diagnosed chronic kidney disease patient.
Simon Greenall, Author

Web Sites

5660 American Association of Kidney Patients

www.aakp.org

Serves the needs and interests of kidney patients, for kidney patients, the purpose of this Association is to help patients and their families cope with the emotional, physical and social impact of kidney disease.

5661 American Kidney Fund

www.akfinc.org/

A nonprofit, national health organization providing direct financial assistance to thousands of Americans who suffer from kidney disease.

5662 Healing Well

www.healingwell.com

An online health resource guide to medical news, chat, information and articles, newsgroups and message boards, books, disease-related web sites, medical directories, and more for patients, friends, and family coping with disabling diseases, disorders, or chronic illnesses.

5663 Health Finder

www.healthfinder.gov

Searchable, carefully developed web site offering information on over 1000 topics. Developed by the US Department of Health and Human Services, the site can be used in both English and Spanish.

5664 Healthlink USA

www.healthlinkusa.com

Links to websites which may include treatment, cures, diagnosis, prevention, support groups, email lists, messageboards, personal stories, risk factors, statistics, research and more.

5665 Helios Health

www.helioshealth.com

Online resource for your health information. Detailed information about specific health topics, access to expert advice from our Medical Advisory Board, and up-to-date health news.

5666 MedicineNet

www.medicinenet.com

An online resource for consumers providing easy-to-read, authoritative medical and health information.

5667 Medscape

www.medscape.com

Medscape offers specialists, primary care physicians, and other health professionals the Web's most robust and integrated medical information and educational tools.

5668 Polycystic Kidney Research Foundation

www.pkdcure.org

Provide information on research into the cause, treatment, and cure of polycystic kidney disease by raising financial support for peer approved biomedical research projects and fostering public awareness among medical professionals, patients and the general public.

5669 **WebMD**

www.webmd.com

Provides credible information, supportive communities, and in-depth reference material about health subjects. A source for original and timely health information as well as material from well known content providers.

Description

5670 Liver Disease

Liver disease covers a wide range of disorders that can result in chronic liver damage, such as scarring (fibrosis) or the development of cirrhosis. An estimated 43,000 Americans die each year from liver disease.

Specific liver diseases that damage the liver include infection (e.g., viral hepatitis), chronic alcoholism or drug abuse, medications and certain systemic illnesses. Severe disease can permanently damage the liver, causing it to fail totally.

Common signs of liver damage are fatigue, loss of appetite, nausea and tea-colored urine. Yellowing of the skin and the whites of the eye (jaundice) is seen in 50 percent of cases. Other symptoms include liver enlargement and tenderness, and fluid collection in the abdominal cavity. A shriveling liver indicates more chronic and severe damage.

Treatment for liver disease depends on the underlying cause. In less severe injury, due to its remarkable capacity to heal itself, the liver can completely recover. Liver transplantation is accepted as appropriate treatment for end-stage liver dysfunction. See also *Hepatitis*.

National Agencies & Associations

5671 American Association for the Study of Liver Diseases
1001 North Fairfax Street 703-299-9766
Alexandria, VA 22314 Fax: 703-299-9622
e-mail: aasld@aasld.org
www.aasld.org
Physicians, researchers, and allied hepatology health professionals.
J. Gregory Fitz, MD, President
Nellie Sarkissian, COO

5672 American Liver Foundation
39 Broadway 212-668-1000
New York, NY 10006 800-GOL-IVER
Fax: 212-483-8179
e-mail: info@liverfoundation.org
www.liverfoundation.org
National, nonprofit organization dedicated to the prevention treatment and cure of hepatitis and other liver diseases through research and advocacy. The ALF offers information, physician referrals, a 24-hour, 7 day-a-week national helpline and support groups.
Thomas F Nealon III, Chairman
David Ticker, Chief Financial Officer

5673 Association for Glycogen Storage Disease
P.O. Box 896 563-514-4022
Durant, IA 52747 e-mail: info@agsdus.org
www.agsdus.org
The Association for Glycogen Storage Disease - AGSD - was established in 1979 in order to create an organization which would be a focus for parents of and individuals with glycogen storage disease (GSD) to communicate, share their successes and concerns, share useful findings, provide support, create an awareness of this condition for the public, and to stimulate research in the various forms of glycogen storage diseases.
Kathy Thelen, President
Matt Peters, Vice President

5674 Association of Cancer Online Resources
173 Duane Street 212-226-5525
New York, NY 10013 e-mail: Feedback@acor.org
www.acor.org

ACOR is a unique collection of online cancer communities designed to provide timely and accurate information in a supportive environment.

5675 Children's Liver Association For Support Services
25379 Wayne Mills Place 661-263-9099
Valencia, CA 91355 877-679-8256
Fax: 661-263-9099
e-mail: admin@classkids.org:
www.classkids.org
C.L.A.S.S. was founded out of the recognized need for an organization dedicated to addressing the emotional, educational and financial needs of families with children affected by liver disease and transplantation.
Diane Sumner, President
Ann Whithead, RN, JD, Vice President

State Agencies & Associations

Arizona

5676 American Liver Foundation Arizona Chapter
4545 E Shea Boulevard 602-953-1800
Phoenix, AZ 85028 866-953-1800
Fax: 602-953-1806
e-mail: mmcracken@liverfoundation.org
www.liverfoundation.org
Melissa McCracken, Executive Director
Ashley Drew, Events Manager

California

5677 American Liver Foundation Greater Los Angeles Chapter
5777 Century Boulevard 310-670-4624
Los Angeles, CA 90045 Fax: 310-670-4672
e-mail: tfantini@liverfoundation.org
www.liverfoundation.org
Taly Fantini, Executive Director

5678 American Liver Foundation Northern CA Chapter
870 Market Street 415-248-1060
San Francisco, CA 94102 800-292-9099
Fax: 415-248-1066
e-mail: gmartin@liverfoundation.org
www.liverfoundation.org
Greg Martin, Executive Director

5679 American Liver Foundation San Diego Chapte r
2515 Camino del Rio S 619-291-5483
San Diego, CA 92108 800-749-2630
Fax: 619-295-7181
e-mail: mdemotto@liverfoundation.org
www.liverfoundation.org
Michele De Motto, Executive Director

Colorado

5680 American Liver Foundation Rocky Mountain Division
1660 S Albion Street 303-988-4388
Denver, CO 80222 Fax: 303-988-4398
e-mail: jmccormack@liverfoundation.org
www.liverfoundation.org
Joe McCormack, Executive Director

Connecticut

5681 American Liver Foundation: Connecticut Chapter
127 Washington Avenue 203-234-2022
N Haven, CT 06473 Fax: 203-234-1386
e-mail: jthompson@liverfoundation.org
www.liverfoundation.org
Offers support for patients and families provides educational meetings and conferences raising vital liver research dollars; encouraging the beautifully unselfish gift of organ donation and the medical miracle of organ transplantation.
12 pages Quarterly
JoAnn Thompson, Executive Director

District of Columbia

5682 Administration for Children and Families
370 L'Enfant Promenade
Washington, DC 20447   www.acf.hhs.gov
The Administration for Children & Families (ACF) is a division of
the U.S. Department of Health & Human Services (HHS). ACF
promotes the economic and social well-being of families, children,
individuals and communities.
Mark Greenberg, Acting Assistant Secretary
Jeff Hild, Chief of Staff

5683 National Institute for Occupational Safety and Health
395 E Street, SW   202-245-0625
Washington, DC 20201   800-232-4636
                                        Fax: 513-533-8347
                                        TTY: 888-232-6348
                                        www.cdc.gov/niosh/
The National Institute for Occupational Safety and Health
(NIOSH) is the U.S. federal agency that conducts research and
makes recommendations to prevent worker injury and illness.
John Howard, MD, Director
Frank Hearl, PE, Chief of Staff

Florida

5684 American Liver Foundation Gulf Coast Chapter
202 S 22nd Street   813-248-3337
Ybor City, FL 33605   Fax: 813-248-3340
                        e-mail: jbourgeois@liverfoundation.org
                                        www.liverfoundation.org
Jennifer Nillias, Executive Director

Georgia

5685 Agency for Toxic Substances and Disease Registry
4770 Buford Hwy NE
Atlanta, GA 30341   800-232-4636
                                        TTY: 888-232-6348
                                        www.atsdr.cdc.gov
The Agency for Toxic Substances and Disease Registry (ATSDR),
based in Atlanta, Georgia, is a federal public health agency of the
U.S. Department of Health and Human Services. ATSDR serves
the public by using the best science, taking responsive public
health actions, and providing trusted health information to prevent
harmful exposures and diseases related to toxic substances.
Patrick Breysse, PhD, CIH, Director
Donna Knutson, PhD, Acting Deputy Director

Illinois

5686 American Liver Foundation Illinois Chapter
67 East Madison Street   312-377-9030
Chicago, IL 60603   Fax: 312-377-9035
                        e-mail: info@illinois-liver.org
                                        www.illinois-liver.org
Kevin Sutton, Executive Director
Kristin Gray, Development Coordinator

Indiana

5687 American Liver Foundation Indiana Chapter
PO BOX 36085   317-635-5074
Indianapolis, IN 46236   877-548-3730
                                        Fax: 317-635-5075
                        e-mail: dsparksunsworth@liverfoundation.org
                                        www.liverfoundation.org
Katrina Marshall, Executive Director

Maryland

5688 Agency for Healthcare Research and Quality
540 Gaither Road
Rockville, MD 20850   301-427-1364
                                        www.ahrq.gov/index.html
The Agency for Healthcare Research and Quality's (AHRQ) mission is to produce evidence to make health care safer, higher quality, more accessible, equitable, and affordable, and to work within
the U.S. Department of Health and Human Services and with other
partners to make sure that the evidence is understood and used.
Richard G. Kronick, PhD, Director, Director
Sharon B. Arnold, PhD, Deputy Director

5689 Centers for Medicare and Medicaid Services
7500 Security Boulevard   410-786-3000
Baltimore, MD 21244   877-267-2323
                                        TTY: 866-226-1819
                        e-mail: Mandy.Cohen@cms.hhs.gov
                                        www.cms.gov
US federal agency which administers Medicare, Medicaid, and the
State Children's Health Insurance Program.
Dr. Mandy Cohen, M.D., MPH, Chief of Staff
Timothy P. Love, Chief Operating Officer

5690 National Center for Complementary and Integrative Health
9000 Rockville Pike
Bethesda, MD 20892   888-644-6226
                                        TTY: 866-464-3615
                        e-mail: nccih-info@mail.nih.gov
                                        nccih.nih.gov
The National Center for Complementary and Integrative Health
(NCCIH) is the Federal Government's lead agency for scientific
research on the diverse medical and health care systems, practices,
and products that are not generally considered part of conventional
medicine.
Josephine P. Briggs, M.D., Director
David Shurtleff, Ph.D., Deputy Director

5691 National Human Genome Research Institute
Building 31, Room 4B09   301-402-0911
Bethesda, MD 20892   Fax: 301-402-2218
                                        www.genome.gov
The National Human Genome Research Institute began as the Na-
tional Center for Human Genome Research (NCHGR), which was
established in 1989 to carry out the role of the National Institutes
of Health (NIH) in the International Human Genome Project
(HGP).
Eric D. Green, M.D., Ph.D., Director
Lawrence Brody, Ph.D., Director, Division of Genomics & Society

5692 National Institute of Biomedical Imaging and Bioengineering
9000 Rockville Pike   301-496-8859
Bethesda, MD 20892   e-mail: info@nibib.nih.gov
                                        www.nibib.nih.gov
The mission of the National Institute of Biomedical Imaging and
Bioengineering (NIBIB) is to improve health by leading the devel-
opment and accelerating the application of biomedical
technologies.
Roderic I. Pettigrew, Ph.D., M.D., Director
Marcella Canada, Administrative Officer

5693 National Institute of General Medical Sciences
45 Center Drive MSC 6200   301-496-7301
Bethesda, MD 20892   e-mail: info@nigms.nih.gov
                                        www.nigms.nih.gov
The National Institute of General Medical Sciences (NIGMS) supports basic research that increases understanding of biological
processes and lays the foundation for advances in disease diagnosis, treatment and prevention.
Jon R. Lorsch, Ph.D., Director
Judith H. Greenberg, Ph.D., Deputy Director

5694 National Institute on Alcohol Abuse and Alcoholism
Bethesda, MD

                                        888-69 -4222
                        e-mail: niaaaweb-r@exchange.nih.gov
                                        www.niaaa.nih.gov
NIAAA supports and conducts research on the impact of alcohol
use on human health and well-being. It is the largest funder of alco-
hol research in the world.
Dr. George Koob, Director
Kenneth R. Warren, Ph.D., Deputy Director

5695 National Institute on Drug Abuse
6001 Executive Boulevard   301-443-1124
Bethesda, MD 20892   e-mail: dd279k@nih.gov
                                        www.drugabuse.gov

NIDA's mission is to lead the Nation in bringing the power of science to bear on drug abuse and addiction.
Nora D. Volkow, M.D., Director
David Daubert, Acting Associate Director for Management

5696 U.S. Food and Drug Administration
10903 New Hampshire Ave 301-796-8240
Silver Spring, MD 20993 888-463-6332
www.fda.gov
FDA is responsible for protecting the public health by assuring the safety, efficacy and security of human and veterinary drugs, biological products, medical devices, our nation's food supply, cosmetics, and products that emit radiation.
Stephen Ostroff, M.D., Acting Commissioner
James Tyler, Chief Financial Officer

Michigan

5697 American Liver Foundation Michigan Chapter
21886 Farmington Road 248-615-5768
Farmington, MI 48336 888-MYL-IVER
Fax: 248-615-5778
e-mail: michigan@liverfoundation.org
www.liverfoundation.org
Jennifer L Stibbe, Executive Director
Meghan Likes, Community Events Coordinator

Minnesota

5698 American Liver Foundation Minnesota Chapter
2626 E 82nd Street 952-854-6181
Bloomington, MN 55425 Fax: 952-854-6956
e-mail: dgirard@liverfoundation.org
www.liverfoundation.org
Dee Girard, Executive Director

Missouri

5699 American Liver Foundation Greater Kansas City Chapter
16 Hampton Village Plaza 314-352-7377
St. Louis, MO 63109 866-455-4837
Fax: 612-892-8442
e-mail: rmattler@liverfoundation.org
www.liverfoundation.org
Richard Mattler, Executive Director

New York

5700 American Liver Foundation Greater New York Chapter
39 Broadway 212-943-1059
New York, NY 10006 877-307-7507
Fax: 212-943-1314
e-mail: greaterny@liverfoundation.org
www.liverfoundation.org
Randa Adib, Director, Development
Stephanie Paul, Gala Director

5701 American Liver Foundation Western New York Chapter
25 Canterbury Road 585-271-2859
Rochester, NY 14607 Fax: 585-271-8642
e-mail: nkoris@liverfoundation.org
www.liverfoundation.org
Nancy Rodwa MNO, Executive Director

North Carolina

5702 National Institute of Environmental Health Sciences
111 T.W. Alexander Drive 919-541-4580
Research Triangle Park, NC 27709 e-mail: carroll1@niehs.nih.gov
www.niehs.nih.gov
The mission of the NIEHS is to discover how the environment affects people in order to promote healthier lives.
Linda S. Birnbaum, Ph.D., Director
Richard Woychik, Ph.D., Deputy Director

Pennsylvania

5703 American Liver Foundation Delaware Valley Chapter
1341 North Delaware Avenue 215-425-8080
Philadelphia, PA 19125 Fax: 215-425-8181
e-mail: iallison@liverfoundation.org
www.liverfoundation.org
Ivory Allison, Executive Director

5704 American Liver Foundation Western Pennsylvania
100 W Station Square Drive 412-434-7044
Pittsburgh, PA 15219 Fax: 412-434-7040
e-mail: samasartis@liverfoundation.org
www.liverfoundation.org
Suzanna Masartis, Executive Director

Tennessee

5705 American Liver Foundation Midsouth Chapter
PO BOX 486 901-766-7668
Ellendale, TN 38029 866-756-7668
Fax: 901-881-3842
e-mail: midsouth@liverfoundation.org
www.liverfoundation.org
Winn Stephenson, Division Founder
Tina Sandoval, Board Chair

Virginia

5706 National Science Foundation
4201 Wilson Blvd 703-292-5111
Arlington, VA 22230 TDD: 703-292-5090
e-mail: info@nsf.gov
www.nsf.gov
NSF is the only federal agency whose mission includes support for all fields of fundamental science and engineering, except for medical sciences.
France A. Córdova, Director
Richard O. Buckius, Chief Operating Officer

Washington

5707 American Liver Foundation Pacific Northwest Chapter
PO BOX 22108 212-668-1000
Seattle, WA 98122 800-465-4837
Fax: 206-443-1511
www.liverfoundation.org
Dr. Stephen Corrigan Rayhill, MD, Director
Dr. Andrew Precht, MD, Director

Wisconsin

5708 American Liver Foundation Wisconsin Chapter
1845 N Farwell Avenue 414-763-3435
Milwaukee, WI 53202 Fax: 414-961-7288
e-mail: dgirard@liverfoundation.org
www.liverfoundation.org
Dee Girard, Executive Director

Research Centers

5709 Clinical Research Center: Pediatrics Children's Hospital Research Foundation
Children's Hospital Research Foundation
Elland & Bethesda Avenues 513-559-4412
Cincinnati, OH 45229 Fax: 513-559-7431
Studies of pediatric acquired diseases including liver disease and Reye's Syndrome.
Dr James G Redeker, Co-director

5710 University of California Liver Research Unit
7601 E Imperial Highway 562-940-8961
Downey, CA 90242 Fax: 562-940-6628
Dr Allan Lee MD Facp, Professor InteRNal Medicine / Director

5711 University of Texas Southwestern Medical Center
5323 Harry Hines Boulevard 214-645-8300
Dallas, TX 75390-9151 Fax: 214-645-7999
www.utsouthwestern.edu
Daniel K Podolsky, MD, President
J. Gregory Fitz, Executive Vice President

5712 University of Texas Southwestern Medical
5323 Harry Hines Boulevard 214-645-8300
Dallas, TX 75390 Fax: 214-645-7999
e-mail: news@utsouthwestern.edu
www.utsouthwestern.edu
Daniel K Podolsky, MD, President
J. Gregory Fitz, Executive Vice President

5713 Yeshiva University Marion Bessin Liver Research Center
Albert Einstein College of Medicine
1300 Morris Park Avenue 718-430-2000
Bronx, NY 10461-1975 Fax: 718-918-0857
www.einstein.yu.edu/centers/liver-resear
Liver disease research and therapy.
Allan W Wolkoff, MD, Director
David A Shafritz, MD, Associate Director

Support Groups & Hotlines

5714 Children's Liver Association for Support S ervices
25379 Wayne Mills Place 661-263-9099
Valencia, CA 91355 877-679-8256
Fax: 661-263-9099
e-mail: admin@classkids.org
www.classkids.org
Dedicated to addressing the emotional, educational, and financial needs of families with children with liver disease or liver transplantation. Telephone hotline, newsletter, parent matching, literature and financial assistance. supports research and educates public about organ donations.
Mark Sumner, Co-Founder
Diane Sumner, Co-Founder

5715 National Gaucher Foundation (NGF)
2227 Idlewood Road
Tucker, GA 30084 800-504-3189
Fax: 770-934-2911
e-mail: ngf@gaucherdisease.org
www.gaucherdisease.org/
The National Gaucher Foundation (NGF), established in 1984, supports and promotes research into the causes of, and a cure for Gaucher Disease. NGF provides information and assistance for those affected by Gaucher disease in addition to education and outreach to increase public awareness. NGF operates the Gaucher Disease Family Support Network.
Brian E Berman, President
Rhonda P Buyers, CEO/Executive Director

5716 National Health Information Center
PO Box 1133 310-565-4167
Washington, DC 20013 800-336-4797
Fax: 301-984-4256
e-mail: info@nhic.org
www.health.gov/nhic
Offers a nationwide information referral service, produces directories and resource guides.
Freudenberger, President
Larry Lasky, Vice President

5717 National Reye's Syndrome Foundation
426 N Lewis Street 419-636-2679
Bryan, OH 43506 800-233-7393
Fax: 419-636-9897
e-mail: nrsf@reyessyndrome.org
www.reyessyndrome.org
Devoted to conquering Reye's syndrome, primarily a children's disease affecting the liver and brain, but can affect all ages. Provides support, information and referrals. Encourages research.
John Symonds, Executive Director

5718 Wilson's Disease Association
5572 North Diversey Boulevard 414-961-0533
Milwaukee, WI 53217 866-961-0533
Fax: 330-264-0974
e-mail: info@wilsonsdisease.org
www.wilsonsdisease.org
Serves as a communications support network for individuals affected by Wilson's disease; distributes information to professionals and the public; makes referrals; and holds meetings.
8 pages
Mary L Graper, President
Stefanie F Kaplan, Vice-President

Books

5719 Liver Cancer
Churchill Livingstone
PO Box 3188 201-319-9800
Secaucus, NJ 07096-3188 800-553-5426
Fax: 201-319-9659
www.churchillmed.com
1997 640 pages Hardcover
ISBN: 0-443054-81-9
Steven A. Curley, Author

5720 Liver Disease in Children
Mosby Year Book
11830 Westline Indus Drv 314-872-8370
Saint Louis, MO 63146-3313 800-325-4177
1993 800 pages
ISBN: 1-556443-77-2
Frederick J. Suchy, Author
Ronald J. Sokol, Author

Magazines

5721 American Association for the Study of Liver Diseases
1729 King Street 703-299-9766
Alexandria, VA 22314 Fax: 703-299-9622
e-mail: aasld@aasld.org
www.aasld.org
Information for professionals interested in disease of the liver and biliary tract.
Sherrie H Cathcart, Executive Director

5722 Hepatology
American Assoc. for the Study of Liver Disease
1729 King Street 703-299-9766
Alexandria, VA 22314 Fax: 703-299-9622
e-mail: aasld@aasld.org
www.aasld.org
Information for professionals interested in disease of the liver and biliary tract.
Sherrie H Cathcart, Executive Director

Newsletters

5723 Children's Liver Association for Support S ervices Newsletter
25379 Wayne Mills Place 661-263-9099
Valencia, CA 91355 877-679-8256
Fax: 661-263-9099
e-mail: SupportSrv@aol.com
www.classkids.org
Dedicated to addressing the emotional, educational, and financial needs of families with children with liver disease or liver transplantation. Telephone hotline, newsletter, parent matching, literature and financial assistance. supports research and educates public about organ donations.
Yearly
Diane Summer, President Board of Directors
Ann Whitehead RN/JD, Vice President Board of Directors

5724 Liver Update
American Liver Foundation

1425 Pompton Avenue
Cedar Grove, NJ 07009-1000

973-256-2550
800-465-4837
Fax: 973-256-3214
e-mail: info@liverfoundation.org
www.liverfoundation.org

Clinical newsletter for physicians.
BiAnnually
Rick Smith, President & CEO
Rebecca Frank, Chief Development Officer

5725 LiverLink
Alagille Syndrome Alliance
10630 SW Garden Park Plc
Tigard, OR 97223-3832

503-639-6217
e-mail: info@liverkink.com
www.liverlink.com

Newsletter for Alagille Syndrome.

5726 Progress
American Liver Foundation
1425 Pompton Avenue
Cedar Grove, NJ 07009-1000

973-256-2550
800-465-4837
Fax: 973-256-3214
e-mail: info@liverfoundation.org
www.liverfoundation.org

Newsletter about liver disease and ALF.
TriAnnually
Rick Smith, President & CEO
Rebecca Frank, Chief Development Officer

Pamphlets

5727 Alcohol and the Liver: Myth vs. Facts
American Liver Foundation
1425 Pompton Avenue
Cedar Grove, NJ 07009-1000

973-256-2550
800-223-0179
e-mail: info@liverfoundation.org
www.liverfoundation.org

Rick Smith, President & CEO
Rebecca Frank, Chief Development Officer

5728 Biliary Atresia
American Liver Foundation
1425 Pompton Avenue
Cedar Grove, NJ 07009-1000

973-857-2626
800-223-0179
e-mail: info@liverfoundation.org
www.liverfoundation.org

Rick Smith, President & CEO
Kazuhiko Bessho, Author

5729 Diet and Your Liver
American Liver Foundation
1425 Pompton Avenue
Cedar Grove, NJ 07009-1000

973-256-2550
800-223-0179
Fax: 973-256-3214
e-mail: info@liverfoundation.org
www.liverfoundation.org

Rick Smith, President & CEO
Rebecca Frank, Chief Development Officer

5730 Facts on Liver Transplantation
American Liver Foundation
1425 Pompton Avenue
Cedar Grove, NJ 07009-1000

973-256-2550
800-223-0179
Fax: 973-256-3214
e-mail: info@liverfoundation.org
www.liverfoundation.org

Rick Smith, President & CEO
Rebecca Frank, Chief Development Officer

5731 Fatty Liver
American Liver Foundation
1425 Pompton Avenue
Cedar Grove, NJ 07009-1000

973-256-2550
800-223-0179
Fax: 987-256-3214
e-mail: info@liverfoundation.org
www.liverfoundation.org

Rick Smith, President & CEO
Sandra Cabot, Author

5732 Gallstones
American Liver Foundation
1425 Pompton Avenue
Cedar Grove, NJ 07009-1000

973-256-2550
800-223-0179
Fax: 973-256-3214
e-mail: info@liverfoundation.org
www.liverfoundation.org

Rick Smith, President & CEO
M. M. Fisher, Author

5733 Getting Help to Hepatitis
American Liver Foundation
1425 Pompton Avenue
Cedar Grove, NJ 07009-1000

973-256-2550
800-223-0179
Fax: 973-256-3214
e-mail: info@liverfoundation.org
www.liverfoundation.org

Rick Smith, President & CEO

5734 Hemochromatosis
American Liver Foundation
1425 Pompton Avenue
Cedar Grove, NJ 07009-1000

973-256-2550
800-223-0179
Fax: 973-256-3214
e-mail: info@liverfoundation.org
www.liverfoundation.org

Rick Smith, President & CEO
James C. Bartonÿ, Author

5735 Hepatitis A, B & C
American Liver Foundation
1425 Pompton Avenue
Cedar Grove, NJ 07009-1000

973-256-2550
800-223-0179
Fax: 973-256-3214
e-mail: info@liverfoundation.org
www.liverfoundation.org

Rick Smith, President & CEO

5736 Hepatitis B: Your Child at Risk
American Liver Foundation
1425 Pompton Avenue
Cedar Grove, NJ 07009-1000

973-256-2550
800-223-0179
Fax: 973-256-3214
e-mail: info@liverfoundation.org
www.liverfoundation.org

Rick Smith, President & CEO

5737 How Can You Love Me
American Liver Foundation
1425 Pompton Avenue
Cedar Grove, NJ 07009-1000

973-857-2626
800-223-0179
Fax: 973-256-3214
e-mail: info@liverfoundation.org
www.liverfoundation.org

Rick Smith, President & CEO

5738 Liver Function Tests
American Liver Foundation
1425 Pompton Avenue
Cedar Grove, NJ 07009-1000

973-256-2550
800-223-0179
Fax: 973-256-3214
e-mail: info@liverfoundation.org
www.liverfoundation.org

Rick Smith, President & CEO

5739 Liver Transplant Fund
American Liver Foundation
1425 Pompton Avenue
Cedar Grove, NJ 07009-1000

973-256-2550
800-223-0179
Fax: 973-256-3214
e-mail: info@liverfoundation.org
www.liverfoundation.org

Rick Smith, President & CEO

5740 Liver Transplantation
American Liver Foundation

1425 Pompton Avenue
Cedar Grove, NJ 07009-1000

973-857-2626
800-223-0179
Fax: 973-256-3214
e-mail: info@liverfoundation.org
www.liverfoundation.org

Rick Smith, President & CEO
Dilip Chakravarty, Author

5741 Viral Hepatitis
American Liver Foundation
1425 Pompton Avenue
Cedar Grove, NJ 07009-1000

973-256-2550
800-223-0179
Fax: 973-256-3214
e-mail: info@liverfoundation.org
www.liverfoundation.org

Rick Smith, President & CEO

5742 Your Liver Lets You Live
American Liver Foundation
1425 Pompton Avenue
Cedar Grove, NJ 07009-1000

973-256-2550
800-223-0179
Fax: 973-256-3214
e-mail: info@liverfoundation.org
www.liverfoundation.org

Rick Smith, President & CEO

Web Sites

5743 American Association for the Study of Liver Diseases
www.aasld.org/
Conducts symposia and educational courses for professionals interested in disease of the liver and biliary tract. The leading organization for advancing the science and practice of hepatology.

5744 Children's Liver Alliance
www.liverkids.org.au/
Empowering the hearts and minds of children with liver disease, their families and the medical professionals who care for them.

5745 Healing Well
www.healingwell.com
An online health resource guide to medical news, chat, information and articles, newsgroups and message boards, books, disease-related web sites, medical directories, and more for patients, friends, and family coping with disabling diseases, disorders, or chronic illnesses.

5746 Health Finder
www.healthfinder.gov
Searchable, carefully developed web site offering information on over 1000 topics. Developed by the US Department of Health and Human Services, the site can be used in both English and Spanish.

5747 Healthlink USA
www.healthlinkusa.com
Health information concerning treatment, cures, prevention, diagnosis, risk factors, research, support groups, email lists, personal stories and much more. Updated regularly.

5748 Helios Health
www.helioshealth.com
Online resource for your health information. Detailed information about specific health topics, access to expert advice from our Medical Advisory Board, and up-to-date health news.

5749 Liver Support
www.liversupport.com
Information about the world's safest, most powerful liver-protecting supplement, milk thistle. Specifically facts about the safe, yet highly potent, Phytosome form.

5750 MedicineNet
www.medicinenet.com
An online resource for consumers providing easy-to-read, authoritative medical and health information.

5751 Medscape
www.medscape.com
Medscape offers specialists, primary care physicians, and other health professionals the Web's most robust and integrated medical information and educational tools.

5752 WebMD
www.webmd.com
Provides credible information, supportive communities, and in-depth reference material about health subjects. A source for original and timely health information as well as material from well known content providers.

Description

5753 **Lung Disease**

The lungs are in intimate contact with a person's environment, so they may be damaged by scores of agents, including dusts, gases and micro-organisms. The majority of lung, or pulmonary, diseases are related to exposure to external irritants, such as cigarette smoke, asbestos, bacteria and viruses. The most common chronic lung diseases of this type are emphysema and chronic bronchitis; both are part of the class of diseases called Chronic Obstructive Pulmonary Disease, or COPD. Most cases are associated with tobacco usage. High-risk occupations for lung disease include mining, farming, building construction and certain types of manufacturing. Lung cancer may be primary (originating in the lung) or secondary (spread, or metastasized, from another area). Bronchogenic cancer accounts for more than 90 percent of all lung tumors; cigarette smoking is the principal cause. Lung cancer is usually seen in people with COPD, because the two conditions have similar causes. Other lung disorders are secondary to clots originating from other sites in the body, systemic illness, and skeletal abnormalities that interfere with chest expansion during breathing.

Symptoms of lung disease may include coughing, sputum production, breathlessness, and sometimes fever or chest pain. In advanced cases, breathlessness is constant, and cyanosis (a bluish discoloration of the lips and fingernails) may occur.

Diagnosis of pulmonary disorders depends on a very careful history, physical examination, chest x-ray and pulmonary function testing, or spirometry. These measures are also important in following disease progression and response to treatment. Other chest imaging techniques, such as computed tomography (CT) scans and MRIs, and examination of fluid in the lung and lung tissue help establish a diagnosis. Recent research indicates that PET (positron emission tomography) scans may be helpful in the earlier diagnosis and treatment of lung cancer. Treatment of lung disease depends on the underlying cause. Management of COPD includes avoiding tobacco or other environmental exposure, antibiotics to control heavy sputum production and drugs to open up the narrowed airways. In advanced cases, breathing oxygen directly by nasal prongs improves quality of life and survival. Lung transplantation has occasionally been attempted, usually when COPD is due to a genetic disorder. Early screening for lung cancer has been disappointing; quitting smoking early is the only meaningful way of reducing one's risk of dying of the disease. Treatment may include surgery, radiation, or chemotherapy; success depends on the stage of the tumor and its precise type as determined by tissue biopsy.

Severe Acute Respiratory Syndrome, known as SARS, is an infectious disease that first appeared in China in 2002. SARS is caused by a corona-virus, which is related to the virus behind the common cold. The symptoms of SARS are a fever, greater than 100.4 degrees, fatigue, headache and chills. It is also accompanied by a dry cough and difficulty breathing, owing to the inflamed lungs. Until effective treatment or a vaccine is developed, prevention in SARS-infected areas includes isolating patients, wearing protective surgical masks, and restricting travel.

National Agencies & Associations

5754 **American Association for Respiratory Care**
9425 N MacArthur Boulevard   972-243-2272
Irving, TX 75063-4706   Fax: 972-484-2720
e-mail: info@aarc.org
www.aarc.org
Committed to enhancing professionalism as a respiratory care practitioner improving your performance on the job and helping to broaden the scope essential for success.
Michael T Amato, Chair
Neil MacIntyre, Vice-Chair

5755 **American Lung Association**
1301 Pennsylvania Avenue NW   202-785-3355
Washington, DC 20004   800-LUN-GUSA
e-mail: lungdc@lung.org
www.lung.org
The mission of the American Lung Association is to prevent lung disease and promote lung health. Founded in 1904 to fight tuberculosis the American Lung Association today fights disease in all its forms with special emphasis on asthma and tobacco control.
Ross P Lanzafame, Chairman
Harold P Wimmer, President & CEO

5756 **Coalition for Pulmonary Fibrosis**
10866 W. Washington Boulevard
Culver City, CA 90232   888-222-8541
Fax: 408-266-3289
e-mail: info@coalitionforpf.org
www.coalitionforpf.org
Founded to further education patient support and research efforts for pulmonary fibrosis specifically idiopathic pulmonary fibrosis.
Marvin I Schwarz, MD, Chairman
Gregory Tino, MD, Vice-Chairman

5757 **National Jewish Medical and Research Center**
1400 Jackson Street   303-398-1565
Denver, CO 80206   877-225-5654
e-mail: allstetterw@njhealth.org
www.nationaljewish.org
Offers comprehensive diagnosis treatment and rehabilitation of people with chronic obstructive pulmonary disease asthma allergies and other respiratory and immune diseases.
Rich Schierburg, Chair
Michael Salem, MD, President & CEO

5758 **Pulmonary Fibrosis Association**
230 East Ohio Street   888-733-6741
Chicago, IL 60611-0004   Fax: 866-587-9158
e-mail: info@pulmonaryfibrosis.org
www.pulmonaryfibrosis.org
Dedicated to finding a cure for and raising awareness of pulmonary fibrosis an often fatal lung disease.
Daniel M Rose, Chief Executive Officer and Chairman of
Patti Tuomey, President and Chief Operating Officer

5759 **Pulmonary Fibrosis Foundation**
230 East Ohio Street   888-733-6741
Chicago, IL 60611   Fax: 866-587-9158
e-mail: info@pulmonaryfibrosis.org
www.pulmonaryfibrosis.org
A non-profit corporation founded in the state of Colorado in 2000 by Albert Rose and Michael Rosenzweig, both of whom were diagnosed with Pulmonary Fibrosis (IPF).
Daniel M Rose, Chief Executive Officer and Chairman of
Patti Tuomey, President and Chief Operating Officer

5760 Pulmonary Hypertension Association
801 Roeder Road   301-565-3004
Silver Spring, MD 20910   800-748-7274
                                                    Fax: 301-565-3994
                                        e-mail: pha@PHAssociation.org
                                              www.PHAssociation.org
A nonprofit organization for pulmonary hypertension patients, families, caregivers and PH-treating medical professionals. The mission of the Pulmonary Hypertension Association (PHA) is to find ways to prevent and cure pulmonary hypertension.
Vallerie McLaughlin, MD, Chair
Rino Aldrighetti, President & CEO

5761 US Environmental Protection Agency: Indoor Environments Division
1200 Pennsylvania Avenue NW   202-343-9370
Washington, DC 20460   Fax: 202-343-2392
                                            e-mail: iaqinfo@aol.com
                                               www.epa.gov/iaq
Responsible for implementing EPA's Indoor Environments Program, a voluntary (non-regulatory) program to address indoor air pollution.
Gina McCarthy, Administrator
Bob Perciasepe, Deputy Administrator

5762 White Lung Association
PO Box 1483   410-243-5864
Baltimore, MD 21203-1483   e-mail: jfite@whitelung.org
                                               www.whitelung.org
A national nonprofit organization dedicated to the education of the public to the hazards of asbestos exposure. The association developed programs of public education and consults with victims of asbestos exposure, school boards, building owners and government representatives.
Jim Perry, Director of Development

State Agencies & Associations

Alabama

5763 American Lung Association of Alabama
PO BOX 2178   601-206-5810
Ridgeland, AL 35244   Fax: 202-452-1805
                              e-mail: inquiries@breathehealthy.org
                            www.lung.org/associations/states/alabama
Robin Robinson, Chair
Sara Dreiling, Chief Executive Officer

Alaska

5764 American Lung Association of Alaska
500 W International Airport Road   907-276-5864
Anchorage, AK 99518-1105   800-LUN-GUSA
                                            Fax: 907-565-5587
                                   e-mail: mstoneking@aklung.org
                              www.lung.org/associations/states/alaska/
Marge Pfeifer, President/CEO

Arizona

5765 American Lung Association of Arizona
102 W McDowell Road   602-258-7505
Phoenix, AZ 85003-1299   800-LUN-GUSA
                                            Fax: 602-258-7507
                                 e-mail: calexander@lungarizona.org
                             www.lung.org/associations/states/arizona
Through research education and advocacy the American Lung Association of Arizona works to prevent lung disease and promote lung health. Our areas of focus are asthma air quality and tobacco control.
Terry Daane, Chair
Stacey Mortenson, Executive Director

Arkansas

5766 American Lung Association of Arkansas
211 Natural Resources Drive   501-224-5864
Little Rock, AR 72205-1539   800-880-5864
                                            Fax: 501-224-5654
                                   e-mail: klackey@lungark.org
                                              www.lungark.org
Karen S Abate, President/CEO
Sylvia Goodin, Secretary

California

5767 American Lung Association of California
424 Pendleton Way   510-638-5864
Oakland, CA 94621-2189   Fax: 510-638-8984
                                     e-mail: cainfo@lung.org
                            www.lung.org/associations/states/califor
A.Linda Hinojosa, Chair
Jane Warner, President/CEO

Colorado

5768 American Lung Association of Colorado
5600 Greenwood Plaza Boulevard   303-388-4327
Greenwood Village, CO 80111   800-LUN-GUSA
                                            Fax: 303-377-1102
                                  e-mail: info@lungcolorado.org
                               http://www.lung.org/associations/states/
Curt Huber˜, Executive Director
Connor Michael, Communications Manager

Connecticut

5769 American Lung Association of Connecticut
45 Ash Street   860-289-5401
E Hartford, CT 06108-3272   800-586-4872
                                            Fax: 860-289-5405
                                     e-mail: bcase@alact.org
                                              www.alact.org
Part of the American Lung Association the oldest voluntary health agency dedicated to fighting a single disease. Highest priorities are asthma tobacco control and clean air.
Lisa Brown, VP Community Outreach
Susan DeNardo, Development Director

Delaware

5770 American Lung Association of Delaware
630 Churchmans Road   302-737-6414
Wilmington, DE 19702-3280   800-LUN-GUSA
                                            Fax: 888-415-5757
                                    e-mail: llyons@lunginfo.org
                            www.lung.org/associations/charters/mid-a
Christopher Carney, Chair
Deborah Brown, CEO

District of Columbia

5771 American Lung Association of the District of Columbia
1301 Pennsylvania Avenue NW   202-785-3355
Washington, DC 20004-2617   e-mail: lungdc@lung.org
                            www.lung.org/associations/charters/distr
Resource for information and programs in the area of lung health, including asthma, tobacco control, air quality, sarcoidosis, and turberculosis.
Dennis C Alexander, Regional Executive Director
Marc Ittelson, Regional Development Director

Florida

5772 American Lung Association of Florida
6852 Belfort Oaks Place   904-743-2933
Jacksonville, FL 32216-5216   800-940-2933
                                            Fax: 904-743-2916
                                     e-mail: alaf@lungfla.org
                            www.lung.org/associations/states/florida

Works for the prevention and control of lung disease through education, advocacy and research.
Marcia Williams, Chairwoman
Martha C Bogdan, President/CEO

5773 Goodwill Industries-Suncoast
Goodwill Industries-Suncoast
10596 Gandy Boulevard   727-523-1512
St. Petersburg, FL 33702   888-279-1988
                                 Fax: 727-563-9300
e-mail: gw.marketing@goodwill-suncoast.com
www.goodwill-suncoast.org
A non-profit community based organization whose purpose is to improve the quality of life for people who are disabled, disadvantaged and/or aged. This mission is accomplished through a staff of over 1,200 employees providing independent living skills, affordable housing, career assessment and planning, job skills, training, placement, and job retention assistance with useful employment. Annually, Goodwill Industries-Suncoast serves over 30,000 people in Citrus, Hernando, Levy, Marion and more.
Oscar J Horton, Chair
Deborah A Passerini, President/CEO

Georgia

5774 American Lung Association of Georgia
2452 Spring Road   770-434-5864
Smyrna, GA 30080-3862   Fax: 770-319-0349
e-mail: alaga@lungga.org
www.lung.org/associations/states/georgia
Marcia Williams, Chairwoman of the Board
Martha C Bogdan, President/CEO

Hawaii

5775 American Lung Association of Hawaii
650 Iwilei Road   808-537-5966
Honolulu, HI 96817   Fax: 808-537-5971
e-mail: lleslie@ala-hawaii.org
www.lung.org/associations/states/hawaii
Lorraine Leslie, Hawaii Director
Debbie Apolo, Tobacco Control Manager

Idaho

5776 American Lung Association of Idaho
1412 W Idaho   208-345-5864
Boise, ID 83702   800-LUN-GUSA
                                 Fax: 208-345-5896
e-mail: jflynn@lungmtpacific.org
www.lung.org/associations/states/idaho/
Wimmer, CEO
Kim Streib, Vice President Finance

Illinois

5777 American Lung Association of Illinois
55 West Wacker Drive   312-781-1100
Chicago, IL 60601   800-LUN-GUSA
                                 Fax: 318-781-9250
e-mail: info@lungil.org
www.lung.org/associations/states/illinoi
Frank Keldermans, Chair
Lewis Bartfield, President/CEO

Indiana

5778 American Lung Association of Indiana
115 W Washington Street   317-819-1181
Indianapolis, IN 46204-1470   800-LUN-GUSA
                                 Fax: 317-819-1187
e-mail: info@lungin.org
www.lung.org/associations/states/indiana
Alan D Rowe, Chair
Lewis Bartfield, President/CEO

Iowa

5779 American Lung Association of Iowa
2530 73rd Street   515-309-9507
Des Moines, IA 50322-1800   800-LUN-GUSA
                                 Fax: 515-334-9564
e-mail: info@lungia.org
www.lung.org/associations/states/iowa/
Alan D Rowe, Chair
Lewis Bartfield, President/CEO

Kansas

5780 American Lung Association of Kansas
6701 W. 64th Street   913-912- 719
Overland Park, KS 66202-2419   800-LUN-GUSA
                                 Fax: 913-912-7206
e-mail: inquiries@breathehealthy.org
www.lung.org/associations/charters/plain
Robin Robinson, Chair
Veena B Antony, Director

Kentucky

5781 American Lung Association of Kentucky
4100 Churchman Avenue   502-363-2652
Louisville, KY 40215-0067   800-LUN-GUSA
                                 Fax: 502-363-0222
e-mail: bgottschalk@midlandlung.org
www.lung.org/associations/states/kentuck
Barry Gottschalk, President/CEO
Robert Singletary, Vice President - Finance & Administratio

Louisiana

5782 American Lung Association of Louisiana
2325 Severn Avenue   504-828-5864
Metairie, LA 70001-6918   800-586-4872
                                 Fax: 504-828-5867
e-mail: inquiries@breathehealthy.org
www.lung.org/associations/charters/plain
Robin Robinson, Chair
Veena B Antony, Director

Maine

5783 American Lung Association of Maine
122 State Street   207-622-6394
Augusta, ME 04330   888-241-6566
                                 Fax: 207-626-2919
e-mail: info@lungne.org
www.lung.org/associations/states/maine/
Ross P Lanzafame, Chairman of the Board
John F Emanuel, Secretary/ Treasurer

Maryland

5784 American Lung Association of Maryland
211 East Lombard Street   443-451-4950
Baltimore, MD 21202   800-LUN-GUSA
                                 Fax: 410-560-0829
e-mail: lungmd@lungusa.org
www.lung.org/associations/states/marylan
Dennis C Alexander, Regional Executive Director
Marc Ittelson, Regional Development Director

Massachusetts

5785 American Lung Association of Massachusetts
5 Mountain Road   781-272-2866
Burlington, MA 01903
Adams, CEO
Nicole Crumpton, Executive Office Manager

Michigan

5786 American Lung Association of Michigan
1475 E 12 Mile Road   248-784-2000
Madison Heights, MI 48071   800-543-LUNG
                                    Fax: 248-784-2008
e-mail: midland@midlandlung.org
www.lung.org/associations/states/michiga
Barry Gottschalk, President/CEO
Robert Singletary, Vice President-Finance & Administration

Minnesota

5787 American Lung Association of Minnesota
490 Concordia Avenue   651-227-8014
Saint Paul, MN 55103-2441   800-LUN-GUSA
                                    Fax: 651-227-5459
e-mail: info@lungmn.org
www.lung.org/associations/states/minneso
Angie Carlson, PhD, Chair
Lewis Bartfield, President/CEO

Mississippi

5788 American Lung Association of Mississippi
PO Box 2178   601-206-5810
Ridgeland, MS 39158   Fax: 601-206-5813
e-mail: inquiries@breathehealthy.org
www.lung.org/associations/charters/plain
Robin Robinson, Chair
Veena B Antony, Director

5789 American Lung Association of Missouri
6701 W. 64th Street   913-912- 719
Overland Park, KS 66202   Fax: 913-912-7206
e-mail: inquiries@breathehealthy.org
www.lung.org/associations/charters/plain
Robin Robinson, Chair
Veena B Antony, Director

Missouri

5790 American Lung Association of Eastern Missouri
1118 Hampton Avenue   314-645-5505
Saint Louis, MO 63139-3196   Fax: 314-645-7128
www.lungusa2.org/missouri/index.html

5791 American Lung Association: Kansas City Office
2400 Troost   816-842-5242
Kansas City, MO 64108   Fax: 816-842-5470
e-mail: qnimrod@breathehealthy.org
www.lungusa2.org/missouri/index.html
National health association dedicated to promoting lung health
and preventing lung disease.

Montana

5792 American Lung Association of Northern Rockies
825 Helena Avenue   406-442-6556
Helena, MT 59601-3459   Fax: 406-442-2346
e-mail: ala-nr@ala-nr.org
www.lungusa.org

Nebraska

5793 American Lung Association of Nebraska
8990 West Dodge   402-502-4950
Omaha, NE 68114   800-LUN-GUSA
                                    Fax: 402-502-3112
e-mail: inquiries@breathehealthy.org
www.lung.org/associations/charters/plain
Robin Robinson, Chair
Veena B Antony, Director

Nevada

5794 American Lung Association of Nevada
10615 Double R Boulevard   775-829-LUNG
Reno, NV 89521   800-LUN-GUSA
                                    Fax: 775-829-5850
e-mail: lgenasci@lungnevada.org
www.lungusa.org
Lisa Genasci, Executive Director
Heather Lunsford, Development & Program Manager

New Hampshire

5795 American Lung Association of New Hampshire
1800 Elm Street   603-369-3977
Manchester, NH 03104   800-83L-UNGS
                                    Fax: 603-369-3978
e-mail: info@lungne.org
www.lung.org/associations/states/new-ham
Ross P Lanzafame, Chairman of the Board
John F Emanuel, Secretary/ Treasurer

New Jersey

5796 American Lung Association of New Jersey
1031 Route 22 West   908-685-8040
Bridgewater, NJ 08807-3410   Fax: 888-415-5757
e-mail: jgrinwald@lunginfo.org
www.lung.org/associations/charters/mid-a
Christopher Carney, Chair
Deborah Brown, CEO

New Mexico

5797 American Lung Association of New Mexico
5911 Jefferson Street NE   505-265-0732
Albuquerque, NM 87109   800-LUN-GUSA
                                    Fax: 505-260-1739
e-mail: info@lungnewmexico.org
www.lung.org/associations/states/new-mex
Support group for adults with lung disease. Also offers lung health
education.
Deborah Hoffman, Executive Director
JoAnna DeMaria, Director of Programs

New York

5798 American Lung Association of New York State
418 Broadway   518-465-2013
Albany, NY 12207-2804   800-499-LUNG
                                    Fax: 781-890-4280
e-mail: info@lungne.org
www.lung.org/associations/charters/north
Brian Simonds, Chair
Jeff Seyler, President/CEO

North Carolina

5799 American Lung Association of North Carolina
514 Daniels Street   919-424-6069
Raleigh, NC 27605   800-586-4872
                                    Fax: 919-856-8530
e-mail: lungnc@lungusa.org
www.lungnc.org
Better breathing clubs for chronic lung disease patients.
Dennis C Alexander, Regional Executive Director
Marc Ittelson, Regional Development Director

North Dakota

5800 American Lung Association of North Dakota
212 N. 2nd Street   701-223-5613
Bismarck, ND 58501   800-252-6325
                                    Fax: 701-223-5727
e-mail: info@lungnd.org
http://www.lung.org/associations/states/
A voluntary health agency whose objective is the conquest of lung
disease and the promotion of lung health. We sponsor Super
Asthma Saturday and open airways for schools events to educate

asthmatics and their families and Dakota Superkids Asthma Camp for kids 8-15 with asthma. Smoking cessation classes for adults and youth.
Alan D Rowe, Chair
Lewis Bartfield, President/CEO

Ohio

5801 American Lung Association of Ohio
1950 Arlingate Lane
Columbus, OH 43228-4102
614-279-1700
800-LUN-GUSA
Fax: 614-279-4940
e-mail: alao@ohiolung.org
www.lung.org/associations/states/ohio/in
Barry Gottschalk, President/CEO
Robert Singletary, Vice President - Finance & Administratio

Oklahoma

5802 American Lung Association of Oklahoma
11212 N May Avenue
Oklahoma City, OK 73120
405-748-4674
800-LUN-GUSA
Fax: 405-748-6274
e-mail: inquiries@breathehealthy.org
www.lung.org/associations/charters/plain
Robin Robinson, Chair
Veena B Antony, Director

Oregon

5803 American Lung Association of Oregon
7420 SW Bridgeport Road
Tigard, OR 97224-7790
503-924-4094
800-LUN-GUSA
Fax: 503-924-4120
e-mail: info@lungmtpacific.org
www.lung.org/associations/states/oregon/

Pennsylvania

5804 American Respiratory Alliance of Western Pennsylvania
201 Smith Drive
Cranberry Township, PA 16066
724-772-1750
800-220-1990
Fax: 724-772-1180
e-mail: info@healthylungs.org
www.healthylungs.org
Dedicated to the prevention and control of lung disease through education training, direct services, research funding and advocacy since 1904.
Christine R Cavan, Director
Robert Petix, Chair/Executive Committee

5805 Breathe Pennsylvania
3001 Old Gettysburg Road
Camp Hill, PA 17011
717-541-5864
800-932-0903
Fax: 888-415-5757
e-mail: dbrown@lunginfo.org
www.lung.org/associations/charters/mid-a
Provide education, research and information on lung disease and lung health, including asthma, tobacco prevention and cessation, chronic obstructive pulmonary disease, indoor and outdoor air quality, children's summer camps, support groups and specialty programs.
Christopher Carney, Chair
Deborah Brown, CEO

Rhode Island

5806 American Lung Association of Rhode Island
260 W Exchange Street
Providence, RI 02903-3700
401-421-6487
800-586-4872
Fax: 401-331-5266
e-mail: info@lungne.org
www.lung.org/associations/charters/north
Brian Simonds, Chair
Jeff Seyler, President/CEO

South Carolina

5807 American Lung Association of South Carolina
44-A Markfield Drive
Charleston, SC 29407-2344
843-556-8451
800-849-5864
Fax: 843-766-3294
e-mail: alasc1@lungsc.org
www.lung.org/associations/states/south-c
Marcia Williams, Chairwoman of the Board
William R Cook, Chair-Elect

South Dakota

5808 American Lung Association of South Dakota
401 East 8th Street
Sioux Falls, SD 57103-0233
605-336-7222
800-873-5864
Fax: 605-336-7227
e-mail: info@lungsd.org
www.lung.org/associations/states/south-d
Alan D Rowe, Chair
Lewis Bartfield, President/CEO

Tennessee

5809 American Lung Association of Tennessee
1 Vantage Way
Nashville, TN 37228
615-329-1151
800-LUN-GUSA
Fax: 615-329-1723
e-mail: gbost@midlandlung.org
www.lung.org/associations/states/tenness
A statewide organization the oldest national health agency in the US. Our mission is to prevent lung disease and to promote lung health. Our program priorities include environmental health asthma education tobacco control for children and finding a cure.
Dr Steven Coulter, Chairman
Barry Gottschalk, President/CEO

Texas

5810 American Lung Association of Texas
5926 Balcones Drive
Austin, TX 78731
512-467-6753
800-252-LUNG
Fax: 512-467-7621
e-mail: inquiries@breathehealthy.org
www.texaslung.org
Robin Robinson, Chair
Veena B Antony, Director

Utah

5811 American Lung Association of Utah
1930 S 1100 E
Salt Lake City, UT 84106-2317
801-484-4456
800-548-8252
Fax: 801-484-5461
e-mail: info@lungutah.org
www.lung.org/associations/states/utah/
Troy Neerings, Chair
W. Glenn Lanham, Executive Director

Virginia

5812 American Lung Association of Virginia
9702 Gayton Road
Richmond, VA 23238
804-955-4910
800-345-5864
Fax: 804-267-5634
e-mail: lungva@lungusa.org
www.lungva.org
Dennis C Alexander, Regional Executive Director
Marc Ittelson, Regional Development Director

Washington

5813   American Lung Association of Washington
822 John Street
Seattle, WA 98109
206-441-5100
800-732-9339
Fax: 206-441-3277
e-mail: info@alaw.org
www.lung.org/associations/states/washing
Marina Crickenberger, Executive Director
Chantal Fields, Assistant Executive Director

West Virginia

5814   American Lung Association of West Virginia
2102 Kanawha Blvd
East Charleston, WV 25311
304-342-6600
800-LUN-GUSA
Fax: 888-415-5757
e-mail: cfields@lunginfo.org
www.lung.org/associations/charters/mid-a
Christopher Carney, Chair
Deborah Brown, CEO

Wisconsin

5815   American Lung Association of Wisconsin
13100 W Lisbon Road
Brookfield, WI 53005-2508
262-703-4200
800-LUN-GUSA
Fax: 262-781-5180
e-mail: info@lungwi.org
www.lung.org/associations/states/wiscons
Alan D Rowe, Chair
Lewis Bartfield, President/CEO

Research Centers

5816   Enzymology Research Laboratory Dept. of Veterans Affairs Medical Center
Dept. of Veterans Affairs Medical Center
150 Muir Road
Martinez, CA 94553
925-228-6800
Studies affecting emphysema in mankind.
Michael C Gaussig, President

5817   National Jewish Center for Immunology
1400 Jackson Street
Denver, CO 80206
303-388-4461
877-225-5654
www.nationaljewish.org
Offers basic and clinical research into the causes and treatments of various lung diseases and respiratory problems.
Rafeul Alam, Division Chief

5818   University of Utah Rocky Mountain Center for Occupational & Environmental Health
University of Utah
391 Chipeta Way
Salt Lake City, UT 84108
801-581-4800
Fax: 801-817-24
TTY: 801-581-7224
e-mail: rmoser@rmcoeh.utah.edu
medicine.utah.edu/rmcoeh/
Provides graduate and continuing education programs in occupational medicine occupational health nursing ergonomics and safety industrial hygiene and hazardous materials. Additionally provides clinical evaluations and consultations in the listed areas.
Dennis Lloyd, Chair
Sen Karen Mayne, Advisory Member

5819   Warren Grant Magnuson Clinical Center
National Institute of Health
10 Center Drive MSC 1078
Bethesda, MD 20892
301-496-3311
800-411-1222
Fax: 301-496-2390
TTY: 866-411-1010
e-mail: mmichael@cc.nih.gov
www.clinicalcenter.nih.gov
Established in 1953 as the research hospital of the National Institutes of Health. Designed so that patient care facilities are close to research laboratories so new findings of basic and clinical scientists can be quickly applied to the treatment of patients. Upon referral by physicians, patients are admitted to NIH clinical studies.
John Mark, Lung Help Line Director

Support Groups & Hotlines

5820   American Lung Association Help Line
American Lung Association
3000 Kelly Lane
Springfield, IL 62711
217-787-5864
800-586-4872
Fax: 217-787-5916
www.helpline.org
Provides information for the lung association of the state in which you make the call. Offers support group referrals.
Michael Salem MD, President/CEO
William Allstetter, Public Affairs/Media

5821   Lung Facts
National Jewish Center for Immunology
1400 Jackson Street
Denver, CO 80206
303-388-4461
877-225-5654
Fax: 303-270-2220
e-mail: allstetterw@njc.org
www.nationaljewish.org
An automated information service with recorded health messages developed by Lung Line Information Service. The information provided on this system offers help and support, as well as medical updates for persons suffering from lung diseases.
Michael

5822   National Health Information Center
PO Box 1133
Washington, DC 20013
310-565-4167
800-336-4797
Fax: 301-984-4256
e-mail: info@nhic.org
www.health.gov/nhic
Offers a nationwide information referral service, produces directories and resource guides.
Austin, PhD

Books

5823   American Lung Association Family Guide to Asthma and Allergies
American Lung Association
1740 Broadway
New York, NY 10019-4315
212-315-8700
e-mail: info@lungusa.org
www.lungusa.org
Norman H. Edelman, Author

5824   Health Consequences of Smoking: Cancer & Chronic Lung Disease in the Workplace
DIANE Publishing Company
330 Pusey Avenue
Darby, PA 19023
610-461-6200
800-782-3833
Fax: 610-461-6130
e-mail: dianepublishing@gmail.com
www.dianepublishing.net
Examines the relationship between cigarette smoking and occupational exposures. Establishes that in order to protect the workers fully, forces of labor, management, insurers and government must become as engaged in attempts to reduce the prevalence of cigarette smoking as they are in occupational exposure. Tables and figure. Extensive bibliography, index.
542 pages Paperback
ISBN: 0-788123-11-4
Herman Baron, Publisher

5825   Management of Acute Exacerbations of Chronic Obstructive Pulmonary Disease
DIANE Publishing Company
330 Pusey Avenue
Darby, PA 19023
610-461-6200
800-782-3833
Fax: 610-461-6130
e-mail: dianepublishing@gmail.com
www.dianepublishing.net
This report describes evidence about the clinical assessment and management of patients presenting with acute exacerbation of

chronic obstructive pulmonary disease, a frequent cause of health care utilization, morality and decreased quality of life.
256 pages Paperback
ISBN: 0-756721-99-7
Herman Baron, Publisher

5826   Seven Steps to a Smoke-Free Life
American Lung Association
1740 Broadway   212-315-8700
New York, NY 10019-4315   800-586-4872
                                          e-mail: info@lungusa.org
                                                 www.lungusa.org

---

Pamphlets

5827   Around the Clock with COPD
American Lung Association
1740 Broadway   212-315-8700
New York, NY 10019-4315   800-586-4872
                                          e-mail: info@lungusa.org
                                                 www.lungusa.org
A booklet with non-medical helpful hints written by persons living with a chronic lung disease for others.

5828   Asbestos in Your Home
American Lung Association
1740 Broadway   212-315-8700
New York, NY 10019-4315   800-586-4872
                                          e-mail: info@lungusa.org
                                                 www.lungusa.org
Offers information on asbestos.

5829   Black Lung
National Jewish Center for Immunology
1400 Jackson Street   303-388-4461
Denver, CO 80206-2762   800-222-5864
Offers information on black lung and the respiratory system.

5830   Emphysema
American Lung Association of Connecticut
45 Ash Street   860-289-5401
East Hartford, CT 06108-3294   800-586-4872
                                           Fax: 860-289-5405
                                                 www.alact.org
Offers information on who gets emphysema, how it attacks, causes, effects, prevention and treatment.
John E Zinn, President/CEO

5831   Exercise Guidelines for the Person with Lung Disease
American Lung Association of Connecticut
45 Ash Street   860-289-5401
East Hartford, CT 06108-3294   800-586-4872
                                           Fax: 860-289-5405
                                                 www.alact.org
Offers exercise information and illustrations for persons with lung disease.
John E Zinn, President/CEO

5832   Facts About AAT Deficiency-Related Emphysema
American Lung Association
1740 Broadway   212-315-8700
New York, NY 10019-4315   800-586-4872
                                          e-mail: info@lungusa.org
                                                 www.lungusa.org
Offers information on this type of emphysema, risk factors, development, symptoms and early detection.

5833   Facts About Asbestos
American Lung Association
1740 Broadway   212-315-8700
New York, NY 10019-4315   800-586-4872
                                          e-mail: info@lungusa.org
                                                 www.lungusa.org
Offers information on lung hazards on the job and what employers can do to protect themselves and the people that work for them.

5834   Facts About Asthma
American Lung Association

1740 Broadway   212-315-8700
New York, NY 10019-4315   800-586-4872
                                          e-mail: info@lungusa.org
                                                 www.lungusa.org

5835   Steps to a Better Understanding of Lung Cancer: A Patient and Family Guide
American Lung Association
1740 Broadway   212-315-8700
New York, NY 10019-4315   800-586-4872
                                          e-mail: info@lungusa.org
                                                 www.lungusa.org
A booklet with non-medical helpful hints written by persons living with a chronic lung disease for others.

5836   Understanding Emphysema
National Jewish Center for Immunology
1400 Jackson Street   303-388-4461
Denver, CO 80206-2762   800-222-5864
Offers information on emphysema, causes, treatments, symptoms and prevention.

Audio & Video

5837   Keeping the Balance
Fanlight Productions
4196 Washington Street   617-469-4999
Boston, MA 02131-1731   800-937-4113
                                           Fax: 617-469-3379
                                        e-mail: fanlight@fanlight.com
                                                 www.fanlight.com
Siblings of children with serious lung disease share their experiences of being the normal child, exploring the frequent conflict between their feelings of love and concern and their resentment over the attention denied to them because of the sibling's illness. Offers advice on how parents can keep the balance between the needs of all of their children.
1993 23 Minutes
ISBN: 1-572950-89-7

5838   Sickle Cell Disease: Faces of Our Children
Fanlight Productions
4196 Washington Street   617-469-4999
Boston, MA 02131-1731   800-937-4113
                                           Fax: 617-469-3379
                                        e-mail: fanlight@fanlight.com
                                                 www.fanlight.com
This program examines the devastating impact of sickle cell disease on these young people and their families and caregivers. It will be an important tool for increasing awareness in the community and among healthcare and social service providers in community clinics, hospitals, and other settings.
1999 14 Minutes
ISBN: 1-572953-05-5

Web Sites

5839   American Lung Association
                                                 www.lungusa.org
Offers research, medical updates, fund-raising, educational materials and public awareness campaigns relating to lung disease causes.

5840   Healing Well
                                                 www.healingwell.com
An online health resource guide to medical news, chat, information and articles, newsgroups and message boards, books, disease-related web sites, medical directories, and more for patients, friends, and family coping with disabling diseases, disorders, or chronic illnesses.

5841   Health Central
                                                 www.healthcenter.com
Provides support group and diagnostic information regarding lung disease.

5842   Health Finder
                                                 www.healthfinder.gov

Searchable, carefully developed web site offering information on over 1000 topics. Developed by the US Department of Health and Human Services, the site can be used in both English and Spanish.

5843   Healthlink USA

www.healthlinkusa.com
Health information concerning treatment, cures, prevention, diagnosis, risk factors, research, support groups, email lists, personal stories and much more. Updated regularly.

5844   Helios Health

www.helioshealth.com
Online resource for your health information. Detailed information about specific health topics, access to expert advice from our Medical Advisory Board, and up-to-date health news.

5845   Lung Disease

www.lungusa.org
The American Lung Association's website, including information on diseases A to Z, living with lung disease, tobacco control, air quality, data, statistics, research, and more.

5846   MedicineNet

www.medicinenet.com
An online resource for consumers providing easy-to-read, authoritative medical and health information.

5847   Medscape

www.medscape.com
Medscape offers specialists, primary care physicians, and other health professionals the Web's most robust and integrated medical information and educational tools.

5848   National Heart, Lung & Blood Institute

www.nhlbi.nih.gov
A website maintained by the National Institute of Health offering general information regarding the heart, lungs, and blood.

5849   WebMD

www.webmd.com
Provides credible information, supportive communities, and in-depth reference material about health subjects. A source for original and timely health information as well as material from well known content providers.

Description

5850 Lupus Erythematosus

Lupus erythematosus refers to two distinct but overlapping conditions. Systemic lupus erythematosus, SLE, is a chronic multi-organ inflammatory illness that may involve the brain, skin, kidneys, joints, bowel, and eyes. Discoid lupus erythematosus, DLE, is a much less serious disease that is limited to the skin. In DLE, patches of skin may turn red and develop white scales, followed by thinning and scarring. About 10 percent of patients with DLE will go on to develop SLE; roughly 25 percent of patients with SLE also have the manifestations of DLE.

Of SLE cases, 90 percent are women, and the disease usually begins during the child-bearing years. Although the cause is unclear, SLE causes its damage through auto-immune mechanisms. The body's own immune system, designed to fight off invasion from micro-organisms, turns against its own tissues, evidence of which can be measured in the blood. Almost any organ system can be affected, and symptoms include fatigue, fever, loss of appetite, skin rash, sensitivity to light (photophobia), joint pain, headaches, personality change, eye irritation, and inflammation of the kidney.

In general, the course of SLE is chronic and relapsing, often with long periods (years) of remission. It may only be mild or progress towards more serious illness and death from infection, kidney failure, or neurologic damage. Survival has improved markedly in the past two decades because, for most patients with SLE, the disease can be controlled with large, prolonged doses of steroids, and other drugs that affect the immune system. Some of these therapies may be associated with long-term complications.

National Agencies & Associations

5851 American Juvenile Arthritis Organization (AJAO)
1330 West Peachtree Street
Atlanta, GA 30309
404-872-7100
800-283-7800
Fax: 440-872-9559
e-mail: help@arthritis.org
www.arthritis.org

A council of the Arthritis Foundation devoted to serving the special needs of children, teens and young adults with childhood rheumatic diseases (including systemic lupus erythematosus) and their families. Provides support groups, information, advocacy, research updates, and conferences.
Daniel T McGowan, Chair
John H Klippel, President & CEO

5852 American Juvenile Arthritis Organization
1330 W Peachtree Street
Atlanta, GA 30309
404-872-7100
800-283-7800
Fax: 440-872-9559
e-mail: help@arthritis.org
www.arthritis.org

A council of the Arthritis Foundation devoted to serving the special needs of children teens and young adults with childhood rheumatic diseases (including systemic lupus erythematosus) and their families. Provides support groups, information and advocacy.
Daniel T McGowan, Chair
John H Klippel, President & CEO

5853 Autoimmune Diseases Association
22100 Gratiot Avenue
E Detroit, MI 48021
586-776-3900
Fax: 586-776-3903
e-mail: aarda@aarda.org
www.aarda.org

Provides mutual support and education for patients with any type of autoimmune disease. Support includes advocacy referral to support groups literature and conferences.
Stanley M Finger, Chair
Virginia T Ladd, President & CEO

5854 Lupus Foundation of America
2000 L Street NW
Washington, DC 20036
202-349-1155
800-558-0121
Fax: 202-349-1156
e-mail: info@lupus.org
www.lupus.org

The Lupus Foundation of America is the nation's leading non-profit voluntary health organization dedicated to finding the causes and cure for lupus. Our mission is to improve the diagnosis and treatment of lupus and support individuals and families affected by this disease.
Peter M Schwab, Chair
Sandra C Raymond, President & CEO

5855 Lupus Network
230 Ranch Drive
Bridgeport, CT 06606
203-372-5795

Seeks to foster better understanding of the disease among patients and the general public educators and professionals through the distribution of educational materials.

State Agencies & Associations

Alaska

5856 Lupus Foundation of America: Alaska Chapter
PO Box 240628
Anchorage, AK 99524
907-338-6332
800-307-5878
Fax: 907-345-0695
e-mail: LFA_Alaska@hotmail.com
www.lupus.org/webmodules/webarticlesnet/
Judy Powell, Chair of the Board
Anna Tillman, Executive Director

Arizona

5857 Lupus Foundation of America: Greater Arizona Chapter
2001 West Camelback Road
Phoenix, AZ 85015-4908
480-201-5334
e-mail: juliano@lupus.org
www.lupus.org/webmodules/webarticlesnet/
David Juliano, Outreach Development Manager

5858 Lupus Foundation of America: Southern Arizona Chapter
2583 North 1st Avenue
Tucson, AZ 85719
480-201-5334
e-mail: juliano@lupus.org
www.lupus.org/webmodules/webarticlesnet/
David Juliano, Outreach Development Manager

Arkansas

5859 Lupus Foundation of America: Arkansas Chapter
220 Mockingbird
Hot Springs, AR 71913
501-525-9380
800-294-8878
Fax: 501-525-9380
e-mail: lupusarkhs@direclynx.net
www.lupus-arkansas.com
Jamesetta Smith, President

California

5860 Bay Area LE Foundation
2635 N 1st Street
San Jose, CA 95134
408-954-8600
800-523-3363
Chapter of the Lupus Foundation of America.

5861 Lupus Foundation of America: California Chapter
18000 Studebaker Road   562-467-8994
Cerritos, CA 90703   800-558-0121
     Fax: 916-973-8124
     e-mail: gray@lupus.org
     www.lupus.org/webmodules/webarticlesnet/
Laurie Gray, National Manager of Walk Development
Luz Maria Hernandez, Health Educator

Colorado

5862 Lupus Foundation of Colorado
1211 S Parker Road   303-597-4050
Denver, CO 80231   800-858-1292
     Fax: 303-597-4054
     e-mail: info@lupuscolorado.org
     www.lupuscolorado.org
Chapter of the Lupus Foundation of America.
Carol Wright, Chair
Debbie Lynch, Chief Executive Officer

Connecticut

5863 Lupus Foundation of America: Connecticut Chapter
270 Farmington Avenue   860-269-6240
Farmington, CT 06032-2402   800-699-6967
     Fax: 860-269-6243
     e-mail: office@lupusct.org
     www.lupus.org/webmodules/webarticlesnet/
A non-profit organization and a National Health Agency established for the purpose of enlightening the public by focusing professional and public attention on Lupus Erythematosus promotes research by providing financial assistance and serves as the support bond for patients and their families.
Ron Marek, Chair
Michael Tommasi, President & CEO

Delaware

5864 Lupus Foundation of America: Delaware Chapter
100 West 10th Street   302-622-8700
Wilmington, DE 19801   800-880-8686
     www.lupus.org/webmodules/webarticlesnet/
Debra L Riegel Jepson, Chair
James Stewart, Treasurer

Florida

5865 Lupus Foundation of America: Northeast Florida Chapter
PO Box 10486   904-645-8398
Jacksonville, FL 32247-0486   800-853-8398
Lee, President
Jon Kagan, Vice President

5866 Lupus Foundation of America: Northwest Florida Chapter
PO Box 17841   904-444-7070
Pensacola, FL 32522-7841   800-458-8211
     e-mail: info@lupus.pensacola.com
     www.lupus.pensacola.com
Brenda Barto, Executive Director
Kathleen Laca, Director of Operations

5867 Lupus Foundation of America: Southeast Florida Chapter
2300 High Ridge Road   561-279-8606
Boynton Beach, FL 33426   855-905-8787
     Fax: 561-935-1435
     e-mail: info@lupusfl.org
     www.lupusfl.com
John Apgar, Chair
Amy Kelly-Yalden, President & CEO

5868 Lupus Foundation of America: Suncoast Chapter
3637 4th Street N   727-447-7075
St Petersburg, FL 33704-7485   800-684-9276
     Fax: 727-447-8925
     e-mail: info@lupusflorida.org
     www.lupusfl.com

5869 Lupus Foundation of America: Tampa Area Chapter
Dibbs Plaza

4119-20A Gunn Highway   813-960-3992
Tampa, FL 33624   800-330-3992
     www.milupus.org/southeast.htm

5870 Lupus Foundation of Florida
535 Central Avenue   727-447-7075
St. Petersburg, FL 33701   800-684-9276
     Fax: 727-447-7075
     e-mail: rmccolllum@lupusflorida.org
     www.hstrial-lupusfoundati.intuitwebsites
Chapter of the Lupus Foundation of America.
Maggi McQueen, Chairman
Rick McCollum, President & CEO

Georgia

5871 Lupus Foundation of America: Columbus Chapter
233 12th Street
Columbus, GA 31901   706-571-8950
     www.milupus.org/southeast.htm

5872 Lupus Foundation of America: Greater Atlanta Chapter
1850 Lake Park Drive   770-333-5930
Smyrna, GA 30080-2203   800-800-4532
     Fax: 770-333-5932
     e-mail: info@lgaga.org
     www.lupus.org/webmodules/webarticlesnet/
Maria Myler, President & CEO
Teri Emond, Program Director

Hawaii

5873 Hawaii Lupus Foundation
1200 College Walk   808-538-1522
Honolulu, HI 96817   800-201-1522
Chapter of the Lupus Foundation of America.

Illinois

5874 Lupus Foundation of America: Illinois Chapter
525 W. Monroe Street   312-542-0002
Chicago, IL 60661   800-258-7872
     Fax: 312-255-8020
     e-mail: charles@lupusil.org
     www.lupus.org/webmodules/webarticlesnet/
Offers support to individuals and families affected by Lupus, and looks to improve the diagnosis of and treatment of Lupus.
Charles Brummell, President & CEO
Mary Dollear, Vice-President

Indiana

5875 Lupus Foundation of America: Northeast Indiana Chapter
5401 Keystone Drive   219-482-8205
Fort Wayne, IN 46825
Largent, Director

5876 Lupus Foundation of America: Northwest Indiana Lupus Chapter
PO Box 2763   219-762-6575
Portage, IN 46368   800-948-8806
     e-mail: lupusnwichapter@aol.com
     www.lupusnwichapter.org
Tammie

5877 Lupus Foundation of Indiana
9302 N. Meridian Street   317-225-4400
Indianapolis, IN 46260   800-948-8806
     e-mail: info@lupusindiana.org
     www.lupus.org/webmodules/webarticlesnet/
Chapter of the Lupus Foundation of America.
Matthew Johnson, Chair
Jan Ferris, Chief Executive Officer

Iowa

5878   Lupus Foundation of America: Iowa Chapter
3839 Merle Hay Road   515-279-3048
Des Moines, IA 50310-1044   888-279-3048
e-mail: info@lupusia.org
www.lupus.org/webmodules/webarticlesnet/
Barb Logue, President
Marilyn Rumsey, Treasurer

Kansas

5879   Lupus Foundation of America: Heartland Chapter
PO Box 12204   316-262-6180
Wichita, KS 67277   e-mail: ruth@lupus.org
www.lupus.org/webmodules/webarticlesnet/
Ruth Busch, Board Chair
Sandy Blaylock, Recording Secretary

Kentucky

5880   Lupus Foundation of Kentuckiana
4004 Hillsboro Pike   615-298-2273
Nashville, TN 37215   877-865-8787
Fax: 615-292-0520
e-mail: info@lupusmidsouth.org
www.lupus.org/webmodules/webarticlesnet/
Chapter of the Lupus Foundation of America.
Tanisha Hall, Chair
Mike Singer, President & CEO

Louisiana

5881   Louisiana Lupus Foundation
7732 Goodwood Boulevard   225-927-8052
Baton Rouge, LA 70806   800-355-7473
www.louisianalupusfoundation.org/
Chapter of the Lupus Foundation of America.
Linda B Perkins, President
Carolyn M Bajoie, Board Member

Maine

5882   Lupus Group of Maine
PO Box 8168
Portland, ME 04104   207-878-8104
www.milupus.org/northeast.htm
Chapter of the Lupus Foundation of America.
Watson, Executive Director
Jessica Gilbart, Health Education Coordinator

Maryland

**5883   Lupus Foundation of America: DC, Maryland and Central &
Northern Virginia**
2000 L Street NW   202-787-5380
Washington, DC 20036   888-787-5380
Fax: 202-787-5399
e-mail: info@lupusgw.org
www.lupus.org/webmodules/webarticlesnet/
Chapter of the Lupus Foundation of America.
Marguerete A Luter, Chair
Jessica Gilbart, President & CEO

Massachusetts

5884   Lupus Foundation of America: Massachusetts Chapter
425 Watertown Street   617-332-9014
Newton, MA 02158   e-mail: info@lupusne.org
www.lupusmass.org

Michigan

5885   Lupus Foundation of America: Michigan Lupus Foundation
26507 Harper Avenue   586-775-8310
Saint Clair Shores, MI 48081   800-705-6677
Fax: 586-775-8494
e-mail: info@milupus.org
www.milupus.org
Judith A Sova, President
Frank Mortl, III, Executive Director

Minnesota

5886   Lupus Foundation of America: Minnesota Chapter
2626 E 82nd Street   952-746-5151
Bloomington, MN 55425   800-645-1131
Fax: 942-746-5155
e-mail: info@lupusmn.org
www.lupusmn.org
Scott Brown, Chair
Jennifer Monroe, President

Mississippi

5887   Lupus Foundation of America: Mississippi Chapter
PO Box 24292   601-366-5655
Jackson, MS 39225-4292   800-866-9606
www.milupus.org/southeast.htm

Missouri

5888   Lupus Foundation of America: Kansas City
4640 Shenandoah Avenue
St Louis, MO 63110   800-958-7876
e-mail: info@LFAheartland.org
www.lupus.org/webmodules/webarticlesnet/
Kevin Cheung, Chair of the Board
Amy Ondr, President & CEO

5889   Lupus Foundation of America: Ozarks Chapter
3150 W Marty Street
Springfield, MO 65807   417-887-1560
www.lupus.org

Montana

5890   Lupus Foundation of America: Montana Chapter
29 1/2 Alderson
Billings, MT 59102   406-254-2082
www.lupus.org

Nebraska

5891   Lupus Foundation of America: Omaha Chapter
Community Health Plaza
7101 Newport Avenue
Omaha, NE 68152   402-572-3150
www.milupus.org/midwest.htm

5892   Lupus Foundation of America: Western Nebraska Chapter
HCR 72 Box 58   308-764-2474
Sutherland, NE 69165

New Hampshire

5893   New Hampshire Lupus Foundation
PO Box 444
Nashua, NH 03061-0444   603-424-0111
www.milupus.org
Chapter of the Lupus Foundation of America.
Beck-Clemens, Interim President and CEO
Adam Gold, Development Associate

New Jersey

5894 Lupus Foundation of America: New Jersey Chapter
150 Morris Avenue, Suite 102   973-379-3226
Springfield, NJ 07081   800-322-5816
                                 Fax: 973-379-1053
                            e-mail: info@lupusnj.org
                www.lupus.org/webmodules/webarticlesnet/
Ranit C Shriky, Chairman
Leonard J Andriuzzi, President & CEO

5895 Lupus Foundation of America: South Jersey Chapter
One Greentree Center   856-988-5444
Marlton, NJ 08053   Fax: 856-596-8359
                          e-mail: lupusinfo@sjlupus.org
                                  www.sjlupus.org

New Mexico

5896 Lupus Foundation of America: New Mexico Chapter
PO Box 9125   505-999-1981
Albuquerque, NM 87119   800-843-9081
                             e-mail: info@lupusnm.org
                www.lupus.org/webmodules/webarticlesnet/
Quinn, Executive Director
Nancy Beder, Director of Resources

New York

5897 Lupus Alliance of America LIQ Affiliate
2255 Centre Avenue   516-783-3370
Bellmore, NY 11710   800-850-9000
                                 Fax: 516-826-2058
                        e-mail: info@lupusliqueens.org
                              www.lupusliqueens.org

Carol Goldklang, President
Kate Anastasia, Executive Director

5898 Lupus Alliance of Upstate New York
3871 Harlem Road   716-835-7161
Cheektowaga, NY 14215   800-300-4198
                                 Fax: 716-835-7251
                       e-mail: info@lupusupstateny.org
                              www.lupusupstateny.org

Lynn Szubinski, President
Honi Kurzeja, Executive Director

5899 Lupus Foundation of America: Bronx Chapter
PO Box 1117
Bronx, NY 10462
                                      718-822-6542
                         www.milupus.org/northeast.htm

5900 Lupus Foundation of America: Central New York Chapter
Pickard Office Building
5858 E Molloy Road
Syracuse, NY 13211   315-454-9886
                      e-mail: cnylupus@dreamscape.com
                         www.milupus.org/northeast.htm

Aman, President/CEO
Bob Stewart, Chairperson

5901 Lupus Foundation of America: Genessee Valley Chapter
500 Helendale Road   585-288-2910
Rochester, NY 14609   Fax: 585-288-1608
                         e-mail: lupusgvc@frontiernet.net
                                  www.lupusgvc.org

Eileen M Arntsen, President/CEO
James E Mitchell Jr, Vice President

5902 Lupus Foundation of America: Westchester
100 S Bedford Road   914-948-1032
Mt Kisco, NY 10549   888-57L-UPUS
                     e-mail: pguidice@stellarishealth.org
                           www.lupushudsonvalley.org

5903 Lupus Foundation of Mid and Northern New York
PO Box 139   315-829-4272
Utica, NY 13503-4303   866-258-7874
                                 Fax: 315-829-4272
                          e-mail: lupusmidny@aol.com
                                   www.nolupus.org

David L Arntsen, Chairman
Kathleen A Arntsen, President/CEO

5904 SLE Foundation
330 Seventh Avenue   212-685-4118
New York, NY 10001   800-74L-UPUS
                                 Fax: 212-545-1843
                           e-mail: lupus@lupusny.org
                                   www.lupusny.org
Chapter of the Lupus Foundation of America.
Bruce Cronstein, Chairman
Richard K DeScherer, President

North Carolina

5905 Lupus Foundation of America: Winston-Triad Lupus Chapter NCLF
2841 Foxwood Lane   910-768-1493
Winston Salem, NC 27103
Ruth John, President/CEO
Ginger Dickerson, Chairman of the Board

5906 Lupus Foundation of America: North Carolin a Chapter
4530 Park Road   704-716-5640
Charlotte, NC 28209   877-849-8271
                                 Fax: 704-716-5641
                            e-mail: info@lupuslinks.org
                www.lupus.org/webmodules/webarticlesnet/
Christine John-Fuller, President/CEO
Lorna Denton, Administrative Assistant

Ohio

5907 Lupus Foundation of America: Greater Ohio Chapter
12930 Chippewa Road   440-717-0183
Brecksville, OH 44141   888-665-8787
                                 Fax: 440-717-0186
                    e-mail: suzanne@lupusgreaterohio.org
                              www.lupuscleveland.org

John Sheldon, Chairman
Suzanne Tierney, President & CEO

Oklahoma

5908 Oklahoma Lupus Association
4100 N Lincoln Boulevard
Oklahoma City, OK 73105   405-427-8787
                                 Fax: 405-427-8778
                            e-mail: oklupus@flash.net
                                   www.oklupus.com
Chapter of the Lupus Foundation of America.
Katherine

Pennsylvania

5909 Lupus Foundation of America: Central Pennsylvania Chapter
Old Liberty Square
4813 Jonestown Road   717-671-9515
Harrisburg, PA 17109   800-800-5776
                           e-mail: hbginfo@lupuspa.org
                                   www.lupuspa.org

Cheston M Berlin, Branch Council
Douglas C Berlin, Branch Council

5910 Lupus Foundation of America: Northeast Pennsylvania Chapter
615 Jefferson Avenue   570-558-2008
Scranton, PA 18510   800-800-5776
                                 Fax: 570-558-2009
                            e-mail: neinfo@lupuspa.org
                                   www.lupuspa.org

Marilyn Deutsch, PhD, Branch Council
Devon Fawcett, Branch Council

5911   Lupus Foundation of America: Northwestern Pennsylvania Chapter
PO Box 885
Erie, PA 16512-0885
724-962-0368
800-800-5776
Fax: 724-962-0368
e-mail: erieinfo@lupuspa.org
www.lupuspa.org

Jane Lippinc Myarick, CEO

5912   Lupus Foundation of America: Western Pennsylvania Chapter
Landmarks Building
100 West Station Square Drive
Pittsburgh, PA 15219
412-261-5886
800-800-5776
Fax: 412-261-5365
e-mail: info@lupuspa.org
www.lupuspa.org

Deborah Nigro, Executive Director
Shelly Tonti, Branch Director

5913   Lupus Foundation of Philadelphia
500 Old York Road
Jenkintown, PA 19046
215-517-5070
866-517-5070
Fax: 215-517-8483
www.lupus.org/webmodules/webarticlesnet/
Chapter of the Lupus Foundation of America.
Debra L Riegel Jepson, Chair
Annette Myarick, CEO

Rhode Island

5914   Lupus Foundation of America: Rhode Island Chapter
#8 Fallon Avenue
Providence, RI 02908
401-421-7227
www.milupus.org

South Carolina

5915   Lupus Foundation of America: South Carolina Chapter
L.E. Support Club
8039 Nova Court
Charleston, SC 29420-8934
843-764-1769
e-mail: hmeisic@awod.com
www.galaxymall.com/commerce/lupus

Nelson, Executive Director

Tennessee

5916   Lupus Foundation of America Memphis Area Chapter
3181 Poplar Avenue
Memphis, TN 38111
901-458-5302
888-915-8787
Fax: 901-217-3193
e-mail: info@memphislupus.org
www.lupus.org/webmodules/webarticlesnet/
To educate and support those affected by lupus and to assist in finsing its cure. The goal is to unite and provide moral support and group strength for those individuals who are suspected of or diagnosed victims of Systemic Lupus Erythematosus and related disorders.
Yvonne D

5917   Lupus Foundation of America: East Tennessee Chapter
5612 Kingston Pike
Knoxville, TN 37919
615-584-5215
e-mail: lupustn@aol.com
www.lupus.org/chapters/southeastern.html

Hammond, Executive Director
Renee Levay Stewart, President

5918   Lupus Foundation of America: Mid-South Area Chapter
4004 Hillsboro Pike
Nashville, TN 37215
615-298-2273
877-865-8787
Fax: 615-292-0520
e-mail: info@lupusmidsouth.org
www.lupus.org/webmodules/webarticlesnet/

Tanisha Hall, Chair
Mike Singer, President & CEO

Texas

5919   Lupus Foundation of America: North Texas Chapter
15660 North Dallas Parkway
Dallas, TX 75248
469-374-0590
866-205-2369
Fax: 469-374-0794
e-mail: tessie@lupus-northtexas.org
www.lupus.org/webmodules/webarticlesnet/

Saundra Finley, Chair
Tessie Holloway, President & CEO

5920   Lupus Foundation of America: South Central Texas Chapter
9330 Corporate Drive
Selma, TX 78154
210-651-9480
866-205-2369
e-mail: salupus@texas.net
www.lupus.org/webmodules/webarticlesnet/

Sylvia Arcos, Chair
Amy Humphrey, Treasurer

5921   Lupus Foundation of America: Texas Gulf Coast Chapter
3701 Kirby Drive
Houston, TX 77098
713-529-0126
800-458-7870
Fax: 713-529-0780
e-mail: info@lupustexas.org
www.lupus.org/webmodules/webarticlesnet/

Tamara Atkins, Chair
Rebecca Kramer, President & CEO

5922   Lupus Foundation of America: West Texas Chapter
1717 Avenue K
Lubbock, TX 79401
806-744-6666
800-580-5878
e-mail: lfawesttx@juno.com
www.milupus.org/southwest.htm

Reymond, Executive Director
Katie Fillnow, President

Utah

5923   Lupus Foundation of America Utah Chapter
352 S Denver Street
Salt Lake City, UT 84111
801-364-0366
800-657-6398
e-mail: info@utahlupus.org
www.lupus.org/webmodules/webarticlesnet/

Noelle Reymond, President & CEO
Annette Lee, Development Director

Vermont

5924   Lupus Foundation of America: Vermont Chapter
57 S Main Street
Waterbury, VT 05676
802-244-5988
877-735-8787
e-mail: lupusvermont@myfairpoint.net
www.lupus.org/webmodules/webarticlesnet/

Virginia

5925   Lupus Foundation of America: Eastern Virginia Chapter
Pembroke One
281 Independence Boulevard
Virginia Beach, VA 23462
757-490-2793
www.lupus.org/webmodules/webarticlesnet/

Fletcher, President
Sarah Guy, Executive Assistant

Washington

5926   Lupus Foundation of America: Pacific Northwest Chapter
800 5th Avenue
Seattle, WA 98104
877-774-2992
Fax: 206-546-8946
e-mail: info@lupuspnw.org
www.lupus.org/webmodules/webarticlesnet/

Kristi Thomsen, President
Celia Y Weisman, CEO

5927 Lupus Foundation of America: Wisconsin Chapter
1109 N Mayfair Road   414-443-6400
Milwaukee, WI 53226   866-LUP-USWI
                                                   Fax: 414-443-6400
                           e-mail: lupuswi@lupuswi.org
                       www.lupus.org/webmodules/webarticlesnet/
Mary E Cronin, MD, Chairperson
Dawn T Thomas-Semanko, Executive Director

Foundations

5928 SLE Lupus Foundation
330 Seventh Avenue   212-685-4118
New York, NY 10001   800-74L-UPUS
                                                   Fax: 212-545-1843
                                e-mail: lupus@lupusny.org
                                        www.lupusny.org
The Foundation helps people with lupus, as well as their families
and friends, cope with the anxieties and frustrations that often accompany daily living with a chronic illness. Sharing information
and networking among patients and their families further helps
dispel myths and provides daily support to those learning to live
with lupus.
Bruce Cronstein, MD, Chairman
Richard K DeScherer, President

Research Centers

5929 Alliance for Lupus Research
28 W 44th Street   212-218-2840
New York, NY 10036   800-867-1743
                           e-mail: info@lupusresearch.org
                                   www.lupusresearch.org
Research foundation dedicated to providing information about
lupus.
Robert Wood Johnson IV, Chairman
Ira Akselrad, Director

**5930 Hahnemann University Lupus Study Center Hahnemann
University Medical Center**
Hahnemann University Medical Center
Broad and Vine Street   215-762-7000
Philadelphia, PA 19102   866-884-4HUH
                                                   Fax: 215-762-8109
                                   www.hahnemannhospital.com

Raphael J Gotthelf, President

5931 Terri Gotthelf Lupus Research Institute
3 Duke Place   800-828-87
S Norwalk, CT 06854   Fax: 203-852-9720
Founded to help millions of lupus victims in the world and to encourage coordinate and direct future progress in the etiology diagnosis and treatment of this disease.
Theodore

Support Groups & Hotlines

5932 National Health Information Center
PO Box 1133   310-565-4167
Washington, DC 20013   800-336-4797
                                                   Fax: 301-984-4256
                                    e-mail: info@nhic.org
                                        www.health.gov/nhic
Offers a nationwide information referral service, produces direc-
tories and resource guides.

Books

5933 Coping with Lupus
Lupus Foundation of America

1300 Piccard Drive   301-670-9292
Rockville, MD 20850-4303   800-558-0121
                                e-mail: lupusinfo@aol.com
                                        www.lupus.org
A practicing psychologist offers sound, meaningful and compas-
sionate advice to individuals who must deal with lupus.
276 pages Paperback
ISBN: 0-895294-75-3

5934 Disability Workbook for Social Security Disability Applicants
Lupus Foundation of America
1300 Piccard Drive   301-670-9292
Rockville, MD 20850-4303   800-558-0121
                                e-mail: lupusinfo@aol.com
                                        www.lupus.org
Helps people get their disability benefits promptly, without unnec-
essary appeals. Tells what you have to prove and how to prove it.
137 pages
Douglas M. Smith, Author

5935 Get to Sleep! How to Sleep Well...Despite Lupus
Lupus Foundation of America
1300 Piccard Drive   301-670-9292
Rockville, MD 20850-4303   800-558-0121
                                e-mail: lupusinfo@aol.com
                                        www.lupus.org
Written in a simple, straightforward style, this easy-to-follow action guide teaches you the most effective strategies for enabling
you to get the sleep you want and need!
17 pages

5936 Lupus Book
Lupus Foundation of America
1300 Piccard Drive   301-670-9292
Rockville, MD 20850-4303   800-558-0121
                                e-mail: lupusinfo@aol.com
                                        www.lupus.org
Packed with useful, easy-to-understand information and practical
guidance for people with lupus, their family members, friends and
physicians. This hardcover book explains virtually every aspect of
the disease and will help people better manage their day-to-day
fight with lupus.

ISBN: 0-195084-43-8
Iris Carden, Author

**5937 Lupus Erythematosus: A Handbook for Physicians, Patients &
Families**
Lupus Foundation of America
1300 Piccard Drive   301-670-9292
Rockville, MD 20850-4303   800-558-0121
                                e-mail: lupusinfo@aol.com
                                        www.lupus.org
Written for physicians, people with lupus, their families and
friends, this is LFA's most popular publication. The handbook provides a brief, but detailed, overview of the disease and guide for
living well with lupus.
60 pages

5938 Lupus: Everything You Need to Know
Lupus Foundation of America
1300 Piccard Drive   301-670-9292
Rockville, MD 20850-4303   800-558-0121
                                e-mail: lupusinfo@aol.com
                                        www.lupus.org
Resource written for patients that want to learn more about lupus
than what their doctors may or may not tell them.
236 pages
Jean Luc, Author

5939 Sick and Tired of Feeling Sick and Tired
Lupus Foundation of America
1300 Piccard Drive   301-670-9292
Rockville, MD 20850-4303   800-558-0121
                                e-mail: lupusinfo@aol.com
                                        www.lupus.org
Written in simple terms, the authors offer all readers- people with
invisible chronic illness (ICI's), spouses, friends, family members,
employers or health care providers, both understanding and practi-

cal guidance. This is a very useful resource for all those who live with ICI's and those who care for and about them.
288 pages
Mary E. E. Siegel, Author
Paul J. Donoghue, Author

5940 We Are Not Alone: Learning to Live with Chronic Illness
Lupus Foundation of America
1300 Piccard Drive   301-670-9292
Rockville, MD 20850-4303   800-558-0121
                                    e-mail: lupusinfo@aol.com
                                              www.lupus.org
Complete and comprehensive, this book is about redesigning your life... about how to live better, not just differently.
335 pages
Sefra Kobrin Pritzele, Author

Children's Books

5941 Embracing the Wolf: A Lupus Victim and Her Family Learn to Live
Cherokee Publishing Company
PO Box 1730   770-438-7366
Marietta, GA 30061-1730   800-653-3952
This book gives a very detailed account of the effects of the disease that include emotions and moods for the victim and the way in which these attributes affect loved ones.
192 pages Hardcover
ISBN: 0-877971-66-8
Kenneth W Boyd, Publisher

5942 In Search of the Sun: A Woman's Courageous Victory Over Lupus
Scribner
866 3rd Avenue   212-702-2000
New York, NY 10022-6221   800-257-5755
This book is a revision of Henrietta Aladjem's book, The Sun Is My Enemy. In this book, with Peter Schur she discusses her fight with this deadly and widespread disease.
Grades 10-12

5943 When Mom Gets Sick
Lupus Foundation of America
1300 Piccard Drive   301-670-9292
Rockville, MD 20850-4303   800-558-0121
                                    e-mail: lupusinfo@aol.com
                                              www.lupus.org
Written and illustrated by a 9-year-old, this is a compelling story based on the experiences of a sensitive and insightful young girl who makes the best from what could be a devastating situation.
27 pages

Newsletters

5944 Heliogram
Lupus Network
230 Ranch Drive   203-372-5795
Bridgeport, CT 06606-1747
Includes book reviews, medical abstracts and resource listings of physicians.
Quarterly
ISBN: 0-887168-0 -
Linda Rosinsky, Editor

5945 Informer
Simon Foundation
PO Box 815   847-864-3913
Wilmette, IL 60091-0815   Fax: 847-864-9758
Offers information and the latest updates concerning incontinence treatments, cures, medical aspects, resources and more.
Quarterly

5946 Lupus Foundation of America Memphis Area Chapter Newsletter
Lupus Foundation of America Memphis Area Chapter

3181 Poplar Avenue   901-458-5320
Memphis, TN 38111   888-915-8787
                                        Fax: 901-217-3193
                            e-mail: info@memphislupus.org
                                           memphislupus.org
Monthly
Yvonne D Nelson, Executive Director

5947 Lupus Informer
Lupus Foundation of America: Arkansas Chapter
220 Mockingbird   501-525-9380
Hot Springs, AR 71913   800-294-8878
                                        Fax: 501-525-9380
                            e-mail: lupusarkhs@direclynx.net
                                        www.lupus-arkansas.com
Lupus Chapter membership dues annually
Jamesetta Smith, President/CEO

5948 Lupus News
Lupus Foundation of America
1300 Piccard Drive   301-670-9292
Rockville, MD 20850-4303   800-558-0121
Provides detailed news for physicians, patients, their families and friends on lupus.
Quarterly

5949 Pennsylvania Lupus News
Lupus Foundation of Pennsylvania
Landmarks Building   412-261-5886
Pittsburgh, PA 15219   Fax: 412-261-5365
                               e-mail: info@lupuspa.org
                                             www.lupuspa.org

Deborah Nigro, Executive Director
Marian Belotti RN, Patient Services Director

5950 The Loop
SLE Lupus Foundation
330 Seventh Avenue   212-685-4118
New York, NY 10001   Fax: 212-545-1843
                                e-mail: lupus@lupusny.org
                                             www.lupusny.org

Richard K DeScherer, President
Margaret G Dowd, Executive Director

Pamphlets

5951 Control Your Pain!
Lupus Foundation of America
1300 Piccard Drive   301-670-9292
Rockville, MD 20850-4303   800-558-0121
                                    e-mail: lupusinfo@aol.com
                                              www.lupus.org
This easy to read booklet offers 144 concrete strategies for reducing and managing the pain of lupus.
48 pages

5952 Facts About Lupus
Lupus Foundation of America
1300 Piccard Drive   301-670-9292
Rockville, MD 20850-4303   800-558-0121
                                    e-mail: lupusinfo@aol.com
                                              www.lupus.org
A series of brochures on a wide range of lupus-related topics including lab tests, medications, joint and muscle involvement, skin involvement, lupus and the kidneys, central nervous system involvement, lupus in men, pregnancy, well/coping, etc.
21 Brochures

5953 Handout on Health: Systemic Lupus Erythematosus
NAMSIC/National Institutes of Health
1 AMS Circle   301-495-4484
Bethesda, MD 20892-0001   877-226-4267
                                        Fax: 301-718-6366
                                        TTY: 301-565-2966
                            e-mail: niamsinfo@mail.nih.gov
                                             www.nih.gov/niams

5954 Living Well, Despite Lupus!
Lupus Foundation of America

1300 Piccard Drive 301-670-9292
Rockville, MD 20850 800-558-0121
e-mail: lupusinfo@aol.com
www.lupus.org

This booklet offers 204 sure-fire strategies for taking charge of
your life to enable you to live well.
1996 50 pages
ISBN: 0-895294-75-3

5955 Lupus Eritematoso (Spanish Booklet)
Lupus Foundation of America
1300 Piccard Drive 301-670-9292
Rockville, MD 20850-4303 800-558-0121
e-mail: lupusinfo@aol.com
www.lupus.org

Written for physicians, people with lupus, their families and
friends, this is LFA's most popular publication. The handbook provides a brief, but detailed, overview of the disease and guide for
living well with lupus.

5956 Lupus Erythematosus
Lupus Foundation of America
1300 Piccard Drive 301-670-9292
Rockville, MD 20850-4303 800-558-0121
e-mail: lupusinfo@aol.com
www.lupus.org

This booklet is intended to help patients understand what lupus is,
how it may affect their lives and what they can do to help themselves and their physician in the management of the illness.
Edmund L. Dubois, Author
Daniel J. Wallace, Author

5957 Lupus Information Package
NAMSIC/National Institutes of Health
1 AMS Circle 301-495-4484
Bethesda, MD 20892-0001 877-226-4267
Fax: 301-718-6366
TTY: 301-565-2966
e-mail: niamsinfo@mail.nih.gov
www.nih.gov/niams

**5958 Many Shades of Lupus: Information for Multicultural
Communities**
NAMSIC/National Institutes of Health
1 AMS Circle 301-495-4484
Bethesda, MD 20892-0001 877-226-4267
Fax: 301-587-4352
TTY: 301-565-2966
e-mail: niamsinfo@mail.nih.gov
www.nih.gov/niams

Audio & Video

5959 For Life: More Stories of Lupus
Marcia Urbin Raymond, author
Fanlight Productions
4196 Washington Street 617-469-4999
Boston, MA 02131 800-937-4113
Fax: 617-469-3349
e-mail: fanlight@fanlight.com
www.fanlight.com

Three years after 'Stories of Lupus', the filmmaker revisits five
people from the earlier film, to explore the day-to-day challenges
and gifts that come to people living with a chronic illness as it
evolves over time.
2002 53 Minutes
ISBN: 1-572954-17-5
Nicole Johnson, Publicity Coordinator

5960 Stories of Lupus
Fanlight Productions
4196 Washington Street 617-469-4999
Boston, MA 02131 800-937-4113
Fax: 617-469-3379
e-mail: fanlight@fanlight.com
www.fanlight.com

Recently diagnosed with lupus, the filmmakers go on the road to
interview others enduring the precarious roller coaster of symptoms, treatment, flare-ups and recoveries which characterize this
complex, mysterious, and often life-threatening disease.
1999 27 Minutes
ISBN: 1-572954-16-7
Nicole Johnson, Publicity Coordinator

Web Sites

5961 Healing Well
www.healingwell.com
An online health resource guide to medical news, chat, information and articles, newsgroups and message boards, books, disease-related web sites, medical directories, and more for patients,
friends, and family coping with disabling diseases, disorders, or
chronic illnesses.

5962 Health Finder
www.healthfinder.gov
Searchable, carefully developed web site offering information on
over 1000 topics. Developed by the US Department of Health and
Human Services, the site can be used in both English and Spanish.

5963 Healthlink USA
www.healthlinkusa.com
Health information concerning treatment, cures, prevention, diagnosis, risk factors, research, support groups, email lists, personal
stories and much more. Updated regularly.

5964 Helios Health
www.helioshealth.com
Online resource for your health information. Detailed information
about specific health topics, access to expert advice from our Medical Advisory Board, and up-to-date health news.

5965 Lupus Foundation of America
www.lupus.org
The LFA mission is to assist local chapters in their efforts to provide supportive services to individuals living with lupus, educate
the public about lupus, and supports research into the cause and
cure of lupus.

5966 MedicineNet
www.medicinenet.com
An online resource for consumers providing easy-to-read, authoritative medical and health information.

5967 Medscape
www.medscape.com
Medscape offers specialists, primary care physicians, and other
health professionals the Web's most robust and integrated medical
information and educational tools.

5968 WebMD
www.webmd.com
Provides credible information, supportive communities, and
in-depth reference material about health subjects. A source for
original and timely health information as well as material from
well known content providers.

Description

5969 Mental Illness/General

Mental illness includes disorders of mood, thinking and behavior, with psychiatry being the branch of medicine responsible for their study, diagnosis, treatment, and prevention. Mental illness may be determined by genetic, physical, chemical, psychological, and social factors. Mental or emotional illness includes such conditions as major depression, schizophrenia, bipolar disorder (i.e., manic depression), panic and other anxiety disorders, substance abuse and dependence, and dementia and other cognitive disorders.

Psychiatric diagnoses generally are based on criteria outlined in *Diagnostic and Statistical Manual of Mental Disorders* (DSM-IV), published by the American Psychiatric Association. DSM-V, due out in May 2013, is thought by many to be one of the most anticipated events in the mental health field. Depending on the specific diagnosis, treatment can include medication, counseling, behavior modification, psychotherapy, and modification of the patient's environment. See also *Mental Illness/Depression* and *Mental Illness/Schizophrenia*.

National Agencies & Associations

5970 Action Autonomie
3958 Rue Dandurand   514-525-5060
Montreal, Quebec, H1X 1-2H2   Fax: 514-525-5580
e-mail: lecollectif@actionautonomie.qc.ca
www.actionautonomie.qc.ca
Community organization set up by people living or having lived with mental health problems who believed in the necessity of uniting their efforts collectively in order to defend their rights.
Hendren, President

5971 American Academy of Child & Adolescent Psychiatry
3615 Wisconsin Avenue NW   202-966-7300
Washington, DC 20016   Fax: 202-966-2891
e-mail: communications@aacap.org
www.aacap.org
A professional organization that represents 7 500 child and adolescent psychiatrists that actively research diagnose and treat psychiatric and mental illness disorders in children and adolescents.
Martin J Drell, MD, President
Kristin Kroeger Ptakowski, Director & Sr. Deputy Executive Director

5972 American Association of Children's Residential Centers
11700 W Lake Park Drive   877-332-2272
Milwaukee, WI 53224   Fax: 877-36A-ACRC
e-mail: info@aacrc-dc.org
www.aacrc-dc.org
Brings professionals together to advance the frontiers of knowledge pertaining to the spectrum of therapeutic living environments for adolescents with behavioral health disorders.
Christopher Bellonci, M.D., President
Kari Sisson, Director

5973 American Association on Intellectual and D evelopmental Disabilities
501 3rd Street NW   202-387-1968
Washington, DC 20001-1512   800-424-3688
Fax: 202-387-2193
e-mail: mnygren@aaidd.org
www.aamr.org
Promotes progressive policies sound research effective practices and universal human rights for people with intellectual and developmental disabilities.
Marc J Tasse, PhD, President
Margaret A Nygren, EdD, Executive Director & CEO

5974 American Psychiatric Association
1000 Wilson Boulevard   703-907-7300
Arlington, VA 22209-3901   888-357-7924
e-mail: apa@psych.org
www.psych.org
Works to promote the best interest of patients and those actually or potentially making use of psychiatric services.
Bray, President

5975 American Psychological Association
750 1st Street NE   202-336-5500
Washington, DC 20002-4242   800-374-2721
TTY: 202-336-6123
TDD: 202-336-6123
e-mail: practice@apa.org
www.apa.org
A scientific and professional organization the represents psychology in the United States. The largest association of psychologists worldwide.
Donald N Bersoff, PhD, JD, President
Norman B Anderson, PhD, Chief Executive Officer and Executive Vi

5976 Calgary Association of Self Help
1019-7th Avenue SW   403-266-8711
Calgary, Alberta, T2P 1-1A8   Fax: 403-266-2478
e-mail: info@calgaryselfhelp.com
www.calgaryselfhelp.com
Calgary Association of Self Help have been assisting people with a mental illness to live full lives within our community since 1973.
Samuel Peter Mckenzie, Chairperson
Marian McGrath, Chief Executive Officer

5977 Canadian Federation of Mental Health Nurse s
1 Concorde Gate   416-426-7029
Toronto, Ontario, M3C 3-3C6   Fax: 416-426-7280
e-mail: info@cfmhn.ca
www.cfmhn.ca
A national voice for psychiatric and mental health (PMH) nursing.
Lorelei Faulkner-Gibson, President
Joanna Lynch, Director of Communication

5978 Canadian Mental Health Association
1110-151 Slater Street   416-484-7750
Ottawa, Ontario, K1P 5-1Z8   Fax: 613-745-5522
e-mail: info@cmha.ca
www.cmha.ca
Promotes the mental health of all and supports the resilience and recovery of people experiencing mental illness.
David Copus, Chair
Peter Coleridge, Chief Executive Officer

5979 Center for Mental Health Services: Knowledge Exchange Network
PO Box 42557
Washington, DC 20015   800-789-2647
Fax: 240-221-4295
TTY: 866-889-2647
TDD: 866-889-2647
e-mail: ken@mentalhealth.org
www.mentalhealth.org
Goal is to provide the treatment and support services needed by adults with mental disorders and children with serious emotional problems.
A Kathryn PsyD, Past President
Donna Colonna, Vice President

5980 Community Access
2 Washington Street   212-780-1400
New York, NY 10004   Fax: 212-780-1412
e-mail: info@communityaccess.org
www.cairn.org
A nonprofit agency providing housing and advocacy for people with psychiatric disabilities.
Stephen H Chase, President
Steve Coe, Chief Executive Officer

5981 Federation of Families for Children's Mental Health
9605 Medical Center Drive   240-403-1901
Rockville, MD 20850   Fax: 240-403-1909
e-mail: ffcmh@ffchm.org
www.ffcmh.org
Provides leadership to develop and sustain a nationwide network of family-run organizations.
Teka Dempson, President
Sandra Spencer, Executive Director

5982 Mental Health America
2000 N Beauregard Street   703-684-7722
Alexandria, VA 22311   800-969-6642
Fax: 703-684-5968
TTY: 800-433-5959
e-mail: info@mentalhealthamerica.net
www.mentalhealthamerica.net
Mental Health America (formerly National Mental Health Association) is dedicated to helping all people live mentally healthier lives. With our more than 320 affiliates nationwide, we represent a growing movement of Americans who promote mental health.
340+ Members
Ann Boughtin, Chair of the Board
Eric Ashton, Vice-Chair

5983 Mental Health America Resource Center
2000 North Beauregard Street   703-684-7722
Alexandria, VA 22311   800-969-6642
Fax: 703-684-5968
TTY: 800-433-5959
e-mail: info@mentalhealthamerica.net
www.mentalhealthamerica.net
The NMHA publishes pamphlets and booklets on many aspects of mental health and mental illnesses. Topics include children and families, recovery, doctor/patient communication, mental health policy, culturally competent services, teen suicide, coping, schizphrenia, stress, depression and many others.
340+ Members
Ann Boughtin, Chair of the Board
Eric Ashton, Vice-Chair

5984 National Alliance for Hispanic Health
1501 16th Street NW   202-387-5000
Washington, DC 20036   Fax: 202-797-4353
e-mail: alliance@hispanichealth.org
www.hispanichealth.org
Members are Spanish-speaking mental health professionals and patients and those interested in the special emotional needs of Hispanics.
Augustine C Baca, Chairperson
Jane L Delgado, PhD, President & CEO

5985 National Alliance for the Mentally Ill
Colonial Place Three
3803 N. Fairfax Drive   703-524-7600
Arlington, VA 22203-3042   800-950-6264
Fax: 703-524-9094
TDD: 703-516-7227
e-mail: bbc@naimi.org
www.nami.org
The leading self-help organization for families and friends of those suffering from serious mental illnesses and those persons themselves. Over 900 affiliate groups nationwide offer support to members, advocate better lives for their loved ones, support research efforts and educate the public to reduce the stigma attached to serious mental illnesses.
Keris Jan Myrick, President
Jim Payne, Vice President

5986 National Association of State Mental Health Program Directors
66 Canal Center Plaza   703-739-9333
Alexandria, VA 22314   Fax: 703-548-9517
e-mail: webmaster@nasmhpd.org
www.nasmhpd.org
Offers referrals to state mental health programs services and physicians for persons with mental illness.
Robert W Glover, PhD, Executive Director
Shina Animasahun, Network Manager

5987 National Association of Therapeutic Wilderness Camps
437 William Avenue Suite 5
Davis, WV 26260   e-mail: natwc@gcol.net
www.natwc.org
Represents nearly fifty therapeutic wilderness camps located all over the US. We believe therapeutic wilderness camps represent the most effective method to help troubled young people change the way they deal with their parents, school and other authorities.
Rick MSW CSW, President/ CEO
Jeannie Campbell, Executive Vice President

5988 National Council for Community Behavior Healthcare
1701 K Street NW   202-684-7457
Washington, DC 20006   Fax: 301-881-7159
e-mail: lindar@thenationalcouncil.org
www.thenationalcouncil.org
Represents community mental health centers working on Capitol Hill to ensure funding for community mental health services. Offers technical support and guidance and serves as a liaison with state organizations and other mental health related organizations.
Linda Rosenb Delgado PhD, President
Adolph Falcon, Vice President for Science and Policy

5989 National Institute of Mental Health
6001 Executive Boulevard   301-443-4513
Bethesda, MD 20892-9663   866-615-6464
Fax: 301-443-4279
TTY: 301-443-8431
e-mail: nimhinfo@nih.gov
www.nimh.nih.gov
A federal agency that supports research nationwide on mental illness and mental health. The Institute provides research, demonstrations and technical assistance concerning the housing and service needs of the homeless mentally ill population.
Thomas R Power MEd, Director
Edward B Searle, Deputy Director

5990 National Mental Health Services Knowledge Exchange Network
PO Box 42557
Washington, DC 20015   800-789-2647
Fax: 240-747-5470
TTY: 866-889-2647
TDD: 866-889-2647
e-mail: nmhic-info@samhsa.hhs.gov
www.mentalhealth.org
The National Mental Health Information Center was developed for users of mental health services and their families, the general public, policy makers, providers and the media.
A Kathryn Muise, President
Joan Edwards-Karmazyn, VP

5991 Obsessive Compulsive Information Center Dean Foundation
Dean Foundation
7617 Mineral Point Road   608-827-2470
Madison, WI 53717-1914   Fax: 608-827-2479
e-mail: mim@miminc.org
www.miminc.org
Provides access to published literature on obsessive compulsive disorder certain obsessive compulsive spectrum disorders and their treatments.

5992 Option Istitute Learning and Training Center
2080 S. Undermountain Road   413-229-2100
Sheffield, MA 01257   800-714-2779
Fax: 413-229-8931
e-mail: happiness@option.org
www.option.org
As the worldwide teaching center for the Option Process(R). The Option Institute offers empowering personal growth programs and seminars using life-changing experiential learning techniques that help people overcome adversity, maximize their success and happiness and greatly improve their health, career, relationships and quality of life.
Barry Neils Kaufman, Co-Founder/ Co-Director
Samahria Lyte Kaufman, Co-Founder/ Co-Director

5993 Texas Mining and Reclamation Association
100 Congress Avenue 512-236-2325
Austin, TX 78701 Fax: 512-236-2002
e-mail: information@tmra.com
www.tmra.com

Serves as a unified voice for mental health patients in consumer social and political affairs. Helps members to live outside a hospital setting by providing assistance in the areas of resocialization, employment and housing.
Greg Shurbet, Chair
Trey G Powers, Executive Director

5994 The Coalition of Behavioral Health Agencies
90 Broad Street 212-742-1600
New York, NY 10004 Fax: 212-742-2080
e-mail: kkrampitz@coalitionny.org
www.coalitionny.org

An umbrella advocacy organization of New York's mental health community representing over 100 non-profit community health agencies that serve more than 300 000 clients in the five boroughs of New York City and its environs.
Tino Hernandez, President
Phillip A Saperia, Chief Executive Officer

5995 World Federation for Mental Health
PO Box 807 703-494-6515
Occoquan, VA 22125 Fax: 703-490-6926
e-mail: info@wfmh.com
www.wfmh.com

WFMH is an international membership organization founded in 1948 to advance among all peoples and nations the prevention of mental and emotional disorders the proper treatment and care of those with such disorders and the promotion of mental health.
Deborah Wan, President
Helen Millar, Treasurer

State Agencies & Associations

Alabama

5996 National Alliance on Mental Illness of Alabama: NAMI Alabama
1401 I-85 Parkway 334-396-4797
Montgomery, AL 36106-1902 800-626-4199
Fax: 334-396-4794
e-mail: wlaird@namialabama.org
www.namialabama.org

Will O'Rear, President
Sue Guffey, 1st Vice President

Alaska

5997 National Alliance on Mental Illness of Alaska
144 W 15th Avenue 907-277-1300
Anchorage, AK 99501-5106 800-478-4462
Fax: 907-277-1400
e-mail: trishmcd@nami.org
www.nami.org/sites/alaska

Scott Owens, Co-President
Pat Dobbins, Co-President

Arizona

5998 Mentally Ill Kids In Distress
2642 E Thomas Road 602-253-1240
Phoenix, AZ 85016-2723 800-35M-IKID
Fax: 602-253-1250
e-mail: Phoenix@MIKID.org
www.mikid.org

Steve Carter, President
Vicki L Johnson, Executive Director

5999 National Alliance on Mental Illness of Arizona
5025 E. Washington Street 602-244-8166
Phoenix, AZ 85034-1604 Fax: 602-252-1349
e-mail: namiaz@namiaz.org
www.namiaz.org

Provides emotional support education and advocacy to persons of all ages who are affected by serious mental illnesses. Supports research to find a cure.
Robert McCabe

6000 Navaho Nation K'E Project: Tuba City Children & Families Advocacy Corp
PO Box 3937 520-283-5415
Tuba City, AZ 86045 Fax: 520-283-5413
Rueben Clark

6001 Navaho Nation K'E Project: Winslow Children & Families Advocacy Corp
HC 63 Box E 520-657-3234
Winslow, AZ 86047 Fax: 520-657-3207
Jayne

Arkansas

6002 Arkansas FFCMH Jane Burgan
Jane Burgan
PO Box 56667 501-374-7218
Little Rock, AR 72115-4023 Fax: 501-374-2711
e-mail: pammarshall7218@sbcglobal.net
www.affcmh.org/

Billie Denney, Board Member
James Wilson, Board Member

6003 NAMI Arkansas
1012 Autumn Road 501-661-1548
Little Rock, AR 72211-2222 800-844-0381
Fax: 501-312-7540
e-mail: nami-ar@namiarkansas.org
www.nami.org

Grassroots organization that focuses on improving mental health services. The mission is three prong: Support, Education, and Advocacy. Support Group meetings are held at 11 locations across the state.
Rick Scott, First Vice President
Karen H Henry, President

California

6004 NAMI California
1851 Heritage Lane 916-567-0163
Sacramento, CA 95815-3218 Fax: 916-567-1757
e-mail: nami.california@namicalifornia.org
www.namicalifornia.org

Dorothy Hendrickson, President
Jessica Cruz, Executive Director

6005 United Advocates for Children of California
2035 Hurley Way 916-643-1530
Sacramento, CA 95825 866-643-1530
Fax: 916-643-1592
e-mail: info@uacf4hope.org
www.uacf4hope.org

Carmen Diaz, President
Mary Jane Gross, Treasurer

Colorado

6006 Colorado FFCMH
2950 Tennyson Street 303-572-0302
Denver, CO 80212 888-569-7500
Fax: 303-433-1605
e-mail: tdillingham@coloradofederation.org
www.coloradofederation.org

6007 FFCMH: Denver/Aurora Chapter
12485 E 13th Avenue 303-343-1019
Aurora, CO 80011 Fax: 720-859-9367
e-mail: **ffcmhda@comcast.net

Carmen Mohr, President
Carol Reynolds, Executive Director

6008 National Alliance for the Mentally Ill of Colorado
2280 S Albion Street
Denver, CO 80222-3334
303-321-3104
888-566-6264
Fax: 303-321-0912
e-mail: admin@namicolorado.org
www.namicolorado.org
The National Alliance for the Mentally Ill Of Colorado is a statewide, grassroots, nonprofit organization whose mission is; To give strength and hope to individuals with mental illness and their families.
Greg C Coleman, President
Scott Glaser, Executive Director

6009 No. Colorado FFCMH
2950 Tennyson Street
Denver, CO 80212
303-572-0302
888-569-7500
Fax: 303-433-1605
e-mail: thefeds@attbi.com
www.coloradofederation.org
Meltz

Connecticut

6010 Families United For CMH, Inc.
PO Box 151
New London, CT 06320
860-537-6125
Fax: 860-537-6130
www.familiesunited.org
Morgan Correll, President
Sheila King, Executive Director

6011 National Alliance for the Mentally Ill of Connecticut
576 Farmington Avenue
Hartford, CT 06105
860-882-0236
800-215-3021
Fax: 860-882-0240
e-mail: membership@namict.org
www.namict.org
Kate Mattias, Executive Director

Delaware

6012 Alliance for the Mentally Ill in Delaware (AMID)
2400 W 4th Street
Wilmington, DE 19805-3306
302-427-0787
888-427-2643
Fax: 302-427-2075
e-mail: namide@namide.org
www.namide.org
Mary Berger, President
John P Smoots, Treasurer

6013 Delaware FFMCH
19 Baltusrol Court
Dover, DE 19904
302-730-0325
866-994-0000
Fax: 302-730-8952
e-mail: marags1@aol.com
www.ffcmh.org
Earline McArthur, Director Development/Communications

6014 Mental Health Association of Delaware
100 W 10th Street
Wilmington, DE 19801
302-654-6833
800-287-6423
Fax: 302-654-6838
e-mail: jlafferty@mhainde.org
www.mhainde.org
Janet M Brown, President
James Lafferty, Executive Director

District of Columbia

6015 DC Threshold Alliance for the Mentally Ill
422 8th Street SE
Washington, DC 20003-2832
202-546-0646
Fax: 202-546-6817
e-mail: namidc@juno.com
www.nami.org/MSTemplate.cfm?MicrositeID=
Lois Fitzgerald, President
Mary J DiPietro, Secretary

6016 Family Advocacy and Support Association
PO Box 74884
Washington, DC 20056
202-234-2325
Fax: 202-576-7154
Lynne M Gladysz, Chair
R Lee Waits, President

Florida

6017 Florida Alliance for the Mentally Ill
1030 E. Lafayette Street
Tallahassee, FL 32301-2646
850-671-4445
877-626-4352
Fax: 850-671-5272
e-mail: Info@namiflorida.org
www.namiflorida.org
James Sleeper, President
Judith Evans, Executive Director

6018 Florida FFCMH: Tampa Chapter
13301 Bruce B Downs Boulevard
Tampa, FL 33612
813-974-7930
Fax: 813-974-7712
e-mail: ffcmh@earthlink.net
www.federationoffamilies.org
Linda M Gladysz, Chair
R Lee Waits, President/CEO

Georgia

6019 Georgia Alliance for the Mentally Ill
3050 Presidential Drive
Atlanta, GA 30340-3916
770-234-0855
800-728-1052
Fax: 770-234-0237
e-mail: namigeorgia@namiga.org
www.namiga.org
Bill Kissel, President
Eric Spencer, Executive Director

Hawaii

6020 NAMI: The Local Affiliate of the National Alliance for the Mentally Ill
770 Kapiolani Boulevard
Honolulu, HI 96813-2025
808-591-1297
Fax: 808-591-2058
e-mail: info@namihawaii.org
namihawaii.org
Members include consumers families health professionals and interested persons/organizations. Programs include advocacy support and education and are free and open to the public. Office has lending library of books and videos. Newsletter is published.
6 pages Quarterly
Carol Kozlovich, President
Kathleen Hasegawa, Executive Director

Idaho

6021 FFCMH: Idaho Chapter
704 North 7th Street
Boise, ID 83702
208-433-8845
800-905-3436
Fax: 208-433-8337
e-mail: info@idahofederation.org
www.idahofederation.org
Stephen Graci, Executive Director
Cindy Shotton, Administrative Assistant

6022 Idaho Alliance for the Mentally Ill
4097 Bottle Bay Road
Sagle, ID 83860-0068
208-242-7430
800-572-9940
Fax: 208-673-6685
e-mail: namiidaho@yahoo.com
www.nami.org/MSTemplate.cfm?MicrositeID=
Douglas McKnight, President
Tom Hanson, Vice President

Illinois

6023 Illinois Alliance for the Mentally Ill
218 W Lawrence Avenue
Springfield, IL 62704-2612

217-522-1403
800-346-4572
Fax: 217-522-3598
e-mail: namiil@sbcglobal.net
il.nami.org

Hugh Brady, President
Brian Allen, Vice President

6024 Illinois Federation of Families
PO Box 413
McHenry, IL 60051

847-265-0500
800-871-8400
Fax: 847-265-0501
e-mail: iffcmh@msn.com
www.iffcmh.net

Cynthia Hamilton

Indiana

6025 FFCMH: Indiana Chapter
2205 Costello Drive
Anderson, IN 46011

765-622-0601
866-247-8547
Fax: 765-622-0643
e-mail: indianafedfam@comcast.net
www.indianafamilies.org/page4.php

Brenda Hamilton

6026 Family Action Network
PO Box 322
Winnetka, IN 60093-2206

765-643-4357
e-mail: info@familyactionnetwork.net
www.familyactionnetwork.net

Susan Rooney, Co-Chair
Lonnie Stonitsch, Co-Chair

6027 NAMI Indiana
PO Box 22697
Indianapolis, IN 46222-0697

317-925-9399
800-677-6442
Fax: 317-925-9398
e-mail: info@namiindiana.org
www.namiindiana.org/

Grass roots advocacy support and educational group for families affected by severe and persistent mental illnesses.
Joshua G Sprunger, Executive Director
Joanne Abbott, Program Director

Iowa

6028 FFCMH: Iowa Chapter
106 S Booth
Anamosa, IA 52205

319-462-2187
888-400-6302
Fax: 319-462-6789
e-mail: help@iffcmh.org
www.iffcmh.org

Lori Reynolds, Executive Director
Heidi Reynolds, Program Director

6029 NAMI Iowa: National Alliance on Mental Illness
5911 Meredith Drive
Des Moines, IA 50322-1903

515-254-0417
800-417-0417
Fax: 515-254-1103
e-mail: info@namiiowa.com
www.namiiowa.com

Dawn Adams

Kansas

6030 Keys for Networking: Kansas FFCMH
900 South Kansas Avenue
Topeka, KS 66612

785-233-8732
800-499-8732
Fax: 785-235-8732
e-mail: jadams@keys.org
www.keys.org

Mary Ellen Conlee, President
Greg Whittaker, Treasurer

6031 NAMI Kansas: Kansas' Voice on Mental Illness
610 SW 10th Ave
Topeka, KS 66612-0675

785-233-0755
800-539-2660
Fax: 785-233-4804
e-mail: info@namikansas.org
www.nami.org/MSTemplate.cfm?Site=NAMI_Ka

John Brennan, President
Mr Richard D Cagan, Executive Director

Kentucky

6032 KY Partnership For Families and Children
207 Holmes Street
Frankfort, KY 40601

502-875-1320
800-369-0533
Fax: 502-875-1399
e-mail: kpfc@kypartnership.org
www.kypartnership.org

Carol W Cecil, Executive Director
Joy Varney, Associate Director

6033 Kentucky Alliance for the Mentally Ill
808 Monticello Street
Somerset, KY 42501-1277

606-451-6935
800-257-5081
Fax: 606-677-4052
e-mail: namiky@nami.org
www.nami.org/MSTemplate.cfm?micrositeID=

Wendy Morris, Chair
Bertha Diaz-Story, 1st Vice Chair

Louisiana

6034 Louisiana Alliance for the Mentally Ill
5534 Galeria Drive
Baton Rouge, LA 70816-2398

225-291-6262
800-437-0303
Fax: 225-926-8773
e-mail: info@namilouisiana.org
www.namilouisiana.org

Stephanie Boyd, President
Mitch Bergeron, Vice President

Maine

6035 Maine Alliance for the Mentally Ill
1 Bangor Street
Augusta, ME 04330-4701

207-622-5767
800-464-5767
Fax: 207-621-8430
e-mail: info@namimaine.org
www.namimaine.org

Valerie Gamache, President
Cathy Kidman, Interim Executive Director

6036 United Families for Children's Mental Health
PO Box 2107
Augusta, ME 04338-2107

207-622-3309
Fax: 207-622-1661

Pat Bellack, Executive Director
Dana Lefko

Maryland

6037 National Alliance for the Mentally Ill: Maryland
10630 Little Patuxent Parkway
Columbia, MD 21044-4486

410-884-8691
877-878-2371
Fax: 410-884-8695
e-mail: amimd@aol.com
md.nami.org

Chris Griffin, President
Kate Farinholt, Executive Director

6038 Parents Supporting Parents of MD
PO Box 30
Kensington, MD 20895-0030

800-498-5551
e-mail: Marge_Samels@umail.umd.edu

Marge Sagalyn, President
Toby Fisher, Director of Public Policy

Massachusetts

6039 Massachusetts Alliance for the Mentally Ill
400 W Cummings Park
Woburn, MA 01801-6528
781-938-4048
800-370-9085
Fax: 781-938-4069
e-mail: helpline@namimass.org
www.namimass.org

Lynda Cutrell, President
Laurie Martinelli, Executive Director

Michigan

6040 Association for Children's Mental Health
6017 W Street Joseph Highway
Lansing, MI 48917
517-372-4016
888-226-4543
Fax: 517-372-4032
e-mail: acmhjane@sbcglobal.net
www.acmh-mi.org

Jane Shank, Interim Executive Director
Mary Porter, Business Manager

6041 JIMHO Affiliated Centers (Justice in Mental Health Organization)
520 Cherry Street
Lansing, MI 48933
517-371-2221
800-831-8035
Fax: 517-371-5770
e-mail: brwellwood@aol.com
www.jimho.org
JIMHO advocates for the rights and dignity that all people suffering from mental or emotional illness deserve.
Huebl, President
Sharon Solomon, Executive Director

6042 Michigan Alliance for the Mentally Ill
921 N Washington Avenue
Lansing, MI 48906-5137
517-485-4049
800-331-4264
Fax: 517-485-2333
e-mail: namimichigan@acd.net
mi.nami.org

Hubert Lloyd, President
Sue Abderholden, Executive Director

Minnesota

6043 Minnesota Alliance for the Mentally Ill
800 Transfer Road
Saint Paul, MN 55114-1146
651-645-2948
888-NAM-IHEL
Fax: 651-645-7379
e-mail: namihelps@namimn.org
www.namihelps.org

Barb Lindberg, President
Sue Abderholden, Executive Director

6044 Minnesota Association for Children's Mental Health
165 Western Avenue
Saint Paul, MN 55102
651-644-7333
800-528-4511
Fax: 651-644-7391
e-mail: info@macmh.org
www.macmh.org

Joel V Oberstar, MD, President
Deborah Saxhaug, Executive Director

Mississippi

6045 Mississippi Alliance for the Mentally Ill
411 Briarwood Drive
Jackson, MS 39206-3058
601-899-9058
800-357-0388
Fax: 601-956-6380
e-mail: stateoffice@namims.org
www.namims.org/

Debbie Waller, President
Hank Rainer, Vice President

6046 Mississippi Families as Allies
5166 Keele Street
Jackson, MS 39206
601-355-0915
800-833-9671
Fax: 601-355-0919
e-mail: info@msfaacmh.org
www.msfaacmh.org

Joy Hogge, PhD, Executive Director
Cynthia Moore-Hardy, MS, Director of Respite Services

Missouri

6047 MO-SPAN
440 Rue Saint Francois
Florissant, MO 63031
314-972-0600
Fax: 314-972-0606
www.mo-span.org

Donna Dittrich, Executive Director
Tina VarVera, Administrative Assistant

6048 Missouri Coalition Alliance for the Mentally Ill
230 W Dunklin Street
Jefferson City, MO 65101-3260
573-634-7727
800-374-2138
Fax: 573-761-5636
e-mail: Keele@aol.com

Keele, Executive Director
Karren Jones, President

6049 NAMI of Missouri
1001 SW Boulevard
Jefferson City, MO 65109-2501
573-634-7727
800-374-2138
Fax: 573-761-5636
e-mail: namimosjf@yahoo.com
www.nami.org/MSTemplate.cfm?MicrositeID=
A nonprofit education adudcacy, referal and support organization serving people with mental illness and their families.
12 pages newsletter
Cinda Holloway, President and Chairman
Cindi Keele, Executive Director

Montana

6050 Family Support Network
1002 10th Street W
Billings, MT 59102
406-256-7783
877-376-4850
Fax: 406-256-9879
e-mail: info@mtfamilysupport.org
www.mtfamilysupport.org

Barbara Milhelish, President
Matt Kuntz, Executive Director

6051 Montana Alliance for the Mentally Ill Mihelish's Residence
Mihelish's Residence
616 Helena Avenue
Helena, MT 59601-6946
406-443-7871
888-280-6264
Fax: 406-862-6352
e-mail: info@namimt.org
www.namimt.org

Matt Kuntz, Executive Director
Carole Denton, President

Nebraska

6052 National Alliance for the Mentally Ill: Nebraska (NAMI)
415 South 25th Avenue
Omaha, NE 68131-2986
402-345-8101
877-463-6264
Fax: 402-346-4070
e-mail: nami.nebraska@nami.org
www.nami.org/sites/ne
NAMI is a nonprofit organization dedicated to providing support, education and advocacy to and for anyone whose life has been touched by a mental illness.
Tim Cuddigan, President
Steve Spelic, Vice President

Nevada

6053 Nevada Alliance for the Mentally Ill
2251 N Rampart Boulevard
Las Vegas, NV 89128
702-310-5764
Fax: 775-329-1618
e-mail: joetyler@sdi.net
www.nami-nevada.org

Joe Abate

New Hampshire

6054 Granite State FFCMH
940 Mammoth Road
Manchester, NH 03104
603-296-0692
e-mail: gsffcmh@aol.com
www.ffcmh.org

Kathleen Cohen, Executive Director
Win Saltmarsh, Development Director

6055 National Alliance for the Mentally Ill: New Hampshire
85 North State Street
Concord, NH 03301-4020
603-225-5359
800-242-6264
Fax: 603-228-8848
e-mail: info@naminh.org
www.naminh.org

Family support and advocacy for consumers and family members.
Michele Grennon, President
Ken Norton, Executive Director

New Jersey

6056 All Access Mental Health
Information
819 Alexander Road
Princeton, NJ 08540
609-452-2088
Fax: 609-452-0627
e-mail: info@aamh.org
www.aamh.org

This organization was founded to create a permanent community support system for mentally ill and developmentally disabled adults and their families living in the Greater Mercer County area of New Jersey.
Cynthia Murphy, President
Lauren Murphy, Vice-President

6057 Community Mental Health Foundation
610 Industrial Avenue
Paramus, NJ 07652
201-986-5070
Fax: 201-265-3543
e-mail: staff@cmhf.org
www.cmhf.org

Perrin, President
Sylvia Axelrod, Executive Director

6058 New Jersey Alliance for the Mentally Ill
1562 Route 130
N Brunswick, NJ 08902-3004
732-940-0991
Fax: 732-940-0355
e-mail: info@naminj.org
www.naminj.org

Mark Perrin, MD, President
Sylvia Axelrod, Executive Director

New Mexico

6059 Navaho Nation K'E Project Children and Families Advocacy Corp
PO Box 309
Tohatchi, NM 87325
505-733-2474
Fax: 505-733-2444
Vera Balwin

6060 Navajo Nation K'E Project: Shiprock Children & Families Advocacy Corp
PO Box 1240
Shiprock, NM 87420
505-368-4479
Fax: 505-368-5582
Evelyn Beckett, President
Elaine Jones, Executive Director

6061 New Mexico Alliance for the Mentally Ill
8015 Mountain Rd NE
Albuquerque, NM 87110-3086
505-260-0154
Fax: 505-260-0342
e-mail: naminm@aol.com
www.nami.org/MSTemplate.cfm?MicrositeID=
Patricia D Romero, President

New York

6062 Children's Mental Health Coalition of WNY, Inc.
814 Kenmore Avenue
Buffalo, NY 14216
716-871-8997
Fax: 716-871-8656
e-mail: mtskorupa@aol.com
www.raisingminds.org

Mary Pierce, Executive Director
Joan Cullen, Program Director/Family Specialist

6063 Families Together in New York State
737 Madison Avenue
Albany, NY 12209
518-432-0333
888-326-8644
Fax: 518-434-6478
e-mail: info@ftnys.org
www.ftnys.org

Vicky McCarthy, President
Paige Pierce, Executive Director

6064 New York Alliance for the Mentally Ill
99 Pine Street
Albany, NY 12207
518-462-2000
800-950-3228
Fax: 518-462-3811
e-mail: info@naminys.org
www.naminys.org

Thomas Easterly, President
Paul A Capofari, 1st Vice President

6065 Parents United Network: Parsons Child Family Center
60 Academy Road
Albany, NY 12208
518-426-2600
Fax: 518-447-5234
e-mail: communications@parsonscenter.org
www.parsonscenter.org

Rose Mary Bailly, President
John Henley, Chief Executive Officer

North Dakota

6066 North Dakota Alliance for the Mentally Ill
PO Box 3215
Minot, ND 58702-6016
701-770-8063
Fax: 701-725-4334
e-mail: l.lund8@hotmail.com
www.namind.org/

Linda Lund, President

6067 North Dakota FFCMH
PO Box 3061
Bismarck, ND 58502-3061
701-222-3310
800-484-2263
Fax: 701-222-3310
e-mail: carlottamccleary@bis.midco.nrt
www.ndffcmh.org/

Carlotta McCleary, Executive Director
Deb Jendro, Parent Coordinator

Ohio

6068 1st Capital FFCMH
394 Chestnut Street
Chillicothe, OH 45601
740-775-2674
Fax: 740-775-7834
e-mail: rmh1@adelphia.net

Rosemary Snider, President
Jim Mauro, Executive Director

6069 Ohio Alliance for the Mentally Ill
1225 Dublin Road
Columbus, OH 43215
614-224-2700
800-686-2646
Fax: 614-224-5400
TTY: 866-924-1478
e-mail: namiohio@namiohio.org
www.namiohio.org

Bob Spada, President
Terry Russell, Executive Director

Oklahoma

6070 Oklahoma Alliance for the Mentally Ill
4200 Perimeter Drive   405-230-1900
Oklahoma City, OK 73112-6200   800-583-1264
                                        Fax: 405-230-1903
                            e-mail: namiok@coxinet.net
                                www.namioklahoma.org/

Paula Walker, President
Traci Cook, Executive Director

6071 Tulsa Unified FFCMH
1022 N Howard   918-838-8033
Tulsa, OK 74115   e-mail: sherryscoobydoo@aol.com
                                        www.ffcmh.org

Sherry Gorger, Education Program Director
Cora Palazzolo, Communications Coordinator

Oregon

6072 NAMI-Oregon
4701 SE 24th Avenue   503-230-8009
Portland, OR 97202-1552   800-343-6264
                                        Fax: 503-230-2751
                        e-mail: namioregon@namior.org
            www.nami.org/MSTemplate.cfm?Site=NAMI_Or
Providing support education and advocacy for people with biological mental illness and their families. The in-state 800 phone number is Oregon's NAMI-Line. Callers to this line are provided with
information about mental illnesses and referrals to support and
treatment services.
Chris Bouneff, Executive Director
Michelle Madison, Events Manager/Outreach Coordinator

6073 Oregon Family Support Network
1300 Broadway Street   503-363-8068
Salem, OR 97301   800-323-8521
                                        Fax: 503-390-3161
                                e-mail: ofsn@ofsn.org
                                        www.ofsn.org

David De Fiebre, Board President
Sandy Bumpus, Executive Director

Pennsylvania

6074 Parents Involved Network
1211 Chestnut Street   215-751-1800
Philadelphia, PA 19107   800-688-4226
                                e-mail: pin@pinofpa.org
                                        www.pinofpa.org

Janet Jordan Jr, Executive Director
Jyoti Shah, President

6075 Pennsylvania Alliance for the Mentally Ill
2149 N 2nd Street   717-238-1514
Harrisburg, PA 17011-1005   800-223-0500
                                        Fax: 717-238-4390
                                        TTY: 800-890-6093
                        e-mail: nami-pa@nami-pa.org
                                        www.nami-pa.org/

Suzanne Vogel-Scibilia, M.D, President
James W Jordan, Jr, Executive Director

Rhode Island

6076 National Alliance for the Mentally Ill of Rhode Island (NAMI)
154 Waterman Street   401-331-3060
Providence, RI 02906-4312   800-749-3197
                                        Fax: 401-274-3020
                            e-mail: chaznami@cox.net
                            www.namirhodeisland.org

Marcia Boyd, Esq, President
Chaz J Gross, Executive Director

South Carolina

6077 NAMI-SC: National Alliance on Mental Illness: South Carolina
PO BOX 1267   803-733-9592
Columbia, SC 29202-1267   800-788-5131
                                        Fax: 803-733-9593
                            e-mail: namisc@namisc.org
                                        www.namisc.org

Advocacy, Education and Support
Joan Herbert, MS, President
Bill Lindsey, Executive Director

South Dakota

6078 NAMI South Dakota
PO Box 88808   605-271-1871
Sioux Falls, SD 57109-1204   800-551-2531
                                        Fax: 605-271-1871
                    e-mail: namisd@midconetwork.com
            www.nami.org/sites/NAMISouthDakota

Shelly Jablonski, President
Sita Diehl, Executive Director

Tennessee

6079 Tennessee Alliance for the Mentally Ill
1101 Kermit Drive   615-361-6608
Nashville, TN 37217-2126   800-467-3589
                                        Fax: 615-361-6698
                        e-mail: rpbaxter@comcast.net
                                        www.namitn.org

Dick Baxter, President
Jeff Fladen, Executive Director

Texas

6080 Central Texas FFCMH
6814 Orange Blossom   512-282-7126
Austin, TX 78744   Fax: 512-282-5817
                    e-mail: mattie_dixon@hotmail.com

Mattie Owens

6081 North Texas FFCMH
722 E Summitt
Sherman, TX 75090   e-mail: patoadv@msn.com
Pat Nazaroff

6082 San Antonio Bexar County FFCMH
2516 Bandara   210-523-2351
San Antonio, TX 78238   Fax: 210-523-2352
                            e-mail: ideasjn@aol.com

Joseph Peyson, Executive Director
Donna Fisher, President

6083 Texas Alliance for the Mentally Ill
Foundtain Park Plaza III   512-693-2000
Austin, TX 78704   800-633-3760
                                        Fax: 512-693-8000
                        e-mail: kjeschke@namitexas.org
                                        www.namitexas.org

Andrea Hazlitt, Board President
Ed Dickey, Vice President

6084 Texas FFCMH
7800 Shoal Creek Road   512-407-8844
Austin, TX 78752   866-893-3264
                                        Fax: 512-407-8266
                        e-mail: PattiDerr@txffcmh.org
                                        www.txffcmh.org

Patti Muller, President
Sherri Wittwer, Executive Director

Utah

6085 **Utah Alliance for the Mentally Ill**
1600 West 2200 South
West Valley City, UT 84119-1701
801-323-9900
877-230-6264
Fax: 801-323-9799
e-mail: rebecca@namiut.org
www.namiut.org

Zara Juillerat, President
Rebecca Glathar, Executive Director

Vermont

6086 **Vermont Alliance for the Mentally Ill**
162 S Main Street
Waterbury, VT 05676-1519
802-244-1396
800-639-6480
Fax: 802-244-1405
e-mail: info@namivt.org
www.nami.org/MSTemplate.cfm?Site=NAMI_Ve

Karen Kelley, Chair
Wendy Beinner, President/CEO

6087 **Vermont FFCMH**
600 Blair Park Road
Williston, VT 05495-0607
802-876-7021
800-639-6071
Fax: 802-329-2135
e-mail: vffcmh@vffcmh.org
www.vffcmh.org

Ted Tighe, President
Kathy Holsopple, Executive Director

Virginia

6088 **Virginia Alliance for the Mentally Ill**
PO Box 8260
Richmond, VA 23226-1903
804-285-8264
888-486-8264
Fax: 804-285-8464
e-mail: namiva@verizon.net
www.namivirginia.org/

Robert Cluck, President
Mira Signer, Executive Director

Washington

6089 **NAMI Washington (National Alliance for the Mentally Ill of Washington)**
7500 Greenwood Avenue North
Seattle, WA 98103-5580
206-783-4288
800-782-9264
e-mail: office@namiwa.org
www.namiwa.org/

Advocacy, support and education for the mentally ill, their families and friends.
Gordon Bopp, President
Jim Bloss, Vice President

6090 **Washington FFCMH**
801 E 141 Street
Tacoma, WA 98445-2768
253-537-2145
Fax: 253-537-2162
e-mail: acvmarge@comcast.net
www.ffcmh.org/

Marge Coleman, President
Terrie Isaly, Fast Track Program Director

West Virginia

6091 **Mountain State/Parents/Children/ Adolescents Network**
1201 Garfield Street
McMechen, WV 26040
304-233-5399
800-CHI-LD35
Fax: 304-233-3847
e-mail: ttoothman@mcpcan.org
www.mspcan.org

Joyce Floyd, President
Hope Coleman, Vice President

6092 **NAMI West Virginia**
PO Box 2706
Charleston, WV 25330-2706
304-342-0497
800-598-5653
Fax: 304-342-0499
e-mail: namiwv@aol.com
www.namiwv.org

Educational advocacy and support for families consumers and friends of people with mental illnesses.
Randal Rutkowski, Co-President
Terence Schnapp, Interim Executive Director

Wisconsin

6093 **Wisconsin Alliance for the Mentally Ill**
4233 W Beltline Highway
Madison, WI 53711-3814
608-268-6000
800-236-2988
Fax: 608-268-6004
e-mail: nami@namiwisconsin.org
www.namiwisconsin.org

Jim Connors, President
Julianne Carbin, Executive Director

6094 **Wisconsin Family Ties**
16 N Carroll Street
Madison, WI 53703
608-267-6888
800-422-7145
Fax: 608-267-6801
e-mail: info@wifamilyties.org
www.wifamilyties.org

Hugh Johnson, President
Deion Hagemeister, Vice-President

Wyoming

6095 **Wyoming Alliance for the Mentally Ill**
133 W 6th Street
Casper, WY 82601-3124
307-265-2573
888-882-4968
Fax: 307-234-0440
e-mail: coem@tctwest.net
www.namiwyoming.org/

Marty Coe, President
Tammy Noel, Executive Director

Libraries & Resource Centers

6096 **Alta Bates Summit Medical Center**
2001 Dwight Way
Berkeley, CA 94704-2608
510-204-4444
www.altabatessummit.org/

Alta Bates Summit Medical Center has made community healthcare a priority. We are proud of our many areas of clinical excellence including cardiovascular, behavioral health, women and infants, orthopedics, rehabilitation, and oncology care.
Carolyn McGee, Medical Librarian

6097 **Central Louisiana State Hospital Medical and Professional Library**
242 West Shamrock Street
Pineville, LA 71360
318-484-6363
Fax: 318-484-6284
e-mail: bentonmcgee@hotmail.com
www.clmlc.org

The Consortium was established to increase and better utilize the health information resources of Central Louisiana. Information offered on psychiatry, psychology and mental health.
Carol Rogers, Director

6098 **National Mental Health Consumer's Self-Help Clearinghouse**
1211 Chestnut Street
Philadelphia, PA 19107
267-507-3810
800-553-4539
Fax: 215-636-6312
e-mail: info@mhselfhelp.org
www.mhselfhelp.org

The National Mental Health Consumers' Self-Help Clearinghouse, the nation's first national consumer technical assistance center, has played a major role in the development of the mental health consumer movement. The consumer movement strives for dignity, respect, and opportunity for those with mental illnesses.
Joseph Rogers, Executive Director
Susan Rogers, Director

6099 **National Mental Health Consumers' Self- Help Clearinghouse**
1211 Chestnut Street
Philadelphia, PA 19107
267-507-3810
800-553-4539
Fax: 215-636-6312
e-mail: info@mhselfhelp.org
www.mhselfhelp.org

The National Mental Health Consumers' Self-Help Clearinghouse, the nation's first national consumer technical assistance center, has played a major role in the development of the mental health consumer movement. The consumer movement strives for dignity, respect, and opportunity for those with mental illnesses. Consumers—those who receive or have received mental health services—continue to reject the label of 'those who cannot help themselves.'

Joseph Rogers, Executive Director
Susan Rogers, Director

Research Centers

6100 Anxiety Disorders Center University of Wisconsin
University of Wisconsin
Department of Psychiatry
Madison, WI 53719-0001
608-263-6100
www.psychiatry.wisc.edu/uwpFacilities.ht
Provides evaluation and treatment for individuals suffering from anxiety disorders as well as training and education for clinicians.
Andy Alexander, PhD, Professor
Ruth Benca, MD, PhD, Professor

6101 Institute of Psychiatry and Human Behavior: University of Maryland
655 West Baltimore Street
410-706-7410
Baltimore, MD 21201-1542
Fax: 410-706-0235
e-mail: alehman@psych.umaryland.edu
www.medschool.umaryland.edu
Studies in psychiatric disorders.
Anthony Lehm MD, Director
Craig Vantyke, Chief Executive Officer

6102 Jane & Terry Semel Institute for Neuroscie nce & Human Behavior
Neuropsychiatric Institute
760 Westwood Plaza
310-825-2631
Los Angeles, CA 90095
800-825-9989
www.semel.ucla.edu
Studies behavior disorders and psychosocial adaptation and the future.
Peter Whybrow, Director
Fawzy Fawzy, Associate Director

6103 Langley Porter Psychiatric Institute University of California
University of California
401 Parnassus Avenue
San Francisco, CA 94143-9911
415-476-7365
www.universityofcalifornia.edu
Conducts clinical studies of psychiatric disorders.
Samuel Barno Faucher, Director

6104 Medical College of Pennsylvania: Eastern Psychiatric Institute
3200 Henry Avenue
215-842-6990
Philadelphia, PA 19129-1137
Offers research into all aspects of mental illness.
Michael Spohn, Director

6105 Menninger Clinic: Department of Research
12301 S. Main Street
713-275-5140
Houston, TX 77035-0829
800-351-9058
Fax: 785-350-5392
www.menningerclinic.com/
Focuses research on mental illness and mental health issues.
B. Christoph Frueh, PhD, Director of Clinical Research
Chris Fowler, PhD, Associate Director of Clinical Research

6106 Mental Illness Research and Education Institute
Eastern State Hospital
PO Box 800
509-299-3121
Medical Lake, WA 99022-800
Fax: 509-997-15
Governmental organization focusing on mental illness research.
Harold David, Director

6107 NIH Clinical Center
National Institute of Health
9000 Rockville Pike
301-496-4000
Bethesda, MD 20892
800-411-1222
Fax: 301-402-2984
TTY: 866-411-1010
e-mail: prpl@mail.cc.nih.gov
www.cc.nih.gov
Established in 1953 as the research hospital of the National Institutes of Health. Designed so that patient care facilities are close to research laboratories so new findings of basic and clinical scientists can be quickly applied to the treatment of patients. Upon referral by physicians patients are admitted to NIH clinical studies.
John I Gallin, MD, Clinical Center Director
David Henderson, MD, Deputy Director for Clinical Care

6108 State University of New York At Stony Brook: Mental Health Research
450 Clarkson Avenue
Brooklyn, NY 11203-2056
718-270-1270
www.stonybrook.edu
Benjamin S Hsiao, Phd, Vice President for Research

6109 Thresholds Psychiatric Rehabilitation
2700 N Ravenswood Avenue
773-281-3800
Chicago, IL 60614-1894
Fax: 773-818-90
e-mail: thresholds@thresholds.org
www.luc.edu
A psychosocial rehabilitation agency serving persons with severe and persistent mental illness.
Tom MD, Director
Peter Whybrow, Director

6110 University of Michigan: Mental Health Research Institute
205 Washtenaw Place
734-763-1817
Ann Arbor, MI 48109
e-mail: UMresearch@umich.edu
www.umich.edu
Focuses on the diagnosis treatment and prevention of mental illnesses and disorders.
Dr Bernard Schulz, Chair of Psychiatry

6111 University of Minnesota Department of Psychiatry
420 Delaware Street SE
612-624-2430
Minneapolis, MN 55455-374
Fax: 612-265-91
www.umn.edu
Behavior and mental illness research.
S Charles PhD, Director

6112 University of Missouri: Columbia Missouri Institute of Mental Health
5247 Fyler Avenue
573-634-8787
Saint Louis, MO 63139-1300
Fax: 314-644-8834
Mental health policy and ethics studies.
Danny Weddin MD, Director

6113 University of Pittsburgh: Western Psychiatric Institute & Clinic
3811 Ohara Street
412-246-6356
Pittsburgh, PA 15213-2593
Fax: 412-246-6350
e-mail: reitzpm@msx.upmc.edu
www.pitt.edu
Advancement of basic and clinical knowledge in mental health and psychiatric care.
Thomas Detre Camarata, Acting Director

6114 Vanderbilt Kennedy Center
Vanderbilt University
110 Magnolia Center
615-322-8240
Nashville, TN 37203-5701
Fax: 615-228-36
e-mail: kc@vanderbilt.edu
www.kc.vanderbilt.edu
Mental health research.
Donna G Eskind, Chair
Cathy S Brown, Past Chair

6115 Veterans Medical Center: Mental Health Clinical Research Center
3801 Miranda Avenue
Palo Alto, CA 94304-1207
650-858-3941
www.va.gov
Jerome Gallin, Director
David Henderson, Deputy Director for Clinical Care

6116 Yeshiva University: Soundview-Throgs Neck Community Mental Health Center
2527 Glebe Avenue   718-904-4400
Bronx, NY 10461-3109   Fax: 718-931-7307
Mental health mental illness and recovery from mental illness research.
Dr Itamar

Support Groups & Hotlines

6117 National Health Information Center
PO Box 1133   310-565-4167
Washington, DC 20013   800-336-4797
                                        Fax: 301-984-4256
                                        e-mail: info@nhic.org
                                        www.health.gov/nhic
Offers a nationwide information referral service, produces directories and resource guides.
Rivers, Federal Program Coordinator

Alabama

6118 Alabama Education of Homeless Children and Youth Program
Alabama State Department of Education
5348 Gordon Persons Building   334-242-8199
Montgomery, AL 36130-3901   Fax: 334-420-9633
                                        e-mail: mrivers@alsde.edu
                                        www.alsde.edu/html/home.asp
The major responsibilities of the Federal Programs Section are to administer all federally funded education programs and to provide technical assistance to local education agencies and schools. These responsibilities include promoting, supervising, and coordinating statewide educational programs with federal programs in addition to assisting schools in developing, revising, and implementing their school wide plans.
Maggie McDonald, Program/Education Director
Augusta Reimer, Leadership Project Coordinator

Alaska

6119 National Alliance for the Mentally Ill (NA MI) Alaska
144 West 15th Avenue   907-227-1300
Anchorage, AK 99501-5106   800-478-4462
                                        Fax: 907-227-1400
                                        e-mail: info@nami-alaska.org
                                        www.nami.org/sites/alaska
NAMI Alaska is a grassroots, 501(c)(3) nonprofit, support, educational and advocacy organization of consumers, families, and friends of people with severe brain disorders such as schizophrenia, schizo-affective disorder, bipolar disorder, major depressive disorder, obsessive-compulsive disorder, panic and anxiety disorders, and attention deficit/hyperactivity disorder. In addition, NAMI provides information and referral services and works with local media on stories about mental illness.
Scott Owens, Co-President
Pat Dobbins, Co-President

Arizona

6120 Navajo Nation Office of Special Education & Rehabilitation Services (OSERS)
PO Box 1420   928-871-6338
Window Rock, AZ 86515   866-341-9918
                                        Fax: 928-871-7865
                                        e-mail: osers@navajo.org
                                        www.osers.navajo-nsn.gov/
Navajo OSERS is a program within the Division of DINE Education, which offers vocational rehabilitation to people with disabilities. Vocational Rehabilitation includes an array of services, which are funded by a grant to the Navajo Nation from the U.S. Department of Education. The goal of vocational rehabilitation is to assist people with disabilities to obtain or maintain employment.
Treva M Roanhorse, Director
Paula S Seanez, Assistant Director

Colorado

6121 Laradon Services for Children and Adults w ith Developmental Disabilities
5100 Lincoln Street   303-296-2400
Denver, CO 80216   866-381-2163
                                        Fax: 303-296-4012
                                        TDD: 7209746821
                                        www.laradon.org/
Laradon specializes in services to children and adults with developmental disabilities, operating 15 programs that are designed to help each individual develop to his or her fullest potential and maximize self-sufficiency.
John Galvin, Chairman
Frank Lucero, PhD, Executive Director

Florida

6122 Florida Institute for Family Involvement (FIFI)
3927 Spring Creek Highway   305-293-7626
Crawfordville, FL 32327   877-926-3514
                                        Fax: 863-582-9358
                                        e-mail: HewFLMOM@aol.com
                                        www.fifionline.org
Florida Institute for Family Involvement (FIFI), an affiliate of Federation of Families for Children's Mental Health (FFCMH), enhances, facilitates, and supports family and consumer involvement in the development of responsive, family centered, and community based systems of care. FIFI works in collaboration with state, federal, and private programs to develop a resource and training information center to enable individuals to advocate for appropriate services and make wise service choices.
Connie Hawke, Co-Director
Tara Bremer, Co-Director

6123 Parent Education Network (PEN) Project Health
Family Network on Disabilities of Florida
2735 Whitney Road   727-523-1130
Clearwater, FL 33760   800-825-5736
                                        Fax: 727-523-8687
                                        e-mail: wilbur@fndfl.org
                                        www.fndfl.org/programs/pen-parent-educat
The PEN Project provides: information on specific disabilities; individual assistance by telephone, email, and in-person; referrals to local, state, and national resources; opportunities for youths with disabilities to be involved in training to parents and students; and, collaboration with Family Network on Disabilities Heart and Hope annual statewide conference for families.
Wilbur Smith, Co-Chief Executive Officer
Anna M McLaughlin, Co-Chief Executive Officer

Georgia

6124 Georgia Parent Support Network (GPSN)
1381 Metropolitan Parkway   404-758-4500
Atlanta, GA 30310   Fax: 404-758-6833
                                        e-mail: rheba.smith@gpsn.org
                                        www.gpsn.org/
Georgia Parent Support Network (GPNS) provides support, education, and advocacy for children and youth with mental illness, emotional disturbances, and behavioral differences and their families.
Kathy Dennis, Board President
Sue L Smith, Ed.D, Chief Executive Officer

Hawaii

6125 Hawaii Families As Allies (HFAA)
99-209 Moanalua Road   808-487-8785
Aiea, HI 96701   866-361-8825
                                        Fax: 808-487-0514
                                        e-mail: hfaa@hfaa.net
                                        www.hfaa.net/
Hawaii Families as Allies (HFAA) is a statewide parent-controlled family network organization that provides support, services and information for families of children and adolescents with emotional and/or behavioral challenges. HFAA is the Hawaii state chapter of the Federation of Families for Children's Mental

Health, a national organization that advocates for service system change so that families are valued and treated as true partners.
Linda Machado, Executive Director
Charlene Daraban, Family Resource Specialist

Illinois

6126 CANDU Parent Group
24W 681 Woodcrest Drive
Naperville, IL 60540   630-983-9027
Cathy Dennis

6127 KALEIDOSCOPE
1340 S. Damen Avenue   773-278-7200
Chicago, IL 60608   Fax: 773-278-5663
                                        TTY: 773-292-4086
                         e-mail: info@kaleidoscope4kids.org
                              www.kaleidoscope4kids.org

William J Binder, Chair
Ivy Walker, Vice Chairman-Secretary

6128 Parents Information Network FFCMH
1926 1700th Avenue
Lincoln, IL 62656   217-735-1662
Bridget Van Gogh, President

Indiana

6129 NAMI Indiana - National Alliance on Mental Illness
PO Box 22697   317-925-9399
Indianapolis, IN 46222-0697   800-677-6442
                                    Fax: 317-925-9398
                           e-mail: info@namiindiana.org
                                   www.namiindiana.org
NAMI Indiana is a non-profit grassroots organization dedicated to improving the lives of people afflicted by serious and persistent mental illness. NAMI Indiana consists of families, consumers, and professionals that are dedicated to helping families through a network of support, education, advocacy, and promotion of research. NAMI Indiana is affiliated with the National Alliance on Mental Illness (NAMI), which is located in Arlington, Virginia.
Joshua G Sprunger, Executive Director
Joanne Abbott, Program Director

Iowa

6130 Iowa Federaion of Families for Children's Mental Health (FFCMH)
106 South Booth   319-462-2187
Anamosa, IA 52205   888-400-6302
                                    Fax: 319-462-6789
                               e-mail: help@iffcmh.org
                                      www.iffcmh.org
The mission of Iowa Federation of Families for Children's Mental Health is to link families to community, county and state partners for needed supports and services; and to promote systems change that will enable families to live in a safe, stable and respectful environment.
Lori Reynolds, Executive Director
Heidi Reynolds, Program Director

Kentucky

6131 Kentucky IMPACT
275 E Main Street
Frankfort, KY 40621   502-564-7610
Sandra Welles, Executive Director

Massachusetts

6132 Parent Professional Advocacy League
45 Bromfield Street   617-542-7860
Boston, MA 02108   866-815-8122
                                    Fax: 617-542-7832
                                 e-mail: info@ppal.net
                                        www.ppal.net

Earl N Stuck, Chair
Lisa Lambert, Executive Director

Minnesota

6133 Emotional Health Anonymous
PO Box 4245   651-647-9712
St Paul, MN 55104-0245   Fax: 651-647-1593
                    e-mail: info2gh99jsd@emotionsanonymous.org
                                www.emotionsanonymous.org
A twelve-step organization, similar to Alcoholics Anonymous. Compsed of people who come together in weekly meetings for the purpose of working toward recovery from emotional difficulties.
Karen Mead, Executive Director

6134 PACER Center
8161 Normandale Boulevard   952-838-9000
Bloomington, MN 55437-1044   800-537-2237
                                    Fax: 952-838-0199
                                    TTY: 952-838-0190
                              e-mail: pacer@pacer.org
                                      www.pacer.org

Paula F Goldberg, Executive Director
Mary Schrock, Chief Operating and Development Officer

Missouri

6135 MO-SPAN Southwest Region
210 W Vine Street
Butler, MO 64730   660-679-5767
Eldonna Dittrich, Executive Director
Tina Vervara, Administrative Assistant

6136 MOSPAN Northwest Region
440 Rue Street Fran‡ois   314-972-0600
Jefferson City, MO 63031   Fax: 314-720-06
                            e-mail: mospan2@fid.net.com
                                      www.mospan.org

Donna Taycher, Executive Director

Nevada

6137 Nevada PEP
2101 S. Jones Boulevard   702-388-8899
Las Vegas, NV 89146   800-216-5188
                                    Fax: 702-388-2966
                             e-mail: KTaycher@nvpep.org
                                      www.nvpep.org
A statewide non-profit helping families who have children with disabilities, and the professionals who work with them. Support groups, training, workshops, lending resource library. Services are provided at no cost.
Karen Taycher, Executive Director
Stephanie Vrsnik, Community Development Director

New Hampshire

6138 National Alliance for the Mentally Ill: New Hampshire
85 North State Street   603-225-5359
Concord, NH 03301   800-242-6264
                                    Fax: 603-228-8848
                                e-mail: info@naminh.org
                                      www.naminh.org
Family support and advocacy for consumers and family members.
Michele Grennon, President
Ken Norton, Executive Director

New Mexico

6139 Navajo Nation Office Special Education & R ehabilitation Services
IHS PO Box 1337   505-722-1454
Gallup, NM 87301   Fax: 505-722-1554
                               e-mail: osers@navajo.org
                              www.osers.navajo-nsn.gov/
Navajo OSERS is a program within the Division of DINE Education, which offers vocational rehabilitation to people with disabilities. Vocational Rehabilitation includes an array of services, which are funded by a grant to the Navajo Nation from the U.S. Department of Education. The goal of vocational rehabilitation is to assist people with disabilities to obtain or maintain employment.
Treva M Roanhorse, Director
Paula S Seanez, Assistant Director

New York

6140 Mental Health Association in Dutchess Coun ty
253 Mansion Street
Poughkeepsie, NY 12601   845-473-2500
     Fax: 845-473-4870
e-mail: mhadc@hvc.rr.com
www.mhadc.com/
The Mental Health Association in Dutchess County promotes mental well-being and advances the recovery from mental illness, provides rehabilitation programs and support services for adults with a history of mental illness and their families.
Joseph Ellman, President
Andrew O'Grady, Executive Director

6141 Mental Health Association in Orange County
Mental Health Association of Orange County
73 James P. Kelly Way   845-342-2400
Middletown, NY 10940-1906   800-832-1200
Fax: 845-343-9665
e-mail: mha@mhaorangeny.com
www.mhaorangeny.com/
Mental Health Association of Orange County/MHA is a private, not-for-profit organization seeking to promote the mental health and emotional well being of Orange County residents. Under the leadership of a volunteer Board of Directors, MHA's staff members, consultants and volunteers provide free mental health services to thousands of Orange County residents each year. Several volunteers answer several hotlines, provide companionship, public education, direct services and assist with fundraisers.
David Goggins, President
Nadia Allen, Executive Director

North Dakota

6142 ND FFCMH Region II
PO Box 3061
Bismarck, ND 58502-3061   701-222-1223
Fax: 701-250-8835
e-mail: carlottamccleary@bis.midco.nrt
www.ffcmh.org
Carlotta Jendro, Executive Director

6143 ND Region V FFCMH Chapter-Federation of Fa milies for Children's Mental Health
1104 2nd Avenue South
Fargo, ND 58103   701-235-9923
Fax: 701-235-9923
e-mail: ndffrgv@nbinternet.com
www.ffcmh.org/who_chapters.php
The FFCMH, a national family-run organization serves to: provide advocacy at the national level for the rights of children and youth with emotional, behavioral and mental health challenges and their families; provide leadership and technical assistance to a nation-wide network of family run organizations; and, collaborate with family run and other child serving organizations to transform mental health care in America.
Deborah Sevart, Executive Director

6144 ND Region VII FFCMH-Federation of Families for Children's Mental Health
2252 La Corte Loop
Bismarck, ND 58503   701-258-1628
Fax: 701-258-1628
www.ffcmh.org/who_chapters.php
The FFCMH, a national family-run organization serves to: provide advocacy at the national level for the rights of children and youth with emotional, behavioral and mental health challenges and their families; provide leadership and technical assistance to a nation-wide network of family run organizations; and, collaborate with family run and other child serving organizations to transform mental health care in America.
Becky Beale Psy.D, Group Programs Director
David J Coleman Ph.D, Director of Psychological Services

Ohio

6145 Child & Adolescent Behavioral Health
919 2nd Street NE
Canton, OH 44704   330-454-7917
Fax: 330-452-8860
e-mail: bsnyder@casrv.org
www.childandadolescent.org/

The Child and Adolescent Service Center (CASC) was founded and incorporated in 1976 by a standing committee of the Stark County Mental Health Foundation. CASC provides dynamic leadership through innovative service, training and evaluation and is committed to providing culturally-sensitive programs and services throughout the community.
Lisa Warburton-Gregory, President
Michael Johnson, Chief Executive Officer

6146 First Ohio Chapter: FFCMH
4505 Quaker Court
Canfield, OH 44406-9131   330-726-9570
Fax: 330-726-9031
e-mail: xuparents@aol.com OR ffcmh@ffcmh.org
www.ffcmh.org/who_chapters.php
The Federation of Families for Children's Mental Health (FFCMH) is a national organization dedicated exclusively to helping children with mental health needs and their families achieve a better quality of life.
Chrysanne Cianon, Executive Director
Brenda Alego, Assistant Director

Rhode Island

6147 Parent Support Network of Rhode Island
1395 Atwood Avenue
Johnston, RI 02919   401-467-6855
     800-483-8844
Fax: 401-467-6903
e-mail: c.ciano@psnri.org
www.psnri.org
Family-run organization whose mission is to provide support, education and advocacy to parents of children at risk for or who have emotional, behavioral, and/or mental health challenges.
Linda Winfield, Board President
Cathy Ciano, Executive Director

South Carolina

6148 Federation of Families of South Carolina
810 Dutch Square Boulevard
Columbia, SC 29210-2344   803-772-5210
     866-779-0402
Fax: 803-772-5212
e-mail: FedFamSC@yahoo.com
www.fedfamsc.org/
Kathleen Scharer, President
Roxann McKinnon, Vice President

Tennessee

6149 Tennessee Voices for Children
701 Bradford Avenue
Nashville, TN 37204   615-269-7751
     800-670-9882
Fax: 615-269-8914
e-mail: tvc@tnvoices.org
www.tnvoices.org
Michele Johnson, President
Paula Sandidge, M.D, Board Secretary

Texas

6150 Harris County FFCMH
431 Breeze Park Drive
Houston, TX 77015   713-455-8962
e-mail: annn@flash.net
Elizabeth Cerar, Executive Director
Karen Greenwell, Community Education Coordinator

Utah

6151 Allies with Families
505 East 200 South
Salt Lake City, UT 84102-2979   801-433-2595
     877-477-0764
Fax: 801-521-0872
e-mail: Allies@AlliesWithFamilies.org
www.allieswithfamilies.org
Allies with Families was created in 1991 to offer practical support and resources for parents and their children and youth who face serious emotional, behavioral and mental health challenges. It was created to support all families in the state of Utah.
Lori Cerar, Executive Director
Karen Greenwell, Project Director and Newsletter Editor

Vermont

6152 Vermont FFCMH
PO Box 1577
Williston, VT 05495-0507

802-244-1955
800-639-6071
Fax: 802-329-2135
e-mail: vffcmh@vffcmh.org
www.ffcmh.org/find-local-chapter

The Federation of Families for Children's Mental Health (FFCMH) is a national organization dedicated exclusively to helping children with mental health needs and their families achieve a better quality of life,
Kathleen Holsopple

Virginia

6153 PACCT
8032 Mechanicsville Turnpike
Mechancsville, VA 23111

804-559-6833
Fax: 804-559-6835

Joyce Scheibe

6154 PACCT of Roanoke Valley
PO Box 21112
Roanoke, VA 24018

703-989-5042
Fax: 703-989-5675
e-mail: scheibe.p@worldnet.att.net

Sue Critchlow, Director
Sandra Spencer, Executive Director Corporate Office (MD)

Washington

6155 Common Voice for Pierce County Parents
10402 Kline Street
Lakewood, WA 98445-2768

253-537-2145
Fax: 253-537-2162
e-mail: nrascon@dadsmove.org
www.ffcmh.org/find-local-chapter

A Common Voice for Pierce County Parents is affiliated with the Federation of Families for Children's Mental Health (FFCMH), a national organization dedicated exclusively to helping children with mental health needs and their families achieve a better quality of life.
Sherry Lyons

Wisconsin

6156 We Are the Children's Hope/Support Group
First Love Outreach Ministries
PO Box 06204
Milwaukee, WI 53206

414-263-1323
Fax: 414-263-1148
e-mail: zelodius@aol.com
www.firstlovelifecoaching.com

Pr Zelodius Gerlosky

Wyoming

6157 Concerned Parent Coalition
1125 Sioux Avenue
Gillette, WY 82718-6529

307-682-6684

Michelle Nikkel, Executive Director
Carla Schroeder, Deputy Director

6158 Uplift
200 W 17th Street
Cheyenne, WY 82003

307-778-8686
888-875-4383
Fax: 307-778-8681
e-mail: uplift@upliftwy.org
www.upliftwy.org

Peggy Logan, President
Richard Yep, Executive Director

Books

6159 Anatomy of a Psychiatric Illness
American Psychiatric Press
1400 K Street NW
Washington, DC 20005-2403

202-682-6268
Fax: 202-789-2648

Answers questions, provides clinical anecdotes, explains what medical science does and does not know about mental illnesses and discusses compassion and hard scientific facts surrounding the psychiatric profession.
230 pages
ISBN: 0-880485-21-3
Keith Russell Ablow, Author

6160 Assessing Psychopathology and Behavior Problems: Mentally Ill Persons
National Clearinghouse for Alcohol and Drug Abuse
PO Box 2345
Rockville, MD 20857-0001

800-729-6686
www.health.org

239 pages

6161 Caring for People with Severe Mental Disorders: A National Plan
Superintendent of Documents
PO Box 371954
Pittsburgh, PA 15250-7954

202-512-2250

This report offers, from three panels of expert consultants, recommendations for strengthening both services research and research resources that should lead to improvement of the standard and provision of care for persons who have severe mental disorders.
80 pages

6162 Complete Mental Health Directory
Grey House Publishing
4919 Route 22
Amenia, NY 12501

518-789-8700
800-562-2139
Fax: 518-789-0545
e-mail: books@greyhouse.com
www.greyhouse.com

Offers critical and comprehensive information on disorders, support groups, clinical management, government agencies, professional conferences, research centers and training.
687 pages
ISBN: 1-930956-06-1
Leslie Mackenzie, Publisher

6163 Creating New Options
Bazelon Center for Mental Health Law
1101 15th Street NW
Washington, DC 20005-5002

202-467-5730
Fax: 202-223-0409
TDD: 202-467-4342
e-mail: pubs@bazelon.org
www.bazelon.org

Training for corrections administrators and staff on access to federal benefits for people with mental illnesses who are leacing jail or prison. Available as a manual ($7.50), a PowerPoint presentation on CD ($5), or both ($11).
2008
Lee Carly, Communications Director

6164 Creating a Circle of Learning: The Church and the Mentally Ill
National Alliance for the Mentally Ill
PO Box 753
Waldorf, MD 20604-0753

301-524-7600
Fax: 301-843-0159
www.NAMI.org

A curriculum designed to sensitize adults in the church to the plight of people with severe mental illnesses and their families. Leaders can teach the study as 12 one-hour lessons or six two-hour lessons. The teaching sessions build on a Biblical-based theological reflection calling congregations to minister to their brothers and sisters with mental illnesses.
1997

6165 Culture and the Restructuring of Community Mental Health
William A Vega, author
Greenwood Publishing Group, Inc.
PO Box 6926
Portsmouth, NH 03802-6926

800-225-5800
Fax: 877-231-6980
e-mail: service@greenwood.com
www.greenwood.com

Examines treatment, organizational planning and research issues and offers a critique of the theoretical and programmatic aspects of

providing mental health services to traditionally undeserved populations.
168 pages
ISBN: 0-313268-87-8
William Vega, Author
John W. Murphy, Author

6166 Dealing with Mental Incapacity
Center for Public Representation
PO Box 260049   608-251-4008
Madison, WI 53726-0049   800-369-0388
                                      Fax: 608-251-1263
This manual contains a comprehensive introduction to the problem of guardianship as well as chapters of financial and health care planning tools, guardianship under Wisconsin law, protective placement and Watts reviews.
Training Manual

6167 Design of Rehabilitation Services in Psychiatric Hospital Settings
American Occupational Therapy Association
PO Box 1725   301-948-9626
Rockville, MD 20849-1725   800-729-2082
Presents a design for constructing a rehabilitation system that will ensure the delivery of quality services to patients in a psychiatric hospital setting.
130 pages
Jeanette Bair, Executive Director

6168 Dimensions of State Mental Health Policy
Greenwood Publishing Group, Inc/Praeger Publishers
PO Box 6926
Portsmouth, NH 03802-6926   800-225-5800
                                      Fax: 877-231-6980
                          e-mail: service@greenwood.com
                                  www.greenwood.com
Introduces students to the emerging field of state mental health policy.
320 pages
ISBN: 0-275932-52-4

6169 Dual Diagnosis of Major Mental Illness and Substance Disorder
National Alliance for the Mentally Ill
PO Box 753   703-524-7600
Waldorf, MD 20604-0753   Fax: 703-524-9094
                                       www.NAMI.org
Written for professionals, readable for families including descriptions of model programs.

6170 Educating Patients and Families About Mental Illness: A Practical Guide
Aspen Publishers
7201 McKinney Circle
Frederick, MD 21704-8356   800-638-8437
Introducing the manual to specifically address educating your patients and their families about mental illness.
496 pages
Cynthia Bisbee, Author

6171 Elderly with Chronic Mental Illness
Springer Publishing Company
536 Broadway   212-431-4370
New York, NY 10012-3955   877-687-7476
                                      Fax: 212-941-7842
                    e-mail: marketing@springerpub.com
                                www.springerpub.com

384 pages Hardcover
ISBN: 0-826172-80-6
Annette Imperati, Marketing Director

6172 Elders Assert Their Rights
Bazelon Center for Mental Health Law
1101 15th Street NW   202-467-5730
Washington, DC 20005-5002   Fax: 202-223-0409
                                      TDD: 202-467-4342
                          e-mail: pubs@bazelon.org
                                    www.bazelon.org
A guide for residents, family members and advocates to the legal rights of elderly people with mental disabilities in nursing homes.
Paperback
Lee Carly, Communications Director

6173 Encyclopedia of Mental Health
Facts on File
11 Penn Plaza   212-967-8800
New York, NY 10001   800-322-8755
                                      Fax: 800-678-3633
Here, readers will find inciseve definitions of theories, syndromes, symptons, treatments, and contemporary issues in easy-to-understand language.
480 pages Hardcover

6174 Encyclopedia of Phobias, Fears, and Anxieties
Facts on File
11 Penn Plaza   212-967-8800
New York, NY 10001   800-322-8755
                                      Fax: 800-678-3633

500 pages Hardcover

6175 Evaluation and Treatment of the Psychogeriatric Patient
Diane Gibson, MS, author
Haworth Press
10 Alice Street   607-722-5857
Binghamton, NY 13904-1580   800-429-6784
                                      Fax: 607-722-0012
                                  www.haworthpress.com
This pertinent book assists occupational therapists and other health care providers in developing up-to-date psychogeriatric programs.
111 pages Hardcover
ISBN: 1-560240-52-1

6176 Family Caregiving in Mental Illness
National Alliance for the Mentally Ill
PO Box 753   301-524-7600
Waldorf, MD 20604-0753   Fax: 301-843-0159
                                       www.NAMI.org
Examines patients' rights and treatment needs from the point of view of all those involved. Focuses on family burden and research and theoretical perspectives that influence mental health professionals.
1996
Amir Ella, Author

6177 Federal Law of the Mentally Handicapped
William Hein & Company
1285 Main Street   716-882-2600
Buffalo, NY 14209-1987
Chronological compilation of all relevant federal laws dealing with the mentally handicapped along with supporting documentation necessary to create a complete legislative history.
42 volumes/set

6178 Focal Group Psychotherapy for Mental Health Professionals
New Harbinger Publications
5674 Shattuck Avenue
Oakland, CA 94609-1662   800-748-6273
                                      Fax: 510-652-5472
                                  www.newharbinger.com
Definitive guide to leading brief, theme-based groups. This book offers an extensive week-by-week description of the basic concepts and interventions for 14 theme or focal groups.
544 pages

6179 Handbook of Mental Health and Mental Disor der Among Black Americans
Greenwood Publishing Group, Inc.
PO Box 6926
Portsmouth, NH 03802-6926   800-225-5800
                                      Fax: 877-231-6980
                          e-mail: service@greenwood.com
                                  www.greenwood.com
In addition to providing a wealth of new data on the mental health status of black communities, this handbook presents analyses of specific social, structural, and cultural conditions that affect the lives of individual black Americans.
352 pages
ISBN: 0-313263-30-2

6180 How to Live with a Mentally Ill Person: A Handbook of Day-to-Day Strategies
National Alliance for the Mentally Ill

PO Box 753
Waldorf, MD 20604-0753 301-524-7600
Fax: 301-843-0159
www.NAMI.org

Offers self-help-styled advice to caregivers. Includes personal experiences, education, stigma, coping, and the mental health system.
1996

6181 Last in Line
Bazelon Center for Mental Health Law
1101 15th Street NW 202-467-5730
Washington, DC 20005-5002 Fax: 202-223-0409
TDD: 202-467-4342
e-mail: pubs@bazelon.org
www.bazelon.org

discusses barriers to community integration of older adults with mental illnesses, and recommendations for change.
2006 72 pages
Lee Carly, Communications Director
James Stewart Bain, Author

6182 Living with Mental Handicaps
Jessica Kingsley Publishers
118 Pentonville Road 071-833-2307
London, England, Fax: 071-837-2917

The focus of this book lies in its insistence that mentally handicapped people make transitions like the rest of us from youth to old age.
176 pages

6183 Madness in the Streets
Free Press
866 3rd Avenue
New York, NY 10022-6221 800-323-7445
Fax: 800-943-9831
www.simonsays.com

How psychiatry and the law abandoned the mentally ill.
436 pages
ISBN: 0-029153-80-8
Virginia C Armat, Author
Rael Jean Isaac, Author

6184 Making Child Welfare Work
Bazelon Center for Mental Health Law
1101 15th Street NW 202-467-5730
Washington, DC 20005-5002 Fax: 202-223-0409
TDD: 202-467-4342
e-mail: pubs@bazelon.org
www.bazelon.org

How the RC lawsuit forged new partnership to protect children and sustain families. The story of systems reform from the bottom up and the rededication of a burocracy to focus on the children and families it is meant to serve.
1998 126 pages
Lee Carly, Communications Director

6185 Managed Mental Health Care
American Psychiatric Press
1400 K Street NW 202-682-6268
Washington, DC 20005-2403 Fax: 202-789-2648

This text presents the collective wisdom of 40 experts experienced in clinical and managerial issues in managed care.
425 pages Hardcover
ISBN: 0-880483-55-5

6186 Managing Managed Care: A Mental Health Practitioner's Survival Guide
American Psychiatric Press
1400 K Street NW 202-682-6268
Washington, DC 20005-2403 Fax: 202-789-2648

Provides an easy-to-learn system for communicating with external reviewers and documenting quality of care.
200 pages Hardcover
ISBN: 0-880483-69-5

6187 Manic Depressive Illness
National Alliance for the Mentally Ill
PO Box 753 703-524-7600
Waldorf, MD 20604-0753 Fax: 703-524-9094
www.NAMI.org

A definitive overview of bipolar disorder.

6188 Medicare Rx Consumer Workbook
Mental Health America
2000 N Beauragard Strt 703-684-7722
Alexandria, VA 22311 800-969-6642
Fax: 703-684-5968
TTY: 800-433-5959
www.mentalhealthamerica.net

This workbook is designed to help you as a mental health consumer to get educated about and get enrolled in the new Medicare prescription drug program. Designed as a pocket folder, the workbook includes basic language explanations, tips for enrollment preparation, questions you should ask regarding plan options, worksheets, and definitions.

6189 Membership Directory
Natl. Council for Community Behavioral Healthcare
12300 Twinbrook Parkway
Rockville, MD 20852 301-984-6200
www.icai.org

6190 Mental Disability Law: A Primer
Commission on The Mentally Disabled
1800 M Street NW 202-331-2240
Washington, DC 20036-5802

An updated and expanded version of the 1984 edition. Addresses the considerations involved in representing clients with mental disabilities.

6191 Mental Health Care in Prisons and Jails
Vance Bibliographies
PO Box 229 217-762-3831
Monticello, IL 61856-0229

A bibliography regarding health care in prisons.
30 pages
ISBN: 0-792006-94-1

6192 Mental Health Concepts and Techniques for the Occupational Therapy Assistant
Raven Press
1185 Ave of the Americas 212-930-9500
New York, NY 10036-2601 800-777-2295

This text offers clear and easily understood explanations of the various theoretical and practice health models. Second edition.
344 pages
ISBN: 0-781700-74-4

6193 Mental Health Law Reporter
Business Publishers, Inc.
PO Box 17592
Baltimore, MD 21297 800-274-6737
e-mail: custserv@bpinews.com
www.bpinews.com

Brings you the most timely, focused and thorough information on the legal issues that concern you in mental health litigation.
monthly
Leonard Eiserer, Publisher

6194 Mental Health: Counseling Services
Vance Bibliographies
PO Box 229 217-762-3831
Monticello, IL 61856-0229

Selected annotated bibliography on counseling services for the mentally handicapped from a black perspective.
23 pages
ISBN: 1-555903-76-2

6195 Mental Illness-Opposing Viewpoints Series
Greenhaven Press
Thomson Gale
Farmington Hills, MI 48333-9187 800-877-4253
Fax: 800-414-5043
e-mail: gale.customerservice@thomson.com
www.gale.com/greenhaven

In-depth overview of the topic written for upper elementary and junior/senior high school students.
2006
ISBN: 1-560061-68-5

6196 Mental and Physical Disability Law Report
American Bar Association
1800 M Street NW   202-331-2240
Washington, DC 20036-5802
Covers case law, legislative and regulatory developments that affect persons with mental or physical disabilities.

6197 Mentally Ill Individuals
Mainstream
1030 5th Street NW   202-898-1400
Washington, DC 20001-2504
Mainstreaming mentally ill individuals into the workplace.
12 pages

6198 Mood Apart: Depression, Mania, and Other Afflictions of the Self
National Alliance for the Mentally Ill
PO Box 753   301-524-7600
Waldorf, MD 20604-0753   Fax: 301-843-0159
                                    www.NAMI.org
Discussion of depression and mania includes the symptoms, human costs, biological underpinnings, and therapies. Uses case histories, appendices, and historical references.
1997

6199 National Plan for Research on Child and Adolescent Mental Disorders
Superintendent of Documents
PO Box 371954   202-512-2250
Pittsburgh, PA 15250-7954
Summarizes the current knowledge about the prevalence and causes of mental disorders among children, identifies the possible treatments and prevention strategies and notes promising areas of research.
64 pages

6200 Occupational Therapy Practice Guidelines for Adults with Mood Disorders
American Occupational Therapy Association
4720 Montgomery Lane   301-652-2682
Bethesda, MD 20824-1220   Fax: 301-652-7711
                               TDD: 800-377-8555
                                    www.aota.org

27 pages
ISBN: 1-569001-10-3
Leslie L. Jackson, Author
Arbesman Marian, Ph.D, Author

6201 Playing Cure
Jason Aronson
PO Box 15100
York, PA 17405-7100   800-782-0015
                                    www.aronson.com

400 pages Hardcover
ISBN: 0-765700-21-2
Donna M. Cangelosi, Author
Heidi Kaduson, Author

6202 Protection and Advocacy Program for the Mentally Ill
US Department of Health and Human Services
5600 Fishers Lane
Rockville, MD 20857-0001   301-443-3667
                                    www.uls-dc.org/
Federal formula grant program to protect and advocate the rights of people with mental illnesses who are in residential facilities and to investigate abuse and neglect in such facilities.
Natalie Reatia, Chief

6203 Somatization Disorder in the Medical Setting
Superintendent of Documents
PO Box 371954   202-512-2250
Pittsburgh, PA 15250-7954
Somatization is a process in which psychological distress is expressed in multiple physical symptoms that have no discernible medical cause.
98 pages

6204 Strengthening the Role of Families in States' Early Intervention Systems
CEC, Department K00757   703-471-9543
Herdon, VA 22091
Policy guide for procedural safeguards for infants and toddlers under Part H of the Individuals with Disabilities Education Act.
213 pages Report

6205 Surviving Mental Illness
National Alliance for the Mentally Ill
14738 72nd Avenue   718-261-3772
Flushing, NY 11367-0753   Fax: 703-524-9094
                               www.survivingmentalillness.net
The subjective experiences of people with multiple diagnoses including schizophrenia, bipolar disorder and manic depression.

6206 Teaching Adults with Mental Handicaps
Sunday School Board of the Southern Baptists
127 9th Avenue N
Nashville, TN 37234-0001   800-458-BSSB
Offers guidelines in methods of teaching adults with mental handicaps, their needs, outreach ideas, curriculum resources, adaptation procedures, and ministry suggestions.

6207 Troubled Journey
National Alliance for the Mentally Ill
PO Box 753   301-524-7600
Waldorf, MD 20604-0753   Fax: 301-843-0159
                                    www.NAMI.org
Long associated with NAMI's former Siblings and Adult Children Network, the authors use their years of listening to stories - plus Marsh's professional experience - to provide a book that offers support to siblings and a caring and heartfelt approach to healing.
1997
Faith Cook, Author

6208 Turning Point
American Psychiatric Press
1400 K Street NW   202-682-6268
Washington, DC 20005-2403   Fax: 202-789-2648
                               www.turningpoint.org.in
The first comprehensive chronicle of the contributions made by conscientious objectors who volunteered for service in America's mental hospitals and state institutions for the developmentally disabled.
314 pages Hardcover
ISBN: 0-880485-60-4
Tiffany Snow, Author

6209 Understanding Depression
Patricia Ainsworth, MD, author
University Press of Mississippi
3825 Ridgewood Road   601-432-6205
Jackson, MS 39211-6492   Fax: 601-432-6217
                         e-mail: kburgess@ihl.state.ms.us
                                 www.upress.state.ms.us
A clear explanation for those who know the illness personally and for those who want to understand them.
2000 120 pages Paperback
ISBN: 1-578061-69-5
J. Raymond DePaulo, Author
Leslie Alan Horvitz, Author

6210 Understanding Mental Retardation
Patricia Ainsworth, MD; Pamela C Baker, PhD, author
University Press of Mississippi
3825 Ridgewood Road   601-432-6205
Jackson, MS 39211-6492   Fax: 601-432-6217
                         e-mail: kburgess@ihl.state.ms.us
                                 www.upress.state.ms.us
A resource for parents, caregivers, and counselors.
2004 192 pages Paperback
ISBN: 1-578066-47-6
Edward Zigler, Author
Robert M. Hodapp, Author

6211 Understanding Panic and Other Anxiety Disorders
Benjamin Root, MD, author
University Press of Mississippi

3825 Ridgewood Road
Jackson, MS 39211-6492

601-432-6205
Fax: 601-432-6217
e-mail: kburgess@ihl.state.ms.us
www.upress.state.ms.us

A patients guide to panic disorders, panic attacks, and other stress-related maladies.
2000 128 pages Paperback
ISBN: 1-578062-45-4
Kathy Burgess, Advertising/Marketing Services Manager
Root Benjamin, Author

6212 Victims of Dementia
Haworth Press
10 Alice Street
Binghamton, NY 13904-1580

607-722-5857
800-429-6784
Fax: 607-722-0012
www.haworthpress.com

Provides an in-depth look at the concept, construction and operation of Wesley Hall, a special living area at the Chelsea United Methodist retirement home in Michigan.
1993 155 pages Hardcover
ISBN: 1-560242-64-0

6213 Way to Go: School Success for Children wit h Mental Health Care Needs
Bazelon Center for Mental Health Law
1101 15th Street NW
Washington, DC 20005-5002

202-467-5730
Fax: 202-223-0409
TDD: 202-467-4342
e-mail: pubs@bazelon.org
www.bazelon.org

A report and fact sheets that document how states and school districts have successfully combined school-wide positive behavior support (PBS) with effective mental health services to foster a school environment that is conducive to learning, and improves children's lives. Order book and fact sheets sheets seperately or together. Pricing according to volume begins at $25 per book, $10 per fact sheet, or $29 for the combination.
1998
Lee Carly, Communications Director

6214 What

6215 What Fair Housing Means for People with Disabilities
Bazelon Center for Mental Health Law
1101 15th Street NW
Washington, DC 20005-5002

202-467-5730
Fax: 202-223-0409
TDD: 202-467-4342
e-mail: pubs@bazelon.org
www.bazelon.org

Explains in plain language how three federal laws protect the housing rights of people with mental or physical disabilities. 2003 edition available as pdf download.
2006 56 pages
Lee Carly, Communications Director
Judge David L. Bazelon, Author

6216 When Madness Comes Home
National Alliance for the Mentally Ill
PO Box 753
Waldorf, MD 20604-0753

301-524-7600
Fax: 301-843-0159
www.NAMI.org

Personal accounts offer first-hand, day-to-day experiences with mental illness of a sibling (mostly) and partner/spouse (briefly) and discuss the effects of growing up in a family whose energies are focused on an ill family member.
1997
Victoria Secunda, Author

6217 When Someone You Love Has a Mental Illness
National Alliance for the Mentally Ill
PO Box 753
Waldorf, MD 20604-0753

703-524-7600
Fax: 703-524-9094
www.NAMI.org

Excellent for families recently stricken with severe mental illness.

Children's Books

6218 Compassion Books, Inc.
7036 State Highway 80 S
Burnsville, NC 28714-7569

828-675-5909
800-970-4220
Fax: 828-675-9687
e-mail: orders@compassionbooks.com
www.compassionbooks.com

Hand picked resources to help people through loss, grief and changes of all kinds. Carry over 400 books and videos on death and dying, bereavement and change, comfort and healing, hope and much more.
Bruce Greene, VP

Magazines

6219 AJMR
American Association on Mental Retardation
444 N Capitol Street NW
Washington, DC 20001-1508

202-387-1968
800-424-3688
Fax: 202-387-2193
e-mail: AAMR@access.digex.net
www.aamr.org

Provides information on the latest program advances, current research, and information on products and services in the developmental disabilities field.
BiMonthly

6220 American Journal of Psychiatry
American Psychiatric Association
1000 Wilson Boulevard
Arlington, VA 22209-2492

703-907-7322
800-368-5777
Fax: 703-907-1091
ajp.psychiatryonline.org

Professional papers on topics in psychiatry.
Monthly
Public Affairs, Division

6221 American Psychologist
American Psychological Association
750 First Street NE
Washington, DC 20002-4242

202-336-5510
800-374-2721
Fax: 202-336-5502
TDD: 202-336-6123
e-mail: books@apa.org
www.apa.org

Articles on current issues in psychology as well as empirical, theoretical and practical articles on broad aspects of psychology.
9x a year

6222 Journal of Clinical Psychology
Clinical Psychology Publishing Company
4 Conant Square
Brandon, VT 05733-1018

802-247-6877

Scholarly research reports in the field of psychology.

6223 Mental Retardation
American Association on Mental Retardation
444 N Capitol Street NW
Washington, DC 20001-1508

202-387-1968
800-424-3688
Fax: 202-387-2193
e-mail: AAMR@access.digex.net
www.aamr.org

Provides information on the latest program advances, current research, and information on products and services in the developmental disabilities field.
BiMonthly
James R. Patton, Author

6224 Psychopharmacology Bulletin
Superintendent of Documents/NIMH Journal
PO Box 371954
Pittsburgh, PA 15250-7954

202-512-2250

Emphasizes rapid, informal dissemination of recent research findings that have not previously appeared in the more formal literature.
Quarterly

6225 Psychosocial Rehabilitation Journal
Int'l Assoc. of Psychosocial Rehab. Services
730 Commonwealth Avenue   617-353-3549
Boston, MA 02215-1209
Discusses issues, programs and research on psychiatric rehabilitation.

Newsletters

6226 ACMH Newsletter
Association for Children's Mental Health
1705 Coolidge Road   517-336-7222
East Lansing, MI 48823-1735   800-782-0883
Offers the latest information, including unmet needs and notices of relevant agency and legislative activities, hearings, public meetings and other opportunities for promoting children's mental health.
Quarterly
Gail Allen, Director
Marla Holle, Parent Advocate

6227 Advocate
National Alliance for the Mentally Ill
200 N Glebe Road   703-524-7600
Arlington, VA 22203-3754   Fax: 703-524-9094
Offers reviews of books, medical information, legislative information and Alliance activities for persons with mental illness, their families and professionals who work with them.
Quarterly

6228 Mental Health Law News
Interwood Publications
PO Box 20241   513-221-3715
Cincinnati, OH 45220-0241
Mental health case law summaries.
6 pages Monthly
ISBN: 0-889017-0 -
Frank J Bardack, Editor

6229 News & Notes
American Association on Mental Retardation
444 N Capitol Street NW   202-387-1968
Washington, DC 20001-1508   800-424-3688
                                              Fax: 202-387-2193
                                  e-mail: AAMR@access.digex.net
                                              www.aamr.org
Covers legislative, program, and research developments of interest to the field, as well as international news, Association activities, job ads and other classifieds, and upcoming events.
BiMonthly

Pamphlets

6230 14 Worst Myths About Recovered Mental Patients
National Institutes of Health
5600 Fishers Lane   301-496-4000
Rockville, MD 20857-0001   Fax: 301-443-6349
                                      e-mail: NIHInfo@nih.gov
                                              www.nih.gov
Refutes false beliefs that stigmatize recovered mental patients and suggests ways that the public can help advance the truth.

6231 Bipolar Disorder
National Institutes of Health
5600 Fishers Lane   301-443-3706
Rockville, MD 20857-0001   Fax: 301-443-6349
                                      e-mail: NIHInfo@nih.gov
                                              www.nih.gov
A short booklet offering a concise description of this disorder, which is also called manic-depressive illness.
Francis Mark Mondimore, Author

6232 Coping with Mental Illness in the Family
National Alliance for the Mentally Ill
PO Box 753   703-524-7600
Waldorf, MD 20604-0753   Fax: 703-524-9094
                                              www.NAMI.org
A handbook for families.

6233 Dual Diagnosis: Substance Abuse and Mental Illness
National Alliance for the Mentally Ill
PO Box 753   703-524-7600
Waldorf, MD 20604-0753   Fax: 703-524-9094
                                              www.NAMI.org
A booklet for families and consumers.

6234 Helping Families Understand PTSD
National Veterans Services Fund
PO Box 2465   203-656-0003
Darien, CT 06820-0465   Fax: 203-656-1957
                                    e-mail: NatVetSvc@aol.com
                                          www.valdezhousing.com
Pamphlet

6235 Let's Talk Facts About Childhood Disorders
American Psychiatric Association
1400 K Street NW   202-682-6220
Washington, DC 20005-2492
Offers information on depression and depressive disorders including the causes, symptoms, treatments, anxiety, and various other phobias.
Public Affairs, Division

6236 Mental Health Problems of Vietnam Veterans
National Veterans Services Fund
PO Box 2465   203-656-0003
Darien, CT 06820-0465   Fax: 203-656-1957
                                    e-mail: NatVetSvc@aol.com
                                          www.valdezhousing.com
Pamphlet

6237 Minority Advocacy Notebook
Bazelon Center for Mental Health Law
1101 15th Street NW   202-467-5730
Washington, DC 20005-5002   Fax: 202-223-0409
                                              TDD: 202-467-4342
                                      e-mail: pubs@bazelon.org
                                              www.bazelon.org
Selected materials and models from our manual on outreach and advocacy for African Americans and Latinos with mental disabilities; includes Impediments to Services and Advocacy for Black and Hispanic People with Mental Illness.
1998
Lee Carly, Communications Director

6238 New Challenge: Responding to Families
Federation for Children with Special Needs
95 Berkeley Street   617-482-2915
Boston, MA 02116-6230   800-331-0688
Addresses the needs of children with emotional, behavioral and mental disorders and their families.

6239 PTSD and the Family: Secondary Traumatization
National Veterans Services Fund
PO Box 2465   203-656-0003
Darien, CT 06820-0465   Fax: 203-656-1957
                                    e-mail: NatVetSvc@aol.com
                                          www.valdezhousing.com
Pamphlet

6240 Plain Talk About...Dealing with the Angry Child
Superintendent of Documents
PO Box 371954   202-512-2250
Pittsburgh, PA 15250-7954
A flyer that offers suggestions for helping children cope with their anger in a healthy and constructive way.

6241 Plain Talk About...Handling Stress
Superintendent of Documents
PO Box 371954   202-512-2250
Pittsburgh, PA 15250-7954
Information on stress and how you can make it work for you rather than against you.

6242 Psychotherapy with Traumatized Vietnam Combatants
National Veterans Services Fund

PO Box 2465
Darien, CT 06820-0465

203-656-0003
Fax: 203-656-1957
e-mail: NatVetSvc@aol.com
www.valdezhousing.com

Pamphlet

6243 Triumph Over Fear
National Alliance for the Mentally Ill
PO Box 753
Waldorf, MD 20604-0753

703-524-7600
Fax: 703-524-9094
www.NAMI.org

Step-by-step treatment plans for the many faces of phobias, panic disorder, obsessive-compulsive disorder, and post-traumatic stress. Includes case histories.
1994 Softcover
Rosalynn Carter, Author
Jerilyn Ross, Author

Audio & Video

6244 And After Tomorrow
G. Allan Roeher Institute
4700 Keele Street
Downsview, ON, M3J 1P3,

416-661-9611

A film about lives of people with a mental handicap and their families, in which parents and friends speak candidly about their personal experiences.
Films

6245 With a Little Help from My Friends
L'institut Roeher Institute
York University
North York, ON, M3J 1P3,

416-661-9611
Fax: 416-661-5701

This three-part video provides insight into inclusive education for people with mental handicaps.

Web Sites

6246 American Psychological Association

www.apa.org

Mission is to advance psychology as a science and professional organization that represents psychology in the United States.

6247 Coalition of Voluntary Mental Health Agencies

www.cvmha.org/

An umbrella advocacy organization of New York's mental health community, representing over 100 non-profit community based mental health agencies that serve more than 300,000 clients in the five boroughs of New York City and its environs.

6248 Community Access

www.cairn.org/

A nonprofit agency providing housing and advocacy for people with psychiatric disabilities.

6249 Federation of Families for Children's Mental Health

www.ffcmh.org/

Providing leadership to develop and sustain a nationwide network of family-run organizations.

6250 Healing Well

www.healingwell.com

An online health resource guide to medical news, chat, information and articles, newsgroups and message boards, books, disease-related web sites, medical directories, and more for patients, friends, and family coping with disabling diseases, disorders, or chronic illnesses.

6251 Health Finder

www.healthfinder.gov

Searchable, carefully developed web site offering information on over 1000 topics. Developed by the US Department of Health and Human Services, the site can be used in both English and Spanish.

6252 Healthlink USA

www.healthlinkusa.com

Health information concerning treatment, cures, prevention, diagnosis, risk factors, research, support groups, email lists, personal stories and much more. Updated regularly.

6253 Helios Health

www.helioshealth.com

Online resource for your health information. Detailed information about specific health topics, access to expert advice from our Medical Advisory Board, and up-to-date health news.

6254 Internet Mental Health

www.mentalhealth.com

A site whose goal is to improve understanding, diagnosis, and treatment of mental illness throughout the world. Includes information on specific disorders, medications, diagnosis, research, news, and other internet links.

6255 MedicineNet

www.medicinenet.com

An online resource for consumers providing easy-to-read, authoritative medical and health information.

6256 Medscape

www.medscape.com

Medscape offers specialists, primary care physicians, and other health professionals the Web's most robust and integrated medical information and educational tools.

6257 Mental Health America (formerly NMHA) Information Center

www.mentalhealthamerica.net

Provides informational materials, lobbies for Federal mental health legislation, stimulates funding of research on the causes and treatment of mental illnesses.

6258 National Alliance for the Mentally Ill

www.nami.org

Over 900 affiliate groups nationwide offer support to members, advocate better lives for their loved ones, support research efforts and educate the public to reduce the stigma attached to serious mental illnesses.

6259 National Mental Health Services Knowledge Exchange Network

www.mentalhealth.org

Leading the national system that delivers mental health services. Provides the treatment and support services neede by adults with mental disorders and children with serious emotional problems.

6260 WebMD

www.webmd.com

Provides credible information, supportive communities, and in-depth reference material about health subjects. A source for original and timely health information as well as material from well known content providers.

6261 World Federation for Mental Health

www.wfmh.com

Mission is to promote, among all people and nations, the highest possible level of mental health in its broadest biological, medical, educational, and social aspects.

Description

6262 Mental Illness/Depression

Depression is a mood disorder that can cause marked impairment of physical and social function and work capacity. It differs from normal grief which occurs in response to a significant separation or loss. It affects twice as many women as men and is more common in people with a family history of depression.

Research is gathering evidence of the relationship between depression and chemical imbalances in the brain. Clinical depression can also be associated with medication or other physical illnesses.

Common symptoms associated with depression include irritability, sleeping problems, changes in appetite, sadness, apathy, loss of interest in previously enjoyed activities and anxiety. Depression frequently disrupts a person's relationship with friends, family members and colleagues. It is also associated with alcohol and substance abuse. Suicide is the cause of death in approximately 15 percent of untreated patients.

Treatment must be tailored to the individual and can include talk therapy and/or medication. Newer groups of antidepressant medications have markedly improved the success of treatment. Patient and family education can play a crucial role. See also *Mental Illness/General and Mental Illness/Schizophrenia.*

National Agencies & Associations

6263 American Counseling Association
5999 Stevenson Avenue
Alexandria, VA 22304
800-347-6647
Fax: 800-473-2329
e-mail: webmaster@counseling.org
www.counseling.org
The American Counseling Association is a non-profit professional and educational organization that is dedicated to the growth and enhancement of the counseling profession. Founded in 1952 ACA is the world's largest such association.
Cirecie A West, President
Robert L Smith, President Elect

6264 American Psychiatric Association
1000 Wilson Boulevard
Arlington, VA 22209-3901
703-907-7300
888-357-7924
e-mail: apa@psych.org
www.psychiatry.org
The American Psychiatric Association is a medical specialty society recognized world wide. Its over 35,000 U.S. and international member physicians work together to ensure humane care and effective treatment for all persons with mental disorders.
Jeffrey Lieberman, MD, President

6265 Anxiety Disorders Association of America
8701 Georgia Avenue
Silver Spring, MD 20910
240-485-1001
Fax: 240-485-1035
e-mail: information@adaa.org
www.adaa.org
The Anxiety Disorders Association (ADAA) is a non profit organization whose mission is to promote the prevention treatment and cure of anxiety disorders and to improve the lives of all people who suffer from them.
Terence M Keane, PhD, President
Alies Muskin, Executive Director

6266 Brain & Behavior Research Foundation
60 Cutter Miller Road
Great Neck, NY 11021-3104
516-829-0091
800-829-8289
Fax: 516-487-6930
e-mail: info@bbrfoundation.org
www.bbrfoundation.org/
NARSAD Information and helpline staff is available to answer basic questions about the symptoms, causes and treatments of psychiatric illnesses. Information on support groups and other mental health organizations can also be provided.
Steve Lieber, Chairman of the Board
Jeffrey Borenstein, M.D., President & CEO

6267 Mental Health America
PO Box 17598
Baltimore, MD 21297-2257
800-239-1265
Fax: 443-782-0739
e-mail: info@ifred.org
www.ifred.org
Founded in 1983 to correct the myths and misconceptions surrounding the illness and help reverse the devastating effects depression has on the individual and our society. NAFDI's purpose is to educate the public and primary health care providers.
Kathryn Goetzke, Founder
Tom Dean, Chairman of the Board

6268 National Alliance On Mental Illness
3803 N. Fairfax Drive
Arlington, VA 22203
703-524-7600
800-950-6264
Fax: 703-524-9094
TDD: 703-516-7227
www.nami.org
Membership organization with over 858 affiliates in 50 states, offers newsletters, a mail-order bookstore and many programs, conferences, symposia and groups meetings for family members and patients.
Keris Jan Myrick, President
Jim Payne, Vice President

6269 National Anxiety Foundation
3135 Custer Drive
Lexington, KY 40517-4001
606-272-7166
www.lexington-on-line.com/naf.html
Offers information and help to persons with panic disorders manic and depressive disorders and mental illness.
Stephen Cox, President
Linda Vernon Blair, Vice-President

6270 National Mental Health Association
2000 N Beauregard Street
Alexandria, VA 22311
703-684-7722
800-969-6642
Fax: 703-684-5968
TTY: 800-433-5959
e-mail: infoctr@nmha.org
www.mentalhealthamerica.net
Serves over 700 affiliates nationally providing information publications and other services.
Ann Boughtin, Chair of the Board
Eric Ashton, Vice-Chair

6271 National Mental Health Information Center
2000 N Beauregard Street
Alexandria, VA 22311
703-684-7722
800-969-6642
Fax: 703-684-5968
TTY: 866-889-2647
TDD: 866-889-2647
e-mail: nmhic-info@samhsa.hhs.gov
www.mentalhealthamerica.net
The Center for Mental Health Services (CMHS) is charged with leading the national system that delivers mental health services. The goal of this system is to provide the treatment and support services needed by adults and children with mental disorders.
Ann Boughtin, Chair of the Board
Eric Ashton, Vice-Chair

6272 Option Institute
2080 S Undermountain Road
Sheffield, MA 01257
413-229-2100
800-714-2779
Fax: 413-229-8931
e-mail: participantsupport@option.org
www.option.org
Self-defeating beliefs, along with attitudes and judgments can lead to depression and a host of physical and psychological challenges. The Option Institute offers programs designed to help uproot self-defeating beliefs and remove roadblocks to happiness.
Barry Neils Kaufman, Co-Founder/ Co-Director
Samahria Lyte Kaufman, Co-Founder/ Co-Director

6273 Screening For Mental Health
Screening For Mental Health
One Washington Street
Wellesley Hills, MA 02481
781-239-0071
Fax: 781-431-7447
e-mail: smhinfo@mentalhealthscreening.org
www.mentalhealthscreening.org
Screening for Mental Health (SHM) is the non-profit organization that first introduced the concept of large-scale mental health screenings with its flagship program National Depression Screening Day in 1991. SHM programs now include both in-person and online.
Douglas George Jacobs, President & Medical Director
Effie Malley, Executive Director

Research Centers

6274 University of Pennsylvania: Depression Research Unit
School of Medicine
Department of Psychiatry
Philadelphia, PA 19104
215-662-3462
Fax: 215-662-6443
Focuses on mental health and depression.
Jay D MD, Chairman
Alex Cabrera, Clinic Manager

6275 University of Texas Mental Health Clinical Research Center
University of Texas
5323 Harry Hines Boulevard
Dallas, TX 75390
214-645-8300
Fax: 214-645-7999
e-mail: news@utsouthwester.edu
www.utsouthwesteRN.edu
Research activity of major and atypical depression.
Daniel K Podolsky, MD, President
J. Gregory Fitz, Executive Vice President

6276 Yale University: Behavioral Medicine Clinic
Yale School of Medicine
333 Cedar Street
New Haven, CT 06510
203-432-7960
www.medicine.yale.edu
Focuses on mental disorders including schizophrenia and depression.
Peter Salovey, President
Richard Belitsky, Deputy Dean for Education

6277 Yale University: Ribicoff Research Facilities/CT Mental Health Center
34 Park Street
New Haven, CT 06511
203-789-7300
Fax: 203-562-7079
Clinical research in the areas of schizophrenia depression and mental disorders.
George Henin Ashenden, President

Support Groups & Hotlines

6278 Depression and Bipolar Support Alliance
730 N Franklin Street
Chicago, IL 60654
312-642-0049
800-826-3632
Fax: 312-642-7243
e-mail: adoederlein@dbsalliance.org
www.dbsalliance.org
Consists of approximately 900 patient groups providing support and direct services to persons with clinical depression and/or bipolar disorder.
Lucinda Jewell, Chair
Allen Doederlein, President

6279 National Health Information Center
PO Box 1133
Washington, DC 20013
310-565-4167
800-336-4797
Fax: 301-984-4256
e-mail: info@nhic.org
www.health.gov/nhic
Offers a nationwide information referral service, produces directories and resource guides.
Steele, President
Paul F Dell PhD, President-Elect

Books

6280 Columbia University Complete Home Guide to Mental Health
Henry Holt & Company
115 W 18th Street
New York, NY 10011-4113
212-886-9200
Fax: 212-633-0748
www.cumc.columbia.edu
A compendium of information on all aspects of mental health; written primarily for the lay reader.
476 pages

6281 Coping with Depression and Mood Disorders
Rosen Publishing Group
29 E 21st Street
New York, NY 10010
212-777-3017
800-237-9932
Fax: 888-436-4643
e-mail: customerservice@rosenpub.com
www.rosenpublishing.com
With an emphasis on life's myriad difficulties, the authors help teens find practical ways to cope with depression.

ISBN: 0-823929-73-6
Lawrence Clayton PhD, Author
Sharon Carter, Author

6282 Depression Sourcebook
Brian P. Quinn, author
McGraw-Hill Companies
Returns Department
Dubuque, IA 52002
877-833-5524
Fax: 614-759-3749
e-mail: pbg.ecommerce_custserv@mcgrw-hill.com
www.mcgraw-hill.com
Everything anyone afflicted with a depressive disorder - or the people who care about them - need to know about unipolar and bipolar depression.
2000 288 pages
ISBN: 0-737303-79-4
Amy L. Sutton, Author

6283 Depression and its Treatment
Warner Books
1271 Ave of the Americas
New York, NY 10020-1300
212-522-7200
A layman's guide to help one understand and cope with America's #1 mental health problem.
157 pages

6284 Depressive Illnesses: Treatments Bring New Hope
Superintendent of Documents
PO Box 371954
Pittsburgh, PA 15250-7954
202-512-2250
Offers the general public an overview of the various depressive illnesses. Topics include causes, symptoms and types of depression, clinical evaluation and treatment, helpful suggestions for family and friends, and other sources of information.
28 pages

6285 Encyclopedia of Depression
Facts on File

11 Penn Plaza
New York, NY 10001

212-967-8800
800-322-8755
Fax: 800-678-3633

This volume defines and explains all terms and topics relating to depression.
170 pages Hardcover

6286 Essential Guide to Psychiatric Drugs
St. Martin's Press
175 5th Avenue
New York, NY 10010-7848

212-674-5151
800-221-7945
Fax: 212-420-9314

Basic information on 123 drugs used for depression, anxiety and bipolar illness.

6287 Everything You Need to Know About Depression
Rosen Publishing Group
29 E 21st Street
New York, NY 10010

212-777-3017
800-237-9932
Fax: 888-436-4643
e-mail: customerservice@rosenpub.com
www.rosenpublishing.com

An important resource for teens who are looking for help with depression.
Grades 7-12
ISBN: 0-823934-39-X
Elanor H Ayer, Author

6288 Inside Manic Depression
Sunnyside Press
PO Box 1717
San Marcos, CA 92079-1717

619-424-3348

The true story of one victim's triumph over despair. A first person account.
176 pages

6289 Medical Management of Depression
EMIS Medical Publishers
PO Box 6100
Durant, OK 74702-1607

580-924-0643
800-225-0694
Fax: 580-924-9414

ISBN: 0-929240-62-6

6290 Mood Apart
Basic Books
10 E 53rd Street
New York, NY 10022-5244

212-207-7057

An overview of the depression and manic depression and the available treatments for them.
363 pages

6291 Overcoming Depression
Harper & Row
10 E 53rd Street
New York, NY 10022-5299

212-207-7000

318 pages Paperback

6292 Panic Disorder in the Medical Setting
Superintendent of Documents
PO Box 371954
Pittsburgh, PA 15250-7954

202-512-2250

This book serves the primary care physicians as a helpful guide in recognizing and treating panic disorder in patients and in identifying those who need psychiatric consultation or rerferrals.
1993 135 pages

6293 Pastoral Care of Depression
The Haworth Press
10 Alice Street
Binghamton, NY 13904-1580

607-722-5857
800-429-6784
Fax: 607-895-0582
e-mail: getinfo@haworth.com
www.haworth.com

Helps caregivers by overcoming the simplistic myths about depressive disorders and probing the real issues.
Paperback
ISBN: 0-789002-65-5

6294 Prozac Nation: Young & Depressed in America: A Memoir
Houghton Mifflin Company

Wayside Road
Burlington, MA 01803

800-225-3362

Struck with depression at 11, now 27, Wurtzel chronicles her struggle with the illness. Witty, terrifying and sometimes funny, it tells the story of a young life almost destroyed by depression.
317 pages

6295 Psychotherapy of Severe and Mild Depression
Jason Aronson
PO Box 15100
York, PA 17405-7100

800-782-0015
Fax: 201-840-7242
www.aronson.com

464 pages Softcover
ISBN: 1-568211-46-5

6296 Questions & Answers About Depression & Its Treatment
Ivan K Goldberg, MD, author
Charles Press Publishers
PO Box 15715
Philadelphia, PA 19103-0715

215-561-2786
Fax: 215-561-0191
e-mail: mailbox@charlespresspub.com
www.charlespresspub.com

All the questions you'd like to ask, asked and answered.
139 pages
ISBN: 0-914783-68-8

6297 Report of the Secretary's Task Force on Youth Suicide, Volume 1
Superintendent of Documents
PO Box 371954
Pittsburgh, PA 15250-7954

202-512-2250

A comprehensive review of information about youth suicide. The task force recommendations are presented in Volume 1.
110 pages

6298 Touched with Fire:- Manic Depressive Illness & the Artistic Temperment
Free Press
866 3rd Avenue
New York, NY 10022-6221

Fax: 800-943-9831
www.simonsays.com

Describing and discussing the markedly increased rates of severe mood disorders and suicides among the artistically creative and the reasons why.
370 pages

6299 Winter Blues
Norman E Rosenthal, author
Guilford Press
72 Spring Street
New York, NY 10012-4019

800-265-7006
Fax: 212-966-6708
e-mail: info@guilford.com
www.guilford.com

Complete information about Seasonal Affective Disorder and its treatment.
2005
ISBN: 1-593852-14-2

6300 Women and Depression
Springer Publishing Company
536 Broadway
New York, NY 10012-3955

212-431-4370
877-687-7476
Fax: 212-941-7842
e-mail: marketing@springerpub.com
www.springerpub.com

This volume examines depression in women within a developmental context. It ranges from issues in childhood and adolescence through premenstrual syndrome and postpartum depression to issues of menopause and aging.
328 pages Hardcover
ISBN: 0-826151-40-X
Annette Imperati, Marketing Director

6301 Yesterday's Tomorrow
Hazelden
15251 Pleasant Valley Rd
Center City, MN 55012-9640

651-257-4010
800-328-9000
Fax: 651-213-4426
www.hazelden.org

A meditation book that shows why and how recovery works, from the author's own experiences.
432 pages Paperback
ISBN: 1-568381-60-3

Children's Books

6302 Compassion Books, Inc.
7036 State Highway 80 S
Burnsville, NC 28714-7569
828-675-5909
800-970-4220
Fax: 828-675-9687
e-mail: orders@compassionbooks.com
www.compassionbooks.com
Hand picked resources to help people through loss, grief and changes of all kinds. Carry over 400 books and videos on death and dying, bereavement and change, comfort and healing, hope and much more.
Bruce Greene, VP

Newsletters

6303 NFDI Newsletter
National Foundation for Depressive Illness
PO Box 2257
New York, NY 10116-2257
212-268-4260
800-248-4344
Fax: 212-268-4434
e-mail: pross@att.net
www.depression.org
To correct the myths and misconceptions surrounding the illness and help reverse the devastating effects depression has on the individual and our society and to inform the public, primary health care providers, other healthcare professionals and corporations about depression and manic depression and to provide the information about correct diagnosis and treatment and the availability of qualified doctors and support groups.
4 pages Quarterly

Pamphlets

6304 Depression is a Treatable Illness: A Patients Guide
Department of Health & Human Services
2101 E Jefferson Street
Rockville, MD 20852-4908
301-217-1245
Tells about major depressive disorder, which is only one form of depressive illness. This booklet answers important questions regarding this disorder and gives information on where to go for more help.

6305 If You're Over 65 and Feeling Depressed...
National Institutes on Mental Health
5600 Fishers Lane
Rockville, MD 20857-0001
301-443-3706
Fax: 301-443-6349
Many older people believe that their age alone is responsible for feelings of exhaustion, helplessness and worthlessness. This brochure discusses the causes of depression in the older years, symptoms, types of treatment and where to go for help.
12 pages

6306 Let's Talk About Depression
Superintendent of Documents
PO Box 371954
Pittsburgh, PA 15250-7954
202-512-2250
Targeted especially for inner-city youth. The colorful design will capture attention and focus on depression in a way that young people will understand and identify with.

6307 Lithium and Manic Depression
Lithium Info. Center-Dean Foundation for Health
8000 Excelsior Drive
Madison, WI 53717-1972
608-836-8070
A guidebook about lithium and its effects on bipolar affective disorders and manic depression.
1992 32 pages

6308 Living Without Depression & Manic Depression: A Workbook
National Alliance for the Mentally Ill

3803 N. Fairfax Drive
Arlington, VA 22203-0753
703-524-7600
800-950-6264
Fax: 703-524-9094
www.NAMI.org
Workbook offering checklists and helpful advice targeted for individuals whose depressive illness is stabilized.
1994
Jim Payne, President
Ralph E. Nelson, Jr., First Vice President

6309 Panic Disorder
National Institutes of Health
5600 Fishers Lane
Rockville, MD 20857-0001
301-443-3706
Fax: 301-443-6349
Written for the lay public, this pamphlet contains a description of panic disorder, gives the symptoms, describes treatment methods, and encourages the person who has the symptoms to seek treatment.

6310 Plain Talk About Depression
Superintendent of Documents
PO Box 371954
Pittsburgh, PA 15250-7954
202-512-2250
A flyer discussing types of depression, major depression, symptoms and causes.

6311 Understanding Panic Disorder
National Institutes of Health
5600 Fishers Lane
Rockville, MD 20857-0001
301-443-3706
Fax: 301-443-6349
Offers information on what an panic disorder is, symptoms, causes, treatment, medications and therapy.

6312 Useful Information on Phobias and Panic
Superintendent of Documents
PO Box 371954
Pittsburgh, PA 15250-7954
202-512-2250
This booklet provides information on both phobias and panic. Symptoms, causes and treatments of these disorders are referred to. If you know someone who is excessively fearful, this booklet will be of great help to them in understanding their problem.
40 pages 50 copies

6313 What to Do When a Friend is Depressed: Guide for Students
Superintendent of Documents
PO Box 371954
Pittsburgh, PA 15250-7954
202-512-2250
Offers information on depression and its symptoms and suggests things a young person can do to guide a depressed friend in finding help.

6314 What to Do When an Employee is Depressed: A Guide for Supervisors
Superintendent of Documents
PO Box 371954
Pittsburgh, PA 15250-7954
202-512-2250
A D/ART program brochure that will enable an employer to recognize the symptoms of depression in an employee and offers suggestions on what to say to the employee to encourage him or her to seek help.

Audio & Video

6315 Four Lives: A Portrait of Manic Depression
Fanlight Productions
4196 Washington Street
Boston, MA 02131-1731
617-469-4999
800-937-4113
Fax: 617-469-3379
e-mail: fanlight@fanlight.com
www.fanlight.com
Four patients, families and psychiatrists share their perspectives on living with manic depression.
1987 60 Minutes
ISBN: 1-572950-29-3

6316 Taking Control of Depression
800-228-2495

Dramatic program offering new hope in the understanding and treatment of depression, with actor Ed Asner and Alan Xenakis, M.D.

6317   When Someone You Love Suffers from Depression
Medcom/Trainex

800-320-1444

Helping family and friends identify depression in a loved one - offers ways to help stop the suffering and get appropriate treatment.

Web Sites

6318   Healing Well

www.healingwell.com

An online health resource guide to medical news, chat, information and articles, newsgroups and message boards, books, disease-related web sites, medical directories, and more for patients, friends, and family coping with disabling diseases, disorders, or chronic illnesses.

6319   Health Finder

www.healthfinder.gov

Searchable, carefully developed web site offering information on over 1000 topics. Developed by the US Department of Health and Human Services, the site can be used in both English and Spanish.

6320   Healthlink USA

www.healthlinkusa.com

Health information concerning treatment, cures, prevention, diagnosis, risk factors, research, support groups, email lists, personal stories and much more. Updated regularly.

6321   Helios Health

www.helioshealth.com

Online resource for your health information. Detailed information about specific health topics, access to expert advice from our Medical Advisory Board, and up-to-date health news.

6322   MedicineNet

www.medicinenet.com

An online resource for consumers providing easy-to-read, authoritative medical and health information.

6323   Medscape

www.medscape.com

Medscape offers specialists, primary care physicians, and other health professionals the Web's most robust and integrated medical information and educational tools.

6324   National Anxiety Foundation

www.lexington-on-line.com/naf.html

Offers information and help to persons with panic disorders, manic and depressive disorders and mental illness.

6325   National Foundation for Depressive Illness

www.ifred.org

iFred engages with individuals and organizations to execute high-impact and effective campaigns that educate the public about support and treatment for depression.

6326   WebMD

www.webmd.com

Provides credible information, supportive communities, and in-depth reference material about health subjects. A source for original and timely health information as well as material from well known content providers.

Description

6327 Mental Illness/Schizophrenia

Schizophrenia is a chronic mental illness that is characterized by disturbances of thinking, feeling, and behavior. It usually begins in late adolescence or early adult life, with a lifetime prevalence between 0.2 to 1 percent. Despite its literal translation of split mind, schizophrenia is not the same as split personality. Although its specific cause is unknown, most cases of schizophrenia are believed to result from a complex interaction between biologic, inherited and environmental factors.

Symptoms of schizophrenia vary in type and severity and may include delusions and auditory hallucinations (hearing voices), incoherent thought patterns, catatonic behavior, and a flat or grossly inappropriate emotional state.

Drug treatment is the cornerstone of managing schizophrenia. When treated early, patients tend to respond quickly and more fully. Effective drugs have been available for several decades, and have revolutionized treatment of the disease. However, these drug treatments may be limited by side effects (especially movement disorders resembling Parkinsons disease) and by the patient's failure or refusal to stay on treatment. Patient non-compliance is sometimes addressed with long-acting injectable medications. A new class of drugs, lacking the Parkinson-like side effects, and sometimes dramatically more effective than previously used drugs, became available during the 1990s. Their use is limited by high costs and the threat of serious blood-related side effects. Treatment includes counseling, social support, rehabilitation, and skills retraining. Poor outcome frequently leads to extensive and long-term disability. Psychological and educational interventions can reduce the rate of relapse. People close to persons with schizophrenia are often very affected by the disease and can be helped by support and advocacy groups. See also *Mental Illness/General and Mental Illness/Depression*.

National Agencies & Associations

6328 International Society for the Study of Dissociation
8400 Westpark Drive
McLean, VA 22102

703-610-9037
Fax: 703-610-0234
e-mail: info@isst-d.org
www.issd.org

A nonprofit professional association that promotes research and training in the identification of treatment of multiple personality, provides professional and public education about multiple personality and initiates international communication among clinicians.
Joan Turkus, President
Philip J Kinsler, PhD, President-Elect

6329 NARSAD: Mental Health Research Association
60 Cutter Miller Road
Great Neck, NY 11021-3104

516-829-0091
800-829-8289
Fax: 516-487-6930
e-mail: info@bbrfoundation.org
www.bbrfoundation.org/

NARSAD Information and helpline staff is available to answer basic questions about the symptoms, causes and treatments of psychi-

atric illnesses. Information on support groups and other mental health organizations can also be provided.
Steve Lieber, Chairman of the Board
Jeffrey Borenstein, M.D., President & CEO

6330 National Alliance for the Mentally Ill
Colonial Place Three
2107 Wilson Boulevard
Arlington, VA 22201-3042

703-524-7600
800-950-6264
Fax: 703-524-9094
TDD: 703-516-7227
e-mail: membership@naminyc.org
www.nami-nyc-metro.org

Nonprofit, self-help, volunteer organization that offers practical support, useful education, advocacy, comfort and understanding to those in the greater New York area who suffer or have family members suffering from mental illnesses. Chapter of the National Alliance for the Mentally Ill and the New York State Alliance for the Mentally Ill.
Charolette Hoffer, MD PhD, President
Elizabeth Plante, Director, Huxley Institute

Research Centers

6331 Huxley Insititute-American Schizophrenic Association
86-B Dorchester Drive
Lakewood, NJ 08701

www.schizohprenia.org

The ASA works to bring effective, low-cost treatment to patients woth schizophrenia and help them in a cooperative effort to cope with the disorder.
Abram Carpenter Jr, Director
Vito J Seskunas, Deputy Director for Administration

6332 Maryland Psychiatric Research Center
655 W. Baltimore Street
Baltimore, MD 21201

410-402-7666
Fax: 410-788-3837
www.mprc.umaryland.edu/default.asp

Providing treatment to patients with schizophrenia and related disorders educating professionals and consumers about schizophrenia and conducting basic and translational research into the manifestations causes and treatment of schizophrenia.
Robert Buchanan, MD, Interim Director
Vito J Seskunas, Deputy Director for Administration

6333 National Alliance for Research on Schizophrenia and Depression
Grants Office
60 Cutter Mill Road
Great Neck, NY 11021

516-829-0091
800-829-8289
Fax: 516-487-6930
e-mail: info@bbrfoundation.org
www.bbrfoundation.org/

Research focusing on varieties of mental illness and mental disorders.
Steve Lieber, Chairman of the Board
Jeffrey Borenstein, M.D., President & CEO

6334 Schizophrenia Research Branch: Division of Clinical and Treatment Research
5600 Fisher Lane, Parklawn Building
Rockville, MD 20857

301-443-4707
Fax: 301-443-6000

Plans, supports, and conducts programs of research, research training, and resource development of schizophrenia and related disorders. Reviews and evaluates research developments in the field and recommends new program directors. Collaborates with organizations in and outside of the National Institue of Mental Health (NIMH) to stimulate work in the field through conferences and workshops.

6335 Tennessee Neuropsychiatric Institute Middle Tennessee Mental Health Institute
Middle Tennessee Mental Health Institute
221 Stewarts Ferry Pike
Nashville, TN 37217

615-902-7535

Michael Eber Andreassen MD, Director

6336 University of Iowa Mental Health Clinical Research Center
University of Iowa Hospitals & Clinics

200 Hawkins Drive
Iowa City, IA 52242

319-356-1553
877-575-2864
Fax: 319-353-8300
www.iowa-mhcrc.psychiatry.uiowa.edu

Schizophrenia studies and other cognitive disorder research.
Nancy C

Support Groups & Hotlines

6337 National Health Information Center
PO Box 1133
Washington, DC 20013

310-565-4167
800-336-4797
Fax: 301-984-4256
e-mail: info@nhic.org
www.health.gov/nhic

Offers a nationwide information referral service, produces directories and resource guides.
Rydell, Executive Director & CEO
Stephen M Sergay, President

Books

6338 Encyclopedia of Schizophrenia and the Psychotic Disorders
Facts on File
11 Penn Plaza
New York, NY 10001

212-967-8800
800-322-8755
Fax: 800-678-3633

This volume details recent theories and research findings on schizophrenia and psychotic disorders, together with a complete overview of the field's history.
368 pages Hardcover

6339 Experiences of Schizophrenia
Guilford Press
72 Spring Street
New York, NY 10012

800-365-7006
Fax: 212-966-6708
e-mail: info@guilford.com
www.guilford.com

This authoritative book presents new information on seasonal affective disorder. It includes remedies such as recent advances in light box therapy, research on the effectiveness of antidepressants, and new recipes to counterbalance unhealthy winter food cravings. This book also helps distinguish various degrees of the disorder ranging from winter blues to full blown SAD, and provides a self test that readers can use to evalutate their own seasonal mood changes.
2005 372 pages
ISBN: 1-593852-14-2

6340 Occupational Therapy Practice Guidelines for Adults with Schizophrenia
American Occupational Therapy Association
4720 Montgomery Lane
Bethesda, MD 20824-1220

301-652-2682
Fax: 301-652-7711
TDD: 800-377-8555
www.aota.org

24 pages
ISBN: 1-569001-53-7

6341 Return from Madness
Jason Aronson
PO Box 15100
York, PA 17405-7100

800-783-0015
www.aronson.com

256 pages Hardcover
ISBN: 1-568216-25-4

6342 Schizophrenia and Primitive Mental States
Jason Aronson
PO Box 15100
York, PA 17405-7100

800-782-0015
Fax: 201-840-7242
www.aronson.com

288 pages Softcover
ISBN: 0-765700-27-1

6343 Schizophrenia: From Mind to Molecule
American Psychiatric Press
1400 K Street NW
Washington, DC 20005-2403

202-682-6268
Fax: 202-789-2648

Presents a change in the scientific understanding and outlook regarding the devastating disorder of schizophrenia. It provides a thorough, up-to-date look at schizophrenia that includes neural behavioral studies, technologies and medical treatments.
274 pages Hardcover
ISBN: 0-880489-50-2

Children's Books

6344 Year it Rained
MacMillan Publishing Company
866 3rd Avenue
New York, NY 10022-6221

212-702-2000
www.mcp.com

The story of a girl traumatized by an alcoholic father and her desire to commit suicide. Hospitalized for schizophrenia, Elizabeth reaches a catharsis and, with the help of a poet, discovers that her talent and therapy may be in writing.
Grades 7-10

Magazines

6345 Dissociation
ISSMP&D
5700 Old Orchard Road
Skokie, IL 60077-1036

847-966-4322
Fax: 847-966-9418

A professional journal offering the latest information about the issues and research into multiple personalities and related disorders.

6346 Schizophrenia Bulletin
Superintendent of Documents/NIMH Journal
PO Box 371954
Pittsburgh, PA 15250-7954

202-512-2250

Serves as a forum for multidisciplinary exchange of information about schizophrenia and is exclusively devoted to the exploration of this severe disorder.
Quarterly

Newsletters

6347 ISSD News
Int'l Society for the Study of Dissociation
8400 Westpark Drive
McLean, VA 22102

703-610-9037
Fax: 703-610-0234
e-mail: info@isst-d.orgÿ
www.isst-d.org

Includes current news from other onzations of interest to members, information about recent articles and books, news from US and international affiliates and the latest issues concerning multiple personality/dissociative states.
17 pages 6 times a year
Lynette S. Danylchuk, President
Christine Forner, Treasurer

Pamphlets

6348 Schizophrenia
National Alliance for the Mentally Ill
3803 N. Fairfax Drive
Arlington, VA 22203-3754

703-524-7600
800-950-6264
Fax: 703-524-9094
www.NAMI.org

Part of the NAMI medical information series offering information on the causes, symptoms and treatments of Schizophrenia.
Jim Payne, President
Ralph E. Nelson, Jr., First Vice President

Web Sites

6349 Healing Well

www.healingwell.com

An online health resource guide to medical news, chat, information and articles, newsgroups and message boards, books, disease-related web sites, medical directories, and more for patients, friends, and family coping with disabling diseases, disorders, or chronic illnesses.

6350 Health Finder

www.healthfinder.gov

Searchable, carefully developed web site offering information on over 1000 topics. Developed by the US Department of Health and Human Services, the site can be used in both English and Spanish.

6351 Healthlink USA

www.healthlinkusa.com

Health information concerning treatment, cures, prevention, diagnosis, risk factors, research, support groups, email lists, personal stories and much more. Updated regularly.

6352 Helios Health

www.helioshealth.com

Online resource for your health information. Detailed information about specific health topics, access to expert advice from our Medical Advisory Board, and up-to-date health news.

6353 International Society for the Study of Dissociation

www.issd.org

Association that promotes research and training in the identification of treatment of multiple personality.

6354 MedicineNet

www.medicinenet.com

An online resource for consumers providing easy-to-read, authoritative medical and health information.

6355 Medscape

www.medscape.com

Medscape offers specialists, primary care physicians, and other health professionals the Web's most robust and integrated medical information and educational tools.

6356 National Alliance for the Mentally Ill

www.nami.org

Mental health organization dedicated to building better lives for the millions of Americans affected by mental illness.

6357 Schizophrenia Therapy Online Resource Center

www.schizophreniatherapy.com

A website which provides effective and lasting alternatives to traditional treatment for individuals suffering with schizophrenia. Offers an effective and full continium of services ranging from psychopharmacology to individual and group psychotherapy to social rehabilitation, supported work experience, assertive community training and supported housing.

6358 WebMD

www.webmd.com

Provides credible information, supportive communities, and in-depth reference material about health subjects. A source for original and timely health information as well as material from well known content providers.

Description

6359 Migraine

Roughly 45 million Americans suffer from chronic headaches, the most disabling of which is migraine. Classified as a vascular headache, migraine headaches are caused by intracranial vasospasm, that is, alternating swelling and constricting of blood vessels on the surface of the brain. The swelling phase brings on intense pain and nausea, while the constricting phase may cause neurologic symptoms such as focal loss of vision or numbness involving one side of the body. Another theory is that migraines are due to a different dysfunction of the neurovascular system that results in the release of a substance that leads to migraine. More than 50 percent of patients have a family history of migraine. They also appear to have a hormonal component, being more common in women and often affected by menstrual cycles or pregnancy.

Management of migraine begins with careful observation for triggering agents like foods, alcohol, or irregular sleep patterns. Acute treatment to stop a migraine involves a class of drugs which antagonize the action of the 5-HT that aggravates the migraine process. They block inflammation and can abort migraine in about 70 percent of patients. Sumatriptan, the prototype, is available in oral and subcutaneous injection forms. Ergot drugs, also available in oral and injectable forms, work by helping the swollen blood vessels constrict down to normal size. If headaches become very frequent, doctors may recommend preventive therapy, which requires daily drug administration. Drugs used in this way include beta-blockers and calcium-channel blockers, which were originally developed for hypertension and heart disease, and certain medicines ordinarily used for depression or seizures.

Pain medication should be used sparingly. Nonsteroidal anti-inflammatory drugs, such as ibuprofen are best for mild to moderate headaches. Narcotic medications should be avoided except under special circumstances and with strict guidelines. Most migraine sufferers can be satisfactorily managed by their primary care physician or a neurologist, but in refractory cases a multi-disciplinary headache center may be of help.

Tension is the other common cause of disabling headaches. They are not migraine and are not considered vascular headache, but are mentioned here because they are so common. Some of the resources listed in this section may be helpful for persons with tension headache.

National Agencies & Associations

6360 American Academy of Neurology
201 Chicago Avenue   612-928-6000
Minneapolis, MN 55415-2311   800-879-1960
                                       Fax: 612-454-2746
e-mail: memberservices@aan.com
www.aan.com

A professional organization representing neurologists worldwide.
Timothy A Pedley, President
Catherine M Rydell, Executive Director & CEO

6361 American Council for Headache Education
19 Mantua Road   856-423-0043
Mount Royal, NJ 08061   800-255-2243
                                       Fax: 856-423-0082
e-mail: achehq@talley.com
www.achenet.org

A not-for-profit alliance of headache sufferers and physicians who are working together to improve the quality of care and the quality of information available to people with chronic or severe headache conditions.
Paul Winner, Chair
Dawn C Buse, PhD, Member of Committee

6362 American Headache Society
19 Mantua Road   856-423-0043
Mount Royal, NJ 08061   Fax: 856-423-0082
e-mail: ahshq@talley.com
www.americanheadachesociety.org/

Professional society of health care providers who study and treat headache and face pain. AHS brings physicians from various fields and specialties together to share concepts and developments about headache and related conditions.
Linda Lucas BA, Director

6363 Help for Headaches
515 Richmond Street   519-434-0008
London, Ontario, N6A 5-5M3 e-mail: brent@helpforheadaches.org
www.headache-help.org

A non-profit organization, and a registered Canadian charity that is committed to educational services for those suffering from and treating headaches.
G Brent Lucas, BA, Director

6364 Migraine Association of Canada
356 Bloor Street E   416-920-4916
Toronto Ontario, M4W   800-663-3557
                                       Fax: 416-920-3677
www.migraine.ca

A registered charity funded through memberships. Activities include a 24 hour telephone information access line the development of materials and assistance for those who start community self-help groups, workplace seminars and awareness programs.
Coleman, President
Terri Miller Burchfield, Exec VP & Legislative Director

6365 Migraine Awareness Group: A National Understanding for Migraineurs
100 N Union Street   703-349-1929
Alexandria, VA 22314   Fax: 703-739-2432
e-mail: comments@migraines.org
www.migraines.org

Works to bring public awareness utilizing the electronic print and artistic mediums to the fact that migraine is a true organic neurological disease.
Michael John Coleman, President & Executive Director
Terri Miller Burchfield, Executive VP & Legislative Director

6366 National Headache Foundation
820 N Orleans   312-274-2650
Chicago, IL 60610-3132   888-NHF-5552
                                       Fax: 312-640-9049
e-mail: info@headaches.org
www.headaches.org

A nonprofit organization established in 1970 dedicated to serve as an information resource to headache sufferers, their families and the healthcare providers who treat them. Promotes research into potential headache causes and treatments.
Seymour Diamond, MD, Founder & Executive Chairman
Arthur H Elkind, MD, President

Research Centers

6367 Baltimore Headache Institute
11 E Chase Street   410-547-0200
Baltimore, MD 21202
Brian E Goldstein, Director

6368 San Francisco Clinical Research Center
909 Hyde Street   415-673-4600
San Francisco, CA 94109   Fax: 415-673-9352
                                    e-mail: SFHACLIN@aol.com
                                           www.sfcrc.com
This research center also specializes in diagnosis of Alzheimer's
related dementia in addition to migraine headaches.
Jerome Goldstein, M.D., Director
Guy Engelmann, M.D., Team Member

Support Groups & Hotlines

6369 National Health Information Center
PO Box 1133   310-565-4167
Washington, DC 20013   800-336-4797
                                    Fax: 301-984-4256
                                    e-mail: info@nhic.org
                                       www.health.gov/nhic
Offers a nationwide information referral service, produces direc-
tories and resource guides.

Books

6370 Conquering Headache
Alan Rapoport, MD, author
B.C Decker, Inc.
50 King Street E, Floor 2   905-522-7017
Ontario, Canada L8N 3K7,   800-568-7281
                                    Fax: 905-522-7839
                                    e-mail: info@bcdecker.com
                                           www.bcdecker.com
Conquering Headache, Fourth Edition provides the information
needed to conquer headaches and improve the quality of life.ÿ
2003 128 pages Paperback
ISBN: 1-550092-33-2
Alan M. Rapoport, Author
Fred D. Sheftellÿ, Author

6371 Freedom from Headaches
Simon & Schuster Order Department
200 Old Tappan Road
Old Tappan, NJ 07675-7095   800-999-5479
Headache pain is unlike any other pain; when your head throbs,
your entire body suffers.

ISBN: 0-671254-04-9
Joel R. Saper, Author

6372 Handbook of Headache Disorders
Essential Medical Information Systems
PO Box 1607   580-924-0643
Durant, OK 74702-1607   800-225-0694
                                    Fax: 580-924-9414
1993 Paperback
ISBN: 0-929240-62-6

**6373 Handbook of Headache Management: A Practic al Guide to
Diagnosis & Treatment**
Williams & Wilkins
351 W Camden Street   301-528-4000
Baltimore, MD 21201-7912   800-638-0672
                                          www.wwilkins.com
1993 224 pages
ISBN: 0-683058-01-0
Paoloÿ Martelletti, Editor
Timothy J Steiner, Editor

6374 Migraine and Other Headaches: Vascular Mechanisms
Raven Press

1185 Ave of the Americas   212-930-9500
New York, NY 10036-2601   800-777-2295
                                          www.raven.com
Leading international experts present new concepts on the mechanisms of migraine and other vascular headaches and detail the latest strategies for diagnosis and treatment of migraine with and
without aura, tension-type headaches, cluster headaches and other
vascular disorders.
368 pages
ISBN: 0-881677-95-7

6375 Migraine: The Complete Guide
American Council for Headache Education
19 Mantua Road   856-423-0258
Mount Royal, NJ 08061   800-255-2243
                                    Fax: 856-423-0082
                                    e-mail: achehq@talley.com
                                           www.achenet.org
A comprehensive resource book for people with migraine, their
families and physicians (updated in 1999) by Lynne M
Constantine, Suzanne Scott and ACHE.
Teriÿ Robert, Chair
Dr. Paul Winner, Co-Chair

6376 Overcoming Headaches & Migraines
Longmeadow Press
19 Mantua Road   856-423-0258
Mount Royal, NJ 08061-1469   800-255-2243
                                    Fax: 856-423-0082
                                    e-mail: achehq@talley.com
                                           www.achenet.org
1993 128 pages Paperback
ISBN: 0-681417-92-7
Teriÿ Robert, Chair
Dr. Paul Winner, Co-Chair

6377 Understanding Migrain and Other Headaches
Stewart J Tepper, MD, author
University Press of Mississippi
3825 Ridgewood Road   601-432-6205
Jackson, MS 39211-6492   Fax: 601-432-6217
                                    e-mail: press@ihl.state.ms.us
                                           www.upress.state.ms.us
A comprehensive overview of causes, diagnoses, and treatments.
2004 112 pages Paperback
ISBN: 1-578065-92-5
Chip Mercer, Sales Representative
Jim Barkley, Sales Representative

6378 Wolff's Headaches & Other Head Pain
Oxford University Press
2001 Evans Road   212-726-6000
Cary, NC 27513-2010   800-445-9714
                                    Fax: 919-677-1303
                                    e-mail: custserv.us@oup.com
                                           www.oup-usa.org
1993
ISBN: 0-195082-50-8

Newsletters

6379 Headache
American Council for Headache Education
19 Mantua Road   856-423-0258
Mount Royal, NJ 08061   800-255-2243
                                    Fax: 856-423-0082
                                    e-mail: achehq@talley.com
                                           www.achenet.org
The ACHE 12 page quarterly newsletter provides valuable and
current information on new treatments, as well as time proven
headache management strategies. All articles are written or reviewed by headache experts from the American Headache Society
(AHS). Recent issues have included articles by headache experts
on drug and nondrug treatment options and information on new
treatments and research is regularly included.
Quarterly
Teriÿ Robert, Chair
Dr. Paul Winner, Co-Chair

6380 NHF Head Lines
National Headache Foundation
820 N Orleans   312-274-2650
Chicago, IL 60610-3132   888-643-5552
                                   Fax: 312-640-9049
                        e-mail: info@headaches.org
                              www.headaches.org

Offers the latest information on headaches, causes and treatments. Contains news on drugs and medical forums, in depth discussions of headaches and preventions and a question and answer section in which physicians respond to reader inquiries and support group information.
16 pages Quarterly
Arthur H. Elkind, President
Vincent Martin, Vice President

Pamphlets

6381 52 Proven Stress Reducers
National Headache Foundation
820 N Orleans   312-274-2650
Chicago, IL 60610   888-643-5552
                                   Fax: 312-640-9049
                        e-mail: info@headaches.org
                              www.headaches.org

Members only.
Suzanne Simons, Executive Director

6382 About Headaches
National Headache Foundation
820 N Orleans   312-274-2650
Chicago, IL 60610   888-643-5552
                                   Fax: 312-640-9049
                        e-mail: info@headaches.org
                              www.headaches.org

Contains an in depth look at headaches, tips on when to seek medical advice, methods of treatment and more.
16 pages
Suzanne Simons, Executive Director

6383 Analgesic Rebound Headaches: Fact Sheet
National Headache Foundation
820 N Orleans   312-274-2650
Chicago, IL 60610   888-643-5552
                                   Fax: 312-640-9049
                        e-mail: info@headaches.org
                              www.headaches.org

Offers information on analgesic agents or drugs used to control pain including migraine and other types of headaches.
Suzanne Simons, Executive Director

6384 Cluster Headache: Fact Sheet
National Headache Foundation
820 N Orleans   312-274-2650
Chicago, IL 60610   888-643-5552
                                   Fax: 312-640-9049
                        e-mail: info@headaches.org
                              www.headaches.org

Offers information on cluster headaches and the treatment available for them. This information sheet can be downloaded from the web site.
Suzanne Simons, Executive Director

6385 Diet and Headache: Fact Sheet
National Headache Foundation
820 N Orleans   312-274-2650
Chicago, IL 60610   888-643-5552
                                   Fax: 312-640-9049
                        e-mail: info@headaches.org
                              www.headaches.org

Offers information on what foods should be avoided and what foods trigger headaches in all migraine sufferers. This information sheet can be dowloaded from the web site.
Suzanne Simons, Executive Director

6386 Headache Facts: What Everyone Should Know
American Council for Headache Education

19 Mantua Road   856-423-0258
Mount Royal, NJ 08061   800-255-2243
                                   Fax: 856-423-0082
                        e-mail: achehq@talley.com
                              www.achenet.org

Teriÿ Robert, Chair
Dr. Paul Winner, Co-Chair

6387 Headache Handbook
National Headache Foundation
820 N Orleans   312-274-2650
Chicago, IL 60610   888-643-5552
                                   Fax: 312-640-9049
                        e-mail: info@headaches.org
                              www.headaches.org

Gives information on causes and types of headaches as well as treatments available.
8 pages
Teriÿ Robert, Chair
Dr. Paul Winner, Co-Chair

6388 Headache in Children: Fact Sheet
National Headache Foundation
820 N Orleans   312-274-2650
Chicago, IL 60610   888-643-5552
                                   Fax: 312-640-9049
                        e-mail: info@headaches.org
                              www.headaches.org

Offers information on vascular headaches, tension-type headaches, traction and inflammatory headaches and treatment. This information sheet can be downloaded from the web site.
Suzanne Simons, Executive Director

6389 Hormones and Migraines: Fact Sheet
National Headache Foundation
820 N Orleans   312-274-2650
Chicago, IL 60610   888-643-5552
                                   Fax: 312-640-9049
                        e-mail: info@headaches.org
                              www.headaches.org

Offers information on the link between hormones and migraines.
Suzanne Simons, Executive Director

6390 How to Talk to Your Doctor About Headaches
National Headache Foundation
820 N Orleans   312-274-2650
Chicago, IL 60610   888-643-5552
                                   Fax: 312-640-9049
                        e-mail: info@headaches.org
                              www.headaches.org

Learn how to keep a headache diary to pinpoint symptoms and effective diagnosis.
Suzanne Simons, Executive Director

6391 Impact of Migraine: A Disabling and Costly Condition
American Council for Headache Education
19 Mantua Road   856-423-0258
Mount Royal, NJ 08061   800-255-2243
                                   Fax: 856-423-0082
                        e-mail: achehq@talley.com
                              www.achenet.org

Teriÿ Robert, Chair
Dr. Paul Winner, Co-Chair

6392 Migraine and Coexisting Conditions: Other Illnesses That May Affect Migraine
American Council for Headache Education
19 Mantua Road   856-423-0258
Mount Royal, NJ 08061   800-255-2243
                                   Fax: 856-423-0082
                        e-mail: achehq@talley.com
                              www.achenet.org

Teriÿ Robert, Chair
Dr. Paul Winner, Co-Chair

6393 Migraine: Fact Sheet
National Headache Foundation

820 N Orleans
Chicago, IL 60610

312-274-2650
888-643-5552
Fax: 312-640-9049
e-mail: info@headaches.org
www.headaches.org

Offers information on migraines and treatments.
Suzanne Simons, Executive Director

6394   Tap the Best Resource
National Headache Foundation
820 N Orleans
Chicago, IL 60610

312-274-2650
888-643-5552
Fax: 312-640-9049
e-mail: info@headaches.org
www.headaches.org

Informational brochure offering facts and statistics on headaches. Everything from muscle contraction, vascular headaches, sinus headaches, TMJ and much more.
Suzanne Simons, Executive Director

6395   Tension-Type Headache: Fact Sheet
National Headache Foundation
820 N Orleans
Chicago, IL 60610

312-274-2650
888-643-5552
Fax: 312-640-9049
e-mail: info@headaches.org
www.headaches.org

Offers information on the least known type of headache, chronic tension-type headaches. This information sheet can be downloaded from the web site.
Teriÿ Robert, Chair
Dr. Paul Winner, Co-Chair

6396   What's the Best Medicine for My Headaches?
American Council for Headache Education
19 Mantua Road
Mount Royal, NJ 08061

856-423-0258
800-255-2243
Fax: 856-423-0082
e-mail: achehq@talley.com
www.achenet.org

Teriÿ Robert, Chair
Dr. Paul Winner, Co-Chair

Audio & Video

6397   Relaxation Tape
National Headache Foundation
820 N Orleans
Chicago, IL 60610

312-274-2650
888-643-5552
Fax: 312-640-9049
e-mail: info@headaches.org
www.headaches.org

Contains techniques to assist the listener in experiencing greater self control and relaxation.
Audio Tape
Suzanne Simons, Executive Director

6398   Stretch and Relax Tape
National Headache Foundation
820 N Orleans
Chicago, IL 60610

312-274-2650
888-643-5552
Fax: 312-640-9049
e-mail: info@headaches.org
www.headaches.org

Based on a series of progressive relaxation techniques which involve the tightening and relaxing of specific muscle groups.
Audio Tape
Suzanne Simons, Executive Director

Web Sites

6399   American Academy of Neurology

www.aan.com/
A professional organization representing neurologists worldwide.

6400   American Council for Headache Education (ACHE)
www.achenet.org

The ACHE website offers an extensive library of headache information, including a searchable database of past articles from our newsletter, discussion forums that provide virtual contact with leading headache specialists and fellow headache sufferers, a searchable database of physicians to find a specialist in your area and more.

6401   American Headache Society
www.americanheadachesociety.org
The American Headache Society (AHS) is a professional society of health care providers dedicated to the study and treatment of headache and face pain. Educating physicians, health professionals and the public and encouraging scientific research are the primary functions of this organization.

6402   American Medical Association
Journal of the American Medical Association
www.ama-assn.org/
An organized web site focusing on treatment options, education and support available to those suffering from migraine headaches.

6403   Cluster Headaches
www.clusterheadaches.com
A web site devoted completely and exclusively to those that suffer from cluster headaches.

6404   Healing Well
www.healingwell.com
An online health resource guide to medical news, chat, information and articles, newsgroups and message boards, books, disease-related web sites, medical directories, and more for patients, friends, and family coping with disabling diseases, disorders, or chronic illnesses.

6405   Health Finder
www.healthfinder.gov
Searchable, carefully developed web site offering information on over 1000 topics. Developed by the US Department of Health and Human Services, the site can be used in both English and Spanish.

6406   Healthlink USA
www.healthlinkusa.com
Health information concerning treatment, cures, prevention, diagnosis, risk factors, research, support groups, email lists, personal stories and much more. Updated regularly.

6407   Helios Health
www.helioshealth.com
Online resource for your health information. Detailed information about specific health topics, access to expert advice from our Medical Advisory Board, and up-to-date health news.

6408   MedicineNet
www.medicinenet.com
An online resource for consumers providing easy-to-read, authoritative medical and health information.

6409   Medscape
www.medscape.com
Medscape offers specialists, primary care physicians, and other health professionals the Web's most robust and integrated medical information and educational tools.

6410   Medsupport
michiganheadache.com
The Michigan Headache Clinic has been evolving in Michigan since 1981 and consists of our centrally located headache clinic, our web-based headache information pages and a working relationship we have developed with many skilled colleagues in different parts of Michigan over the years.

6411   Migraine Awareness Group: A National Understanding for Migraineurs
www.migraines.org/
Works to bring public awareness, utilizing the electronic, print, and artistic mediums, to the fact that migraine is a true organic neurological disease.

6412   National Headache Foundation
www.headaches.org
Information for headache sufferers, their families, and the physicians who treat them.

6413   Neurology Channel

www.healthcommunities.com

Find clearly explained, medically accurate information regarding conditions, including an overview, symptoms, causes, diagnostic procedures and treatment options. On this site it is possible to ask questions and get information from a neurologist and connect to people who have similar health interests.

6414   WebMD

www.webmd.com

Provides credible information, supportive communities, and in-depth reference material about health subjects. A source for original and timely health information as well as material from well known content providers.

Description

6415 Multiple Sclerosis

Multiple sclerosis, MS, is a chronic disease that affects the central nervous system and impairs many of its functions. Over 300,000 Americans have MS. Although its cause is unknown, an immunologic abnormality is suspected. There also appear to be both genetic and environmental factors involved. Interestingly, the incidence of MS increases the further one lives from the equator.

Age of onset is typically between 20 and 40 years, and women are affected somewhat more than men. MS destroys the protective myelin sheath that surrounds nerve fibers. This special sheath normally allows passage of electrical signals through the brain, spinal cord, and nerves of the body. The disease is characterized by remissions and recurring exacerbations. The clinical signs vary depending on the area of demyelination and can include: generalized or focal weakness; difficulty walking; clumsiness; slurred speech; easy fatigability; numbness and tingling; visual loss; incontinence (loss of bladder and bowel control); loss of sexual function; and problems with short-term memory, judgment, or reason.

Significant strides are being made in both treating and understanding MS. Currently there is no curative treatment, but corticosteroids, interferon and other new medications may shorten or prevent relapses.

Supportive treatment includes medications to control muscle spasticity, fatigue and pain. Maintaining a normal lifestyle is recommended, avoiding fatigue and exposure to excessive heat. Physical therapy may also be helpful. Because of the debilitating nature of MS, counseling, psychiatric support, and antidepressant medication may be warranted.

National Agencies & Associations

6416 Multiple Sclerosis Association of America
706 Haddonfield Road
Cherry Hill, NJ 08002-2652
856-488-4500
800-532-7667
Fax: 856-661-9797
e-mail: webmaster@mymsaa.org
www.mymsaa.org/
A national nonprofit organization dedicated to enriching the quality of life for everyone affected by multiple sclerosis.
Robert Manley, Chair
Sue Rehmus, Vice Chair

6417 Multiple Sclerosis Foundation
6350 N Andrews Avenue
Fort Lauderdale, FL 33309
954-776-6805
888-225-6495
Fax: 954-938-8708
e-mail: admin@msfocus.org
www.msfocus.org
Dedicated to helping create a brighter tomorrow for those with MS the foundation offers a wide array of free services including: national toll-free support, educational programs, homecare, support groups, assistive technology and publications.
Jules Kuperberg, Executive Director
Alan Segaloff, Executive Director

6418 National Institute of Neurological Disorders and Stroke
NIH Neurological Institute
Bethesda, MD 20824
301-496-5751
800-352-9424
Fax: 301-402-2186
TTY: 301-468-5981
www.ninds.nih.gov
The mission of NINDS is to reduce the burden of neurological disease - a burden borne by every age group, by every segment of society, by people all over the world.
Story C Landis, PhD, Director
Walter J Koroshetz, M.D., Deputy Director

6419 National Multiple Sclerosis Society
733 3rd Avenue
New York, NY 10017-3288
212-986-3240
800-344-4867
Fax: 212-986-7981
e-mail: nat@nmss.org
www.nationalmssociety.org/
Serves persons with MS, their families, health professionals and the interested public. The Society provides funding for research, public and professional education, advocacy and the design of rehabilitative and psychosocial programs. Direct services to MS persons are provided through local chapters and branches. Among the services offered are counseling, referral, equipment loan and other support activities.
Eli Rubenstein, Chairman of the Board
Cynthia Zagieboylo, President & CEO

6420 Toronto Parents of Multiple Births Associa tion
790 Bay Street
Toronto, Ontario, M5G 1-1N9
416-760-3944
e-mail: info@tpomba.org
www.tpomba.org
A not-for-profit self-help and support organization in Canada for parents of twins, triplets, and more.
Laura Daniel, Chapter President
Taylor Lander, Development Manager

State Agencies & Associations

Alabama

6421 National Multiple Sclerosis Society: Alabama Chapter
813 Shades Creek Parkway
Birmingham, AL 35209
205-879-8881
800-FIG-HTMS
Fax: 205-879-8869
e-mail: alc@nmss.org
www.nationalmssociety.org/alc
Dedicated to serving people with MS and their families by providing programs and services designed to enhance quality of life.
Frank D McPhillips, Chairman
Jan Bell, Chapter President

Alaska

6422 National Multiple Sclerosis Society: Alaska Chapter
511 W 41st Avenue
Anchorage, AK 99503-6643
907-563-1115
800-344-4867
Fax: 907-562-6673
e-mail: aka@nmss.org
www.nationalmssociety.org/aka
Nonprofit organization providing equipment loan, information and referral, leading library, self-help groups, advocacy, education, training, newsletter, educational programs, volunteer opportunities, exercise/aquatics, newly diagnosed support and educational material.
Gary Wells, Regional Development Manager
Pam McElrath, President, All American Chapter

Arizona

6423 National Multiple Sclerosis Society Desert Southwest Chapter
National Multiple Sclerosis Society
5025 E. Washington Street
Phoenix, AZ 85034-2343
480-968-2488
800-344-4867
Fax: 602-966-4049
e-mail: info@aza.nmss.org
www.nationalmssociety.org
Serves Central and Northern Arizona.

Arkansas

6424 National Multiple Sclerosis Society: Arkansas Chapter
Evergreen Place
1100 N University Avenue   501-663-8104
Little Rock, AR 72207-6367   800-344-4867
                                       Fax: 501-666-4355
                                       e-mail: arr@nmss.org
                                       www.nationalmssociety.org/arr
Rick Selig, Division Manager

California

6425 Central California Chapter National Multiple Sclerosis Society
National Multiple Sclerosis Society
334 Shaw Avenue   209-325-9293
Clovis, CA 93612-3839   Fax: 209-325-9295
                                       www.nationalmssociety.org
Dan Dietrich, Development Director
Karen Nunn, Service Director

6426 National Multiple Sclerosis Society: Southern California Chapter
2440 S Sepulveda Boulevard   310-479-4456
Los Angeles, CA 90064   800-344-4867
                                       Fax: 310-479-4436
                                       e-mail: ms@cal.nmss.org
                                       www.nationalmssociety.org
Leon A LeBuffe, President

6427 National Multiple Sclerosis Society Channel Islands Chapter
14 W Valerio Street   805-682-8783
Santa Barbara, CA 93101   800-344-4867
                                       Fax: 805-563-1489
                                       e-mail: can_info@nmss.org
                                       www.nationalmssociety.org
Joan Young, Chapter President

6428 National Multiple Sclerosis Society: Silicon Valley Chapter
2589 Scott Boulevard   408-988-7557
Santa Clara, CA 95050-2508   800-344-4867
                                       Fax: 408-988-1816
                                       e-mail: cau@nmss.org
                                       www.nationalmssociety.org
Funds, researches and supports people with MS and their families
to end the devastating effects of multiple sclerosis.
Carla Hines, Chapter President
Michelle Spam-Allen, Program Director

6429 Northern California Chapter National Multiple Sclerosis Society
National Multiple Sclerosis Society
1700 Owens Street   415-230-6678
San Francisco, CA 94158   800-344-4867
                                       Fax: 415-230-6652
                                       e-mail: can_info@nmss.org
                                       www.nationalmssociety.org
David Hartman, Chapter President
Denise Casey, Director of Chapter Programs

6430 Orange County Chapter National Multiple Sclerosis Society
National Multiple Sclerosis Society
5950 La Place Court   760-448-8400
Carlsbad, CA 92008-5677   800-344-4867
                                       Fax: 949-833-3104
                                       e-mail: msinfo@mspacific.org
                                       www.nationalmssociety.org
Richard V Israel, Chapter President
Karen Hooper, Vice President Programs & Services

6431 San Diego Area Chapter National Multiple Sclerosis Society
National Multiple Sclerosis Society
12121 Scripps Summit Dr   619-974-8640
San Diego, CA 92131-1498   800-486-6762
                                       Fax: 760-804-9266
                                       e-mail: msinfo@mspacific.org
                                       www.nationalmssociety.org
Allan Shaw, Chapter President
Karen Barton, Service Director

Colorado

6432 National MS Society: Colorado Chapter
900 S Broadway   303-698-7400
Denver, CO 80209-3442   800-344-4867
                                       Fax: 303-698-7421
                                       e-mail: co-wyreceptionist@nmss.org
                                       www.nationalmssociety.org/chapters/COC/i
Carrie Nolan, President
Mary Ann Peters, Executive Assistant

Connecticut

6433 National MS Society: Greater Connecticut Chapter
659 Tower Avenue   860-913-2550
Hartford, CT 06112   800-344-4867
                                       Fax: 860-761-2466
                                       e-mail: info@ctfightsMS.org
                                       www.nationalmssociety.org/chapters/CTN/i
Lisa Gerrol, President and Chief Professional Officer
Cheryl Donati, Executive Vice President

Delaware

6434 National MS Society: Delaware Chapter
2 Mill Road   302-655-5610
Wilmington, DE 19806-2175   800-344-4867
                                       Fax: 302-655-0993
                                       e-mail: kate.cowperthwait@msdelaware.org
                                       www.nationalmssociety.org/chapters/DED/i
Provides the encouragement, materials and skills needed to
achieve and maintain a productive lifestyle with multiple sclerosis. The organization is a voluntary, nonprofit entity.
1100 members
Kate Cowperthwait, Chapter President
Helen Serbu, Director of Finance

District of Columbia

6435 National MS Society: National Capital Chapter
1800 M Street   202-296-5363
Washington, DC 20036-1003   800-344-4867
                                       Fax: 202-296-3425
                                       e-mail: INFORMATION@MSandYOU.ORG
                                       www.nationalmssociety.org/chapters/DCW/i
J Christophe Broullire, Chapter President
Kevin Dougherty, Vice President Programs and Services

Florida

6436 Central Florida Chapter
2701 Maitland Center Parkway   407-478-8880
Orlando, FL 32751-6726   800-344-4867
                                       Fax: 407-478-8893
                                       e-mail: INFO@FLC.NMSS.ORG
                                       www.nationalmssociety.org/chapters/FLC/i
Tami Caesar, President
Ryan Bumgardner, Bike MS Manager

6437 Florida Gulf Coast Chapter National Multiple Sclerosis Society
National Multiple Sclerosis Society
4919 Memorial Highway   813-889-8303
Tampa, FL 33634-3540   800-344-4867
                                       Fax: 813-889-8313
                                       www.nationalmssociety.org/chapters/FLC/i
Judy Wilkinson, Service Director
Tim Hanke, Chairman

6438 Goodwill Industries-Suncoast
Goodwill Industries-Suncoast
2421 4th Street North   727-523-1512
St. Petersburg, FL 33704   888-279-1988
                                       Fax: 727-577-2749
                                       www.goodwill-suncoast.org
A nonprofit community based organization whose purpose is to improve the quality of life for people who are disabled, disadvantaged and/or aged. This mission is accomplished through a staff of
over 1,200 employees providing independent living skills, affordable housing, career assessment and planning, job skills, training,
placement, and job retention assistance with useful employment.

Annually, Goodwill Industries-Suncoast serves over 30,000 people in Citrus, Hernando, Levy, Marion and more.
Oscar J.ÿ Horton, Chair
Martin W Gladyszÿ, Sr. Vice Chair

6439   National Multiple Sclerosis Society: North Florida Chapter
4237 Salisbury Road   904-332-6810
Jacksonville, FL 32216-8171   800-344-4867
                                                    Fax: 904-332-0898
                                                    TDD: 800-955-8770
                                        e-mail: msnorfla@fln.nmss.org
                                        www.nationalmssociety.org/fln

Jennifer Lee, Chapter President
Sabrah Witkamp, Client Program Director

6440   South Florida Chapter National Multiple Sclerosis Society
National Multiple Sclerosis Society
3201 W Commercial Boulevard   954-731-4224
Fort Lauderdale, FL 33309-6350   800-344-4867
                                                    Fax: 954-739-1398
                                            e-mail: fls@nmss.org
                                        fls.nationalmssociety.org

Karen Dresbach, Chapter President
Fred Zuckerman, Chairman

Georgia

6441   National MS Society: Georgia Chapter
1117 Perimeter Center W   678-672-1000
Atlanta, GA 30338-3097   800-344-4867
                                                    Fax: 678-672-1015
                                    e-mail: gaa.mailbox@nmss.org
                                    www.nationalmssociety.org/chapters/GAA/i
Roy A Rangel, Chapter President
Nicole Hill, Director of Finance & Administrative

Hawaii

6442   National MS Society: Hawaii Chapter
418 Kuwili Street   808-532-0806
Honolulu, HI 96817   800-344-4867
                                                    Fax: 808-532-0814
                                            e-mail: HIH@NMSS.ORG
                                    www.nationalmssociety.org/chapters/HIH/i
Jeffrey D Peier, Chairman
Pam McElrath, President

Idaho

6443   National MS Society: Idaho Division
6901 W Emerald Street   208-388-4253
Boise, ID 83704   800-344-4867
                                                    Fax: 208-388-1907
                                            e-mail: idi@nmss.org
                                    www.nationalmssociety.org/chapters/IDI/i
Pam McElrath, Chapter President
Suzanne Bland, Executive Vice President

Illinois

6444   National MS Society: Chicago, Greater Illinois Chapter
525 West Monroe Street   312-922-8000
Chicago, IL 60661-3814   800-344-4867
                                                    Fax: 312-922-2752
                                        e-mail: cgic@ild.nmss.org
                                        www.nationalmssociety.org
The Greater Illnois Chapter is comprised of all the Illinoisans whohave chosen to fight MS and the work that they do through the National Multiple Sclerosis Society Volunteers, staff, healthcare workers, researchers, donors, advocated, and partners together represent the Greater Illinoisans Chapter, and all the many ways it's possible to join the fight against multiple sclerosis.
Steven Pratapous, Chapter President

Indiana

6445   National MS Society: Indiana State Chapter
3500 DePauw Blvd.   317-870-2500
Indianapolis, IN 46268   800-344-4867
                                                    Fax: 317-870-2520
                                        e-mail: Indiana@nmss.org
                                    www.nationalmssociety.org/chapters/INI/i
Tiffany Bogard, Chapter President
Lisa Coffman, Director of Chapter Programs

Iowa

6446   National MS Society: Iowa Chapter
8187 University Boulevard   515-270-6337
Clive, IA 50325   800-344-4867
                                                    Fax: 515-270-0337
                                        e-mail: mark.davis@nmss.org
                                    www.nationalmssociety.org/chapters/NTH/a
Brett Ridge, Chapter President
Mark Davis, Area Director

Kansas

6447   National MS Society: Mid-America Chapter
7611 State Line   913-432-3926
Kansas City, KS 64114-2915   800-344-4867
                                                    Fax: 816-361-2369
                                        e-mail: info@nmsskc.org
                                    www.nationalmssociety.org/chapters/KSG/i
The National Multiple Sclerosis Society is a not-for-profit organization serving people with MS in every state. The Mid-America Chapter serves the 25,000 people who are affected by MS in eastern Kansas and western Missouri.
Kay Julian, Chapter President
Amy Goldstein, Program Director

6448   National MS Society: South Central & West Kansas Division
9415 E Harry Street   316-264-7043
Wichita, KS 67211-1515   800-344-4867
                                                    Fax: 316-264-5436
                                        e-mail: KSS@NMSS.ORG
                                    www.nationalmssociety.org/chapters/KSS/i
Cammy Mathews, Donor Relations Coordinator
Becky Kimbell, Regional Programs and Services Manager

Kentucky

6449   National MS Society: Kentucky Chapter
1201 Story Avenue   502-451-0014
Louisville, KY 40206   800-344-4867
                                                    Fax: 502-581-1010
                                        e-mail: KYW@NMSS.ORG
                                        www.nationalmssociety.org
Jeff Hamilton, Chairman
Stacy Funk, Chapter President

Louisiana

6450   National Multiple Sclerosis Society: Louisiana
4613 Fairfield Street   504-832-4013
Metairie, LA 70006   800-344-4867
                                                    Fax: 504-831-7188
                                e-mail: louisianachapter@lam.nmss.org
                                www.nationalmssociety.org/chapters/LAM/i
Brian Berrigon, Chapter President
Crystal Smith, Director of Programs and Services

Maine

6451   National MS Society: Maine Chapter
170 US Route One   800-344-4867
Falmouth, ME 04105   800-344-4867
                                                    Fax: 207-781-7961
                                        e-mail: info@msmaine.org
                                    www.nationalmssociety.org/chapters/MEM/i
The National Multiple Sclerosis Societ is dedicated to enind the devastating the devastating effects of multiple sciersis, a chronic,

disease of the central nervous system often diagnosed in young adults
Robin Doughty, Director of Finance & Operations
Denise Clavette, Chapter President

Maryland

6452 **National MS Society: Maryland Chapter Hunt Valley Business Center**
Hunt Valley Business Center
2219 York Road.   443-641-1200
Timonium, MD 21093   800-344-4867
                              Fax: 443-641-1201
              e-mail: INFO@NMSS-MD.ORG
          www.nationalmssociety.org/chapters/MDM/i
Mark Roeder, Chapter President
Nicole Weedon, Executive Assistant/Office Manager

Massachusetts

6453 **National MS Society: Massachusetts Chapter**
101A 1st Avenue   781-890-4990
Waltham, MA 02451-1160   800-344-4867
                              Fax: 781-890-2089
           e-mail: CommunicationsGNE@nmss.org
          www.nationalmssociety.org/chapters/MAM/i
Linda Guiod, Executive Vice President
Arlyn White, Chapter President & CEO

Michigan

6454 **National MS Society: Michigan Chapter**
21311 Civic Center Drive   248-351-2190
Southfield, MI 48076   800-344-4867
                              Fax: 248-350-0029
              e-mail: info@mig.nmss.org
          www.nationalmssociety.org/mig
Offer a variety of programs and services benefiting people with multiple sclerosis and their family members. Programs include educational seminars, information and referrals, peer support, advocacy, free legal clinic, financial assistance for medical equipment, medical transportation, home care, technical assistance and much more
Elana Sullivan, Chapter President
Melissa Ryan, Executive Administrative Assistant

Minnesota

6455 **National MS Society: Minnesota Chapter**
200 12th Avenue S   612-335-7900
Minneapolis, MN 55415   800-344-4867
                              Fax: 612-335-7997
              e-mail: INFO@MSSOCIETY.ORG
          www.nationalmssociety.org/chapters/MNM/i

Mississippi

6456 **National Multiple Sclerosis Society: Alaba ma-Mississippi Chapter**
145 Executive Drive   601-856-5831
Madison, MS 39110-9198   800-344-4867
                              Fax: 601-856-7173
              e-mail: alc@nmss.org
          www.nationalmssociety.org/alc
Angie Jackson, Area Director
Andi Agnew, Programs and Services Coordinator

Missouri

6457 **National MS Society: Gateway Area Chapter**
1867 Lackland Hill Parkway   314-781-9020
Saint Louis, MO 63146-3545   800-344-4867
                              Fax: 314-781-1440
              e-mail: info@mos.nmss.org
          www.nationalmssociety.org/chapters/MOS/i

Sponsors research and offers educational programs, counseling, lending library, referral services, independent living aids, legislative advocacy and therapeutic recreation for people with MS.
Phyllis Robsham, Chapter President
Kathi Taylor, Executive Assistant

Montana

6458 **National MS Society: Montana Division**
1629 Avenue D   406-252-5927
Billings, MT 59102   800-344-4867
                              Fax: 406-252-5956
              e-mail: MTT@NMSS.ORG
          www.nationalmssociety.org/chapters/MTT/i
Rebecca Wiehe, Regional Programs and Services Manager
Heather Ohs, Regional Development~Manager

Nebraska

6459 **National MS Society: Midlands Chapter Community Health Plaza**
Community Health Plaza
328 S 72nd Street   402-505-4000
Omaha, NE 68114-2153   800-344-4867
                              Fax: 402-572-3002
              e-mail: NEN@NMSS.ORG
          www.nationalmssociety.org/chapters/NEN/i
Lisa Brink, Chapter President
Milton Trabal, Director of Finance

Nevada

6460 **Natioanl Multiple Sclerosis Society Desert Southwest Chapter**
National Multiple Sclerosis Society
6000 S Eastern Avenue   702-736-1478
Las Vegas, NV 89119-3157   800-344-4867
                              Fax: 702-736-2487
              e-mail: NVL@NMSS.ORG
          www.nationalmssociety.org/chapters/NVL/i
Serves southern Nevada & northwest Arizona.
Nicole Rainey, Development Coordinator Special Events
Linda Nowell, Programs and Services Coordinator

6461 **National MS Society: Great Basin Sierra Chapter**
4600 Keitzke Lane   702-329-7180
Reno, NV 89502   800-344-4867
                              Fax: 775-827-3167
              e-mail: nvn@nvn.nmss.org
          www.nationalmssociety.org/chapters/NVN/i
Linda Lott, Regional Development Manager
Danielle Lutzow, Programs and Services Coordinator

New Hampshire

6462 **National MS Society: Central New England Chapter**
101A First Avenue   781-890-4990
Waltham, MA 02451-1115   800-493-9255
                              Fax: 781-490-2089
           e-mail: CommunicationsGNE@nmss.org
              www.nationalmssociety.org
Serving people with MS in Massachusetts and New Hampshire.
Judy Cotton, Director Chapter Services
Arlyn White, Chapter President & CEO

New Jersey

6463 **National MS Society: Greater North Jersey Chapter**
1 Kalisa Way   201-967-5599
Paramus, NJ 07652-3550   800-344-4867
                              Fax: 201-967-7085
              e-mail: Njminfo@nmss.org
          www.nationalmssociety.org/chapters/NJM/i
Michael Elkow, Chapter President
Marianne Maddocks, Vice President of Operations

6464 National MS Society: Mid-Jersey Chapter
246 Monmouth Road   732-660-1005
Oakhurst, NJ 07755   800-344-4867
Fax: 732-660-1388
e-mail: Njminfo@nmss.org
www.nationalmssociety.org/chapters/NJM/i
The National Multiple Sclerosis Society is the only voluntary health agency that supports an international program of scientific research designed to cure, prevent and treat MS.
Michael Elkow, Chapter President
Marianne Maddocks, Vice President of Operations

New Mexico

6465 National MS Society: Rio Grande Division
4125-A Carlisle Boulevard NE   505-243-2792
Albuquerque, NM 87107   800-344-4867
Fax: 505-244-0629
e-mail: NMX@NMSS.ORG
www.nationalmssociety.org/chapters/NMX/i
Maggie Schold, Development Coordinator Special Events
Sheri Wharton, Programs and Services Coordinator

New York

6466 National MS Society: Long Island Chapter
40 Marcus Drive   631-864-8337
Melville, NY 11747   800-344-4867
Fax: 631-864-8342
e-mail: PMASTROTA@NMSSLI.ORG
www.nationalmssociety.org/chapters/NYH/i
The National Multiple Sclerosis Society, Long Island Chapter, is dedicated to helping people with MS and their families live useful and fulfilling lives by opening their minds to opportunities and providing the tools to live with dignity.
Pamela Jones Mastrota, President & CEO
Barbara Travis, Vice President of Donor Development

6467 National MS Society: New York City Chapter
733 Third Avenue   212-463-7787
New York, NY 10017-2098   800-344-4867
Fax: 212-989-4362
e-mail: INFO@MSNYC.ORG
www.nationalmssociety.org/chapters/NYN/i
Committed to providing comprehensive support services to help people with MS and their families cope with the consequences of the disease. The goal is to empower people with MS and their loved ones so that they can better control their lives.
Ruth Brenner, Chapter President
Robin Einbinder, Executive Vice President Programs

6468 National MS Society: Northeastern New York Chapter
421 New Karner Road   585-271-0801
Albany, NY 12205-5156   800-344-4867
Fax: 518-464-1232
e-mail: chapter@msupstateny.org
www.nationalmssociety.org/chapters/NYR/i
Barbara R Milano, Chapter President
Elliey Kiale-Ingalsb, Chapter Chair

6469 National MS Society: Southern New York Chapter
2 Gannett Drive   914-694-1655
White Plains, NY 10604-2145   800-344-4867
Fax: 914-345-3504
e-mail: NYV@NMSS.ORG
www.nationalmssociety.org/chapters/NYV/i
The mission of the National MS Society is to end the devastating effects of multiple sclerosis. The Southern NY Chapter is committed to helping people with MS to live independently.
Andrea Maloney, Interim Chapter President
Christina Szeliga, Administrative Coordinator

6470 National MS Society: Upstate New York Chapter
457 State Street   585-271-0801
Binghamton, NY 13901-2341   800-344-4867
Fax: 607-722-1485
e-mail: chapter@msupstateny.org
www.nationalmssociety.org/chapters/NYR/i
James Ahearn, Chapter President
Jonathan Smith, Program Coordinator

6471 National MS Society: Western New York/ Northwestern Pennsylvania Chapter
4245 Union Road   585-271-0801
Buffalo, NY 14225-5040   800-344-4867
Fax: 716-634-2979
e-mail: chapter@msupstateny.org
www.nationalmssociety.org/chapters/NYR/i
Arthur V Cardella, Chapter President
Betsy Farkas, Director Chapter Programs

6472 National Multiple Sclerosis: Upstate New York Chapter
National Multiple Sclerosis Society
1650 S Avenue   716-271-0801
Rochester, NY 14620-3901   800-344-4867
Fax: 716-442-2817
e-mail: CHAPTER@MSUPSTATENY.ORG
www.nationalmssociety.org/chapters/NYR/i
Randal A Simonetti, President~& CEO
Stephanie Mincer, Senior Vice President of Programs

North Carolina

6473 National MS Society: Central North Carolina Chapter
2211 W Meadowview Road   336-299-4136
Greensboro, NC 27407-3400   800-344-4867
Fax: 336-855-3039
e-mail: NCC@NMSS.ORG
www.nationalmssociety.org/chapters/NCC/i
Elizabeth Green, Chapter President
Davishia Baldwin, Volunteer Coordinator

6474 National MS Society: Eastern North Carolina Chapter
3101 Industrial Drive   919-834-0678
Raleigh, NC 27609-7577   800-344-4867
Fax: 919-834-9822
e-mail: NCT@NMSS.ORG
www.nationalmssociety.org/chapters/NCT/i
Craig Robertson, Interim Chapter President
Debbie Hoffman, Vice President Operations

6475 National Multiple Sclerosis Society
9801-I Southern Pine Boulevard   704-525-2955
Charlotte, NC 28273-5561   800-344-4867
Fax: 704-527-0406
e-mail: mac@nmss.org
www.nationalmssociety.org/mac
The Mid-Atlantic chapter of the National MS Society serves 80,000 people with multiple sclerosis in South Carolina and western North Carolina. The Chapter is dedicated to helping people with MS learn to manage and understand their disease and to achieve maximum independence.
Allison Mertens, Chair Board of Trustees
Jennifer Lee, Chapter President

North Dakota

6476 National MS Society: Dakota Chapter
5990 14th Street S   701-235-2678
Fargo, ND 58104   800-344-4867
Fax: 701-235-6358
www.nationalmssociety.org/chapters/NTH/i
Kelly Boeddeker, Senior Development Manager
Amanda Noce, Programs Manager

Ohio

6477 Columbus Center of the National Multiple Sclerosis Society
National Multiple Sclerosis Society
651 G Lakeview Plaza Boulevard   614-880-2290
Worthington, OH 43229-3626   800-344-4867
Fax: 614-880-2296
www.nationalmssociety.org
Stacey Wilko LSW, Program Coordinator
Tony Bernard LSW, Program Coordinator

6478 National MS Soceity: Western Ohio Chapter The Woolpert Building
The Woolpert Building

409 E Monument Avenue
Dayton, OH 45402-1261

937-461-5232
800-344-4867
Fax: 937-461-3500
e-mail: donnasimpson@ohm.nmss.org
www.nationalmssociety.org

Providing accurate, up-to-date information to individuals with MS, their families and healthcare providers is central to our mission.
12 pages
Karen Joseph, Program Director
Judy LaMusga, Chapter Chair

6479 National MS Society: Southwestern Ohio/Northern Kentucky
4440 Lake Forest Drive
Cincinnati, OH 45242-3755

513-769-4400
800-344-4867
Fax: 513-769-6019
e-mail: OHGinfo@nmss.org
www.nationalmssociety.org

Tena Bunnell, Chapter President
Becky Wiehe, Service Director

6480 National MS Society: Northeast Ohio Chapter
The Hanna Building
6155 Rockside Road
Independence, OH 44131-1901

216-696-8220
800-344-4867
Fax: 216-696-2817
e-mail: WEBMASTER@NMSSOHA.ORG
www.nationalmssociety.org

Janet Kramer, Chapter President
Greg Kovach, Director of Services

6481 National MS Society: Northwest Ohio Chapter
401 Tomahawk Drive
Maumee, OH 43537-1633

419-897-9533
800-344-4867
Fax: 419-897-9733
e-mail: Maureen.Mohney@nmss.org
www.nationalmssociety.org/chapters/OHO/i

Jacque Pratt, Chapter Program Coordinator
Tonya Scherf, Program Director

Oklahoma

6482 National MS Society: Oklahoma Chapter
4604 E 67th Street
Tulsa, OK 74136-4946

918-488-0882
800-344-4867
Fax: 918-488-0913
e-mail: LISA.GRAY@OKE.NMSS.ORG
www.nationalmssociety.org/chapters/OKE/i

Paula Cortner, Chapter President
Denise Allen, Finance/HR Manager

Oregon

6483 National MS Society: Oregon Chapter
5331 SW Macadam Avenue
Portland, OR 97239

503-223-9511
800-344-4867
Fax: 503-223-2912
e-mail: INFO@DEFEATMS.COM
www.nationalmssociety.org/chapters/ORC/i

The Pregon Chapter is aggressively pursuing the mission to end the devastating effects of MS by providing programs designed to enhance the families throughout Oregon and Clark County, Washington.
Wendy Allison, Office Coordinator
Sally Alworth, Director of Finance

Pennsylvania

6484 National MS Society: Central Pennsylvania Chapter
2040 Linglestown Road
Harrisburg, PA 17110-1095

717-652-2108
800-344-4867
Fax: 717-652-2590
e-mail: PAC@NMSS.ORG
www.nationalmssociety.org/chapters/PAC/i

Margie Adelmann, President
Debbie Rios, Executive Vice President

6485 National MS Society: Greater Delaware Valley Chapter
30 South 17th Street
Philadelphia, PA 19103-5519

215-271-1500
800-344-4867
Fax: 215-271-6122
e-mail: PAE@NMSS.ORG
www.nationalmssociety.org/chapters/PAE/i

John H Scott, President
Randee Forstein, VP Programs & Community Outreach

Rhode Island

6486 National MS Society: Rhode Island Chapter
205 Hallene Road
Warwick, RI 02886-2452

401-738-8383
800-344-4867
Fax: 401-738-8469
e-mail: christina.roche@nmss.org
www.nationalmssociety.org/chapters/RIR/i

Provides local programs and services to people with MS and their families. These services include information and referral, equipment loans, purchase assistance, programs for the newly diagnosed and education and support groups.
3M Members
Kathy Mechnig, Chapter President
Catie Dussault, Director of Special Events

South Carolina

6487 National MS Society: South Carolina Branch
2711 Middleburg Drive
Columbia, SC 29204-2413

803-799-7848
800-344-4867
www.nationalmssociety.org/chapters/NCP/i

Tennessee

6488 National MS Society: Southeast Tennessee/North Georgia Chapte
5720 Uptain Road
Chattanooga, TN 37411-5642

423-954-9700
800-344-4867
Fax: 423-855-9667
e-mail: questions@msmidsouth.org
www.nationalmssociety.org

Jeanne Brice, Services Manager

6489 National MS Society: Mid-South Chapter
3100 Walnut Grove Road
Memphis, TN 38111-3530

901-755-4900
800-344-4867
Fax: 901-324-9668
www.nationalmssociety.org

The mission of the National Multiple Sclerosis Society is to end the devastating effects of MS.
Dee Blake, Chapter President
Sherree Wilson, Services Director

6490 National MS Society: Mid-South Chapter, Nashville Office
4219 Hillsboro Road
Nashville, TN 37215-3332

615-269-9055
800-344-4867
Fax: 615-269-9470
e-mail: TNS@NMSS.ORG
www.nationalmssociety.org/chapters/TNS/i

Jim Ward, Chapter President
Beth Smith, Vice President of Client Programs

Texas

6491 National MS Society: North Central Texas Chapter
4086 Sandshell Drive
Fort Worth, TX 76137

817-306-7003
800-344-4867
Fax: 817-877-1205
www.nationalmssociety.org/chapters/TXH/i

Educational programs, self-help groups, and information and referral for persons and families diagnosed with multiple sclerosis.
12 pages Quarterly
Justin Martin, Coordinator Development
Lynette Jarvis-Barre, Senior Manager Programs & Services

6492   National MS Society: Panhandle Chapter
6222 Canyon Drive   806-468-8005
Amarillo, TX 79109-6730   800-344-4867
                                                      Fax: 806-468-8022
                                              e-mail: TXP@NMSS.ORG
                          www.nationalmssociety.org/chapters/TXP/i
Gail Lindsey, Programs and Services Coordinator
April Brownlee, Development Coordinator Special Events

6493   National MS Society: Southern Texas
8111 N Stadium Drive   713-526-8967
Houston, TX 77054   800-344-4867
                                                      Fax: 713-394-7422
                                              e-mail: TXH@NMSS.ORG
                          www.nationalmssociety.org/chapters/TXH/i
Mark Neagli, Chapter President
Deborah Pope, VP - Operations

6494   National MS Society: West Texas Division
1031 Andrews Highway   432-522-2143
Midland, TX 79701-4636   800-344-4867
                                                      Fax: 432-694-7970
                                              e-mail: TXQ@NMSS.ORG
                          www.nationalmssociety.org/chapters/TXQ/i
Sharon Rader, Regional Development Manager
Rona Bowerman, Regional Programs and Services Manager

6495   National MS Socisty: Southeast Texas Chapter
8111 N Stadium Drive   713-526-8967
Houston, TX 77054-4051   800-344-4867
                                                      Fax: 713-394-7422
                                              e-mail: TXH@NMSS.ORG
                                          www.nationalmssociety.org
Mark Neagli, Chapter President
Jim Tidwell, Chairman

Utah

6496   National MS Society: Utah State Chapter
1440 Foothill Drive   801-493-0113
Salt Lake City, UT 84108-3537   800-527-8116
                                                      Fax: 801-493-0122
                                          e-mail: utah.idaho@nmss.org
                                          www.nationalmssociety.org
Our mission is to end the devastating effects of MS. Serving individuals with MS and their families through programs, research, awareness and education.
Annette Royle, Chapter President
Dee Dee Fox, Director of Client Programs and Services

Vermont

6497   National MS Society: Vermont Division
75 Talcott Road   802-864-6356
Williston, VT 05495   800-344-4867
                                                      Fax: 802-864-6509
                                              e-mail: VTN@NMSS.ORG
                          www.nationalmssociety.org/chapters/VTN/i
Committed to ending the devastating effects of MS.
Christine Newberr, Programs and Services Coordinator
Lindsay Going, Development Coordinator Special Events

Virginia

6498   National MS Society: Blue Ridge Chapter
1020 Carrington Place   804-971-8010
Charlottesville, VA 22901   800-344-4867
                                                      Fax: 804-979-4475
                                              e-mail: VAB@NMSS.ORG
                          www.nationalmssociety.org/chapters/VAB/i
Faith Painter, Chapter President
Delton Hanson, Operations Director

6499   National MS Society: Central Virginia Chapter
2112 W Laburnum Avenue   804-353-5008
Richmond, VA 23227   800-344-4867
                                                      Fax: 804-353-5595
                                  e-mail: JUDY.GRIFFIN@NMSS.ORG
                          www.nationalmssociety.org/chapters/VAR/i
Sherri Ellis, Chapter President
Andy Page, Director of Community Development

6500   National MS Society: Hampton Roads Chapter
760 Lynnhaven Parkway   757-490-9627
Virginia Beach, VA 23452-6311   800-344-4867
                                                      Fax: 757-490-1617
                                              e-mail: info@fightms.com
                          www.nationalmssociety.org/chapters/VAX/i
Sharon Grossman, Chapter President
Michelle Derr, Vice President Finance/Administration

Washington

6501   National MS Society: Greater Washington Chapter
192 Nickerson Street   206-284-4254
Seattle, WA 98109   800-344-4867
                                                      Fax: 206-284-4972
                                  e-mail: MSnorthwest@nmsswas.org
                          www.nationalmssociety.org/chapters/WAS/i
Patricia Shepherd-Ba, Chapter President
Erin Poznanski, Vice President Chapter Programs

6502   National MS Society: Inland Northwest Chapter
818 E Sharp Avenue   509-482-2022
Spokane, WA 99202-1935   800-344-4867
                                                      Fax: 509-483-1077
                                              e-mail: WAI@NMSS.ORG
                          www.nationalmssociety.org/chapters/WAI/i
Robert Hansen, Chapter President
Patty Mathias, Office Manager

Wisconsin

6503   National MS Society: Wisconsin Chapter
1120 James Drive   262-369-4400
Hartland, WI 53029   800-344-4867
                                                      Fax: 262-369-4410
                                          e-mail: info.wisms@nmss.org
                          www.nationalmssociety.org/chapters/WIG/i
Colleen Kalt, President & CEO
Melissa Palfery, Executive Assistant

Wyoming

6504   National MS Society: Wyoming Chapter
525 Randall Avenue   307-433-9590
Cheyenne, WY 82001-1627   800-344-4867
                                                      Fax: 307-433-8657
                                              e-mail: WYY@NMSS.ORG
                          www.nationalmssociety.org/chapters/WYY/i
Cheryl Seaberg, Programs and Services Coordinator
Stephanie Batson, Development Coordinator Special Events

Libraries & Resource Centers

6505   Information Resource Center and Library
National Multiple Sclerosis Society
733 Third Avenue   866-675-4787
New York, NY 10017   800-344-4867
                                          www.nationalmssociety.org
The primary venue for educating the community about multiple sclerosis.Offers the latest information about MS information and provides referrals to local MS care centers, physicians and service providers.
Weyman T Johnson, Jr, Chairman
Joyce M Nelson, President/CEO

6506   St. Agnes Hospital Medical: Health Science Library
305 North Street   914-681-4500
White Plains, NY 10605   Fax: 914-328-6408
Labe C Scheinberg MD, Director

Research Centers

6507   Brigham and Women's Hospital: Center for Neurologic Diseases
LMRC Building
75 Francis Street   617-732-5500
Boston, MA 02115   800-294-9999
                                       TTY: 617-732-6458
www.brighamandwomens.org
Offers research relating to Multiple Sclerosis and other autoimmune diseases.
Dennis J. Selkoe, Co-Director
Howard L. Weiner, Co-Director

6508   Center for Neuroimmunology: University of Alabama at Birmingham
1720 7th Ave S   205-934-0683
Birmingham, AL 35294   Fax: 205-996-4039
www.main.uab.edu/neurology
Evaluate and treat acute and chronic neurological and neuromuscular diseases which are caused by autoimmune mechanisms or linked to presumed abnormalities affecting the immune system.
Khurram Bashir, Director

6509   Jimmie Heuga Center
27 Main Street   970-926-1290
Edwards, CO 81632   800-367-3101
                                       Fax: 970-926-1295
e-mail: info@mscando.org
www.mscando.org
Conducts research and studies on multiple sclerosis patients.
Kim Lennox Sharkey, Chief Executive Officer
Carrie Van Beek, Office Coordinator

6510   Neuromuscular Treatment Center: Univ. of Texas Southwestern Medical Center
Department of Neurology
Dallas, TX 75390   214-648-3111
www.utsouthwestern.edu
Basic and clinical studies of myasthenia gravis.
Daniel K Podolsky MD, President
Diane Jeffries, Director

6511   Rush University Multiple Sclerosis Center
1653 W. Congress Parkway   312-942-5000
Chicago, IL 60612   888-352-RUSH
                                       TTY: 312-942-2207
e-mail: complaint@jointcommission.org
www.rush.edu
The Multiple Sclerosis Center combines comprehensive treatment with clinical and laboratory research to provide the highest quality patient care.
Floyd A Davis, Director

Support Groups & Hotlines

6512   MS Toll-Free Information Line
National Multiple Sclerosis Society
733 3rd Avenue
New York, NY 10017-3288   800-344-4867
Offers public and professional information, brochures and referrals to MS patients, their families and health care professionals.

6513   MSWorld
1943 Morrill Street   415-701-1117
Sarasota, FL 34236   877-710-0302
e-mail: msworld@msworld.org
www.msworld.org/
MSWorld is for people with multiple sclerosis their families and friends, offer support via chat, e-mail, message boards, magazines.
Kathleen Wilson, Founder/President

6514   Multiple Sclerosis Action Group
National Multiple Sclerosis Society

733 3rd Avenue   409-883-2282
New York, NY 10017   800-344-4867
e-mail: msag@erasems.com
www.nationalmssociety.org/index.aspx
Richard J Mengel, Treasurer
Fred J Lublin, Director

6515   National Health Information Center
PO Box 1133   310-565-4167
Washington, DC 20013   800-336-4797
                                       Fax: 301-984-4256
e-mail: info@nhic.org
www.health.gov/nhic
Offers a nationwide information referral service, produces directories and resource guides.

6516   Traditional Tibetan Healing
13 Harrison Street   617-666-8635
Sommerville, MA 2143-6504   866-628-6504
e-mail: Kelob@gte.net
www.tibetanherbalhealing.com/
To rid mankind from chronic illnesses using alternative methods.
Keyzon Bhutti, Chief Physician

Books

6517   300 Tips for Making Life with Multiple Sclerosis Easier
Demos Medical Publishing
11 West 42nd Street   212-683-0072
New York, NY 10036   Fax: 212-683-0118
e-mail: orderdept@demospub.com
www.demosmedpub.com
Techniques for better living.
109 pages
ISBN: 1-888799-23-4
Shelley Peterman Schwarzÿ, Author

6518   Alternative Medicine and Multiple Sclerosis
Demos Medical Publishing
11 West 42nd Street   212-683-0072
New York, NY 10036   Fax: 212-683-0118
e-mail: orderdept@demospub.com
www.demosmedpub.com
These therapies are organized alphabetically so that readers can readily pinpoint a specific treatment and learn about its origins, merits, and possible uses in MS
272 pages
ISBN: 1-888799-52-8
Allen C. Bowling, Author

6519   Fall Down Seven Times Get Up Eight
Miramar Communications
PO Box 8987
Malibu, CA 90265-8987   800-543-4116
The second in Dr. Wolf's series on MS management: including chapters on stress and fatigue, planning for serious disability and lots more.
211 pages

6520   Living with Multiple Sclerosis
Demos Medical Publishing
11 West 42nd Street   212-683-0072
New York, NY 10036   Fax: 212-683-0118
e-mail: orderdept@demospub.com
www.demosmedpub.com

ISBN: 1-888799-26-9
Dr. Diana M Schneider

6521   Living with Multiple Sclerosis: A Wellness Approach
Demos Vermande
11 West 42nd Street   212-683-0072
New York, NY 10036-8804   800-532-8663
The book incorporates recent developments in the management of multiple sclerosis and includes strategies for patients who want to

optimize their health through exercise, stress management and good nutrition.
112 pages
ISBN: 1-888799-00-5
George Kraft, Author
Marciỹ Catanzaro,, Author

6522   Meeting the Challenge of Progressive Multiple Sclerosis
Demos Medical Publishing
11 West 42nd Street   212-683-0072
New York, NY 10036   Fax: 212-683-0118
e-mail: orderdept@demospub.com
www.demosmedpub.com
This book is designed specifically for people who have been told they have or are developing the progressive form of multiple sclerosis. It focuses on ways to not only manage the progressive disease and its symptoms but also to cope with the life changes that may accompany it.
128 pages
ISBN: 1-888799-46-3
Patricia K.ỹ Coyle, Author
June Halper, Author

6523   Multiple Sclerosis
Demos Medical Publishing
11 West 42nd Street   212-683-0072
New York, NY 10036   800-532-8663
Fax: 212-683-0118
e-mail: orderdept@demospub.com
www.demosmedpub.com
This new comprehensive review of the many fields of basic and clinical research that impact our understanding of multiple sclerosis has its basis in this premise
224 pages
ISBN: 1-888799-54-4
Robert Herndonỹ, Author

6524   Multiple Sclerosis, The Questions you Have Answers You Need
Demos Medical Publishing
11 West 42nd Street   212-683-0072
New York, NY 10036   Fax: 212-683-0118
e-mail: orderdept@demospub.com
www.demosmedpub.com
The Questions You Have, The Answers You Need continues to be the definitive guide for everyone concerned with this disease those who have MS, those who share their lives with someone who has it, and all healthcare professionals involved with its management
592 pages
ISBN: 1-888799-43-9
Rosalind C.ỹ Kalb, Author

6525   Multiple Sclerosis: A Guide for Families
Demos Medical Publishing
11 West 42nd Street   212-683-0072
New York, NY 10036-8804   800-532-8663
Fax: 212-683-0118
e-mail: orderdept@demospub.com
www.demosmedpub.com
With its complex and unpredictable course, MS affects every area of family life. This book covers a broad range of medical, psychological, social, vocational, economic and legal problems.
1997 207 pages Paperback
ISBN: 1-888799-14-5
Rosalind C.ỹ Kalb, Author

6526   Multiple Sclerosis: A Guide for Patients and Their Families
Raven Press
11 West 42nd Street   212-683-0072
New York, NY 10036-2601   800-777-2295
e-mail: orderdept@demospub.com
www.demosmedpub.com
The Second Edition of this popular and highly acclaimed guide features expanded coverage of the causes, epidemiology, and genetics of multiple sclerosis and contains many new illustrations that make the rehabilitative techniques presented easier for the patient to understand and follow.ỹ
288 pages Paperback
ISBN: 0-881672-55-6
Labe C. Scheinberg, Author
Nancy J. Holland, Editor

6527   Multiple Sclerosis: A Personal Exploration
Demos Vermande
11 West 42nd Street   212-683-0072
New York, NY 10036-8804   800-532-8663
Fax: 212-683-0118
e-mail: orderdept@demospub.com
www.demosmedpub.com
As a doctor and psychiatrist who has MS, the author of this refreshingly frank and practical book is able to draw on personal experience, as well as professional knowledge and insights.
1993 192 pages
ISBN: 0-285650-18-1
Alexander Burnfield, Author

6528   Multiple Sclerosis: Your Legal Rights
Demos Medical Publishing
11 West 42nd Street   212-683-0072
New York, NY 10036   Fax: 212-683-0118
e-mail: orderdept@demospub.com
www.demosmedpub.com
This extensively revised third edition continues to provide reliable basic information and possible solutions to the legal problems that often affect people with multiple sclerosis (MS).
156 pages
ISBN: 1-888799-31-5
Lannyỹ Perkins, Author
Sara Perkins, Author

6529   The Comfort of Home Multiple Sclerosis Edi tion: A Guide for Caregivers
Marie M. Meyer and Paula Derr, RN, author
CareTrust Publications
PO Box 10283
Portland, OR 97296-0283   800-565-1533
Fax: 415-673-2005
e-mail: sales@comfortofhome.com
www.comfortofhome.com
Reviews caregiving options and discusses the financial and legal decisions you may encounterr. Readers will learn how to set up a safe and comfortable home for the person whose needs are changing and abilities declining. Comfort offers guidance through every caregiving stage and most decisions one will face in daily living, as well as in avoiding caregiver burnout. Valuable for the caregiver and the patient.
324 pages
ISBN: 0-966476-76-X
Paula Derr, Author
Maria M. Meyer, Author

6530   Understanding Multiple Sclerosis
Melissa Stauffer, author
University Press of Mississippi
3825 Ridgewood Road   601-432-6205
Jackson, MS 39211-6492   Fax: 601-432-6217
e-mail: kburgess@ihl.state.ms.us
www.upress.state.ms.us
For patients and companions, an overview of all aspects of MS.
2006 144 pages Paperback
ISBN: 1-578068-03-7
Melissa Stauffer, Author

Magazines

6531   Inside MS
National Multiple Sclerosis Society
733 3rd Avenue   212-986-3240
New York, NY 10017-3288   800-344-4867
Fax: 212-986-7981
www.nationalmssociety.org
Full color quarterly magazine on living well with multiple sclerosis. Articles by people with MS; daily living, achievments, news, treatments, research, advocacy, humor, travel, helpful resources, large type. The magazine is a benefit of membership.
64 pages 4x Year
Eliỹ rubenstein, Chairman of the Board
Cynthia Zagieboylo, Chapter President

Newsletters

6532 Inside MS Bulletin
National Multiple Sclerosis Society
733 3rd Avenue   212-986-3240
New York, NY 10017-3288   800-344-4867
                                  Fax: 212-986-7981
                            www.nationalmssociety.org
Newsletter offering information on the organization activities.
Profiles of donors, and reports on MS research programs.
Eliÿ Rubenstein, Chairman of the Board
Cynthia Zagieboylo, Chapter President

6533 MS Connection
National Multiple Sclerosis Society
3101 Industrial Drive   919-834-0678
Raleigh, NC 27609   Fax: 704-527-0406
                            e-mail: mac@nmss.org
                        www.nationalmssociety.org/mac
Provides education, support and information about Chapter activities for people living with multiple sclerosis in South Carolina and western North Carolina.
Quarterly
Eliÿ Rubenstein, Chairman of the Board
Cynthia Zagieboylo, Chapter President

6534 Motivator
Multiple Sclerosis Foundation
6350 N Andrews Avenue   954-776-6805
Fort Lauderdale, FL 33309-2130   800-441-7055
                         e-mail: msfacts@icanect.net
                                     www.msfacts.org
Reports on the latest advancements regarding medical treatments/therapies for MS, inspirational feature stories, coping skills, correspondence from readers, and ongoing MSAA programs, services, and activities.
BiMonthly

6535 Multiple Sclerosis Quarterly Report
Demos Vermande
11 West 42nd Street   212-683-0072
New York, NY 10036-8804   800-532-8663
                                  Fax: 212-683-0118
                       e-mail: orderdept@demospub.com
                             www.demosmedpub.com
This is the definitive newsletter for everyone who has MS, with feature articles, research updates, book reviews, and more. It is developed with the sponsorship of the Eastern Paralyzed Veterans of America and the National Multiple Sclerosis Society. The MSQR will keep you informed of new developments in the management of MS and strategies for living successfully with the disease.
1997 Quarterly

6536 National Multiple Sclerosis Society: Allegheny District Chapter
1501 Reedsdale Street   412-261-6347
Pittsburgh, PA 15233-6220   800-344-4867
                                  Fax: 412-232-1461
                            e-mail: pa@nmss.org
                            www.nationalmssociety.org

12 pages 4 per year
Eliÿ Rubenstein, Chairman of the Board
Cynthia Zagieboylo, President & CEOÿ

Pamphlets

6537 ADA and People with MS
National Multiple Sclerosis Society
733 3rd Avenue   212-986-3240
New York, NY 10017-3288   800-344-4867
                                  Fax: 212-986-7981
                            www.nationalmssociety.org
What the Americans with Disabilities Act means in employment, public accommodations, transportation, and telecommunications.
24 pages
Laura D. Cooper, Author
Mark Stolman, Volunteer

6538 At Home with MS: Adapting Your Environment
National Multiple Sclerosis Society
733 3rd Avenue   212-986-3240
New York, NY 10017-3288   800-344-4867
                                  Fax: 212-986-7981
                            www.nationalmssociety.org
Modify a house or apartment to save energy, compensate for reduced vision or mobility, and live comfortably. Many do-it-yourself changes.
28 pages
Jane E. Harmon, Author
Donna M. Jensen, Assistant Writer

6539 At Our House
National Multiple Sclerosis Society
733 3rd Avenue   212-986-3240
New York, NY 10017-3288   800-344-4867
                                  Fax: 212-986-7981
                            www.nationalmssociety.org
A coloring book for children, ages 5-8, about a Mama Bear with MS. contains some very basic facts with an afterword for parents on how to talk to young children about MS.
20 pages

6540 Chapter Services at a Glance
National Multiple Sclerosis Society
733 3rd Avenue   212-986-3240
New York, NY 10017-3288   800-344-4867
                                  Fax: 212-986-7981
                            www.nationalmssociety.org
A summary of services offerred by local chapters. Contains membership form.

6541 Check Your Multiple Sclerosis Facts
National Multiple Sclerosis Society
733 3rd Avenue   212-986-3240
New York, NY 10017-3288   800-344-4867
                                  Fax: 212-986-7981
                            www.nationalmssociety.org
A brief checklist of MS basics - definition, symptoms, and outlook.

6542 Choosing a Pharmacy Service
National Multiple Sclerosis Society
733 3rd Avenue   212-986-3240
New York, NY 10017-3288   800-344-4867
                                  Fax: 212-986-7981
                            www.nationalmssociety.org
What to look for when choosing a prescription drug provider.
20 pages

6543 Clear Thinking About Alternative Therapies
National Multiple Sclerosis Society
733 3rd Avenue   212-986-3240
New York, NY 10017-3288   800-344-4867
                                  Fax: 212-986-7981
                            www.nationalmssociety.org
Highlights facts and common misconceptions, compares alternative and conventional medicine, and suggests ways to evaluate benefits and risks.

6544 Controlling Spasticity
National Multiple Sclerosis Society
733 3rd Avenue   212-986-3240
New York, NY 10017-3288   800-344-4867
                                  Fax: 212-986-7981
                            www.nationalmssociety.org
An overview of ways to control this common and sometimes disabling MS symtpom. Includes roles of self-help, medications, physical therapists, nurses, and physicians.

6545 Food for Thought: MS and Nutrition
National Multiple Sclerosis Society
733 3rd Avenue   212-986-3240
New York, NY 10017-3288   800-344-4867
                                  Fax: 212-986-7981
                            www.nationalmssociety.org
A guide to healthy eating and coping with symptoms that may affect eating habits.
20 pages

6546 Getting a Grip on Gait
National Multiple Sclerosis Society
733 3rd Avenue   212-986-3240
New York, NY 10017-3288   800-344-4867
                                 Fax: 212-986-7981
                           e-mail: nat@nmss.org
                           www.nationalmssociety.org
Walking problems and how they can be addressed.

6547 Hiring Help at Home?
National Multiple Sclerosis Society
733 3rd Avenue   212-986-3240
New York, NY 10017-3288   800-344-4867
                                 Fax: 212-986-7981
                           e-mail: nat@nmss.org
                           www.nationalmssociety.org
Checklists and worksheets for people who need help at home.
Forms for needs assessment, job description, and employment con-
tract.

6548 Insight Into Eyesight
National Multiple Sclerosis Society
733 3rd Avenue   212-986-3240
New York, NY 10017-3288   800-344-4867
                                 Fax: 212-986-7981
                           e-mail: nat@nmss.org
                           www.nationalmssociety.org
Current therapy for MS-related eye disorders. Discusses low-vi-
sion aids.

6549 Living with MS
National Multiple Sclerosis Society
733 3rd Avenue   212-986-3240
New York, NY 10017-3288   800-344-4867
                                 Fax: 212-986-7981
                           e-mail: nat@nmss.org
                           www.nationalmssociety.org
Answers to 28 questions most often asked when the diagnosis is
MS - from possible causes to advice on coping.
20 pages

6550 Moving with Multiple Sclerosis
National Multiple Sclerosis Society
733 3rd Avenue   212-986-3240
New York, NY 10017-3288   800-344-4867
                                 Fax: 212-986-7981
                           e-mail: nat@nmss.org
                           www.nationalmssociety.org
Step-by-step illustrations of passive and active stretching, balance, and conditioning exercises.
30 pages

6551 Multiple Sclerosis and Your Emotions
National Multiple Sclerosis Society
733 3rd Avenue   212-986-3240
New York, NY 10017-3288   800-344-4867
                                 Fax: 212-986-7981
                           e-mail: nat@nmss.org
                           www.nationalmssociety.org
How to manage some of the emotional challenges created by MS.
32 pages

6552 On the Question of Pregnancy
National Multiple Sclerosis Society
733 3rd Avenue   212-986-3240
New York, NY 10017-3288   800-344-4867
                                 Fax: 212-986-7981
                           e-mail: nat@nmss.org
                           www.nationalmssociety.org
Reassuring answers on pregnancy, delivery, and nursing.

6553 On: Alternative Therapies
National Multiple Sclerosis Society
733 3rd Avenue   212-986-3240
New York, NY 10017-3288   800-344-4867
                                 Fax: 212-986-7981
                           e-mail: nat@nmss.org
                           www.nationalmssociety.org
Checklist for people who are considering an alternative treatment.

6554 On: Diagnosis...Putting the Pieces Together
National Multiple Sclerosis Society
733 3rd Avenue   212-986-3240
New York, NY 10017-3288   800-344-4867
                                 Fax: 212-986-7981
                           e-mail: nat@nmss.org
                           www.nationalmssociety.org
Explains usual steps and tests. Includes how to prepare for an MRI.

6555 On: Energy Management
National Multiple Sclerosis Society
733 3rd Avenue   212-986-3240
New York, NY 10017-3288   800-344-4867
                                 Fax: 212-986-7981
                           e-mail: nat@nmss.org
                           www.nationalmssociety.org
Guidelines for budgeting your energy when it's limited by fatigue
through prioritizing, delegating, and simplifying tasks.

6556 On: Fatigue
National Multiple Sclerosis Society
733 3rd Avenue   212-986-3240
New York, NY 10017-3288   800-344-4867
                                 Fax: 212-986-7981
                           e-mail: nat@nmss.org
                           www.nationalmssociety.org
The mystery of MS fatigue, practical tips for coping, and the medi-
cations sometimes prescribed.

6557 On: Genes
National Multiple Sclerosis Society
733 3rd Avenue   212-986-3240
New York, NY 10017-3288   800-344-4867
                                 Fax: 212-986-7981
                           e-mail: nat@nmss.org
                           www.nationalmssociety.org
Recent information on MS and heredity.

6558 On: Pain
National Multiple Sclerosis Society
733 3rd Avenue   212-986-3240
New York, NY 10017-3288   800-344-4867
                                 Fax: 212-986-7981
                           e-mail: nat@nmss.org
                           www.nationalmssociety.org
Myths and facts about MS pain. Covers types of pain and possible
treatment.

6559 Plaintalk: A Booklet About MS for Families
National Multiple Sclerosis Society
733 3rd Avenue   212-986-3240
New York, NY 10017-3288   800-344-4867
                                 Fax: 212-986-7981
                           e-mail: nat@nmss.org
                           www.nationalmssociety.org
Discusses some of the more difficult physical and emotional problems families may face.
32 pages

6560 Rehab Outlook
National Multiple Sclerosis Society
733 3rd Avenue   212-986-3240
New York, NY 10017-3288   800-344-4867
                                 Fax: 212-986-7981
                           e-mail: nat@nmss.org
                           www.nationalmssociety.org
What rehabilitation can do for mobility, fatigue, driving, speech,
memory, bowel or bladder problems, sexuality, and more.
24 pages

6561 Research Directions in Multiple Sclerosis
National Multiple Sclerosis Society
733 3rd Avenue   212-986-3240
New York, NY 10017-3288   800-344-4867
                                 Fax: 212-986-7981
                           e-mail: nat@nmss.org
                           www.nationalmssociety.org
An overview of current research on key areas of immunology, genetics, virology, and cell biology explained for nonscientists.
16 pages

6562 **Sexual Problems Your Doctor Didn't Mention**
National Multiple Sclerosis Society
733 3rd Avenue   212-986-3240
New York, NY 10017-3288   800-344-4867
                            Fax: 212-986-7981
                      e-mail: nat@nmss.org
                      www.nationalmssociety.org
How MS may affect sexuality and what can be done.

6563 **Solving Cognitive Problems**
National Multiple Sclerosis Society
733 3rd Avenue   212-986-3240
New York, NY 10017-3288   800-344-4867
                            Fax: 212-986-7981
                      e-mail: nat@nmss.org
                      www.nationalmssociety.org
Mental functions most likely to be affected by MS. Suggestions for
self-help and information about cognitive rehabiitation.
20 pages

6564 **Someone You Know Has MS: A Book for Families**
National Multiple Sclerosis Society
733 3rd Avenue   212-986-3240
New York, NY 10017-3288   800-344-4867
                            Fax: 212-986-7981
                      e-mail: nat@nmss.org
                      www.nationalmssociety.org
For children ages 6-12 who have a parent with MS. Provides facts
and explores children's fears and concerns.
32 pages

6565 **Taking Care: A Guide for Well Partners**
National Multiple Sclerosis Society
733 3rd Avenue   212-986-3240
New York, NY 10017-3288   800-344-4867
                            Fax: 212-986-7981
                      e-mail: nat@nmss.org
                      www.nationalmssociety.org
Introduces the concept of carepartnering to balance both partners'
needs. Includes practical suggestions about getting and giving
help.
16 pages

6566 **Taming Stress in Multiple Sclerosis**
National Multiple Sclerosis Society
733 3rd Avenue   212-986-3240
New York, NY 10017-3288   800-344-4867
                            Fax: 212-986-7981
                      e-mail: nat@nmss.org
                      www.nationalmssociety.org
Stress and depression, and how both relate to MS. Tips on simplifying daily life. Instructions on muscle relaxation, deep breathing,
and visualization relaxation.
36 pages

6567 **Things I Wish Someone Had Told Me**
National Multiple Sclerosis Society
733 3rd Avenue   212-986-3240
New York, NY 10017-3288   800-344-4867
                            Fax: 212-986-7981
                      e-mail: nat@nmss.org
                      www.nationalmssociety.org
First-person story. A positive and practical approach to adjusting
to life with MS.
20 pages

6568 **Understanding Bladder Problems in Multiple Sclerosis**
National Multiple Sclerosis Society
733 3rd Avenue   212-986-3240
New York, NY 10017-3288   800-344-4867
                            Fax: 212-986-7981
                      e-mail: nat@nmss.org
                      www.nationalmssociety.org
The three main types of bladder dysfunction explained. Guidelines
for management.
12 pages

6569 **Understanding Bowel Problems in MS**
National Multiple Sclerosis Society

733 3rd Avenue   212-986-3240
New York, NY 10017-3288   800-344-4867
                            Fax: 212-986-7981
                      e-mail: nat@nmss.org
                      www.nationalmssociety.org
An exploration of ways to manage bowel problems in MS.
24 pages

6570 **What Everyone Should Know About Multiple Sclerosis**
National Multiple Sclerosis Society
733 3rd Avenue   212-986-3240
New York, NY 10017-3288   800-344-4867
                            Fax: 212-986-7981
                      e-mail: nat@nmss.org
                      www.nationalmssociety.org
Overview of MS, suitable for the whole family.
16 pages

6571 **What Is Multiple Sclerosis?**
National Multiple Sclerosis Society
733 3rd Avenue   212-986-3240
New York, NY 10017-3288   800-344-4867
                            Fax: 212-986-7981
                      e-mail: nat@nmss.org
                      www.nationalmssociety.org
For the newly diagnosed and others who need an overview of
symptoms, disease patterns, diagnosis, prognosis, treatment, and
research efforts.

6572 **When a Parent Has MS: A Teenager's Guide**
National Multiple Sclerosis Society
733 3rd Avenue   212-986-3240
New York, NY 10017-3288   800-344-4867
                            Fax: 212-986-7981
                      e-mail: nat@nmss.org
                      www.nationalmssociety.org
For older children and teenagers who have a parent with MS. Discusses issues brought up by real kids.
24 pages

6573 **Win-Win Approach to Reasonable Accommodations**
National Multiple Sclerosis Society
733 3rd Avenue   212-986-3240
New York, NY 10017-3288   800-344-4867
                            Fax: 212-986-7981
                      e-mail: nat@nmss.org
                      www.nationalmssociety.org
A practical guide to obtaining workplace accommodations.
20 pages

Audio & Video

6574 **Aqua Exercises for Multiple Sclerosis**
National Multiple Sclerosis Society
733 3rd Avenue   212-986-3240
New York, NY 10017-3288   800-344-4867
                            Fax: 212-986-7981
                      e-mail: nat@nmss.org
                      www.nationalmssociety.org
A workout that cools and supports the body, with exercises to reduce spasticity, build muscles, and improve posture. With water-
proof chart.
20 minutes

6575 **Clinical Trials in Multiple Sclerosis: Searching for New
Therapies**
National Multiple Sclerosis Society
733 3rd Avenue   212-986-3240
New York, NY 10017   800-344-4867
                            Fax: 212-986-7981
                      e-mail: nat@nmss.org
                      www.nationalmssociety.org
Describes studies to determine the safety and efficacy of new drugs
to treat MS. Why studies are essential, how they are conducted, and
the role of participants.
20 minutes

6576 **Now, More Than Ever: Progress in Multiple Sclerosis Research**
National Multiple Sclerosis Society

733 3rd Avenue
New York, NY 10017-3288

212-986-3240
800-344-4867
Fax: 212-986-7981
e-mail: nat@nmss.org
www.nationalmssociety.org

Traces the National Multiple Sclerosis Society's historic role in propelling MS research and explains current approaches for nonscientists.

10 minutes

Web Sites

6577 Healing Well

www.healingwell.com

An online health resource guide to medical news, chat, information and articles, newsgroups and message boards, books, disease-related web sites, medical directories, and more for patients, friends, and family coping with disabling diseases, disorders, or chronic illnesses.

6578 Health Finder

www.healthfinder.gov

Searchable, carefully developed web site offering information on over 1000 topics. Developed by the US Department of Health and Human Services, the site can be used in both English and Spanish.

6579 Healthlink USA

www.healthlinkusa.com

Health information concerning treatment, cures, prevention, diagnosis, risk factors, research, support groups, email lists, personal stories and much more. Updated regularly.

6580 Helios Health

www.helioshealth.com

Online resource for your health information. Detailed information about specific health topics, access to expert advice from our Medical Advisory Board, and up-to-date health news.

6581 MedicineNet

www.medicinenet.com

An online resource for consumers providing easy-to-read, authoritative medical and health information.

6582 Medscape

www.medscape.com

Medscape offers specialists, primary care physicians, and other health professionals the Web's most robust and integrated medical information and educational tools.

6583 Multiple Sclerosis Foundation

www.msfocus.org

Dedicated to helping create a brighter tomorrow for those with MS, the foundation offers a wide array of free services including: national toll-free support, educational programs, homecare, support groups, assitive technology, publications, a comprehensive website and more to improve the quality of life for those affected by MS.

6584 National Multiple Sclerosis Society

www.nmss.org

The Society helps people affected by MS by funding cutting-edge research, driving change through advocacy, facilitating professional education, and providing programs and services that help people with MS and their families move their lives forward.

6585 Neurology Channel

www.healthcommunities.com

Find clearly explained, medically accurate information regarding conditions, including an overview, symptoms, causes, diagnostic procedures and treatment options. On this site it is possible to ask questions and get information from a neurologist and connect to people who have similar health interests.

6586 WebMD

www.webmd.com

Provides credible information, supportive communities, and in-depth reference material about health subjects. A source for original and timely health information as well as material from well known content providers.

Description

6587 Muscular Dystrophy

Muscular dystrophy is a group of genetic disorders marked by progressive weakness and degeneration of the skeletal, or voluntary, muscles that control movement. The muscles of the heart and other involuntary muscles may also affected in some forms of muscular dystrophy, and a few forms of the disease involve other organs as well.

Muscular dystrophy can affect people of all ages. The most common form, Duchenne, appears in childhood, but others may not appear until middle age or later.

Duchenne muscular dystrophy affects males almost exclusively. By age five, those with Duchenne experience progressive weakness and difficulty in climbing, jumping and hopping. By ages eight to ten, leg braces are often required, and eventually walking is impossible. Duchenne is also associated with heart problems, although without symptoms, and intellectual impairment that affects verbal ability more than performance. Death usually occurs in the third decade of life, often as a result of pneumonia.

No specific treatment exists. Daily prednisone provides significant benefit but owing to the medication's numerous side effects, it should be reserved for patients with major functional decline. Other treatment includes physical therapy, which can help minimize the shortening of the muscles that occurs around joints; assistive devices; and avoidance of prolonged immobility. There are now techniques available to detect female carriers of the defective gene, enabling genetic counseling for families and couples considering conception.

Other forms of muscular dystrophy are myotonic, Becker, limb-girdle and facioscapulohumeral. Information about when and where muscle weakness first occurred, and its severity, is very helpful in classifying the type of muscular dystrophy. Studying a small piece of muscle tissue can indicate whether the disorder is muscular dystrophy and which form of the disease it is.

National Agencies & Associations

6588 Muscular Dystrophy Association
3300 E Sunrise Drive   520-529-2000
Tucson, AZ 85718-3299   800-572-1717
e-mail: mda@mdausa.org
www.mda.org
Primary objective of MDA is the support of scientific investigators seeking the causes of and effective treatments for muscular dystrophy and related neuromuscular disorders. The worldwide research program supports over 400 scientific investigations annually.
Robert Ross, President/CEO

6589 Muscular Dystrophy Canada
2345 Yonge Street   866-687-2538
Toronto, Ontario, M4P-2E5   Fax: 416-488-7523
e-mail: info@muscle.ca
www.muscle.ca
Since 1954, Muscular Dystrophy Canada has been committed to improving the quality of life for the tens of thousands of Canadians with neuromuscular disorders and funding leading research for the discovery of therapies and cures for neuromuscular disorders.

6590 Parent Project: Muscular Dystrophy
401 Hackensack Avenue   201-250-8440
Hackensack, NJ 07601   800-714-5437
Fax: 201-250-8435
e-mail: info@parentprojectmd.org
www.parentprojectmd.org
Organization of families around the world who have children diagnosed with DMD/BMD. Our goal is to invest significant amounts of money raised into medical research with clinical application.
Patricia Furlong, President
Kimberly Galberaith, Executive Vice President

6591 Society for Muscular Dystrophy Information International
PO Box 7490   902-685-3961
Bridgewater, Nova Scotia, B4V-2X6 Fax: 902-685-3962
e-mail: smdi@auracom.com
users.auracom.com
A registered Canadian charity founded in 1983 by us, to provide a non-technical worldwide information links via publications and now this web site, for neuromuscular disorders.

Research Centers

6592 Baylor College of Medicine: Jerry Lewis Neuromuscular Disease Research
Methodist Neurological Institute
Department of Neurology   713-798-4333
Houston, TX 77030   Fax: 713-798-3854
e-mail: neurochair@bcm.edu
www.bcm.edu/neurology
Offers research into biochemistry molecular genetics and neuromuscular disorders.
Eli M. Mizrahi, M.D., Chair, Department of Neurology
Travis G. Corwin, Department Administrator

6593 Columbia Presbyterian Medical Center Neurological Institute
Columbia University
710 W 168th Street   212-305-2700
New York, NY 10032   Fax: 212-058-98
www.cumc.columbia.edu
Neuromuscular clinical research center.
Hiroshi Mits MD, Division Head Neuromuscular Division

6594 Columbia University Clinical Research Center for Muscular Dystrophy
College of Physicians & Surgeons
116th and Broadway   212-854-1754
New York, NY 10027   Fax: 212-305-1343
www.columbia.edu

Salvatore DiMauro, Co Director

6595 Hospital of the University of Pennsylvania University of Pennsylvania
University of Pennsylvania
3400 Spruce Street   215-662-4000
Philadelphia, PA 19104   800-789-PENN
Fax: 215-903-09
e-mail: pleasure@email.chop.edu
www.pennhealth.com
Research program centering its efforts on finding better ways to prevent and treat neuromuscular disorders.
David E Pleasure MD, Director

6596 Mayo Clinic and Foundation Mayo Foundation
Mayo Foundation
201 W Center Street   507-284-2511
Rochester, MN 55905   Fax: 507-284-0161
TTY: 507-284-9786
www.mayo.edu
Neuromuscular clinical research center with a primary research interest in neuropathies.
Peter J Dyck MD, Director Nerve Studies
Andrew G Engel MD, Director Muscle Studies

6597 Muscular Dystrophy Association
3300 E Sunrise Drive
Tucson, AZ 85718-3299 520-529-2000
800-572-1717
Fax: 520-529-5300
e-mail: mda@mdausa.org
www.MDausa.org
Fights neuromuscular disease including all muscular dystrophies. Conducts extensive programs of research services and public education including 230 clinics.
Robert Ross, President/CEO

6598 University of Utah Utah Genome Depot University of Utah
University of Utah
20 S 2030 E
Salt Lake City, UT 84112 801-585-7606
Fax: 801-857-7177
e-mail: bob.weiss@genetics.utah.edu
www.genome.utah.edu
Focuses research on human muscular dystrophies.
Robert Weiss, Principal Investigator
Jackie Tyce, Program Coordinator

Support Groups & Hotlines

6599 Facioscapulohumeral Muscular Dystrophy Soc iety (FSH Society)
450 Bedford Street
Lexington, MA 02420 781-860-0501
Fax: 781-860-0599
e-mail: solvefshd@fshsociety.org
www.fshsociety.org
The Facioscapulohumeral Muscular Dystrophy Society (FSH Society) serves as a resource for individuals and families with FSHD, representing them and advocating on their behalf. Purposes of the organization are to accumulate, disseminate and encourage the exchange of information about FSHD, including educating the general public, relevant governmental bodies, and the medical and scientific professions about the existence, diagnosis and treatment of FSHD.
Daniel Paul Perez, President/CEO
June Kinoshita, Executive Director

6600 National Health Information Center
PO Box 1133
Washington, DC 20013 310-565-4167
800-336-4797
Fax: 301-984-4256
e-mail: info@nhic.org
www.health.gov/nhic
Offers a nationwide information referral service, produces directories and resource guides.

Books

6601 Clinical Evaluation and Diagnostic Tests for Neuromuscular Disorders
Butterworth-Heinemann Medical
3255 Bell Helicopter Blvd
Fort Worth, TX 76101 817-280-2011
Fax: 817-280-2321
e-mail: custserv.bh@elsevier.com
www.bellhelicopter.com
Expert advice from leading authorities on how and when to use the numerous evaluation tests now available for diagnosis and management of neuromuscular disorders.
2002

6602 Everyday Life with ALS: A Practical Guide
Muscular Dystrophy Association
3300 E Sunrise Drive
Tucson, AZ 85718-3299 520-529-5317
800-572-1717
Fax: 520-529-5383
e-mail: publications@mdausa.org
www.mda.org
Advice and information addressing degrees of affliction of those with ALS. Ways to conserve energy, to modifying your home space, to medical devices and equipment. Consider using the Guide with your care team.
2005
Christina Medvescek, Director of Editorial Services

6603 Journey of Love: Parent's Guide to Duchenne Muscular Dystrophy
Muscular Dystrophy Association
3300 E Sunrise Drive
Tucson, AZ 85718-3299 520-529-5317
800-572-1717
Fax: 520-529-5383
e-mail: publications@mdausa.org
www.mda.org
Complete guide for parents with children diagnosed with DMD. Information includes explanation of the disease, treatments, research, services provided by MDA, guides to finding assistance and more.
170 pages Paperback
Bob Mackle, Director Public Information
Christina Medvescek, Director of Editorial Services

6604 MDA ALS Caregiver's Guide
Muscular Dystrophy Association
3300 E Sunrise Drive
Tucson, AZ 85718-3299 520-529-5317
800-572-1717
e-mail: publication@mdusa.org
www.mda.org
A comprehensive guide to caring for a person with ALS at home. Covers everything from physical care to psychological and emotional concerns to getting financial assistance. Companion to Everyday Life with ALS: A Practical Guide.
2008 58 pages Paperback
Bob Mackle, Director Public Information
Christina Medvescek, Director of Editorial Services

6605 Moonrise: One Family, Genetic Identity, & Muscular Dystrophy
St. Martin's Press
175 5th Avenue
New York, NY 10010 212-674-5151
Fax: 212-677-7456
us.macmillan.com/smp
A mother writes about her teen-age son who has Duchenne muscular dystrophy, the life he leads, and the one he can look forward to.
2003

6606 Muscular Dystrophy & Other Neuromuscular Diseases: Psychological Issues
Leon Charash, Robert Lovelace, author
Haworth Press
10 Alice Street
Binghamton, NY 13904 607-722-5857
800-429-6784
Fax: 607-722-0012
www.haworthpress.com
Thoughtful book from professionals who assist people with neuromuscular disorders to help them adapt to lifestyle changes accompanying these disorders.
250 pages Hardcover
ISBN: 1-560240-77-0

6607 Muscular Dystrophy in Children: Guide for Families
Demos Medical Publishing
11 West 42nd Street
New York, NY 10036 212-683-0072
800-532-8663
Fax: 212-683-0118
e-mail: support@demosmedical.com
www.demosmedical.com
Addresses emotional as well as physical challenges that families and caregivers will have to face and gives readers information on muscular dystrophy, how to adapt to a child's needs, and present research being conducted. In addition, it gives parents and caregivers sources for additional support and suggestions for further reading.
1999
Beth Kaufman Barry, Publisher
David D'Addona, Acquisitions Editor

6608 Neuromuscular Dis. of Infancy, Childhood & Adolesesce: A Clinician's Approach
Butterworth-Heinemann Medical
3255 Bell Helicopter Blvd
Fort Worth, TX 76101 817-280-2011
Fax: 817-280-2321
e-mail: custserv.bh@elsevier.com
www.bellhelicopter.com

Explains how childhood neuromuscular diseases differ from those in adult patients, and provides clinicians with all the knowledge they need to successfully diagnose and treat pediatric patients.
2003

6609 Noninvasive Mechanical Ventilation
John Bach, MD, author
Elsevier
Book Customer Service Dpt
St. Louis, MO 63146   800-545-2522
                                          Fax: 800-535-9935
                         e-mail: usbkinfo@elsevier.com
                                       www.elsevier.com
Describes the use of inspiratory and expiratory muscle aids to prevent the pulmonary complications of lung disease and conditions with muscle weakness. It also describes treatment and rehabilitation interventions specific for patients with these conditions. This book is unique in presenting the use of entirely noninvasive management alternatives to eliminate respiratory morbidity and avoid the need to resort to tracheostomy for the majority of patients with lung or neuromuscular disease.
2002 348 pages Paperback
ISBN: 1-560535-49-0

6610 Physical Medicine & Rehabilitation
WB Saunders/Elsevier Science/Harcourt
200 Wheeler Road   781-221-2212
Burlington, MA 01803   Fax: 781-221-1615
                         e-mail: custserv.bh@elsevier.com
                                  www.us.elsevierhealth.com
Current aspects of physical medicine and rehabilitation in a single, readable volume. Completely updated and revised edition includes all the latest advances and techniques.
2001

Children's Books

6611 Abby & the South Seas Adventure Series
Tyndale House Publishers
PO Box 80   630-668-8300
Wheaton, IL 60189   Fax: 630-668-3245
                                       www.tyndalecatalog.com
Delightful new series, focusing on the travels of Abby Kendall, who has muscular dystrophy, is a sure-fire hit for 8 to 12 year old girls. Lots of surprises will keep them coming back for each new Abby title.
2000

6612 Heartsongs, Journey Through Heartsongs, Hope Through Heartsongs, Celebrate
Hyperion Books
1344 Crossman Avenue   408-744-9500
Sunnyvale, CA 94089   Fax: 408-744-0400
                                          www.hyperion.com
By the 2002-2003 National Goodwill Ambassador for the Muscular Dystrophy Association. The first two books of inspiring poems were both on the New York Times bestseller list. Mattie's struggle with muscular dystrophy has never kept him from feeling deep love for his family, friends, country and faith — heartfelt emotions that are reflected throughout these pages by a precociously brilliant boy.
2001-2003
Carol Sowell, Director Publications

6613 Muscular Dystrophy
Enslow Publishers
40 Industrial Road
Berkeley Heights, NJ 07922-0398   800-398-2504
                                          Fax: 908-771-0925
                               e-mail: info@enslow.com
                                        www.enslow.com
Written for children, this book follows two families with muscular dystrophy and describes various forms of the disease, who gets it, and how to learn to live with it.
2000

Magazines

6614 Quest Magazine
Muscular Dystrophy Association
3300 E Sunrise Drive   520-529-5317
Tucson, AZ 85718-3299   800-572-1717
                                          Fax: 520-529-5300
                         e-mail: publications@mdusa.org
                                           www.mda.org
Quarterly magazine. Contains stories about vital concerns of people with meuromuscular diseases and their community. Find tips, hobbies, resources, treatments, findings, and products. Available online.
30 pages Paperback
Bob Mackle, Director Public Information
Christina Medvescek, Director of Editorial Services

Pamphlets

6615 Breathe Easy: Respiratory Care with Muscular Dystrophy
Muscular Dystrophy Association
3300 E Sunrise Drive   520-529-5317
Tucson, AZ 85718-3299   800-572-1717
                                          Fax: 520-529-5383
                         e-mail: publications@mdusa.org
                                           www.mda.org
Members of a respiratory care team describe how muscular dystrophy can affect breathing, maintaining respiratory health and types of therapies. Also available in Spanish.
2006
Christina Medvescek, Director of Editorial Services

6616 Everybody's Different Nobody's Perfect
Muscular Dystrophy Association
3300 E Sunrise Drive   520-529-5317
Tucson, AZ 85718-3299   800-572-1717
                                          Fax: 520-529-5300
                         e-mail: publications@mdusa.org
                                           www.mda.org
Children's Book. Explains how muscular dystrophy affects children and describes how people are different from each other in many ways. Emphasizing fun, friendship and caring, this booklet is ideal for heightening awareness and encouraging understanding of persons with disabilities. Also available in Spanish.
1999 11 pages Paperback
Bob Mackle, Director Public Information
Christina Medvescek, Director of Editorial Services

6617 Facts About Charcot-Marie-Tooth Disease
Muscular Dystrophy Association
3300 E Sunrise Drive   520-529-5317
Tucson, AZ 85718-3299   800-572-1717
                                          Fax: 520-529-5383
                         e-mail: publications@mdausa.org
                                           www.mda.org
Covers the forms of the disease and outlines the characteristics and genetic patterns of the CMTs. Research efforts aimed at finding the causes, treatments and cures are also described. Also available in Spanish.
15 pages
Christina Medvescek, Director of Editorial Services

6618 Facts About Duchenne & Becker Muscular Dystrophies
Muscular Dystrophy Association
3300 E Sunrise Drive   520-529-5317
Tucson, AZ 85718-3299   800-572-1717
                                          Fax: 520-529-5383
                         e-mail: publications@mdausa.org
                                           www.mda.org
Introductory booklet describes the two disorders, testing, inheritance and treatments. Also available in Spanish.
Christina Medvescek, Director of Editorial Services

6619 Facts About Facioscapulohumeral Muscular Dystrophy
Muscular Dystrophy Association

3300 E Sunrise Drive
Tucson, AZ 85718-3299
520-529-5317
800-572-1717
Fax: 520-529-5383
e-mail: publications@mdusa.org
www.mda.org

Introductory booklet describes FSHD in easy-to-understand terms and answers commonly asked questions about the disease. Also available in Spanish.
Christina Medvescek, Director of Editorial Services

6620 Facts About Friedreich's Ataxia
Muscular Dystrophy Association
3300 E Sunrise Drive
Tucson, AZ 85718-3299
520-529-5317
800-572-1717
Fax: 520-529-5300
e-mail: publications@mdausa.org
www.mda.org

Explains Friedreich's ataxia in layman's terms and answers commonly asked questions about the disease. Also available in Spanish.
15 pages Paperback
Bob Mackle, Director Public Information
Christina Medvescek, Director of Editorial Services

6621 Facts About Limb-Girdle Muscular Dystrophy
Muscular Dystrophy Association
3300 E Sunrise Drive
Tucson, AZ 85718-3299
520-529-5317
800-572-1717
Fax: 520-529-5383
e-mail: publications@mdausa.org
www.mda.org

Introductory booklet provides basic facts about LGMD and contains information regarding the many forms, diagnostic tests and current treatments. Also available in Spanish.
Christina Medvescek, Director of Editorial Services

6622 Facts About Metabolic Diseases of Muscle
Muscular Dystrophy Association
3300 E Sunrise Drive
Tucson, AZ 85718-3299
520-529-5317
800-572-1717
Fax: 520-529-5300
e-mail: publications@mdusa.org
www.mda.org

Provides an overview of the 11 inheritable metabolic diseases of muscle encompassed by MDA's program. Addresses commonly asked questions and highlights MDA's research efforts aimed at finding the causes of and effective treatments for these disorders. Also available in Spanish.
20 pages Paperback
Bob Mackle, Director Public Information
Christina Medvescek, Director of Editorial Services

6623 Facts About Mitochondrial Myopathies
Muscular Dystrophy Association
3300 E Sunrise Drive
Tucson, AZ 85718-3299
520-529-5317
800-572-1717
Fax: 520-529-5300
e-mail: publications@mdusa.org
www.mda.org

Explains mitochondrial myopathies in layman's terms and answers the most frequently asked questions about this disease. Also available in Spanish.
24 pages Paperback
Bob Mackle, Director Public Information
Christina Medvescek, Director of Editorial Services

6624 Facts About Myasthenia Gravis
Muscular Dystrophy Association
3300 E Sunrise Drive
Tucson, AZ 85718-3299
520-529-5317
800-572-1717
Fax: 520-529-5300
e-mail: publications@mdusa.org
www.mda.org

Explains myasthenia gravis and Lambert-Eaton syndrome in layman's terms and answers the most frequently asked questions about these diseases. Also available in Spanish.
19 pages Paperback
Bob Mackle, Director Public Information
Carol Sowall, Director Publications

6625 Facts About Myopathies
Muscular Dystrophy Association
3300 E Sunrise Drive
Tucson, AZ 85718-3299
520-529-5317
800-572-1717
Fax: 520-529-5300
e-mail: publications@mdusa.org
www.mda.org

Overview of the myopathies encompassed by MDA's program. Addresses commonly asked questions and highlights MDA's research efforts aimed at finding the causes of and effective treatments for these disorders. Also available in Spanish.
18 pages Paperback
Bob Mackle, Director Public Information
Christina Medvescek, Director of Editorial Services

6626 Facts About Myotonic Muscular Dystrophy
Muscular Dystrophy Association
3300 E Sunrise Drive
Tucson, AZ 85718-3299
520-529-5317
800-572-1717
Fax: 520-529-5383
e-mail: publications@mdausa.org
www.mda.org

Introductory booklet provides basic facts about the disorder and explains the causes and effects, as well as tests used to diagnose and MDA's search for treatments and cures. Also available in Spanish.
Christina Medvescek, Director of Editorial Services

6627 Facts About Plasmapheresis
Muscular Dystrophy Association
3300 E Sunrise Drive
Tucson, AZ 85718-3299
520-529-5317
800-572-1717
Fax: 520-529-5300
e-mail: publications@mdusa.org
www.mda.org

Describes plasmapheresis, a plasma exchange procedure often utilized as a treatment for autoimmune disease such as myasthenia gravis and Lambert-Eaton syndrome.
Paperback
Bob Mackle, Director Public Information
Christina Medvescek, Director of Editorial Services

6628 Facts About Polymyostis/Dermatomyositis
Muscular Dystrophy Association
3300 E Sunrise Drive
Tucson, AZ 85718-3299
520-529-5317
800-572-1717
Fax: 520-529-5300
e-mail: publications@mdusa.org
www.mda.org

Outlines these two front forms of inflammatory myopathy. Current approaches to treatment and MDA's efforts in continued research are described. Also available in Spanish.
13 pages Paperback
Bob Mackle, Director Public Information
Christina Medvescek, Director of Editorial Services

6629 Facts About Rare Muscular Dsytrophies
Muscular Dystrophy Association
3300 E Sunrise Drive
Tucson, AZ 85718-3299
520-529-5317
800-572-1717
Fax: 520-529-5300
e-mail: publications@mdusa.org
www.mda.org

This brochure gives basic facts about four forms of muscular dystrophy (Congenital, Distal, Emery-Dreifuss and Oculopharyngeal) and addresses commonly asked questions. Also available in Spanish.
28 pages Paperback
Bob Mackle, Director Public Information
Christina Medvescek, Director of Editorial Services

6630 Facts About Spinal Muscular Atrophy
Muscular Dystrophy Association
3300 E Sunrise Drive
Tucson, AZ 85718-3299
520-529-5317
800-572-1717
Fax: 520-529-5300
e-mail: publications@mdusa.org
www.mda.org

Covers the four forms of the disease and outlines the characteristics and genetic patterns of the SMAs. Research efforts aimed at

finding the causes, treatments and cures are also described. Also available in Spanish.
15 pages Paperback
Bob Mackle, Director Public Information
Christina Medvescek, Director of Editorial Services

6631 Genetics and Neuromuscular Diseases
Muscular Dystrophy Association
3300 E Sunrise Drive
Tucson, AZ 85718-3299
520-529-5317
800-572-1717
Fax: 520-529-5383
e-mail: publications@mdausa.org
www.mda.org
Booklet describes what a genetic disorder is and explains how genetic testing and counseling can help people understand how disorders that may affect them or their children are inherited. Also available in Spanish.
Christina Medvescek, Director of Editorial Services

6632 Hey, I'm Here Too
Muscular Dystrophy Association
3300 E Sunrise Drive
Tucson, AZ 85718-3299
520-529-5317
800-572-1717
Fax: 520-529-5383
e-mail: publications@mdausa.org
www.mda.org
Help for siblings of boys with Duchenne muscular dystrophy. Explores how they feel about themselves, their brothers and their families. Also provides specific answers to some questions that siblings may wonder about. Also available in Spanish.
28 pages
Bob Mackle, Director Public Information
Christina Medvescek, Director of Editorial Services

6633 Learning to Live with Neuromuscular Desease: A Message to Parents
Muscular Dystrophy Association
3300 E Sunrise Drive
Tucson, AZ 85718-3299
520-529-5317
800-572-1717
Fax: 520-529-5383
e-mail: publications@mdausa.org
www.mda.org
Helps parents and families cope with the fact that their child has a neuromuscular disease and with the impact the disease will have on everyday life. Also available in Spanish.
Christina Medvescek, Director of Editorial Services

6634 MDA Camp: A Special Place
Muscular Dystrophy Association
3300 E Sunrise Drive
Tucson, AZ 85718-3299
520-529-5317
800-572-1717
Fax: 520-529-5300
e-mail: publications@mdusa.org
www.mdusa.org
Highlights the activities of MDA dummer camps for youngsters diagnosed with one of the more than 40 diseases in MDA's program. Shares camper and volunteer reactions. Also available in Spanish.
Paperback
Bob Mackle, Director Public Information
Carol Sowall, Director Publications

6635 MDA Fact Sheet
Muscular Dystrophy Association
3300 E Sunrise Drive
Tucson, AZ 85718-3299
520-529-5317
800-572-1717
Fax: 520-529-5383
e-mail: publications@mdausa.org
www.mda.org
Basic information on MDA's origins and purposes; the more than 40 neuromuscular diseases in MDA's program, and brief symptom descriptions by category. Also available in Spanish.
Christina Medvescek, Director of Editorial Services

6636 MDA Services for the Individual, Family and Community
Muscular Dystrophy Association
3300 E Sunrise Drive
Tucson, AZ 85718-3299
520-529-5317
800-572-1717
Fax: 520-529-5383
e-mail: publications@mdausa.org
www.mda.org

Lists the diseases covered by MDA as well as eligibility criteria for MDA's services program, a list of MDA-sponsored clinics nationwide, and the services available through local MDA offices. Also available in Spanish.
Christina Medvescek, Director of Editorial Services

6637 Teacher's Guide to Neuromuscular Disease
Muscular Dystrophy Association
3300 E Sunrise Drive
Tucson, AZ 85718-3299
520-529-5317
Fax: 520-529-5383
e-mail: publications@mdausa.org
www.mda.org
This publication provides a source of guidance and information to teachers, giving details about neuromuscular diseases, how they affect school participation, and ways that teachers can help meet the needs of students affected by these disorders.
2005
Christina Medvescek, Director of Editorial Services

6638 Travis, I Got Lots of Neat Stuff Children Living with Muscular Dystrophy
Muscular Dystrophy Association
3300 E Sunrise Drive
Tucson, AZ 85718-3299
520-529-5317
800-572-1717
Fax: 520-529-5383
e-mail: publications@mdausa.org
www.mda.org
Booklet illustrates that a child with muscular dystrophy can do many things. Adapted for MDA's Hop-a-Thon program, the booklet heightens awareness and understanding of people with disabilities. It's suitable for youngsters in elementary school. Also available in Spanish.
24 pages
Christina Medvescek, Director of Editorial Services

Audio & Video

6639 Muscular Dystrophy
Films for the Humanities & Sciences
Box 2053
Princeton, NJ 08543-2053
609-419-8000
800-257-5126
Fax: 609-275-3767
Video deals with how Muscular Dystrophy sufferers deal with the disease that has no cure. Three life stories dealing with surgery, medicine, therapy and bracing as a means to survive. Dr. Betty Banke discusses the need to find a cure while Richard Nordgren from the Dartmouth-Hitchcock Medical Center discusses treatment.
20 Minutes

Web Sites

6640 Healing Well
www.healingwell.com
An online health resource guide to medical news, chat, information and articles, newsgroups and message boards, books, disease-related web sites, medical directories, and more for patients, friends, and family coping with disabling diseases, disorders, or chronic illnesses.

6641 Health Finder
www.healthfinder.gov
Searchable, carefully developed web site offering information on over 1000 topics. Developed by the US Department of Health and Human Services, the site can be used in both English and Spanish.

6642 Healthlink USA
www.healthlinkusa.com
Health information concerning treatment, cures, prevention, diagnosis, risk factors, research, support groups, email lists, personal stories and much more. Updated regularly.

6643 Helios Health
www.helioshealth.com
Online resource for your health information. Detailed information about specific health topics, access to expert advice from our Medical Advisory Board, and up-to-date health news.

6644 MedicineNet

www.medicinenet.com

An online resource for consumers providing easy-to-read, authoritative medical and health information.

6645 Medscape

www.medscape.com

Medscape offers specialists, primary care physicians, and other health professionals the Web's most robust and integrated medical information and educational tools.

6646 Muscular Dystrophy Association

www.mdausa.org

Information on effective treatments for muscular dystrophy, related neuromuscular disorders and research programs. In addition, MDA offers a comprehensive program of patient and community services, with access to over 230 MDA-supported clinics nationwide.

6647 Parent Project: Muscular Dystrophy

www.parentprojectmd.org

Parent Project Muscular Dystrophy (PPMD) is the largest most comprehensive nonprofit organization in the United States focused on finding a cure for Duchenne muscular dystrophy. There mission is to end Duchenne. They invest deeply in treatments for this generation of young men affected by Duchenne and in research that will benefit future generations.

6648 WebMD

www.webmd.com

Provides credible information, supportive communities, and in-depth reference material about health subjects. A source for original and timely health information as well as material from well known content providers.

Description

6649 Myasthenia Gravis

Myasthenia gravis is a disease of the neuromuscular junction - the structure which carries the nerve's chemical signal that tells the muscle to contract. Circulating antibodies attack this junction, leading to weakness of voluntary muscles and muscle fatigue after exercise. Any muscle may be involved, but muscles in the face and throat are especially susceptible. The disease therefore especially affects chewing, swallowing, coughing and facial expressions. These manifestations fluctuate in intensity over hours to days.

Because this disease is caused by an overactive immune system, most treatments target this system. These include corticosteroids, immunosuppressive drugs such as azathioprine, plasmapheresis (filtration of the blood with retention of the cells and removal of the plasma), intravenous immunoglobulins and surgical removal of the thymus gland. In addition, anticholinesterase drugs like pyridostigmine increase the level of the messenger chemical at the neuromuscular junction, thereby increasing muscle strength.

Because of the progressive weakness associated with this disease, physical therapy and assistive devices are generally required.

National Agencies & Associations

6650 American Association for Pediatric Ophthalmology And Strabismus
655 Beach Street
San Francisco, CA 94109
415-561-8505
Fax: 415-561-8531
e-mail: aapos@aao.org
www.aapos.org

AAPOS is the American Association for Pediatric Ophthalmology and Strabismus.
Sherwin J. Isenberg, MD, President
M. Edward Wilson, MD, Vice President

6651 American Association of Neuromuscular & Electrodiagnostic Medicine
2621 Superior Drive NW
Rochester, MN 55901
507-288-0100
Fax: 507-288-1225
e-mail: aanem@aanem.org
www.aanem.org

The American Association of Neuromuscular & Electrodiagnostic Medicine (AANEM) is a nonprofit membership association dedicated to the advancement of neuromuscular, musculoskeletal, and electrodiagnostic medicine.
Vincent J. Tranchitella, MD, President
Shirlyn A. Adkins, JD, Executive Director

6652 Myasthenia Gravis Association of BC
2805 Kingsway
Vancouver, BC, V5R-5H9   e-mail: mgabc@centreforability.bc.ca
640-451-5511
www.myasthenia.org

Informs members about new treatment thods and research concerning myasthenia gravis.

6653 Myasthenia Gravis Foundation of America, Inc.
355 Lexington Ave.
New York, NY 10017
212-297-2156
800-541-5454
Fax: 212-370-9047
e-mail: mgfa@myasthenia.org
www.myasthenia.org

The mission of the Foundation is to facilitate the timely diagnosis end optimal care of individuals affected by myasthenia gravis and closely related disorders and to improve their lives through programs of patient services, public information and medical reports.
Marcia Lorimer, Executive Committee
Sam Schulhof, Chair

State Agencies & Associations

Alaska

6654 Pacific Northwest Chapter of the Myasthenia Gravis Foundation of America
PO Box 58785
Renton, WA 98058-6562
425-235-1435
877-252-0677
Fax: 425-204-2070
e-mail: washington@myasthenia.org
www.myasthenia.org

Arizona

6655 Jim L Walker: Arizona Chapter of the Myasthenia Gravis Foundation of America
PO Box 34173
Phoenix, AZ 85067-4173
480-451-3060
877-347-7905
Fax: 480-767-7029
e-mail: arizona@myasthenia.org
www.azmgfa.org

Jim LoVecchio, Chairman
Stephane Borsk, Vice Chairman

Connecticut

6656 Connecticut Chapter of the Myasthenia Gravis Foundation of America
P.O. Box 2801
Danbury, CT 06813-2801
203-556-5012
866-329-8784
e-mail: conn@myasthenia.org
www.myasthenia.org/connecticut_nutmeg

Irving Beck ED

Delaware

6657 MD/DC/Delaware Chapter of Myasthenia Gravis Foundation of America
PO Box 186
Pasedena, MD 21123-0186
410-437-1157
866-437-2881
e-mail: maryland@myasthenia.org
www.myasthenia.org/LivingwithMG/MGFAChap

District of Columbia

6658 MD/DC/Delaware Chapter of Myasthenia Gravis Foundation of America
PO Box 186
Pasedena, MD 21113-0186
410-437-1157
866-437-2881
e-mail: maryland@myasthenia.org
www.myasthenia.org/LivingwithMG/MGFAChap

Florida

6659 Florida Chapter of the Myasthenia Gravis Foundation of America
14502 87 Avenue N
Seminole, FL 33776-0623
727-596-1491
877-596-1491
Fax: 727-596-1491
e-mail: wcflorida@myasthenia.org
www.myasthenia.org

Georgia

6660 Georgia Chapter of the Myasthenia Gravis Foundation of America
P.O. Box 889085
Atlanta, GA 30356
770-427-3441
800-743-4339
Fax: 770-973-3269
e-mail: georgia@myasthenia.org
www.mggeorgia.org

Hawaii

6661 **Pacific Northwest Chapter of the Myasthenia Gravis Foundation of America**
PO Box 58785   425-235-1435
Renton, WA 98058-6562   877-252-0677
Fax: 425-204-2070
e-mail: washington@myasthenia.org
www.myasthenia.org

Idaho

6662 **Pacific Northwest Chapter of the Myasthenia Gravis Foundation of America**
PO Box 58785   425-235-1435
Renton, WA 98058-6562   877-252-0677
Fax: 425-204-2070
e-mail: washington@myasthenia.org
www.myasthenia.org

Indiana

6663 **Greater Indianapolis Chapter of the Myasthenia Gravis Foundation of America**
8922 Haverstick Road   317-846-1462
Indianapolis, IN 46240   e-mail: Spknke@aol.com
www.4-mga.org/?

Earl Zimmerman, Chair

Maine

6664 **Connecticut Chapter of the Myasthenia Gravis Foundation of America**
P.O. Box 2801   203-556-5012
Danbury, CT 06813-2801   866-329-8784
e-mail: conn@myasthenia.org
www.myasthenia.org/connecticut_nutmeg

Irving Beck ED

Maryland

6665 **MD/DC/Delaware Chapter of Myasthenia Gravis Foundation of America**
PO Box 186   410-437-1157
Pasadena, MD 21123-0186   866-437-2881
e-mail: maryland@myasthenia.org
www.myasthenia.org

Massachusetts

6666 **Mass./New Hampshire Chapter of the Myasthenia Gravis Foundation of America**
460 S. River St.   508-435-3808
Marshfield, MA 02050   e-mail: massachusetts@myashtenia.org
www.ma-nhmgfa.org

Michigan

6667 **Great Lakes Chapter of the Myasthenia Gravis Foundation of America**
2660 Horizon Drive SE   616-956-0622
Grand Rapids, MI 49546   800-224-9180
Fax: 616-956-9234
e-mail: myasthenia.info@gmail.com
www.myasthenia-mi.org
Autoimmune, neuromuscular disease manifest in weakness of voluntary muscles; arms, legs, eyes, facial expressions, severe cases of breathing.
Susan Richards, Executive Director
Paulus Heule, President

Minnesota

6668 **Minnesota State Chapter of the Myasthenia Gravis Foundation of America**
29234 Piney Way   218-562-4594
Breezy Point, MN 56472-1715   e-mail: minnesota@myasthenia.org
www.myasthenia.org

Montana

6669 **Pacific Northwest Chapter of the Myasthenia Gravis Foundation of America**
PO Box 58785   425-235-1435
Renton, WA 98058-6562   877-252-0677
Fax: 425-204-2070
e-mail: washington@myasthenia.org
www.myasthenia.org

New Hampshire

6670 **Mass./New Hampshire Chapter of the Myasthenia Gravis Foundation of America**
460 S River Street   508-435-3808
Marshfield, MA 02050   e-mail: massachusetts@myasthenia.org
www.ma-nhmgfa.org

Marilyn Buckner, Chair
Virginia Pierce, RN, Treasurer

New Jersey

6671 **Garden State Chapter of the Myasthenia Gravis Foundation of America**
PO Box 4258   973-835-4444
Wayne, NJ 07474-1362   800-437-4949
Fax: 973-835-4452
e-mail: mgnj@mgnj.org
www.mgnj.org

Robert Allen, Chairman
Kelley DeVincentis, Executive Director

New York

6672 **Upstate NY Chapter of the Myasthenia Gravis Foundation of America**
14 Summit Rd.   518-439-5377
Delmar, NY 12054   800-581-5377
Fax: 518-439-8783
e-mail: upstatenewyork@myasthenia.org
www.myasthenia.org

Barry Levine, President/Chair

North Carolina

6673 **Carolinas Chapter of the Myasthenia Gravis Foundation of America**
506 E Forest Hills Boulevard   919-966-4131
Durham, NC 27707-1801   800-842-8711
Fax: 919-489-7564
e-mail: tvassar56@aol.com
www.med.unc.edu/mgfa/mgnc-hom.htm

Oklahoma

6674 **Oklahoma Chapter of the Myasthenia Gravis Foundation of America**
4606 E 67th St S   918-494-4951
Tulsa, OK 74136   Fax: 918-494-4951
e-mail: oklahoma@myasthenia.org
www.myasthenia.org

Peggy Foust, Executive Director
Margret Feller, Vice-President/Treasurer

Oregon

6675 **Pacific Northwest Chapter of the Myasthenia Gravis Foundation of America**
PO Box 58785   425-235-1435
Renton, WA 98058-6562   877-252-0677
Fax: 425-204-2070
e-mail: washington@myasthenia.org
www.myasthenia.org

Rhode Island

6676 Connecticut Chapter of the Myasthenia Gravis Foundation of America
P.O. Box 2801   203-556-5012
Danbury, CT 06813-2801   866-329-8784
e-mail: conn@myasthenia.org
www.myasthenia.org/connecticut_nutmeg
Irving Beck ED

South Carolina

6677 Carolinas Chapter of the Myasthenia Gravis Foundation of America
506 E Forest Hills Boulevard   919-490-2937
Durham, NC 27707-1801   800-842-8711
Fax: 919-489-7564
e-mail: tvassar56@aol.com
www.myasthenia.org

Texas

6678 Northwest Texas Chapter of the Myasthenia Gravis Foundation of America
3406 Manioca Road   806-749-3126
Lubbock, TX 79403   Fax: 915-554-7044
e-mail: nwtexas@myasthenia.org
www.nwtcmg.org

Lowell McBroom, Vice-Chairperson

Vermont

6679 Connecticut Chapter of the Myasthenia Gravis Foundation of America
P.O. Box 2801   203-556-5012
Danbury, CT 06813-2801   866-329-8784
e-mail: conn@myasthenia.org
www.myasthenia.org/connecticut_nutmeg
Irving Beck ED

Washington

6680 Pacific Northwest Chapter of the Myasthenia Gravis Foundation of America
PO Box 58785   425-235-1435
Renton, WA 98058-6562   877-252-0677
Fax: 425-204-2070
e-mail: washington@myasthenia.org
www.myasthenia.org

Wisconsin

6681 Wisconsin Chapter of the Myasthenia Gravis Foundation of America
2474 S 96 Street   262-938-9800
W Allis, WI 53227   800-541-5454
Fax: 262-789-3363
e-mail: wisconsin@myasthenia.org
www.myasthenia.org
The Myasthenia Gravis Foundation of America is the only national volunteer health agency dedicated solely to fight against myasthenoia gravis.
Patricia Lamp, Chairperson
Ellie Burbach, Vice-Chairperson

Wyoming

6682 Pacific Northwest Chapter of the Myasthenia Gravis Foundation of America
PO Box 58785   425-235-1435
Renton, WA 98058-6562   877-252-0677
Fax: 425-204-2070
e-mail: washington@myasthenia.org
www.myasthenia.org

Support Groups & Hotlines

6683 National Health Information Center
US Department of Health and Human Services
PO Box 1133   301-565-4167
Washington, DC 20013-1133   800-336-4797
Fax: 301-984-4256
e-mail: info@nhic.org
www.health.gov/nhic
Offers a nationwide referral service, produces directories and resource guides.

Arizona

6684 Myasthenia Gravis Support Group of Arizona Jim L. Walker Chapter
Phoenix, AZ
520-889-6910
www.myasthenia.org
Serves patients and their families throughout the state. The goal is to help achieve the conquest of Myasthenia Gravis through research, education, public awareness, anf fundraising.

Connecticut

6685 Myasthenia Gravis Support Group of Connect icut (Nutmeg Group)
e-mail: conn@myasthenia.org
www.myasthenia.org
Serves patients and their families throughout the state. The goal is to help achieve the conquest of Myasthenia Gravis through research, education, public awareness, anf fundraising.

Georgia

6686 Myasthenia Gravis Support Group of Atlanta
770-427-3441
e-mail: mg.georgia@yahoo.com
www.myasthenia.org
Serves patients and their families throughout the state. The goal is to help achieve the conquest of Myasthenia Gravis through research, education, public awareness, anf fundraising.

Iowa

6687 Myasthenia Gravis Support Group of Ames
515-708-5386
e-mail: amy.schindel@gmail.com
www.myasthenia.org
Serves patients and their families throughout the state. The goal is to help achieve the conquest of Myasthenia Gravis through research, education, public awareness, anf fundraising.

Kentucky

6688 Myasthenia Gravis Support Group of Louisvi lle
859-967-4117
e-mail: jennifer-howard@hotmail.com
www.myasthenia.org
Serves patients and their families throughout the state. The goal is to help achieve the conquest of Myasthenia Gravis through research, education, public awareness, anf fundraising.

Louisiana

6689 Myasthenia Gravis Support Group of Louisia na
504-376-7474
e-mail: tommy.santora@gmail.com
www.myasthenia.org
Serves patients and their families throughout the state. The goal is to help achieve the conquest of Myasthenia Gravis through research, education, public awareness, anf fundraising.

Massachusetts

6690 Myasthenia Gravis Support Group of Eastern Massachusetts and New Hampshire

508-435-3808
www.ma-nhmgfa.org
Serves patients and their families throughout the state. The goal is to help achieve the conquest of Myasthenia Gravis through research, education, public awareness, anf fundraising.

6691 Myasthenia Gravis Support Group of Western Massachusetts and New Hampshire

508-435-3808
www.ma-nhmgfa.org
Serves patients and their families throughout the state. The goal is to help achieve the conquest of Myasthenia Gravis through research, education, public awareness, anf fundraising.

Minnesota

6692 Myasthenia Gravis Support Group of Mid-Min n

218-563-4594
e-mail: mgcorn@uslink.net
www.myasthenia.org
Serves patients and their families throughout the state. The goal is to help achieve the conquest of Myasthenia Gravis through research, education, public awareness, anf fundraising.

6693 Myasthenia Gravis Support Group of South East Minnesota

507-206-0625
e-mail: mgwalleworld@gmail.com
www.myasthenia.org
Serves patients and their families throughout the state. The goal is to help achieve the conquest of Myasthenia Gravis through research, education, public awareness, anf fundraising.

6694 Myasthenia Gravis Support Group of the Twin Cities

651-633-5465
e-mail: liannema@mac.com
www.myasthenia.org
Serves patients and their families throughout the state. The goal is to help achieve the conquest of Myasthenia Gravis through research, education, public awareness, anf fundraising.

New Hampshire

6695 Myasthenia Gravis Support Group of Eastern Massachusetts and New Hampshire

508-435-3808
www.ma-nhmgfa.org
Serves patients and their families throughout the state. The goal is to help achieve the conquest of Myasthenia Gravis through research, education, public awareness, anf fundraising.

6696 Myasthenia Gravis Support Group of Western Massachusetts and New Hampshire

508-435-3808
www.ma-nhmgfa.org
Serves patients and their families throughout the state. The goal is to help achieve the conquest of Myasthenia Gravis through research, education, public awareness, anf fundraising.

New Mexico

6697 Myasthenia Gravis Support Group of New Mex ico

505-934-2423
e-mail: cormier87@q.com
www.myasthenia.org
Serves patients and their families throughout the state. The goal is to help achieve the conquest of Myasthenia Gravis through research, education, public awareness, anf fundraising.

New York

6698 Myasthenia Gravis Support Group of Manhatt an

e-mail: namerican@myasthenia.org
www.myasthenia.org
Serves patients and their families throughout the state. The goal is to help achieve the conquest of Myasthenia Gravis through research, education, public awareness, anf fundraising.

6699 Myasthenia Gravis Support Group of Upstate New York

518-439-5377
www.myasthenia.org
Serves patients and their families throughout the state. The goal is to help achieve the conquest of Myasthenia Gravis through research, education, public awareness, anf fundraising.

North Carolina

6700 Myasthenia Gravis Support Group of Charlotte

704-536-9572
877-643-2221
e-mail: zebheads@carolin.rr.com
www.cncmg.org
Serves patients and their families throughout the state. The goal is to help achieve the conquest of Myasthenia Gravis through research, education, public awareness, anf fundraising.

6701 Myasthenia Gravis Support Group of Central North Carolina

919-567-9313
e-mail: info@cncmg.org
www.cncmg.org
Serves patients and their families throughout the state. The goal is to help achieve the conquest of Myasthenia Gravis through research, education, public awareness, anf fundraising.

6702 Myasthenia Gravis Support Group of Durham/ Chapel Hill

704-536-9572
877-643-2221
e-mail: mmenold@gmail.com
www.myasthenia.org
Serves patients and their families throughout the state. The goal is to help achieve the conquest of Myasthenia Gravis through research, education, public awareness, anf fundraising.

6703 Myasthenia Gravis Support Group of Fayette ville

877-643-2221
www.myasthenia.org
Serves patients and their families throughout the state. The goal is to help achieve the conquest of Myasthenia Gravis through research, education, public awareness, anf fundraising.

Ohio

6704 Myasthenia Gravis Support Group of Columbu s

e-mail: j.eickholt@aol.com
www.myasthenia.org
Serves patients and their families throughout the state. The goal is to help achieve the conquest of Myasthenia Gravis through research, education, public awareness, anf fundraising.

6705 Myasthenia Gravis Support Group of Summit- Stark

330-628-2148
e-mail: ralberte@neo.rr.com
www.myasthenia.org
Serves patients and their families throughout the state. The goal is to help achieve the conquest of Myasthenia Gravis through research, education, public awareness, anf fundraising.

Oklahoma

6706 Myasthenia Gravis Support Group of Tulsa and Oklahoma City

918-494-4951
e-mail: oklahoma@myasthenia.org
www.myasthenia.org

Serves patients and their families throughout the state. The goal is to help achieve the conquest of Myasthenia Gravis through research, education, public awareness, anf fundraising.

Pennsylvania

6707 Myasthenia Gravis Support Group of Scranto n

570-687-6009
e-mail: vkrewsun@comcast.net
www.myasthenia.org

Serves patients and their families throughout the state. The goal is to help achieve the conquest of Myasthenia Gravis through research, education, public awareness, anf fundraising.

South Carolina

6708 Myasthenia Gravis Support Group of Low Country

843-388-1683
e-mail: mgsupport11@comcast.net
www.myasthenia.org

Serves patients and their families throughout the state. The goal is to help achieve the conquest of Myasthenia Gravis through research, education, public awareness, anf fundraising.

6709 Myasthenia Gravis Support Group of the Mountain and Up Country

828-698-3928
e-mail: wemtglen@bellsouth.net
www.myasthenia.org

Serves patients and their families throughout the state. The goal is to help achieve the conquest of Myasthenia Gravis through research, education, public awareness, anf fundraising.

Virginia

6710 Myasthenia Gravis Support Group of Manassa s

804-742-5149
e-mail: agsteele@hughes.net
www.myasthenia.org

Serves patients and their families throughout the state. The goal is to help achieve the conquest of Myasthenia Gravis through research, education, public awareness, anf fundraising.

Washington

6711 Myasthenia Gravis Support Group of Seattle , Olympia and Poulsbo

425-271-5151
e-mail: nwmg2012@gmail.com
www.myasthenia.org

Serves patients and their families throughout the state. The goal is to help achieve the conquest of Myasthenia Gravis through research, education, public awareness, anf fundraising.

6712 Myasthenia Gravis Support Group of Spokane

509-468-0507
www.myasthenia.org

Serves patients and their families throughout the state. The goal is to help achieve the conquest of Myasthenia Gravis through research, education, public awareness, anf fundraising.

Wisconsin

6713 Myasthenia Gravis Support Group of Fox Valley

262-938-9800
Fax: 262-789-3363
e-mail: wisconsin@myasthenia.org
www.myasthenia.org

Serves patients and their families throughout the state of Wisconsin. The goal is to help achieve the conquest of Myasthenia Gravis through research, education, public awareness, anf fundraising.

6714 Myasthenia Gravis Support Group of Milwauk ee

262-878-3866
Fax: 262-789-3363
e-mail: mmcb1981@yahoo.com
www.myasthenia.org

Serves patients and their families throughout the state of Wisconsin. The goal is to help achieve the conquest of Myasthenia Gravis through research, education, public awareness, anf fundraising.

Newsletters

6715 Alabama Chapter of the Myasthenia Gravis Foundation of America
Alabama Chapter of the Myasthenia Gravis Found
300 Office Park Drive   205-868-1210
Birmingham, AL 35223   Fax: 205-868-1211
e-mail: alchaptermgfa@aol.com

Three to four newsletters per year. Support Group Information, articles about MG and it's treatment, information about chapters operations.

6716 Connecticut Nutmeg
Myasthenia Gravis Foundation
113 Folly Brook Boulevard   860-529-8784
Wethersfield, CT 06109   Fax: 860-529-8784

6717 Conquer
Myasthenia Gravis Foundation of Illinois
2411 New Street   708-385-3888
Blue Island, IL 60406-2328   800-888-6208
Fax: 708-385-0447
e-mail: myastheniaill@aol.com
myastheniagravis.org

A quarterly newsletter containing articles and stories relating to myasthenia gravis.
16 pages Quarterly
Gerald Tarka, Executive Director

6718 East Central Florida Chapter of the Myasthenia Gravis Foundation of America
PO Box 623   904-672-2635
Ormond Beach, FL 32175-0623

Published bi-monthly, and contains information about latest research. area meetings, and topics of concern for our readers.

6719 Facts About Myasthenia Gravis for Patients and Families
Myasthenia Gravis Foundation of America
5841 Cedar Lake Road   952-545-9438
Minneapolis, MN 55416   800-541-5454
Fax: 952-646-2028
e-mail: myastheniagravis@msn.com
www.myasthenia.org

Offers information on the history, clinical symptoms and features, causes, diagnosis, treatment and prognosis of Myasthenia Gravis.
16 pages 4 per year
Debora K Boelz, CEO
Jennifer Heidelberger, Chapter Relations Manager

6720 MG Communicator
Great Lakes Chapter of the Myasthenia Gravis Found
2680 Horizon Drive SE   616-956-0622
Grand Rapids, MI 49546   800-224-9180
Fax: 616-956-9234
e-mail: myasthenia.info@gmail.com
www.myasthenia-mi.org

3x/year
Susan Richards, Executive Director
Paulus Heule, President

6721 Myasthenia Gravis Foundation: Geater South Texas
10592 A Fuqua   281-987-9393
Houston, TX 77089-1402   Fax: 281-328-2430
e-mail: gowens@accesscomm.net

Six issues per year. Support Group Information, articles about MG and it's treatment, information about Chapter operations.
Gary Owens, Chair

6722 Myasthenia Gravis Foundation: Northwest Texas Chapter
281 County Road 135
Ovalo, TX 79541   e-mail: nwtxmg@hotmail.com

A quarterly newsletter containing articles and stories relating myasthenia gravis.
Jenne McVicker, Editor

6723 Puget Sound Chapter Newsletter
PO Box 587853
Renton, WA 98058-1785

206-235-1435
Fax: 206-204-2070

A quarterly newsletter containing the latest articles and stories relating to myasthenia gravis.

Web Sites

6724 Healing Well

www.healingwell.com

An online health resource guide to medical news, chat, information and articles, newsgroups and message boards, books, disease-related web sites, medical directories, and more for patients, friends, and family coping with disabling diseases, disorders, or chronic illnesses.

6725 Health Finder

www.healthfinder.gov

Searchable, carefully developed web site offering information on over 1000 topics. Developed by the US Department of Health and Human Services, the site can be used in both English and Spanish.

6726 Healthlink USA

www.healthlinkusa.com

Health information concerning treatment, cures, prevention, diagnosis, risk factors, research, support groups, email lists, personal stories and much more. Updated regularly.

6727 Helios Health

www.helioshealth.com

Online resource for your health information. Detailed information about specific health topics, access to expert advice from our Medical Advisory Board, and up-to-date health news.

6728 MedicineNet

www.medicinenet.com

An online resource for consumers providing easy-to-read, authoritative medical and health information.

6729 Medscape

www.medscape.com

Medscape offers specialists, primary care physicians, and other health professionals the Web's most robust and integrated medical information and educational tools.

6730 Myasthenia Gravis Foundation of America

www.myasthenia.org

The Myasthenia Gravis Foundation of America (MGFA) is a national volunteer health agency in the United States dedicated solely to the fight against myasthenia gravis. MGFA serves patients, their families and caregivers through a network of chapters, support groups and programs. Each chapter shares the vision of a world without MG.

6731 Neurology Channel

www.healthcommunities.com

Find clearly explained, medically accurate information regarding conditions, including an overview, symptoms, causes, diagnostic procedures and treatment options. On this site it is possible to ask questions and get information from a neurologist and connect to people who have similar health interests.

6732 WebMD

www.webmd.com

Provides credible information, supportive communities, and in-depth reference material about health subjects. A source for original and timely health information as well as material from well known content providers.

Description

6733 Neurofibromatosis

Neurofibromatosis, or von Recklinghausen disease, named after a German pathologist, is an inherited genetic disorder. The more common form occurs once in 4,000 births. The skin and the nervous system are the primary target organs. Characteristic skin lesions are large, flat brown freckles, called cafe au lait spots, owing to their light coffee color. They are apparent at birth or in infancy in more than 90 percent of patients. Flesh-colored tumors appear in late childhood. Abnormal growths may be detectable in the brain, perhaps accounting for the seizures and learning difficulties commonly seen in this syndrome. Tumors may appear on the nerves from the eyes or the ears, sometimes causing hearing loss or visual disturbance.

There is no specific therapy for this condition, but tumors that produce severe symptoms can be surgically removed or irradiated. Genetic counseling is important for the entire family.

National Agencies & Associations

6734 Association for the Neurologically Disable d of Canada
59 Clement Road 416-244-1992
Etobicoke, Ontario, M9R-1Y5 Fax: 416-244-4099
e-mail: info@and.ca
www.and.ca
Provides functional rehabilitation programs to individuals with neurological disabilities.
Basil Ziv, Executive Director
Dr John Unruh, Director of Rehabilitation

6735 BC Centre for Ability
2805 Kingsway 604-451-5511
Vancouver, BC, V5R-5H9 Fax: 604-451-5651
e-mail: home@centreforability.bc.ca
www.centreforability.bc.ca
Founded in 1969 by families who desired alternatives to hospital or institutional-based services. The centre provides education and promotes the rights of individuals with disabilities to participate as valued members of their communities.
Angie Kwok, Executive Director
Moses Gabriel, Director of Resource Development

6736 Children's Tumor Foundation
95 Pine Street 212-344-6633
New York, NY 10005 800-323-7938
Fax: 212-747-0004
e-mail: info@ctf.org
www.ctf.org
Dedicated to health and well being of individuals and families affected by the neurofibromatoses (NF).
Allison Walsh, Communications Officer
John Risner, President

6737 NF Canada
PO Box 5055 888-986-3876
Victoria, V8R 6-2R7 e-mail: infocanada@nfcanada.ca
www.nfcanada.ca
To ensure that all Canadians living with neurofibromatosis benefit from support, understanding, appropriate medical treatment and the hope that a cure is on the horizon.
Inara Kundzins, President

6738 Neurofibromatosis
Po Box 18246 651-225-1720
Minneapolis, MN 55418 800-942-6825
Fax: 301-918-0009
e-mail: info@nfinc.org
www.nfnetwork.org
A national nonprofit organization with independent and regional chapters that provides support and services to NF families. Simulates funds and encourages participation in NF research. Works closely with clinical and research professionals.
Miguel Lessing, President
Rosemary Anderson, Vice President

6739 Neurofibromatosis Society of Ontario
2004 Underhill Court 905-683-0811
Pickering, Ontario, L1X 2-3T2 Fax: 705-685-1409
e-mail: info@nfon.ca
www.nfon.ca
Support individuals and families affected by NF, to educate its members, professionals, and the general public about NF, and support NF research.
Lynne Leyland, Director
Gladys Hamilton, Director

6740 Neurological Science Federation
7015 Macleod Trail SW 403-229-9544
Calgary, AB, T2H-2K6 Fax: 403-229-1661
e-mail: info@cnsfederation.org
www.ccns.org
To promote and encourage all aspects of neurology, including research, education, assessment and accreditation.

State Agencies & Associations

Alabama

6741 NNFF Alabama Affiliate
1205 Branchwater Lane 205-529-8006
Birmingham, AL 35216 e-mail: info@ctf.org
www.ctf.org
Jeff Albright, Chairperson

Arizona

6742 Neurofibromatosis Association of Arizona
Po Box 2718 480-945-9650
Chandler, AZ 85244 Fax: 480-945-9650
e-mail: info@nfaz.org
www.nfaz.org
Nicole Hicks, Executive Director
Michael Sheedy, President

Arkansas

6743 NNFF Arkansas Affilaite
139 Rainbow Lne 501-759-2710
Bigelow, AR 72016 e-mail: info@ctf.org
www.ctf.org
Lesley Oslica, Information and Support

Colorado

6744 NNFF Colorado Chapter
70 N Ranch Road 303-734-9942
Littleton, CO 80127 e-mail: info@ctf.org
www.ctf.org
Mark Ebel, Chapter President

Connecticut

6745 NNFF Connecticut Chapter
8 S Barn Hill Road 860-286-2705
Bloomfield, CT 06002-1622 Fax: 860-286-2705
TTY: 860-286-2705
TDD: 860-286-2705
e-mail: StevenSand@aol.com
Steve Sandler, Chapter President

Florida

6746 **NNFF Florida Chapter**
PO Box 410684
Melbourne, FL 32941

321-253-1622
800-540-5721
e-mail: info@ctf.org
www.ctf.org

Suzanne Earle, Chapter President

Georgia

6747 **NNFF Georgia Affiliate**
5 Ardmore Circle
Cartersville, GA 30120

678-428-9711
e-mail: info@ctf.org
www.ctf.org

Randy Watkins, Chairman

Idaho

6748 **NNFF Idaho Chapter**
4419 E Linden Street
Caldwell, ID 83605-8037
Suzy Crici, Chapter President

208-459-6022

Illinois

6749 **Illinois Midwest Neurofibromatosis**
Neurofibromatosis
473 Dunham Rd
St. Charles, IL 60174

630-945-3562
800-322-6363
Fax: 630-932-8119
e-mail: info@nfmidwest.org
nfmidwest.org

Diana Haberkamp, Executive Director
Jenny Perkins, Development Director/ Great Steps

6750 **NF Center: North Broward Medical Center Neurofibromatosis**
Neurofibromatosis
213 S. Wheaton Ave.
Wheaton, IL 60187-3502

630-510-1115
800-942-6825
Fax: 630-510-8508
e-mail: admin@nfnetwork.org
www.nfnetwork.org

6751 **NNFF Illinois Chapter: Chicago Area**
5604 W Henderson 3 W
Chicago, IL 60634

e-mail: info@ctf.org
www.ctf.org

Debbi Callahan, Vice President

6752 **NNFF Illinois Chapter: Silvis Area**
513 16th Street
Silvis, IL 61282

309-792-4195
e-mail: nfquadcities@juno.com

Sue Rockwell, Patient Information and Support

6753 **NNFF Illinois Chapter: Springfield Area**
5 Twilight Lane
Springfield, IL 62712

217-529-0834
e-mail: info@ctf.org
www.ctf.org

Marcia Miller, Treasurer

6754 **NNFF Illinois Chapter:Peoria Region**
PO Box 213
Emden, IL 62635

217-732-8568
e-mail: info@ctf.org
www.ctf.org

Paul Beach, President

Indiana

6755 **NNFF Indiana Chapter**
1173 Hague Court
Franklinolis, IN 46131

317-736-7577
e-mail: info@ctf.org
www.ctf.org

Dottie Whitehurst, Chapter President

Iowa

6756 **NNFF Iowa Chapter**
321 Glenview Drive
De Moines, IA 50312

515-277-8494
e-mail: info@ctf.org
www.ctf.org

Sheila Drevyanko, Chapter President

Kansas

6757 **NNFF Kansas Affiliate**
12606 E 49th Terrace
Independence, MO 64055

816-737-8378
e-mail: info@ctf.org
www.ctf.org

Annette Novak, Chairperson

6758 **Neurofibromatosis Kansas and Central Plains**
Neurofibromatosis
9218 Metcalf
Overland Park, KS 66212-1792

620-669-8453
800-942-6825
e-mail: nprieb@sbcglobal.net
www.nfnetwork.org

Louisiana

6759 **NNFF Louisiana Chapter**
PO Box 499
Baton Rouge, LA 70821

225-665-3547
e-mail: info@ctf.org
www.ctf.org

Debbie Bouy, Chairperson

Maryland

6760 **Neurofibromatosis: Mid-Atlantic**
Neurofibromatosis
2 Village Square.
Baltimore, MD 21210-2924

443-423-0535
800-942-6825
Fax: 301-577-0016
e-mail: info@nfmidatlantic.org
www.nfmidatlantic.org

Mid-Atlantic Chapter serves the following states: Maryland Virginia District of Columbia Delaware New Jersey Pennsylvania West Virginia and North Carolina.
Barbra Levin, Executive Director
Beverly B Dobson, President

Massachusetts

6761 **Neurofibromatosis: New England**
Neurofibromatosis
9 Bedford Street
Burlington, MA 01803-3702

781-272-9936
Fax: 781-272-9937
e-mail: info@nfincne.org
www.nfincne.org

Karen Peluso, Executive Director
Dr Paul Epstein, President

Minnesota

6762 **Neurofibromatosis: Minnesota**
Neurofibromatosis
PO Box 18246
Minneapolis, MN 55418

651-225-1720
e-mail: JohnE@cipmn.org
www.nfincmn.org

John Everett, President
Steven Schutts, Vice-President

Nevada

6763 **NNFF Nevada Affiliate: Reno Area**
8065 White Falls Drive
Reno, NV 89506

775-972-1882
e-mail: info@ctf.org
www.ctf.org

David Rice, Chairperson

Oregon

6764 **NNFF Oregon Affiliate Kaiser Permanente Northwest**
Kaiser Permanente Northwest

2806 SW Troy
Portland, OR 97227

503-331-6325
Fax: 503-331-6320
e-mail: info@ctf.org
www.ctf.org

Katie Crow, Genetic Counselor

South Carolina

6765 NNFF South Carolina Chapter
111 Oakview Drive
Darlington, SC 29532

843-393-9672
e-mail: info@ctf.org
www.ctf.org

Pat Chrisely, Chairperson

Wisconsin

6766 NNFF Wisconsin Chapter
6562 W Glenbrook Road
Brown Deer, WI 53223

414-362-0211
e-mail: info@ctf.org
www.ctf.org

Elaine Pankow, President

Support Groups & Hotlines

6767 Children's Tumor Foundation
95 Pine Street
New York, NY 10005

212-344-6633
800-323-7938
Fax: 212-747-0004
e-mail: info@ctf.org
www.ctf.org

Sponsors critical research, public awareness and patient support services.
Allison Walsh, Communications Officer

6768 NF Support Group of West Michigan
Spectrum Health
PO Box 6026
Grand Rapids, MI 49516

616-451-3699
e-mail: nfwestmich@aol.com
www.nfsupport.org

Rose Mary Anderson, Patient Advocate

6769 National Health Information Center
PO Box 1133
Washington, DC 20013

310-565-4167
800-336-4797
Fax: 301-984-4256
e-mail: info@nhic.org
www.health.gov/nhic

Offers a nationwide information referral service, produces directories and resource guides.

6770 Neurofibromatosis
9320 Annapolis Road
Lanham, MD 20706-3123

301-918-4600
800-942-6825
Fax: 301-918-0009
e-mail: nfinfo@nfinc.com
www.nfnetwork.org

Dedicated to individuals and families affected by the neurofibromatosis through educational, support, clinical and research programs.
Miguell Lessing, President
Rosemary Anderson, Vice President

6771 Neurofibromatosis Foundation: Colorado
2505 18th Street, Denver
Denver, CO 80211

303-433-8383
800-323-7938
e-mail: UsRKids@aol.com
www.unitedwaydenver.org

Offers a support group to persons affected by neurofibromatosis. Offers panel discussion, sharing, fundraising, and fun activities. Also provides new patient information.
Charles Taylor
Jane Cahn

6772 Neurofibromatosis Support Network
Parents Helping Parents
1400 Parkmoor Avenue
San Jose, CA 95126

408-727-5775
855-727-5775
Fax: 408-286-1116
www.php.com

Helping children with special needs receive the resources, love, hope, respect, health care, education and other services they need to achieve their full potential by providing them with strong families and dedicated professionals to serve them.
Sheri Sobrato, MA/MFC

6773 Neuroscience Institute at Mercy Hospital
4120N W Memorial Road
Oklahoma City, OK 73120

800-996-3729
Fax: 405-752-3977
www.okmercy.net

Mike Patt, Chief Executive Officer

6774 Texas Neurofibromatosis Foundation
3030 Olive Street
Dallas, TX 75219

972-868-794
Fax: 972-868-7626
www.texasnf.org

Cindy Hahn, Executive Director
Emily Deutscher, Development Coordinator

Newsletters

6775 Neurofibromatosis
213 S. Wheaton Ave.
Wheaton, IL 60187-3123

630-510-1115
800-942-6825
Fax: 630-510-8508
e-mail: admin@nfnetwork.org
www.nfnetwork.org

Provides a variety of resources for NF families, professionals and researchers.
SemiAnnual
Gwen Charest, Executive Director

Pamphlets

6776 Child with Neurofibromatosis 1
Children's Tumor Foundation
120 Wall Street
New York, NY 10005-1703

212-344-6633
800-323-7938
e-mail: info@ctf.org
www.ctf.org

Offers information on the prognosis, management, complications, genetic implications, and sources of support for children with neurofibromatosis 1.
Allison Walsh, Communications Officer

6777 Guide for Teens
Children's Tumor Foundation
120 Wall Street
New York, NY 10005-1703

212-344-6633
800-323-7938
e-mail: info@ctf.org
www.ctf.org

Offers information for teenagers on how to face neurofibromatosis on a daily basis.
Allison Walsh, Communications Officer

6778 How NF-1 Affects the Body
Neurofibromatosis
213 S. Wheaton Ave.
Wheaton, IL 60187-3123

630-510-1115
800-942-6825
Fax: 630-510-8508
e-mail: admin@nfnetwork.org
www.nfnetwork.org

A graphic showing the parts of the body where symptoms of NF-1 can occur.
Gwen Charest, Executive Director

6779 How NF-2 Affects the Body
Neurofibromatosis
213 S. Wheaton Ave.
Wheaton, IL 60187-3123

630-510-1115
800-942-6825
Fax: 630-510-8508
e-mail: admin@nfnetwork.org
www.nfnetwork.org

A graphic showing the parts of the body where symptoms of NF-2 can occur.
Gwen Charest, Executive Director

6780   National NF Medical Resource Listing
Neurofibromatosis
213 S. Wheaton Ave.   630-510-1115
Wheaton, IL 60187-3123   800-942-6825
                                  Fax: 630-510-8508
                       e-mail: admin@nfnetwork.org
                                 www.nfnetwork.org
A listing of medical centers in the US where geneticists and NF experts are located.
Gwen Charest, Executive Director

6781   Neurofibromatosis
March of Dimes
1275 Mamaroneck Avenue   914-997-4488
White Plains, NY 10605   Fax: 212-254-3518
                     e-mail: NY639@marchofdimes.com
                               www.marchofdimes.com
Located on the website.

6782   Neurofibromatosis Type 2: Information for Patients and Families
Children's Tumor Foundation
120 Wall Street   212-344-6633
New York, NY 10005-1703   800-323-7938
                               e-mail: info@ctf.org
                                       www.ctf.org
Offers extensive information on what NF2 is and answers the most asked about questions regarding the illness.
Allison Walsh, Communications Officer

6783   Understanding Neurofibromatosis
213 S. Wheaton Ave.   630-510-1115
Wheaton, IL 60187-3123   800-942-6825
                                  Fax: 630-510-8508
                       e-mail: admin@nfnetwork.org
                                 www.nfnetwork.org
A handbook specifically designed for the newly diagnosed NF families.
Gwen Charest, Executive Director

Web Sites

6784   Healing Well
                                www.healingwell.com
An online health resource guide to medical news, chat, information and articles, newsgroups and message boards, books, disease-related web sites, medical directories, and more for patients, friends, and family coping with disabling diseases, disorders, or chronic illnesses.

6785   Health Finder
                               www.healthfinder.gov
Searchable, carefully developed web site offering information on over 1000 topics. Developed by the US Department of Health and Human Services, the site can be used in both English and Spanish.

6786   Healthlink USA
                               www.healthlinkusa.com
Health information concerning treatment, cures, prevention, diagnosis, risk factors, research, support groups, email lists, personal stories and much more. Updated regularly.

6787   Helios Health
                                www.helioshealth.com
Online resource for your health information. Detailed information about specific health topics, access to expert advice from our Medical Advisory Board, and up-to-date health news.

6788   MGH Neurology
                                 www.mgh.harvard.edu
Provides both unmonderated message boards and chat rooms for specific neurological disorders including: amyloidosis, arachnoiditis, cerebellar ataxia, congenital fiber type disproportion, CFS leak, DeMorsiers syndrome, erythromealgia, Lewy body disease, meningitis, meralgia paresthetic, Norrie disease, periodic paralysis, phantom limb pain, Romberg disorder, Syndenhams chorea, tethered cord syndrome, and thoracic outlet syndrome.

6789   MedicineNet
                                 www.medicinenet.com
An online resource for consumers providing easy-to-read, authoritative medical and health information.

6790   Medscape
                                  www.medscape.com
Medscape offers specialists, primary care physicians, and other health professionals the Web's most robust and integrated medical information and educational tools.

6791   Neurology Channel
                            www.healthcommunities.com
Find clearly explained, medically accurate information regarding conditions, including an overview, symptoms, causes, diagnostic procedures and treatment options. On this site it is possible to ask questions and get information from a neurologist and connect to people who have similar health interests.

6792   WebMD
                                     www.webmd.com
Provides credible information, supportive communities, and in-depth reference material about health subjects. A source for original and timely health information as well as material from well known content providers.

Description

6793 Obesity

Obesity refers to a condition in which there is an excessive accumulation of fat in subcutaneous and other tissues of the body. Being obese and being overweight are not necessarily synonymous, as people who are overweight may have increased body size as a result of increased muscle or skeletal tissue mass. Obesity may develop at any age, but peak development periods occur during the first 12 months of life, between the ages of five and six years, and during the adolescent years in children. In adults, obesity may develop at any time, but many people may find that weight gain progresses through the 3rd-6th decade. It is clear from numerous medial, public health and sociologic studies that obesity in the United States occurs in a staggering proportion of the population and many consider it to be an epidemic.

Obesity may result from an increase in the actual number of fat cells or from an increase in the size of the individual fat cells. Researchers believe that fat cells increase in number in proportion to caloric intake increase and that this increase is particularly evident in the first 12 months of life. As children grow, increases in fat cell populations continue at a slower rate. Because the number of fat cells cannot be decreased, except surgically, later weight loss must result from the reduction of fat in individual cells.

Obesity usually results when caloric intake exceeds the energy demands of the body, thus increasing the storage of body fat. Fat accumulation is usually a progressive process, resulting from repeated episodes of food intake exceeding the body's demand for energy (calories). Many factors may influence appetite or obesity. Such factors may include environmental influences; psychosocial disturbances that may be induced by stress or emotional upset or trauma; brain lesions that may involve certain area of the brain such as the hypothalamus or the pituitary gland (both essential to hormone production); an overabundance of insulin in the body (hyperinsulinism); and genetic influences. In addition, in rare instances, obesity may be a feature of certain genetic disorders (see *Prader-Willi syndrome*). the most common cause in North America however, is the excessive intake of calories, particularly those from fats and sugars, and the concomitant lack of physical exercise and activity that uses calories.

Complications of obesity in the child and the adult may include respiratory difficulties such as shortness of breath and increased cardiovascular risk factors such as high blood pressure, elevated total cholesterol levels as well as increased bad or LDL cholesterol and decreased good or HDL cholesterol, and increased levels of fatty acid and glycerol compounds (triglycerides). These are risk factors for the development of coronary artery disease, one of the leading causes of morbidity and the mortality in North America. In addition, obesity may be associated with a resistance to the hormone insulin that aids in the metabolism of glucose, fats, carbohydrates, and proteins. This resistance may lead to excessive levels of circulating insulin in the body (hyperinsulinism); however, the body is not able to appropriately use insulin and high blood sugar (hyperglycemia) may occur. This condition is known as Type II Diabetes Mellitus and its incidence in the population is also increasing dramatically in both children and adults. The diagnosis of obesity in children, adolescents and adults is usually determined through the use of certain screening methods such as measurement of the body mass index (BMI) as well as the triceps skinfold thickness.

Patterns of behavior that may lead to obesity may be established as early as infancy. For example, if parents or caregivers persistently use a bottle to pacify a crying baby, the baby may learn that food is equivalent to relief of stress. Treatment for obesity should include the cooperation and support of the entire family and may be directed toward psychological considerations, as well as proper exercise and nutrition to psychological and emotional needs may include behavior modification, as well as individual and family counseling. See also *Eating Disorders*.

National Agencies & Associations

6794 Active Healthy Kids Canada
77 Bloor Street West
Toronto, Ontario, M5S 1-3C6
416-913-0238
888-446-7432
Fax: 416-913-1541
e-mail: info@activehealthykids.ca
www.activehealthykids.ca
Established in 1994 to advocate the importance of quality, accessible, and enjoyable physical activity participation experiences for children and youth.
Stacie Smith, Communications Manager
Jennifer Crowie-Bonne, Director of Development/Programs

6795 American Obesity Association
1250 24th Street NW
Washington, DC 20037
202-776-7711
Fax: 202-776-7712
e-mail: executive@obesity.org
obesity1.tempdomainname.com
AOA provides obesity awareness and prevention information.
Morgan Downey, Executive Director
Richard L Atkinson, President

6796 Canadian Obesity Network
10240 Kingsway Avenue
Edmonton, AB T5H 3-2X2
780-735-6764
Fax: 780-735-6763
e-mail: info@obesitynetwork.ca
www.obesitynetwork.ca
Focuses the expertise and deciation of more than 1,000 member researchers, clinicans, allied health care providers and other professionals with an interest in obesity in a unified effort to reduce the mental, physical and economic burden of obesity in Canadians.
Dr. Arya M. Sharma, Scientific Director & CEO
Ximena Ramos Salas, Managing Director

6797 National Association to Advance Fat Acceptance
PO Box 4662
Foster City, CA 94404
916-558-6880
Fax: 916-558-6881
e-mail: naafa@naafa.org
www.naafaonline.com/dev2/
NAAFA provides educational information a newsletter and hosts a national conference.
Carole Cullum, Co-Chair
Kara Brewer Allen, Co-Chair

6798 Overeaters Anonymous World Service Office
World Service Office

PO Box 44020
Rio Rancho, NM 87174-4020

505-891-2664
Fax: 505-891-4320
e-mail: info@oa.org
www.oa.org

A fellowship of men and women from all walks of life who meet in order to help solve a common problem - compulsive overeating.
Naomi, Managing Director, Board Administrator

6799 Research Chair on Obesity
2725 Chemin Sainte-Foy
Quebec, Canada, G1V

418-656-8711
Fax: 418-656-4929
e-mail: obesite.chair@crhl.ulaval.ca
http://obesity.chair.ulaval.ca

Provides understanding of the pathophysiology of obesity. Promotes communication and interaction among basic scientists and clinicians, involved in nutrition, energy metabolism, obesity, lipid metabolism and cardiovascular research., Provides continuing education about the best possible knowledge on obesity to health professionals, physicians and to the public at large regarding the causes, the complications and the treatment of obesity.
Paul Boisvert, Coordinator
Denis Richard, Ph. D., Chair

Libraries & Resource Centers

6800 Weight-control Information Network
1 WIN Way
Bethesda, MD 20892-3665

202-828-1025
877-946-4627
Fax: 202-828-1028
e-mail: win@info.niddk.nih.gov
http://win.niddk.nih.gov/

WIN addresses the health information needs of individuals through the production and dissemination of educational materials. In addition, WIN is developing communication strategies for a pilot program to encourage at-risk individuals to achieve and maintain a healthy weight by making changes in their lifestyle.

Research Centers

6801 Harvard Clinical Nutrition Research Center
Harvard Medical School
Boston, MA 02215

617-998-8803
Fax: 617-998-8804
e-mail: allan_walker@hms.harvard.edu
nutrition.med.harvard.edu

Mission is to derive the benefit of continuity in assessing the effectiveness of the Center from year to year while still allowing flexibility for new insights as the Center's activities evolve.
W Allan Walker, Director
George Blackburn, Associate Director

6802 Minnesota Obesity Center
1334 Eckles Avenue
St Paul, MN 55108

763-807-0559
e-mail: mnoc@tc.umn.edu
www.mnoc.umn.edu

Mission is to find ways to prevent weight gain obesity and its complications. The Center incorporates 46 Participating Investigators who are studying the causes and treatments of obesity. Provides the general public with a source of information on the happenings of the Center and on the current developments in the field of obesity.
Catherine C Welch, Program Coordinator

6803 New York Obesity/Nutrition Research Center
31 Center Drive MSC 2560
Bethesda, MD 20892-2560

301-496-3583
www2.niddk.nih.gov

Griffin P Rodgers, Director

6804 Obesity Research Center St. Luke's-Roosevelt Hospital
St. Luke's-Roosevelt Hospital
1090 Amsterdam Avenue
New York, NY 10025

212-523-4196
Fax: 212-523-3416
e-mail: dg108@columbia.edu
www.nyorc.org

The mission of the New York Obesity Research Center is to help reduce the incidence of obesity and related diseases through leadership in basic research clinical research epidemiology and public health patient care and public education.
Dr Xavier Pi-Sunyer, Director
Janet Crane, Dietitians

Support Groups & Hotlines

6805 Greater New York Metro Intergroup of Overeaters Anonymous
Madison Square Station
New York, NY 10159-1235

212-946-4599
e-mail: office@oanyc.org
www.oanyc.org

Tom M, Chairman
Raina M, Vice chairman

6806 Office of Chronic Disease Prevention and Nutrition Services
Obesity Prevention Program
150 N. 18th Avenue
Phoenix, AZ 85007

602-542-1025
Fax: 602-542-0883
www.azdhs.gov/search/index.htm

Mission is to improve the health and quality of life of Arizona residents by reducing the incidence and severity of chronic disease and obesity through physical activity and nutrition interventions.
Renae Cunnien, Program Manager

Books

6807 An Atlas of Obesity and Weight Control
George A. Bray, author

212-216-7800
Fax: 212-564-7854
e-mail: odphpinfo@hhs.gov
www.health.gov/dietaryguidelines/

This informative guide is a clearly written, beautifully illustrated color atlas on obesity, including its etiology, development and treatment. Contains nearly 150 clinical pictures of obesity and its related conditions, as well as many pertinent clinical guidelines and up-to-the-minute data on assessment and treatment.
135 pages

6808 Dietary Guidelines for Americans 2005
U.S. Government Printing Office
200 Indep. Ave, S.W.
Washington, DC 20201

202-619-0257
877-696-6775
e-mail: odphpinfo@hhs.gov
www.health.gov/dietaryguidelines/

80 pages
Tommy G. Thompson, HHS-Secretary
Ann M. Veneman, USDA-Secretary

6809 Encyclopedia of Obesity and Eating Disorders
Facts on File
11 Penn Plaza
New York, NY 10001

212-967-8800
800-322-8755
Fax: 800-678-3633

From abdominoplasty to Zung Rating Scale, this volume defines and explains these disorders, along with medical and other problems associated with them.
272 pages Hardcover

6810 Handbook of Obesity Treatment
Guilford Press
370 Seventh Avenue
New York, NY 10001

800-365-7006
Fax: 212-966-6708
e-mail: info@guilford.com
www.guilford.com

This comprehensive handbook guides mental, medical, and allied health professionals through the process of planning and delivering individualized treatment services for those seeking help for Obesity.
2001 624 pages Hardcover
ISBN: 1-572307-22-6

6811 Obesity
National Academies Press

500 Fifth Street, NW   202-334-3313
Washington, DC 20001   888-624-8373
Fax: 202-334-2451
www.nap.edu

A ground breaking report on childhood obesity providing indepth background and instructive case studies that illustrate just how serious and widespread the problem is; gives honest, authoritive, based advice that consitute our best weapons in this critical battle.
280 pages

6812   Overeaters Anonymous
World Service Office
6075 Zenith Court NE   505-891-2664
Rio Rancho, NM 87144-6807   Fax: 505-891-4320
www.oa.org

World Service Office offers literature, provides information or meetings world wide.
204 pages Hardcover

6813   Preventing Childhood Obesity: Health in the Balance
National Academies Press
500 Fifth Street NW   202-334-3313
Washington, DC 20001   888-624-8373
Fax: 202-334-2451
www.nap.edu

Provides a broad-based examination of the nature, extent, and consequences of obesity. Also explores the underlying causes of this serious health problem and the actions needed to initiate support, and sustain the societal and lifestyle changes that can reverse the trend among our children and youth.
436 pages
ISBN: 0-309091-96-9

6814   Shape Up America!
6707 Democracy Boulevard
Bethesda, MD 20817   www.shapeup.org
A high profile national initiative to promote healthy weight and increased physical activity in America. Involves a broad based coalition of industry, medical/health, nutrition, physical fitness, and related organizations and experts.
C. Everett Koop, Founder
Barbara J. Moore, President And CEO

6815   Understanding Childhood Obesity
J Clinton Smith, MD, author
University Press of Mississippi
3825 Ridgewood Road   601-432-6205
Jackson, MS 39211-6492   800-737-7788
Fax: 601-432-6217
e-mail: press@ihl.state.ms.us
www.upress.state.ms.us

A clear explanation of causes, diagnosis, and treatment of childhood obesity.
1999 120 pages Paperback
ISBN: 1-578061-34-2
Kathy Burgess, Advertising/Marketing Services Manager

6816   Understanding Obesity: The Five Medical Causes
Lance Levy, author
Firefly Books Ltd
50 Staples Avenue   416-499-8412
Richmond Hill, Ontario, L4B-1H1   Fax: 416-499-1142
www.fireflybooks.com

An authoritative book that focuses on the causes of, and the treatment for, obesity. Obesity is usually related to other health problems and treatment for them is the first step.
200 pages

Children's Books

6817   I Was a Fifteen-Year-Old Blimp
Harper & Row
10 E 53rd Street   212-207-7000
New York, NY 10022-5299
This story focuses on Gabby, a teenage girl who overhears others discuss her weight and takes radical steps to become popular.
Grades 6-9

Magazines

6818   CheckUp
Medical University of South Carolina
67 President Street   843-792-2273
Charleston, SC 29425   800-424-6872
Fax: 843-792-5432
www.muschealth.com/weight

Provides health information about screenings, treatments, medical advances and services available through MUSC, as well as advice about nutrition and prevention.
Susan Kammeraad-Campbell, Managing Editor
Damon Simmons, Art Director

6819   Official Journal of NAASO
NAASO
8757 Georgia Avenue   301-563-6526
Silver Spring, MD 20910   Fax: 301-563-6595
e-mail: teffk!niddk.nih.gov
www.obesity.org

Promotes research, education and advocacy to better understand, prevent and treat obesity and improve the lives of those affected.
Barbara E. Corkey, Editor-In-Chief
Deborah Moskowitz, Managing Editor

6820   Progress Notes
Medical University of South Carolina
67 President Street   843-792-2273
Charleston, SC 29425   800-922-5250
Fax: 843-792-5432
www.muschealth.com/weight

Designed to inform the medical community developments at the Medical University of South Carolina and as a continuing medical education resource for practicing physicians and faculty.
Susan Kammeraad-Campbell, Managing Editor
Lynne Barber Associate Editor, Alex Sargent, Associate Editor

Newsletters

6821   Trim & Fit
Obesity Foundation
5600 S Quebec Street   303-850-0328
Englewood, CO 80111-2202
Offers nutrition facts and articles, low-fat recipes, medical information on heart disease and cancer relating to nutrition and more.
James F Merker CAE, Editor

Pamphlets

6822   About Overeaters Anonymous
Metro Intergroup of Overeaters Anonymous
6075 Zenith Court NE   212-206-8621
Rio Rancho, NM 87144-6807   Fax: 505-891-4320
www.oa.org

World Service Office offers literature, provides information or meetings world wide.

6823   An Inside View
Metro Intergroup of Overeaters Anonymous
6075 Zenith Court NE   212-206-8621
Rio Rancho, NM 87144-6807   Fax: 505-891-4320
www.oa.org

World Service Office offers literature, provides information or meetings world wide.

6824   Anonymity
Metro Intergroup of Overeaters Anonymous
6075 Zenith Court NE   212-206-8621
Rio Rancho, NM 87144-6807   Fax: 505-891-4320
www.oa.org

World Service Office offers literature, provides information or meetings world wide.

6825   Before You Take That First...
Metro Intergroup of Overeaters Anonymous

6075 Zenith Court NE
Rio Rancho, NM 87144-6807

212-206-8621
Fax: 505-891-4320
www.oa.org

World Service Office offers literature, provides information or meetings world wide.

6826 Compulsive Overeaters in the Military
Metro Intergroup of Overeaters Anonymous
6075 Zenith Court NE
Rio Rancho, NM 87144-6807

212-206-8621
Fax: 505-891-4320
www.oa.org

World Service Office offers literature, provides information or meetings world wide.

6827 Compulsive Overeating & Overaters Anonymous
Metro Intergroup of Overeaters Anonymous
6075 Zenith Court NE
Rio Rancho, NM 87144-6807

212-206-8621
Fax: 505-891-4320
www.oa.org

World Service Office offers literature, provides information or meetings world wide.

6828 For the Obese Employee
Metro Intergroup of Overeaters Anonymous
6075 Zenith Court NE
Rio Rancho, NM 87144-6807

212-206-8621
Fax: 505-891-4320
www.oa.org

World Service Office offers literature, provides information or meetings world wide.

6829 Guide to the 12 Steps for You
Metro Intergroup of Overeaters Anonymous
6075 Zenith Court NE
Rio Rancho, NM 87144-6807

212-206-8621
Fax: 505-891-4320
www.oa.org

World Service Office offers literature, provides information or meetings world wide.

6830 Hazelden Step Pamphlets for Overeaters
Hazelden
15251 Pleasant Valley Rd
Center City, MN 55012-9640

651-213-4200
800-328-9000
Fax: 651-213-4793
e-mail: customersupport@hazelden.org
www.hazelden.org

A 12 pamphlet collection that offers one person's interpretation of the Twelve Steps for overeaters.

6831 If God Spoke to Overeaters Anonymous
Metro Intergroup of Overeaters Anonymous
6075 Zenith Court NE
Rio Rancho, NM 87144-6807

212-206-8621
Fax: 505-891-4320
www.oa.org

World Service Office offers literature, provides information or meetings world wide.

6832 Many Symptoms, One Disease
Metro Intergroup of Overeaters Anonymous
6075 Zenith Court NE
Rio Rancho, NM 87144-6807

212-206-8621
Fax: 505-891-4320
www.oa.org

World Service Office offers literature, provides information or meetings world wide.

6833 Members in Relapse
Metro Intergroup of Overeaters Anonymous
6075 Zenith Court NE
Rio Rancho, NM 87144-6807

212-206-8621
Fax: 505-891-4320
www.oa.org

World Service Office offers literature, provides information or meetings world wide.

6834 One Day at a Time
Metro Intergroup of Overeaters Anonymous
6075 Zenith Court NE
Rio Rancho, NM 87144-6807

212-206-8621
Fax: 505-891-4320
www.oa.org

World Service Office offers literature, provides information or meetings world wide.

6835 Overeaters Anonymous Cares
Metro Intergroup of Overeaters Anonymous
6075 Zenith Court NE
Rio Rancho, NM 87144-6807

212-206-8621
Fax: 505-891-4320
www.oa.org

World Service Office offers literature, provides information or meetings world wide.

6836 Overeaters Anonymous is Not a Diet Club
Metro Intergroup of Overeaters Anonymous
6075 Zenith Court NE
Rio Rancho, NM 87144-6807

212-206-8621
Fax: 505-891-4320
www.oa.org

World Service Office offers literature, provides information or meetings world wide.

6837 Person to Person
Metro Intergroup of Overeaters Anonymous
6075 Zenith Court NE
Rio Rancho, NM 87144-6807

212-206-8621
Fax: 505-891-4320
www.oa.org

World Service Office offers literature, provides information or meetings world wide.

6838 Program of Recovery
Metro Intergroup of Overeaters Anonymous
6075 Zenith Court NE
Rio Rancho, NM 87144-6807

212-206-8621
Fax: 505-891-4320
www.oa.org

World Service Office offers literature, provides information or meetings world wide.

6839 Questions and Answers
Metro Intergroup of Overeaters Anonymous
6075 Zenith Court NE
Rio Rancho, NM 87144-6807

212-206-8621
Fax: 505-891-4320
www.oa.org

World Service Office offers literature, provides information or meetings world wide.

6840 So You've Reached Goal Weight
Metro Intergroup of Overeaters Anonymous
6075 Zenith Court NE
Rio Rancho, NM 87144-6807

212-206-8621
Fax: 505-891-4320
www.oa.org

World Service Office offers literature, provides information or meetings world wide.

6841 Think First...
Metro Intergroup of Overeaters Anonymous
6075 Zenith Court NE
Rio Rancho, NM 87144-6807

212-206-8621
Fax: 505-891-4320
www.oa.org

World Service Office offers literature, provides information or meetings world wide.

6842 To the Family
Metro Intergroup of Overeaters Anonymous
6075 Zenith Court NE
Rio Rancho, NM 87144-6807

212-206-8621
Fax: 505-891-4320
www.oa.org

World Service Office offers literature, provides information or meetings world wide.

6843 To the Man
Metro Intergroup of Overeaters Anonymous
6075 Zenith Court NE
Rio Rancho, NM 87144-6807

212-206-8621
Fax: 505-891-4320
www.oa.org

World Service Office offers literature, provides information or meetings world wide.

6844 To the Newcomer
Metro Intergroup of Overeaters Anonymous
6075 Zenith Court NE
Rio Rancho, NM 87144-6807

212-206-8621
Fax: 505-891-4320
www.oa.org

World Service Office offers literature, provides information or meetings world wide.

6845 To the Teen
Metro Intergroup of Overeaters Anonymous
6075 Zenith Court NE
Rio Rancho, NM 87144-6807
212-206-8621
Fax: 505-891-4320
www.oa.org
World Service Office offers literature, provides information or meetings world wide.

6846 Tools of Recovery
Metro Intergroup of Overeaters Anonymous
6075 Zenith Court NE
Rio Rancho, NM 87144-6807
212-206-8621
Fax: 505-891-4320
www.oa.org
World Service Office offers literature, provides information or meetings world wide.

6847 Twelve Traditions of Overeaters Anonymous
Metro Intergroup of Overeaters Anonymous
6075 Zenith Court NE
Rio Rancho, NM 87144-6807
212-206-8621
Fax: 505-891-4320
www.oa.org
World Service Office offers literature, provides information or meetings world wide.

6848 Welcome Back
Metro Intergroup of Overeaters Anonymous
6075 Zenith Court NE
Rio Rancho, NM 87144-6807
212-206-8621
Fax: 505-891-4320
www.oa.org
World Service Office offers literature, provides information or meetings world wide.

Audio & Video

6849 Obesity Online
NAASO

301-563-6526
www.obesity-online.com
Educational resource for clinicians, researchers and educators with an interest in obesity and its related disorders.
Samuel Klein, Editor
Christie M. Ballantyne, Editor

Web Sites

6850 Boston Obesity Nutrition Research Center (BONRC)
www.bmc.org
Provides resources and support for studies in the area of obesity and nutrition. Comprised of four research cores located within the Boston area. In the areas of adipocytes, epidemiology and statistics, body composition, energy expenditure and genetic analyses, and transgenic animal models.

6851 Center for Human Nutrition
www.uchsc.edu/nutrition
A interdisciplinary team encompassing basic and clinical research, post-graduate training and career development of nutrition professionals, and commuity outreach. The research conducted at the CHN focuses on obesity prevention and treatment, nutrient metabolism, and micronutrient status in children. Activities conducted aim to improve the quallity of life by promoting physical activity and nutritional awareness.

6852 Clinical Nutrition Research Unit (CNRU)
depts.washington.edu/uwnorc
Promotes and enhances the interdisciplinary nutrition research and education at the Univerity of Washington. By providing a number of Core Facilities, the CNRU attempts to integrate and coordinate the abundant ongoing activities with the goals of fostering new interdiscilinary research collaborations, stimulating new research activities, improving nutrition education at multiple levels, and facilitating the nutritional management of patients.

6853 MedicineNet
www.medicinenet.com
An online resource for consumers providing easy-to-read, authoritative medical and health information.

6854 New York Obesity/Nutrition Research Center (ONRC)
www.niddk.nih.gov
Funded by the National Institute of Diabetes and Digestive and Kidney Diseases (NIDDK). A combined effort of Columbia ane Cornell Universities. Provides participating investigators of funded projects relevant to obesity research with valuable laboratory, technical, and educational services that otherwise would not be available to them, thereby improving the productivity an efficiency of their operations.

6855 North American Association for the Study of Obesity
www.obesity.org
The leading scientific society dedicated to the study of obesity. Committed to encouraging research on the causes and treatment of obesity, and to keeping the medical community and public informed of new advances.

6856 Research Chair on Obesity
2725 Chemin Sainte Foy
Quebec,Canada,
418-656-8711
e-mail: obesite.chair@crhl.ulaval.ca
obesity.chair.ulaval.ca
Ever since 1997, the Research Chair in Obesity is dedicated to support and launch initiatives leading to a better understanding of obesity through research on the mechanisms of body weight regulation, to facilitate communication between researchers, to promote the training of highly qualified personnel, to contribute to continuing education for health professionals, and to inform the public on the causes, consequences, treatments, and prevention of obesity.

6857 University of Pittsburgh Obesity/Nutrition Research Center
www.pitt.edu/~mdm2/ONRCWeb
Goal is to develop more effective interventions for the prevention and treatment of obesity. Exists to support research functions for investigators studying the broad areas of obesity and nutrition. Focuses on behavioral aspects of obesity and behavioral treatment of this disease.

6858 Vanderbilt Clinical Nutrition Research Unit (CNRU)
www.vanderbilt.edu/nutrition/index.html
A core center grant funded by the National Institute of Diabetes and Digestive and Kidney Diseases (NIDDK). Nutrition research is carried out by faculty members i most academic departments and extends from basic laboratory research to clinical and applied research. Maintains service facilities to support both basic and clinical research. Supports research cores that bring nutrition investigators together to discuss their work.

6859 Weight-control Information Network
www.niddk.nih.gov
The Weight-control Information Network (WIN) was established in 1994 to provide the general public, health professionals, and the media with up-to-date, science-based information on obesity, weight control, physical activity, and related nutritional issues. WIN provides tip sheets, fact sheets, and brochures for a range of audiences. Some of WIN's content is available in Spanish.

Description

6860 Osteogenesis Imperfecta

Osteogenesis imperfecta, OI, often called "brittle bone" disease, is actually is a group of serious genetic disorders that are characterized by abnormally fragile bones that break or fracture easily. There are at least four distinct forms of the disorder, with neonatal (congenital) being the most severe. A person with OI has either less collagen, the major protein of the connective tissue, including bone, or a poorer quality collagen. Infants born with OI may have multiple bone fractures and hearing loss, and routine vaginal delivery may lead to significant bone fracture, hemorrhage into the brain and other major problems. Survivors develop shortened extremities and other bony abnormalities. If no injury to the brain occurs then mental and intellectual function should be unaffected. Hearing loss may occur.

At present, there is no effective treatment for this disorder. Careful handling of these infants is essential. Gentle exercise and physical therapy are directed at preventing fractures and increasing function. Surgical implants can provide stability to the skeletal structure. Genetic counseling is also important.

National Agencies & Associations

6861 NIH Osteoporosis and Related Bone Diseases - National Resource Center
2 AMS Circle
Bethesda, MD 20892-3676

301-496-8190
877-226-4267
Fax: 301-480-2814
TTY: 301-565-2966
e-mail: niamsboneinfo@mail.nih.gov
www.niams.nih.gov

Provides patients, health professionals and the public with an important link to resources and information on osteoporosis, Paget's disease of bone, osteogenesis imperfecta, and other metabolic bone diseases. The National Resource Center's mission is to expand awareness and enhance knowledge and understanding of the prevention, early detection, and treatment of these diseases.

6862 National Institute of Child Health and Human Development
National Institutes of Health
31 Center Drive
Bethesda, MD 20892-0001

301-496-5133
Fax: 301-496-7107

Supports several basic and clinical research projects on osteogenesis imperfecta.
Duane Alexander, Director

6863 Osteogenesis Imperfecta Foundation
804 W Diamond Avenue
Gaithersburg, MD 20878-1414

301-947-0083
800-981-2663
Fax: 301-947-0456
TTY: 202-466-4315
TDD: 202-466-4315
e-mail: BoneLink@oif.org
www.oif.org

Support and resources for families and medical professionals dealing with osteogeneis imperfecta.
Mary Beth Huber, Information/Resource Director
Tracy Smith Hart, CEO

Libraries & Resource Centers

6864 NIH Osteoporosis and Related Bone Diseases - National Resource Center
2 AMS Circle
Bethesda, MD 20892-3676

202-223-0344
800-624-2663
Fax: 202-293-2356
TTY: 202-466-4315
e-mail: niamsboneinfo@mail.nih.gov
www.osteo.org

Provides patients, health professionals and the public with an important link to resources and information on osteoporosis, Paget's disease of bone, osteogenesis imperfecta, and other metabolic bone diseases. The National Resource Center's mission is to expand awareness and enhance knowledge and understanding of the prevention, early detection, and treatment of these diseases.

Research Centers

6865 American Society for Bone and Mineral Research
2025 M Street NW
Washington, DC 20036-3309

202-367-1161
Fax: 202-672-2161
e-mail: asbmr@asbmr.org
www.asbmr.org

The mission of the ASBMR is to be the premier society in the field of bone and mineral metabolism through promoting excellence in bone and mineral research fostering integration of clinical and basic science and facilitating the translation of that science to health care and clinical practice.
Ann Elderkin, Executive Director
Douglas Fesler, Associate Executive Director

6866 Children's Brittle Bone Foundation
7701 95th Street
Pleasant Pride, WI 53158

773-236-2223
866-694-2223
Fax: 262-947-0724
e-mail: info@cbbf.org
www.cbbf.org

The mission of the Children's Brittle Bone Foundation is to provide for research into the causes diagnosis treatment prevention a eventual cure for Osteogenesis Imperfecta (OI) while supporting programs which improve the quality of life for people afflicted.

Support Groups & Hotlines

6867 National Health Information Center
PO Box 1133
Washington, DC 20013

310-565-4167
800-336-4797
Fax: 301-984-4256
e-mail: info@nhic.org
www.health.gov/nhic

Offers a nationwide information referral service, produces directories and resource guides.

6868 Osteogenesis Imperfecta Foundation
804 W Diamond Avenue
Gaithersburg, MD 20878

301-947-0083
800-981-2663
Fax: 301-947-0456
TDD: 202-466-4315
e-mail: BoneLink@oif.org
www.oif.org

Support and resources for families and medical professional dealing with osteogeneis imperfecta.
Marybeth Huber, Information Resource Director
Bill Bradner, Director Communication/Events

Books

6869 Children with Ostegogenesis Imperfecta: St raties to Enhance Performance
Holly Lea Cintas, Lynn Gerber, author
Osteogenesis Imperfecta Foundation

804 W Diamond Avenue
Gaithersburg, MD 20878

301-947-0083
800-981-2663
Fax: 301-947-0456
e-mail: BoneLink@oif.org
www.oif.org

This guide covers the same issues, but has been written especially for elementary school readers.
252 pages Paperback
ISBN: 0-964218-95-X
Mary Beth Huber, Information/Resource Director

6870   Growing Up with OI: A Guide for Children
Ellen Painter Dollar, author

Osteogenesis Imperfecta Foundation
804 W Diamond Avenue
Gaithersburg, MD 20878

301-947-0083
800-981-2663
Fax: 301-947-0456
e-mail: bonelink@oif.org
www.oif.org

This guide covers the same issues as the adult book, Growing Up with OI: A Guide for Families and Caregivers, but has been written especially for elementary school readers.
122 pages Paperback
ISBN: 0-964218-92-5
Mary Beth Huber, Information/Resource Director

6871   Growing Up with OI: A Guide for Families a nd Caregivers
Ellen Painter Dollar, author

Osteogenesis Imperfecta Foundation
804 W Diamond Avenue
Gaithersburg, MD 20878-1414

301-947-0083
800-981-2663
Fax: 301-947-0456
e-mail: BoneLink@oif.org
www.oif.org

This guide covers common questions parents, family members and caregivers have about raising a child with OI. The focus is on maximizing abilities and proactive problem solving. Chapters cover medical, financial, emotional and school related issues.
295 pages Paperback
ISBN: 0-964218-91-7
Mary Beth Huber, Information/Resource Director

6872   Managing Osteogenesis Imperfecta: A Medical Manual
Priscilla Wacaster, MD, author

Osteogenesis Imperfecta Foundation
804 W Diamond Avenue
Gaithersburg, MD 20878-1414

301-947-0083
800-981-2663
Fax: 301-947-0456
e-mail: BoneLink@oif.org
www.oif.org

The manual is designed for physicians, physical and occupational therapists, orthopedic technologists, early intervention providers and others who come in contact with persons with OI. It covers a broad range of topics including genetics, diagnosis, pregnancy, arthritis, osteoperosis and rodding.
Mary Beth Huber, Information/Resource Director

6873   Therapeutic Strategies: A Guide for Occupational & Physical Therapists
Ellen Painter Dollar, author

Osteogenesis Imperfecta Foundation
804 W Diamond Avenue
Gaithersburg, MD 20878-1414

301-947-0083
800-981-2663
Fax: 301-947-0456
e-mail: BoneLink@oif.org
www.oif.org

This booklet is intended for medical professionals, or for families to use as a resource while working with a medical professional.
14 pages
Mary Beth Huber, Information/Resource Director

Newsletters

6874   Breakthrough
Osteogenesis Imperfecta Foundation

804 W Diamond Avenue
Gaithersburg, MD 20878-1414

301-947-0083
800-981-2663
Fax: 301-947-0456
e-mail: BoneLink@oif.org
www.oif.org

Newsletter of the Osteogenesis Imperfecta Foundation that provides information on current research and OIF fundraising activities as well as support features.
15 pages Quarterly
Mary Beth Huber, Information/Resource Director

Pamphlets

6875   Caring for Infants and Children with Osteogenesis Imperfecta
Osteogenesis Imperfecta Foundation
804 W Diamond Avenue
Gaithersburg, MD 20878-1414

301-947-0083
800-981-2663
Fax: 301-947-0456
e-mail: BoneLink@oif.org
www.oif.org

A companion to the videotape You Are Not Alone. Presents some basic information and unique tips on caring for a baby with OI. Available in Spanish.
24 pages
Mary Beth Huber, Information/Resource Director

6876   Osteogenesis Imperfecta: A Guide for Medic al Professionals, Individuals & Families
Osteogenesis Imperfecta Foundation
804 W Diamond Avenue
Gaithersburg, MD 20878-1414

301-947-0083
800-981-2663
Fax: 301-947-0456
e-mail: BoneLink@oif.org
www.oif.org

This pamphlet contains basic information about the types of OI, inheritance factors, diagnosis and treatment.
10 pages Paperback
Mary Beth Huber, Information/Resource Director

Audio & Video

6877   Going Places and Plan for Success: An Educ ator's Guide to Students with OI
Osteogenesis Imperfecta Foundation
804 W Diamond Avenue
Gaithersburg, MD 20878-1414

301-947-0083
800-981-2663
Fax: 301-947-0456
e-mail: BoneLink@oif.org
www.oif.org

A 15-minute video with booklet that guides educators and parents through planning steps that will help children with OI fully participate in school activities.
Mary Beth Huber, Information/Resource Director

6878   Within Reach
Osteogenesis Imperfecta Foundation
804 W Diamond Avenue
Gaithersburg, MD 20878-1414

301-947-0083
800-981-2663
Fax: 301-947-0456
TDD: 202-466-4315
e-mail: BoneLink@oif.org
www.oif.org

This 50-minute video features in-depth interviews with adults living with OI. They talk candidly about how they have achieved independent and satisfying lives, addressing such issues as travel, career, marriage and family.
VHS/DVD
Mary Beth Huber, Information/Resource Director

6879   You Are Not Alone
Osteogenesis Imperfecta Foundation
804 W Diamond Avenue
Gaithersburg, MD 20878-1414

301-947-0083
800-981-2663
Fax: 301-947-0456
TDD: 202-466-4315
e-mail: BoneLink@oif.org
www.oif.org

Explores the emotional turmoil of dealing with the diagnosis of OI and offers practical and uplifting solutions for caring for infants with Type II to severe Type III OI. Also valuable for new families with the more mild forms of OI. Available open captioned or with Spanish subtitles (specify if needed). Add $5.00 per video for Canadian orders and $11.00 per video for overseas orders.

Mary Beth Huber, Information/Resource Director

Web Sites

6880 Healing Well

www.healingwell.com

An online health resource guide to medical news, chat, information and articles, newsgroups and message boards, books, disease-related web sites, medical directories, and more for patients, friends, and family coping with disabling diseases, disorders, or chronic illnesses.

6881 Health Finder

www.healthfinder.gov

Searchable, carefully developed web site offering information on over 1000 topics. Developed by the US Department of Health and Human Services, the site can be used in both English and Spanish.

6882 Healthlink USA

www.healthlinkusa.com

Health information concerning treatment, cures, prevention, diagnosis, risk factors, research, support groups, email lists, personal stories and much more. Updated regularly.

6883 Helios Health

www.helioshealth.com

Online resource for your health information. Detailed information about specific health topics, access to expert advice from our Medical Advisory Board, and up-to-date health news.

6884 MedicineNet

www.medicinenet.com

An online resource for consumers providing easy-to-read, authoritative medical and health information.

6885 Medscape

www.medscape.com

Medscape offers specialists, primary care physicians, and other health professionals the Web's most robust and integrated medical information and educational tools.

6886 Osteogenesis Imperfecta Foundation

www.oif.org

A website for those who want to learn more about Osteogenesis Imperfecta, the OI Foundation, and what they do.

6887 Osteoporosis and Related Bone Diseases: National Resource Center (NIGH)

www.niams.nih.gov/Health_Info/Bone

Provides patients, health professionals and the public with an important link to resources and information on osteoporosis and other metabolic bone diseases.

6888 WebMD

www.webmd.com

Provides credible information, supportive communities, and in-depth reference material about health subjects. A source for original and timely health information as well as material from well known content providers.

Description

6889 Osteoporosis

Osteoporosis is a general term for many conditions which result in a reduction in bone mass. Most cases occur in post-menopausal women because estrogen loss is associated with decreased bone mass. These women are at risk for fractures of the wrist, spine and hip. Post-menopausal osteoporosis may also cause marked reduction in a woman's height, as multiple vertebral bodies in the spine compress downwards over the years. Risk factors for osteoporosis include white race, cigarette smoking, thin body build and early menopause. Men can develop a similar condition, but it is generally much less severe. Excessive activity of the adrenal glands (Cushing's syndrome), the thyroid gland (thyrotoxicosis), the parathyroid glands (hyperparathyroidism), and the pituitary gland (hyperprolactinemia) cause bones to thin, as does underactivity of the testes or ovaries. Anorexia nervosa and prolonged administration of cortisone or heparin will also thin the bones.

Treatment is in part nonspecific, and can include surgery or other immobilization to treat fractures of the hip or wrist, control of pain with medications and physical therapy to encourage return to pre-fracture function. Specific therapy includes calcium and Vitamin D supplementation and weight-bearing exercises. Biphosphonates, such as alendronate, have been approved for osteoporosis and other new therapies are being developed.

National Agencies & Associations

6890 American Association of Clinical Endocrinologists
245 Riverside Avenue 904-353-7878
Jacksonville, FL 32202 Fax: 904-353-8185
www.aace.com

The American Association of Clinical Endocrinologists is a professional community of physicians specializing in endocrinology, diabetes, and metabolism committed to enhancing the ability of its members to provide the highest quality of patient care.
Donald C. Jones, Chief Executive Officer
Dan Kelsey, MS,MBA,CAE, Deputy CEO

6891 American Medical Directors Association
11000 Broken Land Parkway 410-740-9743
Columbia, MD 21044 800-876-2632
Fax: 410-740-4572
e-mail: info@amda.com
www.amda.com

AMDA - The Society for Post-Acute and Long-Term Care Medicine is dedicated to excellence in patient care and provides education, advocacy, information and professional development to promote the delivery of quality post-acute and long-term care medicine.
Naushira Pandya, MD, FACP, CMD, President
Heidi K. White, Vice President

6892 American Physical Therapy Association
1111 North Fairfax Street 703-684-2782
Alexandria, VA 22314 800-999-2782
Fax: 703-684-7343
TDD: 703-683-6748
e-mail: memberservices@apta.org
www.apta.org

APTA is an individual membership professional organization representing more than 90,000 member physical therapists, physical therapist assistants, and students.
J. Michael Bowers, Chief Executive Officer
Justin Moore, PT, DPT, Chief Public Affairs Officer

6893 National Association of Chronic Disease Directors
2200 Century Parkway
Atlanta, GA 30345 770-458-7400
www.chronicdisease.org

The National Association of Chronic Disease Directors (NACDD) is a non-profit Public Health organization committed to serve the chronic disease program directors of each state and U.S. jurisdiction.
Schwanna Lakine, MBA, Director of Finance and Operations
Stephanie Mathews, MPH, CHES, Professional Development Coordinator

6894 National Osteoporosis Foundation
1232 22nd Street NW 202-223-2226
Washington, DC 20037-1292 800-223-9994
Fax: 202-223-2237
e-mail: communications@nof.org
www.nof.org

The nation's leading resource for people seeking up-to-date medically sound information on the causes prevention detection and treatment of osteoporosis.
Leo Schargorodski, Executive Director
Ethel Siris, President

6895 Osteoporosis Canada
1090 Don Mills Road 416-696-2663
Toronto, Ontario, M3C-3R6 800-463-6842
Fax: 416-696-2673
e-mail: info@osteoporosis.ca
www.osteoporosis.ca

A registered charity, is the only national organization serving people who have, or are at risk for, osteoporosis.
Cheryl Baldwin, Chairman
Emliy Bartens, Vice chairman

District of Columbia

6896 National Association of Nurse Practitioners In Women's Health
505 C Street, Northeast 202-543-9693
Washington, DC 20002 e-mail: info@npwh.org
www.npwh.org

The National Association of Nurse Practitioners in Women's Health (NPWH) was founded in 1980. NPWH's mission is to ensure the provision of quality primary and specialty healthcare to women of all ages by women's health and women's health focused nurse practitioners.
Gay Johnson, Chief Executive Officer
Carol Wiley, Director of Membership

Libraries & Resource Centers

6897 NIH Osteoporosis and Related Bone Diseases - National Resource Center
2 AMS Circle 202-223-0344
Bethesda, MD 20892-3676 800-624-2663
Fax: 202-293-2356
TTY: 202-466-4315
e-mail: niamsboneinfo@mail.nih.gov
www.osteo.org

Provides patients, health professionals and the public with an important link to resources and information on osteoporosis, Paget's disease of bone, osteogenesis imperfecta, and other metabolic bone diseases. The National Resource Center's mission is to expand awareness and enhance knowledge and understanding of the prevention, early detection, and treatment of these diseases.

Research Centers

6898 Medical College of Pennsylvania Center for the Mature Woman
3300 Henry Avenue 215-842-6000
Philadelphia, PA 19129

our purpose is to provide consumers information to help them get high quality services and products at the best possible prices.
Jon Schneider,MD, Director

6899 Osteoporosis Center Memorial Hospital/Advanced Medical Diagn
Memorial Hospital/Advanced Medical Diagnostic
1700 Coffee Road
Modesto, CA 95355   209-526-4500
www.memorialmedicalcenter.org
Memorial Medical Center is part of Memorial Hospitals Association a not-for-profit organization that exists to maintain and improve the health status of citizens in the greater Stanislaus County.
David Benn, Director
Bev Finley, Director

6900 Regional Bone Center Helen Hayes Hospital
Helen Hayes Hospital
51-55 Route 9W   845-786-4000
W Haverstraw, NY 10993   1 8-8 7- 734
Fax: 845-947-3097
TTY: 845-947-3187
e-mail: info@helenhayeshospital.org
www.helenhayeshospital.org
The mission of the Regional Bone conduct a broad-based research program focused on the elucidation of cellular mechanisms underlying metabolic bone disease and the development of new treatments for bone disease.
David W Dempster PhD, Director
Adrienne Tewksbury, Grants Administrator

6901 University of Connecticut Osteoporosis Center
263 Farmington Avenue   860-679-2000
Farmington, CT 06030   800-535-6232
Fax: 860-679-1258
www.uchc.edu

Jay R Lieberman, Director

Support Groups & Hotlines

6902 National Health Information Center
PO Box 1133   310-565-4167
Washington, DC 20013   800-336-4797
Fax: 301-984-4256
e-mail: info@nhic.org
www.health.gov/nhic
Offers a nationwide information referral service, produces directories and resource guides.

6903 National Osteoporosis Foundation (NOF)
1232 22nd Street NW   202-223-2226
Washington, DC 20037-1292   Fax: 202-223-2237
e-mail: webmaster@nof.org
www.nof.org
Dedicated to reducing the widespread prevalence of osteoporosis through programs of research, education and advocacy. Provides referrals to existing support groups, as well as free resources, training and materials to assist people to start groups.
Amy Porter, Executive Director& CEO
Robert R Recker, Chairman of the Board

Books

6904 One-Hundred-Fifty Most Asked Questions About Osteoporosis
Hearst Books
1350 Ave of the Americas   212-261-6500
New York, NY 10016   Fax: 212-261-6595
1993
ISBN: 0-688123-34-1

6905 Preventing & Reversing Osteoporosis: Every Woman's Guide
Prima Publishing
PO Box 1260
Rocklin, CA 95677-1260   916-624-5718
www.primapub.com

1993 275 pages
ISBN: 1-559582-98-7

6906 Preventing and Managing Osteoporosis
Springer Publishing Company
11 West 42nd Street   212-431-4370
New York, NY 10036-3955   877-687-7476
Fax: 212-941-7842
e-mail: cs@springerpub.com
www.springerpub.com
This book will raise awareness and inform health professionals about this often preventable and treatable disease. Written by a team of authors from medicine, nursing, nutrition, exercise physiology, and physical therapy, the book provides an overview of the disease process.
216 pages Hardcover
ISBN: 0-826113-18-4
M Susan Burke MD, Editor
Helen Wright PhD, Editor

Newsletters

6907 Osteoporosis Report
National Osteoporosis Foundation
1150 17th Street, NW   202-223-2226
Washington, DC 20036-1292   800-221-4222
Fax: 202-223-2237
e-mail: communications@nof.org
www.nof.org
A benefit to members of the National Osteoporosis Foundation (NOF), the Osteoporosis Report includes updates on recent research, strategies for bone health and other information. NOF is the only nonprofit, voluntary health organization dedicated to reducing the widespread prevalence of osteoporosis through programs of research, education and advocacy. Contact the foundation for membership information.
Quarterly

Pamphlets

6908 Boning Up on Osteoporosis
National Osteoporosis Foundation
1150 17th Street, NW   202-223-2226
Washington, DC 20036-1292   800-221-4222
Fax: 202-223-2237
e-mail: info@nof.org
www.nof.org
Risk factor card.

6909 How Strong Are Your Bones?
1150 17th Street, NW   202-223-2226
Washington, DC 20036-1292   800-221-4222
Fax: 202-223-2237
e-mail: info@nof.org
www.nof.org
Describes the various methods for determining bone mass, including types of equipment and how bone density testing is used in the diagnosis and treatment of osteoporosis.
12 pages

6910 Living with Osteoporosis
1150 17th Street, NW   202-223-2226
Washington, DC 20036-1292   800-221-4222
Fax: 202-223-2237
e-mail: info@nof.org
www.nof.org
A guide to preventing falls in the home and to protecting yourself from injury during your daily routine.

6911 Medications and Bone Loss
1150 17th Street, NW   202-223-2226
Washington, DC 20036-1292   800-221-4222
Fax: 202-223-2237
e-mail: info@nof.org
www.nof.org
Designed for women dealing with menopause, this brochure provides information of estrogen replacement therapy and its relationship to bone health and osteoporosis prevention and treatment.

6912 Men with Osteoporosis: In Their Own Words
1150 17th Street, NW
Washington, DC 20036-1292
202-223-2226
800-221-4222
Fax: 202-223-2237
e-mail: info@nof.org
www.nof.org

6913 Official Prevention Month Poster
1150 17th Street, NW
Washington, DC 20036-1292
202-223-2226
800-221-4222
Fax: 202-223-2237
e-mail: info@nof.org
www.nof.org

Poster promotes public awareness about osteoporosis. It can be used as a compliment to the education kit, or by itself for exhibits, health fairs or community programs.

6914 Official Prevention Week Poster
1150 17th Street, NW
Washington, DC 20036-1292
202-223-2226
800-221-4222
Fax: 202-223-2237
e-mail: info@nof.org
www.nof.org

Poster promotes public awareness about osteoporosis. It can be used as a compliment to the education kit, or by itself for exhibits, health fairs or community programs.

6915 Osteoporosis Education Kit
1150 17th Street, NW
Washington, DC 20036-1292
202-223-2226
800-221-4222
Fax: 202-223-2237
e-mail: info@nof.org
www.nof.org

This kit is designed for preparing public and patient education programs. Updated annually and includes age-targeted materials, nutrition information and osteoporosis fact sheets that are easily duplicated.

6916 Osteoporosis Education Poster
1150 17th Street, NW
Washington, DC 20036-1292
202-223-2226
800-221-4222
Fax: 202-223-2237
e-mail: info@nof.org
www.nof.org

Ideal for health care settings, the poster clearly illustrates the effect of osteoporosis on bone tissue and common fracture sites.

6917 Osteoporosis Information Package
NAMSIC/National Institutes of Health
1 AMS Circle
Bethesda, MD 20892-0001
301-495-4484
877-226-4267
Fax: 301-718-6366
TTY: 301-565-2966
e-mail: niamsinfo@mail.nih.gov
www.nih.gov/niams

The National Institute of Arthritis and Musculoskeletal and Skin Diseases Information Clearinghouse serves the public, patients, and health professionals
19 pages

6918 Osteoporosis International
1150 17th Street, NW
Washington, DC 20036-1292
202-223-2226
800-221-4222
Fax: 202-223-2237
e-mail: info@nof.org
www.nof.org

An international multidisciplinary, clinically oriented journal for the exchange of ideas concerning osteoporosis.

6919 Osteoporosis in Men Information Package
NAMSIC/National Institutes of Health
1 AMS Circle
Bethesda, MD 20892-0001
301-495-4484
877-226-4267
Fax: 301-715-6366
TTY: 301-565-2966
e-mail: niamsinfo@mail.nih.gov
www.nih.gov/niams

The National Institute of Arthritis and Musculoskeletal and Skin Diseases Information Clearinghouse serves the public, patients, and health professionals
19 pages

6920 Osteoporosis: Clinical Updates
1150 17th Street, NW
Washington, DC 20036-1292
202-223-2226
800-221-4222
Fax: 202-223-2237
e-mail: info@nof.org
www.nof.org

NOF's health profession newsletter provides an in depth focus on varying clinical topics.

6921 Osteoporosis: The Silent Disease-Slide Lecture Presentation
1150 17th Street, NW
Washington, DC 20036-1292
202-223-2226
800-221-4222
Fax: 202-223-2237
e-mail: info@nof.org
www.nof.org

This 42-slide presentation is ideal for community, patient and worksite education progams. It covers basic bone biology, osteoporosis risk factors, diagnosis, prevention and treatment and concludes with a patient case history. A question and answer document is also provided to assist the presenter with audience questions.
Slide set

6922 Patient Education Sample Pack
1150 17th Street, NW
Washington, DC 20036-1292
202-223-2226
800-221-4222
Fax: 202-223-2237
e-mail: info@nof.org
www.nof.org

This pack contains one of each of NOF's patient education brochures and a catalog; health professionals can select the brochures appropriate for their audience.
Ten brochures

6923 Risk Factor Card: Can It Happen to You?
National Osteoporosis Foundation
1150 17th Street, NW
Washington, DC 20036-1292
202-223-2226
800-221-4222
Fax: 202-223-2237
e-mail: info@nof.org
www.nof.org

Explains osteoporosis, the causes, symptoms and preventions and high risk persons.

6924 Stand Up to Osteoporosis
National Osteoporosis Foundation
1150 17th Street, NW
Washington, DC 20036-1292
202-223-2226
800-221-4222
Fax: 202-223-2237
e-mail: info@nof.org
www.nof.org

One of 25 educational brochures on all aspects of this chronic and debilitating disease. The National Osteoporosis Foundation (NOF) is the nation's only private, nonprofit organization dedicated to education, advocacy and public services. Memberships are available to health professionals and public. Quarterly newsletter and physician's guide.

6925 Strategies for People with Osteoporosis
1150 17th Street, NW
Washington, DC 20036-1292
202-223-2226
800-221-4222
Fax: 202-223-2237
e-mail: info@nof.org
www.nof.org

This series of articles from NOF's newsletter helps patients learn how to cope with osteoporosis. Articles cover hip, vertebrae and wrist fracture recovery, fall-proofing your home, finding the right doctor, what to do after you've been diagnosed and more.

Audio & Video

6926 Be BoneWise: Exercise
National Osteoperosis Foundation
1150 17th Street, NW
Washington, DC 20036-1292
202-223-2226
800-221-4222
Fax: 202-223-2237
e-mail: info@nof.org
www.nof.org

Take steps toward better bones, health, flexibility and balance with the offical weight bearing and strength training exercise video.

6927 Osteoperosis: The Silent Disease
National Osteoperosis Foundation
1150 17th Street, NW
Washington, DC 20036-1292
202-223-2226
800-221-4222
Fax: 202-223-2237
e-mail: info@nof.org
www.nof.org

A scripted, visual presentation covers basic bone biology, osteoperosis risk factors, diagnosis, prevention and treatment. Available as a slide presentation or power point CD Rom.

6928 Patient Education Video
National Osteoperosis Foundation
1150 17th Street, NW
Washington, DC 20036-1292
202-223-2226
800-221-4222
Fax: 202-223-2237
e-mail: info@nof.org
www.nof.org

Discusses treatment, exercise, nutrition and coping strategies for those already diagnoses with osteoporosis.
15 minutes

Web Sites

6929 Healing Well
www.healingwell.com
An online health resource guide to medical news, chat, information and articles, newsgroups and message boards, books, disease-related web sites, medical directories, and more for patients, friends, and family coping with disabling diseases, disorders, or chronic illnesses.

6930 Health Finder
www.healthfinder.gov
Searchable, carefully developed web site offering information on over 1000 topics. Developed by the US Department of Health and Human Services, the site can be used in both English and Spanish.

6931 Healthlink USA
www.healthlinkusa.com
Health information concerning treatment, cures, prevention, diagnosis, risk factors, research, support groups, email lists, personal stories and much more. Updated regularly.

6932 Helios Health
www.helioshealth.com
Online resource for your health information. Detailed information about specific health topics, access to expert advice from our Medical Advisory Board, and up-to-date health news.

6933 MedicineNet
www.medicinenet.com
An online resource for consumers providing easy-to-read, authoritative medical and health information.

6934 Medscape
www.medscape.com
Medscape offers specialists, primary care physicians, and other health professionals the Web's most robust and integrated medical information and educational tools.

6935 NIH Osteoporosis and Related Bone Disease
www.niams.nih.gov/Health_Info/Bone
Provides patients, health professionals, and the public with an important link to resources and information on metabolic bone diseases. The center is dedicated to increasing the awareness, knowledge, and understanding of physicians, health professionals, patients, underserved and at-risk populations, and the general public about the prevention, early detection, and treatment of osteoporosis and related bone diseases.

6936 National Osteoporosis Foundation
www.nof.org
The National Osteoporosis Foundation is dedicated to preventing osteoporosis, promoting strong bones, and reducing human suffering through education, advocacy and research.

6937 WebMD
www.webmd.com
Provides credible information, supportive communities, and in-depth reference material about health subjects. A source for original and timely health information as well as material from well known content providers.

Description

6938 Paget's Disease

Paget's disease is a disorder of the bone, which typically results in enlarged and deformed bones in one or more regions of the skeleton. Excessive bone breakdown and formation cause new bone to be dense but fragile. Paget's disease occurs most frequently in the spine, skull, pelvis, and legs.

Early symptoms of Paget's disease include bone and joint pain and fatigability, as well as headaches and hearing loss, when the skull is affected. Deformities of bone such as enlargement of the forehead, bowing of a limb, and curvature of the spine may occur as the disease progresses.

The cause of Paget's disease is unknown. It is sometimes familial, but a specific genetic pattern is unclear.

The course of the disease varies greatly and may range from complete stability to rapid progression. Generally, symptoms progress slowly in affected bones with usually no spread to normal ones.

Although there is no cure for Paget's disease at the present, treatments include drugs that suppress disease activity. Orthopedic surgery for joint replacement or stabilization may also be beneficial.

National Agencies & Associations

6939 American Skin Association
6 East 43rd Street
New York, NY 10017
212-889-4858
800-499-SKIN
Fax: 212-889-4959
e-mail: info@americanskin.org
www.americanskin.org
A unique collaboration of patients, families, advocates, physicians and scientists, American Skin Association has evolved over the past two decades as a leading force in efforts to defeat melanoma, skin cancer and disease.
Philip G. Prioleau, MD, President
Kathleen Reichert, Executive Vice President

6940 Arthritis Foundation
1330 W Peachtree Street
Atlanta, GA 30309
404-872-7100
800-283-7800
Fax: 404-872-0457
e-mail: help@arthritis.org
www.arthritis.org
A nonprofit organization that depends on volunteers to provide services to help people with arthritis. Supports research to find ways to cure and prevent arthritis and provides services to improve the quality of life for those affected by arthritis.
Daniel T. McGowen, Chair
John H Klippel MD, President and CEO

6941 Paget Foundation for Paget's Disease of Bone & Related Disorders
120 Wall Street
New York, NY 10005-4001
212-509-5335
800-237-2438
Fax: 212-509-8492
e-mail: PagetFdn@aol.com
www.paget.org
Private voluntary health agency that provides information to patients and health professionals on several bone disorders including: Paget's disease of bone, primary hyperparathyroidism, fibrous dysplasia, osteoporosis (not osteoporosis) and complications of these conditions.
Teresa A. Guise, Chair
Christal Sumpter, Administrator & Web Manager

Support Groups & Hotlines

6942 National Health Information Center
PO Box 1133
Washington, DC 20013
310-565-4167
800-336-4797
Fax: 301-984-4256
e-mail: info@nhic.org
www.health.gov/nhic
Offers a nationwide information referral service, produces directories and resource guides.

Newsletters

6943 Update
Paget Foundation
120 Wall Street
New York, NY 10005-4001
212-509-5335
800-237-2438
Fax: 212-509-8492
e-mail: PagetFdn@aol.com
www.paget.org
Provides information for consumers and health professionals on the following disorders: paget's disease of bone, primary hyperparathyroidism, fibrous dysplasia, osteopetrosis (not osteoporosis) and the complications of breast and prostate cancer metastic to the bone.
3 per year
Charlene Waldman, Executive Director

Pamphlets

6944 Questions & Answers About Paget's Disease of Bone
Paget Foundation
120 Wall Street
New York, NY 10005-4001
212-509-5335
800-237-2438
Fax: 212-509-8492
e-mail: pagetfdn@aol.com
www.paget.org

The Paget Foundation provides this and other question and answer booklets and fact sheets on Paget's disease of bone, primary hyperparathyroidism,, fibrous dysplasia, osteopetrosis (not osteoporosis) and breast and prostate cancer metastic to bone. These publications are available on the foundation websit and in print.
Charlene Waldman, Executive Director

Web Sites

6945 Healing Well
www.healingwell.com
An online health resource guide to medical news, chat, information and articles, newsgroups and message boards, books, disease-related web sites, medical directories, and more for patients, friends, and family coping with disabling diseases, disorders, or chronic illnesses.

6946 Health Finder
www.healthfinder.gov
Searchable, carefully developed web site offering information on over 1000 topics. Developed by the US Department of Health and Human Services, the site can be used in both English and Spanish.

6947 Healthlink USA
www.healthlinkusa.com
Health information concerning treatment, cures, prevention, diagnosis, risk factors, research, support groups, email lists, personal stories and much more. Updated regularly.

6948 Helios Health
www.helioshealth.com

Online resource for your health information. Detailed information about specific health topics, access to expert advice from our Medical Advisory Board, and up-to-date health news.

6949 MedicineNet

www.medicinenet.com

An online resource for consumers providing easy-to-read, authoritative medical and health information.

6950 Medscape

www.medscape.com

Medscape offers specialists, primary care physicians, and other health professionals the Web's most robust and integrated medical information and educational tools.

6951 Paget Foundation for Paget's Disease of Bone & Related Disorders

www.paget.org

Includes information for patients and health professionals on Paget's disease of bone, primary hyperparathyroidism, fibrous dysplasia, osteopetrosis (not osteoporosis) and the complications of certain cancers on the skeleton.

6952 WebMD

www.webmd.com

Provides credible information, supportive communities, and in-depth reference material about health subjects. A source for original and timely health information as well as material from well known content providers.

Description

6953 ## Parkinson Disease

Parkinson disease is a neurological condition characterized by slow and decreased movement. It affects about 1 percent of those over age 65. The cause of Parkinson disease is unknown, but both genetic and environmental factors may play a role. In a minority of cases, Parkinson disease develops after repeated head trauma, carbon monoxide poisoning, drug use, or viral infections that affect the brain.

In about 50 percent to 80 percent of patients, Parkinson disease begins with a slight tremor in the hands, resembling "pill-rolling." With fatigue and stress, the tremor becomes more pronounced. As the disease progresses, voluntary movements, such as walking and eating, become more and more difficult. Rigidity and postural instability (difficulty standing up) develop. Dementia affects approximately one third of patients with advanced Parkinson disease.

Because Parkinson disease is characterized by reduced levels of neurotransmitter chemicals, notably dopamine, in certain parts of the brain, therapy has focused on restoring these levels to normal. Monoamine oxidase type B inhibitors given early in the disease, may protect the cells that secrete these chemicals, and thus delay the need for other therapy. When it is necessary to directly manipulate the chemical levels because of progression of the disease, levodopa, related to dopamine, is the mainstay of treatment and is associated with improvement of all Parkinson symptoms. Anticholinergic medications are especially helpful in treating tremor.

Parkinson disease is the subject of intense research, and experimental surgical or drug treatments are frequently available to patients whose response to standard therapy has been unsatisfactory. General supportive care should not be neglected, and includes physical therapy and an exercise program to help optimize mobility.

National Agencies & Associations

6954 **American Parkinson Disease Association**
135 Parkinson Avenue — 718-981-8001
Staten Island, NY 10305-1943 — 800-223-2732
Fax: 718-981-4399
e-mail: apda@apdaparkinson.org
www.apdaparkinson.org
Funds research towards finding the cause(s) and cure for Parkinson's Disease, patient education, information, support groups nationwide.
Lesli A. Chambers, President&CEO
Fred Greene, Chairman of the Board

6955 **Michael J. Fox Foundation for Parkinson's Research**
Grand Central Station
New York, NY 10163 — 800-708-7644
www.michaeljfox.org
The Michael J. Fox Foundation is dedicated to ensuring the development of a cure for Parkinson's disease within this lifetime through an aggressively funded research center.
Deborah W Brooks, Co-Founder
Todd Sherer, CEO

6956 **National Health Information Center**
PO Box 1133 — 310-565-4167
Washington, DC 20013 — 800-336-4797
Fax: 301-984-4256
e-mail: info@nhic.org
www.health.gov/nhic
Offers a nationwide information referral service, produces directories and resource guides.

6957 **National Institute of Neurological Disorders and Stroke**
NIH Neurological Institute — 301-496-5751
Bethesda, MD 20824 — 800-352-9424
Fax: 301-402-2186
TTY: 301-468-5981
www.ninds.nih.gov
The mission of NINDS is to reduce the burden of neurological disease - a burden borne by every age group, by every segment of society, by people all over the world.
Story C Landis PhD, Director
Walter J Koroshetz, Deputy Director

6958 **National Parkinson Foundation**
1501 NW 9th Avenue — 305-243-6666
Miami, FL 33136-1407 — 800-327-4545
Fax: 305-243-6073
e-mail: contact@parkinson.org
www.parkinson.org
A nonprofit organization dedicated to research, diagnosis, treatment and care for men and women suffering from Parkinson's and other related neurological diseases. The Foundation also supports the Bob Hope research and rehabilitation center.
Bernard J. Fogel, Chairman
Joyce A Oberdorf, President and Chief Executive Officer

6959 **Parkinson Society Canada**
4211 Yonge Street — 416-227-9700
Toronto, Ontario, M2P-2A9 — 800-565-3000
Fax: 416-227-9600
e-mail: info@parkinson.ca
www.parkinson.ca
A not-for-profit, national charitable organization. The Society raises money through corporate sponsorships, public donations, and planned gifts. Finding the cause and cure for Parkinson's disease remains our mission.
Bruce Ireland, President/CEO
Jean Pascal Souque, Vice President

6960 **Parkinson's Action Network (PAN)**
1025 Vermont Avenue NW — 202-638-4101
Washington, DC 20005 — 800-850-4726
Fax: 202-638-7257
e-mail: info@parkinsonsaction.org
www.parkinsonsaction.org
The Parkinson's Action Network is the unified voice of the Parkinson's disease community-advocating for more than one million Americans and their families.
Ronald H Galowich, Chair
Ed Weidenfield, Vice Chair

6961 **Parkinson's Institute**
675 Almanor Avenue — 408-734-2800
Sunnyvale, CA 94085-1605 — 800-655-2273
Fax: 408-734-8455
e-mail: info@thepi.org
www.thepi.org
The mission of the Parkinson's Institute is to find the cause(s) and a cure for Parkinson's Disease and provide the best possible treatment to those afflicted with the disease.
Thomas D Follet, Chair
Thomas E Bailard, Secretary of Board

6962 **WE MOVE**
5731 Mosholu Avenue — 212-875-8312
New York, NY 10471 — e-mail: wemove@wemove.org
www.wemove.org
WE MOVE's mission is to raise awareness of neurologic movement disorder among healthcare professionals, patients and families and the public.
Susan B Bressman, President
Mo Moadeli, Vice President

State Agencies & Associations

Arizona

6963 Arizona Chapter of the National Parkinson Foundation
20280 N 59th Avenue   480-607-1960
Glendale, AZ 85308-6182   866-637-8772
                                    Fax: 480-607-1957
                                    e-mail: info@aznpf.org
                                    www.aznpf.org
Affiliate chapter of The National Parkinson Foundation Inc.
Alan Marks, President
Kenneth Larkin, Vice President

California

6964 Los Angeles Alliance Against Parkinson's Disease
3251 Oakley Drive   323-851-3230
Los Angeles, CA 90068-1315   e-mail: Millard@millardtipp.com
                              www.parkinson.org/chapters.htm#
Affiliate of the National Parkinson Foundation.

6965 National Parkinson Foundation: California Office
4929 Wilshire Boulevard   323-442-8434
Los Angeles, CA 90010-3899

6966 National Parkinson Foundation: Orange County Chapter
PO Box 2207   949-945-6200
Newport Beach, CA 92659   Fax: 949-548-4624
                                    e-mail: info@yahoo.com
                                    www.npfocc.org
Affiliate of The National Parkinson Foundation.
George Strickland, President
Janet Buell, Vice president

6967 Northstate Parkinson's Chapter
1003 Yuba Street
Redding, CA 96001   530-229-0878
                                    www.parkinson.org
Affiliate of The National Parkinson Foundation, Inc.
Craig Boyer

6968 Parkinson Association of the Sacramento Valley
900 Fulton Avenue   916-534-7279
Sacramento, CA 96825-4502   800-473-4636
                                    Fax: 916-489-0241
                                    e-mail: parkanc@sbcglobal.net
                                    www.parkinsonsacramento.org
Bernardine Ford, President
George Johnston, 2nd Vice President

6969 Parkinson Network of Mount Diablo
Po Box 3127   925-284-2189
Walnut Creek, CA 94598-0127   e-mail: mmhansell@hotmail.com
                              www.parkinson.org
Affiliate of the National Parkinson Foundation.
Mary Hansell

Colorado

6970 Colorado Parkinson Foundation
1155 Kelly Johnson Boulevard   719-884-0103
Colorado Springs, CO 90920-1494   800-327-4545
                                    Fax: 719-495-909
                                    e-mail: rpfarrer@msn.com
                                    colorado.parkinson.org
The mission of the National Parkinson Foundation if to find the cause of the cure for Parkinson disease through research. To improve the quality if life for persons with Parkinson and their caregivers. To also educate persons with Parkinson their carecar
Ric Pfarrer, Chairperson

Florida

6971 Alzheimer/Parkinson Association of Indian River County
2300 5th Avenue   772-563-0505
Vero Beach, FL 32960   e-mail: alzsupport@fastmail.fm
                              www.parkinson.org
Toni Teresi, Chairperson

6972 Goodwill Industries-Suncoast
Goodwill Industries-Suncoast
10596 Gandy Boulevard   727-523-1512
St. Petersburg, FL 37023   888-279-1988
                                    Fax: 727-563-9300
                                    e-mail: gw.marketing@goodwill-suncoast.org
                                    www.goodwill-suncoast.org
A nonprofit community based organization whose purpose is to improve the quality of life for people who are disabled, disadvantaged and/or aged. This mission is accomplished through a staff of over 1,200 employees providing independent living skills, affordable housing, career assessment and planning, job skills, training, placement, and job retention assistance with useful employment. Annually, Goodwill Industries-Suncoast serves over 30,000 people in Citrus, Hernando, Levy, Marion and more.
R Lee Waits, President/CEO
Martin W Gladysz, Chair

6973 Parkinson Association of Greater Daytona Beach
111 North Frederick Avenue   386-252-8959
Daytona Beach, FL 32114   e-mail: goatie@cfl.rr.com
                              www.parkinson.org
Nancy Dawson, Chairperson

6974 Parkinson Association of Southwest Florida
1048 Goodlette-Frank Road   239-417-3465
Naples, FL 34102   Fax: 239-417-3469
                                    e-mail: pasfi@aol.com
                                    www.pasfi.org
Affiliate of the National Parkinson Foundation.
Scott Leamon, Chair
Chris Spine, Executive Director

6975 South Palm Beach County Chapter of NFP
PO Box 880145
Boca Raton, FL 33433-0145   561-482-2867
                                    www.parkinson.org
Irving Layton, Chairperson

6976 Southeast Parkinson Disease Association
6530 Metrowest Boulevard   407-489-4124
Orlando, FL 32835-6520   e-mail: srh_pres@sepda.org
                              www.sepda.org
Steve Hochberger, Chairperson

Georgia

6977 Northwest Georgia Parkinson Disease Association
708 Glen Milner Boulevard   706-235-3164
Rome, GA 30161   e-mail: webmaster@gaparkinsons.org
                              www.gaparkinsons.org
James Trussel, Chairperson

Hawaii

6978 Hawaii Parkinson Association Gwendolyn A Montibon President
Gwendolyn A Montibon, President
3375 Koapaka St.,   808-734-9398
Honolulu, HI 96817   Fax: 808-528-1897
                                    e-mail: kekim@hawaii.edu
                                    www.parkinson.org
Affiliate of The National Parkinson Foundation.

Kansas

6979 Northeast Kansas Parkinson Association
PO Box 251
Topeka, KS 66601   785-228-1337
                                    www.parkinson.org
Mary Hatke, Chairperson

6980 Parkinson Association of Greater Kansas City
8900 State Line Road   913-341-8828
Leawood, KS 66206   Fax: 913-341-8885
                                    e-mail: meg@parkinsonheartland.org
                                    www.parkinsonheartland.org
Affiliate of The National Parkinson Foundation.
Kirk Gutekunst, President
Mary Lee Shucart, Secretary

Louisiana

6981 Eljay Foundation for Parkinson Syndrome Awareness
715 Ryan Street   337-310-0083
Lake Charles, LA 70601   e-mail: info@eljayfd.org
www.eljayfd.org

Eligha Guillory, President
Anna C. Drake, Secretary

Massachusetts

6982 Cape Cod Chapter National Parkinson Foundation
33 Ships Way   508-385-2333
Buzzards Bay, MA 02532-0584   e-mail: meacapecod@yahoo.com
www.parkinson.org
Affiliate of The National Parkinson Foundation.
Joseph Wimbrow, President

6983 National Parkinson Foundation:Cape Cod Chapter
33 Ships Way   508-385-2333
Buzzards Bay, MA 02532-0584   e-mail: meacapecod@yahoo.com
www.parkinson.org

Garland Smith, Chairperson

6984 Northeast Parkinson's and Caregivers
27 Sutcliffe Road   508-756-7721
Brimfield, MA 01010   e-mail: rstake@northeastparkinsons.com
www.northeastparkinsons.com

Richard Stake, Chairperson

Minnesota

6985 Parkinson Association of Minnesota
5905 Golden Valley Road,   763-545-1272
Golden Valley, MN 55422-4602   800-327-4545
e-mail: info@parkinsonmn.org
www.parkinsonmn.org
Affiliate of The National Parkinson Foundation.
Paul Blom, President
Collen Crane, Therapy Representative

New Jersey

6986 Parkinson Alliance
PO Box 308   609-688-0870
Kingston, NJ 08528   800-579-8440
Fax: 609-688-0875
e-mail: admin@parkinsonalliance.net
www.parkinsonalliance.net
The Princeton-New Jersey based Parkinson Alliance is a National nonprofit organization dedicated to raising funds to help finance the most promising research to find the cause and curefor Parkinson's disease.
Martin Tuchman, Chairman
Margaret Tuchman, President

New York

6987 National Parkinson Foundation: New York Office
122 E 42nd Street
New York, NY 10017-5622   800-457-6676
www.parkinson.org/

6988 Parkinsons Wellness Group of Western New York
5140 Main Street   716-218-1027
Depew, NY 14221   e-mail: coach71395@aol.com
http://www.npfwny.org/
Site changed
Robert J Plunket, President
Gary Kurdziel, Vice President

Oklahoma

6989 Parkinson Foundation of the Heartland Oklahoma Branch
1000 W Wilshire   405-810-0695
Oklahoma City, OK 73116   e-mail: jimk@parkinsonheartland.org
www.parkinson.org
Satellite office of the Kansas Chapter
Jim Keating, Chairperson

Oregon

6990 Parkinsons Resources of Oregon
3975 Mercantile Drive   503-594-0901
Lake Oswego, OR 97035   800-426-6806
Fax: 503-594-0547
e-mail: info@parkinsonsresources.org
www.parkinsonsresources.org
Holly Chaimov, Executive Director

Pennsylvania

6991 Parkinson Chapter of Greater Pittsburgh
6507 Wilkins Avenue   412-365-2086
Pittsburgh, PA 15217   e-mail: info@pfwpa.org.
www.parkinsonpittsburgh.org

Doreen Grasso, Chairperson
Maggie Schmidt, Executive Director

6992 Parkinson Council
111 Presidential Boulevard   610-668-4292
Bala Cynwyd, PA 19004   Fax: 610-668-4275
e-mail: info@theparkinsoncouncil.org
www.theparkinsoncouncil.org
The Parkinson Council is dedicated to promoting research initiating to find the causes and cure for Parkinson Disease educating patients their caregivers healthcare professionals and the general public about Parkinson's and improving the quality of lif
Jeff Keefer, President
Jo Ann Zoll, Vice President

South Dakota

6993 Parkinson Association of South Dakota
PO Box 87952   605-328-4227
Sioux Falls, SD 57109-9938   Fax: 605-328-7150
e-mail: info@parkinsonsd.org
www.parkinsonsd.org
Affiliate of The National Parkinson Foundation.
Elaine Spader, President
Lori Jones, Vice President

Virginia

6994 Parkinson Foundation of the National Capitol Area
7700 Leesburg Pike,   703-734-1017
Falls church, VA 22043-4201   Fax: 703-734-1241
e-mail: pfnca@parkinsonfoundation.org
www.parkinsonfoundation.org
Daniel M Lewis, Chairperson
Donna Schena, Vice Chairman

Wisconsin

6995 Wisconsin Parkinson Association
945 N 12th Street   414-219-7061
Milwaukee, WI 53233   800-972-5455
Fax: 414-219-6564
www.wiparkinson.org
Chapter of The National Parkinson Foundation.
Keith Brewer, President

Foundations

6996 Parkinsons Disease Foundation
1359 Broadway   212-923-4700
New York, NY 10018   800-457-6676
Fax: 212-923-4778
e-mail: info@pdf.org
www.pdf.org
The foundation has been one of teh leaders in subsidizing research into Parkinson's Disease. Offers many services including The Summer Fellowship Program, The Postdoctoral Fellowship Program, support groups nationwide, grants for clinical and laboratory studies, public awareness and government promotion of the disease.
Howard D. Morgan, chair/Co Preident
Constance Woodruff atwell, Vice Chair

Libraries & Resource Centers

6997 Parkinson's Resource Organization
74090 El Paseo   760-773-5628
Palm Desert, CA 92260-4135   877-775-4111
                                         Fax: 760-773-9803
                     e-mail: info@parkinsonsresource.org
                                www.parkinsonsresource.org
Our mission is to help families affected by Parkinson's forge through the journey of the disease's progression with as much quality as life can provide. Working so no one is isolated because of Parkinson's
Jo Rosen, Visionary, President, Founder
William R Remery, Treasurer

Research Centers

6998 California Institute for Medical Research
2260 Clove Drive   408-998-4554
San Jose, CA 95128   Fax: 408-998-2723
                                        e-mail: admin@clmr.org
                                                www.cimr.org
Medical research including infectious diseases stroke and cancer specializing in Parkinson's Disease related studies.
David A Stevens, President
John Hotson, Vice President

6999 Texas Tech University Tarbox Parkinson's Disease Institute
3601 4th Street
Lubbock, TX 79430   806-743-1000
                                                www.ttuhsc.edu
The current objectives of the Tarbox Institute are to provide services for Parkinson's disease patients and their families in the underserved West Texas area; to maintain a Parkinson's Disease Information and Referral Center to enable both healthcare professionals and affected families to obtain the latest information on services available new developments in research support groups and educational literature.
Tedd L Mitchell, President
Pureza Martinez, Chief of Staff

7000 University of Alabama at Birmingham Parkinsons Disease Center
1720 7th Avenue S   205-934-4011
Birmingham, AL 35294   Fax: 205-346-78
                                         TDD: 205-934-4642
                                        e-mail: apda@uab.edu
                                                www.uab.edu
Offers educational emotional and political support to Parkinson disease patients and their families.
Ray Watts, Interim CEO
David G Standaert, Director

7001 William T Gossett Parkinson's Disease Center
Henry Ford Hospital
Department of Neurology   313-972-1693
Detroit, MI 48202
Jay M Gorell MD, Director

Support Groups & Hotlines

California

7002 Parkinson's Disease Association of San Die go (PDASD)
8555 Areo Drive   858-273-6763
San Diego, CA 92123-1746   877-737-7576
                                         Fax: 858-273-6764
                                        e-mail: info@pdasd.org
                                                www.pdasd.org
Information and referral research center for Parkinson's disease patients and their families.
Jerry Henberger, Executive Director
Rick Brydges, President

Florida

7003 Greater Daytona Area Parkinson Support Group
Bishop's Glen Retirement Center   904-322-4748
Daytona, FL   e-mail: boba@n-jcenter.com
                                                www.parkinson.org
Affiliate of the National Parkinson Foundation.

7004 National Parkinson Foundation Hotline
National Parkinson Foundation
1501 NW 9th Avenue Bob Hope Road   305-243-6666
Miami, FL 33136   800-327-4545
                                         Fax: 305-243-5595
                                                www.parkinson.org
Offers support and emergency information for persons with Parkinson's and their families.
Jose Garcia Pebrosa, Director

7005 Pembroke Pines Parkinson Support Group
Century Village, Club House
Pembroke Pines, FL 33027   954-433-0947
                                                www.parkinson.org
Affiliate of the National Parkinson Foundation.

Hawaii

7006 Kuakini Parkinson Disease (PD) Information & Referral
Kuakini Medical Center
347 North Kuakini Street   808-536-2236
Honolulu, HI 96817   800-570-1101
                                         Fax: 808-528-1897
                                        e-mail: pr@kuakini.org
                                        www.kuakini.org/SiteMap.asp
The Kuakini Parkinson Disease (PD) Information & Referral Office provides referrals to neurologists and other special services for Parkinson disease patients; provides information about community services to assist PD patients and their caregivers in finding optimal care; distributes educational materials; conducts educational conferences and other activities; and assists with support groups for PD patients and caregivers.
Gary K Kajiwara, President/Chief Executive Officer
Gregg Oishi, SVP/Chief Operating Officer

Illinois

7007 Rockford Parkinson's Support Group
5415 Watson Road   815-654-0614
Rockford, IL 61108   800-972-5455
Affiliate of The National Parkinson Foundation, Inc.

Maryland

7008 Parkinson Support Groups of America
11376 Cherry Hill Road   301-937-1545
Beltsville, MD 20705
Offers support networks and groups for persons with Parkinson's disease, families, friends and professionals.

Missouri

7009 APDA Center for Advanced Parkinson Disease Research
Washington University School of Medicine
660 South Euclid   314-362-6909
St Louis, MO 63110   Fax: 314-362-0168
                                       e-mail: joel@npg.wustl.edu
                                       www.neuro.wustl.edu/parkinson/
Information and referral research center for Parkinson's disease patients and their families.
David m Holtzman, Chairman
Brad a Racette, Vice Chairman

7010 Ozarks Parkinson Support Group
Po Box 50595
Springfield, MO 65805   417-885-9595
                               www.parkinson.org/shell/areacode.pl
Affiliate of the National Parkinson Foundation.
Monty Montgomery, Contact

New Jersey

7011 New Jersey Parkinson's Disease Information Center
Robert Wood Johnson University Hospital
One Robert Wood Johnson Place   732-828-3000
New Brunswick, NJ 08901   Fax: 732-745-3114
e-mail: elizabeth.schaaf@rwjuh.edu
www.rwjuh.edu/medical_services/
The New Jersey Parkinson's Disease Information and Referral Center reaches out to persons affected by Parkinson's disease, including patients, families and healthcare professionals. This Information and Referral Center is committed to providing community education and information as well as support groups for caregivers and persons with Parkinson's disease.
Elizabeth Schaaf, Parkinson's Disease Center Coordinator

New York

7012 American Parkinson Disease Association Hotline
1250 Hylan Boulevard
Staten Island, NY 10305   800-908-2732
Fax: 718-981-4399
www.attaparkinson.org
Offers information and physician referrals to patients and their families.
Joel Gerstel, Director

7013 New York College of Osteopathic Medicine
PO Box 8000   516-686-3747
Old Westbury, NY 11568-8000   800-345-6948
Fax: 516-686-7613
e-mail: Barbara
http://www.nyit.edu/medicine/
Information and referral research center for Parkinson's disease patients and their families.
Rosslee , Vice President

7014 Parkinson's Support Group of Upstate New York
PO Box 23204
Rochester, NY 14692-3204   716-377-6718
www.parkinson.org/upstate.htm
Affiliate of The National Parkinson Foundation, Inc.
David Look, President

7015 St. John's Episcopal Hospital
327 Beach 19th street
Smithtown, NY 11691   718-869-7000
www.ehs.org
Information and referral research center for Parkinson's disease patients and their families.
Nelson toebbe, Chief Executive Officer
Richard A Brown, Chief Operating Officer

7016 University of Rochester
500 Wilson Boulevard   585-275-3221
Rochester, NY 14627   888-822-2256
www.rochester.edu/
Information and referral research center for Parkinson's disease patients and their families.

Oregon

7017 Oregon Health Sciences University
3181 SW Sam Jackson Park Road   503-494-5285
Portland, OR 97239   888-222-6478
www.ohsu.edu
Information and referral research center for Parkinson's disease patients and their families.

Pennsylvania

7018 University of Pittsburgh
4200 Fifth avenue   412-624-4141
Pittsburgh, PA 15260   Fax: 412-383-2264
e-mail: webmaster@pitt.edu
www.pitt.edu
Information and referral research center for Parkinson's disease patients and their families.
Patricia E. Beeson, Vice Chancellor
John P Elliott, Director of Internal Affairs

Texas

7019 Presbyterian Hospital of Dallas
612 E. Lamar Boulevard
Arlington, TX 76011   214-345-6789
www.texashealth.org
Information and referral research center for Parkinson's disease patients and their families.
Phillip Moroneso, Chair
Brock Campton, Vice Chair

7020 University of Texas HSC at San Antonio
7703 Floyd Curl Drive
San Antonio, TX 78229-3900   210-567-7000
www.uthscsa.edu/
Information and referral research center for Parkinson's disease patients and their families.

Washington

7021 University of Washington
Box 355840   206-543-5369
Seattle, WA 98195-5840   e-mail: uwvic@u.washington.edu
www.washington.edu/
Information and referral research center for Parkinson's disease patients and their families.

Books

7022 Coping with Parkinson's Disease
American Parkinson's Disease Association
135 Parkinson Avenuey   718-981-8001
Staten Island, NY 10305-1944   800-223-2732
Fax: 718-981-4399
e-mail: apda@apdaparkinson.org
www.apdaparkinson.org
Offers information on the illness, incidence, treatments, education and support for both patients and professionals.
88 pages

7023 Living with Parkinson's Disease
Demos Medical Publishing
386 Park Avenue S   212-683-0072
New York, NY 10016-8804   800-532-8663
Fax: 212-683-0118
e-mail: orderdept@demospub.com
www.demospub.com
Written specifically for anyone who has been diagnosed with Parkinson's disease, as well as family members and friends.
1996 150 pages
ISBN: 1-888799-10-2
Dr. Diana M Schneider, President

7024 Parkinson's - A Personal Story of Acceptance
Branden Publishing Company
17 Station Street Box 843   617-734-2045
Wellesley, MA 02482   Fax: 617-734-2046
www.brandenbooks.com
1993 162 pages Paperback
ISBN: 0-828319-49-9

7025 Parkinson's Disease & Movement Disorders
Williams & Wilkins
351 W Camden Street   301-528-4000
Baltimore, MD 21201-7912   800-638-0672
1993 640 pages
ISBN: 0-683043-80-3

7026 Parkinson's Disease Handbook
National Parkinson Foundation
200 SE 1st Street   305-547-6666
Miami, FL 33131-1407   800-473-4636
Fax: 305-537-9901
e-mail: contact@parkinson.org
www.parkinson.org
A guide for patients and their families regarding the illness of Parkinson's.
Paperback

7027 Parkinson's Disease: A Guide for Patient and Family
Raven Press
1185 Ave of the Americas   212-930-9500
New York, NY 10036-2601   800-777-2295
Recommended by patients, the medical community and the leading medical journals, this guide offers information on the most recent medical advances in the field of Parkinson's disease and answers the patients most frequently asked questions about the illness.
224 pages Hardcover
ISBN: 0-781703-12-3

7028 Parkinsonian Syndromes
John H Dekker & Sons
2941 Clydon Avenue SW   616-538-5160
Grand Rapids, MI 49509-2403   Fax: 616-538-0720
1993 584 pages
ISBN: 0-824788-38-9

7029 The Comfort of Home for Parkinson Disease: A Guide for Caregivers
Marie Meyer & Paula Derr, RN with Susa Imke, RN/MS, author
CareTrust Publications
PO Box 10283
Portland, OR 97296-0283
                                            800-565-1533
                                       Fax: 415-673-2005
                         e-mail: sales@comfortofhome.com
                                      www.comfortofhome.com
Comfort will help caregivers be equipped with information about everything from the importance of and noticing wearing off signs to making difficult decisions to travel, equipment options, therapies and dietary guidelines. It offers caregivers mental and emotional support in coping with their challenging role, as well.
2007 298 pages
ISBN: 0-966476-77-8

Children's Books

7030 Journey to Almost There
Clarion Books
215 Park Avenue S
New York, NY 10003-1603   212-420-5800
An interesting tale that surrounds the relationship of Alison and her Granfather O'Brien when Alison's mother feels that he should enter an elderly home.
Grades 6-9

Newsletters

7031 APDA Newsletter
American Parkinson Disease Association
135 Parkinson Avenue   718-981-8001
Staten Island, NY 10305-1943   800-223-2732
                                       Fax: 718-981-4399
                           e-mail: apda@apdaparkinson.org
                                     www.apdaparkinson.org
Current information on matters of interest for PD patients and families.
Joel A Miele, President
Joel Gerste, Executive Director

7032 American Parkinson Disease Association Newsletter
60 Bay Street   718-981-8001
Staten Island, NY 10301-2514   800-223-2732
Offers information on the association activities and events, convention and legislative information, medical updates and research reports for the Parkinson's patient and their families.
Quarterly

7033 News & Review
Parkinsons Disease Foundation
1359 Broadway   212-923-4700
New York, NY 10018   800-457-6676
                                       Fax: 212-923-4778
                                   e-mail: info@pdf.org
                                            www.pdf.org
In each issue we include reports on scientific research and discoveries, treatments and therapies, commentary from physicians and

insight from Parkinson's specialists. We also provide practical suggestions, tips and articles from people who live with the disease and wish to share their experiences.
Quarterly
Lewis P Rowland, MD, President
Robin A Elliott, Executive Director

7034 Parkinson Report
National Parkinson Foundation
200 SE 1st Street   305-547-6666
Miami, FL 33131-1407   800-473-4636
                                       Fax: 305-537-9901
                          e-mail: contact@parkinson.org
                                       www.parkinson.org
Offers association news and events, conference and symposia news, legislative and medical updates, research reports and more for the Parkinson's patient, their families and the general public.
Quarterly

7035 Parkinson's Disease Foundation Newsletter
Parkinson's Disease Foundation
650 W 168th Street   212-923-4700
New York, NY 10032-3702   800-457-6676
Provides information on Parkinson's Disease Foundation events, news stories of research findings, and technical advances in the field of patient care.

Pamphlets

7036 A One-Stop Shop for Parkinson's Informatio n
Parkinsons Disease Foundation
1359 Broadway   212-923-4700
New York, NY 10018   800-457-6676
                                       Fax: 212-923-4778
                                   e-mail: info@pdf.org
                                            www.pdf.org
An explanation of PDF's services and resources that are available to answer your most important questions about Parkinson's disease. These services include a toll-free helpline, our Ask the Expert web service and print/video materials.
Lewis P Rowland, MD, President
Robin A Elliott, Executive Director

7037 Adjustment, Adaptation and Accomodation: Psychological Approaches
National Parkinson Foundation
200 SE 1st Street   305-547-6666
Miami, FL 33131-1407   800-473-4636
                                       Fax: 305-537-9901
                          e-mail: contact@parkinson.org
                                       www.parkinson.org
Coping strategies for Parkinson's disease.

7038 Akathisia in Parkinson's Disease
Parkinson United Foundation
833 W Washington Blvd   312-733-1893
Chicago, IL 60607
1990

7039 Answering Your Questions About PROPATH
525 Middlefield Road
Menlo Park, CA 94025-3447   800-776-7284
This brochure explains and offers an introduction to PROPATH, a program for Parkinson's disease patients.

7040 Autonomic Failure and Parkinson's Disease
United Parkinson Foundation
833 W Washington Blvd   312-733-1893
Chicago, IL 60607-2316
1990

7041 Balance Disturbances and Parkinson's Disease
United Parkinson Foundation
833 W Washington Blvd   312-733-1893
Chicago, IL 60607-2316
1990

7042 Basic Information About Parkinson's Disease
American Parkinson's Disease Association

135 Parkinson Avenueÿ
Staten Island, NY 10305-1944

718-981-8001
800-223-2732
Fax: 718-981-4399
e-mail: apda@apdaparkinson.org
www.apdaparkinson.org

Offers information on the illness, incidence, treatments, education and support for both patients and professionals.

7043 Deep Brain Stimulation for Parkinson's Disease
Parkinsons Disease Foundation
1359 Broadway
New York, NY 10018

212-923-4700
800-457-6676
Fax: 212-923-4778
e-mail: info@pdf.org
www.pdf.org

This booklet addresses the newest area of surgical options in the treatment of PD symptoms _ deep brain stimulation (or DBS) surgery _ while also describing older surgical approaches used to treat PD.
Lewis P Rowland, MD, President
Robin A Elliott, Executive Director

7044 Dental Care for the Patient with Parkinson's Disease
United Parkinson Foundation
833 W Washington Blvd
Chicago, IL 60607-2316
1987

312-733-1893

7045 Depression and Dementia in Parkinson's Disease
United Parkinson Foundation
833 W Washington Blvd
Chicago, IL 60607-2316
1993

312-733-1893

7046 Diagnosis Parkinson's Disease: You Are Not Alone
Parkinsons Disease Foundation
1359 Broadway
New York, NY 10018

212-923-4700
800-457-6676
Fax: 212-923-4778
e-mail: info@pdf.org
www.pdf.org

Designed for the person newly diagnosed with Parkinson's, this informational booklet serves as a reference for the many questions that may arise. It shares resources, medical expert testimony and the experiences of people who have dealt with the diagnosis of Parkinson's disease.
Booklet
Lewis P Rowland, MD, President
Robin A Elliott, Executive Director

7047 Dietary Considerations for Parkinson's Disease Patients
United Parkinson Foundation
833 W Washington Blvd
Chicago, IL 60607-2316

312-733-1893

7048 Differential Diagnosis of Parkinsonism
United Parkinson Foundation
833 W Washington Blvd
Chicago, IL 60607-2316
1984

312-733-1893

7049 Driving and the Parkinson's Disease Patient: Some Considerations
United Parkinson Foundation
833 W Washington Blvd
Chicago, IL 60607-2316
1994

312-733-1893

7050 Efficacy of Antiparkinson Medications
United Parkinson Foundation
833 W Washington Blvd
Chicago, IL 60607-2316
1983

312-733-1893

7051 Equipment and Suggestions for Persons with Parkinson's Disease
American Parkinson's Disease Association
135 Parkinson Avenueÿ
Staten Island, NY 10305-1944

718-981-8001
800-223-2732
Fax: 718-981-4399
e-mail: apda@apdaparkinson.org
www.apdaparkinson.org

Offers information on the illness, incidence, treatments, education and support for both patients and professionals.
19 pages

7052 Eyes and Parkinson's Disease
United Parkinson Foundation
833 W Washington Blvd
Chicago, IL 60607-2316
1986

312-733-1893

7053 Fighting Back Against PD: One Women's Story
National Parkinson Foundation
200 SE 1st Street
Miami, FL 33131-1407

305-547-6666
800-473-4636
Fax: 305-537-9901
e-mail: contact@parkinson.org
www.parkinson.org

One woman's battle against Parkinson's disease.

7054 Fulfilling the Hope: Our Commitment to the Parkinson's Community
Parkinsons Disease Foundation
1359 Broadway
New York, NY 10018

212-923-4700
800-457-6676
Fax: 212-923-4778
e-mail: info@pdf.org
www.pdf.org

This brochure provides an overview of Parkinsons Disease Foundations services and programs.
Lewis P Rowland, MD, President
Robin A Elliott, Executive Director

7055 Good Nutrition in Parkinson's Disease
American Parkinson Disease Association
60 Bay Street
Staten Island, NY 10301-2514

800-223-2732

Offers information on diet, nutrients, proteins and recipes for people with Parkinson's disease.

7056 How to Start a Parkinson's Disease Support Group
American Parkinson's Disease Association
135 Parkinson Avenueÿ
Staten Island, NY 10305-1944

718-981-8001
800-223-2732
Fax: 718-981-4399
e-mail: apda@apdaparkinson.org
www.apdaparkinson.org

Offers information on the illness, incidence, treatments, education and support for both patients and professionals.
42 pages

7057 MR Imaging in Parkinson's Disease
United Parkinson Foundation
833 W Washington Blvd
Chicago, IL 60607-2316
1990

312-733-1893

7058 Micrographia
United Parkinson Foundation
833 W Washington Blvd
Chicago, IL 60607-2316
1991

312-733-1893

7059 Neuropsychology and Parkinson's Disease
United Parkinson Foundation
833 W Washington Blvd
Chicago, IL 60607-2316
1992

312-733-1893

7060 Neurotrophic Factors in Parkinson's Disease
United Parkinson Foundation
833 W Washington Blvd
Chicago, IL 60607-2316
1992

312-733-1893

7061 One Step at a Time Brochure
United Parkinson Foundationon
833 W Washington Blvd
Chicago, IL 60607-2316

312-733-1893

An exercise manual for the Parkinsonian patient.
1985

7062 Pain Syndromes and Parkinson's Disease
United Parkinson Foundation
833 W Washington Blvd   312-733-1893
Chicago, IL 60607-2316
1990

7063 Parkinson Handbook: A Guide for Patients and Their Families
National Parkinson Foundation
200 SE 1st Street   305-547-6666
Miami, FL 33131-1407   800-473-4636
Fax: 305-537-9901
e-mail: contact@parkinson.org
www.parkinson.org
Offers informative, up-to-date information on exercises, hobbies, treatments, speech impairments and psychological aspects.

7064 Parkinson's Advocacy: The Keys to Empowerment
Parkinsons Disease Foundation
1359 Broadway   212-923-4700
New York, NY 10018   800-457-6676
Fax: 212-923-4778
e-mail: info@pdf.org
www.pdf.org
Use this informational brochure to learn how to harness your power as a person living with Parkinson's and join the fight for a cure.
Lewis P Rowland, MD, President
Robin A Elliott, Executive Director

7065 Parkinson's Disease Handbook
American Parkinson's Disease Association
135 Parkinson Avenue̎   718-981-8001
Staten Island, NY 10305-1944   800-223-2732
Fax: 718-981-4399
e-mail: apda@apdaparkinson.org
www.apdaparkinson.org
Offers information on the illness, incidence, treatments, education and support for both patients and professionals.
40 pages

7066 Parkinson's Disease Q&A: A Guide for Patients
Parkinsons Disease Foundation
1359 Broadway   212-923-4700
New York, NY 10018   800-457-6676
Fax: 212-923-4778
e-mail: info@pdf.org
www.pdf.org
This booklet answers the most frequently asked questions about Parkinson's disease. Movement disorder specialists from the Columbia University Medical Center address topics ranging from signs of Parkinson's to treatment options to daily living issues.
Booklet
Lewis P Rowland, MD, President
Robin A Elliott, Executive Director

7067 Parkinson's Disease and the Menstrual Cycle
United Parkinson Foundation
833 W Washington Blvd   312-733-1893
Chicago, IL 60607-2316
1990

7068 Parkinson's Disease: The Patient Experience
United Parkinson Foundation
833 W Washington Blvd   312-733-1893
Chicago, IL 60607-2316
Booklet designed for patients with Parkinson's disease and their families to explain medical terminology and offer suggestions on how to deal with the disease more easily.
1986

7069 Parkinson's Patient: What You and Your Family Should Know
National Parkinson Foundation
200 SE 1st Street   305-547-6666
Miami, FL 33131-1407   800-473-4636
Fax: 305-537-9901
e-mail: contact@parkinson.org
www.parkinson.org
Offers a brief overview of Parkinson's Disease causes, symptoms and treatments as well as offering an insight into statistical information on the illness.

7070 Patient Perspectives on Parkinson's
National Parkinson Foundation
200 SE 1st Street   305-547-6666
Miami, FL 33131-1407   800-473-4636
Fax: 305-537-9901
e-mail: contact@parkinson.org
www.parkinson.org
Offers a brief overview of Parkinson's disease, the onset of the illness, depression, sexuality, exercise, sleep and nutrition information for daily living.
45 pages

7071 Perioperative Management of Parkinson's Disease
United Parkinson Foundation
833 W Washington Blvd   312-733-1893
Chicago, IL 60607-2316
1989

7072 Pet Scans: A New Look at Parkinson's Disease
United Parkinson Foundation
833 W Washington Blvd   312-733-1893
Chicago, IL 60607-2316
1989

7073 Podiatry and Parkinson's Disease
United Parkinson Foundation
833 W Washington Blvd   312-733-1893
Chicago, IL 60607-2316
1983

7074 Postural Hypotension
United Parkinson Foundation
833 W Washington Blvd   312-733-1893
Chicago, IL 60607-2316
1988

7075 Practical Pointers for Parkinson Patients
National Parkinson Foundation
200 SE 1st Street   305-547-6666
Miami, FL 33131-1407   800-473-4636
Fax: 305-537-9901
e-mail: contact@parkinson.org
www.parkinson.org
Offers a brief overview of Parkinson's disease, the onset of the illness, depression, sexuality, exercise, sleep and nutrition information for daily living.

7076 Role of Physical Therapy in Parkinson's Disease
United Parkinson Foundation
833 W Washington Blvd   312-733-1893
Chicago, IL 60607-2316
1985

7077 Sexual and Bladder Difficulties in Parkinson's Disease
United Parkinson Foundation
833 W Washington Blvd   312-733-1893
Chicago, IL 60607-2316
1988

7078 Sleep Problems with Parkinson's Disease
United Parkinson Foundation
833 W Washington Blvd   312-733-1893
Chicago, IL 60607-2316
1992

7079 Speech & Swallowing Problems for Parkinsonians
National Parkinson Foundation
200 SE 1st Street   305-547-6666
Miami, FL 33131-1407   800-473-4636
Fax: 305-537-9901
e-mail: contact@parkinson.org
www.parkinson.org
Offers a brief overview of Parkinson's disease, the onset of the illness, depression, sexuality, exercise, sleep and nutrition information for daily living.

7080 Speech Problems & Swallowing Problems in Parkinson's Disease
American Parkinson Disease Association
60 Bay Street
Staten Island, NY 10301-2514   800-223-2732

Offers information on speech problems, swallowing problems, hearing impairments and facial mobility for the person with Parkinson's.

7081 Speech and Voice Impairment
United Parkinson Foundation
833 W Washington Blvd   312-733-1893
Chicago, IL 60607-2316
1983

7082 Stages of Parkinson's Disease
United Parkinson Foundation
833 W Washington Blvd   312-733-1893
Chicago, IL 60607-2316
1983

7083 Suggested Exercise Program for People with Parkinson's Disease
American Parkinson Disease Association
60 Bay Street
Staten Island, NY 10301-2514   800-223-2732
Exercise program pamphlet with full illustrations explaining each exercise.
23 pages

7084 Treatment of Parkinson's Disease with Carbidopa-Levodopa
National Parkinson Foundation
200 SE 1st Street   305-547-6666
Miami, FL 33131-1407   800-473-4636
                              Fax: 305-537-9901
                   e-mail: contact@parkinson.org
                              www.parkinson.org
Offers information on treating Parkinson's Disease.

Audio & Video

7085 Diagnosis Parkinson's Disease: You Are Not Alone
Parkinsons Disease Foundation
1359 Broadway   212-923-4700
New York, NY 10018   800-457-6676
                              Fax: 212-923-4778
                        e-mail: info@pdf.org
                              www.pdf.org
Designed for the person newly diagnosed with Parkinson's, this informational booklet and video serve as a reference for the many questions that may arise. It shares resources, medical expert testimony and the experiences of people who have dealt with the diagnosis of Parkinson's disease.
Video & Booklet
Lewis P Rowland, MD, President
Robin A Elliott, Executive Director

7086 Motivating Moves for People with Parkinson's
Parkinsons Disease Foundation
1359 Broadway   212-923-4700
New York, NY 10018   800-457-6676
                              Fax: 212-923-4778
                        e-mail: info@pdf.org
                              www.pdf.org
Motivating Moves is a unique program of 24 seated exercises designed especially for people with Parkinson's. Exercises address typical Parkinson's symptoms such as stability, flexibility, posture, vocal range and facial expressivity. The video is divided into three sections, How to Do Motivating Moves (45 minutes), The Exercise Class (36 minutes) and Practical Tips for Daily Living (4 minutes).
Video
Lewis P Rowland, MD, President
Robin A Elliott, Executive Director

7087 PDF Exercise Program
Parkinsons Disease Foundation
1359 Broadway   212-923-4700
New York, NY 10018   800-457-6676
                              Fax: 212-923-4778
                        e-mail: info@pdf.org
                              www.pdf.org
This program consists of three sets of exercises specifically designed for PD patients. Each exercise is clearly illustrated in a 3-ring binder with flip-chart pages and includes two cassette tapes, which provide verbal cues and music for timing.
Cassettes
Lewis P Rowland, MD, President
Robin A Elliott, Executive Director

7088 Parkingson's: Lynda's Story
David Tucker, author
Fanlight Productions
32 Court Street   718-488-8900
Brooklyn, NY 11201   800-876-1710
                              Fax: 718-488-8642
                   e-mail: info@fanlight.com
                              www.fanlight.com
Parkingson's disease is robbing Lynda McKenzie of normal coordination and movement. She's prepared to participate in a clinical study of surgery to transplant fetal cells directly into her brain, but she will have to live for a year not knowing whether she has received the actual cells or a placebo.
1999 46 Minutes
ISBN: 1-572954-22-1
Nicole Johnson, Publicity Coordinator

Web Sites

7089 Healing Well
                              www.healingwell.com
An online health resource guide to medical news, chat, information and articles, newsgroups and message boards, books, disease-related web sites, medical directories, and more for patients, friends, and family coping with disabling diseases, disorders, or chronic illnesses.

7090 Health Finder
                              www.healthfinder.gov
Searchable, carefully developed web site offering information on over 1000 topics. Developed by the US Department of Health and Human Services, the site can be used in both English and Spanish.

7091 Healthlink USA
                              www.healthlinkusa.com
Health information concerning treatment, cures, prevention, diagnosis, risk factors, research, support groups, email lists, personal stories and much more. Updated regularly.

7092 Helios Health
                              www.helioshealth.com
Online resource for your health information. Detailed information about specific health topics, access to expert advice from our Medical Advisory Board, and up-to-date health news.

7093 MedicineNet
                              www.medicinenet.com
An online resource for consumers providing easy-to-read, authoritative medical and health information.

7094 Medscape
                              www.medscape.com
Medscape offers specialists, primary care physicians, and other health professionals the Web's most robust and integrated medical information and educational tools.

7095 National Parkinson Foundation
                              www.parkinson.org
Information on research, diagnosis, treatment and care for men and women suffering from parkinson's and other related neurological diseases.

7096 Neurology Channel
                              www.healthcommunities.com
Find clearly explained, medically accurate information regarding conditions, including an overview, symptoms, causes, diagnostic procedures and treatment options. On this site it is possible to ask questions and get information from a neurologist and connect to people who have similar health interests.

7097 WebMD
                              www.webmd.com

Provides credible information, supportive communities, and
in-depth reference material about health subjects. A source for
original and timely health information as well as material from
well known content providers.

Description

7098 Post-Polio Syndrome

Post-Polio syndrome, PPS, also known as the late effects of polio or post polio sequelae, is characterized by new symptoms that occur in people with a history of polio after a long period of stability during which whatever strength they had recovered remained unchanged. PPS affects approximately 60 percent of polio survivors, 20 to 40 years after the initial episode. The hallmark of PPS is new weakness. Other symptoms include fatigue, pain, difficulty breathing and swallowing, intolerance to cold, and new muscle atrophy.

While the cause of PPS is not clearly understood, two theories exist. One suggests that it is caused by normal muscle loss that accompanies aging. The other is that PPS is caused by the repeated over use of muscle groups. In both cases, muscle groups not previously known to have been affected by polio are weakened, and it is this weakness that is the major indicator of PPS. A polio survivor with an affected leg may find that his or her arms are newly affected. Whether the arm problems are a result of undetected muscle damage that occurred at the time of the original polio or newer damage resulting from the over use of the remaining good muscles, or a combination of the two, is not clearly understood.

PPS is frequently emotionally difficult for polio survivors. Many feel they have triumphed over their initial polio, or have come to terms with their resulting disabilities. To think that the polio is coming back is often terrifying. These emotional issues are frequently made more difficult by the fact that PPS is often mis-diagnosed as other conditions or normal aging. Also, patients are often given misinformation about PPS.

Post-polio syndrome, like most diseases classified as syndromes, does not have a specific diagnostic test, but a diagnosis of exclusion. This means that other medical conditions that may present with symptoms similar to those found in PPS should be considered and excluded, if possible. Once diagnosis of PPS is determined, treatment is individualized by primary symptoms and may include medications, supervised therapy, injections and, in some cases, surgery.

National Agencies & Associations

7099 American Association of Neuromuscular & Electrodiagnostic Medicine
2621 Superior Drive NW 507-288-0100
Rochester, MN 55901 Fax: 507-288-1225
e-mail: aanem@aanem.org
www.aanem.org
The American Association of Neuromuscular & Electrodiagnostic Medicine (AANEM) is a nonprofit membership association dedicated to the advancement of neuromuscular, musculoskeletal, and electrodiagnostic medicine.
Vincent J. Tranchitella, MD, President
Shirlyn A. Adkins, JD, Executive Director

7100 Chronic Syndrome Support Association
801 Riverside Drive
Lumberton, NC 28358 www.cssa-inc.org
The Chronic Syndrome Support Association, Inc., is a 501(c)3 non-profit corporation. It was founded in 1997 in order to educate the general population and health-care professionals who lack current knowledge of the research being done, and potential research that needs to be done, on these serious, yet invisible, Chronic Immunological and Neurological Disorders.

7101 Orthopaedic Rehabilitation Association
8290 University Ave. NE. 763-957-5310
Fridley, MN 55432 Fax: 763-786-3320
e-mail: debfinch@oppamn.com
www.orthorehabassoc.org
At the 1989 annual meeting of the American Academy of Orthopaedic Surgeons (AAOS) in New Orleans, a group of Orthopedic surgeons met and founded the Orthopedic Rehabilitation Association (ORA). These surgeons were interested in the orthopaedic care of patients with complex musculoskeletal problems, which were global in nature and were not being addressed by other specialty societies.

7102 Polio Survivors Association
12720 La Reina Avenue 562-862-4508
Downey, CA 90242 Fax: 562-862-4508
e-mail: info@polioassociation.org
www.polioassociation.org
The Polio Survivors Association was formed in 1975 as a 501(c)(3) non-profit corporation to promote the well being and improve the quality of life for these severely disabled polio survivors.
Richard Daggett, President

7103 Post Polio Awareness and Support Society o f British Columbia
#2-2630 Ross Lane 250-477-8244
Victoria, BC, V8T-5L5 Fax: 250-477-8287
e-mail: ppass@ppass.bc.ca
www.ppass.bc.ca
A non-profit society that links area groups, through our board and our provincial office in Victoria.
Joan Toone, President

Support Groups & Hotlines

7104 PostPolio Health International
4207 Lindell Boulevard 314-534-0475
Saint Louis, MO 63108-2915 Fax: 314-534-5070
e-mail: info@postpolio.org
www.post-polio.org/
Post-Polio Health International's mission is to enhance the lives and independence of polio survivors and home ventilator users through education, advocacy, research and networking.
Willism G Stothers, President
Saul J Morse, Legal counsel

Books

7105 Managing Post-Polio: A Guide for Polio Survivors and Their Families
Yale University Press
4207 Lindell Boulevard 314-534-0475
St. Louis, MO 63108-9040 Fax: 314-534-5070
e-mail: info@post-polio.org
www.post-polio.org
Diagnosis and management of polio-related health problems . Essential resources for polio survivors, their families and health care providers.

7106 Managing Post-Polio: A Guide to Living Well with Post-Polio Syndrome
ABI Professional Publications
PO Box 5243 703-525-5488
Arlington, VA 22205 Fax: 703-524-4105
Practical information resulting from a combination of professional knowledge and personal experience. A comprehensive array of topics are addressed: the diagnostic process, finding expert medical care, energy conservation, psychosocial aspects of disability,

support groups, vocational strategies, managed care concerns, Social Security benefits, and internet resources.
256 pages

Newsletters

7107 Polio Network News
Post-Polio Health International
4207 Lindell Boulevard
St. Louis, MO 63108-2915

314-534-0475
Fax: 314-534-5070
e-mail: info@ventusers.org
www.ventusers.org

The newsletter of the International Ventilator Users Network, an affiliate of Post-Polio Health International.
Joan Headley, Executive Director

7108 Post-Polio Health
Post-Polio Health International
4207 Lindell Boulevard
Saint Louis, MO 63108-2915

314-534-0475
Fax: 314-534-5070
e-mail: info@ventusers.org
www.ventusers.org

The newsletter of the International Ventilator Users Network, an affiliate of Post-Polio Health International.
12 pages Quarterly
Joan Headley, Executive Director

7109 Post-Polio Health International
Joan L Headley, author

4207 Lindell Boulevard
St. Louis, MO 63108-2915

314-534-0475
Fax: 314-534-5070
e-mail: info@post-polio.org
www.post-polio.org

Provides educational materials, advocacy, networking and support research to enhance the lives and independence of polio survivors and users of home mechanical ventilators. Minimum $25.00 with membership.
12 pages
Joan Headley, Executive Director

7110 Ventilator-Assisted Living
Joan L Headley, author

4207 Lindell Boulevard
St. Louis, MO 63108-2915

314-534-0475
Fax: 314-534-5070
e-mail: info@post-polio.org
www.post-polio.org

Provides educational materials, advocacy, networking and support research to enhance the lives and independence of polio survivors and users of home mechanical ventilators. Minimum $25.00 with membership.
12 pages
Joan Headley, Executive Director

7111 Ventilator: Assisted Living
Post-Polio Health International
4207 Lindell Boulevard
St. Louis, MO 63108-2915

314-534-0475
Fax: 314-534-5070
e-mail: info@ventusers.org
www.ventusers.org

The newsletter of the International Ventilator Users Network, an affiliate of Post-Polio Health International.
12 pages Newsletter
Joan Headley, Executive Director

Pamphlets

7112 Guidelines for People Who Have Had Polio
March of Dimes
PO Box 1657
Wilkes-Barre, PA 18703

717-820-8104
800-367-6630
Fax: 570-825-1987

Located on website as a PDF file. Information based on March of Dimes International Conference on Post-Polio Syndrome.

7113 Post-Polio Syndrome: Identifying Best Practices in Diagnosis and Care
March of Dimes

1275 Mamaroneck Avenue
White Plains, NY 10605

914-997-4488
Fax: 212-254-3518
e-mail: NY639@marchofdimes.com
www.marchofdimes.com

Located on website as PDF file.

Web Sites

7114 EMedicine

emedicine.medscape.com

EMedicine was launched in 1996 and is the largest and most current clinical knowledge base available to physicians and health professionals.

7115 International Rehabilitation Center for Polio

www.polioclinic.org

International Rehabilitation Center for Polio (IRCP) at Spaulding Rehabilitation HOspital website offers information about PPS and resources for polio survivors and others with an interest in post-polio syndrome.

7116 MedicineNet

www.medicinenet.com

An online resource for consumers providing easy-to-read, authoritative medical and health information.

7117 Polio Experience Network

www.polionet.org

The Polio Experience Network offers information, inspiration, ideas and resources for polio survivors and those seeking information on post-polio syndrome.

7118 Social Security Administration

www.ssa.gov/agency

Social Security delivers a broad range of services online at socialsecurity.gov and through a nationwide network of over 1,400 offices that include regional offices, field offices, card centers, teleservice centers, processing centers, hearing offices, the Appeals Council, and our State and territorial partners, the Disability Determination Services.

Description

7119 Post-Traumatic Stress Disorder

Post-Traumatic Stress Disorder, or PTSD, is one of the Anxiety Disorders receiving particular attention because it affects a significant number of individuals returning from war zones, as well as those affected by terrorism and natural disasters. PTSD has been recognized for at least a hundred years. During and after World War I, traumatized soldiers' symptoms of hypersensitivity, avoidance, and other characteristics of what we now call PTSD were called 'shell shock' in the past.

PTSD continues to be identified with military service, but it is not limited to members of the military. It can affect adults and children exposed to terrifying and dangerous events in any circumstances: natural disasters, physical and/or sexual attacks, acts of terrorism and accidents, for example. By definition, the precipitating event must be outside the bounds of everyday human experience and the individual must feel helpless to protect him or herself from the event. Women appear to be somewhat more vulnerable to PTSD than men.

National Agencies & Associations

7120 AMSUS
9320 Old Georgetown Road
Bethesda, MD 20814
301-897-8800
800-761-9320
Fax: 301-530-5446
e-mail: membership@amsus.org
www.amsus.org
Organized in 1891 and chartered by Congress in 1903, AMSUS is a non-profit, 501(c)3, organization for federal and international health professionals.
VADM Mike Cowan, MC, USN (Ret.), Executive Director
CDR John Class, MSC, USN (Ret.), Deputy Executive Director

7121 African American Post Traumatic Stress Disorder Association
9129 Veterans DR SW
Lakewood, WA 98498
253-589-0766
Fax: 253-589-0769
e-mail: tacomaptsd@earthlink.net
www.aaptsdassn.org
The African American Post Traumatic Stress Disorder Association (AA PTSD Assn.) is a non-partisan, non-profit, 501(c) 3, National Veteran's Service Organization. We are dedicated to the service of All Veterans and the family members of veterans in the achievement and education of Veterans Benefits as provided in Public Laws, Chapter 38 Code of Federal Regulations (CFR) and Title 38 United States Code (USC).
Sidney A. Lee, President
Donald Curtis, Vice President

7122 American Academy of Child and Adolescent Psychiatry
3615 Wisconsin Avenue, NW
Washington, DC 20016
202-966-7300
Fax: 202-966-2891
e-mail: communications@aacap.org
www.aacap.org
The mission of AACAP is to promote the healthy development of children, adolescents, and families through advocacy, education, and research, and to meet the professional needs of child and adolescent psychiatrists throughout their careers.
Paramjit T. Joshi, MD, President
David G. Fassler, MD, Treasurer

7123 American Medical Association
330 N Wabash Ave.
Chicago, IL 60611
800-262-3211
www.ama-assn.org/ama

AMA is dedicated to ensuring sustainable physician practices that result in better health outcomes for patients.
James L. Madara, MD, CEO/EVP
Bernard L. Hengesbaugh, Chief Operating Officer

7124 American Psychiatric Association
1000 Wilson Boulevard
Arlington, VA 22209
703-907-7300
888-35-7924
e-mail: apa@psych.org
www.psychiatry.org
It is a medical specialty society representing growing membership of more than 36,000 psychiatrists.

7125 American Psychological Association
750 First St. NE
Washington, DC 20002
202-336-5500
800-374-2721
TTY: 202-336-6123
www.apa.org
The mission is to advance the creation, communication and application of psychological knowledge to benefit society and improve people's lives.
Norman B. Anderson, PhD, CEO/EVP
L. Michael Honaker, PhD, Deputy Chief Executive Officer

7126 American Public Health Association
800 I Street, NW
Washington, DC 20001
202-777-2742
Fax: 202-777-2534
TTY: 202-777-2500
www.apha.org
APHA champions the health of all people and all communities. They aim to strengthen the public health profession and speak out for public health issues and policies backed by science.
Georges C. Benjamin, MD, Executive Director
Kemi Oluwafemi, MBA, CPA, Chief Financial Officer

7127 American Trauma Society
201 Park Washington Court
Falls Church, VA 22046
703-538-3544
800-556-7890
Fax: 703-241-5603
e-mail: info@amtrauma.org
www.amtrauma.org
American Trauma Society (ATS) is dedicated to the elimination of needless death and disability from injury.
Ian Weston, Executive Director
Kathy Robinson, Associate Director

7128 Anxiety Disorders Association of America
8701 Georgia Ave.
Silver Spring, MD 20910
240-485-1001
www.adaa.org
ADAA is a national nonprofit organization dedicated to the prevention, treatment, and cure of anxiety, depression, OCD, PTSD, and related disorders and to improving the lives of all people who suffer from them through education, practice, and research.
Mark H. Pollack, MD, President
Alies Muskin, Executive Director

7129 Anxiety and Depression Association of America
8701 Georgia Ave.
Silver Spring, MD 20910
240-485-1001
Fax: 240-485-1035
www.adaa.org
ADAA is a national nonprofit organization dedicated to the prevention, treatment, and cure of anxiety, depression, OCD, PTSD, and related disorders and to improving the lives of all people who suffer from them through education, practice, and research.
Mark H. Pollack, MD, President
Alies Muskin, Executive Director

7130 Association for Behavioral and Cognitive Therapies
305 7th Avenue
New York, NY 10001
212-647-1890
www.abct.org
The Association for Behavioral and Cognitive Therapies is a multidisciplinary organization committed to the advancement of scientific approaches to the understanding and improvement of human functioning through the investigation and application of behavioral, cognitive, and other evidence-based principles to the

assessment, prevention, treatment of human problems, and the enhancement of health and well-being.
Mary Jane Eimer, CAE, Executive Director
David Teisler, CAE, Director of Communications

7131 Association for Traumatic Stress Specialists
5000 Old Buncombe Road   864-294-4337
Greenville, SC 29617   e-mail: admin@atss.info
www.atss.info
ATSS is a professional membership organization of individuals engaged in and committed to excellence in trauma services, response, and treatment.
Chrys Harris, Ph.D., CTS, President
Bill Mc Dermott, Vice President

7132 Depression and Bipolar Support Alliance
55 E. Jackson Blvd
Chicago, IL 60604   800-826-3632
Fax: 312-642-7243
www.dbsalliance.org
DBSA provides hope, help, support, and education to improve the lives of people who have mood disorders.
Katee Crawford, Development Manager
Angie Day, Chapter Relations Coordinator

7133 Freedom From Fear
308 Seaview Avenue   718-351-1717
Staten Island, NY 10305   e-mail: help@freedomfromfear.org
www.freedomfromfear.org
Freedom From Fear is a national not-for-profit mental health advocacy organization. Mary Guardino founded FFF in 1984 as an outgrowth of her own personal experiences having suffered from anxiety and depressive illnesses for more than 25 years. The mission of FFF is to impact, in a positive way, the lives of all those affected by anxiety, depressive and related disorders through advocacy, education, research and community support.
Mary Guardino, Founder/Executive Director

7134 International Society for Traumatic Stress Studies
111 Deer Lake Road   847-480-9028
Deerfield, IL 60015   Fax: 847-480-9282
e-mail: info@istss.org
www.istss.org
The International Society for Traumatic Stress Studies is dedicated to sharing information about the effects of trauma and the discovery and dissemination of knowledge about policy, program and service initiatives that seek to reduce traumatic stressors and their immediate and long-term consequences.
Miranda Olff, PhD, President
Julian Ford, PhD, Vice President

7135 International Society for the Study of Trauma And Dissociation
8400 Westpark Drive   703-610-9037
McLean, VA 22102   Fax: 703-610-0234
e-mail: info@isst-d.org
www.isst-d.org
The International Society for the Study of Trauma and Dissociation is an international, non-profit, professional association organized to develop and promote comprehensive, clinically effective and empirically based resources and responses to trauma and dissociation and to address its relevance to other theoretical constructs.
Lynette S. Danylchuk, PhD, President
Philip J. Kinsler, PhD, ABPP, Past President

7136 National Alliance on Mental Illness
3803 N. Fairfax Drive   703-524-7600
Arlington, VA 22203   800-950-6264
Fax: 703-524-9094
e-mail: info@nami.org
www.nami.org
NAMI, the National Alliance on Mental Illness, is the nation's largest grassroots mental health organization dedicated to building better lives for the millions of Americans affected by mental illness.
Jim Payne, J.D., President
Ralph E. Nelson, Jr., M.D., First Vice President

7137 National Association of Social Workers
750 First Street, NE   202-408-8600
Washington, DC 20002   e-mail: membership@naswdc.org
www.socialworkers.org
The National Association of Social Workers (NASW) is the largest membership organization of professional social workers in the world, with 132,000 members. NASW works to enhance the professional growth and development of its members, to create and maintain professional standards, and to advance sound social policies.
Darrell P. Wheeler, PhD, MPH, ACSW, President
Angelo McClain, PhD, LICSW, Chief Executive Officer

7138 National Institute of Mental Health
6001 Executive Boulevard   301-443-4536
Rockville, MD 20852   Fax: 301-443-4279
e-mail: NIMHinfo@mail.nih.gov
www.nimh.nih.gov
The mission of NIMH is to transform the understanding and treatment of mental illnesses through basic and clinical research, paving the way for prevention, recovery, and cure.

7139 Posttraumatic Stress Disorder (PTSD) Alliance
www.ptsdalliance.org
The Posttraumatic Stress Disorder (PTSD) Alliance is a group of professional and advocacy organizations that have joined forces to provide educational resources to individuals diagnosed with PTSD and their loved ones; those at risk for developing PTSD; and medical, healthcare and other frontline professionals.

State Agencies & Associations

District of Columbia

7140 Administration for Children and Families
370 L'Enfant Promenade
Washington, DC 20447   www.acf.hhs.gov
The Administration for Children & Families (ACF) is a division of the U.S. Department of Health & Human Services (HHS). ACF promotes the economic and social well-being of families, children, individuals and communities.
Mark Greenberg, Acting Assistant Secretary
Jeff Hild, Chief of Staff

7141 Administration for Community Living
One Massachusetts Avenue   202-619-0724
Washington, DC 20001   800-677-1116
Fax: 202-357-3555
e-mail: aclinfo@acl.hhs.gov
www.acl.gov
ACL brings together the efforts and achievements of the Administration on Aging, the Administration on Intellectual and Developmental Disabilities, and the HHS Office on Disability to serve as the Federal agency responsible for increasing access to community supports, while focusing attention and resources on the unique needs of older Americans and people with disabilities across the lifespan.
Kathy Greenlee, Administrator
Sharon Lewis, Principal Deputy Administrator

7142 Federal Emergency Management Agency
500 C Street S.W.   202-646-2500
Washington, DC 20472   800-621-3362
TTY: 800-427-5593
www.fema.gov
FEMA's mission is to support the citizens and first responders to ensure that as a nation we work together to build, sustain and improve our capability to prepare for, protect against, respond to, recover from and mitigate all hazards.
W. Craig Fugate, Administrator
Michael Coen, Jr., Chief of Staff

7143 U.S. Department of Health and Human Services
200 Independence Ave, SW
Washington, DC 20201   877-696-6775
www.hhs.gov
The U.S. Department of Health and Human Services (HHS) is the U.S. government's principal agency for protecting the health of all

Americans and providing essential human services, especially for those who are least able to help themselves.
Sylvia M. Burwell, Secretary
Mary K. Wakefield, Acting Deputy Secretary

Georgia

7144 Agency for Toxic Substances and Disease Registry
4770 Buford Hwy NE
Atlanta, GA 30341   800-232-4636
                                                    TTY: 888-232-6348
                                                    www.atsdr.cdc.gov
The Agency for Toxic Substances and Disease Registry (ATSDR), based in Atlanta, Georgia, is a federal public health agency of the U.S. Department of Health and Human Services. ATSDR serves the public by using the best science, taking responsive public health actions, and providing trusted health information to prevent harmful exposures and diseases related to toxic substances.
Patrick Breysse, PhD, CIH, Director
Donna Knutson, PhD, Acting Deputy Director

Maryland

7145 Agency for Healthcare Research and Quality
540 Gaither Road
Rockville, MD 20850   301-427-1364
                                                    www.ahrq.gov/index.html
The Agency for Healthcare Research and Quality's (AHRQ) mission is to produce evidence to make health care safer, higher quality, more accessible, equitable, and affordable, and to work within the U.S. Department of Health and Human Services and with other partners to make sure that the evidence is understood and used.
Richard G. Kronick, PhD, Director, Director
Sharon B. Arnold, PhD, Deputy Director

7146 Center for Mental Health Services
Room 6-1057
Rockville, MD 20857   240-276-1310
                                                    www.samhsa.gov
The Center for Mental Health Services leads federal efforts to promote the prevention and treatment of mental disorders. Congress created CMHS to bring new hope to adults who have serious mental illness and children with emotional disorders.
Paolo del Vecchio, M.S.W., Director
Elizabeth Lopez, Ph.D., Deputy Director

7147 Centers for Medicare & Medicaid Services
7500 Security Boulevard   410-786-3000
Baltimore, MD 21244   877-267-2323
                                                    TTY: 866-226-1819
                                                    e-mail: Mandy.Cohen@cms.hhs.gov
                                                    www.cms.gov
US federal agency which administers Medicare, Medicaid, and the State Children's Health Insurance Program.
Dr. Mandy Cohen, M.D., MPH, Chief of Staff
Timothy P. Love, Chief Operating Officer

7148 National Center for Complementary and Integrative Health
9000 Rockville Pike
Bethesda, MD 20892   888-644-6226
                                                    TTY: 866-464-3615
                                                    e-mail: nccih-info@mail.nih.gov
                                                    nccih.nih.gov
The National Center for Complementary and Integrative Health (NCCIH) is the Federal Government's lead agency for scientific research on the diverse medical and health care systems, practices, and products that are not generally considered part of conventional medicine.
Josephine P. Briggs, M.D., Director
David Shurtleff, Ph.D., Deputy Director

7149 National Human Genome Research Institute
Building 31, Room 4B09   301-402-0911
Bethesda, MD 20892   Fax: 301-402-2218
                                                    www.genome.gov
The National Human Genome Research Institute began as the National Center for Human Genome Research (NCHGR), which was established in 1989 to carry out the role of the National Institutes

of Health (NIH) in the International Human Genome Project (HGP).
Eric D. Green, M.D., Ph.D., Director
Lawrence Brody, Ph.D., Director, Division of Genomics & Society

7150 National Institute of General Medical Sciences
45 Center Drive MSC 6200   301-496-7301
Bethesda, MD 20892   e-mail: info@nigms.nih.gov
                                                    www.nigms.nih.gov
The National Institute of General Medical Sciences (NIGMS) supports basic research that increases understanding of biological processes and lays the foundation for advances in disease diagnosis, treatment and prevention.
Jon R. Lorsch, Ph.D., Director
Judith H. Greenberg, Ph.D., Deputy Director

North Carolina

7151 National Institute of Environmental Health Sciences
111 T.W. Alexander Drive   919-541-4580
Research Triangle Park, NC 27709 e-mail: carroll1@niehs.nih.gov
                                                    www.niehs.nih.gov
The mission of the NIEHS is to discover how the environment affects people in order to promote healthier lives.
Linda S. Birnbaum, Ph.D., Director
Richard Woychik, Ph.D., Deputy Director

Virginia

7152 National Science Foundation
4201 Wilson Blvd   703-292-5111
Arlington, VA 22230   TDD: 703-292-5090
                                                    e-mail: info@nsf.gov
                                                    www.nsf.gov
NSF is the only federal agency whose mission includes support for all fields of fundamental science and engineering, except for medical sciences.
France A. Córdova, Director
Richard O. Buckius, Chief Operating Officer

Libraries & Resource Centers

7153 Anxiety Resource Center
312 Grandville Ave.   616-356-1614
Grand Rapids, MI 49503 e-mail: director@anxietyresourcecenter.org
                                                    anxietyresourcecenter.org
The Anxiety Resource Center, Inc. of Grand Rapids, Michigan, was founded to educate the public and professional communities about anxiety disorders, including Obsessive-Compulsive Disorder and OCD Spectrum Disorders; to reduce the stigma associated with these illnesses; and to provide a place that offers support, hope and inspiration.

7154 Brain Injury Resource Center
P.O.BOX 84151   206-621-8558
Seattle, WA 98124   e-mail: brain@headinjury.com
                                                    www.headinjury.com
Providing wealth of information, creative solutions and leadership on issues related to brain injury since 1985.

7155 BrainLine.org
2775 South Quincy Street   703-998-2020
Arlington, VA 22206   e-mail: info@BrainLine.org
                                                    www.brainline.org
BrainLine is a national multimedia project offering information and resources about preventing, treating, and living with TBI.
Noel Gunther, Executive Director
Christian Lindstrom, Director, Learning Media

7156 Center for the Study of Traumatic Stress
4301 Jones Bridge Road
Bethesda, MD 20814   e-mail: cstsinfo@usuhs.mil
                                                    www.cstsonline.org
There sustained mission is to advance scientific and academic knowledge, interventions, educational resources and outreach to mitigate the impact of trauma from exposure to war, disasters, terrorism, community violence and public health threats.
Robert J. Ursano, MD, Director

7157 Gift From Within
16 Cobb Hill Rd.
Camden, ME 4843
207-236-8858
Fax: 207-236-2818
e-mail: JoyceB3955@aol.com
www.giftfromwithin.org
PTSD Resources for Survivors and Caregivers.

7158 Institute on Violence, Abuse and Trauma
10065 Old Grove Road
San Diego, CA 92131
858-527-1860
Fax: 858-527-1743
e-mail: ivat@alliant.edu
www.ivatcenters.org
The Institute on Violence, Abuse and Trauma (IVAT) is an international resource and training center at Alliant International University.
Robert Geffner, Ph.D., President
Sandi Capuano Morrison, M.A., Executive Director

7159 National Center for PTSD
802-296-6300
e-mail: ncptsd@va.gov
www.ptsd.va.gov
The National Center for PTSD is dedicated to research and education on trauma and PTSD.

7160 National Center for Victims of Crime
2000 M Street NW
Washington, DC 20036
202-467-8700
Fax: 202-467-8701
e-mail: webmaster@ncvc.org
www.victimsofcrime.org
The mission of the National Center for Victims of Crime is to forge a national commitment to help victims of crime rebuild their lives. They are dedicated to serving individuals, families, and communities harmed by crime.
Mai Fernandez, Executive Director
Jeffrey R. Dion, Deputy Executive Director

7161 National Headache Foundation
820 N. Orleans
Chicago, IL 60610
312-274-2650
e-mail: info@headaches.org
www.headaches.org
The mission at the National Headache Foundation has been to further awareness of headache and migraine as legitimate neurobiological diseases.
Arthur H. Elkind, M.D., President
Vincent Martin, M.D., Vice President

7162 National Sexual Violence Resource Center
123 North Enola Drive
Enola, PA 17025
717-909-0710
877-739-3895
Fax: 717-909-0714
TTY: 717-909-0715
e-mail: resources@nsvrc.org
www.nsvrc.org
The NSVRC's Mission is to provide leadership in preventing and responding to sexual violence through collaboration, sharing and creating resources, and promoting research.

7163 Posttraumatic Stress Disorder (PTSD) Alliance
www.ptsdalliance.org
The Posttraumatic Stress Disorder (PTSD) Alliance is a group of professional and advocacy organizations that have joined forces to provide educational resources to individuals diagnosed with PTSD and their loved ones; those at risk for developing PTSD; and medical, healthcare and other frontline professionals.

7164 RNtoBSN.org
1001 McKinney St.
Houston, TX 77002
505-221-6056
e-mail: contact@rntobsn.org
www.rntobsn.org
RNtoBSN.org's mission is plain: Further the education of new and established nurses.
Caroline Porter Thomas, BSN, RN, Expert

7165 Sidran Institute
PO Box 436
Brooklandville, MD 21022
410-825-8888
Fax: 410-560-0134
e-mail: help@sidran.org
www.sidran.org
Sidran (SID-run) began in 1986 out of a family tragedy when a beloved family member who had been abused in childhood was subsequently diagnosed with serious, debilitating psychiatric problems and a related life-threatening medical disorder.
Esther Giller, President/ Director
Tracy Howard, Book Sales/ Office Manager

7166 Suicide Prevention Resource Center
43 Foundry Avenue
Waltham, MA 2453
877-438-7772
Fax: 617-969-9186
TTY: 617-964-5448
e-mail: info@sprc.org
www.sprc.org
SPRC is the nation's only federally supported resource center devoted to advancing the National Strategy for Suicide Prevention.
Jerry Reed, PhD, MSW, Director
Chris Miara, MS, Director of Operations & Resources

7167 Trauma Center
1269 Beacon Street
Brookline, MA 2446
617-232-1303
Fax: 617-232-1280
www.traumacenter.org
The Trauma Center is a program of Justice Resource Institute (JRI), a large nonprofit organization dedicated to social justice by offering hope and promise of fulfillment to children, adults, and families who are at risk of not receiving effective services essential to their safety, progress, and/or survival.
Dr. Bessel van der Kolk, Founder
Margaret Blaustein, Ph.D, Director of Training and Education

7168 Women's Resource Center
113 W. Wayne Avenue
Wayne, PA 19087
610-687-6391
Fax: 610-687-2967
e-mail: info@womensrc.org
womensresourcecenter.net
Women's Resource Center (WRC) is a registered 501c3 nonprofit that supports women, strengthens families and builds communities through information, referral, counseling, legal, and educational services.
Shelley Potente, MA, President
Virginia Bowden, Vice President

Research Centers

7169 ChildTrauma Academy
866-943-9779
Fax: 713-513-5465
e-mail: cta@childtrauma.org
childtrauma.org
CTA is a not-for-profit organization based in Houston, Texas working to improve the lives of high-risk children through direct service, research and education.
Bruce D. Perry, M.D., Ph.D., Founder/ Senior Fellow
Jana Rosenfelt, M.Ed., Executive Director

7170 National Center for PTSD
802-296-6300
e-mail: ncptsd@va.gov
www.ptsd.va.gov
The National Center for PTSD is dedicated to research and education on trauma and PTSD.

Arizona

7171 Mayo Clinic
13400 E. Shea Blvd.
Scottsdale, AZ 85259
480-301-8000
800-446-2279
www.mayoclinic.org
Mayo Clinic is a not-for-profit organization and proceeds from Web advertising help support our mission. Mayo Clinic does not endorse any of the third party products and services advertised.
Sandhya Pruthi, M.D., Medical Director
Kenneth G. Berge, M.D., Senior Medical Editor

California

7172 Synergy Clinical Research Center
1908 Sweetwater Road
National City, CA 91950
888-539-0282
Fax: 619-327-0163
www.synergyresearchcenters.com
Synergy is dedicated to providing comprehensive and exemplary clinical research services to advance the science of medicine.
Dr. Bari , Medical Director, Principal Investigator
Dr. Ishaque , Medical Director, Principal Investigator

7173 The Center for Culture, Trauma and Mental Health Disparities
760 Westwood Plaza
Los Angeles, CA 90024
310-794-9929
www.semel.ucla.edu/cctmhd
The Center for Culture, Trauma, and Mental Health Disparities is a multi-ethnic and multi-disciplinary group promoting interdisciplinary research examining the prevalence and impact of traumatic experiences on PTSD, depression and concomitant cognitive/emotional, behavioral, psychological and biological processes in ethnic minority populations.
Gail Wyatt, Director

7174 UCLA Anxiety Disorders Research Center
Department of Psychology
Los Angeles, CA 90094
310-825-9312
e-mail: rose@psych.ucla.edu
anxiety.psych.ucla.edu
The purpose of The ADRC is to further our understanding of the factors that place individuals at risk for developing phobias, anxiety disorders and related conditions, and to develop more effective treatments that have long lasting effects and are cost effective.
Michelle G. Craske, Ph.D., Director
Raphael Rose, Ph.D., Associate Director

Connecticut

7175 Yale Child Study Center
230 South Frontage Rd.
New Haven, CT 6519
203-785-2540
childstudycenter.yale.edu
At our core is the mission to improve the lives of children and families through research, service, and training.
Dr. Linda Mayes, Interim Director

District of Columbia

7176 Center for Mind-Body Medicine
5225 Connecticut Avenue
Washington, DC 20015
202-966-7338
cmbm.org
The Center for Mind-Body Medicine creates communities of hope and healing.
James S. Gordon, MD, President
James S. Gordon, MD, Founder/ Director

Florida

7177 Center for the Study of Emotion and Attention
University of Florida
Gainesville, FL 32611
Fax: 352-392-6047
csea.phhp.ufl.edu
The Center for the Study of Emotion & Attention is a facility for the scientific study of human emotion, highlighting emotion's foundation on survival circuits in the mammalian brain, and its motivational significance for attentional engagement and response mobilization.

Georgia

7178 Mood and Anxiety Disorders Program of Emory University
12 Executive Park Dr., NE
Atlanta, GA 30329
404-778-6663
e-mail: studies@emoryclinicaltrials.com
www.psychiatry.emory.edu
The Mood and Anxiety Disorders Program of Emory Univeristy's School of Medicine is a dedicated research program within Emory's Department of Psychiatry and Behavioral Sciences.
Boadie Dunlop, M.D., Assistant Professor
Jeff Rakofsky, M.D., Associate Professor

Illinois

7179 International Society for Traumatic Stress Studies
111 Deer Lake Road
Deerfield, IL 60015
847-480-9028
Fax: 847-480-9282
e-mail: info@istss.org
www.istss.org
The International Society for Traumatic Stress Studies is dedicated to sharing information about the effects of trauma and the discovery and dissemination of knowledge about policy, program and service initiatives that seek to reduce traumatic stressors and their immediate and long-term consequences.
Miranda Olff, PhD, President
Julian Ford, PhD, Vice President

Indiana

7180 GoldPoint Clinical Research
8902 North Meridian Strt.
Indianapolis, IN 46260
317-229-6202
Fax: 317-218-3347
goldpointcr.com
GoldPoint Clinical Research of Indianapolis' team has 20 years of experience conducting more than 250 Phase II, III & IV neuroscience clinical trials. As one of the Midwest's leading research study centers, GoldPoint is led by medical director and board-certified addiction psychiatrist, Richard Saini, MD. - See more at: http://goldpointcr.com/about-us/leadership/#sthash.oaNpLa69.dpuf
Mary Newkerk, Director of Operations

Maryland

7181 Center for the Study of Traumatic Stress
Uniformed Services Uni.
Bethesda, MD 20814
e-mail: cstsinfo@usuhs.mil
www.cstsonline.org
Robert J. Ursano, MD, Director

7182 National Institute of Mental Health
6001 Executive Boulevard
Rockville, MD 20852
301-443-4536
Fax: 301-443-4279
e-mail: NIMHinfo@mail.nih.gov
www.nimh.nih.gov
The mission of NIMH is to transform the understanding and treatment of mental illnesses through basic and clinical research, paving the way for prevention, recovery, and cure.

Massachusetts

7183 Center for Anxiety and Related Disorders at Boston University
648 Beacon St.
Boston, MA 2215
617-353-9610
e-mail: bonnieb@bu.edu
www.bu.edu/card
The Center for Anxiety and Related Disorders (CARD) is an internationally known clinical and research center dedicated to advancing knowledge and providing care for anxiety, mood, eating, sleep, and related disorders.
David H. Barlow, Ph.D., Founder and Director Emeritus
Timothy A. Brown, Psy.D., Director of Research and Research Admin

7184 Trauma Center
1269 Beacon Street
Brookline, MA 2446
617-232-1303
Fax: 617-232-1280
www.traumacenter.org
The Trauma Center is a program of Justice Resource Institute (JRI), a large nonprofit organization dedicated to social justice by offering hope and promise of fulfillment to children, adults, and families who are at risk of not receiving effective services essential to their safety, progress, and/or survival.
Dr. Bessel van der Kolk, Founder
Margaret Blaustein, Ph.D, Director of Training and Education

New York

7185 The Dana Foundation
505 Fifth Avenue
New York, NY 10017
212-223-4040
Fax: 212-317-8721
e-mail: danainfo@dana.org
www.dana.org

The Dana Foundation is a private philanthropic organization that supports brain research through grants, publications, and educational programs.
Edward F. Rover, Chairman/ President
Burton M. Mirsky, EVP, Finance

Virginia

7186 Samueli Institute
1737 King Street
Alexandria, VA 22314
703-299-4800
Fax: 703-535-6752
e-mail: communications@siib.org
www.samueliinstitute.org
Samueli Institute is advancing the science of healing worldwide by applying academic rigor to research on healing, well-being and re-silience; translating evidence into action for the U.S. Military and large-scale health systems; and fostering wellness through self-care to create a flourishing society.
Susan Samueli, PhD, Co-Founder
Wayne B. Jonas, MD, President/ CEO

Washington

7187 Center for Anxiety and Traumatic Stress
Guthrie Annex 2
Seattle, WA
206-685-3617
faculty.washington.edu/zoellner/
Lori A. Zoellner, PhD, Director
Richard Ries, MD, Medical Director

Wisconsin

7188 Injury Research Center
8701 Watertown Plank Rd.
Milwaukee, WI 53226
414-955-7670
Fax: 414-955-6470
e-mail: irc@mcw.edu
www.mcw.edu
The Injury Research Center (IRCInjury Research Center at the Medical College of Wisconsin) at the Medical College was established as a comprehensive federally funded injury control research center to address the burden of injury in the Great Lakes Region of the Midwest (WI, MN, IL, IN, MI and OH).
Stephen Hargarten, MD, MPH, Director
E. Brook Lerner, PhD, Deputy Director

Support Groups & Hotlines

7189 American Self-Help Group Clearinghouse
e-mail: admin@selfhelpgroups.org
www.selfhelpgroups.org
American Self-Help Group Clearinghouse has a keyword-search-able database of over 1,100 national, international, model and on-line self-help support groups for addictions, bereavement, health, mental health, disabilities, abuse, parenting, caregiver concerns and many other stressful life situations.

7190 COPLINE
501 Iron Bridge Rd.
Freehold, NJ 7728
800-267-5463
e-mail: Copline@optonline.net
www.copline.org
Copline is the first national law enforcement officers hotline in the country that is manned by retired law enforcement officers. Re-tired law enforcement officers are trained in active listening and bring the knowledge and understanding of the many psychosocial stre
Stephanie Samuels, M.A., MSW, LCSW, President/ Creator/ Founder
Dennis Cronin, Vice President

7191 Child Help
4350 E. Camelback Road
Phoenix, AZ 85018
480-922-8212
800-422-4453
www.childhelp.org

Michael Medoro, Child Development Officer
Jon Taylor, Chief Financial Officer

7192 Crime Survivors
PO Box 54552
Irvine, CA 92619
949-872-7895
844-853-4673
e-mail: crimesurvivors@aol.com
www.crimesurvivors.org
Crime Survivors vision is for victims of crime to recover from their experience mentally, physically, emotionally, and financially, by receiving the respect, support, and protection from law enforce-ment, the judicial system, and the community.
Patricia Wenskunas, Founder / CEO
Janet Wilson Irving, Chairperson

7193 Heal My PTSD with Michele Rosenthal
healmyptsd.com
Offers information anyone would need to discover what there is to know about symptoms of PTSD, treatment options and the path to feeling better.
Michele Rosenthal, Founder

7194 MDJunction
800-273-8255
www.mdjunction.com
MDJunction is a meeting place for people who deal with health challenges, a comfort zone to help and get help by people who are in your spot.

7195 Mental Health America
2000 N. Beauregard Street
Alexandria, VA 22311
703-684-7722
800-969-6642
Fax: 703-684-5968
www.mentalhealthamerica.net
Mental Health America (MHA) - founded in 1909 - is the nation's leading community-based non-profit dedicated to helping all Americans achieve wellness by living mentally healthier lives.
Paul Gionfriddo, President/ CEO
Nathaniel Counts, Senior Policy Associate

7196 Out of the Storm
cptsd.org
Out of the Storm is a discussion group and resource site for those whose lives have been affected by Complex Post Traumatic Disor-der (CPTSD).

7197 PTSD Family Support Group
2133 Upton Drive
Virginia Beach, VA 23454
757-222-2247
e-mail: info@love4vets.org
love4vets.org
Love4Vets will ambitiously, humbly, and respectfully aim to be-come a proactive organization throughout the nation that military veterans will have as a first choice for empowerment and support.
April Krowel, Chairman
Ela Kelly, Founder/ CEO

7198 PTSD Hotline
800-273-8255
e-mail: Info@PTSDHotline.Com
www.ptsdhotline.com/index.html
This Website deals primarily with PTSD as it relates to Veterans.

7199 PTSDanonymous.org
e-mail: ptsda@comcast.net
www.ptsdanonymous.org
A nationwide network of community based, non-clinical, veteran lead support group meetings for those suffering from military trauma and seeking the fellowship of their peers.

7200 Pandora's Aquarium
www.pandys.org
A rape, sexual assault, and sexual abuse survivor message board and chat room.

7201 Panic Survivor
www.panicsurvivor.com
A community to sove anxiety disorder problem.

7202 Rape, Abuse & Incest National Network
1220 L Street, NW   202-544-3064
Washington, DC 20005   Fax: 202-544-3556
e-mail: info@rainn.org
rainn.org
RAINN (Rape, Abuse & Incest National Network) is the nation's largest anti-sexual violence organization and was named one of America's 100 Best Charities by Worth magazine.
Scott Berkowitz, President/ Founder
Regan Burke, Chairperson

7203 Recovery International
105 W. Adams St.   312-337-5661
Chicago, IL 60603   866-221-0302
Fax: 312-726-4446
e-mail: Christine@recoveryinternational.org
www.recoveryinternational.org
Recovery International offers meetings to men and women of all ages that ease the suffering from mental health issues by gaining skills to lead more peaceful and productive lives. In the last 76 years RI has equipped over 1 million people with tools to control behavior and change attitudes.
Christine Lewis, Executive Director
Caitlin Fahey, Project Coordinator

7204 Suicide.org

800-784-2433
e-mail: Kevin@Suicide.org
www.suicide.org
If you are suicidal, have attempted suicide, or are a suicide survivor, you will find help, hope, comfort, understanding, support, love, and extensive resources here.
Kevin Caruso, Founder
Adam Sutherland, Vice President

7205 Support4Hope
PO Box 184
Deer Lodge, TN 37726   e-mail: Admin@Support4hope.com
www.support4hope.com
Support4Hope is dedicated to support of various mental health issues such as Bipolar Disorder, Depression, Anxiety Disorders, Schizophrenia, Post Traumatic Stress Disorder (PTSD) and the problems that arise from them along with other problems such as Domestic Abuse.

7206 United States 211 Information and Referral Systems
www.211.org
Helps connect to a community resource specialist in an area to get in touch with local organizations that provide critical services.

7207 Veterans Crisis Line

800-273-8255
www.veteranscrisisline.net
The Veterans Crisis Line connects Veterans in crisis and their families and friends with qualified, caring Department of Veterans Affairs responders through a confidential toll-free hotline, online chat, or text.

7208 Vetwives Living With PTSD
livingwithptsd.yuku.com
Forum for people suffering with PTSD.

Books

7209 A Practical Guide to PTSD Treatment: Pharmacological & Psychotheraputic Approach
750 First St. NE   202-336-5500
Washington, DC 20002   800-374-2721
TTY: 202-336-6123
TDD: 202-336-6123
www.apa.org
The book is suitable for psychologists and social workers who may be unfamiliar with pharmacological approaches to PTSD, as well as psychiatrists and other medical personnel who may be less familiar with the best empirically-validated forms of psychotherapy.
Matthew J. Friedman, MD, PhD, Editor
Nancy C. Bernardy, PhD, Editor

7210 Caring for Veterans With Deployment-Related Stress Disorders
750 First St. NE   202-336-5500
Washington, DC 20002   800-374-2721
TTY: 202-336-6123
TDD: 202-336-6123
www.apa.org
Caring for Veterans With Deployment-Related Stress Disorders explores the myriad causes and consequences of these peculiar war-zone disorders, yet its emphasis is on prevention and treatment through better assessment, psychopharmacological and psychotherapeutic interventions (including couple/family therapy), and appropriate evidence-based treatments.
Matthew J. Friedman, MD, PhD, Editor
Jennifer J. Vasterling, PhD, Editor

7211 EMDR as an Integrative Psychotherapy Approach
750 First St. NE   202-336-5500
Washington, DC 20002   800-374-2721
TTY: 202-336-6123
TDD: 202-336-6123
www.apa.org
In EMDR as an Integrative Psychotherapy Approach, EMDR originator Francine Shapiro explores the latest developments and theoretical perspectives on, and clinical implications of, this complex psychotherapy approach originally developed to treat posttraumatic stress disorder.
Francine Shapiro, PhD, Editor

7212 Ethnocultural Aspects of Post-traumatic Stress Disorder: Issues, Research, Clinical Applications
750 First St. NE   202-336-5500
Washington, DC 20002   800-374-2721
TTY: 202-336-6123
TDD: 202-336-6123
www.apa.org
This richly documented, edited volume is the first systematic examination of ethnocultural aspects of PTSD. Leaders in the field of PTSD research and practice explore both universal and culture-specific reactions to trauma, and discusses implications for research, treatment, and prevention.
Raymond M. Scurfield, Editor
Ellen T. Gerrity, Editor

7213 Hope for Recovery: Understanding Post-traumatic Stress Disorder
www.ptsdalliance.org
In clear and sympathetic language, Hope for Recovery seeks to dispel the myths about PTSD that keep many people from recognizing the problem and obtaining help.

7214 Personality-Guided Therapy for Post-traumatic Stress Disorder
750 First St. NE   202-336-5500
Washington, DC 20002   800-374-2721
TTY: 202-336-6123
TDD: 202-336-6123
www.apa.org
In Personality-Guided Therapy for Posttraumatic Stress Disorder, George S. Everly, Jr. and Jeffrey M. Lating shed light on the role personality factors play in the genesis and treatment of posttraumatic stress disorder (PTSD).
Jeffrey M. Lating, PhD, Editor
George S. Everly, Jr., PhD, Editor

7215 Psychological Assessment Of Adult Post Traumatic States: Phenomenolgy, Diagnosis & Measurement
750 First St. NE   202-336-5500
Washington, DC 20002   800-374-2721
TTY: 202-336-6123
TDD: 202-336-6123
www.apa.org
This book is the second edition of the well-known Psychological Assessment of Adult Posttraumatic States, published in 1997. A major update from the first edition, it presents a detailed, yet practical summary of the major issues and instruments involved in the assessment of posttraumatic disturbance.
John Briere, PhD, Editor

7216   Psychology in the Service of National Security
750 First St. NE
Washington, DC 20002
202-336-5500
800-374-2721
TTY: 202-336-6123
TDD: 202-336-6123
www.apa.org
This volume highlights the diverse contributions of military psychologists toward U.S. security and toward the discipline of psychology itself.
A. David Mangelsdorff, PhD, Author

7217   Taking Control of Anxiety: Small Steps for Getting The Best Of Worry,Stress&Fear
750 First St. NE
Washington, DC 20002
202-336-5500
800-374-2721
TTY: 202-336-6123
TDD: 202-336-6123
www.apa.org
This straightforward guide, filled with compelling case examples and easy to use techniques, will teach you to identify, reduce, eliminate, and prevent the negative effects of anxiety.
Bret A. Moore, PsyD, Author

7218   Trauma Services for Women in Substance Abuse Treatment: An Integrated Approach
750 First St. NE
Washington, DC 20002
202-336-5500
800-374-2721
TTY: 202-336-6123
TDD: 202-336-6123
www.apa.org
This book is a hands-on guide for clinicians seeking to treat women who suffer from both a history of trauma and the effects of substance abuse.
Aimee Campbell, MSSW, Author
Gloria M. Miele, PhD, Author

7219   Trauma & Health:Physical Health Consequences of Exposure To Extreme Stress
750 First St. NE
Washington, DC 20002
202-336-5500
800-374-2721
TTY: 202-336-6123
TDD: 202-336-6123
www.apa.org
This volume provides a comprehensive summary of existing literature and a refreshing look at current empirical work. It will stimulate research and support clinical practice by providing clinicians with solid information that can inform their work with patients. Trauma and Health clearly shows that poor physical health should be recognized, along with poor mental health as an outcome of traumatic exposure.
Bonnie L. Green, PhD, Editor
Paula P. Schnurr, PhD, Editor

7220   Trauma & Substance Abuse: Causes, Consequences and Treatment of Comorbid Disorders
750 First St. NE
Washington, DC 20002
202-336-5500
800-374-2721
TTY: 202-336-6123
TDD: 202-336-6123
www.apa.org
Trauma and Substance Abuse: Causes, Consequences, and Treatment of Comorbid Disorders, Second Edition offers a broad overview of current trends in the field of co-occurring substance abuse and PTSD from both clinical and research perspectives.
Jennifer P. Read, PhD, Editor
Paige Ouimette, PhD, Editor

7221   Treating PTSD With Cognitive-Behavioral Therapies: Interventions That Work
750 First St. NE
Washington, DC 20002
202-336-5500
800-374-2721
TTY: 202-336-6123
TDD: 202-336-6123
www.apa.org
Explaining each approach's theoretical underpinnings as well as its step-by-step implementation, the authors cover both trauma-focused techniques such as prolonged exposure, cognitive processing therapy, and stress inoculation training, and non-trauma-focused or present-centered techniques such as breathing training, relaxation training, and positive self-talk. The

book also addresses depression and social isolation, symptoms that often accompany PTSD.
Philippe Shnaider, Author
Candice M. Monson, PhD, Author

7222   Wheels Down: Adjusting to Life After Deployment
750 First St. NE
Washington, DC 20002
202-336-5500
800-374-2721
TTY: 202-336-6123
TDD: 202-336-6123
www.apa.org
This book, written by military psychologists Moore and Kennedy, is a down-to-earth guide that's full of practical advice. The authors talk straight about both the joys and challenges of returning home, advising that one size does NOT fit all when it comes to making the transition. They share thoughtful, constructive tips for dealing with unwanted surprises like relationship break-ups, financial problems, and kids who are suddenly strangers.
Carrie H. Kennedy, PhD, ABPP, Author
Bret A. Moore, PsyD, ABPP, Author

7223   Why Are You So Scared? A Child's Book About Parents With PTSD
750 First St. NE
Washington, DC 20002
202-336-5500
800-374-2721
TTY: 202-336-6123
TDD: 202-336-6123
www.apa.org
When a parent has PTSD, children can often feel confused, scared, or helpless. Why Are You So Scared? explains PTSD and its symptoms in nonthreatening, kid-friendly language, and is full of questions and exercises that kids and parents can work through together.
Beth Andrews, LCSW, Author

7224   Your Life After Trauma
500 Fifth Avenue
New York, NY 10110
212-354-5500
Fax: 212-869-0856
books.wwnorton.com
In this book, the author applies her personal experience and professional wisdom to offer readers an invaluable roadmap to overcoming their own trauma, in particular the loss of sense of self that often accompanies it.
Michele Rosenthal, Author

Newsletters

7225   PTSD Research Quarterly
802-296-6300
e-mail: ncptsd@va.gov
www.ptsd.va.gov
Each RQ contains a review article written by guest experts on a specific topic related to PTSD.

7226   The Post-Traumatic Gazette
P.O. Box 2757
High Springs, FL 32655
352-215-9251
www.patiencepress.com
Offers new perspectives, new ideas, new treatments, new resources and encourage people to find what works for people suffering with PTSD.

7227   The Post-Traumatic Stress Disorder Relationship
800-289-0963
e-mail: DrDianeEngland@PTSDRelationship.com
www.ptsdrelationship.com

Pamphlets

7228   PTSD: A Guide for the Frontline
www.ptsdalliance.org
This free, 20-page booklet is designed as a primer for "frontline" professionals who interact with trauma survivors and people suffering from Posttraumatic Stress Disorder.

Web Sites

7229 Aces Too High

acestoohigh.com

ACESTooHigh is a news site that reports on research about adverse childhood experiences, including developments in epidemiology, neurobiology, and the biomedical and epigenetic consequences of toxic stress.

7230 AdvocateWeb
P.O. Box 240
Newton, MA 2468

www.advocateweb.org

AdvocateWeb is a nonprofit organization providing information and resources to promote awareness and understanding of the issues involved in the exploitation of persons by trusted helping professionals.
Stanley J. Spero, President/CEO/Director
Kevin Gourley, Founder

7231 AfterTheInjury.org

e-mail: aftertheinjury@email.chop.edu
www.aftertheinjury.org

This website was developed by an interdisciplinary team of researchers and practitioners with expertise in pediatric injury, child health care, and traumatic stress.

7232 Athealth.com
7829 Center Blvd SE
Snoqualmie, WA 98065

425-292-0329
888-284-3258
Fax: 623-322-0498
e-mail: support@athealth.com
athealth.com

Athealth.com was founded in 1997 by a psychiatrist to provide mental health information and services for mental health professionals and those they serve.

7233 Bright Side, The

www.the-bright-side.org

The Bright Side was created as a means of support - whether you are dealing with depression, grief, suicide, mental illness, emotional crisis, or are just feeling overwhelmed with life, you are not alone!

7234 David Baldwin's Trauma Information Pages

www.trauma-pages.com

These Trauma Pages focus primarily on emotional trauma and traumatic stress, including PTSD (Post-traumatic Stress Disorder) and dissociation, whether following individual traumatic experience(s) or a large-scale disaster.

7235 Family of a Vet

e-mail: Info@FamilyofaVet.com
www.familyofavet.com

Family Of a Vet was started by the proud wife of an OIF Veteran who suffers from PTSD (Post Traumatic Stress Disorder) and TBI (Traumatic Brain Injury).

7236 Gift From Within
16 Cobb Hill Rd.
Camden, ME 4843

207-236-8858
Fax: 207-236-2818
e-mail: JoyceB3955@aol.com
www.giftfromwithin.org

PTSD Resources for Survivors and Caregivers.

7237 Healing From Complex Trauma & PTSD/CPTSD

www.healingfromcomplextraumaandptsd.com

Assists people in their healing from complex trauma journey.
Lilly Hope Lucario, Survivor/Author/Writer/Blogger

7238 Hope for Healing.Org

865-471-8366
hopeforhealing.org

7239 Make the Connection

800-273-8255
maketheconnection.net

Make the Connection is a public awareness campaign by the U.S. Department of Veterans Affairs (VA) that provides personal testimonials and resources to help Veterans discover ways to improve their lives.

7240 Mental Health Matters
19206 65th Pl NE
Kenmore, WA 98028

mental-health-matters.com

MHMatters was founded to supply information and resources to mental health consumers, professionals, students and supporters.

7241 Mental Health Today

mental-health-today.com

The purpose of Mental Health Today is to help stop the pain caused by mental health disorders.
Patty Fleener M.S.W., Owner/ Operator

7242 MentalHelp.net

800-273-TALK
www.mentalhelp.net

They provide online mental health and wellness education.

7243 MyPTSD

www.myptsd.com

PTSD Forum launched on the 06th Sep, 2005, with one simple aim, to provide quality PTSD information and support to all concerned.

7244 PTSD Support Services

888-335-8699
www.ptsdsupport.net

7245 PTSDinfo.org

www.ptsdinfo.org

7246 Psychguides.com

855-900-6733
www.psychguides.com

There goal is to shed light on psychological disorders, allowing you to recognize, understand and cope with these challenging diagnoses in yourself, friends and family members.

Description

7247 ## Prader-Willi Syndrome

Prader-Willi syndrome, PWS, is a group of abnormalities first described by Drs. Prader, Labart, and Willi in 1956. This uncommon condition occurs in about one in every 20,000 births. In about 50 percent of PWS patients, there is a missing piece (deletion) of part of chromosome 15.

PWS is characterized by obesity, short stature, small penis and testicles (hypogonadism), small hands and feet, mental retardation and decreased muscle tone. During the toddler years, many patients begin to overeat. Some persons with PWS may show signs of obsessive-compulsive disorder, apart from their obsessions with food. In addition to insatiable hunger, other behavioral features include emotional highs and lows, poor motor skills and cognitive impairment. Sexual development is halted, and facial and skeletal abnormalities develop.

Therapies for PWS are aimed at symptoms with an emphasis on specialized diets and customized exercise programs and support.

National Agencies & Associations

7248 **Foundation for Prader-Willi Research**

888-322-5487
Fax: 888-559-4105
e-mail: info@fpwr.org
www.fpwr.org

The mission of FPWR is to eliminate the challenges of Prader-Willi syndrome through the advancement of research.
Susan Hedstrom, Executive Director
Hannah Berger, Director of Development

7249 **National Institute of Child Health and Human Development**
9000 Rockville Pike
Bethesda, MD 20892
301-496-5133
Fax: 301-496-7101
www.nih.gov
Offers reprints, articles and various information on Prader-Willi Syndrome in children and adults.
Dr Francis Collin, Director

7250 **Prader-Willi Syndrome Association (USA)**
Prader-Willi Syndrome Association (USA)
17777 S. W. 285 Street
Homestead, FL 33030
305-245-6484
800-926-4797
Fax: 941-312-0142
e-mail: webmaster1@pwsausa.org
www.pwsausa.org

Provides to parents and professionals a national and international network of information, support services and research endeavors to expressly meet the needs of affected children and adults and their families. Offers 31 state chapters and published materials.
Janalee Heinemann, Executive Director

State Agencies & Associations

Arizona

7251 **Prader-Willi Syndrome Arizona Association: Phoenix Area**
Prader-Willi Syndrome Association
3920 East Bronco Trail
Phoenix, AZ 85044
602-481-5314
e-mail: shemc@netzero.net
www.pwsausa.org

Sheila McMahon, President

7252 **Prader-Willi Syndrome Arizona Association**
Prader-Willi Syndrome Association

13839 N Bentwater Drive
Tucson, AZ 85737
602-481-5314
e-mail: p.penta@comcast.net
www.pwsausa.org

Tammie Penta, President

Arkansas

7253 **Prader-Willi Arkansas Association Prader-Willi Syndrome Association**
Prader-Willi Syndrome Association
107 Jessica Drive
Sherwood, AR 72120-4245
501-920-6768
e-mail: jpattpnlr@msn.com
www.pwsausa.org

Jim Patton, President

California

7254 **Prader-Willi California Foundation**
514 N Prospect Avenue
Redondo Beach, CA 90277
310-372-5053
800-400-9994
Fax: 310-372-4329
e-mail: PWCF1@aol.com
www.pwsausa.org

Lisa Graziano, Executive Director

Colorado

7255 **Prader-Willi Colorado Association**
Prader-Willi Syndrome Association
8290 S Yukon Way
Littleton, CO 80128
303-973-4780
e-mail: hosler@dynamicsolutions.com
www.pwsausa.org

Lynette Hosler, President

Connecticut

7256 **Prader-Willi Connecticut Association**
Prader-Willi Syndrome Association
129 Way Road
Salem, CT 06420-3306
203-239-9902
e-mail: pwsactchapter@yahoo.com
www.pwsausa.org

Vicki Knoph, President

Delaware

7257 **Prader-Willi Delaware Association**
Prader-Willi Syndrome Association
300 Bethel Circle Millwood
Middletown, DE 19709
302-378-7385
e-mail: swede455@aol.com
www.pwsausa.org

Karen Swanson, President

Florida

7258 **Prader-Willi Florida Association**
Prader-Willi Syndrome Association
17777 S W 285 Street
Homestead, FL 33030
305-245-6484
e-mail: pwfa2000@aol.com
www.pwsausa.org

Debbie Stallings, Co-President
John Stallings, Co-President

Georgia

7259 **Prader-Willi Georgia Association**
Prader-Willi Syndrome Association
562 Lakeland Plaza
Cumming, GA 30040
770-886-2334
877-866-2334
Fax: 770-886-2335
e-mail: pwsaga@earthlink.net
www.pwsausa.org

Debbie Lang, Executive Director
Greg Talley, President

Hawaii

7260 **Prader-Willi Hawaii Association**
Prader-Willi Syndrome Association

269 Kaha Street
Hailua, HI 96734

808-263-8177
e-mail: susanlundh@yahoo.com
www.pwsausa.org

Susan Lundh, President

Idaho

7261 Prader-Willi Idaho Association
Prader-Willi Syndrome Association
550 Lodgepole Road
Athol, ID 83801

208-683-2993
e-mail: idaho4ts@aol.com
www.pwsausa.org

Susan Lundh, President
Gene Todhunter, Local Contact

Illinois

7262 Prader-Willi Illinois Association
Prader-Willi Syndrome Association
2128 N Sedgwick Street
Chicago, IL 60614

773-281-9170
e-mail: illinois@pwsausa.org
www.pwsausa.org

Jeffrey Fender, President

Indiana

7263 Prader-Willi Indiana Association
Prader-Willi Syndrome Association
7536 Moonbeam Drive
Indianapolis, IN 46259

317-527-9173
e-mail: pwsain@yahoo.com
www.pwsausa.org

Jacque McGuire, President

Iowa

7264 Prader-Willi Iowa Association
Prader-Willi Syndrome Association
15130 Holcomb Avenue
Clive, IA 50325-9695

515-987-0288
e-mail: ktcaedav@netins.net
www.pwsausa.org

Tammi Davis, President
Edie Bogaczyk, President

Kentucky

7265 Prader-Willi Kentucky Association
Prader-Willi Syndrome Association
9213 Reigate Court
Louisville, KY 40222

502-339-7872
e-mail: national@pwsausa.org
www.pwsausa.org

Frank Beckles, President
Rick Settles

Massachusetts

7266 Prader-Willi New England Association
Prader-Willi Syndrome Association
Andover, MA 01757

978-475-5570
e-mail: pwsane@aol.com
www.pwsausa.org

Eileen Rullo, President

Michigan

7267 Prader-Willi Michigan Association
2155 Ascot Rd
Ann Arbor, MI 48103

734-998-3507
e-mail: chrishendrick@cablespeed.com
www.pwsausa.org

Jon Hendrick, Co-Chairperson
Chris Hendrick, Co-Chairperson

Minnesota

7268 Prader-Willi Minnesota Association
Prader-Willi Syndrome Association
7209 Oaklawn Avenue
Woodbury, MN 55105

952-893-9318
e-mail: national@pwsausa.org
www.pwsausa.org

Jey Behnken, President

Missouri

7269 Prader-Willi Missouri Association
Prader-Willi Syndrome Association
1465 S Grand Boulevard Missouri Str
Louis, MO 63104

314-268-4027
Fax: 314-935-7461
e-mail: national@pwsausa.org
www.pwsausa.org

Barbara Whitman, President

Nebraska

7270 Prader-Willi Nebraska Association
Prader-Willi Syndrome Association
302 S 49th Avenue
Omaha, NE 68132

402-551-9168
e-mail: national@pwsausa.org
www.pwsausa.org

Jennifer Varner, Local Contact

New Jersey

7271 Prader-Willi New Jersey Association
Prader-Willi Syndrome Association
514 Gatewod Road
Cherry Hill, NJ 08003

856-795-4229
e-mail: national@pwsausa.org
www.pwsausa.org

Sybil Cohen, President
Judy Livny, Vice-President

New York

7272 Prader-Willi New York Association
Prader-Willi Syndrome Association
PO Box 1114
Niagara Falls, NY 14304

716-276-2211
800-442-1655
e-mail: alliance@prader-willi.org
www.prader-willi.org

Nina Roberto, Executive Director
Amy McDougall, President

North Carolina

7273 Prader-Willi North Carolina Association
Prader-Willi Syndrome Association
1404 Sutton Drive
Kinston, NC 28501

252-527-1813
e-mail: national@pwsausa.org
www.pwsausa.org

Becky Smith, President

North Dakota

7274 Prader-Willi North Dakota Association
Prader-Willi Syndrome Association
2902 S University Drive
Fargo, ND 58103-6032

701-232-3301
Fax: 701-237-5775
e-mail: fraser@fraserltd.org
www.fraserltd.org

Sandra leyland, Executive Director
Michael Kirk, Vice President

Ohio

7275 Prader-Willi Ohio Association
Prader-Willi Syndrome Association
4075 W 226 Street
Fairview Park, OH 44126

440-716-0552
e-mail: pwsaohio@aol.com
www.pwsausa.org

Jennifer Bolander, President

Oklahoma

7276 Prader-Willi Oklahoma Association
Prader-Willi Syndrome Association
3816 SE 89th Street
Oklahoma City, OK 74135-6222

405-677-8089
e-mail: national@pwsausa.org
www.pwsausa.org

Daphne Mosley, President

Oregon

7277 Prader-Willi Oregon Association
Prader-Willi Syndrome Association
303 E Historic Columbia   503-669-7191
Troutdale, OR 97060   e-mail: national@pwsausa.org
                                             www.pwsausa.org

Lennae Elkington, President

Pennsylvania

7278 Prader-Willi Pennsylvania Association
Prader-Willi Syndrome Association
104 Persimmon Place   724-779-4415
Cranberry Township, PA 16066   e-mail: national@pwsausa.org
                                             www.pwsausa.org

Debbie Fabio, President

South Carolina

7279 Prader-Willi South Carolina Association
Prader-Willi Syndrome Association
912 Lake Spur Lane   803-345-1379
Chapin, SC 29036   e-mail: national@pwsausa.org
                                             www.pwsausa.org

Rhett Eleazer, Local Contact

Tennessee

7280 Prader-Willi Tennessee Association
Prader-Willi Syndrome Association
1200 Villa Place   615-790-6659
Nashville, TN 37212   e-mail: national@pwsausa.org
                                             www.pwsausa.org

Misti Love, President

Texas

7281 Prader-Willi Texas Association
Prader-Willi Syndrome Association
14427 Perchin Drive   210-946-6789
San Antonio, TX 78247   e-mail: national@pwsausa.org
                                             www.pwsausa.org

Amber Robenson, President

Utah

7282 Prader-Willi Utah Association
Prader-Willi Syndrome Association
2652 Nottingham Way   801-582-0998
Salt Lake City, UT 84108   Fax: 801-768-3924
                                e-mail: national@pwsausa.org
                                             www.pwsausa.org

Lisa Thornton, President

Washington

7283 Prader-Willi Washington Association
Prader-Willi Syndrome Association
16208 SE 46th Place   206-285-7679
Bellevue, WA 98006   e-mail: jlubderwood@juno.com
                                             www.pwsausa.org

Joanne Underwood, Co-President
Susan Lundh, Co-President

Wisconsin

7284 Prader-Willi Wisconsin Association
Prader-Willi Syndrome Association
2701 N Alexander Street   920-882-6371
Appleton, WI 54911-2512   866-797-2947
                              e-mail: wisconsion@pwsausa.org
                                             www.pwsausa.org

Mary Lynn Larson, Program Director
Mike Larson, President

Support Groups & Hotlines

7285 National Health Information Center
PO Box 1133   310-565-4167
Washington, DC 20013   800-336-4797
                                        Fax: 301-984-4256
                                   e-mail: info@nhic.org
                                       www.health.gov/nhic

Offers a nationwide information referral service, produces directories and resource guides.

7286 PraderWilli Syndrome Association
PraderWilli Syndrome Association
5700 Midnight Pass Road   941-312-0400
Sarasota, FL 34242   800-926-4797
                                        Fax: 941-312-0142
                               e-mail: pwsuasa@aol.com
                                             www.pwsausa.org

John Heybatch, Co-Chair
Julie Doherty, Secretary

Books

7287 Child with Prader-Willi Syndrome: Birth to Three
Prader-Willi Syndrome Association (USA)
8588 Potter Park Drive   941-312-0400
Sarasota, FL 34238   800-926-4797
                                        Fax: 941-312-0142
                                e-mail: info@pwsausa.org
                                             www.pwsausa.org

Discusses the common concerns of the first three years and offers specific recommendations for early intervention strategies. A helpful and positive resource for families, physicians, early intervention workers and other care providers. Booklet
2004 34 pages
Craig Pulhemus, Executive Director

7288 Early Years
Prader-Willi Syndrome Association (USA)
8588 Potter Park Drive   941-312-0400
Sarasota, FL 34238   800-926-4797
                                        Fax: 941-312-0142
                                e-mail: info@pwsausa.com
                                             www.pwsausa.org

Collection of articles regarding young children with PWS — many from a parent's perspective.
1998 37 pages
Craig Polhemus, Executive Director

7289 Growing Up with Prader-Willi Syndrome: Personal Reflections of a Mother
Prader-Willi Syndrome Association (USA)
8588 Potter Park Drive   941-312-0400
Sarasota, FL 34238   800-926-4797
                                        Fax: 941-312-0142
                                e-mail: info@pwsausa.org
                                             www.pwsausa.org

Collection of 15 articles. Tips for managing family life on a practical level. Booklet
2003 37 pages
Craig Polhemus, Executive Director

7290 Growth Hormone & Prader-Willi Syndrome: A Reference for Familes & Care Providers
Linda S. Keder, author
Prader-Willi Syndrome Association (USA)
8588 Potter Park Drive   941-312-0400
Sarasota, FL 34238   800-926-4797
                                        Fax: 941-312-0142
                                e-mail: info@pwsausa.com
                                             www.pwsausa.org

Reference for families and care providers.
2001 52 pages
Craig Polhemus, Executive Director

7291 Handbook for Parents
Shirley Neason, author
Prader-Willi Syndrome Association (USA)

8588 Potter Park Drive
Sarasota, FL 34238
941-312-0400
800-926-4797
Fax: 941-312-0142
e-mail: info@pwsausa.org
www.pwsausa.org

Parent-to-Parent handbook for understanding and managing issues related to PWS, from birth to adulthood.
1999 75 pages
Craig Polhemus, Executive Director

7292 Nutrition Care for Children with PWS: Infants and Toddlers
J. Hovasi & D. Doorlag, with J. Loker & C. Loker, author
Prader-Willi Syndrome Association (USA)
8588 Potter Park Drive
Sarasota, FL 34238
941-312-0400
800-926-4797
Fax: 941-312-0142
e-mail: info@pwsausa.com
www.pwsausa.org

Provides answers to frequently asked questions about nutrition and feeding infants and toddlers with PWS.
2004 62 pages
Craig Polhemus, Executive Director

7293 Sometimes I'm Mad, Sometimes I'm Glad - A Sibling Booklet
Sarah Heinemann, author
Prader-Willi Syndrome Association (USA)
8588 Potter Park Drive
Sarasota, FL 34238
941-312-0400
800-926-4797
Fax: 941-312-0142
e-mail: info@pwsausa.com
www.pwsausa.org

Explains sibling relationships and how they are affected by Prader-Willi syndrome. Written in the voice of a sibling of someone with PWS. Ages 5-13
32 pages
Craig Polhemus, Executive Director

7294 Supporting Adults with Prader-Willi Syndro me in a Residential Setting
B.J. Goff, Ed.D, author
Prader-Willi Syndrome Association (USA)
8588 Potter Pass Drive
Sarasota, FL 34238
941-312-0400
800-926-4797
Fax: 941-312-0142
e-mail: info@pwsausa.com
www.pwsausa.org

Filling a large gap for care givers of those with Prader-Willi Sydrome, this is an extensive manual covering residential care issues; including management strategies, specifics for phase of life, and a number of additional ideas.
2002 121 pages
Craig Polhemus, Executive Director

Newsletters

7295 Gathered View
Prader-Willi Syndrome Association (USA)
8588 Potter Park Drive
Sarasota, FL 34238
941-312-0400
800-926-4797
Fax: 941-312-0142
e-mail: info@pwsausa.com
www.pwsausa.org

The official newsletter of PWSA, mailed 6 time/year to members. Offers current research findings, behavior and weight management techniques, educational news, articles and more.
BiMonthly
Craig Polhemus, Executive Director

Pamphlets

7296 An Early Prader-Willi Syndrome Diagnosis & How to Make it Easier on Parents
Prader-Willi Foundation

40 Holly Lane
Roslyn Hts, NY 11577-1533
516-944-8136
800-253-7993
Fax: 516-944-3173
e-mail: foundation@prader-willi.inter.net
www.prader-willi.org

A parent of a child with PWS and an advocate for others with the afflication speaks.
Rachel Johnson, President and Author

7297 Behavior Management: Collection of Articless
Prader-Willi Syndrome Association (USA)
8588 Potter Park Drive
Sarasota, FL 34238
941-312-0400
800-926-4797
Fax: 941-312-0142
e-mail: info@pwsausa.com
www.pwsausa.org

Includes general articles of behavior concerns, use of psychotropic medications, skin picking and teaching social skills.
2003 49 pages
Craig Polhemus, Executive Director

7298 Educational Choices for Children with PWS
Prader-Willi Foundation
40 Holly Lane
Roslyn Hts, NY 11577-1533
516-944-8136
800-253-7993
Fax: 516-944-3173
e-mail: foundation@prader-willi.inter.net
www.prader-willi.org

Parents of young children with Prader-Willi syndrome discuss their individual philosophies of educational choice - inclusion vs. specialized setting.
Rachel Johnson, President and Author

7299 Nutrition Care for Adolescents and Adults with PWS
Karenn H. Borgie, MA, RD, author
Prader-Willi Syndrome Association (USA)
8588 Potter Park Drive
Sarasota, FL 34238
941-312-0400
800-926-4797
Fax: 941-312-0142
e-mail: info@pwsausa.com
www.pwsausa.org

covers essential diet information for families, caregivers, and residential service providers.
Craig Polhemus, Executive Director

7300 Nutrition Care for Children with PWS, Ages 3-9
Karen H. Borgie, MA, RD, author
Prader-Willi Syndrome Association (USA)
8588 Potter Park Drive
Sarasota, FL 34238
941-312-0400
800-926-4797
Fax: 941-312-0142
e-mail: info@pwsausa.com
www.pwsausa.org

Discusses calorie needs, supplements, diet planning, food management, and exchange lists. Softvcover.
Craig Polhemus, Executive Director

7301 What Educators Should Know About Prader-Willi Syndrome
Prader-Willi Syndrome Association (USA)
8588 Potter Park Drive
Sarasota, FL 34238
941-312-0400
800-926-4797
Fax: 941-312-0142
e-mail: info@pwsausa.com
www.pwsausa.org

Offers guidelines and strategies for helping the student with PWS stay focused, develop skills and knowledge, and minimize problems associated with the syndrome in the school setting.
Craig Polhemus, Executive Director

Audio & Video

7302 Prader-Willi Syndrome: An Overview for Health Professionals
Prader-Willi Syndrome Association
5700 Midnight Pass Road
Sarasota, FL 34242-3000
941-312-0400
800-926-4797
Fax: 941-312-0142
e-mail: info@pwsausa.com
www.pwsausa.org

Essential viewing for all health care professionals who are not experts on prader-willi syndrome. It deals with all major genetics and health care issues of the child with PWS.
2002

7303   Prader-Willi Syndrome: the Early Years
Prader-Willi Syndrome Association
5700 Midnight Pass Road
Sarasota, FL 34242-3000

941-312-0400
800-926-4797
Fax: 941-312-0142
e-mail: info@pwsausa.com
www.pwsausa.org

Offers help and practical suggestions for those families with a young child newly diagnosed with PWS. Genetics, medical, early intervention and family issues are presented, personalized with family interviews. Although focusing on young children, this video is a wonderful resource for schools and families with children of all ages.
2002

Web Sites

7304   Healthlink USA

www.healthlinkusa.com

Health information concerning treatment, cures, prevention, diagnosis, risk factors, research, support groups, email lists, personal stories and much more. Updated regularly.

7305   MedicineNet

www.medicinenet.com

An online resource for consumers providing easy-to-read, authoritative medical and health information.

7306   Medscape

www.medscape.com

Medscape offers specialists, primary care physicians, and other health professionals the Web's most robust and integrated medical information and educational tools.

Description

7307 Raynaud's Disease

Raynaud's disease is the spasm of blood vessels to fingers and toes, resulting in restricted blood supply in response to cold or emotional upset. Symptoms include tingling and numbness. During an episode, which can last from minutes to hours, the arteries contract briefly and the skin, deprived of oxygen, turns pale and then blue. As arteries relax and blood begins to flow, reddening, tingling, or swelling may occur. While hands and feet are most commonly affected, the nose and ears can also be subject to Raynaud's.

Raynaud's most commonly affects women under 40, accounting for perhaps 90 percent of all cases. When the classic symptoms are present, without other complaints, the condition is referred to as Raynaud's disease (primary Raynaud's), and generally results in no serious consequences. The second form, Raynaud's phenomenon (secondary Raynaud's), is the result of other underlying medical conditions, including scleroderma, vascular disease, rheumatoid arthritis and lupus.

Certain drugs can also trigger Raynaud's, including ergotamine and a number of beta-blocking drugs that are used in the treatment of heart disease. About 10 percent of Raynaud's cases are related to specific repetitive stress activities such as the operation of pneumatic drills and other hand-held vibrating machinery. In most Raynaud's cases, symptoms are discomforting but not serious. In extreme cases, Raynaud's can result in tissue atrophy and gangrene. Preventative measures include protection from cold, even when taking food out of the refrigerator or freezer, and avoiding behavior that disrupts bloodflow, for instance, smoking cigarettes.

Medical treatment of Raynaud's is directed toward improving blood flow to the extremities. In many cases, simple exercises are prescribed, and relaxation techniques, such as biofeedback, teach the body to ignore trivial or transient signals of cold. In other cases, vasodilator drugs which are designed to relax and open blood vessels to improve blood flow are prescribed. In the most extreme cases, surgery may be performed to cut nerves that may be inappropriately triggering the contraction of arteries, although relief may last only 1 to 2 years. Herbal remedies have been used in the treatment of Raynaud's and other circulatory conditions, especially the Chinese herb Dong quai. There is also evidence that foods rich in vitamin E, and fish oils, may help to reduce or moderate the vascular spasms that produce Raynaud's symptoms.

National Agencies & Associations

7308 **Arthritis Foundation**
1330 W Peachtree Street
Atlanta, GA 30309
404-872-7100
800-283-7800
Fax: 404-872-0457
e-mail: help@arthritis.org
www.arthritis.org

A nonprofit organization that depends on volunteers to provide services to help people with arthritis. Supports research to find ways to cure and prevent arthritis and provides services to improve the quality of life for those affected by arthritis.
Daniel T Mcgowen, Chair
Rowland W chang, Vice Chair

7309 **Raynaud's Foundation**
11 Topstone Road
Redding, CT 06896-6176
773-622-9220
Fax: 773-622-9221
www.raynauds.org

The Raynaud's Foundation is a non-profit dedicated to the promotion of education and research Raynaud's Phenomenon and related diseases, both autoimmune and non-autoimmune.
Ida Therese Jablanovec, Executive Director

7310 **United Scleroderma Foundation**
300 Rosewood Drive
Danvers, MA 01923-0350
978-463-5843
800-722-4673
Fax: 978-463-5809
www.scleroderma.org

Offers materials and referrals conducts workshops and support groups for those with Raynaud's and their families.
Mary Ann Berman, Office Assistant
Liz Dorsett, Communications Manager

Libraries & Resource Centers

7311 **Arizona Telemedicine Program**
University of Arizona, Health Science Center
PO Box 245105
Tucson, AZ 85724-5105
520-626-2493
Fax: 520-626-4774
e-mail: kerps@email.arizona.edu
www.telemedicine.arizona.edu/index.html

The Arizona Telemedicine Program is a large, multidisciplinary, university-based program that provides telemedicine services, distance learning, informatics training, and telemedicine technology assessment capabilities to communities throughout Arizona, the sixth largest state in the United States, in square miles.
Ronald S Weinstein, MD, Director
Ana Maria Lopez, Medical Director

Support Groups & Hotlines

7312 **National Health Information Center**
PO Box 1133
Washington, DC 20013
310-565-4167
800-336-4797
Fax: 301-984-4256
e-mail: info@nhic.org
www.health.gov/nhic

Offers a nationwide information referral service, produces directories and resource guides.

Books

7313 **Raynaud's Phenomenon**
Oxford University Press
PO Box 7669
Atlanta, GA 30357
404-872-7100
800-283-7800
Fax: 404-872-0457

This is a detailed and technical work on the physiology finger circulation, and on diagnosis and treatment of Raynaud's Phenomenon and Raynaud's Disease. Includes a chapter on Acrocyanosis and Livedo reticularis.
186 pages
ISBN: 0-195057-56-2

Pamphlets

7314 **Raynaud's Phenomenon**
Arthritis Foundation
PO Box 7669
Atlanta, GA 30357-0669
404-872-7100
800-283-7800
Fax: 404-872-0457

Web Sites

7315 Health Finder

www.healthfinder.gov

Searchable, carefully developed web site offering information on over 1000 topics. Developed by the US Department of Health and Human Services, the site can be used in both English and Spanish.

7316 MedicineNet

www.medicinenet.com

An online resource for consumers providing easy-to-read, authoritative medical and health information.

7317 United Scleroderma Foundation

www.scleroderma.org

Offers materials and referrals, conducts workshops and support groups for those with Raynaud's and their families.

Description

7318 ## Sarcoidosis

Sarcoidosis is a chronic disease that can affect almost any part of the body. It is characterized by the deposit of small masses of tissue (granulomas) in multiple organs. The cause is unknown, although it is speculated to be related to an immunologic defect or infection. Incidence varies widely between countries. In the United States, sarcoidosis is 10- to 18-fold higher in African Americans than in whites. Most cases start between the ages of 30 and 50 years.

Clinical features vary considerably, depending on the site and extent of involvement. Systemic symptoms may include fatigue, weight loss, loss of appetite and fever. Local symptoms may involve any organ, but the most commonly affected are the lungs, skin, eyes and lymph nodes. If the disease becomes severe and life-threatening, it is usually because of lung involvement. Patients develop cough, wheeze, chest pain and difficulty breathing.

Both the severity and the long-term outlook are extremely variable. In most patients, the disease regresses within 2 years and does not recur. In approximately 25 percent of patients, the disease progresses and causes serious disability. If progressive symptoms require treatment, corticosteroids are usually given. If these are not effective or tolerated, immuno suppressive drugs such as methotrexate or azathioprine may be tried. Approximately 5 percent of patients die of respiratory failure.

National Agencies & Associations

7319 **Autoimmune Advocacy Alliance**

509-630-5344
e-mail: info@a3autoimmunity.org
www.a3autoimmunity.org
The Autoimmune Advocacy Alliance (A3) is a collective effort to achieve clarity, understanding and support for the needs of those living with autoimmune diseases.

7320 **National Sarcoidosis Family Aid and Research Foundation**
1400 Parkmoor Avenue
San Jose, CA 95126   www.php.com
Provides information on a rare disease involving inflammation in lymph nodes and other body tissues, usually in young adults.
Suzanne Cistulli, Board Chair
Joyce Uggla, Board Secretary

7321 **National Sarcoidosis Resource Center**
PO Box 1593   732-463-0497
Piscataway, NJ 08855-1593   Fax: 732-463-0467
www.nsrc-global.net
The center provides a national computer database with statistical information and studies, telephone support for patients, subscriptions to national magazines and newsletters and public information provided by mail.
Sandra Conroy, President

7322 **Sarcoid Networking Association**
12619 S. Wilderness Way
Molalla, OR 97038   541-905-2092
www.sarcoidosisnetwork.org
The association was founded in 1992 to educate individuals, provide information and heighten public awareness about Sarcoidosis.

Research Centers

7323 **Sarcoidosis Center**
6005 Park Avenue   901-761-5877
Memphis, TN 38119   866-727-2643
Fax: 901-761-2280
e-mail: sarcoid@sarcoidcenter.com
www.sarcoidcenter.com
A nonprofit tax exempt organization dedicated to increasing knowledge of the disease sarcoidosis. This broad goal encompasses three main areas: Disseminating information to professionals who assist with treatment of the disease obtaining and dispersing funds to assist with investigation into the cause and treatment of the disease and providing support for individuals afflicted with the disease.

7324 **Sarcoidosis Treatment and Research Center Thomas Jefferson University Hospital**
Thomas Jefferson University Hospital
111 S 11th Street   215-955-6840
Philadelphia, PA 19107-5092   Fax: 215-923-5828
www.jeffersonhospital.org

Stephen K klasko, President/CEO
Sergio Jimen MD, Professor

Support Groups & Hotlines

7325 **Better Breather's Clubs**
American Lung Association of Virginia
1301 Pennsylvania Ave.   202-785-3355
Richmond, DC 20004   Fax: 202-452-1805
e-mail: chamm@lungva.org
www.lungusa.srg
Support Groups for those suffering from chronic obstructive pulmonary disease (COPD) such as emphysema, chronic bronchitis and asthma. In these meetings members give and receive support, and learn more about chronic lung disease from health care professionals who share trends in therapy, medication and other topics, or simply answer members' questions.
Catherine G Hamm, President/Chief Excutive Officer
Michelle LaRose, Development Director

7326 **Let's Breathe Sarcoidosis Support Group**
2225 Foster Street   708-328-9410
Evanston, IL 60201-3353   e-mail: bharris354@aol.com
Brenda Harris, Facilitator

7327 **Middle Tennessee Sarcoidosis Support Group**
PO Box 1342
Cookesville, TN 38503   931-528-7826
www.tennesseesarcoidisawareness.org
Becky Robertson, Group Leader

7328 **Mount Sinai Sarcoidosis Support Group**
One Gustave L. Levy Place   212-241-6500
New York, NY 10029   86- 67- 372
www.mountsinai.org

7329 **National Health Information Center**
PO Box 1133   310-565-4167
Washington, DC 20013   800-336-4797
Fax: 301-984-4256
e-mail: info@nhic.org
www.health.gov/nhic
Offers a nationwide information referral service, produces directories and resource guides.

7330 **Pacific NW Support Group**
Providence Hospital
PO Box 58785   42- 2-5 14
Renton, WA 98058   877- 25- 067
Fax: 42- 2-4 20
e-mail: washington@myasthenia.org
www.myasthenia.org

Ed Girvan, Facilitator

7331 Sarcoidosis HelpNet
PO Box 022642
Brooklyn, NY 11202
732-463-0497
Fax: 732-463-0467
www.nsrc-gllobal.net

Soneni B Smith, Contact

7332 Sarcoidosis Research Institute (SRI)
3475 Central Avenue
Memphis, TN 38111
901-766-6951
Fax: 901-774-7294
e-mail: sarcoid@sarcoidcenter.com
www.sarcoidcenter.com/saradd.htm

The Sarcoidosis Research Institute is a non-profit, tax-exempt organization dedicated to increasing knowledge of the disease sarcoidosis. This broad goal encompasses three main areas: Disseminating information to professionals who assist with treatment of the disease; Obtaining and dispersing funds to assist with investigation into the cause and treatment of the disease; and, providing support for individuals afflicted with the disease.
Paula Yette Polite, Board of Directors President
Wayne Crook, Vice President Board of Directors

7333 Sarcoidosis Self-Help Group: New York
Nassau County Medical Center
2201 Hempstead Turnpike
East Meadow, NY 11554
516-483-2666
Robert Schoenfeld, Facilitator

7334 Sarcoidosis Self-Help Group: Virginia
American Lung Association of Northern Virginia
9735 Main Street
Fairfax, VA 22031
703-591-4131
Carolyn Thomas, Facilitator

7335 Sarcoidosis Support Group Delaware
American Lung Association of Delaware
1021 Gilpin Avenue
Wilmington, DE 19806
302-655-7258
800-548-8252
Fax: 302-655-8546
e-mail: dbrown@alade.org
www.alade.org
Peter Shanley, Chairman
Harold P. Wimmer, President/CEO

7336 Sarcoidosis Support Group: New Jersey
268 Dr. ML King Boulevard
Newark, NJ 07106
201-374-7570
Jean Curlin-Miller, Facilitator

7337 Sarcoidosis Support Group: Washington DC
110 Irving Street
Washington, DC 20010
202-877-6286
Fax: 202-877-5779

7338 Triangle Area Sarcoidosis Support Group
Soapstone UM Church
12837 Norwood Road
Raleigh, NC 27613
919-676-6498
e-mail: fairleyl@bellsouth.net
Priscilla Fairley, Facilitator

7339 Understanding Sarcoidosis Self-Help Group
2112 Highland Avenue
New Castle, PA 16105
412-652-6089

7340 University of North Carolina Sarcoidosis Support Group
UNC Chapel Hill Healthcare
130 Mason Farm Road
Chapel Hill, NC 27599
919-966-2531
e-mail: sharikia_burt@med.unc.edu
Sharikia Burt, Clinical Coordinator

7341 West Tennessee Sarcoidosis Support Group
1670 McLemoresville Road
Huntington, TN 38344
731-986-9832
www.tennesseesarcoidosisawareness.org
Patricia Coleman, Group Leader

Books

7342 Sarcoidosis Resource Guide and Directory
PC Publications

PO Box 1593
Piscataway, NJ 08855-1593
732-699-0733
800-223-6429
Fax: 732-699-0882
www.nsrc-global.net

1993 304 pages Paperback
ISBN: 0-963122-25-8

Newsletters

7343 Online Sarcoidosis Newsletter
National Sarcoidosis Resource Center
PO Box 1593
Piscataway, NJ 08855-1593
732-699-0733
800-223-6429
Fax: 732-699-0882
www.nsrc-global.net

Offers information on the center's activities and events, medical and legislative updates for the patients and their families.
Quarterly

Pamphlets

7344 Anemia of Sarcoidosis
PC Publications
PO Box 1593
Piscataway, NJ 08855-1593
732-699-0733
800-223-6429
Fax: 732-699-0882
www.nsrc-global.net

7345 Bronchoalveolar Lymphocytes in Sarcoidosis
PC Publications
PO Box 1593
Piscataway, NJ 08855-1593
732-699-0733
800-223-6429
Fax: 732-699-0882
www.nsrc-global.net

7346 Case Report: MR Imaging of Myocardial Sarcoidosis
PC Publications
PO Box 1593
Piscataway, NJ 08855-1593
732-699-0733
800-223-6429
Fax: 732-699-0882
www.nsrc-global.net

7347 Case Report: Osseous Sarcoidosis and Chronic Polyarthritis
PC Publications
PO Box 1593
Piscataway, NJ 08855-1593
732-699-0733
800-223-6429
Fax: 732-699-0882
www.nsrc-global.net

7348 Case Report: Overlap of Granulomatous Vasculitis and Sarcoidosis
PC Publications
PO Box 1593
Piscataway, NJ 08855-1593
732-699-0733
800-223-6429
Fax: 732-699-0882
www.nsrc-global.net

7349 Case Report: Rapidly Dev. Confusion, Impaired Memory and Unsteady Gait
PC Publications
PO Box 1593
Piscataway, NJ 08855-1593
732-699-0733
800-223-6429
Fax: 732-699-0882
www.nsrc-global.net

7350 Coping with Sarcoidosis
National Sarcoidosis Resource Center
PO Box 1593
Piscataway, NJ 08855-1593
732-699-0733
800-223-6429
Fax: 732-699-0882
www.nsrc-global.net

A pamphlet offering information on how to manage and live with sarcoidosis.

7351 Disability Law: A Legal Primer
PC Publications

PO Box 1593
Piscataway, NJ 08855-1593

732-699-0733
800-223-6429
Fax: 732-699-0882
www.nsrc-global.net

7352 Drugs That Have Been Used for the Treatment of Sarcoidosis
PC Publications
PO Box 1593
Piscataway, NJ 08855-1593

732-699-0733
800-223-6429
Fax: 732-699-0882
www.nsrc-global.net

7353 Effect of Corticosteroid or Methotrexate Therapy on Lung Lymphocytes
PC Publications
PO Box 1593
Piscataway, NJ 08855-1593

732-699-0733
800-223-6429
Fax: 732-699-0882
www.nsrc-global.net

7354 Effects of Sarcoid and Steroids on Angiotensin-Converting Enzyme
PC Publications
PO Box 1593
Piscataway, NJ 08855-1593

732-699-0733
800-223-6429
Fax: 732-699-0882
www.nsrc-global.net

7355 Evaluation of the Efficacy and Toxicity of the Cyclosporine
PC Publications
PO Box 1593
Piscataway, NJ 08855-1593

732-699-0733
800-223-6429
Fax: 732-699-0882
www.nsrc-global.net

7356 Gastrointestinal Presentation of Churg Strauss Syndrome
PC Publications
PO Box 1593
Piscataway, NJ 08855-1593

732-699-0733
800-223-6429
Fax: 732-699-0882
www.nsrc-global.net

7357 Governor New Jersey Proclamation: Sarcoidosis Awareness Day
PC Publications
PO Box 1593
Piscataway, NJ 08855-1593

732-699-0733
800-223-6429
Fax: 732-699-0882
www.nsrc-global.net

7358 How to Get the Most Out of Your Doctor: A Neurologist's Perspective
PC Publications
PO Box 1593
Piscataway, NJ 08855-1593

732-699-0733
800-223-6429
Fax: 732-699-0882
www.nsrc-global.net

7359 Ideas and Considerations for Starting a Self-Help Mutual Aid Group
PC Publications
PO Box 1593
Piscataway, NJ 08855-1593

732-699-0733
800-223-6429
Fax: 732-699-0882
www.nsrc-global.net

7360 Masqueraders of Sarcoidosis
PC Publications
PO Box 1593
Piscataway, NJ 08855-1593

732-699-0733
800-223-6429
Fax: 732-699-0882
www.nsrc-global.net

7361 Mayor Piscataway, NJ Proclamation: Sarcoidosis Awareness Day
PC Publications
PO Box 1593
Piscataway, NJ 08855-1593

732-699-0733
800-223-6429
Fax: 732-699-0882
www.nsrc-global.net

7362 Multidisciplinary Clinico-Pathologic Conference
PC Publications

7363 National Sarcoidosis Resource Center
PC Publications
PO Box 1593
Piscataway, NJ 08855-1593

732-699-0733
800-223-6429
Fax: 732-699-0882
www.nsrc-global.net

A booklet offering a brief introduction to the illness and offers information on the role of the Center in finding a cure and educating the public on Sarcoidosis.

7364 Neurosarcoidosis
PC Publications
PO Box 1593
Piscataway, NJ 08855-1593

732-699-0733
800-223-6429
Fax: 732-699-0882
www.nsrc-global.net

7365 Neurosarcoidosis or Multiple Sclerosis?
National Sarcoidosis Resource Center
PO Box 1593
Piscataway, NJ 08855-1593

732-699-0733
800-223-6429
Fax: 732-699-0882
www.nsrc-global.net

7366 Paranoid Psychosis Due to Neurosarcoidosis
PC Publications
PO Box 1593
Piscataway, NJ 08855-1593

732-699-0733
800-223-6429
Fax: 732-699-0882
www.nsrc-global.net

7367 Patient Information Package
National Sarcoidosis Resource Center
PO Box 1593
Piscataway, NJ 08855-1593

732-699-0733
800-223-6429
Fax: 732-699-0882
www.nsrc-global.net

Contains various brochures and pamphlets offering information about Sarcoidosis.

7368 Physician Listings
PC Publications
PO Box 1593
Piscataway, NJ 08855-1593

732-699-0733
800-223-6429
Fax: 732-699-0882
www.nsrc-global.net

7369 Possible Association of Rheumatoid Arthritis & Sarcoidosis
PC Publications
PO Box 1593
Piscataway, NJ 08855-1593

732-699-0733
800-223-6429
Fax: 732-699-0882
www.nsrc-global.net

7370 Presidential Proclamation - National Sarcoidosis Awareness Day
PC Publications
PO Box 1593
Piscataway, NJ 08855-1593

732-699-0733
800-223-6429
Fax: 732-699-0882
www.nsrc-global.net

7371 Psychological Factors in Sarcoidosis
PC Publications
PO Box 1593
Piscataway, NJ 08855-1593

732-699-0733
800-223-6429
Fax: 732-699-0882
www.nsrc-global.net

7372 Public Law 102-94
PC Publications
PO Box 1593
Piscataway, NJ 08855-1593

732-699-0733
800-223-6429
Fax: 732-699-0882
www.nsrc-global.net

7373 Pulmonary Sarcoidosis: Evaluation with High Resolution
PC Publications

PO Box 1593
Piscataway, NJ 08855-1593

732-699-0733
800-223-6429
Fax: 732-699-0882
www.nsrc-global.net

7374 Pulmonary Sarcoidosis: What We Are Learning
PC Publications
PO Box 1593
Piscataway, NJ 08855-1593

732-699-0733
800-223-6429
Fax: 732-699-0882
www.nsrc-global.net

7375 Questionnaire Responses for Demographics and Symptoms from 1000 Patients
PC Publications
PO Box 1593
Piscataway, NJ 08855-1593

732-699-0733
800-223-6429
Fax: 732-699-0882
www.nsrc-global.net

7376 Right & Left Ventricular Function at Rest in Patients with Sarcoidosis
PC Publications
PO Box 1593
Piscataway, NJ 08855-1593

732-699-0733
800-223-6429
Fax: 732-699-0882
www.nsrc-global.net

7377 Role of Magnetic Resonance Imaging in Neurosarcoidosis
PC Publications
PO Box 1593
Piscataway, NJ 08855-1593

732-699-0733
800-223-6429
Fax: 732-699-0882
www.nsrc-global.net

7378 Sarcoidosis
PC Publications
PO Box 1593
Piscataway, NJ 08855-1593

732-699-0733
800-223-6429
Fax: 732-699-0882
www.nsrc-global.net

Offers information on the illness, causes, symptoms and treatments.

7379 Sarcoidosis Diagnosed in a Patient with Known HIV Infection
PC Publications
PO Box 1593
Piscataway, NJ 08855-1593

732-699-0733
800-223-6429
Fax: 732-699-0882
www.nsrc-global.net

7380 Sarcoidosis Patient Questionnaire
PC Publications
PO Box 1593
Piscataway, NJ 08855-1593

732-699-0733
800-223-6429
Fax: 732-699-0882
www.nsrc-global.net

7381 Sarcoidosis Questionnaire: Demographics and Symptomatology-The Patients Respond
PC Publications
PO Box 1593
Piscataway, NJ 08855-1593

732-699-0733
800-223-6429
Fax: 732-699-0882
www.nsrc-global.net

7382 Sarcoidosis and Pregnancy: Clinical Observation
PC Publications
PO Box 1593
Piscataway, NJ 08855-1593

732-699-0733
800-223-6429
Fax: 732-699-0882
www.nsrc-global.net

7383 Sarcoidosis and You: A Listing of Possible Symptoms
PC Publications
PO Box 1593
Piscataway, NJ 08855-1593

732-699-0733
800-223-6429
Fax: 732-699-0882
www.nsrc-global.net

7384 Sarcoidosis in India: A Review of 125 Biopsy-Proven Cases from India
PC Publications
PO Box 1593
Piscataway, NJ 08855-1593

732-699-0733
800-223-6429
Fax: 732-699-0882
www.nsrc-global.net

7385 Sarcoidosis of the Liver
PC Publications
PO Box 1593
Piscataway, NJ 08855-1593

732-699-0733
800-223-6429
Fax: 732-699-0882
www.nsrc-global.net

7386 Sarcoidosis: A Multisystem Disease
PC Publications
PO Box 1593
Piscataway, NJ 08855-1593

732-699-0733
800-223-6429
Fax: 732-699-0882
www.nsrc-global.net

Explains the effects of the illness on the lungs and joints.

7387 Sarcoidosis: International Review
PC Publications
PO Box 1593
Piscataway, NJ 08855-1593

732-699-0733
800-223-6429
Fax: 732-699-0882
www.nsrc-global.net

7388 Sarcoidosis: Pleural Involvement Mimicking a Coin Lesson
PC Publications
PO Box 1593
Piscataway, NJ 08855-1593

732-699-0733
800-223-6429
Fax: 732-699-0882
www.nsrc-global.net

7389 Sarcoidosis: Usual and Unusual Manifestations
PC Publications
PO Box 1593
Piscataway, NJ 08855-1593

732-699-0733
800-223-6429
Fax: 732-699-0882
www.nsrc-global.net

7390 Seasonal Clustering of Sarcoidosis
National Sarcoidosis Resource Center
PO Box 1593
Piscataway, NJ 08855-1593

732-699-0733
800-223-6429
Fax: 732-699-0882
www.nsrc-global.net

7391 Successful Treatment of Myocardial Sarcoidosis with Steriods
PC Publications
PO Box 1593
Piscataway, NJ 08855-1593

732-699-0733
800-223-6429
Fax: 732-699-0882
www.nsrc-global.net

7392 Support Group Listing
PC Publications
PO Box 1593
Piscataway, NJ 08855-1593

732-699-0733
800-223-6429
Fax: 732-699-0882
www.nsrc-global.net

7393 Use of Low Dose Methotrexate in Refractory Sarcoidosis
PC Publications
PO Box 1593
Piscataway, NJ 08855-1593

732-699-0733
800-223-6429
Fax: 732-699-0882
www.nsrc-global.net

7394 World Association Sarcoidosi Other Granulatomous
PC Publications
PO Box 1593
Piscataway, NJ 08855-1593

732-699-0733
800-223-6429
Fax: 732-699-0882
www.nsrc-global.net

Audio & Video

7395 Dialogue with Doris
PC Publications
PO Box 1593
Piscataway, NJ 08855-1593
732-699-0733
800-223-6429
Fax: 732-699-0882
www.nsrc-global.net

7396 Help with a Hidden Disease Update
PC Publications
PO Box 1593
Piscataway, NJ 08855-1593
732-699-0733
800-223-6429
Fax: 732-699-0882
www.nsrc-global.net

7397 Of Their Own: Person to Person Show
PC Publications
PO Box 1593
Piscataway, NJ 08855-1593
732-699-0733
800-223-6429
Fax: 732-699-0882
www.nsrc-global.net

7398 Sarcoidosis Conference 2
PC Publications
PO Box 1593
Piscataway, NJ 08855-1593
732-699-0733
800-223-6429
Fax: 732-699-0882
www.nsrc-global.net

7399 Sarcoidosis Conference 3
PC Publications
PO Box 1593
Piscataway, NJ 08855-1593
732-699-0733
800-223-6429
Fax: 732-699-0882
www.nsrc-global.net

7400 Sarcoidosis and Lyme Disease
PC Publications
PO Box 1593
Piscataway, NJ 08855-1593
732-699-0733
800-223-6429
Fax: 732-699-0882
www.nsrc-global.net

7401 Sarcoidosis: What's That?
PC Publications
PO Box 1593
Piscataway, NJ 08855-1593
732-699-0733
800-223-6429
Fax: 732-699-0882
www.nsrc-global.net

7402 XIV International World Conference on Sarcoidosis: Patient Symposium
PC Publications
PO Box 1593
Piscataway, NJ 08855-1593
732-699-0733
800-223-6429
Fax: 732-699-0882
www.nsrc-global.net
Cassette.

Web Sites

7403 Healing Well
www.healingwell.com
An online health resource guide to medical news, chat, information and articles, newsgroups and message boards, books, disease-related web sites, medical directories, and more for patients, friends, and family coping with disabling diseases, disorders, or chronic illnesses.

7404 Health Finder
www.healthfinder.gov
Searchable, carefully developed web site offering information on over 1000 topics. Developed by the US Department of Health and Human Services, the site can be used in both English and Spanish.

7405 Healthlink USA
www.healthlinkusa.com
Health information concerning treatment, cures, prevention, diagnosis, risk factors, research, support groups, email lists, personal stories and much more. Updated regularly.

7406 Helios Health
www.helioshealth.com
Online resource for your health information. Detailed information about specific health topics, access to expert advice from our Medical Advisory Board, and up-to-date health news.

7407 MedicineNet
www.medicinenet.com
An online resource for consumers providing easy-to-read, authoritative medical and health information.

7408 Medscape
www.medscape.com
Medscape offers specialists, primary care physicians, and other health professionals the Web's most robust and integrated medical information and educational tools.

7409 National Sarcoidosis Resource Center
www.nsrc-global.net
Provides the general public with sarcoidosis information, for patients to obtain medical and emotional help and to provide government officials with the information they need.

7410 WebMD
www.webmd.com
Provides credible information, supportive communities, and in-depth reference material about health subjects. A source for original and timely health information as well as material from well known content providers.

Description

7411 Scleroderma

Scleroderma, literally 'hard skin', is a form of systemic sclerosis, a generalized disturbance of connective and vascular tissue which leads to scarring (sclerosis). Scleroderma is a rare disease, with about 5,000 new cases in the United States each year. Women are 3 or 4 times as likely as men to get the disease, which typically begins between the ages of 30 and 50 years. It is comparatively rare in children. The cause of the disease is unknown.

Since almost any organ may be involved, the list of possible symptoms is extensive. Important ones include weakness, fatigue, stiffness, weight loss, shortness of breath, abdominal bloating and pain, diarrhea and irritation of the eyes. Kidney involvement usually causes abrupt acceleration of high blood pressure. A very characteristic symptom, although not unique to this disease, is Raynaud's phenomenon. On exposure to cold, the arteries of the patient's hands and feet contract, causing the skin color to change from red, to white (blanch), to blue (cyanosis), accompanied by pain and numbness.

If the disease is limited to the skin the outlook is good, but involvement of lung and kidney in the systemic form may be fatal. Use of the ACE inhibitor class of anti-hypertensive drugs has helped preserve kidney function. Many immunosuppressive drugs have been tried without clear success. Clinical trials of new agents are often available to patients. When end-stage kidney disease cannot be prevented, dialysis and transplant can be used, although the death rate remains high.

National Agencies & Associations

7412 Canadian Dermatology Association
1385 Bank Street
Ottawa, Ontario, K1H-8N4   613-738-1748
                                   800-267-3376
                              Fax: 613-738-4695
          e-mail: contact.cda@dermatology.ca
                         www.dermatology.ca
Ensure the Canadian public has equal access to timely and exemplary dermatologic care, by advocating on dermatologic issues, providing leadership in continuing medical and public education, and promoting and disseminating dermatologic knowledge and research.
Dr Richard Langley, President of the Board
Chantal Courchesne, Executive Director

7413 Raynaud's Association
11 Topstone Road
Redding, CT 6896   800-280-8055
                   e-mail: info@raynauds.org
                           www.raynauds.org
A 501c3 non-profit organization providing support and education to the many sufferers of Raynaud's Phenomenon - an exaggerated sensitivity to cold temperatures.

7414 Scleroderma Foundation
462 Boston Street
Topsfield, MA 01983   978-887-0658
                                   800-722-4673
                              Fax: 978-463-5809
          e-mail: newengland@scleroderma.org
                         www.scleroderma.org
A national nonprofit organization serving the interests of persons with Scleroderma. The Foundation's 26 chapters and 135 support

groups nationwide help to carry out its three-fold mission of support, education and research.
Joseph Camerino, Chair
Carol Feghali-Bostwi, Vice Chair

7415 Scleroderma Society of Ontario
393 University Avenue   905-544-0343
Toronto, Ontario, M5G-1E6   Fax: 416-979-8366
                       www.sclerodermaontario.ca
Committed to promoting increased public awareness, advancing patient wellness and supporting research in scleroderma.
Brian Hinchey, Treasurer
Maureen Sauve, President of the Board

State Agencies & Associations

Arizona

7416 Scleroderma Foundation: Arizona Chapter
18402 N 19th Avenue   623-847-3757
Phoenix, AZ 85023   e-mail: carolnader@cox.net
                           www.scleroderma.org
Local chapter of the national Scleroderma Foundation in Byfield, Massachusetts. Please contact this group for information on area support groups.
Carol Nader, President

California

7417 Scleroderma Foundation: Greater San Diego Chapter
PO Box 502948   619-655-4342
San Diego, CA 92150   e-mail: kellyd.sclerosd@gmail.com
                           www.scleroderma.org
Local chapter of the national Scleroderma Foundation in Byfield, Massachusetts. Please contact this group for information on area support groups.
Fletcher Diehl, President
Carol Ireland, Vice President

7418 Scleroderma Foundation: Northern California Chapter
PO Box 601313   916-832-1102
Sacramento, CA 95860 e-mail: NoCAchapter@scleroderma.org
                           www.scleroderma.org
Local chapter of the national Scleroderma Foundation in Byfield, Massachusetts. Please contact this group for information on area support groups.
Cathy Eddy, President
Cheryl George, Vice President

7419 Scleroderma Foundation: Southern California Chapter
10319 Jefferson Blvd.   310-287-0793
Culver City, CA 90232   877-443-5755
                              Fax: 310-477-8774
          e-mail: SoCAchapter@scleroderma.org
                           www.scleroderma.org
Local chapter of the national Scleroderma Foundation in Byfield, Massachusetts. Please contact this group for information on area support groups.
Brian Ross Adams, Executive Director
Dan Furst, President

Colorado

7420 Scleroderma Foundation: Colorado Chapter
2280 S Albion Street   303-806-6686
Denver, CO 80222-0940 e-mail: COchapter@scleroderma.org
                           www.scleroderma.org
Local chapter of the national Scleroderma Foundation in Danvers, Massachusetts. Please contact this group for information on area support groups.
Rita Miller, President
Fran Penk, Vice President

District of Columbia

7421 Scleroderma Foundation: Greater Washington DC Chapter
2010 Corporate Ridge   202-999-4562
McLean, VA 22102   888-233-4779
e-mail: GWDCchapter@scleroderma.org
www.scleroderma.org
Local chapter of the national Scleroderma Foundation in Byfield, Massachusetts. Please contact this group for information on area support groups.
Carol Sodetz, President

Florida

7422 Scleroderma Foundation: Southeast Florida Chapter
3930 Oaks Clubhouse Drive   954-798-1854
Pompano Beach, FL 33069-3913   Fax: 954-255-8081
e-mail: sclerodermasefl@gmail.com
www.scleroderma.org
Local chapter of the national Scleroderma Foundation in Byfield, Massachusetts. Please contact this group for information on area support groups.
Berna Falkoff, President
Ruth Greenspan, Vice - Chair

Georgia

7423 Scleroderma Foundation: Georgia Chapter Scleroderma Foundation
Scleroderma Foundation
PO Box 522   770-925-7037
Liburn, GA 30048   800-722-4673
e-mail: GAchapter@scleroderma.org
www.scleroderma.org
Local chapter of the national Scleroderma Foundation in Byfield, Massachusetts. Call the national office for contact information on the Georgia Chapter. Please contact this group for information on area support groups.
Stacy Wright, Contact
Mary Haulk, Contact

Illinois

7424 Scleroderma Foundation: Greater Chicago Chapter
134 N. LaSalle St.   312-660-1131
Chicago, IL 60602   Fax: 312-660-1133
e-mail: GCchapter@scleroderma.org
www.scleroderma.org
Local chapter of the national Scleroderma Foundation. Please contact group for information on area support groups.
Mike Robbins, President

Maine

7425 Scleroderma Foundation: New England Chapter
462 Boston Street   978-887-0658
Topsfield, MA 01983   888-525-0658
Fax: 978-887-0659
e-mail: newengland@scleroderma.com
www.scleroderma.org
Local chapter of the national Scleroderma Foundation in Byfield, Massachusetts. Please contact this group for information on area support groups. Includes MA, ME, NH, VT, & RI.
Marie Coyle, President
Peter L. Hart, Treasurer

Massachusetts

7426 Scleroderma Foundation: New England Chapter
462 Boston Street   978-887-0658
Topsfield, MA 01983   888-525-0658
Fax: 978-887-0659
e-mail: newengland@scleroderma.com
www.scleroderma.org
Local chapter of the national Scleroderma Foundation in Byfield, Massachusetts. Please contact this group for information on area support groups.
Marie Coyle, President
Peter L. Hart, Treasurer

Michigan

7427 Scleroderma Foundation: Michigan Chapter
23999 Telegraph   248-595-8526
Southfield, MI 48033   800-716-6554
Fax: 248-595-8586
e-mail: MIchapter@scleroderma.org
www.scleroderma.org
Local chapter of the national Scleroderma Foundation in Danvers, Massachusetts. Please contact this group for information on area support groups, medical referrals, confrence dates and fund raising activities.
Duane Maladecki, President
Paul Rybicki, Vice President

Minnesota

7428 Scleroderma Foundation: Minnesota Chapter
PO Box 385246   877-794-0347
Bloomington, MN 55438   877-794-0347
e-mail: MNChapter@scleroderma.org
www.scleroderma.org
Local chapter of the national Scleroderma Foundation in Byfield, Massachusetts. Please contact this group for information on area support groups.
Bonnie Handmacher, President
Jordana Schmidt, Vice President

Missouri

7429 Scleroderma Foundation: Missouri Chapter
PO Box 4123   417-887-3269
Springfield, MO 65808   e-mail: MOchapter@scleroderma.org
www.scleroderma.org
Local chapter of the national Scleroderma Foundation in Byfield, Massachusetts. Please contact this group for information on area support groups.
Mary Blades, President
Rhonda Costa, Vice President

Nevada

7430 Scleroderma Foundation: Nevada Chapter
6760 Surrey Street   702-368-1572
Las Vegas, NV 89119   e-mail: NVchapter@scleroderma.org
www.scleroderma.org
Local chapter of the national Scleroderma Foundation in Byfield, Massachusetts. Please contact this group for information on area support groups.
Barbara Dempsey, President
Sheila Gray, VP Support Group

New Hampshire

7431 Scleroderma Foundation: New England Chapter
462 Boston Street   978-887-0658
Topsfield, MA 01983   888-525-0658
Fax: 978-887-0659
e-mail: newengland@scleroderma.com
www.scleroderma.org
Local chapter of the national Scleroderma Foundation in Byfield, Massachusetts. Please contact this group for information on area support groups.
Marie Coyle, President
Peter L. Hart, Treasurer

New York

7432 Scleroderma Foundation: Tri-State Chapter
59 Front Street   800-867-0885
Binghamton, NY 13905   800-867-0885
Fax: 607-723-2039
e-mail: chribar@scleroderma.org
www.scleroderma.org
Local chapter of the national Scleroderma Foundation in Byfield, Massachusetts. Please contact this group for information on area support groups.
Jeff Mace, President
Bruce Cowen, Vice President

7433 **Scleroderma Foundation: Western New York Chapter**
PO Box 708 716-627-2283
Hamburg, NY 14075 877-969-2478
e-mail: wnychpt@aol.com
www.scleroderma.org
Local chapter of the national Scleroderma Foundation in Byfield,
Massachusetts. Please contact this group for information on area
support groups.
Laura Henry, Co-President

Ohio

7434 **Scleroderma Foundation: Ohio Chapter**
PO Box 105 614-334-0846
Worthington, OH 43085-0846 866-849-9030
e-mail: OHchapter@scleroderma.org
www.scleroderma.org
Local chapter of the national Scleroderma Foundation in Byfield,
Massachusetts. Please contact this group for information on area
support groups.
Debbie Metz, President
Garry Lazenby, Vice President

Oregon

7435 **Scleroderma Foundation: Oregon Chapter**
PO Box 19296 503-245-4588
Portland, OR 97280-0296 e-mail: ORchapter@scleroderma.org
www.scleroderma.org
Local chapter of the national Scleroderma Foundation in Byfield,
Massachusetts. Please contact this group for information on area
support groups.
Liz Orem-Bedel, President
Richard Bates, Vice President

Pennsylvania

7436 **Scleroderma Foundation: Western Pennsylvania Chapter**
3500 Terrace Street 800-603-8960
Pittsburgh, PA 15261 800-722-4673
e-mail: WPAchapter@scleroderma.org
www.scleroderma.org
Local chapter of the national Scleroderma Foundation in Byfield,
Massachusetts. Please contact this group for information on area
support groups.
Betty Aquino, President
Thomas A Medsger Jr, Treasurer

Rhode Island

7437 **Scleroderma Foundation: New England Chapter**
462 Boston Street 978-887-0658
Topsfield, MA 01983 888-525-0658
Fax: 978-887-0659
e-mail: newengland@scleroderma.com
www.scleroderma.org
Local chapter of the national Scleroderma Foundation in Byfield,
Massachusetts. Please contact this group for information on area
support groups.
Marie Coyle, President
Peter L. Hart, Treasurer

South Carolina

7438 **Scleroderma Foundation: South Carolina Chapter**
713-D east Greenvile Street 864-617-0237
Anderson, SC 29621 866-557-3729
e-mail: SCchapter@scleroderma.org
www.scleroderma.org
Local chapter of the national Scleroderma Foundation in Byfield.
Massachusetts. Please contact this group for information on area
support groups.
Susan Melvin, President
Karen Kemper, Vice President

Tennessee

7439 **Scleroderma Foundation: Tennessee Chapter**
PO Box 281977 615-792-4610
Nashville, TN 37228 800-497-5193
Fax: 615-792-4610
e-mail: TNchapter@scleroderma.org
www.scleroderma.org
Local chapter of the national Scleroderma Foundation in Byfield,
Massachusetts. Please contact this group for information on area
support groups.
April Simpkins, President
Charles Cowell, Vice President

Texas

7440 **Scleroderma Foundation: Bluebonnet Chapter**
PO Box 1836 972-396-9400
Allen, TX 75013-1894 866-532-7673
Fax: 972-649-7910
e-mail: TXchapter@scleroderma.org
www.scleroderma.org
Local chapter of the national Scleroderma Foundation in Byfield,
Massachusetts. Please contact this group for information on area
support groups.
Cindi Brannum, President
Peggy Brown, Vice President

Vermont

7441 **Scleroderma Foundation: New England Chapter**
462 Boston Street 978-887-0658
Topsfield, MA 01983 888-525-0658
Fax: 978-887-0659
e-mail: newengland@scleroderma.com
www.scleroderma.org
Local chapter of the national Scleroderma Foundation in Byfield,
Massachusetts. Please contact this group for information on area
support groups.
Marie Coyle, President
Peter L. Hart, Treasurer

Virginia

7442 **Scleroderma Foundation: Greater Washington DC Chapter**
2010 Corporate Ridge 202-999-4562
McLean, VA 22102 888-233-4779
e-mail: GWDCchapter@scleroderma.org
www.scleroderma.org
Local chapter of the national Scleroderma Foundation in Byfield,
Massachusetts. Please contact this group for information on area
support groups.
Carol Sodetz, President
Solomon reed, Treasurer

Washington

7443 **Scleroderma Foundation: Evergreen Chapter**
PO Box 84506 206-285-9822
Seattle, WA 98124-5806 e-mail: WAchapter@scleroderma.org
www.scleroderma.org
Local chapter of the national Scleroderma Foundation in Byfield,
Massachusetts. Please contact this group for information on area
support groups.
Bunny Garthe, President
Nic Evans, Vice President

Foundations

7444 **Juvenile Scleroderma Network**
1204 W 13th Street 310-519-9511
San Pedro, CA 90731 866-338-5892
e-mail: OutreachJSDN@jsdn.org
www.jsdn.org

Organization that is working to provide educational programs about JSD, and to help children and their families to gain a better understanding.
Jerry Gaither, Chairman
Kathy Gaither, President

Research Centers

7445 Boston University University Medical Center
University Medical Center
One Boston Medical Center Place
Boston, MA 02118
617-638-8000
www.bmc.org
Ongoing clinical trials and studies in scleroderma. Office hours by appointment.
Kate Walsh, President/CEO
Melynn Nuite RN, Clinical Trails Contact

7446 Center for Rheumatology
1367 Washington Avenue
518-489-4471
Albany, NY 12206
e-mail: cbarr@joint-docs.com
www.joint-docs.com
This is a committed research facility as well as a medical practice. Our research practice is made up of seven physicians a certified physician's assistant and four research coordinators. We may have as many as 20 ongoing trails at a time in various indications within the study of rheumatology. Investigational treatment of interstitial lung disease associated with systemic sclerosis.
Norman R Romanoff, Practitioner
Joel M Kremer, Practitioner

7447 Georgetown University Hospital: Department of Rheumatology
3800 Reservoir Road NW
202-444-8233
Washington, DC 20007
Fax: 202-444-7584
www.medicine.georgetown.edu
Research is based on clinical trials and special interest in scleroderma and kidney pulmonary hypertension pregnancy epidemiology and natural history of scleroderma subsets.
Sherry Magrudar, Executive Assistant
Ann Nichols, Senior Adminstrator

7448 Johns Hopkins University: Scleroderma Center
Johns Hopkins Bayview Medical Center
5501 Hopkins Bayview Circle
410-550-7715
Baltimore, MD 21224
Fax: 410-550-1363
www.scleroderma.jhmi.edu
Specializes in the management of systemic sclerosis (scleroderma) Raynaud's phenomenon and related disorders. In addition to patient care the center is involved in both basic and clinical research projects.
Frederick M Wigley MD, Director
Sheila Friend, medical office coordinatorÿ

7449 Mayo Clinic Scottsdale Center for Scleroderma Care & Research
Mayo Clinic
13400 E Shea Boulevard
480-301-8000
Scottsdale, AZ 85259
800-446-2279
Fax: 480-301-7006
e-mail: newsbureau@mayo.edu
www.mayoclinic.org/rheumatology
Integrates multiple medical as well as surgical specialties under the direction of the Division of Rheumatology to provide coordinated and comprehensive evaluations and treatment. New clinical trails are in development.
John H. Noseworthy MD, President/CEO
April Chang-Miller, Assistant Professor of Medicine

7450 Medical University of South Carolina Medical University of South Carolina
Medical University of South Carolina
171 Ashley Avenue
843-792-1414
Charleston, SC 29425
800-424-6872
Fax: 843-792-2601
e-mail: wickman@musc.edu
www.musc.edu
Actively engaged in basic and clinical research of scleroderma.
Raymond S Greenburg, President
Dr. Mark Sothman, Vice President

7451 Scleroderma Clinical & Research Center State University of New York at Stonybro
State University of New York at Stonybrook
26 Research Way
631-444-0580
E Setauket, NY 01173-9260
Fax: 631-444-0562
www.scleroderma.org
Ongoing research of scleroderma.
Joseph Camerino, chair
Carol Feghali-Bostwick, Vce Chair

7452 Scleroderma Research Foundation
220 Montgomery Street
415-834-9444
San Francisco, CA 94104
800-637-4005
Fax: 415-834-9177
e-mail: info@sclerodermaresearch.org
www.srfcure.org
Mission is to find a cure for scleroderma a life threatening and degenerative illness by funding and facilitating the most promising highest quality research and placing the disease and its need for a cure in the public eye.
Alex Gonzalez, Director of Development
Amy Hewitt, Executive Director

7453 Thomas Jefferson University Hospital
111 S 11th Street
215-955-6840
Philadelphia, PA 19107
Fax: 215-923-5828
www.jeffersonhospital.org
Provides diagnostic evaluations treatment and access to the latest research studies for more than one thousand patients with scleroderma and related diseases.
Stephen K klasko, President/CEO
Sergio Jimen MD, Professor

7454 University of Alabama Birmingham
1720 second Av Soyth
Birmingham, AL 35294
205-934-4011
www.uab.edu
Located in the Clinical Immunology and Rheumatology department Oral Type 1 Collagen in Scleroderma is studied.
Carol Garrison, President
William Ferniany, CEO

7455 University of Chicago Center for Advanced Medicine Duchossis Center
University of Chicago hospital
5841 S Maryland Avenue
773-702-1000
Chicago, IL 60637
888-824-0200
Fax: 773-028-02
e-mail: orogers@medicine.bsd.uchicago.edu
www.uchospitals.com
Scleroderma clinic.
Michael Ellm MD, Clinic Contact
Ornery Rogers, Clinic Contact

7456 University of Illinois at Chicago Medical Center Outpatient Clinical Center
University of Illinois
600 S Hoyne Avenue
312-996-7000
Chicago, IL 60612
800-842-1002
Fax: 312-633-3434
TTY: 312-413-0123
e-mail: info@iMDc.org
www.uic.edu
Scleroderma clinic held on the first and third Thursdays of every month.
Paula Allen Meares, Chancellor
Lon S. Kauffman, Vice Chancellor

7457 University of Pittsburgh
4200 Fifth avenue
412-624-4141
Pittsburgh, PA 15260
Fax: 412-383-2264
e-mail: webmaster@pitt.edu
www.pitt.edu
Clinic and research of scleroderma.
Patricia E. Beeson, Vice Chancellor
John P Elliott, Director of Internal Affairs

7458 University of Tennessee Medical Group
956 Court Avenue
Memphis, TN 38103
901-866-8383
Fax: 901-866-8380
www.utmedicalgroup.com
Ongoing research protocols.
Charles E. Woeppel MD, CEO

7459 University of Texas Health Science Center
7000 Fannin
Houston, TX 77030
713-500-4472
Fax: 713-500-3026
e-mail: sclerodermaregister@uth.tmc.edu
www.uthouston.edu
Clinic research and clinical trials concerning scleroderma.
Giuseppe N. Colasurdo, President

Support Groups & Hotlines

7460 National Health Information Center
PO Box 1133
Washington, DC 20013
310-565-4167
800-336-4797
Fax: 301-984-4256
e-mail: info@nhic.org
www.health.gov/nhic
Offers a nationwide information referral service, produces directories and resource guides.

7461 Rhode Island Scleroderma Support Group
18 Talbot Manor
Cranston, RI 02905
401-781-5013
e-mail: scleroderma@hotmail.com
www.angelfire.com/ri/scleroderma
Meets on the fourth Wednsday of every month at Roger Williams Hospital.
Carole Cowell, President

7462 Scleroderma Support Groups
Scleroderma Foundation
12 Kent Way
Byfield, MA 01922
978-463-5843
800-722-4633
Fax: 978-463-5809
e-mail: sfinfo@scleroderma.org
www.scleroderma.org
Please contact the Scleroderma Foundation or visit our web site for a listing of support groups in your area.

Books

7463 Best of the Beacon
Scleroderma Foundation
12 Kent Way
Byfield, MA 01922
978-463-5843
800-722-4673
Fax: 978-463-5809
e-mail: sfinfo@scleroderma.org
www.scleroderma.org
Interesting, readable and highly practical collection of articles of particular interest to those living with scleroderma. This mini encyclopedia includes 11 medical articles, 358 most frequently asked questions, 34 sharing stories, 62 articles of special interest on a variety of useful topics and a glossary that defines 240 words you may encounter when reading about scleroderma.
Marie Coyle, Editor
Bianca Podesta, Author

7464 Handout on Health: Scleroderma
NAMSIC/National Institutes of Health
9000 Rockville Pike
Bethesda, MD 20892-0001
301-495-4484
877-226-4267
Fax: 301-718-6366
TTY: 301-565-2966
e-mail: niamsinfo@mail.nih.gov
www.nih.gov
143 pages

7465 Helpful Hints for Living with Scleroderma
Scleroderma Foundation

12 Kent Way
Byfield, MA 01922
978-463-5843
800-722-4673
Fax: 978-463-5809
e-mail: sfinfo@scleroderma.org
www.scleroderma.org
Booklet of helpful suggestions from our chapters and members, for the comfort and convienience of others who share the same challenges.
57 pages
Marie Coyle, Editor

7466 Perspectives on Living with Scleroderma
Scleroderma Foundation
12 Kent Way
Byfield, MA 01922
978-463-5843
800-722-4673
Fax: 978-463-5809
e-mail: sfinfo@scleroderma.org
www.scleroderma.org
Insightful articles on coping with scleroderma come from not only from Dr. Flapan's counseling and volunteer work, but also from his personal experience as a scleroderma patient.
233 pages

7467 Scleroderma Book
Scleroderma Foundation
12 Kent Way
Byfield, MA 01922
978-463-5843
800-722-4673
Fax: 978-463-5809
e-mail: sfinfo@scleroderma.org
www.scleroderma.org
Definitive guide to scleroderma for patients and their families, with easy to understand explanations.
182 pages
Maureen D. Mayes, Author

7468 Scleroderma: Surviving a Seventeen-Year Itch
Scleroderma Foundation

978-463-5809
800-722-4673
Fax: 978-463-5809
e-mail: sfinfo@scleroderma.org
www.scleroderma.org
Self-help manual including history, diagnosis, daily routines and exercise programs for persons with scleroderma.

7469 Scleroderma: a New Role for Patients and Families
Scleroderma Foundation
12 Kent Way
Byfield, MA 01922
978-463-5843
800-722-4673
Fax: 978-463-5809
e-mail: sfinfo@scleroderma.org
www.scleroderma.org
Provides an overview of key issues and offers resources that enable patients and their families to find more resources on thier own.
168 pages
Michael Brown, Author

7470 Understanding & Managing Scleroderma
Scleroderma Foundation
12 Kent Way
Byfield, MA 01923
978-463-5843
800-722-4633
Fax: 978-463-5809
e-mail: sfinfo@scleroderma.org
www.scleroderma.org
Booklet intended to help persons with scleroderma, their families and others interested in scleroderma to better understand what scleroderma is, what effects it may have, and what those with scleroderma can do to help themselves and their physicians manage the disease. It answers some of the most frequently asked questions about scleroderma.

Magazines

7471 Scleroderma Voice
Scleroderma Foundation

12 Kent Way
Byfield, MA 01922

978-463-5843
800-722-4673
Fax: 978-463-5809
e-mail: sfinfo@scleroderma.org
www.scleroderma.org

Feeatures the latest information available on scleroderma treatments and research. Subscription to the Voice includes a one-year membership in the Scleroderma Foundation.
Quarterly

Pamphlets

7472   If You Have Scleroderma You Need Not Feel Alone
Scleroderma Foundation
12 Kent Way
Byfield, MA 01922

978-463-5843
800-722-4673
Fax: 978-463-5809
e-mail: sfinfo@scleroderma.org
www.scleroderma.org

Scleroderma Foundation's membership brochure. Free of charge, also available in Spanish.

7473   Scleroderma: an Overview
Scleroderma Foundation
12 Kent Way
Byfield, MA 01922

978-463-5843
Fax: 978-463-5809
e-mail: sfinfo@scleroderma.org
www.scleroderma.org

Concise genral overview of sytemic scleroderma. Also available in Spanish, and downloadable in Portugese.

7474   What Causes Scleroderma?
Scleroderma Foundation
12 Kent Way
Byfield, MA 01922

978-463-5843
800-722-4673
Fax: 978-463-5809
e-mail: sfinfo@scleroderma.org
www.scleroderma.org

Discusses the puzzling nature of scleroderma. Also available in Spanish, and downloadable in Portugese.

Web Sites

7475   Healing Well

www.healingwell.com

An online health resource guide to medical news, chat, information and articles, newsgroups and message boards, books, disease-related web sites, medical directories, and more for patients, friends, and family coping with disabling diseases, disorders, or chronic illnesses.

7476   Health Finder

www.healthfinder.gov

Searchable, carefully developed web site offering information on over 1000 topics. Developed by the US Department of Health and Human Services, the site can be used in both English and Spanish.

7477   Healthlink USA

www.healthlinkusa.com

Health information concerning treatment, cures, prevention, diagnosis, risk factors, research, support groups, email lists, personal stories and much more. Updated regularly.

7478   Helios Health

www.helioshealth.com

Online resource for your health information. Detailed information about specific health topics, access to expert advice from our Medical Advisory Board, and up-to-date health news.

7479   MedicineNet

www.medicinenet.com

An online resource for consumers providing easy-to-read, authoritative medical and health information.

7480   Medscape

www.medscape.com

Medscape offers specialists, primary care physicians, and other health professionals the Web's most robust and integrated medical information and educational tools.

7481   Scleroderma Foundation

www.scleroderma.org

501 (c)3 national nonprofit organization serving the interests of persons with scleroderma. The Foundation's 26 chapters and 135 support groups nationwide help to carry out its three-fold mission of support, education and research. The Scleroderma Foundation is a leading nonprofit supporter of scleroderma research — funding over $1 million of new grants each year to find the cause and cure of scleroderma.

7482   WebMD

www.webmd.com

Provides credible information, supportive communities, and in-depth reference material about health subjects. A source for original and timely health information as well as material from well known content providers.

Description

7483 Scoliosis

Scoliosis is a lateral curvature of the spine, with 60 to 80 percent of the cases occurring in girls. It may first be suspected when one of the teenager's shoulders appears higher than the other or clothes don't hang straight. The spinal curve is more pronounced when the adolescent bends forward. More than 80 percent of scoliosis is idiopathic, that is, there is no known cause.

Symptoms include prominent shoulder blades, uneven hip levels, and fatigue in the lower back after sitting or standing for prolonged periods of time. In many cases there are no symptoms unless the scoliosis is severe.

The prognosis depends on the site and severity of the curve, and the age of onset of symptoms. Early detection through school screening provides more treatment options, and prompt referral to an orthopedist is indicated. The majority of cases require only observation for progression. Approximately 20 percent of those with scoliosis will require an orthopedic brace or spinal fusion surgery.

National Agencies & Associations

7484 American Academy of Orthopaedic Surgeons
6300 N River Road
Rosemont, IL 60018-4238
847-823-7186
800-346-2267
Fax: 847-823-8125
e-mail: custserv@aaos.org
www.aaos.org

The American Academy of Orthopaedic Surgeons provides education and practice management services for orthopaedic surgeons and allied health professionals. The Academy also serves as an advocate for improved patient care and informs the public.
Joshua J. Jacobs, President
Andrew N. Pollack, Treasurer

7485 International Federation of Spine Associations
Howard M Shulman
9908 Cape Scott Court
Raleigh, NC 27614-9025
919-846-2204
www.scoliosisrx.com

IFOSA is a federation of various national Spine Associations from countries in North America Europe and Australia. These organizations principally represent the spine patients and their families.

7486 National Scoliosis Foundation
5 Cabot Place
Stoughton, MA 02072
781-341-6333
800-673-6922
Fax: 781-341-8333
e-mail: NSF@scoliosis.org
www.scoliosis.org

Promotes school screening offers public awareness materials to promote public education maintains a resource center for professional information conducts scoliosis conferences and offers support groups to people affected by the disease.
Joseph P O'Brien, President/CEO
Dennis J Fusco, Treasurer

7487 Scoliosis Association
PO Box 811705
Boca Raton, FL 33481-1705
561-994-4435
800-800-0669
Fax: 561-994-2455
e-mail: normlipin@aol.com
www.scoliosis-assoc.org

Sponsors and encourages spinal screening programs. Disseminates information throughout the country and raises funds for scoliosis research. Membership fee includes subscription to newsletter. Videos and printed information available.

Research Centers

7488 Scoliosis Research Society
555 E Wells Street
Milwaukee, WI 53202
414-289-9107
Fax: 414-276-3349
e-mail: info@srs.org
www.srs.org

This society provides an international forum for those interested in the management of spinal deformities. It holds a yearly meeting at which health professionals meet to share observations and results and to explore new avenues of research.
Kamal N. Ibrahim, President
Hubert Labelle, Treasurer

7489 Shriners Hospital for Crippled Children Chicago Unit
Chicago Unit
2211 N Oak Park Avenue
Chicago, IL 60707
813-281-0300
Fax: 773-855-88
www.shrinershospitalsforchildren.org

A 60-bed orthopedic hospital providing comprehensive spinal cord injury care to children. Provides care for spinal deformities Cerebral Palsy Osteoeneisis Imperfecta and Scoliosis as well as others.
John A. Cinotto, Chairman
Diether Sturm, Chief of Staff

Support Groups & Hotlines

7490 National Health Information Center
PO Box 1133
Washington, DC 20013
310-565-4167
800-336-4797
Fax: 301-984-4256
e-mail: info@nhic.org
www.health.gov/nhic

Offers a nationwide information referral service, produces directories and resource guides.

Books

7491 Adult Scoliosis Surgery...It Can Be Done
St. Luke's Spine Center
555 East Wells Street
Milwaukee, WI 53202-3805
414-289-9107
Fax: 414-276-3349
e-mail: info@srs.org
www.srs.org

21 pages
Ashtin Neuschaefer, Administrative Manager
Lily Atonio, Education and Program Manager

7492 Coalition Index
American School Health Association
7918 Jones Branch Drive
McLean, VA 22102
703-506-7675
800-445-2742
Fax: 703-506-3266
e-mail: info@ashaweb.org
www.ashaweb.org

Linda Morse, President
Ty Oehrtman, Vice President

7493 Getting Ready, Getting Well
National Scoliosis Foundation
5 Cabot Place
Stoughton, MA 02072
781-341-6333
800-673-6922
Fax: 781-341-8333
e-mail: NSF@scoliosis.org
www.scoliosis.org

73 pages
Joseph P O'Brien, President/CEO

7494 Handbook of Scoliosis
Scoliosis Research Society

555 East Wells Street
Milwaukee, WI 53202

414-289-9107
Fax: 414-276-3349
e-mail: info@srs.org
www.srs.org

Ashtin Neuschaefer, Administrative Manager
Lily Atonio, Education and Program Manager

7495 Stopping Scoliosis
National Scoliosis Foundation
5 Cabot Place
Stoughton, MA 02072

781-341-6333
800-673-6922
Fax: 781-341-8333
e-mail: NSF@scoliosis.org
www.scoliosis.org

Joseph P O'Brien, President/CEO

7496 Twenty Years at Hull House
New American Library
375 Hudson Street
New York, NY 10014
Grades 7-12

212-366-2000

Children's Books

7497 Deenie
Bradbury Press
866 3rd Avenue
New York, NY 10022-6221

212-702-2000
800-257-5755

Deenie, a beautiful thirteen-year-old girl, had a mother who was pushing her to become a model. The agency representatives told Deenie she had the looks but walked differently. Deenie's main wish was to become a cheerleader. Her close friend, Janet, made the cheerleading squad but Deenie didn't make the finalist list. After this her gym teacher noticed her posture and called her family. After seeing therapists, the diagnosis of adolescent idiopathic scoliosis was made.
159 pages Hardcover
ISBN: 0-027110-20-6

7498 Tina's Story...Scoliosis and Me
Alfred I DuPont Institute
555 East Wells Street
Milwaukee, WI 53202

414-289-9107
Fax: 414-276-3349
e-mail: info@srs.org
www.srs.org

Ashtin Neuschaefer, Administrative Manager
Lily Atonio, Education and Program Manager

7499 What Young People and Parents Need to Know about Scoliosis
American Physical Therapy Association
5 Cabot Place
Stoughton, MA 02072

781-341-6333
800-673-6922
Fax: 781-341-8333
e-mail: NSF@scoliosis.org
www.scoliosis.org

A physical therapist's perspective.

Newsletters

7500 Backtalk
Scoliosis Association
5 Cabot Place
Stoughton, MA 02072-1705

781-341-6333
800-673-6922
Fax: 781-341-8333
e-mail: NSF@scoliosis.org
www.scoliosis.org

Information for families, patients and health care professionals.

Pamphlets

7501 1 in Every 10 Persons Has Scoliosis
National Scoliosis Foundation
5 Cabot Place
Stoughton, MA 02072

781-341-6333
800-673-6922
Fax: 781-341-8333
e-mail: NSF@scoliosis.org
www.scoliosis.org

Explains what scoliosis is and illustrates how to screen for it. It also contains facts about the Foundation.
Joseph P O'Brien, President/CEO

7502 Adolescent Idiopathic Scoliosis: Prevelance, Natural History, Treatments
National Scoliosis Foundation
5 Cabot Place
Stoughton, MA 02072

781-341-6333
800-673-6922
Fax: 781-341-8333
e-mail: NSF@scoliosis.org
www.scoliosis.org

Expert overview of a condition that affects many young people.
Joseph P O'Brien, President/CEO

7503 Boston Bracing System for Idiopathic Scoliosis
National Scoliosis Foundation
5 Cabot Place
Stoughton, MA 02072

781-341-6333
800-673-6922
Fax: 781-341-8333
e-mail: NSF@scoliosis.org
www.scoliosis.org

Explaination of an available option.
Joseph P O'Brien, President/CEO

7504 Brace & Her Brace is No Handicap
National Scoliosis Foundation
5 Cabot Place
Stoughton, MA 02072

781-341-6333
800-673-6922
Fax: 781-341-8333
e-mail: NSF@scoliosis.org
www.scoliosis.org

Contains two illustrated short stories, each about a teenage girl coping successfully with scoliosis.
Joseph P O'Brien, President/CEO

7505 Getting a Second Opinion
National Scoliosis Foundation
5 Cabot Place
Stoughton, MA 02072

781-341-6333
800-673-6922
Fax: 781-341-8333
e-mail: NSF@scoliosis.org
www.scoliosis.org

Reprinted from Health Tips.
Joseph P O'Brien, President/CEO

7506 Going Home
University Hospital Spine Center
2074 Abington Road
Cleveland, OH 44106

216-844-1616

Instructions for pediatric and adult patients who have had a spinal fusion.

7507 Medical Update Column
National Scoliosis Foundation
5 Cabot Place
Stoughton, MA 02072

781-341-6333
800-673-6922
Fax: 781-341-8333
e-mail: NSF@scoliosis.org
www.scoliosis.org

Reprints from past issues of the Spinal Connections Medical Update Column available on various topics.
Joseph P O'Brien, President/CEO

7508 NSF Packets
National Scoliosis Foundation
5 Cabot Place
Stoughton, MA 02072

781-341-6333
800-673-6922
Fax: 781-341-8333
e-mail: NSF@scoliosis.org
www.scoliosis.org

Packet contains information for parents and young people, adults, and healthcare professionals.
Joseph P O'Brien, President/CEO

7509 Patient with Scoliosis
Educational Services, Division of AJV Company
555 East Wells Street
Milwaukee, WI 53202-2925

414-289-9107
Fax: 414-276-3349
e-mail: info@srs.org
www.srs.org

A reprint from the American Journal of nursin.
Ashtin Neuschaefer, Administrative Manager
Lily Atonio, Education and Program Manager

7510   Postural Screening Program
National Scoliosis Foundation
5 Cabot Place
Stoughton, MA 02072   781-341-6333
                                              800-673-6922
                                         Fax: 781-341-8333
                               e-mail: NSF@scoliosis.org
                                         www.scoliosis.org

Guidelines for physicians and school nurses.
Joseph P O'Brien, President/CEO

7511   Questions Most Often Asked the NSF
National Scoliosis Foundation
5 Cabot Place
Stoughton, MA 02072   781-341-6333
                                              800-673-6922
                                         Fax: 781-341-8333
                               e-mail: NSF@scoliosis.org
                                         www.scoliosis.org

Answers the most frequently asked questions about scoliosis and
the foundation in general.
Joseph P O'Brien, President/CEO

7512   Scoliosis
Scoliosis Research Society
555 East Wells Street
Milwaukee, WI 53202   414-289-9107
                                         Fax: 414-276-3349
                                   e-mail: info@srs.org
                                              www.srs.org

Brochure describing scoliosis, kyphosis, lordosis; causes, preven-
tion, treatment and adult scoliosis.
Ashtin Neuschaefer, Administrative Manager
Lily Atonio, Education and Program Manager

7513   Scoliosis Patient Becomes a Model
National Scoliosis Foundation
5 Cabot Place
Stoughton, MA 02072   781-341-6333
                                              800-673-6922
                                         Fax: 781-341-8333
                               e-mail: NSF@scoliosis.org
                                         www.scoliosis.org

Reprinted from Children's Today.
Joesph P O'Brien, President/CEO

7514   Scoliosis Road Map
University Hospital Spine Center
555 East Wells Street
Milwaukee, WI 53202   414-289-9107
                                         Fax: 414-276-3349
                                   e-mail: info@srs.org
                                              www.srs.org

Written for teenagers affected by this illness.
Ashtin Neuschaefer, Administrative Manager
Lily Atonio, Education and Program Manager

7515   Scoliosis Screening: The Carlsbad Program
National Scoliosis Foundation
5 Cabot Place
Stoughton, MA 02072   781-341-6333
                                              800-673-6922
                                         Fax: 781-341-8333
                               e-mail: NSF@scoliosis.org
                                         www.scoliosis.org

Exceptional scoliosis screening program.
Joseph P O'Brien, President/CEO

7516   Scoliosis Surgery, What's It All About?
University Hospital Spine Center
555 East Wells Street
Milwaukee, WI 53202   414-289-9107
                                         Fax: 414-276-3349
                                   e-mail: info@srs.org
                                              www.srs.org

This pamphlet answers many of the questions patients ask before
having surgery.
Ashtin Neuschaefer, Administrative Manager
Lily Atonio, Education and Program Manager

7517   Scoliosis and Kyphosis
Scoliosis Research Society
555 East Wells Street
Milwaukee, WI 53202   414-289-9107
                                         Fax: 414-276-3349
                                      e-mail: info@srs.org
                                              www.srs.org

Information and advice from parents.
Ashtin Neuschaefer, Administrative Manager
Lily Atonio, Education and Program Manager

7518   Scoliosis, Me?
North Dallas Scoliosis Center
555 East Wells Street
Milwaukee, WI 53202-3525   414-289-9107
                                         Fax: 414-276-3349
                                    e-mail: info@srs.org
                                              www.srs.org

Detailed answers to questions most asked by parents and teens.
Ashtin Neuschaefer, Administrative Manager
Lily Atonio, Education and Program Manager

7519   Scoliosis... Now it Can Be Treated in Adults as Well as Children
National Scoliosis Foundation
5 Cabot Place
Stoughton, MA 02072   781-341-6333
                                              800-673-6922
                                         Fax: 781-341-8333
                               e-mail: NSF@scoliosis.org
                                         www.scoliosis.org

Reprinted from Cleveland Magazine.
Joseph P O'Brien, President/CEO

7520   Scoliosis: Handbook for Patients
National Scoliosis Foundation
5 Cabot Place
Stoughton, MA 02072   781-341-6333
                                              800-673-6922
                                         Fax: 781-341-8333
                               e-mail: NSF@scoliosis.org
                                         www.scoliosis.org

Information on detection and treatment of adolescent scoliosis,
kyphosis and lordosis and adult scoliosis.
Joseph P O'Brien, President/CEO

7521   Screening Procedure Guidelines for Spinal Deformity
Scoliosis Research Society
555 East Wells Street
Milwaukee, WI 53202   414-289-9107
                                         Fax: 414-276-3349
                                    e-mail: info@srs.org
                                              www.srs.org

Seven page brochure covers reasons, organizations and procedures for spinal screening. Signs of spinal deformity, as seen in
both standing and forward bending positions are illustrated and
discussed. Includes sample screening form.
7 pages
Ashtin Neuschaefer, Administrative Manager
Lily Atonio, Education and Program Manager

7522   Spinal Deformity: Congenital Scoliosis and Kyphosis
Scoliosis Research Society
555 East Wells Street
Milwaukee, WI 53202   414-289-9107
                                         Fax: 414-276-3349
                                    e-mail: info@srs.org
                                              www.srs.org

Discusses signs and causes of congenital spinal deformities, associated conditions, treatment options and a glossary of terms.
12 pages
Ashtin Neuschaefer, Administrative Manager
Lily Atonio, Education and Program Manager

7523   Spinal Deformity: Scoliosis and Kyphosis
Scoliosis Research Society
555 East Wells Street
Milwaukee, WI 53202   414-289-9107
                                         Fax: 414-276-3349
                                    e-mail: info@srs.org
                                              www.srs.org

Twelve page brochure discusses signs and causes of scoliosis and
kyphosis, indications for treatment, treatment options, commonly
asked questions and a glossary of terms.
12 pages
Ashtin Neuschaefer, Administrative Manager
Lily Atonio, Education and Program Manager

7524 What Young People & Their Parents Need to Know About Scoliosis
American Physical Therapy Association
555 East Wells Street
Milwaukee, WI 53202-1488
414-289-9107
Fax: 414-276-3349
e-mail: info@srs.org
www.srs.org

A physical therapists' perspective.
Ashtin Neuschaefer, Administrative Manager
Lily Atonio, Education and Program Manager

7525 What if You Need an Operation for Scoliosis?
St. Luke's Spine Center
555 East Wells Street
Milwaukee, WI 53202-3805
414-289-9107
Fax: 414-276-3349
e-mail: info@srs.org
www.srs.org

Ashtin Neuschaefer, Administrative Manager
Lily Atonio, Education and Program Manager

7526 When the Spine Curves
National Scoliosis Foundation
5 Cabot Place
Stoughton, MA 02072
781-341-6333
800-673-6922
Fax: 781-341-8333
e-mail: NSF@scoliosis.org
www.scoliosis.org

Joseph P O'Brien, President/CEO

7527 You and Your Brace
University Hospital Spine Center
152 South Street
Bridgewater, MA 02324 e-mail: smilemaker@archorthodontics.com
www.archorthodontics.com

Audio & Video

7528 Cutting Edge Medical Report
National Scoliosis Foundation
5 Cabot Place
Stoughton, MA 02072
781-341-6333
800-673-6922
Fax: 781-341-8333
e-mail: NSF@scoliosis.org
www.scoliosis.org
As seen on the Discovery Channel, this video is an indepth examination of the latest developments in the diagnosis and treatment of scoliosis.
Joseph P O'Brien, President/CEO

7529 Growing Straighter and Stronger
National Scoliosis Foundation
5 Cabot Place
Stoughton, MA 02072
781-341-6333
800-673-6922
Fax: 781-341-8333
e-mail: NSF@scoliosis.org
www.scoliosis.org
Fifteen-minute presentation available in VHS video format, for the pre-screening education of students in grades 5 through 7.
Videotape
Joseph P O'Brien, President/CEO

7530 Preparing Yourself for Spinal Surgery for Teenagers with Severe Scoliosis
National Scoliosis Foundation
5 Cabot Place
Stoughton, MA 02072
781-341-6333
800-673-6922
Fax: 781-341-8333
e-mail: NSF@scoliosis.org
www.scoliosis.org
Patient education video helping to reduce anxiety for teenagers facing surgery by giving a sense of what to expect before, during, and after surgery.
Joseph P O'Brien, President/CEO

7531 School Screening with Dr. Robert Keller
National Scoliosis Foundation

5 Cabot Place
Stoughton, MA 02072
781-341-6333
800-673-6922
Fax: 781-341-8333
e-mail: NSF@scoliosis.org
www.scoliosis.org
Training video that teaches the proper technique for doing spinal screening. Defines scoliosis and kyphosis. Four teenagers, three with curves and one without, are examined and the findings explained.
Videotape
Joseph P O'Brien, President/CEO

7532 Scoliosis: An Adult Perspective
National Scoliosis Foundation
5 Cabot Place
Stoughton, MA 02072
781-341-6333
800-673-6922
Fax: 781-341-8333
e-mail: NSF@scoliosis.org
www.scoliosis.org
Dr. Blackman and five women patients provide an overall perspective of what scoliosis is, who gets it, the types of devices, myths about the disorder, and options for treatment.
Joseph P O'Brien, President/CEO

7533 Sharing Scoliosis: You're Not Alone
National Scoliosis Foundation
5 Cabot Place
Stoughton, MA 02072
781-341-6333
800-673-6922
Fax: 781-341-8333
e-mail: NSF@scoliosis.org
www.scoliosis.org
The Missouri chapter of the NSF, shares their experience with scoliosis including diagnosis, wearing a brace, surgery, and recovery. It is a good source of support for patients of all ages and their families.
Joseph P O'Brien, President/CEO

7534 Spinal Screening Program
Scoliosis Research Society
555 East Wells Street
Milwaukee, WI 53202
414-289-9107
Fax: 414-276-3349
e-mail: info@srs.org
www.srs.com
Twenty minute videotape designed to instruct screeners in the spinal screening program. It demonstrates methods of screening, showing adolescents with normal and abnormal spines. Includes sample screening form.
VHS Video Tape
Ashtin Neuschaefer, Administrative Manager
Lily Atonio, Education and Program Manager

7535 Taking the Mystery Out of Spinal Deformities
Children's Hospital of LA, Div. of Orthopaedics
1300 N. Vermont
Los Angeles, CA 90027
213-660-2450
800-841-7439
e-mail: RWETZEL@chla.usc.edu
www.answers4families.org
Answers questions most often asked by screeners, patients and parents.
Videotape

7536 Understanding Scoliosis
National Scoliosis Foundation
5 Cabot Place
Stoughton, MA 02072
781-341-6333
800-673-6922
Fax: 781-341-8333
e-mail: NSF@scoliosis.org
www.scoliosis.org
Kaiser Permanente's educational video clearly and positively addresses the patient community. In this video four teenagers at various stages of treatment talk about their life with scoliosis.
Joseph P O'Brien, President/CEO

7537 What's This Thing Called Scoliosis
National Scoliosis Foundation
5 Cabot Place
Stoughton, MA 02072
781-341-6333
800-673-6922
Fax: 781-341-8333
e-mail: NSF@scoliosis.org
www.scoliosis.org

Comprehensive overview of scoliosis using the latest computer technology. The anatomical spine and animated model work together to truly show the 3D aspects of scoliosis and the corresponding impact on the patient.
Joseph P O'Brien, President/CEO

7538 You Are Not Alone
Minnesota Spine Center
606 24th Avenue S
Minneapolis, MN 55454-1438   612-332-3843
A video presenting two women's experiences with surgery. Personal life, concerns, hospital experience, recovery and improved lifestyle are openly discussed.
Videotape

Web Sites

7539 American Association of Neurological Surgeons
www.neurosurgery.org/
Official web site of the American Association of Neurological Surgeons and Congress of Neurological Surgeons. Whether you are a patient, physician, health care professional, or member of the media, this site is your online resource for neurosurgical information.

7540 British Scoliosis Research Society
www.ndos.ox.ac.uk/pzs/
This site contains: background to the meeting, Scoliosis Research Society review papers on the aetiology of idiopathic scoliosis, a list of participants, abstracts classified by discussion group and the chairman's conclusions for each group.

7541 Healing Well
www.healingwell.com
An online health resource guide to medical news, chat, information and articles, newsgroups and message boards, books, disease-related web sites, medical directories, and more for patients, friends, and family coping with disabling diseases, disorders, or chronic illnesses.

7542 Health Finder
www.healthfinder.gov
Searchable, carefully developed web site offering information on over 1000 topics. Developed by the US Department of Health and Human Services, the site can be used in both English and Spanish.

7543 Healthlink USA
www.healthlinkusa.com
Health information concerning treatment, cures, prevention, diagnosis, risk factors, research, support groups, email lists, personal stories and much more. Updated regularly.

7544 Helios Health
www.helioshealth.com
Online resource for your health information. Detailed information about specific health topics, access to expert advice from our Medical Advisory Board, and up-to-date health news.

7545 MedicineNet
www.medicinenet.com
An online resource for consumers providing easy-to-read, authoritative medical and health information.

7546 Medscape
www.medscape.com
Medscape offers specialists, primary care physicians, and other health professionals the Web's most robust and integrated medical information and educational tools.

7547 Patients Rate Their Scoliosis Doctors
This web site is a free internet service for communicating subjective impressions of medical doctor (MD) reputations among scoliosis patients. Please use this system to learn some of the subjective impressions of the treatment other patients have received from their doctors.

7548 Scoliosis Association
www.sauk.org.uk/
The Scoliosis Association (UK) was founded in 1981. It is the only independent support group for scoliosis in the UK. SAUK aims to

provide information about scoliosis, eliminate fear and stigma, and offer contacts for shared experiences.

7549 WebMD
www.webmd.com
Provides credible information, supportive communities, and in-depth reference material about health subjects. A source for original and timely health information as well as material from well known content providers.

Description

7550 Seizure Disorders

There are two types of seizure disorders: an isolated, nonrecurring attack, such as may occur with high fevers in children, head trauma, or from other diseases (metabolic abnormalities or brain tumor) and epilepsy, which is characterized by recurrent, sudden, rapid changes in brain function caused by abnormalities in the electrical activity of the brain. Roughly 2 million Americans suffer from epilepsy, with half of the cases found in children and adolescents.

Seizures can be classified as generalized, affecting the whole brain at once, or partial, affecting a part of the brain. Absence (petit mal) attacks are generalized seizures in which there is only a brief (10-30 second) loss of consciousness, with eye and muscle fluttering but no loss of muscle tone. A generalized tonic-clonic seizure (grand mal) usually lasts 1-2 minutes, and includes loss of consciousness, falling, and involuntary contractions of the arms and legs. Some patients report that they see flashing lights and experience a heightened sense of taste and smell (known as an aura) that indicates they are about to have a seizure.

In many cases there is no apparent cause of the disorder, and it is therefore called idiopathic epilepsy.

Treatment aims primarily to control seizures. Causative or precipitating factors should be eliminated. Drug treatment is the mainstay of therapy for most types of seizures. In order to limit toxic effects, an attempt is made to use only a single drug. Some patients may need to take more than one drug. In most cases, acceptable control can be achieved with medications alone. Rarely, seizures will not respond to drugs, and surgery on the brain will be recommended. In this procedure, the surgeon tries to identify and destroy the part of the brain that is triggering the seizures.

National Agencies & Associations

7551 American Epilepsy Society
342 N Main Street   860-586-7505
W Hartford, CT 06117-2500   Fax: 860-568-7550
e-mail: ctubby@aesnet.org
www.aesnet.org
Fosters treatment of epilepsy in its biological clinical and social phases.
M Suzanne C Berry, Executive Director
Cheryl-Ann Tubby, Assistant Executive Director

7552 Epilepsy Foundation
8301 Professional Place   866-330-2718
Landover, MD 20785   800-332-1000
Fax: 301-459-1569
e-mail: postmaster@efa.org
www.epilepsyfoundation.org
A national charitable nonprofit volunteer agency in the US dedicated to the welfare of people with epilepsy. Its goals are the prevention and cure of seizure disorders, the alleviation of their effects and the promotion of independence.
Lee Gaston, CFO
Phil Gattone, President & CEO

7553 National Association of Epilepsy Centers
5775 Wayzata Boulevard   202-484-1100
Minneapolis, MN 55416-1222   888-525-6232
Fax: 202-484-1244
e-mail: info@naec-epilepsy.org
www.naec-epilepsy.org
A nonprofit organization that encourages and supports professional and technical education in the treatment of epilepsy. Over 50 centers nationwide are members of the trade association which will make referrals to its member centers.
David M. Labiner, President
Nathan B. Fountain, VP

7554 National Institute of Neurological Disorders and Stroke
NIH Neurological Institute   301-496-5751
Bethesda, MD 20824   800-352-9424
Fax: 301-402-2186
TTY: 301-468-5981
www.ninds.nih.gov
The mission of NINDS is to reduce the burden of neurological disease - a burden borne by every age group, by every segment of society, by people all over the world.
Story C Landis PhD, Director
Walter J Koroshetz, Deputy Director

State Agencies & Associations

California

7555 Epilepsy Foundation of Northern California
5700 Stoneridge Mall Road   415-677-4011
Pleasanton, CA 94588-2824   800-632-3532
Fax: 415-677-4190
e-mail: efnca@epilepsynorcal.org
www.epilepsynorcal.org
Nonprofit organization serving families affected by epilepsy.
Katherine Keene, President & CEO
Mary Lee Cascino, Programme Manager

District of Columbia

7556 Administration for Children and Families
370 L'Enfant Promenade
Washington, DC 20447   www.acf.hhs.gov
The Administration for Children & Families (ACF) is a division of the U.S. Department of Health & Human Services (HHS). ACF promotes the economic and social well-being of families, children, individuals and communities.
Mark Greenberg, Acting Assistant Secretary
Jeff Hild, Chief of Staff

7557 National Institute for Occupational Safety and Health
395 E Street, SW   202-245-0625
Washington, DC 20201   800-232-4636
Fax: 513-533-8347
TTY: 888-232-6348
www.cdc.gov/niosh/
The National Institute for Occupational Safety and Health (NIOSH) is the U.S. federal agency that conducts research and makes recommendations to prevent worker injury and illness.
John Howard, MD, Director
Frank Hearl, PE, Chief of Staff

Florida

7558 Epilepsy Association of Big Bend
1215 Lee Avenue   850-222-1777
Tallahassee, FL 32303-2651   Fax: 850-222-7440
e-mail: epilepsyassoc@embarqmail.com
www.epilepsyassoc.org
Services include: Case management, prevention education, counseling and advocacy, information and referral.

7559 Epilepsy Foundation of South Florida
7300 N Kendall Drive   305-670-4949
Miami, FL 33156-7840   Fax: 305-670-0904
e-mail: information@epilepsysofla.org
www.epilepsyfound.org

A twenty five year old nonprofit community based organization dedicated to enhancing the personal and social adjustments of individuals with seizure disorders and their families.
Karen Basha Egozi, Executive Director
Ana Alfonso, Executive Administrator

7560   Epilepsy Services Foundation
4618 N Armenia Avenue   813-374-8907
Tampa, FL 33603-2706   Fax: 813-443-5546
                                      e-mail: info@epilepsysf.org
                                             www.epilepsysf.org
Information on medical and supportive services for persons affected by epilepsy living in West Central Florida. Raise funds to provide medical and supportive services and to build an endowment to make a difference in the lives of generations to come.
Thomas Orth, Executive Director

7561   Epilepsy Services of North Central Florida
11200 NW 8th Avenue   352-392-6449
Gainesville, FL 32601-4946   800-330-9746
                                           Fax: 352-392-5792
                            e-mail: jlyons@college.med.ufl.edu
                         www.floridaepilepsy.org/northcentral.htm
Jim Lyons, Program Director
Mike Dorsey, PE Coordinator

7562   Epilepsy Services of Northeast Florida
5209 San Jose Boulevard   904-731-3751
Jacksonville, FL 32207-2267   e-mail: epilepsy@bellsouth.net
Services include: Program case management, program prevention and education, employment services, children's summer camp, counseling and advocacy, and information and referrals.

7563   Epilepsy Services of Southwest Florida
1900 Main Street   941-953-5988
Sarasota, FL 34236   Fax: 941-366-5890
                            www.epilepsyservicesofswfl.org
Dedicated to providing case management and medical services for individuals with seizure disorders who meet eligibility criteria. Provides employment education for individuals and families affected by seizure disorders and prevention education to the com
Thomas Garrity, Executive Director

7564   Manattee County Office Epilepsy Services of Southwest Florida
1701 14th Street W   941-746-6488
Bradenton, FL 34205-7132   Fax: 941-746-8382
                            e-mail: bardentonep@aol.com
Brian Larocque, Social Worker

Georgia

7565   Agency for Toxic Substances and Disease Registry
4770 Buford Hwy NE
Atlanta, GA 30341
                                               800-232-4636
                                          TTY: 888-232-6348
                                             www.atsdr.cdc.gov
The Agency for Toxic Substances and Disease Registry (ATSDR), based in Atlanta, Georgia, is a federal public health agency of the U.S. Department of Health and Human Services. ATSDR serves the public by using the best science, taking responsive public health actions, and providing trusted health information to prevent harmful exposures and diseases related to toxic substances.
Patrick Breysse, PhD, CIH, Director
Donna Knutson, PhD, Acting Deputy Director

Maryland

7566   Agency for Healthcare Research and Quality
540 Gaither Road
Rockville, MD 20850
                                               301-427-1364
                                         www.ahrq.gov/index.html
The Agency for Healthcare Research and Quality's (AHRQ) mission is to produce evidence to make health care safer, higher quality, more accessible, equitable, and affordable, and to work within the U.S. Department of Health and Human Services and with other partners to make sure that the evidence is understood and used.
Richard G. Kronick, PhD, Director, Director
Sharon B. Arnold, PhD, Deputy Director

7567   Centers for Medicare and Medicaid Services
7500 Security Boulevard   410-786-3000
Baltimore, MD 21244   877-267-2323
                                          TTY: 866-226-1819
                              e-mail: Mandy.Cohen@cms.hhs.gov
                                                  www.cms.gov
US federal agency which administers Medicare, Medicaid, and the State Children's Health Insurance Program.
Dr. Mandy Cohen, M.D., MPH, Chief of Staff
Timothy P. Love, Chief Operating Officer

7568   National Center for Complementary and Integrative Health
9000 Rockville Pike
Bethesda, MD 20892   888-644-6226
                                          TTY: 866-464-3615
                             e-mail: nccih-info@mail.nih.gov
                                              nccih.nih.gov
The National Center for Complementary and Integrative Health (NCCIH) is the Federal Government's lead agency for scientific research on the diverse medical and health care systems, practices, and products that are not generally considered part of conventional medicine.
Josephine P. Briggs, M.D., Director
David Shurtleff, Ph.D., Deputy Director

7569   National Human Genome Research Institute
Building 31, Room 4B09   301-402-0911
Bethesda, MD 20892   Fax: 301-402-2218
                                             www.genome.gov
The National Human Genome Research Institute began as the National Center for Human Genome Research (NCHGR), which was established in 1989 to carry out the role of the National Institutes of Health (NIH) in the International Human Genome Project (HGP).
Eric D. Green, M.D., Ph.D., Director
Lawrence Brody, Ph.D., Director, Division of Genomics & Society

7570   National Institute of Biomedical Imaging an Bioengineering
9000 Rockville Pike   301-496-8859
Bethesda, MD 20892   e-mail: info@nibib.nih.gov
                                             www.nibib.nih.gov
The mission of the National Institute of Biomedical Imaging and Bioengineering (NIBIB) is to improve health by leading the development and accelerating the application of biomedical technologies.
Roderic I. Pettigrew, Ph.D., M.D., Director
Marcella Canada, Administrative Officer

7571   National Institute of General Medical Sciences
45 Center Drive MSC 6200   301-496-7301
Bethesda, MD 20892   e-mail: info@nigms.nih.gov
                                             www.nigms.nih.gov
The National Institute of General Medical Sciences (NIGMS) supports basic research that increases understanding of biological processes and lays the foundation for advances in disease diagnosis, treatment and prevention.
Jon R. Lorsch, Ph.D., Director
Judith H. Greenberg, Ph.D., Deputy Director

7572   U.S. Food and Drug Administration
10903 New Hampshire Ave   301-796-8240
Silver Spring, MD 20993   888-463-6332
                                                  www.fda.gov
FDA is responsible for protecting the public health by assuring the safety, efficacy and security of human and veterinary drugs, biological products, medical devices, our nation's food supply, cosmetics, and products that emit radiation.
Stephen Ostroff, M.D., Acting Commissioner
James Tyler, Chief Financial Officer

New Jersey

7573 **Epilepsy Foundation of New Jersey**
429 River View Plaza
Trenton, NJ 08611-3420
800-336-5843
800-336-5843
Fax: 609-392-5621
TTY: 800-852-7899
TDD: 800-852-7899
e-mail: efnj@efnj.com
www.efnj.com

Robert L. D'Avanzo, President
Michael P. Rinaldo, Chairman of the Board

New York

7574 **Epilepsy Foundation of Long Island**
506 Stewart Avenue
Garden City, NY 11530-4700
516-739-7733
888-672-7154
Fax: 516-794-2180
e-mail: info@epil.org
www.efli.org

Jeffrey L. Nagel, President
Henry Klosowski, Vice President

North Carolina

7575 **National Institute of Environmental Health Sciences**
111 T.W. Alexander Drive
919-541-4580
Research Triangle Park, NC 27709 e-mail: carroll1@niehs.nih.gov
www.niehs.nih.gov
The mission of the NIEHS is to discover how the environment affects people in order to promote healthier lives.
Linda S. Birnbaum, Ph.D., Director
Richard Woychik, Ph.D., Deputy Director

Pennsylvania

7576 **Epilepsy Foundation of Western Pennsylvania**
1323 Forbes Avenue
Pittsburgh, PA 15219-4725
412-261-5880
Fax: 412-261-5361
e-mail: staff@efwp.org
www.efwp.org

Judith K. Painter, Executive Director
Peggy Beem, Associate Director

Virginia

7577 **National Science Foundation**
4201 Wilson Blvd
Arlington, VA 22230
703-292-5111
TDD: 703-292-5090
e-mail: info@nsf.gov
www.nsf.gov
NSF is the only federal agency whose mission includes support for all fields of fundamental science and engineering, except for medical sciences.
France A. Cŕdova, Director
Richard O. Buckius, Chief Operating Officer

Washington

7578 **Epilepsy Foundation of North West Washington**
2311 N 45th Street
Seattle, WA 98103
206-547-4551
800-752-3509
Fax: 206-547-4557
e-mail: mail@epilepsynw.org
www.epilepsyfoundation.org

Brent Herrmann, President/CEO
Alta C Hancock, Associate Director

Research Centers

7579 **Baylor College of Medicine: Epilepsy Research Center**
Texas Medical Center
6550 Fannin
Houston, TX 77030
713-798-4333
Fax: 713-798-7533
e-mail: neurochair@bcm.edu
www.bcm.edu/neurology

The clinical program at Baylor College of Medicine for the comprehensive evaluation of those with epilepsy or those suspected of having seizures or epilepsy.
Eli Mizrahi MD, Director

7580 **Duke University Center for the Advanced Study of Epilepsy**
Duke Neuroscience Clinic
200 Trent Drive
Durham, NC 27710
919-668-7600
888-ASK-DUKE
www.dukehealth.org
Clinical and research unit that experiments in limbic epilepsy.
James McNama MD, Director
William B Gallentine

7581 **Neurology Research Center Helen Hayes Hospital**
Helen Hayes Hospital
53-55 Route 9W
W Haverstraw, NY 10993
845-786-4535
888-70R-EHAB
Fax: 845-947-3097
e-mail: info@helenhayeshospital.org
www.helenhayeshospital.org

Robert Linds MD, Chief Internal medicine
Jason P Greenberg, Assistant Clinical Professor of Neurolog

7582 **University of Illinois at Chicago Consultation Clinic for Epilepsy**
912 S Wood Street
Chicago, IL 60612-7330
312-996-7000
800-842-1002
Fax: 312-633-3434
TTY: 312-413-0123
e-mail: neu50@uic.edu
www.uic.edu

Paula Allen Meares, Chancellor
Lon S. Kauffman, Vice Chancellor

7583 **University of Tennessee: Center for Neuroscience**
875 Monroe Avenue
Memphis, TN 38163-0001
901-448-5960
Fax: 901-448-4685
www.uthsc.edu/neuroscience/

Epilepsy research and studies.
William E Armstrong, Director
Anton J Reiner, Co-Director

7584 **University of Wisconsin Madison Neurophysiology Laboratory**
UW Hospital and Clinics
600 Highland Avenue
Madison, WI 53792
608-263-6400
800-323-8942
Fax: 608-265-5512
www.uwhealth.org
Epilepsy research.
Thomas P Sutula, Chairman of Neurology
Paul A Rutecki, Vice Chairman of Neurology

Support Groups & Hotlines

7585 **Epilepsy Foundation of America Helpline**
Epilepsy Foundation of America
4351 Garden City Drive
Landover, MD 20785-7223
866-330-1000
800-332-1000
Fax: 301-459-1569
e-mail: postmaster@esa.org
www.epilepsyfoundation.org

A toll free information and referral service staffed by specially trained people who will answer questions and discuss concerns about seizure disorders and their treatment. Staff will direct callers to local affiliates of the EFA and tell about a broad range of medical services that respond to the needs of people with seizure disorders.
Phil Gattone, Chief Executive Officer

7586 **National Health Information Center**
PO Box 1133
Washington, DC 20013
310-565-4167
800-336-4797
Fax: 301-984-4256
e-mail: info@nhic.org
www.health.gov/nhic

Offers a nationwide information referral service, produces directories and resource guides.

Books

7587 **Americans with Disabilities Act**
Epilepsy Foundation of America
200 Constitution Ave., NW
Washington, DC 20210-2267
301-459-3700
866-487-2365
Fax: 301-577-9056
www.dol.gov
Learn how the Americans With Disabilities Act of 1990 can benifit you. Excellent comprehensive resource for individuals with seizure disorders.
46 pages Softcover
ISBN: 0-802774-65-2

7588 **Bomb in the Brain: A Heroic Tale of Science, Surgery and Survival**
MacMillan Publishing Company
3651 Peachtree Parkway
Suwanee, GA 30024
678-802-1922
Fax: 678-802-1922
www.paperbackswap.com
The autobiographical account of this author's struggle with epilepsy and the debilitating effects it has on health, emotions, and mental stability.
Grades 10-12
Richard Pickering, Founder & President

7589 **Brainstorms: Epilepsy in Our Words**
8301 Prof PlaceÿE
Landover, MD 20785-2267
301-459-3700
800-332-1000
Fax: 301-459-1569
e-mail: ContactUs@efa.org
www.epilepsy.com
Patients describe their experiences with seizures. Sixty-eight in-depth personal accounts of actual seizures are followed by a short section on how epilepsy affects the lives of the patients.
197 pages Paperback
ISBN: 0-802774-65-2

7590 **Children with Epilepsy**
Epilepsy Foundation of America
8301 Prof PlaceÿE
Landover, MD 20785-2267
301-459-3700
800-332-1000
Fax: 301-459-1569
e-mail: ContactUs@efa.org
www.epilepsy.com
Offers direction and support to parents of a child with epilepsy, by first educating them about epilepsy and then helping them cope with the effects this disorder will have on their child and family.
314 pages Paperback
ISBN: 0-933149-19-0

7591 **Does Your Child Have Epilepsy?**
8301 Prof PlaceÿE
Landover, MD 20785-2267
301-459-3700
800-332-1000
Fax: 301-459-1569
e-mail: ContactUs@efa.org
www.epilepsy.com
This book establishes Ten Basic Rules for parents of children with epilepsy.
201 pages Softcover

7592 **Embrace the Dawn**
Epilepsy Foundation of America
8301 Prof PlaceÿE
Landover, MD 20785-2267
301-459-3700
800-332-1000
Fax: 301-459-1569
e-mail: ContactUs@efa.org
www.epilepsy.com
A moving biographical account of one person's lifelong experience with epilepsy.
127 pages Softcover

7593 **Epilepsy A to Z**
8301 Prof PlaceÿE
Landover, MD 20785-2267
301-459-3700
800-332-1000
Fax: 301-459-1569
e-mail: ContactUs@efa.org
www.epilepsy.com
This book is designed to give health-care personnel a convenient way to find brief answers to questions about epilepsy. It includes definitions of terms, ranging all the way from abdominal epilepsy to Zonisimide.
322 pages Softcover

7594 **Epilepsy Diet Treatment: An Introduction to the Ketogenic Diet**
Epilepsy Foundation of America
8301 Prof PlaceÿE
Landover, MD 20785-2267
301-459-3700
800-332-1000
Fax: 301-459-1569
e-mail: ContactUs@efa.org
www.epilepsy.com
The only book devoted exclusively to the ketogenic diet - a rigid, mathematically calculated, doctor-supervised diet that is high in fat and low in carbohydrate and protein with strictly limited calories and liquid intake. Gives all the facts about the diet, plus quotes from parents showing what the experience is really like and 30 sample recipes.
1996 200 pages
ISBN: 0-939957-86-8

7595 **Epilepsy Surgery**
Raven Press
Landover, MD 20785-2601
301-459-3700
800-332-1000
Fax: 301-459-1569
e-mail: ContactUs@efa.org
www.epilepsy.com
The most complete and current references on surgical treatments of the epilepsies.
880 pages
ISBN: 0-881678-21-0

7596 **Epilepsy and the Family: A New Guide**
Harvard University Press
79 Garden Street
Cambridge, MA 02138
800-448-2242
www.hup.harvard.edu/catalog/LECEPF.html

ISBN: 0-674258-97-5

7597 **Epilepsy: 199 Answers**
Demos Medical Publishing
11 West 42nd Street
New York, NY 10016-8804
212-683-0072
800-532-8663
Fax: 212-683-0118
e-mail: support@demosmedical.com
www.demosmedpub.com
Addresses the needs of everyone with epilepsy. A helpful guide to the most common questions asked by people with epilepsy and will help the reader to work with his physician and take charge of the epilepsy.
1996 152 pages
ISBN: 1-888799-09-9
Dr. Diana M Schneider, President

7598 **Epilepsy: A Behavior Medicine Approach to Assessment & Treatment in Children**
Hogrefe & Huber Publications
PO Box 51
Lewiston, NY 14092-0051
716-282-1610
Fax: 716-484-4200
1993 200 pages
ISBN: 0-889371-06-7

7599 **Epilepsy: Current Approaches to Diagnosis and Treatment**
Raven Press
919 South Univ Ave
Ann Arbor, MI 48109-2601
212-930-9500
catalog.hathitrust.org

288 pages
ISBN: 0-881676-15-2

7600 **Epilepsy: I Can Live with That**
Landover, MD 20785-2267
301-459-3700
800-332-1000
Fax: 301-577-9056
e-mail: ContactUs@efa.org
www.epilepsy.com
The experience of epilepsy as recorded by a group of ordinary men and women living in Australia. Each story focuses on personal

growth, triumph over disability and emphasizes individual courage and hope.
Softcover
ISBN: 0-802774-65-2

7601 Epilepsy: Models, Mechanisms & Concepts
Cambridge University Press
40 W 20th Street   212-924-3900
New York, NY 10011-4211   800-221-4512
Fax: 212-691-3239
e-mail: customerservice@cup.org
www.cup.org

1993 400 pages
ISBN: 0-521392-98-5
Alice Ra, Assistant Marketing Manager

7602 Epilepsy: Patient and Family Guide
O Devinsky, MD, author
FA Davis Company
1915 Arch Street   215-568-2172
Philadelphia, PA 19103   800-523-4049
Fax: 215-568-5065
e-mail: info@fadavis.com
www.fadavis.com
Epilepsy expert Dr. Orrin Devinsky provides an easy-to-read guide to understanding the disease so that patients can achieve — and maintain — a higher quality of life. This book will educate recently-diagnosed patients, as well as those who have been living with epilepsy for years.
434 pages Paperback
ISBN: 0-803604-98-X
Michael Torso, Marketing Manager

7603 Equal Partners
Epilepsy Foundation of America
7, Market Street   356-212-0400
Floriana, MT 1083-2267   800-332-1000
Fax: 356-212-0397
e-mail: info@equalpartners.org.mt
www.equalpartners.org.mt
This book tells the story of a young Harvard-trained doctor whose experiences with seizures, brain surgery and subsequent epilepsy turns her from physician to patient.
257 pages Hardcover
ISBN: 0-802774-65-2
Louise Pisani, President
Elena Tanti Burlo, VP

7604 Guide to Understanding and Living with Epilepsy
8301 Prof PlaceÿE   301-459-3700
Landover, MD 20785-2267   800-332-1000
Fax: 301-577-9056
e-mail: ContactUs@efa.org
www.epilepsy.com
Easy-to-understand resource for people with epilepsy and their families. Covers a wide range of medical, social and legal issues. Topics include expanation of seizures and epilepsy; information about medication, side effects and risks; and getting the best medical care.

7605 Ketogenic Diet: A Treatment for Epilepsy
Demos Medical Publishing
11 West 42nd Street   212-683-0072
New York, NY 10036   Fax: 212-683-0118
e-mail: support@demosmedical.com
www.demosmedpub.com

256 pages
ISBN: 1-888799-39-0
Dr. Diana M Schneider

7606 Living Well with Epilepsy
Epilepsy Foundation of America
8301 Prof PlaceÿE   301-459-3700
Landover, MD 20785-2267   800-332-1000
Fax: 301-459-1569
e-mail: ContactUs@efa.org
www.epilepsy.com
Designed to help both health-care professionals and patients to understand all aspects of diagnosis and of pharmacologic and surgical management; to enable patients to participate more

knowledgeably in interactions with their health care team and to help steer them toward a more normal, fulfilling life.
166 pages Softcover
ISBN: 1-888799-11-0

7607 Managing Seizure Disorder
Epilepsy Foundation of America
8301 Prof PlaceE   301-459-3700
Landover, MD 20785-2267   800-332-1000
Fax: 301-459-1569
e-mail: ContactUs@efa.org
www.epilepsy.com
Provides health professionals with detailed information, on a variety of subjects, designed to help them help people with epilepsy live the kind of life they desire.
276 pages Softcover
ISBN: 0-802774-65-2

7608 Miles to Go Before I Sleep
Epilepsy Foundation of America
8301 Prof PlaceÿE   301-459-3700
Landover, MD 20785-2267   800-332-1000
Fax: 301-459-1569
e-mail: ContactUs@efa.org
www.epilepsy.com
This book tells the story of a hijacking in which the author sustained a severe brain injury that, among other things, affected her vision, her memory, and left her with epilepsy.
230 pages Hardcover
ISBN: 0-802774-65-2

7609 Students with Seizures: A Manual for School Nurses
Epilepsy Foundation of America
8301 Prof PlaceÿE   301-459-3700
Landover, MD 20785-2267   800-332-1000
Fax: 301-459-1569
e-mail: ContactUs@efa.org
www.epilepsy.com
A professional text with the sole purpose of creating a more accepting and understanding school environment for children with seizure disorders.
131 pages Paperback

Children's Books

7610 Dotty the Dalmatian has Epilepsy
Epilepsy Foundation of America
8301 Prof PlaceÿE   301-459-3700
Landover, MD 20785-2267   800-332-1000
Fax: 301-459-1569
e-mail: ContactUs@efa.org
www.epilepsy.com
This is the story of Dotty the Dalmatian who discovers she has epilepsy.
16 pages Softcover
ISBN: 0-802774-65-2

7611 Epilepsy
Franklin Watts Grolier
8301 Prof PlaceÿE   301-459-3700
Landover, MD 20785-0001   800-332-1000
Fax: 301-459-1569
e-mail: ContactUs@efa.org
www.epilepsy.com
This book explains what epilepsy is, causes of epileptic seizures, diagnosis and treatments.
96 pages Grades 7-12
ISBN: 0-531108-07-4

7612 Lee the Rabbit with Epilepsy
8301 Prof PlaceÿE   301-459-3700
Landover, MD 20785-2267   800-332-1000
Fax: 301-459-1569
e-mail: ContactUs@efa.org
www.epilepsy.com
Written for children ages 3-6, this illustrated picture book follows the adventures of a small rabbit who has seizures during a fishing trip with her Grandpa.
23 pages Hardcover

7613 Season of Secrets
Little, Brown & Company
3 Center Plz — 617-227-0730
Boston, MA 02108 — 800-759-0190
Fax: 800-286-9471
Grades 4-6

Newsletters

7614 Epilepsia: Journal of the International League Against Epilepsy
Blackwell Publishing, Inc.
Commerce Place — 201-748-6000
Hoboken, NJ 07030 — 800-862-6657
Fax: 201-748-6088
e-mail: info@wiley.com
www.blackwellpublishing.com
The leading international journal on the epilepsies for more than 30 years, Epilepsia provides comprehensive coverage of current clinical and research results.

7615 Epilepsy Services Foundation Newsletter
4618 N Armenia Avenue — 813-870-3414
Tampa, FL 33603-2706 — Fax: 813-870-1321
e-mail: eswcf@epilepsyservices.com
www.epilepsyservices.com
Information on medical and supportive services for persons affected by epilepsy living in West Central Florida. Raise funds to provide medical and supportive services to build and endowment to make a difference in the lives of generations to come.
2 pages 2-3 x/year
Thomas Orth, Executive Director

Pamphlets

7616 Child with Epilepsy at Camp
Epilepsy Foundation of America
8301 Prof PlaceÿE — 301-459-3700
Landover, MD 20785-2267 — 800-332-1000
Fax: 301-459-1569
e-mail: ContactUs@efa.org
www.epilepsy.com
Helps to explain why the child with epilepsy should be included in the camping experience.
14 pages Pamphlet

7617 Children and Seizures: Information for Babysitters
Epilepsy Foundation of America
8301 Prof PlaceÿE — 301-459-3700
Landover, MD 20785-2267 — 800-332-1000
Fax: 301-459-1569
e-mail: ContactUs@efa.org
www.epilepsy.com
Explains seizures, routine and special care, emergency aid and first aid to babysitters. Also offers a graph to write down important information about the child with seizure disorders for a quick reference.

7618 Epilepsy Medicines and Dental Care
Epilepsy Foundation of America
8301 Prof PlaceÿE — 301-459-3700
Landover, MD 20785-2267 — 800-332-1000
Fax: 301-459-1569
e-mail: ContactUs@efa.org
www.epilepsy.com
Explains dental care and includes instructions for brushing and flossing.

7619 Epilepsy: Legal Rights, Legal Issues
Epilepsy Foundation of America
8301 Prof PlaceÿE — 301-459-3700
Landover, MD 20785-2267 — 800-332-1000
Fax: 301-459-1569
e-mail: ContactUs@efa.org
www.epilepsy.com
Offers persons diagnosed with epilepsy information on their legal rights in employment, education, insurance and general disability benefits.
9 pages

7620 Epilepsy: Part of Your Life Series
Epilepsy Foundation of America
8301 Prof PlaceÿE — 301-459-3700
Landover, MD 20785-2267 — 800-332-1000
Fax: 301-459-1569
e-mail: ContactUs@efa.org
www.epilepsy.com
Provides information for staying healthy, describes various tests and diagnostic procedures, includes information for parents of children with epilepsy and provides general answers to questions about epilepsy.
Series of 4

7621 Epilepsy: You and Your Child, a Guide for Parents
Epilepsy Foundation of America
8301 Prof PlaceÿE — 301-459-3700
Landover, MD 20785-2267 — 800-332-1000
Fax: 301-459-1569
e-mail: ContactUs@efa.org
www.epilepsy.com
This instructional booklet offers information on emotional aspects of epilepsy, how to handle seizures, medication, diet and nutrition, and offers referral organizations for parents.

7622 Epilepsy: You and Your Treatment
Epilepsy Foundation of America
8301 Prof PlaceÿE — 301-459-3700
Landover, MD 20785-2267 — 800-332-1000
Fax: 301-459-1569
e-mail: ContactUs@efa.org
www.epilepsy.com
Reviews medical tests and diagnostic procedures used by physicians in diagnosing epilepsy.

7623 Facts About Epilepsy
Epilepsy Foundation of America
8301 Prof PlaceÿE — 301-459-3700
Landover, MD 20785-2267 — 800-332-1000
Fax: 301-459-1569
e-mail: ContactUs@efa.org
www.epilepsy.com
Designed for use by physicians and other health professionals with an interest in or who deal with the problems of people with epilepsy.
16 pages Softcover

7624 Finding Out About Seizures: A Guide to Medical Tests
Epilepsy Foundation of America
8301 Prof PlaceÿE — 301-459-3700
Landover, MD 20785-2267 — 800-332-1000
Fax: 301-459-1569
e-mail: ContactUs@efa.org
www.epilepsy.com
Introduces adults and children with epilepsy to the types of tests they may have to undergo.

7625 Kits for Adults with Epilepsy
Epilepsy Foundation of America
8301 Prof PlaceÿE — 301-459-3700
Landover, MD 20785-2267 — 800-332-1000
Fax: 301-459-1569
e-mail: ContactUs@efa.org
www.epilepsy.com
A variety of informative pamphlets for persons with epilepsy or seizure disorders.

7626 Management by Common Sense
Epilepsy Foundation of America
8301 Prof PlaceÿE — 301-459-3700
Landover, MD 20785-2267 — 800-332-1000
Fax: 301-459-1569
e-mail: ContactUs@efa.org
www.epilepsy.com
Promotes the employability of people with seizure disorders. Provides employers with information about epilepsy, customer/client reactions, workers' compensation issues, side effects of medication and other information relevant to employing a person with epilepsy.
46 pages Paperback
ISBN: 0-802774-65-2

7627   Me and My World Packet for Children
Epilepsy Foundation of America
8301 Prof PlaceÿE   301-459-3700
Landover, MD 20785-2267   800-332-1000
                                                        Fax: 301-459-1569
                                                    e-mail: ContactUs@efa.org
                                                         www.epilepsy.com
Collection of pamphlets designed for children with epilepsy.

7628   Medicines for Epilepsy
Epilepsy Foundation of America
8301 Prof PlaceÿE   301-459-3700
Landover, MD 20785-2267   800-332-1000
                                                        Fax: 301-459-1569
                                                    e-mail: ContactUs@efa.org
                                                         www.epilepsy.com
Offers information on medication and treatments, generic drugs, side effects, drug abuse and more. Contains a color chart with picyures of the most common medications for epilepsy.

7629   Mom I Have a Staring Problem
Epilepsy Foundation of America
8301 Prof PlaceÿE   301-459-3700
Landover, MD 20785-2267   800-332-1000
                                                        Fax: 301-459-1569
                                                    e-mail: ContactUs@efa.org
                                                         www.epilepsy.com
Tiffany, a seven-year-old, describes her experience with petit mal seizures; her feelings, wishes and fears. Written to help adults recognize a hidden problem that could be occuring with a child who has learning problems.
24 pages Softcover
ISBN: 0-802774-65-2

7630   My Brother Matthew
Woodbine House
8301 Prof PlaceÿE   301-459-3700
Landover, MD 20785-2267   800-332-1000
                                                        Fax: 301-459-1569
                                                    e-mail: ContactUs@efa.org
                                                         www.epilepsy.com
A picture and text book for children who have a brother or sister with developmental delay.
25 pages Harcoverr
ISBN: 0-802774-65-2

7631   My Friend Emily
Epilepsy Foundation of America
8301 Prof PlaceÿE   301-459-3700
Landover, MD 20785-2267   800-332-1000
                                                        Fax: 301-459-1569
                                                    e-mail: ContactUs@efa.org
                                                         www.epilepsy.com
A story about Emily and her best friend Katy. Emily, a self confident child who enjoys life, shows that kids with epilepsy are just like other kids.
35 pages Softcover
ISBN: 0-802774-65-2

7632   Patient's Guide to Everyday Life
Epilepsy Foundation of America
8301 Prof PlaceÿE   301-459-3700
Landover, MD 20785-2267   800-332-1000
                                                        Fax: 301-459-1569
                                                    e-mail: ContactUs@efa.org
                                                         www.epilepsy.com
Provides information for the newly diagnosed individual with epilepsy.

7633   Preventing Epilepsy
Epilepsy Foundation of America
8301 Prof PlaceÿE   301-459-3700
Landover, MD 20785-2267   800-332-1000
                                                        Fax: 301-459-1569
                                                    e-mail: ContactUs@efa.org
                                                         www.epilepsy.com
Examines some known causes of seizures and suggests precautionary measures which may prevent the occurrence of epilepsy.
16 pages

7634   Recognizing the Signs of Childhood Seizures
Epilepsy Foundation of America
8301 Prof PlaceÿE   301-459-3700
Landover, MD 20785-2267   800-332-1000
                                                        Fax: 301-459-1569
                                                    e-mail: ContactUs@efa.org
                                                         www.epilepsy.com
Explains what seizures are and what to look for in your child.

7635   Seizure Recognition and First Aid
Epilepsy Foundation of America
8301 Prof PlaceÿE   301-459-3700
Landover, MD 20785-2267   800-332-1000
                                                        Fax: 301-459-1569
                                                    e-mail: ContactUs@efa.org
                                                         www.epilepsy.com
Helps you recognize a seizure when it happens and give basic first aid.

7636   Surgery for Epilepsy
Epilepsy Foundation of America
8301 Prof PlaceÿE   301-459-3700
Landover, MD 20785-2267   800-332-1000
                                                        Fax: 301-459-1569
                                                    e-mail: ContactUs@efa.org
                                                         www.epilepsy.com
Describes current surgical treatment and the testing that precedes it.
12 pages

7637   Talking to Your Doctor About Seizure Disorders
Epilepsy Foundation of America
8301 Prof PlaceÿE   301-459-3700
Landover, MD 20785-2267   800-332-1000
                                                        Fax: 301-459-1569
                                                    e-mail: ContactUs@efa.org
                                                         www.epilepsy.com
Designed to help the patient talk with medical personnel about treatment of epilepsy.
Pamphlet

7638   Teacher's Role, A Guide for School Personnel
Epilepsy Foundation of America
8301 Prof PlaceÿE   301-459-3700
Landover, MD 20785-2267   800-332-1000
                                                        Fax: 301-459-1569
                                                    e-mail: ContactUs@efa.org
                                                         www.epilepsy.com
Provides tips on recognizing seizures and handling a seizure in the classroom.
14 pages

Audio & Video

7639   Comprehensive Clinical Management of the Epilepsies
Epilepsy Foundation of America
8301 Prof PlaceÿE   301-459-3700
Landover, MD 20785-2267   800-332-1000
                                                        Fax: 301-459-1569
                                                    e-mail: ContactUs@efa.org
                                                         www.epilepsy.com
Excellent reference on the treatment of epilepsy.
17 minutes

7640   How to Recognize and Classify Seizures
Epilepsy Foundation of America
8301 Prof PlaceÿE   301-459-3700
Landover, MD 20785-2267   800-332-1000
                                                        Fax: 301-459-1569
                                                    e-mail: ContactUs@efa.org
                                                         www.epilepsy.com
Discusses the classification of seizures and epileptic syndromes.
25 minutes

7641   Just Like You and Me
TASH

2013 H Street NW
Washington, DC 20006

202-540-9020
Fax: 202-637-0138
e-mail: btrader@tash.org
www.tash.org/index.html

A video/print package on successful living with epilepsy.
Ralph Edwards, President
Jean Trainor, Vice President

7642 Meeting the Challenge: Employment Issues and Epilepsy
Epilepsy Foundation of America
8301 Prof PlaceÿE
Landover, MD 20785-2267

301-459-3700
800-332-1000
Fax: 301-459-1569
e-mail: ContactUs@efa.org
www.epilepsy.com

This video answers the fquestions most often asked by emloyers. It covers issues such as driving, absenteeism, productivity, accidents and first aid, and emphasized that most people with epilepsy can be gainfully employed.
9 minutes

7643 Rest of the Family
Epilepsy Foundation of America
8301 Prof PlaceÿE
Landover, MD 20785-2267

301-459-3700
800-332-1000
Fax: 301-459-1569
e-mail: ContactUs@efa.org
www.epilepsy.com

Presents the feelings and concerns of other family members including siblings, of children with epilepsy.
Video cassette

7644 Seizure First Aid
Epilepsy Foundation of America
8301 Prof PlaceÿE
Landover, MD 20785-2267

301-459-3700
800-332-1000
Fax: 301-459-1569
e-mail: ContactUs@efa.org
www.epilepsy.com

This video combines footage of real seizures with reenactments to demonstrate proper first aid procedures. In addition, people with epilepsy talk about how they feel when they have a seizure, discuss how they would like friends, family and the general public to react when a seizure occurs.
10 minutes

7645 Understanding Seizure Disorders
Epilepsy Foundation of America
8301 Prof PlaceÿE
Landover, MD 20785-2267

301-459-3700
800-332-1000
Fax: 301-459-1569
e-mail: ContactUs@efa.org
www.epilepsy.com

Provides an explanation of seizure disorders in everyday language and dispels many misconceptions about epilepsy with medically accurate information.
Video cassette

7646 Voices from the Workplace
Epilepsy Foundation of America
8301 Prof PlaceÿE
Landover, MD 20785

301-459-3700
800-332-1000
Fax: 301-459-1569
e-mail: ContactUs@efa.org
www.epilepsy.com

Inspirational tape to help people with epilepsy cope with employment challenges. Individuals with epilepsy describe personal and social challenges in the workplace. They explain how they cope with their seizures and the reactions of co-workers and the public.

Web Sites

7647 American Epilepsy Society

www.aesnet.org

The Society seeks to promote interdisciplinary communications, scientific investigation and exchange of clinical information about epilepsy.

7648 Epilepsy Foundation of America

www.efa.org

Information on the prevention and cure of seizure disorders, the alleviation of their effects, and the promotion of independence and optimal quality of life for people who have these disorders.

7649 Healing Well

www.healingwell.com

An online health resource guide to medical news, chat, information and articles, newsgroups and message boards, books, disease-related web sites, medical directories, and more for patients, friends, and family coping with disabling diseases, disorders, or chronic illnesses.

7650 Health Finder

www.healthfinder.gov

Searchable, carefully developed web site offering information on over 1000 topics. Developed by the US Department of Health and Human Services, the site can be used in both English and Spanish.

7651 Healthlink USA

www.healthlinkusa.com

Health information concerning treatment, cures, prevention, diagnosis, risk factors, research, support groups, email lists, personal stories and much more. Updated regularly.

7652 Helios Health

www.helioshealth.com

Online resource for your health information. Detailed information about specific health topics, access to expert advice from our Medical Advisory Board, and up-to-date health news.

7653 MedicineNet

www.medicinenet.com

An online resource for consumers providing easy-to-read, authoritative medical and health information.

7654 Medscape

www.medscape.com

Medscape offers specialists, primary care physicians, and other health professionals the Web's most robust and integrated medical information and educational tools.

7655 National Institute of Neurological Disorders and Stroke

www.ninds.nih.gov

The mission of NINDS is to seek fundamental knowledge about the brain and nervous system and to use that knowledge to reduce the burden of neurological disease.

7656 Neurology Channel

www.healthcommunities.com

Find clearly explained, medically accurate information regarding conditions, including an overview, symptoms, causes, diagnostic procedures and treatment options. On this site it is possible to ask questions and get information from a neurologist and connect to people who have similar health interests.

7657 WebMD

www.webmd.com

Provides credible information, supportive communities, and in-depth reference material about health subjects. A source for original and timely health information as well as material from well known content providers.

Description

7658 Sexually Transmitted Diseases

Sexually transmitted diseases, STDs, are among the most common infectious diseases in the U.S. More than 20 STDs have been identified, and roughly 13 million persons are affected. Fortunately, most STDs are curable with prompt treatment, and do not become chronic. These include bacterial vaginosis, gonorrhea, syphilis, trichomoniasis and chlamydia. People who suffer from these diseases over long periods almost always do so because of re-infection rather than treatment failure. HIV and hepatitis B are commonly transmitted through sexual intercourse; see also *AIDS* and *Hepatitis*.

Fortunately, behavioral changes in sexual practices can drastically reduce the risk of STDs. Abstinence from intercourse or having a long-term mutually faithful monogamous relationship with an uninfected partner give essentially complete protection. Risk rises with multiple partners, unprotected intercourse between males, anonymous sex and contact with high-risk individuals, such as prostitutes. Barrier methods, notably condoms, give significant but not complete protection.

Until recently, no vaccines were available for any common STD except hepatitis B. However, researchers developed a vaccine for human papilloma virus (HPV) that is, amazingly, 100 percent effective. The vaccine is such a critical discovery because one specific type of HPV causes cervical cancer. Common STDs which may become chronic despite treatment are described below.

Genital herpes is a virus of the herpes family characterized by blisters (vesicles) in the genital area. The appearance of the blisters is often preceded by low-grade fever and by burning pain in the affected area. The first episode is often the most painful. Specific anti-viral therapy will shorten the duration and intensity of an attack. Herpes infections are self-limited but recurrent because the virus chronically infects nerves that radiate from the spinal column. Under certain conditions, such as febrile illness and physical or emotional stress, the virus reactivates and causes another outbreak. People with frequent recurrences can lower the risk of repeat attacks by taking a low dose of the anti-viral medication every day.

Genital warts are caused by the human papilloma virus (HPV.) There are roughly 750,000 new cases each year in the United States. The warts may appear anywhere in the genital and rectal area, making transmission difficult to prevent with a condom. Genital warts in the male, unless quite large, are often just a cosmetic nuisance, although a wart inside the urinary passage may cause discomfort. Women with genital warts not only need to have the warts removed, but to be observed for pre-cancerous changes in the cervix. Warts are generally destroyed by application of chemicals, but doctors have also used laser beams, freezing and electrical currents to destroy them. Recurrence after treatment is common, even in the absence of re-infection.

Pelvic inflammatory disease (PID) is not always sexually transmitted, but it is included here because chlamydia and gonorrhea, which are sexually transmitted, are commonly the cause of PID. In this condition, the sensitive pelvic reproductive organs are attacked, leading to fever and lower abdominal pain and occasionally collection of pus in a pelvic abscess. Even after the attack is treated with high doses of antibiotics, residual scarring may lead to chronic pelvic pain, pain with intercourse, infertility and ectopic pregnancy, in which the fertilized egg implants in other pelvic structures outside the uterus. Prompt recognition and vigorous treatment of the acute attack of PID are important.

National Agencies & Associations

7659 American Foundation for the Prevention of Venereal Disease
799 Broadway
New York, NY 10003   212-759-2069
www.chclibrary.org
Encourages every individual to assume responsible sexual relations and proper personal hygiene.
Mary O'Connell, Secretary

7660 American Social Health Association
PO Box 13827   919-361-8400
Research Triangle Park, NC 27709-3827 800-227-8922
Fax: 919-361-8425
www.ashastd.org
Provides resources to local communities to improve STD control programs through citizen action.
Lynn Barclay, President CEO
Deborah Arrindell, Vice President Health Policy

7661 American Venereal Disease Association
PO Box 1753
Baltimore, MD 21203-1753   301-955-3150
www.alternativemedicine.com
Primary interest of this organization is in the reduction of the prevalence of the diseases.
Edward Hook III MD, Secretary

7662 Centers for Disease Control and Prevention
1600 Clifton Road   404-639-3534
Atlanta, GA 30333   800-232-4636
TTY: 888-232-6348
e-mail: cdcinfo@cdc.gov
www.cdc.gov
An information awareness resource produced by the Division of Adolescent and School Health. The database offers descriptions of various educational resources for professionals relevant to the education of children and youth about HIV infection and AIDS.
Thomas R. Frieden, Director
Ileana Arias, Principal Deputy Director

7663 Citizens Alliance for VD Awareness
5002 W Madison   773-379-1000
Chicago, IL 60644   Fax: 773-379-1342
e-mail: info@cfhcn.org
www.circlefamilycare.org
Seeks to increase commitment of health professionals to venereal disease and AIDS control.
Bruce Peoples, President/CEO
Patrick C Nwaezeigwe, CFO

7664 Herpes Resource Center
PO Box 13827   919-361-8400
Research Triangle Park, NC 27709-3827 800-227-8922
Fax: 919-361-8425
www.ashastd.org

Gives emotional support to individuals and provides information to the public about herpes.
Carolyn Mabry, Coordinator
Lynn Barclay, President CEO

7665 National Institute of Allergy and Infectious Diseases
6610 Rockledge Drive
Bethesda, MD 20892-6612
301-496-5717
866-284-4107
Fax: 301-402-3573
www.niaid.nih.gov

Dr. Anthony Fauci, Director

Research Centers

7666 Herpes Resource Center
PO Box 13827
Research Triangle Park, NC 27709
919-361-8400
800-227-8922
Fax: 919-361-8425
www.ashastd.org
Offers information and referrals for persons affected by herpes and other sexually transmitted disease prevention.
Lynn Barclay, President and Chief Executive Officer
Deborah Arrindell, Vice President Health Policy

7667 International Union Against Venereal Diseases
New York Hospital - Cornell Medical Center
1153 York Avenue
New York, NY 10021
212-746-1200
Fax: 212-746-1202
e-mail: ajacobso@myp.org
Encourages campaigns medical and social against venereal disease.
Lewis Drusin MD, Director

7668 University of Chicago Committee on Virology
Marjorie B Kovler Viral Oncology Laboratories
910 E 58th Street
Chicago, IL 60637
773-702-1620
Fax: 773-702-1631
mgcb.bsd.uchicago.edu
Focuses research into the area of sexually transmitted disease.
Bernard Roizman, Chairman
Olaf Schneewind, Professor and Chairman

Support Groups & Hotlines

7669 National Health Information Center
PO Box 1133
Washington, DC 20013
310-565-4167
800-336-4797
Fax: 301-984-4256
e-mail: info@nhic.org
www.health.gov/nhic
Offers a nationwide information referral service, produces directories and resource guides.

Books

7670 Herpes and Papilloma Viruses Volume I & II
Raven Press
1600 Clifton Road
Atlanta, GA 30329-2601
212-930-9500
800-232-4636
www.cdc.gov
382 pages
ISBN: 0-881671-95-9

7671 Sexually Transmitted Diseases
Raven Press
1600 Clifton Road
Atlanta, GA 30329-2601
212-930-9500
800-232-4636
www.cdc.gov
Focuses on the clinically important subject of the immune response to sexually transmitted diseases.
350 pages
ISBN: 0-881678-82-1

7672 Understanding Helps
University Press of Mississippi

3825 Ridgewood Road
Jackson, MS 39211-6492
601-432-6205
800-737-7788
Fax: 601-432-6217
e-mail: press@ihl.state.ms.us
www.upress.state.ms.us
This book is for people who wish to learn about herpes simplex viruses, two remarkably complex microbes capable of causing a wide variety of infections. These include genital herpes, a very common chronic sexually transmitted disease.
120 pages Hardcover
ISBN: 1-578060-40-0
Kathy Burgess, Advertising Manager/Marketing Assistant

7673 Understanding Herpes: Revised Second Edition
Lawrence R Stanberry, MD; PhD, author
University Press of Mississippi
3825 Ridgewood Road
Jackson, MS 39211-6492
601-432-6205
Fax: 601-432-6217
e-mail: kburgess@ihl.state.ms.us
www.upress.state.ms.us
A concise overview of advances and resources.
2006 144 pages Paperback
ISBN: 1-578068-68-1
Kathy Burgess, Advertising/Marketing Services Manager

7674 Women at Risk
Bristol Publishing
2790 44th St. SW
Wyoming, MI 49519-0811
415-895-4461
Fax: 415-895-4459
https://warinternational.org
1993 159 pages
ISBN: 0-917851-62-5

Children's Books

7675 Teen Guide to Safe Sex
Franklin Watts Grolier
90 Old Sherman Tpke
Danbury, CT 06816-0001
203-797-3500
800-621-1115
Fax: 203-797-3197
www.grolier.com
A basic book about sexually transmitted diseases. Describes what they are, what causes them, how to recognize them and how teenagers can protect against them.
64 pages Grades 9-12
ISBN: 0-531105-92-0

Newsletters

7676 Sexually Transmitted Diseases: Journal
Julius Schachter, PhD, author
Lippincott Wiliiams & Wilkins
2700 Lake CookÿRoad
Riverwoods, IL 60015-1600
847-580-5000
800-638-3030
Fax: 301-223-2400
e-mail: orders@lww.com
www.lww.com
This timely, scholarly journal publishes original, peer-reviewed articles on clinical, laboratory, immunologic, epidemiologic, sociologic, and historical topics pertaining to sexually transmitted diseases and related fields.
Monthly

7677 Step Perspective
Seattle Treatment Education Project
127 Broadway E
Seattle, WA 98102-5711
206-329-4857
800-869-7837
www.quick-step.in
A publication of the Seattle Treatment Education Project. Published three times a year.
Michael Auch, Executive Director

Pamphlets

7678 AIDS...What We Need To Know Pamphlet
March of Dimes

1275 Mamaroneck Avenue

White Plains, NY 10605

914-997-4488

Fax: 212-254-3518

e-mail: NY639@marchofdimes.com

www.marchofdimes.com

Discusses the facts about HIVÆinfection and AIDS and how you can reduce your risk.

Pkg of 50

ISBN: 0-923500- -

7679 Chlamydial Infection

National Institute of Allergy/Infectious Diseases

Nat Institutes of Health

Bethesda, MD 20892-0001

301-496-5717

www.nih.gov

Offers information on diagnosis, treatment, effects, prevention and research.

7680 Genital Herpes

National Institute of Allergy/Infectious Diseases

Nat Institutes of Health

Bethesda, MD 20892-0001

301-496-5717

www.nih.gov

Offers information on symptoms, causes, diagnosis and reccurences.

7681 Genital Herpes Fact Sheet

March of Dimes

1275 Mamaroneck Avenue

White Plains, NY 10605

914-997-4488

Fax: 212-254-3518

e-mail: NY639@marchofdimes.com

www.marchofdimes.com

Fact Sheets: one to two page review written for the general public.

7682 Gonorrhea

National Institute of Allergy/Infectious Diseases

Nat Institutes of Health

Bethesda, MD 20892-0001

301-496-5717

www.nih.gov

Offers information on the symptoms, diagnosis, treatment, complications, prevention and research.

7683 Human Papillomavirus and Genital Warts

National Institute of Allergy/Infectious Diseases

Nat Institutes of Health

Bethesda, MD 20892-0001

301-496-5717

www.nih.gov

Offers information on diagnosis, treatment, complications and prevention of the diseases.

7684 Introduction to Sexually Transmitted Diseases

National Institute of Allergy/Infectious Diseases

Nat Institutes of Health

Bethesda, MD 20892-0001

301-496-5717

www.nih.gov

Offers information on STDs, various types and symptoms, research, and referral services.

7685 Other Important STD's

National Institute of Allergy/Infectious Diseases

Nat Institutes of Health

Bethesda, MD 20892-0001

301-496-5717

www.nih.gov

Lists over ten of the most common sexually transmitted diseases. Offers information on what they are, the causes and treatments, research being done in these areas and referral numbers of where to call for more information on the diseases.

7686 Pelvic Inflammatory Disease

National Institute of Allergy/Infectious Diseases

Nat Institutes of Health

Bethesda, MD 20892-0001

301-496-5717

www.nih.gov

Offers information on the causes, symptoms, risk factors, diagnosis, treatment, and prevention.

7687 Syphilis

National Institute of Allergy/Infectious Diseases

Nat Institutes of Health

Bethesda, MD 20892-0001

301-496-5717

www.nih.gov

Offers information on what syphilis is, the symptoms, complications, diagnosis, prevention and treatment methods available.

7688 Vaginal Infections

National Institute of Allergy/Infectious Diseases

Nat Institutes of Health

Bethesda, MD 20892-0001

301-496-5717

www.nih.gov

Lists three specific types of vaginitis, with information on their symptoms, prevention, complications and treatments.

Web Sites

7689 American Social Health Association

www.ashasexualhealth.org

The American Sexual Health Association promotes the sexual health of individuals, families and communities by advocating sound policies and practices and educating the public, professionals and policy makers, in order to foster healthy sexual behaviors and relationships and prevent adverse health outcomes.

7690 Centers for Disease Control

www.cdc.gov

Offers reprints, reports, public awareness and educational materials and research on sexually transmitted diseases.

7691 Healing Well

www.healingwell.com

An online health resource guide to medical news, chat, information and articles, newsgroups and message boards, books, disease-related web sites, medical directories, and more for patients, friends, and family coping with disabling diseases, disorders, or chronic illnesses.

7692 Health Finder

www.healthfinder.gov

Searchable, carefully developed web site offering information on over 1000 topics. Developed by the US Department of Health and Human Services, the site can be used in both English and Spanish.

7693 Healthlink USA

www.healthlinkusa.com

Health information concerning treatment, cures, prevention, diagnosis, risk factors, research, support groups, email lists, personal stories and much more. Updated regularly.

7694 Helios Health

www.helioshealth.com

Online resource for your health information. Detailed information about specific health topics, access to expert advice from our Medical Advisory Board, and up-to-date health news.

7695 MedicineNet

www.medicinenet.com

An online resource for consumers providing easy-to-read, authoritative medical and health information.

7696 Medscape

www.medscape.com

Medscape offers specialists, primary care physicians, and other health professionals the Web's most robust and integrated medical information and educational tools.

7697 WebMD

www.webmd.com

Provides credible information, supportive communities, and in-depth reference material about health subjects. A source for original and timely health information as well as material from well known content providers.

Description

7698 Sickle Cell Disease

Sickle cell disease (also called sickle cell anemia) is an inherited defect of hemoglobin, the oxygen-carrying element in the blood. Under some circumstances, the normally disc-shaped red blood cell takes on a crescent or sickle shape. It then becomes lodged in small capillaries and prevents normal oxygen flow to the tissues. This oxygen deprivation can cause sickle cell crises, with symptoms of severe pain in the back, joints, hands, and feet, and may even include neurologic changes. Severe abdominal pain and vomiting may also occur.

Sickle cell anemia occurs almost exclusively in African Americans. There are approximately 55,000 people in the United States with this condition. These children have sickle cell trait, occurring when one receives a copy of the sickle cell gene from only one parent. Only if a child receives a copy of the defective gene from both parents will the full-blown disease develop.

Therapy for sickle cell disease is aimed at preventing and treating infections, maintaining an adequate diet and fluid intake, and managing acute attacks with painkillers, oxygen, antibiotics and blood transfusion. Hydroxyurea has been shown to reduce the number of attacks by 50 percent as well as the need for transfusion. In the past, death typically occurred because of overwhelming infection or from organ destruction brought about by multiple sickling crises. Modern therapy has improved life expectancy dramatically, but some level of disability is common. Geneticcounseling is important for the patient and all family members.

National Agencies & Associations

7699 American Sickle Cell Anemia
10300 Carnegie Avenue
Cleveland, OH 44106-0171

216-229-8600
Fax: 216-229-4500
e-mail: irabragg@ascaa.org
www.ascaa.org

Provides education testing counseling and supportive services for sickle cell anemia and its hemoglobinopathy variants.
Ira Bragg-Grant, Executive Director
Leslie Carter, Newborn Screening Coordinator

7700 Comprehensive Sickle Cell Center
80 Jesse Hill Jr Drive SE
Atlanta, GA 30303

404-616-3572
Fax: 404-616-5998
e-mail: aplatt@emory.edu
www.scinfo.org

The mission of Sickle Cell Information Center is to provide sickle cell patient and professional education, news, research updates and world wide sickle cell resources, as well as world class compassionate care.
James R Eckman, Medical Director
Lewis Hsu, Interim Director

7701 Sickle Cell Anemia Foundation
503 S Center Street
Statesville, NC 28687

704-878-0732

This program is designed to provide information about sickle cell disease symptoms available treatments and service facilities by distributing literature and dispatching foundation members to address organizations church or school groups.
Priscilla Dudley

7702 Sickle Cell Association of Ontario
3199 Bathurst Street
Toronto, Ontario, M6A-2B2

416-789-2855
Fax: 416-789-1903
e-mail: sicklecell@look.ca
www.sicklecellontario.com

A voluntary, non-profit, charitable organization which is funded by donations from individuals, organizations and employee charitable funds.
John Kirya, President

7703 Sickle Cell Disease Association of America
231 E Baltimore Street
Baltimore, MD 21202

410-528-1555
800-421-8453
Fax: 410-528-1495
e-mail: scdaa@sicklecelldisease.org
www.sicklecelldisease.org

Purpose is to promote leadership on a national level in order to create awareness in all circles of the impact of sickle cell disease on emotional and economic well-being of families and the individual.
Christopher Hollins, Chair
Jeannine Knight, Executive Assistant to the President/COO

7704 Sickle Cell Information Center Grady Memorial Hospital
Grady Memorial Hospital
80 Jesse Hill Jr Drive SE
Atlanta, GA 30303

404-616-3572
Fax: 404-616-5998
e-mail: aplatt@emory.edu
www.SCInfo.org

Our mission is to provide sickle cell patient and professional education news research updates and world wide sickle cell resources. It is the mission of our organizations to provide world class compassionate care.
James R Eckman, Medical Director
Lewis Hsu, Interim Director

Foundations

7705 James R Clark Memorial Sickle Cell Foundation
1420 Gregg Street
Columbia, SC 29201

803-765-9916
800-506-1273
Fax: 803-799-6471
e-mail: sicklecell@sc.rr.com

Genetic Blood Disorder Disease.
Melodie A Hunnicutt, Executive Director
Saundra Kidwell, Director Finance

7706 Northeast Louisiana Sickle Cell Anemia Foundation
1604 Winnsboro Road
Monroe, LA 71202

318-322-0896
Fax: 318-387-4740
e-mail: sickle@bayou.com

The Foundation is a community-based non-profit, tax-exempt organization whose purpose is to provide services to sickle cell patients and their families, as well as be a resource in the communities we serve (12 northeast parishes) We provide education, trait counseling, patient assistance and social services. Our services are free.
Lasandre R Starks, Executive Director
Cheryl Minor, Registered Social Worker

7707 Sickle Cell Foundation of Georgia
2391 Benjamin E Mays Drive
Atlanta, GA 30311

404-755-1641
800-326-5287
Fax: 404-755-7955
e-mail: n_nichols@sicklecellatlaga.org
www.sicklecellatlaga.org

Our mission is dedicated to providing education, screening and counseling programs for Sickle Cell and other abnormal hemoglobin.
D Jean Brannan, President
Nesby Gibson, Project Director

7708 Sickle Cell Foundation of Greater Montgomery
3180 US Highway 8 West
Montgomery, AL 36108

334-286-9122
800-742-5534
e-mail: sicklec2@aol.com
www.scfgm.org

The main objectives of the Foundation are to give accurate information about sickle cell disease and related hemoglobinopathies, to provide testing and diagnostic services to interested persons, to

counsel individuals with positive test results so they can make informed decisions about their lives and to provide supportive services for clients and their family members.
Willie Owens, Executive Director

Research Centers

7709   Boston Sickle Cell Center Boston Medical Center
Boston Medical Center
88 E Newton Street   617-414-1020
Boston, MA 02118-2999   Fax: 617-414-1021
                                               e-mail: mhsteinb@bu.edu
                                                    www.bu.edu/sicklecel
The treatment facility of choice for Boston-area patients with sickle cell disease. The Center also promotes interactive basic and clinical research and patient and professional educational activities.
Martin Steinberg, Director
Shawn H Eung, Program Manager

7710   Columbia University: Comprehensive Sickle Cell Center
Harlem Hospital
506 Lenox Avenue
New York, NY 10037-1000   212-939-1426
                     www.nyc.gov/html/hhc/html/facilities/har
Research into sickle cell disease.
Dr Jeanne Smith, Director

7711   Comprehensive Sickle Cell Center Children's Hospital Research Foundation
Children's Hospital Research Foundation
3333 Burnet Avenue   513-636-4541
Cincinnati, OH 45229   800-344-2462
                                               Fax: 513-636-5562
                                               e-mail: blood@cchmc.org
                                               www.cincinnatichildrens.org
Offers research and statistical information in the area of sickle cell disease.
Clinton Joiner, Director
Karen Kalinyak, Clinical Director

7712   Howard University Center for Sickle Cell Disease
1840 7th Street NW   202-865-8284
Washington, DC 20001   Fax: 202-232-6719
                                               e-mail: sicklecell@howard.edu
                                               www.sicklecell.howard.edu

Victor R Gordeuk, Director
Catherine Nwokolo, Clinical Staff Member

7713   Medical College of Georgia: Sickle Cell Center
1521 Pope Avenue   706-721-2171
Augusta, GA 30912-0002   Fax: 706-721-4575
                                               www.mcg.edu/centers/sicklecel
Offers research into sickle cell disease.
Abdullah Kutlar, Director
Kavita Natarajan

7714   Philadelphia Biomedical Research Institute
100 Ross and Royal Road   610-962-0615
King of Prussia, PA 19406   Fax: 610-254-9332
                                               e-mail: stohmishi@aol.com
                                  members.aol.com/stohinishi/phila_biomed
Study on the management of sickle cell anemia through nutrition.
S Tsuyoshi Ohinishi PhD, Director

7715   SUNY Health Science Center at Brooklyn Sickle Cell Center
450 Clarkson Avenue   718-270-1000
Brooklyn, NY 11203   Fax: 718-270-7592
                                               www.hscbklyn.edu

John C LaRosa, President
Paul J Davis, Interim Chief Financial Officer

7716   Sickle Cell Anemia Research Foundation
2625 3rd Street   913-588-5000
Alexandria, VA 71309   877-722-7370
                                               Fax: 318-487-9990
                                       e-mail: scarf@sicklecelldisease.org
                                                        www.kumc.edu

The Sickle Cell Anemia Research Foundation provides a comprehensive program on Sickle Cell Disease. We offer education training counseling and help with prescriptions.

7717   Sickle Cell Association of the Texas Gulf Coast
2626 S Loop W   713-666-0300
Houston, TX 77054-2649   Fax: 713-660-17
Rebecca Jasso, Executive Director

7718   University of California Northern Comprehensive Sickle Cell Center
Childrens Hospital Research Center
747 50 2nd Street   510-428-3651
Oakland, OK 94609-3594
Sickle cell disease research.
Elliot Vichinsky, Director

7719   University of Southern California: Comprehensive Sickle Cell Center
2025 Zonal Avenue   213-342-1259
Los Angeles, CA 90033-1034
Dr Cage S Johnson, Director

7720   University of Texas Southwestern Medical Center/Sickle Cell Management
Southwestern Medical Center
1935 Medical District Drive   214-456-7000
Dallas, TX 75235-7701   Fax: 214-648-3122
                                       e-mail: jsquires@childmed.dallas.tx.us
                                                        www.childrens.com
Focuses on the prevention of disease complications and management using the newest treatment strategies including hydroxyurea chronic transfusions stem cell (bone marrow) transplantation and state-of-the-art approaches to infection prevention pain management and treatment of specific organ-related complications (chest syndrome priapism avascular necrosis of the femoral head etc.).
George Bucha MD, Director
James F Amatruda

7721   Wayne State University: Comprehensive Sickle Cell Center
Curricular Affairs Office
Scott Hall   313-577-2424
Detroit, MI 48201   Fax: 313-577-8777
                                                           wayne.edu

Charles F Whitten MD, President

Support Groups & Hotlines

7722   Keon Paschal Perry Sickle Cell Anemia Disease Awareness
7510 Granby Street, Perry Building
Norfolk, VA 23505   888-406-5111
                                               e-mail: keon4u@aol.com
International Sickle Cell Anemia Disease Awareness Campaign.
Roy L Perry-Bey, CEO/Executive Director

7723   Lehigh Valley Sickle Cell Support Group
PO Box 1711   610-706-0636
Allentown, PA 18105-1711   e-mail: SororW@aol.com
                                       www.members.aol.com/SororW/index.html
Anyone affected/effected by Sickle Cell and all interested persons. Our mission is to educate the local community about Sickle Cell.

7724   National Health Information Center
PO Box 1133   310-565-4167
Washington, DC 20013   800-336-4797
                                               Fax: 301-984-4256
                                               e-mail: info@nhic.org
                                               www.health.gov/nhic
Offers a nationwide information referral service, produces directories and resource guides.

7725   Sickle Cell Anemia Association of Austin: Marc Thomas Chapter
PO Box 201092   512-335-2306
Austin, TX 78720-1092   e-mail: llthomas@austin.cc.tx.us
                                               www.tdh.state.tx.us
To raise awareness, resources and support for clients with sickle cell disease.
Linda L Thomas

7726 **Sickle Cell Disease Association of America Philadelphia/Delaware Valley Chapter**
4601 Market Street
Philadelphia, PA 19139
215-471-8686
Fax: 215-471-7441
e-mail: scdaa.pdvc@verizon.net
www.sicklecelldisorder.com

The Philadelphia/Delaware Valley Chapter of the Sickle Cell Disease Association of America (SCDAA/PDVC) assists the sickle cell community by serving as a vehicle and resource center for the psycho-social and social service needs of those individuals affected by the disease through the following services: case management; counseling; hospital/clinic visits; advocacy; career/vocational assistance; newborn screening follow-up; transportation; and outreach/community education.

Stanley A Simpkins, Executive Director
Karin Darius, Program Director

Pamphlets

7727 **Sickle Cell Disease**
March of Dimes
1275 Mamaroneck Avenue
White Plains, NY 10605
914-997-4488
Fax: 212-254-3518
e-mail: NY639@marchofdimes.com
www.marchofdimes.com

Fact Sheets: one to two page review written for the general public.

Web Sites

7728 **American Sickle Cell Anemia**

www.ascaa.org

Comprehensive services through diagnostic testing, evaluation, counseling and supportive services to individuals and families at risk for Sickle Cell Disease.

7729 **Healing Well**

www.healingwell.com

An online health resource guide to medical news, chat, information and articles, newsgroups and message boards, books, disease-related web sites, medical directories, and more for patients, friends, and family coping with disabling diseases, disorders, or chronic illnesses.

7730 **Health Finder**

www.healthfinder.gov

Searchable, carefully developed web site offering information on over 1000 topics. Developed by the US Department of Health and Human Services, the site can be used in both English and Spanish.

7731 **Healthlink USA**

www.healthlinkusa.com

Health information concerning treatment, cures, prevention, diagnosis, risk factors, research, support groups, email lists, personal stories and much more. Updated regularly.

7732 **Helios Health**

www.helioshealth.com

Online resource for your health information. Detailed information about specific health topics, access to expert advice from our Medical Advisory Board, and up-to-date health news.

7733 **MedicineNet**

www.medicinenet.com

An online resource for consumers providing easy-to-read, authoritative medical and health information.

7734 **Medscape**

www.medscape.com

Medscape offers specialists, primary care physicians, and other health professionals the Web's most robust and integrated medical information and educational tools.

7735 **Sickle Cell Disease Association of America**

sicklecelldisease.org

Purpose is to promote leadership on a national level in order to create awareness in all circles of the impact of sickle cell disease on emotional and economic well-being of families and the individual.

7736 **WebMD**

www.webmd.com

Provides credible information, supportive communities, and in-depth reference material about health subjects. A source for original and timely health information as well as material from well known content providers.

Description

7737 Sjogren's Syndrome

Sjogren's syndrome (also called sicca syndrome) is an autoimmune disorder characterized by dryness of the mouth, eyes and mucous membranes. Variable enlargement of the lacrimal (tear) or salivary gland can occur. The disorder has no known cause, but many researchers believe that it has a genetic basis. Sjogren's syndrome is divided into primary (affecting only the eyes and mouth) and secondary (generalized) forms which may be associated with connective tissue diseases such as rheumatoid arthritis, systemic lupus erythematosus, polymyositis or scleroderma.

Patients who suffer from Sjogren's syndrome often complain initially of a gritty sensation in the eyes or severe dryness of the mouth. Patients may develop kidney, skin, neurologic, pulmonary or joint problems.

Treatment for Sjogren's is mainly symptomatic in the form of artificial tears, sipping fluids throughout the day, chewing gum and using special mouthwash. Pilocarpine may be used to stimulate saliva production. Severe cases, especially if they affect parts of the body outside of the glands, may require corticosteroid therapy. Dental caries (cavities) are a complication of dry mouth, so close dental follow-up is important.

National Agencies & Associations

7738 National Sjogren's Syndrome Foundation NSSA
NSSA
5815 N Blk Canyon Highway
Phoenix, AZ 85015-2200

301-530-4420
800-395-6772
Fax: 301-530-4415
e-mail: NSSA@aol.com
www.sjogrens.org

Provides educational materials to members about medical developments and research concerning SS nationally and internationally. Membership also includes assorted discounts on additional materials and events.
S. Lance Forstot, Chairman
Sheriese DeFruscio, Vice President of Development

7739 Sjogren's Syndrome Foundation
6707 Democracy Boulevard
Bethesda, MD 20817-2025

301-530-4420
800-475-6473
Fax: 301-530-4415
e-mail: tms@sjogrens.org
www.sjogrens.org

A non-profit voluntary health organization whose purposes are to educate patients and their families about Sjogren's syndrome and help them cope with the problems and frustrations of living with Sjogren's syndrome and to increase public and medical awareness.
Philip C Fox, President
Steven Taylor, CEO

Support Groups & Hotlines

7740 National Health Information Center
PO Box 1133
Washington, DC 20013

310-565-4167
800-336-4797
Fax: 301-984-4256
e-mail: info@nhic.org
www.health.gov/nhic

Offers a nationwide information referral service, produces directories and resource guides.

Books

7741 New Sjogren's Syndrome Handbook
Sjogren's Syndrome Foundation
6707 Democracy Boulevard
Bethesda, MD 20817-2025

301-530-4420
800-475-6473
Fax: 301-530-4415
www.sjogrens.org

An authoritative guide for patients and health care providers on the many aspects of Sjogren's syndrome written by renowned experts, plus practical suggestions for living more comfortably with this chronic illness.
Hardcover
ISBN: 0-195117-24-7
Kenneth Economou, Chairman
Stephen Cohen, Chairman-Elect

Newsletters

7742 Moisture Seekers Newsletter
Sjogren's Syndrome Foundation
6707 Democracy Boulevard
Bethesda, MD 20817-2025

301-530-4420
800-475-6473
Fax: 301-530-4415
www.sjogrens.org

Contains up-to-date information on Sjogren's syndrome including new treatments, new products, and clinical trails; also features articles on the ways members cope with this chronic disease.
9x Year
Kenneth Economou, Chairman
Stephen Cohen, Chairman-Elect

Pamphlets

7743 Dry Eyes? Dry Mouth? Dry Nose? Arthritis? If Two or More: Sjogren's Syndrome
Sjogren's Syndrome Foundation
1 AMS Circle
Bethesda, MD 20892-3136

301-495-4484
877-226-4267
Fax: 301-718-6366
TTY: 301-565-2966
e-mail: NIAMSinfo@mail.nih.gov
www.niams.nih.gov

Offers a brief overview of what the illness is, a history, statistical information, causes, symptoms and treatments.

7744 Sjogren's Syndrome
NAMSIC/National Institutes of Health
1 AMS Circle
Bethesda, MD 20892-0001

301-495-4484
877-226-4267
Fax: 301-718-6366
TTY: 301-565-2966
e-mail: NIAMSinfo@mail.nih.gov
www.nih.gov/niams/

14 pages

Audio & Video

7745 SjoGren's Syndrome Survival Guide
6707 Democracy Boulevard
Bethesda, MD 20817

301-530-4420
800-475-6473
Fax: 301-530-4415
e-mail: staylor@sjogrens.org
www.sjogrens.org

A complete resource for Sjogren's sufferers providing the newest medical information, research results, and treatment methods available, as well as the most effective and practical self-help strategies. Sjogren's syndrome is an autoimmune disease in which the body's immune system mistakenly attacks its own moisture producing glands.
Kenneth Economou, Chairman
Stephen Cohen, Chairman-Elect

Web Sites

7746 Healing Well

www.healingwell.com

An online health resource guide to medical news, chat, information and articles, newsgroups and message boards, books, disease-related web sites, medical directories, and more for patients, friends, and family coping with disabling diseases, disorders, or chronic illnesses.

Peter Waite, Founder & CEO

7747 Health Finder

www.healthfinder.gov

Searchable, carefully developed web site offering information on over 1000 topics. Developed by the US Department of Health and Human Services, the site can be used in both English and Spanish.

7748 Healthlink USA

www.healthlinkusa.com

Health information concerning treatment, cures, prevention, diagnosis, risk factors, research, support groups, email lists, personal stories and much more. Updated regularly.

7749 Helios Health

www.helioshealth.com

Online resource for your health information. Detailed information about specific health topics, access to expert advice from our Medical Advisory Board, and up-to-date health news.

7750 MedicineNet

www.medicinenet.com

An online resource for consumers providing easy-to-read, authoritative medical and health information.

7751 Medscape

www.medscape.com

Medscape offers specialists, primary care physicians, and other health professionals the Web's most robust and integrated medical information and educational tools.

7752 National Sjogren's Syndrome Association

www.sjogrens.org

Provides educational materials to members about medical developments and research concerning SS nationally and internationally. Membership also includes assorted discounts on additional materials and events.

7753 Sjogren's Syndrome Foundation

www.sjogrens.org

Information on Sjogren's Syndrome, the SS Foundation, and links to other related sites.

7754 WebMD

www.webmd.com

Provides credible information, supportive communities, and in-depth reference material about health subjects. A source for original and timely health information as well as material from well known content providers.

Description

7755 Skin Disorders

The three most common chronic skin disorders are acne, psoriasis and eczema. Although these conditions do not shorten one's life, or cause significant disability, they can have a profound effect on one's quality of life and self-esteem.

Acne is probably the most common skin disorder, and can affect all age groups. It typically occurs in adolescents and young adults. Acne involves the sebaceous glands - glands that produce sebum, a substance that preserves the skin's natural oiliness. In acne, the glands' pores become plugged, trapping the sebum and bacteria. Inflammation follows, resulting in small red tender bumps with a corresponding blackhead or whitehead. These lesions can become pus-filled or even cystic ranging from 1 mm to 5 mm. Acne is seen most commonly on the face, neck, back and shoulders. Treatment starts with keeping affected areas clean. Locally-applied creams include retinoic acid, benzoyl peroxide and various antibiotics. Oral antibiotics (tetracycline) are especially effective for large, deep pimples. Oral tretinoin (Accutane) is very affective, but causes birth defects and other side effects and should be used only as a last resort and in consultation with a dermatologist. Oral contraceptives are often helpful in young women.

Psoriasis usually begins in early adult life, and affects 2 to 4 percent of the white population. A family history is common. The disease is characterized by scaly patches, some as small rain drop, others a few inches in diameer. Typical locations are the scalp, knees and elbows, but any part of the body may be affected. The patches are extremely itchy, and compulsive scratching may further damage the skin. In roughly 10 percent there is an associated arthritis. Milder cases are treated with steroid creams applied to skin and tar preparations or oral psoralen drugs, is effective in more severe cases. The most severe cases require immunomodulating drugs like methotrexate or cyclosporine.

Eczema is a catchall term for many diseases which involve skin inflammation in response to some irritant. The irritant may be a direct one, such as contact dermatitis from the metal in a belt buckle, or an indirect one, as in atopic dermatitis triggered by various environmental agents (inhalants) and factors (certain foods). Atopic dermatitis is frequently associated with a personal or family history of allergic disorders (hay fever, asthma). For either situation, treatment consists of identifying and eliminating the offending agent(if possible) and local application of corticosteroid creams or nonspecific soothing and hydrating substances. Topical tacrolimus, approved by the FDA in 2000, is an immunosuppressive ointment effective for severe eczema without damaging the skin in the way that long-term topical steroids sometimes do.

National Agencies & Associations

7756 American Academy of Dermatology
PO Box 4014
Schaumburg, IL 60168-4014

847-240-1280
866-503-7546
Fax: 847-240-1859
e-mail: volunteer@aad.org
www.aad.org

The largest, most influential dermatologic association in the world. The Academy is committed to the highest quality standards in continuing medical education and plays a major role in formulating socioeconomic solutions.
Cyndi Del Boccio, Board of Director
Barbara Greenan, Advisory Board

7757 American Board of Dermatology American Society for Dermatologic Surger
American Society for Dermatologic Surgery
5550 Meadowbrook Drive
Rolling Meadows, IL 60008

847-956-0900
Fax: 847-956-0999
e-mail: info@asds.net
www.asds.net

Sole mission is to ensure competence for patients with cutaneous diseases through board representation.
Timothy Flynn, President
Debra Kennedy, Associate Executive Director

7758 American Dermatological Association University of Iowa Hospital and Clinics
University of Iowa Hospital and Clinics
5550 Meadowbrook Drive
Rolling Meadows, IL 60008

847-956-0900
Fax: 847-956-0999
e-mail: info@asds.net
www.asds-net.org

Professional society of physicians specializing in dermatology. Promotes teaching, practice, public education and research into dermatology.
Katherine J Svedman, Executive Director
Debra Kennedy, Associate Executive Director

7759 American Society for Dermatologic Surgery
5550 Meadowbrook Drive
Rolling Meadows, IL 60008-2005

847-956-0900
Fax: 847-956-0999
e-mail: info@asds.net
www.asds.net

Seeks to improve the quality of abnormal skin conditions especially the structural changes produced by skin cancer and other disease.
Katherine J Svedman, Executive Director
Robert A Weiss, President

7760 American Society of Plastic and Reconstructive Surgeons
444 E Algonquin Road
Arlington Heights, IL 60005-4654

847-228-9900
800-475-2784
e-mail: media@plasticsurgery.org
www.plasticsurgery.org

This Society sends free information about various surgical procedures and also provides the names of board certified plastic surgeons in a patient's area.
Dr.Gregory evans, President

7761 Dermatology Foundation
1560 Sherman Avenue
Evanston, IL 60201-4808

847-328-2256
Fax: 847-328-0509
e-mail: dfgen@dermatologyfoundation.org
www.dermfnd.org

Raises funds for the control of skin diseases through research improved education and better patient care. Supports basic clinical investigations.
Michael D tharp, President
Bruce U Wintroub, Chairman

7762 Eczema Association for Science and Education
4460 Redwood Highway
San Rafael, CA 94903

415-499-3474
800-818-7546
Fax: 415-472-5345
e-mail: info@nationaleczema.org
www.nationaleczema.org

Offers research and information to persons with eczema and other skin disorders.
Susan Tofte, Secretary
jamie Huber, Chair

7763 International Society of Dermatology
2323 N State Street 386-437-4405
Bunnell, FL 32110-0001 Fax: 386-437-4427
e-mail: info@intsocderm.org
www.intsocderm.org
Promotes interest education and research in dermatology.
Sigfrid A Muller MD, President
Mark Davis, Vice President

7764 National Arthritis and Musculoskeletal & Skin Diseases
Information Clearinghouse
National Institutes of Health
1 AMS Circle 301-495-4484
Bethesda, MD 20892-2350 Fax: 301-718-6366
TTY: 301-565-2966
e-mail: niamsinfo@mail.nih.gov
www.niams.nih.gov
Our mission is to support research into the causes, treatment and prevention of arthritis and musculoskeletal and skin diseases, the training of basic and clinical scientists to carry out this research and the dissemination of information on research.
Stephen I Katz MD PhD, Director

7765 National Institute of Arthritis and Musculoskeletal and Skin
Disease (NIAMS)
1 AMS Circle 301-495-4484
Bethesda, MD 20892 877-226-4267
Fax: 301-718-6366
TTY: 301-565-2966
e-mail: niamsinfo@mail.nih.gov
www.niams.nih.gov
The NIAMS Information Clearinghouse provides free information about various forms of arthritis and rheumatic disease and bone, muscle and skin diseases. It distributes patient and professional education materials and refers people to other sources of information.
Stephen I Katz MD PhD, Director

Foundations

7766 National Psoriasis Foundation
6600 SW 92nd Avenue 503-244-7404
Portland, OR 97223-7195 800-723-9166
Fax: 503-245-0626
e-mail: getinfo@psoriasis.org
www.psoriasis.org
Misson: To find a cure for psoriasis arthritis and to eliminate their devastating effects through research, advocacy, and education. Provides: patient services; public and professional education; community services; government affairs; research.
Randy Beranek, President/CEO
Bill Cardmon, Chief Field Operations

Research Centers

7767 Agromedicine Program Medical University of South Carolina
Medical University of South Carolina
171 Ashley Av. 843-792-1414
Charleston, SC 29425-0100 Fax: 843-792-1798
www.musc.edu
Does research into the effects of pesticides on humans including epidemiology and skin diseases.
Dr Stanley Schuman, Director
W Stuart Smith, Vice President for Clinical Operations a

7768 Duke University Plastic Surgery Research Laboratories
Medical Center
Box 3974 919-681-8555
Durham, NC 27710-1 e-mail: elizabeth.yundt@duke.edu
plastic.surgery.duke.edu

Conducts studies on skin cancer and aging skin.
Gregory Georgiade, Chief Division of Plastic and Reconstru
Detlev Erdmann, Associate Professor of Surgery

7769 Laboratory of Dermatology Research Memorial Sloane-Kettering
Cancer Center
Memorial Sloane-Kettering Cancer Center
1275 York Avenue 212-639-2000
New York, NY 10065-6007 Fax: 212-717-3363
www.mskcc.org/mskcc
Specific studies on the identification of skin disorders and dermatology.
Allan C Halpern, Chief Dermatology Service

7770 Massachusetts General Hospital: Harvard Cutaneous Biology
Research Center
Massachusetts General Hospital
55 Fruit Street 617-726-5254
Boston, MA 02114 Fax: 617-726-1875
TTY: 617-724-8800
www.massgeneral.org
Dermatology research.
Peter L Flavin, President
John R Hinghman, Secretary

7771 Orentreich Foundation for the Advancement of Science
855 Route 301 212-606-0836
Cold Spring, NY 10516-4155 Fax: 845-265-4210
e-mail: ofas@orentreich.org
http://www.orentreich.org/team
Conducts biomedical research on dermatology.
Norman Orentreich, Founder and Co-Director
David S Orentreich, Co-Director

7772 Psoriasis Research Institute
6600 SW 92nd Avenue 503-244-7404
Portland, OR 97223 800-723-9166
Fax: 503-245-0626
e-mail: getinfo@psoriasis.org
www.psoriasis.org
Studies the causes symptoms and treatments of psoriasis.
Randy Beranek, President/CEO
Bill Cardmon, Chief Field Operations

7773 Rockefeller University Laboratory for Investigative Dermatology
Rockefeller University
1230 York Avenue 212-327-7458
New York, NY 10021-6399 Fax: 212-570-8232
www.rockefeller.edu
Research into skin disorders and the whole specialty of dermatology in general.
D Martin Carter MD, PhD, Head

7774 Rockefeller University, Laboratory for Investigative Dermatology
1230 York Avenue 212-327-7458
New York, NY 10021-6399 Fax: 212-570-8232
www.rockefeller.edu

D Martin Carter MD, PhD, Head

7775 Scripps Clinic and Research Foundation: Autoimmune Disease
Center
10550 N Torrey Pines Road 858-784-1000
La Jolla, CA 92037-1092 Fax: 619-554-6805
www.scripps.edu
Research into dermatomyostis and polymyositis.
Eng Tan, Professor Emeritus

7776 Sulzberger Institute for Dermatologic Education
PO Box 94020 847-330-0230
Palatine, IL 60094-4020 Fax: 847-330-0050
http://www.aad.org/
A nonprofit research center whose sole goal is to enhance patient care through the development and promotion of quality educational programs on the care and disorders of the skin, hair, nails and mucous membranes.
Dirk M. Elston, President
Lisa A.ÿ Garner, Vice president

7777 Sulzberger Institute for Dermatologic Educ
PO Box 94020 847-330-0230
Palatine, IL 60094 Fax: 847-330-0050
http://www.aad.org/
A nonprofit research center whose sole goal is to enhance patient care through the development and promotion of quality educational programs on the care and disorders of the skin hair nails and mucous membranes.
Dirk M. Elston, President
Lisa A.ÿ Garner, Vice president

7778 University of California: San Francisco Dermatology Drug Research
515 Spruce 415-476-2001
San Francisco, CA 94143-0001 Fax: 415-221-4751
www.ucsf.edu
Conducts clinical testing of new or existing pharmalogic agents used in the treatment of skin disorders.
John Koo MD, Director
Susan Desmond, Chancellor

7779 University of Texas: Southwestern Medical Center at Dallas, Immunodermatology
5323 Harry Hines Boulevard 214-648-3111
Dallas, TX 75390-7208 Fax: 214-688-8275
www.utsouthwestern.edu
Provides a focus for research into the causes prevention and management of diseases such as immune deficiencies and infections. Studies are aimed at increasing basic-level understanding of immunologic skin diseases.
Daniel K Podolsky MD, President
Diane Jeffries, Director

Support Groups & Hotlines

7780 National Health Information Center
PO Box 1133 310-565-4167
Washington, DC 20013 800-336-4797
Fax: 301-984-4256
e-mail: info@nhic.org
www.health.gov/nhic
Offers a nationwide information referral service, produces directories and resource guides.

Books

7781 Managing Your Psoriasis
MasterMedia
P.O. Box 4014 847-240-1280
Schaumburg, IL 60168 866-503-7546
Fax: 847-240-1859
www.aad.org
1993 Paperback
ISBN: 0-942361-83-0

7782 Psoriasis and Psoriatic Arthritis Pocket G uide
National Psoriasis Foundation
6600 SW 92nd Avenue 503-244-7404
Portland, OR 97223-7195 800-723-9166
Fax: 503-245-0626
e-mail: getinfo@psoriasis.org
www.psoriasis.org
The Pocket Guide includes algorithms for therapy_including combination and biologic treatments_based on patient types. This second edition was revised to provide guidance for managing patients with severe psoriasis and to put the roll of new biologics into perspective.
2005 79 pages
Krista Kellogg, Chair
Pete Redding, Vice-Chair

7783 Q&A's About Psoriasis
NAMSIC/National Institutes of Health

1 AMS Circle 301-495-4484
Bethesda, MD 20892-0001 877-226-4267
Fax: 301-718-6366
TTY: 301-565-2966
e-mail: niamsinfo@mail.nih.gov
www.nih.gov/niams
Offers various information for the psoriasis patient and their family regarding treatments, risks, nutrition and more.
24 pages

7784 Therapy of Moderate-to-Severe Psoriasis
National Psoriasis Foundation
6600 SW 92nd Avenue 503-244-7404
Portland, OR 97223-7195 800-723-9166
Fax: 503-245-0626
e-mail: getinfo@psoriasis.org
www.psoriasis.org
Edited by Gerald D. Weinstein, MD, and Alice Gottlieb, MD, PhD, this book includes information on state-of-the-art clinical management through contributions from national experts on psoriasis.
2002
Krista Kellogg, Chair
Pete Redding, Vice-Chair

7785 Treatment Guide for the Health Insurance Industry
National Psoriasis Foundation
6600 SW 92nd Avenue 503-244-7404
Portland, OR 97223-7195 800-723-9166
Fax: 503-245-0626
e-mail: getinfo@psoriasis.org
www.psoriasis.org
This easy-to-read general overview is a valuable tool for the insurer or any health professional interested in detailed information about psoriasis and psoriatic arthritis, patient quality of life issues, and many available treatments.
Krista Kellogg, Chair
Pete Redding, Vice-Chair

Magazines

7786 International Journal of Dermatology
International Society of Dermatology
200 1st Street SW
Rochester, MN 55905-0001 507-284-3736
onlinelibrary.wiley.com
Focuses on information for dermatologists and the whole specialty of dermatology research and education.
10x Year

7787 Journal of Dermatologic Surgery and Oncology
International Society for Dermatologic Surgery
930 N Meachan Road 847-240-1005
Schaumburg, IL 60173 Fax: 847-240-0101
www.aad.org
Focuses on medical updates and information on dermatology.
Monthly
Terrie Duhadway, Executive Publisher

7788 Journal of the Academy of Dermatology
American Academy of Dermatology
930 E. Woodfield Road 847-240-1005
Schaumburg, IL 60173-4020 Fax: 847-240-0101
www.aad.org
A scientific publication serving the clinical needs of the specialty and provides a wide selection of articles on various topics important to continuing medical education of Academy members and the international dermatologic community.
Monthly
Terrie Duhadway, Executive Publisher

7789 Psoriasis Advance
National Psoriasis Foundation
6600 SW 92nd Avenue 503-244-7404
Portland, OR 97223-7195 800-723-9166
Fax: 503-245-0626
e-mail: getinfo@npfusa.org
www.psoriasis.org
Written especially for the psoriatis community four times a year. Provides current articles to keep you up to date with treatmetnt and

research information, pave the way to empowerment, and connect you with others.
40 pages BiMonthly
Krista Kellogg, Chair
Pete Redding, Vice-Chair

7790 Psoriasis Forum
National Psoriasis Foundation
6600 SW 92nd Avenue   503-244-7404
Portland, OR 97223-7195   800-723-9166
                       Fax: 503-245-0626
             e-mail: getinfo@psoriasis.org
                         www.psoriasis.org
Dedicated to providing up-to-date and practical information to health care providers on the frontline of psoriasis treatment. Professional Members only.
Quarterly
Krista Kellogg, Chair
Pete Redding, Vice-Chair

Newsletters

7791 Dermatology Focus
Dermatology Foundation
1560 Sherman Avenue   847-328-2256
Evanston, IL 60201-4808   Fax: 847-328-0509
       e-mail: dfgen@dermatologyfoundation.org
                         www.dermfnd.org
Designed to communicate to practitioners the latest advances in medical and surgical dermatology. The publication also serves as the Foundation's newsletter, recognizing the accomplishments and activities of the many dermatologists who give not only their monetary support, but countless hours to develop the research and teaching careers of future leaders throughout the specialty.
Quarterly
Michael D. Tharp, President
Bruce U. Wintroub, Chairman

7792 Dermatology Focus
Dermatology Foundation
1560 Sherman Avenue   847-328-2256
Evanston, IL 60201-4808   Fax: 847-328-0509
       e-mail: dfgen@dermatologyfoundation.org
                         www.dermfnd.org
Designed to communicate to practitioners the latest advances in medical and surgical dermatology. The publication also serves as the Foundation's newsletter recognizing the accomplishments and activities of the many dermatologists who give not only their monetary support, but countless hours to develop the research and teaching careers of future leaders throughout the specialty.
Quarterly
Michael D. Tharp, President
Bruce U. Wintroub, Chairman

7793 Dermatology World
American Academy of Dermatology
P.O. Box 4014   847-240-1280
Schaumburg, IL 60168-4020   866-503-7546
                    Fax: 847-240-1859
                         www.aad.org
Offers Academy members information outside the clinical realm. It carries news of government actions, reports of socioeconomic issues, societal trends and other events which impinge on the practice of dermatology.
Monthly

7794 Progress in Dermatology
Dermatology Foundation
1560 Sherman Avenue   847-328-2256
Evanston, IL 60201-4808   Fax: 847-328-0509
       e-mail: dfgen@dermatologyfoundation.org
                         www.dermfnd.org
The journal provides in-depth coverage of clinically relevant topics as well as basic scientific advances affecting all of dermatology. Distributed exclusively to members of the Foundation.
Quarterly
Michael D. Tharp, President
Bruce U. Wintroub, Chairman

7795 Psoriasis Newsletter
Psoriasis Research Institute
6600 SW 92nd Avenue   503-244-7404
Portland, OR 97223   800-723-9166
                     Fax: 503-245-0626
             e-mail: getinfo@psoriasis.org
                         www.psoriasis.org
Offers information and medical updates on the disease of psoriasis, events, fundraising and more.
4 pages Quarterly
Krista Kellogg, Chair
Pete Redding, Vice-Chair

Pamphlets

7796 Acne
American Academy of Dermatology
PO Box 4014   847-240-1280
Schaumburg, IL 60168-4014   866-503-7546
                    Fax: 847-240-1859
                         www.aad.org
Explains the causes of acne. Treatments are explored, including diet, medications, antibiotics, and sun exposure. Available in Spanish.
1996

7797 Allergic Contact Rashes
American Academy of Dermatology
PO Box 4014   847-240-1280
Schaumburg, IL 60168-4014   866-503-7546
                    Fax: 847-240-1859
                         www.aad.org
Lists the common causes of skin rashes, including jewelry and hidden ingredients in fabrics and household products.
1997

7798 Athlete's Foot
American Academy of Dermatology
PO Box 4014   847-240-1280
Schaumburg, IL 60168-4014   866-503-7546
                    Fax: 847-240-1859
                         www.aad.org
This common fungal infection is not only a problem for athletics. Discusses what causes it and how to treat it.
1994

7799 Black Skin
American Academy of Dermatology
PO Box 4014   847-240-1280
Schaumburg, IL 60168-4014   866-503-7546
                    Fax: 847-240-1859
                         www.aad.org
Explains the skin diseases common with black skin and how they are diagnosed and treated.
1996

7800 Conception, Pregnancy & Psoriasis
National Psoriasis Foundation
6600 SW 92nd Avenue   503-244-7404
Portland, OR 97223-7195   800-723-9166
                    Fax: 503-245-0626
                         www.aad.org
Explains pregnancy factors for persons with psoriasis.

7801 Cosmetics & Skin Care
American Academy of Dermatology
PO Box 4014   847-240-1280
Schaumburg, IL 60168-4014   866-503-7546
                    Fax: 847-240-1859
                         www.aad.org
Discusses skin reactions to fragrances, makeup, and bath and body care products.
1994

7802 Darker Side of Tanning
American Academy of Dermatology

PO Box 4014
Schaumburg, IL 60168-4014

847-240-1280
866-503-7546
Fax: 847-240-1859
www.aad.org

Discusses the dangers of ultraviolet radiation from the sun, tanning beds, and sun lamps. Includes descriptions of the different skin types and tips to help minimize the sun's damage to the skin and eyes.
1996

7803 Eczema/Atopic Dermatitis
American Academy of Dermatology
PO Box 4014
Schaumburg, IL 60168-4014

847-240-1280
866-503-7546
Fax: 847-240-1859
www.aad.org

Explains how to recognize and treat dermatitis.
1995

7804 For Parents
National Psoriasis Foundation
6600 SW 92nd Avenue
Portland, OR 97223-7195

503-244-7404
800-723-9166
Fax: 503-245-0626
e-mail: getinfo@npfusa.org
www.psoriasis.org

Offers advice and resources on how to educate yourself about psoriasis and your child, as well as treatment information and summer camps.

7805 Genital Psoriasis
National Psoriasis Foundation
6600 SW 92nd Avenue
Portland, OR 97223-7195

503-244-7404
800-723-9166
Fax: 503-245-0626
e-mail: getinfo@npfusa.org
www.psoriasis.org

Introduces the reader to the basics of genital psoriasis, and treatment options.

7806 Hand Eczema
American Academy of Dermatology
PO Box 4014
Schaumburg, IL 60168-4014

847-240-1280
866-503-7546
Fax: 847-240-1859
www.aad.org

Shows examples of hand rashes, explains causes, lists protective measures and treatments.
1993

7807 Hives
American Academy of Allergy, Asthma and Immunology
555 East Wells Street
Milwaukee, WI 53202-3889

414-272-6071
800-822-2762
Fax: 414-272-6070
www.aaaai.org

This brochure offers information on what causes hives, what is Angioedema, and how hives can be treated.

7808 Home Phototherapy
National Psoriasis Foundation
6600 SW 92nd Avenue
Portland, OR 97223-7195

503-244-7404
800-723-9166
Fax: 503-245-0626
e-mail: getinfo@npfusa.org
www.psoriasis.org

Talks about the use of a home UVB unit to treat psoriasis.

7809 Methotrexate (MTX)
National Psoriasis Foundation
6600 SW 92nd Avenue
Portland, OR 97223-7195

503-244-7404
800-723-9166
Fax: 503-245-0626
e-mail: getinfo@npfusa.org
www.psoriasis.org

An introductions to MTX treatment.

7810 Oral Retinoid Therapy (Soriatane)
National Psoriasis Foundation

6600 SW 92nd Avenue
Portland, OR 97223-7195

503-244-7404
800-723-9166
Fax: 503-245-0626
e-mail: getinfo@npfusa.org
www.psoriasis.org

Explains Soriatane treatment options.

7811 PUVA (Psoralen Plus Ultraviolet Light A)
National Psoriasis Foundation
6600 SW 92nd Avenue
Portland, OR 97223-7195

503-244-7404
800-723-9166
Fax: 503-245-0626
e-mail: getinfo@npfusa.org
www.psoriasis.org

Explains PUVA treatment options, pros, cons, and potential side-effects.

7812 Pityriasis Rosea
American Academy of Dermatology
PO Box 4014
Schaumburg, IL 60168-4014

847-240-1280
866-503-7546
Fax: 847-240-1859
www.aad.org

Discusses the appearance, symptoms, and causes of this common rash. Diagnosis and treatment are also explained.
1996

7813 Psoriasis on Specific Skin Sites
National Psoriasis Foundation
6600 SW 92nd Avenue
Portland, OR 97223-7195

503-244-7404
800-723-9166
Fax: 503-245-0626
e-mail: getinfo@npfusa.org
www.psoriasis.org

Including nails, ears, eyelids, face, mouth and lips, hands and feet.

7814 Psoriasis: How It Makes You Feel
National Psoriasis Foundation
6600 SW 92nd Avenue
Portland, OR 97223-7195

503-244-7404
800-723-9166
Fax: 503-245-0626
e-mail: getinfo@npfusa.org
www.psoriasis.org

7815 Psoriatic Arthritis
National Psoriasis Foundation
6600 SW 92nd Avenue
Portland, OR 97223-7195

503-244-7404
800-723-9166
Fax: 503-245-0626
e-mail: getinfo@npfusa.org
www.psoriasis.org

7816 Rosacea
American Academy of Dermatology
PO Box 4014
Schaumburg, IL 60168-4014

847-240-1280
866-503-7546
Fax: 847-240-1859
www.aad.org

The condition, do's and don'ts for rosacea patients, and treatment are explained.
1995

7817 Scabies
American Academy of Dermatology
PO Box 4014
Schaumburg, IL 60168-4014

847-240-1280
866-503-7546
Fax: 847-240-1859
www.aad.org

Explains the nature of the scabies parasite, symptoms, at-risk groups, individual and large group treatments. Available in Spanish.
1997

7818 Scalp Psoriasis
National Psoriasis Foundation
6600 SW 92nd Avenue
Portland, OR 97223-7195

503-244-7404
800-723-9166
Fax: 503-245-0626
e-mail: getinfo@npfusa.org
www.psoriasis.org

7819 Seborrheic Dermatitis
American Academy of Dermatology
PO Box 4014
Schaumburg, IL 60168-4014

847-240-1280
866-503-7546
Fax: 847-240-1859
www.aad.org

Answers the most frequently asked questions about this common, easily treatable skin condition.
1995

7820 Seborrheic Keratoses
American Academy of Dermatology
PO Box 4014
Schaumburg, IL 60168-4014

847-240-1280
866-503-7546
Fax: 847-240-1859
www.aad.org

Describes seborrheic keratosis growths, causes, and treatments.
1997

7821 Skin Cancer
American Academy of Dermatology
PO Box 4014
Schaumburg, IL 60168-4014

847-240-1280
866-503-7546
Fax: 847-240-1859
www.aad.org

Warning signs and how to perform self-examinations are discussed.
1994

7822 Skin Conditions Related to AIDS
American Academy of Dermatology
PO Box 4014
Schaumburg, IL 60168-4014

847-240-1280
866-503-7546
Fax: 847-240-1859
www.aad.org

What AIDS is, who's at risk, and other important information about this major health problem are discussed.
1997

7823 Specific Forms of Psoriasis
National Psoriasis Foundation
6600 SW 92nd Avenue
Portland, OR 97223-7195

503-244-7404
800-723-9166
Fax: 503-245-0626
e-mail: getinfo@npfusa.org
www.psoriasis.org

Pustular, Guttate, Inverse, and Erythrodermic.

7824 Spider Veins, Varicose Vein Therapy
American Academy of Dermatology
PO Box 4014
Schaumburg, IL 60168-4014

847-240-1280
866-503-7546
Fax: 847-240-1859
www.aad.org

Discusses the latest methods for removing unsightly and unwanted blood vessels that appear mostly on the legs.
1995

7825 Sun & Water Therapy
National Psoriasis Foundation
6600 SW 92nd Avenue
Portland, OR 97223-7195

503-244-7404
800-723-9166
Fax: 503-245-0626
e-mail: getinfo@npfusa.org
www.psoriasis.org

7826 Sun Protection for Children
American Academy of Dermatology
PO Box 4014
Schaumburg, IL 60168-4014

847-240-1280
866-503-7546
Fax: 847-240-1859
www.aad.org

Teaches parents how to protect their children from the sun's harmful rays.
1996

7827 Sun and Your Skin
American Academy of Dermatology
PO Box 4014
Schaumburg, IL 60168-4014

847-240-1280
866-503-7546
Fax: 847-240-1859
www.aad.org

Information on acute sunburn, premature aging of the skin, allergies, and skin cancer. Tips on how to be sun smart.
1994

7828 Sunlight, Ultraviolet Radiation and the Skin
National Cancer Institute
149 Madison Avenue
New York, NY 10016-0001

212-725-5176
800-422-6237
www.skincancer.org

7829 Tinea Versicolor
American Academy of Dermatology
PO Box 4014
Schaumburg, IL 60168-4014

847-240-1280
866-503-7546
Fax: 847-240-1859
www.aad.org

Discusses the symptoms, diagnosis, and treatment of this often misunderstood fungal infection.
1995

7830 Treatment Overview
National Psoriasis Foundation
6600 SW 92nd Avenue
Portland, OR 97223-7195

503-244-7404
800-723-9166
Fax: 503-245-0626
e-mail: getinfo@npfusa.org
www.psoriasis.org

Discusses a number of available psoriasis treatments, what is considered by the doctor when developing a treatment plan, and treatment resources.

7831 Vascular Birthmarks
American Academy of Dermatology
PO Box 4014
Schaumburg, IL 60168-4014

847-240-1280
866-503-7546
Fax: 847-240-1859
www.aad.org

Includes descriptions and treatments for most common types of vascular birthmarks - macular stains, hemangiomas, and port-wine stains.
1997

7832 Vitiligo
American Academy of Dermatology
PO Box 4014
Schaumburg, IL 60168-4014

847-240-1280
866-503-7546
Fax: 847-240-1859
www.aad.org

Discusses lost skin pigmentation and what can be done about it, including repigmentation therapy.
1994

7833 Young People and Psoriasis
National Psoriasis Foundation
6600 SW 92nd Avenue
Portland, OR 97223-7195

503-244-7404
800-723-9166
Fax: 503-245-0626
e-mail: getinfo@npfusa.org
www.psoriasis.org

Infancy through adolescence.

7834 Your Diet & Psoriasis
National Psoriasis Foundation
6600 SW 92nd Avenue
Portland, OR 97223-7195

503-244-7404
800-723-9166
Fax: 503-245-0626
e-mail: getinfo@npfusa.org
www.psoriasis.org

A discussion of particular diets, foods and supplements and the effect they have on psoriasis.

7835 Your Skin and Your Dermatologist
American Academy of Dermatology
PO Box 4014
Schaumburg, IL 60168-4014

847-240-1280
866-503-7546
Fax: 847-240-1859
www.aad.org

Explains why a dermatologist is the appropriate specialist for the care of diseases of the skin, hair, nails, and mucous membranes.
1997

Audio & Video

7836   Allergic Skin Reactions
American Academy of Allergy, Asthma and Immunology
555 East Wells Street   414-272-6071
Milwaukee, WI 53202-3889   800-822-2762
                                      Fax: 414-272-6070
                                          www.aaaai.org

In some people, allergy symptoms include itching redness, rashes, or hives. This video describes the symptoms, triggers, and treatment for common skin reactions such as dermatitis, hives and angioedema.
10-13 minutes

7837   Basic Science Series
American Academy of Dermatology
PO Box 4014   847-240-1280
Schaumburg, IL 60168-4014   866-503-7546
                                      Fax: 847-240-1859
                                           www.aad.org

Combines high-quality 35mm slides and accompanying narration on audiocassette and features topics that underline and support clinical dermatology. The series is useful for residents in training as well as practicing dermatologists.
Slides

7838   CME Video Library
American Academy of Dermatology
PO Box 4014   847-240-1280
Schaumburg, IL 60168-4014   866-503-7546
                                      Fax: 847-240-1859
                                           www.aad.org

A series of video programs developed by AAD experts recognized for their continued efforts in dermatologic advancement.
Videotapes

7839   Facts About Acne
American Academy of Dermatology
PO Box 4014   847-240-1280
Schaumburg, IL 60168-4014   866-503-7546
                                      Fax: 847-240-1859
                                           www.aad.org

The etiology of acne and treatment choices are explained by consultants, with patient encounters.
13 minutes

7840   Mystery of Contact Dermatitis
American Academy of Dermatology
PO Box 4014   847-240-1280
Schaumburg, IL 60168-4014   866-503-7546
                                      Fax: 847-240-1859
                                           www.aad.org

The causes and treatment of some common forms of contact dermatitis are shown with consultation and commentary.
10 minutes

7841   National Library of Dermatologic Teaching Slides
American Academy Of Dermatology
PO Box 94020   847-240-1280
Palatine, IL 60094-4020   866-503-7546
                                      Fax: 847-240-1859
                                           www.aad.org

A collection of dermatologic teaching slides offering the most comprehensive series ever assembled. Each set offers a realistic presentation of classic clinical skin conditions encountered by the dermatologist.

7842   Skin Cancer: The Undeclared Epidemic
American Academy of Dermatology
PO Box 4014   847-240-1280
Schaumburg, IL 60168-4014   866-503-7546
                                      Fax: 847-240-1859
                                           www.aad.org

Examples of skin cancer lesions, interviews with patients at screenings, and comments from Academy members.
9 minutes

7843   Skin Care Under the Sun
American Academy of Dermatology
PO Box 4014   847-240-1280
Schaumburg, IL 60168-4014   866-503-7546
                                      Fax: 847-240-1859
                                           www.aad.org

Dramatization of the dangers of overexposure to the sun, providing explanations of the effects of ultraviolet radiation on the skin.
7 minutes

Web Sites

7844   American Academy of Dermatology
                                           www.aad.org
Promotes and advances the science and art of medicine and surgery related to the skin, promotes the highest possible standards in clinical practice, education and research.

7845   American Society of Plastic and Reconstructive Surgeons
                                     www.plasticsurgery.org
The mission of ASPS is to advance quality care to plastic surgery patients by encouraging high standards of training, ethics, physician practice and research in plastic surgery. The Society is a strong advocate for patient safety and requires its members to operate in accredited surgical facilities that have passed rigorous external review of equipment and staffing.

7846   Derma Doctor
                                       www.dermadoctor.com
The most informative skin care site on the Web. An extensive library of newsletters to help answer your questions.

7847   Dermatology Foundation
                                           www.dermfnd.org
Raises funds for the control of skin diseases through research, improved education and better patient care. Supports basic clinical investigations.

7848   Healing Well
                                        www.healingwell.com
An online health resource guide to medical news, chat, information and articles, newsgroups and message boards, books, disease-related web sites, medical directories, and more for patients, friends, and family coping with disabling diseases, disorders, or chronic illnesses.

7849   Health Finder
                                        www.healthfinder.gov
Searchable, carefully developed web site offering information on over 1000 topics. Developed by the US Department of Health and Human Services, the site can be used in both English and Spanish.

7850   Healthlink USA
                                       www.healthlinkusa.com
Health information concerning treatment, cures, prevention, diagnosis, risk factors, research, support groups, email lists, personal stories and much more. Updated regularly.

7851   Helios Health
                                        www.helioshealth.com
Online resource for your health information. Detailed information about specific health topics, access to expert advice from our Medical Advisory Board, and up-to-date health news.

7852   MedicineNet
                                        www.medicinenet.com
An online resource for consumers providing easy-to-read, authoritative medical and health information.

7853   Medscape
                                          www.medscape.com
Medscape offers specialists, primary care physicians, and other health professionals the Web's most robust and integrated medical information and educational tools.

7854 Nat'l Arthritis and Musculoskeletal Skin

www.niams.nih.gov
The mission of the National Institute of Arthritis and
Musculoskeletal and Skin Diseases is to support research into the
causes, treatment, and prevention of arthritis and musculoskeletal
and skin diseases; the training of basic and clinical scientists to
carry out this research; and the dissemination of information on research progress in these diseases.

7855 Nat'l Institute of Arthritis

www.niams.nih.gov
The mission of the National Institute of Arthritis and
Musculoskeletal and Skin Diseases is to support research into the
causes, treatment, and prevention of arthritis and musculoskeletal
and skin diseases; the training of basic and clinical scientists to
carry out this research; and the dissemination of information on research progress in these diseases.

7856 National Psoriasis Foundation

www.psoriasis.org
The National Psoriasis Foundation (NPF) is a non-profit, voluntary health agency dedicated to curing psoriatic disease and improving the lives of those affected.

7857 Skin Store

www.skinstore.com
Carries over 500 of the finest skincare products, available at the
lowest prices, delivered immediately to your home.

7858 WebMD

www.webmd.com
Provides credible information, supportive communities, and
in-depth reference material about health subjects. A source for
original and timely health information as well as material from
well known content providers.

Description

7859 # Sleep Disorders

Sleep disorders are defined as disturbances that affect the ability to fall or stay asleep, that involve sleeping too much, or that result in abnormal sleep-related behavior. They can be categorized into primary sleep disorders; sleep disorders related to another mental disorder or a general medical condition; and substance induced sleep disorder. The two conditions discussed here, narcolepsy and obstructive sleep apnea, are both primary sleep disorders.

Narcolepsy is a rare disorder of abnormal and irresistible daytime drowsiness. Excessive daytime sleepiness with involuntary daytime sleep episodes, disturbed nighttime sleep, and cataplexy (sudden weakness or loss of muscle tone, often triggered by emotion), are the most common symptoms of narcolepsy. Generally, symptoms appear between the onset of puberty and age 25, and worsen as the patient ages. There are 100,000 people in the US with this condition.

Although the exact cause of narcolepsy is unknown, there appears to be a genetic link.

Oral medication, including stimulant agents, as well as specific sleep schedules and other forms of behavioral therapy are also prescribed.

Obstructive sleep apnea is a serious and common sleep disorder that features heavy snoring and breathing irregularities. It is chronic and relapsing, and varies in severity from mild to lethal. Almost 90 percent of the estimated 12 million sleep apnea sufferers are male. Obstructive sleep apnea is biomechanical and usually occurs when tissues in the back of the throat collapse and close the breathing passage. Sufferers experience heavy snoring, periods during sleep when breathing halts for 10 seconds or more, and many short awakenings which they do not remember. In the worst cases, sufferers may cease breathing for more than half of total sleeping time, which can result in daytime fatigue, oxygen deprivation and hypertension.

Signs of sleep apnea or a related sleeping disorder include loud, habitual snoring, fatigue on waking, daytime sleepiness, and choking, gasping or holding one's breath while asleep. Overweight persons and smokers are more prone to develop this disorder. Heavy eating, late-night snacking, sedative use, and alcohol consumption are often contributing factors.

The diagnosis of sleep apnea often requires a polysomnography, or sleep study, which monitors brain waves, muscle tension, eye movement, respiration and blood-oxygen levels. Obviously, a partner can easily help to confirm these symptoms; single people can arrange for sleep observation in a hospital or clinic setting. Behavior modification is frequently sufficient to reduce or eliminate many snoring problems, as is sleep-ing on one's side and/or without a pillow. In addition to behavioral changes, mild cases are often responsive to oral devices that help to keep airways open by bringing the jaw forward, elevating the soft palate, or repositioning the tongue. More severe cases can be treated with a C-PAP (continuous positive airway pressure) machine, or a Bi-Level (Bi-PAP) machine, both of which blow air into the patient's airways in a regulated manner. Surgery is sometimes indicated, when facial or oral irregularities, such as jaw irregularities, small throat openings, enlarged tonsils, a large tongue or other tissue in front of the airway, or a deviated septum, impede proper airflow.

National Agencies & Associations

7860 **American Narcolepsy Association**
129 Waterwheel Lane
North Kingstown, RI 02852-6230   800-222-6085
http://www.narcolepsynetwork.org/
Offers help and information to persons with narcolepsy and their families.

7861 **American Sleep Apnea Association**
6856 E Avenue   202-293-3650
Washington, DC 20012   Fax: 202-293-3656
e-mail: asaa@sleepapnea.org
www.sleepapnea.org
Offers help and information to persons with sleep apnea and their families.
Michael P Coppola MD, President and Chief Medical Officer
Nancy Rothstein, Secretary

7862 **Association of Professional Sleep Societies**
One Westbrook Corporate Center   708-492-0930
Westchester, IL 60154   Fax: 708-273-9354
www.apss.org
Works to facilitate the research and development of sleep disorders medically by encouraging exchange of information among members.
Jerome A Barrett, Executive Director
Jennifer Markkanen, Assistant Executive Director

7863 **Lung Association**
6856 E Avenue   202-293-3650
Washington, DC 20012-6K2   Fax: 202-293-3656
e-mail: asaa@sleepapnea.org
www.sleep-apnea-ab.ca
The Lung Association - Sleep Apnea (LASA) is a patient and professional coalition providing support through improved care for patients with respiratory disorders of sleep.

7864 **NIH/National Institute of Neurological Disorders and Stroke**
PO Box 5801   301-496-5751
Bethesda, MD 20824   800-352-9424
TTY: 301-468-5981
www.ninds.nih.gov
Mission is to reduce the burden of neurological disease, a burden borne by every age group, by every segment of society, by people all over the world.
Story C Landis, Director
Walter J Koroshetz, Deputy Director

7865 **Narcolepsy Institute/Montefiore Medical Center**
111 E 210th Street   718-920-6799
Bronx, NY 10467-2490   Fax: 718-654-9580
e-mail: MGoswami@aol.com
www.montefiore.org
Offers services such as screening, information on narcolepsy, counseling and referrals for individuals and their families with problems arising as a consequence of narcolepsy, and adult and teenage support groups to help individuals develop positive self-images.
Dr Meeta Goswami, Director

7866 National Sleep Foundation
1522 K Street NW
Washington, DC 20005-1253
202-347-3471
Fax: 202-347-3472
e-mail: nsf@sleepfoundation.org
www.sleepfoundation.org
The National Sleep Foundation (NSF) is an independent nonprofit organization dedicated to improving public health and safety by achieving understanding of sleep and sleep disorders and by supporting education sleep-related research and advocacy.
Meir H Kryger, Chairman
Thomas J Balkin, Vice Chairman

7867 Sleep Research Society American Academy of Sleep Medicine
American Academy of Sleep Medicine
One Westbrook Corporate Center
Westchester, IL 60154
708-492-1093
Fax: 708-492-0943
e-mail: ncekosh@srsnet.org
www.sleepresearchsociety.org
Facilitates communication among research workers in this field but does not sponsor research investigations on its own.
Michael V Vitiello, President
Ronald Szymusiak, Secretary/Treasurer

Research Centers

7868 Baylor College of Medicine: Sleep Disorder and Research Center
6620 Main St
Houston, TX 77030-3498
713-798-1000
800-229-5671
Fax: 713-796-9718
e-mail: baylorclinicweb@bcm.edu
www.baylorclinic.com
Internal unit of the College that focuses on research into sleep and sexual dysfunction in males.
Shyam Subramanian, Medical Director
Charlie Lan, Assistant Professor of Medicine

7869 Capital Regional Sleep-Wake Disorders Center
St. Peter's Hospital and Albany Medical Center
25 Hackett Boulevard
Albany, NY 12208-3420
518-436-9253
Cheryl Carlu MD

7870 Center for Narcolepsy Research at the University of Illinois at Chicago
University of Illinois
845 S Damen Avenue
Chicago, IL 60612-7350
312-996-5176
Fax: 312-996-7008
e-mail: CNSHR@listserv.uic.edu
uic.edu/depts/cnr
Provides information to health professionals and people with sleep disorders regarding diagnosis and treatment. Maintain national network with sleep professionals throughout the US.
6-8 pages 2 per year
David W Carley, Director
Julie Law, Center Administrator

7871 Center for Research in Sleep Disorders Affiliated with Mercy Hospital
Mercy Hospital of Hamilton/Fairfield
1275 E Kemper Road
Cincinnati, OH 45246
513-671-3101
Martin Schar PhD

7872 Center for Sleep & Wake Disorders: Miami Valley Hospital
One Wyoming Street
Dayton, OH 45409-2722
937-208-8000
www.miamivalleyhospital.org
Offering the largest variety of sleep disorder testing available in the area it also offers comprehensive sleep care and care of related issues with a sleep lab clinical treatment pulmonary treatment and behavioral treatment in the same facility.
Kevin Huban, Director
Amy Cline, Administrative Director

7873 Center for Sleep Medicine of the Mount Sinai Medical Center
One Gustave L.Levy Place
New York, NY 10029-6500
212-241-6500
Fax: 212-875-84
www.mountsinai.org

The Center for Sleep Medicine at The Mount Sinai Medical Center is a comprehensive program dedicated to the diagnosis and treatment of all aspects of sleep pathology including breathing related sleep disorders periodic limb movements in sleep insomnia and narcolepsy. Mechanical (CPAP BiPAP ventilator) surgical dental and pharmacologic therapies are available.
E Neil Schachter, Professor
Gwen S Skloot, Associates Professor

7874 Geisinger Wyoming Valley Medical Center: Sleep Disorders Center
1000 E Mountain Drive
Wilkes-Barre, PA 18711
570-819-5770
www.geisinger.org

Our dedicated sleep team operates service sleep centers and laboratories to diagnose and treat a broad range of sleep disorders.˜ Geisinger sleep centers are conveniently located in Danville Bloomsburg Shamokin Wilkes-Barre and Mt. Pocono.
Andrew Paul Matragrano, Director
Stephanie Schaefer, Nurse Practitioner

7875 Johns Hopkins University: Sleep Disorders Francis Scott Key Medical Center
Francis Scott Key Medical Center
601 N Caroline Street
Baltimore, MD 21287
410-550-0545
www.hopkinshospital.org
The Johns Hopkins University Sleep Disorders Center is a tertiary care center for patients with sleep/wake disorders and medical disorders associated with sleep.
Phillip L Smith, Director

7876 Knollwoodpark Hospital Sleep Disorders Center
5600 Girby Road
Mobile, AL 36693-3398
251-660-5120
Fax: 251-660-5245
e-mail: 71054.2530@compuserve.com
www.southalabama.edu/usakph

7877 Knollwoodpark Hospital Sleep Disorders Cen
5600 Girby Road
Mobile, AL 36693
251-660-5120
Fax: 251-660-5245
e-mail: 71054.2530@compuserve.com
www.southalabama.edu/usakph

7878 Loma Linda University Sleep Disorders Clinic
VA Hospital Medical Services Center
11201 Benton Street
Loma Linda, CA 92357-1
909-825-7084
800-741-8387
Fax: 909-963-64
www.lom.med.va.gov
Ralph Downey III MD, Director

7879 Methodist Hospital Sleep Center Winona Memorial Hospital
Rehab Centers
6565 Fannin Street
Houston, TX 77030-8126
713-441-7854
Fax: 713-790-2612
www.methodisthealth.com
Marc L Boom, President & CEO
David M Underwood, Vice Chairman

7880 MidWest Medical Center: Sleep Disorders Center
Winona Memorial Hospital
Indianapolis, IN 46208-4688
317-927-2100
Fax: 317-927-2914

7881 Northwest Ohio Sleep Disorders Center Toledo Hospital
Toledo Hospital
2142 N Cove Boulevard
Toledo, OH 43606-3896
419-471-5629
Frank O Horton III MD, Director

7882 Ohio Sleep Medicine Institute
4975 Bradenton Avenue
Dublin, OH 43017-3521
614-766-0773
Fax: 614-766-2599
e-mail: info@sleepmedicine.com
www.sleepmedicine.com
A comprehensive accredited sleep disorders center that is dedicated to excellence in sleep medicine care. Offer evaluation, diagnosis and treatment for adults and children with sleep apnea, insomnia, restless legs syndrome, narcolepsy, parasomnias, circa-

dian rhythms disorders, shift work, fatigue and other sleep problems.
Betty Palmer, Director

7883 Penn Center for Sleep Disorders: Hospital of the University of Pennsylvania
3400 Spruce Street 215-662-7772
Philadelphia, PA 19104-4204 Fax: 215-349-8038
Joanne Getsy MD, Director

7884 Presbyterian-University Hospital: Pulmonary Sleep Evaluation Center
DeSoto At O'Hara Street 412-647-3475
Pittsburgh, PA 15213
Mark Sanders MD, Director

7885 Scripps Clinic Sleep Disorders Center Scripps Clinic
Scripps Clinic
10666 N Torrey Pines Road 858-455-9100
La Jolla, CA 92037-1027 Fax: 858-828-64
e-mail: malcoRN@scrippsclinic.com
www.scripps.org
The Scripps Clinic Sleep Center provides evaluation diagnosis and treatment of a full range of sleep disorders such as Circadian rhythm disorders Insomnia Narcolepsy Night terror Nightmares Restless legs syndrome Sleep apnea Sleepwalking and Snoring.
Dan Dworsky MD, Medical Director
Merrill M Mitler MD, Scientific Director

7886 Sleep Alertness Center: Lafayette Home Hospital
2400 S Street 765-447-6811
Lafayette, IN 47904-3027 e-mail: glenda.eberhard@glhsi.org
Frederick Ro MD

7887 Sleep Center: Community General Hospital
750 East Adams Street
Syracuse, NY 13210-5100 315-464-5540
www.cgh.org
The Sleep Center at Community General Hospital is a specialized facility providing accurate diagnosis and recommending treatment of sleep-related problems.
Robert Westl MD, Medical Director
Antonio Cule MD, Neurology Consultant

7888 Sleep Disorders Center Bethesda Oak Hospital
619 Oak Street
Cincinnati, OH 45206-1613 513-569-5400
www.trihealth.com

Milton Krame MD

7889 Sleep Disorders Center Columbia Presbyterian Medical Center
The University Hospital of Columbia & Cornell
161 Fort Washington Avenue 212-305-1860
New York, NY 10032 Fax: 212-305-5496
e-mail: inquire@sleepNYP.com
www.sleepnyp.com
A Highly specialized outpatient facility for the evaluation and treatment of patients with problems related to sleep and wakefulness.
Neil B Kavey, Medical Director
Andrew Tucker, Director

7890 Sleep Disorders Center Dartmouth Hitchcock Medical Center
Darthmouth Hitchcock medical Center
One Rope Ferry Road 603-650-1200
Hanover, NH 03755-1 877-367-1797
Fax: 603-650-1202
e-mail: Joanne.MacQuarrie@dartmouth.edu
dms.dartmouth.edu
Provides consultation and testing for all varieties of sleep-related disturbances including snoring sleep apnea narcolepsy restless legs syndrome periodic limb movement disorder insomnia parasomnias and circadian rhythm disorders.
Glen Greenough, Fellowship Director
Michael Sate MD, Director

7891 Sleep Disorders Center Lankenau Hospital
100 E Lancaster Avenue 610-645-3400
Wynnewood, PA 19096-3498 Fax: 610-645-2291

7892 Sleep Disorders Center Ohio State University Medical Center
410 W.10th Ave 614-257-2500
Columbus, OH 43210-1228 800-293-5123
Fax: 614-257-2551
e-mail: webmaster@osumc.edu
medicalcenter.osu.edu
Ulysses J Magalang MD, Medical Director

7893 Sleep Disorders Center at California: Pacific Medical Center
2340 Clay Street 415-923-3336
San Francisco, CA 94115-1932 Fax: 415-923-3584
e-mail: 76307.2221@compuserve.com

7894 Sleep Disorders Center at California: Paci
2340 Clay Street 415-923-3336
San Francisco, CA 94115 Fax: 415-923-3584
e-mail: 76307.2221@compuserve.com

7895 Sleep Disorders Center of Metropolitan Toronto
500 Alden Road 905-475-5155
Markham Ontario, CA M6B-4H6 888-401-5155
Fax: 647-436-7607
e-mail: sleep@compuserve.com
www.sdc.ca
Jeffrey Lips MD, Director

7896 Sleep Disorders Center of Rochester: St. Mary's Hospital
2110 Clinton Avenue S 716-442-4141
Rochester, NY 14618-2616
Donald Green MD

7897 Sleep Disorders Center of Western New York Millard Fillmore Hospital
726 Exchange Street 716-859-5600
Buffalo, NY 14210-1120 Fax: 716-887-5332
gates.kaleidahealth.org
Daniel Rifkin, Director

7898 Sleep Disorders Center: Cleveland Clinic Foundation
9500 Euclid Avenue 216-636-5860
Cleveland, OH 44195-0001 800-223-2273
Fax: 216-445-1022
TTY: 216-444-0261
my.clevelandclinic.org
Accredited by the American Academy of Sleep Medicine the Cleveland Clinic Sleep Disorders Center is staffed by physicians specializing in sleep disorders from a variety of disciplines including adult and child neurology pulmonary and critical care medicine psychology psychiatry otolaryngology and dentistry.
Nancy Foldva Schaefer DO, Director
Petra Podmor RPSGT, Laboratory Manager

7899 Sleep Disorders Center: Community Medical Center
1822 Mulberry Street 717-969-8931
Scranton, PA 18510-2375
John Goodnow, Director

7900 Sleep Disorders Center: Crozer-Chester Medical Center
Sleep Disorders Center
175 E Chester Pike
Ridley Park, PA 19078-3975 610-447-2689
www.crozer.org
A multidisciplinary facility for the investigation and treatment of sleep problems
Calvin Staff MD, Medical Director

7901 Sleep Disorders Center: Good Samaritan Medical Center
1020 Franklin Street 814-533-1661
Johnstown, PA 15905-4109
Richard Parc DO, Director

7902 Sleep Disorders Center: Kettering Medical Center
3935 Southern Boulevard 937-395-8805
Kettering, OH 45439-1295 Fax: 937-395-8821
www.kmcnetwork.org

Donna Arand PhD, Clinical Director
George G Burton MD, Medical Director

7903 Sleep Disorders Center: Medical College of Pennsylvania
3200 Henry Avenue   215-842-4250
Philadelphia, PA 19129-1137
June M Fry MD PhD, Director

7904 Sleep Disorders Center: Newark Beth Israel Medical Center
201 Lyons Avenue at Osborne Terrace
Newark, NJ 07112-2027   973-926-2973
www.sbhcs.com
Evaluates a wide range of disorders including sleep apnea snoring insomnia narcolepsy sleep-wake schedule disorders and male impotency. The center also provides board-certified consultants in sleep medicine neurology urology endocrinology psychiatry cardiology and ear nose and throat surgery in addition to certified sleep technologists.
Monroe S Karetzky MD

7905 Sleep Disorders Center: Rhode Island Hospital
70 Catamore Boulevard   401-431-5420
E Providence, RI 02914   Fax: 401-431-5429
www.lifespan.org
Richard Mill MD, Director

7906 Sleep Disorders Center: St. Vincent Medical Center
2213 Cherry Street   419-321-4980
Toledo, OH 43608-2691
Joseph Schaf PhD, Director

7907 Sleep Disorders Center: University Hospital, SUNY at Stony Brook
240 Middle Country Road   631-444-2500
Smithtown, NY 11787-0001   Fax: 631-444-2580
uhmc-xweb1.uhmc.sunysb.edu/sleepdisorder
Wallace Mend MD

7908 Sleep Disorders Center: Winthrop, University Hospital
259 First Street
Mineola, NY 11501-3808   516-663-0333
www.winthrop.org
Steven H Feinsilver MD

7909 Sleep Disorders Unit Beth Israel Deaconess Medical Center
330 Brookline Avenue
Boston, MA 02215-5400   617-667-3237
www.bidmc.org
Jean K Matheson MD

7910 Sleep Laboratory St Joseph's Hospital
St Joseph's Hospital
301 Prospect Ave   315-703-2138
Syracuse, NY 13203   888-785-6371
Fax: 315-755-77
www.sjhsyr.org
The Sleep Lab focuses on diagnosing and treating Obstructive Sleep Apnea and sleep-related breathing disorders and has the largest number of sleep-credentialed physicians and registered sleep technologists of any sleep lab in the area.
Edward T Downing, Director

7911 Sleep Laboratory, Maine Medical Center
22 Bramhall Street   207-871-2279
Portland, ME 04102-3134

7912 Sleep Medicine Associates of Texas
5477 Glen Lakes Drive   214-750-7776
Dallas, TX 13210-4353   Fax: 214-750-4621
e-mail: smat@sleepmed.com
www.sleepmed.com
First largest and longest standing accredited sleep center in North Texas.
Philipp Becker, President and Founding Partner
Andrew O Jamieson MD, Chairman of the Board and Founding Partn

7913 Sleep Research Foundation
170 Morton Street   617-522-9270
Boston, MA 02130-3735
Ernest Hartm MD, Director

7914 Sleep Wake Disorders Center Montefiore Sleep Disorders Center
111 E 210th Street   718-920-4321
Bronx, NY 10467-2401   Fax: 718-798-4352
www.montefiore.org
Provide outstanding clinical care for patients with disorders that affect the sleep-wake cycle and are committed to performing high quality research and to making outstanding contributions to the areas of clinical research that includes the entire spectrum of sleep medicine.
Michael J Thorpy MD, Director
Karen Ballab MD, Associate Director

7915 Sleep and Chronobiology Center: Western Psychiatric Institute and Clinic
3811 Ohara Street   412-624-2246
Pittsburgh, PA 15213-2593
Charles F Reynolds III MD, Director

7916 Sleep-Wake Disorders Center: New York Hospital-Cornell Medical Center
520 E 70th Street   212-746-2623
New York, NY 10021-1504   Fax: 212-746-5509
www.weillcornell.org
Charles Poll MD, Director

7917 Sleep/Wake Disorders Center: Community Hospitals of Indianapolis
1500 N Ritter Avenue   317-355-4275
Indianapolis, IN 46219-3027   Fax: 317-351-2785
e-mail: mevollmer@pol.net
Marvin E Vollmer MD

7918 Sleep/Wake Disorders Center: Hampstead Hospital
E Road   603-329-5311
Hampstead, NH 03841
Deborah Sewi PhD

7919 Stanford University Center for Narcolepsy Dept of Psychiatry & Behavioral Sciences
450 Broadway Street   650-725-6517
Redwood City, CA 94063-5102   Fax: 650-498-7761
e-mail: jck@stanford.edu
med.stanford.edu
Dr Emanuel Mignot, Director
Marlene Iry, Admin Associate

7920 Thomas Jefferson University: Sleep Disorders Center
Jefferson Medical College
1020 Walnut Street   215-955-6000
Philadelphia, PA 19107-5083   800-JEF-FNOW
Fax: 215-955-9783
www.jefferson.edu
A comprehensive clinical research and educational program in sleep and sleep disorders medicine.
Karl Doghram MD, Medical Director

7921 University of Texas Sleep/Wake Disorders Center
Southwestern Medical Center
5323 Harry Hines Boulevard   214-648-7350
Dallas, TX 75390-9070   Fax: 214-487-59
Studies sleep/wake disorders including insomnia apnea and narcolepsy.
Howard Roffw MD, Director

Support Groups & Hotlines

7922 Narcolepsy Institute/Montefiore Medical Center
111 E 210th Street   718-920-6799
Bronx, NY 10467-2490   Fax: 718-654-9580
e-mail: MGoswami@aol.com
www.narcolepsyinstitute.org
The Narcolepsy Institute provides psychosocial support services for narcolepsy.
Dr. Meeta Goswami, Director

7923 Narcolepsy Network
129 Waterwheel Lane
North Kingstown, RI 02852   401-667-2523
   888-292-6522
Fax: 401-633-6567
e-mail: narnet@narcolepsynetwork.org
www.narcolepsynetwork.org
Provides advocacy and education, supports research. Newsletter, conferences, phone support and group development guidelines.
Patricia Higgins, President
Eveline V. Honig, Md, MPh, Executive Director

7924 National Health Information Center
PO Box 1133
Washington, DC 20013   310-565-4167
   800-336-4797
Fax: 301-984-4256
e-mail: info@nhic.org
www.health.gov/nhic
Offers a nationwide information referral service, produces directories and resource guides.

Books

7925 ABC of ZZZs
National Sleep Foundation
1010 N. Glebe Road
Arlington, VA 22201-1235   703-243-1697
Fax: 202-347-3472
e-mail: nsf@sleepfoundation.org
www.sleepfoundation.org
A primer on sleep basics, including getting enough sleep, why sleep is important, and ' sleep stealers.'
Charles A. Czeisler, Chairman
Max Hirshkowitz, Vice Chairman

7926 Doctor, I Can't Sleep: Insomnia Training Manual
Narcolepsy Network
1010 N. Glebe Road
Arlington, VA 22201-0460   703-243-1697
Fax: 513-891-9936
e-mail: nsf@sleepfoundation.org
www.sleepfoundation.org
Comprehensive course manual for primary care physicians and the public. Outlines basic facts about epidemiology, sleep hygiene, relaxation techniques, diagnosis, and treatment.
100+ pages
Charles A. Czeisler, Chairman
Max Hirshkowitz, Vice Chairman

7927 International Classification of Sleep Disorders
American Academy of Sleep Medicine
2510 North Frontage Road
Darien, IL 60561   630-737-9700
Fax: 630-737-9790
www.aasmnet.org
A comprehensive manual for physicians and other healthcare professionals containing information on 84 sleep disorders. The extensive text describes the diagnostic features of each disorder and includes specific diagnostic and severity criteria for each disorder.
396 pages Paperback
Timothy I. Morgenthaler, President
Nathaniel F. Watson, President-Elect

7928 Living with Narcolepsy
National Sleep Foundation
1010 N. Glebe Road
Arlington, VA 22201-1235   703-243-1697
Fax: 513-891-9936
e-mail: nsf@sleepfoundation.org
www.sleepfoundation.org
Defines and describes narcolepsy and what can be expected after diagnosis, including effects on education, career, social and family life.
Charles A. Czeisler, Chairman
Max Hirshkowitz, Vice Chairman

7929 Melatonin: The Basic Facts
National Sleep Foundation
1010 N. Glebe Road
Arlington, VA 22201-1235   703-243-1697
Fax: 513-891-9936
e-mail: nsf@sleepfoundation.org
www.sleepfoundation.org
If you're curious about melatonin, it's not suprising. There has been a lot of attention paid to the hormone in popular magazines

and books, scholarly journals, and advertisements. You may habe heard claims that malatonin cures everything from jet lag to insomnia to aging.
Charles A. Czeisler, Chairman
Max Hirshkowitz, Vice Chairman

7930 Narcolepsy Primer
Meeta Goswami, Michael Thorpy, author
Narcolepsy Institute/Montefiore Medical Center
111 E 210th Street   718-920-6799
Bronx, NY 10467-2401   Fax: 718-654-9580
e-mail: MGsowami@aol.com
narcolepsyinstitute.org
A guide for physicians, patients and their families on the affects, causes and prevention of narcolepsy.
Dr. Meeta Goswami, Director

7931 Narcolepsy Primer Package
Meeta Goswami, Michael Thorpy, author
Narcolepsy Institute/Montefiore Medical Center
111 E 210th Street   718-920-6799
Bronx, NY 10467-2401   Fax: 718-654-9580
e-mail: MGsowami@aol.com
narcolepsyinstitute.org
The package includes: Narcolepsy Primer; Manuel on Narcolepsy and A Counseling Service for Narcolepsy: A Sociomedical Model.
Dr. Meeta Goswami, Director

7932 Pain and Sleep
National Sleep Foundation
1010 N. Glebe Road
Arlington, VA 22201-1235   703-243-1697
Fax: 513-891-9936
e-mail: nsf@sleepfoundation.org
www.sleepfoundation.org
Whether pain results from headache, backache, arthritis, or other conditions, it frequently occurs with sleep difficulty. This overview of the pain and sleep connection describes behavioral and pharmacological approaches to pain management.
Charles A. Czeisler, Chairman
Max Hirshkowitz, Vice Chairman

7933 Sleep Aids: Everything You Wanted To Know But Were Too Tired To Ask
National Sleep Foundation
1010 N. Glebe Road
Arlington, VA 22201-1235   703-243-1697
Fax: 513-891-9936
e-mail: nsf@sleepfoundation.org
www.sleepfoundation.org
If you have trouble falling or staying asleep, or you wake up feeling unrefreshed, you may be suffering from insomnia. Insomnia is a symptom. It may be caused by stress, anxiety, depression, disease, pain, medications, sleep disorders or poor sleep habits.
Charles A. Czeisler, Chairman
Max Hirshkowitz, Vice Chairman

7934 Sleep Apnea
National Sleep Foundation
1010 N. Glebe Road
Arlington, VA 22201-1235   703-243-1697
Fax: 513-891-9936
e-mail: nsf@sleepfoundation.org
www.sleepfoundation.org
A brochure about sleep apnea, a breathing disorder characterized by brief interruptions of breathing during sleep. Brochure explains what it is, who gets it, and how it is diagnosed and treated.
Charles A. Czeisler, Chairman
Max Hirshkowitz, Vice Chairman

7935 Snoring and Sleep Apnea
Demos Medical Publishing
11 West 42nd Street   212-683-0072
New York, NY 10036   Fax: 212-683-0118
e-mail: orderdept@demopub.com
www.demosmedpub.com
A straightforward, jargon-free approach to dealing with snoring and sleep problems.
222 pages
ISBN: 1-888799-29-3
Dr. Diana M Schneider, President

7936 You Don't LOOK Sick!: Living Well with Invisible Chronic Illness
Joy Selak, Steven Overman, author
Haworth Press
10 Alice Street
Binghamton, NY 13904-1580
607-722-5857
800-429-6784
Fax: 607-722-0012
www.haworthpress.com

Chronicles a patient's true-life stories and her physician's compassionate commentary as they take a journey through the three stages of chronic illness - Getting Sick, Being Sick, and Living Well. Hardcover $29.95 (ISBN): 978-0-7890-2488-0, Paperback $14.95 (ISBN): 978-0-7890-2499-7.
145 pages Hrdcover/Ppbck

Magazines

7937 SleepMatters
National Sleep Foundation
1010 N. Glebe Road
Arlington, VA 22201-1235
703-243-1697
Fax: 513-891-9936
e-mail: nsf@sleepfoundation.org
www.sleepfoundation.org

Covering hot sleep news, profiles, advice from experts and much more!
Quarterly
Charles A. Czeisler, Chairman
Max Hirshkowitz, Vice Chairman

Newsletters

7938 Eye Opener
American Narcolepsy Association
425 Cal Strt, Suite 201
San Francisco, CA 94126-6230
415-788-4793

Offers information on sleep disorders including a question and answer column for persons suffering from disorders.

7939 Narcolepsy Institute/Montefiore Medical Center
Meeta Goswami, author
Narcolepsy Institute
111 E 210th Street
Bronx, NY 10467-2490
718-920-6799
Fax: 718-654-9580
e-mail: MGsowami@aol.com
narcolepsyinstitute.org

The Narcolepsy Institute provides psychosocial support services for narcolepsy and has a newsletter, a video, and a primer on narcolepsy.
8 pages Bi-Annual
Dr. Meeta Goswami, Director

7940 Sleep Medicine Alert
Nationa Sleep Foundation
1010 N. Glebe Road
Arlington, VA 22201-1235
703-243-1697
Fax: 513-891-9936
e-mail: nsf@sleepfoundation.org
www.sleepfoundation.org

This quearterly newsletter is for healthcare professionals. It offers updates on sleep research and its clinical implications, information on diagnosing and treating a variety of sleep disorders.
Charles A. Czeisler, Chairman
Max Hirshkowitz, Vice Chairman

7941 Wake-Up Call
American Sleep Apnea Association
1717 Penn Ave, NW
Washington, DC 20006
202-293-3650
888-293-3650
Fax: 202-293-3656
e-mail: asaa@sleepapnea.org
www.sleepapnea.org

Contains information of interest to APNEA patients and their families.
Quarterly
Michael P Coppola MD, President and Chief Medical Officer
Nancy Rothstein, Secretary

Pamphlets

7942 Get the Facts About Sleep Apnea
American Sleep Apnea Association
1717 Penn Ave, NW
Washington, DC 20006
202-293-3650
888-293-3650
Fax: 202-293-3656
e-mail: asaa@sleepapnea.org
www.sleepapnea.org

7943 Helping Yourself to a Good Night's Sleep
Nantional Sleep Foundation
1010 N. Glebe Road
Arlington, VA 22201-1253
703-243-1697
Fax: 513-891-9936
e-mail: nsf@sleepfoundation.org
www.sleepfoundation.org

About half of Americans report sleep difficulty at least occasionally, according to National Sleep Foundation surveys. These woescalled insomnia by doctors-have far reaching effects. This brochure details the many things you can do to improve your sleep.
Charles A. Czeisler, Chairman
Max Hirshkowitz, Vice Chairman

7944 Narcolepsy
American Academy of Sleep Medicine
2510 North Frontage Road
Darien, IL 60561
630-737-9700
Fax: 630-737-9790
www.aasmnet.org

Describes the causes, symptoms and treatments of a disorder characterized by excessive sleepiness.
Lot of 50
Timothy I. Morgenthaler, President
Nathaniel F. Watson, President-Elect

7945 Sleep Diary
National Sleep Foundation
1010 N. Glebe Road
Arlington, VA 22201-1235
703-243-1697
Fax: 513-891-9936
e-mail: nsf@sleepfoundation.org
www.sleepfoundation.org

It includes sections on sleep schedules, quality and quantity of sleep, sleep disturbances, sleep hygiene and daytime sleepiness. It enables people to identify their sleep and health habits and note any sleep problems they may have.
Charles A. Czeisler, Chairman
Max Hirshkowitz, Vice Chairman

7946 Sleep Strategies for Shift Workers
National Sleep Foundation
1010 N. Glebe Road
Arlington, VA 22201-1235
703-243-1697
Fax: 513-891-9936
e-mail: nsf@sleepfoundation.org
www.sleepfoundation.org

This brochure outlines the common effects of shift work on health, workplace alertness and productivity and offers tips about diet, sleep environment, medications, light therapy and sleep hygiene.
Charles A. Czeisler, Chairman
Max Hirshkowitz, Vice Chairman

7947 Wake Up! Brochure
National Sleep Foundation
1010 N. Glebe Road
Arlington, VA 22201-1235
703-243-1697
Fax: 513-891-9936
e-mail: nsf@sleepfoundation.org
www.sleepfoundation.org

A blooklet dedicated to the drowsy driving problem, including the risks, the myths, the danger signals and recommendations.
Charles A. Czeisler, Chairman
Max Hirshkowitz, Vice Chairman

7948 When You Can't Sleep
Narcolepsy Network
1010 N. Glebe Road
Arlington, VA 22201-0460
703-243-1697
888-292-6522
Fax: 513-891-9936
e-mail: nsf@sleepfoundation.org
www.sleepfoundation.org

A primer on sleep basics, including getting enough sleep, why sleep is important, and sleep stealers. Plus a sleep quotient quiz.

Charles A. Czeisler, Chairman
Max Hirshkowitz, Vice Chairman

7949   Women and Sleep
National Sleep Foundation
1010 N. Glebe Road   703-243-1697
Arlington, VA 22201-1235   Fax: 513-891-9936
                                        e-mail: nsf@sleepfoundation.org
                                        www.sleepfoundation.org

A brochure dealing with the effects of sleep on women which explores reasons for tiredness, increased accidents, problems concentrating, and poor performance on the job and in school, and possible increased sickness.

Charles A. Czeisler, Chairman
Max Hirshkowitz, Vice Chairman

Audio & Video

7950   Narcolepsy
American Academy of Sleep Medicine
2510 North Frontage Road   630-737-9700
Darien, IL 60561   Fax: 630-737-9790
                                        www.aasmnet.org

Addresses the etiology, pathophysiology, diagnosis and management of narcolepsy.

58 slides
Timothy I. Morgenthaler, President
Nathaniel F. Watson, President-Elect

7951   Narcolepsy: Fanlight Productions
Jason Margolis, author

Fanlight Productions
4196 Washington Street   617-469-4999
Boston, MA 02131-1731   800-937-4113
                                          Fax: 617-469-3379
                                        e-mail: fanlight@fanlight.com
                                        www.fanlight.com

This remarkable film presents the experiences of three individuals whose lives and relationships have been disrupted by narcolepsy.

2000 25 Minutes
ISBN: 1-572953-23-2

7952   Video on Narcolepsy
Narcolepsy Institute/Montefiore Medical Center
111 E 210th Street   718-920-6799
Bronx, NY 10467   Fax: 718-654-9580
                                        e-mail: MGsowami@aol.com
                                        www.narcolepsyinstitute.org

Clinical symptoms, genetics, diagnosis, effects of Narcolepsy, support groups.

Dr. Meeta Goswami, Director

Web Sites

7953   American Sleep Apnea Association
                                        www.sleeppapnea.org

The American Sleep Apnea Association, founded in 1990, is a 501(c)(3) nonprofit organization that promotes awareness of sleep apnea, works for continuing improvements in treatments for this serious disorder, and advocates for the interests of sleep apnea patients.

7954   American Sleep Disorders Association
Provides full diagnostic and treatment services to improve the quality of care for patients with all types of sleep disorders.

7955   Healing Well
                                        www.healingwell.com

An online health resource guide to medical news, chat, information and articles, newsgroups and message boards, books, disease-related web sites, medical directories, and more for patients, friends, and family coping with disabling diseases, disorders, or chronic illnesses.

7956   Health Finder
                                        www.healthfinder.gov

Searchable, carefully developed web site offering information on over 1000 topics. Developed by the US Department of Health and Human Services, the site can be used in both English and Spanish.

7957   Healthlink USA
                                        www.healthlinkusa.com

Health information concerning treatment, cures, prevention, diagnosis, risk factors, research, support groups, email lists, personal stories and much more. Updated regularly.

7958   Helios Health
                                        www.helioshealth.com

Online resource for your health information. Detailed information about specific health topics, access to expert advice from our Medical Advisory Board, and up-to-date health news.

7959   MGH Neurology WebForums
Online. Provides both unmoderated message boards and chat rooms for specific neurological disorders.

7960   MedicineNet
                                        www.medicinenet.com

An online resource for consumers providing easy-to-read, authoritative medical and health information.

7961   Medscape
                                        www.medscape.com

Medscape offers specialists, primary care physicians, and other health professionals the Web's most robust and integrated medical information and educational tools.

7962   National Sleep Foundation
                                        www.sleepfoundation.org

Information for millions of Americans who suffer from sleep disorders, and to prevent the catastrophic accidents that are related to poor or disordered sleep through research, education and the dissemination of information.

7963   Neurology Channel
                                        www.healthcommunities.com

Find clearly explained, medically accurate information regarding conditions, including an overview, symptoms, causes, diagnostic procedures and treatment options. On this site it is possible to ask questions and get information from a neurologist and connect to people who have similar health interests.

7964   Sleep Research Society
                                        www.sleepresearchsociety.org

Facilitates communication among research workers in this field, but does not sponsor research investigations on its own.

7965   WebMD
                                        www.webmd.com

Provides credible information, supportive communities, and in-depth reference material about health subjects. A source for original and timely health information as well as material from well known content providers.

Description

7966 Spina Bifida

Spina bifida refers to conditions which result in an incomplete closure of the spinal column during fetal development. It is the most serious of a group of disorders called neural tube defects. The severity of spina bifida ranges from mild to severe.

Spina bifida occulta is an opening in one or more vertebrae without damage to the spinal cord. Meningocele is when the protective covering around the spinal cord (meninges) has protruded into the vertebrae, with little, if any, damage. Myelomeningocele, the most severe form of spina bifida, is when part of the actual spinal cord pushes through the back and exposes nerves and tissues.

The effects of spina bifida, in its most extreme state, are serious. They can include paralysis, loss of bowel and bladder control and hydrocephalus. Other inherited abnormalities may be present. Open spina bifida can be diagnosed in utero by finding elevations of a specific protein in maternal amniotic fluid. Prevention involves supplementation with folic acid. Treatments for spina bifida require a united effort by a team of specialists, and depend on the severity of the defects. With proper care, many children with spina bifida live fairly normal lives. See also *Birth Defects*.

National Agencies & Associations

7967 Canadian & American Spinal Research Organi zation
120 Newkirk Road
Richmond Hill, ON, L4C-9S7
905-508-4000
800-361-4004
Fax: 905-508-4002
e-mail: info@csro.com
www.csro.com
Dedicated to the improvement of the physical quality of life for persons with a spinal cord injury and those with related neurological deficits, through targeted medical and scientific research.
Barry Munro, Chair
Dave Lostchuk, Treasurer

7968 Easter Seals
233 South Wacker Drive
Chicago, IL 60606-4703
312-726-6200
800-221-6827
Fax: 312-726-1494
TTY: 312-726-4258
e-mail: info@easter-seals.org
www.easter-seals.org
Provides serves to children and adults with disabilities as well as support to their families.
Reenie Kavalar, VP Medical/Rehabilitation Services

7969 March of Dimes Birth Defects Foundation
1275 Mamaroneck Avenue
White Plains, NY 10605
914-949-7166
www.marchofdimes.com
Our mission is to improve the health of babies by preventing birth defects premature birth and infant mortality. The March of Dimes carries out this mission through programs of research community services education and advocacy to save babies' lives.

7970 Spina Bifida Association of America
4590 Macarthur Boulevard NW
Washington, DC 20007-4226
202-944-3285
800-621-3141
Fax: 202-944-3295
e-mail: sbaa@sbaa.org
www.sbaa.org

The association works for people with spina bifida and their families through education advocacy research and service. There is also an annual conference and publications available.
Cindy Brownstein, CEO
Maya House, Resource Center Manager

7971 Spina Bifida and Hydrocephalus Association of Canada
#977-167 Lombard Avenue
Winnipeg, Manitoba, R3B-0V3
204-925-3650
800-565-9488
Fax: 204-925-3654
e-mail: spinab@mts.net
www.sbhac.ca
To improve the quality of life of all individuals with spina bifida and/or hydrocephalus and their families, through awareness, education, research, and advocacy, and to reduce the incidence of neural tube defects.
Lorelei Fletcher, President
Gene Layton, VP

State Agencies & Associations

Alabama

7972 Spina Bifida Association of Alabama
PO Box 13254
Birmingham, AL 35202-0538
256-617-1414
e-mail: info@sbaofal.org
www.sbaofal.org
Betsy Hopson, President
Steven Horne, Vice President

Arizona

7973 Spina Bifida Association of Arizona
1001 E Fairmount Avenue
Phoenix, AZ 85014-4806
602-274-3323
Fax: 602-274-7632
e-mail: office@sbglobal.net
www.sbaaz.org
Benjaman D Scanlan, President
Ron Whiteside, Treasurer

California

7974 Spina Bifida Association of Greater San Diego
PO Box 232272
San Diego, CA 92193-2272
619-491-9018
Fax: 619-275-3361
e-mail: sbaofgsd@hotmail.com
www.spinabifidasandiego.com
Erika Jorquera, President

Colorado

7975 Spina Bifida Association of Colorado
PO Box 22994
Denver, CO 80222-0994
303-797-7870
Fax: 303-730-8032
e-mail: sbacolorado@gmail.com
www.coloradospinabifida.org
Chris Mestas, Chairman
Lavon Birney, Executive Director

Connecticut

7976 Spina Bifida Association of Connecticut
370 Osgood Avenue
New Britain, CT 06053-2545
860-839-0115
800-574-6274
Fax: 860-832-6260
e-mail: sbac@sbac.org
www.sbac.org
Mary Attardo, President
Kiley J Carlson, Executive Director

Delaware

7977 Spina Bifida Association of Delaware
PO Box 807
Wilmington, DE 19899-0807
302-478-4805
e-mail: kbasar@aol.com
www.angelfire.com/de/sbaofde/
Blake Heath, Vice President
Andy Anderso Jr, Treasurer

Florida

7978 Spina Bifida Association of Florida Space Coast
100 W Lucerne Circle
Orlando, FL 32801-2549
407-248-9210
Fax: 321-454-9737
e-mail: sbafscearthlink.com
www.sbacentralflorida.org

Rob Roy, Chairman
Melisa Portnoy, Secretary

7979 Spina Bifida Association of Jacksonville
807 Childrens Way
Jacksonville, FL 32207-8426
904-697-3686
800-722-6355
Fax: 904-390-3466
e-mail: sbaj@sbaj.org
www.sbaj.org

Michael Erhard, Chairperson

7980 Spina Bifida Association of Tampa
100 W Lucerne Circle
Orlando, FL 32801-1038
407-248-9210
Fax: 813-872-9845
e-mail: sbatampabay@aol.com
www.sbatampabay.org

Dianne Gore, President

Georgia

7981 Spina Bifida Association of Georgia
1448 Mclendon Drive
Decatur, GA 30033
770-939-1044
Fax: 770-939-1049
e-mail: info@spinabifidaga.org
www.spinabifidaofgeorgia.org
Provides referrals, evaluation, treatment and therapeutic activities for children and teens afflicted with spina bifida. The goal of this center is to help children or teenagers prepare for life.
William Turnispeed, President
Judy Thibadeau, Vice President

Illinois

7982 Illinois Spina Bifida Association
8765 W Higgins Road
Chicago, IL 60631-1693
773-444-0305
800-969-4722
Fax: 630-637-1066
e-mail: info@i-sba.org
www.sbail.org
Dedicated to improving the quality of life of people with spina bifida through direct services, information and referral and public awareness. Direct services include a residential summer camp for children with spina bifida over the age of seven.
Scott J Munkvold, President
Amy Maggio, CEO

Indiana

7983 Spina Bifida Association of Central Indiana
PO Box 19814
Indianapolis, IN 46279-0814
317-592-1630
Fax: 317-351-2010
e-mail: pres@sbaci.org
www.sbaci.org

James Zetzl, President

Iowa

7984 Spina Bifida Association of Iowa
8525 Douglas Avenue
Urbandale, IA 50322-1456
515-278-7013
e-mail: contact@sbaia.org
www.spinabifidaia.com

Rod Tressel, President

Kentucky

7985 Spina Bifida Association of Kentucky
Kosair Charities Center
982 Eastern Parkway
Louisville, KY 40217-1568
502-637-7363
866-340-7225
Fax: 502-637-1010
e-mail: sbak@sbak.org
www.sbak.org

Angela Cosby, President
Patty Dissell, Executive Director

Louisiana

7986 Spina Bifida Association of Greater New Orleans
PO Box 1346
Kenner, LA 70063-1346
504-737-5181
Fax: 504-538-9046
e-mail: sbagno@sbagno.com
www.sbagno.org

Al Hitt, President
Judy Otto, Vice-President

Maryland

7987 Spina Bifida Association of Maryland
2416 Lampost Lane
Baltimore, MD 21234-1460
410-665-1543
Fax: 410-833-1700
e-mail: sbamaryland@comcast.net ~
www.home.comcast.net/~sbamaryland

7988 Spina Bifida Association of the Eastern Shore
316 Prospect Avenue
Easton, MD 21601-4046
410-822-8609
Fax: 410-822-5455
www.spinabifidaassociation.org

Massachusetts

7989 Spina Bifida Association of Massachusetts
321 Fortune Boulevard
Milford, MA 01757-2741
617-742-2574
888-479-1900
Fax: 978-649-8725
e-mail: bsullivan@sbaMass.org
www.msbaweb.org

Brendan Sullivan, President
Cara Packard, Vice President

Michigan

7990 Spina Bifida Association of Grand Rapids
235 Wealthy Street SE
Grand Rapids, MI 49503-5299
616-240-9672
Fax: 616-222-1541
e-mail: WMiSBA@hotmail.com~
www.spinabifida.org

Carol Carpenter, President

7991 Spina Bifida Association of Upper Peninsula Michigan
1220 N 3rd Street
Ishpeming, MI 44849-1108
906-485-5127
Fax: 906-225-7230
e-mail: cbengson@nmu.edu
www.sba-up.8m.com

Lois Bengson, President

7992 Spina Bifida and Hydrocephalus Association of Southwestern Michigan
PO Box 212
Mattawan, MI 49071-0212
269-385-3959
Fax: 269-392-9765
e-mail: marenhorkness@yahoo.com
Richard Benthnin, President

Minnesota

7993 Spina Bifida Association of Minnesota
PO Box 29323
Minneapolis, MN 55429-0212
651-222-6395
Fax: 952-591-0246
e-mail: sbamn@hotmail.com
www.sbamn.com

Wendy Swanson, President
Jim Thayer, Executive Director

Missouri

7994 Spina Bifida Association of Greater St. Louis
8050 Watson Road   314-843-2244
Saint Louis, MO 63119-2000   800-784-0983
                                Fax: 314-353-1446
                                e-mail: sbastl@charter.net
                                www.sbstl.com

Mark Abbott, President

Nebraska

7995 Spina Bifida Association of Nebraska
7612 Maple Street   402-932-5826
Omaha, NE 68134-2153   Fax: 402-572-3002
                                www.spinabifidanebraska.org

LeAnn Karman, President

New Jersey

7996 Spina Bifida Association of the Tri-State Region
84 Park Avenue   908-782-7475
Flemington, NJ 08822-1174   877-722-8774
                                Fax: 908-782-6102
                                e-mail: info@thesbrn.org
                                www.sbatsr.org
Serves New Jersey, New York Metro Area and Southern Connecticut.
Jane Horowitz, Executive Director and President
K David Holmes, Chairman of the Board

New Mexico

7997 Spina Bifida Association of New Mexico
1127 University Boulevard NE
Albuquerque, NM 87102-1740
                                505-242-1184
                                www.sbanm.com

Rey Garduno, Executive Director
Ann Beddingfield, Interim Treasurer

New York

7998 Spina Bifida Association of Albany/Capital District
100 Spring   518-399-9151
Scotia, NY 12302-3312   e-mail: sbaalbany102@aol.com
                                www.abaalbany.org

Kevin Chamberlain, Co-President
Vanessa Chamberlain, Co-President

7999 Spina Bifida Association of Greater Rochester
PO Box 3   585-381-5471
Fairport, NY 14450-0003   Fax: 585-264-9547
                                e-mail: jarmst4459@aol.com

JoAnn Armstrong, President

8000 Spina Bifida Association of Nassau County
12 Hampton Road   631-821-9028
Sound Beach, NY 11789   e-mail: kid3418@optonline.net
                                www.spinabifidaassociation.org

Leslieann Sussman, President

North Carolina

8001 Spina Bifida Association of North Carolina
3915 Grace Court   704-882-0988
Indian Trail, NC 28079   800-847-2262
                                Fax: 704-882-0988
                                e-mail: sbanc@mindspring.com
                                www.spinabifidaassociation.org

Julie Yindra, President
Kin Gates, Executive Director

Ohio

8002 Spina Bifida Association of Canton
S Cherokee Trail   330-863-2531
Malvern, OH 44644   Fax: 330-863-1172
                                e-mail: cmgriffin@nero.rr.com
                                www.spinabifidasupport.com

Connie Griffin, President

8003 Spina Bifida Association of Central Ohio
7239 Upper Cambridge Way   614-818-3840
Westerville, OH 43082   e-mail: sbaco@sbaco.net
                                www.sbaco.net

Laurie Schulze, Treasurer
Chrissy Zepfel, President

8004 Spina Bifida Association of Cincinnati
644 Linn Street   513-923-1378
Cincinnati, OH 45203-0152   e-mail: sbacincy@sbacincy.org
                                www.sbacincy.org

Brady Sellet, President
Diane Burns, Executive Director

8005 Spina Bifida Association of Greater Dayton
4801 Springfield Street   937-236-1122
Dayton, OH 45431   Fax: 937-434-4899
                                e-mail: mvspinabifida@yahoo.com
                                www.sbadayton.org

David Skinner, President
Lisa Maas, Vice President

8006 Spina Bifida Association of Northwest Ohio
302 Conant St   419-794-0561
Maumee, OH 43537   Fax: 419-533-3952
                                e-mail: sba@sbaofnorthwestohio.org
                                www.sbaofnorthwestohio.org

Ginnette Clark, President
Julie Harley, Vice President

Pennsylvania

8007 Spina Bifida Association of Central Pennsylvania
209 E State Street   717-786-9280
Quarryville, PA 17566-1242   888-770-SBPA
                                Fax: 717-786-8821
                                e-mail: SBAofPA@aol.com
                                www.geocities.com/sbaofgpa

Patricia Fulvio, President
Amy Graver, Chairman

8008 Spina Bifida Association of Delaware Valley
Havertown, PA 19083-0289   610-584-5530
                                800-223-0222
                                Fax: 215-412-9396
                                e-mail: info@sbadv.org
                                www.sbadv.org
Spina Bifida is the most common permanently disabling birth defect in the United States. An average of 8 babies every day are born with Spina Bifida or a similar birth defect of the brain and spine. There are over 60 million women in the U.S. who could become pregnant and each one is at risk of having a baby born with Spina Bifida. The mission of the Spina Bifida Association of Delaware Valley is to promote the prevention of Spina Bifida and to enhance the lives of all affected.
Marilyn Lieb, President
Keri Mascaro, Executive Director

8009 Spina Bifida Association of Greater Pennsylvania
209 E State Street   717-786-9280
Quarryville, PA 17566-9614   Fax: 717-786-8821
                                e-mail: sbaofpa@aol.com
                                www.spinabifidaresource.weebly.com
The Spina Bifida Resource was started in the 1970's, when a group of Moms met while their children had therapy. As the needs and issues were discussed, the group decided to band together for support. Thus the Spina Bifida Association of Lancaster County was born. Our first public meeting had 45 parents and concerned professionals in attendance. After about 20 years, the Board felt the need to change our name to reflect all those we served in and around Pennsylvania. Thus we became the Spina
Amy Graver, President
Patricia Fulvio, Executive Director

Rhode Island

8010 Spina Bifida Association of Rhode Island
Warwick, RI 02887-6948   401-732-7862
                                Fax: 401-732-7862
                                www.spinabifidaassociation.org

Tennessee

8011 **Spina Bifida Association of Tennessee**
Nashville, TN 37202-5529
615-791-8117
Fax: 615-791-1518
e-mail: lynnhess56@comcast.net
www.spinabifidasupport.com

Lynn Cook, President

Texas

8012 **Spina Bifida Association of Austin**
9301 Bradner Drive
Austin, TX 78748
512-292-6317
Fax: 512-479-3845
e-mail: austinspinabifida@yahoo.com
www.spinabifidasupport.com

Kelley Hively, President

8013 **Spina Bifida Association of Dallas**
705 W Avenue B
Garland, TX 75040
972-238-8755
Fax: 972-414-3772
e-mail: sbdal@aol.com
www.sbdallas.org

Robin Lee¯, President
Ryan McCoy, Vice President

8014 **Spina Bifida Association of Texas, Gulf Coast**
440 Benmar
Houston, TX 77060-2460
281-447-2707
Fax: 281-997-2278
e-mail: fandfsports@sbcglobal.net
www.sbahgc.org
The mission of Spina Bifida Houston Gulf Coast is to promote public awareness and enrich the lives of individuals and families living with spina bifida.
Jennifer Franklin, Vice President
Joan Peck, Treasurer

Washington

8015 **Spina Bifida Association of Washington State**
611 2nd Street
Snohomish, WA 98290
253-589-3700
888-289-3702
Fax: 775-766-1654
e-mail: sbaws@yahoo.com
www.sbaws.org
The Spina Bifida Association of Washington State is an affiliated chapter of the national Spina Bifida Association.
Jason Lane, Chair
Ryan Callaway, Director

Wisconsin

8016 **Spina Bifida Association of Northern Wisconsin**
Schofield, WI 54476-0421
715-798-3944
e-mail: dtackley@chegnet.net

David Blanchard, President

8017 **Spina Bifida Association of Southeastern Wisconsin**
830 N 109th Street
Wauwatosa, WI 53226
414-607-9061
Fax: 414-607-9602
e-mail: sbawi@sbawi.org
www.sbawi.org
Spina Bifida occurs when the spine of the baby fails to close. This creates an opening, or lesion, on the spinal column. Because of the opening on the spinal column, the nerves in the spinal column may be damaged and not work properly. This results in some degree of paralysis. The higher the lesion is on the spinal column, the greater the likelihood of increased paralysis. Surgery to close the spine is generally done within hours after birth. The surgery helps reduce the risk of infection and pr
Karen Drzewiecki, President
David G. Tucker, MSW, Executive Director

8018 **Spina Bifida Association of the Greater Fox Valley**
325 N John Street
Kimberly, WI 54136
920-687-0801
e-mail: fus1234@athenet.net
www.spinabifidasupport.com

Kelly Richard, President

Support Groups & Hotlines

8019 **National Health Information Center**
Washington, DC 20013
310-565-4167
800-336-4797
Fax: 301-984-4256
e-mail: info@nhic.org
www.health.gov/nhic
Offers a nationwide information referral service, produces directories and resource guides.

Books

8020 **Answering Your Questions About Spina Bifida**
Spina Bifida Association of America
1600 Wilson Blvd.
Arlington, VA 22209-4226
202-944-3285
800-621-3141
Fax: 202-944-3295
e-mail: sbaa@sbaa.org
www.sbaa.org
Provides information to help people understand the basic medical, educational and social issues which commonly affect people with Spina Bifida.
Megan Sorensen, Chair
Wilson Neyland, Chair-Elect

8021 **Bowel Continence and Spina Bifida**
Spina Bifida Association of America
1600 Wilson Blvd.
Arlington, VA 22209-4226
202-944-3285
800-621-3141
Fax: 202-944-3295
e-mail: sbaa@sbaa.org
www.sbaa.org
An excellent book aimed at anyone (infant or adult) trying to attain bowel continence. Focuses on continence programs, bowel management development and techniques.
Megan Sorensen, Chair
Wilson Neyland, Chair-Elect

8022 **Clinic Directory**
Spina Bifida Association of America
1600 Wilson Blvd.
Arlington, VA 22209-4226
202-944-3285
800-621-3141
Fax: 202-944-3295
e-mail: sbaa@sbaa.org
www.sbaa.org
A directory of health care clinics throughout the United States for children and adults with spina bifida.
200 pages 3-Ring Binder
Megan Sorensen, Chair
Wilson Neyland, Chair-Elect

8023 **Complete IEP Guide: How to Advocate for Your Special Ed Child**
Spina Bifida Association
1600 Wilson Blvd.
Arlington, VA 22209-4226
202-944-3285
800-621-3141
e-mail: sbaa@sbaa.org
www.sbaa.org
This all-in-one guide will help you understand special education law, identify your child's needs, prepare for meetings, develop the IEP and resolve disputes.
Megan Sorensen, Chair
Wilson Neyland, Chair-Elect

8024 **Confronting the Challenges of Spina Bifida**
Spina Bifida Association of America
1600 Wilson Blvd.
Arlington, VA 22209-4226
202-944-3285
800-621-3141
Fax: 202-944-3295
e-mail: sbaa@sbaa.org
www.sbaa.org
A group curriculum addressing self-care, self-esteem, and social skills in 8 to 13 year olds.
Megan Sorensen, Chair
Wilson Neyland, Chair-Elect

8025 **Healthcare Guidelines**
Spina Bifida Association of America

1600 Wilson Blvd. 202-944-3285
Arlington, VA 22209-4226 800-621-3141
Fax: 202-944-3295
e-mail: sbaa@sbaa.org
www.sbaa.org

Megan Sorensen, Chair
Wilson Neyland, Chair-Elect

8026 Learning Disabilities and the Person with Spina Bifida
Spina Bifida Association of America
1600 Wilson Blvd. 202-944-3285
Arlington, VA 22209-4226 800-621-3141
Fax: 202-944-3295
e-mail: sbaa@sbaa.org
www.sbaa.org

Megan Sorensen, Chair
Wilson Neyland, Chair-Elect

8027 Negotiating the Special Education Maze: A Guide for Parents and Teachers
Spina Bifida Association
1600 Wilson Blvd. 202-944-3285
Arlington, VA 22209-4226 800-621-3141
e-mail: sbaa@sbaa.org
www.sbaa.org

An excellent aid for the development of an effective special education program.
Megan Sorensen, Chair
Wilson Neyland, Chair-Elect

8028 New Language of Toys: Teaching Communication Skills to Children...
Spina Bifida Association
1600 Wilson Blvd. 202-944-3285
Arlington, VA 22209-4226 800-621-3141
e-mail: sbaa@sbaa.org
www.sbaa.org

A guide for parents and teachers, this reader-friendly resource guide provides a wealth of information on how play activities affect a child's language development (with a focus on special needs) and where to get the toys and materials to use in these activities.
Megan Sorensen, Chair
Wilson Neyland, Chair-Elect

8029 Nick Joins In
Spina Bifida Association
1600 Wilson Blvd. 202-944-3285
Arlington, VA 22209-4226 800-621-3141
e-mail: sbaa@sbaa.org
www.sbaa.org

When Nick, who is in a wheelchair, enters a regular classroom, for the first time he realizes that he has much to contribute.
Megan Sorensen, Chair
Wilson Neyland, Chair-Elect

8030 Princess Pooh
Spina Bifida Association
1600 Wilson Blvd. 202-944-3285
Arlington, VA 22209-4226 800-621-3141
e-mail: sbaa@sbaa.org
www.sbaa.org

Jealous of her disabled sister's royal treatment as she sits on her throne with wheels, Patty Jean borrows it and discovers that life in a wheelchair isn't so easy.
Megan Sorensen, Chair
Wilson Neyland, Chair-Elect

8031 SBAA General Information Packet
Spina Bifida Association of America
1600 Wilson Blvd. 202-944-3285
Arlington, VA 22209-4226 800-621-3141
Fax: 202-944-3295
e-mail: sbaa@sbaa.org
www.sbaa.org

Megan Sorensen, Chair
Wilson Neyland, Chair-Elect

8032 Sexuality and the Person with Spina Bifida
Spina Bifida Association of America

1600 Wilson Blvd. 202-944-3285
Arlington, VA 22209-4226 800-621-3141
Fax: 202-944-3295
e-mail: sbaa@sbaa.org
www.sbaa.org

Focuses on sexuality, sexual development, sexual activity, and other important issues.
Megan Sorensen, Chair
Wilson Neyland, Chair-Elect

8033 Social Development and the Person with Spina Bifida
Spina Bifida Association of America
1600 Wilson Blvd. 202-944-3285
Arlington, VA 22209-4226 800-621-3141
Fax: 202-944-3295
e-mail: sbaa@sbaa.org
www.sbaa.org

Megan Sorensen, Chair
Wilson Neyland, Chair-Elect

8034 Steps to Independence: Teaching Everyday Skills to Children with Special Needs
Spina Bifida Association
1600 Wilson Blvd. 202-944-3285
Arlington, VA 22209-4226 800-621-3141
e-mail: sbaa@sbaa.org
www.sbaa.org

A guide to help parents teach life skills to their disabled child.
Megan Sorensen, Chair
Wilson Neyland, Chair-Elect

8035 Taking Charge
Spina Bifida Association of America
1600 Wilson Blvd. 202-944-3285
Arlington, VA 22209-4226 800-621-3141
Fax: 202-944-3295
e-mail: sbaa@sbaa.org
www.sbaa.org

Teenagers talk about life and physical disabilities.
Megan Sorensen, Chair
Wilson Neyland, Chair-Elect

8036 Unlocking Potential: College and Other Choices for People with LD and AD/HD
Spina Bifida Association
1600 Wilson Blvd. 202-944-3285
Arlington, VA 22209-4226 800-621-3141
e-mail: sbaa@sbaa.org
www.sbaa.org

An indispensible tool for high school students with learning disabilities and AD/HD. Includes a comprehensive listing of resources.
Megan Sorensen, Chair
Wilson Neyland, Chair-Elect

Children's Books

8037 Margaret's Moves
Dutton Children's Books
2620 S. 7th St 502-584-5234
Louisville, KY 40216-3658 Fax: 502-371-0615
e-mail: info@margaretsmoving.com
margaretsmoving.com

This story deals with all the nuances and impairments that children afflicted with spina bifida must encounter and succeed in overcoming.
Grades 4-6

8038 Rolling Along with Goldilocks and the Three Bears
Spina Bifida Association
1600 Wilson Blvd. 202-944-3285
Arlington, VA 22209-4226 800-621-3141
e-mail: sbaa@sbaa.org
www.sbaa.org

The familiar folktale with a special-needs twist.
Megan Sorensen, Chair
Wilson Neyland, Chair-Elect

8039 **Views from Our Shoes: Growing Up with a Brother or Sister with Special Needs**
Spina Bifida Association
1600 Wilson Blvd.   202-944-3285
Arlington, VA 22209-4226   800-621-3141
e-mail: sbaa@sbaa.org
www.sbaa.org

A balanced view of the positives and negatives of living with a disabled sibling. Written for siblings ages nine and up.
Megan Sorensen, Chair
Wilson Neyland, Chair-Elect

Newsletters

8040 **Insights Into Spina Bifida**
Spina Bifida Association of America
1600 Wilson Blvd.   202-944-3285
Arlington, VA 22209-4226   800-621-3141
Fax: 202-944-3295
e-mail: sbaa@sbaa.org
www.sbaa.org

Includes articles on the latest research, the latest up-dates on legislation, features and emotional aspects specific to Spina Bifida, educational information and information on the Association's national conference.
BiMonthly
Megan Sorensen, Chair
Wilson Neyland, Chair-Elect

8041 **NASS News**
1400 Indpndc Ave., SW   847-698-1628
Washington, DC 20250-4037   800-727-9540
e-mail: nass@nass.usda.gov
www.nass.usda.gov

Association activities newsletter.
Sue King, Public Affairs Office Director
Kissy Young, Senior Public Affairs Specialist

Pamphlets

8042 **Educational Issues Among Children with Spina Bifida**
Spina Bifida Association of America
1600 Wilson Blvd.   202-944-3285
Arlington, VA 22209-4226   800-621-3141
Fax: 202-944-3295
e-mail: sbaa@sbaa.org
www.sbaa.org

1995
Megan Sorensen, Chair
Wilson Neyland, Chair-Elect

8043 **Learning Among Children with Spina Bifida**
Spina Bifida Association of America
1600 Wilson Blvd.   202-944-3285
Arlington, VA 22209-4226   800-621-3141
Fax: 202-944-3295
e-mail: sbaa@sbaa.org
www.sbaa.org

1995
Megan Sorensen, Chair
Wilson Neyland, Chair-Elect

8044 **Monetary Allowance, Health Care and Vocational Training**
National Veterans Services Fund
PO Box 2465   203-656-0003
Darien, CT 06820-0465   Fax: 203-656-1957
e-mail: NatVetSvc@aol.com
Monetary allowance, health care and vocational training and rehabilitation for Vietnam Veterans' children with spine bifida.
Pamphlet

8045 **Sexual Issues in Spina Bifida**
Spina Bifida Association of America

1600 Wilson Blvd.   202-944-3285
Arlington, VA 22209-4226   800-621-3141
Fax: 202-944-3295
e-mail: sbaa@sbaa.org
www.sbaa.org

1993
Megan Sorensen, Chair
Wilson Neyland, Chair-Elect

8046 **Urologic Care of the Child with Spina Bifida**
Spina Bifida Association of America
1600 Wilson Blvd.   202-944-3285
Arlington, VA 22209-4226   800-621-3141
Fax: 202-944-3295
e-mail: sbaa@sbaa.org
www.sbaa.org

1994
Megan Sorensen, Chair
Wilson Neyland, Chair-Elect

Audio & Video

8047 **Protecting Against Latex Allergy**
Spina Bifida Association of America
1600 Wilson Blvd.   202-944-3285
Arlington, VA 22209-4226   800-621-3141
Fax: 202-944-3295
e-mail: sbaa@sbaa.org
www.sbaa.org

Audio-visual resource focusing on the awareness of latex allergies.
Audio-Visual
Megan Sorensen, Chair
Wilson Neyland, Chair-Elect

8048 **Raising a Child with Spina Bifida: An Introduction**
Ajn Company
New York, NY 10019   212-582-8820
800-226-6256
Fax: 212-586-5462
Offers information parents need when their child is born with spina bifida. Uses clear explanations to define spina bifida and discuss its implications for the child. Covers procedures the child may face, such as a ventricular shunt. Emphasizes the importance of early intervention and contains footage of happy and healthy children and interviews with parents.
29 minutes

8049 **The Challenge**
Spina Bifida Association of America
1600 Wilson Blvd.   202-944-3285
Arlington, VA 22209-4226   800-621-3141
Fax: 202-944-3295
e-mail: sbaa@sbaa.org
www.sbaa.org

A human look of how people come to grips with and overcome the challenges related to living with Spina Bifida.
14 minutes
Megan Sorensen, Chair
Wilson Neyland, Chair-Elect

Web Sites

8050 **Healing Well**
www.healingwell.com
An online health resource guide to medical news, chat, information and articles, newsgroups and message boards, books, disease-related web sites, medical directories, and more for patients, friends, and family coping with disabling diseases, disorders, or chronic illnesses.

8051 **Health Finder**
www.healthfinder.gov
Searchable, carefully developed web site offering information on over 1000 topics. Developed by the US Department of Health and Human Services, the site can be used in both English and Spanish.

8052 Healthlink USA

www.healthlinkusa.com

Health information concerning treatment, cures, prevention, diagnosis, risk factors, research, support groups, email lists, personal stories and much more. Updated regularly.

8053 Helios Health

www.helioshealth.com

Online resource for your health information. Detailed information about specific health topics, access to expert advice from our Medical Advisory Board, and up-to-date health news.

8054 March of Dimes Birth Defects Foundation

www.modimes.org

Information on the treatment and prevention of birth defects, including spina bifida.

8055 MedicineNet

www.medicinenet.com

An online resource for consumers providing easy-to-read, authoritative medical and health information.

8056 Medscape

www.medscape.com

Medscape offers specialists, primary care physicians, and other health professionals the Web's most robust and integrated medical information and educational tools.

8057 Spina Bifida Association of America

www.sbaa.org

The Spina Bifida Association (SBA) serves adults and children who live with the challenges of Spina Bifida. Since 1973, SBA has been a national voluntary health agency solely dedicated to enhancing the lives of those with Spina Bifida and those whose lives are touched by this challenging birth defect. Its tools are education, advocacy, research, and service.

8058 WebMD

www.webmd.com

Provides credible information, supportive communities, and in-depth reference material about health subjects. A source for original and timely health information as well as material from well known content providers.

Description

8059 **Spinal Cord Injuries**

Spinal cord injury results from trauma to or disease of the spinal cord. Depending on where the spinal cord was injured, paraplegia (paralysis affecting the legs and lower part of the body) or quadriplegia (paralysis affecting all muscles below the neck and therefore all four limbs), may occur. Bladder and/or sexual function may be damaged. Each year, 12,000 people, mostly teenage males, sustain a spinal cord injury as a result of motor vehicle or sports-related accidents, or violent crimes.

Modern medical and surgical care has dramatically increased both long-term survival and quality of life in victims of spinal cord injury. This improvement reflects intensive medical care and appropriate surgical stabilization at the time of the injury, and in later years, attention to preventing the complications, such as skin breakdown, bladder infection and lung dysfunction. One of the greatest challenges is helping persons with spinal cord injuries to live as productive and independent a life as possible. Rehabilitation should begin as soon as possible after the injury. It usually starts with several weeks at a specialized inpatient facility, then transitions to family-assisted or independent living, depending on the extent of the disability. The multidisciplinary team provides education, emotional support, physical and occupational therapy, assistive devices, braces, and beds, and helps arrange special vans or modifications to the patient's home. Many voluntary societies and government agencies can help with the transition to life in the community.

National Agencies & Associations

8060 **American Association of Spinal Cord Injury Nurses**
801 18th Street NW
Washington, DC 20006   202-416-7704
                                Fax: 202-416-7641
                        e-mail: aascin@pva.org
                                www.aascin.org
Comprised of nurses who specialize in spinal cord research nursing and education.
Maurice L Jordan, Acting Executive Director
Sara Lerman MPH, Program Manager

8061 **American Paraplegic Society**
801 18th Street NW   202-416-7704
Washington, DC 20006-1131   Fax: 202-416-7641
                        e-mail: aps@pva.org
                                www.apssci.org
A professional membership organization for physicians scientists and allied health care professionals.
Maurice L Jordan, Acting Executive Director
Brenda Finkel, Administrative Assistant

8062 **American Spinal Cord Injury Association**
2020 Peachtree Road NW   404-355-9772
Atlanta, GA 30309   Fax: 404-355-1826
                        e-mail: ASIA_Office@shepherd.org
                                www.asia-spinalinjury.org
Promotes and establishes standards of excellence for all aspects of health care of individuals with spinal cord injury from onset throughout life.
Michael Haak, M.D, President
Mary . Jane Mulcahey, PhD., O.T, President-Elect

8063 **American Spinal Injury Association (ASIA)**
2020 Peachtree Road NW   404-355-9772
Atlanta, GA 30309   Fax: 404-355-1826
                        e-mail: ASIA_Office@shepherd.org
                                www.asia-spinalinjury.org
Promotes and establishes standards of excellence for all aspects of health care of individuals with spinal cord injury from onset throughout life.
Michael Haak, M.D, President
Mary . Jane Mulcahey, PhD., O.T, President-Elect

8064 **Association of Spinal Cord Injury Psychologists and Social Workers**
801 18th Street NW   202-416-7704
Washington, DC 20006-1131   Fax: 202-416-7641
                        e-mail: aascipsw@epua.org
                                www.aascipsw.org
Formed in 1986 to provide a forum for the exchange of ideas and information with assistance of the Eastern Paralyzed Veterans Association.
Maurice L Jordan, Acting Executive Director
Brenda Finkel, Administrative Assistant

8065 **Christopher & Dana Reeve Foundation Paralysis Resource Center**
636 Morris Turnpike   973-467-8270
Short Hills, NJ 07078   800-225-0292
                        e-mail: info@paralysis.org
                                www.christopherreeve.org
The Reeve Foundation is dedicated to curing spinal cord injury by funding innovative research, and improving the quality of life for people living with paralysis through grants, information and advocacy.
John M. Hughes, Chairman
John E. McConnell, Vice Chairman

8066 **Eastern Paralyzed Veterans Association of America**
7520 Astoria Boulevard   718-803-3782
E Elmhurst, NY 11370-1177   800-444-0120
                                Fax: 718-803-0414
Dedicated to serving veterans with a spinal cord injury or disease in New York New Jersey Connecticut or Pennsylvania. Based in New York City EPVA is the leader in funding SCI research and care.
Angela Wu, Director of Library Information

8067 **FES Information Center WO Walker Industrial Rehabilitation Cent**
WO Walker Industrial Rehabilitation Center
11000 Cedar Avenue
Cleveland, OH 44106-3052   800-666-2353
FES offers technology to persons with neuromuscular disorders resulting from spinal cord injury, head injury or stroke. The most widely known use of FES in the spinal community is for exercise.

8068 **International Medical Society of Paralegia: US Office**
T Giles
1333 Moursend Avenue   713-797-5910
Houston, TX 77030   Fax: 713-799-7017
National non-profit organization offers information resources and research for people with spinal cord injury or dysfunction. Professional organization for physicians.

8069 **International Spinal Cord Regeneration Center**
PO Box 451   619-463-5350
Bonita, CA 91908   Fax: 619-460-2699
                        e-mail: spinal@mailutopia.net
                                www.spinal.siteutopia.net
Specializes in spinal cord regeneration as well as Embryonic Cell Transplant Therapy.
Fernando C Ramirez del Rio, Medical Director
Wolfram W Kuhnau, Associate

8070 **Kent Waldrep National Paralysis Foundation Main Office**
Main Office
16415 Addison Road   972-248-7100
Addison, TX 75001   800-925-2873
                                Fax: 972-248-7313

National non-profit organization offers information referral resources and research for people with spinal cord injury their family members or service providers.

8071 **National Spinal Cord Injury Association: Metropolitan Washington Chapter**
6701 Democracy Boulevard   301-214-4006
Bethesdae, MD 20817   800-962-9629
                                    Fax: 301-881-9817
                              e-mail: stevetowle@cs.com
The mission of the National Spinal Cord Injury Association is to enable people with spinal cord injury and disease to achieve their highest level of indepedence, health, and personal fulfillment by providing resources, services, and peer support.
Harley Thomas, President

8072 **National Spinal Cord Injury Statistical Center**
University of Alabama, Dept. of Physical Medicine
1717 6th Ave South   205-934-3342
Birmingham, AL 35233   Fax: 205-975-4691
                                    TDD: 205-934-4642
                               e-mail: nscisc@uab.edu
                                     www.nscisc.uab.edu
The UAB Department of Physical Medicine and Rehabilitation is funded by the National Institute on Disability and Rehabilitation Research (NIDRR) to operate the National Spinal Cord Injury Statistical Center (NSCISC). NSCISC supports and directs the collection, management and analysis of the world's largest and longest spinal cord injury research database. Organizationally, NSCISC is currently at the hub of a network of 14 NIDRR-sponsored and 5 subcontract-funded Spinal Cord Injury Model Systems
Yuying Chen, MD, PhD, Director
Pam Mott, Director Research Services

8073 **Paralyzed Veterans of America**
801 18th Street NW   202-872-1300
Washington, DC 20006-3517   800-424-8200
                                    Fax: 202-785-4452
                                    TTY: 800-795-4327
                                  e-mail: info@pva.org
                                          www.pva.org
For more than 67 years, Paralyzed Veterans of America has been on a mission to change lives and build brighter futures for our seriously injured heroes-to empower these brave men and women with what they need to achieve the things they fought for: freedom and independence.
Bill Lawson, National President
Al Kovach, Jr., National Senior Vice President

8074 **Rick Hansen Foundation**
300-3820 Cessna Drive   604-295-8149
Richmond, V7B 0-1A1   800-213-2131
                                    Fax: 604-295-8159
                            e-mail: info@rickhansen.com
                                    www.rickhansen.com
The Rick Hansen Foundation unifies organizations and leaders to work in partnership towards positive change for a healthy and inclusive world, with a key focus of improving the lives of those with spinal cord injuries.Through Rick's leadership, the Foundation has leveraged the $26 million raised during the original Tour to more than $280 million in investments toward SCI research, rehabilitation and quality of life initiatives.
Doramy Ehling, Executive Vice President
Colin Ewart, Vice President of Strategic Relations

8075 **Spinal Cord Injury Network International**
3911 Princeton Drive   707-577-8796
Santa Rosa, CA 95405-7013   800-548-2673
                                    Fax: 707-577-0605
                               e-mail: spinal@sonic.net
                                    www.spinalcordinjury.org
Spinal Cord Injury Network International was founded in 1986 by Lennice Ambrose after her son suffered a spinal cord injury in a car accident. She soon came to the realization that there was a lack of collected resources for those seeking help. Starting the organization at her home in Santa Rosa, California; the organization has grown to be recognized internationally for being dedicated to helping injured persons and their families reach the best possible care and knowledgable information. Our o
Lennice Ambrose, Executive Director
Sharon E Hunt, Medical Librarian

8076 **Spinal Cord Society**
19051 County Highway 1   218-739-5252
Fergus Falls, MN 56537   Fax: 218-739-5262
                                          www.scsus.org
Funds research for spinal cord injuries and provides physician referrals.

State Agencies & Associations

Arizona

8077 **Arizona Spinal Cord Injury Association**
Samaritan Rehab Institute R-2
5025 E Washington St   602-507-4209
Phoenix, AZ 85034   888-889-2185
                                    Fax: 602-507-4214
                               e-mail: info@azspinal.org
                                          www.azspinal.org
The Arizona Spinal Cord Injury Association is a nonprofit organization dedicated to enhancing the lives of individuals with spinal cord injuries. We also offer support and education to family members, professionals, and community members.
Don Price, President
Donna Powers, Vice President

California

8078 **National Spinal Cord Injury Association: San Diego County Chapter**
6645 Alvarado Road   619-229-7001
San Diego, CA 92120   e-mail: rehabdsg@gte.net
                                          www.users.erols.com
Organization dedicated to improving the quality of life for persons with spinal cord injury and related disorders and their families. Seeks to fufill this mission by raising awareness about spinal cord injury through education, injury prevention, improvement of medical, rehabilitative and supportive services, research and public policy formulation.
Royce Hamrick

8079 **National Spinal Cord Injury Association: Los Angeles Chapter**
311 Robertson Boulevard   310-553-4833
Beverly Hills, CA 90211   Fax: 310-659-5040
                                          www.users.erols.com
Organization dedicated to improving the quality of life for persons with spinal cord injury and related disorders and their families. Seeks to fufill this mission by raising awareness about spinal cord injury through education, injury prevention, improvement of medical, rehabilitative and supportive services, research and public policy formulation.
Paul Berns MD, President

Connecticut

8080 **National Spinal Cord Injury Association: Connecticut Chapter**
Wallingford, CT 06492   203-284-1045
                               e-mail: nscia@sciact.org
                                          www.users.erols.com
Organization dedicated to improving the quality of life for persons with spinal cord injury and related disorders and their families. Seeks to fufill this mission by raising awareness about spinal cord injury through education, injury prevention, improvement of medical, rehabilitative and supportive services, research and public policy formulation.
Bill Mancini, President
Liza Ethier, Contact

Florida

8081 **Goodwill Industries-Suncoast**
Goodwill Industries-Suncoast

10596 Gandy Boulevard
Saint Petersburg, FL 33702

727-523-1512
888-279-1988
Fax: 727-579-0850
TTY: 727-579-1068
e-mail: gw.marketing@goodwill-suncoast.com
www.goodwill-suncoast.org

Goodwill-Suncoast was founded in October 1954 in downtown St. Petersburg. We began by assisting a handful of people with disabilities to gain work skills and paychecks. Now we help thousands of people overcome a variety of barriers to employment through employment programs, five subsidized apartment buildings, work activities centers for adults with developmental disabilities, as well as rehabilitative community corrections facilities. To support these services, Goodwill-Suncoast operates 15 ret

Oscar J. Horton, Chair
Martin W. Gladysz, Sr. Vice Chair

Georgia

8082 **Shepherd Center**
2020 Peachtree Road NW
Atlanta, GA 30309

404-352-2020
e-mail: admissions@shepherd.org
www.shepherd.org

Shepherd Center is a 152-bed facility. Last year Shepherd had 965 admissions to its inpatient programs and 571 to its day patient programs. In addition, Shepherd sees more than 6,600 people annually on an outpatient basis.

Gary R. Ulicny, Ph.D, President/CEO
Brock K Bowman, Assistant Medical Director

Illinois

8083 **Spinal Cord Injury Association of Illinois**
1032 S LaGrange Road
LaGrange, IL 60525

708-352-6223
877-373-0301
Fax: 708-352-9065
e-mail: sciinjury@aol.com
www.sci-illinois.org

Spinal Cord Injury Association of Illinois (formerly NSCIA, Illinois Chapter) is a 501(c)3 non-profit organization providing information and support resources for people paralyzed by trauma and medical conditions, family members, and health care and related professionals that serve the SCI community. Our office is located in LaGrange, IL, a suburb of Chicago, but we serve the entire state.

Kim Eberhardt Muir, MS, OTR, President
Vic Myers, Vice President

Indiana

8084 **National Spinal Cord Injury Association: Central Indiana Chapter**
2109 Cleveland Street
Garyanapolis, IN 46404

219-944-8037
Fax: 317-329-2530
e-mail: rjackson@ci.gary.in.us

Organization dedicated to improving the quality of life for persons with spinal cord injury and related disorders and their families. Seeks to fufill this mission by raising awareness about spinal cord injury through education, injury prevention, improvement of medical, rehabilitative and supportive services, research and public policy formulation.

Lucille Hightower

Kentucky

8085 **National Spinal Cord Injury Association: Derby City Area Chapter**
Center for Accessible Living
305 W. Broadway
Louisville, KY 40202

502-588-8574
e-mail: dallgood@calky.org
www.derbycityspinalcord.org

Derby City Area Spinal Cord Injury Association, the Louisville Kentucky Chapter of the (N.S.C.I.A.) National Spinal Cord Injury Association. Derby City Area Spinal Cord Injury Association is a organization for individuals with spinal cord injuries, their families, and health professionals across Kentucky. Founded in 1984 as a Charter Member of the N.S.C.I.A., it was incorporated under IRS Section 501 (c) 3 as a not for profit organization.

David Allgood, President
Adam Ford, Vice President

Louisiana

8086 **National Spinal Cord Injury Association: Louisiana Chapter**
3650 18th Street
Metairie, LA 70002

504-455-1178
Fax: 504-455-7315

Organization dedicated to improving the quality of life for persons with spinal cord injury and related disorders and their families. Seeks to fufill this mission by raising awareness about spinal cord injury through education, injury prevention, improvement of medical, rehabilitative and supportive services, research and public policy formulation.

Yadi Mark

Massachusetts

8087 **National Spinal Cord Injury Association**
545 Concord Avenue
Cambridge, MA 02138-1173

301-588-6959
800-962-9629
Fax: 301-588-9414
e-mail: nscia2@aol.com
www.spinalcord.org

Organization dedicated to improving the quality of life for persons with spinal cord injury and related disorders and their families. Seeks to fufill this mission by raising awareness about spinal cord injury through education, injury prevention, improvement of medical, rehabilitative and supportive services, research and public policy formulation.

8088 **National Spinal Cord Injury Association: Greater Boston Chapter**
New England Rehabilitation Hospital
Two Rehabilitation Way
Woburn, MA 01801

781-933-8666
Fax: 781-933-0043
e-mail: sciboston@aol.com
www.sciboston.com

Organization dedicated to improving the quality of life for persons with spinal cord injury and related disorders and their families. Seeks to fulfill this mission by raising awareness about spinal cord injury through education and injury prevention.

Dave Estrada, Director
Kevin Gibson, Coordinator

New Hampshire

8089 **New Hampshire Chapter NSCIA**
Northeast Rehabilitation Hospital
21 Chenell Drive
Concord, NH 03301-3974

603-479-0560
800-826-3700
Fax: 928-438-9607
e-mail: debbie@gsil.org
www.spinalcord.org

Lisa Thompson, President

New York

8090 **Greater Rochester Area Chapter NSCIA**
Rochester, NY 14602-0076

585-234-3269
e-mail: rochesternscia@yahoo.com
www.spinalcord.org

Karen Genet, Contact
Cathy Flanagan, Contact

8091 **National Spinal Cord Injury Association**
75-20 Astoria Blvd
Jackson Heights, NY 11370

718-803-3782
800-962-9629
Fax: 301-990-0445
e-mail: nscia2@aol.com
www.spinalcord.org

National Spinal Cord Injury Association, the membership division of United Spinal, was founded in 1948 to improve the lives of all paralyzed Americans. Our mission is to improve the quality of life of all people living with a spinal cord injury or disease. We provide active-lifestyle information, peer support and advocacy that empower individuals to achieve their highest potential in all facets of life

Steven A Towle, Contact

Pennsylvania

8092 Shriners Hospital for Children
3551 N Broad Street   215-430-4000
Philadelphia, PA 19140   800-281-4050
Fax: 215-430-4079
e-mail: tdiamond@shrinenet.org
www.shrinershospitalsforchildren.org
Studies and research done on children with spinal cord injuries.
Scott . Kozin, M.D, Chief of Staff
Terry Diamond, Development Officer

8093 Spinal Cord Injury Program at Harmarville Rehabilitation Center
Pittsburgh, PA 15238   412-828-1300
800-624-4673
Most comprehensive center for the treatment of spinal cord injury and disease.

Texas

8094 Rio Grande Chapter: NSCIA Rio Vista Rehabilitation Hospital
Rio Vista Rehabilitation Hospital
1395 George Dieter   915-298-7241
El Paso, TX 79936-2901   e-mail: riograndenscia@aol.com
www.spinalcord.org

Sukie Armendariz, Contact
Ron Prieto, Contact

Virginia

8095 Old Dominion Area Chapter: NSCIA
5206 Markel Road   804-726-4990
Richmond, VA 23226   Fax: 888-752-7857
e-mail: info@odcnscia.org
www.odcnscia.org
Our mission is to enable people with spinal cord injuries and disease to achieve their highest level of health, independence and quality of life. We educate public officials, community leaders, and citizens to the needs of persons with spinal cord injury and disease, and the importance of creating an environment of greater independence for all. We offer a variety of services and a wealth of knowledge towards unlocking the door for active living with SCI.
Steve Fetrow, President
Craig Fabian, Vice President

Wisconsin

8096 Southeastern Wisconsin Chapter of the Nati onal Spinal Cord Injury Association
Sacred Heart Rehabilitation Hospital
540 South 1st Street   414-384-4022
Milwaukee, WI 53204-1993   Fax: 414-384-7820
e-mail: office@spinalcordwi.org
www.spinalcord.org
The mission of the NSCIA-SWC is to assist people who have some degree of paralysis through injury or disease with a goal of returning them to a life of dignity, self-confidence and independence in a community that is all inclusive.
John Dzicwa, President

Research Centers

8097 Miami Project to Cure Paralysis
1095 NW 14th Terrace   305-243-6001
Miami, FL 33101   800-STA-NDUP
Fax: 205-243-6017
e-mail: miamiproject@med.miami.edu
www.miamiproject.miami.edu
In 1985, Barth A. Green, M.D. and NFL Hall of Fame linebacker Nick Buoniconti helped found TheMiami Projectto Cure Paralysis after Nick's son, Marc, sustained a spinal cord injury during a college football game. Today, The Miami Project is the world's most comprehensive spinal cord injury research center, and is a designated Center of Excellence at the University of Miami Miller

School of Medicine. The Miami Project's international team is housed in the Lois Pope LIFE Center and includes more t
Barth A. Green, M.D., Co-Founder and Chairman
Marc A Buoniconti, President

8098 Pushin On: RRTC on Secondary Conditions of Spinal
UAB Office of Research Services
1717 6th Avenue South   205-934-3283
Birmingham, AL 35249-7330   Fax: 205-975-4691
TDD: 205-934-4642
e-mail: sciweb@uab.edu
www.spinalcord.uab.edu
Pushin' On is an enewsletter published to provide persons with SCI and their families with information of interest. The newsletter is offered 2 times per year and sent electronically to subscribers to the UAB-SCIMS Email List, and it is posted online for our follows on facebook and twitter.
8 pages 2 per year
Amie B McLain, MD., Program Director
Phil Klebine, Editor

8099 RRTC on Aging with a Disability Los Amigos Research and Education Instit
Los Amigos Research and Education Institute
7601 E Imperial Highway   562-401-7402
Downey, CA 90242-3456   Fax: 562-401-7011
e-mail: lcarrothers@agingwithdisability.org
www.agingwithdisability.org
A federally funded rehabilitation research and training center.
Bryan Kemp PhD, Director
Leanne Carro Pt PhD, Training Director

Support Groups & Hotlines

8100 Georgia National Spinal Cord Injury Association Support Group Network
Columbus, GA 31920
800-422-3352
Support group dedicated to improving the quality of life for persons with spinal cord injury and related disorders and their families. Seeks to fufill this mission by raising awareness about spinal cord injury through rehabilitative and supportive services, research and public policy formulation.
Andy Harp

8101 HEALTHSOUTH Rehabilitation Hospital of Tal lahassee
1675 Riggins Road   850-656-4800
Tallahassee, FL 32308   Fax: 850-656-4809
www.healthsouthtallahassee.com
Our hospital provides a wide range of physical rehabilitation services, a vast network of highly-skilled, independent private practice physicians and HealthSouth therapists and nurses, and the most innovative equipment and rehabilitation technology, ensuring that all patients have access to the highest quality care. Designed with our patient's care in mind, HealthSouth Rehabilitation Hospital of Tallahassee offers semi-private rooms, which promote social interaction and support throughout the re
Dale Neely, Chief Executive Officer
Robert Rowland, M.D., Medical Director

8102 Maryland National Spinal Cord Injury Association Support Group Network
Kerman Hospital
2200 Kerman Drive   410-448-6307
Baltimore, MD 21207   800-962-9629
e-mail: mhenley@kernan.umm.edu
www.spinalcord.org
Open group for all caregivers and does not focus on a specific disability, disease or condition.

8103 National Health Information Center
Washington, DC 20013   310-565-4167
800-336-4797
Fax: 301-984-4256
e-mail: info@nhic.org
www.health.gov/nhic
Offers a nationwide information referral service, produces directories and resource guides.

8104 **National Spinal Cord Injury Support Goups**
Florida Rehabilitation and Sports Medicine
5165 Adanson Street   407-895-7991
Orlando, FL 32804
Support group dedicated to improving the quality of life for persons with spinal cord injury and related disorders and their families. Seeks to fufill this mission by raising awareness about spinal cord injury through rehabilitative and supportive services, research and public policy formulation.

8105 **VIVA!**
Health Enhancement Learning Programs
Dallas, TX 75354-3065   972-986-2977
                                       800-334-4403
A computer-based patient education system on spinal cord injury.

8106 **National Spinal Cord Injury Support Groups**
Healthsouth Central Georgia Rehab Hospital
777 Hemlock Street   478-633-1000
Macon, GA 31201   800-491-3550
                                  Fax: 478-633-5134
              e-mail: tamboli.sara@mccg.org
                     www.centralgarehab.com/
Support group dedicated to improving the quality of life for persons with spinal cord injury and related disorders and their families. Seeks to fufill this mission by raising awareness about spinal cord injury through rehabilitative and supportive services, research and public policy formulation.
Connie Cater, President
Starr H. Purdue, Chairman

8107 **National Spinal Cord Injury Support Groups**
HEALTHSOUTH, Sea Pines Rehabilitation Hospital
101 E Florida Avenue   407-984-4600
Melbourne, FL 32901   e-mail: laura.leitz@healthsouth.com
                                  www.spinalcord.org
In a support group, members provide each other with various types of help for shared purposes. The help can take the form of providing and evaluating relevant information, relating personal experiences, listening to and accepting others' experiences, educating and guiding, or for providing sympathetic understanding and establishing social networks. Support Groups may each have their own way of accomplishing their mission but all of them share the same goal of improving the lives of participants.

8108 **National Spinal Cord Injury Support Groups**
115 Alpine Street   334-456-1768
Chickasaw, AL 36611
Support group dedicated to improving the quality of life for persons with spinal cord injury and related disorders and their families. Seeks to fufill this mission by raising awareness about spinal cord injury through rehabilitative and supportive services, research and public policy formulation.

Books

8109 **Body Silent: An Anthropologist Embarks into the World of the Disabled**
WW Norton Publishing
500 Fifth Avenue   212-354-5500
New York, NY 10110   Fax: 212-869-0856
                                  www.wwnorton.com
Diagnosed at midlife in the early 1980s with an inoperable (and, at the time, untreatable) ependymona of the spine, an anthropologist frankly discusses his progressive disability.

ISBN: 0-393307-02-6

8110 **Climbing Back**
Miramar Communications
PO Box 8987
Malibu, CA 90265-8987   800-543-4116
The author broke his back after a climbing fall. With his sights at the top of the mountain he climbs back in this inspiring story.
256 pages Hardcover

8111 **Occupational Therapy Practice Guidelines for Adults with Spinal Cord Injury**
American Occupational Therapy Association

4720 Montgomery Lane   301-652-6611
Bethesda, MD 20814-1220   Fax: 240-762-5150
                                  TDD: 800-377-8555
                                       www.aota.org

31 pages
ISBN: 1-569001-54-5

8112 **Options: Spinal Cord Injury and the Future**
National Spinal Cord Injury Association
120-34 Queens Blvd.   718-803-3782
Kew Gardens, NY 11415-3243   800-404-2898
                                  Fax: 718-803-0414
                     e-mail: info@unitedspinal.org
                                  www.spinalcord.org
A collection of conversations with people who have had spinal cord injuries who share some of their experiences and emotions.
150 pages
David C. Cooper, Chairman
Joseph Gaskins, President & CEO

8113 **Spinal Cord Injury Home Care Manual**
Santa Clara Valley Medical Center
751 S Bascom Avenue
San Jose, CA 95128-2699   408-885-5000
                                  www.scvmed.org
Provides people with spinal cord injury, their families and professionals with information about physical care, independent living, psychosocial issues, attendant care and supplies.
Paul E. Lorenz, Chief Executive Officer
Benita McLarin, Chief Operating Officer

8114 **Spinal Network**
Miramar Communications
120-34 Queens Blvd.   718-803-3782
Kew Gardens, NY 11415   800-404-2898
                                  Fax: 718-803-0414
                     e-mail: info@unitedspinal.org
                                  www.spinalcord.org
Total wheelchair resource book.
David C. Cooper, Chairman
Joseph Gaskins, President & CEO

Children's Books

8115 **Follow Your Dreams**
National Spinal Cord Injury Association
120-34 Queens Blvd.   718-803-3782
Kew Gardens, NY 11415-3243   800-404-2898
                                  Fax: 718-803-0414
                     e-mail: info@unitedspinal.org
                                  www.spinalcord.org
JT, born with spina bifida, goes on an adventure. Written for and by children with SCI, for children ages 9-12.
30 pages
David C. Cooper, Chairman
Joseph Gaskins, President & CEO

8116 **Tell it Like it is**
National Spinal Cord Injury Association
120-34 Queens Blvd.   718-803-3782
Kew Gardens, NY 11415-3243   800-404-2898
                                  Fax: 718-803-0414
                     e-mail: info@unitedspinal.org
                                  www.spinalcord.org
Written by teenagers with SCI for teenagers with SCI.
David C. Cooper, Chairman
Joseph Gaskins, President & CEO

Magazines

8117 **SCI Life**
National Spinal Cord Injury Association
120-34 Queens Blvd.   718-803-3782
Kew Gardens, NY 11415-3243   800-404-2898
                                  Fax: 718-803-0414
                     e-mail: info@unitedspinal.org
                                  www.spinalcord.org

Official magazine of NSCIA. Updates on topics such as research, medical issues, prevention, new products, books, and Association activities.
Quarterly
David C. Cooper, Chairman
Joseph Gaskins, President & CEO

8118 **Spinal Column**
Shepherd Spinal Center
7075 Veterans Blvd.
Burr Ridge, IL 60527-1465   630-230-3600
                                            www.spine.org
This quarterly magazine from the spinal center offers information on the newest treatments, therapies, referral centers, assistive devices and much more for persons living with spina bifida, multiple sclerosis and other chronic physical ailments.
Quarterly
Heidi Prather, President
Christopher Bono, First Vice President

Newsletters

8119 **Progress in Research**
American Paralysis Association
4400 Fifth Avenue   412-268-1062
Pittsburgh, PA 15213-1020   800-225-0292
                                            Fax: 973-912-9433
                                            http://www.chem.cmu.edu
Offers information on the association, news, reviews, books, and information on the latest medical and technological advances in spinal cord injury research.
Quarterly
Susan P Howley, Research Director
Mitchell R Stoller, President/CEO

8120 **Pushing on: University of Alabama**
Christopher Reeve Association
4400 Fifth Avenue   412-268-1062
Pittsburgh, PA 15213   800-225-0292
                                            Fax: 973-912-9433
                                            http://www.chem.cmu.edu
A research newsletter regarding spinal cord injuries.
Quarterly
Mitchell R Stoller, President/CEO

8121 **Spinal Cord Society Newsletter**
Spinal Cord Society
19051 County Highway 1   218-739-5252
Fergus Falls, MN 56537   Fax: 218-739-5262
                                            www.members.aol.com/scsweb
Offers medical reports, articles, convention news, chapter news and more for persons with spinal cord injury.
Monthly

8122 **Walking Tomorrow: University of Alabama**
Christopher Reeve Association
4400 Fifth Avenue   412-268-1062
Pittsburgh, PA 15213-1020   800-225-0292
                                            Fax: 973-912-9433
                                            http://www.chem.cmu.edu
A research newsletter regarding spinal cord injuries.
Quarterly
Mitchell R Stoller, President/CEO

Pamphlets

8123 **Autonomic Dysreflexia**
National Spinal Cord Injury Association
120-34 Queens Blvd.   718-803-3782
Kew Gardens, NY 11415-3243   800-404-2898
                                            Fax: 718-803-0414
                                            e-mail: info@unitedspinal.org
                                            www.spinalcord.org
David C. Cooper, Chairman
Joseph Gaskins, President & CEO

8124 **Choosing A Spinal Cord Injury Rehabilitation Program**
National Spinal Cord Injury Association
120-34 Queens Blvd.   718-803-3782
Kew Gardens, NY 11415-3243   800-404-2898
                                            Fax: 718-803-0414
                                            e-mail: info@unitedspinal.org
                                            www.spinalcord.org
Includes a listing of programs accredited by CARF & Model Centers designated by NIDRR.
David C. Cooper, Chairman
Joseph Gaskins, President & CEO

8125 **Fun and Games**
National Spinal Cord Injury Association
120-34 Queens Blvd.   718-803-3782
Kew Gardens, NY 11415-3243   800-404-2898
                                            Fax: 718-803-0414
                                            e-mail: info@unitedspinal.org
                                            www.spinalcord.org
David C. Cooper, Chairman
Joseph Gaskins, President & CEO

8126 **Functional Electrical Stimulation: Clinical Applications**
National Spinal Cord Injury Association
120-34 Queens Blvd.   718-803-3782
Kew Gardens, NY 11415-3243   800-404-2898
                                            Fax: 718-803-0414
                                            e-mail: info@unitedspinal.org
                                            www.spinalcord.org
David C. Cooper, Chairman
Joseph Gaskins, President & CEO

8127 **Importance of Basic Science in Research**
National Spinal Cord Injury Association
120-34 Queens Blvd.   718-803-3782
Kew Gardens, NY 11415-3243   800-404-2898
                                            Fax: 718-803-0414
                                            e-mail: info@unitedspinal.org
                                            www.spinalcord.org
David C. Cooper, Chairman
Joseph Gaskins, President & CEO

8128 **Male Reproductive Function After Spinal Cord Injury**
National Spinal Cord Injury Association
120-34 Queens Blvd.   718-803-3782
Kew Gardens, NY 11415-3243   800-404-2898
                                            Fax: 718-803-0414
                                            e-mail: info@unitedspinal.org
                                            www.spinalcord.org
David C. Cooper, Chairman
Joseph Gaskins, President & CEO

8129 **Medical Facilities and Resources for Ventilator Users**
National Spinal Cord Injury Association
120-34 Queens Blvd.   718-803-3782
Kew Gardens, NY 11415-3243   800-404-2898
                                            Fax: 718-803-0414
                                            e-mail: info@unitedspinal.org
                                            www.spinalcord.org
David C. Cooper, Chairman
Joseph Gaskins, President & CEO

8130 **Reading Resources on Spinal Cord Injury**
National Spinal Cord Injury Association
120-34 Queens Blvd.   718-803-3782
Kew Gardens, NY 11415-3243   800-404-2898
                                            Fax: 718-803-0414
                                            e-mail: info@unitedspinal.org
                                            www.spinalcord.org
David C. Cooper, Chairman
Joseph Gaskins, President & CEO

8131 **Sexuality After Spinal Cord Injury**
National Spinal Cord Injury Association
120-34 Queens Blvd.   718-803-3782
Kew Gardens, NY 11415-3243   800-404-2898
                                            Fax: 718-803-0414
                                            e-mail: info@unitedspinal.org
                                            www.spinalcord.org
David C. Cooper, Chairman
Joseph Gaskins, President & CEO

8132 Spinal Cord Injury Awareness
National Spinal Cord Injury Association
120-34 Queens Blvd.   718-803-3782
Kew Gardens, NY 11415-3243   800-404-2898
                                  Fax: 718-803-0414
                        e-mail: info@unitedspinal.org
                                   www.spinalcord.org
Understanding the importance of language and images.
David C. Cooper, Chairman
Joseph Gaskins, President & CEO

8133 Spinal Cord Injury: Statistical Information
National Spinal Cord Injury Association
120-34 Queens Blvd.   718-803-3782
Kew Gardens, NY 11415-3243   800-404-2898
                                  Fax: 718-803-0414
                        e-mail: info@unitedspinal.org
                                   www.spinalcord.org

David C. Cooper, Chairman
Joseph Gaskins, President & CEO

8134 Starting a Support Group
National Spinal Cord Injury Association
120-34 Queens Blvd.   718-803-3782
Kew Gardens, NY 11415-3243   800-404-2898
                                  Fax: 718-803-0414
                        e-mail: info@unitedspinal.org
                                   www.spinalcord.org

David C. Cooper, Chairman
Joseph Gaskins, President & CEO

8135 Tendon Transfer Surgery
National Spinal Cord Injury Association
120-34 Queens Blvd.   718-803-3782
Kew Gardens, NY 11415-3243   800-404-2898
                                  Fax: 718-803-0414
                        e-mail: info@unitedspinal.org
                                   www.spinalcord.org

David C. Cooper, Chairman
Joseph Gaskins, President & CEO

8136 Travel After Spinal Cord Injury
National Spinal Cord Injury Association
120-34 Queens Blvd.   718-803-3782
Kew Gardens, NY 11415-3243   800-404-2898
                                  Fax: 718-803-0414
                        e-mail: info@unitedspinal.org
                                   www.spinalcord.org

David C. Cooper, Chairman
Joseph Gaskins, President & CEO

8137 Understanding Spinal Muscular Atrophy
Families of Spinal Muscular Atrophy
PO Box 196   847-367-7620
Libertyville, IL 60048-0196   800-886-1762
                                  Fax: 847-367-7623
                              e-mail: info@fsma.org
                                   www.curesma.com
Offers a brief overview of Spinal Muscular Atrophy, causes, treatments, symptoms and unknowns.
Kenneth Hobby, President
Richard Rubenstein, Chair

8138 What is Spinal Cord Injury?
National Spinal Cord Injury Association
120-34 Queens Blvd.   718-803-3782
Kew Gardens, NY 11415-3243   800-404-2898
                                  Fax: 718-803-0414
                        e-mail: info@unitedspinal.org
                                   www.spinalcord.org

David C. Cooper, Chairman
Joseph Gaskins, President & CEO

8139 What is a Physiatrist?
National Spinal Cord Injury Association

120-34 Queens Blvd.   718-803-3782
Kew Gardens, NY 11415-3243   800-404-2898
                                  Fax: 718-803-0414
                        e-mail: info@unitedspinal.org
                                   www.spinalcord.org

David C. Cooper, Chairman
Joseph Gaskins, President & CEO

8140 What's New in Spinal Cord Injury Research?
National Spinal Cord Injury Association
120-34 Queens Blvd.   718-803-3782
Kew Gardens, NY 11415-3243   800-404-2898
                                  Fax: 718-803-0414
                        e-mail: info@unitedspinal.org
                                   www.spinalcord.org

David C. Cooper, Chairman
Joseph Gaskins, President & CEO

Audio & Video

8141 Living with Spinal Cord Injury
Barry Corbet, author
Fanlight Productions
4196 Washington Street   617-469-4999
Boston, MA 02131-1731   800-937-4113
                                  Fax: 617-469-3379
                        e-mail: fanlight@fanlight.com
                                    www.fanlight.com
A series of three videos produced by an individual who has experienced spinal cord injury himself. Changes is about coming to terms with spinal cord injury and beginning rehabilitation. Outside looks at the life-long process by which some injured people have created active and rewarding lives. Survivors explores the problems of growing old with a disability.
1973 84 Minutes

8142 SCI and Lower Extremity Orthoses
Health Enhancement Learning Programs
292 Washington Ave, Ext   518-452-6898
Albany, NY 12203-3065   800-334-4403
                                    lermagazine.com
A video presenting an overview of indications and use of HKAFO, KAFO and AFO. Perfect resource for medical presentations and professional workshops.
Richard Dubin, Founder and Publisher
Jordana Bieze Foster, Editor

8143 Spinal Cord Injury Video Access
Spinal Cord Injury Access International
292 Washington Ave, Ext   518-452-6898
Albany, NY 12203   800-548-2673
                                    lermagazine.com
Offers informational videotapes on spinal cord injury.
Richard Dubin, Founder and Publisher
Jordana Bieze Foster, Editor

8144 Spinal Injury Slide Series
Health Enhancement Learning Programs
292 Washington Ave, Ext   518-452-6898
Albany, NY 12203-3065   800-334-4403
                                    lermagazine.com
A slide series based on the VIVA program, a patient education system on spinal cord injury.
Richard Dubin, Founder and Publisher
Jordana Bieze Foster, Editor

Web Sites

8145 American Association of Spinal Cord Injury Nurses
                                     www.aascin.org
Comprised of nurses who specialize in spinal cord research, nursing and education.

8146 American Paraplegic Society
                                      www.apssci.org
A professional membership organization for physicians, scientists and allied health care professionals.

8147 **Christopher Reeve Paralysis Foundation**

www.christopherreeve.org

The Reeve Foundation is dedicated to curing spinal cord injury by funding innovative research, and improving the quality of life for people living with paralysis through grants, information and advocacy.

8148 **Healing Well**

www.healingwell.com

An online health resource guide to medical news, chat, information and articles, newsgroups and message boards, books, disease-related web sites, medical directories, and more for patients, friends, and family coping with disabling diseases, disorders, or chronic illnesses.

8149 **Health Finder**

www.healthfinder.gov

Searchable, carefully developed web site offering information on over 1000 topics. Developed by the US Department of Health and Human Services, the site can be used in both English and Spanish.

8150 **Healthlink USA**

www.healthlinkusa.com

Health information concerning treatment, cures, prevention, diagnosis, risk factors, research, support groups, email lists, personal stories and much more. Updated regularly.

8151 **Helios Health**

www.helioshealth.com

Online resource for your health information. Detailed information about specific health topics, access to expert advice from our Medical Advisory Board, and up-to-date health news.

8152 **MedicineNet**

www.medicinenet.com

An online resource for consumers providing easy-to-read, authoritative medical and health information.

8153 **Medscape**

www.medscape.com

Medscape offers specialists, primary care physicians, and other health professionals the Web's most robust and integrated medical information and educational tools.

8154 **Miami Project to Cure Paralysis**

www.miamiproject.miami.edu

Science and clinical research to restore function after spinal cord injury. The primary emphasis is on basic science research, under the direction of Dr. Richard Bunge, an eminent researcher.

8155 **Sexual Health Network**

www.sexualhealth.com

Informative site dealing with disability, sexuality and fertility.

8156 **Spinal Cord Injury Information Network Center**

www.spinalcord.uab.edu

The University of Alabama at Birmingham Spinal Cord Injury Model System (UAB-SCIMS) maintains this Information Network as a resource to promote knowledge in the areas of research, health and quality of life for people with spinal cord injuries, their families, and SCI-related professionals. Here, you will find our educational materials and information on research activities of the UAB-SCIMS along with links to outside (Internet) information.

8157 **Spinal Cord Injury Network International**

www.sonic.net/~spinal

A non-profit organization that provides information and referral services and lends videos.

8158 **University of Alabama, (UAB)**

www.spinalcord.uab.edu

The University of Alabama at Birmingham Spinal Cord Injury Model System (UAB-SCIMS) maintains this Information Network as a resource to promote knowledge in the areas of research, health and quality of life for people with spinal cord injuries, their families, and SCI-related professionals. Here, you will find our educational materials and information on research activities of the UAB-SCIMS along with links to outside (Internet) information.

8159 **WebMD**

www.webmd.com

Provides credible information, supportive communities, and in-depth reference material about health subjects. A source for original and timely health information as well as material from well known content providers.

Description

8160 Stroke

Strokes are caused by an interruption of blood flow in the brain, and usually — 80 percent of cases — are the result of a blocked blood vessel. The incidence increases with age, is higher in men than in women, and is higher in blacks than in whites. Depending on the severity and location of the damage, symptoms of stroke may include sudden weakness or paralysis (especially on one side of the body), blurred vision, difficulty speaking, slurred speech, dizziness and falling, extreme headache, stiff neck, altered level of alertness, and loss of bladder control. High blood pressure, atherosclerosis (fatty deposits), heart disease, diabetes, cigarette smoking, and heavy alcohol use are the major risk factors predisposing someone to stroke.

Preventive therapy is aimed at treatment of high blood pressure, heart disease, and diabetes. If someone has had a stroke they may be treated with blood thinning agents and/or other medication to prevent brain swelling. Research has shown that patients who are given one of these agents within three hours of stroke symptoms may have some or total restoration of neurologic function. To that end, the Golden Hour program was developed in which emergency medical personnel can initiate therapy in certain patients on the way to the hospital. Rehabilitation after the stroke involves physical and occupational therapy. Many stroke survivors experience depression and difficulty regaining independence, so it is important to provide emotional support for both survivors and their families.

National Agencies & Associations

8161 American Heart Association
7272 Greenville Avenue
Dallas, TX 75231
214-373-6300
800-242-8721
www.heart.org

The American Heart Association is the nation's oldest, largest voluntary organization devoted to fighting cardiovascular diseases and stroke. Founded by six cardiologists in 1924, our organization now includes more than 22.5 million volunteers and supporters working tirelessly to eliminate these diseases. We fund innovative research, fight for stronger public health policies and provide life-saving tools and information to save and improve lives.
Bernie Dennis, Chairman
Mariell Jessup, President

8162 American Stroke Association
7272 Greenville Avenue
Dallas, TX 75231
888-478-7653
www.heart.org

Created in 1997, the American Stroke Association is dedicated to prevention, diagnosis and treatment to save lives from stroke - America's No. 4 killer and a leading cause of serious disability. We fund scientific research, help people better understand and avoid stroke, encourage government support, guide healthcare professionals and provide information to enhance the quality of life for stroke survivors. To learn more, call 1-888-4-STROKE or browse strokeassociation.org.
Gordon F. Tomaselli, President

8163 Heart and Stroke Foundation of Canada
222 Queen Street
Ottawa, Ontario, K1P 5-5V9
613-569-4361
Fax: 613-569-3278
www.heartandstroke.com

The Foundation's health promotion and advocacy programs across the country are saving lives every day. Working together, our employees, volunteers, donors and world-class researchers have made the Heart and Stroke Foundation what we are today: Canada's most widely recognized and trusted authority on cardiovascular health. Our mission is to create healthy lives free of heart disease and stroke. Together, we will make it happen.
Douglas B. Clement, CM, MD, Chair
Mark R. Andrews, Director

8164 National Heart, Lung & Blood Institute
PO Box 301051
Bethesda, MD 20824
301-592-8573
Fax: 301-592-8563
TTY: 240-629-3255
e-mail: nhlbiinfo@nhlbi.nih.gov
www.nhlbi.nih.gov

The NHLBI stimulates basic discoveries about the causes of disease, enables the translation of basic discoveries into clinical practice, fosters training and mentoring of emerging scientists and physicians, and communicates research advances to the public. It creates and supports a robust, collaborative research infrastructure in partnership with private and public organizations, including academic institutions, industry, and other government agencies. The Institute collaborates with patients, f
Gary H. Gibbons, MD, Director
Susan B. Shurin, MD, Chief of Staff

8165 National Institute of Neurological Disorders and Stroke
PO Box 5081
Bethesda, MD 20824
301-496-5751
800-352-9424
Fax: 301-402-2186
TTY: 301-468-5981
e-mail: webManagers@ninds.nih.gov
www.ninds.nih.gov

The mission of NINDS is to reduce the burden of neurological disease - a burden borne by every age group, by every segment of society, by people all over the world.
Story C Landis PhD, Director
Walter J Koroshetz, Deputy Director

8166 National Institute of Neurological Disorde rs and Stroke
PO Box 5801
Bethesda, MD 20824
301-496-5751
800-352-9424
Fax: 301-402-2186
TTY: 301-468-5981
e-mail: webManagers@ninds.nih.gov
www.ninds.nih.gov

The mission of NINDS is to reduce the burden of neurological disease - a burden borne by every age group, by every segment of society, by people all over the world.
Story C Landis PhD, Director
Walter J Koroshetz, Deputy Director

8167 National Stroke Association
9707 E Easter Lane
Centennial, CO 80112-3747
303-649-9299
800-787-6537
Fax: 303-649-1328
e-mail: Info@stroke.org
www.stroke.org

A national organization whose sole purpose is to reduce the incidence and impact of stroke through prevention treatment rehabilitation and research and support for stroke survivors and their families.
Jamie Charbonneau, Director, Corporate Alliances
James Baranski, Chief Executive Officer

8168 Stroke Recovery Canada
10 Overlea Boulevard
Toronto, Ontario, M4H 1-1A4
416-425-3463
800-263-3463
Fax: 416-425-1920
e-mail: info@marchofdimes.ca
www.marchofdimes.ca

Stroke Recovery Canadar is a national service offering support, education and community programs for stroke survivors, their caregivers and families. Stroke Recovery Canada will connect you with a network of support that can help you reclaim your independence, your sense of community and your ability to thrive.
Andria Spindel, President/Chief Executive Officer
Jerry Lucas, Vice President, Programs

Foundations

8169 American Stroke Foundation
5916 Dearborn   913-649-1776
Mission, KS 66202   866-549-1776
                                   Fax: 913-649-6661
                                   www.americanstroke.org
The vision of the American Stroke Foundation is to reach out to stroke survivors and their families across America and empower them to reclaim hope for life after stroke
Joan McDowd, Executive Director
Jen Creed, Director of Programs and Outreach

Research Centers

8170 Bowman Gray School of Medicine
Medical Center Boulevard   919-716-7461
Winston Salem, NC 27157-0001   Fax: 919-716-5639
                                        www.web.bgsm.edu
James Toole MD, Professor

8171 Cerebral Blood Flow Laboratories Veterans Administration Medical Center
Veterans Administration Medical Center
2002 Holcombe Boulevard   713-795-5807
Houston, TX 77030-4211   Fax: 713-957-01
Offers research in cerebrovascular disorders and risk factors for stroke.
John S Meyer MD, Director

8172 Comprehensive Stroke Center of Oregon University of Oregon Health Sciences Cen
University of Oregon Health Sciences Center
3181 SW Sam Jackson Park Road
Portland, OR 97239-3098   503-494-7225
                                        www.ohsu.edu
The Oregon Stroke Center (OSC) was established over 20 years ago to provide comprehensive treatment and prevention services to stroke patients throughout the Northwest. Recognized as a national leader in acute stroke treatment, the OSC mobile stroke team provides novel stroke treatments to multiple Portland hospitals. In addition to clinical care, the OSC is actively involved in clinical and basic research and provides extensive stroke related education to the public and providers. Quick action
Wayne Clark, M.D., Professor
Helmi Lutsep, M.D., Professor

8173 Departments of Neurology & Neurosurgery: University of California, San Francisco
UCSF Medical Center
505 Parnassus Avenue   415-476-1537
San Francisco, CA 94143   Fax: 415-476-0616
                           e-mail: bill.dillon@radiology.ucsf.edu
                                        www.radiology.ucsf.edu
The Department of Radiology & Biomedical Imaging at the University of California, San Francisco combines clinical excellence, trailblazing research, and outstanding education in a leading academic health sciences institution. Our faculty includes some of the foremost names in diagnostic and interventional radiology today.
Dr. Ronald Arenson, Chairman
Catherine Garzio, Director of Administration

8174 Hospital of the University of Pennsylvania
3400 Spruce Street   215-662-4000
Philadelphia, PA 19104   800-789-PENN
                                   Fax: 215-903-09
                           e-mail: pleasure@email.chop.edu
                                        www.pennmedicine.org
The Hospital of the University of Pennsylvania (HUP) is world-renowned for its clinical and research excellence, forging the way for newer and better ways to diagnose and treat illnesses and disorders. The world-class faculty and staff of the Hospital of the University of Pennsylvania are dedicated to superior patient care, education and research for a better, healthier future. Their significant and groundbreaking contributions to medicine are recognized both nationally and internationally. The
David E Pleasure MD, Director

8175 Massachusetts General Departments of Neurology and Neurosurgery
Massachusetts General Hospital
55 Fruit Street
Boston, MA 02114   617-726-2000
                                        www.massgeneral.org
Guided by the needs of our patients, our mission is to be the preeminent academic neurology department in the US by: providing outstanding clinical care while rapidly discovering new treatments to reduce and eliminate the devastating impact of neurological disorders; training the very best neurologists and scientists of the future, and improving the health and well-being of the diverse communities we serve.
Peter Slavin, Director
Robert Ackerman, Doctor

8176 Stroke Research and Treatment Center UAB Medical Center
Medical Center
1530 3rd Ave S   205-934-9999
Birmingham, AL 35294-7   800-822-6478
                                   Fax: 205-996-4039
                                   www.main.uab.edu/neurology
The nationally-ranked UAB Department of Neurology is home to eight comprehensive divisions and seven centers offering an array of clinical activities. Over 26,000 patients are cared for annually through state-of-the-art subspecialty care and innovative treatments. Our residents have the opportunity to work in various neurology fields with 50 clinical and research faculty members.
Andrei V Alexandrov MD, Director and Professor
Andrei V. Alexandrov, M.D., Director, Comprehensive Stroke Research

8177 University of Iowa College of Medicine
451 Newton Road   319-335-6707
Iowa City, IA 52242   e-mail: webmaster@mail.medicine.uiowa.edu
                                        www.medicine.uiowa.edu
The Roy J. and Lucille A. Carver College of Medicine is a highly ranked medical school where students learn to become accomplished clinicians and top-flight researchers and educators. Students come to Iowa to study medicine in a program that uses case-based learning as the basis of their education. With its emphasis on problem-solving skills, early exposure to patients, and enhanced community-based experiences, UI medical students typically earn impressive scores on Step 1 of the U.S. Medical Li
Debra A. Schwinn, MD, Dean
Donna L. Hammond, PhD, Executive Associate Dean

8178 University of Maryland Center for Studies of Cerebrovascular Disease & Stroke
16 S Utah Street   410-328-4323
Baltimore, MD 21201   Fax: 410-328-1149
Thomas R Price MD, Principal Investor

8179 University of Miami School of Medicine Department of Neurology
1120 NW 14th Street   305-243-6732
Miami, FL 33136   877-243-4340
                                   Fax: 305-243-1632
                           e-mail: RSacco@med.miami.edu
                                        www.med.miami.edu
Ralph L Sacco MD, Chairman-Department of Neurology
Myron D Ginsberg MD, Professor

8180 Wake Forest University: Cerebrovascular Research Center
Department of Neurology
300 S Hawthorne Road   336-748-2338
Winston-Salem, NC 27103-2732   Fax: 336-748-5477
Cerebrovascular research.
Dr James Toole, Director

8181 Washington University School of Medicine
660 S Euclid Avenue   314-362-5000
Saint Louis, MO 63110-1016   e-mail: web@medicine.wustl.edu
                                        www.medicine.wustl.edu
Washington University School of Medicine is a leader in improving human health throughout the world. As noted leaders in patient care, research and education, our outstanding faculty members have contributed many discoveries and innovations to the field of science since the founding of the School of Medicine in 1891. The

School of Medicine is one of seven schools of Washington University in St. Louis.
Larry J. Shapiro, M.D, Executive Vice Chancellor for Medical Af

Support Groups & Hotlines

8182 National Health Information Center
Washington, DC 20013
310-565-4167
800-336-4797
Fax: 301-984-4256
e-mail: info@nhic.org
www.health.gov/nhic
Offers a nationwide information referral service, produces directories and resource guides.

8183 Stroke Clubs International
805 12th Street
Galveston, TX 77550
409-762-1022
e-mail: strokeclubs@earthlink.net
www.ninds.nih.gov
Organization of persons who have experienced strokes, their families and friends for the purpose of mutual support, education, social and recreational activities. Provides information and assistance to Stroke Clubs (which are usually sponsored by local organizations).
Ellis Williamson

Books

8184 Alzheimer's, Stroke and 29 Other Neurological Disorders Sourcebook
Omnigraphics
155 West Congress
Detroit, MI 48226-3993
313-961-1340
800-234-1340
Fax: 800-875-1340
e-mail: contact@omnigraphics.com
omnigraphics.com
Provides vital information for the nontechnical reader focusing on Alzheimer's disease, stroke and various neurological disorders. Answers thousands of questions related to afflications of the central nervous system with each chapter reviewing a particular disorder and offers in-depth discussions.

8185 Courage: Poems & Positive Thoughts for Stroke Survivors
National Stroke Association
9707 E Easter Lane
Centennial, CO 80112-3747
303-649-9299
800-787-6537
Fax: 303-649-1328
e-mail: info@stroke.org
www.stroke.org
Words of inspiration from survivors and caregivers.
83 pages
Matt Lopez, Chief Executive Officer
Sharon Januchowski, Executive Vice President

8186 Discovery Circles
National Stroke Association
9707 E Easter Lane
Centennial, CO 80112-3747
303-649-9299
800-787-6537
Fax: 303-649-1328
e-mail: info@stroke.org
www.stroke.org
NSA's guide to organizing and facilitating stroke support groups. This detailed manual describes the support group structure and the facilitator's role.
213 pages
Matt Lopez, Chief Executive Officer
Sharon Januchowski, Executive Vice President

8187 Magic of Humor in Caregiving
National Stroke Association
9707 E Easter Lane
Centennial, CO 80112-3747
303-649-9299
800-787-6537
Fax: 303-649-1328
e-mail: info@stroke.org
www.stroke.org

A dynamic researching tool focusing on the necessity of humor in daily caregiving interaction.
Matt Lopez, Chief Executive Officer
Sharon Januchowski, Executive Vice President

8188 November Days
National Stroke Association
9707 E Easter Lane
Centennial, CO 80112-3747
303-649-9299
800-787-6537
Fax: 303-649-1328
e-mail: info@stroke.org
www.stroke.org
A caregiver's story of her struggle with a loved one's stroke.
225 pages
Matt Lopez, Chief Executive Officer
Sharon Januchowski, Executive Vice President

8189 Occupational Therapy Practice Guidelines for Adults with Stroke
American Occupational Therapy Association
4720 Montgomery Lane
Bethesda, MD 20814-1220
301-652-6611
Fax: 240-762-5150
TDD: 800-377-8555
www.aota.org
15 pages
ISBN: 1-569001-55-3

8190 Stroke Book
William Morrow & Company
P.O. Box 1181
Bloomington, IN 47402-4702
212-261-6500
mystrokeofinsight.com
1993
ISBN: 0-688090-55-9

8191 Stroke: A Clinical Approach
Butterworth-Heinemann
P.O. Box 1181
Bloomington, IN 47402-2079
617-928-2500
800-366-2665
mystrokeofinsight.com
1993 584 pages
ISBN: 0-750691-81-6

8192 Stroke: A Guide for Patient and Family
Raven Press
5323 Harry Hines Blvd
Dallas, TX 75390-2601
214-648-3111
e-mail: info@strokecenter.org
www.strokecenter.org
224 pages
ISBN: 0-881672-79-3

8193 Stroke: Your Complete Exercise Guide
Human Kinetics Publishers
9707 E Easter Lane
Centennial, CO 80112-5076
217-351-1549
800-747-4457
Fax: 217-351-5076
e-mail: info@stroke.org
www.stroke.org
Part of the Cooper Clinic and Research Institute Fitness Series providing exercise rehabilitation for persons suffering from strokes.
126 pages Paperback
ISBN: 0-873224-28-0
Matt Lopez, Chief Executive Officer
Sharon Januchowski, Executive Vice President

8194 Ted's Stroke: The Caregiver's Story
National Stroke Association
9707 E Easter Lane
Centennial, CO 80112-3747
303-649-9299
800-787-6537
Fax: 303-649-1328
e-mail: info@stroke.org
www.stroke.org
Personal experiences, guidance and tips for caregivers.
175 pages
ISBN: 0-962487-61-9
Matt Lopez, Chief Executive Officer
Sharon Januchowski, Executive Vice President

8195 The Comfort of Home for Stroke: A Guide fo r Caregivers
Marie Meyer & Paula Derr, RN with Jon Caswell, author
CareTrust Publications

PO Box 10283
Portland, OR 97296-0283

800-565-1533
Fax: 415-673-2205
e-mail: sales@comfortofhome.com
www.comfortofhome.com

Comfort guides readers through every caregiving stage, from understanding personality changes, preparing the home, equipment, the healthcare team, and the activities of daily living. It helps take the fear out of home care and assists caregivers in maintaining peace of mind.
2007 344 pages
ISBN: 0-966476-78-6

8196 **Women in Your Life: Protect Yourself, Protect Your Family**
National Stroke Association
9707 E Easter Lane
Centennial, CO 80112-3747

303-649-9299
800-787-6537
Fax: 303-649-1328
e-mail: info@stroke.org
www.stroke.org

Valuable information about the unique toll stroke takes on women.
Matt Lopez, Chief Executive Officer
Sharon Januchowski, Executive Vice President

Magazines

8197 **Stroke Connection**
American Stroke Foundation
5916 Dearborn St
Mission, KS 66202

913-649-1776
Fax: 913-649-6661
www.americanstroke.org

Official magazine of the American Stroke Foundation. Supports stroke survivors, their families, caregivers and friends by providing resources, services, education and information that improves the quality of life.
Richard March, Chair
David Marshall, Vice Chairman

Pamphlets

8198 **African-Americans and Stroke**
National Stroke Association
9707 E Easter Lane
Centennial, CO 80112-3747

303-649-9299
800-787-6537
Fax: 303-649-1328
e-mail: info@stroke.org
www.stroke.org

Matt Lopez, Chief Executive Officer
Sharon Januchowski, Executive Vice President

8199 **Aneurysm Answers**
National Stroke Association
9707 E Easter Lane
Centennial, CO 80112-3747

303-649-9299
800-787-6537
Fax: 303-649-1328
e-mail: info@stroke.org
www.stroke.org

Matt Lopez, Chief Executive Officer
Sharon Januchowski, Executive Vice President

8200 **Check Your Pulse, America: Atrial Fibrillation**
National Stroke Association
9707 E Easter Lane
Centennial, CO 80112-3747

303-649-9299
800-787-6537
Fax: 303-649-1328
e-mail: info@stroke.org
www.stroke.org

Matt Lopez, Chief Executive Officer
Sharon Januchowski, Executive Vice President

8201 **Cholesterol and Stroke**
National Stroke Association

9707 E Easter Lane
Centennial, CO 80112-3747

303-649-9299
800-787-6537
Fax: 303-649-1328
e-mail: info@stroke.org
www.stroke.org

Matt Lopez, Chief Executive Officer
Sharon Januchowski, Executive Vice President

8202 **Facts on Heart Disease, Heart Attack, Stroke and Risk Factors**
American Heart Association
1600 Clifton Road
Atlanta, GA 30329-5129

214-373-6300
800-232-4636
Fax: 214-706-1341
www.cdc.gov

Offers information on how to recognize a heart attack or stroke, recovery and rehabilitation techniques and risk factors.

8203 **High Blood Pressure and Stroke**
National Stroke Association
9707 E Easter Lane
Centennial, CO 80112-3747

303-649-9299
800-787-6537
Fax: 303-649-1328
e-mail: info@stroke.org
www.stroke.org

Matt Lopez, Chief Executive Officer
Sharon Januchowski, Executive Vice President

8204 **Mobility: Issues Facing Stroke Survivors and Their Families**
National Stroke Association
9707 E Easter Lane
Centennial, CO 80112-3747

303-649-9299
800-787-6537
Fax: 303-649-1328
e-mail: info@stroke.org
www.stroke.org

Matt Lopez, Chief Executive Officer
Sharon Januchowski, Executive Vice President

8205 **Recurrent Stroke**
National Stroke Association
9707 E Easter Lane
Centennial, CO 80112-3747

303-649-9299
800-787-6537
Fax: 303-649-1328
e-mail: info@stroke.org
www.stroke.org

Matt Lopez, Chief Executive Officer
Sharon Januchowski, Executive Vice President

8206 **Smoking Cessation: Be Smoke Free in 3 Minutes**
National Stroke Association
9707 E Easter Lane
Centennial, CO 80112-3747

303-649-9299
800-787-6537
Fax: 303-649-1328
e-mail: info@stroke.org
www.stroke.org

Matt Lopez, Chief Executive Officer
Sharon Januchowski, Executive Vice President

8207 **Stroke: Hope Through Research**
Office of Scientific & Health Reports
P.O. Box 5801
Bethesda, MD 20824-0001

301-496-5751
800-352-9424
www.ninds.nih.gov

Offers information on stroke, research and advances in treatments and rehabilitation programs to help patients.

8208 **Transient Ischemic Attack**
National Stroke Association
9707 E Easter Lane
Centennial, CO 80112-3747

303-649-9299
800-787-6537
Fax: 303-649-1328
e-mail: info@stroke.org
www.stroke.org

Matt Lopez, Chief Executive Officer
Sharon Januchowski, Executive Vice President

Audio & Video

8209 **Secret Life of the Brain**
PBS Home Video

PO Box 751089
Charlotte, NC 28275   877-727-7467
                                        Fax: 703-739-8131
                        www.pbs.org/wnet/brain/about.html
Reveals the facinating processes involved in brain development across a lifetime. The five-part series informs viewers of exciting new information in the brain sciences, introduces the foremost researchers in the field, and utilizes dynamic visual imagry and compelling human stories to help a general audience understand otherwise difficult scientific concepts.
5 Tapes
Paula Kerger, President/CEO
Wayne Godwin, Chief Operating Officer

8210   Stroke: Touching the Soul of Your Family
National Stroke Association
9707 E Easter Lane
Centennial, CO 80112-3747   303-649-9299
                                             800-787-6537
                                        Fax: 303-649-1328
                                   e-mail: info@stroke.org
                                           www.stroke.org
Fifteen minute video chronicling three stroke survivors and their courageous struggle to overcome daily challenges and educate others about stroke.
Matt Lopez, Chief Executive Officer
Sharon Januchowski, Executive Vice President

Web Sites

8211   American Heart Association
                        www.heart.org/HEARTORG
A national organization whose primary concern is the reduction of death and disability due to cardiovascular diseases and stroke.

8212   Healing Well
                            www.healingwell.com
An online health resource guide to medical news, chat, information and articles, newsgroups and message boards, books, disease-related web sites, medical directories, and more for patients, friends, and family coping with disabling diseases, disorders, or chronic illnesses.

8213   Health Finder
                            www.healthfinder.gov
Searchable, carefully developed web site offering information on over 1000 topics. Developed by the US Department of Health and Human Services, the site can be used in both English and Spanish.

8214   Healthlink USA
                            www.healthlinkusa.com
Health information concerning treatment, cures, prevention, diagnosis, risk factors, research, support groups, email lists, personal stories and much more. Updated regularly.

8215   Helios Health
                            www.helioshealth.com
Online resource for your health information. Detailed information about specific health topics, access to expert advice from our Medical Advisory Board, and up-to-date health news.

8216   MedicineNet
                            www.medicinenet.com
An online resource for consumers providing easy-to-read, authoritative medical and health information.

8217   Medscape
                            www.medscape.com
Medscape offers specialists, primary care physicians, and other health professionals the Web's most robust and integrated medical information and educational tools.

8218   National Heart, Lung & Blood Institute
                            www.nhlbi.nih.gov
Primary responsibility of this organization is the scientific investigation of heart, blood vessel, lung and blood disorders. Oversee research, demonstration, prevention, education and training activities in these fields and emphasizes the control of stroke.

8219   National Institute of Neurological Disorders and Stroke
                            www.ninds.nih.gov

The mission of NINDS is to seek fundamental knowledge about the brain and nervous system and to use that knowledge to reduce the burden of neurological disease.

8220   National Stroke Association
                            www.stroke.org
A national organization whose sole purpose is to reduce the incidence and impact of stroke through prevention, treatment, rehabilitation and research, and support for stroke survivors and their families. Educational resources on all aspects of stroke available on website.

8221   Neurology Channel
                        www.healthcommunities.com
Find clearly explained, medically accurate information regarding conditions, including an overview, symptoms, causes, diagnostic procedures and treatment options. On this site it is possible to ask questions and get information from a neurologist and connect to people who have similar health interests.

8222   WebMD
                            www.webmd.com
Provides credible information, supportive communities, and in-depth reference material about health subjects. A source for original and timely health information as well as material from well known content providers.

Description

8223 Substance Abuse

Substance abuse is a broad term that refers to any illegal, dangerous or destructive use of some substance. This use may be legal (binge drinking by an adult) or illegal (smoking marijuana). Abused substances include alcohol, nicotine, marijuana, heroin, prescription painkillers and tranquilizers, stimulants such as amphetamines and cocaine, and hallucinogens such as LSD. The abuse may be a danger to the user, family members, business associates, close friends or even total strangers. Substance dependence refers to a state of strong compulsion to use the substance, in many cases accompanied by physical withdrawal symptoms if the substance is not regularly available.

The cause of substance abuse is very complex, and involves an interplay between the individual's behavioral choices, their genetic background and past and present social environment. Some substance abusers also have a definable psychiatric disorder such as depression or schizophrenia; treatment of these dual-disorder patients is especially challenging.

The consequences of substance abuse are well-known, and include job loss, arrest, family breakup, automobile and other accidents, birth defects (fetal alcohol syndrome), direct toxic effects (cirrhosis of the liver from alcohol or lung cancer from smoking), and infections (HIV or hepatitis B from sharing needles). Substance abuse, unless it occurs in extremely isolated persons, greatly affects family members and loved ones. Family members often deny the reality of the abuse, and may help, or enable, the abuser to cover up the problem and avoid its consequences.

There is no quick and universally effective treatment for substance abuse. Options range from inexpensive peer-based organizations such as Alcoholics Anonymous to very expensive long-term inpatient programs. Some peer-based programs appeal to a niche defined by sex, race, age or religious affiliation. Treatment is much more likely to succeed if it is freely chosen by the individual rather than mandated by a court. Dropout during treatment and relapse after initial success are common, but many people do achieve life-long cures with abstinence from further substance abuse. Family members should look for education and support through groups like Al-Anon, which bring them together with people facing similar situations.

National Agencies & Associations

8224 AAA Foundation for Traffic Safety
607 14th Street NW
Washington, DC 20005-6001 202-638-5944
Fax: 202-638-5943
e-mail: info@aaafoundation.org
www.aaafoundation.org
This national organization publishes drinking and traffic safety programs for K-6 and junior high students. Courses offered are taught by school district teachers who have participated in two-hour in-service training seminars.
J Peter Kissinger, President
Kristin Backstrom, Senior Manager Development

8225 African American Family Services
2616 Nicollet Avenue
Minneapolis, MN 55408 612-871-7878
Fax: 612-871-2567
e-mail: contact@aafs.net
www.aafs.net
African American Family Services works with individuals, families and communities affected by addiction and mental illness. From our holistic standpoint, we provide culturally-specific chemical and mental health services that impact family preservation and promote community-based change and wellness.
Terry J Ticey, Chairman of the Board
Thomas Adams, PhD (ABD), MSW, Chief Executive Officer

8226 Al-Anon Family Group Headquarters
1600 Corporate Landing Parkway
Virginia Beach, VA 23454-5617 757-563-1600
888-425-2666
Fax: 757-563-1655
e-mail: wso@al-anon.org
www.al-anon.alateen.org
At Al-Anon Family Group meetings, the friends and family members of problem drinkers share their experiences and learn how to apply the principles of the Al-Anon program to their individual situations.
Robert Schneider, Director of Communications

8227 Alateen Al-Anon Family Group Headquarters
Al-Anon Family Group Headquarters
1600 Corporate Landing Parkway
Virginia Beach, VA 23454-5617 757-563-1600
800-425-2666
Fax: 757-563-1655
e-mail: wso@al-anon.org
www.al-anon.alateen.org
A part of the Al-Anon program Alateen is for teenagers who have been affected by someone else's drinking whether it be a family member or a friend.
Robert Schneider, Director Communications

8228 Alcoholics Anonymous General Service Office/Grand Central Sta
General Service Office/Grand Central Station
Grand Central Station
New York, NY 10163-0459 212-870-3400
Fax: 212-870-3003
e-mail: international@aa.org
www.aa.org
Alcoholics Anonymousr is a fellowship of men and women who share their experience, strength and hope with each other that they may solve their common problem and help others to recover from alcoholism. The only requirement for membership is a desire to stop drinking. There are no dues or fees for AA membership; we are self-supporting through our own contributions.

8229 American Council for Drug Education
50 Jay Street
Brooklyn, NY 11201-2301 718-222-6641
877-769-9698
Fax: 212-595-2553
e-mail: hlozada@phoenixhouse.org
www.phoenixhouse.org
The Career Academy guides clients as they work toward their personal and professional goals. Residents live, learn, and work in an environment specifically tailored to meet their needs. Our specialized programs provide training in such high-demand fields as building maintenance and repairs and culinary arts.
J David Hawkins, Director
Herman Lozada, Contact

8230 American Council on Alcohol Problems
1000 E Indian School Road
Phoenix, AZ 85014 602-264-7897
800-527-5344
Fax: 602-264-7403
e-mail: info@aca-usa.com
www.aca-usa.com
The American Council on Alcoholism (ACA) is a national non-profit 501(c)3 health organization dedicated to educating the public about the effects of alcohol, alcoholism and alcohol abuse,

and the need for prompt, effective, readily-available, and afford-able alcoholism treatment.
Lloyd R. Vocovsky, Chairman
Jeff Becker, Vice Chairman

8231   American Dental Association Department of Library Services
Department of Library Services
211 E Chicago Avenue   312-440-2500
Chicago, IL 60611-2637   Fax: 312-440-2822
e-mail: affiliates@ada.org
www.ada.org
Founded in 1859, the not-for-profit ADA is the nation's largest dental association, representing 157,000 dentist members. Since then, the ADA has grown to become the leading source of oral health related information for dentists and their patients. Learn more about the ADA's mission and vision, and our commitment to the public's oral health, ethics, science and professional advancement and access to care for all Americans.
Linda Kittel MS RN, Manager
Brandon R Maddox, Representative

8232   Associate Administrator for Alcohol Prevention and Treatment Policy
Substance Abuse & Mental Health Services Offices
200 Independance Avenue   301-443-8956
Washington, DC 20201-0001   e-mail: info@samhsa.gov
www.samhsa.gov
Promotes monitors evaluates and coordinates programs for the prevention and treatment of alcoholism and alcohol abuse.

8233   Association of Halfway House Alcoholism Programs of North America
401 E Sangamon Avenue   217-523-0527
Springfield, IL 62702   Fax: 217-698-8234
e-mail: president@ahhap.org
www.ahhap.org
Acts as a clearinghouse of the latest literature on alcoholism assists chemical dependency counselors in placing post treatment individuals in halfway houses and helps in setting up halfway houses.
Olivia Howard, President
David Logan, Vice President

8234   BACCHUS of the US
PO Box 938   303-871-0901
Littleton, CO 80160   Fax: 303-871-0907
e-mail: admin@bacchusnetwork.org
www.bacchusnetwork.org
BACCHUS develops cutting edge tools for campuses consisting of student-friendly training programs, resource manuals, posters, and pamphlets. Currently there are 120 educational resources and training materials offered by our organization. In addition, each affiliate group receives health issue campaigns that, when used in combination, lay the foundation for a year-round prevention program.
Janet Cox, MA, President/CEO
Ann . Quinn-Zobeck, Ph.D, Director of Education and Training

8235   CSAP State Liason Program CSAP Division of Communications Programs
CSAP Division of Communications Programs
7200 Wisconsin Avenue
Bethesda, MD 20857-0001   301-941-8500
www.covesoft.com/csap.html
This program is designed to support alcohol and other drug abuse prevention efforts in the States.

8236   Center for Substance Abuse Prevention
Substance Abuse and Mental Health Services Admin.
PO Box 2345
Rockville, MD 20847-2345   800-279-6686
TTY: 800-487-4886
TDD: 800-487-4886
e-mail: info@health.org.
www.ncadi.samhsa.gov
This organization's goal is to connect people and resources with innovative ideas strategies and programs designed to encourage creative and effective efforts aimed at reducing and eliminating alcohol tobacco and other drug problems in our society.

8237   Chemical People Project Public Television Outreach Alliance
Public Television Outreach Alliance

4802 5th Avenue   412-391-0900
Pittsburgh, PA 15213-2957
The project supplies information in the form of tapes literature and seminars.

8238   Cocaine Anonymous: World Service Office
3740 Overland Avenue   310-559-5833
Los Angeles, CA 90049-6337   800-999-9951
Fax: 310-559-2554
e-mail: webservant@ca.org
www.ca.org
The best way to reach someone is to speak to them on a common level. The members of C.A. are all recovering addicts who maintain their individual sobriety by working with others. We come from various social, ethnic, economic and religious backgrounds, but what we have in common is addiction.

8239   Drug Abuse Resistance Education of America
PO Box 512090   310-215-0575
Los Angeles, CA 90051-0090   800-223-3273
Fax: 310-215-0180
www.dare.com
Provides information, resources, tips, warning signs and other information for parents and kids to help keep children off drugs.
Francisco X Pegueros, President/CEO
Thomas Hazelton, President of Development

8240   Drugs Anonymous
PO Box 473   212-874-0700
New York, NY 10023
A twelve-step program that holds more than 30 meetings for drug addicts in the Greater New York Area including several in hospitals and institutions.

8241   Families Anonymous
PO Box 3475   310-815-8010
Culver City, CA 90231-3475   800-736-9805
Fax: 310-815-9682
e-mail: famanon@familiesanonymous.org
www.familiesanonymous.org
Addresses the needs of families who are concerned about a relative with a drug problem and with related behavioral problems. Offers informational packets meetings and support networks for these families.

8242   Families in Action National Drug Information Center
2957 Clairmont Road NE   404-248-9676
Atlanta, GA 30333   Fax: 404-248-1312
e-mail: nfia@nationalfamilies.org
www.nationalfamilies.org
National Families in Action is a 501 (c) (3) nonprofit organization that was founded in Atlanta, Georgia in 1977. The organization obtained the nation's first state laws banning the sale of drug paraphernalia. It led a national effort to help parents replicate Georgia's laws in other states to prevent the marketing of drugs and drug use to children and helped them form parent groups to protect children's health.
Sue Rusche, President
Carol S. Reeder, Treasurer

8243   Hazelden
PO Box 11   651-213-4200
Center City, MN 55012-0011   800-257-7810
Fax: 651-213-4411
e-mail: info@hazeldon.org
www.hazelden.com
Hazelden helps individuals, families, and communities struggling with alcohol abuse, substance abuse, and drug addiction transform their lives. Our locations across the United States help people at all stages of the treatment and recovery process, supporting them with our Twelve Step-based model that is the modern standard for addiction treatment and recovery services.
Mark Mishek, President/CEO
Ann Bray, General Counsel/Vice President of Strate

8244   Indian Health Service
801 Thompson Avenue
Rockville, MD 20852-1627   605-226-7456
www.ihs.gov

Charged with providing a comprehensive program of alcoholism and substance abuse prevention and treatment for Native Americans and Alaskan natives.

8245 Lawyers Concerned for Lawyers
2550 University Avenue W   651-646-5590
Saint Paul, MN 55114-4127   866-525-6466
                                                Fax: 651-646-2364
                                                e-mail: help@mnlcl.org
                                                www.mnlcl.org
A nonprofit organization of recovering lawyers and judges and concerned others. Educates lawyers and judges about the disease of chemical dependency assists in assessments and arranging interventions and offers lawyer-only AA meetings.
Joan Bibelhausen, Executive Director
Ellen Murphy-Fritsch, Case Manager

8246 Marijuana Anonymous: World Services
Marijuana Anonymous World Services
PO Box 7807
Terrance, CA 90504-2318   800-766-6779
                                e-mail: office@marijuana-anonymous.org
                                www.marijuana-anonymous.org
A fellowship of men and women who share our experience strength and hope with each other that we may solve our common problem and help others to recover from marijuana addiction.

8247 Mothers Against Drunk Driving (MADD)
511 E John Carpenter Freeway   214-744-6233
Irving, TX 75062   877-275-6233
                                                Fax: 972-869-2206
                                                www.madd.org
Founded by a small group of mothers and has turned into one of the largest crime victims organizations in the world.
Janet Withers, President
Debbie Wier, CEO

8248 Narcotics Anonymous World Service Office
World Service Office
PO Box 9999
Van Nuys, CA 91409-9099   818-773-9999
                                                Fax: 818-700-0700
                                                e-mail: fsmail@na.org
                                                www.na.org
Similar to Alcoholics Anonymous this program is a fellowship of men and women who meet to help one another with their drug dependency problems.

8249 National Association for Children of Alcoholics
11426 Rockville Pike   301-468-0985
Rockville, MD 20852-3007   888-554-2627
                                                Fax: 301-468-0987
                                                e-mail: nacoa@nacoa.org
                                                www.nacoa.org
Advocates for all children and families affected by alcohol and other drug dependencies.
Sis Wenger, President/CEO
Judy Galloway, Coordinator-Affiliate Services

8250 National Association for Native American Children of Alcoholics
Seattle Indian Health Board
1402 Third Avenue   206-467-7686
Seattle, WA 98114-3364   800-322-5601
                                                Fax: 206-467-7689
                                                e-mail: nanacoa@aol.com
Formed to facilitate positive change in individuals and communities in order to break the intergenerational cycle of addiction among Native Americans.

8251 National Association of Alcoholism and Drug Abuse Counselors
1001 N Fairfax Street   703-741-7686
Alexandria, VA 22314   800-548-0497
                                                Fax: 703-741-7698
                                                e-mail: naadac2@naadac.org
                                                www.naadac.org
Largest membership organization serving addiction counselors educators and other addiction-focused health care professionals who specialize in addiction prevention treatment and education.
Cynthia Tuhoy, Executive Director
Shirley Mikell, Director of Certification and Education

8252 National Association on Drug Abuse Problems
Director of Corporate and Community Services
355 Lexington Avenue   212-986-1170
New York, NY 10017   Fax: 212-697-2939
                                                e-mail: info@nadap.org
                                                www.nadap.org
Provides skills evaluation job training and job placement to recovering drug addicts in the metropolitan New York area.
John A Darin, President/CEO
Gary Stankowski, Senior Vice President

8253 National Clearinghouse for Alcohol and Drug Information
11420 Rockville Pike   301-468-2600
Rockville, MD 20847-2345   800-729-6686
                                                Fax: 240-221-4292
                                                TTY: 800-487-4889
                                                TDD: 800-487-4889
                                                e-mail: webmaster@health.org
                                                www.health.org
Nation's one-stop resource for information about substance abuse prevention and addiction treatment.

8254 National Council on Alcoholism and Drug Dependence
217 Broadway   212-269-7797
New York, NY 10007-3128   800-622-2255
                                                Fax: 212-269-7510
                                                e-mail: national@ncadd.org
                                                www.ncadd.org
The National Council on Alcoholism and Drug Dependence, Inc and it's Affiliate Network is a voluntary health organization dedicated to fighting the Nation's #1 health problem-alcholism, drug addiction and the devestating consequences of alcohol and other drugs on individuals, families and communities.
Robert Lindsey, President
Leah Brock, Director of Affiliate Relations

8255 National Crime Prevention Council
2001 Jefferson Davis Highway   202-466-6272
Arlington, VA 22202   Fax: 202-296-1356
                                                www.ncpc.org
This organization works to prevent crime and drug use in many ways including developing materials for parents and children.
Alfonso E Lenhardt, President/CEO
David A Dean, Executive Committee Chair

8256 National Families in Action
2957 Clairmont Rd   404-248-9676
Atlanta, GA 30329   Fax: 404-248-1312
                                                e-mail: nfia@nationalfmailies.org
                                                www.nationalfamilies.org
Mission is to help families and communities prevent drug use among children by promoting policies based on science.
William F. Carter, Chairman
Sue Rusche, President & CEO

8257 National Organization on Fetal Alcohol Syndrome
1200 Eton Court NW   202-785-4585
Washington, DC 20007   800-666-6327
                                                Fax: 202-466-6456
                                                e-mail: information@nofas.org
                                                www.nofas.org
Dedicated to eliminating birth defects caused by alcohol consumption during pregnancy and to improving the quality of life for those affected individuals and families.
Kate Boyce, Chair
Tom Donaldson, President

8258 Office of Applied Studies Substance Abuse & Mental Health Services
Substance Abuse & Mental Health Services Offices
5600 Fishers Lane
Rockville, MD 20857-0001   301-443-8956
                                                www.samhsa.gov
Provides the leadership needed for collecting data on mental illness and substance abuse including incidence and prevalence studies.

8259 Office of Substance Abuse Prevention
5600 Fishers Lane
Rockville, MD 20857-0001 301-443-0373
www.samhsa.gov
Reviews the government's alcohol and drug abuse policy operates a grant program supports development of model programs and conducts prevention workshops.

8260 Office of Women's Services Substance Abuse & Mental Health Services
Substance Abuse & Mental Health Services Offices
5600 Fishers Lane 301-443-8956
Rockville, MD 20857-0001
Provides leadership and guidance in creating and maintaining an agency-wide focus for addressing the substance abuse and mental health needs of women.

8261 Office on Smoking and Health: CDCP
Centers for Disease Control And Prevention
1600 Clifton Road 404-639-3311
Atlanta, GA 30333 800-232-4636
TTY: 888-232-6348
e-mail: tobaccoinfo@cdc.gov
www.cdc.gov/tobacco
Offers reference services to researchers through the Technical Information Center. Publishes and distributes a number of titles in the field of smoking and health.

8262 PRIDE Youth Programs
707 West Main Street 231-924-1662
Fermont, MI 49412 800-668-9277
Fax: 231-924-5663
e-mail: info@prideyouthprograms.org
www.prideyouthprograms.org
A provider of prevention services in the area of alcohol and other drugs. Mission is to build a drug-free America.
Jay Dewispelaere, President/CEO
Lou Anne Wheater, Membership Coordinator

8263 Partnership for a Drug-Free America
352 Park Avenue South 212-922-1560
New York, NY 10010-0002 Fax: 212-922-1570
www.drugfree.org
Non-profit coalition of communication health medical and educational professionals working to reduce illicit drug use and help people live health drug-free lives.
Stephen J Pasierb, President & CEO
Robert Caruso, CFO

8264 Remove Intoxicated Drivers (RID-USA)
Schenectady, NY 12301 518-372-0034
877-823-9235
Fax: 518-310-4917
e-mail: dwi@rid-usa.org
rid-usa.org
Volunteers working to deter impaired driving, to help its victims obtain justice, restitution and peace of mind when faced with the maze of criminal justice systems, and to curb the alcohol abuse which leads to drunken driving.
Doris Aiken, Founder/President
Bill Aiken, VP/Manager

8265 Safe Homes
4 Mann Street 508-755-0333
Worcester, MA 01602-0702 Fax: 508-836-5560
e-mail: safehomes@thebridgecm.org
www.safehomesma.org
This national organization encourages parents to sign a contract stipulating that when parties are held in one another's homes they will adhere to a strict no-alcohol/no-drug-use rule.
Laura Farnsworth, Director of Safe Homes & Worcester PFLAG
Michael S Petracca, Clinician

8266 Students Against Destructive Decisions
255 Main Street 508-481-3568
Marlborough, MA 01752 877-723-3462
Fax: 508-481-5759
e-mail: info@sadd.org
www.sadd.org

To provide students with the best prevention tools possible to deal with the issues of underage drinking, other drug use, risky and impaired driving, and other destructive decisions.
Larry Bailin, Founder/CEO
Ovidio B. Bermudez MD, Chairman/Chief Medical Officer

8267 Substance Abuse and Mental Health Services Administration
1 Choke Cherry Road 877-726-4727
Rockville, MD 20857-0001 877-696-6775
TTY: 800-487-4889
www.samhsa.gov
The goal of this organization is to reduce incidence and prevalence of mental disorders and substance abuse and improve treatment outcomes for persons suffering from addictive and mental health problems and disorders.

8268 Workplace Program CSAP Division of Communication Programs
CSAP Division of Communication Programs
5600 Fishers Lane 301-443-9936
Rockville, MD 20857-0001
This program sets standards for drug testing in workplace settings.

State Agencies & Associations

Alabama

8269 Division of Mental Illness and Substance Abuse Community Programs
Department of Mental Health
Montgomery, AL 36130-1410 334-242-3454
800-367-0955
Fax: 334-242-0725
e-mail: Alabama.DMH@mh.alabama.gov
www.mh.alabama.gov
Kent Hunt, Associate Commissioner Substance Abuse
Susan P Chambers, Associate Commissioner Mental Illness

Alaska

8270 Office of Alcohol and Substance Abuse Department of Health and Social Services
Department of Health and Social Services
350 Main Street 907-465-3030
Juneau, AK 99811 800-465-4828
Fax: 907-465-3068
e-mail: Stacy.Toner@Alaska.gov
dhss.alaska.gov/Pages/default.aspx
William J. Streuss, Commissioner
Tara Horton, Special Assistant

Arizona

8271 Alcoholism and Drug Abuse: Office of Community Behavioral Health
Department of Health Services
150 N 18th Avenue 602-364-4558
Phoenix, AZ 85007-3228 Fax: 602-364-4570
e-mail: cancerlr@azdhs.gov
www.azdhs.gov
The Arizona Department of Health Services promotes and protects the health of Arizona's children and adults. Its mission is to set the standard for personal and community health through direct care, science, public policy, and leadership.
January Contreras, Acting Director

Arkansas

8272 Office of Alcohol and Drug Abuse Prevention
305 South Palm Street 501-686-9866
Little Rock, AR 72205 877-726-4727
Fax: 501-686-9035
e-mail: linda.baker@arkansas.gov
www.captus.samhsa.gov/grantee-organizati
SAMHSA's mission is to reduce the impact of substance abuse and mental illness on America's communities.

California

8273 California Women's Commission on Alcohol and Drug Dependencies
14622 Victory Boulevard 818-376-0470
Van Nuys, CA 91411
Dedicated to improving the quality and increasing the quantity of services to women with alcohol-related problems.

8274 Department of Alcohol and Drug Programs
1700 K Street 916-445-0834
Sacramento, CA 95811-4037 800-879-2772
Fax: 916-323-1270
e-mail: resourcecenter@adp.state.ca.us
www.colorado.gov/CDHS

Kathryn P Jett, Director

Colorado

8275 Alcohol and Drug Abuse Division Department of Human Services
Department of Human Services
4055 S Lowell Boulevard 303-866-7480
Denver, CO 80236-3120 Fax: 303-866-7481
e-mail: jaqueline.enriques@state.co.us
www.cdhs.state.co.us

Janet Wood, Director
Mary McCann, Acting Manager

Connecticut

8276 Connecticut Alcohol and Drug Abuse Commission
410 Capitol Avenue 860-418-7000
Hartford, CT 06134 800-446-7348
Fax: 860-418-6780
TTY: 860-418-6707
e-mail: ronna.keil@pa.state.ct.us
www.dmhas.state.ct.us

The mission of the Department of Mental Health and Addiction Services is to improve the quality of life of the people of Connecticut by providing an integrated network of comprehensive, effective and efficient mental health and addiction services that foster self-sufficiency, dignity and respect.
Patricia Rehmer, Commissioner

Delaware

8277 Delaware Division of Alcoholism, Drug Abuse and Mental Health
Alcohol And Drug Services
1901 North DuPont Highway 302-255-9399
New Castle, DE 19720 Fax: 302-255-4427
e-mail: DHSSInfor@state.de.us
www.dhss.delware.gov
Our mission is to promote health and recovery by ensuring that Delawareans have access to quality prevention and treatment for mental health, substance use, and gambling conditions.
Renata J. Henry, Director

District of Columbia

8278 Health Planning and Development
825 N Capitol Street NE 202-727-8473
Washington, DC 20002 Fax: 202-727-8411
e-mail: doh@dc.gov
doh.dc.gov/service/doh-substance-abuse

Florida

8279 Alcohol and Drug Abuse Program Department Of Children And Families
Department Of Children And Families
1317 Winewood Boulevard 850-487-2920
Tallahassee, FL 32399-6570 Fax: 850-414-7474
www.dcf.state.fl.us/mentalhealth/sa
The Substance Abuse and Mental Health (SAMH) Program, within the Florida Department of Children and Families, is the single state authority on substance abuse and mental health as designated by the federal Substance Abuse and Mental Health Services Administration (SAMHSA). The Department's SAMH Program oversees a statewide system of care for the prevention, treatment, and recovery of children and adults with serious mental illnesses and/or substance abuse disorders.
Cynthea Panzarino, Director

Georgia

8280 Alcohol and Drug Services Addictive Diseases Program
Addictive Diseases Program
Two Peachtree Street NW 404-657-2331
Atlanta, GA 30303-3171 Fax: 404-657-2160
www.mhddad.dhr.georgia.gov
DBHDD contracts with providers in all 6 regions to provide outpatient and residential substance abuse treatment to men and women who are struggling with the disease of addiction
Frank Berry, Commissioner

Hawaii

8281 Alcohol and Drug Abuse Division Department of Health
Department of Health
601 Kamokila Boulevard 808-692-7506
Kapoleiu, HI 96707 Fax: 808-692-7521
e-mail: ATRINFO@doh.hawaii.gov
www.hawaii.gov/health
The mission of the Department of Health is to protect and improve the health and environment for all people in Hawai'i .
Loretta J. Fuddy, Director
Keith Yamamoto, Asst. Director

Idaho

8282 Department of Health and Welfare Department Of Health And Welfare
Department Of Health And Welfare
1720 Westgate Drive 208-334-6747
Boise, ID 83704-0036 800-926-2588
Fax: 208-334-6738
e-mail: rossil@dhw.idaho.gov
www.healthandwelfare.idaho.gov

Landis Rossi, Regional Director
Richard Armstrong, Director

Illinois

8283 Department of Alcoholism and Substance Abuse
Department Of Human Services
100 W Randolph Street 312-814-3840
Chicago, IL 60601 800-843-6154
Fax: 312-814-2419
TTY: 800-447-6404
e-mail: dhsas16@dhs.state.il.us
www.dhs.state.il.us

Theodora Binion-Tayl, Director

8284 Illinois Church Action on Alcohol Problems
1132 W Jefferson Street 217-546-6871
Springfields, IL 62702 Fax: 217-546-2814
e-mail: ilcaaap@sbcglobal.net
www.ilcaaap.org
An interdenominational Christian agency representing church groups in Illinois. Works to prevent alcohol and other drug-related problems through education legislative action and public awareness.

8285 Parkside Medical Services Corporation
205 W Touhy Avenue 847-698-9866
Park Ridge, IL 60068-4256 800-727-5723
This establishment offers treatment and hope for the alcoholic/substance abuser. A resource center that provides information books and resources pertaining to substance abuse and offers treatment facilities in various states across the country.

Indiana

8286 Division of Addiction Services Department of Mental Health
Department of Mental Health

402 W Washington Street
Indianapolis, IN 46204-3614

317-232-7800
800-662-4357
Fax: 317-233-3472
www.in.gov/fssa

Gina Eckart, Director
Alma Burrus, Operations Manager

Iowa

8287 Department of Public Health: Division of Substance Abuse and Health
Lucas State Office Building
321 E 12th Street
Des Moines, IA 50319-0075

515-281-7689
866-227-9878
Fax: 515-281-4535
e-mail: jzwick@idphstate.ia.us
www.idph.state.ia.us

The Iowa Department of Public Health (IDPH) partners with local public health, policymakers, health care providers, business and many others to fulfill our mission of promoting and protecting the health of Iowans.
Kathy Stone, Director

Kansas

8288 Alcohol and Drug Abuse Services
915 Harrison Street
Topeka, KS 66612

785-296-3959
800-586-3690
Fax: 785-296-7275
TTY: 785-296-1491
e-mail: dxmd@srskansas.org
www.srskansas.org

Don Jordan, Secretary
Laura Howard, Deputy Secretary/CFO

Kentucky

8289 Division of Substance Abuse: Department of Mental Health
Department For MH/MR Services
100 Fair Oaks Lane
Frankfort, KY 40621

502-564-2880
Fax: 502-564-7152
TTY: 502-564-5777
www.mhmr.ky.gov

Louisiana

8290 Office of Human Services: Division of Alcohol and Drug Abuse
628 N 4th Street
Baton Rouge, LA 70802-2790

225-342-9500
855-229-6848
Fax: 225-342-3875
TTY: 225-342-5568
e-mail: dhhwebinfo@la.gov
www.dhh.louisiana.gov

Maine

8291 Office of Alcohol and Drug Abuse Prevention
Ofice Of Substance Abuse
AMHI Complex, Marquardt Building
Augusta, ME 04333-0159

207-289-2595
Fax: 207-287-4334
e-mail: osa.ircosa@state.me.us
www.maine.gov/dhhs/samhs/osa/

Kimberly A. Johnson, Director

Maryland

8292 Maryland State Alcohol and Drug Abuse Administration
55 Wade Avenue
Catonsville, MD 21228

410-402-8600
Fax: 410-402-8601
e-mail: adaainfo@dhmh.state.md.us
www.maryland-adaa.org

The Alcohol and Drug Abuse Administration is committed to providing access to a quality and effective substance abuse prevention, intervention and treatment service system for the citizens of Maryland.
Kathleen Rebbert-Fra, Acting Director
Steve Bocian, Acting Deputy Director

Massachusetts

8293 Division of Substance Abuse
250 Washington Street
Boston, MA 02108-4619

617-624-5111
800-327-5050
Fax: 617-624-5185
TTY: 888-448-8321
e-mail: bsas.questions@state.ma.us
www.mass.gov/eohhs/gov/departments/dph/p

Michael Botticelli, Director

Michigan

8294 Office of Substance Abuse Services Department of Public Health
Department of Public Health
320 S Walnut Street
Lansing, MI 48913

517-373-4700
888-736-0253
Fax: 517-335-2121
TTY: 517-373-3573
www.michigan.gov/mdch

Yvonne Blackmond, Director

Minnesota

8295 Chemical Dependency Program Division Department of Human Services
Department of Human Services
Saint Paul, MN 55164-3899

651-431-2460
800-627-3529
Fax: 651-582-1865
e-mail: dhs.info@state.mn.us
mn.gov/dhs/about-dhs/

The Minnesota Department of Human Services, working with many others, helps people meet their basic needs so they can live in dignity and achieve their highest potential.

8296 Dentists Concerned for Dentists
450 N Syndicate
Saint Paul, MN 55104

651-641-0730
www.medhelp.org/amshc/amshc53.htm

A nonprofit organization for chemically dependent Minnesota dentists and concerned others.

Mississippi

8297 Division of Alcohol & Drug Abuse: Mississippi
Department of Mental Health
1101 Robert E Lee Building
Jackson, MS 39201

601-359-1288
877-210-8513
Fax: 601-359-6295
TTY: 601-359-6230
www.dmh.state.ms.us

Supporting a better tomorrow by making a difference in the lives of Mississippians with mental illness, substance abuse problems and intellectual/developmental disabilities one person at a time.
Rose Roberts, Chair
Jim Herzog, Vice Chair

8298 Division of Alcohol & Drug Abuse: South Department of Mental Health
1101 Robert E Lee Building
Jackson, MS 39201

601-359-1288
877-210-8513
Fax: 601-359-6295
TTY: 601-359-6230
www.dmh.state.ms.us

Supporting a better tomorrow by making a difference in the lives of Mississippians with mental illness, substance abuse problems and intellectual/developmental disabilities one person at a time.
Rose Roberts, Chair
Jim Herzog, Vice Chair

Missouri

8299 Missouri Division of Alcohol and Drug Abuse
Department of Mental Health

1706 E Elm Street
Jefferson City, MO 65102

573-751-4942
800-575-7480
Fax: 573-751-8224
TTY: 573-526-1201
e-mail: dmhmail@dmh.mo.gov
dmh.mo.gov/ada/

Keith Schafer, Director
Heidi DiBiaso, Administrative Assistant

Montana

8300 Department of Institutions, Alcohol and Drug Abuse Division
Helena, MT 59620-2905

406-444-3964
Fax: 406-444-9389
e-mail: jcassidy@mt. gov
www.dphhs.st.mt.us

Nebraska

8301 Department of Public Instruction: Division of Alcoholism and Drug Abuse
Division Of Behavioral Health
Lincoln, NE 68509-8925

402-471-7818
800-648-4444
Fax: 402-479-5162
e-mail: richard.deliberty@hhss.ne.gov
www.hhs.state.ne.us

Scot Adams, Director
GibsonBlaine Shaffer, CEO

Nevada

8302 Alcohol and Drug Abuse Bureau: Department of Human Resources
4126 Technology Way
Carson City, NV 89706

775-684-5943
Fax: 775-684-5964
e-mail: MHDS@MHDS.NV.GOV
www.mhds.nv.gov

Maria Canfield, Chief

New Hampshire

8303 Office of Alcohol and Drug Abuse Prevention
State Office Park South
129 Pleasant Street
Concord, NH 03301-3852

800-804-0909
Fax: 603-271-6105
e-mail: rosemary.shannon@dhhs.sate.nh.us
www.dhhs.state.nh.us

New Jersey

8304 Department of Health
120 S Stockton Street
Trenton, NJ 08625-0362

609-292-7837
800-367-6543
Fax: 609-292-3816
e-mail: georgene.rhodunda@dhs.state.nj.us
www.state.nj.us

Heather Howard, Commissioner
Mary E O'Dowd, Chief of Staff

8305 Division of Narcotic and Drug Abuse Control
120 S Stockton Street
Trenton, NJ 08625-0362

609-292-5760
800-238-2333
Fax: 609-292-3816
www.state.nj.us/humanservices

Jeffers, Director

New Mexico

8306 Substance Abuse Bureau
1190 Saint Francis Drive
Santa Fe, NM 87502

505-827-2601
800-362-2013
Fax: 505-827-0097
www.nmcares.org

New York

8307 Division of Substance Abuse Services
Substance Abuse Services
1450 Western Avenue
Albany, NY 12203-3526

518-473-3460
877-846-7369
Fax: 518-457-5474
e-mail: communications@oasas.ny.gov
www.oasas.ny.gov

Karen M Carpenter-Palumbo, Commissioner
Kathleen Caggiano-Si, Executive Deputy Commissioner

North Carolina

8308 Alcohol and Drug Abuse Section
Division of Mental Health & Mental Retardation
2001 Mail Service Center
Raleigh, NC 27699-3007

919-733-7011
800-662-7030
Fax: 919-508-0951
www.dhhs.state.nc.us

Leza Wainwright, Director
Michael S Lancaster, Director

North Dakota

8309 Division of Alcoholism & Drug Abuse: Department of Human Services
Department Of Human Services
1237 W Divide Avenue
Bismarck, ND 58501

701-328-8920
800-755-2719
Fax: 701-328-8969
e-mail: dhsmhsas@nd.gov
www.nd.gov/dhs/services/mentalhealth/

The Mental Health and Substance Abuse Services Division provides leadership for the planning, development, and oversight of a system of care for children, adults, and families with severe emotional disorders, mental illness, and/or substance abuse issues.

Ohio

8310 Bureau on Alcohol Abuse and Recovery Ohio Department of Health
Ohio Department of Health
30 East Broad Street
Columbus, OH 43215-2550

614-466-3445
Fax: 614-752-8645
e-mail: info@ada.ohio.gov
www.odadas.state.oh.us

The mission of the Ohio Department of Mental Health and Addiction Services (OhioMHAS) is to provide statewide leadership of a high-quality mental health and addiction prevention, treatment and recovery system that is effective and valued by all Ohioans.
Tracy J. Plouck, Director
Orman Hall, Director of the Governor's Cabinet Opiat

8311 Bureau on Drug Abuse: Ohio Department of Health
Ohio Department of Health
30 East Broad Street
Columbus, OH 43215

614-466-3445
Fax: 614-752-8645
e-mail: info@ada.ohio.gov
www.odadas.state.oh.us

The mission of the Ohio Department of Mental Health and Addiction Services (OhioMHAS) is to provide statewide leadership of a high-quality mental health and addiction prevention, treatment and recovery system that is effective and valued by all Ohioans.
Tracy J. Plouck, Director
Orman Hall, Director of the Governor's Cabinet Opiat

Oklahoma

8312 Oklahoma Department of Mental Health and Substance Abuse Services
Substance Abuse Program

1200 NE 13th Street
Oklahoma City, OK 73117-3277

405-522-3908
800-522-9054
Fax: 405-522-3650
TTY: 405-522-3851
e-mail: jglover@odmhsas.org
www.odmhsas.org

J. Andy Sullivan, Chairperson
Larry McCauley, Vice Chair

Oregon

8313   Office of Alcohol and Drug Abuse Programs
500 Summer Street NE
Salem, OR 97301-1118

503-945-5763
Fax: 503-378-8467
TTY: 800-375-2863
e-mail: omhas.web@state.or.us
www.oregon.gov/DHS/addiction/index.shtml

Pennsylvania

8314   Drug and Alcohol Programs Department Of Health
Department Of Health
02 Kline Plaza
Harrisburg, PA 17104-0090

717-783-8200
877-724-3258
Fax: 717-787-6285
e-mail: rkauffman@state.pa.us
www.ddap.pa.gov

Gary Tennis, Secretary
Kim Bowman, Deputy Secretary

Rhode Island

8315   Division of Substance Abuse: Department of Mental Health and Hospitals
Department Of Mental Health And Retardation
14 Harrington Road
Cranston, RI 02920-0944

401-462-2339
800-622-7422
Fax: 401-462-3204
e-mail: CStenning@bhddh.ri.gov
www.mhrh.state.ri.us

Committed to assuring access to quality services and supports for Rhode Islanders with developmental disabilities, mental health and substance abuse issues, and chronic long term medical and psychiatric conditions. Our mission includes addressing the stigma attached to these disabilities as well as planning for the development of new services and prevention activities.
Craig S Stenning, Executive Director

South Carolina

8316   South Carolina Commission on Alcohol and Drug Abuse
Department Of Alcohol And Drug Abuse Services
2414 Bull Street
Columbia, SC 29201-9498

803-896-5555
Fax: 803-896-5557
www.daodas.org

The department's mission is to ensure the provision of quality services to prevent or reduce the negative consequences of substance use and addictions.
Bob Toomey, Director
Kaitlin Blanco-Silva, Project Manager

South Dakota

8317   Division of Alcohol & Drug Abuse: South Dakota
Department Of Human Services
3800 E Highway 34
Pierre, SD 57501-5070

605-773-5990
800-265-9684
Fax: 605-773-5483
TTY: 605-773-6412
e-mail: infodhs@state.sd.us
www.dhs.sd.gov

Gilbert Sudbeck, Director

Tennessee

8318   Department of Mental Health and Mental Retardation, Alcohol & Drug Service
Bureau Of Alcohol And Drug Abuse Services

601 Mainstream Drive
Nashville, TN 37243-4401

615-532-6500
800-560-5767
Fax: 615-532-2419
e-mail: oca.mhdd@tn.gov
www.state.tn.us

Michael A. Rabin, Director and Meida Contact
Lorene Lambert, Publications & Web Management

Texas

8319   Texas Commission on Alcohol and Drug Abuse Department Of State Health
Department Of State Health
Austin, TX 78714

512-206-5000
866-378-8440
Fax: 512-458-7477
TTY: 800-735-2989
TDD: 800-735-2989
e-mail: web.master@dshs.state.tx.us
www.dshs.state.tx.us/mhsa/

Mission is to improve health and well-being in Texas.
David L. Lakey, Commissioner

Utah

8320   Department of Social Services: Division of Substance Abuse
Department Of Human Services
195 North 1950 West
Salt Lake City, UT 84116

801-538-3939
Fax: 801-538-9892
e-mail: jemarrott@utah.gov
www.hsdsa.utah.gov

The Utah Division of Substance Abuse and Mental Health is the State agency responsible for ensuring that prevention and treatment services for substance abuse and mental health are available statewide. If you, a friend, or family member is struggling with a mental health problem or a problem with alcohol, tobacco, or other drugs there is help available. Hope and recovery are possible.
Paula Bell, Chairperson
Darryl Wagner, Vice Chairman

Vermont

8321   Alcohol and Drug Abuse Programs of Vermont Department Of Health
Department Of Health
108 Cherry Street
Burlington, VT 05402-1531

802-651-1550
Fax: 802-651-1573
e-mail: vtadap@vdh.state.vt.us
www.healthvermont.gov

Virginia

8322   Substance Abuse Services Office of Virginia
Department of Mental Health & Mental Retardation
1220 Bank Street
Richmond, VA 23218-1797

804-786-3921
800-451-5544
Fax: 804-371-6638
TTY: 804-371-8977
e-mail: wglover@co.dmhmrsas.virginia.gov
www.dmhmrsas.virginia.gov

Available to citizens statewide, Virginia's public mental health, intellectual disability and substance abuse services system is comprised of 16 state-operated facilities and 40 locally-run community services boards (CSBs) The CSBs and facilities serve children and adults who have-or who are at risk of-mental illness, serious emotional disturbance, intellectual disabilities, or substance abuse disorders.
Jim Stewart, Commissioner
Olivia Garland, Deputy Commissioner

Washington

8323   Washington Department of Social and Health Services, Alcohol and Drug Prog.
Department Of Social And Health Services

Olympia, WA 98504-5330

877-301-4557
800-737-0617
Fax: 360-438-8078
TTY: 877-301-4557
e-mail: starkkd@dshs.wa.gov
www1.dshs.wa.gov

West Virginia

8324 West Virginia Division of Alcohol & Drug Abuse
Department Of Health And Human Resources
350 Capitol Street
Charleston, WV 25304-3702

304-356-4811
Fax: 304-558-1008
e-mail: obhs@wvdhhr.org
www.dhhr.wv.gov

The Division on Alcoholism and Drug Abuse, an operating division of the Bureau for Behavioral Health and Health Facilities (BBHHF) within the West Virginia Division of Health and Human Services is charged in code with being the Single State Authority (SSA) primarily responsible for prevention, control, treatment, rehabilitation, educational research and planning for substance abuse related services
Craig A. Richards, Deputy Commissioner

Wisconsin

8325 Office of Alcohol and Other Drug Abuse
1 W Wilson Street
Madison, WI 53703-7851

608-266-1865
Fax: 608-266-1533
TTY: 608-267-7371
e-mail: dhswebmaster@wisconsin.gov
www.dhfs.state.wi.us

John Easterday, Administrator
Susan Gadacz, Contact

Wyoming

8326 Alcohol & Drug Abuse Programs of Wyoming Department Of Health
Department Of Health
401 Hathaway Building
Cheyenne, WY 82002-0480

307-777-7656
866-571-0944
Fax: 307-777-7439
e-mail: aburde@state.wy.us
health.wyo.gov/default.aspx

Thomas O. Forslund, Director
Lee Clabots, Deputy Director

Libraries & Resource Centers

8327 National Clearinghouse for Alcohol and Drug Information
Rockville, MD 20847-2345

240-221-4019
800-729-6686
Fax: 240-221-4292
TDD: 800-487-4889
e-mail: info@health.org
www.ncadi.samhsa.gov

A resource for alcohol and other drug information. It carries a wide variety of publications dealing with alcohol and other drug abuse.
John Noble, Director

8328 Parents Resource Institute for Drug Education
160 Vanderbilt Court
Bowling Green, KY 42103

800-279-6361
Fax: 270-746-9598
e-mail: info@pridesurveys.com
www.pridesurveys.com

Offers national information and educational materials pertaining to alcohol and drug dependency.
Thomas J Gleaton, EdD, President
Janie Pitcock, President

Research Centers

8329 Alcohol Disease Foundation
33 Eglantine Avenue
Pennington, NJ 08534-2308

609-737-0088

Founded in 1988 to promote research on testing systems that could diagnose the metabolic aspects of alcoholism. Seeks to educate the public on the validity of the disease concept of alcoholism.

8330 Alcohol Research Group Public Health Institute
Public Health Institute
6475 Christie Avenue
Emeryville, CA 94608-1324

510-597-3440
Fax: 510-985-6459
e-mail: info@arg.org
www.arg.org

The Alcohol Research Group (ARG) of the Public Health Institute was established in 1959 to conduct and disseminate high-quality research in epidemiology of alcohol consumption and problems including alcohol use disorders, alcohol-related health services research, and analyses of alcohol policy and its impacts.
Dominique La MPH, Executive Director
Thomas K. Greenfield, Scientific Director

8331 Boston University Laboratory of Neuropsychology
Dept of Behavioral Neuroscience
80 E Concord Street M9
Boston, MA 02118

617-638-4803
Fax: 617-638-4806
www.bu.edu

Offers research and studies into the effects of Alcoholism pertaining to aphasia apraxia dementia memory disorders and various other neurological malfunctions.
Marlene Osca Berman PhD, Director

8332 Center for Alcohol & Addiction Studies Brown University
Brown University
121 South Main Street
Providence, RI 02903-0001

401-863-6600
Fax: 401-863-6697
e-mail: caas@brown.edu
www.caas.brown.edu

The Center for Alcohol and Addiction Studies through its affiliation with the Brown Medical School occupies a unique position within the University. The Center brings together more that 90 faculty and professional staff members from 11 University departments and eight affiliated hospitals to promote the identification prevention and effective treatment of alcohol and other substance abuse.
Peter M Monti PhD, Center Director
Suzanne Colby Ph. D, Associate Director

8333 Cornerstone Medical Arts Center Hospital
Medical Arts Center Hospital
159-05 Union Turnpike
Fresh Meadows, NY 11366-2802

718-906-6700
800-233-9999
Fax: 718-906-6840
e-mail: admin@cornerstoneny.com
www.cornerstoneny.com

Offers a complete integrated program for alcohol assessment alcohol and drug rehabilitation continuing care community education and comprehensive family recovery.
Norine Hurtado, Senior Vice President of Human Resources

8334 Do it Now Foundation
PO Box 27658
Tempe, AZ 85285-7658

480-736-0599
Fax: 480-736-0599
e-mail: info@dci-dcitnaw.com
www.doitnow.org

An information clearinghouse for service providers that publishes well-written pamphlets booklets and materials on chemical dependency and recovery.

8335 Dorothea Dix Hospital Clinical Research Unit
809 Ruggles Drive
Raleigh, NC 27603

919-733-5227
866-349-5627
Fax: 919-733-5351
www.med.unc.edu

Researches the biological risk factors of alcoholism using young adults without the disease but with history of familial alcoholism.
Terry Spell, Director
William L Roper, CEO

8336 Ernest Gallo Clinic and Research Center
5858 Horton Street
Emeryville, CA 94608

510-985-3100
Fax: 510-985-3101
e-mail: ngreen@gallo.ucsf.edu
www.galloresearch.org

Alcoholism studies with a special emphasis on genetics.
John A. De Luca PHD, Chairman of the Board/President
Joseph E Gallo, President/Chief Executive Officer

8337   Families in Action National Drug Abuse Center
National Drug Abuse Center
PO Box 3553   252-237-1242
Wilson, NC 27895
                                          Fax: 252-237-6544
                             e-mail: phil@familiesinaction.org
                                         www.familiesinaction.org
Publish prevention materials and serves as an information clearinghouse for families with a member suffering from a drug or alcohol addiction.
Phillip A Mooring, Executive Director
Anna Godwin, Coordinator

8338   Friends Medical Science Research Center
1229 West Mount Royal Avenue   410-752-4218
Baltimore, MD 21217   Fax: 310-477-9601
                                              www.wellness.com

Studies narcotic addictions.
John Valenty, President
Rob Greenstein, President

8339   Hahnemann University Laboratory of Human Pharmacology
Department of Pharmacology
Broad and Vine   215-762-7000
Philadelphia, PA 19102   Fax: 215-762-8109
                                         www.hahnemannhospital.com
Hahnemann University hospital is committed to providing quality patient care in an academic setting.
Benjamin Cal MD, Director

8340   Harvard Cocaine Recovery Project
1493 Cambridge Street   617-498-1000
Cambridge, MA 02139-1099   Fax: 617-642-58
Six-year study of relapse and recovery in cocaine addicts.
William McAu MD, Principal Investigator

8341   Interdisciplinary Program in Cell and Molecular Pharmacology
Medical University of South Carolina
173 Ashley Avenue BSB 358   843-792-8975
Charleston, SC 29425   Fax: 843-792-0481
                                              www.musc.edu/pharm
Research into pharmacology and toxicology.
Kenneth D Tew, Ph.D., D.Sc., Professor and Chairman
Michelle Shorter, Administrative Coordinator

8342   Johns Hopkins University: Behavioral Pharmacology Research Unit
John Hopkins Bay View Campus
5510 Nathan Shock Drive   410-955-5000
Baltimore, MD 21224-2735   Fax: 410-550-0030
                                    e-mail: bigelow@jhmi.edu
                                         www.hopkinsmedicine.org
An internationally recognized center of excellence in research on psychoactive drugs. As the name implies BPRU's orientation is behavioral and pharmacological emphasizing a behavioral analysis of drug action.
George E Bigelow PhD, Scientific Director
Eric C Strain MD, Medical Director

8343   Kettering-Scott Magnetic Resonance Laboratory
Wright State University, School of Medicine
PO Box 927
Dayton, OH 45435-0927   937-775-2934
                                              www.med.wright.edu
No information found on the website.
Marjorie Bowman, MD and Dean
Betty Kangas, Assistant to the dean

8344   Marin Institute
24 Belvedere Street   415-456-5692
San Rafael, CA 94901-4817   Fax: 415-456-0491
                                              www.marinInstitute.org
The mission of this Institute is to reduce the toll of alcohol and other drug problems on Marin County and society in general. The Institute fulfills this mission by developing implementing evaluat-

ing and disseminating innovative approaches to prevention locally nationally and internationally.
Bruce Lee Livingston MPP, Executive Director
Michele Simo JD MPH, Research & Policy Director

8345   Narcotic and Drug Research
11 Beach Street   212-966-8700
New York, NY 10013-2429   Fax: 212-334-8058
Nonprofit organization that is devoted to drug abuse education treatment and prevention.
Douglas S Lipton PhD, Director

8346   National Center on Addiction and Substance Abuse
Columbia University
633 3rd Avenue   212-841-5200
New York, NY 10017-6706   800-622-4357
                                          Fax: 212-956-8020
                                              www.casacolumbia.org
The only nation-wide organization that brings together under one roof all the professional disciplines needed to study and combat abuse of all substances - alcohol nicotine as well as illegal prescription and performance enhancing drugs - in all sectors of society.
Lee C. Bollinger, President
Ursula M. Burns, Chairman and CEO

8347   National Prevention Resource Center CSAP Division of Communications Programs
CSAP Division of Communications Programs
5600 Fishers Lane   301-443-9936
Rockville, MD 20857-0001
Supports an array of prevention program evaluation approaches including individual grantee evaluations program evaluations and a National Evaluation Project. Also offers a National Data Base to provide information on programs for prevention of substance abuse.

8348   National Treatment Consortium for Alcohol and Other Drugs
PO Box 1294
Washington, DC 20013   202-434-4780
                                              www.ntc-usa.org

8349   National Volunteer Training Center for Substance Abuse Prevention
CSAP Division of Communications Programs
5600 Fishers Lane   301-443-9936
Rockville, MD 20857
Volunteers are always on hand to provide answers, information, referrals and resources pertaining to alcohol, drugs and substance abuse.

8350   National Volunteer Training Center for Sub CSAP Division of Communications Programs
5600 Fishers Lane   301-443-9936
Rockville, MD 20857
Volunteers are always on hand to provide answers information referrals and resources pertaining to alcohol drugs and substance abuse.

8351   Ohio State University Clinical Pharmacology Division
College of Medicine
370 Western 9th Avenue   614-292-2220
Columbus, OH 43210-1239   800-252-3636
                                          Fax: 614-292-4293
                                    e-mail: medicine@osu.ede
                                              www.medicine.osu.edu
Substance abuse and alcohol related research.
Robert Bornstein PHD, Vice dean for academic affairs
Glen Apsloss, Director

8352   RADAR Network National Clearinghouse for Alcohol & Dru
National Clearinghouse for Alcohol & Drug Info
PO Box 2345   301-468-2600
Rockville, MD 20847-2345   800-729-6686
                                          Fax: 240-221-4292
                                          TTY: 800-487-4889
                                          TDD: 800-487-4889
                                              ncadi.samhsa.gov
Consists of state clearinghouses specialized information centers of national organizations and the Department of Education Re-

gional Training Centers. Each RADAR member can offer the public a variety of information services.
John Noble, Director

8353 Research Institute on Alcoholism State University of New York at Buffalo
State University of New York at Buffalo
1021 Main Street 716-887-2566
Buffalo, NY 14203 Fax: 716-872-52
e-mail: connors@ria.buffalo.edu
www.ria.buffalo.edu
Integral part of the New York State Division of Alcoholism and Alcohol Abuse.
Kenneth E Leonard, PhD, Director
Kimberly S Walitzer, PhD, Deputy Director

8354 Rockefeller University Laboratory of Biology
1230 York Avenue 212-327-8000
New York, NY 10065 Fax: 212-327-7974
www.rockefeller.edu

Marc Tessier Lavigne, President

8355 Rutgers University Center of Alcohol Studies
Busch Campus
607 Allison Road 732-445-2190
Piscataway, NJ 08854 Fax: 732-445-3500
e-mail: alclib@rci.rutgers.edu
alcoholstudies.rutgers.edu
Causes and treatment of alcoholism.
Robert Pandi PhD, Director

8356 Rutgers University: Controlled Drug- Delivery Research Center
College of Pharmacy
PO Box 789 732-932-3834
Piscataway, NJ 08855-0789 Fax: 732-932-5767
Yie W Chien, Director

8357 Ruth E Golding Clinical Pharmacokinetics Laboratory
College of Pharmacy
1703 E Mabel 520-626-1938
Tucson, AZ 85721-1427 e-mail: webmaster@pharmacy.arizona.edu
www.pharmacy.arizona.edu
Conducts studies of drugs in humans and animals.
Michael Maye MD, Head

8358 Southern California Research Institute
7065 Hayvenhurst Avenue 310-390-8481
Van Nuys, CA 90066 Fax: 310-390-8482
www.scri.org
Effects of alcohol and drugs on behavior studies.
Dary Fiorent PhD, Executive Director
Bergetta Die BA, Research Associate

8359 Stanford Center for Research in Disease Prevention
Stanford University School of Medicine
1070 Arastradero Road 650-723-6254
Palo Alto, CA 94304 Fax: 650-723-6254
prevention.stanford.edu
Prevention and control of alcohol and drug abuse related disorders.
John P.A Loannidis, MD, DSc, Director

8360 State University of New York at Buffalo Toxicology Research Center
3435 Main Street 716-831-2125
Buffalo, NY 14214 Fax: 716-829-2806
www.smbs.buffalo.edu
Toxicology-related research and services including the development of tests to evaluate toxins chemicals and drugs.
Michale E. Cain, Director
Dr James R Olson, Assistant Director

8361 University of California: Los Angeles Alcohol Research Center
405 Hilgard Ave 310-825-4321
Los Angeles, CA 90095-8353 Fax: 310-206-7309
www.ucla.edu

Causes of alcoholism including genetics.
Dr Ernest Noble, Director

8362 University of Michigan: Alcohol Research Center
400 E Eisenhower Parkway 734-764-1817
Ann Arbor, MI 48108-3318 Fax: 734-998-7994
www.umich.edu
Alcohol abuse studies among the elderly including the relationship between alcohol and aged disorders.
Robert A Zucker PhD, Contact

8363 University of Michigan: Psychiatric Center
4250 Plymouth road 734-936-5900
Ann Arbor, MI 48109-0001 Fax: 734-936-9761
www.umich.edu
Psychiatric disease research pertaining to the effects of alcoholism and drug abuse.
Gregory W Dalack, MD

8364 University of Minnesota: Program on Alcohol/Drug Control
Stadium Gate 27 612-624-6861
Minneapolis, MN 55455
Alcohol tobacco and drug research.
Dr James Schaefer, Director

8365 University of Missouri: Kansas City Drug Information Service
2464 Charlotte 816-235-5490
Kansas City, MO 64108-2640 Fax: 816-235-5491
e-mail: umkcdruginformation@umkc.edu
dic.umkc.edu
Literature research and evaluation of clinical drug problems and questions.
Pat Bryant PhD, Director
Heather A Pace PhD, Assistant Director

8366 University of Tennessee Drug Information Center
875 Monroe Avenue 901-528-5555
Memphis, TN 38163-1 Fax: 901-448-5419
e-mail: utdic@utmem.edu
dop.utmem.edu/dic

Katie Suda, Director
Camille Thornton, Assistant Professor

8367 University of Texas Health Science Center Neurophysiology Research Center
Speech & Hearing Institute
7000 Fannin 713-500-4472
Houston, TX 77030-3405 Fax: 713-792-4513
Conducts clinical and animal studies aimed at combating alcohol drug and tobacco dependence.
Giuseppe N Colasurdo, Director

8368 University of Texas at Austin: Drug Synamics Institute
1 University Station 512-475-9746
Austin, TX 78712 Fax: 512-471-2746
www.utexas.edu

Pharmaceutical and drug research.
Janet C Walkow PhD, Director
Carla Van Den Berg PhD, Associate Professor

8369 University of Utah: Center for Human Toxicology
30 South 2000 East 801-581-6731
Salt Lake City, UT 84112-1210 Fax: 801-581-3716
e-mail: dwilkins@alanine.pharm.utah.edu
www.pharmacy.utah.edu
Clinical forensic and toxicology research.
Chris M . Ireland PHd, Dean
Dennis Crouch, Director

8370 University of Wisconsin Milwaukee Medicinal Chemistry Group
University of Wisconsin
PO Box 413
Milwaukee, WI 53201-413 414-229-1122
www4.uwm.edu
Research on drugs including studies of valium receptors.
Michael R. Lovell, Chancellor

Support Groups & Hotlines

8371 Al-Anon Alateen Family Group Hotline
1600 Corporate Landing Parkway 757-563-1600
Virginia Beach, VA 23454-970 888-425-2666
Fax: 757-563-1655
e-mail: wso@alanon.org
www.al-anon.alateen.org
A mutual peer-to-peer support program with groups meeting worldwide to provide hope and help to the families of alcoholics. Although a seperate entity from Alcoholics Anonymous, our program is based upon the Twelve Steps.
Ric Buchanan, Executive Director

8372 Alcohol Drug Treatment Referral
1316 South Coast Highway
Laguna Beach, CA 92651-3118 800-454-8966
Fax: 949-281-1933
National Help and Referral Network, a nonprofit organization available 24 hours a day to assist people troubled by drug or alcohol abuse. Here to provide information on addiction treatment and support services and to help save lives and mend broken dreams.
Mike Cohan, Director

8373 Alcoholics Anonymous World Services
PO Box 459 212-870-3400
New York, NY 10163-4059 Fax: 212-870-3003
www.aa.org
Alcoholics Anonymous is a fellowship of men and women who share their experience, strength and hope with each other that they may solve their common problem and help others to recover from alcoholism. The only requirement for membership is a desire to stop drinking. There are no dues or fees for AA membership; they are self-supporting through their own contributions.
Greg M, General Manager

8374 Drug Free Workplace Hotline
Division of Workplace Programs
Samhsa Diagonal CSAP 1 Choke Cherry 240-276-2612
Rockville, MD 20857 877-726-4727
Fax: 240-276-1210
TDD: 800-457-4889
e-mail: webmaster@samhsa.hhs.gov
www.drugfreeworkplace.gov
A hotline for businesses to obtain information on a wide range of drug abuse related problems, issues and services.
Robert Stephenson II, Director

8375 Friday Night Live
California Dept of Drug & Alcohol Programs
1700 K Street 916-445-7456
Sacramento, CA 95814 Fax: 916-230-59
e-mail: laura@tcoe.org
www.communitycounseling.org/fnl
These groups, located in California, are all run by students with a faculty adviser. They arrange local alcohol and drug free events, from dances and movies to visiting hospitalized children. Students not only have fun but they learn to have fun sober.
Jim Kooler, Administrator
Laura Purcellabuzo, Project Coordinator

8376 Images Within: A Child's View of Parental Alcoholism
Children of Alcoholics Foundation
PO Box 4185 212-595-5810
New York, NY 10163-4185 800-359-2623
e-mail: coaf@phoenixhouse.org
www.coaf.org
An innovative program designed to teach all children about family alcoholism. Middle-school-aged children learn how to get help for themselves or give help to their friends.

8377 International Lawyers in Alcoholics Anonymous
39 Smith Neck Road 860-529-7474
Old Lyme, CT 6371 e-mail: bert@bertwitehead.com
www.ilaa.org
Provides 40 independent local groups.
Scoot Huyghebaert, Chairman

8378 National Health Information Center
PO Box 1133 310-565-4167
Washington, DC 20013 800-336-4797
Fax: 301-984-4256
e-mail: info@nhic.org
www.health.gov/nhic
Offers a nationwide information referral service, produces directories and resource guides.

8379 ToughLove International
PO Box 1069 215-348-7090
Doylestown, PA 18901-0019 800-333-1069
www.toughlove.org
This national self-help group for parents, children and communities emphasizes cooperation, personal initiative and action. Publishes books, brochures and promotional information and holds workshops and seminars across the country.

8380 WFS' New Life Program
Women for Sobriety
PO Box 618 215-536-8026
Quakertown, PA 18951-0618 Fax: 215-538-9026
e-mail: newlife@nni.com
www.womenforsobriety.org
A self-help program for women that can be used independent from AA or with AA. Groups are in many states in the United States. Donations suggested.
Rebecca M Fenner, Director

Books

8381 AA Comes of Age
Alcoholics Anonymous
PO Box 459 212-870-3400
New York, NY 10163-0459 Fax: 212-870-3137
www.aa.org
Tells how AA was started, how the Steps and Traditions evolved and how the AA Fellowship grew and spread overseas.

8382 AA in Prison: Inmate to Inmate
Alcoholics Anonymous
PO Box 459 212-870-3400
New York, NY 10163-0459 Fax: 212-870-3137
www.aa.org
Thirty-two stories that share the experience of men and women who found AA while in prison.
128 pages

8383 Accepting Ourselves & Others
Hazelden
15251 Pleasant Valley Rd 651-213-4200
Center City, MN 55012-9640 800-257-7810
Fax: 651-213-4426
www.hazelden.org
Fully revised and expanded second edition. Examines recovery as it affects the gay, lesbian, and bisexual community, as well as their friends, family, and therapists. Addresses the relationship between substance abuse and being a sexual minority, and discusses the impact of other issues such as anxiety, depression, sexual abuse, and learning disabilities.
379 pages Paperback
ISBN: 1-568381-20-4
Sharon Birnbaum, Corporateÿ Director of Human Resources
Jim Blaha, VP CFO and CAO

8384 Addiction and Responsibility
The Crossroad Publishing Company
1001 N. Fairfax St. 703-741-7686
Alexandria, VA 22314-6503 800-548-0497
Fax: 703-741-7698
e-mail: naadac@naadac.org
www.naadac.org
Anyone who has wrestled with such basic questions about addiction such as: Is drug addiction a behavior disorder or a character flaw? Is it genetic or learned? What is it like to be addicted? will find welcome answers in this groundbreaking philosophical in-

quiry into the addictive mind. The author helps readers understand addiction.
192 pages
ISBN: 0-824513-65-7
Kirk Bowden, President
Gerry Schmidt, President-Elect

8385 Addictions Counseling
The Crossroad Publishing Company
1001 N. Fairfax St.   703-741-7686
Alexandria, VA 22314-6503   800-548-0497
                                   Fax: 703-741-7698
                            e-mail: naadac@naadac.org
                                      www.naadac.org
A practical guide to counseling people with chemical and other addictions.
144 pages Paperback
ISBN: 0-824513-86-0
Kirk Bowden, President
Gerry Schmidt, President-Elect

8386 Addictive Personality
Hazelden
15251 Pleasant Valley Rd   651-213-4200
Center City, MN 55012-9640   800-257-7810
                                   Fax: 651-213-4426
                                      www.hazelden.org
Understanding how an individual becomes an addict through examination of addiction's causes, stages of development, and consequences. Second edition further refines these ideas and includes the most recent information on the addictive process, cultural influences on addictive behaviors, recovery, genetic factors in addiction, mental health issues, and new research findings.
130 pages Paperback
ISBN: 1-568381-29-8
Sharon Birnbaum, Corporateÿ Director of Human Resources
Jim Blaha, VP CFO and CAO

8387 Addictive Thinking Understanding Self-Deception
Hazelden
15251 Pleasant Valley Rd   651-213-4200
Center City, MN 55012-9640   800-257-7810
                                   Fax: 651-213-4426
                                      www.hazelden.org
Illustrates the irrational perspective and complicated, contradictory thinking patterns of addictive thinking, and demonstrates how they lead to low self-esteen, addiction, and relapse. Revised edition includes expanded information on depression and affective disorders, the relationship between addictive thinking and relapse, and the new research related to the origins of addictive thinking.
140 pages Paperback
ISBN: 1-568381-38-7
Sharon Birnbaum, Corporateÿ Director of Human Resources
Jim Blaha, VP CFO and CAO

8388 Adult Children of Alcoholics
Hazelden
15251 Pleasant Valley Rd   651-213-4200
Center City, MN 55012-9640   800-257-7810
                                   Fax: 651-213-4426
                                      www.hazelden.org
Written to and for adult children of dysfunctional families.
138 pages Paperback
Sharon Birnbaum, Corporateÿ Director of Human Resources
Jim Blaha, VP CFO and CAO

8389 Al-Anon Family Groups
Al-Anon Family Group Headquarters
1600 Corp Landing Pkwy   757-563-1600
Virginia Beach, VA 23454-5617   800-425-2666
                                   Fax: 757-563-1655
                             e-mail: wso@al-anon.org
                                 www.al-anon.alateen.org
Basic book that explains the purpose of fellowship, how it works and how it is held in unity. Includes real life stories by husbands, wives, parents and children of those who suffer from alcoholism.
177 pages
ISBN: 0-910034-54-0
Caryn Johnson, Director Communications

8390 Al-Anon's Twelve Steps and Twelve Traditions
Al-Anon Family Group Headquarters
1600 Corp Landing Pkwy   757-563-1600
Virginia Beach, VA 23454-5617   800-425-2666
                                   Fax: 757-563-1655
                             e-mail: wso@al-anon.org
                                 www.al-anon.alateen.org
Written for people whose lives have been affected by alcoholism.
142 pages Hardcover
ISBN: 0-910034-24-9
Caryn Johnson, Director Communications

8391 Alateen: A Day at a Time
Al-Anon Family Group Headquarters
1600 Corp Landing Pkwy   757-563-1600
Virginia Beach, VA 23454-5617   800-425-2666
                                   Fax: 757-563-1655
                             e-mail: wso@al-anon.org
                                 www.al-anon.alateen.org
A collection of positive, daily sharings written by teenagers around the world.
384 pages
ISBN: 0-910034-53-2
Caryn Johnson, Director Communications

8392 Alateen: Hope for Children of Alcoholics
Al-Anon Family Group Headquarters
1600 Corp Landing Pkwy   757-563-1600
Virginia Beach, VA 23454-5617   800-425-2666
                                   Fax: 757-563-1655
                             e-mail: wso@al-anon.org
                                 www.al-anon.alateen.org
A gold mine of information written by Alateens themselves. It covers the history of Alateen, understanding alcoholism and personal stories.
115 pages
ISBN: 0-910034-20-6
Caryn Johnson, Director Communications

8393 Alcohol and Other Drug Services: Dir. of California's Community Services
Department of Alcohol and Drug Programs
1501 Capitol Avenue
Sacramento, CA 95899-4022   916-332-7012
                                      www.dhcs.ca.gov
A directory listing agencies, alcohol and drug providers, county 504 coordinators and county program administrators for the state of California.
136 pages

8394 Alcohol, Drug and Other Addictions: A Directory of Treatment Centers
Oryx Press
3100 East Commercial Blvd   602-265-2651
Fort Lauderdale, FL 33308-3397   800-279-4663
                                      www.recovery.org
Lists 18,000 federal, state and local addiction treatment regimens that include public and private centers.

8395 Alcohol, Tobacco and Other Drugs May Harm the Unborn
National Clearinghouse for Alcohol and Drug Info.
PO Box 2345
Rockville, MD 20847-2345   800-729-6686
Presents the most recent findings of basic research and clinical studies conducted on the effects of alcohol, drugs and tobacco on the unborn.

8396 Alcoholics Anonymous
Alcoholics Anonymous
PO Box 459   212-870-3400
New York, NY 10163-0459   Fax: 212-870-3137
                                      www.aa.org
Third edition of the Big Book, basic text of AA. Chapters describe the AA recovery program and personal histories have been added.

8397 Alcoholics Anonymous: The Big Book
Hazelden

15251 Pleasant Valley Rd
Center City, MN 55012-9640
651-213-4200
800-257-7810
Fax: 651-213-4426
www.hazelden.org
Classic text that guides Alcoholics Anonymous programs and describes how millions of men and women have recovered from alcoholism.
575 pages Paperback
Sharon Birnbaum, Corporateÿ Director of Human Resources
Jim Blaha, VP CFO and CAO

8398 American Academy of Psychiatrists in Alcoholism and Addiction Directory
400 Massasoit Avenue
East Providence, RI 02914
401-524-3076
Fax: 401-272-0922
www.aaap.org
Lists 900 member professionals who are concerned with drug and alcohol abuse.
Laurence M. Westreich, President
John A. Renner, Jr., President-Elect

8399 An Annotated Bibliography of Recent Empirical Research In Methadone
National Clearinghouse for Alcohol and Drug Info.
PO Box 2345
Rockville, MD 20847-2345
800-729-6686
Provides guidelines and suggestions to investigators engaged in the demanding and essential task of followup research on intravenous drug users who have contracted AIDS.
97 pages

8400 As Bill Sees It
Alcoholics Anonymous
PO Box 459
New York, NY 10163-0459
212-870-3400
Fax: 212-870-3137
www.aa.org
This collection of Bill W's writings offers a daily source of comfort and inspiration.

8401 As We Understood...
Al-Anon Family Group Headquarters
1600 Corp Landing Pkwy
Virginia Beach, VA 23454-5617
757-563-1600
800-425-2666
Fax: 757-563-1655
e-mail: wso@al-anon.org
www.al-anon.alateen.org
Al-Anon members share their understanding of a higher power, fellowship, spiritual awakening, prayer, meditation and letting go.
269 pages
ISBN: 0-910034-56-7
Caryn Johnson, Director Communications

8402 Black, Beautiful and Recovering
African American Family Services
2616 Nicollet Avenue S
Minneapolis, MN 55408
612-871-7878
A helpful guide for Black people who are in the process of recovering from alcohol or other substance abuse problems.
10 pages

8403 Body, Mind, and Spirit
Hazelden
15251 Pleasant Valley Rd
Center City, MN 55012-9640
651-213-4200
800-257-7810
Fax: 651-213-4426
www.hazelden.org
Addressing such issues as self-esteem, fear, anger, and spirituality, these 366 daily meditations and affirmations integrate the physical, mental, and spiritual aspects of healing from addiction.
410 pages Paperback
ISBN: 1-568380-77-1
Sharon Birnbaum, Corporateÿ Director of Human Resources
Jim Blaha, VP CFO and CAO

8404 Came to Believe
Alcoholics Anonymous
PO Box 459
New York, NY 10163-0459
212-870-3400
Fax: 212-870-3137
www.aa.org

A collection of stories by AA members who write about what the phrase spiritual awakening means to them.
120 pages

8405 Chemically Dependent Older Adults
Hazelden
15251 Pleasant Valley Rd
Center City, MN 55012-9640
651-213-4200
800-257-7810
Fax: 651-213-4426
www.hazelden.org
Reviews the importance of considering the older adult's health, living conditions and social and economic resources when developing treatment and aftercare plans.
136 pages Paperback
Sharon Birnbaum, Corporateÿ Director of Human Resources
Jim Blaha, VP CFO and CAO

8406 Childhood and Adolescent Drug Abuse: A Physician's Guide
American Council on Drug Education
6001 Executive Boulevard
Bethesda, MD 20892-4425
301-443-1124
800-488-3784
www.drugabuse.gov
A scientific monograph which educates and sensitizes doctors to the dimensions of drug problems.
68 pages

8407 Circle of Hope
Hazelden
15251 Pleasant Valley Rd
Center City, MN 55012-9640
651-213-4200
800-257-7810
Fax: 651-213-4426
www.hazelden.org
Spirituality, acceptance, and living one day at a time are show through personal stories of individuals living with HIV and AIDS and dealing with adiction and recovery.
364 pages Paperback
ISBN: 0-894866-10-9
Sharon Birnbaum, Corporateÿ Director of Human Resources
Jim Blaha, VP CFO and CAO

8408 Citizen's Alcohol and Other Drug Prevention Directory
National Clearinghouse for Alcohol and Drug Info.
PO Box 2345
Rockville, MD 20847-2345
800-729-6686
National directory of over 3,000 state, local and government agencies dealing with alcohol and other drug-related topics.
276 pages

8409 Cocaine Today
American Council on Drug Education
6001 Executive Boulevard
Bethesda, MD 20892-4425
301-443-1124
800-488-3784
www.drugabuse.gov
A recent revision of this popular book. Cocaine Today takes a new look at cocaine and its derivative, crack.

8410 Codependent No More
Hazelden
15251 Pleasant Valley Rd
Center City, MN 55012-9640
651-213-4200
800-257-7810
Fax: 651-213-4793
e-mail: info@hazelden.org
www.hazelden.org
Explains codependent behaviors in clear, simple terms.
208 pages Paperback
Mark Mishek, President and Chief Executive Officer
Joe Jaksha, Publisher

8411 Color of Light
Hazelden
15251 Pleasant Valley Rd
Center City, MN 55012-9640
651-213-4200
800-257-7810
Fax: 651-213-4793
e-mail: info@hazelden.org
www.hazelden.org
These 366 meditations speak to both the practical and spiritual journey of living with HIV/AIDS, and demonstrate how to inte-

grate personal values with those offered in chemical dependency recovery and the Twelve Steps.
400 pages Paperback
ISBN: 0-894865-11-0
Mark Mishek, President and Chief Executive Officer
Joe Jaksha, Publisher

8412   Confusion is a State of Grace
Hazelden
15251 Pleasant Valley Rd   651-213-4200
Center City, MN 55012   800-257-7810
                                          Fax: 651-213-4793
                                  e-mail: info@hazelden.org
                                          www.hazelden.org
Compilation of quotes that captures the wisdom, humor, and healing found in Al-Anon and other Twelve Step groups.
153 pages Paperback
ISBN: 1-568380-89-5
Mark Mishek, President and Chief Executive Officer
Joe Jaksha, Publisher

8413   Courage to Be Me: Living with Alcoholism
Al-Anon Family Group Headquarters
1600 Corp Landing Pkwy   757-563-1600
Virginia Beach, VA 23454-5617   800-425-2666
                                          Fax: 757-563-1655
                                   e-mail: wso@al-anon.org
                                       www.al-anon.alateen.org
Written for and by Alateens of all ages who will treasure the honesty and strength of recovery shown.
326 pages
ISBN: 0-910034-30-3
Caryn Johnson, Director Communications

8414   Daily Reflections: A Book of Reflections by AA Members for AA Members
Alcoholics Anonymous
PO Box 459   212-870-3400
New York, NY 10163-0459   Fax: 212-870-3137
                                               www.aa.org
AAs reflect on favorite quotations from A.A. literature. A reading for each day of the year.

8415   Day at a Time: Daily Reflections for Recovering People
Hazelden
15251 Pleasant Valley Rd   651-213-4200
Center City, MN 55012-9640   800-257-7810
                                          Fax: 651-213-4793
                                  e-mail: info@hazelden.org
                                          www.hazelden.org
Offers inspiration and hope for people recovering from chemical dependency or other addictions. Each daily passage reinforces the message of Twelve Step recovery.
384 pages Paperback
ISBN: 1-568380-36-4
Mark Mishek, President and Chief Executive Officer
Joe Jaksha, Publisher

8416   Day by Day
Hazelden
15251 Pleasant Valley Rd   651-213-4200
Center City, MN 55012   800-257-7810
                                          Fax: 651-213-4793
                                  e-mail: info@hazelden.org
                                          www.hazelden.org
A book of daily meditations for recovering addicts that reinforce Narcotics Anonymous principles and objectives.
400 pages Paperback
Mark Mishek, President and Chief Executive Officer
Joe Jaksha, Publisher

8417   Days of Healing, Days of Joy
Hazelden
15251 Pleasant Valley Rd   651-213-4200
Center City, MN 55012-9640   800-257-7810
                                          Fax: 651-213-4793
                                  e-mail: info@hazelden.org
                                          www.hazelden.org

Three hundred and sixty-six daily quotes, meditations and affirmations to help adult children in their search for serenity.
400 pages Paperback
Mark Mishek, President and Chief Executive Officer
Joe Jaksha, Publisher

8418   Developing Chemical Dependency Services for Black People
African American Family Services
2616 Nicollet Avenue S   612-871-7878
Minneapolis, MN 55408
This manual has been developed to address many of the questions asked by new or expanding programs as they establish new culturally specific initiatives for African-American clients.
78 pages

8419   Dilemma of the Alcoholic Marriage
Al-Anon Family Group Headquarters
1600 Corp Landing Pkwy   757-563-1600
Virginia Beach, VA 23454-5617   800-425-2666
                                          Fax: 757-563-1655
                                   e-mail: wso@al-anon.org
                                       www.al-anon.alateen.org
This book explores the problem of alcoholism in marriage and includes questions for applying the twelve steps to relationships.
100 pages
ISBN: 0-910034-18-4
Caryn Johnson, Director Communications

8420   Dr. Bob and the Good Oldtimers
Alcoholics Anonymous
PO Box 459   212-870-3400
New York, NY 10163-0459   Fax: 212-870-3137
                                               www.aa.org
The life story of the fellowship's co-founder, interwoven wth recollections of early AA in the Midwest.

8421   Drug Abuse and Addiction Information/Treatment Programs
American Business Directories
5711 S 86th Circle   402-593-4600
Omaha, NE 68127-4146   Fax: 402-331-1505
Number of entries is 9,425.

8422   Drug Use Among American High School Seniors, College Students & Youth
National Clearinghouse for Alcohol and Drug Info.
PO Box 2345
Rockville, MD 20847-2345   800-729-6686
Comprehensive reports presenting the results of the 16th national survey of the drug use and related attitudes of American high school seniors.
199 pages Volumes I & II

8423   Drugs and Pregnancy: It's Not Worth the Risk
American Council on Drug Education
204 Monroe Street
Rockville, MD 20850   800-488-3784
A scientific monograph for health care providers which teaches them to identify alcohol and drug problems in their patients.
48 pages

8424   Dual Diagnosis
Hazelden
15251 Pleasant Valley Rd   651-213-4200
Center City, MN 55012-9640   800-257-7810
                                          Fax: 651-213-4793
                                  e-mail: info@hazelden.org
                                          www.hazelden.org
Focuses on the issues surrounding the treatment of clients with co-existing chemical dependency and psychiatric conditions.
191 pages Paperback
Mark Mishek, President and Chief Executive Officer
Joe Jaksha, Publisher

8425   Dual Disorders
Hazelden
15251 Pleasant Valley Rd   651-213-4200
Center City, MN 55012-9640   800-257-7810
                                          Fax: 651-213-4793
                                  e-mail: info@hazelden.org
                                          www.hazelden.org

Presents case histories and analyses of psychiatric disorders.
140 pages Paperback
Mark Mishek, President and Chief Executive Officer
Joe Jaksha, Publisher

8426   Dual Disorders Recovery Book
Hazelden
15251 Pleasant Valley Rd   651-213-4200
Center City, MN 55012-9640   800-257-7810
                                      Fax: 651-213-4793
                          e-mail: info@hazelden.org
                                      www.hazelden.org
Helps individuals with dual disorders develop a plan for daily liv-
ing through a specially-designed Twelve-Step program.
242 pages Paperback
ISBN: 1-568380-34-8
Mark Mishek, President and Chief Executive Officer
Joe Jaksha, Publisher

8427   Each Day a New Beginning
Hazelden
15251 Pleasant Valley Rd   651-213-4200
Center City, MN 55012-9640   800-257-7810
                                      Fax: 651-213-4793
                          e-mail: info@hazelden.org
                                      www.hazelden.org
Promotes the development of a significant spiritual core for recov-
ery that can be enhanced throughout the rest of life.
400 pages Paperback
Mark Mishek, President and Chief Executive Officer
Joe Jaksha, Publisher

8428   Elephant in the Living Room: A Leader's Guide
Hazelden
15251 Pleasant Valley Rd   651-213-4200
Center City, MN 55012-9640   800-257-7810
                                      Fax: 651-213-4793
                          e-mail: info@hazelden.org
                                      www.hazelden.org
The adult companion to the classic children's book. Caretakers
learn how to explain addiction and its effect on the family to small
children who's parents or siblings are chemically dependent.
129 pages Paperback
ISBN: 1-568380-34-8
Mark Mishek, President and Chief Executive Officer
Joe Jaksha, Publisher

8429   Encyclopedia of Drug Abuse
Facts on File
11 Penn Plaza   212-967-8800
New York, NY 10001   800-322-8755
                                      Fax: 800-678-3633
                                      www.ncjrs.gov
More that 500 entries explore: specific drugs, countries, organizations, treatment programs, laws, medical terms, and psychosocial
concepts.
496 pages Hardcover

8430   Ethics for Addiction Professionals
Hazelden
15251 Pleasant Valley Rd   651-213-4200
Center City, MN 55012-9640   800-257-7810
                                      Fax: 651-213-4793
                          e-mail: info@hazelden.org
                                      www.hazelden.org
Probes crucial, complex ethical issues including counselor re-
lapse, paid referrals and discrimination.
60 pages
Mark Mishek, President and Chief Executive Officer
Joe Jaksha, Publisher

**8431   Extent and Adequacy of Insurance Coverage for Substance
Abuse I & II**
National Clearinghouse for Alcohol and Drug Info.
PO Box 2345
Rockville, MD 20847-2345   800-729-6686
These volumes examine the extent to which the cost of alcohol and
other drug treatments is covered by private insurance, public fi-
nancing and other sources.

8432   Eye Opener
Hazelden
15251 Pleasant Valley Rd   651-213-4200
Center City, MN 55012-9640   800-257-7810
                                      Fax: 651-213-4793
                          e-mail: info@hazelden.org
                                      www.hazelden.org
Daily meditations about understanding the Alcoholics Anony-
mous program, writen by a favorite early AA member and author.
380 pages Cloth
ISBN: 0-894860-23-2
Mark Mishek, President and Chief Executive Officer
Joe Jaksha, Publisher

**8433   Fact Is...Hispanic Parents Can Help Their Children Avoid
Alcohol/Drugs**
National Clearinghouse for Alcohol and Drug Info.
PO Box 2345
Rockville, MD 20852-2345   800-729-6686

8434   Feeding the Hungry Heart, the Experience of Compulsive Eating
Gurze Books
PO Box 2238
Carlsbad, CA 92018-2238   888-346-8205
                                     Fax: 760-434-5476
                          e-mail: gzcatl@aol.com
                                     www.bulimia.com
This is a widely respected, extremely readable book from Ms. Roth
and the many participants of early breaking free workshops. It is an
intimate, vulnerable sharing of experiences which continues to
touch and change lives.
212 pages Paperback

8435   Food for Thought: Daily Meditations for Overeaters
Hazelden
15251 Pleasant Valley Rd   651-213-4200
Center City, MN 55012-9640   800-257-7810
                                      Fax: 651-213-4793
                          e-mail: info@hazelden.org
                                      www.hazelden.org
Offers guidance in the early days of living a Twelve Step program.
400 pages Paperback
ISBN: 0-894860-90-9
Mark Mishek, President and Chief Executive Officer
Joe Jaksha, Publisher

8436   Forum Favorites: Volumes 1, 2, 3 & 4
Al-Anon Family Group Headquarters
1600 Corp Landing Pkwy   757-563-1600
Virginia Beach, VA 23454-5617   800-425-2666
                                      Fax: 757-563-1655
                          e-mail: wso@al-anon.org
                                     www.al-anon.alateen.org
Personal sharings show how the fundamentals of the Al-Anon pro-
grams are applied to everyday situations.
428 pages Set of 4
ISBN: 0-910034-51-6
Caryn Johnson, Director Communications

8437   Freedom from Smoking at Work Program
American Lung Association
55 W. Wacker Drive   312-801-7630
Chicago, IL 60601   800-548-8252
                                      Fax: 202-452-1805
                                      www.lungusa.org
ALA program for organizations interested in creating a healthier
workplace environment through a comprehensive,
multicomponent smoking education, cessation and policy devel-
opment program designed for the workplace.
Kathryn A. Forbes, Chairman
Harold Wimmer, President and CEO

8438   Future by Design/A Community Framework
National Clearinghouse for Alcohol and Drug Info.
PO Box 2345
Rockville, MD 20847-2345   800-729-6686
Provides communities with a manageable framework for getting
involved in alcohol and other drug prevention.
234 pages

8439 Gentle Path Through the Twelve Steps
Hazelden
15251 Pleasant Valley Rd
Center City, MN 55012-9640
651-213-4200
800-257-7810
Fax: 651-213-4793
e-mail: info@hazelden.org
www.hazelden.org
This workbook provides a unique set of structured forms and exercises to help recoving people integrate the Twelve Steps in all aspects of their lives.
224 pages Paperback
ISBN: 1-568380-58-5
Mark Mishek, President and Chief Executive Officer
Joe Jaksha, Publisher

8440 Getting Started in AA
Hazelden
15251 Pleasant Valley Rd
Center City, MN 55012-9640
651-213-4200
800-257-7810
Fax: 651-213-4793
e-mail: info@hazelden.org
www.hazelden.org
Practical suggestions for staying sober, summaries of AA principles, concepts, and slogans, and a historical overview to help the reader understand the spirit of the program.
211 pages Paperback
ISBN: 1-568380-91-7
Mark Mishek, President and Chief Executive Officer
Joe Jaksha, Publisher

8441 Getting Tough on Gateway Drugs: A Guide for the Family
American Council On Drug Education
204 Monroe Street
Rockville, MD 20850-4425
301-294-0603
800-488-3784
Gateway drugs including marijuana, alcohol and tobacco are those which open doors into all drug abuse. This family survival guide helps parents understand the consequences of drug dependence and suggests actions the family can take to prevent and solve drug problems.
332 pages
William F Current, Executive Director

8442 Getting it Together: Promoting Drug Free Communities
National Clearinghouse for Alcohol and Drug Info.
PO Box 2345
Rockville, MD 20847
800-729-6686
Provides resources and step-by-step information on how local communities and organizations can work effectively with young people who are committed to preventing alcohol and other drug abuse.
71 pages

8443 God Grant Me the Laughter: A Treasury of Twelve Step Humor
Hazelden
15251 Pleasant Valley Rd
Center City, MN 55012-9640
651-213-4200
800-257-7810
Fax: 651-213-4793
e-mail: info@hazelden.org
www.hazelden.org
Hearty cartoons and humorous anecdotes clearly demonstrate how readers' lives today contrast with their drinking and drug using in the past.
200 pages Paperback
ISBN: 1-568380-38-0
Mark Mishek, President and Chief Executive Officer
Joe Jaksha, Publisher

8444 Good First Step
Hazelden
15251 Pleasant Valley Rd
Center City, MN 55012-9640
651-213-4200
800-257-7810
Fax: 651-213-4793
e-mail: info@hazelden.org
www.hazelden.org
Features a structured format and emphasis on the meaning of the First Step to help build a solid foundation for recovery.
60 pages Paperback
ISBN: 1-568381-13-1
Mark Mishek, President and Chief Executive Officer
Joe Jaksha, Publisher

8445 Goodbye Hangovers, Hello Life
Women for Sobriety
PO Box 618
Quakertown, PA 18951-0618
215-536-8026
Fax: 215-536-9026
e-mail: newlife@nni.com
www.womenforsobriety.org
A book about recovery - how it happens, what problems arise and how to overcome these problems.
250 pages Paperback

8446 Grateful to Have Been There
Hazelden
15251 Pleasant Valley Rd
Center City, MN 55012
651-213-4200
800-257-7810
Fax: 651-213-4793
e-mail: info@hazelden.org
www.hazelden.org
Aide and executive secretary to AA's co-founder Bill W. for 20 years, Wing shares her memories and impressions of 42 years of involvement with the Fellowship.
150 pages Paperback
ISBN: 0-942421-44-2
Mark Mishek, President and Chief Executive Officer
Joe Jaksha, Publisher

8447 Growing Up Drug Free: A Parent's Guide to Prevention
National Clearinghouse for Alcohol and Drug Info.
400 Maryland Ave, SW
Washington, DC 20202
202-260-3954
800-729-6686
www.jtnn.org
Offers information on what parents can do to prevent their child from becoming a substance abuser/alcoholic. Focuses on counseling, peer pressure issues, education, school-parent cooperation and offers an introduction to each drug, symptoms and how to spot the warning signs of drug addiction.
47 pages

8448 Handle with Care
Hazelden
15251 Pleasant Valley Rd
Center City, MN 55012-9640
651-213-4200
800-257-7810
Fax: 651-213-4793
e-mail: info@hazelden.org
www.hazelden.org
A comprehensive look at how parents, teachers and other care givers of children ages 10 and younger can identify and meet their special needs.
Mark Mishek, President and Chief Executive Officer
Joe Jaksha, Publisher

8449 Help for Helpers: Daily Meditations for Counselors
Hazelden
15251 Pleasant Valley Rd
Center City, MN 55012-9640
651-213-4200
800-257-7810
Fax: 651-213-4793
e-mail: info@hazelden.org
www.hazelden.org
Written by addiction treatment center staff members from across the country, these daily meditations encourage, comfort, and challenge helpers to understand others and themselves.
400 pages Paperback
ISBN: 1-568380-61-5
Mark Mishek, President and Chief Executive Officer
Joe Jaksha, Publisher

8450 Helping Homeless People with Alcohol and Other Drug Problems
National Clearinghouse for Alcohol and Drug Info.
PO Box 2345
Rockville, MD 20847
800-729-6686
Developed by professionals who work directly with homeless people, this manual provides basic information about homeless people with AOD problems.
50 pages

8451 Helping Your Students Say No Teacher's Guide
National Clearinghouse for Alcohol and Drug Info.
PO Box 2345
Rockville, MD 20847-2345
800-729-6686
TDD: 800-487-4489

Explains the effects of alcohol on the body, why children start to drink, how teachers can help their students refuse alcohol and deal with the first signs of drinking.
13 pages
Lynn Hallard, Author

8452 **How to Manage Your Drug-Free Workplace Programs**
American Council on Drug Education
204 Monroe Street
Rockville, MD 20850-4425   800-488-3784
                                                 www.ascicorp.com
Step-by-step process for introducing and managing a drug awareness program that includes a variety of additional tips to complement messages in the drug awareness pamphlet series.
48 pages

8453 **I'm Black and I'm Sober**
Hazelden
15251 Pleasant Valley Rd   651-213-4200
Center City, MN 55012-9640   800-257-7810
                                            Fax: 651-213-4793
                                    e-mail: info@hazelden.org
                                            www.hazelden.org
An autobiography written by a recovering African American woman who discusses the impact of discrimination and the obstacles faced through the journey back to sobriety.
279 pages Paperback
ISBN: 1-568380-71-2
Mark Mishek, President and Chief Executive Officer
Joe Jaksha, Publisher

8454 **If Only I Could Quit**
Hazelden
15251 Pleasant Valley Rd   651-213-4200
Center City, MN 55012-9640   800-257-7810
                                            Fax: 651-213-4793
                                    e-mail: info@hazelden.org
                                            www.hazelden.org
Promotes the Twelve Step process for recovery from nicotine addiction.
320 pages Paperback
Mark Mishek, President and Chief Executive Officer
Joe Jaksha, Publisher

8455 **In God's Care**
Hazelden
15251 Pleasant Valley Rd   651-213-4200
Center City, MN 55012-9640   800-257-7810
                                            Fax: 651-213-4793
                                    e-mail: info@hazelden.org
                                            www.hazelden.org
Excellent relaxation and education tool for clients working on their Second and Third Steps.
400 pages Paperback
Mark Mishek, President and Chief Executive Officer
Joe Jaksha, Publisher

8456 **Keep Quit**
Hazelden
15251 Pleasant Valley Rd   651-213-4200
Center City, MN 55012-9640   800-257-7810
                                            Fax: 651-213-4793
                                    e-mail: info@hazelden.org
                                            www.hazelden.org
Daily motivational guide to help the new nonsmoker understand the craving for nicotine and learn how to break the rituals and patterns associated with relapse.
300 pages Paperback
ISBN: 1-568381-04-2
Mark Mishek, President and Chief Executive Officer
Joe Jaksha, Publisher

8457 **Keep it Simple**
Hazelden
15251 Pleasant Valley Rd   651-213-4200
Center City, MN 55012-9640   800-257-7810
                                            Fax: 651-213-4793
                                    e-mail: info@hazelden.org
                                            www.hazelden.org

Daily prayers that help clients learn to ask for help and to turn their self-will over to a Higher Power.
400 pages Paperback
Mark Mishek, President and Chief Executive Officer
Joe Jaksha, Publisher

8458 **Learning to Live Drug Free: A Curriculum Model for Prevention**
National Clearinghouse for Alcohol and Drug Info.
PO Box 2345
Rockville, MD 20847-2345   800-729-6686
Provides a flexible framework for classroom-based prevention efforts for kindergarten through grade 12.
52 pages

8459 **Let's Talk About Alcohol Abuse**
Rosen Publishing Group's PowerKids Press
29 East 21st Street   212-777-3017
New York, NY 10010   800-237-9932
                                            Fax: 888-436-4643
                        e-mail: customerservice@rosenpub.com
                                        www.rosenpublishing.com
In gentle and sensitive terms this book talks about when a parent drinks and what alcohol can do to the body. Kids are told about the illegality of drinking as minors. Recommended for grade K-4.

ISBN: 0-823923-03-7
Marianne Johnston, Author

8460 **Life of My Own: Daily Meditations on Hope and Acceptance**
Hazelden
15251 Pleasant Valley Rd   651-213-4200
Center City, MN 55012-9640   800-257-7810
                                            Fax: 651-213-4793
                                    e-mail: info@hazelden.org
                                            www.hazelden.org
Offers daily access to strength, serenity, and insight in our relationships with chemically dependent people.
400 pages Paperback
ISBN: 0-894868-63-2
Mark Mishek, President and Chief Executive Officer
Joe Jaksha, Publisher

8461 **Little Red Book**
Hazelden
15251 Pleasant Valley Rd   651-213-4200
Center City, MN 55012-9640   800-257-7810
                                            Fax: 651-213-4793
                                    e-mail: info@hazelden.org
                                            www.hazelden.org
A primer for members of Alcoholics Anonymous. Each page acts as a study guide to the Big Book and its teachings.
164 pages Paperback
ISBN: 0-894869-85-X
Mark Mishek, President and Chief Executive Officer
Joe Jaksha, Publisher

8462 **Living Sober**
Hazelden
15251 Pleasant Valley Rd   651-213-4200
Center City, MN 55012-9640   800-257-7810
                                            Fax: 651-213-4793
                                    e-mail: info@hazelden.org
                                            www.hazelden.org
Offers clients sound advice about how to stay sober.
88 pages Paperback
Mark Mishek, President and Chief Executive Officer
Joe Jaksha, Publisher

8463 **Lois Remembers**
Al-Anon Family Group Headquarters
1600 Corp Landing Pkwy   757-563-1600
Virginia Beach, VA 23454-5617   800-425-2666
                                            Fax: 757-563-1655
                                    e-mail: wso@al-anon.org
                                    www.al-anon.alateen.org

The memoirs of a co-founder of Al-Anon. Lois tells her personal story and recalls the eventful years before and after the founding of AA and Al-Anon.
204 pages
ISBN: 0-910034-23-0
Caryn Johnson, Director Communications

8464   Marijuana
Branden Publishing Company
PO Box 812094   617-734-2045
Wellesley, MA 02482   Fax: 617-734-2046
                                                                        www.branden.com
Paperback
ISBN: 0-828319-49-9

8465   Marijuana Smoking Prevention Program for Schools
American Lung Association
1740 Broadway
New York, NY 10017   212-315-8700
                                                education.drugfreeworld.org
Cast of the TV show FAME enlivens highly motivational program to inform parents about the dangers of pot and discourages 9-11 year olds from using it.

8466   Marijuana Today
American Council on Drug Education
204 Monroe Street   301-762-0505
Rockville, MD 20850-4425   800-488-3784
                                                                Fax: 301-762-0080
                                            e-mail: info@armstrongcheris.com
                                                        www.armstrongcheris.com
A revision of the long time bestseller, this book examines the history of marijuana, its use, the risks associated with use and the short and long-term effects of use.

8467   Marijuana and Reproduction
American Council on Drug Education
204 Monroe Street   301-762-0505
Rockville, MD 20850-4425   800-488-3784
                                                                Fax: 301-762-0080
                                            e-mail: info@armstrongcheris.com
                                                        www.armstrongcheris.com
A scientific monograph for physicians which describes marijuana, profiles the users and discusses the effects on the reproductive system.
30 pages

8468   Marketing Booze to Blacks
African American Family Services
2616 Nicollet Avenue S   612-871-7878
Minneapolis, MN 55408
This controversial book details how liquor industries target the black population with its advertising.
55 pages

8469   Mistaken Beliefs About Relapse
Hazelden
15251 Pleasant Valley Rd   651-213-4200
Center City, MN 55012-9640   800-257-7810
                                                                Fax: 651-213-4793
                                                    e-mail: info@hazelden.org
                                                                www.hazelden.org
Examines mistaken beliefs people have about relapse.
30 pages Paperback
Mark Mishek, President and Chief Executive Officer
Joe Jaksha, Publisher

8470   My Mind is Out to Get Me: Humor and Wisdom in Recovery
Hazelden
15251 Pleasant Valley Rd   651-213-4200
Center City, MN 55012   800-257-7810
                                                                Fax: 651-213-4793
                                                    e-mail: info@hazelden.org
                                                                www.hazelden.org
Five hundred inspirational sayings and slogans that reflect both the lighter side of living a sober life and the profound wisdom of-

fered in recovery. Each quote has been drawn from the wisdom of Alcoholics Anonymous.
180 pages Paperback
ISBN: 1-568380-10-0
Mark Mishek, President and Chief Executive Officer
Joe Jaksha, Publisher

8471   Narcotics Anonymous
Hazelden
15251 Pleasant Valley Rd   651-213-4200
Center City, MN 55012-9640   800-257-7810
                                                                Fax: 651-213-4793
                                                    e-mail: info@hazelden.org
                                                                www.hazelden.org
Men and women describe the N.A. program and how it works.
289 pages Paperback
Mark Mishek, President and Chief Executive Officer
Joe Jaksha, Publisher

8472   National Conference on Drug Abuse Researcg & Practice
National Clearinghouse for Alcohol and Drug Info.
PO Box 2345
Rockville, MD 20847   800-729-6686
Offers summaries of workshops, forums, dinner speeches and sessions presented at the National Conference on Drug Abuse Research and Practice.
275 pages
Alan I Leshner, Director
Donna E Shalala, secretary

8473   National Directory of Drug Abuse and Alcoholism Treatment and Programs
US National Institute On Drug Abuse
6001 Executive Boulevard   301-443-1124
Bethesda, ML 20892   e-mail: NIDANEWS@list.nih.gov
                                                                www.nida.nih.gov
Eleven thousand listings of agencies that administer treatment and services on the federal, state and local levels.
Nora D. Volkow, Director

8474   Night Light: A Book of Nighttime Meditations
Hazelden
15251 Pleasant Valley Rd   651-213-4200
Center City, MN 55012-9640   800-257-7810
                                                                Fax: 651-213-4793
                                                    e-mail: info@hazelden.org
                                                                www.hazelden.org
Three hundred and sixty-six meditations designed to help relax and encourage prayer. Reminds readers to look to their Higher Power for strength, reassurance, comfort, and guidance.
400 pages Paperback
ISBN: 0-894863-81-9
Mark Mishek, President and Chief Executive Officer
Joe Jaksha, Publisher

8475   Not God: A History of Alcoholics Anonymous
Hazelden
15251 Pleasant Valley Rd   651-213-4200
Center City, MN 55012-9640   800-257-7810
                                                                Fax: 651-213-4793
                                                    e-mail: info@hazelden.org
                                                                www.hazelden.org
Documenting AA's philosophical and social development within the larger context of American culture, this book follows the remarkable story of the evolution of a small group of Depression-era alcoholics into a worldwide movement.
436 pages Paperback
ISBN: 0-894860-65-8
Mark Mishek, President and Chief Executive Officer
Joe Jaksha, Publisher

8476   Occupational Therapy Practice Guidelines for Adults with Substance Use Disorders
American Occupational Therapy Association

4720 Montgomery Lane
Bethesda, MD 20814-1220
301-652-6611
800-729-2682
Fax: 240-762-5150
TDD: 800-377-8555
e-mail: praota@aota.org.
www.aota.org

22 pages
ISBN: 1-569001-60-X

8477   Of Course You're Angry
Hazelden
15251 Pleasant Valley Rd
Center City, MN 55012-9640
651-213-4200
800-257-7810
Fax: 651-213-4793
e-mail: info@hazelden.org
www.hazelden.org
Revised edition dealing with the nature and resolution of anger. Demonstrates how to make anger work in a positive and effective way that can ease, rather than exacerbate, the challenges of early recovery.
120 pages Paperback
ISBN: 1-568381-41-7
Mark Mishek, President and Chief Executive Officer
Joe Jaksha, Publisher

8478   One Day at a Time in Al-Anon
Al-Anon Family Group Headquarters
1600 Corp Landing Pkwy
Virginia Beach, VA 23454-5617
757-563-1600
800-425-2666
Fax: 757-563-1655
e-mail: wso@al-anon.org
www.al-anon.alateen.org
Inspirational daily readings cover various aspects of the Al-Anon philosopha and relate it to everyday situations.
376 pages
ISBN: 0-910034-21-4
Caryn Johnson, Director Communications

8479   Operation PAR
National Clearinghouse for Alcohol and Drug Info.
PO Box 2345
Rockville, MD 20847-2345
800-729-6686
Describes successful community alcohol and other drug abuse prevention and treatment programs.
40 pages

8480   Parent Training is Prevention
National Clearinghouse for Alcohol and Drug Info.
PO Box 2345
Rockville, MD 20847-2345
800-729-6686
www.sdsalarms.com
Contains information to help communities identify and carry out programs on parenting.
184 pages

8481   Pass it On
Alcoholics Anonymous
Grand Central Station
New York, NY 10163
212-870-3400
Fax: 212-870-3137
www.aa.org
The story of Bill Wilson, the co-founder of AA and the development of the Fellowship.

8482   Passages Through Recovery
Hazelden
15251 Pleasant Valley Rd
Center City, MN 55012-9640
651-213-4200
800-257-7810
Fax: 651-213-4793
e-mail: info@hazelden.org
www.hazelden.org
Guides clients through the six stages of recovery.
130 pages Paperback
Mark Mishek, President and Chief Executive Officer
Joe Jaksha, Publisher

8483   Peer Pressure Reversal
Human Resource Development Press
22 Amherst Road
Amherst, MA 01002-9730
413-253-3488

8484   Pregnancy and Exposure to Alcohol and Other Drug Use
National Clearinghouse for Alcohol and Drug Info.
PO Box 2345
Rockville, MD 20847-2345
800-729-6686
www.health.org
This report is for health care professionals presenting the state-of-the-art information about preventing ATOD use among women of childbearing age.

8485   Preparing for the Drug-Free Years: A Family Activity Book
Developmental Research and Programs
130 Nickerson Street
Seattle, WA 98145-1746
206-286-1805
800-736-2630
Fax: 206-286-1462
www.drp.org

8486   Presence at the Center
Hazelden
15251 Pleasant Valley Rd
Center City, MN 55012-9640
651-213-4200
800-257-7810
Fax: 651-213-4793
e-mail: info@hazelden.org
www.hazelden.org
About a new way of life that addresses transformation, change, the presence of a Higher Power, letting go of reluctance and fear, and the freedom commitment can bring.
76 pages Paperback
ISBN: 1-568380-01-1
Mark Mishek, President and Chief Executive Officer
Joe Jaksha, Publisher

8487   Prevention Plus II: Tools for Creating & Sustaining a Drug-Free Community
National Clearinghouse for Alcohol and Drug Info.
PO Box 2345
Rockville, MD 20847-2345
800-729-6686
www.health.org
Provides a framework for organizing or expanding community alcohol and other drug problem prevention activities for youth into a coordinated, complimentary system.
541 pages

8488   Prevention Plus III: Assessing Alcohol & Other Prevention Programs
National Clearinghouse for Alcohol and Drug Info.
PO Box 2345
Rockville, MD 20847-2345
800-729-6686
www.health.org
Provides tools and techniques for alcohol and other drug prevention, planning and implementation.
470 pages

8489   Prevention Resource Guide: Alcohol and Other Drug Related Periodicals
National Clearinghouse for Alcohol and Drug Info.
PO Box 2345
Rockville, MD 20847-2345
800-729-6686
www.health.org
Provides a concise annotated bibliography of journals, newsletters and other publications related to the AOD prevention field.
12 pages

8490   Prevention Resource Guide: American Indian/Native Alaskans
National Clearinghouse for Alcohol and Drug Info.
PO Box 2345
Rockville, MD 20847-2345
800-729-6686
www.health.org
This resource guide is a survey of current data on alcohol abuse among American Indians and Native Alaskans.
24 pages

8491   Prevention Resource Guide: Asian and Pacific Islander Americans
National Clearinghouse for Alcohol and Drug Info.
PO Box 2345
Rockville, MD 20847-2345
800-729-6686
www.health.org
Contains facts and figures about Asian and Pacific Islander Americans and alcohol and other drug prevention.
13 pages

8492 Prevention Resource Guide: Elementary Youth
National Clearinghouse for Alcohol and Drug Info.
PO Box 2345
Rockville, MD 20847-2345   800-729-6686
                                 www.health.org
This resource guide includes materials specifically developed for
youth that may be used in an elementary school setting.
23 pages

**8493 Prevention Resource Guide: Pregnant Postpartum Women and
Their Infants**
National Clearinghouse for Alcohol and Drug Info.
PO Box 2345
Rockville, MD 20847-2345   800-729-6686
                                 www.health.org
This resource guide targets health care providers, prevention pro-
gram planners and counselors of pregnant and postpartum women
between the ages of 15 and 44.
30 pages

8494 Prevention Resource Guide: Secondary School Students
National Clearinghouse for Alcohol and Drug Info.
PO Box 2345
Rockville, MD 20847-2345   800-729-6686
                                 www.health.org
This resource guide targets teachers, administrators and program
leaders who come in contact with secondary school youth.
27 pages

8495 Prevention Resource Guide: Women
National Clearinghouse for Alcohol and Drug Info.
PO Box 2345
Rockville, MD 20847-2345   800-729-6686
                                 www.health.org
This resource guide provides the latest information about the ef-
fects of drugs and alcohol on women.
32 pages

8496 Prevention in Action
National Clearinghouse for Alcohol and Drug Info.
PO Box 2345
Rockville, MD 20847-2345   800-729-6686
Provides descriptions selected by representatives of national orga-
nizations and State alcohol and drug agency representatives.
20 pages

8497 Program for You
Hazelden
15251 Pleasant Valley Rd   651-213-4200
Center City, MN 55012-9640   800-257-7810
                                 Fax: 651-213-4793
                                 e-mail: info@hazelden.org
                                 www.hazelden.org
Study guide interpreting the original AA program as described in
Alcoholics Anonymous and helps apply the wisdom to everyday
life.
183 pages Paperback
ISBN: 0-894867-41-5
Mark Mishek, President and Chief Executive Officer
Joe Jaksha, Publisher

8498 Promise of a New Day: A Book of Daily Meditations
Hazelden
15251 Pleasant Valley Rd   651-213-4200
Center City, MN 55012-9640   800-257-7810
                                 Fax: 651-213-4793
                                 e-mail: info@hazelden.org
                                 www.hazelden.org
Simple, inspiring wisdom about creating and maintaining inner
peace. Each of the 366 daily meditations expresses the essence of
Twelve Step spirituality without the program jargon.
400 pages Paperback
ISBN: 0-894862-03-0
Mark Mishek, President and Chief Executive Officer
Joe Jaksha, Publisher

8499 Quit & Stay Quit: A Personal Program to Stop Smoking
Hazelden

15251 Pleasant Valley Rd   651-213-4200
Center City, MN 55012-9640   800-257-7810
                                 Fax: 651-213-4793
                                 e-mail: info@hazelden.org
                                 www.hazelden.org
Guide to nicotine recovery offerring an effective long-term pro-
gram to quit by showing readers how smoking has subtly shaped
their values, attitudes, and lives.
196 pages Paperback
ISBN: 1-568381-09-3
Mark Mishek, President and Chief Executive Officer
Joe Jaksha, Publisher

8500 Quit Smoking Manual
American Lung Association
1740 Broadway   212-315-8700
Silver Spring, MD 20907-4315   800-358-9295
                                 www.tobaccoprogram.org
Original self-help smoking cessation manual showing the public
how to quit smoking in 20 days.
64 pages

8501 Recovery Journal for Exploring Who I Am
Hazelden
15251 Pleasant Valley Rd   651-213-4200
Center City, MN 55012-9640   800-257-7810
                                 Fax: 651-213-4793
                                 e-mail: info@hazelden.org
                                 www.hazelden.org
Introduces clients to journal writing as an effective therapeutic ad-
junct for addiction recovery.
48 pages
Mark Mishek, President and Chief Executive Officer
Joe Jaksha, Publisher

8502 School Answers Back: Responding to Student Drug Use
American Council on Drug Education
204 Monroe Street
Rockville, MD 20850   800-488-3784
Provides teachers, counselors, administrators and parents with a
model for schools to use in confronting drug and alcohol abuse.
145 pages

8503 Search for Serenity
Hazelden
15251 Pleasant Valley Rd   651-213-4200
Center City, MN 55012-9640   800-257-7810
                                 Fax: 651-213-4793
                                 e-mail: info@hazelden.org
                                 www.hazelden.org
Provides clients with practical inspiration to change their feelings
toward people and situations.
152 pages Paperback
Mark Mishek, President and Chief Executive Officer
Joe Jaksha, Publisher

8504 Shame Faced
Hazelden
15251 Pleasant Valley Rd   651-213-4200
Center City, MN 55012-9640   800-257-7810
                                 Fax: 651-213-4793
                                 e-mail: info@hazelden.org
                                 www.hazelden.org
Discusses the relationship between shame and chemical depend-
ency.
28 pages
Mark Mishek, President and Chief Executive Officer
Joe Jaksha, Publisher

8505 Skeptic's Guide to the 12 Steps
Hazelden
15251 Pleasant Valley Rd   651-213-4200
Center City, MN 55012-9640   800-257-7810
                                 Fax: 651-213-4793
                                 e-mail: info@hazelden.org
                                 www.hazelden.org

Investigates each of the 12 steps to gain a deeper understanding of a Higher Power.
241 pages Paperback
Mark Mishek, President and Chief Executive Officer
Joe Jaksha, Publisher

8506 **Smoking and Pregnancy Kit for Health Care Providers**
American Lung Association
1740 Broadway   212-315-8700
New York, NY 10019-4315
A program kit for health care providers designed to educate pregnant women not to smoke and to help them kick the habit.

8507 **Smoking, Drinking & Illicit Drug Use**
National Clearinghouse for Alcohol and Drug Info.
PO Box 2345
Rockville, MD 20847-2345   800-729-6686
www.healthieryou.com
Comprehensive reports representing the results of the 12th national survey on drug use and analyzing data collected from young Americans from 1975-1991.

8508 **Sober But Stuck**
Hazelden
15251 Pleasant Valley Rd   651-213-4200
Center City, MN 55012-9640   800-257-7810
Fax: 651-213-4793
e-mail: info@hazelden.org
www.hazelden.org
Collection of personal stories by men and women who are long-time members of Alcoholics Anonymous. Each story shares the anecdotes and resources which helped members break through the barriers that limited their enjoyment of a sober life.
215 pages Paperback
ISBN: 1-568380-78-X
Mark Mishek, President and Chief Executive Officer
Joe Jaksha, Publisher

8509 **Social Policy Prevention Handbook**
African American Family Services
2616 Nicollet Avenue S   612-871-7878
Minneapolis, MN 55408
A manual that details IBCA's community based approach to the development of alcohol and drug abuse prevention strategies.
24 pages

8510 **Staying Clean**
Hazelden
15251 Pleasant Valley Rd   651-213-4200
Center City, MN 55012-9640   800-257-7810
Fax: 651-213-4793
e-mail: info@hazelden.org
www.hazelden.org
Each section focuses on one of 33 proven ideas for staying drug-free, such as professional help, prayer, support groups and meditation.
76 pages Paperback
Mark Mishek, President and Chief Executive Officer
Joe Jaksha, Publisher

8511 **Staying Sober**
Hazelden
15251 Pleasant Valley Rd   651-213-4200
Center City, MN 55012-9640   800-257-7810
Fax: 651-213-4793
e-mail: info@hazelden.org
www.hazelden.org
Discusses addictive diseases and its physical, psychological and social effects.
228 pages Paperback
Mark Mishek, President and Chief Executive Officer
Joe Jaksha, Publisher

8512 **Step Zero: Getting to Recovery**
Hazelden
15251 Pleasant Valley Rd   651-213-4200
Center City, MN 55012-9640   800-257-7810
Fax: 651-213-4793
e-mail: info@hazelden.org
www.hazelden.org

Explains the concepts of Step Zero, when clients drop their defenses, begin to face themselves and start to assess their behavior and the reasons for it.
170 pages Paperback
Mark Mishek, President and Chief Executive Officer
Joe Jaksha, Publisher

8513 **Stools and Bottles**
Hazelden
15251 Pleasant Valley Rd   651-213-4200
Center City, MN 55012-9640   800-257-7810
Fax: 651-213-4793
e-mail: info@hazelden.org
www.hazelden.org
Depicts the first Three steps using a three-legged stool and eight whiskey bottles representing character defects revealed when working Step Four.
160 pages Hardcover
Mark Mishek, President and Chief Executive Officer
Joe Jaksha, Publisher

8514 **Substance Abuse and Physical Disability**
Allen Heinemann, PhD, author
Haworth Press
9400 Universal Boulevard   607-722-5857
Orlando, FL 32819-1580   866-860-1971
Fax: 607-722-0012
www.haworthpress.com
This book offers information on alcohol and drug abuse being a contributing factor in traumatic and disabling injuries.
1993 289 pages Hardcover
ISBN: 1-560242-89-3
Amie Gilmore, Show Director
Kerry Cree, Sales Manager

8515 **Success Stories from Drug-Free Schools**
National Clearinghouse for Alcohol and Drug Info.
PO Box 2345
Rockville, MD 20847-2345   800-729-6686
www.health.org
Salutes the 107 schools honored by the US Department of Education's Drug-Free Recognition Program.
59 pages

8516 **Tackling Alcohol Problems on Campus: Tools for Media Advocacy**
National Clearinghouse for Alcohol and Drug Info.
PO Box 2345
Rockville, MD 20857-2345   800-729-6686
www.nacoa.org
Reviews the role of alcohol on campus and shows how to use the media to get attention and support.
38 pages
Stephanie Loebs, Chairman
Peter Palanca, Vice Chairman

8517 **Team Up for Drug Prevention with America's Young Athletes**
Drug Enforcement Administration, Demand Reduction
1405 I Street NW
Washington, DC 20537-0001   202-307-5550
www.dea.gov
Michele M. Leonhart, DEA Administrator

8518 **Ten Steps to Help Your Child Say No: A Parent's Guide**
National Clearinghouse for Alcohol and Drug Info.
PO Box 2345
Rockville, MD 20847-2345   800-729-6686

8519 **Things My Sponsors Taught Me**
Hazelden
15251 Pleasant Valley Rd   651-213-4200
Center City, MN 55012-9640   800-257-7810
Fax: 651-213-4793
e-mail: info@hazelden.org
www.hazelden.org
Features AA philosophy, quotes, slogans and refreshing reminders.
76 pages Paperback
Mark Mishek, President and Chief Executive Officer
Joe Jaksha, Publisher

8520 **Today I Will Do One Thing: Daily Readings for Awareness & Hope**
Hazelden
15251 Pleasant Valley Rd　　　　　　651-213-4200
Center City, MN 55012-9640　　　　　800-257-7810
　　　　　　　　　　　　　　　　Fax: 651-213-4793
　　　　　　　　　　　　e-mail: info@hazelden.org
　　　　　　　　　　　　　　　www.hazelden.org
Specially designed to integrate recovery from addiction with the treatment of emotional or psychiatric illness. Each meditation focuses on a task or goal to be completed each day.
400 pages Paperback
ISBN: 1-568380-83-6
Mark Mishek, President and Chief Executive Officer
Joe Jaksha, Publisher

8521 **Today's Gift**
Hazelden
15251 Pleasant Valley Rd　　　　　　651-213-4200
Center City, MN 55012-9640　　　　　800-257-7810
　　　　　　　　　　　　　　　　Fax: 651-213-4793
　　　　　　　　　　　　e-mail: info@hazelden.org
　　　　　　　　　　　　　　　www.hazelden.org
Inspiring meditations bringing families together and strengthening family bonds.
400 pages Paperback
Mark Mishek, President and Chief Executive Officer
Joe Jaksha, Publisher

8522 **Touchstones**
Hazelden
15251 Pleasant Valley Rd　　　　　　651-213-4200
Center City, MN 55012-9640　　　　　800-257-7810
　　　　　　　　　　　　　　　　Fax: 651-213-4793
　　　　　　　　　　　　e-mail: info@hazelden.org
　　　　　　　　　　　　　　　www.hazelden.org
A book of daily meditations for men in the Twelve-Step program.
400 pages Paperback
Mark Mishek, President and Chief Executive Officer
Joe Jaksha, Publisher

8523 **Turnabout**
Women for Sobriety
14488 Old Stage Road
Lenoir City, TN 37772-0618　　　　Fax: 215-536-8026
　　　　　　　　　　　　e-mail: WFSobriey@aol.com
　　　　　　　　　　　　　　www.mediapulse.com
This is the story of the founder of Women for Sobriety and her struggle to quit drinking.
183 pages

8524 **Turning Awareness Into Action: What Your Community Can Do About Drug Use**
National Clearinghouse for Alcohol and Drug Info.
PO Box 2345
Rockville, MD 20847-2345　　　　　800-729-6686
　　　　　　　　　　　　　　　　www.health.org
This bilingual booklet is designed to show leaders at the grassroots level how to make the most of their talents and their community's resources.
73 pages

8525 **Twelve Step Sponsorship: How it Works**
Hazelden
15251 Pleasant Valley Rd　　　　　　651-213-4200
Center City, MN 55012-9640　　　　　800-257-7810
　　　　　　　　　　　　　　　　Fax: 651-213-4793
　　　　　　　　　　　　e-mail: info@hazelden.org
　　　　　　　　　　　　　　　www.hazelden.org
Complete handbook for working with a newcomer. Based on Twelve Step traditions and knowledge passed orally through the generations, this working manual defines the sponsorship role and guides sponsors through the rewards and pitfalls of reaching out to help new program members.
260 pages Paperback
ISBN: 1-568381-22-0
Mark Mishek, President and Chief Executive Officer
Joe Jaksha, Publisher

8526 **Twelve Steps and Traditions**
Hazelden
15251 Pleasant Valley Rd　　　　　　651-213-4200
Center City, MN 55012-9640　　　　　800-257-7810
　　　　　　　　　　　　　　　　Fax: 651-213-4793
　　　　　　　　　　　　e-mail: info@hazelden.org
　　　　　　　　　　　　　　　www.hazelden.org
Outlines the core principles by which AA members recover and by which the fellowship functions.
192 pages Paperback
Mark Mishek, President and Chief Executive Officer
Joe Jaksha, Publisher

8527 **Twelve Steps and Twelve Traditions**
Alcoholics Anonymous
PO Box 459　　　　　　　　　　　　212-870-3400
New York, NY 10163-0459　　　　　　800-328-9000
　　　　　　　　　　　　　　　　Fax: 212-870-3137
　　　　　　　　　　　　e-mail: info@hazelden.org
　　　　　　　　　　　　　　　www.hazelden.org
Twenty-four essays on the Steps and Traditions that discuss the principles of individual recovery and group unity.

8528 **Twelve Steps and Twelve Traditions for Alateen**
Al-Anon Family Group Headquarters
1600 Corp Landing Pkwy　　　　　　757-563-1600
Virginia Beach, VA 23454-5617　　　　800-425-2666
　　　　　　　　　　　　　　　　Fax: 757-563-1655
　　　　　　　　　　　　e-mail: wso@al-anon.org
　　　　　　　　　　　　www.al-anon.alateen.org
Questions, discussions and personal reflections of Alateen members.
60 pages
Caryn Johnson, Director Communications

8529 **Twelve Steps for Everyone...Who Really Wants Them**
Hazelden
15251 Pleasant Valley Rd　　　　　　651-213-4200
Center City, MN 55012-9640　　　　　800-257-7810
　　　　　　　　　　　　　　　　Fax: 651-213-4793
　　　　　　　　　　　　e-mail: info@hazelden.org
　　　　　　　　　　　　　　　www.hazelden.org
A basic primer outlining how spiritual and emotional health can be found by working and living the Twelve Steps. Emphasizes that the Twelve Steps are for anyone who wants to change.
208 pages Paperback
ISBN: 1-568380-47-X
Mark Mishek, President and Chief Executive Officer
Joe Jaksha, Publisher

8530 **Twelve Steps of Alcoholics Anonymous**
Hazelden
15251 Pleasant Valley Rd　　　　　　651-213-4200
Center City, MN 55012-9640　　　　　800-257-7810
　　　　　　　　　　　　　　　　Fax: 651-213-4793
　　　　　　　　　　　　e-mail: info@hazelden.org
　　　　　　　　　　　　　　　www.hazelden.org
A series of short discussions that interpret each of the Twelve Steps, from admission of individual powerlessness outlined in Step One to the moral inventory of Step Four and the spiritual awakening of Step Twelve.
130 pages Paperback
ISBN: 0-894869-04-3
Mark Mishek, President and Chief Executive Officer
Joe Jaksha, Publisher

8531 **Twenty Four Hours a Day**
Hazelden
15251 Pleasant Valley Rd　　　　　　651-213-4200
Center City, MN 55012-9640　　　　　800-257-7810
　　　　　　　　　　　　　　　　Fax: 651-213-4793
　　　　　　　　　　　　e-mail: info@hazelden.org
　　　　　　　　　　　　　　　www.hazelden.org
Offers a resource that serves as a solid foundation in a spiritual program. Simple, yet effective resource that helps clients relate to the Twelve-Step program.
400 pages Paperback
Mark Mishek, President and Chief Executive Officer
Joe Jaksha, Publisher

8532 Walk in Dry Places
Hazelden
15251 Pleasant Valley Rd
Center City, MN 55012-9640
651-213-4200
800-257-7810
Fax: 651-213-4793
e-mail: info@hazelden.org
www.hazelden.org

Core-recovery book filled with practical spiritual advice and time-honored Twelve Step philosophy. Insightful explorations of the deeper issues of living in recovery address the daily concerns of those new to life without alcoholism, as well as those with long-term sobriety.
400 pages Paperback
ISBN: 1-568381-27-1
Mark Mishek, President and Chief Executive Officer
Joe Jaksha, Publisher

8533 Wasted Tales of a Gen X Drunk
Hazelden
15251 Pleasant Valley Rd
Center City, MN 55012-9640
651-213-4200
800-257-7810
Fax: 651-213-4793
e-mail: info@hazelden.org
www.hazelden.org

Cynicism and black humor underscore this hard-edged memoir of a young journalist's alcoholism and subsequent recovery. Captures the ethos of a generation often suspicious and alienated by the Twelve-Step approach.
250 pages Cloth
ISBN: 1-568381-42-5
Mark Mishek, President and Chief Executive Officer
Joe Jaksha, Publisher

8534 What Works: Schools Without Drugs
National Clearinghouse for Alcohol and Drug Info.
PO Box 2345
Rockville, MD 20847-2345
800-729-6686

8535 What You Can Do About Drug Use in America
National Clearinghouse for Alcohol and Drug Info.
PO Box 2345
Rockville, MD 20847-2345
301-468-2600
800-729-6686
www.health.org

Offers information on what parents and professionals can do to prevent drug use in America.

8536 Why Am I Afraid to Tell You Who I Am?
Hazelden
15251 Pleasant Valley Rd
Center City, MN 55012-9640
651-213-4200
800-257-7810
Fax: 651-213-4793
e-mail: info@hazelden.org
www.hazelden.org

Outlines types of interpersonal relationships.
Mark Mishek, President and Chief Executive Officer
Joe Jaksha, Publisher

8537 Woman's Way Through the Twelve Steps
Hazelden
15251 Pleasant Valley Rd
Center City, MN 55012-9640
651-213-4200
800-257-7810
Fax: 651-213-4793
e-mail: info@hazelden.org
www.hazelden.org

How women understnad and work the Twelve Steps of AA, including reflections of spirituality, powerlessness, and the emergence of a sense of the feminine soul.
228 pages Paperback
ISBN: 0-894869-93-0
Mark Mishek, President and Chief Executive Officer
Joe Jaksha, Publisher

8538 Young Teens: Who They Are and How to Talk to Them About Alcohol & Drugs
National Clearinghouse for Alcohol and Drug Info.
PO Box 2345
Rockville, MD 20847-2345
800-729-6686
e-mail: www.coaf.org

Offers information on how parents, educators and concerned citizens can work together to help youngsters avoid alcohol and other drugs by understanding the risks and dangers.
57 pages

Children's Books

8539 Alcoholism
Franklin Watts Grolier
90 Old Sherman Turnpike
Danbury, CT 06816-0001
203-797-3500
800-621-1115
Fax: 203-797-3197
www.grolier.com

This comprehensive overview describes the different types of alcoholism, the addictive personality and the warning signs.
112 pages Grades 7-12
ISBN: 0-531108-79-1

8540 Alcoholism and the Family
Franklin Watts Grolier
90 Old Sherman Turnpike
Danbury, CT 06816-0001
203-797-3500
800-621-1115
Fax: 203-797-3197
www.grolier.com

This book, after discussing what alcoholism is, its effects on health and behavior modifications through alcohol, starts addressing one of the most important aspects of alcoholism, the effects on the family.
32 pages Grades 3-5
ISBN: 0-531125-48-3

8541 America's War on Drugs
Franklin Watts Grolier
90 Old Sherman Turnpike
Danbury, CT 06816
203-797-3500
800-621-1115
Fax: 203-797-3197
www.grolier.com

An overview of the United States' attempts to combat illegal drugs on the supply side, from stopping the supply of drugs into the country.
160 pages Grades 7-12
ISBN: 0-531109-54-2

8542 Buzzy's Rebound
National Clearinghouse for Alcohol and Drug Info.
PO Box 2345
Rockville, MD 20847-2345
800-729-6686
www.sdsalarms.com

A Fat Albert comic book that describes the pressure on a new kid in town to drink.
18 pages

8543 Caffeine and Nicotine
Hazelden
15251 Pleasant Valley Rd
Center City, MN 55012-9640
651-213-4200
800-257-7810
Fax: 651-213-4793
e-mail: info@hazelden.org
www.hazelden.org

Simple, clear, and accurate presentation of nicotine and caffeine dependency. How to avoid these addictions, and why teens ought to do so.
64 pages Paperback
ISBN: 1-568381-68-9
Mark Mishek, President and Chief Executive Officer
Joe Jaksha, Publisher

8544 Christy's Chance
Crestridge Corporate Center
10155 York Road
Hunt Valley, MD 21030
410-628-0390
Fax: 410-628-0398
e-mail: cboyce@networkpub.com
www.networkpub.com

A story geared to younger teens that allows the reader to make a nonuse decision about marijuana.

8545 Cocaine
Hazelden

15251 Pleasant Valley Rd
Center City, MN 55012-9640

651-213-4200
800-257-7810
Fax: 651-213-4793
e-mail: info@hazelden.org
www.hazelden.org

The information that teens need to stay drug-free, promoting understanding of the ramifications, both social and personal.
64 pages Paperback
ISBN: 1-568381-64-6
Mark Mishek, President and Chief Executive Officer
Joe Jaksha, Publisher

8546 Coping with Codependency
Hazelden
15251 Pleasant Valley Rd
Center City, MN 55012-9640

651-213-4200
800-257-7810
Fax: 651-213-4793
e-mail: info@hazelden.org
www.hazelden.org

Explains the cycle of codependency, describes its destructive effects on all involved, and suggests ways to break free and live in more healthy relationships.
64 pages Paperback
ISBN: 1-568381-85-9
Mark Mishek, President and Chief Executive Officer
Joe Jaksha, Publisher

8547 Coping with Depression
Hazelden
15251 Pleasant Valley Rd
Center City, MN 55012-9640

651-213-4200
800-257-7810
Fax: 651-213-4793
e-mail: info@hazelden.org
www.hazelden.org

Practical ways to cope with depression. Provides clear suggestions for handling life's downers, and encourages readers to seek professional help when they feel they can't deal with problems themselves.
64 pages Paperback
ISBN: 1-568381-79-4
Mark Mishek, President and Chief Executive Officer
Joe Jaksha, Publisher

8548 Coping with Drinking and Driving
Hazelden
15251 Pleasant Valley Rd
Center City, MN 55012-9640

651-213-4200
800-257-7810
Fax: 651-213-4793
e-mail: info@hazelden.org
www.hazelden.org

Addressing teens' illusion of invulnerability, the author describes exactly how alcohol affects the body and one's driving skills, emphasizing that teens are not immune to alcohol's effects.
64 pages Paperback
ISBN: 1-568381-80-8
Mark Mishek, President and Chief Executive Officer
Joe Jaksha, Publisher

8549 Coping with Peer Pressure
Hazelden
15251 Pleasant Valley Rd
Center City, MN 55012-9640

651-213-4200
800-257-7810
Fax: 651-213-4793
e-mail: info@hazelden.org
www.hazelden.org

Discussion of the positive and negative effects that members of a peer group can have on each other and explores ways teens can handle the pressure they face.
64 pages Paperback
ISBN: 1-568381-83-2
Mark Mishek, President and Chief Executive Officer
Joe Jaksha, Publisher

8550 Coping with Stress
Hazelden
15251 Pleasant Valley Rd
Center City, MN 55012-9640

651-213-4200
800-257-7810
Fax: 651-213-4793
e-mail: info@hazelden.org
www.hazelden.org

Outlines positive strategies to help teens learn to cope more effectively with stress, rather than turning to destructive outlets such as drugs and even suicide.
64 pages Paperback
ISBN: 1-568381-76-X
Mark Mishek, President and Chief Executive Officer
Joe Jaksha, Publisher

8551 Coping with a Drug-Abusing Parent
Hazelden
15251 Pleasant Valley Rd
Center City, MN 55012-9640

651-213-4200
800-257-7810
Fax: 651-213-4793
e-mail: info@hazelden.org
www.hazelden.org

Describes steps that teens, powerless to stop a drug-abusing parent from continuing on that destructive path, can take to to learn to take better care of themselves. Includes coping strategies and who to call for help.
64 pages Paperback
ISBN: 1-568381-78-6
Mark Mishek, President and Chief Executive Officer
Joe Jaksha, Publisher

8552 Crack Down on Drugs
National Clearinghouse for Alcohol and Drug Info.
PO Box 2345
Rockville, MD 20847

800-729-6686
www.healthieryou.com

Coloring book for children featuring McGruff, the crime dog, that teaches young children the importance of refusing alcohol and drug abuse.
Ages 5-8

8553 Different Like Me: A Book for Teens Who Worry About Their Parents' Using
Johnson Institute
Ohms Lane
Edina, MN

612-831-1630
www.kineticvideo.com

Provides support and information for teens who are concerned, confused, scared and angry because their parents abuse alcohol and other drugs.
110 pages

8554 Drug Abuse: The Impact on Society
Franklin Watts Grolier
90 Old Sherman Turnpike
Danbury, CT 06816

203-797-3500
800-621-1115
Fax: 203-797-3197
www.grolier.com

Discusses all major aspects of illegal drug usage and the health and personality effects they cause.
144 pages Grades 7-12
ISBN: 0-531105-79-2

8555 Drugs and AIDS
Hazelden
15251 Pleasant Valley Rd
Center City, MN 55012-9640

651-213-4200
800-257-7810
Fax: 651-213-4793
e-mail: info@hazelden.org
www.hazelden.org

Covers many topics through case studies, including the effects of the disease on the body, transmission, homosexuality, condom use, drug treatment, and peer pressure.
64 pages Paperback
ISBN: 1-568381-72-7
Mark Mishek, President and Chief Executive Officer
Joe Jaksha, Publisher

8556 Drugs and Anger
Hazelden
15251 Pleasant Valley Rd
Center City, MN 55012-9640

651-213-4200
800-257-7810
Fax: 651-213-4793
e-mail: info@hazelden.org
www.hazelden.org

True-to-life scenarios and practical techniques found here can help teens cope constructively with their anger.
64 pages Paperback
ISBN: 1-568381-73-5
Mark Mishek, President and Chief Executive Officer
Joe Jaksha, Publisher

8557   Drugs and Depression
Hazelden
15251 Pleasant Valley Rd   651-213-4200
Center City, MN 55012-9640   800-257-7810
                                         Fax: 651-213-4793
                              e-mail: info@hazelden.org
                                          www.hazelden.org
Describes positive ways of handling depression, as well as suggesting resources for receiving assistance.
64 pages Paperback
ISBN: 1-568381-74-3
Mark Mishek, President and Chief Executive Officer
Joe Jaksha, Publisher

8558   Drugs and Domestic Violence
Hazelden
15251 Pleasant Valley Rd   651-213-4200
Center City, MN 55012-9640   800-257-7810
                                         Fax: 651-213-4793
                              e-mail: info@hazelden.org
                                          www.hazelden.org
Describes valuable coping tactics that can help teens stay safe in situations involving domestic violence and drug use.
64 pages Paperback
ISBN: 1-568381-75-1
Mark Mishek, President and Chief Executive Officer
Joe Jaksha, Publisher

8559   Drugs and Your Friends
Hazelden
15251 Pleasant Valley Rd   651-213-4200
Center City, MN 55012-9640   800-257-7810
                                         Fax: 651-213-4793
                              e-mail: info@hazelden.org
                                          www.hazelden.org
Helps teens make sound decisions on vital choices and provides many suggestions for resisting peer pressure.
64 pages Paperback
ISBN: 1-568381-70-0
Mark Mishek, President and Chief Executive Officer
Joe Jaksha, Publisher

8560   Drugs and Your Parents
Hazelden
15251 Pleasant Valley Rd   651-213-4200
Center City, MN 55012-9640   800-257-7810
                                         Fax: 651-213-4793
                              e-mail: info@hazelden.org
                                          www.hazelden.org
Practical advice for teenage children of parents addicted to alcohol or other drugs. How to cope initially with the situation as well as long-term survival strategies.
64 pages Paperback
ISBN: 1-568381-71-9
Mark Mishek, President and Chief Executive Officer
Joe Jaksha, Publisher

8561   Drugs in the Body: Effects of Abuse
Franklin Watts Grolier
90 Old Sherman Turnpike   203-797-3500
Danbury, CT 06816   800-621-1115
                                         Fax: 203-797-3197
                                          www.grolier.com
Traces the effects of cocaine and crack, opium, morphine, heroine, marijuana and hashish, LSD and PCP in a person's system. Special emphasis is placed on long-term adverse effects in the body.
144 pages Grades 7-12
ISBN: 0-531125-07-6

8562   Elephant in the Living Room: The Children's Book
Hazelden

15251 Pleasant Valley Rd   651-213-4200
Center City, MN 55012-9640   800-257-7810
                                         Fax: 651-213-4793
                              e-mail: info@hazelden.org
                                          www.hazelden.org
An activity book to help children understand and cope with the problem of chemical dependency in the family.
88 pages Paperback
ISBN: 1-568380-35-6
Mark Mishek, President and Chief Executive Officer
Joe Jaksha, Publisher

8563   Facts on Alcohol
Franklin Watts Grolier
90 Old Sherman Turnpike   203-797-3500
Danbury, CT 06816   800-621-1115
                                         Fax: 203-797-3197
                                          www.grolier.com
Offers various information on alcohol so young children can have an opportunity to form their own opinions and the ability to make their own decisions when it comes to alcoholism.
32 pages Grades 5-7
ISBN: 0-531108-21-0

8564   Facts on the Crack and Cocaine Epidemic
Franklin Watts Grolier
90 Old Sherman Turnpike   203-797-3500
Danbury, CT 06816   800-621-1115
                                         Fax: 203-797-3197
                                          www.grolier.com
Offers young children information on these deadly drugs to help them become informed.
32 pages Grades 5-7
ISBN: 0-531108-22-8

8565   Feed Your Head
Hazelden
15251 Pleasant Valley Rd   651-213-4200
Center City, MN 55012-9640   800-257-7810
                                         Fax: 651-213-4793
                              e-mail: info@hazelden.org
                                          www.hazelden.org
Offers practical guidance for young people.
137 pages Paperback
Mark Mishek, President and Chief Executive Officer
Joe Jaksha, Publisher

8566   Gangs and Drugs
Hazelden
15251 Pleasant Valley Rd   651-213-4200
Center City, MN 55012-9640   800-257-7810
                                         Fax: 651-213-4793
                              e-mail: info@hazelden.org
                                          www.hazelden.org
Encouraging and helpful message that goes beyond Just say no.
240 pages Paperback
ISBN: 1-568381-35-2
Mark Mishek, President and Chief Executive Officer
Joe Jaksha, Publisher

8567   How to Say No and Keep Your Friends
Hazelden
15251 Pleasant Valley Rd   651-213-4200
Center City, MN 55012-9640   800-257-7810
                                         Fax: 651-213-4793
                              e-mail: info@hazelden.org
                                          www.hazelden.org
Ideas to help teens deal with negative peer pressure.
112 pages
Mark Mishek, President and Chief Executive Officer
Joe Jaksha, Publisher

8568   I Can Talk About What Hurts
Hazelden
15251 Pleasant Valley Rd   651-213-4200
Center City, MN 55012-9640   800-257-7810
                                         Fax: 651-213-4793
                              e-mail: info@hazelden.org
                                          www.hazelden.org

Written and illustrated for children whose lives have been affected by someone else's chemical dependency.
56 pages Paperback
Mark Mishek, President and Chief Executive Officer
Joe Jaksha, Publisher

8569   I Wish Daddy Didn't Drink So Much
Judith Vigna, author

Albert Whitman & Company
250 South NW Highway   847-232-2800
Park Ridge, IL 60068-2723   800-255-7675
                                           Fax: 847-581-0039
                              e-mail: mail@awhitmanco.com
                                       www.albertwhitman.com
A young girl shres her feelings and frustrations about her alcoholic father's behavior.
1993 32 pages Grades P-3
ISBN: 0-807535-23-0
Pat McPartland, Sales
Joe Campbell, Customer Service

8570   If Drugs Are So Bad, Why Do So Many People Use Them?
Hazelden
15251 Pleasant Valley Rd   651-213-4200
Center City, MN 55012-9640   800-257-7810
                                           Fax: 651-213-4793
                              e-mail: info@hazelden.org
                                       www.hazelden.org
Uses direct language to explain drugs and their effects.
29 pages Grades 5-9
Mark Mishek, President and Chief Executive Officer
Joe Jaksha, Publisher

8571   In a Perfect World
Hazelden
15251 Pleasant Valley Rd   651-213-4200
Center City, MN 55012-9640   800-257-7810
                                           Fax: 651-213-4793
                              e-mail: info@hazelden.org
                                       www.hazelden.org
Kevin thinks his world will be perfect when his father stops drinking, but Kevin is in for a few surprises.
160 pages Softcover
Mark Mishek, President and Chief Executive Officer
Joe Jaksha, Publisher

8572   Inhalants
Hazelden
15251 Pleasant Valley Rd   651-213-4200
Center City, MN 55012-9640   800-257-7810
                                           Fax: 651-213-4793
                              e-mail: info@hazelden.org
                                       www.hazelden.org
Clear, straightforward explanation of the dangers and consequences of using seemingly harmless chemicals, such as model airplane glue, hair spray, whipping cream, and cleaning and lighter fluids, as well as sources of help for those who need it.
64 pages Paperback
ISBN: 1-568381-69-7
Mark Mishek, President and Chief Executive Officer
Joe Jaksha, Publisher

8573   Inside Out
Hazelden
15251 Pleasant Valley Rd   651-213-4200
Center City, MN 55012-9640   800-257-7810
                                           Fax: 651-213-4793
                              e-mail: info@hazelden.org
                                       www.hazelden.org
Offers open-ended sentences for readers to fill in their responses.
97 pages Paperback
Mark Mishek, President and Chief Executive Officer
Joe Jaksha, Publisher

8574   Kids and Alcohol: Get High on Life
Health Communications
1721 Blount Road
Pompano Beach, FL 33069   954-360-0909
                                       www.hoffmanestates.com

A workbook designed to help children make important decisions in their lives and feel good about themselves.
Ages 11-14
Jamie Rattray, Author

8575   Let's Talk About Drug Abuse
Rosen Publishing Group's PowerKids Press
29 East 21st Street   212-777-3017
New York, NY 10010   800-237-9932
                                           Fax: 888-436-4643
                       e-mail: customerservice@rosenpub.com
                                       www.rosenpublishing.com
A first step in a child's education about the dangers of drugs. Recommended for grade K-4.

ISBN: 0-823923-02-9
Anna Kreiner, Author

8576   McGruff's Surprise Party
National Clearinghouse for Alcohol and Drug Info.
PO Box 2345
Rockville, MD 20847-2345   800-729-6686
                                           files.eric.ed.gov
A comic book that helps children understand the importance of refusing alcohol and other drugs.
14 pages Ages 8-10
Paula Stauffer, Author

8577   My Body is My House
Hazelden
15251 Pleasant Valley Rd   651-213-4200
Center City, MN 55012   800-257-7810
                                           Fax: 651-213-4793
                              e-mail: info@hazelden.org
                                       www.hazelden.org
A coloring book about alcohol, drugs and health.
16 pages
Mark Mishek, President and Chief Executive Officer
Joe Jaksha, Publisher

8578   Sad Story of Mary Wanna or How Marijuana Harms You
Woodmere Press
PO Box 20190   A coloring book for children that contains pictures of the damage that
New York, NY 10025   marijuana does to the body.
40 pages Grades 1-4

8579   Should Drugs Be Legalized?
Franklin Watts Grolier
90 Old Sherman Turnpike   203-797-3500
Danbury, CT 06816-0001   800-621-1115
                                           Fax: 203-797-3197
                                           www.grolier.com
Presents a discussion of this controversial subject.
160 pages Grades 7-12

8580   Smoking-At Issues Series
Greenhaven Press
10650 Toebben Drive
Independence, KY 41051-9187   800-354-9706
                                           Fax: 800-487-8488
                      e-mail: order.samples@cengage.com
                              solutions.cengage.com/greenhaven
Written in a straightforward manner, this book answers questions most young adults are asking regarding smoking and health.

ISBN: 0-737701-57-9

8581   Stand Strong
African American Family Services
2616 Nicollet Avenue S   612-871-7878
Minneapolis, MN 55408   888-786-6798
                                           www.rehabs.com
Comic book prevention for young adults. Profiles two African-American teens as they go through the hazards and risks of drug use and sexual behavior.
16 pages

8582   Summer of Sassy Jo
Houghton Mifflin

Wayside Road
Burlington, MA 01803   800-225-3362
A story of a thirteen-year-old girl faced with reconciliation with
her recovered alcoholic mother after eight years of abandonment.
192 pages Grades 7+
ISBN: 0-395669-56-1

8583   Teen Alcoholism-Teen Issues
Lucent Books
Thomson Gale
San Diego, CA 48333-9187   800-877-4253
                                             Fax: 800-414-5043
                            e-mail: gale.customerservice@thomson.com
                                          www.gale.com/lucent
Offers readable interviews for reports and answers the most fre-
quently asked questions about alcohol.

ISBN: 1-590185-01-3

8584   Teen Guide to Pregnancy, Drugs and Smoking
Franklin Watts Grolier
90 Old Sherman Turnpike   203-797-3500
Danbury, CT 06816-0001   800-621-1115
                                             Fax: 203-797-3197
                                               www.grolier.com
Outlines the risks of smoking and drug taking while pregnant and
answers teenagers' questions about the use of legal, illegal and prescription drugs.
64 pages Grades 9-12
ISBN: 0-531108-35-0

8585   Understanding Drugs
Franklin Watts Grolier
90 Old Sherman Turnpike   203-797-3500
Danbury, CT 06816-0001   800-621-1115
                                             Fax: 203-797-3197
                                               www.grolier.com
This series of books explains the current drug phenomenon at a
high-interest, low-vocabulary level. Gives in-depth information
about all aspects of commonly abused substances, including their
negative mental, physical and social effects. Each book features
photographs, diagrams, a glossary, an index and list of addresses
for futher information and help. Set of seven volumes.
Grades 5-7

8586   Violence and Drugs
Franklin Watts Grolier
90 Old Sherman Turnpike   203-797-3500
Danbury, CT 06816-0001   800-621-1115
                                             Fax: 203-797-3197
                                               www.grolier.com
This informative book studies the fascinating link between drug
use and violent behavior.
112 pages Grades 9-12
ISBN: 0-531108-18-0

8587   What's Drunk Mama?
Al-Anon Family Group Headquarters
1600 Corp Landing Pkwy   757-563-1600
Virginia Beach, VA 23454-5617   800-425-2666
                                             Fax: 757-563-1655
                                            e-mail: wso@al-anon.org
                                          www.al-anon.alateen.org
Large print illustrated booklet for use as a shared reading experi-
ence to help younger children understand alcoholism.
32 pages
Caryn Johnson, Director Communications

8588   Whiskers Says No to Drugs
Weekly Reader Skills Books
245 Long Hill Road
Jefferson City, MO 65102-4063   860-446-3355
                                           Fax: 800-724-4911
                                             www.weeklyreader.com
This book contains stories and follow-up activities for students to
provide information and form attitudes before they face peer pres-
sure to experiment.
Grades 2-3

8589   Why Do People Drink Alcohol?
Franklin Watts Grolier

90 Old Sherman Turnpike   203-797-3500
Danbury, CT 06816-0001   800-621-1115
                                             Fax: 203-797-3197
                                               www.grolier.com
Answers young children's questions about alcoholism.
32 pages Grades 3-5
ISBN: 0-531171-34-5

8590   Why Do People Smoke?
Franklin Watts Grolier
90 Old Sherman Turnpike   203-797-3500
Danbury, CT 06816-0001   800-621-1115
                                             Fax: 203-797-3197
                                               www.grolier.com
Raises and answers questions of specific interest to seven-to-ten
year olds about smoking.
32 pages Grades 3-5
ISBN: 0-531171-92-2

8591   Why Do People Take Drugs?
Franklin Watts Grolier
90 Old Sherman Turnpike   203-797-3500
Danbury, CT 06816-0001   800-621-1115
                                             Fax: 203-797-3197
                                               www.grolier.com
Raises important questions and offers some answers for young
children on the aspects and everyday living with a drug addiction.
32 pages Grades 3-5
ISBN: 0-531171-13-2

8592   Winning the Battle Against Drugs: Rehabilitation Programs
Franklin Watts Grolier
90 Old Sherman Turnpike   203-797-3500
Danbury, CT 06816-0001   800-621-1115
                                             Fax: 203-797-3197
                                               www.grolier.com
Programs contained in this book will help adolescents see that drug
and alcohol addiction can be successfully treated.
160 pages Grades 7-12
ISBN: 0-531110-63-0

8593   Young Person's Guide to the Twelve Steps
Hazelden
15251 Pleasant Valley Rd   651-213-4200
Center City, MN 55012-9640   800-257-7810
                                             Fax: 651-213-4793
                                          e-mail: info@hazelden.org
                                               www.hazelden.org
Explains the Twelve Steps in the best way young people can under-
stand: in their own language.
168 pages Paperback
Mark Mishek, President and Chief Executive Officer
Joe Jaksha, Publisher

8594   Young, Sober & Free
Hazelden
15251 Pleasant Valley Rd   651-213-4200
Center City, MN 55012-9640   800-257-7810
                                             Fax: 651-213-4793
                                          e-mail: info@hazelden.org
                                               www.hazelden.org
Features young peoples' personal experiences of living with addic-
tion.
137 pages Paperback
Mark Mishek, President and Chief Executive Officer
Joe Jaksha, Publisher

Magazines

8595   ACAP Recap
American Council on Alcohol Problems
3426 Bridgeland Drive
Bridgeton, MO 63044-2603   314-739-5944
                                             Fax: 314-739-0848
                                           www.lifemanagement.com
Offers information on organization activities and events, updates
on resources and publications and legislative information for affil-
iate executives.
Monthly
Dr. Curt Scarborough, Executive Director

8596 American Issue
American Council on Alcohol Problems
3426 Bridgeland Drive   314-739-5944
Bridgeton, MO 63044-2603   Fax: 314-739-0848
www.lifemanagement.com
Offered to contributors of the organization.
Monthly
Dr. Curt Scarborough, Executive Director

8597 Drug Abuse Update
2296 Henderson Mill Road   770-934-6364
Atlanta, GA 30345-2739
A journal of news and information for persons interested in drug prevention.
Quarterly

8598 Forum Magazine
Al-Anon Alateen Family Group Headquarters
1600 Corp Landing Pkwy   757-563-1600
Virginia Beach, VA 23454-970   888-425-2666
Fax: 757-563-1655
e-mail: wso@alanon.org
www.al-anon.alateen.org
Contains many personal stories of inspiration, some of which are maade available each month on the Internet by authorization of Al-Anon Family Group Headquarters, Inc.
Ric Buchanan, Executive Director

8599 Lead Line
Grapevine
PO Box 1980   212-870-3400
New York, NY 10163-1980   Fax: 212-870-3301
AA members all over the world communicate with each other through the pages of this magazine. It contains: insight into how AAs stay sober; readers' views; old-timers corner, beginners meeting, youth enjoying sobriety, and spotlight on service.
Monthly

Newsletters

8600 ADPA Professional
Alcohol/Drug Problems Association of North America
307 N Main Street   314-589-6702
St. Charles, MO 63301   Fax: 314-940-2358
Offers information to members on events, conferences and activities, reviews the newest resources and technology pertaining to alcoholism and drug addiction.

8601 Drug-Free Workplace Educator
American Council on Drug Education
204 Monroe Street   301-294-0600
Rockville, MD 20850-4425   800-488-3784
www.ascicorp.com
Offers continuing education for employers and their supervisors responsible for substance abuse prevention. Practical articles feature information to help employers design, implement and maintain a drug-free workplace.
BiMonthly

8602 Just Say Notes
Just Say No International
2101 Webster Street   510-451-6666
Oakland, CA 94612-3065   800-258-2766
Offers information on the organizations, activities, programs, conferences and events.
BiMonthly

8603 RID-USA Newsletter
Remove Intoxicated Drivers (RID-USA)
PO Box 520   518-393-4357
Schenectady, NY 12301-0520   888-283-5144
Fax: 518-370-4917
www.rid-usa.org
Membership news.
3x Year
Doris Aiken, President & CEO

8604 Sobering Thoughts
Women for Sobriety

PO Box 618   215-536-8026
Quakertown, PA 18951-0618   800-333-1606
Fax: 215-536-9026
e-mail: newlife@nni.com
www.womenforsobriety.org
A monthly membership newsletter for women with an addiction problem who wish for recovery and start a new life.
16 pages Monthly
Rebecca Fenner, Director

8605 Substance Abuse Funding News
CD Publications
2222 Sedwick Drive   301-588-6380
Durham, NC 27713-4571   855-237-1396
Fax: 800-508-2592
e-mail: info@cdpublications.com
www.cdpublications.com
Detailed coverage of private and federal funding opportunities for alcohol, tobacco and drug abuse programs. Plus advice on successful grantseeking strategies and news affecting your programs.
18 pages BiWeekly
Mary Compton, Publisher
Amy Bernstein, Editor

Pamphlets

8606 AA Member: Medications and Other Drugs
Alcoholics Anonymous
PO Box 459   212-870-3400
New York, NY 10163-0459   Fax: 212-870-3137
www.aa.org
Report from a group of doctors in Alcoholics Anonymous.

8607 AA Service Manual: Twelve Concepts for World Service
Alcoholics Anonymous
PO Box 459   212-870-3400
New York, NY 10163-0459   Fax: 212-870-3137
www.aa.org
This manual opens with a history of AA services.

8608 AA and the Armed Services
Alcoholics Anonymous
PO Box 459   212-870-3400
New York, NY 10163-0459   Fax: 212-870-3137
www.aa.org
Personal stories tell how men and women in the military can beat a drinking problem.

8609 AA and the Gay/Lesbian Alcoholic
Alcoholics Anonymous
PO Box 459   212-870-3400
New York, NY 10163-0459   Fax: 212-870-3137
www.aa.org
Excerpts from experience, strength and hope of sober gay and lesbian alcoholics.

8610 AA as a Resource for Health Care Professionals
Alcoholics Anonymous
PO Box 459   212-870-3400
New York, NY 10163-0459   Fax: 212-870-3137
www.aa.org
Information about the Fellowship and describes some approaches that health care professionals use in referring problem drinkers to AA.

8611 AA for the Native North American
Alcoholics Anonymous
PO Box 459   212-870-3400
New York, NY 10163-0459   Fax: 212-870-3137
www.aa.org
Addressed to and contains stories by Native American AA members.

8612 AA for the Woman
Alcoholics Anonymous
PO Box 459   212-870-3400
New York, NY 10163-0459   Fax: 212-870-3137
www.aa.org

Relates the experiences of alcoholic women, all ages and from all walks of life.

8613   AA in Correctional Facilities
Alcoholics Anonymous
PO Box 459   212-870-3400
New York, NY 10163-0459   Fax: 212-870-3137
                                                      www.aa.org
Experience based on the functioning of AA groups in prisons, with institutional opinions recommending AA as a helpful ally.

8614   AA in Treatment Facilities
Alcoholics Anonymous
PO Box 459   212-870-3400
New York, NY 10163-0459   Fax: 212-870-3137
                                                      www.aa.org
Shares experiences of treatment facility administrators and of AA's who have carried the message into these facilities.

8615   Acceptance
Hazelden
15251 Pleasant Valley Rd   651-213-4200
Center City, MN 55012-9640   800-257-7810
                                             Fax: 651-213-4793
                                    e-mail: info@hazelden.org
                                             www.hazelden.org
Addresses issues such as facing life, the kindness of God, suffering and contentment.
Mark Mishek, President and Chief Executive Officer
Joe Jaksha, Publisher

8616   Adult Children of Alcoholics Newcomer Packet
Al-Anon Family Group Headquarters
1600 Corp Landing Pkwy   757-563-1600
Virginia Beach, VA 23454-5617   800-425-2666
                                          Fax: 757-563-1655
                                    e-mail: wso@al-anon.org
                                          www.al-anon.alateen.org
For those who have grown up with parental alcoholism, this is a loving introduction to Al-Anon and the twelve steps.
9 pieces
Caryn Johnson, Director Communications

8617   African Americans in Treatment
Hazelden
15251 Pleasant Valley Rd   651-213-4200
Center City, MN 55012   800-257-7810
                                             Fax: 651-213-4793
                                    e-mail: info@hazelden.org
                                             www.hazelden.org
Helps African American clients understand treatment from a cultural standpoint.
23 pages
Mark Mishek, President and Chief Executive Officer
Joe Jaksha, Publisher

8618   Al-Anon Newcomers Packet
Al-Anon Family Group Headquarters
1600 Corp Landing Pkwy   757-563-1600
Virginia Beach, VA 23454-5617   800-425-2666
                                          Fax: 757-563-1655
                                    e-mail: wso@al-anon.org
                                          www.al-anon.alateen.org
Material specifically for the newcomer to Al-Anon packed in a handsome sleeve.
8 pieces
Caryn Johnson, Director Communications

8619   Al-Anon Spoken Here
Al-Anon Family Group Headquarters
1600 Corp Landing Pkwy   757-563-1600
Virginia Beach, VA 23454-5617   800-425-2666
                                          Fax: 757-563-1655
                                    e-mail: wso@al-anon.org
                                          www.al-anon.alateen.org
Why are Al-Anon meetings the way they are? Questions and answers that lead to a better understanding of the importance of keeping Al-Anon principles.
8 pages
Caryn Johnson, Director Communications

8620   Al-Anon is for Men
Al-Anon Family Group Headquarters
1600 Corp Landing Pkwy   757-563-1600
Virginia Beach, VA 23454-5617   800-425-2666
                                          Fax: 757-563-1655
                                    e-mail: wso@al-anon.org
                                          www.al-anon.alateen.org
Straight forward questions to help men identify their reactions to alcoholism in another person.
6 pages
Caryn Johnson, Director Communications

8621   Al-Anon, You and the Alcoholic
Al-Anon Family Group Headquarters
1600 Corp Landing Pkwy   757-563-1600
Virginia Beach, VA 23454-5617   800-425-2666
                                          Fax: 757-563-1655
                                    e-mail: wso@al-anon.org
                                          www.al-anon.alateen.org
Answers the most frequently asked questions about Al-Anon and how it helps families deal with problems brought about by alcoholism.
12 pages
Caryn Johnson, Director Communications

8622   Alateen Newcomer Packet
Al-Anon Family Group Headquarters
1600 Corp Landing Pkwy   757-563-1600
Virginia Beach, VA 23454-5617   800-425-2666
                                          Fax: 757-563-1655
                                    e-mail: wso@al-anon.org
                                          www.al-anon.alateen.org
Helpful leaflets assembled in a sleeve ready to give to the new young member.
13 pieces
Caryn Johnson, Director Communications

8623   Alateen Talk
Al-Anon Family Group Headquarters
1600 Corp Landing Pkwy   757-563-1600
Virginia Beach, VA 23454-5617   800-425-2666
                                          Fax: 757-563-1655
                                    e-mail: wso@al-anon.org
                                          www.al-anon.alateen.org
Al-Anon is a mutual support group of peers who share their experience in applying the Al-Anon principles to problems related to the effects of a problem drinker in their lives. It is not group therapy and is not led by a counselor or therapist
Robert Schneider, Director Communications

8624   Alcohol Alert #11: Estimating the Cost of Alcohol Abuse
National Clearinghouse for Alcohol and Drug Info.
1101 Wootton Parkway
Rockville, MD 20852-2345   800-729-6686
                                             Fax: 240-453-8282
                                    e-mail: odphpinfo@hhs.gov
                                             www.health.org
Discusses the various problems of estimating the cost of alcohol abuse.

8625   Alcohol Alert #15: Alcohol and AIDS
National Clearinghouse for Alcohol and Drug Info.
1101 Wootton Parkway
Rockville, MD 20852-2345   800-729-6686
                                             Fax: 240-453-8282
                                    e-mail: odphpinfo@hhs.gov
                                             www.health.org
Discusses the relationship between alcohol consumption and HIV infection and AIDS.

8626   Alcohol Alert #16: Moderate Drinking
National Clearinghouse for Alcohol and Drug Info.
1101 Wootton Parkway
Rockville, MD 20852-2345   800-729-6686
                                             Fax: 240-453-8282
                                    e-mail: odphpinfo@hhs.gov
                                             www.health.org
Defines moderate drinking and explores the benefits and risks associated with moderate drinking.

8627 Alcohol Alert #17: Treatment Outcome Research
National Clearinghouse for Alcohol and Drug Info.
1101 Wootton Parkway
Rockville, MD 20852-2345   800-729-6686
                                        Fax: 240-453-8282
                              e-mail: odphpinfo@hhs.gov
                                            www.health.org
Discusses purpose, methodology, randomization, blinding, followup and what treatment outcome research reveals.

8628 Alcohol Alert #18: The Genetics of Alcoholism
National Clearinghouse for Alcohol and Drug Info.
1101 Wootton Parkway
Rockville, MD 20852-2345   800-729-6686
                                        Fax: 240-453-8282
                              e-mail: odphpinfo@hhs.gov
                                            www.health.org
Presents the results of studies that investigate the role of genes and the environment in the development of alcoholism.

8629 Alcohol Alert #21: Alcohol and Cancer
National Clearinghouse for Alcohol and Drug Info.
1101 Wootton Parkway
Rockville, MD 20852-2345   800-729-6686
                                        Fax: 240-453-8282
                              e-mail: odphpinfo@hhs.gov
                                            www.health.org
The Office of Disease Prevention and Health Promotion (ODPHP) plays a vital role in keeping the Nation healthy. Learn more about our work by exploring our national health initiatives

8630 Alcohol Alert #23: Alcohol and Minorities
National Clearinghouse for Alcohol and Drug Info.
1101 Wootton Parkway
Rockville, MD 20852-2345   800-729-6686
                                        Fax: 240-453-8282
                              e-mail: odphpinfo@hhs.gov
                                            www.health.org
The Office of Disease Prevention and Health Promotion (ODPHP) plays a vital role in keeping the Nation healthy. Learn more about our work by exploring our national health initiatives

8631 Alcohol Alert #24: Animal Models in Alcohol Research
National Clearinghouse for Alcohol and Drug Info.
1101 Wootton Parkway
Rockville, MD 20852-2345   800-729-6686
                                        Fax: 240-453-8282
                              e-mail: odphpinfo@hhs.gov
                                            www.health.org
The Office of Disease Prevention and Health Promotion (ODPHP) plays a vital role in keeping the Nation healthy. Learn more about our wso work by exploring our national health initiatives

8632 Alcohol Alert #25: Alcohol-Related Impairment
National Clearinghouse for Alcohol and Drug Info.
1101 Wootton Parkway
Rockville, MD 20852-2345   800-729-6686
                                        Fax: 240-453-8282
                              e-mail: odphpinfo@hhs.gov
                                            www.health.org
The Office of Disease Prevention and Health Promotion (ODPHP) plays a vital role in keeping the Nation healthy. Learn more about our work by exploring our national health initiatives

8633 Alcohol Alert #26: Alcohol and Hormones
National Clearinghouse for Alcohol and Drug Info.
1101 Wootton Parkway
Rockville, MD 20852-2345   800-729-6686
                                        Fax: 240-453-8282
                              e-mail: odphpinfo@hhs.gov
                                            www.health.org
The Office of Disease Prevention and Health Promotion (ODPHP) plays a vital role in keeping the Nation healthy. Learn more about our work by exploring our national health initiatives

8634 Alcohol Alert #27: Alcohol Medication Interactions
National Clearinghouse for Alcohol and Drug Info.
1101 Wootton Parkway
Rockville, MD 20852-2345   800-729-6686
                                        Fax: 240-453-8282
                              e-mail: odphpinfo@hhs.gov
                                            www.health.org
The Office of Disease Prevention and Health Promotion (ODPHP) plays a vital role in keeping the Nation healthy. Learn more about our work by exploring our national health initiatives

8635 Alcohol and Drug Abuse in Black America: A Guide for Community Action
African American Family Services
2616 Nicollet Avenue S   612-871-7878
Minneapolis, MN 55408   855-522-3013
                                          findthebestrehab.org
A booklet giving a description of the history and the current manifestations of alcohol and drug problems in Black America with a discussion of strategies for fundamental change.
24 pages

8636 Alcohol and Pregnancy
March of Dimes
233 Park Avenue South   212-353-8353
New York, NY 10003   Fax: 212-254-3518
                          e-mail: NY639@marchofdimes.com
                                       www.marchofdimes.com

8637 Alcoholics Anonymous and Employee Assistance Program
Alcoholics Anonymous
PO Box 459   212-870-3400
New York, NY 10163-0459   Fax: 212-870-3137
                                              www.aa.org
Of interest to management and union officials, this pamphlet gives concise descriptions of the help AA can offer to the alcoholic employee.

8638 Alcoholism Tends to Run in Families
National Clearinghouse for Alcohol and Drug Info.
1101 Wootton Parkway
Rockville, MD 20852-2345   800-729-6686
                                        Fax: 240-453-8282
                              e-mail: odphpinfo@hhs.gov
                                            www.health.org
Provides answers and questions about how to help children of alcoholics and where to find resources for additional information.

8639 Alcoholism: A Merry-Go-Round Named Denial
Al-Anon Family Group Headquarters
1600 Corp Landing Pkwy   757-563-1600
Virginia Beach, VA 23454-5617   800-425-2666
                                        Fax: 757-563-1655
                                 e-mail: wso@al-anon.org
                                    www.al-anon.alateen.org
Dramatic explanations that help family members and friends see the roles they play in the problems of alcoholism.
18 pages
Caryn Johnson, Director Communications

8640 Alcoholism: The Family Disease
Al-Anon Family Group Headquarters
1600 Corp Landing Pkwy   757-563-1600
Virginia Beach, VA 23454-5617   800-425-2666
                                        Fax: 757-563-1655
                                 e-mail: wso@al-anon.org
                                    www.al-anon.alateen.org
A treasury of information and inspiration with the purpose of the Al-Anon program, actual stories of people who found serenity in Al-Anon, questions/answers, slogans, evaluations and thoughts to live by.
48 pages
Caryn Johnson, Director Communications

8641 Anabolic Steroids: A Threat to Body and Mind
National Clearinghouse for Alcohol and Drug Info.
PO Box 2345
Rockville, MD 20847   800-729-6686
                                          files.eric.ed.gov
Summarizes the findings of recent studies on the use of anabolic steroids in the United States.
11 pages

8642 Anonymity
Al-Anon Family Group Headquarters
1600 Corp Landing Pkwy   757-563-1600
Virginia Beach, VA 23454-5617   800-425-2666
                                         Fax: 757-563-1655
                              e-mail: wso@al-anon.org
                                  www.al-anon.alateen.org
Offers information on Al-Anon and Alateen traditions and what a
big factor anonymity plays for members.
6 pages
Caryn Johnson, Director Communications

8643 Are You Concerned About Someone's Drinking
Al-Anon Family Group Headquarters
1600 Corp Landing Pkwy   757-563-1600
Virginia Beach, VA 23454-5617   800-425-2666
                                         Fax: 757-563-1655
                              e-mail: wso@al-anon.org
                                  www.al-anon.alateen.org
Al-Anon is a mutual support group of peers who share their experience in applying the Al-Anon principles to problems related to the
effects of a problem drinker in their lives. It is not group therapy
and is not led by a counselor or therapist
12 pages
Caryn Johnson, Director Communications

8644 Be Kind to Nonsmokers
American Lung Association
1740 Broadway   212-315-8700
New York, NY 10019-4315
Explains why smoke hurts nonsmokers.

8645 Best of Public Outreach
Al-Anon Family Group Headquarters
1600 Corp Landing Pkwy   757-563-1600
Virginia Beach, VA 23454-5617   800-425-2666
                                         Fax: 757-563-1655
                              e-mail: wso@al-anon.org
                                  www.al-anon.alateen.org
Helps groups, committees and individuals carry out their PI institutions and CPC activities; includes suggested activities and open
letters to various professionals.
24 pages
Caryn Johnson, Director Communications

8646 Black, Beautiful and Recovering
Hazelden
15251 Pleasant Valley Rd   651-213-4200
Center City, MN 55012-9640   800-257-7810
                                         Fax: 651-213-4793
                              e-mail: info@hazelden.org
                                       www.hazelden.org
Hazelden, a part of the Hazelden Betty Ford Foundation, has been
saving lives and restoring families from substance abuse and ad-
diction for more than 60 years
20 pages
Mark Mishek, President and Chief Executive Officer
Joe Jaksha, Publisher

8647 Chemical Dependency and the African American
Hazelden
15251 Pleasant Valley Rd   651-213-4200
Center City, MN 55012-9640   800-257-7810
                                         Fax: 651-213-4793
                              e-mail: info@hazelden.org
                                       www.hazelden.org
Reviews the impact alcohol and other drug abuse has on African
American communities.
66 pages
Mark Mishek, President and Chief Executive Officer
Joe Jaksha, Publisher

8648 Chemical Dependency: An Acceptable Disease
Hazelden
15251 Pleasant Valley Rd   651-213-4200
Center City, MN 55012-9640   800-257-7810
                                         Fax: 651-213-4793
                              e-mail: info@hazelden.org
                                       www.hazelden.org

Help persons identify and acknowledge their chemical dependency.
14 pages
Mark Mishek, President and Chief Executive Officer
Joe Jaksha, Publisher

8649 Chew or Snuff is Real Bad Stuff
National Cancer Institute
Building 31
Bethesda, MD 20892   301-496-4000
                                       www.killthecan.org
A pamphlet describing the hazards of using smokeless tobacco.
8 pages

8650 Cigarette Smoking
American Lung Association
1740 Broadway   212-315-8700
New York, NY 10019-4315
Leaflet presenting the facts about how cigarette smoke is related to
lung disease.

8651 Communication Skills
Hazelden
15251 Pleasant Valley Rd   651-213-4200
Center City, MN 55012-9640   800-257-7810
                                         Fax: 651-213-4793
                              e-mail: info@hazelden.org
                                       www.hazelden.org
Helps clients discover how to become better listeners.
Mark Mishek, President and Chief Executive Officer
Joe Jaksha, Publisher

8652 Community Campaign Brochure
National Clearinghouse for Alcohol and Drug Info.
PO Box 2345
Rockville, MD 20847-2345   800-729-6686
                                           files.eric.ed.gov
Information and promotional brochure discusses key prevention
concepts and messages and details how to plan campaign events.

8653 Crack
Hazelden
15251 Pleasant Valley Rd   651-213-4200
Center City, MN 55012-9640   800-257-7810
                                         Fax: 651-213-4793
                              e-mail: info@hazelden.org
                                       www.hazelden.org
Explains history, use and effects of crack cocaine.
Mark Mishek, President and Chief Executive Officer
Joe Jaksha, Publisher

8654 Crack Cocaine: The Big Lie
National Clearinghouse for Alcohol and Drug Info.
1101 Wootton Parkway
Rockville, MD 20852-2345   800-729-6686
                                         Fax: 240-453-8282
                              e-mail: odphpinfo@hhs.gov
                                          www.health.org
Offers information on what crack and cocaine are, how strong the
addictions are from these drugs, how they affect the body and other
risks in taking cocaine and crack.

8655 Crossing the Line Between Social Drinking and Alcoholism
Hazelden
15251 Pleasant Valley Rd   651-213-4200
Center City, MN 55012-9640   800-257-7810
                                         Fax: 651-213-4793
                              e-mail: info@hazelden.org
                                       www.hazelden.org
Hazelden, a part of the Hazelden Betty Ford Foundation, has been
saving lives and restoring families from substance abuse and ad-
diction for more than 60 years
20 pages
Mark Mishek, President and Chief Executive Officer
Joe Jaksha, Publisher

8656 Denial
Hazelden

15251 Pleasant Valley Rd
Center City, MN 55012-9640

651-213-4200
800-257-7810
Fax: 651-213-4793
e-mail: info@hazelden.org
www.hazelden.org

Describes denial and its role in the five-stage acceptance process.
Mark Mishek, President and Chief Executive Officer
Joe Jaksha, Publisher

8657 Depression and Recovery from Chemical Dependency
Hazelden
15251 Pleasant Valley Rd
Center City, MN 55012-9640

651-213-4200
800-257-7810
Fax: 651-213-4793
e-mail: info@hazelden.org
www.hazelden.org

Outlines depression's warning signs.
Mark Mishek, President and Chief Executive Officer
Joe Jaksha, Publisher

8658 Detaching with Love
Hazelden
15251 Pleasant Valley Rd
Center City, MN 55012-9640

651-213-4200
800-257-7810
Fax: 651-213-4793
e-mail: info@hazelden.org
www.hazelden.org

Addresses the essential recovery tools clients need to cope with addiction and detach from the problem.
Mark Mishek, President and Chief Executive Officer
Joe Jaksha, Publisher

8659 Detachment
Al-Anon Family Group Headquarters
1600 Corp Landing Pkwy
Virginia Beach, VA 23454-5617

757-563-1600
800-425-2666
Fax: 757-563-1655
e-mail: wso@al-anon.org
www.al-anon.alateen.org

Everything you always wanted to know about detachment in an easy-to-use leaflet.
Caryn Johnson, Director Communications

8660 Did You Grow Up with a Problem Drinker?
Al-Anon Family Group Headquarters
1600 Corp Landing Pkwy
Virginia Beach, VA 23454-5617

757-563-1600
800-425-2666
Fax: 757-563-1655
e-mail: wso@al-anon.org
www.al-anon.alateen.org

Twenty personal questions help individuals decide if they can benefit from Al-Anon.
Caryn Johnson, Director Communications

8661 Do You Think You're Different?
Alcoholics Anonymous
PO Box 459
New York, NY 10163-0459

212-870-3400
Fax: 212-870-3137
www.aa.org

Speaks to newcomers who may wonder how AA can work for someone different.

8662 Don't Let Your Dreams Go Up in Smoke
American Lung Association
1740 Broadway
New York, NY 10019-4315

212-315-8700

Photos, testimonials and clear language to deliver the message that everyone can and should stop smoking.

8663 Don't Lose a Friend to Drugs
National Crime Prevention Council
1201 Connecticut Ave NW
Washington, DC 20036-3802

202-466-6272
Fax: 202-296-1356
www.ncpc.org

Offers practical advice to teenagers on how to say no to drugs, how to help a friend who uses drugs and how to initiate community efforts to prevent drug use.
Ann M. Harkins, President and Chief Executive Officer

8664 Drinking Alcohol During Pregnancy
March of Dimes

1275 Mamaroneck Avenue
White Plains, NY 10605

212-353-8353
Fax: 212-254-3518
e-mail: NY639@marchofdimes.com
www.marchofdimes.com

Fact Sheets: one to two page review written for the general public. Also available electronically from the website www.marchofdimes.com

8665 Drug Free Zones: A Manual
African American Family Services
2616 Nicollet Avenue S
Minneapolis, MN 55408

612-871-7878

This booklet describes a variety of strategies concerned citizens are using to reclaim their neighborhoods from rampant drug abuse and dealing.
24 pages

8666 Drugs and Pregnancy
March of Dimes
1275 Mamaroneck Avenue
White Plains, NY 10605

212-353-8353
Fax: 212-254-3518
e-mail: NY639@marchofdimes.com
www.marchofdimes.com

Brochures: 3 panel color brochures written for the general public.
pkg 50

8667 Employer's Guide to Dealing with Substance Abuse
National Clearinghouse for Alcohol and Drug Info.
1101 Wootton Parkway
Rockville, MD 20852-2345

800-729-6686
Fax: 240-453-8282
e-mail: odphpinfo@hhs.gov
www.health.org

Instructs employers in setting up comprehensive alcohol and other drug programs in the workplace.
18 pages

8668 Enabling
Hazelden
15251 Pleasant Valley Rd
Center City, MN 55012-9640

651-213-4200
800-257-7810
Fax: 651-213-4793
e-mail: info@hazelden.org
www.hazelden.org

Describes problems families encounter when they focus their lives on their chemically dependent family member.
Mark Mishek, President and Chief Executive Officer
Joe Jaksha, Publisher

8669 Facts About Alateen
Al-Anon Family Group Headquarters
1600 Corp Landing Pkwy
Virginia Beach, VA 23454-5617

757-563-1600
800-425-2666
Fax: 757-563-1655
e-mail: wso@al-anon.org
www.al-anon.alateen.org

Offers information on Alateen member services.
4 pages
Caryn Johnson, Director Communications

8670 Facts About Alcohol Abuse
Medical Arts Center Hospital
57 W 57th Street
New York, NY 10019-2802

212-838-2169
Fax: 212-755-0200

A question and answer pamphlet that offers information on alcohol abuse and the effects the abuse has on the family unit.

8671 Family Denial
Hazelden
15251 Pleasant Valley Rd
Center City, MN 55012-9640

651-213-4200
800-257-7810
Fax: 651-213-4793
e-mail: info@hazelden.org
www.hazelden.org

Describes ways for families to recognize denial, examine common fears that cause denial and develop methods for overcoming it.
Mark Mishek, President and Chief Executive Officer
Joe Jaksha, Publisher

8672 Fetal Alcohol Syndrome
Hazelden

15251 Pleasant Valley Rd
Center City, MN 55012-9640

651-213-4200
800-257-7810
Fax: 651-213-4793
e-mail: info@hazelden.org
www.hazelden.org

A source of information about the effects of drinking while pregnant.
Mark Mishek, President and Chief Executive Officer
Joe Jaksha, Publisher

8673 Fight Drug Abuse at Home, Work, School and in the Community
American Council for Drug Education
204 Monroe Street
Rockville, MD 20850-4425

800-488-3784
www.hoffmanestates.com

A catalog of print and video materials pertaining to substance abuse, alcoholism and drugs.

8674 For a Strong and Healthy Baby
National Clearinghouse for Alcohol and Drug Info.
1101 Wootton Parkway
Rockville, MD 20852-2345

800-729-6686
Fax: 240-453-8282
e-mail: odphpinfo@hhs.gov
www.health.org

Recommends that women not drink or use other drugs if pregnant or planning to become pregnant.

8675 Free to Care
Hazelden
15251 Pleasant Valley Rd
Center City, MN 55012-9640

651-213-4200
800-257-7810
Fax: 651-213-4793
e-mail: info@hazelden.org
www.hazelden.org

Explores today's definition of family and new attitudes about gender, technology, single-parents, relatives and friends.
Mark Mishek, President and Chief Executive Officer
Joe Jaksha, Publisher

8676 Freedom from Despair
Al-Anon Family Group Headquarters
1600 Corp Landing Pkwy
Virginia Beach, VA 23454-5617

757-563-1600
800-425-2666
Fax: 757-563-1655
e-mail: wso@al-anon.org
www.al-anon.alateen.org

A message of hope for those faced with a problem they can't solve alone.
4 pages
Caryn Johnson, Director Communications

8677 Freedom from Smoking Flyer
American Lung Association
1740 Broadway
New York, NY 10019-4315

212-315-8700

4 color flyer describing all FFS programs.

8678 Getting in Touch with Al-Anon/Alateen
Al-Anon Family Group Headquarters
1600 Corp Landing Pkwy
Virginia Beach, VA 23454-5617

757-563-1600
800-425-2666
Fax: 757-563-1655
e-mail: wso@al-anon.org
www.al-anon.alateen.org

A listing of Al-Anon information services throughout the world. Helps members, the public and professionals located nearby Al-Anon or Alateen groups.
Caryn Johnson, Director Communications

8679 Grieving
Hazelden
15251 Pleasant Valley Rd
Center City, MN 55012-9640

651-213-4200
800-257-7810
Fax: 651-213-4793
e-mail: info@hazelden.org
www.hazelden.org

Outlines the five-phase grieving process for clients and the significance of each.
Mark Mishek, President and Chief Executive Officer
Joe Jaksha, Publisher

8680 Guidance on Our Journeys
Hazelden
15251 Pleasant Valley Rd
Center City, MN 55012-9640

651-213-4200
800-257-7810
Fax: 651-213-4793
e-mail: info@hazelden.org
www.hazelden.org

Examines the relationship between the recovering person and his or her sponsor.
Mark Mishek, President and Chief Executive Officer
Joe Jaksha, Publisher

8681 Guide for the Family of the Alcoholic
Al-Anon Family Group Headquarters
1600 Corp Landing Pkwy
Virginia Beach, VA 23454-5617

757-563-1600
800-425-2666
Fax: 757-563-1655
e-mail: wso@al-anon.org
www.al-anon.alateen.org

A clear and realistic look at alcoholism, problems encountered by those close to the alcoholic and choices available to the family.
16 pages
Caryn Johnson, Director Communications

8682 Have Fun! Figure Out the Smoking Puzzle
American Lung Association
1740 Broadway
New York, NY 10019-4315

212-315-8700

Crossword puzzles make stimulating points on the effects of smoking.

8683 Healthy Beginning, Promotional Flyers
American Lung Association
1740 Broadway
New York, NY 10019-4315

212-315-8700

Flyer offers tips to help protect newborn and young children from the harmful effects of passive smoking.

8684 Help a Friend to Stop Smoking
American Lung Association
1740 Broadway
New York, NY 10019-4315

212-315-8700

This original guide to helping family members and friends support a smoker who is trying to quit smoking.
12 pages

8685 Helping Smokers Get Ready to Quit
American Lung Association
1740 Broadway
New York, NY 10019-4315

212-315-8700

Offers suggestions on how to get smokers to think about quitting and how to open up a dialogue on the issue.

8686 Helping Your Child Say No: A Parent's Guide
National Clearinghouse for Alcohol and Drug Info.
PO Box 2345
Rockville, MD 20847-2345

800-729-6686
www.hoffmanestates.com

Explains to parents how alcohol affects the body, how to tell if your child has been drinking and why children start to drink.

8687 Homeward Bound
Al-Anon Family Group Headquarters
1600 Corp Landing Pkwy
Virginia Beach, VA 23454-5617

757-563-1600
800-425-2666
Fax: 757-563-1655
e-mail: wso@al-anon.org
www.al-anon.alateen.org

A booklet designed to help beginners make the transition from the family treatment setting to Al-Anon. Contains forty members' personal sharings, a basic glossary of Al-Anon terms, brief explanations of Al-Anon slogans and helpful suggestions for newcomers.
48 pages
Caryn Johnson, Director Communications

8688 How Can I Help My Children?
Al-Anon Family Group Headquarters
1600 Corp Landing Pkwy   757-563-1600
Virginia Beach, VA 23454-5617   800-425-2666
                                        Fax: 757-563-1655
                                    e-mail: wso@al-anon.org
                                        www.al-anon.alateen.org
Parents can help their children achieve a healthier attitude. Improving our own attitudes and behavior will help the entire family.
20 pages
Caryn Johnson, Director Communications

8689 How Drug Abuse Takes Profit Out of Business
National Clearinghouse for Alcohol and Drug Info.
PO Box 2345
Rockville, MD 20847-2345   800-729-6686
                                    www.hoffmanestates.com
Answers employers questions about substance abuse in the workplace.

8690 How to Get the Most Out of Group Therapy
Hazelden
15251 Pleasant Valley Rd   651-213-4200
Center City, MN 55012-9640   800-257-7810
                                        Fax: 651-213-4793
                                    e-mail: info@hazelden.org
                                        www.hazelden.org
Answers clients' questions about going to and getting help from group therapy.
Mark Mishek, President and Chief Executive Officer
Joe Jaksha, Publisher

8691 How to Help a Friend Quit Smoking
American Lung Association
1740 Broadway
New York, NY 10019-4315   212-315-8700
Discusses how friends, family and co-workers can assist smokers with their concerns about quitting smoking.

8692 How to Take Care of Your Baby Before Birth
National Clearinghouse for Alcohol and Drug Info.
1101 Wootton Parkway
Rockville, MD 20852-2345   800-729-6686
                                        Fax: 240-453-8282
                                    e-mail: odphpinfo@hhs.gov
                                        www.health.org
A low-literacy brochure aimed at pregnant women that describes what they should and should not do during pregnancy.

8693 I Can't Be Addicted Because...
Hazelden
15251 Pleasant Valley Rd   651-213-4200
Center City, MN 55012-9640   800-257-7810
                                        Fax: 651-213-4793
                                    e-mail: info@hazelden.org
                                        www.hazelden.org
Focuses on denial and elaborates on its most common forms.
Mark Mishek, President and Chief Executive Officer
Joe Jaksha, Publisher

8694 Ice Storm
Hazelden
15251 Pleasant Valley Rd   651-213-4200
Center City, MN 55012-9640   800-257-7810
                                        Fax: 651-213-4793
                                    e-mail: info@hazelden.org
                                        www.hazelden.org
Prepares treatment professionals for the complications of one of the most recently synthesized drugs - ice.
Mark Mishek, President and Chief Executive Officer
Joe Jaksha, Publisher

8695 If Someone Close to You Has a Problem with Alcohol or Other Drugs
National Clearinghouse for Alcohol and Drug Info.
1101 Wootton Parkway
Rockville, MD 20852-2345   800-729-6686
                                        Fax: 240-453-8282
                                    e-mail: odphpinfo@hhs.gov
                                        www.health.org

This booklet is aimed at the general public and gives support and suggestions on coping with someone close who has an alcohol or drug problem.

8696 If You Are a Professional, AA Wants to Work with You
Alcoholics Anonymous
PO Box 459   212-870-3400
New York, NY 10163-0459   Fax: 212-870-3137
                                        www.aa.org
Directed at professionals of all types who deal with alcoholics.

8697 If Your Parents Drink Too Much
Al-Anon Family Group Headquarters
1600 Corp Landing Pkwy   757-563-1600
Virginia Beach, VA 23454-5617   800-425-2666
                                        Fax: 757-563-1655
                                    e-mail: wso@al-anon.org
                                        www.al-anon.alateen.org
Alateen's cartoon booklet.
24 pages
Caryn Johnson, Director Communications

8698 Illicit Drug Use During Pregnancy
March of Dimes
1275 Mamaroneck Avenue   212-353-8353
White Plains, NY 10605   Fax: 212-254-3518
                            e-mail: NY639@marchofdimes.com
                                        www.marchofdimes.com
Fact Sheets: one to two page review for the general public. Also available electronically from the website www.marchofdimes.com

8699 Index to Alcoholics Anonymous
Hazelden
15251 Pleasant Valley Rd   651-213-4200
Center City, MN 55012-9640   800-257-7810
                                        Fax: 651-213-4793
                                    e-mail: info@hazelden.org
                                        www.hazelden.org
Features page and line references to the topics discussed in Alcoholics Anonymous, the Big Book.
Mark Mishek, President and Chief Executive Officer
Joe Jaksha, Publisher

8700 Is AA for Me?
Alcoholics Anonymous
PO Box 459   212-870-3400
New York, NY 10163-0459   Fax: 212-870-3137
                                        www.aa.org
An illustrated easy to read version of the 12 questions in Is AA for You? pamphlet.
32 pages

8701 Is AA for You?
Alcoholics Anonymous
PO Box 459   212-870-3400
New York, NY 10163-0459   Fax: 212-870-3137
                                        www.aa.org
Symptoms of alcoholism are summed up in 12 questions most AA's had answered to identify themselves as alcoholics.

8702 Is There a Safe Tobacco?
American Lung Association
1740 Broadway   212-315-8700
New York, NY 10019-4315
Offers information on the health risks of cigarette smoking, pipes and cigars.

8703 Is There an Alcoholic in Your Life?
Alcoholics Anonymous
PO Box 459   212-870-3400
New York, NY 10163-0459   Fax: 212-870-3137
                                        www.aa.org
Explains the AA program as it affects anyone close to an alcoholic.

8704 It Happened to Alice
Alcoholics Anonymous
PO Box 459   212-870-3400
New York, NY 10163-0459   Fax: 212-870-3137
                                        www.aa.org
Easy to read comic-book style format for women alcoholics.

8705 **It Sure Beats Sitting in a Cell**
Alcoholics Anonymous
PO Box 459   212-870-3400
New York, NY 10163-0459   Fax: 212-870-3137
                                                       www.aa.org
An illustrated pamphlet which presents the experience of seven in-
mates who found AA while in prison. It also offers suggested dos
and don'ts for staying sober after release.

8706 **Kids and Drugs: A Handbook for Parents & Professionals**
PANDAA Press
4111 Watkins Trl
Annandale, VA 22003-2051   703-750-9285
                                                   www.sdsalarms.com

8707 **Let's Solve the Smokeword Puzzle**
American Lung Association
1740 Broadway   212-315-8700
New York, NY 10019-4315
Fifth graders will love getting an antismoking message through
solving a crossword puzzle.

8708 **Let's Talk**
Hazelden
15251 Pleasant Valley Rd   651-213-4200
Center City, MN 55012-9640   800-257-7810
                                                Fax: 651-213-4793
                                       e-mail: info@hazelden.org
                                                  www.hazelden.org
Offers 12 guidelines to promote effective communication between
parent and child.
Mark Mishek, President and Chief Executive Officer
Joe Jaksha, Publisher

8709 **Letter to a Woman Alcoholic**
Alcoholics Anonymous
PO Box 459   212-870-3400
New York, NY 10163-0459   Fax: 212-870-3137
                                                       www.aa.org
Describes with sensitive understanding the problem of the alco-
holic woman.

8710 **Letting Go of the Need to Control**
Hazelden
15251 Pleasant Valley Rd   651-213-4200
Center City, MN 55012-9640   800-257-7810
                                                Fax: 651-213-4793
                                       e-mail: info@hazelden.org
                                                  www.hazelden.org
Discusses how control issues are common among chemically de-
pendent people.
Mark Mishek, President and Chief Executive Officer
Joe Jaksha, Publisher

8711 **Lifetime of Freedom from Smoking: Maintenance Manual**
American Lung Association
1740 Broadway   212-315-8700
New York, NY 10019-4315
Companion manual helps persons stay quit once they have stopped
smoking.
28 pages

8712 **Little More About Alcohol**
Alcohol Research Information Service
1120 E Oakland Avenue   517-485-9900
Lansing, MI 48906-5513   Fax: 517-485-1928
          e-mail: alcoholisadrugtoo@yoyoger.net
                                        www.hoffmanestates.com
A cartoon character explains the facts about alcohol and its effects
on the body.

8713 **Living Sober**
Alcoholics Anonymous
PO Box 459   212-870-3400
New York, NY 10163-0459   Fax: 212-870-3137
                                                       www.aa.org
Practical book demonstrating through simple examples, how AA
members throughout the world live and stay sober one day at a
time.
88 pages

8714 **Living in a Shelter?**
Al-Anon Family Group Headquarters
1600 Corp Landing Pkwy   757-563-1600
Virginia Beach, VA 23454-5617   800-425-2666
                                                Fax: 757-563-1655
                                       e-mail: wso@al-anon.org
                                            www.al-anon.alateen.org
Al-Anon is a mutual support group of peers who share their experience in applying the Al-Anon principles to problems related to the
effects of a problem drinker in their lives. It is not group therapy
and is not led by a counselor or therapist
100 pieces
Caryn Johnson, Director Communications

8715 **Look at Cross-Addiction**
Hazelden
15251 Pleasant Valley Rd   651-213-4200
Center City, MN 55012-9640   800-257-7810
                                                Fax: 651-213-4793
                                       e-mail: info@hazelden.org
                                                  www.hazelden.org
Discusses cross-addiction, denial, coping skills and avoidance.
Mark Mishek, President and Chief Executive Officer
Joe Jaksha, Publisher

8716 **Look at Relapse**
Hazelden
15251 Pleasant Valley Rd   651-213-4200
Center City, MN 55012-9640   800-257-7810
                                                Fax: 651-213-4793
                                       e-mail: info@hazelden.org
                                                  www.hazelden.org
Addresses emotional consequences of relapse, such as decreased
feelings of self-esteem and self-confidence.
Mark Mishek, President and Chief Executive Officer
Joe Jaksha, Publisher

8717 **Managing Cocaine Cravings**
Hazelden
15251 Pleasant Valley Rd   651-213-4200
Center City, MN 55012-9640   800-257-7810
                                                Fax: 651-213-4793
                                       e-mail: info@hazelden.org
                                                  www.hazelden.org
Offers clients hands-on plan to help them stay away from cocaine.
Mark Mishek, President and Chief Executive Officer
Joe Jaksha, Publisher

8718 **Marijuana**
Hazelden
15251 Pleasant Valley Rd   651-213-4200
Center City, MN 55012-9640   800-257-7810
                                                Fax: 651-213-4793
                                       e-mail: info@hazelden.org
                                                  www.hazelden.org
Outlines the physical and psychological effects of marijuana
unique to episodic and chronic use.
65 pages
Mark Mishek, President and Chief Executive Officer
Joe Jaksha, Publisher

8719 **Media Kit**
Al-Anon Family Group Headquarters
1600 Corp Landing Pkwy   757-563-1600
Virginia Beach, VA 23454-5617   800-425-2666
                                                Fax: 757-563-1655
                                       e-mail: wso@al-anon.org
                                            www.al-anon.alateen.org
An attractive silver folder containing information necessary to
work with radio and TV stations.
Caryn Johnson, Director Communications

8720 **Member's Eye View of Alcoholics Anonymous**
Alcoholics Anonymous
PO Box 459   212-870-3400
New York, NY 10163-0459   Fax: 212-870-3137
                                                       www.aa.org
Designed to explain to people in the helping professionals how AA
works.
30 pages

659

8721   Members of the Clergy Ask About Alcoholics Anonymous
Alcoholics Anonymous
PO Box 459   212-870-3400
New York, NY 10163-0459   Fax: 212-870-3137
www.aa.org
Introduction to AA for members of the clergy unfamiliar with the Fellowship.

8722   Memo to an Inmate Who May Be an Alcoholic
Alcoholics Anonymous
PO Box 459   212-870-3400
New York, NY 10163-0459   Fax: 212-870-3137
www.aa.org
A message from AA's who have themselves been inmates. Their personal stories offer a new outlook to inmate alcholics who want to know who AA can help.

8723   Men Newcomer Packet
Al-Anon Family Group Headquarters
1600 Corp Landing Pkwy   757-563-1600
Virginia Beach, VA 23454-5617   800-425-2666
Fax: 757-563-1655
e-mail: wso@al-anon.org
www.al-anon.alateen.org
For men who are not sure Al-Anon is for them, this collection offers a realistic look at alcoholism and straight forward answers to frequently asked questions.
8 pieces
Caryn Johnson, Director Communications

8724   Message to Correctional Facilities Administrators
Alcoholics Anonymous
PO Box 459   212-870-3400
New York, NY 10163-0459   Fax: 212-870-3137
www.aa.org
Information about what AA is and can do, and how groups function in correctional facilities.

8725   Message to Teenagers
Alcoholics Anonymous
PO Box 459   212-870-3400
New York, NY 10163-0459   Fax: 212-870-3137
www.aa.org
This brochure offers a simple, 12-question quiz designed to help teenagers decide when drinking is becoming a problem in their lives.

8726   Military Packet
Al-Anon Family Group Headquarters
1600 Corp Landing Pkwy   757-563-1600
Virginia Beach, VA 23454-5617   800-425-2666
Fax: 757-563-1655
e-mail: wso@al-anon.org
www.al-anon.alateen.org
For those in the armed services with loved ones or colleagues who are alcoholic, here's a collection that says, Al-Anon can help.
7 pieces
Caryn Johnson, Director Communications

8727   Moment to Reflect on Codependency
Hazelden
15251 Pleasant Valley Rd   651-213-4200
Center City, MN 55012-9640   800-257-7810
Fax: 651-213-4793
e-mail: info@hazelden.org
www.hazelden.org
A collection of four booklets offering meditations that emphasize and reinforce self-esteem for young people recovering from addiction.
Mark Mishek, President and Chief Executive Officer
Joe Jaksha, Publisher

8728   Moment to Reflect on Self-Esteem
Hazelden
15251 Pleasant Valley Rd   651-213-4200
Center City, MN 55012-9640   800-257-7810
Fax: 651-213-4793
e-mail: info@hazelden.org
www.hazelden.org

Focuses on the fundamental recovery issue of self-esteem.
4 Booklets
Mark Mishek, President and Chief Executive Officer
Joe Jaksha, Publisher

8729   Moving On! From Alateen to Al-Anon
Al-Anon Family Group Headquarters
1600 Corp Landing Pkwy   757-563-1600
Virginia Beach, VA 23454-5617   800-425-2666
Fax: 757-563-1655
e-mail: wso@al-anon.org
www.al-anon.alateen.org
Former Alateen members experience the joy of continued recovery in Al-Anon.
12 pages
Caryn Johnson, Director Communications

8730   NIDA Capsules
National Clearinghouse for Alcohol and Drug Info.
1101 Wootton Parkway
Rockville, MD 20852-2345   800-729-6686
Fax: 240-453-8282
e-mail: odphpinfo@hhs.gov
www.health.org
The Office of Disease Prevention and Health Promotion (ODPHP) plays a vital role in keeping the Nation healthy. Learn more about our work by exploring our national health initiatives

8731   Newcomer Asks
Alcoholics Anonymous
PO Box 459   212-870-3400
New York, NY 10163-0459   Fax: 212-870-3137
www.aa.org
Gives straightforward answers on 15 points that once puzzled many of us.

8732   Nicotine Addiction and Cigarettes
American Lung Association
1740 Broadway   212-315-8700
New York, NY 10019-4315
Offers information on nicotine and cigarette smoking.

8733   No Smoking Coloring Book
American Lung Association
1740 Broadway   212-315-8700
New York, NY 10019-4315
Preschool and primary grade children will enjoy drawing and coloring while getting an antismoking message.

8734   No Smoking: Lungs At Work
American Lung Association
1740 Broadway   212-315-8700
New York, NY 10019-4315
Describes how lungs work and how they are affected by smoking.

8735   Now What Do I Do for Fun?
Hazelden
15251 Pleasant Valley Rd   651-213-4200
Center City, MN 55012-9640   800-257-7810
Fax: 651-213-4793
e-mail: info@hazelden.org
www.hazelden.org
Explores the dilemma of finding new interests in recovery after completing treatment.
Mark Mishek, President and Chief Executive Officer
Joe Jaksha, Publisher

8736   Older Adults After Treatment
Hazelden
15251 Pleasant Valley Rd   651-213-4200
Center City, MN 55012-9640   800-257-7810
Fax: 651-213-4793
e-mail: info@hazelden.org
www.hazelden.org
Discusses aftercare issues, such as family relations, health, medication and relapse.
Mark Mishek, President and Chief Executive Officer
Joe Jaksha, Publisher

8737   Older Adults in Treatment
Hazelden

15251 Pleasant Valley Rd
Center City, MN 55012-9640

651-213-4200
800-257-7810
Fax: 651-213-4793
e-mail: info@hazelden.org
www.hazelden.org

Examines past beliefs about addiction and defines chemical dependency as a disease.
Mark Mishek, President and Chief Executive Officer
Joe Jaksha, Publisher

8738 On the Air: A Guide to Creating A Smoke-Free Workplace
American Lung Association
1740 Broadway
New York, NY 10019-4315

212-315-8700

A step-by-step guide for organizations interested in developing and implementing a successful workplace smoking control policy.
24 pages

8739 Parents Newcomer Packet
Al-Anon Family Group Headquarters
1600 Corp Landing Pkwy
Virginia Beach, VA 23454-5617

757-563-1600
800-425-2666
Fax: 757-563-1655
e-mail: wso@al-anon.org
www.al-anon.alateen.org

For parents who realize their child is an alcoholic, this is a compassionate and reassuring welcome to Al-Anon.
9 pieces
Caryn Johnson, Director Communications

8740 Points for Parents Perplexed About Drugs
Hazelden
15251 Pleasant Valley Rd
Center City, MN 55012-9640

651-213-4200
800-257-7810
Fax: 651-213-4793
e-mail: info@hazelden.org
www.hazelden.org

Clear guidelines to help adults recognize, evaluate and deal with adolescent drug abuse.
16 pages
Mark Mishek, President and Chief Executive Officer
Joe Jaksha, Publisher

8741 Preventing Relapse
Hazelden
15251 Pleasant Valley Rd
Center City, MN 55012-9640

651-213-4200
800-257-7810
Fax: 651-213-4793
e-mail: info@hazelden.org
www.hazelden.org

Offers practical information and personal stories to help clients better understand the relapse process.
28 pages
Mark Mishek, President and Chief Executive Officer
Joe Jaksha, Publisher

8742 Program Booklet
Women for Sobriety
PO Box 618
Quakertown, PA 18951-0618

215-536-8026
Fax: 215-536-8026
e-mail: newlife@nni.com
www.womenforsobriety.org

Purse size booklet that explains the Thirteen Statements of Dr. Kirkpatrick's New Life program, statement by statement.

8743 Put on the Brakes Bulletin: Take a Look at College Drinking
National Clearinghouse for Alcohol and Drug Info.
1101 Wootton Parkway
Rockville, MD 20852-2345

800-729-6686
Fax: 240-453-8282
e-mail: odphpinfo@hhs.gov
www.health.org

This second edition continues CSAP's campaign to raise awareness about the problems of college drinking.

8744 Q&A About Smoking and Health
American Lung Association
1740 Broadway
New York, NY 10019-4315

212-315-8700

Gives fact-crammed answers to questions on smoking and health.

8745 Quick List to Build Pride in Your Communities
National Clearinghouse for Alcohol and Drug Info.
PO Box 2345
Rockville, MD 20847-2345

800-729-6686
www.hoffmanestates.com

This parent guide is an adaptation of CSAP's Be Smart! Quick List: 10 Steps to Help Your Child Say No.

8746 Reducing the Health Risks of Secondhand Smoke
American Lung Association
1740 Broadway
New York, NY 10019-4315

212-315-8700

What a person can do at home, work and in public places to reduce the health risks of secondhand smoke.

8747 Relapse and the Addict
Hazelden
15251 Pleasant Valley Rd
Center City, MN 55012-9640

651-213-4200
800-257-7810
Fax: 651-213-4793
e-mail: info@hazelden.org
www.hazelden.org

Identifies specific stages and triggers of relapse.
Mark Mishek, President and Chief Executive Officer
Joe Jaksha, Publisher

8748 Releasing Anger
Hazelden
15251 Pleasant Valley Rd
Center City, MN 55012-9640

651-213-4200
800-257-7810
Fax: 651-213-4793
e-mail: info@hazelden.org
www.hazelden.org

Discusses anger as a normal feeling and how anger can endanger recovery.
Mark Mishek, President and Chief Executive Officer
Joe Jaksha, Publisher

8749 Research on Drugs and the Workplace
National Clearinghouse for Alcohol and Drug Info.
PO Box 2345
Rockville, MD 20847-2345

800-729-6686
www.hoffmanestates.com

Discusses prevalence and costs to society of drug use in the workplace, along with information on employee assistance programs, drug testing, grants and additional resources.

8750 Secondhand Smoke
American Lung Association
1740 Broadway
New York, NY 10019-4315

212-315-8700

Documents the effects of tobacco smoke on nonsmokers.

8751 Seven Reasons Not to Use Drugs and Alcohol
American Council On Drug Education
204 Monroe Street
Rockville, MD 20850-4425

800-488-3784
www.hoffmanestates.com

A series of five pamphlets offering information on the hazards of alcohol, crack, cocaine, steroids and tobacco products.
Grades 4-6

8752 Sexual Intimacy and the Alcoholic Relationship
Al-Anon Family Group Headquarters
1600 Corp Landing Pkwy
Virginia Beach, VA 23454-5617

757-563-1600
800-425-2666
Fax: 757-563-1655
e-mail: wso@al-anon.org
www.al-anon.alateen.org

Sex and alcohol? Al-Anon members face this personal problem when they apply to the Al-Anon program indexed.
48 pages
Caryn Johnson, Director Communications

8753 Should Tobacco Advertising and Promotion Be Banned?
American Lung Association
1740 Broadway
New York, NY 10019-4315

212-315-8700

Answers many questions about tobacco advertising and promotion, and explains how ads are targeted to vulnerable populations.

8754 Smoke Free Family Promotional Leaflet
American Lung Association
1740 Broadway   212-315-8700
New York, NY 10019-4315
Leaflet and order form describe an entire range of ALA's smoking-related materials.

8755 Smokeless Tobacco: No Way
American Lung Association
1740 Broadway   212-315-8700
New York, NY 10019-4315
Written for junior and senior high school students, this booklet presents the facts about health risks of smokeless tobacco use.

8756 Smoking and Pregnancy
American Lung Association
1740 Broadway   212-315-8700
New York, NY 10019-4315
Written in a question/answer format, this pamphlet discusses many issues relating to smoking and pregnancy.

8757 Stop Smoking, Stay Trim
American Lung Association
1740 Broadway   212-315-8700
New York, NY 10019-4315
Outlines how to avoid gaining weight while quitting smoking.

8758 Stop Smoking: A Guide to Your Options
American Lung Association
1740 Broadway   212-315-8700
New York, NY 10019-4315
Describes a variety of approaches to smoking cessation. Offers guidance on how to choose a program.

8759 Straight Back Home
Hazelden
15251 Pleasant Valley Rd   651-213-4200
Center City, MN 55012-9640   800-257-7810
                                  Fax: 651-213-4793
                            e-mail: info@hazelden.org
                                   www.hazelden.org
Written for adolescents completing inpatient treatment and returning home.
Mark Mishek, President and Chief Executive Officer
Joe Jaksha, Publisher

8760 Stress in Recovery
Hazelden
15251 Pleasant Valley Rd   651-213-4200
Center City, MN 55012-9640   800-257-7810
                                  Fax: 651-213-4793
                            e-mail: info@hazelden.org
                                   www.hazelden.org
Outlines methods for clients to overcome stress in their daily lives.
Mark Mishek, President and Chief Executive Officer
Joe Jaksha, Publisher

8761 This Is AA
Alcoholics Anonymous
PO Box 459   212-870-3400
New York, NY 10163-0459   Fax: 212-870-3137
                                          www.aa.org
A pamphlet offering an introduction to the AA recovery program.

8762 Three Talks to Medical Societies
Alcoholics Anonymous
PO Box 459   212-870-3400
New York, NY 10163-0459   Fax: 212-870-3137
                                          www.aa.org
Contains Bill Wilson's, the co-founder of AA, principles borrowed from medicine and religion and a summary of AA's first 23 years.

8763 Time to Start Living
Alcoholics Anonymous
PO Box 459   212-870-3400
New York, NY 10163-0459   Fax: 212-870-3137
                                          www.aa.org
Addresses the older alcoholic, with nine stories of men and women who came to AA after the age of 60 (large print edition is also available).

8764 Too Many Young People Drink and Know Too Little About the Consequences
National Clearinghouse for Alcohol and Drug Info.
PO Box 2345
Rockville, MD 20847-2345   800-729-6686
                               www.hoffmanestates.com
Provides up-to-date resources and statistics on the widespread use of alcohol by youth under 21 years of age.

8765 Too Young?
Alcoholics Anonymous
PO Box 459   212-870-3400
New York, NY 10163-0459   Fax: 212-870-3137
                                          www.aa.org
This cartoon pamphlet speaks to teenagers in their own language, telling the varied drinking stories of six youn people (13 to 18).

8766 Treating Nicotine Addiction
Hazelden
15251 Pleasant Valley Rd   651-213-4200
Center City, MN 55012-9640   800-257-7810
                                  Fax: 651-213-4793
                            e-mail: info@hazelden.org
                                   www.hazelden.org
Describes the success of one chemical dependency treatment center that began treating nicotine as an addiction.
Mark Mishek, President and Chief Executive Officer
Joe Jaksha, Publisher

8767 Twelve Steps Illustrated
Alcoholics Anonymous
PO Box 459   212-870-3400
New York, NY 10163-0459   Fax: 212-870-3137
                                          www.aa.org
An easy-to-read version of AA's twelve steps.

8768 Twelve Steps for Tobacco Users
Hazelden
15251 Pleasant Valley Rd   651-213-4200
Center City, MN 55012-9640   800-257-7810
                                  Fax: 651-213-4793
                            e-mail: info@hazelden.org
                                   www.hazelden.org
Presents the Surgeon General's findings that classify nicotine as an addictive substance.
25 pages
Mark Mishek, President and Chief Executive Officer
Joe Jaksha, Publisher

8769 Understanding Depression and Addiction
Hazelden
15251 Pleasant Valley Rd   651-213-4200
Center City, MN 55012-9640   800-257-7810
                                  Fax: 651-213-4793
                            e-mail: info@hazelden.org
                                   www.hazelden.org
Hazelden, a part of the Hazelden Betty Ford Foundation, has been saving lives and restoring families from substance abuse and addiction for more than 60 years
29 pages
Mark Mishek, President and Chief Executive Officer
Joe Jaksha, Publisher

8770 Understanding Major Anxiety Disorders and Addiction
Hazelden
15251 Pleasant Valley Rd   651-213-4200
Center City, MN 55012-9640   800-257-7810
                                  Fax: 651-213-4793
                            e-mail: info@hazelden.org
                                   www.hazelden.org
Hazelden, a part of the Hazelden Betty Ford Foundation, has been saving lives and restoring families from substance abuse and addiction for more than 60 years
36 pages
Mark Mishek, President and Chief Executive Officer
Joe Jaksha, Publisher

8771 Understanding Ourselves and Alcoholism
Al-Anon Family Group Headquarters

1600 Corp Landing Pkwy
Virginia Beach, VA 23454-5617
757-563-1600
800-425-2666
Fax: 757-563-1655
e-mail: wso@al-anon.org
www.al-anon.alateen.org

Explains how compulsion, obsession and denial affect those close to an alcoholic as well as the alcoholic.
6 pages
Caryn Johnson, Director Communications

8772   Understanding Personality Problems and Addiction
Hazelden
15251 Pleasant Valley Rd
Center City, MN 55012-9640
651-213-4200
800-257-7810
Fax: 651-213-4793
e-mail: info@hazelden.org
www.hazelden.org

Describes common features of personality problems, such as self-centeredness and setting boundaries.
28 pages
Mark Mishek, President and Chief Executive Officer
Joe Jaksha, Publisher

8773   Understanding Post-Traumatic Stress Disorder and Addiction
Hazelden
15251 Pleasant Valley Rd
Center City, MN 55012-9640
651-213-4200
800-257-7810
Fax: 651-213-4793
e-mail: info@hazelden.org
www.hazelden.org

Hazelden, a part of the Hazelden Betty Ford Foundation, has been saving lives and restoring families from substance abuse and addiction for more than 60 years
17 pages
Mark Mishek, President and Chief Executive Officer
Joe Jaksha, Publisher

8774   Unpuffables Promotional Brochure
American Lung Association
1740 Broadway
New York, NY 10019-4315
212-315-8700

Describes the ALA Unpuffables program.

8775   What Are the Signs of Alcoholism?
Hazelden
15251 Pleasant Valley Rd
Center City, MN 55012-9640
651-213-4200
800-257-7810
Fax: 651-213-4793
e-mail: info@hazelden.org
www.hazelden.org

Self-test for clients to review the role of alcohol in their lives.
Mark Mishek, President and Chief Executive Officer
Joe Jaksha, Publisher

8776   What Happened to Joe?
Alcoholics Anonymous
PO Box 459
New York, NY 10163-0459
212-870-3400
Fax: 212-870-3137
www.aa.org

Dramatic story of a young construction worker and his drinking problem, told in brightly colored comic book style.

8777   What Happens After Treatment?
Al-Anon Family Group Headquarters
1600 Corp Landing Pkwy
Virginia Beach, VA 23454-5617
757-563-1600
800-425-2666
Fax: 757-563-1655
e-mail: wso@al-anon.org
www.al-anon.alateen.org

Al-Anon is a mutual support group of peers who share their experience in applying the Al-Anon principles to problems related to the effects of a problem drinker in their lives. It is not group therapy and is not led by a counselor or therapist
100 pieces
Caryn Johnson, Director Communications

8778   What is AA?
Hazelden

15251 Pleasant Valley Rd
Center City, MN 55012-9640
651-213-4200
800-257-7810
Fax: 651-213-4793
e-mail: info@hazelden.org
www.hazelden.org

Answers the basic questions about Alcoholics Anonymous.
Mark Mishek, President and Chief Executive Officer
Joe Jaksha, Publisher

8779   What is NA?
Hazelden
15251 Pleasant Valley Rd
Center City, MN 55012-9640
651-213-4200
800-257-7810
Fax: 651-213-4793
e-mail: info@hazelden.org
www.hazelden.org

Helps clients evaluate their addiction to narcotics and answers their questions about N.A.
Mark Mishek, President and Chief Executive Officer
Joe Jaksha, Publisher

8780   What's Your Cigarette Smoking IQ?
American Lung Association
1740 Broadway
New York, NY 10019-4315
212-315-8700

Brief true-or-false quiz that tests a person's knowledge of the effects of smoking.

8781   When You Go Back to Work
Hazelden
15251 Pleasant Valley Rd
Center City, MN 55012-9640
651-213-4200
800-257-7810
Fax: 651-213-4793
e-mail: info@hazelden.org
www.hazelden.org

Stories demonstrating co-workers' attitudes clients may face upon their return to work.
Mark Mishek, President and Chief Executive Officer
Joe Jaksha, Publisher

8782   When Your Teen is in Treatment
Hazelden
15251 Pleasant Valley Rd
Center City, MN 55012-9640
651-213-4200
800-257-7810
Fax: 651-213-4793
e-mail: info@hazelden.org
www.hazelden.org

A guide for parents.
Mark Mishek, President and Chief Executive Officer
Joe Jaksha, Publisher

8783   Where Do I Go from Here?
Alcoholics Anonymous
PO Box 459
New York, NY 10163-0459
212-870-3400
Fax: 212-870-3137
www.aa.org

For people leaving treatment facilities, single-sheet flyer tells of continuing help offered by outside AAs.

8784   Why Anonymity in Al-Anon?
Al-Anon Family Group Headquarters
1600 Corp Landing Pkwy
Virginia Beach, VA 23454-5617
757-563-1600
800-425-2666
Fax: 757-563-1655
e-mail: wso@al-anon.org
www.al-anon.alateen.org

Al-Anon is a mutual support group of peers who share their experience in applying the Al-Anon principles to problems related to the effects of a problem drinker in their lives. It is not group therapy and is not led by a counselor or therapist
12 pages
Caryn Johnson, Director Communications

8785   Workers at Risk: Drugs and Alcohol on the Job
National Clearinghouse for Alcohol and Drug Info.
PO Box 2345
Rockville, MD 20847-2345
800-729-6686
www.hoffmanestates.com

Gives facts about drugs in the workplace and suggests appropriate behavior for employees who are confronted with a coworker's use of alcohol or other drugs.

8786   You Can Help Your Community Get Rid of Drugs
National Clearinghouse for Alcohol and Drug Info.
PO Box 2345
Rockville, MD 20847-2345   800-729-6686
                                            www.hoffmanestates.com
Supports drug abuse treatment and explains how drug use can create problems for your community.

8787   Young Children and Drugs: What Parents Can Do
Wisconsin Clearinghouse
1954 E Washington Avenue
Madison, WI 53704-5275   www.hoffmanestates.com
100 Brochures

8788   Youth and the Alcoholic Parent
Al-Anon Family Group Headquarters
1600 Corp Landing Pkwy   757-563-1600
Virginia Beach, VA 23454-5617   800-425-2666
                                            Fax: 757-563-1655
                                            e-mail: wso@al-anon.org
                                            www.al-anon.alateen.org
Questions and suggestions to help young people improve their own lives.
12 pages
Caryn Johnson, Director Communications

Audio & Video

8789   AA: Rap with Us
Alcoholics Anonymous
PO Box 459   212-870-3400
New York, NY 10163-0459   Fax: 212-870-3137
                                            www.aa.org
Features four anonymous young AA members. Rap music and lyrics bridge these four young people's stories of alcoholic despair and A.A. recovery.
16 minutes

8790   Al-Anon Video
Al-Anon Family Group Headquarters
1600 Corp Landing Pkwy   757-563-1600
Virginia Beach, VA 23454-5617   800-425-2666
                                            Fax: 757-563-1655
                                            e-mail: wso@al-anon.org
                                            www.al-anon.alateen.org
Al-Anon is a mutual support group of peers who share their experience in applying the Al-Anon principles to problems related to the effects of a problem drinker in their lives. It is not group therapy and is not led by a counselor or therapist
12 pages
Caryn Johnson, Director Communications

8791   Al-Anon is for African Americans...and All People of Color
Al-Anon Family Group Headquarters
1600 Corp Landing Pkwy   757-563-1600
Virginia Beach, VA 23454-5617   800-425-2666
                                            Fax: 757-563-1655
                                            e-mail: wso@al-anon.org
                                            www.al-anon.alateen.org
Al-Anon is a mutual support group of peers who share their experience in applying the Al-Anon principles to problems related to the effects of a problem drinker in their lives. It is not group therapy and is not led by a counselor or therapist
12 pages
Caryn Johnson, Director Communications

8792   Al-Anon's Path to Recovery: Al-Anon is for Americans/Aboriginals
Al-Anon Family Group Headquarters
1600 Corp Landing Pkwy   757-563-1600
Virginia Beach, VA 23454-5617   800-425-2666
                                            Fax: 757-563-1655
                                            e-mail: wso@al-anon.org
                                            www.al-anon.alateen.org

Al-Anon is a mutual support group of peers who share their experience in applying the Al-Anon principles to problems related to the effects of a problem drinker in their lives. It is not group therapy and is not led by a counselor or therapist
12 pages
Caryn Johnson, Director Communications

8793   Alcoholics Anonymous: An Inside View
Alcoholics Anonymous
PO Box 459   212-870-3400
New York, NY 10163-0459   Fax: 212-870-3137
                                            www.aa.org
Depicts alcoholics, recovering in A.A., going about their daily lives, attending A.A. meetings, and other gatherings.
28 minutes

8794   Art of Living with Change: Turning Your Good Intentions Into Progress...
Hazelden
15251 Pleasant Valley Rd   651-213-4200
Center City, MN 55012-9640   800-257-7810
                                            Fax: 651-213-4793
                                            e-mail: info@hazelden.org
                                            www.hazelden.org
Hazelden, a part of the Hazelden Betty Ford Foundation, has been saving lives and restoring families from substance abuse and addiction for more than 60 years
45 minutes
ISBN: 0-894868-40-3
Mark Mishek, President and Chief Executive Officer
Joe Jaksha, Publisher

8795   Bill Discusses the Twelve Traditions
Alcoholics Anonymous
PO Box 459   212-870-3400
New York, NY 10163-0459   Fax: 212-870-3137
                                            www.aa.org
Bill W. tells how the principles safe-guarding A.A. unity developed.
60 minutes

8796   Bill's Own Story
Alcoholics Anonymous
PO Box 459   212-870-3400
New York, NY 10163-0459   Fax: 212-870-3137
                                            www.aa.org
Co-founder Bill W. tells of his drinking and recovery.
60 minutes

8797   Caring for Ourselves: Hope for Healthy Relationships
Hazelden
15251 Pleasant Valley Rd   651-213-4200
Center City, MN 55012-9640   800-257-7810
                                            Fax: 651-213-4793
                                            e-mail: info@hazelden.org
                                            www.hazelden.org
Hazelden, a part of the Hazelden Betty Ford Foundation, has been saving lives and restoring families from substance abuse and addiction for more than 60 years
50 minutes
ISBN: 0-894866-38-9
Mark Mishek, President and Chief Executive Officer
Joe Jaksha, Publisher

8798   Hope: Alcoholics Anonymous
Alcoholics Anonymous
PO Box 459   212-870-3400
New York, NY 10163-0459   Fax: 212-870-3137
                                            www.aa.org
Explains the principles of AA: what it is, steps, traditions, sponsorship, and basic recovery tools.
15 minutes

8799   It Sure Beats Sitting in a Cell
Alcoholics Anonymous
PO Box 459   212-870-3400
New York, NY 10163-0459   Fax: 212-870-3137
                                            www.aa.org

Filmed inside correctional facilities in the United States and Canada, this film tells the story of four young AA's who were in prison as a result of drinking, yet today are sober.
17 minutes

8800 Markings on the Journey
Alcoholics Anonymous
PO Box 459   212-870-3400
New York, NY 10163-0459   Fax: 212-870-3137
                                                            www.aa.org
Videocassette depicts 45 years of AA history, using rare materials from our archives.
35 minutes

8801 Men's Work: How to Stop the Violence that Tears Our Lives Apart
Hazelden
15251 Pleasant Valley Rd   651-213-4200
Center City, MN 55012-9640   800-257-7810
                                                      Fax: 651-213-4793
                                          e-mail: info@hazelden.org
                                                     www.hazelden.org
Hazelden, a part of the Hazelden Betty Ford Foundation, has been saving lives and restoring families from substance abuse and addiction for more than 60 years
50 minutes
ISBN: 0-894868-28-4
Mark Mishek, President and Chief Executive Officer
Joe Jaksha, Publisher

8802 Secret to a Satisfied Life: The Way You Encounter Life Can Bring Happiness...
Hazelden
15251 Pleasant Valley Rd   651-213-4200
Center City, MN 55012-9640   800-257-7810
                                                      Fax: 651-213-4793
                                          e-mail: info@hazelden.org
                                                     www.hazelden.org
Hazelden, a part of the Hazelden Betty Ford Foundation, has been saving lives and restoring families from substance abuse and addiction for more than 60 years
45 minutes
ISBN: 0-894868-17-9
Mark Mishek, President and Chief Executive Officer
Joe Jaksha, Publisher

8803 Women: Coming Out of the Shadows
Elyse A Williams, author
Fanlight Productions
32 Court Street   718-488-8900
Brooklyn, NY 11201-1731   718-488-8642
                                                      Fax: 718-488-8642
                                          e-mail: info@fanlight.com
                                                     www.fanlight.com
Fanlight Productions is a leading distributor of innovative film and video works on the social issues of our time
1991 27 Minutes
ISBN: 1-572950-84-6

8804 Young People and AA
Alcoholics Anonymous
PO Box 459   212-870-3400
New York, NY 10163-0459   Fax: 212-870-3137
                                                            www.aa.org
Four young AA members describe what it is like drinking, what happened to bring them to AA, and what their lives are like sober today.
28 minutes

Web Sites

8805 AAA Foundation for Traffic Safety
                                                www.aaafoundation.org
The AAA Foundation for Traffic Safety was founded in 1947 by AAA to conduct research to address growing highway safety issues. The organization's mission is to identify traffic safety problems, foster research that seeks solutions and disseminate information and educational materials.

8806 Al-Anon
                                                    www.al-anon.alateen.org
The single purpose of this organization is to help families and friends of alcoholics, whether the alcoholic is still drinking or not.

8807 Alateen
                                                    www.al-anon.org/for-alateen
A part of the Al-Anon program, Alateen is for teenagers who have been affected by someone else's drinking, whether it be a family member or a friend.

8808 American Council for Drug Education
                                                            www.acde.org/
This organization provides information on drug use, publishes books and offers films and curriculum materials for prevention.

8809 CSAP State Liason Program
                                                            www.samhsa.gov
This program is designed to support alcohol and other drug abuse prevention efforts in the States.

8810 Center for Substance Abuse Prevention
                                                            www.samhsa.gov
The mission of the Center for Substance Abuse Prevention is to improve behavioral health through evidence-based prevention approaches.

8811 Cocaine Anonymous
                                                            www.ca.org
A support group based on the twelve steps of Alcoholics Anonymous that focuses specifically on problems of cocaine addiction.

8812 Dentists Concerned for Dentists
                                          www.medhelp.org/amshc/amshc53.htm
A nonprofit organization for chemically dependent Minnesota dentists and concerned others.

8813 Families Anonymous
                                                    www.familiesanonymous.org/
Addresses the needs of families who are concerned about a relative with a drug problem and with related behavioral problems.

8814 Hazelden
                                                            www.hazelden.com
Organization dedicated to providing quality rehabilitation, education and professional services for chemical dependency and related addictive behaviors.

8815 Healing Well
                                                            www.healingwell.com
An online health resource guide to medical news, chat, information and articles, newsgroups and message boards, books, disease-related web sites, medical directories, and more for patients, friends, and family coping with disabling diseases, disorders, or chronic illnesses.

8816 Health Finder
                                                            www.healthfinder.gov
Searchable, carefully developed web site offering information on over 1000 topics. Developed by the US Department of Health and Human Services, the site can be used in both English and Spanish.

8817 Healthlink USA
                                                            www.healthlinkusa.com
Health information concerning treatment, cures, prevention, diagnosis, risk factors, research, support groups, email lists, personal stories and much more. Updated regularly.

8818 Helios Health
                                                            www.helioshealth.com
Online resource for your health information. Detailed information about specific health topics, access to expert advice from our Medical Advisory Board, and up-to-date health news.

8819 Indian Health Service
                                                            www.ihs.gov
Charged with providing a comprehensive program of alcoholism and substance abuse prevention and treatment for Native Americans and Alaskan natives.

8820 Lawyers Concerned for Lawyers
                                                            www.mnlcl.org/

Lawyers Concerned for Lawyers provides free, confidential peer and professional assistance to Minnesota lawyers, judges, law students, and their immediate family members on any issue that causes stress or distress.

8821 MedicineNet

www.medicinenet.com

An online resource for consumers providing easy-to-read, authoritative medical and health information.

8822 Medscape

www.medscape.com

Medscape offers specialists, primary care physicians, and other health professionals the Web's most robust and integrated medical information and educational tools.

8823 National Clearinghouse for Alcohol and Drug Information

www.health.org

8824 National Council on Alcoholism and Drug Dependence

www.ncadd.org

Provides education, information, help and hope in the fight against addictions. Nationwide network of affiliates, advocates prevention, intervention and treatment, and is committed to ridding the disease of its stigma and its sufferers of their denial and shame.

8825 National Crime Prevention Council

www.ncpc.org

This organization works to prevent crime and drug use in many ways, including developing materials for parents and children.

8826 Office on Smoking and Health

www.cdc.gov/tobacco/

Offers reference services to researchers through the Technical Information Center. Publishes and distributes a number of titles in the field of smoking and health.

8827 Safe Homes

www.yescap.org/safehomes/safehomes.htm

This national organization encourages parents to sign a contract stipulating that when parties are held in one another's homes they will adhere to a strict no-alcohol/no-drug-use rule.

8828 Substance Abuse and Mental Health Services Administration

www.samhsa.gov

The goal of this organization is to reduce incidence and prevalence of mental disorders and substance abuse and improve treatment outcomes for persons suffering from addictive and mental health problems and disorders.

8829 WebMD

www.webmd.com

Provides credible information, supportive communities, and in-depth reference material about health subjects. A source for original and timely health information as well as material from well known content providers.

Description

8830 Sudden Infant Death Syndrome

Sudden Infant Death Syndrome, SIDS, is the sudden death of an infant or young child that is unexpected and for which there is no demonstrable cause. It is the most common cause of death in children between 1 and 12 months of age, with a peak incidence between the second and fourth month of life. Almost all SIDS deaths occur when the infant is thought to be sleeping.

Despite extensive research, no cause for SIDS has been found, although evidence suggests that it may be related to malfunction of the mechanisms that control the heart function and breathing process. The diagnosis cannot be made without an adequate investigation of the infant after its death. The incidence of SIDS is greater in babies born to mothers who are young, unwed, smoke, have had many births, did not complete high school and have had poor prenatal care. Other possible factors include exposure to cigarette smoke, cold months, soft bedding (lamb's wool), waterbed mattresses, an overheated environment, and being a sibling of a SIDS victim.

Recent studies have indicated that having babies sleep on their backs reduces the risks of SIDS. The American Academy of Pediatrics recommends that infants be placed on their back for sleep. It further advises to avoid overwrapping the infant, remove soft bedding, and avoid smoking during and after pregnancy. In 1994, the Back to Sleep Campaign was launched, a national campaign that encourages that infants be placed to sleep on their backs. Between 1992 and 1996,the rate of SIDS dropped 38 percent and has continued to decrease since then.

Parents who lose a child to SIDS are grief-stricken and, because no definitive cause can be found for their seemingly healthy baby's death, usually have excessive guilt feelings. Bereavement support is necessary not only during the days immediately following the infant's death, but also for at least several months.

National Agencies & Associations

8831 American SIDS Institute
509 Augusta Drive 770-426-8746
Marietta, GA 30067-8657 800-232-7437
Fax: 770-426-1369
e-mail: prevent@sids.org
www.sids.org
Dedicated to the prevention of sudden infant death and the promotion of infant health through research clinical services education and family support.
Betty McEnti PhD, Executive Director
Marc Peterzell, Chairman

8832 Center for Research for Mothers & Children
National Institute of Child Health & Development
PO Box 3006 800-370-5947
Rockville, MD 20847 800-370-2943
Fax: 866-760-5947
TTY: 888-320-6942
e-mail: NICHDinformationresourcecenter@mail.nih
www.nichd.nih.gov
Mission is to ensure that every person is born healthy and wanted, that women suffer no harmful effects from reproductive processes, and that all children have the chance to achieve their full potential for healthy and productive lives free from disease.
Duane F Alexander, Director
Christine Ma Banks, Secretary

8833 Compassionate Friends
PO Box 3696 630-990-0010
Oak Brook, IL 60522 877-969-0010
Fax: 630-990-0246
e-mail: nationaloffice@compassionatefriends.org
www.compassionatefriends.org
A national organization that offers 600 local chapters that give support to parents and siblings who have experienced the death of a child. Offers monthly support meetings to get through the difficult times and learn how to cope.
Patricia Loder, Executive Director

8834 National Center for Education in Maternal and Child Health
Georgetown University
Box 571272 202-784-9770
Washington, DC 20057-1272 Fax: 202-784-9777
e-mail: mchlibrary@ncemch.org
www.ncemch.org
Provides national leadership to the maternal and child health community in three key areas—program development education and state-of-the-art knowledge—to improve the health and well-being of the nation's children and families.
Rochelle Mayer Ed. D, Director

8835 National Organization for Rare Disorders (NORD)
55 Kenosia Avenue 203-744-0100
Danbury, CT 06810-1968 800-999-6673
Fax: 203-798-2291
TDD: 203-797-9590
e-mail: orphan@rarediseases.org
www.rarediseases.org
The NORD is a unique federation of voluntary health organizations dedicated to helping people with rare orphan diseases and assisting the organizations that serve them.
E Michael D. Scott, Chair
Carolyn Asbury, PhD, Vice Chair

8836 Parent Care
9041 Colgate Street
Indianapolis, IN 46268-1210 Fax: 317-872-5464
This organization was formed in 1982 to improve the neonatal intensive care experience for families and care providers. Provides leadership to promote the development of effective parent support services at the local level.
Sarah Killion, Administrative Director

8837 Share Pregnancy and Infant Loss Support, Inc.
The National Share Office
402 Jackson Street 636-947-6164
St. Charles, MO 63301 800-821-6819
Fax: 636-947-7486
e-mail: info@nationalshare.org
www.nationalshare.org
Offers support, resources and education on miscarriage, stillborn and newborn death.
Meridith Byers, MD
Rose Carlson, Program Director

8838 Sudden Infant Death Syndrome (SIDS) Network
PO Box 520 86 -89 -704
Ledyard, CT 06339 Fax: 860-887-7309
e-mail: sidsnet1@sids-network.org
www.sids-network.org
Dedicated to eliminate Sudden Infant Death Syndrome through the support of SIDS research projects. Provides support for those who have been touched by the tragedy of Sudden Infant Death Syndrome and to raise public awareness of this event.
Chuck Mihalko, Co-founder and President

8839 Sudden Infant Death Syndrome Alliance
2105 Laurel Bush Road 443-640-1049
Baltimore, MD 21015-6605 800-221-7437
Fax: 410-653-8709
e-mail: info@firstcandle.org
www.sidsalliance.org

The purpose of the Alliance is to help parents educate the community about SIDS and to support SIDS research. The Alliance assists parents to organize local chapters and provides services including a newsletter and other literature.
Marian Sokol, President
Deborah Boyd, Executive Director

State Agencies & Associations

Alabama

8840 Bureau of Family Health Services: Alabama Department of Public Health
19 South Jackson Street
201 Monroe Street   334-206-5300
Montgomery, AL 36104   800-252-1818
                                                Fax: 334-269-5200
                                              e-mail: llee@aap.net
                                                     www.adph.org
Linda P Lee, Executive Director

Alaska

8841 SIDS Information and Counseling Program: Alaska Department of Health
350 Main Street, Room 404   907-465-3030
Juneau, AK 99811-3553   Fax: 907-465-3068
                                  e-mail: william.hogan@alaska.gov
                                                www.dhss.alaska.gov
Alaska Pioneer Homes assist older Alaskans to have the highest quality of life by providing assisted living in a safe home setting which promotes positive relationships, meaningful activities, physical, emotional and spiritual growth.
William J Streur, Commissioner
Jay Butler, Chief Medical Officer

Arizona

8842 Arizona SIDS Founation
PO Box 1111   520-297-6013
Phoenix, AZ 85001   800-597-7437
                                              e-mail: info@azsidf.org
                                                     www.azsidf.org
Vanessa Seaney, President

8843 Office of Womens And Childrens Health: Alabama Department of Health
State Dapartment of Healths Services
150 N 18th Avenue   602-542-1025
Phoenix, AZ 85007-2602   Fax: 602-542-0883
                                        e-mail: newbers@azdhs.gov
                                                     www.azdhs.gov
The Arizona Department of Health Services promotes and protects the health of Arizona's children and adults. Its mission is to set the standard for personal and community health through direct care, science, public policy, and leadership.
Susan Newber RN, Manager

Arkansas

8844 Arkansas Department of Health: SIDS Information & Counseling Program
4815 W Markham Street
Little Rock, AR 72205-3866   501-661-2000
                                              www.healthyarkansas.com
To protect and improve the health and well-being of allÿÿArkansans
Nathaniel Smith, MD, MPH
Dawn Graziani

California

8845 California SIDS Program
11344 Coloma Road   916-851-7437
Gold River, CA 95670-6052   800-369-7437
                                               Fax: 916-851-5937
                                       e-mail: info@californiasids.com
                                                www.californiasids.com

IT is designed to serve the many individuals affected by a SIDS death, and to educate the public about SIDS.
Gwen Edelstein RN,PNP,MPA, Program Director
Cheryl McBride, Program Manager

8846 SIDS Alliance Of Northern California
1547 Palos Verdes Mall   925-274-1109
Walnut Creek, CA 94597   877-938-7437
                                                e-mail: info@sidsnc.org
                                                       www.sidsnc.org
A non-profit, completely volunteer group of SIDS parents and professionals dedicated to family support and community education regarding SIDS.
Lorie Gehrke, President

8847 SIDS Foundation of Southern California
10811 Washington Boulevard   310-558-4511
Culver City, CA 90232   Fax: 310-558-7075
                                         e-mail: sidsfsc@aol.com
                                    sidsfoundationofsoutherncalifornia.org
Margot Stern Bennett, Executive Director

Colorado

8848 Colorado SIDS Program
425 S Cherry Street   303-320-7771
Denver, CO 80224   888-285-7437
                                               Fax: 303-320-7827
                                         e-mail: rlouie@hrsa.gov
                                                 www.coloradosids.org
Tena Saltzman, Executive Director

8849 Colordao Department of Health and Environment
4300 Cherry Creek Drive S   303-692-2000
Denver, CO 80246-1530   800-886-7689
                                               Fax: 303-782-5576
                                              TTY: 303-691-7700
                              e-mail: cdphe.information@state.co.us
                                                 www.cdphe.state.co.us
Martha Rudolph, Director
Karin McGowan, Interim Executive Director

Connecticut

8850 Connecticut SIDS Alliance
PO Box 486   860-626-1542
Torrington, CT 06790   866-574-7437
                                               Fax: 860-496-9919
                                        e-mail: ctsids@aol.com
                                                     www.ctsids.org
Shannon Strandberg, Secretary

8851 SIDS Program: Connecticut Department of Health
410 Capitol Avenue   860-509-8074
Hartford, CT 06134   Fax: 860-509-7720
                             e-mail: marilyn.binns@po.state.ct.us
                                    sidsfoundationofsoutherncalifornia.org
Marilyn Binns, Program Coordinator

Delaware

8852 SIDS Information & Counseling: Division of Public Health
1901 N DuPont Highway   302-255-9040
New Castle, DE 19720   Fax: 302-255-4429
                                  e-mail: dhssinfo@state/de/us
                                                www.dhss.delaware.gov
To improve the quality of life for Delaware's citizens by promoting health and well-being, fostering self-sufficiency, and protecting vulnerable populations.
Elaine Marke LCSW BCD, Program Coordinator

District of Columbia

8853 DC Department of Health Maternal and Family Health Administration
Maternal And Family Health Administration

899 North Capitol Street NE
Washington, DC 20002

202-442-5955
Fax: 202-442-4795
TTY: 711
e-mail: doh@dc.gov
www.dchealth.dc.gov

The Mission of the Department of Health is to promote and protect the health, safety and quality of life of residents, visitors and those doing business in the District of Columbia.
Saul M. Levin, M.D., M.P.A., Interim Director
Rosie McLaren, Program Manager

8854 Department of Health and Human Services
200 Independence Avenue SW
Washington, DC 20201

919-715-8430
877-696-6775
e-mail: april.ellis@ncmail.net
www.hhs.gov

The Department of Health and Human Services (HHS) is the United States government's principal agency for protecting the health of all Americans and providing essential human services, especially for those who are least able to help themselves.
April Ellis, SIDS Program Manager

8855 Region III Office Program: Consultants for Maternal and Child Health
Public Ledger Building
2115 Wisconsin Avenue NW
Washington, DC 20007-3309

202-784-9771
Fax: 202-784-9777
e-mail: OHRCinfo@georgetown.edu
www.mchoralhealth.org

The purpose of the National Maternal and Child Oral Health Resource Center (OHRC) is to respond to the needs of states and communities in addressing current and emerging public oral health issues. OHRC supports health professionals, program administrators, educators, policymakers, and others with the goal of improving oral health services for infants, children, adolescents, and their families.
Jolene Bertness, Health Education Specialist
Katrina Holt, Director

8856 Region IV Office Program Consultants for Maternal and Child Health
2115 Wisconsin Avenue
Washington, DC 20007-8909

202-784-9771
Fax: 202-784-9777
e-mail: OHRCinfo@georgetown.edu
www.mchoralhealth.org

The purpose of the National Maternal and Child Oral Health Resource Center (OHRC) is to respond to the needs of states and communities in addressing current and emerging public oral health issues.
E Joseph Alderman DDS MPH, Oral Health Consultant

8857 Region IX Office Program Consultants for Maternal and Child Health
2115 Wisconsin
Washington, DC 94103

202-784-9771
Fax: 202-784-9777
e-mail: OHRCinfo@georgetown.edu
www.mchoralhealth.org

Katrina Holt, Director

8858 Region VIII Office Program Consultants for Maternal and Child Health
2115 Wisconsin Avenue
Washington, DC 80294-1961

202-784-9771
Fax: 202-784-9777
e-mail: OHRCinfo@georgetown.edu
www.mchoralhealth.org

The purpose of the National Maternal and Child Oral Health Resource Center (OHRC) is to respond to the needs of states and communities in addressing current and emerging public oral health issues
Valerie Orla RDH BS, Oral Health Consultant

Florida

8859 Children's Medical Services Program: Florida SIDS Program
4052 Bald Cypress Way
Tallahassee, FL 32399

850-245-4444
Fax: 904-488-2341
e-mail: Health@doh.state.fl.us
www.doh.state.fl.us

To protect, promote & improve the health of all people in Florida through integrated state, county, & community efforts.
Susan Potts, Coordinator

8860 Florida Department of Health
4052 Bald Cypress Way
Tallahassee, FL 32399

850-245-4444
Fax: 850-245-4047
e-mail: Health@doh.state.fl.us
www.doh.state.fl.us

To protect, promote & improve the health of all people in Florida through integrated state, county, & community efforts.
Susan Potts, Coordinator

8861 Florida SIDS Alliance
4044 W Lake Mary Boulevard
Lake Mary, FL 32746

305-232-1640
800-SID-SFLA
Fax: 407-444-5208
e-mail: sidsfla@yahoo.com
www.flasids.com

Steve Bonwit, Officer
Roy Bagley, President

Georgia

8862 Georgia Department of Human Resources: Center for Family Resource Planning
2 Peach Tree Street NW
Atlanta, GA 30303

404-657-3550
Fax: 404-463-6729
e-mail: kotto@dhr.state.ga.us

Provides grief support for parents.
Katherine Ottoel, Coordinator

8863 Georgia Department of Human Resources: Infant and Child Health
2 Peach Tree Street NW
Atlanta, GA 30303

404-651-7371
Fax: 404-463-6729
e-mail: kotto@dhr.state.ga.us

Katherine Otto, Coordinator

8864 Georgia SIDS Project
4112-2 E Ponce De Leon Avenue
Clarkston, GA 30021

678-342-3360
Fax: 404-296-7211
e-mail: gasids@mindspring.com
www.sidsga.org

Sudden Infant Death Syndrome is the sudden death of an infant under one year of age which remains unexplained after a thorough case investigation.
Diane Manheim, Director

Hawaii

8865 Hawaii Department of Health: Family Health Division
Child Wellness Program
1250 Punchbowl Street
Honolulu, HI 96813

808-586-4400
Fax: 808-733-9032
e-mail: gwen.palmer@fshd.health.state.hi.us
ww.hawaii.gov/health

Gwen Palmer, Coordinator

Idaho

8866 Idaho Department of Health and Welfare
590 W Washington Street
Boise, ID 83720

208-334-4000
800-632-8000
Fax: 208-334-4015
e-mail: gainord@idhw.state.id.us
www.healthandwelfare.idaho.gov

We offer programs that deal with complex social, economic and individual issues, often helping people in crisis situations. Our programs are designed to strengthen families and promote self-reliance.
Richard Armstrong, Director

Illinois

8867 **SIDS of Illinois**
6010 Route 53
Lisle, IL 60532
630-541-3901
Fax: 630-541-8246
e-mail: pam@sidsillinois.org
www.sidsillinois.org

Marsha Cooper, President
Anita L. Jordan Johnson, Vice President

8868 **Statewide SIDS Program: Illinois Department of Public Health**
500 E Monroe Street
Springfield, IL 62761
217-557-2931
Fax: 217-524-2831
e-mail: bbreiden@idph.state.il.us
Babara Breidenbaugh, Program Specialist

Indiana

8869 **Indiana State Department of Health Maternal And Child Health Services**
Maternal And Child Health Services
2 N Meridian Street
Indianapolis, IN 46204
317-233-1325
800-457-8283
Fax: 317-233-1300
e-mail: bmjohnso@isdh.state.in.us
www.in.gov/hpb

Beth Johnson, Nurse Consultant

8870 **SIDS Center of Indiana**
1810 Broad Ripple Avenue
Indianapolis, IN 46220
317-254-9255
Fax: 317-254-9266
e-mail: sidscenter@insids.org
Our mission is to be a resource center that supports parents, families and friends in communities across the state whose lives are touched by sudden, unexpected infant death.ÿ
John Schutt, Chairperson

Iowa

8871 **Iowa SIDS Alliance**
406 SW School Street
Ankeny, IA 50023
515-965-7655
866-480-4741
Fax: 515-964-7506
e-mail: info@iowasids.org
www.iowasids.org
The Iowa Sudden Infant Death Syndrome Foundation is a statewide, non-profit, voluntary health organization dedicated to providing emotional support to SIDS and SUID familiesÿresidingÿin Iowa, educating professionals and the general public about SIDS and risk reduction, and funding medical research into the causes of SIDS.
Patty Keeley, Executive Director
Jennifer Atzen, President

8872 **Iowa SIDS Program Iowa Department of Public Health**
Iowa Department of Public Health
321 E 12th Street
Des Moines, IA 50319-0075
515-281-7689
866-227-9878
www.idph.state.ia.us
Promoting and protecting the health of Iowans
Jane Borst, Bureau Chief
Sally Clausen

Kansas

8873 **Kansas Department of Health & Environment Bureau of Family Health**
Bureau Of Children, Youth And Families
1000 SW Jackson Street
Topeka, KS 66612-1274
786-296-1500
800-332-6262
Fax: 785-296-6553
e-mail: info@kdheks.gov
www.kdheks.gov
To protect and improve the health and environment of all Kansans.
Robert Moser, Director
Kobi Gomel, Administrative Specialist

8874 **SIDS Network of Kansas**
1148 S Hillside
Wichita, KS 67211
316-682-1301
866-399-7437
Fax: 316-682-1274
e-mail: info@sidsks.org
www.kidsks.org

Christy Schunn, LSCSW, Executive Director
Amanda Yoder, Communications Assistant

Kentucky

8875 **Department of Public Health: Adult and Child Health Division**
275 E Main Street
Frankfort, KY 40621
502-564-3236
800-372-2973
Fax: 502-564-8389
TTY: 800-627-4702
e-mail: marcia.burkow@ky.gov

Marcia Burkow, SIDS Coordinator

8876 **SIDS Network of Kentucky**
PO Box 186
Caneyville, KY 42721-3555
800-928-7437
Fax: 859-245-0717
e-mail: info@sidsky.org
www.sidsky.org
Supporting family members and others who have been touched by the tragedy of a sids or other infants death.
Adrienne Grizzell, Executive Director

Louisiana

8877 **Office of Public Health**
628 N 4th Street
Baton Rouge, LA 70802
225-342-9500
Fax: 225-342-5568
e-mail: hhwebadmin@la.gov
www.dhh.louisiana.gov/offices/?ID=79

Tracy Hubbard, Coordinator

8878 **Public Health Services of Louisiana**
628 N 4th Street
Baton Rouge, LA 70802-0629
225-342-9500
Fax: 225-342-5568
e-mail: dhhwebadmin@la.gov
www.dhh.state.la.us/
The mission of the Department of Health and Hospitals is to protect and promote health and to ensure access to medical, preventive and rehabilitative services for all citizens of the State of Louisiana.
Jamie Roques RNC, SIDS Coordinator
Courtney Phillips, Deputy Secretary

Maine

8879 **Department of Human Services**
221 State Street
Augusta, ME 04333-0001
207-287-3707
Fax: 207-287-3005
TTY: 800-606-0215
www.state.me.us/dhs/

Brenda Harvey, Commissioner

8880 **Maine SIDS Foundation**
14 Charlonate Drive
Gray, ME 04039
207-657-2220
Fax: 207-657-3737
e-mail: roybagley@aol.com
www.sidsalliance.org

Roy Bagley, Chairperson

8881 **Maine SIDS Program Department Of Human Services**
Department Of Human Services
200 Main Street
Lewiston, ME 04240
207-795-4450
Fax: 207-795-4445
e-mail: luanne.crinion@maine.gov
Luanne Crinion, Program Coordinator

Maryland

8882 **First Candle**
2105 Laurel Bush Road
Bel Air, MD 21015
Fax: 651-310-2106
TTY: 800-221-7437
e-mail: info@firstcandle.org
www.sidsalliance.org

First Candle is a leading national nonprofit organization dedicated to safe pregnancies and the survival of babies through the first years of life. Current priorities are to eliminate Stillbirth, Sudden Infant Death Syndrome (SIDS) and other Sudden Unexpected Infant Deaths (SUID) with programs of research, education and advocacy

Michael J. Schaffer, President
Kelly Neal Mariotti, Chief Executive Officer

8883 Maryland SIDS Information & Counseling Program
22 S Green Street   410-328-8667
Baltimore, MD 21201   800-492-5538
                                TTY: 410-328-9600
                                TDD: 410-328-9600
                        e-mail: webmaster@umm.edu
                              www.marylandsids.com
UMMC exists to serve the state and region as a tertiary/quaternary care center, to serve the local community with a full range of care options, to educate and train the next generation of health care providers, and to be a site for world-class clinical research.
Jeffrey A Rivest, President and Chief Executive Officer
R Keith Allen, Senior Vice President

Massachusetts

8884 Region I Office Program: Consultants for Maternal and Child Health
John F Kennedy Building   617-899-1355
Boston, MA 02203   Fax: 202-833-8288
                        e-mail: Mary.Foley@mcphs.edu
                              www.mchoralhealth.org
Mary Foley RDH MPH, Oral Health Consultant

Michigan

8885 Apnea Identification Program Children's Ho spital of Michigan
Children's Hospital of Michigan
3901 Beaubien Street   313-745-5437
Detroit, MI 48201-2196   888-DMC-2500
                              www.childrensdmc.org
To provide the highest quality of care for children, to inform that care through research innovations, and to ensure that children have access to the care they need.
Karen Branif RN MSW, Nurse Specialist

8886 Genesee County Health Department
630 S Saignaw Street   810-257-3612
Flint, MI 48502-3915   Fax: 810-257-3147
                        e-mail: gchd-info@gchd.us
                                       www.gchd.us

Kay Doerr, Chairperson
Brenda Clack, Vice-Chairperson

8887 Kent County Health Department
300 Monroe Avenue NE
Grand Rapids, MI 49503-1996   616-632-7590
                                  www.accesskent.com
The mission of Kent County government is to be an effective and efficient steward in delivering quality services for our diverse community. Our priority is to provide mandated services, which may be enhanced and supplemented by additional services to improve the quality of life for all our citizens within the constraints of sound fiscal policy.
Colleen Jill RN, SIDs Coordinator
David Kraker

8888 Michigan Department of Community Health
3423 MLK Boulevard   517-373-1820
Lansing, MI 48909   Fax: 517-373-2129
                        e-mail: lauberc@michigan.gov
                                    www.michigan.gov

Cheryl Lauber, Coordinator

8889 Oakland County Health Division: SIDS Project
1200 N Telegraph   248-858-1280
Pontiac, MI 48341-0482   800-774-4542
                                Fax: 248-858-0178
                                TTY: 248-452-2247
                                TDD: 248-452-2247
                    e-mail: oakllbph@oakland.lib.mi.us
                                     www.oakgov.com

David Conklin, Librarian
George J Miller Jr MA, Director

8890 SIDS LEAD: Children's Special Health Care Services
Michigan Department of Public Health
201 Townsend Street   517-373-3740
Lansing, MI 48913-2934   TTY: 517-373-3573
                                TDD: 517-373-3573
                        e-mail: norris@michigan.gov
                              www.michigan.gov/mdch
Improving the experience of care, improving the health of populations, and reducing per capita costs of health care
Janet Olszewski, Director
Ed Dore, Chief Deputy Director

Minnesota

8891 Minnesota Sudden Infant Death Center Minneapolis Children's Medical Center
Minneapolis Children's Medical Center
2525 Chicago Avenue   612-813-6000
Minneapolis, MN 55404-4518   Fax: 612-813-7344
                e-mail: kathleen.fernbach@childreansHC.org
                www.childrensmn.org/Communities/SIDs.asp
Sara Schumacher, Project Coordinator

Mississippi

8892 Mississippi SIDS Alliance
5454 I-55 North
Jackson, MS 39211-2170   877-471-7437
                        e-mail: mssids@jam.rr.com
                                 www.sidsalliance.org

Scott Parrish, President
Brian Roach, Vice President

8893 Mississippi State Department of Health and Child Health Services
570 E Woodrow Wilson   601-576-7400
Jackson, MS 39216   866-458-4948
                                Fax: 601-576-7498
                e-mail: Linda.Proctor@msdh.state.ms.us
                              www.msdh.state.ms.us

Linda Proctor, Coordinator

Missouri

8894 Region VII Office Program: Consultants for Maternal and Child Health
Federal Building
10031 Perry Drive   913-888-1377
Overland Park, KS 66212-2826   Fax: 816-426-3633
                        e-mail: lwalker17@kc.rr.com
                              www.mchoralhealth.org
Lawrence Wal DDS MPH, Oral Health Consultant

8895 SIDS Resources
1120 S Sixth Street   314-822-2323
Saint Louis, MO 63104   800-421-3511
                                Fax: 314-588-0850
                        e-mail: lahrens@sidsresources.org
                                 www.sidsresources.org
The mission of SIDS Resources, Inc. is to promote safe practices which reduce the risk of infant death and to provide bereavement support for families who have lost babies.
Lori Behrens, Executive Director
Ellen Reynolds, Program Coordinator

8896 Western Region SIDS Resources
4051 Broadway
Kansas City, MO 64111
816-569-6956
Fax: 816-753-6906
e-mail: slogan@sidsresources.org
www.sidsalliance.org
Provides free supportive services and education to those affected by the sudden and unexpected death of an infant - birth through 12 months. Provides education and support to professionals and communities regarding healthy and safe infant care practices and safe sleep for infants
Shay Logan, Program Coordinator

Montana

8897 Department of Public Health and Human Services
1400 Broadway
Helena, MT 59620
406-444-3565
800-232-4636
Fax: 406-444-2606
e-mail: WMcGraw@state.mt.us
www.dphhs.mt.gov

Richard H. Opper, Director
Peggy Baker, Administrative Aide

Nebraska

8898 Nebraska Department of Health Perinatal Child and Adolescent Health
301 Centennial Mall South
Lincoln, NE 68509
402-471-0165
Fax: 402-471-7049
e-mail: jan.heusinkvelt@hhss.ne.gov
Jan Heusinkvelt, RN, BSN, Community Health Nurse

8899 Nebraska SIDS Foundation University of Nebraska Medical Center
University of Nebraska Medical Center
PO Box 460905
Papillion, NE 68046
402-431-8076
e-mail: board@nesids.org
www.nesids.com

Nevada

8900 Nevada State Health Division Bureau of Family Health Services
Bureau Of Family Health Services
3427 Goni Road
Carson City, NV 89706
775-684-4285
Fax: 775-684-4245
e-mail: chuth@nvhd.state.nv.us
www.health2k.state.nv.us
Cynthia Huthht, Health Program Specialist

New Hampshire

8901 New Hampshire SIDS Program
New Hampshire Division of Public Health Services
29 Hazen Drive
Concord, NH 03301
603-271-4536
Fax: 603-271-4519
e-mail: sidsnet1@sids-network.org
www.sids-network.org
Audrey Knigh MSN CPNP, SIDS Coordinator

New Jersey

8902 New Jersey Department of Health: Child Health Program
PO Box 360
Trenton, NJ 08625
609-292-7837
800-367-6543
e-mail: lindajones@doh.state.nj.us
www.state.nj.us/health
The mission of the department of health is to improve health through leadership and innovation.
Linda Jones Hicks, Director
Shirley White-Walker, Chair

8903 New Jersey SIDS Alliance
15 Meadowbrook Road
Boonton Township, NJ 07005
973-299-6523
e-mail: njsids@yahoo.com
www.sidsalliance.org
Genny Elias-Warren, Chairperson

8904 SIDS Center of New Jersey
1 Robert Wood Johnson Place
New Brunswick, NJ 08903-1766
732-249-2160
800-704-7437
Fax: 732-235-6609
e-mail: hegyith@umdnj.edu
www2.umdnj.edu/sids
Provide public health education to reduce the risk of sudden infant death
Thomas Hegyi MD, Co-Medical Director
Barbara Ostf PhD, Program Director

New Mexico

8905 New Mexico SIDS Information and Counseling Program
University of New Mexico School of Medicine
2500 Marble NE
Albuquerque, NM 87131
505-277-3053
Fax: 505-272-3601
e-mail: sidsnet1@sids-network.org
www.sids-network.org
Beverly Whit RN MS, Director

New York

8906 NYS Center for Sudden Infant Death: Eastern Satellite Office
Albany Medical College
47 New Scotland Avenue
Albany, NY 12208
518-262-5918
Fax: 518-262-7237
e-mail: whittrm@mail.amc.edu
Mary Whittredge, Regional Coordinator

8907 New York City Center for SIDS
New York City Satellite Office
520 1st Avenue
New York, NY 10016
212-686-8854
800-522-5006
Fax: 212-532-6564
e-mail: evelyne.longchamp@sids1.ssw.sunysb.edu
Judith Gaine CSW PhD, SIDS Program Director

8908 New York State Center for SIDS: School of Social Welfare
Stony Brook University
101 Nicolls Road
Stony Brook, NY 11794-0001
631-444-4000
800-336-7437
Fax: 631-444-6475
e-mail: marie.chandick@stonybrook.edu
www.hsc.stonybrook.edu
Stony Brook Medicine expresses our shared mission of research, clinical care and education - a mission embraced by our faculty, staff, researchers, and students. It is the embodiment of everything we do on behalf of the health of patients - not only here in our community, but also in the region and worldwide.
Marie Chandi CSW, Associate Project Director

8909 Region II Office Program: Consultants for Maternal and Child Health
345 E 24th Street
New York, NY 10010-0004
212-998-9654
Fax: 212-995-4364
e-mail: ngh1@nyu.edu
www.mchoralhealth.org
Neal Herman DDS, Oral Health Consultant

8910 WNYS Center for SIDS
3580 Harlem Road
Buffalo, NY 14215
716-837-5189
Fax: 716-836-1578
e-mail: jwalkden@palliativecare.org
www.sidsalliance.org
Jan Walkden, Family Service Coordinator

North Carolina

8911 SIDS Alliance of the Carolinas
306 Lucas Park Drive
Greensboro, NC 27455
336-545-3348
e-mail: sandylkennedy@hotmail.com
www.sidsalliance.org
Sandy Kennedy, Chairperson

North Dakota

8912 **North Dakota SIDS Alliance**
128 Apollo Avenue
Bismarck, ND 58503
701-530-2507
Fax: 701-223-0440
e-mail: ndsids@btinet.net
www.sidsalliance.org

Barb Delvo, Chairperson

8913 **North Dakota SIDS Management Program**
Division of Maternal and Child Health
600 E Boulevard Avenue
Bismarck, ND 58505-0200
701-328-2372
800-472-2286
Fax: 701-328-4727
e-mail: kchintz@nd.gov
www.ndhealth.gov

Provides support education and follow-up to parents/caregivers family and childcare providers suffering a sudden infant death
Kjersti Hintz, Program Director
Terry Dwelle, MD

Ohio

8914 **District Board of Health: Mahoning County**
50 Westchester Drive
Youngstown, OH 44515
330-270-2855
800-873-MCHD
Fax: 330-270-2860
TTY: 800-750-0750
e-mail: mchealth@cboss.com
www.mahoning-health.org

The mission of the District Board of Health is to promote and protect the health of individuals and communities, to create a safer, healthier environment, and to improve quality of life
Lisa Weiss MD, Forum Health
Bev Fisher, Manager

8915 **Ohio Department of Health**
Child Fatality Review
246 N High Street
Columbus, OH 43215
614-466-3543
866-634-7654
Fax: 614-564-2433
e-mail: SmkInfo@odh.ohio.gov˜
www.odh.ohio.gov

Theodore E. Wymyslo, Director
Frances Veverka, RS MPH, Ohio Health Commissioners

8916 **SIDS Network of Ohio**
421 Graham Road
Cuyahoga Falls, OH 44221
800-477-7437
Fax: 330-929-0593
e-mail: SIDNetwork@sidsohio.org
www.sidsohio.org

The SID Network of Ohio promotes infant safety in an effort to reduce the rate of SIDS and Sudden Unexpected Infant Death (SUID).ÿ We accomplish this through the promotion of infant health and wellness, community education and medical research.ÿ We also provide supportive services to those who have been affected by the sudden loss of a child age 2 and under.
Leslie Redd, Executive Director
Jennifer Connolly, Development Coordinator

Oklahoma

8917 **Oklahoma State Department of Health: Maternal and Child Health Services**
1000 NE 10th Street
Oklahoma City, OK 73117-1207
405-524-3468
800-955-3468
Fax: 405-271-9202
e-mail: paulaw@health.ok.gov
www.ok.gov

As the official Internet gateway of Oklahoma, we are committed to providing citizens and businesses with efficient online access to government.
Paula Wood, Executive Assistant
Suzanna Dooley

Oregon

8918 **Oregon Department of Human Services**
500 Summer Street NE
Salem, OR 97301
503-945-5944
Fax: 503-378-2897
TTY: 503-945-6214
e-mail: dhs.info@state.or.us
www.oregon.gov

Joyce Edmonds, Public Nurse Consultant

Pennsylvania

8919 **Pennsylvania Department of Health Bureau of Family Health**
Bureau of Family Health
625 Forster Street
Harrisburg, PA 17120
717-772-2762
877-PAH-EALT
Fax: 717-772-0323
e-mail: bcaboot@state.pa.us
www.dsf.health.state.pa.us

Robert Torres, Deputy Secretary for Administration
Michael Wolf, Secretary

8920 **SIDS of Pennsylvania**
810 River Avenue
Pittsburgh, PA 15212
412-322-5680
800-721-7437
Fax: 412-481-5968
e-mail: sidspa@aol.com
www.cribsforkids.org

Cribs for Kidsr has been making an impact on the rates of babies dying of accidental death due to unsafe sleeping environmentsÿby educating parents on the importance of safe sleep practices and by providing Graco Pack 'n Play portable cribs to families who, otherwise, cannot otherwise afford a safe place for their babies to sleep.
Judith A Bannon, Executive Director
Joseph T Dominick, RN, Chairman

Rhode Island

8921 **Rhode Island Department of Health**
3 Capitol Hill
Providence, RI 02908
401-222-5960
800-942-7434
Fax: 401-222-6548
TTY: 711
e-mail: DOH@health.ri.gov
www.health.state.ri.us

David R Gifford MD MPH, Director
Donald L Carcieri, Governor

South Carolina

8922 **Division of Perinatal Systems Mills Jarret Complex**
Mills Jarret Complex
Box 101106
Columbia, SC 29211
803-898-0734
Fax: 803-898-2065
e-mail: swansokm@dhec.sc.gov

Kathy Swanson, State FIMR Director

South Dakota

8923 **South Dakota Department of Health**
Health Building
600 E Capitol Avenue
Pierre, SD 57501
605-773-3361
800-738-2301
Fax: 605-773-5509
e-mail: DOH.info@state.sd.us
www.doh.sd.gov

Nancy Shoup, Program Coordinator

Tennessee

8924 **Tenessee Department of Health**
Division of Maternal & Child Health
425 5th Avenue N
Nashville, TN 37243-4701
615-741-3111
Fax: 615-741-1063
e-mail: tn.health@tn.gov
health.state.tn.us

The Department of Health works to promote, protect and improve the health and well-being of Tennesseans
John J. Dreyzehner, MD, MPH, Commissioner

8925 **Tennessee SIDS Alliance**
373 Woodcrest Drive
Kingsport, TN 37663
423- 23- 821
e-mail: lisasids@cs.com
ww.sidsalliance.org
The SID Alliance of TN's mission is as a volunteer. non-profit organization dedicated to the support and service of all Tennessee SIDS families and friends.
Lisa Hunt, Chairperson

Texas

8926 **Department of State Health Offices**
Title V And Health Resources
100 West 49th Street
Austin, TX 78756
512-776-7111
888-963-7111
Fax: 512-458-7650
e-mail: chan.mcdermott@dshs.state.tx.us
www.dshs.state.tx.us
To improve health and well-being in Texas
David L. Lakey, MD

8927 **Greater Houston Chapter SIDS Alliance**
916 Satsuma Street
Pasadena, TX 77506
713-924-1419
Fax: 281-541-5340
e-mail: anita.carmona@us.rhodia.com
www.sidsalliance.org
Anita Carmona, Chairperson

8928 **Harris County Public Health and Environmental Services**
2223 W Lop S
Houston, TX 77027
713-439-6000
e-mail: publicinfo@hd.co.harris.tx.us
www.hcphes.org
Promoting a Healthy and Safe Community.
Herminia Palacio, Executive Director

8929 **Region VI Office Program Consultants for Maternal and Child Health**
1301 Young Street
Dallas, TX 75202-4325
214-767-3003
Fax: 214-767-3038
e-mail: geurink@zeecon.com
www.mchoralhealth.org
Kathy Geurin RDH BS MA, Oral Health Consultant

8930 **Southwest SIDS Research Institute**
Brazosport Memorial Hospital
230 Parking Way
Lake Jackson, TX 77566
979-297-2101
www.swsids.com
Our mission is to end unexpected infant mortality through education, support, medical servicesÿandÿresearch.

ISBN: 9-792992-81-4
Richard A. Hardoin, MD
Judith A. Henslee, LMSW, Executive Director

Utah

8931 **Utah Department of Health**
Child Adolescent & School Health Program
288 N 1460 W
Salt Lake City, UT 84116-3231
801-538-6003
Fax: 801-538-6200
www.health.utah.gov
The mission of the Utah Department of Health is to protect the public's health through preventing avoidable illness, injury, disability and premature death; assuring access to affordable, quality health care; and promoting healthy lifestyles.
David Sundwa MD, Executive Director
A Richard Melton, Deputy Director

8932 **Utah SIDS Alliance**
1760 American Park Circle
W Valley City, UT 84119
801-487-7800
Fax: 801-487-4477
e-mail: lisa.hughes@fnwmail.com
www.sidsalliance.org
Lisa Hughes, President
Troy Hughes, Co-President

Vermont

8933 **Vermont Department of Health: SIDS Information and Counseling Program**
108 Cherry Street
Burlington, VT 05402
802-652-2000
Fax: 802-652-2005
TTY: 800-253-0191
e-mail: kkelehe@vdh.state.vt.us
healthvermont.gov
Kathy Keleher, Assistant Director Public Health

Virginia

8934 **SIDS Mid-Atlantic**
PO Box 799
Haymarket, VA 20168
703-955-6899
Fax: 703-933-9101
e-mail: bconnal@aol.com
www.sidsma.org
Betty Connal, Executive Director

8935 **Virginia SIDS Alliance**
PO Box 752
Mechanicsville, VA 23111
Fax: 757-548-7074
e-mail: mail@vasids.org
www.vasids.org
Terri Newman, President
Mark Ferraro, Vice President

8936 **Virginia SIDS Program: Virginia Department of Health**
Virginia Department of Health
109 Governor Street
Richmond, VA 23219
804-846-7772
Fax: 804-973-9498
e-mail: WomensAndInfantsHealth@vdh.virginia.gov
www.vdh.virginia.gov
Virginia Health Information' is a resource for patients and consumers looking to learn about and compare options on everything from obstetrical services, to heart care, to pricing information on commonly performed medical procedures.ÿ
Robert Stroube, Commissioner
Rosanne Kolesar, Deputy Commissioner Public Health

Washington

8937 **Region X Office Program Consultants for Maternal and Child Health**
2201 Sixth Avenue
Seattle, WA 98121-1857
206-615-2518
Fax: 206-615-2500
e-mail: rslayton@acf.hhs.gov
www.mchoralhealth.org
Rebecca Slay DDS PhD, Oral Health Consultant

8938 **SIDS Foundation of Washington**
4649 Sunnyside Avenue N
Seattle, WA 98103
206-548-9290
800-533-0376
Fax: 206-548-9445
e-mail: info@nwsids.org
www.nisa-sids.org
The Northwest Infant Survival & SIDS Alliance is dedicated to reducing the risk of sudden unexpected infant death through education and supporting research while providing bereavement services.
Krista Cossa Sandberg, Executive Director
Lindsey Hulet, Office Administrator

8939 **SIDS Northwest Regional Center**
Washington Department of Health
111 Israel Rd SE
Olympia, WA 98501-7880
360-236-3502
800-533-0376
Fax: 360-236-2323
e-mail: mch.support@doh.wa.gov
www.doh.wa.gov
The Department of Health works to protect and improve the health of people in Washington State.
Lorrie Grevstad

West Virginia

8940 **Office of Maternal, Child & Family Health**
Bureau For Public Health

350 Capitol Street
Charelston, WV 25301

304-558-7997
Fax: 304-558-3510
e-mail: annmunson@wvdhhr.org

Ann Munson, SIDS Coordinator

Wisconsin

8941 Infant Death Center of Wisconsin
Childrens Hospital Of Wisconsin
620 S. 76th St
Milwaukee, WI 53214

414-292-4000
Fax: 414-213-4952
e-mail: aharvieux@chw.org
www.idcw.org

Karen Ordinana, Executive Director
Matt Crespin, Associate Director

Wyoming

8942 Wyoming Department of Health
Community & Family Health Section
401 Hathaway Building
Cheyenne, WY 82002

307-777-7656
Fax: 307-777-7439
e-mail: mirandie.peterson@health.wyo.gov
wdh.state.wy.us

Our mission is to promote, protect, and enhance the health of all Wyoming citizens. The Wyoming Department of Health is the primary state agency for providing health and human services. We administer programs maintaining the health and safety of all citizens of Wyoming and our primary approach in solving health problems is prevention.

Thomas O. Forslund, Director
Heather Babbitt, Senior Administrator

Research Centers

8943 Massachusetts Sudden Infant Death Syndrome Boston City Hospital
Boston City Hospital
1 Boston Medical Center Place
Boston, MA 02118

617-638-8000
Fax: 617-534-5555
www.bmc.org

A joint program of Boston City Hospital and Children's Hospital. Services provided include around-the-clock availability for consultation to health professionals and families counseling of families parent group meetings and supportive home visits.

8944 Pediatric Pulmonary Unit Massachusetts General Hospital
Massachusetts General Hospital
55 Fruit Street
Boston, MA 02114

617-726-2000
Fax: 617-242-03
TTY: 617-724-8800
www.massgeneral.org

Sudden infant death syndrome and childhood disorders research.
Paul S Russell, MD

8945 Sudden Infant Death Syndrome Institute of the University of Maryland
22 S Green Street
Baltimore, MD 21201

410-538-3363
800-492-5538
www.umm.edu

Dr M John O'Brien MB, Director
Jeffrey A Rivest, FACHE, President and Chief Executive Officer

8946 USC: Neonatology Research Units
1240 Mission Road
Los Angeles, CA 90033

213-226-3408
Fax: 213-226-3440

Focuses on clinical problems of the newborn and premature infant.
Paul YK Wu MD, Director

Support Groups & Hotlines

8947 National Center for the Prevention of SIDS
1314 Bedford Avenue
Baltimore, MD 21208-6605

800-638-7437

Offers medical updates and information on prevention of SIDS and other disorders to parents and professionals.

8948 National Health Information Center
PO Box 1133
Washington, DC 20013

310-565-4167
800-336-4797
Fax: 301-984-4256
e-mail: info@nhic.org
www.health.gov/nhic

Offers a nationwide information referral service, produces directories and resource guides.

8949 Parents Helping Parents A Family Resource Center
1400 Parkmoor Avenue
San Jose, CA 95126

408-727-5775
855-727-5775
Fax: 408-286-1116
www.php.com

A group of parents and professionals committed to alleviating some of the problems, hardships and concerns of families with children having special needs.
Mary Ellen Peterson, Director

8950 SIDS Information and Referral Hotline
SIDS Alliance
2105 Laurel Bush Road
Baltimore, MD 21015

443-640-1049
800-221-7437
Fax: 410-653-8709
www.firstcandle.org

Twenty-four hour information and referral line for parents who wish to discuss their concerns with a SIDS counselor, request additional information about SIDS and to receive referrals to the local SIDS affiliate in their area.
Deborah Boyd, Director

8951 SIDS Support Group
Massachusetts Center for SIDS
Boston Medical Center
Boston, MA 02118

617-638-8000
800-641-7437
www.bmc.org

Aids in the resolution of the early trauma of grief experienced by parents following the sudden unexpected death of their infant. The purposes are to provide a safe environemnt for parents to express their feelings, to provide contact with others who share their grief and are at various stages of resolution, to provide a reliable source of information about SIDS and to provide the opportunity to go on to help others.

Books

8952 Apparent Life-Threatening Event and Sudden Infant Death Syndrome
National Maternal and Child Health Clearinghouse
2070 Chain Bridge Road
Vienna, VA 22182-2588

703-442-9051
888-275-4772
Fax: 703-821-2098
e-mail: ask@hrsa.gov
www.ask.hrsa.gov

Provides information about ALTE and its relationship to SIDS.

8953 Hospice Care for Children
Oxford University Press
2001 Evans Road
Cary, NC 27513-2010

212-726-6000
800-445-9714
Fax: 919-677-1303
e-mail: custserv.us@oup.com
www.oup-usa.org

A comprehensive book offering the most inclusive and up-to-date information about caring for terminally ill children and their families.
304 pages
ISBN: 0-195073-12-6
Ann Armstrong-Dailey, Editor

8954 Professional's Role in Sudden Infant Death Syndrome
National Maternal and Child Health Clearinghouse
2070 Chain Bridge Road
Vienna, VA 22182-2588

703-442-9051
888-275-4772
Fax: 703-821-2098
e-mail: ask@hrsa.gov
www.ask.hrsa.gov

Contains abstracts of articles on the role of professionals in SIDS.

8955   Smoking and Sudden Infant Death Syndrome
National Maternal and Child Health Clearinghouse
2070 Chain Bridge Road   703-442-9051
Vienna, VA 22182-2588   888-275-4772
                                           Fax: 703-821-2098
                                          e-mail: ask@hrsa.gov
                                              www.ask.hrsa.gov
Contains abstracts of materials about tobacco use, its relationship to SIDS and the dangers to the unborn and the newly born from passive and secondary smoking.

Newsletters

8956   Newsletter: SIDS
Massachusetts Center For SIDS
1 Boston Medical Ctr Plc
Boston, MA 02118-2905   617-638-8000
                                                  www.bmc.org
Boston Medical Center (BMC) is a 482-bed academic medical center located in Boston's historic South End
Monthly

8957   Parent Care News Brief
Parent Care
303 Watts Branch Parkway   301-294-9338
Rockville, MD 20850-1210   Fax: 301-294-8848
                                      e-mail: drscott@parentcare.com
                                              www.parentcare.com
Features articles and medical updates pertaining to the care of the critically ill child.
Quarterly

Pamphlets

8958   Crib Death: The Sudden Infant Death Syndrome
US Department Of Health & Human Services
202 Indp Avenue SW   202-619-0257
Washington, DC 20201-0001   877-696-6775
                                       e-mail: hhsmail@os.dhhs.gov
                                                www.os.dhhs.gov
Offers information on the most frequently asked questions pertaining to SIDS and crib death.
Kristen Brett
Kathy McKnight

8959   Developmental Delays and Developmental Disorders
National Maternal and Child Health Clearinghouse
2070 Chain Bridge Road   703-442-9051
Vienna, VA 22182-2588   888-275-4772
                                           Fax: 703-821-2098
                                          e-mail: ask@hrsa.gov
                                              www.ask.hrsa.gov
Contains abstracts of selected articles on developmental delays and developmental disorders and the relationship to SIDS.
1997

8960   Facts About SIDS
Sudden Infant Death Syndrome Alliance
1227 Malvern Road   410-653-8226
Malvern, 3144-6605   800-221-7437
                                           Fax: 410-653-8709
                                     e-mail: yvonne@sidsandkids.org
                                              www.sidsandkids.org
Offers information on basic facts, answers to the most frequently asked questions about SIDS and information on numbers to call and referral centers for more help.
Graham Henderson, Chairman
Mr Craig Heatley, Deputy Chairman

8961   Grief of Children After the Loss of a Sibling or Friend
National Maternal and Child Health Clearinghouse
2070 Chain Bridge Road   703-442-9051
Vienna, VA 22182-2588   888-275-4772
                                           Fax: 703-821-2098
                                          e-mail: ask@hrsa.gov
                                              www.ask.hrsa.gov

Discusses some of the common expressions of childrens grief and offers ways adults can help during the grieving process.
1995

8962   Infant Positioning and Sudden Infant Death Syndrome
National Maternal and Child Health Clearinghouse
2070 Chain Bridge Road   703-442-9051
Vienna, VA 22182-2588   888-275-4772
                                           Fax: 703-821-2098
                                          e-mail: ask@hrsa.gov
                                              www.ask.hrsa.gov
Contains abstracts of selected articles on the topic of sleep position and SIDS.
1994

8963   Nationwide Survey of Sudden Infant Death Syndrome (SIDS) Service
National Maternal and Child Health Clearinghouse
2070 Chain Bridge Road   703-442-9051
Vienna, VA 22182-2588   888-275-4772
                                           Fax: 703-821-2098
                                          e-mail: ask@hrsa.gov
                                              www.ask.hrsa.gov
Analysis of availability of SIDS services.
1994

8964   Parents and the Grieving Process
National Maternal and Child Health Clearinghouse
2070 Chain Bridge Road   703-442-9051
Vienna, VA 22182-2588   888-275-4772
                                           Fax: 703-821-2098
                                          e-mail: ask@hrsa.gov
                                              www.ask.hrsa.gov
Defines grief, presents common reactions and emotions expressed by the bereaved.
1992

8965   SIDS Information for the EMT
National Maternal and Child Health Clearinghouse
2070 Chain Bridge Road   703-442-9051
Vienna, VA 22182-2588   888-275-4772
                                           Fax: 703-821-2098
                                          e-mail: ask@hrsa.gov
                                              www.ask.hrsa.gov
Provides suggestions for first response of emergency medical technicians and others at the time of sudden infant death.
1983

8966   SIDS Research: An Analysis in Three Parts
National Maternal and Child Health Clearinghouse
2070 Chain Bridge Road   703-442-9051
Vienna, VA 22182-2588   888-275-4772
                                           Fax: 703-821-2098
                                          e-mail: ask@hrsa.gov
                                              www.ask.hrsa.gov
Contains articles from a three part series on SIDS research.
1993

8967   SIDS: Toward Prevention and Improved Infant Health
American SIDS Institute
528 Raven Way   239-431-5425
Naples, FL 34110-8657   800-232-7437
                                           Fax: 239-431-5536
                                       e-mail: prevent@sids.org
                                                  www.sids.org
the American SIDS Institute, a national nonprofit health care organization, is dedicated to the prevention of sudden infant death and the promotion of infant health
Marc Peterzell, Chairman

8968   Selected Book on Sudden Infant Death Syndrome
National Maternal and Child Health Clearinghouse
2070 Chain Bridge Road   703-442-9051
Vienna, VA 22182-2588   888-275-4772
                                           Fax: 703-821-2098
                                          e-mail: ask@hrsa.gov
                                              www.ask.hrsa.gov
Provides a list of selected titles on SIDS covering topics such as research, support information and the professionals role.
1993

8969 Selected Resources for Children Grieving the Loss of Another Child
National Maternal and Child Health Clearinghouse
2070 Chain Bridge Road   703-442-9051
Vienna, VA 22182-2588   888-275-4772
                                  Fax: 703-821-2098
                              e-mail: ask@hrsa.gov
                                  www.ask.hrsa.gov
Provides a list of materials suitable for grieving children and teenagers.
1995

8970 Sudden Infant Death Syndrome and Risk Reduction
National Maternal and Child Health Clearinghouse
2070 Chain Bridge Road   703-442-9051
Vienna, VA 22182-2588   888-275-4772
                                  Fax: 703-821-2098
                              e-mail: ask@hrsa.gov
                                  www.ask.hrsa.gov
Contains abstracts of selected articles on risk reduction.
1997

8971 What Every Parent Should Know About SIDS
SIDS Alliance
1227 Malvern Road   410-653-8226
Malvern, 3144-6605   800-221-7437
                                  Fax: 410-653-8709
                          e-mail: yvonne@sidsandkids.org
                                  www.sidsandkids.org
Pamphlet offering information on what SIDS is, causes, prevention techniques and what parents can do.
Graham Henderson, Chairman
Mr Craig Heatley, Deputy Chairman

8972 What is SIDS?
National Maternal and Child Health Clearinghouse
2070 Chain Bridge Road   703-442-9051
Vienna, VA 22182-2588   888-275-4772
                                  Fax: 703-821-2098
                              e-mail: ask@hrsa.gov
                                  www.ask.hrsa.gov
Provides basic facts about SIDS and answers some of the most commonly asked questions.
1993

8973 When Sudden Infant Death Syndrome Occurs in Childcare Settings
National Maternal and Child Health Clearinghouse
2070 Chain Bridge Road   703-442-9051
Vienna, VA 22182-2588   888-275-4772
                                  Fax: 703-821-2098
                              e-mail: ask@hrsa.gov
                                  www.ask.hrsa.gov
Presents information about SIDS for child care providers.
1993

Web Sites

8974 American SIDS Institute
                                        sids.org/
Dedicated to the prevention of sudden infant death and the promotion of infant health through research, clinical services, education and family support.

8975 Center for Research for Mothers & Children
                                   cdrwww.who.ch/
Mission is to make sure everyone is born healthy and wanted, that women suffer no harmful effects from reproductive processes, and that all children have the chance to achieve their full potential for healthy and productive lives, free from disease or disability, and to ensure the health, productivity, independence, and well-being of all people through optimal rehabilitation.

8976 Compassionate Friends
                             www.compassionatefriends.org
The Compassionate Friends provides highly personal comfort, hope, and support to every family experiencing the death of a son or a daughter, a brother or a sister, or a grandchild, and helps others better assist the grieving family.

8977 Healing Well
                                   www.healingwell.com
An online health resource guide to medical news, chat, information and articles, newsgroups and message boards, books, disease-related web sites, medical directories, and more for patients, friends, and family coping with disabling diseases, disorders, or chronic illnesses.

8978 Healthlink USA
                                   www.healthlinkusa.com
Health information concerning treatment, cures, prevention, diagnosis, risk factors, research, support groups, email lists, personal stories and much more. Updated regularly.

8979 Helios Health
                                   www.helioshealth.com
Online resource for your health information. Detailed information about specific health topics, access to expert advice from our Medical Advisory Board, and up-to-date health news.

8980 MedicineNet
                                   www.medicinenet.com
An online resource for consumers providing easy-to-read, authoritative medical and health information.

8981 Medscape
                                   www.medscape.com
Medscape offers specialists, primary care physicians, and other health professionals the Web's most robust and integrated medical information and educational tools.

8982 National Center for Education in Maternal and Child Health
                                   www.ncemch.org
The National Center for Education in Maternal and Child Health provides national leadership to the maternal and child health community in three key areas - program development, policy analysis and education, and state-of-the-art knowledge to improve the health and well-being of the nation's children and families.

8983 WebMD
                                   www.webmd.com
Provides credible information, supportive communities, and in-depth reference material about health subjects. A source for original and timely health information as well as material from well known content providers.

Description

8984 Tay-Sachs Disease

Tay-Sachs disease results from an absence of an enzyme (hexosaminidase A) which leads to an accumulation of fat (lipid) in the specific brain tissues (cerebral neurons). The disease is genetic and is autosomal recessive; if two carriers have children, the disease would have a 1 in 4 chance of being passed on. The disease is most prevalent in those of Jewish families, particularly those of Eastern European (Ashkenazi) background.

Symptoms usually present between 3-6 months of age. Early symptoms include mild muscle weakness, muscle spasms, and feeding difficulties. As the disease progresses, the patient may experience vision loss, seizures and eventually paralysis. Death usually occurs by the age of 4 years.

Treatment for Tay-Sachs disease is supportive and there is no cure. Genetic and premarital counseling is important to those at high risk.

National Agencies & Associations

8985 National Foundation for Jewish Genetic Diseases
One Gustave L.
New York, NY 10029
212-241-6500
Fax: 212-241-6947
www.mssm.edu/jewish_genetics
Offers information and support for persons suffering from Tay-Sachs Disease as well as their families and professionals working with them. The Foundation supports research into all areas of genetic disorders.
R J Desnick PhD MD, Center Director

8986 National Institute of Child Health and Human Development
31 Center Drive
Bethesda, MD 20892
301-496-5133
800-370-2943
Fax: 866-760-5947
TTY: 888-320-6942
e-mail: NICHDInformationResourceCenter@mail.nih.
www.nichd.nih.gov
Offers reprints, articles and various information on Tay-Sachs Disease for patients and professionals.
Duane Alexan MD, Director
John McGrath, Coordinator

8987 National Institute of Neurological Disorders and Stroke
NIH Neurological Institute
Bethesda, MD 20824
301-496-5751
800-352-9424
Fax: 301-402-2186
TTY: 301-468-5981
www.ninds.nih.gov
The mission of NINDS is to reduce the burden of neurological disease - a burden borne by every age group, by every segment of society, by people all over the world.
Story C Landis PhD, Director
Walter J Koroshetz, Deputy Director

8988 National Organization for Rare Disorders
55 Kenosia Avenue
Danbury, CT 06813-1968
203-744-0100
800-999-6673
Fax: 203-798-2291
TDD: 203-797-9590
e-mail: orphan@rarediseases.org
www.rarediseases.org
Serves as a clearinghouse for information about rare disorders and brings together families with similar disorders for mutual support; fosters communication among rare disease voluntary agencies, Government agencies, industry scientific researchers and academia.
E. Michael D Scott, Chair
Carolyn Asbury, PhD, Vice Chair

8989 National Tay-Sachs and Allied Diseases Association (NTSAD)
2001 Beacon Street
Brighton, MA 02135
617-277-4463
800-906-8723
Fax: 617-277-0134
e-mail: info@ntsad.org
www.ntstad.org
Offers programs of public and professional education prevention services testing research and family services and promotion of TSD genetic screening programs nationally.
Fran Berkwits, MS, Director
Kevin Romer, President

Foundations

8990 National Tay-Sachs and Allied Diseases Association (NTSAD)
2001 Beacon Street
Brighton, MA 02135
617-277-4463
800-906-8723
Fax: 617-277-0134
e-mail: info@ntsad.org
www.ntsad.org
Dedicated to the treatment and preventin of Tay Sachs, Canavan, and related diseases, and to provide information and support services to individuals and families affected by these diseases, as well as the public at large.
Fran Berkwits, MS, Director
Kevin Romer, President

Support Groups & Hotlines

8991 National Health Information Center
PO Box 1133
Washington, DC 20013
310-565-4167
800-336-4797
Fax: 301-984-4256
e-mail: info@nhic.org
www.health.gov/nhic
Offers a nationwide information referral service, produces directories and resource guides.

8992 National Tay-Sachs Association: Delaware Valley (NTSAD-DV)
720 Greenwood Avenue
Jenkintown, PA 19046
215-887-0877
877-599-9293
Fax: 215-887-1931
e-mail: NTSAD@aol.com
www.tay-sachs.org

Rebecca Tantala, Executive Director

8993 National TaySachs & Allied Diseases
2001 Beacon Street
Boston, MA 2135
617-277-4463
800-906-8723
Fax: 617-277-0134
e-mail: info@ntsad.org
www.ntsad.org
A mutual support group coordinated by staff and volunteers who are parents of affected children or affected adults. One of several programs supported and sponsored by the association.
Fran Berkwits, MS, Director
Kevin Romer, President

Books

8994 Home Care Book
National Tay-Sachs and Allied Diseases Association
2001 Beacon Street
Brighton, MA 02135
617-277-4463
800-906-8723
Fax: 617-277-0134
e-mail: info@ntsad.org
www.ntsad.org

Written by parents for parents and professionals, the Home Care Book is a guide to caring for children with progressive neurological disorders at home.
Shari Ungerleider, President
Merle Adelman, Vice President Development

8995   Home-Care Book
National Tay-Sachs and Allied Diseases Association
2001 Beacon Street   617-277-4463
Brookline, MA 02146   800-906-8723
                              Fax: 617-277-0134
                         e-mail: info@ntsad.org
                                 www.ntsad.org
National Tay-Sachs & Allied Diseases Association (NTSAD) is one of the oldest patient advocacy groups in the country. We focus on funding research, supporting over 500 families and individuals worldwide, and raising awareness to prevent disease
Shari Ungerleider, President
Merle Adelman, Vice President Development

8996   Late Onset Tay-Sachs Disease Medical Bibliography
National Tay-Sachs and Allied Diseases Association
2001 Beacon Street   617-277-4463
Brookline, MA 02146   800-906-8723
                              Fax: 617-277-0134
                         e-mail: info@ntsad.org
                                 www.ntsad.org
National Tay-Sachs & Allied Diseases Association (NTSAD) is one of the oldest patient advocacy groups in the country. We focus on funding research, supporting over 500 families and individuals worldwide, and raising awareness to prevent disease
Shari Ungerleider, President
Merle Adelman, Vice President Development

8997   Lifting of Canavan's Carrier Testing Facilities
National Tay-Sachs and Allied Diseases Association
2001 Beacon Street   617-277-4463
Brookline, MA 02146   800-906-8723
                              Fax: 617-277-0134
                         e-mail: info@ntsad.org
                                 www.ntsad.org
National Tay-Sachs & Allied Diseases Association (NTSAD) is one of the oldest patient advocacy groups in the country. We focus on funding research, supporting over 500 families and individuals worldwide, and raising awareness to prevent disease
Shari Ungerleider, President
Merle Adelman, Vice President Development

8998   Monograph on Canavan's Disease
National Tay-Sachs and Allied Diseases Association
2001 Beacon Street   617-277-4463
Brookline, MA 02146   800-906-8723
                              Fax: 617-277-0134
                         e-mail: info@ntsad.org
                                 www.ntsad.org
National Tay-Sachs & Allied Diseases Association (NTSAD) is one of the oldest patient advocacy groups in the country. We focus on funding research, supporting over 500 families and individuals worldwide, and raising awareness to prevent disease
Shari Ungerleider, President
Merle Adelman, Vice President Development

8999   Tay-Sachs Carrier Testing Directory
National Tay-Sachs and Allied Diseases Association
2001 Beacon Street   617-277-4463
Brookline, MA 02146   800-906-8723
                              Fax: 617-277-0134
                         e-mail: info@ntsad.org
                                 www.ntsad.org
National Tay-Sachs & Allied Diseases Association (NTSAD) is one of the oldest patient advocacy groups in the country. We focus on funding research, supporting over 500 families and individuals worldwide, and raising awareness to prevent disease
Shari Ungerleider, President
Merle Adelman, Vice President Development

9000   Tay-Sachs: The Dreaded Inheritance
National Tay-Sachs and Allied Diseases Assocation

2001 Beacon Street   617-277-4463
Brighton, MA 02135   800-906-8723
                              Fax: 617-277-0134
                         e-mail: info@ntsad.org
                                 www.ntsad.org
Descriptive narrative on caring for a child with Tay-Sachs Disease.
Shari Ungerleider, President
Merle Adelman, Vice President Development

9001   There is Only One Child
National Tay-Sachs and Allied Diseases Association
2001 Beacon Street   617-277-4463
Brookline, MA 02146   800-906-8723
                              Fax: 617-277-0134
                         e-mail: info@ntsad.org
                                 www.ntsad.org
National Tay-Sachs & Allied Diseases Association (NTSAD) is one of the oldest patient advocacy groups in the country. We focus on funding research, supporting over 500 families and individuals worldwide, and raising awareness to prevent disease
Shari Ungerleider, President
Merle Adelman, Vice President Development

9002   What Every Family Should Know Sixth Edition
National Tay-Sachs & Allied Diseases Association
2001 Beacon Street   617-277-4463
Brighton, MA 02135   800-906-8723
                              Fax: 617-277-0134
                         e-mail: info@ntsad.org
                                 www.ntsad.org
Detailing lysosomal storage and leukodystrophy disorders, with sections on Tay-Sachs, Sandhoff, Niemann-Pick, Gaucher, Canavan, Fabry, Pompe, therapeutic approaches and unique disease table.
50 pages
Shari Ungerleider, President
Merle Adelman, Vice President Development

Newsletters

9003   Breakthrough
National Tay-Sachs and Allied Diseases Association
2001 Beacon Street   617-277-4463
Boston, MA 02135   800-906-8723
                              Fax: 617-277-0134
                         e-mail: info@ntsad.org
                                 www.ntsad.org
Each year NTSAD publishes a newsletter for friends and supporters that focuses on the latest advances in research, profiles of families and individuals helped by NTSAD and disease profiles.
Annual
Shari Ungerleider, President
Merle Adelman, Vice President Development

9004   Late Onset Community Newsletter
National Tay-Sachs and Allied Diseases Association
2001 Beacon Street   617-277-4463
Brighton, MA 02135   800-906-8723
                              Fax: 617-277-0134
                         e-mail: info@ntsad.org
                                 www.ntsad.org
PSG members dealing with chronic forms of the allied diseases receive this newsletter focused specifically on the issues and perspectives unique to adults struggling with long-term disability issues. Public editions of the newsletter are also available.
Bi-Monthly
Shari Ungerleider, President
Merle Adelman, Vice President Development

9005   Lifeline
National Tay-Sachs and Allied Diseases Association
2001 Beacon Street   617-277-4463
Brighton, MA 02135   800-906-8723
                              Fax: 617-277-0134
                         e-mail: info@ntsad.org
                                 www.ntsad.org
The editorial content is wide ranging: symptom management and home health care; new product reviews; guidance in benefits and services advocacy for families and affected individuals of all ages;

science and medical research updates; coverage of NTSAD events, fundraising, programs and administrative activities. Members only.
Quarterly
Shari Ungerleider, President
Merle Adelman, Vice President Development

Pamphlets

9006 Late Onset Tay-Sachs Fact Sheet
National Tay-Sachs and Allied Diseases Association
2001 Beacon Street   617-277-4463
Brighton, MA 02135   800-906-8723
                                                 Fax: 617-277-0134
                                          e-mail: info@ntsad.org
                                                  www.ntsad.org
This quick reference information sheet on the chronic or late onset form of Tay-Sachs is available for no charge.
Shari Ungerleider, President
Merle Adelman, Vice President Development

9007 Services to Families
National Tay-Sachs and Allied Diseases Association
2001 Beacon Street   617-277-4463
Brookline, MA 02146   800-906-8723
                                                 Fax: 617-277-0134
                                          e-mail: info@ntsad.org
                                                  www.ntsad.org
National Tay-Sachs & Allied Diseases Association (NTSAD) is one of the oldest patient advocacy groups in the country. We focus on funding research, supporting over 500 families and individuals worldwide, and raising awareness to prevent disease
Shari Ungerleider, President
Merle Adelman, Vice President Development

9008 Tay-Sachs Information Sheet
March of Dimes
1275 Mamaroneck Avenue   212-353-8353
White Plains, NY 10605   Fax: 212-254-3518
                                   e-mail: NY639@marchofdimes.com
                                              www.marchofdimes.com
Offers a brief overview of the illness, causes, symptoms and treatments are covered. Availabe electronically on the website: www.marchofdimes.com

9009 Tay-Sachs is
National Tay-Sachs and Allied Diseases Association
2001 Beacon Street   617-277-4463
Brookline, MA 02146   800-906-8723
                                                 Fax: 617-277-0134
                                          e-mail: info@ntsad.org
                                                  www.ntsad.org
National Tay-Sachs & Allied Diseases Association (NTSAD) is one of the oldest patient advocacy groups in the country. We focus on funding research, supporting over 500 families and individuals worldwide, and raising awareness to prevent disease
Shari Ungerleider, President
Merle Adelman, Vice President Development

9010 Understanding Lysosomal Storage Diseases
National Tay-Sachs and Allied Diseases Association
2001 Beacon Street   617-277-4463
Brookline, MA 02146   800-906-8723
                                                 Fax: 617-277-0134
                                          e-mail: info@ntsad.org
                                                  www.ntsad.org
National Tay-Sachs & Allied Diseases Association (NTSAD) is one of the oldest patient advocacy groups in the country. We focus on funding research, supporting over 500 families and individuals worldwide, and raising awareness to prevent disease
Shari Ungerleider, President
Merle Adelman, Vice President Development

9011 What is Canavan Disease?
National Tay-Sachs and Allied Diseases Association

2001 Beacon Street   617-277-4463
Brighton, MA 02135   800-906-8723
                                                 Fax: 617-277-0134
                                          e-mail: info@ntsad.org
                                                  www.ntsad.org
The educational pamphlet describing Canavan Disease.
Shari Ungerleider, President
Merle Adelman, Vice President Development

9012 What is Tay-Sachs? Russian Translation
National Tay-Sachs and Allied Diseases Association
2001 Beacon Street   617-277-4463
Brighton, MA 02135   800-906-8723
                                                 Fax: 617-277-0134
                                          e-mail: info@ntsad.org
                                                  www.ntsad.org
This informative educational pamphlet describing Infantile Tay-Sachs, its inheritance and prevention is available for no charge.
Shari Ungerleider, President
Merle Adelman, Vice President Development

Audio & Video

9013 For My Sister, Elyssa
National Tay-Sachs & Allied Diseases Assocation
2001 Beacon Street   617-277-4463
Brighton, MA 02135   800-906-8723
                                                 Fax: 617-277-0134
                                          e-mail: info@ntsad.org
                                                  www.ntsad.org
Moving and informative 15 minute presentation told by a teenager who baby siter died from Tay-Sachs Disease. Contains information on Tay-Sachs Disease and simple steps each individual can take to prevent the tragedy of Tay-Sachs.
Shari Ungerleider, President
Merle Adelman, Vice President Development

Web Sites

9014 Healing Well
                                              www.healingwell.com
An online health resource guide to medical news, chat, information and articles, newsgroups and message boards, books, disease-related web sites, medical directories, and more for patients, friends, and family coping with disabling diseases, disorders, or chronic illnesses.

9015 Health Finder
                                              www.healthfinder.gov
Searchable, carefully developed web site offering information on over 1000 topics. Developed by the US Department of Health and Human Services, the site can be used in both English and Spanish.

9016 Healthlink USA
                                             www.healthlinkusa.com
Health information concerning treatment, cures, prevention, diagnosis, risk factors, research, support groups, email lists, personal stories and much more. Updated regularly.

9017 Helios Health
                                              www.helioshealth.com
Online resource for your health information. Detailed information about specific health topics, access to expert advice from our Medical Advisory Board, and up-to-date health news.

9018 MedicineNet
                                              www.medicinenet.com
An online resource for consumers providing easy-to-read, authoritative medical and health information.

9019 Medscape
                                                www.medscape.com
Medscape offers specialists, primary care physicians, and other health professionals the Web's most robust and integrated medical information and educational tools.

9020 WebMD
www.webmd.com
Provides credible information, supportive communities, and in-depth reference material about health subjects. A source for original and timely health information as well as material from well known content providers.

Description

9021 Thyroid Disease

Thyroid Disease refers to a number of conditions that affect the thyroid, a small, butterfly-shaped gland located in the middle of the lower neck. Hormones T3 and T4, produced by the thyroid, deliver energy to cells of the body, thus controlling the body's metabolism. Conditions that result from an imbalance of these hormones are Hypothyroidism — not enough hormones that results in the body using energy slower than it should, and Hyperthyroidism — too much hormones that results in the body using energy faser than it should. These conditions can be caused by an inflammation of the thyroid gland, too much or too little iodine (used to produce thyroid hormones), or autoimmune disease, in which antibodies gradually either destroy the thyroid gland or speed up its function. Other thyroid conditions are Goiter — an enlarged thyroid; Thyroid Nodules — cysts, lumps, bumps and tumors that can be cancerous or benign; and Thyroiditis — inflammation of the thyroid gland. More than 20 million Americans have thyroid disease, and it affects many more women than men. Treatment includes synthetic hormone medication to replace missing hormones, radioactive iodine to deactivate the thyroid, and surgery for some goiters and cancerous nodules. Early diagnosis is often the key in prescribing treatment even before the onset of symptoms. Although thyroid disease is a chronic condition, careful disease management allows affected individuals to live healthy, normal lives.

National Agencies & Associations

9022 American Thyroid Association
6066 Leesburg Pike   703-998-8890
Falls Church, VA 22041   800-479-7634
Fax: 703-998-8893
e-mail: thyroid@thyroid.org
www.thyroid.org
Promotes excellence and innovation in clinical care research education and public policy.
Barbara R. Smith, CAE, Executive Director

9023 National Women's Health Resource Center
157 Broad Street   877-986-9472
Red Bank, NJ 07701   877-986-9472
Fax: 732-530-3347
e-mail: snelson@healthwomen.org
www.healthywomen.org
NWHRC develops and distributes up-to-date and objective women's health information based on the latest advances in medical research and practice.
JoAnn V. Pinkerton, Director
Elizabeth Ba Cahill, Executive Director

9024 Thyroid Federation International
797 Princess Street   613-544-8364
Kingston, Ontario, K7L-1G1   Fax: 613-544-9731
e-mail: tfi@on.aibn.com
www.thyroid-fed.org
Aims to work for the benefit of those affected by thyroid disorders throughout the world.
Yvonne Andersson, President, Board of Directors
Peter Lakwijk, VP, Board of Directors

9025 Thyroid Foundation of Canada
797 Princess Street   613-544-8364
Kingston, Ontario, K7L-1G1   800-267-8822
Fax: 613-544-9731
www.thyroid.ca
Thyroid Foundation of Canada is a registered charity.
Katherine Keen, National Office Coordinator

Books

9026 Autoimmune Connection: Essential Informati on for Women on Diagnosis, Treatment
National Women's Health Resource Center
157 Broad Street   917-428-1321
Red Bank, NJ 07701   877-986-9472
Fax: 732-530-3347
e-mail: info@healthywomen.org
www.healthywomen.org
Readers learn about the recent groundbreaking discovery of the links between the different autoimmune diseases and why women are more likely to develop them.
Elizabeth Battaglino Cahill, Executive Director
Beth Battaglino, Chief Executive Officer

9027 The Thyroid Gland
Joel I Hamburger MD & Michael M Kaplan, author
Thyroid Foundation of Canada
P.O. Box 298   613-544-8364
Bath, -1G1   800-267-8822
Fax: 613-544-9731
www.thyroid.ca
The Thyroid Foundation of Canada is a non-profit registered volunteer organization whose mission is to support thyroid patients across Canada through awareness, education, and research
Donna Miniely, President
Rinda Hartner, Treasurer

9028 Thyroid Balance
National Women's Health Resource Center
157 Broad Street   917-428-1321
Red Bank, NJ 07701   877-986-9472
Fax: 732-530-3347
e-mail: info@healthywomen.org
www.healthywomen.org
An authoritative guide to treating thyroid issues-using both traditional and alternative methods.
Elizabeth Battaglino Cahill, Executive Director
Beth Battaglino, Chief Executive Officer

9029 Thyroid Disease: The Facts
RIS Bayliss & WMG Tunbridge MD, author
Thyroid Foundation of Canada
P.O. Box 298   613-544-8364
Bath, -1G1   800-267-8822
Fax: 613-544-9731
www.thyroid.ca
The Thyroid Foundation of Canada is a non-profit registered volunteer organization whose mission is to support thyroid patients across Canada through awareness, education, and research
Donna Miniely, President
Rinda Hartner, Treasurer

9030 Thyroid Power: Ten Steps to Total Health
Richard Shames & Karilee H Shames, author
National Women's Health Resource Center
157 Broad Street   917-428-1321
Red Bank, NJ 07701   877-986-9472
Fax: 732-530-3347
e-mail: info@healthywomen.org
www.healthywomen.org
Discusses the labyrinth of diagnostic and treatment issues a patient must endure.
Beth Battaglino, Chief Executive Officer

9031 Thyroid Solution: A Mind-Body Program for Beating Depression and Regaining Health
National Women's Health Resource Center

157 Broad Street
Red Bank, NJ 07701

917-428-1321
877-986-9472
Fax: 732-530-3347
e-mail: info@healthywomen.org
www.healthywomen.org

This book explains the link between stress and thyroid imbalance; how thyroid imbalance affects your emotions, sex life, and relationships; and how to cope with the effects of this imbalance.
Elizabeth Battaglino Cahill, Executive Director
Beth Battaglino, Chief Executive Officer

9032 Thyroid Sourcebook
Thyroid Foundation of Canada
P.O. Box 298
Bath, -1G1

613-544-8364
800-267-8822
Fax: 613-544-9731
www.thyroid.ca

The Thyroid Foundation of Canada is a non-profit registered volunteer organization whose mission is to support thyroid patients across Canada through awareness, education, and research
Donna Miniely, President
Rinda Hartner, Treasurer

9033 Your Thyroid: A Home Reference
Lawrence Wood MD & David S Cooper MD, author
Thyroid Foundation of Canada
P.O. Box 298
Bath, -1G1

613-544-8364
800-267-8822
Fax: 613-544-9731
www.thyroid.ca

The Thyroid Foundation of Canada is a non-profit registered volunteer organization whose mission is to support thyroid patients across Canada through awareness, education, and research
Donna Miniely, President
Rinda Hartner, Treasurer

Magazines

9034 Clinical Thyroidology
American Thyroid Association
6066 Leesburg Pike
Falls Church, VA 22041

703-998-8890
800-849-7634
Fax: 703-998-8893
e-mail: thyroid@thyroid.org
www.thyroid.org

An online publication, available monthly, this is a broad-ranging look at clinical and preclinical thyroid literature. The Editor searches the world literature for excellent thyroid studies and then summarizes them along side his expert commentary.
Robert C. Smallridge, President
John C. Morris, Secretary/Chief Operating Officer

9035 THYROID
American Thyroid Association
6066 Leesburg Pike
Falls Church, VA 22041

703-998-8890
800-849-7643
Fax: 703-998-8893
e-mail: thyroid@thyroid.org
www.thyroid.org

The Associations monthly journal that touches on topics from the molecular biology of the thyroid gland to clinical management of thyroid disorders. All Association members receive a suvscription, and it is available to non-members.
Robert C. Smallridge, President
John C. Morris, Secretary/Chief Operating Officer

9036 Clinical Thyroidology for Patients
American Thyroid Association
6066 Leesburg Pike
Falls Church, VA 22041

703-998-8890
800-849-7634
Fax: 703-998-8893
e-mail: thyroid@thyroid.org
www.thyroid.org

A collection of summaries of recently published articles fromt the medical literature that covers the broad spectrum of thryroid disorders. Notes descxribing published research studies were prepared by THYROID Editor, Ernest Mazzaferri, MD.
Robert C. Smallridge, President
John C. Morris, Secretary/Chief Operating Officer

Newsletters

9037 SIGNAL
American Thyroid Association
6066 Leesburg Pike
Falls Church, VA 22041

703-998-8890
800-849-7643
Fax: 703-998-8893
e-mail: thyroid@thyroid.org
www.thyroid.org

Covers Association news, meetings, policies, leaders, and important thyroid-related issues.
Robert C. Smallridge, President
John C. Morris, Secretary/Chief Operating Officer

Pamphlets

9038 Hypothyroidism Web Booklet
American Thyroid Association
6066 Leesburg Pike
Falls Church, VA 22041

703-998-8890
800-489-7643
Fax: 703-998-8893
e-mail: thyroid@thyroid.org
www.thyroid.org

This online booklet introduces the thryoid and hypothyroidism to the reader, explains symptoms, treatments, causes, who's at risk, and more.
2003 25 pages
Robert C. Smallridge, President
John C. Morris, Secretary/Chief Operating Officer

Web Sites

9039 American Thyroid Association

www.thyroid.org

Promotes excellence and innovation in clinical care, research, education, and public policy.
David S Cooper MD, President
Gregory A Brent MD, Secretary

9040 MedicineNet

www.medicinenet.com

An online resource for consumers providing easy-to-read, authoritative medical and health information.

9041 National Women's Health Resource Center

www.healthywomen.org

NWHRC developes and distributes up-to-date and objective women's health information based on the latest advances in medical research and practice.
Elizabeth Battaglino Cahill, RN, Executive Director
Maria Bushee, Director of Marketing & Communications

9042 Thyroid Federation International

www.thyroid-fed.org

Aims to work for the benefit of those affected by thyroid disorders throughout the world.

9043 Thyroid Foundation of Canada

www.thyroid.ca

The Thyroid Foundation of Canada is a non-profit registered volunteer organization whose mission is to support thyroid patients across Canada through awareness, education, and research.

Description

9044 Tick-Borne Disease

Ticks transmit disease to humans by being carriers for a variety of microorganismns. The most common tick-borne illness is Lyme disease, first recognized and so named in 1975 because of a cluster of cases found in Lyme, Connecticut. It is a bacterial infection spread by the bite of an infected deer tick. The disease in its earliest stages causes an expanding red rash in at least 75 percent of patients. Flu-like symptoms—headaches, fever, fatigue—are common. The rash may be followed by progressive joint pain and swelling. Dysfunction of the heart (8 percent) and nervous system (15 percent) develop weeks to months later. Further progression causes arthritis and more serious neurologic problems.

Although only one third of patients remember a tick bite, greater than 60 percent do develop the tell-tale rash. Diagnosis requires a blood test to confirm the physical symptoms.

Oral antibiotics may be sufficient for the disease caught in the early stages. Long-standing, disseminated disease responds best to intravenous antibiotics.

Rocky Mountain spotted fever, also known as tick fever, is transmitted by a bite from either a dog tick or wood tick, depending on the part of the country. Like Lyme disease, it begin with flu-like symptoms — chills, fever and loss of appetite. A rash of small, reddish bumps, which gives the disease its name, begins on the wrist and ankle and spreads to the rest of the body. Aggressive antibotic treatment should begin as early as possible. If left untreated, Rocky Mountain spotted fever has a mortality rate of 10 to 80 percent.

Prevention of tick-borne disease requires avoidance of tick bites, by using insect repellants and protective clothing, plus daily checks for ticks during periods of exposure. A vaccine may provide partial protection from Lyme disease for those regularly engaged in high-risk activities (i.e. property maintenance), although other conditions may complicate this treatment.

National Agencies & Associations

9045 Infections Disease Society of America
1300 Wilson Blvd
Arlington, VA 22209
703-299-0200
Fax: 703-299-0204
www.idsociety.org
The Infectious Diseases Society of America (IDSA) represents physicians, scientists and other health care professionals who specialize in infectious diseases.
Stephen B. Calderwood, MD, FIDSA, President
William G. Powderly, MD, FIDSA, Vice President

9046 Lyme Disease Association
PO Box 1438
Jackson, NJ 8527
888-366-6611
Fax: 732-938-7215
www.lymediseaseassociation.org
It was formed by several patients and doctorsÄthe Fordyce and Drulle Families were particularly instrumental Äwho saw the need

to organize and fund research and educate people. It had first a regional then state focus.
Patricia V. Smith, BA, President
Pamela Lampe, Vice President/ Treasurer

9047 Lyme Disease Foundation
PO Box332
Tolland, CT 06084-0332
860-870-0070
800-886-5963
Fax: 860-870-0080
e-mail: info@lyme.org
www.lyme.org
Provides a wide range of services including information and referral network on Lyme Disease, distribution of educational videos to state libraries, educational materials for public and professionals, national public forums and training for community education.
John F Anderson, Board of Director
Willy Burgdorfer, Board of Director

9048 National Capital Lyme Disease Association
P.O. Box 8211
McLean, VA 22106
703-821-8833
www.natcaplyme.org
The National Capital Lyme Disease Association is an all volunteer not-for-profit organization that is committed to helping patients diagnosed with tick-borne illnesses.
Monte Skall, Executive Director
Gregg Skall, Legal Counsel

9049 Tick-Borne Disease Alliance
244 Fifth Avenue
New York, NY 10001
646-450-4882
Fax: 914-967-7744
tbdalliance.org
Dynamic, inclusive and passionate, the Tick-Borne Disease Alliance (TBDA) is dedicated to raising awareness, promoting advocacy, and supporting initiatives to find a cure for tick-borne diseases, including Lyme.
Staci Grodin, President
Drew Goldman, Vice President

Libraries & Resource Centers

9050 California Lyme Disease Association
PO Box 1352
Chico, CA 95927
e-mail: info@lymedisease.org
www.lymedisease.org
The California Lyme Disease Association (CALDA) is an affiliate of the Lyme Disease Association, Inc. CALDA, a non-profit organization, was originally founded in 1990 as The Lyme Disease Resource Center (LDRC). We provide services for Lyme disease patients, their families and friends; provide a forum for physicians and health professionals for the exchange of ideas and information about symptoms, diagnosis, and treatment of Lyme disease.
Marilynn Barkley, Board of Directors
Barbara Barsoschinni, Board of Directors

Research Centers

9051 Ball State University Public Health Entomology Laboratory
2000 University Avenue
Muncie, IN 47306
765-289-1241
800-382-8540
TTY: 7
www.bsu.edu
Offers information on mosquitoes and mosquito-born diseases specializing in Lyme Disease.
Bob Pinger, Director
Jeffrey Clark, Department Chair and Professor

9052 Centers for Disease Control Division of Vector Borne Infectious Diseases
US Public Health Service
1600 Clifton Rd.
Atlanta, GA 30333
800-232-4636
Fax: 970-216-76
TDD: 888-232-6348
www.cdc.gov
Research done into lyme disease tularemia bubonic plague and all vector-borne infectious diseases — including west nile virus.
Dr.Tom Frieden, Director

Support Groups & Hotlines

9053 Advocates 4 Health: Tick-borne Disease Self-Help Group
PALS
PO Box 1271   805-544-0984
San Luis Obispo, CA 93406 e-mail: advocates4heatlh@yahoo.com
Advocacy and support group increasing awareness, education and
understanding of tick-borne disorders and other zoonotic diseases.
This group fosters a supportive network between human/animal
sufferers, caregivers, health care professionals and the general
community.
Sheryl Glidden

9054 American Lyme Disease Foundation
2518 Ridge Court   785-248-3504
Lawrence, CT 66046   e-mail: Inquire@aldf.com
                                             www.aldf.com
Supports research and plays a key role in providing reliable and
scientifically accurate information to the public and health care
providers.
David L Weld, Executive Director
Jeffery Black, Partner

9055 Lyme Alliance
PO Box 454
Concord, MI 49237   517-563-3582
                                       www.lymealliance.org
Lyme Alliance volunteers will address your questions concerning
the newsletter, website, or questions about doctor referrals, medi-
cal treatment options, or information about Lyme disease.

9056 Lyme Disease Network
43 Winton Road   651-644-7239
East Brunswick, NJ 08816
Lynn M Olivier

**9057 Lyme Disease Network Support Group of Alabama: Mobile
Chapter**
Mobile, AL 35758   256-772-6482
                              e-mail: alabamalyme@usa.com
                             www.lymnet.org/supportgroups
Support information, and referrals for victims of Lyme disease and
their families.
Kara Tyson

9058 Lyme Disease Network of New Jersey
43 Winton Road
East Brunswick, NJ 08816   e-mail: carol@lymenet.org
                                        www.lymenet.org
Support information, and referrals for victims of Lyme disease and
their families. Maintains comuter information system.
Bill Stolow, President

9059 Lyme Disease Network of South Carolina
Po Box 6634   803-798-5963
Columbia, SC 29260-6634   e-mail: lyme@sc-lyme.org
                                         www.sc-lyme.org
Sue Fox

9060 National Health Information Center
PO Box 1133   240-453-8280
Washington, DC 20013   800-336-4797
                                         Fax: 240-453-8282
                                     e-mail: info@nhic.org
                                     www.health.gov/nhic
Offers a nationwide information referral service, produces direc-
tories and resource guides.

Books

9061 Coping with Lyme Disease: A Practical Guide
Henry Holt & Company
115 W 18th Street   212-886-9200
New York, NY 10011-4113   Fax: 212-633-0748
1993 288 pages Paperback
ISBN: 0-805026-50-9

9062 Ecology & Environment Management of Lyme Disease
Rutgers University Press

109 Church Street   201-932-7762
New Brunswick, NJ 08901-1242
1993 224 pages
ISBN: 0-813519-28-4

9063 Everything You Need to Know About Lyme Disease
John Wiley & Sons Publishing
111 River Street   212-850-6000
Hoboken, NJ 07030-0012   800-225-5945
                                         Fax: 201-748-6088
                                     e-mail: info@wiley.com
                                             www.wiley.com
Wiley's Professional Development business creates products and
services that help customers become more effective in the work-
place and achieve career success
237 pages
ISBN: 0-471160-61-X
Stephen M. Smith, President and Chief Executive Officer
John Kritzmacher, Executive Vice President

9064 Let's Talk About Having Lyme Disease
Rosen Publishing Group's PowerKids Press
29 East 21st Street   212-777-3017
New York, NY 10010   800-237-9932
                                         Fax: 888-436-4643
                          e-mail: customerservice@rosenpub.com
                                     www.rosenpublishing.com
Kids are taught to take precautions when walking in the woods and
how to inspect themselves for ticks. The illness and recovery are
also explained.
Grades K-4
ISBN: 0-823950-29-8
Elizabeth Weitzman, Author

Children's Books

9065 Lyme Disease
Franklin Watts Grolier
90 Old Sherman Turnpike   203-797-3500
Danbury, CT 06816-0001   800-621-1115
                                         Fax: 203-797-3197
                                             www.grolier.com
This book discusses the symptoms, prevention, treatments and the
role of the tick. This source will not only help readers become
aware of Lyme Disease, it will help them become informed.
64 pages Grades 5-7
ISBN: 0-531109-31-3

9066 Lyme Disease and Other Pest-Borne Illnesses
Franklin Watts Grolier
90 Old Sherman Turnpike   203-797-3500
Danbury, CT 06816-0001   800-621-1115
                                         Fax: 203-797-3197
                                             www.grolier.com
Scientific, without being technical, this book explains what Lyme
Disease is, symptoms, causes and what a person can do if they con-
tract it.
112 pages Grades 7-12
ISBN: 0-531125-23-8

Magazines

9067 Vector Borne & Zoonotic Diseases
Mary Ann Liebert
140 Huguenot Street   914-740-2100
New Rochelle, NY 10801-1961   800-654-3238
                                         Fax: 914-740-2101
                                     www.liebertpub.com/vbz
Essential multidisiplinary journal dedicated to all aspects of hu-
man diseases that occur as zoonoses or are transmitted by
invertibrate vectors.
Quarterly

Newsletters

9068 Lymelight Newsletter
Lyme Disease Foundation
1 Financial Plaza   860-525-2000
Hartford, CT 06103-2608   800-886-5963
                                                     Fax: 860-525-8425
Newsletter offering up to date information on Lyme Disease and related disorders, Foundation activities, conference and fund-raising information and resources.
4x Year

Pamphlets

9069 Frequently Asked Questions
Lyme Disease Foundation
1 Financial Plaza   860-525-2000
Hartford, CT 06103-2608   800-886-5963
                                                     Fax: 860-525-8425
Overview of testing, treatment, transmission, and pregnancy.

9070 Guide to Lyme Disease
Lyme Disease Foundation
1 Financial Plaza   860-525-2000
Hartford, CT 06103-2608   800-886-5963
                                                     Fax: 860-525-8425
Detailed information about Lyme disease and the LDF.

9071 Guide to Tick Spread Diseases
Lyme Disease Foundation
1 Financial Plaza   860-525-2000
Hartford, CT 06103-2608   800-886-5963
                                                     Fax: 860-525-8425
                                                     www.lyme.org
Symptoms, diagnosis and treatment for a variety of diseases.
16 pages

9072 Guide to Tick-Borne Disorders
Lyme Disease Foundation
1 Financial Plaza   860-525-2000
Hartford, CT 06103-2608   800-886-5963
                                                     Fax: 860-525-8425
Symptoms, diagnosis, and treatment for a variety of diseases.

9073 LD Alert Card
Lyme Disease Foundation
1 Financial Plaza   860-525-2000
Hartford, CT 06103-2608   800-886-5963
                                                     Fax: 860-525-8425
LD symptoms and prevention information.

9074 LD Awareness Packet
Lyme Disease Foundation
1 Financial Plaza   860-525-2000
Hartford, CT 06103-2608   800-886-5963
                                                     Fax: 860-525-8425
Educational letter-size posters, brochures listed above, case counts, Spanish information, insurance problem information, General Diagnostic poster, & more.

9075 Lyme Disease & Pets
Lyme Disease Foundation
1 Financial Plaza   860-525-2000
Hartford, CT 06103-2608   800-886-5963
                                                     Fax: 860-525-8425
                                                     e-mail: lymefna@aol.com
                                                     www.lyme.org
Offers information on Lyme Disease and other tick-borne disorders, through pets and animal transmission.
T Forchaser, Executive Director

9076 Quick Guide to Lyme Disease
American Lyme Disease Foundation
Post Office Box 466   914-277-6970
Lyme, CT 06371   Fax: 914-277-6974
                                                     e-mail: Executivedir@aldf.com
                                                     www.aldf.com

Epidemiology, the cause of the disease, recognizing the symptoms, what to do if you are bitten, treatment, vaccine and other tick-borne diseases are all covered. One free copy, quantity prices vary.
Phillip J. Baker, Executive Director
Robert A. Proctor, Managing Director

9077 Self-Help (S-H) Program
Lyme Disease Foundation
1 Financial Plaza   860-525-2000
Hartford, CT 06103-2608   800-886-5963
                                                     Fax: 860-525-8425
How to establish and conduct a S-H Group. Video, instruction manual, brochure masters, posters, and more.
28 minutes

9078 Understanding Lyme Disease: Entendiendo Lyme Disease
American Lyme Disease Foundation
Post Office Box 466   914-277-6970
Lyme, CT 06371   Fax: 914-277-6974
                                                     e-mail: Executivedir@aldf.com
                                                     www.aldf.com
Only available in Spanish, this brochure is for children ages 10-15 years old. Includes a basic desription of Lyme disease, symptoms, diagnosis, prevention and proper tick removal. One free copy, quantity prices vary.
Phillip J. Baker, Executive Director
Robert A. Proctor, Managing Director

9079 Understanding Ticks and Lyme Disease
American Lyme Disease Foundation
Post Office Box 466   914-277-6970
Lyme, CT 06371   Fax: 914-277-6974
                                                     e-mail: Executivedir@aldf.com
                                                     www.aldf.com
For children 10-15 years old, basic description of Lyme disease, symptoms, diagnosis, prevention and proper tick removal. One free copy, quantity prices vary.
Phillip J. Baker, Executive Director
Robert A. Proctor, Managing Director

Audio & Video

9080 Case of the Great Imitator
American Lyme Disease Foundation
Post Office Box 466   914-277-6970
Lyme, CT 06371   Fax: 914-277-6974
                                                     e-mail: Executivedir@aldf.com
                                                     www.aldf.com
For children ages 9-14 years old. Educational video made in cooperation with the Centers for Disease Control and Prevention.
Phillip J. Baker, Executive Director
Robert A. Proctor, Managing Director

9081 LD: Diagnosis & Treatment
Lyme Disease Foundation
1 Financial Plaza   860-525-2000
Hartford, CT 06103-2608   800-886-5963
                                                     Fax: 860-525-8425
Physicians discuss the challenges of diagnosing and treating LD.
60 minutes

9082 LD: Facts for Kids
Lyme Disease Foundation
1 Financial Plaza   860-525-2000
Hartford, CT 06103-2608   800-886-5963
                                                     Fax: 860-525-8425
Targeted toward kindergarten to fourth grade children, these videos educate youngsters about Lyme Disease and ticks.

9083 Lyme Disease: What You Should Know
Lyme Disease Foundation
1 Financial Plaza   860-525-2000
Hartford, CT 06103-2608   800-886-5963
                                                     Fax: 860-525-8425
Diagnosis, treatment, transmission, prevention, and research. Interviews with patients, doctors, school officials, researchers, and health department officials.
60 minutes

9084 Tick Talk
American Lyme Disease Foundation
Post Office Box 466   914-277-6970
Lyme, CT 06371   Fax: 914-277-6974
                                  e-mail: Executivedir@aldf.com
                                                  www.aldf.com
For children ages 5-8 years old. Educational video made in cooperation with the Centers for Disease Control and Prevention.
Phillip J. Baker, Executive Director
Robert A. Proctor, Managing Director

Web Sites

9085 America's Doctor Online Consulting
                                        www.americasdoctor.com
Provides pharmaceutical and biotech companies and contract research organizations an exclusive source for conducting phase II-IV clinical research.

9086 American Lyme Disease Foundation
                                                  www.aldf.com
Provides a wide range of information, both in English and in Spanish, on the diagnosis, treatment, prevention and control of lyme disease and other tick-borne infections.

9087 CDC Intro to Lyme Disease
                          www.cdc.gov/ncidod/dvbid/lyme/incex.htm
Accurate, evidence based information on symptoms, diagnosis, treatment and prevention of Lyme disease and other tick-borne illnesses. Includes vaccine information, late-braking news, frequently asked questions and related links.

9088 Healing Well
                                               www.healingwell.com
An online health resource guide to medical news, chat, information and articles, newsgroups and message boards, books, disease-related web sites, medical directories, and more for patients, friends, and family coping with disabling diseases, disorders, or chronic illnesses.

9089 Health Finder
                                               www.healthfinder.gov
Searchable, carefully developed web site offering information on over 1000 topics. Developed by the US Department of Health and Human Services, the site can be used in both English and Spanish.

9090 Healthlink USA
                                               www.healthlinkusa.com
Health information concerning treatment, cures, prevention, diagnosis, risk factors, research, support groups, email lists, personal stories and much more. Updated regularly.

9091 Helios Health
                                               www.helioshealth.com
Online resource for your health information. Detailed information about specific health topics, access to expert advice from our Medical Advisory Board, and up-to-date health news.

9092 Lyme Disease Foundation
                                                    www.lyme.org
Provides a wide range of services including information and referral network on Lyme disease.

9093 MGH Neurology WebForums
Provides both unmoderated message board and chat rooms for specific neurological disorders including: amyloidosis, asachnoiditis, cerebellar ataxia, congenital fiber type disproportion, CFS leak, DeMorsiers syndrome, erythomelalgia, Lewy body disease, meningitis, meralgia paresthetic, Norrie disease, periodic paralysis, phantom limb pain, Romber disorder, Syndenhams chorea, tethered cord syndrome, and thoracic outlet syndrome.

9094 MedicineNet
                                               www.medicinenet.com
An online resource for consumers providing easy-to-read, authoritative medical and health information.

9095 Medscape
                                               www.medscape.com

Medscape offers specialists, primary care physicians, and other health professionals the Web's most robust and integrated medical information and educational tools.

9096 Neurology Channel
                                      www.healthcommunities.com
Find clearly explained, medically accurate information regarding conditions, including an overview, symptoms, causes, diagnostic procedures and treatment options. On this site it is possible to ask questions and get information from a neurologist and connect to people who have similar health interests.

9097 Pubmed
                                      www.ncbi.nlm.nih.gov/PubMed
National institutes of Health search engine for published medical and scientific research.

9098 University of Rhode Island Tick Research Laboratory
                                               www.tickencounter.org
The TickEncounter Resource Center promotes tick-bite protection and tickborne disease prevention by engaging, educating, and empowering people to take action.

9099 WebMD
                                                    www.webmd.com
Provides credible information, supportive communities, and in-depth reference material about health subjects. A source for original and timely health information as well as material from well known content providers.

Description

9100 Tourette Syndrome

Tourette syndrome, TS, is a neurological disorder characterized by tics - involuntary, rapid, sudden movements or vocalizations that occur repeatedly in the same way. Onset of the disorder occurs before 18 years of age, and usually before the age of 12. Roughly one person in 2000 will demonstrate this behavior at some time in his life. Boys are 3 or 4 times as likely as girls to develop TS.

Multiple motor and vocal tics can appear separately or simultaneously as part of the syndrome. Tics may occur many times daily, or intermittently, with periodic changes in their number, frequency, type and location. Sometimes they may disappear for weeks.

Over time, symptoms can range from hand jerking and throat clearing in the syndrome's early stages to jumping and vocalizing socially unacceptable phrases. Movements may also occur in combination with each other.

Although the cause of TS is unknown, researchers have identified factors which may be involved in producing the disease. Persons with TS may show subtle abnormalities in the structure of certain parts of the brain. The disease may reflect abnormal metabolism of a neurotransmitter (a chemical that brain cells use to signal one another) called dopamine; drugs affecting dopamine levels may reduce symptoms. Relatives of affected persons have an increased risk of disease, suggesting a genetic component. Finally, in some cases the brain's function may be affected by antibodies triggered by infection with a bacterium called Group A Strep. Children who are not bothered by their tics should not be treated with drugs. Medications are reserved for those whose tics lead to symptoms which impair behavioral, physiologic or social function. Simple tics respond to benzodiazepines (tranquilizers). For more severe cases, haloperidol, an antipsychotic, may be used, but should be started slowly. Unfortunately, it sometimes causes other movement disorders after prolonged use. Whether drug treatment is used or not, patients and their families may need counseling to deal with the disease's secondary effects, which may include bullying at school or conflict within the family. Fortunately, the condition often becomes much less severe, without any treatment, after 10 or 15 years.

National Agencies & Associations

9101 American Academy of Neurology: Tourette Syndrome

201 Chicago Avenue
Minneapolis, MN 55415-2311
800-879-1960
800-879-1960
Fax: 612-454-2746
e-mail: memberservices@aan.com
www.aan.com

A medical specialty society established to advance the art and science of neurology and thereby promote the best possible care for patients wit neurological disorders.
Catherine Rydell, Executive Director

9102 National Institute of Neurological Disorders and Stroke

NIH Neurological Institute
Bethesda, MD 20824
301-496-5751
800-352-9424
Fax: 301-402-2186
TTY: 301-468-5981
www.ninds.nih.gov

The mission of NINDS is to reduce the burden of neurological disease - a burden borne by every age group, by every segment of society, by people all over the world.
Story C Landis PhD, Director
Walter J Koroshetz, Deputy Director

9103 Tourette Syndrome Association

42-40 Bell Boulevard
Bayside, NY 11361
718-224-2999
888-486-8738
Fax: 718-279-9596
e-mail: grantadministrator@tsa-usa.org
www.tsa-usa.org

The only national organization exclusively devoted to the research, diagnosis, education and treatments for persons with Tourette Syndrome.
Judit Ungar, President
Sue Levi-Pearl, VP Meical & Scientific Programs

9104 Tourette Syndrome Foundation of Canada

5945 Airport Rd
Mississauga, Ontario, 1R9-2B7
905-673-2255
800-361-3120
Fax: 800-387-0120
e-mail: tsfc@tourette.ca
www.tourette.ca

National voluntary organization dedicated to improving the quality of life for those with or affected by Tourette Syndrome through programs of education, advocacy, self-help and the promotion of research.
Rosie Wartecker, Executive Director

Research Centers

9105 Tourette Syndrome Clinic Yale Child Study Center

Yale Child Study Center
300 George St.
New Haven, CT 06511
203-785-6396
Fax: 203-785-6196
www.medicine.yale.edu

Clinical care center offering research solely into the causes symptoms and treatments for persons with Tourette Syndrome.
Diane B Findley, Associate Research Scientist and Clinic
Robert King, Medical Director

Support Groups & Hotlines

9106 National Health Information Center

PO Box 1133
Washington, DC 20013
310-565-4167
800-336-4797
Fax: 301-984-4256
e-mail: info@nhic.org
www.health.gov/nhic

Offers a nationwide information referral service, produces directories and resource guides.

Books

9107 Children with Tourette Syndrome

Woodbine House
6510 Bells Mill Road
Bethesda, MD 20817-1636
800-843-7323

This book offers parents information on Tourette Syndrome, causes, symptoms and medications, as well as the other disorders which are commonly linked with it. Other chapters include information on family life, education, advocacy and legal rights.
340 pages Paperback
ISBN: 0-933149-44-1

9108 Children with Tourette Syndrome: A Parent's Guide

Adam Ward Seligman, Echolalia Press

35158 Annapolis Road
Annapolis, CA 95412-9713

707-886-1972
888-766-4233
Fax: 707-547-2199
e-mail: seligman@sonic.net
www.sonic.net/echolaliapress/

It Publishes and Distributes Books, Music and TwoOn-Line Magazines for the Following Healing Communities
Adam Ward Seligman, Publisher and Co-editor
John S Hilkevich, Co-editor

9109 Living with Tourette Syndrome
Simon & Schuster
611 W Bay Street
Tampa, FL 33606-2703   800-999-5479

Provides valuable advice for children and adults with TS, their families, co-workers, teachers and friends. Describes the symptoms and related disorders, exposes many myths surrounding the disease, and advises adults on business and personal relationships.
256 pages
ISBN: 0-684811-60-0

9110 Ryan: A Mother's Story of her TS/ADHD Child
Adam Ward Seligman, Echolalia Press
35158 Annapolis Road
Annapolis, CA 95412-9713

707-886-1972
888-766-4233
Fax: 707-547-2199
e-mail: seligman@sonic.net
www.sonic.net

It Publishes and Distributes Books, Music and TwoOn-Line Magazines for the Following Healing Communities
Softcover
Adam Ward Seligman, Publisher and Co-editor
John S Hilkevich, Co-editor

9111 Teaching the Tiger: An Educator's Guide to TS/OCD/ADHD
Adam Ward Seligman, Echolalia Press
35158 Annapolis Road
Annapolis, CA 95412-9713

707-886-1972
888-766-4233
Fax: 707-547-2199
e-mail: seligman@sonic.net
www.sonic.net

It Publishes and Distributes Books, Music and TwoOn-Line Magazines for the Following Healing Communities
Workbook
Adam Ward Seligman, Publisher and Co-editor
John S Hilkevich, Co-editor

9112 Tourette Syndrome and Human Behavior
Adam Ward Seligman, Echolalia Press
35158 Annapolis Road
Annapolis, CA 95412-9713

707-886-1972
888-766-4233
Fax: 707-547-2199
e-mail: seligman@sonic.net
www.sonic.net

It Publishes and Distributes Books, Music and TwoOn-Line Magazines for the Following Healing Communities
Softcover
Adam Ward Seligman, Publisher and Co-editor
John S Hilkevich, Co-editor

9113 Tourette Syndrome: Advances in Neurology
Tourette Syndrome Association
42-40 Bell Boulevard
Bayside, NY 11361-2861

718-224-2999
888-480-8737
Fax: 718-279-9596
www.tsa-usa.org

In this single-volume reference, more than 90 of the foremost research and clinical leaders in the field review the current state of knowledge about this disorder.
400 pages
Thomas N Chase MD, Editor
Arnold J Friedhoff MD, Editor

9114 What Makes Ryan Tic?
Adam Ward Seligman, Echolalia Press
35158 Annapolis Road
Annapolis, CA 95412-9713

707-886-1972
888-766-4233
Fax: 707-547-2199
e-mail: seligman@sonic.net
www.sonic.net

It Publishes and Distributes Books, Music and TwoOn-Line Magazines for the Following Healing Communities
Softcover
Adam Ward Seligman, Publisher and Co-editor
John S Hilkevich, Co-editor

Children's Books

9115 Adam and the Magic Marble
Adam Ward Seligman, Echolalia Press
35158 Annapolis Road
Annapolis, CA 95412-9713

707-886-1972
888-766-4233
Fax: 707-547-2199
e-mail: seligman@sonic.net
www.sonic.net

It Publishes and Distributes Books, Music and TwoOn-Line Magazines for the Following Healing Communities
Adam Ward Seligman, Publisher and Co-editor
John S Hilkevich, Co-editor

9116 Hi! I'm Adam!
Adam Ward Seligman, Echolalia Press
35158 Annapolis Road
Annapolis, CA 95412-9713

707-886-1972
888-766-4233
Fax: 707-547-2199
e-mail: seligman@sonic.net
www.sonic.net

It Publishes and Distributes Books, Music and TwoOn-Line Magazines for the Following Healing Communities
Adam Ward Seligman, Publisher and Co-editor
John S Hilkevich, Co-editor

9117 Matthew and the Tics
Tourette Syndrome Association
42-40 Bell Boulevard
Bayside, NY 11361-2861

718-224-2999
888-480-8738
Fax: 718-279-9596
www.tsa-usa.org

A story for young children with TS and their peers.
2 pages

Newsletters

9118 Tourette Syndrome Association Newsletter
42-40 Bell Boulevard
Bayside, NY 11361

718-224-2999
888-480-8738
Fax: 718-279-9596
e-mail: ts@tsa-usa.org
www.tsa-usa.org

Offers information, articles and news on the latest technology and advancements for persons with Tourette Syndrome.
Quarterly

Pamphlets

9119 Commentary on Alternative Therapies for TS
Tourette Syndrome Association
42-40 Bell Boulevard
Bayside, NY 11361-2861

718-224-2999
888-480-8738
Fax: 718-279-9596
www.tsa-usa.org

Summarizes physician/patient reports of symptom management through non-pharmacological interventions.
2 pages

9120 Consumer's Guide to TS Medications
Tourette Syndrome Association
42-40 Bell Boulevard
Bayside, NY 11361-2861

718-224-2999
888-480-8738
Fax: 718-279-9596
www.tsa-usa.org

Covers common medications used for the control of TS motor and vocal ties as well as those traditionally prescribed for associated behaviors.
1992 12 pages

9121 Coping with TS in the Classroom
Tourette Syndrome Association
42-40 Bell Boulevard   718-224-2999
Bayside, NY 11361-2820   Fax: 718-279-9596
www.tsa-usa.org
Includes practical guidelines for education developed from a study
about cognitive effects on learning.
18 pages

9122 Coping with TS, A Parent's Viewpoint
Tourette Syndrome Association
42-40 Bell Boulevard   718-224-2999
Bayside, NY 11361-2861   888-480-8738
Fax: 718-279-9596
www.tsa-usa.org
An accalaimed medical writer and mother of three children with
TS, the author sensitively addresses common concerns and feel-
ings of parents.
1994 23 pages

9123 Coping with Tourette Syndrome in Early Adulthood
Tourette Syndrome Association
42-40 Bell Boulevard   718-224-2999
Bayside, NY 11361-2861   888-480-8738
Fax: 718-279-9596
www.tsa-usa.org
Focuses on two fundamental challenges facing adults with TS: employment and interpersonal relationships. Provides specific techniques for overcoming barriers.

9124 Current Pharmacology of TS
Tourette Syndrome Association
42-40 Bell Boulevard   718-224-2999
Bayside, NY 11361-2861   888-480-8738
Fax: 718-279-9596
www.tsa-usa.org
Covers all current medications used to treat TS with specific information about clinical evaluations and diagnosis.
12 pages

9125 Dental Treatment of Patients with Gilles de la Tourette Syndrome
Tourette Syndrome Association
42-40 Bell Boulevard   718-224-2999
Bayside, NY 11361-2861   888-480-8738
Fax: 718-279-9596
www.tsa-usa.org
Discusses TS movements and possible adverse interactions of dentistry and TS medications.
5 pages

9126 Development of Behavioral and Emotional Problems in TS
Tourette Syndrome Association
42-40 Bell Boulevard   718-224-2999
Bayside, NY 11361-2861   888-480-8738
Fax: 718-279-9596
www.tsa-usa.org
Using the Child Behavior Checklist, 78 male children were as-
sessed for a variety of behavioral problems. Relation to tic severity
covered.
1989 3 pages

9127 Discipline and the Child with TS
Tourette Syndrome Association
42-40 Bell Boulevard   718-224-2999
Bayside, NY 11361   888-480-8738
Fax: 718-279-9596
www.tsa-usa.org
Helps children redirect impulses and compulsions through teaching cause and effect relationships.
15 pages

9128 Educator's Guide to Tourette Syndrome
Tourette Syndrome Association
42-40 Bell Boulevard   718-224-2999
Bayside, NY 11361-2861   888-480-8738
Fax: 718-279-9596
www.tsa-usa.org
Covers symptoms, treatments and techniques for classroom management, attentional, writing and language problems.
16 pages

**9129 Genetics of Tourette's Syndrome: Who it Affects and How it
Occurs in Families**
Tourette Syndrome Association
42-40 Bell Boulevard   718-224-2999
Bayside, NY 11361-2861   888-480-8738
Fax: 718-279-9596
www.tsa-usa.org
TSA, founded in 1972, is dedicated to education, service, and research to identify the cause of, find the cure for, and control the effects of Tourette Syndrome
10 pages

9130 Getting Into College: Strategies for the Student with TS
Tourette Syndrome Association
42-40 Bell Boulevard   718-224-2999
Bayside, NY 11361   888-480-8738
Fax: 718-279-9596
www.tsa-usa.org
TSA, founded in 1972, is dedicated to education, service, and research to identify the cause of, find the cure for, and control the effects of Tourette Syndrome
10 pages

9131 Gift of Hope
Tourette Syndrome Association
42-40 Bell Boulevard   718-224-2999
Bayside, NY 11361-2861   888-480-8738
Fax: 718-279-9596
www.tsa-usa.org
TSA Brain Bank Program registration information. Includes donor
cards.

9132 Grandparents Club
Tourette Syndrome Association
42-40 Bell Boulevard   718-224-2999
Bayside, NY 11361-2861   888-480-8738
Fax: 718-279-9596
www.tsa-usa.org
A flyer describing how to join with other grandparents to support
TS research to benefit future generations.

9133 Guide to Diagnosis & Treatment
Tourette Syndrome Association
42-40 Bell Boulevard   718-224-2999
Bayside, NY 11361-2861   888-480-8738
Fax: 718-279-9596
www.tsa-usa.org
Covers symptoms, pharmacology and clinical assessments.
30 pages

9134 Guide to Housing for Adults with TS
Tourette Syndrome Association
42-40 Bell Boulevard   718-224-2999
Bayside, NY 11361-2861   888-480-8738
Fax: 718-279-9596
www.tsa-usa.org
A guide to finding housing, housing laws that help people with TS
and ways to maximize living environments.
1991 16 pages

9135 Health Insurance & Tourette Syndrome
Tourette Syndrome Association
42-40 Bell Boulevard   718-224-2999
Bayside, NY 11361-2861   888-480-8738
Fax: 718-279-9596
www.tsa-usa.org
Detailed, up-to-date packet of medical information for obtaining
health insurance as well as information for submission to insurance carriers.

9136 Helpful Techniques to Aid the Student with TS
Tourette Syndrome Association
42-40 Bell Boulevard   718-224-2999
Bayside, NY 11361-2861   888-480-8738
Fax: 718-279-9596
www.tsa-usa.org
Helpful hints for teacher with specific suggestions for test taking,
math computation, and note taking.
1 pages

9137 Learning Problems & the Child with TS
Tourette Syndrome Association
42-40 Bell Boulevard   718-224-2999
Bayside, NY 11361-2861   888-480-8738
Fax: 718-279-9596
www.tsa-usa.org
Report on learning problems identified through a study of 200 children with TS.
1 pages

9138 Need to Know
Tourette Syndrome Association
42-40 Bell Boulevard   718-224-2999
Bayside, NY 11361-2861   888-480-8738
Fax: 718-279-9596
www.tsa-usa.org
Recollections of a young woman who was diagnosed with TS in her 20s.
4 pages

9139 Neuropsychological Performance in Adults with TS
Tourette Syndrome Association
42-40 Bell Boulevard   718-224-2999
Bayside, NY 11361-2861   888-480-8738
Fax: 718-279-9596
www.tsa-usa.org
Describes clinical and neuropsychological testing on learning and memory with TS adults.
7 pages

9140 Peer Problems in Tourette's Disorder
Tourette Syndrome Association
42-40 Bell Boulevard   718-224-2999
Bayside, NY 11361-2861   888-480-8738
Fax: 718-279-9596
www.tsa-usa.org
Detailed research findings of peer problems in children with TS. Includes statistical results obtained from these studies.
1991 7 pages

9141 Pharmacotherapy of TS and Associated Disorders
Tourette Syndrome Association
42-40 Bell Boulevard   718-224-2999
Bayside, NY 11361-2861   888-480-8738
Fax: 718-279-9596
www.tsa-usa.org
Overview with emphasis on the complexities of prescribing TS medications.
19 pages

9142 Problem Behaviors & TS
Tourette Syndrome Association
42-40 Bell Boulevard   718-224-2999
Bayside, NY 11361-2861   888-480-8738
Fax: 718-279-9596
www.tsa-usa.org
Describes recent research and what is now known about the relationship of a variety of behaviors and TS.
21 pages

9143 Recognizing TS in the Classroom
Tourette Syndrome Association
42-40 Bell Boulevard   718-224-2999
Bayside, NY 11361-2861   888-480-8738
Fax: 718-279-9596
www.tsa-usa.org
Provides an overview offering detailed symptoms checklist, post-diagnosis advice and covers special education needs.
4 pages

9144 Risperidone as a Treatment for TS
Tourette Syndrome Association
42-40 Bell Boulevard   718-224-2999
Bayside, NY 11361-2861   888-480-8738
Fax: 718-279-9596
www.tsa-usa.org
TSA, founded in 1972, is dedicated to education, service, and research to identify the cause of, find the cure for, and control the effects of Tourette Syndrome
6 pages

9145 Specific Classroom Strategies and Techniques for Students with TS
Tourette Syndrome Association
42-40 Bell Boulevard   718-224-2999
Bayside, NY 11361-2861   888-480-8738
Fax: 718-279-9596
www.tsa-usa.org
An educator with TS spells out concrete methods for managing students with TS. She outlines many valuable classroom interventions to help youngsters deal with tic symptons, ADHD, visual motor and fine motor integration, and behavioral difficulties.
1994 2 pages

9146 TS and Other Tic Disorders
Tourette Syndrome Association
42-40 Bell Boulevard   718-224-2999
Bayside, NY 11361-2861   888-480-8738
Fax: 718-279-9596
www.tsa-usa.org
Comprehensive overview of the complexities of TS. Includes tic syndrome classifications, epidemiology, genetics, behavioral aspects, and summary.
17 pages

9147 TS and the School Nurse
Tourette Syndrome Association
42-40 Bell Boulevard   718-224-2999
Bayside, NY 11361-2861   888-480-8738
Fax: 718-279-9596
www.tsa-usa.org
Comprehensive professional guide to educational, social and medical implications.
19 pages

9148 TS and the School Psychologist
Tourette Syndrome Association
42-40 Bell Boulevard   718-224-2999
Bayside, NY 11361-2861   888-480-8738
Fax: 718-279-9596
www.tsa-usa.org
The role of the school psychologist is covered including testing procedures, counseling strategies and social implications.
1993 (rev.) 14 pages

9149 TS: A Look at the Interface Between TS & the Law
Tourette Syndrome Association
42-40 Bell Boulevard   718-224-2999
Bayside, NY 11361-2861   888-480-8738
Fax: 718-279-9596
www.tsa-usa.org
Summarizes important legislation protecting the rights of students with TS. Also covers resources and hints about how to prepare for dealing successfully with educators and school systems.
1 pages

9150 TSA Medical Letters
Tourette Syndrome Association
42-40 Bell Boulevard   718-224-2999
Bayside, NY 11361-2861   888-480-8738
Fax: 718-279-9596
www.tsa-usa.org
Annual publication of TSA's Medical Committe covering recent, significant findings from scientific articles.
16 pages

9151 Teens and Tourette Syndrome
Tourette Syndrome Association
42-40 Bell Boulevard   718-224-2999
Bayside, NY 11361-2820   Fax: 718-279-9596
e-mail: ts@tsa-usa.org
www.tsa-usa.org
Covers self esteem, friends, dating, drugs and alcohol, stress, depression, academic and vocational planning, sibling relationships and medication.
16 pages

9152 Tourette Syndrome and the School Nurse
Tourette Syndrome Association

42-40 Bell Boulevard
Bayside, NY 11361-2820

718-224-2999
Fax: 718-279-9596
e-mail: ts@tsa-usa.org
www.tsa-usa.org

Includes symptoms, epidemiology, associated beviors, developmental consequences, causes, treatments, role of the school nurse and additional resources.
20 pages

9153 Tourette: The Man and His Times
Tourette Syndrome Association
42-40 Bell Boulevard
Bayside, NY 11361-2861

718-224-2999
888-480-8738
Fax: 718-279-9596
www.tsa-usa.org

Rare historical biography of the famous French neurologist G. Gilles De La Tourette.
9 pages

9154 What School Bus Drivers Need to Know About Students with Tourette Syndrome
Tourette Syndrome Association
42-40 Bell Boulevard
Bayside, NY 11361-2820

718-224-2999
Fax: 718-279-9596
e-mail: ts@tsa-usa.org
www.tsa-usa.org

Includes a description of the disorder, as well as related disorders and suggestions as to what school bus drivers can do for students with TS.
1 pages

Audio & Video

9155 A Regular Kid That's Me: Inservice Film for Educators
Tourette Syndrome Association
42-40 Bell Boulevard
Bayside, NY 11361

718-224-2999
888-480-8738
Fax: 718-279-9596
e-mail: ts@tsa-usa.org
www.tsa-usa.org

Nineteen students with TS (ages 7-17) along with several educators are seen interacting in classroom settings. Includes the basic criteria for diagnosis, discussions of common associated behaviors, e.g. ADD with or without hyperactivity, obsessive compulsive symptoms and specific learning disabilities. Professionals describe the impact of having TS on educational placement and specific classroom strategies are presented. 45 minutes. May be purchased as part of a curriculum or separately. #AV-2
VHS 1/2 inch

9156 After the Diagnosis...the Next Steps
42-40 Bell Boulevard
Bayside, NY 11361

718-224-2999
888-480-8738
Fax: 718-279-9596
e-mail: ts@tsa-usa.org
www.tsa-usa.org

When the diagnosis is Tourette Syndrome, what do you do first? How do you sort out the complexities of the disorder? Whose advice do you follow? What steps do you take to lead a normal life? Six people with TS—as different as any six people can be—relate the sometimes difficult, but finally triumphant path each took to lead the rich, fulfilling life they now enjoy. Narrated by Academy Award-winning actor, Richard Dreyfuss, the stories are blends of poignancy, fact and inspiration.

9157 Clinical Counseling: Towards a Better Understanding of TS
Tourette Syndrome Association
42-40 Bell Boulevard
Bayside, NY 11361

718-224-2999
888-480-8738
Fax: 718-279-9596
e-mail: ts@tsa-usa.org
www.tsa-usa.org

Targeted to counselors, social workers, educators, psychologists and families, this video features expert physicians, allied professionals and several families summarizing key issues that can arise when counseling families with TS. 15 minutes. #AV-10A

9158 Complexities of TS Treatment: A Physician's Round Table
Tourette Syndrome Association

42-40 Bell Boulevard
Bayside, NY 11361

718-224-2999
888-480-8738
Fax: 718-279-9596
e-mail: ts@tsa-usa.org

Three internationally recognized TS experts provide colleagues with valuable information about the complexities of treating and advising families with TS. Emphasis is on different clinical approaches to patients with a broad range of symptom severity. Co-morbid and associated conditions are covered. 15 minutes. #AV-10

9159 Educator's In-Service Program
Tourette Syndrome Association
42-40 Bell Boulevard
Bayside, NY 11361

718-224-2999
888-480-8738
Fax: 718-279-9596

A curriculum designed to train educators to recognize and understand TS and guide students with TS and associated disorders in a classroom setting. Developed by the Tourette Syndrome Association for the training of all educational personnel. Includes 2 videos, a particpant's guide, a set of 20 transparencies, 2 scripted curriculum modules and a comprehensive teacher's guide. Discounted for members.

9160 Gift of Hope
Tourette Syndrome Association
42-40 Bell Boulevard
Bayside, NY 11361

718-224-2999
888-480-8738
Fax: 718-279-9596
e-mail: ts@tsa-usa.org
www.tsa-usa.org

The cause of TS lies in the brain. Because their are no animal models to study this disorder, human brain tissue is of vital importance for progress in research. Increased brain bank registration is a prime objective of the TSA. VHS 1/2 inch. 14 minutes. Available for shipping cost only. #AV- 7

9161 Guide to Diagnosis
Tourette Syndrome Association
42-40 Bell Boulevard
Bayside, NY 11361-2861

718-224-2999
888-480-8738
Fax: 718-279-9596
www.tsa-usa.org

A video and companion guide for interested medical professionals who have not seen a substantial number of TS patients.
30 minutes

9162 I'm a Person Too
Tourette Syndrome Association
42-40 Bell Boulevard
Bayside, NY 11361

718-224-2999
888-480-8738
Fax: 718-279-9596
e-mail: ts@tsa-usa.org
www.tsa-usa.org

Narrated by Cliff Robertson, this video features 5 people with TS; 2 elementary school students and 3 adults from diverse social backgrounds. They talk about a broad variety of symptoms and their personal experiences living with the disorder. VHS 1/2 inch. 22 minutes. #AV1

9163 Panel of Experts
Tourette Syndrome Association
42-40 Bell Boulevard
Bayside, NY 11361-2861

718-224-2999
888-480-8738
Fax: 718-279-9596
www.tsa-usa.org

Five leading authorities bring their in-depth knowledge and experience to bear in a wide-ranging discussion that covers current strategies in TS diagnosis, and medication.
30 minutes

9164 Parent's Perspective: Diplomacy in Action
Tourette Syndrome Association
42-40 Bell Boulevard
Bayside, NY 11361-2861

718-224-2999
888-480-8738
Fax: 718-279-9596
www.tsa-usa.org

The child with TS faces a set of special problems in school. The level of achievement reached in large measure is dependent on the attitude of teachers and administrators. Therefore, educating the educators becomes a high priority with the parent.
45 minutes

9165   Stop It!... I Can't!
Tourette Syndrome Association
42-40 Bell Boulevard
Bayside, NY 11361

718-224-2999
888-480-8738
Fax: 718-279-9596
e-mail: ts@tsa-usa.org
www.tsa-usa.org

Narrated by William Shatner, this video promotes sensitivity, education, acceptance and confidence for children with TS. Produced in the 1970's, but provides a valuable and classic message. VHS 1/2 inch. 13 minutes.

9166   TS-The Parent's Perspective: Diplomacy in Action
Tourette Syndrome Association
42-40 Bell Boulevard
Bayside, NY 11361

718-224-2999
888-480-8738
Fax: 718-279-9596
e-mail: ts@tsa-usa.org
www.tsa-usa.org

The child with TS faces a set of special problems in school. The level of achievement reached in large measure is dependent on the attitude of teachers and administrators. Therefore educating the educators becomes a high priority for the parent. Special education professionals provide firm guidance to famillies on school advocacy issues. Concrete suggestions are offered to smooth the road to success in school for the student with TS. VHS 1/2 inch. 45 minutes. #AV-6

9167   TS: A Panel of Experts
Tourette Syndrome Association
42-40 Bell Boulevard
Bayside, NY 11361

718-224-2999
888-480-8738
Fax: 718-279-9596
e-mail: ts@tsa-usa.org
www.tsa-usa.org

Five leading authorities bring their in-depth knowledge and experience to bear in a wide-ranging discussion that covers current strategies in TS diagnosis and medication, behavioral problems, predicted course and other aspects of this disorder. VHS 1/2 inch. 30 minutes. # AV-5

9168   Talking About Tourette Syndrome
Tourette Syndrome Association
42-40 Bell Boulevard
Bayside, NY 11361

718-224-2999
888-480-8738
Fax: 718-279-9596
e-mail: ts@tsa-usa.org
www.tsa-usa.org

When the professional is also the patient, a unique perspective emerges. A psychiatrist leads a candid probing discussion with a brother and sister- all have Tourette syndrome. This free-wheeling exchange brings to the viewer many instructive and often surprising observations about TS and obsessive compulsive symptoms. VHS 1/2 inch. 45 minutes. #AV-8

9169   Tourette Syndrome: Guide to Diagnosis
Tourette Syndrome Association
42-40 Bell Boulevard
Bayside, NY 11361

718-224-2999
888-480-8738
Fax: 718-279-9596
e-mail: ts@tsa-usa.org
www.tsa-usa.org

Video for interested medical professionals who have not seen substantial numbers of TS patients. Presents 7 patients with TS who exhibit the full range of movements, vocalizations and behavioral patterns associated with the disorder. Descriptions and demonstrations of other movement disorders are also presented for the purpose of differential diagnosis. VHS 1/2 inch. 30 minutes. A 29 page companion piece by Drs. Ruth Brunn, Donald Cohen and James Leckman is available at $6.00/3.50 shipping.#AV4

9170   Family Life with Tourette Syndrome... Personal Stories: Professor Peter
Tourette Syndrome Association

42-40 Bell Boulevard
Bayside, NY 11361

718-224-2999
888-480-8738
Fax: 718-279-9596
e-mail: ts@tsa-usa.org
tsa-usa.org

Now a world class scientific research expert and a professor of biology at Harvard and Purdue, Professor Hollenbeck talks about growing up positively with TS, never hesitating to have children, and offering good advice for newly diagnosed families. 7 minutes, 27 seconds. If purchased together, the six videos in this series are $50.00. #AV-11A

9171   Family Life with Tourette Syndrome... Personal Stories: Reverend Mike
Tourette Syndrome Association
42-40 Bell Boulevard
Bayside, NY 11361

718-224-2999
888-480-8738
Fax: 718-279-9596
e-mail: ts@tsa-usa.org
tsa-usa.org

Mike Higgins did not receive a diagnosis of TS until he was in the army! Mike overcame significant symptoms and childhood teasing. Reverend Mike talks about the value of strong family life, faith, support groups and acceptance of the person, and not the disorder as a good way to live positively with TS. If purchased together, the six videos in this series are $50.00. #AV-11B

9172   Family Life with Tourette Syndrome... Personal Stories: Rachel
Tourette Syndrome Association
42-40 Bell Boulevard
Bayside, NY 11361

718-224-2999
888-480-8738
Fax: 718-279-9596
e-mail: ts@tsa-usa.org
www.tsa-usa.org

Challenged by TS, ADHD and OCD Rachel and her family endured difficult reactions, behavioral episodes, and at times, a great loss of hope. Now seventeen years old, Rachel and family overcame stresses and strains by sticking together through the highs and lows to find Rachel today a confident and happy teen. 10 minutes. If purchased together, the six videos in this series are $50.00. #AV-11C

9173   Family Life with Tourette Syndrome... Personal Stories: The Turners
Tourette Syndrome Association
42-40 Bell Boulevard
Bayside, NY 11361

718-224-2999
888-480-8738
Fax: 718-279-9596
www.tsa-usa.org

Three of the four Turner daughters have TS in varying degrees. The family wondered how their symptoms came to be, how to dispense attention fairly, what to say to teachers and friends. They learned how to deal with sibling issues and low self esteem among the sisters. This determined family never gave up! 12 minutes. If purchased together, the six videos in this series are $50.00.#AV-11D

9174   Family Life with Tourette Syndrome... Personal Stories: Ryan
Tourette Syndrome Association
42-40 Bell Boulevard
Bayside, NY 11361

718-224-2999
888-480-8738
Fax: 718-279-9596
e-mail: ts@tsa-usa.org
www.tsa-usa.org

Ryan's family first thought his behavior was a deliberate way to get attention. A school principal was harshly critical. The family soon learned to educate themselves and others about Ryan's TS. Things turned around as a result. A good teacher took a great interest, friends began to seek him out and Ryan grew into a young man with a positive outlook. 11 minutes, 28 seconds. If purchased together, the six videos in this series are $50.00. #AV-11E

9175   Family Life with Tourette Syndrome... Personal Stories: Dakota
Tourette Syndrome Association
42-40 Bell Boulevard
Bayside, NY 11361

718-224-2999
888-480-8738
Fax: 718-279-9596
e-mail: ts@tsa-usa.org
www.tsa-usa.org

A happy 11 year old baseball playing, video game whiz, Dakota was initially diagnosed as having a brain tumor! He was actually affected by TS and AHD. This is a story of a child who developed a strong confidence and a good attitude, learning to believe in himself. He says the love of his grandparents was a special help! 7 minutes, 12 seconds. If purchased together, the 6 videos in this series are $50.00. #AV-11F

Web Sites

9176 American Academy of Neurology: Tourette Syndrome

www.aan.com

The American Academy of Neurology (AAN) is a worldwide professional association of more than 17,000 neurologists and neuroscience professionals dedicating to providing the best possible care for patients with neurological disorders.

9177 Healing Well

www.healingwell.com

An online health resource guide to medical news, chat, information and articles, newsgroups and message boards, books, disease-related web sites, medical directories, and more for patients, friends, and family coping with disabling diseases, disorders, or chronic illnesses.

9178 Health Finder

www.healthfinder.gov

Searchable, carefully developed web site offering information on over 1000 topics. Developed by the US Department of Health and Human Services, the site can be used in both English and Spanish.

9179 Healthlink USA

www.healthlinkusa.com

Health information concerning treatment, cures, prevention, diagnosis, risk factors, research, support groups, email lists, personal stories and much more. Updated regularly.

9180 Helios Health

www.helioshealth.com

Online resource for your health information. Detailed information about specific health topics, access to expert advice from our Medical Advisory Board, and up-to-date health news.

9181 MedicineNet

www.medicinenet.com

An online resource for consumers providing easy-to-read, authoritative medical and health information.

9182 Medscape

www.medscape.com

Medscape offers specialists, primary care physicians, and other health professionals the Web's most robust and integrated medical information and educational tools.

9183 National Institute of Neurological Disorders and Stroke

www.ninds.nih.gov

The mission of NINDS is to seek fundamental knowledge about the brain and nervous system and to use that knowledge to reduce the burden of neurological disease.

9184 WebMD

www.webmd.com

Provides credible information, supportive communities, and in-depth reference material about health subjects. A source for original and timely health information as well as material from well known content providers.

Description

9185 Transplant-Related Conditions

In recent decades, transplantation of solid organs (heart, liver, lung, kidney), bone marrow and stem cells has become an established part of medical care for advanced diseases in many patients who otherwise face end-organ failure and poor prognosis. While on one hand, transplantation may serve to cure the underlying disease it nonetheless often entails chronic medical therapy that will likely include the use of immunosuppressants, complications from chronic medications, frequent and long-term medical follow-up and diagnostic testing which may be invasive.

A number of clinical management protocols are utilized in the care of post-transplantation patient, and these vary depending on the type of transplant undertaken, the extent of the tissue match between donor and recipient, and the experience of the given transplantation center. In general however, most patients who receive a transplanted organ or cells will require some chronic therapy (short or long-term) with immunosuppressive medications. These can be several or many and are given in an effort to control the patient's own immunologic response to receiving an organ or cells from another person. The body's natural response after recognizing such an exposure is to "fight" these cells and tissues with its own defense cells, which are designed to attack and kill foreign material. The immunosuppressive medications help modulate this response so that the transplanted organ is not damaged, injured or "rejected" by the recipient who needs the organ or cells to function in a healthier manner. Immunosuppressive therapy and protection of the transplanted organ must be balanced against the adverse creation of an immunocompromised state in the patient placing him at greater risk for contracting infections that can be serious and even life threatening. Given these circumstances, transplant patients require close working relationships with their medical team along with a true commitment to be compliant with these potentially difficult and complicated medical regimens.

In addition to the medical therapy for patients who have received transplants, one must also consider the significant psychological and social aspects of having undergone such procedures. Strong social support systems and close attention to a healthy emotional and psychological status are important for successful management of these patients. Many transplant centers have extensive support services available to patients from which they and their families can benefit.

National Agencies & Associations

9186 American Society of Transplantation (AST)
15000 Commerce Parkway
Mount Laurel, NJ 08054
856-439-9986
Fax: 856-439-9982
e-mail: ast@ahint.com
www.a-s-t.org
The American Society of Transplantation is an international organization of transplant professionals dedicated to advancing the field of transplantation through the promotion of research education advocacy and organ donation to improve patient care.
Libby McDannell, CAE, Executive Director
Susan J Nelson, Executive Vice President

9187 Association of Organ Procurement Organizations (AOPO)
8500 Leesburg Pike
Vienna, VA 22182
703-556-4242
Fax: 703-556-4852
e-mail: aopo@aopo.org
www.aopo.org
Organization involved in helping people find and obtain the organs they need for transplantation.
Ellingÿ Eidbo, Executive Director
Sue Dunn, President/CEO

9188 Children's Organ Transplant Association (COTA)
2501 COTA Drive
Bloomington, IN 47403
700-366-2682
800-366-2682
Fax: 812-336-8885
e-mail: cota@cota.org
www.cota.org
Not-for-profit national chairty dedicated to helping families and communities raise the necessary funds for transplant expenses.
Rick Lofgren, President/CEO
Lisa Fulkerson, VP/CFO

9189 Donate Life America
700 N Fourth Street
Richmond, VA 23219
804-782-4920
Fax: 804-782-4643
e-mail: coalition@donatelife.net
www.donatelife.net
A not-for-profit alliance of national organizations and local coalitions across the United States that have joined forces to educate the public about organ, eye and tissue donation, correcting misconceptions about donation and creating a greater willingness to donate.
Sara Pace Jones, Chairwoman
Bruce Wilson, Director of Organ Procurement

9190 Health Resources and Services Administration (HRSA)
5600 Fishers Lane
Rockville, MD 20857
301-443-7577
e-mail: comments@hrsa.gov
www.hrsa.gov
Envisions optimal health for all, supported by a health care system that assures access to comprehensive, culturally competant, quality care. Provides national leadership, program resources and services needed to improve access to culturally competant, quality health care.
Elizabeth M Duke PhD, Administrator
Dennis P Williams PhD MA, Deputy Administrator

9191 Jewish Hospital Transplant Center
200 Abraham Flexner Way
Louisville, KY 40202
502-587-4011
www.jewishhospital.com
An elite group approved to perform five solid organ transplants and has been named a Federally Designated Medicare Heart Lung Kidney Liver and Pancreas Transplant Center.
Robert L Shircliff, President/CEO
Barbara Mackovic, Senior Manager

9192 National Foundation for Transplants
5350 Poplar Avenue
Memphis, TN 38119
901-684-1697
800-489-3863
Fax: 901-684-1128
e-mail: info@transplants.org
www.transplants.org
Mission is to reach out to help those who seek a new life through transplantation by providing healthcare and financial support services and patient advocacy for transplant candidates families nationwide.
Jackie D Hancock, President
Connie Gonitzke, Vice President

9193 National Institute of Allergy and Infectious Diseases (NIAID)
6610 Rockledge Drive
Bethesda, MD 20892-6612
301-496-2263
Fax: 301-402-0120
www.niaid.nih.gov
Conducts and supports basic and applied research to better understand, treat, and ultimately prevent infectious, immunologic and allergic diseases. Research has led to new therapies, vaccines, di-

agnostic tests, and other technologies that have improved the health of millions of people in the United States and around the world.
Anthony S. Fauci, Director

9194   National Transplant Assistance Fund (NTAF)
150 N. Radnor Chester Rd.   800-642-8399
Radnor, PA 19087   800-642-8399
Fax: 610-353-6106
e-mail: ntaf@transplantfund.org
www.transplantfund.org
Helps to raise funds for transplant and catastrophic injury patients by providing compassionate support education and expertise to them their families and communities.
Lynne Coughl Samson, Executive Director
Fred Kauffman, Managing Director

9195   Organ Procurement and Transplantation Network (OPTN)
700 N 4th Street   804-782-4800
Richmond, VA 23219   888-TXI-NFO1
Fax: 804-782-4994
www.optn.org
A unified transplant network established by the United States Congress under the National Organ Transplant Act (NOTA) of 1984. A unique public-private partnership that links all of the professionals involved in the donation and transplantation system.
Kenneth Andreoni, MD
Carl Berg, Vice President

9196   United Network for Organ Sharing (UNOS)
700 N 4th Street   804-782-4800
Richmond, VA 23219   Fax: 804-782-4817
www.unos.org
Non-profit scientific and educational organization that administers the nation's only Organ Procurement and Transplantation Network (OPTN). Mission is to advance organ availability and transplantation by uniting and supporting our communities.
Walter K Graham, Executive Director
Marcia D Manning, Director of Community Affairs

9197   United Organ Transplant Association (UOTA)
3405 Arlington Avenue
Riverside, CA 92506   e-mail: pres@uota.org
www.uota.org
Non-profit charitable corporation dedicated to providing educational emotional and financial support to pre- and post- transplant patients.
Don Goss, Founder

State Agencies & Associations

Alabama

9198   Alabama Organ Center
500 S 22 Street S
Birmingham, AL 35233   205-731-9200
800-252-3677
Fax: 205-731-9250
e-mail: Rebecca.davis@ccc.uab.edu
alabamaorgancenter.org
A non-profit, independent organ procurement organization (OPO) serving the population of the Southeastern United States.
Devin E Eckhoff, Director
R Alan Hicks MPH CPTC, Associate Director

Arizona

9199   Donor Network of Arizona
201 W Coolidge
Phoenix, AZ 85013   602-222-2200
800-94D-ONOR
Fax: 602-222-2202
e-mail: Contact.Us@dnaz.org
www.dnaz.org
Participates in the equitable distribution of organs, tissues, and corneas for transplant. Also offers donor family support services, community and health care education, and presentations.
Sara Pace Jones, Public Education Contact
Tim Brown, Chief executive officer

Arkansas

9200   Arkansas Regional Organ Recovery Agency
1701 Aldersgate Road   501-907-9150
Little Rock, AR 72205   800-727-6726
Fax: 501-372-6279
e-mail: info@arora.org
www.arora.org
Makes every effort to provide organs and tissues for life-saving and life-enhancing transplantation. Goal will be accomplished through continuous hospital involvement which includes hospital training community involvement andpublic education.
Audrey Brown, Director of Community Education
Boyd Ward, Executive Director

California

9201   California Transplant Donor Network
1000 Broadway   888-570-9400
Oakland, CA 94607   888-570-9400
Fax: 510-444-8501
e-mail: info@ctdn.org
www.ctdn.org
Helps patients in Northern and Central California and Northern Nevada receive organ and tissue transplants. Recovers organs from donors and matches them with the more than 6 000 people who are currently waiting for transplants in this region.
Cynthia Siljestrom, Chief Executive Officer
Sonia Salloum, Community Outreach Coordinator

9202   Golden State Donor Services
1760 Creekside Oaks Drive   916-567-1600
Sacramento, CA 95833   877-401-2546
Fax: 916-567-8300
e-mail: info@gsds.org
www.gsds.org
Support, enhance, and provide for the recovery and allocation of anatomical gifts. Also work to educate the public regarding the critical need for organ and tissue doors.
Katherine Doolittle, Senior Public Education Coordinator
Helen Nelson, Executive Director

9203   LifeSharing Community Organ & Tissue Donation
3465 Camino Del Rio S   619-521-1983
San Diego, CA 92108   Fax: 619-521-2833
e-mail: info@lifesharing.org
www.lifesharing.org
Non-profit unique and creative organ procurement organization that has centers at the University of California at San Diego Medical Center, Green Hospital of Scripps Clinic, Sharp Hospital.
Sharie Shipley, Public Education Contact
Bill Dawson, Chairman of Volunteer Action Committee

9204   One Legacy Transplant Donor Network
221 S Figueroa Street   213-229-5600
Los Angeles, CA 90012   800-786-4077
Fax: 213-229-5601
e-mail: tmone@onelegacy.org
www.onelegacy.org
One Legacy is dedicaated to achieving the donation of life saving and life enhancing organs and tissues for those in need of transplants and to providing a sense of purpose and comfort to those families we serve.
Sandra Walla Blaydow, Human Resources Manager
Thomas Mone, Chief Executive Officer/EVP

Colorado

9205   Donor Alliance
720 S Colorado Boulevard   303-329-4747
Denver, CO 80246   888-868-4747
Fax: 303-321-0366
www.donoralliance.org
In cooperation with others Donor Alliance facilitates the donation and recovery of organs and tissues for people needing transplantation. Donor Alliance is one of 58 not-for-profit organ recovery organizations federally designated by the U.S..
Jennifer Moe, Director of Community Relations/PR
Nancy Williams, Chairman

Connecticut

9206   NorthEast Organ Procurement Organization
80 Seymour Street   860-545-5000
Hartford, CT 06102-5037   Fax: 860-545-5066
www.harthosp.org/NEOPO/index.html
Assures that comprehensive organ and tissue donation services are provided to the community in an efficient and professional manner.
Ginger Van Nostrand, Public Education Contact

Florida

9207   LifeLink of Florida
409 Bayshore Boulevard   813-253-2640
Tampa, FL 33606   800-262-5775
Fax: 813-348-0634
e-mail: info@lifelinkfound.org
www.lifelinkfound.org
Independent, nonprofit community service organization dedicated to the recovery and transplantation of organs and tissues. Operates under the authority of the Social Security Act, and in accordance with the National Organ Transplant Act passed by Congress.
Dennis F Heinrichs, President
Dana L Shires Jr, Chairman of the Board

9208   LifeLink of Southwest Florida
409 Bayshore Boulevard   813-253-2640
Tampa, FL 33906   800-262-5775
Fax: 813-348-0634
e-mail: info@lifelinkfound.org
www.lifelinkfound.org
LifeLink of Southwest Florida and Florida Gulf Coast University joined forces to develop a survey instrument to assss student attitudes and opinions about donation. Worked to conduct and evaluate the impact of the multifaceted education campaign.
Dennis F Heinrichs, President
Dana L Shires Jr, Chairman of the Board

9209   TransLife/Florida Hospital
1560 Orange Avenue   407-644-3770
Winter Park, FL 32789   800-443-6667
Fax: 407-303-2473
www.translife.org
Works closely with hospitals and donor families to coordinate the gift of life in Central Florida. Also a critical link between donors and possible recipients.
Carol Rumsey, Public Education Contact

Georgia

9210   LifeLink of Georgia
2875 Northwoods Parkway   770-225-5465
Norcross, GA 30071   800-544-6667
e-mail: info@lifelinkfound.org
www.lifelinkfound.org/georgia/ga.html
The Foundation atempts to work in a sensitive diligent and compassionate manner with donor families to facilitate the donation of desperately needed organs and tissues for waiting patients.
Dennis F Heinrichs, President
Dana L Shires, Chairman of the Board

Hawaii

9211   Organ Donor Center of Hawaii
1149 Bethel Street   808-599-7630
Honolulu, HI 96813   877-855-0603
Fax: 808-599-7631
e-mail: info@organdonorhawaii.com
www.organdonorhawaii.com
Non-profit organ procurement organization.
Stephen A Kula, Executive Director
Christine L Bogee, Administrative Services Director

Illinois

9212   Regional Organ Bank of Illinois, Inc.
5 Spring Lake Drive   312-431-3600
Chicago, IL 60607   888-307-3668
Fax: 312-803-7643
e-mail: info@robi.org
www.robi.org
ROBI'S mission is to save and enhance the lives of as many people as possible through organ and tissue donation.
Kim McCullough, Public Education Contact

Indiana

9213   Indiana Organ Procurement Organization,
3760 Guion Road   317-685-0389
Indianapolis, IN 46222-1816   888-275-4676
Fax: 317-685-1687
e-mail: info@iopo.org
www.iopo.org
Non-profit organ procurement organization designed to recover and distribute organ and tissues for transplantation.
Sam Davis, Director of Professional Services
Lynn Driver, President and CEO

Iowa

9214   Iowa Donor Network
550 Madison Avenue   319-665-3787
N Liberty, IA 52317   800-831-4131
Fax: 319-665-3788
www.iowadonornetwork.org
Iowa Donor Network is dedicated to serving donow families potentialdonors and candidates doe transplantation through identifying potential donorssupporting and respecting donation decisions and maximizing the recovery of transplantable organs and tissues.
John Watson, Chair
Sara Drobnich, Vice-Chair

Kansas

9215   Midwest Transplant Network & Organ Bank
1900 W 47th Place   913-262-1668
Westwood, KS 66205   Fax: 913-262-5130
e-mail: info@mwob.org
www.mwtn.org
Provides quality transplantation related services that will maximize the availability of organs and tissues to the comunities we serve. Provides procurement services for organ and tissue and laboratory services for HLA.
A. Michael Borkon, MD
Gary Duncan, CEO

Kentucky

9216   Kentucky Organ Donor Affiliates
106 E Broadway   502-581-9511
Louisville, KY 40202   800-525-3456
Fax: 502-589-5157
e-mail: info@kyorgandonor.org
www.kyorgandonor.org
Non-profit organ donor center that retrieves and distributes organs to qualified recipients.

Louisiana

9217   Louisiana Organ Procurement Agency
3545 N. I-10 Service Rd   800-521-4483
Metairie, LA 70002-3626   800-521-GIVE
Fax: 504-837-3587
e-mail: info@lopa.org
www.lopa.org
Non-profit organ procurement organization federally-designated to increase the number of transplantable organs by providing families an opportunity to donate organs and tissues to support these families regardless of their decision.
John Egan, Public Education Contact

Maryland

9218 Transplant Resource Center of Maryland
1730 Twin Springs Road   410-242-7000
Baltimore, MD 21227   800-641-HERO
Fax: 410-242-1871
e-mail: communications@TheLLF.org
www.mdtransplant.org
Provides organ and tissue donation and recovery services hospital
donor program development and community education to 42 hospitals and the citizens living in Maryland.
Ann Bromery, Chief Financial Officer
Charles Alexander, President & Chief Executive Officer

Massachusetts

9219 New England Organ Bank Massachusetts
One Gateway Center
Newton, MA 02158   800-446-NEOB
Fax: 617-244-8755
e-mail: info@neob.com
www.neob.org
Independent, not-for-profit agency whose mission is to recover,
preserve, and distribute human organs and tissues for transplantation. A federally-designated organ procurement organization for
all or part of the six New England states, it serves 177 acute care
hospitals and 14 transplant centers.
Sean Fitzpatrick, Public Education Contact

Michigan

9220 Transplantation Society of Michigan
3861 Research Park Drive   734-973-1577
Ann Arbor, MI 48108   800-482-4881
Fax: 734-973-3133
e-mail: info@giftoflifemichigan.org
www.giftoflifemichigan.org
Nonprofit independent corporation certified by Medicare and designated by the Centers for Medicare and Medicaid Services as an
organ recovery organization for Michigan.
Tammie Harvermahl, Public Education Contact

Minnesota

9221 LifeSource, Upper Midwest Organ Procurement Organization, Inc.
2550 University Avenue West   651-603-7800
St. Paul, MN 55114-1904   Fax: 651-603-7801
e-mail: info@life-source.org
www.life-source.org
Nonprofit, federally-designated organ procurement organization
for the Upper Midwest, managing all organ donation activities in
Minnesota.
Jill Halimi, Donor Family Services

Mississippi

9222 Mississippi Organ Recovery
12 River Bend Place   601-933-1000
Flowood, MS 39232   800-690-8878
Fax: 601-933-1006
www.msora.org
Not-for-profit organization coordinates the recovery of human organs for transplantation by working with and providing education
to medical professionals donor families and the people of
Mississippi.
Kelly Nations, Community Education Coordinator
Kevin Stump, Chief Executive Officer

Missouri

9223 Mid-America Transplant Services
1110 Highlands Plaza Drive E   314-735-8200
Saint Louis, MO 63110-3205   Fax: 314-991-2805
e-mail: info@mts-stl.org
www.mts-stl.org
Community based not-for-profit organ procurement organization
dedicated to enhancing the quality of human life. Coordinates the
procurement of vital organs tissues and eyes in hospitals throughout its service area.
Diane Brockmeier, COO
Dean F Kappel, President and CEO

Nebraska

9224 Nebraska Organ Retrieval System
8502 W Center Road   402-733-1800
Omaha, NE 68124   877-633-1800
Fax: 402-733-9142
www.NEdonation.org
Responsible for retrieving the proper organs and distrbuting them
to the recipients.
Kyle Herber, Executive Director
John Stallabaum, Client Services Manager

Nevada

9225 Nevada Donor Network
2059 E Sahara Avenue   702-384-7616
Las Vegas, NV 89104   Fax: 702-796-4225
e-mail: ksatcher@nvdonor.org
www.nvdonor.org
Improving the quality of human life through the recovery of all
available organs and tissues for transplantation education and research while maintaining the dignity of the donors and their
families.
Liliana Arredondo, Public Education Coordinator
Ken Richardson, Executive Director

New Jersey

9226 Sharing Network Organ Tissue Donation Services
691 Central Avenue   908-516-5400
New Providence, NJ 07974   800-742-7365
Fax: 908-516-5501
e-mail: tsn@sharenj.org
www.sharenj.org
Federally certified state-approved organ procurement organization responsible for recovering organ and tissue for New Jersey
residents currently awaiting transplants.
Vito Pulito, Chair
Bruce I. Goldstein, Vice Chair

New Mexico

9227 New Mexico Donor Services
1609 University Blvd NE   505-843-7672
Albuquerque, NM 87102   877-401-2511
Fax: 505-343-1828
e-mail: info@donatelifenm.org
www.donatelifenm.org
Transplant centers in the service area are: University of New Mexico Hospitals Presbyterian Hospital.
Wayne Dunlap, Interim Executive Director
Maria Sanders, Community Relations

New York

9228 Center for Donation & Transplantation
218 Great Oaks Boulevard   518-262-5606
Albany, NY 12203   800-256-7811
Fax: 518-262-5427
e-mail: dfloeser@cdtny.org
www.cdtny.org
Dedicated to increasing organ and tissue donation by following
procurement and equitable distribution of medically suitable organs and tissue for transplantation.
Michael Thiabault, Executive Director
Martin benoit, Director

9229 Finger Lakes Donor Recovery Network
Corporate Woods of Brighton   585-272-4930
Rochester, NY 14623   800-810-5494
Fax: 585-272-4956
e-mail: info@donorrecovery.org
www.donorrecovery.org

Nonprofit organization that covers the Finger Lakes Region Central and Upstate New York for transplant centers.
Diane Ashley, Executive Director
Julius Gene Lattore, Vice Chair

9230 New York Organ Donor Network, Inc
132 West 31st Street   646-291-4444
New York, NY 10001   Fax: 646-291-4600
                                                                www.nyodn.org
The New York Organ Donor Network is dedicated to the recovery of organs and tissues for people in need of life-saving and life-improvving transplants.
Elaine Berg, President/CEO

9231 Upstate New York Transplant Services, Inc.
110 Broadway   716-853-6667
Buffalo, NY 14203   800-227-4771
                                                          Fax: 716-853-6674
                                                   e-mail: info@unyts.org
                                                                www.unyts.org
An independent nonprofit organization that encourages and coordinates the donation of human organs and tissue for transplantation.
Richard A Grimm, Chairman
Michael Beecher, Vice Chairman

North Carolina

9232 Life Share of the Carolinas
5000 D Airport Center Parkway   704-512-3303
Charlotte, NC 28208   800-932-4483
                                                          Fax: 704-512-3056
                                            e-mail: lifeshare@carolinas.org
                                                   www.lifesharecarolinas.org
Mission is to improve the quality of human life through the provision of organs and tissues for transplantation and to serve our hospitals and their respective communities by rpoviding educational support services which enhance the donation process.
Dan Hayes, Medical Director
David Ugland, Bank Medical Director

Ohio

9233 Life Connection of Ohio
3661 Briarfield Boulevard   419-893-1618
Maumee, OH 43537   800-262-5443
                                                          Fax: 419-893-1827
                                             e-mail: ksteele@lcotro.org
                                            www.lifeconnectionofohio.org
Life Connection of Ohio is committed to serving humanity by ending the wait for organ and tissue transplants in a manner that is beneficial to patients, donor families, health care professionals and the public.
Kara Steele, Director of Community Relations (Toledo)
Cathi Arends, Director of Community Relations (Dayton)

9234 LifeBanc
4775 Richmond Road,   216-752-5433
Cleveland, OH 44128-5343   888-558-LIFE
                                                          Fax: 216-751-4204
                                                 e-mail: info@lifebanc.org
                                                                www.lifebanc.org
Non-profit organization that covers all of Northeast Ohio.
Monica Morgan, Public Education Contact

9235 Lifeline of Ohio Organ Procurement Agency, Inc.
770 Kinnear Road   614-291-5667
Columbus, OH 43212   800-525-5667
                                                          Fax: 614-291-0660
                                                   www.lifelineofohio.org
Lifeline of Ohio (LOOP) is an independent non-profit organization whose purpose is to promote and coordinate the donation of human organs and tissue dor transplantation.
Roger L Walker, Chairperson
Mark E Brainbridge, Treasurer

9236 Ohio Valley LifeCenter
2925 Vernon Place   513-558-5555
Cincinnati, OH 45219-2430   800-981-5433
                                                          Fax: 513-558-5556
                                           e-mail: info@lifepassiton.org
                                                                www.lifecnt.org
Encourages amd coordinates the donation of human organs and tissues in the Greater Cincinnati area. Provides educational and motivational progams to healthcare professionals regarding their important role in the donation of organs and tissues for transplant.
Mark Sommerville, Public Education Contact
Michael Edwards, Chairman

Oklahoma

9237 Oklahoma Organ Sharing Network
5801 N Broadway
Oklahoma City, OK 73118   888-580-5680
                                                          Fax: 405-840-9748
                                             e-mail: philvs@oosn.org ˜
                                                                www.oosn.org
LifeShare Transplant Donor Services of Oklahoma is committed to providing a better quality of life for those people who require organ or tissue transplantation while respecting and honoring those families who share the gift of life.
Harlan Wright, President

Oregon

9238 Pacific NW Transplant Bank
2611 SW 3rd Avenue   503-494-5560
Portland, OR 97201-4952   800-344-8916
                                                          Fax: 503-494-4725
                                                 e-mail: pntb@ohsu.edu
                                                                www.pntb.org
Federally designated nonprofit organ procurement organization serving Oregon southwest Washington and western Idaho.
Mike Seeley, Executive Director
Craig Van De Walker, Director Of Operation

Pennsylvania

9239 Center for Organ Recovery & Education
RIDC Park
Pittsburgh, PA 15238   800-366-6777
                                                          Fax: 412-963-3563
                                            e-mail: hbulvony@core.org
                                                                www.core.org
Continues its efforts to lead the procurement field by becoming a full-service OPO.
Susan A Stuart, President & CEO
Karen Zumba, Executive Adminstratve Director

9240 Gift of Life Donor Program Pennsylvania
401 North 3rd Street   215-557-8090
Philadelphia, PA 19123-3813   888-366-6771
                                                          Fax: 215-963-0587
                                              e-mail: info@donors1.org
                                                                www.donors1.org
Formerly (Delaware Valley Transplant Program) is the region's nonprofit organ and tissue donor program serving eastern half of Pennsylvania, southern New Jersey and the state of Delaware. Also, considered a model program in the United States.
Glen D Moffet, Chair
Gerad J. Fulda, Vice Chair

Tennessee

9241 Mid-South Transplant Foundation, Inc. Tennessee
8001 Centerview Parkway   901-328-4438
Corodova, TN 38018   877-228-LIFE
                                                          Fax: 901-448-8126
                                                   www.midsouthtransplant.org
Mission is to provide the option of donation to all families of potential organ donors and to protect their rights and interest throughout the donation process.
Louis G Britt, President
Kenneth D Sellers, Medical Director

9242 Tennessee Donor Services
1600 Hayes Street
Nashville, TN 37203 423-915-0808
888-562-3774
Fax: 901-448-8126
e-mail: info@donatelifetn.org
donatelifetn.org
Mission is to represent the interests of the people of our service area in the formulation of policies procedures and regulations concerning organ donation and transplantation.
Lisa Peoples, Public Education Contact
Jennifer Jenks, Contact

Utah

9243 Intermountain Donor Services
230 S 500 E
Salt Lake City, UT 84102 801-521-1755
800-833-6667
Fax: 801-364-8815
e-mail: debbie@idslife.org
www.idslife.org
Provides high quality organ and tissue procurement services to the medical and public communities. Educating medical professionals and the public sector on the benefits of organ and tissue donation.
Alex McDonald, Public Education Director
Tracy C Schmidt, Executive Director

Virginia

9244 LifeNet
1864 Concert Drive
Virginia Beach, VA 23453 ÿ75- 46- 476
800-847-7831
Fax: 757-301-6582
e-mail: lifenet@trans.org
www.lifenet.org
An organ procurement agency and the largest full-service tissue bank in the United States providing musculoskeletal and cardiovascular tissues for transplant on a national and international basis.
Becky Lawson, Public Education Contact

9245 Washington Regional Transplant Consortium
7619 Little River Turnpike
Annandale, VA 22003 703-641-0100
866-232-3666
Fax: 703-658-0711
e-mail: contactwrtc@wrtc.org
www.wrtc.org
Recently partnered with fellow Mid-Atlantic Coalition on Donation members and a company called Sports America to sponsor the second annual DeMatha Invitational. WRTC is the official link between organ and tissue donors and the patients who are waiting for transplant.
Sara Idler, Public Education Contact

Washington

9246 LifeCenter Northwest
11245 SE 6th Street
Bellevue, WA 98004 425-201-6563
877-275-5269
Fax: 425-688-7641
e-mail: info@lcnw.org
www.lcnw.org
LifeCenter Northwest Organ Donation Network is a nonprofit organization that facilitates organ donation for a population of over 7.5 million people throughout Washington Montana Alasks and Nothern Idaho. Our mission is to fund education and outreach programs.
Megan Erwin, Vice President Community Relations
Diana Clark, President & CEO

Wisconsin

9247 University of Wisconsin Organ Procurement Organization
University of Wisconsin Hospital and Clinics
600 Highland Ave.
Madison, WI 53972-1735 608-265-0356
Fax: 608-262-9099
e-mail: uwhcopo@uwhealth.org
www.uwhcopo.org

Located within a major academic center and is recognized as one of the most successful organ procurement programs in the nation.
Jill Ellefson, Public Education Contact

9248 Wisonsin Donor Network
638 North 18th Street?
Milwaukee, WI 53233 41- 9-7 61
1 -77 -32 4
Fax: 414-259-8059
e-mail: labinfo@bcw.edu
www.bcw.edu
Recovers organs for transplant as well as provides public and professional education about the tremendous need for organ and tissue donors.
Richard S. Gallaghar, Chairman
Peter D. Zegler, Vice Chair

Foundations

9249 Musculoskeletal Transplant Foundation
125 May Street
Edison, NJ 08837 732-661-0202
800-946-9008
Fax: 732-661-2298
e-mail: information@mtf.org
www.mtf.org
Non-profit service organization dedicated to providing quality tissue through a commitment to excellence in education, research, recovery and care for recipients, donors, and their families.
Bruce W Stroever, President/CEO
Martha Anderson, Executive Vice President

Research Centers

9250 Georgetown University Hospital Transplant Institute
3800 Reservoir Road, NW
Washington, DC 20007 202-444-2000
www.georgetownuniversityhospital.org
Founded to promote health through education, research, and patient care.

Books

9251 History of Organ and Cell Transplantation
Imperial College Press
57 Shelton St.
Lomdon, UK 207-836- 888
Fax: 207-836- 020
e-mail: sales@wspc.co.uk
www.icpress.co.uk
Our aim is to create the highest quality, knowledge-based products and to enable continuous learning for the global scientific and professional communities
464 pages Hardcover
ISBN: 1-860942-09-1

9252 Legal and Ethical Aspects of Organ Transplantation
David P T Price, author
Cambridge University Press
40 West 20th Street
New York, NY 10011-4221 212-924-3900
Fax: 212-691-3239
www.cambridge.org/us
A comprehensive analysis of existing laws and policies governing transplantation practices around the world. Examines the meaning of death, cadaver organ procurement policies, use of living donors, trading in human organs, experimental transplant procedures and xenotransplantation.
507 pages Hardcover
ISBN: 0-521651-64-6

9253 Organ Procurement and Transplantation:
Intitute of Medicine, author
National Academies Press
500 Fifth Street NW
Washington, DC 20001 202-334-3313
800-624-6242
Fax: 202-334-2451
e-mail: Customer_Service@nap.edu
www.nap.edu

This book assesses the potential impact of the Final Rule on organ transplantation. Presents new, original data, and assesses medical practices, social and economic observations, and other information.
232 pages Hardcover

9254 Organ Transplants from Executed Prisoners:
Louis J Palmer, author

McFarland & Company
960 NC Hwy 88W   336-246-4460
Jefferson, NC 28640   800-253-2187
Fax: 336-246-5018
e-mail: info@mcfarlandpub.com
www.mcfarlandpub.com

A study of the utilitarian creation of death sentence organ removal statutes that would make legal the harvesting of transplantable organs from the cadavers of executed capital murders.
156 pages
ISBN: 0-786406-73-9

9255 Transplantation Ethics
Robert M. Veatch, author

Georgetown University Press
3240 Prospect Street, NW   202-687-5889
Washington, DC 20007   Fax: 202-687-6340
e-mail: gupress@georgetown.edu
www.press.georgetown.edu

The first complete and systematic account of the ethical and policy controversies surrounding organ transplants.
2000 448 pages Paperback
ISBN: 0-878408-12-2
Richard Brown, Director
Donald Jacobs, Senior Acquisitions Editor

9256 Twice Dead: Organ Transplants and the Reinvention of Death
Margaret Lock, author

University of California Press
1445 Lower Ferry Road   609-883-1759
Ewing, NJ 08618   800-777-4726
Fax: 800-999-1958
e-mail: orders@cpfsinc.com
www.ucpress.edu/index.html

Raises critically important questions about life and death in the modern world.
429 pages Paperback
ISBN: 0-520228-14-6
Alison Mudditt, Director

9257 US Organ Procurement System: A Prescription for Reform
David L. Kaserman, A.H. Barnett, author

American Enterprise Institute
1150 Seventeenth St, NW   202-862-5800
Washington, DC 20036   Fax: 202-862-7177
e-mail: custserv@nbnbooks.com
www.aei.org

Isolates the procurement issue from others to make a compelling and persuasive case for markets in cadaveric organs.
177 pages Paperback
ISBN: 0-844741-71-X
Tully M. Friedman, Chairman and CEO
Daniel A. D'Aniello, Vice Chairman

Magazines

9258 Encore: Another Chance for Life
Chronimed Pharmacy
Po Box 59032
Minneapolis, MN 55459-9686   800-888-5753
www.transplantawareness.org

Published exclusively for transplant patients, their families, and friends, this publication provides a broad look at many issues surrounding transplantation and encourages personal stories and feedback from readers.
Quarterly

9259 Renalife
The American Association of Kidney Patients

100 S. Ashley Drive
Tampa, FL 33260   800-749-2257
e-mail: aakpaz@enet.net

Provides articles, news items, and information of interest to kindey patients and their families, individuals, and organizations in the renal health care field.
3 Year

9260 Stadtlanders LifeTIMES
Stadtlanders Pharmacy
600 Penn Center Boulevard
Pittsburgh, PA 15235-5810   800-238-7828
www.statlander.com/transplant/#resource

Designed to be an educational, informative and supportive, focusing on a variety of health-care issues of concern to patients (including transplant patients).

Newsletters

9261 Advocate
National Foundation for Transplants
5350 Poplar Ave   901-684-1697
Memphis, TN 38119   800-489-3863
Fax: 901-684-1128
e-mail: info@transplants.org
www.transplants.org

Linda J. Evans, Chairman
Matthew Schneider, Vice-Chairman

9262 Children's Organ Transplant Association (COTA)
2501 COTA Drive   800-366-2682
Bloomington, IN 47403   Fax: 812-336-8885
e-mail: cota@cota.org
www.cota.org

Provides fundraising assistance to children and young adults needing life-saving transplants and promotes organ, marrow and tissue donation.
Rick Lofgren, President/CEO
Lisa Fulkerson, VP/CFO

9263 New Start News
National Transplant Assistance Fund (NTAF)
3475 West Chester Pike   610-353-9684
Newtown Square, PA 19073   800-642-8399
Fax: 610-353-1616
e-mail: ntaf@transplantfund.org
m.helphopelive.org

Sidney P. Constien, Editor
Judy Walker, Editor

Web Sites

9264 American Society of Transplantation (AST)
www.a-s-t.org

An organization of transplant professionals dedicated to research, education, advocacy and patient care in transplantation science and medicine.

9265 Association of Organ Procurement Organizations (AOPO)
www.aopo.org

Organization involved in helping people find and obtain the organs they may need for transplantation.

9266 Children's Organ Transplant Association (COTA)
www.cota.org

Not-for-profit national chairty dedicated to helping families and communities raise the necessary funds for transplant expenses.

9267 Donate Life America
www.donatelife.net

A not-for-profit alliance of national organizations and local coalitions across the United States that have joined forces to educate the public about organ, eye and tissue donation, correcting misconceptions about donation and creating a greater willingness to donate.

9268 Georgetown University Hospital Transplant Institute
www.georgetownuniversityhospital.org

Founded to promote health through education, research, and patient care.

9269   Health Resources and Services Administration (HRSA)

www.hrsa.gov

Envisions optimal health for all, supported by a health care system that assures access to comprehensive, culturally competant, quality care. Provides national leadership, program resources and services needed to improve access to culturally competant, quality health care.

9270   Jewish Hospital Transplant Center

www.jhsmh.org

An elite group approved to perform five solid organ transplants and has been named a Federally Designated Medicare Heart, Lung, Kidney, Liver and Pancreas Transplant Center.

9271   MedicineNet

www.medicinenet.com

An online resource for consumers providing easy-to-read, authoritative medical and health information.

9272   National Foundation for Transplants

www.transplants.org

Mission is to reach out to help those who seek a new life through transplantation, by providing healthcare and financial support services and patient advocacy for transplant candidates families nationwide.

9273   National Transplant Assistance Fund (NTAF)

www.transplantfund.org

Helps to raise funds for transplant and catastrophic injury patients by providing compassionate support, education and expertise to them, their families and communities.

9274   Organ Procurement and Transplantation Network (OPTN)

www.optn.org

A unified transplant network established by the United States Congress under the National Organ Transplant Act (NOTA) of 1984. A unique public-prvate partnership that links all of the professionals nvolved in the donation and transplantation system.

9275   Transweb: All About Transplantation and Donation

www.transweb.org

Non-profit educational website serving the world transplant community. Features news and events, real peoples experinces, the top 10 myths about donation, a donation quiz, and a large collection of questions and answers, as well as a reference area with everything from articles to videos.

9276   United Network for Organ Sharing (UNOS)

www.unos.org

Non-profit, scientific and educational organization that administers the nation's only Organ Procurement and Transplantation Network(OPTN). Mission is to advance organ availability and transplantation by uniting and supporting our communities for the benefit of patients through education, technology and policy development.

9277   United Organ Transplant Association (UOTA)

www.uota.org

Non-profit charitable Corporation dedicated to providing educational, emotional and financial support to pre- and post- transplant patients.

Description

9278 Tuberculosis

Tuberculosis, TB, is an infectious disease caused by mycobacteria. It is spread through the air and normally affects the lungs (pulmonary tuberculosis). Extremely common in the United States early in the twentieth century, tuberculosis declined dramatically after 1950. This trend reversed itself after about 1985, due to immigration, the HIV epidemic, and the development of drug resistance by the germ responsible for the disease.

The usual symptoms of TB infection of the lungs include persistent cough, chest pain and coughing up blood. TB infection can cause weight loss, night sweats and fatigue. Left untreated, TB may spread to the spine, causing bone breakdown with deformity, to the lining of the brain, causing tuberculous meningitis, or, in fact, to any organ of the body (extrapulmonary TB).

People who are otherwise healthy, and who are infected with a strain of mycobacterium that is sensitive to standard drugs, can almost always be cured after 6-9 months of therapy. Persons infected with HIV, because of their lowered resistance to disease, have trouble clearing their TB infection, even if they use effective drugs faithfully. Therefore, they should be treated for one year. Regardless of length of treatment, during this time the germ may become resistant to the drug being used. Therefore treatment includes at least 2 drugs, so that a bacterium that develops resistance to one drug will still be killed by another one. Incomplete or interrupted treatment often leads to drug resistance. Germs that are resistant to multiple drugs may be passed to others, and are now a serious public health menace. Unfortunately, the HIV-infected patient is an ideal breeding ground for drug-resistant TB germs.

Persons with drug-sensitive TB who are otherwise healthy and will cooperate with treatment are generally treated by community physicians. Those with complicated medical status (HIV, drug-resistant organisms) or social difficulties (alcoholism, substance abuse, homelessness) generally require specialized public health clinics that can combine medical expertise with nursing and social outreach support.

Many persons who have been infected by TB keep it successfully contained by their own immune systems. There is some risk of the contained germ, however, even years later, overcoming the body's resistance and causing active disease. The tuberculin skin test (PPD) is used to widely screen certain high-risk populations, particularly those who have been exposed to an infectious individual. Prior, adequately treated infection may be diagnosed by a positive PPD, and is sometimes treated with antibiotics to reduce the risk of future disease.

National Agencies & Associations

9279 American Lung Association
1301 Pennsylvania Avenue NW   202-785-3355
Washington, DC 20004   Fax: 202-452-1805
www.lungusa.org
The mission of the American Lung Association is to prevent lung disease and promote lung health. Founded in 1904 to fight tuberculosis the American Lung Association today fights disease in all its forms, with special emphasis on asthma and tobacco control.
Linn Bilingsly, Director
John F. Emanuel, Secretary

9280 Centers for Disease Control and Prevention National Center for Prevention Services
National Center for Prevention Services
1600 Clifton Road   404-639-8135
Atlanta, GA 30333   800-CDC-INFO
TTY: 888-232-6348
e-mail: cdcinfo@cdc.gov
www.cdc.gov
CDC has been dedicated to protecting health and promoting quality of life through the prevention and control of disease, injury and disability.
Tom Friedan, Director
Ileana Arias, Principle Deputy Director

9281 National Institute of Allergy and Infectious Diseases
6610 Rockledge Drive   301-496-5717
Bethesda, MD 20892-6621   866-284-4107
Fax: 301-402-3573
TTY: 800-877-8339
e-mail: afauci@niaid.nih.gov
www.niaid.nih.gov
Conducts and supports basic and applied research to better understand, treat and ultimately prevent infectious, immunologic and allergic diseases.
Anthony S Fauci MD, Director
H Clifford Lane MD, Acting Deputy Director

9282 New Jersey Medical School: National Tuberculosis Center
225 Warren Street   973-972-3270
Newark, NJ 07101-1709   800-482-3627
Fax: 973-972-3268
www.umdnj.edu/ntbcweb/tbsplash.html
Provides expert medical consultation, trains health care providers and other health related professionals, utilize innovative educational methodologies such as standardized patients, develop linkages with health care delivery systems and collaborate with health care professionals.
Lee B Reichman, Executive Director
Reynard J McDonald, Medical Director

9283 Occupational Safety & Health Administration
200 Constitution Avenue Northwest
Washington, DC 20210   800-321-6742
TTY: 877-889-5627
www.osha.gov
OSHA's mission is to assure the safety and health of America's workers by setting and enforcing standards, providing training, outreach and education, establishing partnerships and encouraging continual improvement in workplace safety and health.
Doug Kalinowski, Director
M. Lucero Oritiz, Chief of Staff

State Agencies & Associations

Alabama

9284 American Lung Association of Alabama
PO Box 3188   205-933-8821
Bessemer, AL 35023   800-LUN-GUSA
Fax: 205-930-1717
e-mail: kperry@alabamalung.org
www.alabamalung.org

Kim Perry, Director of Development

Alaska

9285 American Lung Association of Alaska
500 W International Airport Road
Anchorage, AK 99518

907-276-5864
800-LUN-GUSA
Fax: 907-565-5587
e-mail: mlarson@aklung.org
www.aklung.org

Marge Larson, Director

Arizona

9286 Northern Arizona Branch:Phoenix Area
102 W McDowell Road
Phoenix, AZ 85003-1299

602-258-7505
800-LUN-GUSA
Fax: 602-258-7507
e-mail: infophoenix@lungaz.org
www.lungarizona.org

Nancy Cohrs, Executive Director
Evelyn Frear, Office Manager

9287 Southern Arizona Branch: Tucson Area
2819 E Broadway
Tuscon, AZ 85716

520-323-1812
800-LUN-GUSA
Fax: 520-323-1816
e-mail: infotucson@lungaz.org
www.lungarizona.org

Keith Kaback, Chairman
Heidi Miller, Vice Chairman

Arkansas

9288 American Lung Association of Arkansas
217 W 2nd Street
Little Rock, AR 72201-1539

501-957-0758
Fax: 501-978-5138
e-mail: inquiries@breathehealthy.org
www.lung.org

California

9289 American Lung Association of California
424 Pendleton Way
Oakland, CA 94621-2189

510-638-LUNG
800-LUN-GUSA
Fax: 510-638-8984
e-mail: veronica.cuevas@lung.org
www.lung.org

Linda Hinojosa, Chairman
Laura Keegan Boudreau, Acting CEO

Colorado

9290 American Lung Association of Colorado
5600 Greenwood Plaza Boulevard
Greenwood Village, CO 80111-2305

303-388-4327
800-LUN-GUSA
Fax: 303-377-1102
e-mail: cmichael@lungcolorado.org
www.lung.org

Curt Huber, Executive Director
Connor Michael, Communications Manager

Connecticut

9291 American Lung Association of Connecticut
45 Ash Street
E Hartford, CT 06108-3272

860-289-5401
800-992-2263
Fax: 860-289-5405
e-mail: info@lungne.org
www.lung.org

Margaret LaCroix, Vice President Communications

Delaware

9292 American Lung Association of Delaware
630 Churchmans Rd
Newark, DE 19806-3280

302-737-6414
Fax: 302-737-126
e-mail: llyons@lunginfo.org
www.lung.org

Peter Shanley, Chairman

District of Columbia

9293 American Lung Association of Washington
1301 Pennsylvania Ave NW
Washington, DC 20004

202-785-3355
800-732-9339
Fax: 206-441-3277
e-mail: alaw@alaw.org
www.lung.org

Vivian Echavarria, Chair
Rick Weems, Secretary

9294 American Lung Association of the District of Columbia
1301 Pennsylvania Ave NW
Washington, DC 20004-2617

202-785-3355
Fax: 202-682-5607
e-mail: info@aladc.org
www.lung.org

Jan Morgan, Special Events Director
Phoebe Robinson, Administrative Coordinator

Florida

9295 American Lung Association of Florida
6852 Belfort Oaks Place
Jacksonville, FL 32216-5216

904-743-2933
800-940-2933
Fax: 904-743-2916
e-mail: alaf@lungfla.org
www.lung.org

Michael Diamond, President
Marilin K Glassberg, President-Elect

Georgia

9296 American Lung Association of Georgia
2452 Spring Road
Smyrna, GA 30080

770-434-5864
800-586-4872
Fax: 770-319-0349
e-mail: mail@alaga.org
www.lung.org

Charles J White, Chief Executive Officer
June Deen, VP Public Affairs

Hawaii

9297 American Lung Association of Hawaii
650 Iwilei Road
Honolulu, HI 96817

808-537-5966
Fax: 808-537-5971
e-mail: lung@ala-hawaii.org
www.lung.org

Karen J Lee, President, Executive Director

Illinois

9298 American Lung Association of Illinois-Iowa
55 W Upper Wacker Dr
Chicago, IL 60601

312-781-1100
800-586-4872
Fax: 217-787-5916
e-mail: info@lungil.org
www.lung.org

Harold Wimmer, CEO
Lori Younker, Manager

Indiana

9299 American Lung Association of Indiana: State Office & Support Office
9445 Delegates Row,
Indianapolis, IN 46240

317-573-3900
800-LUN-GUSA
Fax: 317-819-1187
e-mail: info@lungin.org
www.lung.org

Dana Pitts, VP Communications/Marketing

Kansas

9300 **American Lung Association of Kansas**
6701 W 64th Street   913-912-7190
Overland Park, KS 66202-2419   Fax: 866-575-1761
e-mail: menisam@kylung.org
www.lung.org

Judy Keller, Executive Director

Kentucky

9301 **American Lung Association of Kentucky**
4100 Churchman Avenue   502-363-2652
Louisville, KY 40209-0067   800-LUN-GUSA
Fax: 502-363-0222
e-mail: info@kylung.org
www.lung.org

Todd Adams, Development Director
Laura Collins, Executive Assistant

Louisiana

9302 **American Lung Association of Louisiana**
2325 Severn Avenue   504-828-5864
Metairie, LA 70001-6918   800-LUN-GUSA
Fax: 504-828-5867
e-mail: info@louisianalung.org
www.lung.org

Aline Palmisano-Vita, Deputy Executive Director
Thomas P Lotz, Chief Executive Officer

Maine

9303 **American Lung Association of Maine**
122 State Street   207-622-6394
Augusta, ME 04330   800-LUN-GUSA
Fax: 639-426-2919
e-mail: info@lungme.org
www.lung.org

Lee Scott, President of Health Promotion
Edward Miller, Executive Director/SVP

Maryland

9304 **American Lung Association of Maryland**
211 East Lombard St   443-451-4950
Baltimore, MD 21202   Fax: 410-560-0829
e-mail: info@marylandlung.org
www.lung.org

Melina Davis-Martin, President and CEO
Krista Jennings, Chief Operations Officer

Massachusetts

9305 **American Lung Association of Massachusetts**
460 Totten Pond Road   781-890-4262
Waltham, MA 02451   Fax: 781-890-4280
e-mail: info@lungma.org
www.lung.org

Michigan

9306 **American Lung Association of Michigan**
1475 E 12 Mile Road   248-784-2000
Madison Heights, MI 48071   800-543-5864
Fax: 248-784-2008
e-mail: alam@alam.org
www.lung.org

Colette Scholzen, President

Minnesota

9307 **American Lung Association of Minnesota**
490 Concordia Avenue   651-227-8014
Saint Paul, MN 55103-2441   800-LUN-GUSA
Fax: 651-227-5459
e-mail: info@alamn.org
www.lung.org

Bill Westhoff, President

Mississippi

9308 **American Lung Association of Mississippi**
731 Pear Orchard Road   601-206-5810
Ridgeland, MS 39158   800-586-4872
Fax: 601-206-5813
www.lung.org

Greg Wynne, Chairman
Jennifer Cofer, Deputy Executive Director

Missouri

9309 **American Lung Association of Missouri**
1118 Hampton Avenue   314-645-5505
Saint Louis, MO 63139   Fax: 314-645-7128
e-mail: inquiries@breathehealthy.org
www.lung.org

Lori Pickens, Chief Executive Officer
Barry Freedman, VP Community Initiatives

Montana

9310 **American Lung Association of the Northern Rockies: Montana and Wyoming**
825 Helena Avenue   406-442-6556
Helene, MT 59601-3459   Fax: 406-442-2346
e-mail: ala-nr@ala-nr.org
www.lung.org

Nebraska

9311 **American Lung Association of Nebraska**
8990 W Dodge Rd   402-502-4950
Omaha, NE 68114   Fax: 402-502-3012
e-mail: jegerton@breathehealthy.org
www.lung.org

Nevada

9312 **American Lung Association of Idaho/Nevada**
10615 Double R Boulevard   775-829-LUNG
Reno, NV 89521-7056   800-LUN-GUSA
Fax: 775-829-5850
e-mail: lmartin@lungnevada.org
www.lung.org

Louise Martin, Executive Director
Gwen Bourne, Development Manager - Events

New Hampshire

9313 **American Lung Association of New Hampshire**
1800 Elm St   603-369-3977
Manchester, NH 03104   Fax: 603-369-3978
e-mail: info@nhlung.org
www.lung.org

Jeff Seyler, President & CEO
David Ales, Senior Vice President

New Jersey

9314 **American Lung Association of New Jersey**
1031 Route 22 West   908-685-8040
Bridgewater, NJ 08807-3407   800-LUN-GUSA
Fax: 908-851-2625
e-mail: jgrinwald@lunginfo.org
www.lung.org

John A Rutkowski, President

New Mexico

9315 **New Mexico Branch**
7001 Menaul Boulevard NE   505-265-0732
Albuquerque, NM 87110   800-LUN-GUSA
Fax: 505-260-1739
e-mail: ronh@alanm.org
www.lungusa.org

New York

9316 American Lung Association of Mid New York
155 Washington Avenue   518-465-2013
Albany, NY 12210   Fax: 518-465-2926
                                e-mail: info@alany.org
                                          www.lung.org
The mission of the American Lung Association and the American
Lung Association of New York State is to prevent lung disease and
promote lung health. The American Lung Association is the oldest
voluntary health organization in the United States.
Deborah Carioto, President
Michael Seilback, Vice President Public Policy

North Carolina

9317 American Lung Association of North Carolina
514 Daniels St.   919-424-6069
Raleigh, NC 27605   800-892-5650
                                Fax: 919-856-8530
                                e-mail: lungnc@lungusa.org
                                          www.lung.org

Deborah C. Bryan, President

North Dakota

9318 American Lung Association of North Dakota
212 N 2nd Street   701-223-5613
Bismarck, ND 58502   Fax: 919-856-8530
                                e-mail: dbryan@lungnc.org
                                          www.lung.org

Deborah C Bryan, VP Advocacy & Donor Value
Mendi Nieters, Regional VP Development

Ohio

9319 American Lung Association of Ohio
1950 Arlingate Lane   614-279-1700
Columbus, OH 43228   800-LUN-GUSA
                                Fax: 614-279-4940
                                e-mail: alao@ohiolung.org
                                          www.lung.org

Tracy Ross, President / CEO

Oklahoma

9320 American Lung Association of Oklahoma
1010 E 8th Street   918-747-3441
Tulsa, OK 74120   Fax: 918-747-4629
                                          www.lung.org

Sara Dreiling, Chief Executive Officer
Edward C Rosentel, Chief Financial and Operating Officer

Oregon

9321 American Lung Association of Oregon
7420 SW Bridgeport Road   503-924-4094
Tigard, OR 97224   Fax: 503-924-4120
                                e-mail: info@lungoregon.org
                                          www.lung.org

Jan Jensen, President
Dana Kaye, Executive Director

Pennsylvania

9322 American Lung Association of Pennsylvania
3001 Old Gettysburg Road   717-541-5864
Camp Hill, PA 17011   800-LUN-GUSA
                                Fax: 888-415-5757
                                e-mail: dbrown@lunginfo.org
                                          www.lung.org

South Carolina

9323 American Lung Association of South Carolina
1817 Gadsen Street   803-779-5864
Columbia, SC 29201-2392   800-849-5864
                                Fax: 803-254-2711
                                e-mail: alasc@lungsc.org
                                          www.lung.org

South Dakota

9324 American Lung Association of South Dakota
108 E 38th Street   605-336-7222
Sioux Falls, SD 57105   Fax: 803-254-2711
                                e-mail: shelps@alase.org
                                          www.lung.org

Amanda Strickland, Regional Manager Special Events
Sharon Helps, Regional Manager Programs

Tennessee

9325 American Lung Association of Tennesse
One Vantage Way   615-329-1151
Nashville, TN 37228   800-LUN-GUSA
                                Fax: 615-329-1723
                                e-mail: alastaff@alatn.org
                                          www.lung.org

Texas

9326 American Lung Association of Texas
8150 Brookriver Drive   512-467-6753
Dallas, TX 75247-0460   800-252-5864
                                Fax: 512-467-7621
                                e-mail: inquiries@breathehealthy.org
                                          www.lung.org

Phillip J Hanson, Senior VP Resource Development
Margaret Crump, Senior VP Community Initiatives

Utah

9327 American Lung Association of Utah
1930 S 1100 E   801-484-4456
Salt Lake City, UT 84106-2317   Fax: 801-484-5461
                                e-mail: info@utahlung.org
                                          www.lung.org

Vermont

9328 American Lung Association of Vermont
372 Hurricane Lane   802-876-6500
Williston, VT 05495-6196   Fax: 802-876-6505
                                e-mail: info@vtlung.org
                                          www.lung.org

Erin Hickey, Senior Manager Development
Margaret LaCroix, VP Marketing\Communications

Virginia

9329 American Lung Association of Virginia
9702 Gayton Rd   804-955-4910
Richmond, VA 23238   Fax: 804-267-5634
                                e-mail: lungva@lungusa.org
                                          www.lung.org

Melina Davis-Martin, President and CEO
Krista Jennings, Chief Operating Officer

West Virginia

9330 American Lung Association of West Virginia
2102 Kanawha Blvd   304-342-6600
East Charleston, WV 25311-3980   Fax: 304-342-6096
                                e-mail: cfields@lunginfo.org
                                          www.lung.org

Sara Crickenberger, Executive Director

9331 American Lung Association of Wisconsin
13100 W Lisbon Road   262-703-4200
Brookfield, WI 53005-2508   800-586-4872
                                              Fax: 262-781-5180
                                        e-mail: info@lungwi.org
                                                   www.lung.org

Susan Gloede Swan, Executive Director
Dona Wininsky, Director of Public Policy

Research Centers

9332 University of Illinois at Chicago Lions
2035 W Taylor St   312-355-1715
Chicago, IL 60612   Fax: 312-355-2693
                          www.uic.edu/pharmacy/research/itr
The Institute for Tuberculosis Research is comprised of approximately 30 individuals: biologists chemists pharmacologists and support staff - ~ all working towards a single goal - the discovery of new drugs for tuberculosis.
Scott Franzblau, Director
Lorna Haubrich, ITR General Information

9333 University of Illinois at Chicago: Institute for Tuberculosis Research
833 S. Wood Street   312-355-1715
Chicago, IL 60612-7631   Fax: 312-355-2693
                          www.uic.edu/pharmacy/research/itr
Scott Franzblau, Director
Lorna Haubrich, ITR General Information

Support Groups & Hotlines

9334 National Health Information Center
PO Box 1133   310-565-4167
Washington, DC 20013   800-336-4797
                                              Fax: 301-984-4256
                                        e-mail: info@nhic.org
                                            www.health.gov/nhic
Offers a nationwide information referral service, produces directories and resource guides.

Pamphlets

9335 Classification of Tuberculosis and Other Mycobacterial Diseases
American Lung Association
1740 Broadway   212-315-8700
New York, NY 10019-4315
Chart listing different classes of tuberculosis and other mycobacterial diseases.

9336 Facts About Tuberculosis
American Lung Association
1740 Broadway   212-315-8700
New York, NY 10019-4315
Primary public information leaflet on TB as well as on its impact and treatment.
8 pages

9337 TB Skin Test
American Lung Association
1740 Broadway   212-315-8700
New York, NY 10019-4315
Primary public information leaflet on the TB skin test.
8 pages

9338 TB: What You Should Know
American Lung Association of Connecticut
45 Ash Street   860-289-5401
East Hartford, CT 06108-3294   800-586-4872
                                              Fax: 860-289-5405
                                                   www.alact.org
Offers a brief overview of tuberculosis, how transmission is possible, and TB skin testing.
John E Zinn, President/CEO

9339 This is Mr. TB Germ
American Lung Association
1740 Broadway   212-315-8700
New York, NY 10019-4315
Lively booklet of drawings and very brief text giving a basic description of TB and its treatments.
20 pages

Web Sites

9340 American Lung Association
                                                   www.lung.org
Offers research, medical updates, fund-raising, educational materials and public awareness campaigns relating to lung disease and related disorders.

9341 Healing Well
                                              www.healingwell.org
An online health resource guide to medical news, chat, information and articles, newsgroups and message boards, books, disease-related web sites, medical directories, and more for patients, friends, and family coping with disabling diseases, disorders, or chronic illnesses.

9342 Health Finder
                                              www.healthfinder.gov
Searchable, carefully developed web site offering information on over 1000 topics. Developed by the US Department of Health and Human Services, the site can be used in both English and Spanish.

9343 Healthlink USA
                                              www.healthlinkusa.com
Health information concerning treatment, cures, prevention, diagnosis, risk factors, research, support groups, email lists, personal stories and much more. Updated regularly.

9344 Helios Health
                                              www.helioshealth.com
Online resource for your health information. Detailed information about specific health topics, access to expert advice from our Medical Advisory Board, and up-to-date health news.

9345 MedicineNet
                                              www.medicinenet.com
An online resource for consumers providing easy-to-read, authoritative medical and health information.

9346 Medscape
                                              www.medscape.com
Medscape offers specialists, primary care physicians, and other health professionals the Web's most robust and integrated medical information and educational tools.

9347 National Institute of Allergy & Inf. Dis.
                                              www.niaid.nih.gov
NIAID conducts and supports basic and applied research to better understand, treat, and ultimately prevent infectious, immunologic, and allergic diseases.

9348 WebMD
                                                   www.webmd.com
Provides credible information, supportive communities, and in-depth reference material about health subjects. A source for original and timely health information as well as material from well known content providers.

Description

9349 ## Tuberous Sclerosis

Tuberous sclerosis is a genetic disorder that causes benign, (non-cancerous) tumors to form in different locations - primarily in the brain, skin, kidneys, heart, lungs and even eyes. The name is derived from tuber-like growths on the brain that become hard. It usually shows itself in infancy or early childhood, and may cause seizures and/or mental retardation. It is inherited through chromosome 9 or 16. Disease severity is highly variable, even within the same family. Those with tuberous sclerosis can have mental retardation as well as seizures.

There are various skin abnormalities that may provide a clue to the diagnosis when an infant or young child exhibits seizures or delayed development. The first is an area of decreased skin pigmentation, called an ash-leaf spot because of its shape. Multiple ash-leaf spots may appear on the trunk and limbs during infancy. At age 3 or 4, tiny red bumps, adenoma sebaceum, resembling acne may appear on the nose and cheeks. Finally, a roughened spot with the consistency of orange peel, shagren patch, may appear over the lower spine.

There is no cure so treatment is based on symptoms and can include anti-epileptic drugs for seizures, removal of skin lesions, treatment of high blood pressure caused by kidney problems, special education and, in some instances, surgery to remove growing tumors.

National Agencies & Associations

9350 **National Tuberous Sclerosis Association**
801 Roeder Road
Sliver Spring, MD 20910
301-562-9890
800-225-6872
Fax: 301-562-9870
e-mail: info@tsalliance.org
www.ntsa.org
A voluntary nonprofit organization that is dedicated to fostering and supporting tuberous sclerosis research; to provide education of the public educators and health care professionals; and to providing support of individuals with tuberous sclerosis.
Kari Luther Carlson, President & Chief Executive Officer
Gail Alexander, Senior Manager of Operations

9351 **Rare Cancer Alliance**
www.rare-cancer.org
RCA's primary purpose is to disseminate information and provide support to all pediatric (childhood) and adult rare cancer patients.

9352 **Tuberous Sclerosis Alliance**
801 Roeder Road
Silver Spring, MD 20910
301-562-9890
800-225-6872
Fax: 301-562-9870
e-mail: info@tsalliance.org
www.tsalliance.org
Tuberous sclerosis complex (TSC) is a genetic disorder that causes non-malignant tumors to form in many different organs, primarily in the brain, eyes, heart, kidney, skin and lungs.
Kari Luther Rosbeck, President/ CEO
Richard Gollub, Controller/ CFO

9353 **Tuberous Sclerosis Complex International**
801 Roeder Road
Silver Spring, MD 20708
301-562-9890
e-mail: ksmith@tsalliance.org
www.tscinternational.org
Tuberous Sclerosis Complex International (TSCi) is a world-wide consortium of existing tuberous sclerosis complex associations and organizations, serving as an avenue to empower those affected by tuberous sclerosis complex (TSC), including individuals, families, caregivers, educators and health care providers.

Support Groups & Hotlines

9354 **National Health Information Center**
PO Box 1133
Washington, DC 20013
310-565-4167
800-336-4797
Fax: 301-984-4256
e-mail: info@nhic.org
www.health.gov/nhic
Offers a nationwide information referral service, produces directories and resource guides.

Books

9355 **Tuberous Sclerosis**
Oxford University Press
2001 Evans Road
Cary, NC 27513
800-445-9714
Fax: 919-677-1303
e-mail: custserv.us@oup.com
www.oup-usa.org
A revision offering up-to-date medical information to families, researchers, and professionals on TS.

ISBN: 0-195122-10-0

Newsletters

9356 **NTSA Perspective**
National Tuberous Sclerosis Association
801 Roeder Road
Silver Spring, ML 20910-2226
301-562-9890
800-225-6872
Fax: 301-562-9870
e-mail: info@tsalliance.org
www.ntsa.org
Offers the latest research and medical information on tuberous sclerosis to physicians and health care professionals.
Quarterly
Laura Lubbers, Chair
David Fitzmaurice, Vice Chair

Web Sites

9357 **Healing Well**
www.healingwell.com
An online health resource guide to medical news, chat, information and articles, newsgroups and message boards, books, disease-related web sites, medical directories, and more for patients, friends, and family coping with disabling diseases, disorders, or chronic illnesses.

9358 **Health Finder**
www.healthfinder.gov
Searchable, carefully developed web site offering information on over 1000 topics. Developed by the US Department of Health and Human Services, the site can be used in both English and Spanish.

9359 **Healthlink USA**
www.healthlinkusa.com
Health information concerning treatment, cures, prevention, diagnosis, risk factors, research, support groups, email lists, personal stories and much more. Updated regularly.

9360 **Helios Health**
www.helioshealth.com
Online resource for your health information. Detailed information about specific health topics, access to expert advice from our Medical Advisory Board, and up-to-date health news.

9361 **MedicineNet**
www.medicinenet.com
An online resource for consumers providing easy-to-read, authoritative medical and health information.

9362 Medscape

www.medscape.com

Medscape offers specialists, primary care physicians, and other health professionals the Web's most robust and integrated medical information and educational tools.

9363 National Tuberous Sclerosis Association

www.ntsa.org

The Tuberous Sclerosis Alliance is dedicated to finding a cure for tuberous sclerosis complex (TSC) while improving the lives of those affected.

9364 WebMD

www.webmd.com

Provides credible information, supportive communities, and in-depth reference material about health subjects. A source for original and timely health information as well as material from well known content providers.

Description

9365 Turner Syndrome

Turner syndrome is a genetic disorder that occurs in 1 in 2,500 to 10,000 live female births. It only affects females because, rather than having two female sex (X) chromosomes, Turner syndrome patients have only one. The disease usually hinders sexual development and produces small stature and varying degrees of mental retardation. There may be associated anomalies such as webbed neck and defects of the heart or aorta, which may occur in up to 25 percent of individuals.

Turner syndrome cannot be cured, but hormonal treatment may give the patient a more normal life. Growth hormone injections can help the patient reach a taller adult height, and estrogen replacement can encourage breast development and other sex characteristics. A few patients will develop menstrual periods spontaneously, and a few have become pregnant; most, however, are infertile. Psychological support for the patient and her family is important.

National Agencies & Associations

9366 Human Growth Foundation: Turner Syndrome Division
997 Glen Cove Avenue
Glen Head, NY 11545-1554
800-451-6434
Fax: 516-671-4055
e-mail: hgf1@hgfound.org
www.hgfound.org
A nonprofit, national organization committed to expanding and accelerating research into growth and growth disorders, provides education and support to those affected by growth disorders and their families and fosters the exchange of information.
Pisit PITUKCHEEWANONT,, President
Emily Germain-Lee, Vice President

9367 MAGIC Foundation for Children's Growth: Turner's Syndrome Division
6645 W N Avenue
708-383-0808
Oak Park, IL 60302-1376
800-362-4423
Fax: 708-383-0899
e-mail: dianne@magicfoundation.org
www.magicfoundation.org
A national nonprofit organization created to provide support services for the families of children afflicted with a wide variety of chronic and/or critical disorders that affect a child's growth.
Rich Buckley, Chairman
Ken Dickard, Vice Chairman

9368 Turner's Syndrome Society of Canada
323 Chapel Street
613-321-2267
Ottawa, K1N
800-465-6744
Fax: 613-321-2268
e-mail: tssincan@web.net
www.turnersyndrome.ca
International society providing support services, educational information and activities to persons with Turner's Syndrome, their families and the professionals who work with them.

9369 Turner's Syndrome Society of the United States
11250 W Road
832-912-6006
Houston, TX 77065
800-365-9944
Fax: 832-912-6446
e-mail: tssus@turnersyndrome.org
www.turnersyndrome.org
Through this society members have available a host of informational and support services including consultation services a resource center offering access to the most recently published articles on Turner's Syndrome conferences and advocacy.
Cindy Scurlock, Executive Director
Deborah Rios, Member Services Director

State Agencies & Associations

California

9370 Bay Area Turner Syndrome Society
Moraga, CA 94556
925-846-0608
e-mail: jenakiko@aol.com
www.turnersyndrome.org

Jennifer Saito, Contact

Colorado

9371 Turner's Syndrome Society of Rocky Mountain
Longmount, CO 80501
303-774-0720
e-mail: bpblick@earthlink.net
www.turnersyndrome.org

Brian Blick, President

Florida

9372 Florida Southwest Turner Syndrome Society
Orlando, FL 33919
407-859-3131
e-mail: cjubelt@affirmativemanagement.com
www.turnersyndrome.org

Lauren Jubelt, Leader

9373 Turner's Syndrome Society of South Florida
5215 N Dixie Highway
945-815-9100
Oakland Park, FL 33334
e-mail: tigger3927@aol.com
www.turnersyndrome.org

Rachel Nowak, Leader

Georgia

9374 Georgia Atlanta Turner Syndrome Society
10635 Jones Bridge Road
770-918-3120
Alpharetta, GA 30022
e-mail: jbrownlee@rockdale.org
www.turnersyndrome.org

Judy Brownlee, Contact

Illinois

9375 Metro Chicago Turner Syndrome Society
5467 S Ingleside #3E
773-667-1364
Chicago, IL 60615
e-mail: sgfhoff@sbcglobal.net
www.turnersyndrome.org

Susan Hoffman, President

Indiana

9376 Indiana Chapter Turner Syndrome Society
2030 S Odell Street
317-858-9398
Brownsburg, IN 46112
e-mail: candjgarland@yahoo.com
www.turnersyndrome.org

Connie Garland, Contact

Iowa

9377 Turner's Syndrome Society of Iowa
2615 Meadow Glen Road
515-292-2757
Ames, IA 50014-8238
e-mail: mkepolashek@msn.com
www.turnersyndrome.org

Mary Kay Polashek, Leader

Massachusetts

9378 Southern New England Turner Syndrome Society
1034 Maple Street
401-732-2136
Mansfield, MA 02048
e-mail: deb_pomerantz@hotmail.com
www.turnersyndrome.org

Deborah Pomerantz, Leader

Michigan

9379 Michigan Chapter: Southeast
146 Meadow Lane Circle
Rochester Hills, MI 48307   248-608-6127
e-mail: ksemrau@aol.com
www.turnersyndrome.org

Kim Semrau, President

Minnesota

9380 MN Chapter of the Turner Syndrome Society
1531 American Blvd E
Bloomington, MN 55425   952-854-1224
e-mail: jleon101@hotmail.com
www.tssminnesota.org

Julie Leon, Contact

Missouri

9381 Kansas/Missouri- Turner Syndrome Society
Chapter Headquarters
6721 E 127th Street
Grandview, MO 64030   816-763-9550
Fax: 816-763-8884
e-mail: tsskc@hotmail.com
www.tsskc.com

Dennis McKenzie, Co-President
Carolyn McKenzie, Vice-President

9382 Missouri/St. Louis Turner Syndrome Society
8831 Madge
Brentwood, MO 63144   314-963-0565
e-mail: loch5@juno.com
www.turnersyndrome.org

Mary Jo Lochmoeller, Co-President

New Hampshire

9383 Northern New England Turner Society
38 Beaman Street
Laconia, NH 03246   603-524-6011
e-mail: tssnnepa@hotmail.com
www.turnersyndrome.org

Lori Ann Pawlowski, Leader

New Jersey

9384 New Jersey Metroplitan Turner Syndrome Society Association
107 Crabapple Lane
Franklin Park, NJ 08823   732-217-3021
e-mail: tssusnj@turnersyndromenj.com
www.turnersyndrome.org

Laura Fasciano, Contact

New York

9385 Turner Syndrome Support Group of Central New York
476 Ford Hill Road
Berkshire, NY 13736   607-223-4142
e-mail: tlkwwjd@frontiernet.net
www.turnersyndrome.org

Tammy Kozak, President

9386 Turner's Syndrome Society New York - Metro
215 E 95th Street #24M
New York, NY 10128   607-223-4142
e-mail: tlkwwjd@frontiernet.net
www.turnersyndrome.org

Tammy Kozak, Contact

North Carolina

9387 North Carolina Turner Syndrome Society
1223 Pine Springs Drive
Hendersonville, NC 28739   828-699-1088
e-mail: inmydna@charter.net
www.turnersyndrome.org

Cheryl Tuttle, Contact

Ohio

9388 Turner Syndrome Chapter of Ohio
3333 Burnet Avenue ML 5006
Cincinnati, OH 45229   513-697-0941
e-mail: lwestcott@fuse.net
www.turnersyndrome.org

Leslie Westcott, Contact

Oklahoma

9389 Turner Syndrome Chapter of Oklahoma
5904 E Lattimer
Tulsa, OK 74115-6728   918-838-7355
www.turnersyndrome.org

Jean Radtke, Contact

Pennsylvania

9390 Philadelphia Turner Syndrom Society
169 Trappe Lane
Langhorne, PA 19047   215-752-4405
e-mail: wolfepac5@comcast.net
www.turnersyndrome.org
This society covers the 5 surrounding counties of Philadelphia, along with Eastern Pennsylvania, Delaware and Southern New Jersey.
Eileen Wolfe, President

9391 SW Pennsylvania Turner Syndrome Support Gr oup
3110 Westchester
Pittsburgh, PA 15238   412-767-4321
e-mail: fay_larkin@pghcorning.com
www.turnersyndrome.org

Fay Larkin, Contact

Rhode Island

9392 Rhode Island Turner Syndrome Society
24 Turner Street
Warwick, RI 02886   401-732-2136
e-mail: deb_pomerantz@hotmail.com
www.turnersyndrome.org

Debbie Pomerantz, Contact

South Carolina

9393 South Carolina Palmetto Turner Syndrome So ciety
153 Gannet Point Road
Beaufort, SC 29902   843-521-4461
e-mail: auntrobin74@yahoo.com
www.turnersyndrome.org

Robin Butler, Contact

Texas

9394 Turner's Syndrome Society
11250 W Road
Houston, TX 77065   832-912-6006
800-365-9944
Fax: 832-912-6446
e-mail: tssus@turnersyndrome.org
www.turnersyndrome.org

Cindy Scurlock, Executive Director
Deborah Rios, Member Services Director

9395 Turner's Syndrome Society of Texas
11250 W Road
Houston, TX 77065   832-912-6006
800-365-9944
Fax: 832-912-6446
e-mail: tssus@turnersyndrome.org
www.turnersyndrome.org

Cindy Scurlock, Executive Director
Deborah Rios, Member Services Director

Washington

9396 Washington Puget Sound Turner Syndrome Society
12321 22nd Street NE
Seattle, WA 98125   206-417-6776
e-mail: pugetsoundtss@gmail.com
www.turnersyndrome.org

Larin Amos, President

Libraries & Resource Centers

9397 Turner Syndrome Society Resource Center
Turner Syndrome Society of the United States
11250 W Road
Houston, TX 77065   832-912-6006
800-365-9944
Fax: 832-912-6446
e-mail: tssus@turnersyndrome.org
www.turnersyndrome.org

The Turner Syndrome Society of the US creates awareness, promotes research, and provides support for all persons touched by Turner Syndrome.
Cindy Scurlock, Executive Director
Deborah Rios, Member Services Director

Support Groups & Hotlines

9398 National Health Information Center
PO Box 1133
Washington, DC 20013
310-565-4167
800-336-4797
Fax: 301-984-4256
e-mail: info@nhic.org
www.health.gov/nhic
Offers a nationwide information referral service, produces directories and resource guides.

Newsletters

9399 Turner's Syndrome News
Turner's Syndrome Society of the United States
11250 West Road
Houston, TX 77065-4509
832-912-6006
800-365-9944
Fax: 832-912-6446
www.turner-syndrome-us.org
Includes articles addressing current issues in Turner's Syndrome, updates on national and local activities and letters from girls and women with Turner's syndrome and their families.
Quarterly
Trudy McCarthy, President
Emily Havrilak, Secretary

Pamphlets

9400 Answers to Some Commonly Asked Questions
Turner's Syndrome Society of the United States
11250 West Road
Houston, TX 77065-4509
832-912-6006
800-365-9944
Fax: 832-912-6446
www.turner-syndrome-us.org
Offers information on the Society's activities and the role they play in supporting people with Turner's syndrome.
Trudy McCarthy, President
Emily Havrilak, Secretary

9401 Facing the Challenges of Turner's Syndrome Together
Turner's Syndrome Society of the United States
11250 West Road
Houston, TX 77065-4509
832-912-6006
800-365-9944
Fax: 832-912-6446
www.turner-syndrome-us.org
A brochure offering information on Turner's syndrome, statistics on how widespread the disease is and the Society's role in conquering this disease and supporting their members.
Trudy McCarthy, President
Emily Havrilak, Secretary

9402 Facts About Turner's Syndrome
Turner's Syndrome Society of the United States
11250 West Road
Houston, TX 77065-4509
832-912-6006
800-365-9944
Fax: 832-912-6446
www.turner-syndrome-us.org
Offers statistical and factual information on the disease of Turner's syndrome, causes, symptoms, prevention and treatment.
Trudy McCarthy, President
Emily Havrilak, Secretary

9403 How to Start a Turner's Syndrome Support Group
Turner's Syndrome Society of the United States
11250 West Road
Houston, TX 77065-4509
832-912-6006
800-365-9944
Fax: 832-912-6446
www.turner-syndrome-us.org
Offers information to the lay person on how to obtain material from medical professionals, publicity aspects and funding aspects in pertaining to starting a support group.
Trudy McCarthy, President
Emily Havrilak, Secretary

9404 Turner's Syndrome Society Resource Bibliographies
Turner's Syndrome Society of the United States
11250 West Road
Houston, TX 77065-4509
832-912-6006
800-365-9944
Fax: 832-912-6446
www.turner-syndrome-us.org
These fact sheets offer information on books, videos and other resources available on Turner's syndrome.
Trudy McCarthy, President
Emily Havrilak, Secretary

9405 Turner's Syndrome: A Guide for Families
Turner's Syndrome Society of the United States
11250 West Road
Houston, TX 77065-4509
832-912-6006
800-365-9944
Fax: 832-912-6446
www.turner-syndrome-us.org
Offers information to parents on the causes, symptoms, diagnosis and prognosis of Turner'syndrome, includes resources of where to go for help and support.
Trudy McCarthy, President
Emily Havrilak, Secretary

9406 Turner's Syndrome: A Personal Perspective
Turner's Syndrome Society of the United States
11250 West Road
Houston, TX 77065-4509
832-912-6006
800-365-9944
Fax: 832-912-6446
www.turner-syndrome-us.org
A reprint from the Adolescent and Pediatric Gynecology Journal offering a personal account of a woman with Turner's syndrome and her experiences.
Trudy McCarthy, President
Emily Havrilak, Secretary

9407 Turner's Syndrome: Hows and Whys of the Missing X Chromosome
Human Growth Foundation
997 Glencove Ave
Glen Head, NY 11545-1554
516-671-4041
800-451-6434
Fax: 516-671-4055
e-mail: hgf1@hgfound.org
www.hgfound.org
Provides a brief overview for parents about Turner's Syndrome.
Pisit Pitukcheewanont, President
Patricia D Costa, Executive Director

Web Sites

9408 Healing Well
www.healingwell.com
An online health resource guide to medical news, chat, information and articles, newsgroups and message boards, books, disease-related web sites, medical directories, and more for patients, friends, and family coping with disabling diseases, disorders, or chronic illnesses.

9409 Health Finder
www.healthfinder.gov
Searchable, carefully developed web site offering information on over 1000 topics. Developed by the US Department of Health and Human Services, the site can be used in both English and Spanish.

9410 Healthlink USA
www.healthlinkusa.com
Health information concerning treatment, cures, prevention, diagnosis, risk factors, research, support groups, email lists, personal stories and much more. Updated regularly.

9411 Helios Health
www.helioshealth.com

Online resource for your health information. Detailed information about specific health topics, access to expert advice from our Medical Advisory Board, and up-to-date health news.

9412 Human Growth Foundation

hgfound.org

The focus and emphasis of the Foundation objectives vary with the opportunities to provide support, services, and education to children with disorders of growth and adults with growth hormone deficiency, and to the medical profession; and, with the availability of funding and communications media to support the programs and activities, and general office operations necessary to provide them.

9413 MAGIC Foundation for Children's Growth: Turner's Syndrome Division

www.magicfoundation.org

National organization created to provide support services for the families of children afflicted with a wide variety of chronic and/or critical disorders that affect a child's growth.

9414 MedicineNet

www.medicinenet.com

An online resource for consumers providing easy-to-read, authoritative medical and health information.

9415 Medscape

www.medscape.com

Medscape offers specialists, primary care physicians, and other health professionals the Web's most robust and integrated medical information and educational tools.

9416 Turner's Syndrome Society of the United States

www.turner-syndrome-us.org

Through this society, members have available a host of informational and support services including consultation services, a resource center offering access to the most recently published articles on Turner's syndrome, conferences, advocacy, information and referral services and public relations activities.

9417 WebMD

www.webmd.com

Provides credible information, supportive communities, and in-depth reference material about health subjects. A source for original and timely health information as well as material from well known content providers.

Description

9418 Ulcerative Colitis

Ulcerative colitis is an inflammatory condition of the large bowel, or colon. The cause is unknown, but there is a strong genetic association. First degree relatives have a 3 to 9 percent lifetime risk of the disease, and the illness is much more common in certain racial groups.

Inflammation of the wall of the bowel leads to ulcerations of its surface. Symptoms include weight loss, fatigue, abdominal pain, and diarrhea, which may be bloody. Ulcerative colitis in patients who have a specific antibody in their system (HLA-B27) has a strong association with an arthritis called ankylosing spondylitis. Several kinds of liver and biliary tract disease, inflammation of the eye, and certain characteristic skin rashes may occur.

Treatment depends on the severity of symptoms. Mild cases may respond to simple anti-diarrheal medicines. More severe cases are treated with either rectal or oral forms of 5-ASA, marketed under several trade names. Corticosteroids are sometimes necessary. Disease confined to the rectum can generally be managed with steroid enemas. Extensive disease requires oral steroid medication. Immunosuppressive drugs like azathioprine and 6-mercaptopurine are sometimes given if the disease is resistant to steroids or if steroid side effects are unacceptable. Twenty percent of patients will eventually have their entire colon removed, which cures the disease.

After many years of active ulcerative there is an increased risk of colon cancer. It is usually preceded by warning signs visible on colonoscopy, so physicians generally begin an aggressive surveillance program after 8 to 10 years of disease.

National Agencies & Associations

9419 American Gastroenterological Association
4930 Del Ray Avenue
Bethesda, MD 20814
301-654-2055
Fax: 301-654-5920
e-mail: member@gastro.org
www.gastro.org
Dedicated to the mission of advancing the science and practice of gastroenterology. As the oldest specialty medical society in the United States the membership includes physicians and scientists who research diagnose and treat disorders.
Anil K. Rustgi, President
Michael H Camillarie, Vice President

9420 Crohn's & Colitis Foundation of America
386 Park Avenue S
New York, NY 10016-8804
212-685-3440
800-932-2423
Fax: 212-779-4098
e-mail: info@ccfa.org
www.ccfa.org
Supports basic and clinical research into a cure and prevent Crohn's disease and ulcerative colitis; conducts professional and patient education activities; produces public service programs and a wide variety of literature about inflammatory bowel disease.
Maura Breen, Chairperson
Vance Gibbs, General Council

9421 National Institute of Diabetes and Digestive Disorders
5 Information Way
31 Center Drive MSC 2560
Bethesda, MD 20892-3568
301-496-3583
800-860-8747
www2.niddk.nih.gov
Offers information and referrals to persons afflicted with ulcerative colitis.
Griffin P. Rodgers, President
Adil Abdalla, Staff

9422 Reach Out for Youth with Ileitis and Colitis
84 Northgate Circle
Melville, NY 11747
631-293-3102
e-mail: info@reachourforyouth.org
www.reachoutforyouth.org
Provides educational seminars and individual and group support to patients and their families. Fundraising efforts support the Center's programs clinical and laboratory research and purchase of state-of-the-art equipment.
Irwin Maltz, President

9423 United Ostomy Association
PO Box 512
Northfield, MN 55057
800-826-0826
Fax: 507-645-5168
e-mail: info@uoaa.org
www.uoa.org
A national network for bowel and urinary diversion support groups in the United States. Its goal is to provide a nonprofit association that will serve to unify and strengthen its member support groups, which are organized for the benefit of people who have, or will have intestinal or urinary diversions and their caregivers.
David Rudzin, President
Susan Burns, Vice Presdient

Support Groups & Hotlines

9424 National Health Information Center
PO Box 1133
Washington, DC 20013
310-565-4167
800-336-4797
Fax: 301-984-4256
e-mail: info@nhic.org
www.health.gov/nhic
Offers a nationwide information referral service, produces directories and resource guides.

Books

9425 Alive and Kicking
Rolf Benirschke Enterprises
PO Box 9922
Rancho Santa Fe, CA 92067-4922
800-571-4770
www.obrien.ie
Football star writes of his struggle with ulcerative colitis.

9426 Ask Audrey
7466 Pebble Lane
West Bloomfield, MI 48322-3521
248-626-6960
A compilation of material and the personal story of a medical psychotherapist who has inflammatory bowel disease. Includes practical tips on issues such as handling diarrhea, sexuality, relationships, traveling, coping with hospital stays, ostomies, and TPN.

9427 IBD Nutrition Book
John Wiley & Sons
1 Wiley Drive
Somerset, NJ 08873-1222
800-225-5945
Clinical dietitian/nutritionist's overview of the role of diet in IBD, including recipes and meal plans.

9428 Inflammatory Bowel Disease
Williams & Wilkins
351 W Camden Street
Baltimore, MD 21201-7912
410-528-4398
800-638-0672
Fax: 215-701-2407
e-mail: liana.watson@wolterskluwer.com
www.wkadcenter.com

Detailed information on every aspect of IBD. Topics include medical and surgical management, epidemiology, fertility and pregnancy, psychosocial factors, and diagnostic techniques. Written for medical professionals and laypersons who are comfortable with medical terminology.
Liana Watson, Production Associate

Children's Books

9429 You're Bigger Than it
Hotel Dieu Hospital   613-544-3310
Ontario, Canada,
This cartoon book offers a lively, brief introduction to the basics of living with IBD. Contact can be reached at extension 2400.

Magazines

9430 Phoenix Magazine
United Ostomy Association of America
PO Box 512
Northfield, MN 55057   800-826-0826
                                             Fax: 507-645-5168
                                         e-mail: info@uoaa.org
                                                  www.uoa.org
America's leading ostomy patient magazine providing colostomy, ileostomy, urostomy and continent diversion information, management techniques, new products and much more.
Quarterly
Susan Burns, President

Newsletters

9431 Inner Circle
Reach Out for Youth with Ileitis and Colitis
540 E. Canfield   631-293-3102
Detroit, MI 48025   e-mail: bmawsu@gmail.com
                                         www.reachoutforyouth.org
Newsletter for youth with ileitis and colitis.
Irwin Maltz, President
Carolyn King, Co-Founder

Pamphlets

9432 Bleeding in the Digestive Tract
Nat'l Digestive Diseases Information Clearinghouse
9000 Rockville Pike
Bethesda, MD 20892-0001   301-496-6344
                                               www.medhelp.org
Informational fact sheet.

9433 Inside Story
Reach Out for Youth with Ileitis and Colitis
540 E. Canfield   631-293-2102
Detroit, MI 48025   e-mail: bmawsu@gmail.com
                                         www.reachoutforyouth.org
Educational brochure for youth with illeitis and colitis.
Irwin Maltz, President
Carolyn King, Co-Founder

9434 Ulcerative Colitis
National Organization For Rare Disorders
55 Kenosia Avenue   203-744-0100
Danbury, CT 06810-8923   Fax: 203-798-2291
                                  e-mail: orphan@rarediseases.org
                                           www.rarediseases.org
The National Organization for Rare Disorders (NORD), a 501(c)(3) organization, is the leading voice of the rare disease community
Peter L. Saltonstall, President & CEO
Pamela Gavin, Chief Operating Officer

Web Sites

9435 Crohn's & Colitis Foundation of America
                                                  www.ccfa.org
Supports basic and clinical research into a cure and prevent Crohn's disease and ulcerative colitis; conducts professional and patient education activities; produces public service programs and a wide variety of literature about inflammatory bowel disease for patients and their families, professionals and the public; and sponsors chapters nationwide.

9436 Healing Well
                                             www.healingwell.com
An online health resource guide to medical news, chat, information and articles, newsgroups and message boards, books, disease-related web sites, medical directories, and more for patients, friends, and family coping with disabling diseases, disorders, or chronic illnesses.

9437 Health Finder
                                             www.healthfinder.gov
Searchable, carefully developed web site offering information on over 1000 topics. Developed by the US Department of Health and Human Services, the site can be used in both English and Spanish.

9438 Healthlink USA
                                             www.healthlinkusa.com
Health information concerning treatment, cures, prevention, diagnosis, risk factors, research, support groups, email lists, personal stories and much more. Updated regularly.

9439 Helios Health
                                             www.helioshealth.com
Online resource for your health information. Detailed information about specific health topics, access to expert advice from our Medical Advisory Board, and up-to-date health news.

9440 MedicineNet
                                             www.medicinenet.com
An online resource for consumers providing easy-to-read, authoritative medical and health information.

9441 Medscape
                                              www.medscape.com
Medscape offers specialists, primary care physicians, and other health professionals the Web's most robust and integrated medical information and educational tools.

9442 United Ostomy Association
                                                  www.uoa.org
A national network for bowel and urinary diversion support groups in the United States. Its goal is to provide a nonprofit association that will serve to unify and strengthen its member support groups, which are organized for the benefit of people who have, or will have intestinal or urinary diversions and their caregivers.

9443 WebMD
                                                 www.webmd.com
Provides credible information, supportive communities, and in-depth reference material about health subjects. A source for original and timely health information as well as material from well known content providers.

Description

9444 Visual Impairment

Visual impairment encompasses a wide variety of disorders of the eye. It includes damage to the cornea or retina (macular degeneration or secondary to diabetes), cataracts, glaucoma, muscular imbalance, infections, congenital disorders and those associated with premature birth. Occasionally visual impairment reflects a disease behind the eye, involving some part of the brain that receives and processes images from the eyes.

Visual impairment covers a continuum from decreased visual acuity correctible by refractive means (glasses and contact lenses) to legal blindness, indicating less than 20/200 vision in the better eye, or an extremely limited field of vision. Totally blind represents the complete loss of sight.

Many health problems and eye injuries lead to visual impairment. Half a million Americans are visually impaired, and an additional 50,000 lose their sight each year. Cataracts account for one third of all visual impairments and cause 16 persons to lose their sight every day. Glaucoma causes vision impairment in 2 million persons. One thousand eye injuries resulting in some level of vision impairment occur in the workplace or home each day. Diabetic retinopathy is one of the leading causes of the new cases of blindness. Retinitis pigmentosa, a degeneration of the light-sensing tissue at the back of the eye, also causes vision (especially night vision) deterioration.

Depending on the cause of vision loss, the condition may be fully or partially correctible through surgery or visual aids. Sometimes treatment will not reverse prior losses, but will slow the progression of vision loss. When the visual loss cannot be reversed, a variety of supportive devices and services, improved over the past twenty years, can greatly enhance the person's functional status and quality of life.

Technology has played an increasing role in helping the visually impaired function in their daily lives. Recently, doctors implanted the first artificial retina, and relatively new laser technology allows eye specialists to surgically treat extreme degrees of nearsightedness and astigmatism (blurred vision caused by uneven curvature of the eye).

National Agencies & Associations

9445 ACB Radio Amateurs
2200 Wilson Boulevard
Arlington, VA 22201

202-467-5081
800-424-8666
Fax: 703- 46- 508
e-mail: info@acb.org
www.acb.org

A radio amateur network of blind, visually impaired and sighted members who gather and share common problems and solutions to help members improve radio amateurs in getting started, provides access to educational materials in special media and publishes a newsletter.
Mitch Pomerantz, President
Kim Charlson, First Vice President

9446 Alliance for Aging Research
750 17th St.,
Washington, DC 20006

202-293-2856
Fax: 202-785-8574
e-mail: info@agingresearch.org
www.agingresearch.org

Alliance for Aging Research is the nation's leading citizen advocacy organization for improving the health and independence of Americans as they age. It was founded to promote medical and behavioral research into the aging process.
Daniel P Perry, Executive Director
Sarah Rhyne, Executive Coordinator

9447 American Academy of Ophthalmology
655 Beach St.
San Francisco, CA 94109-7424

415-561-8500
Fax: 415-561-8533
e-mail: customer_service@aao.org
www.aao.org

Sponsors National Eye Care Project that gives free eye care to the elderly.

9448 American Association of the Deaf-Blind
PO Box 2831
Kensington, MD 20891-4500

301-495-4403
Fax: 301-495-4404
TTY: 301-495-4402
e-mail: AADB-Info@aadb.org
www.aadb.org

Promotes better opportunities and services for deaf-blind people. The mission of this organization is to assure that a comprehensive coordinated system of services is accessible to all deaf-blind people, enabling them to achieve their maximum potential.
35-50 pages 600 Members
Jamie McNama Pope, Executive Director
Elizabeth Spiers, Director of Information Services

9449 American Coucnil of the Blind Impairment
1155 15th Street NW Suite 1004
Washington, DC 20005

202-467-5081
800-424-8666
Fax: 202-467-5085
e-mail: cindybur@comcast.net
www.acb.org

A network of blind or visually impaired people that offers support and outreach, shares experiences and exchanges information.
Cindy Burgett, President

9450 American Council of Blind Lions
148 Vernon Avenue
Louisville, KY 40206

502-897-1472
Fax: 502-721-9929
e-mail: adam148@bellsouth.net
www.acb.org/acbl

The American Council of Blind Lions (ACBL) is a specially chartered Lions club. The goal of this club is to assist other Lions clubs in understanding the issues surrounding people who are blind or visually impaired.
Adam Ruschival, President

9451 American Council of the Blind
2200 Wilson Boulevard
Arlington, VA 22201-2706

202-467-5081
800-424-8666
Fax: 703-465-5085
e-mail: info@acb.org
www.acb.org

A national membership organization whose members are visually impaired and fully sighted individuals who are concerned about dignity and well-being of blind people throughout America. Formed in 1961, the Council has become the largest organization of blind individuals.
Mitch Pomerantz, President

9452 American Foundation for the Blind
2 Penn Plaza
New York, NY 10121

212-502-7600
800-232-5463
Fax: 888-545-8331
e-mail: afbinfo@afb.net
www.afb.org

AFB is the cause and organization to which Helen Keller dedicated more than 40 years of her life. In addition to being a national information consultative and advocacy resource engaged in a wide variety of initiatives AFB is home to the Helen Keller Arch.
Carl R Augusto, President/CEO
Richard J O'Brien, Chair

9453 American Foundation for the Blind: National Employment Center
2 Penn Plaza   212-502-7600
New York, NY 10121   Fax: 888-545-8331
                                       e-mail: afbinfo@afb.net
                                                www.afb.org

Leads initiatives in the area of employment. Nationally offers consultation, technical assistance and support and undertakes local and national efforts such as training programs and public education in the area of employment. Responds to inquiries from blind and visually impaired people and thier families, service providers and the general public in the region and nationally.
Richard J O'Brien, Chair
John T Bourger, Vice Chair

9454 American Foundation for the Blind: SE National Literacy Center
100 Peachtree Street   404-525-2303
Atlanta, GA 30303   Fax: 646-478-9260
                                       e-mail: literacy@afb.net
                                                www.afb.org

Leads initiatives in the area of literacy. Offers consultation technical assistance and support and undertakes local and national efforts such as training programs and public education in the area of literacy. Offers training and in-service opportunities.

9455 American Optometric Association
243 N Lindbergh Boulevard   314-991-4100
Saint Louis, MO 63141-7881   800-365-2219
                                       Fax: 314-991-4101
                                       e-mail: PHKehoe@aoa.org
                                               www.aoa.org/?

The AOA and affiliates work to provide the public with quality vision and eye care. It sets professional standards helping its members conduct patient care efficiently and effectively. It also lobbies government and other organizations on behalf of the visually impaired population.
Peter H Kehoe, President
Joe E Ellis, Vice President

9456 American Printing House for the Blind
1839 Frankfort Avenue   502-895-2405
Louisville, KY 40206-0085   800-223-1839
                                       Fax: 502-899-2284
                                       e-mail: info@aph.org
                                                www.aph.org

The oldest nonprofit organization of its kind in the US that creates education, workplace and lifestyle products for visually impaired people. This organization promotes the independence of blind persons by providing special media, tools and materials.
Tuck Tinsley III, President
Bob Brasher, Vice President Advisory Services

9457 Assoc. for Education & Rehabilitation of the Blind & Visually Impaired
1703 N Beauregard Street   703-671-4500
Alexandria, VA 22311   877-492-2708
                                       Fax: 703-671-6391
                                       e-mail: lou@aerbvi.org
                                                www.aerbvi.org

The only professional membership organization dedicated to the advancement of education and rehabilitation of blind and visually impaired children and adults.
Lou Tutt, Executive Director
Ginger Croce, Senior Director, Marketing & Office Oper

9458 Associated Services for the Blind
919 Walnut Street   215-627-0600
Philadelphia, PA 19107-5237   Fax: 215-922-0692
                                       e-mail: asbinfo@asb.org
                                                www.asb.org

Limited funding is available to assist aspiring visually impaired users in the purchase of helpful high tech equipment.
Patricia C Johnson, President/CEO
Derby Ewing, Director, Human Services

9459 Association for Macular Diseases
210 E 64th Street   212-605-3719
New York, NY 10065-7480   Fax: 212-605-3795
                              e-mail: association@retinal-research.org
                                                www.macula.org

A nonprofit corporation to promote education and research in this scarcely-explored field. A nationwide support group for individuals and their families to adjust to the restrictions and changes brought about by macular disease.
Bernard Landou, President
Mary Fern Breheney, Board of Director

9460 Blinded Veterans Association
477 H Street NW   202-371-8880
Washington, DC 20001-2694   800-669-7079
                                       Fax: 202-371-8258
                                       e-mail: bva@bva.org
                                                www.bva.org

The organization seeks and identifies legally blind veterans who need services linking them to appropriate benefits training and opportunities in both the public and the private sectors. It represents blinded veterans before congress.
Paperback
Samuel Huhn, National President
Mark Cornell, National Vice President

9461 Braille Institute of America Library
741 North Vermont Avenue   323-663-1111
Los Angeles, CA 90029-3594   800-272-4553
                                       Fax: 323-663-0867
                                   e-mail: la@brailleinstitute.org
                                            www.brailleinstitute.org

Discs, cassettes, braille, Optacon, home visits, braille writer, reference materials on blindness and other handicaps. Closed-circuit TV, Optacon, braille writer, and large print copier also available. Home visits and cassette books are part of special services offered.
Adama Dyoniziak, Regional Program Director

9462 Canine Companions for Independence
2965 Dutton Ave   707-577-1000
Santa Rosa, CA 95407   800-572-2275
                                       TTY: 707-577-1756
                                       e-mail: info@cci.org
                                                www.cci.org

A non-profit organization that enhances the lives of people with disabilities by providing highly trained assistance dogs and ongoing support to ensure quality partnerships.
Corey Hudson, CEO
Kathy Pierson, Northwest Regional Executive Director

9463 Canine Helpers for the Disabled
5699 Ridge Road   716-433-4035
Lockport, NY 14094   716-433-4035
                                   e-mail: chhdogs@aol.com
                                            www.caninehelpers.org

A non-profit organization devoted to training dogs to assist people with disabilities to lead more independent, secure lives.

9464 Catholic Guild for the Blind Catholic Charities of the Archdiocese of
Catholic Charities of the Archdiocese of New York
65 E. Wacker Place   312-236-8569
Chicago, IL 60601-7463   Fax: 312-236-8128
                              e-mail: info@guildfortheblind.org
                                            www.second-sense.org

A nonprofit organization under the sponsorship of the Catholic Charities of the Archdiocese of New York. Daily living skills, orientation and mobility training, communication skills and bilingual preparation for high school equivalency diplomas are among things covered.
Kathy Austin, Coordinator of Adult Rehabilitation
Lauri Dishman, Manager of Career Services

9465   Council for Exceptional Children
2900 Crystal Drive   703-620-3660
Arlington, VA 22202   888-232-7733
                                      Fax: 703-264-9494
                                      TTY: 866-915-5000
                           e-mail: service@cec.sped.org
                                       www.cec.sped.org
Advocates appropriate policies standards and development for individuals with special needs. Provides professional development for special educators.
Stephanie Ineh, Customer Service Manager
Anitra Davis, Senior Customer Services Representative

9466   Council of Citizens with Low Vision International
1155 15th Street NW   714-630-8098
Washington, DC 20005   800-733-2258
                           e-mail: president@cclvi.org
                                          www.cclvi.org
Affiliated with American Council of the Blind. Promotes the concept that persons with partial sight/low vision are not blind and should have every right to maximize the use of their residual vision.
John Horst, President
Richard Rueda, 1st Vice President

9467   Fidelco Guide Dog Foundation
103 Vision Way   860-243-5200
Bloomfield, CT 06002-0142   Fax: 860-243-7215
                            e-mail: info@fidelco.org
                                          www.fidelco.org
Fidelco breeds raises trains and places German shepherd guide dogs with men and women who are visually impaired primarily in the Northeast. The pioneer of in-community training in this country the visually impaired individual can remain independent.
Roberta C Kaman, Chairman
George J Salpietro, Executive Director

9468   Fight for Sight
381 Park Avenue S   212-679-6060
New York, NY 10016   Fax: 212-679-4466
                          e-mail: info@fightforsight.com
                                     www.fightforsight.com
Voluntary health organization that works to conquer defective sight and blindness. Provides grants to accredited medical colleges and institutions to help supply equipment technical assistance and materials for research projects.
Mary Prudden, Executive Director
Kenneth R Barasch MD, President

9469   Foundation Fighting Blindness
7168 Columbia Gateway Drive   410-423-0600
Columbia, MD 21046   800-683-5555
                                      Fax: 410-872-0438
                                      TTY: 410-363-7139
                                      TDD: 800-683-5551
                       e-mail: info@FightBlindness.org
                                        www.blindness.org
Mission is to drive the research that will provide preventions, treatments, and cures for people affected by retinitis pigmentosa, macular degeneration, Usher syndrome and the entire spectrum of retinal degenerative diseases.
William T Schmidt, CEO

9470   Foundation for Glaucoma Research
251 Post Street   415-986-3162
San Francisco, CA 94108   800-826-6693
                                      Fax: 415-986-3763
                        e-mail: question@glaucoma.org
                                         www.glaucoma.org
A national organization dedicated to protecting the sight of people with glaucoma through research and education. The Foundation conducts and supports research that contributes to improved patient care and a better understanding of the disease process.
Andrew Jackson, Director of Communications
Thomas M Brunner, President and CEO

9471   Foundation for the Advancement of the Blind
4058 Moore Street   310-301-0344
Los Angeles, CA 90066-5118
Helps blind people attain and retain employment.

9472   Friends-In-Art
4317 Vermont Court   573-445-5564
Columbia, MO 65203   800-424-8666
                                      Fax: 202-467-5085
                      e-mail: paltschul@centurytel.net
                                       www.friendsinart.com
Aims to enlarge the art experience of blind people encourages blind people to visit museums galleries concerts the theater etc. offers consultation to program planners in establishing accessible art and museum exhibits.
Peter Altschul, President
Gordon Kent, Board Member

9473   Guide Dog Users
4851 N. Cedar Ave.
Fresno, CA 93726-2245   866-799-8436
                            e-mail: president@gdui.org
                                            www.gdui.org
Promotes the acceptance of blind people and their dogs works for enforcement and expansion of laws admitting guide dogs into public places advocates for quality training and follow-up services.
Laurie Mehta, President
Mary Beth Randall, First Vice President

9474   Guide Dogs for the Blind
PO Box 151200   415-499-4000
San Rafael, CA 94915   800-298-4050
                                      Fax: 415-499-4035
                     e-mail: information@guidedogs.com
                                         www.guidedogs.com
Offers educational materials, transportation seminars, and newsletters for the blind providing 2 field offices.
Etta Allen, Board Chair
Morgan Watkins, Interim CEO

9475   Helen Keller National Center's National Parent Network
141 Middle Neck Road   516-944-8900
Sands Point, NY 11050-1218   Fax: 516-944-7302
                                      TTY: 516-944-8637
                            e-mail: hkncinfo@hknc.org
                                            www.hknc.org
Establishes a coalition of state parent organizations to promote the exchange of information among parents of deaf-blind youth. Provides training to parents to develop their legislative advocacy skills, empowers parents and their families to obtain needed services.
Kathy Mezack, Coordinator of Vocational Services

9476   Independent Visually Impaired Enterprises
230 Robinhood Lane
McMurray, PA 15317   e-mail: lengual@concentric.net
                                             www.acb.org
Strives to broaden vocational opportunities in business for the visually impaired. Works to improve rehabilitation facilities for all types of business enterprises and publicizes the capabilities of blind and visually impaired business persons.
Carla Hayes, President

9477   International Agency for the Prevention of Blindness
National Eye Institute
31 Center Drive MSC 2510
Bethesda, MD 20892-3655   301-496-5248
                                            www.nei.nih.gov
Ophthalmic societies and committees for the prevention of blindness whose members include ophthalmologists public health officers nutritionists geneticists and other health workers. Coordinates international research into the causes of impaired vision.
Carl Kupfer, Volunteer
Paul A Sieving, Director

9478   Library Users of America
2200 Wilson Boulevard   202-467-5081
Arlington, VA 22201   800-424-8666
                                      Fax: 703-465-5085
                              e-mail: info@acb.org
                                             www.acb.org
Provides for chapters in states through the US to encourage the development acquisition and use of technology which enables blind

and visually impaired persons to use printed material independently in library settings and elsewhere.
Barry Levine, President

9479 Lighthouse International Headquarters
111 E 59th Street   212-821-9200
New York, NY 10022-1202   800-821-0500
                                                                  Fax: 212-821-9707
                                                                  TTY: 212-821-9713
                                                     e-mail: info@lighthouse.org
                                                                  www.lighthouse.org

A leading resource worldwide on vision impairment and vision rehabilitation. Pioneer in vision rehabilitation services, education, research and advocacy enabling people of all ages who are blind or partially sighted to lead independent and productive lives.
Roger O Goldman, Chairman
Tara A Cortes, President/CEO

9480 Lions World Services for the Blind Lions Clubs International
Lions Clubs International
2811 Fair Park Boulevard   501-664-7100
Little Rock, AR 72204   800-248-0734
                                                                  Fax: 501-664-2743
                                                     e-mail: training@lwsb.org
                                                                  www.lwsb.org

Lions World Services for the Blind was founded in 1947 to serve people who are blind and visually impaired who needed to learn independent living skills or job training skills that considered the special requirements of their individual visual impairments.
Ramona Sangalli, President and Chief Executive Officer
Larry Morgan, Vice President for Development

9481 Macular Degeneration Foundation
PO Box 515   413-268-7660
Northampton, MA 01061-0515   888-622-8527
                                                     e-mail: amdf@macular.org
                                                                  www.macular.org

The American Macular Degeneration Foundation is committed to the prevention and cure of macular degeneration and offers hope and support to those afflicted and their families.
Chip Goehring, President and Trustee
Mark E Torrey, Vice President and Trustee

9482 National Alliance of Blind Students
2200 Wilson Boulevard   202-467-5081
Arlington, VA 22201   800-424-8666
                                                                  Fax: 703-465-5085
                                                     e-mail: info@acb.org
                                                                  www.acb.org

Works to facilitate progress toward full accessibility of college programs and facilities provides opportunities for discussion of issues important to students and assists with National Student Seminars.
Rebecca Bridges, President

9483 National Association for Parents of the Visually Impaired
PO Box 317   617-972-7441
Watertown, MA 02471-0317   800-562-6265
                                                                  Fax: 781-972-7444
                                                     e-mail: napvi@perkins.org
                                                                  www.napvi.org

The only national organization that strives to serve families of children of all ages and ranges with visual loss. It is a community based organization whose members include parents parent organizations agencies and other persons with common objectives.
Susan LaVenture, Executive Director
Doug Halverson, President

9484 National Association for Visually Handicapped
22 West 21st Street   212-889-3141
New York, NY 10010   888-205-5951
                                                                  Fax: 212-727-2931
                                                     e-mail: navh@navh.org
                                                                  www.navh.org

NAVH ensures that those with limited vision do not lead limited lives. We offer emotional support; training in the use of and access to a wide variety of optical aids and lighting; a large print, nationwide, free-by-mail loan library; large print educational materials;

quarterly newsletter; referrals; self-help groups and educational outreach.
Cesar Gomez, Executive Director

9485 National Association for Visually Hand.
22 W 21st Street   212-889-3141
New York, NY 10010   Fax: 212-727-2931
                                                     e-mail: navh@navh.org
                                                                  www.navh.org

NAVH ensures that those with limited vision do not lead limited lives. We offer emotional support; training in the use of and access to a wide variety of optical aids and lighting and a large print, nationwide, free-by-mail loan library.
Lorraine H Marchi, Founder & CEO
Miriam Rosen, Executive Director

9486 National Association of Blind Educators Sheila Koenig
Sheila Koenig
2200 University Avenue West   651-642-0500
St. Paul, MN 55114   800-652-9000
                                          e-mail: jsanders.nfb@comcast.net
                                                                  www.nfb.org

Membership organization of blind teachers professors and instructors in all levels of education. Provides support and information regarding professional responsibilities classroom techniques national testing methods and career obstacles.
Judy Sanders, President

9487 National Association of Blind Lawyers Scott LaBarre
Scott LaBarre
1660 S Albion Street   303-504-5979
Denver, CO 80222-4046   Fax: 303-757-3640
                                          e-mail: slabarre@labarrelaw.com
                                                                  www.nfb.org

Membership organization of blind attorneys law students judges and others in the law field. Provides support and information regarding employment techniques used by the blind, advocacy, laws affecting the blind and current information about the American legal system.
Scott LaBarre, President

9488 National Association of Blind Musicians Linda Mentink
Linda Mentink
6210 Walker Avenue   402-465-5468
Lincoln, NE 68507-0952   e-mail: amy.buresh74@gmail.com
                                                                  www.nfb.org

Blind persons dedicated to advancing employment and entertainment opportunities in various music fields. Offers support and information regarding copyright publishing promotion and other career details.
Linda Mentik, Chairperson
Amy Buresh, President

9489 National Association of Blind Office Professionals
Lisa Hall
P.O. Box 82055   614-935-6965
Columbus, OH 43202-6104   e-mail: eduffy@pobox.com
                                                                  www.nfb.org

Membership organization of blind secretaries and transcribers at all levels including medical and paralegal transcription office workers customer-service personnel and many other similar fields. Addresses issues such as technology, accommodation and caregivers.
Lisa Hall, President
Eric Duffy, President

9490 National Association of Blind Students Angela Wolf
Angela Wolf
314 E. Highland Mall Boulevard   512-323-5444
Austin, TX 78752-1803   e-mail: kflores@nfbtx.org
                                                                  www.nfb.org

For over 30 years this national organization of blind students has provided support information and encouragement to blind college and university students. Leads the way in offering resources in issues such as national testing and accessible textbooks.
Kimberly Flores, President

9491 National Association of Guide Dog Users Priscilla Ferris
Priscilla Ferris

1003 Papaya Drive
Tampa, FL 33619-3714

813-626-2789
800-558-8261
e-mail: president@nagdu.org
www.nagdu.org

Provides information and support for guide dog users and works to secure high standards in guide dog training. Addresses issues of discrimination of guide dog users and offers public education about guide dog use.
Marion Gwizdala, President

9492 National Association to Promote the Use of Braille
Nadine Jacobson
2200 University Avenue West
St. Paul, MN 55114-1819

651-642-0500
800-652-9000
e-mail: nadine.jacobson@visi.com
www.nfb.org

Dedicated to securing improved Braille instruction increasing the number of Braille materials available to the blind and providing information about the importance of Braille in securing independence education and employment for the blind.
Nadine Jacobson, President

9493 National Braille Association
95 Allens Creek Road
Rochester, NY 14618-2513

585-427-8260
Fax: 585-427-0263
e-mail: nbaoffice@nationalbraille.org
www.nationalbraille.org

Provides transcription service for and maintains a depository of braille books.
Diane Spence, President
Jan Carroll, Vice President

9494 National Braille Press
88 Saint Stephen Street
Boston, MA 02115-4302

617-266-6160
888-965-8965
Fax: 617-437-0456
www.nbp.org

The guiding purposes of National Braille Press are to promote the literacy of blind children through braille and to provide access to information that empowers blind people to actively engage in work family and community affairs.
Paul Parravano, Chair
Gayle L Yarnall, Clerk

9495 National Center for Vision and Aging Lighthouse
Lighthouse
111 E 59th Street
New York, NY 10022-1202

212-821-9200
800-829-0500
Fax: 212-821-9707
TTY: 212-821-9713
TDD: 212-821-9713
e-mail: info@lighthouse.org
www.lighthouse.org

The National Center for Vision and Aging provides information on eye conditions and visual impairment of all ages resources education and professionally prepared multimedia and print material for community education lectures.
Roger O Goldman, Chairman
Tara A Cortes, President and Chief Executive Officer

9496 National Center for Vision and Child Development
Lighthouse
111 E 59th Street
New York, NY 10022

212-821-9200
800-829-0500
Fax: 212-821-9707
TTY: 212-821-9713
e-mail: info@lighthouse.org
www.lighthouse.org

Our mission is to overcome vision impairment for people of all ages through worldwide leadership in rehabilitation services education research prevention and advocacy.
Roger O Goldman, Chairman
Tara A Cortes PhD RN, President and Chief Executive Officer

9497 National Diabetes Action Network for the Blind
National Federation of the Blind
1026 East 36th Street
Baltimore, MD 21218-7337

410-645-0632
Fax: 410-685-5653
e-mail: melissa@riccobono.us
www.nfb.org

Leading support and information organization of persons losing vision due to diabetes. Provides personal contact and resource information with other blind diabetics about non-visual techniques of independently managing diabetes and monitoring glucose levels.
Melissa Riccobono, President
Fredric Schroeder, First Vice President

9498 National Eye Institute National Institutes of Health
National Institutes of Health
31 Center Drive MSC 2510
Bethesda, MD 20892-3655

301-496-5248
www.nei.nih.gov

Mission is to discover safe and effective methods to prevent diagnose and treat diseases and disorders of the visual system. In this way the Institute helps to prevent reduce and possibly eliminate blindness and visual impairment.
Paul A Sieving, Director
Carl Kupfer, Volunteer

9499 National Federation of the Blind
1026 East 36th Street
Baltimore, MD 21218

410-645-0632
Fax: 410-685-5653
e-mail: melissa@riccobono.us
www.nfb.org

The largest consumer membership organization for the blind founded in 1940 it has 50 000 members nationwide in 52 affiliates and over 700 local chapters. Provides public education about blindness, support services to the newly blinded and scholarships.
50M Members
Melissa Riccobono, President
Fredric Schroeder, First Vice President

9500 National Federation of the Blind in Computer Science
Curtis Chong
2721 34th Street
Des Moines, IA 50310-4256

515-771-8348
Fax: 515-281-1361
e-mail: michael.NFBI@gmail.com
www.nfb.org

National organization of blind persons knowledgeable in the computer science and technology fields. Works to develop new technologies, to secure access to current technology and to develop new ways of using current or new technologies by the blind.
Curtis Chong, President

9501 National Federation of the Blind: Blind/Deaf Division
Robert Eschbach
9014 East Bellevue Street
Tucson, AZ 85715-5440

520-733-5894
e-mail: krezguy@cox.net
www.nfb.org

Deaf-blind persons working nationally to improve services, training and independence for the deaf-blind. Offers personal contact with other deaf-blind individuals knowledgeable in advocacy, education, employment, technology, discrimination and other issues surrounding deaf-blindness.
Bob Kresmer, President

9502 National Federation of the Blind: Blind Industrial Workers of America
National Federation of the Blind
1026 East 36th Street
Baltimore, MD 21218-4998

410-645-0632
Fax: 410-685-5653
e-mail: melissa@riccobono.us
www.nfb.org

Membership organization of blind persons employed in industrial and manufacturing work or in government job programs for the blind. Dedicated to protecting the rights of blind workers in salary, job stability, advancement and labor issues.
Melissa Riccobono, President

9503 National Federation of the Blind: Human Services Division
Melissa Riccobono
1026 E 36th Street
Baltimore, MD 21218

410-645-0632
e-mail: melissa@riccobono.us
www.nfb.org

Membership organization of blind persons working in counseling personnel psychology social work psychiatry rehabilitation and other social science and human resource fields. Dedicated to im-

proving employment opportunities and advancement for blind persons.
Melissa Riccobono, President

9504   National Federation of the Blind: Masonic Square Club
Fred Flowers
1026 East 36th Street   410-645-0632
Baltimore, MD 21218-4766   e-mail: melissa@riccobono.us
                                                      www.nfb.org
Blind individuals committed to sharing of Masonic experiences goals and history.
Melissa Riccobono, President

9505   National Federation of the Blind: Public Employees Division
Ivan Weich
3101 Northeast 87th Avenue   360-576-5965
Vancouver, WA 98662-3009   e-mail: k7uij@panix.com
                                                      www.nfb.org
Organization of blind persons holding local state or federal jobs. Focuses on issues such as changes in governmental hiring and retention practices new job skills needed for the future, government employment downsizing, new electronic means of finding employment and more.
Michael Freeman, President

9506   National Federation of the Blind: Science and Engineering Division
John Miller
3934 Kern Court   925-462-8575
Pleasanton, CA 94588-1920   e-mail: j8miller@soe.ucsd.edu
                                                      www.nfb.org
Blind persons with expertise and experience in fields such as genetics, telecommunications, biology, chemistry, physics and nuclear physics or mechanical electronic and chemical engineering. This is a strong support group to encourage blind persons to excel in science and engineering.
John Miller, President

9507   National Federation of the Blind: Writers Division
Tom Stevens
504 S 57th Street   402-556-3216
Omaha, NE 68106-0809   e-mail: newmanrl@cox.net
                                              www.nfb-writers-division.org
Blind writers in all styles including poetry short story fiction non-fiction magazine writing and theatrical work offer encouragement and support to blind writers and authors. Issues cover various aspects of this business including selling your work.
Robert L Newman, President

9508   National Industries for the Blind
1310 Braddock Place   703-310-0500
Alexandria, VA 22314-1727   Fax: 703-998-8268
                              e-mail: communications@nib.org
                                                      www.nib.org
A nonprofit organization that represents over 100 associated industries serving people who are blind in thirty-six states. These agencies serve people who are blind or visually impaired and help them to reach their full potential.
Kevin Lynch, President/CEO
Steve Brice, Vice President/CFO

9509   National Library Service for the Blind and Physically Handicapped
Library of Congress
1291 Taylor Street NW   202-707-5100
Washington, DC 20011   888-657-7323
                                              TTY: 202-707-0744
                                              TDD: 202-707-0744
                                              e-mail: nls@loc.gov
                                                      www.loc.gov/nls
Administers a national library service that provides braille and recorded books and magazines on free loan to anyone who cannot read standard print because of visual or physical disabilities who are eligible residents of the United States.
12 pages Quarterly
Frank Kurt Cylke, Director
Michael M Moodie, Research and Development Officer

9510   National Organization of Parents of Blind Children
Barbara Cheadle

1026 East 36th Street   410-645-0632
Baltimore, MD 21218-4998   Fax: 410-685-5653
                                      e-mail: melissa@riccobono.us
                              www.nfb.org/nfb/Parents_and_Teachers.asp
Support information and advocacy organization of parents of blind or visually impaired children. Addresses issues ranging from help to parents of a newborn blind infant, mobility and Braille instruction, education, social and community participation.
Melissa Riccobono, President

9511   New Eyes for the Needy
549 Milburn Avenue   973-376-4903
Short Hills, NJ 07078   Fax: 973-376-3807
                          e-mail: neweyesfortheneedy@yahoo.com
                                      www.neweyesfortheneedy.org/
Provides new glasses for those with low vision who may not be able to afford them.
Jean Gajano, Executive Director

9512   Prevent Blindness America
211 W Wacker Drive
Chicago, IL 60606-5624   800-331-2020
                                  e-mail: info@preventblindness.org
                                                  www.preventblindness.org
Information and referral services provided on specific eye disorders. Publishes literature and supports community screening and testing programs.
Hugh R Parry, President/CEO

9513   Randolph-Sheppard Vendors of America
940 Parc Helene Drive   504-328-6373
Marrero, LA 70072-4104   800-467-5299
                                                  Fax: 504-328-6372
                                      e-mail: kim.venable@att.net
                                                  www.randolph-sheppard.org
Protects the interests of blind vendors seeks proper implementation of the Randolph-Sheppard Act and encourages facility locations in more visible and profitable areas.
Charles Glaser, President
John Gordon, First Vice President

9514   Recording for the Blind and Dyslexic
20 Roszel Road
Princeton, NJ 08540-6294   866-RFB-D585
                                                  www.randolph-sheppard.org
Provides materials for all people who cannot effectively read standard print because of a visual perceptual or other physical disability.

9515   Research to Prevent Blindness
645 Madison Avenue   212-752-4333
New York, NY 10022-1010   800-621-0026
                                                  Fax: 212-688-6231
                                      e-mail: inforequest@rpbusa.org
                                                  www.rpbusa.org
National voluntary health foundation supported by foundations corporations and voluntary gifts and bequests from individuals. Established to stimulate basic and applied research into the causes prevention and treatment of blinding eye diseases.
David Weeks, Chairman
Diane S Swift, President

9516   Seeing Eye
PO Box 375   973-539-4425
Morristown, NJ 07963-0375   Fax: 973-539-0922
                                      e-mail: info@seeingeye.org
                                                  www.seeingeye.org
A training school for dogs to guide qualified blind persons.
James A Kutsch, President and Chief Executive Officer

9517   Smith-Kettlewell Eye Research Foundation
2318 Fillmore Street   415-345-2000
San Francisco, CA 94115   Fax: 415-345-8455
                                              TTY: 415-345-2290
                                                  www.ski.org
Dedicated to research on human vision founded to encourage a productive collaboration between the medical clinic and the scientific laboratories.

9518 Taping for the Blind
3935 Essex Lane
Houston, TX 77027-5113
713-622-2767
Fax: 713-622-2772
www.tapingfortheblind.org
Records reading material on audiotape copied onto cassettes for use by blind and physically handicapped persons. Promotes increased interest in and use of free audio materials. Books textbooks and technical manuals are recorded and sent to libraries.
Kari Musgrove, Executive Director
Mary Farish Johnston, President

9519 United States Association for Blind Athletes
1 Olympic Plaza
Colorado Springs, CO 80909-3508
719-630-0422
Fax: 719-630-0616
e-mail: mlucas@usaba.org
www.usaba.org
Athletic association for blind athletes this association is the national governing body for the United States visually impaired athletes.
Dave Bushland, President
Tracie Foster, Vice President

9520 Vision World Wide
5707 Brockton Drive
Indianapolis, IN 46220-5481
317-254-1332
800-431-1739
Fax: 317-251-6588
e-mail: info@visionenhancement.org
www.visionww.org
Believing there is hope when vision fails. It disseminates relevant information on a variety of topics through its information and referral helpline website e-mail announce list and journal Vision Enhancement all designed to encourage and support individuals with vision impairments.
Patricia Price, Editor-In-Chief
William Corbin, Board Chairman

9521 Washington Ear
12061 Tech Road
Silver Spring, MD 20904-2437
301-681-6636
Fax: 301-625-1986
e-mail: information@washear.org
www.washear.org
A nonprofit organization providing reading and information services for the blind visually impaired and physically disabled persons who cannot effectively read print see plays watch television programs or view museum exhibits.
Margaret Pfanstiehl, President
George Long, Vice President

9522 National Federation of the Blind: Blind Merchants Division
Kevin Worley
1837 S. Nevada Avenue
Colorado Springs, CO 80905-3591
71- 4-3 23
88- 6-1 18
Fax: 303-695-1828
e-mail: kevinworley@blindmerchants.org
www.blindmerchants.org
Membership organization of blind persons employed in either self-employment work or the Randolph-Sheppard vending program. Provides information regarding rehabilitation social security tax and other issues which directly affect blind merchants.
Kevin Worley, President

State Agencies & Associations

Alabama

9523 Alabama Council of the Blind
1018 E Street S
Talladega, AL 35160
256-362-5649
e-mail: dart1018@charter.net
www.acbalabama.org
David Trott, President

9524 National Federation of the Blind: Alabama
4905 Brooke Court
Mobile, AL 36618-2708
251-344-7960
e-mail: mwkoger21@bellsouth.net
www.nfbofalabama.org
Minnie K Walker, President

Alaska

9525 National Federation of the Blind: Alaska
1169 Hess Avenue
Fairbanks, AK 99709
907-479-6118
e-mail: jnhburton@gci.net
www.nfb.org
Jim Burton, President

Arizona

9526 Arizona Center for the Blind and Visually Impaired
3100 E Roosevelt Street
Phoenix, AZ 85008-5036
602-273-7411
Fax: 602-273-7410
e-mail: jlamay@acbvi.org
www.acbvi.org
Provides services for individuals to enhance the quality of life of people who are blind or otherwise visually impaired. Services are available to adults who are either legally blind or visually impaired as well as those who have a degenerative eye condition.
Steve Walker, Chair
Stanton Stipes, Vice Chair

9527 Arizona Industries for the Blind
515 N 51st Avenue
Phoenix, AZ 85043
602-771-9100
Fax: 602-353-5703
e-mail: LHudspeth@azdes.gov
www.azdes.gov/aib
Arizona Industries for the Blind was established in 1952 to provide employment and training opportunities for Arizonans who are legally blind.
Lorraine Hudspeth, Controller
Letty Cerpa, Senior Accountant

9528 National Federation of the Blind: Arizona
9014 E Bellevue Street
Tucson, AZ 85715-5652
520-733-5894
e-mail: krezguy@cox.net
www.nfbarizona.com
Bob Kresmer, President
Vicki Hodges, 1st Vice President

9529 Region 6 of the National Association for Parents of the Visually Impaired
Walnut Creek, CA 85282-5724
602-730-8282
e-mail: mebphillips@comcast.net
www.spedex.com/napvi
Susan LaVenture, Executive Director
Julie Urban, President

Arkansas

9530 Arkansas Lighthouse for the Blind
6818 Murray Street
Little Rock, AR 72209-2666
510-562-2222
Fax: 501-568-5275
e-mail: bjohnson@arkansaslighthouse.org
www.arkansaslighthouse.org
Pat Smith, President
Jim Shenep, Vice President

9531 National Federation of the Blind: Arkansas
2360 Wedington Drive
Fayetteville, AR 72701-2304
479-582-0091
e-mail: tosheeler@cox.net
www.nfb.org
Terry Sheeler, President

California

9532 Lighthouse for the Blind and Visually Impaired
Lighthouse Industries
214 Van Ness Avenue
San Francisco, CA 94102
415-431-1481
Fax: 415-863-7568
TTY: 415-431-4572
e-mail: info@lighthouse-sf.org
www.lighthouse-sf.org
The LightHouse promotes the independence, equality and self-reliance of people who are blind or visually impaired through rehabilitation training and relevant services, such as access to employment, education, government, information, recreation and transportation.
Chuck Godwin, Executive Support
Anthony Fletcher, Associate Executive Director and COO

9533 National Federation of the Blind: California
3934 Kern Court
Pleasonton, CA 94588

818-342-6524
877-558-6524
Fax: 818-344-7930
e-mail: nfbcal@sbcglobal.net
http://www.nfbcal.org/

Mary Willows, President
Ever Lee Harriston, Vice President

9534 Northwest Regional Training Center: Canine Companions for Independence
2965 Dutton Avenue
Santa Rosa, CA 95407-0446

707-577-1000
800-572-2275
TTY: 707-577-1756
e-mail: info@cci.org
www.cci.org

Canine Companions for Independence is a non-profit organization that enhances the lives of people with disabilities by providing highly trained assistance dogs and ongoing support to ensure quality partnerships.
Corey Hudson, CEO
Kathy Pierson, Northwest Regional Executive Director

9535 Southwest Regional Training Center: Canine Companions for Independence
124 Rancho del Oro Drive
Oceanside, CA 92057

760-901-4300
800-572-2275
Fax: 760-901-4350
TTY: 760-901-4326
TDD: 760-901-4350
www.cci.org

Canine Companions for Independence is a non-profit organization that enhances the lives of people with disabilities by providing highly trained assistance dogs and ongoing support to ensure quality partnerships.
Linda Valliant, Executive Director
Chuck Contreras, Director of Development

Colorado

9536 National Federation of the Blind: Colorado
2233 W Shepperd Avenue
Littleton, CO 80120

303-778-1130
800-401-4NFB
e-mail: slabarre@labarrelaw.com
www.nfbco.org

Scott LaBarre, President
Kevan Worley, 1st Vice President

Connecticut

9537 National Federation of the Blind: Connecticut
477 Connecticut Boulevard,
East Hartford, CT 06108-3579

860-289-1971
e-mail: aldelucia@nfbct.org
http://www.nfbct.org/

Alfonse DeLucia, President

9538 Prevent Blindness Tri-State
101 Whitney Avenue
New Haven, CT 06510

800-850-2020
e-mail: info@preventblindnesstristate.org
www.preventblindness.org/tristate

Kathryn Garre-Ayars, President & CEO
Maria Giarratana, Grants Manager

Delaware

9539 Delaware Assocation for the Blind Department of Health & Social Services
Department of Health & Social Services
2915 Newport Gap Pike
Wilmington, DE 19801-1526

302-655-2111
888-777-3925
Fax: 302-655-1442
e-mail: contact@dabdel.org
www.dabdel.org

9540 National Federation of the Blind: Delaware
2215 Bradmoor Road
Wilmington, DE 19803-2646

302-652-6761
e-mail: lynne.majewski@gmail.com
www.nfb.org

Lynne Majewski, President

District of Columbia

9541 American Foundation for the Blind: Governmental Relations
1660 L Street, NW
Washington, DC 20036

202-469-6831
Fax: 646-478-9260
e-mail: afbgov@afb.net
www.afb.org

Advocates on behalf of people who are blind or visually impaired before Congress and Executive Branch offices, and participates in advocacy-related coalitions and initiatives nationwide.
Paul W Schroeder, Vice President, Governmental Relations
Barbara Jackson LeMoine, Legislative Assistant

9542 Columbia Lighthouse for the Blind
1825 K Street NW
Washington, DC 20006

301-589-0894
877-324-5252
Fax: 877-595-9228
e-mail: info@clb.org
www.clb.org

Columbia Lighthouse for the blind offers programs and services that enable individuals who are blind or visually impaired to obtain and maintain independence at home, school and in the community.
Anthony Cancelosi, President/CEO

9543 National Federation of the Blind: DC
2354 13th Place, N.E.
Washington, DC 20018-1841   e-mail: callaway.shawn@gmail.com

202-352-1511
www.nfb.org

Shawn M. Callaway, President

Florida

9544 Goodwill Industries-Suncoast
Goodwill Industries-Suncoast
10596 Gandy Boulevard
Saint Petersburg, FL 33702

727-523-1512
888-279-1988
Fax: 727-579-0850
TTY: 727-579-1068
e-mail: gw.marketing@goodwill-suncoast.com
www.goodwill-suncoast.org

A non-profit community based organization whose purpose is to improve the quality of life for people who are disabled, disadvantaged and/or aged. This mission is accomplished through a staff of over 1,200 employees providing independent living skills.
R Lee Waits, President/Chief Executive Officer
Chris Ward, Marketing and Media Relations Manager

9545 National Federation of the Blind: Florida
3708 West Bay to Bay Blvd
Tampa, FL 33629-4266

386-677-6886
888-282-5972
e-mail: president@nfbflorida.org
www.nfbflorida.org

Dan Hicks, President
Gloria Mills Hicks, Treasurer

9546 Southeast Regional Center: Canine Companions for Independence
Anheuser-Busch/SeaWorld Campus
8150 Clarcona Ocoee Road
Orlando, FL 32818-0388

407-522-3300
Fax: 407-522-3347
e-mail: mager@cci.org
www.cci.org

Canine Companions for Independence is a non-profit organization that enhances the lives of people with disabilities by providing highly trained assistance dogs and ongoing support to ensure quality partnerships.
Margaret S Ager, Executive Director
Nancy Baumann, President

9547 Tampa Lighthouse for the Blind
1106 W Platt Street
Tampa, FL 33606-2142

813-251-2407
866-251-2407
Fax: 813-254-4305
e-mail: TLH@tampalighthouse.org
www.tampalighthouse.org

Tampa Lighthouse for the Blind provides comprehensive rehabilitation programs for persons who are blind or visually impaired.
Cliff Olstrom, Executive Director

Georgia

9548 Georgia Industries for the Blind
700 Faceville Highway
Bainbridge, GA 39818-0218   229-248-2666
www.vocrehabga.org
The primary mission of the Georgia Industries for the Blind (GIB) is to provide employment opportunities for people who are visually impaired or blind.

9549 National Federation of the Blind: Georgia
315 Ponce de Leon Avenue   404-371-1000
Decatur, GA 30030   Fax: 404-371-1002
e-mail: gscott@nfbga.org
www.nfb.org

Garrick Scott, President

9550 Southeastern Region: Helen Keller National Center
1003 Virginia Avenue   404-766-9625
Atlanta, GA 30354-1365   Fax: 404-766-3447
TTY: 404-766-2820
e-mail: bc4hknc@aol.com
www.hknc.org

Barbara Chandler, Regional Representative

Hawaii

9551 Division of Vocational Rehabilitation and Services for the Blind
Department of Human Services
601 Kamokila Boulevard   808-692-7715
Kapolei, HI 96707   Fax: 808-692-7727
TTY: 808-692-7715
e-mail: info@hawaiivr.org
www.hawaiivr.org
The American Macular Degeneration Foundation is committed to the prevention and cure of macular degeneration and offers hope and support to those afflicted and their families. The Foundation is a major voice in establishing national research.
Joe Cordova, Administrator

9552 Ho'opono Workshop for the Blind
1901 Bachelor Street   808-586-5286
Honolulu, HI 96817   Fax: 808-586-5288
TTY: 808-586-5269
e-mail: hoopono@hawaiivr.org
www.hawaiivr.org

Dave Eveland, Administrator

9553 National Federation of the Blind: Hawaii
PO Box 4482   808-391-1214
Honolulu, HI 96812   e-mail: nanifife@aol.com
hawaii.nfb.org

Nani Fife, President
Charlene Ota, Vice-President

Idaho

9554 National Federation of the Blind: Idaho
300 Willard Avenue   208-377-9825
Pocatello, ID 83201   Fax: 208-232-5416
e-mail: ElsieLamp@yahoo.com
www.nfbidaho.org

Elsie H Lamp, President

Illinois

9555 Aid to the Aged, Blind or Disabled
Department of Human Services
100 South Grand Avenue, East
Springfield, IL 62762   800-252-8635
TTY: 800-447-6404
www.macular.org/stagency/state_il.html
The American Macular Degeneration Foundation is committed to the prevention and cure of macular degeneration and offers hope and support to those afflicted and their families. The Foundation will be a major voice in establishing the national research agenda for macular degeneration through promoting an alliance among the scientific community, government, and victims of the disease and their families to ensure the prevention and cure of the disease.

9556 Chicago Lighthouse for People Who are Blind and Visually Impaired
1850 W Roosevelt Road   312-666-1331
Chicago, IL 60608-1298   Fax: 312-243-8539
TTY: 312-666-8874
TDD: 312-666-8874
e-mail: helpdesk@chicagolighthouse.org
www.thechicagolighthouse.org
The Chicago Lighthouse is a comprehensive private rehabilitation and educational facility dedicated exclusively to assisting children youth and adults who are blind visually impaired or multi-disabled.
Janet P Szlyk, Executive Director
William L Conaghan, Chairman

9557 Helen Keller National Center Regional Representatives
485 Avenue of the Cities   309-755-0018
E Moline, IL 61244   Fax: 309-755-0025
TTY: 309-755-0018
TDD: 309-755-0021
e-mail: HKNC5LJT@aol.com
www.hknc.org

Laura J Thomas, Regional Representative

9558 National Federation of the Blind: Illinois
6919 W Berwyn Avenue   773-307-6440
Chicago, IL 60656-2040   e-mail: president@nbfofillinois.org
www.nfbofillinois.org

Patti Gregory-Chang, President
Deborah Kent Stein, First Vice-President

Indiana

9559 Bosma Industries for the Blind
8020 Zionsville Road   317-684-0600
Indianapolis, IN 46268-3876   800-362-5463
Fax: 317-684-1946
e-mail: info@bosma.org
www.bosma.org
It is the mission of Bosma Industries for the Blind to enhance opportunities for individuals who are blind or visually impaired to achieve their potential in vocational, economic, social and personal independence.
Lou Moneymaker, CEO
Connie F Campbell, CFO/COO

9560 National Federation of the Blind: Indiana
6010 Winnpeny Lane   317-205-9226
Indianapolis, IN 46220-5253   e-mail: rb15@iquest.net
www.nfb.org

Ron Brown, President

Iowa

9561 National Federation of the Blind: Iowa
2721 34th Street   515-771-8348
Des Moines, IA 50310   e-mail: m.barber@mchsi.com
www.nfb.org

Michael D Barber, President
April Enderton, First Vice-President

Kansas

9562 Kansas Industries for the Blind
425 MacVicar Street   785-296-3211
Topeka, KS 66606   Fax: 785-296-0728

9563 National Federation of the Blind: Kansas
11405 W Grant   913-339-9341
Wichita, KS 67209-3621   e-mail: donnajwood@cox.net
www.nfbks.org

Donna Wood, President
Susan L Stanzel, First Vice President

Kentucky

9564 Kentucky Industries for the Blind
1900 Brownsboro Road   502-893-0211
Louisville, KY 40206-2102   Fax: 502-893-3885

9565 National Federation of the Blind: Kentucky
210 Cambridge Drive
Louisville, KY 40214-2809

502-366-2317
e-mail: cathyj@iglou.com
www.nfbky.org

Cathy Jackson, President
Pamela Roark-Glisson, Vice President

Louisiana

9566 Industries for the Blind and Visually Impaired of Louisiana
PO Box 366
Delhi, LA 71232-0366

318-878-8171

9567 Louisiana Association for the Blind
1750 Claiborne Avenue
Shreveport, LA 71103

318-635-6471
877-913-6471
Fax: 318-635-8902
e-mail: labstore@lablind.com
www.lablind.com

LAB employs people who are blind in manufacturing administrative training and a variety of job positions that match an individual's goals and potential.
Shelly Taylor, President/CEO
Doug Young, Vice President Administration

9568 National Federation of the Blind: Louisana
605 University Boulevard
Ruston, LA 71270-4862

318-251-1511
800-234-4166
e-mail: pallenp@lcb-ruston.com
www.nfbla.org

Pam Allen, President

Maine

9569 Maine Center for the Blind and Visually Impaired
189 Park Avenue
Portland, ME 04102-2909

207-774-6273
Fax: 207-774-0679
e-mail: info@theiris.org
www.theiris.org

Leonard Cole, Chairman
Katherine Ray, Vice Chair

9570 National Federation of the Blind: Maine
33 Morse Avenue
Lewiston, ME 04240-9707

207-212-1455
e-mail: leonproctorjr@yahoo.com
www.nfb.org

Leon Proctor, Jr, President

Maryland

9571 Blind Industries and Services of Maryland
3345 Washington Boulevard
Baltimore, MD 21227

410-737-2600
888-322-4567
Fax: 410-737-2665
www.bism.org

Blind Industries and Services of Maryland provides innovative rehabilitation services training and stable employment opportunities to our state's citizens who are blind or visually impaired.
Don Morris, Chairperson
Walter Brown, Vice-Chairperson

9572 National Federation of the Blind: Maryland
1026 E 36th Street
Baltimore, MD 21218

41- 6-5 06
e-mail: president@nfbmd.org
www.nfbmd.org/

Melissa Riccobono, President
Debbie Brown, First Vice President

Massachusetts

9573 Carroll Center for the Blind
770 Centre Street
Newton, MA 02458-2597

617-969-6200
800-852-3131
Fax: 617-969-6204
TTY: 617-969-6204
e-mail: info@carroll.org
www.carroll.org

Assists blind and visually impaired adults and adolescents to adjust to loss of vision. The goal of this dynamic program is to en-

courage independence, restore self-confidence, prepare for employment and improve the quality of life.
Dina Rosenbaum, Marketing Director

9574 Massachusetts Commission for the Blind
600 Washington St.
Boston, MA 02111-4718

617-748-2000
www.state.ma.us/mcb

Provides services to blind citizens of Massachusetts, enabling them to lead more fulfilling and independent lives. Offers vocational rehabilitation, independent living, social services, home care and respite assistance, radio reading programs and print resources.
Cheryl Standley, Contact
Janet LaBreck, Commissioner

9575 National Federation of the Blind: Massachusetts
140 Wood Street
Somerset, MA 02726-5225

508-679-8543
e-mail: nfbmass@earthlink.net
http://www.nfbmass.org/

Priscilla Ferris, President

9576 New England Region: Helen Keller National Center
152 Lincoln Road
Lincoln, MA 01773

781-259-7100
Fax: 781-259-4014
e-mail: hknc1meb@comcast.net
www.hknc.org

Mary Ellen Barbiasz, Regional Representative
Peg Ouellette, Administrative Assistant

9577 Region 1 of the National Association for Parents of the Visually Impaired
Hudson, MA 06016-9560

860-623-4129
e-mail: sue.rawley@verizon.net
www.spcdex.com/napvi

Michigan

9578 Association for the Blind & Visually Impaired
456 Cherry Southeast
Grand Rapids, MI 49503

616-458-1187
800-466-8084
Fax: 616-458-7113
e-mail: abvi@abvimichigan.org
www.abvimichigan.org

To advance the independence of people who are visually impaired and to promote the prevention of blindness.
Richard A Stevens, Executive Director
George Kremer, Director of Rehabilitation Services

9579 Greater Detroit Agency for the Blind and Visually Impaired
16625 Grand River Avenue
Detroit, MI 48227-1419

313-272-3900
Fax: 313-272-6893
e-mail: information@gdabvi.org
www.gdabvi.org

We are a non-profit organization dedicated to preventing blindness reducing the impact of blindness and advocating for those with severe vision loss.
Frederick J Simpson, Chairman
Charles L Cone, Vice Chair

9580 National Federation of the Blind: Michigan
1212 N Foster Avenue
Lansing, MI 48912-3309

517-482-1800
e-mail: f.wurtzel@comcast.net
www.nfbmi.org

Fred Wurtzel, President
Mary Ann Rojek, State Braille Coin Project Coordinator

Minnesota

9581 Duluth Lighthouse for the Blind
4505 W Superior Street
Duluth, MN 55807-2728

218-624-4828
800-422-0833
Fax: 218-624-4479
e-mail: info@lighthousefortheblind-duluth.org
www.lighthousefortheblind-duluth.org

The LightHouse for the blind is a teaching facility providing employment, training and rehab instruction for blind and visually-impaired individuals.
Mary Junnila, Executive Director
Debbie , Book keeper

9582 National Federation of the Blind: Minnesota
100 East 22nd street
Minneapolis, MN 55404-2217 612-872-9363
e-mail: joyce.scanlan@earthlink.net
http://www.nfbmn.org/

Jennifer Dunmann, President

Mississippi

9583 Mississippi Industries for the Blind
2501 N W Street
Jackson, MS 39216-4417 601-984-3200
866-859-4461
Fax: 601-987-3892
e-mail: bcoy@msblind.org
www.msblind.org
The Mississippi Industries for the Blind seeks to provide jobs for the blind and visually-impaired.
Michael Chew, Executive Director
Bob Coy, Sales Manager

9584 National Federation of the Blind: Mississippi
PO Box 1515
Jackson, MS 39215-5431 601-969-3352
e-mail: samgleese@earthlink.net
www.nfbofmississippi.org

rev Sam Gleese, President
Barbara Hadnot, Vice President

Missouri

9585 Alphapointe Association for the Blind
7501 Prospect
Kansas City, MO 64132 816-421-5848
Fax: 816-237-2019
e-mail: sliptak@alphapointe.org.
www.alphapointe.org
The Alphapointe Association for the Blind has a Braille library a Senior Adult Services Program and a dedication to finding employment for the blind and visually-impaired.
Paulette Markel, Chairman
Ken Roberson, Secretary

9586 Kansas City Association for the Blind
1844 Broadway Street
Kansas City, MO 64108-2007 816-333-2173

9587 National Federation of the Blind: Missouri
3910 Tropical Lane
Columbia, MO 65202-6205 573-874-1774
e-mail: info@nfbmo.org
www.nfbmo.org

Gary Wunder, President
Shelia Wright, First Vice President

Montana

9588 National Federation of the Blind: Montana
408 W Sussex Avenue
Missoula, MT 59801 406-546-8546
e-mail: burk.dall@gmail.com
www.mt-blind.org

Daniel Burke, President
Dick Howse, 1st Vice President

Nebraska

9589 National Federation of the Blind: Nebraska
1033 O Street
Lincoln, NE 68508-2468 402-477-7711
866-254-6347
e-mail: amy.buresh@ncbvi.ne.gov
nfbn.inebraska.com

Amy Buresh, President
Jeff Altman, First Vice President

Nevada

9590 National Federation of the Blind: Nevada
1344 N. Jones Boulevard
Las Vegas, NV 89108 702-228-4217
e-mail: realhappygirl1@gmail.com
ww.nfb.org

Terri Rupp, President

9591 Southern Nevada Sightless
1001 N Bruce Street
Las Vegas, NV 89101-1247 702-642-6000
Fax: 702-649-6739
e-mail: info@blindcenter.org
www.blindcenter.org

Neal Marek, Chairman
Veronica Wilson, President/CEO

New Hampshire

9592 National Federation of the Blind: New Hampshire
12 Summer St.
Keene, NH 03431 603-357-4080
e-mail: cemcnabb21@yahoo.com
www.nfbnh.org/

Marie Johnson, President

New Jersey

9593 Bestwork Industries for the Blind
801 E Clements Bridge Road
Runnemede, NJ 08078 856-939-5220
800-370-9560
Fax: 856-939-5022
e-mail: bestwork@bestworkindustries.org
www.bestworkindustries.org
Bestwork Industries for the Blind is dedicated to providing employment opportunities for those with visual impairments.
James Varsaci, Founder

9594 National Federation of the Blind: New Jersey
254 Spruce Street
Bloomfield, NJ 07003 973-743-0075
e-mail: nfbnj@yahoo.com
http://www.nfbnj.org/

Joe Ruffalo, President

New Mexico

9595 National Federation of the Blind: New Mexico
10315 Props dr. NE
Albuquerque, NM 87112 505-268-3895
e-mail: blindart@myfreedombox.com
http://www.nfbnm.org/

Arthur Schreiber, President

9596 New Mexico Industries for the Blind
2200 Yale Boulevard SE
Albuquerque, NM 87106-4212 505-841-8844
888-513-7958
Fax: 505-841-8850
e-mail: Greg.Trapp@state.nm.us
www.state.nm.us/cftb

Greg Trapp, Executive Director
Dallas Allen, Commissioner

9597 State of New Mexico Commission for the Blind
2905 Rodeo Park Drive E
Santa Fe, NM 87505 505-476-4479
888-513-7968
e-mail: Greg.Trapp@state.nm.us
www.state.nm.us/cftb
The mission of the New Mexico Commission for the Blind is to encourage and enable blind citizens to achieve vocational economic and social equality. It provides career preparation and training in the skills of blindness.
Greg Trapp, Executive Director
Arthur A Schreiber, Chairman

New York

9598 Association for the Blind & Visually Impaired of Greater Rochester
422 South Clinton Avenue
Rochester, NY 14620-1198 585-232-1111
www.raen.org
Our mission is to assist people who are blind or visually impaired to achieve their highest level of independence in all aspects of their lives.
A Gidget Hopf, EdD, President/CEO

9599 Blind Association of Western New York
1170 Main Street
Buffalo, NY 14209-2331
716-882-1025
e-mail: guildcarebuffalo@jgb.org
www.olmstedcenter.org

Patricia Clabeaux, Chairwomen
Phil Catanese, Vice Chairman

9600 Blind Work Association
55 Washington Street
Binghamton, NY 13901-3770
607-724-2428
Fax: 607-771-8045
e-mail: bobh@clarityconnect.com
www.co.tompkins.ny.us

9601 Central Association for the Blind and Visually Impaired
507 Kent Street
Utica, NY 13501-2317
315-797-2233
877-719-9996
Fax: 315-797-2244
e-mail: info@cabui.org
www.cabvi.org

Edward P. Welsch, Chairman
James B. Turnbill IV, Vice Chairman

9602 National Federation of the Blind: New York
PO Box 205666
Brooklyn, NY 11220-4617
718-567-7821
Fax: 718-765-1843
e-mail: office@nfbny.org
www.nfbny.org

Carl Jacobsen, President
Mindy Jacobson, Vice President

9603 Northeastern Association of the Blind of Albany
301 Washington Avenue
Albany, NY 12206-3012
518-463-1211
Fax: 51- 4-3 35
e-mail: info@naba-vision.org
www.naba-vision.org

NABA offers a wide range of services to those with visual impairments from its free vision screening service for children to training and placing legally blind adults in professional employment. Also provides rehabilitation services to seniors with age-related conditions.
Mark J McKarthy, Chair
david P. Quinn, Vice Chairman

9604 Southern Tier Association for the Visually Impaired
719 Lake Street
Elmira, NY 14901-2538
607-734-1554
Fax: 607-734-9467
e-mail: info@st-avi.org
www.st-avi.org

Brian Bleiler, President
John Luce, Vice President

North Carolina

9605 Lions Industries for the Blind
4126 Berkeley Avenue
Kinston, NC 28504-8321
252-523-1019
Fax: 252-523-7090
e-mail: customerser@lionsindustries.org
www.lionsindustries.com

The Lions Industries for the Blind provides employment opportunities for the blind and visually-impaired.
ray Amette, Executive Director
Marc Camnitz, General Manager

9606 National Federation of the Blind: North Carolina
128 Summerlea Drive
Charlotte, NC 28214-1324
704-491-1486
Fax: 704-391-3204
e-mail: tjnc2@carolina.rr.com
http://www.nfbofnc.org/

Gary Ray, President

9607 Winston-Salem Industries for the Blind
7730 N Point Drive
Winston-Salem, NC 27106-3310
336-759-0551
800-242-7726
Fax: 336-759-0990
e-mail: info@wsifb.com
www.wsifb.com

The Winston-Salem Industries for the Blind provides employment opportunities for the blind and visually-impaired.
david Byler, Chair
Mike Faircloth, Vice Chairman

North Dakota

9608 National Federation of the Blind: North Dakota
301 4th St. East
Williston, ND 58101
701-572-3477
e-mail: diverson@midco.net
www.nfb.org

Duane Iverson, President

Ohio

9609 Cincinnati Association for the Blind
2045 Gilbert Avenue
Cincinnati, OH 45202-1490
513-221-8558
888-687-3935
Fax: 513-221-2995
e-mail: info@cincyblind.org
www.cincyblind.org

Persons who are blind visually impaired or print impaired may choose from a wide range of services to help them live more independently. Our services are provided by qualified certified instructors and staff with highly specialized skills.
John Mitchell, Executive Director
Ginny Backschreider, Director of Program services

9610 Cleveland Sight Center
1909 E 101st Street
Cleveland, OH 44106-8696
216-791-8118
Fax: 216-791-1101
e-mail: sfriedman@clevelandsightcenter.org
www.clevelandsightcenter.org

Mission is to enable people with vision impairment to reach their full potential and assure that adequate services are available to make a normal life possible.
William L. Spring, Chair
Thomas P. Furnas, Vice Chairman

9611 Cleveland Skilled Industries
2239 E 55th Street
Cleveland, OH 44103-4451
216-431-8085
Fax: 216-431-5123

9612 National Federation of the Blind: Ohio
P.O. Box 82055,
Columbus, OH 43202-1517
440-775-2216
e-mail: bbpierce@pobox.com
www.nfbohio.org

Duffy Eric, President
Payne Richard, Vice President

Oklahoma

9613 National Federation of the Blind: Oklahoma
457 N. Blackwelder Avenue
Edmond, OK 73034
405-600-0695
e-mail: jmassay1@cox.net
www.nfb.org

Jeannie Massay, President

9614 Oklahoma League for the Blind
501 N Douglas Avenue
Oklahoma City, OK 73106
405-232-4644
Fax: 405-236-5438
e-mail: swright@newviewoklahoma.org
www.newviewoklahoma.org

The mission of the Oklahoma League for the Blind is to facilitate independence and improve the quality of life for people who are blind or vision impaired by providing employment opportunities and services.
Thomas Larson, Director
Elijha Straw, Business Manager

Oregon

9615 Blind Enterprises of Oregon
6540 SE Foster Road
Portland, OR 97206
503-774-6387
Fax: 503-774-0585
e-mail: blindent@aol.com
www.blindenterprises.com

Tami Foss, Executive Director
Bill Smith, Operator

9616 National Federation of the Blind: Oregon
5005 Main Street
Springfield, OR 97478
541-726-6924
800-422-7093
e-mail: admin@mainstreetmontessori.org
www.nfb.org

Carla McQuillan, President

Pennsylvania

9617 Association for the Blind & Visually Impaired of Lehigh County
845 Wyoming Street
Allentown, PA 18103-2199
610-433-6018
Fax: 610-433-4856
e-mail: info@abvi.org
www.abvi.org

The ABVI mission is to strive to be our community's foremost provider and coordinator of preventative, educational, social and rehabilitative programs concerning vision loss. Our goal is to assist each individual and his/her family to achieve their greatest potential.
Kathleen Meckes, Executive Director

9618 Beaver County Association for the Blind
616 Fourth Street
Beaver Falls, PA 15010
724-843-1111
Fax: 724-843-8886
e-mail: bcab@forcomm.net
bcab2.tripoid.com

The Beaver County Association for the Blind conducts educational programs about blindness or vision problems by request and provides opportunities to learn experience share and celebrate in the lives of the blind and visually impaired in Beaver County.
Fay Lentz, Executive Director
Linda Borghi, Controller/Business Manager

9619 Cambria County Association for the Blind and Handicapped
211 Central Avenue
Johnstown, PA 15902
814-536-3531
Fax: 814-539-3270
e-mail: ccabh@ccabh.com
www.ccabh.com

The mission of the Cambria County Association for the Blind and Handicapped is to develop and support an environment for persons with disabilities which promotes vocational and employment training, independence and community involvement through rehabilitative programs.
Richard C Bosserman, President

9620 Chester County Association for the Blind
71 S First Avenue
Coatesville, PA 19320
610-384-2767
Fax: 610-384-8005
e-mail: info@chescoblind.org
www.chescoblind.org

Anita Cavuto, Executive Director
John W Esworthy, President

9621 Delaware County Branch of the Pennsylvania Association for the Blind
100-106 W 15th Street
Chester, PA 19013
610-874-1476
Fax: 610-874-6454
e-mail: delcosce@liberty.org
www.libertynet.org

9622 Greater Wilkes-Barre Association for the Blind
1825 Wyoming Avenue
Exeter, PA 18643
570-693-3555
877-693-3555
Fax: 570-823-4841
e-mail: info@wilkesbarreblind.com
www.wilkesbarreblind.com

Our mission is to address the needs of those with limited vision and we also take an active role in the prevention of blindness.
Ronald V Petrilla, Executive Director
Denise Culver, Office Manager

9623 Indiana County Association for the Blind
31 S 10th Street
Indiana, PA 15701-2649
724-465-5549

9624 Keystone Blind Association
1230 Stambaugh Avenue
Sharon, PA 16146
724-347-5501
800-837-4122
Fax: 724-347-2204
e-mail: kba@keystoneblind.org
www.keystoneblind.org

The Keystone Blind Association is dedicated to maintaining and improving the quality of life for blind and/or visually impaired persons preventing blindness and providing employment opportunities and advocacy for persons who are disabled.
Jonathan G Fister, President/CEO
Perry Templeton, Vice President of Operations

9625 Lancaster County Association for the Blind
244 N Queen Street
Lancaster, PA 17603-3512
717-291-5951
e-mail: info@sfblind.org
www.sfblind.org

Dennis L Steiner, President/CEO
Kay L Macsi, VP Rehabilitation and Education

9626 Montgomery County Association for the Blind
212 N Main Street
North Wales, PA 19454-3117
215-661-9800
Fax: 215-661-9888
e-mail: mcab@mcab.org
www.mcab.org

MCAB's mission is to enhance the quality of life and independence of people coping with blindness and vision impairment through rehabilitation education support and advocacy.
Douglas Yingling, Executive Director
Sharon Zislis, Director of Development

9627 National Federation of the Blind: Pennsylvania
42 South 15th Street
Philadelphia, PA 19102-2206
215-988-0888
Fax: 215-988-0879
e-mail: nfbofpa@att.net
http://www.nfbp.org/

James Antonacci, President

9628 North Central Sight Services
2121 Reach Road
Williamsport, PA 17701-0292
570-323-9401
866-320-2580
Fax: 570-323-8194
e-mail: ncss@ncsight.org
www.ncsight.org

Our agency philosophy focuses on helping people help themselves and emphasizes the abilities and capabilities of the blind and visually impaired people we serve.
Robert B Garrett, President/CEO
Barbara Snauffer, Administrative Assistant

9629 Pittsburgh Vision Services
1800 W Street
Homestead, PA 15120
412-368-4400
800-706-5050
Fax: 412-368-4090
TTY: 412-368-4095
e-mail: info&ref@pghvis.org
www.bvrspittsburgh.org/

Pittsburgh Vision Services is a private non-profit United Way agency whose mission is to reduce the limitations that may result from loss of vision.
Dennis J Farkos, Chairman
louis A Lobes, Vice Chairman

9630 Somerset County Blind Center
748 S Center Avenue
Somerset, PA 15501
814-445-1310
Fax: 814-445-3184
e-mail: rob@somersetblind.org
www.somersetblind.org

The Somerset Blind Center offers a number of services to those who are blind or visually impaired, including work opportunities, eyeglass prescription programs, free vision screenings, and training facilities.
Rob Stemple, Executive Director
Anna Hope, Finance Manager

9631 Tri-County Association for the Blind
1130 S 19th Street
Harrisburg, PA 17104-2200
717-238-2531
Fax: 717-238-0710
e-mail: info@vrocp.org
www.vrocp.org/

The Tri-County Association for the Blind works to improve the quality of life for people who are visually-impaired in the Tri-County region, by helping each person achieve his or her full potential and maximum independence.
Danette Blank, Executive Director
Laurie Thompson, Public Relations/Development Director

9632 VIABL Services of Northampton County
845 West Wyoming Street
Allentown, PA 18103
610-433-6018
Fax: 610-866-8730
e-mail: viabl@viablservices.org
www.viablservices.org
Our mission is to promote the social economic and physical self-sufficiency of blind deaf-blind and visually impaired individuals by providing them with the resources and skills needed to live rewarding productive and independent lives.
Jan Leon, Executive Director

9633 Washington-Greene County Branch for the Pennsylvania Association for Blind
555 Gettysburg Pike,
Mechanicsberg, PA 17055-3720
71- 7-6 20
Fax: 71- 7-6 20
e-mail: neal.carrigan@pablind.org
www.pablind.org

Neal J Carrigan, President/CEO
Willard D Brown, Vice-President for Finance

9634 York Industries for the Blind: Division of York County Blind Center
A Division of York County Blind Center
1380 Spahn Avenue
York, PA 17403-5711
717-848-1690
Fax: 717-845-3889
www.forsight.org

William H Rhinesmith, President

Rhode Island

9635 IN-SIGHT
43 Jefferson Boulevard
Warwick, RI 02888
401-941-3322
Fax: 401-941-3356
e-mail: insighttri@gmail.com
www.in-sight.org
IN-SIGHT is a private non-profit agency which has been serving the blind and visually impaired since 1925.
Gerard Goulet, President
Eleanor Acton, Director of Communications

9636 National Federation of the Blind: Rhode Island
PO Box 14404
East Providence, RI 02914
401-433-2606
Fax: 877-383-3682
e-mail: info@nfbri.org
www.nfbri.org

Richard Gaffney, President

South Carolina

9637 National Federation of the Blind: South Carolina
1293 Professional Drive
Myrtle Beach, SC 29577
803-254-3777
e-mail: parnell@sccoast.net
http://www.nfbsc.net/

Parnell Diggs, President

South Dakota

9638 National Federation of the Blind: South Dakota
903 Fulton Street
Rapid City, SD 57701
605-791-3939
e-mail: President@nfb-south-dakota.org
www.nfb-south-dakota.org

Kenneth Rollman, President

Tennessee

9639 Ed Lindsey Industries of the Blind
4110 Charlotte Avenue
Nashville, TN 37209-3749
615-627-4012
Fax: 615-741-5024
www.elifortheblind.org/

Allen Broughton, Executive Vice President
Patrick Broughton, Administrative Assistant

9640 National Federation of the Blind: Tennessee
1226 Goodman Circle West
Memphis, TN 38111-6524
901-452-6596
e-mail: michael.seay@ssa.gov
http://www.nfb-tennessee.org/

Michael Seay, President

Texas

9641 American Foundation for the Blind
11030 Ables Lane
Dallas, TX 75229
214-352-7222
Fax: 646-478-9260
e-mail: dallas@afb.net
www.afb.org
Leads initiatives in the areas of aging and education. Nationally offers consultation, technical assistance and support and undertakes local and national efforts such as training programs, public education and coalition building in the areas of aging and elder care.

9642 American Foundation for the Blind: National Aging Center
11030 Ables Lane
Dallas, TX 75229
214-352-7222
Fax: 646-478-9260
e-mail: dallas@afb.net
www.afb.org
Leads initiatives in the areas of aging and education. Nationally offers consultaion, technical assistance and support and undertakes local and national efforts such as training programs, public education and coalition building in the areas of aging and education. Responds to inquiries from blind and visually impaired people and their families, service providers and the general public in the region and nationally.

9643 Dallas Lighthouse for the Blind
4306 Capitol Avenue
Dallas, TX 75204
214-821-2375
Fax: 214-824-4612
www.dallaslighthouse.org
The Dallas Lighthouse for the Blind provides work opportunities for the blind and visually impaired.
Nancy J Perkins, President/CEO
Gordon Spark, Executive Vice president

9644 East Texas Lighthouse for the Blind
500 N Bois D'Arc
Tyler, TX 75702
903-595-3444
888-595-3444
Fax: 903-595-3447
e-mail: customerservice@horizonind.com
www.horizonind.com

9645 El Paso Lighthouse for the Blind
200 Washington Street
El Paso, TX 79905
915-532-4495
Fax: 915-532-6338
e-mail: htyler@elp.rr.com
www.lighthouse-elpaso.com
Lighthouse is guided by the unwavering belief that its rehabilitative and employment services can help any person overcome his or her disability and enable them to reach their fullest potential for self-sufficiency and independence.
Harry Tyler, President/CEO
Rusty Hooten, CFO

9646 Lighthouse for the Blind of Houston
3602 W Dallas
Houston, TX 77019-0435
713-527-9561
Fax: 713-284-8451
e-mail: houstonlighthouse@houstonlighthouse.org
ww.houstonlighthouse.org
Founded in 1839 the Lighthouse of Houston is a private nonprofit rehabilitation center dedicated to helping blind and visually impaired people live independently.
Gibson M DuTerroil, President

9647 Lighthouse of the Blind of Fort Worth
912 W Broadway Street
Fort Worth, TX 76104
817-332-3341
Fax: 817-332-3456
e-mail: plattallen@lighthousefw.org.
www.lighthousefw.org
The Lighthouse of the Blind of Fort Worth offers many services including skills assessment orientation and mobilty training assisted employment and senior services.
Dr. Shannon Ship, Chairman
W.B. Zim Zimmerman, Vice Chair

9648 National Federation of the Blind: Texas
314 E Highland Mall Boulevard
Austin, TX 78752-3123
512-323-5444
866-636-3289
Fax: 512-420-8160
e-mail: president@nfbtx.org
www.nfb-texas.org

Tommy Craig, President

9649 South Texas Lighthouse for the Blind
PO Box 9697
Corpus Christi, TX 78469
361-883-6553
888-255-8011
Fax: 361-883-1041
e-mail: Regisb@stlb.net
www.stlb.net

Regis Barber, President/CEO
Nicky Ooi, VP/COO

9650 Texas Association of Retinitis Pigmentosa
PO Box 8388
Corpus Christi, TX 78468-8388
361-852-8515
Fax: 361-852-8515
e-mail: tarpmail@homebiz101.com
www.geocities.com/HotSprings/7815
A nonprofit organization based in Texas serving as a national information-sharing center to provide human services to persons with progressive vision loss from retinitis pigmentosa and other retinal degenerative disorders.
Dorothy H Stiefel, Executive Director

9651 Travis Association for the Blind
2307 Business Center Drive
Austin, TX 78764-3297
512-442-2329
Fax: 512-442-5498
e-mail: info@austinlighthouse.org
www.austinlighthouse.org
Travis Association for the Blind (aka Austin Lighthouse) is a service oriented non-profit organization with the mission to assist people who are blind or vision impaired to attain the skills they need to become gainfully employed in the community.
Jerry A Mayfield, Executive Director
Benny Galloway, Chief Financial Officer

9652 West Texas Lighthouse for the Blind
2001 Austin Street
San Angelo, TX 76903-8705
325-653-4231
Fax: 325-657-9367
e-mail: customerservice@lighthousefortheblind.or
www.lighthousefortheblind.org
The West Texas Lighthouse for the Blind is a sheltered facility providing employment for blind and visually impaired individuals.
Steve Cecil, Chairman
Barbara Rogers, Vice Chair

Utah

9653 National Federation of the Blind: Utah
1751 Park St
Salt Lake City, UT 84105-7634
801-631-8108
801-463-6632
Fax: 801-294-6000
e-mail: Baconev@yahoo.com
www.nfbutah.org

Everrete Bacon, President
Cheralyn Bra Creer, First Vice President

9654 Utah Industries for the Blind
PO Box 258
Salt Lake Cty, UT 84110-1258
801-533-9689

Vermont

9655 National Federation of the Blind: Vermont
561 East Hill Rd.
Middlesex, VT 05602
802-272-0087
e-mail: deannaljones@comcast.net
www.nfbvt.org

Franklin Shiner, President

Virginia

9656 National Federation of the Blind: Virginia
3230 Grove Avenue
Richmond, VA 23221
703-319-9226
e-mail: fschroeder@sks.com
www.nfbv.org

Fredric K Schroeder, President
Seville Allen, First Vice President

9657 Virginia Industries for the Blind
1102 Monticello Road
Charlottesville, VA 22902
434-295-5168
Fax: 434-977-0122
e-mail: Robert.Berrang@dbvi.virginia.gov
www.vdbvi.org/vib

Our mission is to be a self-sufficient and self-supporting industry enhance the quality of life for blind and visually impaired individuals through providing gainful employment; and provide opportunities in career development and employment related services.
Robert C Berrang, Deputy Commissioner
Richard C Bohrer, Plant Manager

Washington

9658 Lighthouse for the Blind of Washington
2501 South Plum Street
Seattle, WA 98114
206-322-4200
Fax: 206-329-3397
www.seattlelighthouse.org

Kirk Adams, President
Tami berk, Director

9659 Northwestern Region: Helen Keller National Center
1620 18th Avenue
Seattle, WA 98122-6501
206-324-9120
Fax: 206-324-9159
TTY: 206-324-1133
e-mail: nwhknc@juno.com
www.hknc.org

Dorothy Walt, Regional Representative

9660 Washington State Department of Services for the Blind
402 Legion Way
Olympia, WA 98504-0933
360-725-3830
800-552-7103
Fax: 360-407-0679
e-mail: information@dsb.wa.gov
www.dsb.wa.gov
The Washington State Department of Services for the Blind (DSB) is a state rehabilitation agency that offers assistance to persons who are blind or visually impaired. We also provide various services for employers interested in accomodating or hiring workers with visual impairments.
Bill Palmer, Director

West Virginia

9661 AFB Technology & Employment Center
1000 Fifth Avenue
Huntington, WV 25701
304-523-8651
800-824-2184
Fax: 646-478-9260
e-mail: AFBTECH@afb.net
www.afb.org
AFB Technology runs AFB's CareerConnect and the AFB TECH Product Evaluation Laboratory. Nationally offers consultation, technical assistance and support and undertakes local and national efforts in employment and technology.
Brad Hodges, National Technology Associate

9662 National Federation of the Blind: West Virginia
401 East Olive Street,
Bridgeport, WV 26330
304-622-0626
e-mail: cs.nfbwv@verizon.net
www.nfbwv.org

Charlene Smyth, President

Wisconsin

9663 National Federation of the Blind: Wisconsin
27824 Nuthatch Road
Kendall, WI 54638
608-758-4800
e-mail: johnfritz@centurytel.net
www.nfbwis.org/

John Fritz, President

9664 National Federation of the Blind: Writers
27824 Nuthatch Road
Kendall, WI 54638
608-758-4800
e-mail: johnfritz@centurytel.net
www.nfbwis.org

John Fritz, President

9665 Wiscraft: Wisconsin Enterprises for the Blind
5316 W State Street
Milwaukee, WI 53208-2686
414-778-5800
Fax: 414-778-5805
e-mail: sales@wiscraft.com
www.wiscraft.com
Wiscraft provides long-term supportive employment for people who are blind. It is a manufacturing company that operates as a

non-profit with the clear mission of employing people who are blind by sellng blind-made products and services.
Jim Kerlin, President
Ron Hutchinson, Chair

Wyoming

9666   National Federation of the Blind: Wyoming
4808 Ontario Ave.   307-421-8522
Cheyenne, WY 82009-0347   e-mail: kthornbury@bresnan.net
www.nfb.org

Kelly Thornbury, President

Foundations

9667   Foundation Fighting Blindness
7168 Columbia Gateway Drive,   410-568-0150
Columbia, MD 21046-2220   800-683-5555
TDD: 800-683-5551
e-mail: info@FightBlindness.org
www.fightblindness.org
For a $25.00 annual membership fee, FFB offers information and referral services for affected individuals and their families as well as for doctors and eye care professionals. The Foundation also provides comprehensive information kits on retinitis pigmentosa, macular degeneration, and usher syndrome. Their newsletter, InFocus, and their e-newsletter, InSight, present articles on coping research updates, and Foundation news. A national conference is usually held every other year.
Gordon Gund, Chairman
Edward H. Gollob, President

9668   Glaucoma Research Foundation
251 Post Street   415-986-3162
San Francisco, CA 94108   800-826-6693
Fax: 415-986-3763
e-mail: question@glaucoma.org
www.glaucoma.org
The Glaucoma Research Foundation is a nationa nonprofit dedicated to curing glaucoma. We receive no government funding. Your contribution is tax-deductible as allowed by law.
Thomas M Brunner, President/CEO

Libraries & Resource Centers

9669   District of Columbia Public Library Librarian for the Deaf Community
901 G Street North West
Washington, DC 20001   202-727-1111
www.dclibrary.org
Offers reference services through TDD, portable TDD for public use at pay phone, signers for library programs, sign language classes, information about deafness, print and non-print materials for persons who are deaf.
John W Hill, Jr, President
James W Lewis, Vice President

Alabama

9670   Alabama Radio Reading Service Network
WBHM
650 11th Street South   205-934-2606
Birmingham, AL 35233-4530   800-444-9246
Fax: 205-934-5075
e-mail: philip@wbhm.org
www.wbhm.org/ARRS
Services and readings are relayed over the radio to three-quarters of Alabama for the benefit of the visually impaired.
sarah Delia, producer
Will Dahlberg, Manager

9671   Alabama Regional Library for the Blind and Physically Handicapped
Alabama Public Library Service

6030 Monticello Drive   334-213-3906
Montgomery, AL 36130-6000   800-392-5671
Fax: 334-213-3993
e-mail: fzaleski@apls.state.al.us
http://statelibrary.alabama.gov
To promote and support equitable access to library and information resources and services to enable all Alabamians to satisfy their educational, working, cultural, and leisure-time interests. These resources and services will be provided through APLS's statewide programs and through direct grants and assistance to libraries and library systems to meet user's needs.
Fara Zaleski, Regional Librarian
Rebecca Mitchell, Director (APLS)

9672   Houston Love Memorial Library
212 West Burdeshaw Street   334-793-9767
Dothan, AL 36303   e-mail: bforbus@yahoo.com
www.houstonlovelibrary.org
Offers magnifiers, summer reading programs and more for the blind and physically handicapped. Scanner, software and jaws for windows.
Steve Roy, Chair
Cindy Aman, Board

9673   Huntsville Subregional Library for the Blind and Physically Handicapped
P.O. Box 443   256-532-5980
Huntsville, AL 35804   Fax: 256-532-5994
e-mail: bphdept@hpl.lib.al.us
www.hpl.lib.al.us/departments/bph
The Subregional Library for the Blind and Physically Handicapped is located in the Main branch of the Huntsville-Madison County Public Library. It is also part of a Library of Congress administered nationwide network of libraries serving persons who cannot use conventional printed materials.
Joyce Welch, Librarian

9674   Library and Resource Center for the Blind and Physically Handicapped
Alabama Institute for Deaf and Blind
205 South Street   256-761-3237
Talladega, AL 35160   800-848-4722
Fax: 256-761-3561
e-mail: lacy.teresa@aidb.state.al.us
http://www.aidb.org
Using federal and state funds, the Resource Center purchases or produces braille textbooks and other necessary materials for students. The Resource Center also loans equipment, like braillewriters, to help students learn alternative methods of communication.
Dr,John Macia, President
Dr. Freida Meichan, Vice President

9675   Tuscaloosa Subregional Library for the Blind & Physically Handicapped
1801 Jack Warner Parkway   205-345-5820
Tuscaloosa, AL 35401   Fax: 205-752-8300
e-mail: bjordan@tuscaloosa-library.org
www.tuscaloosa-library.org
Provide talking books to patrons who are unable to use standard print because of a visual or physical limitation. Deliver playback equipment to qualified patrons. Provides reference and referral service to this special population also.
Dr. Horace Allen, Chairman
Dr. Marcia Burke, Vice Chair

Alaska

9676   Alaska State Library Talking Book Center
National Library Services
344 W 3rd Avenue   907-269-6575
Anchorage, AK 99501-2337   800-776-6566
Fax: 907-269-6580
TDD: 907-269-6575
e-mail: tbc@eed.state.ak.us
www.library.state.ak.us
The Alaska State Library Talking Book Center is a cooperative effort between the National Library Service and the Alaska State Li-

brary to provide print handicapped Alaskans with talking book and Braille service.
Bev Griffin, Library Assistant II
Stephanie Schott, Administrative Clerk I

Arizona

9677 Arizona State Braille and Talking Book Library
1030 N 32nd Street
Phoenix, AZ 85008-5108
602-255-5578
800-255-5578
Fax: 602-255-4312
e-mail: btbl@lib.az.us
www.lib.az.us
Closed-circuit TV, summer reading programs, volunteer-produced cassette books, braille writer, films, large-print photocopier and more.
Catherine May, Chair
Ruth Solomon, Vice Chair

9678 Flagstaff City Coconino County Public Library
300 W Aspen Avenue
Flagstaff, AZ 86001-5304
520-779-7670
www.flagstaffpubliclibrary.org
Reference materials on blindness and other handicaps, braille writer, magnifiers and large-print photocopier.

9679 Phoenix Public Library: Special Needs Section
Burton Barr Central Library
1221 North Central Avenue
Phoenix, AZ 85004
602-262-4636
TDD: 602-254-8205
e-mail: specialneeds@phxlib.org
www.phoenixpubliclibrary.org
The Special Needs Center is designed to make the services and resources of the Phoenix Public Library accessible to people with disabilities.
Toni Garvey, City Librarian

Arkansas

9680 Arkansas Regional Library for the Blind and Physically Handicapped
900 W Capitol
Little Rock, AR 72201-1049
501-682-2053
866-660-0885
Fax: 501-682-1529
TDD: 501-682-1002
e-mail: nlsbooks@asl.lib.ar.us
www.asl.lib.ar.us
Public library books in recorded or braille format. Popular fiction and nonfiction books for all ages, books and players are on free loan, sent to patrons by mail and may be returned postage free. Anyone who cannot see well enough to read regular print with glasses on or who has a disability that makes it difficult to hold a book or turn the pages is eligible.
John D Hall, Coordinator

9681 Library for the Blind and Handicapped, Southwest
Columbia County Library
2057 North Jackson St
Magnolia, AR 71754
870-234-0399
866-234-8273
Fax: 870-234-5077
e-mail: lbph@hotmail.com
www.youseemore.com/columbia
The mission of the Columbia County Library is to help the people of our community in their pursuits of information and education, as well as vocational and recreational endeavors, by providing current materials, services, and programs. Our inviting public libraries are the cornerstone of our diverse communities where all people, regardless of age, race, or socio-economic circumstances can experience personal enrichment and literary growth.
Laura Cleaveland, Director
Dana Thornton, Assistant Director

California

9682 Blind Childrens Center
4120 Marathon Street
Los Angeles, CA 90029-3584
323-664-2153
Fax: 323-665-3828
www.blindchildrenscenter.org
The Blind Childrens Center is a family-centered agency which serves children with visual impairments from birth to school-age.

The center-based and home-based programs and services help the children acquire skills and build their independence. The Center utilizes its expertise and experience to serve families and professionals worldwide through support services, education, and research.
Midge Horton, Executive Director
Muriel Scharf, Director Development

9683 Braille Institute Library Services
741 North Vermont Avenue
Los Angeles, CA 90029-3594
323-663-1111
800-808-2555
Fax: 323-662-2440
TDD: 323-660-3880
e-mail: dls@braillelibrary.org
www.braillelibrary.org
The Braille Institute is a non-profit organization whose mission is to eliminate barriers to a fulfilling life caused by blindness and severe sight loss. The Institute provides an environment of hope and encouragement for people who are blind and visually impaired through integrated educational, social and recreational services and programs.
Henry C. Chang, Librarian

9684 California State Library Braille and Talking Book Library
National Library Service
PO Box 942837
Sacramento, CA 94237-0001
916-654-0640
800-952-5666
Fax: 916-654-1119
e-mail: btbl@library.ca.gov
www.library.ca.gov
Library services in braille and recorded formats. Free to residents of Northern California who are unable to read ordinary print on hold a printed book.
Michael Marlin, Manager
Mary Jane Kayes, Outreach Coordinator

9685 Fresno County Public Library: Talking Book Library for the Blind
2420 Mariposa Street
Fresno, CA 93721-3640
559-488-3217
800-742-1011
Fax: 559-488-1971
TDD: 559-488-1642
e-mail: wendy.eisenberg@fresnolibrary.org
www.fresnolibrary.org/tblb
We provide books and magazines on cassette tape and in Braille to people of all ages who are blind, visually impaired, or have physical disabilities preventing the reading of standard print.
Karen Bosch Cobb, County Librarian
Wendy Eisenberg, Librarian

9686 San Francisco Public Library for the Blind and Print Disabled
100 Larkin Street
San Francisco, CA 94102-4733
415-557-4253
TTY: 415-557-4433
e-mail: citylibrarian@sfpl.org
www.sfpl.lib.ca.us
Foreign-language books on cassette, children's books on cassettes and more.
Luis Herrera, City Librarian
Marcia Schneider, Chief, Communications/Adult Services

9687 San Jose State University Library
1 Washington Square
San Jose, CA 95192-0001
408-924-1000
www.library.sjsu.edu
Information on physical disabilities, accessibility and learning disabilities.

Colorado

9688 Boulder Public Library
1001 Arapahoe Avenue
Boulder, CO 80302-1326
303-441-3100
Fax: 303-442-1808
e-mail: ask@boulder.lib.co.us
www.boulder.lib.co.us
Offers braille books, cassettes, talking books, large print photocopier, large print books and more for the visually impaired.
Tony Tallent, Library & Arts Director

9689   Colorado Talking Book Library
201 East Colfax Ave.   303-727-9277
Denver, CO 80203-8101   800-685-2136
                                               Fax: 303-727-9281
                                  e-mail: ctbl.info@cde.state.co.us
                                             www.cde.state.co.us
Take advantage of the services offered by the Colorado Talking
Book Library (CTBL). CTBL provides postage-free recorded,
braille, and large print library materials to eligible residents in
Colorado.
Debbi MacLeod, Director

Connecticut

**9690   Connecticut State Library for the Blind and Physically
Handicapped**
198 W Street   860-721-2020
Rocky Hill, CT 06067-3554   800-842-4516
                                               Fax: 860-721-2056
                                          e-mail: lbph@cslib.org
                                           www.cslib.org/lbph.htm
Free audio cassettes and braille books and magazines along with
reference materials on blindness and other handicaps. Necessary
playback equipment for eligible residents of Connecticut.
Carol Taylor, Director

Delaware

**9691   Delaware Division of Libraries: Library for the Blind and
Physically Handicapped**
43 South DuPont Highway   302-739-4748
Dover, DE 19901   800-282-8676
                                               Fax: 302-739-6787
                                               TDD: 302-739-4847
                                 e-mail: john.phillos@state.de.us
                                              www.state.lib.de.us
Since 1971, the Delaware Library for the Blind and Physically
Handicapped has provided books in Braille and audio books on re-
cord and cassette for the blind and physically handicapped resi-
dents of Delaware.
John Phillos, Librarian

District of Columbia

9692   Council of Families with Visual Impairment
American Council of the Blind
1155 15th Street NW   202-467-5081
Washington, DC 20005   800-424-8666
                                               Fax: 202-467-5085
                                             e-mail: info@acb.org
                                                   www.acb.org
Members are sighted parents of blind or visually impaired children. Offers a forum for support and outreach, sharing of experiences in parent-child relationships, and educational and cultural
information about child development. Monitors developments in
technical and legislative arenas.
Melanie Brunson, Executive Director

9693   DC Public Library Adaptive Services Division
901 G Street NW, Room 215   202-727-2142
Washington, DC 20001   Fax: 202-727-1129
                                               TTY: 202-727-2255
                                               TDD: 202-727-1129
                                        e-mail: lbph.dcpl@dc.gov
                                                www.dclibrary.org
The DC Public Library has a special Adaptive Technology Program to help older adults, the deaf, and those with visual and physi-
cal disabilities use library materials and resources.
Venetia V. Demson, Librarian

**9694   National Library Service for the Blind and Physically
Handicapped**
1291 Taylor Street,   202- 70- 510
Washington, DC 20011   Fax: 202-707-0712
                                               TDD: 202-707-0744
                                            e-mail: raj@loc.gov
                                                  www.loc.gov/nls
The NLS, Library of Congress, administers the free programs that
loans recorded and braille books and magazines, music scores in

braille and large print, and specially designed playback equipment
to residents of the United States who are unable to read or use standard print materials due to visual or physical impairment.
Yealuri Rathan Raj, Librarian

Florida

9695   Brevard County Libraries: Talking Books Library
2725 Judge Fran Jamieson Wayÿ   32- 6-3 20
Viera, FL 32940-7781   Fax: 32- 9-2 63
                                             e-mail: dmartin@brev.org
                                                    www.brev.org
The Talking Books/Homebound Services has many devices and
special materials to assist blind, physically handicapped and/or
homebound citizens to access library services.
Debra A. Martin, Librarian

9696   Broward County Talking Book Library
100 S Andrews Avenue   954-357-7555
Fort Lauderdale, FL 33301-1830   Fax: 954-577-20
                              e-mail: talkingbooks@browardlibrary.org
                                 www.broward.org/library/talkingbooks
Reference materials on blindness and other handicaps, closed-circuit TV, Talking Book cassettes, print/Braille and descriptive
videos.
William Forbes, Librarian

9697   Florida Bureau of Braille and Talking Book Library Services
421 Platt Street   386-239-6000
Daytona Beach, FL 32114-2803   800-226-6075
                                               Fax: 386-239-6069
                                 e-mail: mike.gunde@dbs.fldoe.org
                                 dbs.myflorida.com/library/index.php
The Florida Bureau of Braille and Talking Book Library Services
provides information and reading materials needed by Florida residents who are unable to use standard print as the result of visual,
physical, or reading disabilities.
Michael Gunde, Librarian

9698   Hillsborough County Talking Book Library
Jan Kaminis Platt Regional Library
900 N ashley drive   813-273-3652
Tampa, FL 33602-1214   TTY: 813-273-3610
                                               TDD: 813-273-3610
                            e-mail: talkingbooks@hillsboroughounty.org
                                                   www.hcplc.org
This free program provides recorded and braille books and maga-
zines to people who are blind, visually impaired or physically
handicapped.
Ann Palmer, Librarian
Ann Palmer, Librarian

9699   Jacksonville Public Library
303 North Laura Street
Jacksonville, FL 32202   904-630-2665
                                                  http//jpl.coj.net
Discs, cassettes, reference materials on blindness and other handi-
caps and children's books on cassettes.
Dr Brenda Simmons Hutchins, Chairperson
Erin Skinner, Vice Chair

9700   Lee County Talking Books Library
13240 North Cleveland Avenue, #5-6   239-995-2665
North Ft. Myers, FL 33903-4855   800-854-8195
                                               Fax: 239-995-1681
                                               TDD: 2399952665
                                  e-mail: talkingbooks@leegov.com
                                            www.lee-county.com/library
Talking Books are books and magazines that are recorded for people who need to hear their reading. The books are played on special
players provided free by the National Library Service for the Blind
and Physically Handicapped.
Sheldon Kaye, Librarian

9701   Miami Dade Talking Book Library
Miami Dade Public Library System

101 W flagler street
Miami, FL 33130
305- 37- 266
800-451-9544
Fax: 305-757-8401
TDD: 305-474-7258
e-mail: talkingbooks@mdpls.org
www.mdpls.org

The Talking Books Library loans books and magazines on cassette tapes or in Braille FREE by mail to persons who have difficulty seeing or using standard small print.
Raymond Santiago, Director
Barbara Moyer, Librarian

9702 Orange County Library System: Orlando Public Library
101 E Central Boulevard
Orlando, FL 32801-2462
407-835-7323
Fax: 407-425-6779
www.ocls.info

The library's collection consists of a wide variety of print materials, including fiction, nonfiction, world languages, genealogy, and special materials that comprise the Florida and Disney collections. The library also has audiovisual materials and electronic resources to meet customer needs.
Mary Anne Hodel, Library Director/CEO

9703 Palm Beach County Library Annex: Talking Books
Mil-Lake Plaza
3650 Summit Blvd.
West Palm Beach,, FL 33406
561-233-2600
888-780-5151
Fax: 561-233-2627
e-mail: talkingbooks@pbclibrary.org
www.pbclibrary.org

The Talking Books Library is a special service of the Palm Beach County Library and a part of the Library of Congress National Library Service for the Blind and Physically Handicapped.
Pat Mistretta, Librarian

9704 Pinellas Talking Book Library for the Blind and Physically Handicapped
1330 Cleveland Street
Clearwater, FL 33755-5103
727-441-9958
86- 6-9 95
Fax: 727-441-9068
TDD: 727-441-3168
www.pplc.us/tbl/

The Pinellas Talking Book Library's mission is to encourage and support reading by providing free library services to Pinellas County residents for whom conventional print is a barrier. The Pinellas Talking Book Library is part of a nationwide network of cooperating libraries serving people who have difficulty using or reading regular print.
Marilyn Stevenson, Access Services Librarian

9705 Sub Regional Talking Book Library
1755 Edgewood Avenue West
Jacksonville, FL 32208-7206
904-765-5588
Fax: 904-768-7822
TDD: 904-768-7822
e-mail: jerryco@j.net

Susan V Arthur, Librarian
Laurie Baumgardner, Librarian

9706 West Florida Public Library: Talking Book Library
239 North Spring Street
Pensacola, FL 32502-4822
850-436-5060
Fax: 850-436-5039
e-mail: talkingbooks@ci.pensacola.fl.us
www.cityofpensacola.com/library

As a subregional Talking Book Library, the Pensacola Public Library offers free service by mail to blind and physically handicapped adults and children who have difficulty reading ordinary print or holding or turning the pages of a book.
Rodney L Kendig, Chairman
Dr. Rebecca Temple, Vice Chairman

Georgia

9707 Albany Library for the Blind and Physically Handicapped
Dougherty County Public Library
1180 Washington Avenue
Macon, GA 31201
478-744-0840
800-805-7613
Fax: 478-744-0840
e-mail: lbph@docolib.org
www.docolib.org/libblind.html

The Library for the Blind and Physically Handicapped provides resources to individuals who are blind, visually impaired, physically handicapped or learning disabled in a thirteen-county area.
Kathryn Sinquefield, Librarian

9708 Atlanta Metro Subregional Library
1800 Century Place
Atlanta, GA 30345
404-235-7200
800-248-6701
Fax: 404-756-4618
e-mail: glass@georgialibraries.org
www.georgialibraries.org/public.glass

Through Georgia's Regional Library for the Blind and Physically Handicapped and cooperating local libraries, Georgians have access to a free national library program that offers books and magazines on cassette tape and in Braille.
Linda B Stetson, Director

9709 Augusta Regional Library Talking Book Center
425 James Brown Boulevard
Augusta, GA 30901
706-821-2625
Fax: 706-724-5403
e-mail: talkbook@ecgrl.org
www.ecgrl.public.lib.ga.ua/lbph.htm

Through the Georgia Library for Accessible Services, Georgians have access to a free national library program that offers books and magazines on cassette tape and in Braille.
Gary Swint, Librarian

9710 Bainbridge Subregional Library for the Blind and Physically Handicapped
Southwest Georgia Regional Library
301 South Monroe Street
Bainbridge, GA 39819-4029
229-248-2680
800-795-2680
Fax: 229-248-2670
TDD: 229-248-2665
e-mail: lbph@swgrl.org
www.swgrl.org

The library houses a large collection of recorded materials as well as reference materials.
Susan S. Whittle, Director

9711 Columbus Library for Accessible Services (CLASS)
The Columbus Public Library
3000 Macon Road
Columbus, GA 31906-2201
706-243-2686
800-652-0782
Fax: 706-243-2710
e-mail: sbarnes@cvrls.net
www.thecolumbuslibrary.org

CLASS serves as one of the Georgia subregional distribution centers for books and magazines on audiocassettes published by the National Library Service for the Blind and Physically Handicapped.
Suzanne Barnes, Librarian

9712 Georgia Library for Accessible Services (GLASS)
1800 Century Place
Atlanta, GA 30345-3803
404-235-7200
800-248-6701
Fax: 404-756-4618
e-mail: glass@georgialibraries.org
www.georgialibraries.org

Georgians have access to a free national library program that offers books and magazines on cassette tape and in Braille. These materials are provided by the Library of Congress, National Library Service for the Blind & Physically Handicapped (NLS),), to eligible persons with a visual or physical disability. All reading material and playback equipment is sent to borrowers and returned by postage-free mail.
Linda B Stetson, Director

9713 Hall County Library System: East Hall Branch and Special Needs Library
2434 Old Cornelia Highway
Gainesville, GA 30507
770-532-3311
Fax: 770-531-2502
TDD: 770-531-2530
e-mail: kevans@hallcountylibrary.org
www.hallcountylibrary.org/ehmap.htm

The East Hall Branch and Special Needs Library goal is to provide excellent service to those with disabilities including the blind, handicapped, mobility impaired and deaf.
Kathy Evans, Branch Manager

9714 Middle Georgia Subregional Library for the Blind and Physically Handicapped
Washington Memorial Library
1180 Washington Avenue   478-744-0877
Macon, GA 31201-1790   800-805-7613
Fax: 478-744-0840
e-mail: mgrltbc2@bibblib.org
www.co.bibb.ga.us/library/TBC.htm
Books, magazines, newspapers, radio programs and various publications are available. Assistive technology equipment is also available at the library.
Thomas Jones, Director
Karen Monroe, Finance Officer

9715 Oconee Regional Library for the Blind and Physically Handicapped
801 Bellevue Avenue   478-275-5382
Dublin, GA 31040   800-453-5541
Fax: 478-275-3821
e-mail: wdaniel@ocrl.org
www.laurens.public.lib.ga.us
Through the Georgia Library for Accessible Services and cooperating local libraries, Georgians have access to a free national library program which offers braille and recorded materials.
Wanda Daniel, Librarian

9716 Rome Subregional Library for People with Disabilities
205 Riverside Parkway NE   706-236-4618
Rome, GA 30161-2911   888-263-0769
Fax: 706-236-4631
TDD: 706-236-4618
e-mail: dhickman@rome-lpd.org
www.rome-lpd.org
Provides free library service to the disabled in eleven counties of Northwest Georgia.
Delana Hickman, Coordinator

9717 Special Needs Library of Northeast Georgia
Athens-Clarke County Regional Library
2025 Baxter Street   706-613-3655
Athens, GA 30606-6331   800-531-2063
Fax: 706-613-3660
TDD: 706-613-3655
e-mail: specialneedslibrary@athenslibrary.org
www.clarke.public.lib.ga.us/specneeds
The Special Needs Library of Northeast Georgia provides free library services for patrons with visual, physical, and reading disabilities.
Claudia L. Markov, Librarian

9718 Subregional Library for the Blind and Physically Handicapped
Live Oak Public Libraries, Thunderbolt Branch
2002 Bull Street   912-652-3600
Savannah, GA 31401   800-342-4455
Fax: 912-354-5534
e-mail: stokesl@liveoakpl.org
www.liveoakpl.org
Library for the blind and physically handicapped.
LaTrelle Mobley, Manager

9719 Three Rivers Regional Library
Brunswick-Glynn County Regional Library
208 Gloucester Street   912-267-1212
Brunswick, GA 31520-5324   866-833-2878
Fax: 912-267-9597
e-mail: bransom@trrl.org
www.threeriverslibraries.org
The Talking Book Center serves 12 counties with over 1200 patrons. The center provides talking books which are recorded at a slower speed which requires the use of a special player.
Betty D. Ransom, Librarian

9720 Valdosta Talking Book Library
South Georgia Regional Library
300 Woodrow Wilson Drive   229-333-0086
Valdosta, GA 31602-2592   800-246-6515
Fax: 229-333-7669
e-mail: djernigan@sgrl.org
www.sgrl.org

The Talking Book Center is available to blind persons with visual difficulty or physical handicaps which prevent them from using printed material.
Diane Jernigan, Librarian

Hawaii

9721 Hawaii State Library for the Blind and Physically Handicapped
402 Kapahulu Avenue   808-733-8444
Honolulu, HI 96815   800-559-4096
Fax: 808-733-8449
TDD: 808-733-8444
e-mail: olbcirc@librarieshawaii.org
www.librarieshawaii.org
The Library for the Blind and Physically Handicapped serves as the regional library and machine lending agency for the blind and physically disabled throughout the state and the outlying Pacific Islands in cooperation with the Library of Congress and the National Library Service for the Blind and Physically Handicapped.
Fusako Miyashiro, Librarian

Idaho

9722 Idaho Commission for Libraries Talking Book Service
325 West State Street   208-334-2150
Boise, ID 83702-6072   800-458-3271
Fax: 208-334-4016
TDD: 800-377-1363
e-mail: talkingbooks@libraries.idaho.gov
http://libraries.idaho.gov/tbs
The Idaho Talking Book Service provides books and magazines in cassette format for individuals who are unable to read standard print.
Sue Walker, Librarian

Illinois

9723 Catholic Guild for the Blind
65 E. Wacker Place   312-236-8569
Chicago, IL 60601   Fax: 312-236-8128
e-mail: info@guildfortheblind.org
www.second-sense.org
The Guild's adult rehabilitation services include a program geared towards seniors experiencing new vision loss called New Visions. This program promotes independence within the home and community by providing participants with the information, techniques, and tools they need to successfully adjust to their new lives with impaired sight. Two workshop series are available to beginners or to those ready for more advanced topics.
David J Tabak, Executive Director
Polly Abbott, Manager Adult Rehabilitation Services

9724 Illinois State Library Talking Book and Braille Service
401 East Washington   217-782-9435
Springfield, IL 62701-1207   800-665-5576
Fax: 217-558-4723
TDD: 888-261-7863
The Illinois State Library Talking Book and Braille Service plays a supporting rols for the Illinois Network of Libraries Serving the Blind and Physically Handicapped.

9725 Mid-Illinois Talking Book Center
125 Tower Drive   217-224-6619
Burr Ridge, IL 60527   800-426-0709
Fax: 217-224-9818
e-mail: info@illinoistalkingbooks.org
www.illinoistalkingbooks.org
We provide free library service for anyone unable to read regular print because of low vision, blindness, or a physical disability. We provide recorded and Braille books and popular magazines. There are over 60,000 titles available including popular fiction and non-fiction, bestsellers, classics, history, biographies, children's books and more.
Karen Bershe, Director
Valerie Brandon, PR/Outreach Coordinator

9726 Shawnee Library System: Southern Illinois Talking Book Center
607 South Greenbriar Road   618-985-8375
Carterville, IL 62918   800-445-2665
Fax: 618-985-4211
TDD: 618-985-8375
e-mail: imsastaff@imsa.lib.il.us
www.imsa.lib.il.us/

The Talking Book Program is a free library service for anyone who has difficulty reading print or holding books and turning pages due to any visual or physical limitation or medically diagnosed reading disability. Participants are loaned cassette players along with unabridged books and magazines on tape and in Braille.
Diana Brawley Sussman, Director/Librarian

9727 Skokie Accessible Library Services
Skokie Public Library
5215 Oakton Street   847-673-7774
Skokie, IL 60077-3634   Fax: 847-673-7797
e-mail: anthe@skokie.library.info
www.skokie.lib.il.us

Library services for people with disabilities, including electronic aids, materials in special formats, programs and special services, and access to the North Suburban Library System.
Carolyn A Anthony, Director

9728 Voices of Vision Talking Book Center
125 Tower Drive   630-208-0398
Burr Ridge, IL 60527   800-426-0709
Fax: 630-208-0399
e-mail: info@illinoistalkingbooks.org
www.illinoistalkingbooks.org.

Voices of Vision is part of a statewide and national network of libraries which provide the talking book and braille service. We provide free library service to persons unable to read or use conventional print material due to a visual or physical disability. There is no cost to eligible readers.
Karen Odean, Director

Indiana

9729 Bartholomew County Public Library
National Library Services
536 Fifth Street   812-379-1255
Columbus, IN 47201   800-685-0524
Fax: 812-791-75
e-mail: talkingbooks@barth.lib.in.us
www.barth.lib.in.us

Talking Books for the Blind and Physically Handicapped is a free library service for visually or physically challenged persons of all ages. Anyone who is unable to use regular printed materials as the result of a temporary or permanent visual or physical limitation is eligible.
Sharon Thompson, Librarian

9730 Evansville-Vanderburgh County Public Library
200 SE Martin Luther King Jr Blvd   812-428-8200
Evansville, IN 47713   Fax: 812-428-8397
www.evpl.org

The Evansville-Vanderburgh County Public Library, an essential provider of shared information and a core community service, promotes reading, lifelong learning, and economic vitality through its resources, services and programs to the residents of Vanderburgh County.
Mike Russ, President
Brenda Schiedler, Vice President

9731 Indiana Talking Book & Braille Library
315 West Ohio Street   317-232-3697
Indianapolis, IN 46202   800-622-4970
e-mail: lbph@statelib.lib.in.us
www.in.gov/library/tbbl.htm

The TBBL provides large print books, braille books, and books on tape to Indiana residents who are unable to read regular print.
Roberta L Brooker, Interim Director

9732 Lake County Public Library
1919 W 81st Street   219-769-3541
Merrillville, IN 46410   Fax: 219-769-0690
www.lcplin.org/

Talking books provides cassette books, descriptive videos, magazines and large print books to people who are blind and physically handicapped. Materials are sent through the mail and the service is free to those who qualify.
Renee Lewis, Director

Iowa

9733 Iowa Department for the Blind
524 Fourth Street   515-281-1333
Des Moines, IA 50309-2364   800-362-2587
Fax: 515-281-1263
TTY: 515-281-1355
e-mail: information@blind.state.ia.us
www.blind.state.ia.us/?

Our program offers the specialized, integrated services that blind and severely visually impaired Iowans need to live independently and work competitively.
Allen Harris, Director

Kansas

9734 CKLS Headquarters
1409 Williams Street   620-792-4865
Great Bend, KS 67530-4090   800-362-2642
Fax: 620-793-7270
e-mail: jswan@ckls.org
www.ckls.org

Offers direct services to rural residents and those who need special services because of disability.
Chris Rippel, Department Head Continuing Education
Kathy Rippel, Department Head

9735 Manhattan Subregional Library of the Kansas Talking Books Service
629 Poyntz Avenue   785-776-4741
Manhattan, KS 66502-6006   800-432-2796
Fax: 785-776-1545
e-mail: annp@manhattan.lib.ks.us
www.manhattan.lib.ks.us

Books and magazines in braille and recorded format and playback equipment are provided to any Kansas citizen residing in the twelve county area of the North Central Kansas Libraries System who is unable to use standard print as a result of temporary or permanent visual or physical impairments.
Ann Pearce, Department Manager
Wandean Rivers, Assistive Technology Center Instructor

9736 Northwest Kansas Library System
Northwest Kansas Library System
2 Washington Square   785-877-5148
Norton, KS 67654   800-432-2858
Fax: 785-877-5697
www.nwkls.mykansaslibrary.org/

The Kansas Library Network for the Blind and Physically Handicapped, in cooperation with the Library of Congress, National Library Service for the Blind and Physically Handicapped, provides library services and materials to Kansans unable to use conventional print.
Leslie Bell, Director
Clarice Howard, BPH Librarian

9737 South Central Kansas Library System
321A North Main Street   620-663-3211
South Hutchinson, KS 67505   800-234-0529
Fax: 313-663-9797
e-mail: phawkins@sckls.info
www.sckls.info/

Summer reading programs, braille writer, magnifiers, closed-circuit TV, large-print photocopier, cassette books and magazines, children's books on cassette, home visits and other reference materials on blindness and other handicaps.
Paul Hawkins, Director
Tram Nguyen, Technology Services Coordinator

9738 Talking Books Service
Topeka and Shawnee County Public Library

1515 SW 10th Avenue
Topeka, KS 66604-1304

785-580-4530
800-432-2925
Fax: 785-580-4530
e-mail: tbooks@tscpl.lib.ks.us
www.tscpl.org/services/talkingbooks

Summer reading programs, braille writer, magnifiers, closed-circuit TV, large-print photocopier, cassette books and magazines, children's books on cassette, home visits and other reference materials on blindness and other handicaps.
Suzanne Bundy, Librarian

9739   Wichita Public Library
223 S Main
Wichita, KS 67202

316-261-8500
Fax: 316-262-4540
TDD: 316-262-3972
e-mail: admin@wichita.lib.ks.us
www.wichita.lib.ks.us

Talking books provides cassette books, descriptive videos, magazines adn large print books to people who are blind and physically handicapped. Materials are sent through the mail and the service is free to those who qualify.
Brad Reha, Talking Books Manager

Kentucky

9740   Kentucky Talking Book Library
PO Box 537
Frankfort, KY 40602-0537

502-564-8300
800-372-2968
Fax: 502-564-5773
e-mail: katherine.kimball@ky.gov
www.kdla.ky.gov

Our mission is to provide library service to individuals who have a visual or physical disability that prevents them from using standard print materials. We send books on tape and Braille books through the mail at no cost to our patrons.
Katherine K. Adelberg, E-Rate Coordinator,Field Services
Jackie Arnold, Local Records Regional Administrator

9741   Louisville Talking Book Library for the Blind and Physically Handicapped
301 York Street
Louisville, KY 40203-2205

502-574-1611
www.lfpl.org/tbl

The Louisville Talking Book Library offers recorded books and other materials to eligible visually and physically handicapped Jefferson County, KY residents. All recorded books & equipment may be sent to borrowers and returned by postage-free mail.
Linda Atzinger, Supervisor Accessibility Services

9742   Northern Kentucky Talking Book Library
502 Scott Boulevard
Covington, KY 41011

859-962-4095
866-491-7610
Fax: 859-962-4096
www.kenton.lib.ky.us

Our library provides books and magazines on specially recorded cassettes for people who are visually impaired and/or physically handicapped and live in Boone, Campbell, Carroll, Gallatin, Grant, Kenton, Owen and Pendleton counties.
Dave Schroeder, Director

Louisiana

9743   State Library of Louisiana
701 N 4th Street
Baton Rouge, LA 70802

225-342-4913
Fax: 225-219-4804
e-mail: admin@state.lib.la.us
www.state.lib.la.us

Talking books provides cassette books, descriptive videos, magazines and large print books to people who are blind and physically handicapped. Materials are sent through the mail and the service is free to those who qualify.

Maine

9744   Bangor Public Library
145 Harlow Street
Bangor, ME 04401-4900

207-947-8336
Fax: 207-945-6694
e-mail: bplill@bpl.lib.me.us
www.bpl.lib.me.us

Summer reading programs, braille writer, magnifiers, closed-circuit TV, large-print photocopier, cassette books and magazines, children's books on cassette, home visits and other reference materials on blindness and other handicaps.
Barbara McDade, Director

9745   Cary Library
107 Main Street
Houlton, ME 04730-2196

207-532-1302
Fax: 207-532-4350
www.cary.lib.me.us

Summer reading programs, braille writer, magnifiers, closed-circuit TV, large-print photocopier, cassette books and magazines, children's books on cassette, home visits and other reference materials on blindness and other handicaps.
Linda Faucher, Librarian

9746   Lewiston Public Library
200 Lisbon Street
Lewiston, ME 04240-7203

207-513-3004
Fax: 207-784-3011
TTY: 207-784-3123
e-mail: lplweb@lplonline.org
www.lplonline.org

Summer reading programs, braille writer, magnifiers, closed-circuit TV, large-print photocopier, cassette books and magazines, children's books on cassette, home visits and other reference materials on blindness and other handicaps.
Rick Speer, Director
Jake Paris, Adult Services Librarian

9747   Maine State Library
64 State House Station
Augusta, ME 04333-0064

207-287-5650
800-452-8793
Fax: 207-287-5624
www.state.me.us/msl

Large Print Books is a service through Outreach Services for residents of Maine who are certified as visually impaired and public libraries who serve the visually impaired.
Chris Boynton, Outreach/Special Services Coordinator
Alan Fecteau, Media Coordinator

9748   Portland Public Library
5 Monument Square
Portland, ME 04101-4072

207-871-1700
Fax: 207-871-1715
e-mail: reference@portland.lib.me.us
www.portlandlibrary.com

Portland Public Library's Outreach Services brings library resources to those who are unable to visit the library in person. For people living in nursing homes or assisted living facilities, or for those confined to home due to illness or disability, the library will deliver print and audio books right to your doorstep.
Stephen J Podgajny, Director

9749   Waterville Public Library
73 Elm Street
Waterville, ME 04901-6027

207-872-5433
Fax: 207-873-4779
www.watervillelibrary.org

Summer reading programs, braille writer, magnifiers, closed-circuit TV, large-print photocopier, cassette books and magazines, children's books on cassette, home visits and other reference materials on blindness and other handicaps.
Sarah Sugden, Director

Maryland

9750   American Action Fund for Blind Children and Adults
1800 Johnson Street, Suite 100
Baltimore, MD 21230

410-659-9315
e-mail: actionfund@actionfund.org
www.actionfund.org

Our mission is to assist blind persons in securing reading matter, to educate the public about blindness, to give aid to the deaf-blind, to provide specialized aids and appliances to the blind, to give consultation to governmental and private agencies serving the blind, to offer assistance to older blind persons, to offer services to blind children and their parents, and to do any other lawful thing which it can to improve the quality of life for blind persons.
Barbara Loos, President
Ramona Walhof, First Vice President

9751 Disability Resource Center of Montgomery County Public Libraries
Rockville Library
21 Maryland Avenue 240-777-0311
Rockville, MD 20850 TTY: 240-773-3556
e-mail: county.council@montgomerycountymd.gov
www.montgomerycountymd.gov
The Disability Resource Center (DRC) is the focal point within the Montgomery County Public Libraries (MCPL) for library and literacy services to people with disabilities, their families, caretakers and professionals.
Kay Bowman, Agency Manager

9752 International Braille and Technology Center for the Blind
National Federation of the Blind
1026 East 36th Street 410-645-0632
Baltimore, MD 21218-4998 Fax: 410-685-5653
e-mail: melissa@riccobono.us
www.nfb.org
A comprehensive and complete evaluation and demonstration center for assistive technology used by the blind worldwide. Includes all Braille, synthetic speech, print-to-speech scanning, internet and portable devices and programs. Available for tours by appointment to blind persons, employers, technology manufacturers, teachers, parents and those working in the assistive technology field.
Melissa Riccobono, President

9753 Maryland State Library for the Blind and Physically Handicapped
415 Park Avenue 410-230-2424
Baltimore, MD 21201 800-964-9209
Fax: 410-333-2095
TTY: 800-934-2541
www.lbph.lib.md/us
The basic mission of the Maryland State Library for the Blind and Physically Handicapped is to provide comprehensive library services to the eligible blind and physically handicapped residents of the State of Maryland.
Jill Lewis, Director

9754 Prince George's County Memorial Library: Talking Book Center
6532 Adelphi Road 301-699-3500
Hyattsville, MD 20782-2098 TTY: 301-808-2061
e-mail: kathleen.teaze@pgcmls.info
www.prge.lib.md.us
Talking books provides cassette books, descriptive videos, magazines and large print books to people who are blind and physically handicapped. Materials are sent through the mail and the services are free to those who qualify.
Kathleen Teaze, Director

Massachusetts

9755 Caption Center
125 Western Avenue 617-492-9225
Allston, MA 02134-1008 Fax: 617-562-0590
Provides closed captioning for videos, including training, safety, instructional and educational films. Maintains a consumer information service for overcoming communications barriers in the workplace.
Lori Kay, Co-Director
Tom Apone, Co-Director

9756 Laboure College Library
2120 Dorchester Avenue 617-296-8300
Boston, MA 02124-5617 e-mail: library@laboure.edu
www.laboure.edu
Offers information on physical disabilities, independent living, peer counseling and advocacy.
Maryann O'Toole, Director

9757 Perkins Braille and Talking Book Library
175 N Beacon Street 617-924-3434
Watertown, MA 02472-2751 800-852-3133
Fax: 617-972-7315
TTY: 617-972-7690
e-mail: Info@Perkins.org
www.perkins.org

The Perkins Braille & Talking Book Library, funded in part by the Massachusetts Board of Library Commissioners, provides free services to Massachusetts residents of any age who are unable to read traditional print materials due to a visual or physical disability.
Kim Charlson, Director

9758 Talking Book Library at Worcester Public Library
3 Salem Square 508-799-1655
Worcester, MA 1608-2074 800-762-0085
Fax: 508-799-1676
e-mail: talkbook@cwmars.org/talkingbook
www.cwmars.org/talkingbook
Adapted computers, braille embosser, magnifiers, closed circuit TV, large print books, cassette books and magazines, children's books on cassette, reference materials on blindness and other disabilities. Summer reading programs.
James L Izatt, Librarian

Michigan

9759 Detroit Subregional Library for the Blind and Physically Handicapped
Detroit Public Library
3666 Grand River Avenue 313-833-5494
Detroit, MI 48208 Fax: 313-325-97
TDD: 313-833-5492
e-mail: dmiddle@detroitpubliclibrary.org
www.detroit.lib.mi.us
Talking books along with talking book machines are available to eligible residents who live in a 14 ZIP code area of Detroit and Highland Park. Loans of the books and machines are made to individuals and to institutions such as schools, nursing homes and senior residences. Over 45,000 books are available. Magazines available in recorded format include Ebony, Good Housekeeping, and Sports Illustrated.
Dori V. Middleton, LBPH Specialist

9760 Grand Traverse Area Library for the Blind and Physically Handicapped
322 6th Street 616-935-6520
Traverse City, MI 49684-2414 Fax: 616-922-0904
TDD: 616-922-0901

Evelyn Welty

9761 Kent County Library for the Blind
775 Ball Avenue NE 616-336-3250
Grand Rapids, MI 49503-1397 Fax: 616-336-3256
e-mail: kdlem@lakeland.lib.mi.us
Summer reading programs, braille writer, magnifiers, closed-circuit TV, large-print photocopier, cassette books and magazines, children's books on cassette, home visits and other reference materials on blindness and other handicaps.
Claudya Muller, Librarian

9762 Library of Michigan Service for the Blind
PO Box 30007 517-373-5614
Lansing, MI 48909-7507 Fax: 517-735-65
e-mail: sbph@michigan.gov
www.michigan.gov/sbth

Braille writer, magnifiers, closed circuit TV, large print photocopier, cassette books and magazines, children's books on cassette, reference materials on blindness and other handicaps. Books on cassette and braille books and cassette players will be loaned and sent through the mail at no charge. For blind and those physically unable to read standard print or turn the pages.
Susan Thinault, Manager

9763 Macomb Library for the Blind and Physically Handicapped
35891 South Gratiot 586-226-5072
Clinton Township, MI 48035-1132 Fax: 810-286-0634
TDD: 8102869940
e-mail: macbld@libcoop.net
www.cmpl.org/MLBPH/?
Summer reading programs, braille writer, closed-circuit TV, cassette books and magazines, children's books on cassette, reference materials on blindness and other handicaps.
Beverlee Babcock, Librarian

9764 Midwestern Michigan Library Cooperative
G4195 West Pasadena Avenue   810-732-1120
Flint, MI 48504   Fax: 810-321-15
                                    www.mideasteRN.lib.mi.us
Roger Mendell, Director

9765 Muskegon County Library for the Blind
635 Ottawa Street   616-724-6248
Muskegon, MI 49442-1016   Fax: 616-724-6675
                                    TDD: 616-722-4103
Summer reading programs, braille typewriter, magnifiers, closed-circuit TV, large-print photocopier, cassette books and magazines, children's books on cassette, home visits and other reference materials on blindness and other handicaps, The Reading Edge, Perkins Brailler and large print books.
Linda Clapp, Librarian

9766 Northland Library Cooperative
220 W. Clinton St.   231-855-2206
Charlevoix, MI 49720-2892   Fax: 517-354-3939
                                    e-mail: webmaster@nlc.lib.mi.us
                                    www.nlc.lib.mi.us/
Summer reading programs, braille writer, magnifiers, closed-circuit TV, large-print photocopier, cassette books and magazines, children's books on cassette, home visits and other reference materials on blindness and other handicaps.
Catherine Glomski, Librarian

9767 Oakland County Library for the Visually and Physically Impaired
1200 N Telegraph Road   248-858-5050
Pontiac, MI 48341-1032   800-774-4542
                                    Fax: 248-858-9313
                                    e-mail: lVPi@co.oakland..mi.us
                                    www.co.oakland.mi.us/lVPi
Free cassette book service to eligible visually or physically impaired Oakland County residents; demonstrations, CCTV and hand held magnifiers and a large print collection.
David Conklin, Head Librarian

9768 St. Clark County Library for the Blind and Physically Handicapped
210 McMorran Boulevard   810-982-3600
Port Huron, MI 48060-4014   800-272-8570
                                    Fax: 810-987-7327
                                    e-mail: lbph@sccl.lib.mi.us
                                    www.sccl.lib.mi.us/LBPH.aspx
Offers library services to the blind and visually impaired.
Jackie Skinner, Librarian

9769 Upper Peninsula Library for the Blind and Physically Handicapped
1615 Presque Isle Avenue   906-228-7697
Marquette, MI 49855-2811   Fax: 906-285-27
                                    e-mail: uproc.lib.mi.us
                                    www.michigan.gov/sbth
Summer reading programs, braille writer, magnifiers, closed-circuit TV, large-print photocopier, cassette books and magazines, children's books on cassette, home visits and other reference materials on blindness and other handicaps.
Susan Thinault, Manager

9770 Washtenaw County Library for the Blind and Physically Disabled
PO Box 8645   734-971-6059
Ann Arbor, MI 48107-8645   Fax: 734-971-3892
                                    e-mail: lbpd@co.washtennaw.mi.us
                                    comnet.org/cgi-bin/helpnet/viewitem?290+
Book lovers club.adaptive technology,cassette equipment, cassette books and magazines, described videos, low vision aids reference and referral services.
Margaret Wolfe, Cordinator

9771 Wayne County Regional Library for the Blind and Physically Handicapped
41365 Vincenti Court   248-536-3100
Novi, MI 48375-5310   888-968-2737
                                    Fax: 248-536-3098
                                    TDD: 313-326-3008
                                    e-mail: werlbph@tln.lib.mi.us
                                    www.tln.lib.mi.us
Summer reading programs, braille writer, magnifiers, closed-circuit TV, large-print photocopier, cassette books and magazines, children's books on cassette, home visits and other reference materials on blindness and other handicaps.
Pat Klemans, Librarian

Minnesota

9772 Duluth Public Library
City of Duluth Department
520 W Superior Street   218-730-4200
Duluth, MN 55802-1578   Fax: 218-233-15
                                    e-mail: webmail@duluthmn.gov
                                    www.duluth.lib.mn.us
Adapted access to Apple computer, adapted toys and adapted library equipment.
Randall Deth Kelly, Director

9773 Minnesota Library for the Blind
1500 Highway 36 West   507-333-4828
Roseville, MN 55113   800-722-0550
                                    Fax: 507-333-4832
                                    e-mail: mn.lbph@state.mn.us
                                    www.education.state.mn.us
Summer reading programs, braille writer, magnifiers, closed-circuit TV, large-print photocopier, cassette books and magazines, children's books on cassette, home visits and other reference materials on blindness and other handicaps.
Catherine Durivage, Director

Mississippi

9774 Christian Resource for People Who Are Blind
Care Ministries Inc
PO Box 1830   662-323-4999
Starkville, MS 39760-1830   800-366-2232
                                    e-mail: careministries@bellsouth.net
                                    www.careministries.org
Offers braille and large print books and cassettes for the visually impaired.
B J LeJeune, Director

9775 Mississippi Library Commission
3881 Eastwood Drive   601-432-4486
Jackson, MS 39211-7328   800-647-7542
                                    Fax: 601-961-4113
                                    TDD: 601-354-6411
                                    e-mail: mslib@mic.lib.ms.us
                                    www.mlc.lib.ms.us
Summer reading programs, braille writer, magnifiers, closed-circuit TV, large-print photocopier, cassette books and magazines, children's books on cassette, home visits and other reference materials on blindness and other handicaps.
Larry Mc Millan, Director

Missouri

9776 Adriene Resource Center for Blind Children
Assembly of God Center for Blind
1445 Boonville Avenue   417-862-2781
Springfield, MO 65802   Fax: 417-625-20
                                    e-mail: info@ag.org
                                    www.blind.ag.org
Offers braille and cassette lending library, braille and cassette Sunday school materials for all ages, braille and cassette periodicals and resource assistance, and resources for blind children and children of blind parents.
Paul Weingariner, Director
Caryl Weingariner, Co-Director

9777 Assemblies of God National Center for the Blind
1445 Boonville Avenue   417-831-1964
Springfield, MO 65802   Fax: 417-627-66
                                                  e-mail: blind@ag.org
Offers braille and cassette lending library, braille and cassette
Sunday school materials for all ages, braille and cassette periodi-
cals and resource assistance, and resources for blind children and
children of blind parents.
Paul Weingariner, Director

9778 Church of the Nazarene
Nazarene Publishing House
PO Box 419527   816-931-1900
Kansas City, MO 64141-6527   800-877-0700
                                          e-mail: NPH@direct.nph.com
                                                         www.nph.com
Offers braille and large print books. Also offers a lending library
and cassettes for the blind.

9779 Lutheran Library for the Blind
Lutheran Church - Missouri Synod
1333 S Kirkwood Road   314-965-9000
Saint Louis, MO 63122-7295   800-248-1930
                                                 Fax: 314-996-1016
                                          e-mail: infocenter@lcms.org
                                                        www.lcms.org
Offers braille and large print books and cassettes for the blind and
visually impaired.

9780 Whitney Library for the Blind: Assemblies of God
1445 N Boonville Avenue   417-862-2781
Springfield, MO 65802-1894   800-641-4310
                                                 Fax: 417-862-5881
                                              www.gospelpublishing.com
Offers braille and cassette lending library, braille and cassette
Sunday school materials for all ages, braille and cassette periodi-
cals and resource assistance.
Paul Weingariner, Librarian

9781 Wolfner Memorial Library for the Blind
PO Box 387   573-751-8720
Jefferson City, MO 65102-387   800-392-2614
                                                 Fax: 573-526-2985
                                                 TDD: 800-347-1379
                                          e-mail: wolfner@sos.mo.gov
                                              www.sos.mo.gov/wolfner
Summer reading programs, braille writer, closed circuit TV, large
print photocopier, cassette books and magazines, children's books
on cassette, home visits and other reference materials on blindness
and other handicaps.
Richard J Smith, Director Wolfner Library
Debbie Musselman, Administrative Program Coordinator

Montana

9782 Montana State Library
1515 E 6th Avenue   406-444-3009
Helena, MT 59620-1800   Fax: 406-444-0266
                                           home.montanastatelibrary.org/?
Summer reading programs, braille writer, magnifiers, closed-circuit TV, large-print photocopier, cassette books and magazines,
children's books on cassette, home visits and other reference materials on blindness and other handicaps.
Darlene Staffeldt, Director

Nebraska

9783 Nebraska Library Commission Talking Book and Braille Services
1200 N Street, Suite 120   402-471-4038
Lincoln, NE 68508-2023   800-742-7691
                                      e-mail: nlc.talkingbook@nebraska.gov
                                              www.nlc.nebraska.gov/tbbs
Free loan of books and magazines on flash cartridge, cassette, and
in Braille, including children's materials, along with specially designed playback equipment. Summer reading program for children
and young adults, Braille embossing, closed circuit TV,large-print
copier. Reference materials on blindness and other disabilities.
David Oertli, Director
Kay Goehring, Reader Services Coordinator

9784 North Platte Public Library
120 W 4th Street   308-535-8036
North Platte, NE 69101-3901   Fax: 308-535-8296
                                      e-mail: library@ci.north-platte.ne.us
                                           www.ci.north-platte.ne.us/library
Summer reading programs, braille writer, magnifiers, closed-circuit TV, large-print photocopier, cassette books and magazines,
children's books on cassette, home visits and other reference materials on blindness and other handicaps.
Cecelia Lawrence, Library Director

Nevada

9785 Las Vegas Clark County Library District
7060 W. Windmill Lane
Las Vegas, NV 89113-5256   702-734-7323
                                                     www.lvccld.org
Summer reading programs, braille writer, magnifiers, closed circuit TV, large-print photocopier, cassette books and magazines,
children's books on cassette, home visits and other reference materials on blindness and other handicaps.
Daniel Walters, Executive Directors

9786 Nevada State Library and Archives
100 North Stewart Street   775-684-3360
Carson City, NV 89701-4285   800-922-2880
                                                 Fax: 775-684-3330
                                                 TDD: 775-687-8338
                                          e-mail: nslref@clan.lib.nv.us
                                              www.nsla.nevadaculture.org
Summer reading programs, braille writer, magnifiers, closed-circuit TV, large-print photocopier, cassette books and magazines,
children's books on cassette, home visits and other reference materials on blindness and other handicaps.
Kevin E Putnam, Librarian

New Hampshire

9787 New Hampshire State Library
117 Pleasant Street   603-271-3429
Concord, NH 03301-3852   Fax: 603-271-8370
                                       e-mail: talking@lilac.nhsh.lib.nh.us
                                                         www.nh.us
Summer reading programs, braille writer, magnifiers, closed-circuit TV, large-print photocopier, cassette books and magazines,
children's books on cassette, home visits and other reference materials on blindness and other handicaps.
Eileen Keim, Librarian

9788 Voices for the Blind
PO Box 781   603-332-9355
Barrington, NH 3825
Tape library and depository for people with visual and learning
disabilities. Recording services available by request.
Connie Hindman, Director

New Jersey

9789 New Jersey Library for the Blind and Handicapped
2300 Stuyvesant Avenue   609-530-4000
Trenton, NJ 08618-3226   800-792-8322
                                                 Fax: 609-530-6384
                                                 TDD: 877-882-5593
                                          e-mail: nglbh@njstatelib.org
                                           www2.njstatelib.org/lbh/index.htm
Summer reading programs, large print, cassette, braille books and
magazines, children's books on cassette and brailles and other ref-
erence materials on blindness and other handicaps.
Deborah Toomey, Director

New Mexico

9790 New Mexico State Library for the Blind and Physically Handicapped
National Library Services

1209 Camino Carlos Rey
Santa Fe, NM 87507

505-476-9770
800-456-5515
Fax: 505-476-9776
e-mail: lbph@state.nm.us
www.nmstatelibrary.org/lbph?

Summer reading programs, braille writer, magnifiers, closed-circuit TV, large-print photocopier, cassette books and magazines, children's books on cassette, home visits and other reference materials on blindness and other handicaps.
John Mugford, Library Manager

New York

9791 Choice Magazine Listening
85 Channel Drive
Port Washington, NY 11050-2216

516-883-8280
888-724-6423
Fax: 516-944-6849
e-mail: choicemag@aol.com
www.choicemagazinelistening.org

A free recorded spoken word magazine anthology for anyone college level and older unable to read large print because of visual or physical handicaps. Produced on special speed cassette format, playable on free library of congress player.
Sondra Mochson, Editor

9792 JGB Cassette Library International
Jewish Guild for the Blind
15 W 65th Street
New York, NY 10023-6601

212-769-6331
Fax: 212-769-6266
e-mail: bemass@aol.com

Summer reading programs, braille writer, magnifiers, closed-circuit TV, large-print photocopier, cassette books and magazines, children's books on cassette, home visits and other reference materials on blindness and other handicaps.
Bruce Massis

9793 Nassau Library System
900 Jerusalem Avenue
Uniondale, NY 11553-3039

516-292-8920
Fax: 516-481-4777
e-mail: nls@lilrc.org
www.nassaulibrary.org/?

Summer reading programs, braille writer, magnifiers, closed-circuit TV, large-print photocopier, cassette books and magazines, children's books on cassette, home visits and other reference materials on blindness and other handicaps.
Dorothy Pruyear, Librarian

9794 New York State Talking Book & Braille Library, New York State Library, DOE
Empire State Plaza, CEC
Albany, NY 12230-0001

518-474-5935
800-342-3688
Fax: 518-486-2142
e-mail: tbbl@mail.nysed.gov
www.nysl.nysed.gov/tbbl/

Books on audio cassette, cassette players, braille books, summer reading programs, braille writer, magnifiers, closed-circuit TV, large-print photocopier, cassette books and magazines, children's books on cassette, reference materials on blindness and other disabilities. Library is part of the National Service Network serving those with print disabilities. Available: audio and braille books sent post-free by mail, euipment loans, services to schools and institutions. Serves 55 New York counties.
Sharon B. Phillips, Program Director

9795 Suffolk Cooperative Library System
627 N Sunrise Service Road
Bellport, NY 11713-9000

631-286-1600
Fax: 631-286-1647
gateway.suffolklibrarysystem.org

Talking books services.
Julie Klauber, Adjunct Professor

9796 Xavier Society for the Blind
154 E 23rd Street
New York, NY 10010-4501

212-473-7800
800-637-9193
Fax: 212-473-7801
e-mail: info@xaviersocietyfortheblind.org
www.XavierSocietyfortheBlind.org

Provides spiritual and inspirational reading material to visually impaired persons in suitable format: Braille, large print and cassette, throughout the USA and Canada. Services provided by way of regular periodicals which are non-returnable, and through our lending library where books are returned. All services are provided free of charge, and interested persons can write or phone.
Fr. John R. Sheehan, SJ, Chairman
Margie Montenegro, Client Services Representative

North Carolina

9797 North Carolina Library for the Blind
1841 Capital Boulevard
Raleigh, NC 27635

919-733-4376
888-388-2460
Fax: 919-733-6910
TDD: 919-733-1462
e-mail: nclbph@ncdcr.gov
statelibrary.ncdcr.gov/lbph

A general interest library offering books and magazines at no cost in large print, in braille on audio cassette for anyone who cannot use regular print in North Carolina due to physical or visual disability. Summer reading programs, braille writer, magnifiers, closed circuit TV, large print photocopier, cassette books and magazines, children's books on cassette, digital, cartridges and large print and other reference materials.
Carl Keehn, Director

North Dakota

9798 North Dakota State Library Services for the Disabled
North Dakota State Library
604 E Boulevard Avenue
Bismarck, ND 58505-800

701-328-4622
800-843-9948
Fax: 701-328-2040
TDD: 800-892-8622
e-mail: statelib@nd.gov
www.library.nd.gov

Stella Cone, Regional Librarian

9799 Services for the Visually Impaired
8720 Georgia Avenue
Silver, MD 20910

301-589-0894
Fax: 301-589-7281
www.servicesvi.org

Eligible readers of North Dakota receive library service from the regional library in Pierre, South Dakota.
Betty Bender

Ohio

9800 Case Western Reserve University
10900 Euclid Avenue
Cleveland, OH 44117-2620

216-368-2000
www.cwru.edu

Research in electrical stimulation and rehabilitation technology.
Barbara R. Snyder, President
W. A. Bud Baeslack III, Executive Vice President

9801 Ohio Regional Library for the Blind and Physically Handicapped
800 Vine Street
Cincinnati, OH 45202

513-369-6999
800-528-0335
Fax: 513-369-3111
TDD: 513-369-6072
www.cincinatilibrary.org/main/lb.asp

Summer reading programs, braille writer, magnifiers, closed-circuit TV, large-print photocopier, cassette books and magazines, children's books on cassette, home visits and other reference materials on blindness and other handicaps.
Donna Foust, Librarian

9802 State Library of Ohio Talking Book Program
274 E First Avenue
Columbus, OH 43201-3673

614-644-6895
800-686-1531
Fax: 614-995-2186
winslo.state.oh.us/services

A machine-lending agency for the visually impaired.
Roger Verney, Head Supervisor

Oklahoma

9803 Oklahoma Library for the Blind and Physically Handicapped
300 NE 18th Street
Oklahoma City, OK 73105-3212

405-521-3514
Fax: 405-214-82
www.state.ok.us/~library

Summer reading programs, braille writer, magnifiers, closed-circuit TV, large-print photocopier, cassette books and magazines, children's books on cassette, home visits and other reference materials on blindness and other handicaps.
Geraldine Adams, Director

9804 Tulsa City: County Library System
400 Civic Center 918-596-7977
Tulsa, OK 74103-3830 Fax: 918-596-7990
www.tulsalibrary.org
Summer reading programs, braille writer, magnifiers, closed-circuit TV, large-print photocopier, cassette books and magazines, children's books on cassette, home visits and other reference materials on blindness and other handicaps.
Ellen Ontko, Librarian

Oregon

9805 Oregon State Library
250 Winter Street NE 503-378-4243
Salem, OR 97301-3950 800-452-0292
Fax: 503-588-7119
TDD: 503-378-4276
www.oregon.gov/osl
Summer reading programs, braille writer, magnifiers, closed-circuit TV, large-print photocopier, cassette books and magazines, children's books on cassette, home visits and other reference materials on blindness and other handicaps.
Jim Scheppke, Head Librarian

Pennsylvania

9806 Carnegie Library of Pittsburgh
4724 Baum Boulevard 412-687-2440
Pittsburgh, PA 15213-1321 800-242-0586
Fax: 412-687-2442
e-mail: lbph@carneigelibrary.org
www.clpgh.org/clp/LBPH
Provides on loan recorded books and magazines, large print books, and described videos to Western Pennsylvannia residents unable to use standard printed materials due to visual, physical, or physically-based reading disabilities. Also loans special cassette and disc machines; does not loan equipment to play described videos. Information about disabilities and related agencies is also available.
Sue Murdock, Director
Kathleen Kappel, Assistant Director

9807 Free Library of Philadelphia
919 Walnut Street 215-925-3213
Philadelphia, PA 19107-5237 Fax: 215-928-0856
e-mail: flpblind@library.phila.gov
Summer reading programs, braille writer, magnifiers, closed-circuit TV, large-print photocopier, cassette books and magazines, children's books on cassette, home visits and other reference materials on blindness and other handicaps.
Vickie Lange Collins, Librarian

Rhode Island

9808 Rhode Island Department of State Library for the Blind and Physically Handicapped
1 Capitol Hl 401-277-2726
Providence, RI 02908-5803 Fax: 401-277-4195
e-mail: richard@dsl.rhilinet.gov
Offers information and services for the visually impaired including reference materials, braille printers, braille writers, large-print books and more.
Richard Ledue, Librarian

South Carolina

9809 South Carolina State Library
PO Box 11469 803-734-8666
Columbia, SC 29202-0821 Fax: 803-734-8676
TDD: 803-734-7298
e-mail: guynell@leo.scsl.state.sc.us
www.state.sc.us/scsl

Summer reading programs, braille writer, magnifiers, closed-circuit TV, large-print photocopier, cassette books and magazines, children's books on cassette, home visits and other reference materials on blindness and other handicaps.
Guynell Williams, Librarian

South Dakota

9810 South Dakota State Library
800 Governors Drive 605-773-3131
Pierre, SD 57501-2235 Fax: 605-734-50
TDD: 605-773-4950
e-mail: daRN@stlib.state.sd.us
www.sdstatelibrary.com
Summer reading programs, braille writer, magnifiers, closed-circuit TV, large-print photocopier, cassette books and magazines, children's books on cassette, home visits and other reference materials on blindness and other handicaps.
Daniel Boyd, Librarian

Tennessee

9811 LRC for Students with Disabilities
MSU Library Reference Department
Memphis State University 901-678-2208
Memphis, TN 38152-0001 800-669-2267
Fax: 901-678-3070
www.memphis.edu
Information on physical disabilities, blindness and visual impairments.
Ross Johnson, Reference Librarian

9812 Tennessee Library for the Blind and Physically Handicapped
National Library Services
403 7th Avenue N 615-741-3915
Nashville, TN 37243-1409 800-342-3308
Fax: 615-532-8856
e-mail: tlbph@mail.state.tn/sos/statelib/LBPH/
www.state.tn.us
Offers free public library services to those unable to hold, read, or turn the pages of books and magazines due to physical or visual impairment. Collections include books and magazines in large print, braille and audio format. Players loaned for the audio books and magazines. All items are delivered and returned via the US Postal Service free matter mailing.
Ruth Hemphill, Director
Janie Murphee, Assistant Director

Texas

9813 Houston Public Library Access Center
500 McKinney Street 832-393-1313
Houston, TX 77002-2534 Fax: 832-931-83
e-mail: website@hpl.lib.tx.us
www.houstonlibrary.org
Offers Kurzweil Reading Machine 400, closed-circuit TV, braille writer, reference materials on visual impairments and other handicaps.
Heidi Miller, Supervisor

9814 Texas State Library
1201 Brazos Street 512-463-5460
Austin, TX 78711-2927 800-252-9605
Fax: 512-936-0685
TDD: 512-463-5449
e-mail: dale.propp@tsl.state.tx.us
www.tsl.state.tx.us
Summer reading programs, braille writer, magnifiers, closed-circuit TV, large-print photocopier, cassette books and magazines, children's books on cassette, home visits and other reference materials on blindness and other handicaps.
Dale Propp, Librarian

9815 Texas State Library: Talking Book Program
1201 Brazos Street 512-463-5460
Austin, TX 78711-2927 800-252-9605
Fax: 512-936-0685
e-mail: tbp.services@tsl.state.tx.us
www.tsl.state.tx.us

Part of the free National Library Services. Provides equipment and books in alternate formats to qualified individuals who cannot read standard print. Certified applications required. Disabilities and information referral services available.
Ava Smith, Librarian
Dina Abramson, Disabilities/Information Referral

Utah

9816 Utah State Library Division
Program for the Blind and Disabled
250 North 1950 West, Suite A   801-715-6789
Salt Lake City, UT 84116-7901   800-662-5540
                                     Fax: 801-715-6767
                                     TDD: 801-715-6721
                                     e-mail: blind@utah.gov
                                     http://blindlibrary.utah.gov
Library providing services to individuals with visual impairments who cannot read standard print.
Bessie Y. Oakes, Director

Vermont

9817 Vermont Department of Libraries Special Services Unit
109 State Street   80- 8-8 32
montpelier, VT 05609   800-479-1711
                                     Fax: 802-828-2199
                                     e-mail: ssu@mail.dol.state.vt.us
                                     dol.state.vt.us
Summer reading programs, braille writer, magnifiers, closed-circuit TV, large-print photocopier, cassette books and magazines, children's books on cassette, home visits and other reference materials on blindness and other handicaps.
Theresa Faust, Librarian

Virginia

9818 Arlington County Department of Libraries
1015 N Quincy Street   703-228-5959
Arlington, VA 22201-4603   Fax: 703-358-5962
                                     TDD: 703-358-6320
                                     www.library.arlingtonva.us/
Summer reading programs, braille writer, magnifiers, closed-circuit TV, large-print photocopier, cassette books and magazines, children's books on cassette, home visits and other reference materials on blindness and other handicaps.
Roxanne Barnes, Librarian

9819 Central Rappahannock Regional Library
1201 Caroline Street   540-372-1144
Fredericksburg, VA 22401-3701   Fax: 540-373-9411
                                     TDD: 540-371-9165
                                     e-mail: nschiff@hq.crrl.org
Offers reference materials on blindness and other disabilities.
Nancy Schiff, Librarian

9820 Division for the Visually Handicapped
2900 Crystal Drive   703-620-3660
Arlington, VA 22202   888-232-7733
                                     Fax: 703-264-9494
                                     TTY: 866-915-5000
                                     e-mail: service@cec.sped.org
                                     www.cec.sped.org
Members are teachers, college faculty members, administrators, supervisors and others concerned with the education and welfare of visually handicapped and blind children and youth. This is a division of the Council For Exceptional Children.
Stephanie Ineh, Customer Service Manager
Anitra Davis, Senior Customer Services Representative

9821 Fairfax County Public Library
12000 Government Center Parkway   703-660-6943
Fairfax, VA 22035-0012   Fax: 703-765-5893
                                     TDD: 703-660-8524
                                     e-mail: sjapikse@leo.vsla.edu
                                     www.co.fairfax.va.us.
Summer reading programs, braille writer, magnifiers, closed-circuit TV, large-print photocopier, cassette books and magazines,
children's books on cassette, home visits and other reference materials on blindness and other handicaps.
Jeanette Studley, Librarian

9822 Hampton Subregional Library for the Blind
4207 Victoria Blvd.ÿ   75- 7-7 11
Hampton, VA 23669-4243   Fax: 75- 7-7 11
                                     www.hamptonpubliclibrary.org
Summer reading programs, braille writer, magnifiers, closed-circuit TV, large-print photocopier, cassette books and magazines, children's books on cassette, home visits and other reference materials on blindness and other handicaps.
Douglas Perry, Director

9823 Newport News Public Library System
110 Main Street   757-591-4858
Newport News, VA 23601-4105   Fax: 757-591-7425
                                     e-mail: shalswin@leo.vsla.edu
                                     www.newport-news.va.us
Summer reading programs, braille writer, magnifiers, closed-circuit TV, large-print photocopier, cassette books and magazines, children's books on cassette, home visits and other reference materials on blindness and other handicaps.
Sue Balswin, Librarian

9824 Roanoke City Public Library System
2607 Salem Tpke NW   540-853-2648
Roanoke, VA 24017-5333   Fax: 540-853-1030
Summer reading programs, braille writer, magnifiers, closed-circuit TV, large-print photocopier, cassette books and magazines, children's books on cassette, home visits and other reference materials on blindness and other handicaps.
Rebecca Cooper, Librarian

9825 Staunton Public Library: Talking Book Center
1291 Taylor Street,   20- 7-7 51
Washington, DC 20011-3229   20- 7-7 07
                                     Fax: 540-332-3906
                                     e-mail: talkingbook@ci.staunton.via.us
                                     www.loc.gov/nls
Sub-regional library for those who are unable to use standard print materials due to visual, physical, or reading disability.
Oakley Pearson, Librarian

9826 University Library Services
Virginia Commonwealth University
901 Park Avenue   804-828-1105
Richmond, VA 23284-2033   Fax: 804-828-0150
                                     www.ucu.edu
Library services for the visually disabled.
Sally Jacobs, Reference Librarian

9827 Virginia Beach Public Library
936 Independence Boulevard   757-460-7518
Virginia Beach, VA 23455-6006   Fax: 757-460-6741
                                     e-mail: vb311@vbgov.com
                                     vbgov.com/libraries
Summer reading programs, braille writer, magnifiers, closed-circuit TV, large-print photocopier, cassette books and magazines, children's books on cassette, home visits and other reference materials on blindness and other handicaps.
Susan Head, Librarian

Washington

9828 Washington Talking Book & Braille Library
2021 9th Avenue   206-615-0400
Seattle, WA 98121   Fax: 206-615-0437
                                     TTY: 206-615-0418
                                     e-mail: wtbbl@spl.lib.wa.us
                                     www.wtbbl.org
Summer reading programs, braille writer, magnifiers, closed-circuit TV, large-print photocopier, cassette books and magazines, children's books on cassette, home visits and other reference materials on blindness and other handicaps.
Danielle Miller, Director

9829   Cabell County Public Library
455 9th Street
Huntington, WV 25701-1417   304-528-5700
                                         Fax: 304-285-5701
                            e-mail: tbooks@cabell.libwv.us
                                         www.cabell.lib.wv.us
Summer reading programs, braille writer, magnifiers, Arkenstone
reader/scanner, cassette books and magazines, children's books on
cassette, home visits and other reference materials on blindness
and other handicaps.
Judy K Ruke, Director
Angela Strait, Assistant Director

9830   Kanawha County Public Library
1900 Kanawha Boulevard E
Charleston, WV 25305-2609   304-558-2041
                                         800-642-9021
                                         Fax: 304-558-2044
                                         kanawha.lib.wv.us
Summer reading programs, braille writer, magnifiers, closed-circuit TV, large-print photocopier, cassette books and magazines,
children's books on cassette, home visits and other reference materials on blindness and other handicaps.
Francis Fesenmainer, Librarian

**9831   Ohio County Public Library Services for the Blind and Physically
Handicapped**
52 16th Street
Wheeling, WV 26003-3671   304-232-0244
                                         Fax: 304-232-6848
                            e-mail: llnicholson@hotmail.com
Lori Nicholson, Subregional Librarian BIPH

9832   Parkersburg and Wood County Public Library
3100 Emerson Avenue
Parkersburg, WV 26104-2414   304-420-4587
                                         800-642-8674
                                         Fax: 304-420-4589
                         e-mail: raitzb@hp9k.park.lib.wv.us
                                         parkersburg.lib.wv.us
Services for the bind and physically handicapped.
Michael Hickman

9833   West Virginia Library Commission
1900 Kanawha Boulevard E
Charleston, WV 25305-0009   304-558-2041
                                         800-642-9021
                                         Fax: 304-558-2044
                            e-mail: web_one@wvlc.lib.wv.us
                                         librarycommission.lib.wv.us
Summer reading programs, braille writer, magnifiers, closed-circuit TV, large-print photocopier, cassette books and magazines,
children's books on cassette, home visits and other reference materials on blindness and other handicaps.
Francis Fesenmainer, Librarian

9834   West Virginia School for the Blind
301 E Main Street
Romney, WV 26757-1828   304-822-4800
                                         Fax: 304-822-3377
                         e-mail: cjohn@access.mountain.net
Summer reading programs, braille writer, magnifiers, closed-circuit TV, large-print photocopier, cassette books and magazines,
children's books on cassette, home visits and other reference materials on blindness and other handicaps.
Cynthia Johnson, Librarian

9835   Brown County Library
P.O box 23600
Green Bay, WI 54305-5194   920-448-4035
                                         Fax: 920-448-4036
                                         www.co.brown.wi.us
Summer reading programs, braille writer, magnifiers, closed-cir-
cuit TV, large-print photocopier, cassette books and magazines,
children's books on cassette, home visits and other reference mate-
rials on blindness and other handicaps.
Moyninhan Jr Patrick, Chair
Lund Thomas, Vice Chair

9836   Wisconsin Regional Library for the Blind Talking Book Program
813 W Wells Street   414-286-3045
Milwaukee, WI 53233-1436   800-242-8822
                                         Fax: 414-286-3102
                                         TDD: 414-286-3548
                                         e-mail: mvalne@mpl.org
                                         www.regionallibrary.wi.gov
Circulates recorded materials, playback equipment and braille ma-
terials to print-handicapped Wisconsin residents.
Marsha Valance, Regional Librarian

9837   Wyoming Services for the Visually Disabled
State Department of Education
2300 Capitol Avenue Hathaway Buildi   307-777-7690
Cheyenne, WY 82002-50   Fax: 307-776-34
                                         www.k12.wy.us
Eligible readers of Wyoming receive library service from the re-
gional library in Salt Lake City, Utah.
Duane Edmonds, Chairman
Ruby Calvert, Vice Chairman

Research Centers

9838   Baylor College of Medicine: Cullen Eye Institute
6565 Fannin   713-798-6100
Houston, TX 77030-2703   800-229-5676
                                         Fax: 713-798-4231
                                         e-mail: ant@bcm.edu
                                         www.bcm.edu/eye
Research activities focus on restoring vision and preventing blind-
ness through a better understanding of the disease.
Dan B Jones, Professor and Chair
Milton Boniuk, Professor

9839   BermanGund Laboratory for the Study of Retinal Degenerations
Massachusetts Eye & Eye Infirmary
243 Charles Street   617-573-3600
Boston, MA 02114-3002   Fax: 617-733-44
                         e-mail: directors@meei.harvard.edu
                 www.masseyeandear.org/research/ophthalmo
The Berman-Gund Laboratory for the Study of Retinal Degenera-
tions of Harvard Medical School continues multidisciplined re-
search on retinitis pigmentosa, Usher syndrome, macular
degeneration, and other related degenerative diseases of the retina.
Eliot L. Berson, M.D.,, Director
Eric A. Pierce, M.D., Ph.D.,, Associate Director

9840   Braille Institute Desert Center
70-251 Ramon Rd   760-321-1111
Rancho Mirage, CA 92270-5203   800-212-4533
                                         Fax: 760-321-9715
                             e-mail: dc@brailleinstitute.org
                                         www.brailleinstitute.org
Dedicated to providing blind and visually impaired men women
and children with the training programs and services they need to
enjoy productive lives. Services offered include child development youth programs library services and adult education.
Leslie E Stocker Jr, President
Sally H Jameson, VP of Programs and Services

9841   Braille Institute Orange County Center
527 N Dale Avenue   714-821-5000
Anaheim, CA 92801-4899   Fax: 714-527-7621
                             e-mail: oc@brailleinstitute.org
                                         www.brailleinstitute.org
Offers services publications information and programs to blind
and visually impaired persons.
Sheila F Daily, Orange County Regional Director
Gene Mathiowetz, Assistant Regional Director

**9842   Braille Institute Santa Barbara Center Braille Institute of Los
Angeles**
Braille Institute of Los Angeles

2031 De La Vina Street
Santa Barbara, CA 93105-3895

805-682-6222
800-272-4553
Fax: 805-687-6141
e-mail: sb@brailleinstitute.org
www.brailleinstitute.org

Offers classes type library services and information for persons with visual impairments.
Angela Nowlin, Assistant Regional Director
Michael Lazarovits, Santa Barbara Regional Director

9843 Braille Institute Sight Center
741 N Vermont Avenue
Los Angeles, CA 90029

323-663-1112
800-272-4553
Fax: 323-663-0867
e-mail: la@brailleinstitute.org
www.brailleinstitute.org/los_angeles

Offers help programs services and information to the blind and visually impaired children and adults.
Dr Henry C Chang, Director of Library Services
Anita Wright, Los Angeles Regional Program Director

9844 Braille Institute Youth Center
741 N Vermont Avenue
Los Angeles, CA 90029-1381

323-663-1112
800-272-4553
Fax: 323-663-0867
e-mail: la@brailleinstitute.org
www.brailleinstitute.org/los_angeles

Offers various youth programs and services for the blind and visually impaired youngster.
Leslie E Stocker Jr, President
Sally H Jameson, Vice President of Programs and Services

9845 Braille Textbook Assignment Service National Braille Association
National Braille Association
95 Allens Creek Road
Rochester, NY 14618-2537

585-427-8260
Fax: 585-427-0263
e-mail: nbaoffice@nationalbraille.org
www.nationalbraille.org

National Braille Association, founded in 1945, is a non-profit organization dedicated to providing continuing education to those who prepare braille, and to providing braille materials to persons who are visually impaired.
Jan Carroll, President
David W Shaffer, Executive Director

9846 Carroll Center for the Blind
770 Centre Street
Newton, MA 02458-2597

617-969-6200
800-852-3131
Fax: 617-969-6204
TTY: 617-969-6204
e-mail: info@carroll.org
www.carroll.org

The Carroll Center serves the needs of blind and visually-impaired persons by providing rehabilitation, skills training, and educational opportunities to achieve independence, self-sufficiency, and self-fulfillment and by educating the public regarding the potential of persons who are blind and visually-impaired.
Joseph Abely, President
Brian Charlson, Director of Computer Training Services

9847 Clearinghouse for Specialized Media and Translation
California Department of Education/CSMT
1430 N Street
Sacramento, CA 95814

916-445-5103
Fax: 916-323-9732
e-mail: csmt@cde.ca.gov
www.cde.ca.gov/re/pn/sm

Assists schools and students in the identification and acquisition of textbooks reference books and study materials in aural media, braille, large print, and electronic media access technology.
Tom Torlakson, State Superintendent of Public Instructi
Jonn Paris-Salb, Administrator

9848 Clovernook Center for the Blind and Visually Impaired
7000 Hamilton Avenue
Cincinnati, OH 45231-5240

513-522-3860
888-234-7156
Fax: 513-728-3946
www.clovernook.org

Innovative programs including community living support and a youth initiative with a focus on developing the skills people with visual impairments need to become independent in the community.

An array of employment services help individuals maximize their earning potential and job satisfaction, both on site in our manufacturing center and in the local job market.
Robin L Usalis, President/CEO
Jacqueline L Conner, VP of Multi-State Center East

9849 Dean A McGee Eye Institute
608 Stanton L Young Boulevard
Oklahoma City, OK 73104-5065

405-271-6060
800-787-9012
Fax: 405-271-4442
www.dmei.org

The Dean McGee Eye Institute is the first center in Oklahoma to offer a new treatment for dry eyes that can last up to a year and frees patients from time-consuming warm compresses and lubricating eye drops. The LipiFlow Thermal Pulsation System combines precisely administered heat and pressure to open and clear clogged oil glands in the eyelids, allowing lubricating oils to flow naturally again.
Edward L. Gaylord, Professor and Chair
Gregory L. Skuta, MD, President

9850 Emory University: Laboratory for Ophthalmic Research
1365B Clifton Road, N.E.
Atlanta, GA 30322-1013

404-778-2020
www.eyecenter.emory.edu

Various studies into the aspects of blindness.
Timothy W. Olsen, MD, Chair/Director
Joy H. Bell, Director of Public Relations

9851 Florida Ophthalmic Institute
7106 NW 11th Pl
Gainesville, FL 32605-3157

352-331-2020
Fax: 352-331-2019
e-mail: afn22025@gmail.com
www.sites.google.com/site/flophthalmicin

Nonprofit organization that understands and treats ocular diseases including glaucoma.
Norman S Levy MD, Director
Trudy K. Ramjattan, MD, Surgeon

9852 Glaucoma Laser Trabeculoplasty Study Sinai Hospital of Detroit
Sinai Hospital of Detroit
6767 W Outer Drive
Detroit, MI 48235-2899

313-966-3256
Fax: 313-966-4296

Examines the effectiveness and safety of the treatments of glaucoma.
Hugh Beckman, Chairman

9853 Glaucoma Research Foundation
251 Post Street
San Francisco, CA 94108

415-986-3162
800-826-6693
Fax: 415-986-3763
e-mail: question@glaucoma.org
www.glaucoma.org

Our mission is to prevent vision loss from glaucoma by investing in innovative research, education, and support with the ultimate goal of finding a cure.
Thomas M Brunner, Chief Executive Officer/President
Nancy Graydon, Executive Director of Development

9854 Harvard University Howe Laboratory of Ophthalmology
Massachusetts Eye & Ear Infirmary
243 Charles Street
Boston, MA 02114-3002

617-523-7900
www.masseyeandear.org

Established in 1926, the Howe Laboratory is comprised of investigators working on both basic research, focused on retinal development, structure and function in various organisms, and translational research, focused on developing treatments for glaucoma and conditions affecting the cornea.
Dr. Mack Cheney, Director
Wendy Williams, Associate Director

9855 Helen Keller International
352 Park Avenue S
New York, NY 10010

212-532-0544
877-535-5374
Fax: 212-532-6014
e-mail: info@hki.org
www.hki.org

Nonprofit organization for the blind.
Kathy Spahn, President/CEO
Shawn K Baker, VP/Regional Director-Africa

9856 Helen Keller National Center for Deaf/Blind Youths and Adults
141 Middle Neck Road   516-944-8900
Sands Point, NY 11050-1299   Fax: 516-944-7302
                                                        TTY: 516-944-8637
                                e-mail: hkncinfo@hknc.org
                                                        www.hknc.org
We enable all those who are deaf-blind to live and work in the community of their choice. We provide comprehensive vocational rehabilitation training at our headquarters in NY and assistance with job and residential placements when training is completed.
Joseph McNulty, Executive Director

9857 Institute for Visual Sciences
1 E 71st Street   212-305-2919
New York, NY 10021-4102
Ophthalmology with emphasis on the development of care for the eye.
Melissa Mount, Executive Director

9858 Institute of Ophthalmology and Visual Scie nce New Jersey Medical School
New Jersey Medical School
PO Box 1709   973-972-2036
Newark, NJ 07101-2425   Fax: 973-723-94
                                e-mail: churchbf@umdnj.edu
                                                www.njms.rutgers.edu
The Institute comprises ophthalmic surgeons, researchers, ophthalmic surgeons-in-training, administrators, and ancillary staff (such as ophthalmic technicians). We are dedicated to providing outstanding compassionate patient care, teaching current and future providers of eye care, and developing cures for blindness. This site provides comprehensive information on our faculty members, eye-care professionals, patient-care services, research, residency training programs, and continuing education cu
Marco A Zarbin, MD, PhD, FACS, Chair
Robert D. Fechtner, Professor

9859 Jerusalem Center for Multi-Handicapped Blind Children
350 7th Avenue   212-279-4070
New York, NY 10001-7903   Fax: 212-279-4043
                                e-mail: info@keren-or.org
                                                        keren-or.org
Maintains the Keren-Or Center for the Multiply Handicapped Blind Child in Jerusalem for rehabilitation and training. Funds acquired through contributions bequests and legacies.
Madelyn Cohen, Executive Director
Tamara Silberberg, Director Keren-Or Center

9860 Johns Hopkins University: Dana Center for Preventive Ophthalmology
Wilmer Ophthalmology Institute
600 N Wolfe Street
Baltimore, MD 21287-0001   410-955-2777
                www.hopkinsmedicine.org/wilmer/danacente
Research at the Dana Center focuses on national and international public health prevention of blinding eye disease.
Harry A Quigley, Director

9861 New Beginnings: The Blind Children's Center
4120 Marathon Street   213-664-2153
Los Angeles, CA 90029-3505   800-222-3566
The purpose of the Center is to turn initial fears into hope. Helps children and their families become independent by creating a climate of safety and trust. Children learn to develop self confidence and to master a wide range of skills. Services include an infant stimulation program, educational preschool, interdisciplinary assessment services, family services, correspondence program, toll free national hotline and a publication and research service.

9862 New Beginnings: The Blind Children's Cente
4120 Marathon Street   323-664-2153
Los Angeles, CA 90029   800-222-3566
                                                        Fax: 323-665-3828
                                www.blindchildrenscenter.org
The purpose of the Center is to turn initial fears into hope. Helps children and their families become independent by creating a cli-

mate of safety and trust. Children learn to develop self confidence and to master a wide range of skills. Services include an infant stimulation program educational preschool interdisciplinary assessment services family services correspondence program toll free national hotline and a publication and research service.

9863 Oregon Health Sciences University: Elk's Children's Eye Clinic
Casey Eye Institute
3375 SW Terwilliger Boulevard   503-494-3000
Portland, OR 97239-4197   Fax: 503-494-5347
                                                        www.ohsucasey.com
Our mission at the Casey Eye Institute is to provide excellent eye care in a quality cost-effective environment that combines education research clinical leadership and service to the community.
Earl Palmer, Director

9864 Reader-Transcriber Registry National Braille Association
National Braille Association
3 Townline Circle   716-427-8260
Rochester, NY 14623-2537
Certified braillists fill requests for college textbooks and other technical works through this service of the National Braille Association.

9865 Smith-Kettlewell Eye Research Institute
2318 Fillmore Street   415-345-2000
San Francisco, CA 94115-1821   Fax: 415-345-8455
                                                        www.ski.org
Dedicated to research on human vision. The Institute was founded to encourage a productive collaboration between the medical clinic and scientific laboratory. Research is conducted with clinical studies which relate directly to the diagnosis and treatment of eye diseases the development of devices and vocational programs to aid the partially sighted and basic research to understand how the eye and brain work for both the clinical and rehabilitation programs.
Arthur Jampolsky, Executive Director
Ruth S Poole, COO

9866 University of Illinois Eye and Ear Infirma ry
1855 W Taylor Street   312-996-6591
Chicago, IL 60612-7242   Fax: 312-996-7770
                                e-mail: eyeweb@uic.edu
                                                www.uic.edu/com/eye
Offers help support information and research for persons with vision problems including Retinitis Pigmentosa.
Dr. Rohit Verma, Department Chair
Elmer Tu, Director of Cornea Service

9867 University of Illinois at Chicago Lions of Illinois Eye Research Institute
UIC Eye Center
1905 W Taylor Street   312-996-1466
Chicago, IL 60612-7245   Fax: 312-355-4248
                                                www.uic.edu/com/eye/Lions
Visual impairments and blindness research including glaucoma studies.
Janet Szlyk, President~
Julie Daraska, Secretary

9868 University of Miami: Bascom Palmer Eye Institute
Department of Ophthalmalogy
900 NW 17th Street   305-326-6000
Miami, FL 33136-1015   800-329-7000
                                                        Fax: 305-326-6306
                                www.bpei.med.miami.edu/site/default.asp
Clinical and basic research into blindness and visual impairments.
John G Clarkson, Dean Emeritus

9869 Visually Impaired Center
1422 W Court Street   810-767-4014
Flint, MI 48503   Fax: 810-767-0020
                                e-mail: info@vicflint.org
                                                        www.vicflint.org
A private non-profit agency which offers special programs and some very practical help to people who are blind or partially sighted. Offers rehabilitation low vision aids orientation and mobility vocational training reading and information recreation counseling services volunteer services and community awareness.
Fharon Reigle, Director

9870 **Warren Grant Magnuson Clinical Center National Institute of Health**
National Institute of Health
9000 Rockville Pike 301-496-4000
Bethesda, MD 20892 800-411-1222
Fax: 301-480-9793
TTY: 866-411-1010
e-mail: prpl@mail.cc.nih.gov
www.cc.nih.gov
Established in 1953 as the research hospital of the National Institutes of Health. Designed so that patient care facilities are close to research laboratories so new findings of basic and clinical scientists can be quickly applied to the treatment of patients. Upon referral by physicians patients are admitted to NIH clinical studies.
John I Gallin, Director
David Henderson, Deputy Director for Clinical Care

9871 **Yale University: Vision Research Center**
330 Cedar Street 203-785-5687
New Haven, CT 06510-3218 800-395-7949
Fax: 203-785-7401
e-mail: sarah.gelo@yale.edu
visionresearch.med.yale.edu
Vision including studies on growth and development.
Bruce Shields, Chair
Sarah Gelo, Administrator

Kansas

9872 **Kansas Services for the Blind and Visually Impaired**
Social Rehabilitation Services
915 SW Harrison 785-368-7471
Topeka, KS 66612-2445 800-547-5789
Fax: 785-368-7467
TTY: 785-368-7478
e-mail: rehab@srs.ks.gov
www.srskansas.org/rehab/text/SBVI.htm
Instructional employment oriented services for blind adults.
Laura Howard, Deputy Secretary and Chief Financial Off
Theresa Addington, Accounting and Administrative Operations

Support Groups & Hotlines

9873 **1-800-BRAILLE**
Braille Institute
741 N Vermont Avenue 323-663-1111
Los Angeles, CA 90029-3594 800-272-4553
Fax: 323-663-0867
e-mail: la@brailleinstitute.org
www.brailleinstitute.org
A toll free information and referral service where callers can obtain information about community programs and referrals to organizations serving the blind in their local areas.
Lester M. Straussman, Director
James B. Boyle, Boardmember

9874 **AFB Toll-Free Hotline**
American Foundation for the Blind
2 Penn Plaza 212-502-7600
New York, NY 10121-2018 800-232-5463
Fax: 888-545-8331
e-mail: afbinfo@afb.net
www.afb.org
Supplies information on visual impairment and blindness, answers queries regarding AFB services, products, publications, technology, the Careers and Technology Information Bank (a national data bank) and much more.
Carl R. Augusto, President & CEO
Rick Bozeman, CFO

9875 **American Foundation for the Blind Information Center**
11 Penn Plaza 212-502-7600
New York, NY 10001 800-232-5463
Fax: 212-502-7777
e-mail: afbinfo@afb.net
www.afb.org
Nationally recognized information clearinghouse on blindness and visual impairment. Serves people who are blind or visually im-

paired, professionals in the field of blindness and visual impairment — including the staff at AFB, business and government organizations and the general public. Provides a toll-free information line available 24 hours a day, online information and referral services, professional library and archival services.

9876 **Aurora of Central New York**
518 James Street 315-422-7263
Syracuse, NY 13203 Fax: 315-422-4792
TTY: 315-422-9746
TDD: 315-422-9746
e-mail: auroracny@auroraofcny.org
www.auroraofcny.org/
Professional counseling services to assist individuals and their families deal with the trauma of hearing or vision loss.
Earleen Foulk, President Board of Directors
Debra Chaiken, Executive Director

9877 **Carroll Center for the Blind**
770 Centre Street 617-969-6200
Newton, MA 2458-2597 800-852-3131
Fax: 617-969-6204
www.carroll.org
We have developed many methods for people with low vision to learn the skills to be independent in their homes, in class settings, and in their work places. Our services for the blind include vision rehabilitation services, vocational and transition programs, assistive technology training, educational support and recreation opportunities for individuals who are visually impaired of all ages
Dina Rosenbaum, VP Marketing

9878 **Department of Ophthalmology Information Line**
Illinois Eye & Ear Infirmary
1855 W Taylor Street m/c 648 312-996-6500
Chicago, IL 60612-7242 Fax: 312-996-7770
e-mail: eyeweb@uic.edu
www.uic.edu/com/eye/
Offers eye clinic and physician referrals to persons suffering from vision disorders as well as offers emergency information.
Dimitri Azar, Director

9879 **Job Opportunities for the Blind**
National Federation of the Blind
200 E Wells St 410-659-9314
Baltimore, MD 21230-4998 Fax: 410-685-5653
e-mail: nfb@nfb.org
www.nfb.org
A specialized service that provides free support, resources and information to blind persons seeking employment and to employers interested in hiring the blind. A partnership program with the US Department of Labor, this is the most successful program of it's kind in helping blind persons find competitive work.
Anthony Cobb, Dircetor

9880 **National Association for Parents of the Visually Impaired**
Watertown, MA 2471 617-972-7441
800-562-6265
Fax: 617-972-7444
e-mail: napvi@perkins.org
www.napvi.org
Susan Laventure, Executive Director

9881 **National Center for Sight**
National Society to Prevent Blindness
211 Wacker Drive 312-363-6001
Chicago, IL 60606 800-331-2020
Fax: 312-363-6052
A toll-free line offering information on a broad range of vision, eye health and safety topics including sports eye safety, lazy eye, diabetic retinopathy, glaucoma, cataracts, children's eye disorders, and more.

9882 **National Eye Health Education Program**
1855 W Taylor Street 312-996-6590
Chicago, IL 60612-7242 800-786-3937
Fax: 312-996-9967
www.uic.edu
Offers information and support for persons with vision disorders, including Retinitis Pigmentosa.
Mary Go, Supervisor

9883 National Health Information Center
PO Box 1133
Washington, DC 20013

310-565-4167
800-336-4797
Fax: 301-984-4256
e-mail: info@nhic.org
www.health.gov/nhic

Offers a nationwide information referral service, produces directories and resource guides.

9884 National Service Dog Center
Delta society
875 124th Avenue, NE
Bellevue, WA 98005

425-679-550
Fax: 425-679-5539
e-mail: info@petpartners.org
www.petpartners.org

Pet Partners is the leader in demonstrating and promoting positive human-animal interaction to improve the physical, emotional and psychological lives of those we serve.
Brenda Bax, Chair
Mary Craig, Vice Chair/Treasurer

9885 PXE International
4301 Connecticut Avenue NW
Washington, DC 20008-2369

202-362-9599
Fax: 202-966-8553
e-mail: info@pxe.org
www.pxe.org

Initiates, funds and conducts research; provides support for individuals and families affected by pseudoxanthoma elasticum; and provides resrouces for healthcare professionals.
Sharon Terry, CEO
Terry Dermaid, Executive Director

9886 Recorded Periodicals
Associated Services for the Blind
919 Walnut Street
Philadelphia, PA 19107-5237

215-627-0600
Fax: 215-922-0692
e-mail: asbinfo@asb.org
www.asb.org

A subscription service of Associated Services for the Blind, these periodicals provide 21 magazines through this subscription service. A magazine list can be sent, in both large print and on audio cassette.
Richard Forsythe, Director
David Goldfield, Computer Instructor

9887 Recording for the Blind Helpline
20 Roszel Road
Princeton, NJ 08540-6294

609-750-1830
800-221-4792
e-mail: PrincetonStudio@LearningAlly.org
www.learningally.org

An organization dedicated to helping people with print disabilities.
Andrew Friedman, President & CEO
Jim Halliday, Executive VP

9888 Vision Use in Employment
Carroll Center for the Blind
770 Centre Street
Newton, MA 02458-2597

617-969-6200
800-852-3131
Fax: 617-969-6204
www.carroll.org

We have developed many methods for people with low vision to learn the skills to be independent in their homes, in class settings, and in their work places. Our services for the blind include vision rehabilitation services, vocational and transition programs, assistive technology training, educational support and recreation opportunities for individuals who are visually impaired of all ages
Joseph Abely, President
Diana Rosenbaum, Director of Marketing

9889 Washington Connection
American Council of the Blind
1155 15th Street NW
Washington, DC 20005-2706

202-467-5081
800-424-8666
Fax: 202-467-5085
e-mail: info@acb.org
www.acb.org

Coverage of issues affecting blind people via legislative information, participates in law-making, legislative training seminars and networking of support resources across the US.
Melanie Brunson, Executive Director

Books

9890 AFB Directory of Services for Blind/Vis. Impaired Persons in the US & Canada
AFB Press: American Foundation for the Blind
2 Penn Plaza
New York, NY 10121

212-502-7600
800-232-3044
Fax: 888-545-8331
e-mail: literacy@afb.net
www.afb.org/store

Provides the most comprehensive collection of information available on services for blind and visually impaired individuals. Over 800 pages of revised and updated information on more than 1,500 agencies and 45 new indexes. Includes complete descriptions of services offered by organizations and web sites and e-mail addresses. Available online on a subscription basis.
Carl R Augusto, President & CEO
Rick Bozeman, Chief Financial Officer

9891 APH Catalog of Accessible Books for People Who are Visually Impaired
American Printing House for the Blind
1839 Frankfort Avenue
Louisville, KY 40206-3148

502-895-2405
800-223-1839
Fax: 502-899-2284
e-mail: info@aph.org
www.aph.org

Offers thousands of selections and publishers of large type and braille books for persons with visual impairments.

9892 Access to Mass Transit for Blind & Visually Impaired Travelers
AFB Press: American Foundation for the Blind
2 Penn Plaza
New York, NY 10121

212-502-7600
800-232-3044
Fax: 888-545-8331
e-mail: literacy@afb.net
www.afb.org/store

Addresses several travel issues vital to the independence of blind and visually impaired persons from serveral perspectives — those of the blind and visually impaired persons who use mass transit, orientation and mobility instructors and transportation professionals. Focusing on national and international issues, this information filled manual covers approaches to making mass transit available in several cities in the US and Canada, the United Kingdom and Japan.
192 pages Paperback
ISBN: 0-891281-66-5
Carl R Augusto, President & CEO
Rick Bozeman, Chief Financial Officer

9893 An Orientation and Mobility Primer for Families and Young Children
American Foundation for the Blind
2 Penn Plaza
New York, NY 10121-2018

212-502-7600
800-232-3044
Fax: 888-545-8331
e-mail: literacy@afb.net
www.afb.org

Practical information for helping a child learn about his or her environment right from the start. Covers sensory training, concept development and orientation skills.
48 pages Papberback
ISBN: 0-891281-57-6
Carl R Augusto, President & CEO
Rick Bozeman, Chief Financial Officer

9894 Art Beyond Sight: Resource Guide to Art, Creativity and Visual Impairment
AFB Press: American Foundation for the Blind
2 Penn Plaza
New York, NY 10121

212-502-7600
800-232-3044
Fax: 888-545-8331
e-mail: literacy@afb.net
www.afb.org/store

AFB and Art Education for the Blind have joined together to co-publish this one-of-a-kind resource that provides vital information on all aspects of exploring art and creativity by people who are blind or visually impaired. Includes a section of reproducible pages for classroom or workshop activities.
504 pages Paperback
ISBN: 0-891288-50-3
Carl R Augusto, President & CEO
Rick Bozeman, Chief Financial Officer

9895 Art and Science of Teaching Orientation to the Visually Impaired
AFB Press: American Foundation for the Blind
2 Penn Plaza   212-502-7600
New York, NY 10121   800-232-3044
                                             Fax: 888-545-8331
                                   e-mail: literacy@afb.net
                                         www.afb.org/store

Updated and comprehensive description of the techniques of teaching orientation and mobility, presented along with strategies for sensitive and effective teaching. Such factors as individual needs, environmental features and ethical issues are discussed in this important text.
200 pages Paperback
ISBN: 0-891282-59-9
Carl R Augusto, President & CEO
Rick Bozeman, Chief Financial Officer

9896 Beginning with Braille: Balanced Approach to Literacy
AFB Press: American Foundation for the Blind
2 Penn Plaza   212-502-7600
New York, NY 10121   800-232-3044
                                             Fax: 888-545-8331
                                   e-mail: literacy@afb.net
                                         www.afb.org/store

Exciting resource from a skilled practitioner, this book provides a wealth of effective activitoes for promoting literacy at the early stages of braille instruction. The text includes creative and practical strategies for designing and delivering quality braille instruction and offers teacher-friendly suggestions for many areas, such as reading aloud to young children, selecting and making early tactile books and teaching tactile and hand movement skills. Tips on lessons and worksheets.

ISBN: 0-891283-23-4
Carl R Augusto, President & CEO
Rick Bozeman, Chief Financial Officer

9897 Behavioral Vision Approaches for Persons with Physical Disabilities
William V. Padula, author
Optometric Extension Program Foundation
1921 E. Carnegie Ave.   949-250-8070
Santa Ana, CA 92705-5510   Fax: 949-250-8157
                                   e-mail: Kelin.Kushin@oep.org
                                                 www.oepf.org

A discussion of the behavioral vision/neuro-motor approach to providing directions for prescriptive and therapeutic services for the visually handicapped child or adult.
197 pages
ISBN: 0-943599-04-0
Paul A. Harris, President
Robin Lewis, Vice President

9898 Blindness and Early Childhood Development
AFB Press: American Foundation for the Blind
2 Penn Plaza   212-502-7600
New York, NY 10121   800-232-3044
                                             Fax: 888-545-8331
                                   e-mail: literacy@afb.net
                                         www.afb.org/store

Reviews knowledge of motor and locomotor development, language and cognitive processes and social, emotional and personality development. It is a classic resource for teachers and those who work with children who are blind or visually impaired.
384 pages Paperback
ISBN: 0-891281-23-1
Carl R Augusto, President & CEO
Rick Bozeman, Chief Financial Officer

9899 Braille Book Bank: Music Catalog
National Braille Association
95 Allens Creek Road   585-427-8260
Rochester, NY 14618   Fax: 585-427-0263
                                 e-mail: NBAOffice@nationalbraille.org
                                         www.nationalbraille.org
Offers hundreds of musical titles in print form, braille and on cassette.
62 pages
Whitney Williams, President
Jana Hertz, Vice President

9900 Building Blocks: Foundations for Learning for Young Blind & Vis. Impaired Children
AFB Press: American Foundation for the Blind
2 Penn Plaza   212-502-7600
New York, NY 10121   800-232-3044
                                             Fax: 888-545-8331
                                   e-mail: literacy@afb.net
                                         www.afb.org/store
Available in English and Spanish, this work presents the essential components of a successful early intervention program, including collaboration with family members, positive relationships between parents and professionals, public education, and attention to important programming components such as space exploration, braille readiness, orientation and mobility, play, cooking and music. VHS video also available.
149 pages Paperback
ISBN: 0-891281-87-8
Carl R Augusto, President & CEO
Rick Bozeman, Chief Financial Officer

9901 Burns Braille Transcription Dictionary
AFB Press: American Foundation for the Blind
2 Penn Plaza   212-502-7600
New York, NY 10121   800-232-3044
                                             Fax: 888-545-8331
                                   e-mail: literacy@afb.net
                                         www.afb.org/store
A handy, portable guide that is a quick reference for anyone who needs to check print-to-braille and braille-to-print meanings and symbols. This easy-to-use listing provides readers with the essential alphabet, contractions, punctuation and signs and symbols for braille, as well as brief descriptions of rules for thier use. Organized into four clear sections aimed at providing information at a glance, this valuable tool is an ideal reference for teachers, rehabilitation professionals and others.
96 pages Paperback
ISBN: 0-891292-32-7
Carl R Augusto, President & CEO
Rick Bozeman, Chief Financial Officer

9902 Business Owners Who Are Blind or Visually Impaired
AFB Press: American Foundation for the Blind
2 Penn Plaza   212-502-7600
New York, NY 10121   800-232-3044
                                             Fax: 888-545-8331
                                   e-mail: literacy@afb.net
                                         www.afb.org/store
Demonstrates the wide range of careers and talents that can be pursued by persons with visual impairments. Each profile features a successful individual who has accomplised his or her dream of business ownership and who shares important insights. Available in paperback, audio cassette or ASCII disk.
148 pages
ISBN: 0-891283-24-2
Carl R Augusto, President & CEO
Rick Bozeman, Chief Financial Officer

9903 Career Perspectives: Interviews with Blind & Visually Impaired Professionals
AFB Press: American Foundation for the Blind
2 Penn Plaza   212-502-7600
New York, NY 10121   800-232-3044
                                             Fax: 888-545-8331
                                   e-mail: literacy@afb.net
                                         www.afb.org/store
Profiles of 20 successful archivers who describe in their own words what it takes to pursue and attain professional success in a sighted world. From all around the country and representing a wide

range of professions, including law, science, journalism, management and medicine, the blind and visually impaired individuals featured serve as role models for others who wnat to follow career paths.
96 pages Paperback
ISBN: 0-891281-70-3
Carl R Augusto, President & CEO
Rick Bozeman, Chief Financial Officer

9904 Childhood Glaucoma: A Reference Guide for Families
NAPVI
15 West 65th Street   212-769-7819
New York, NY 10023-0317   800-284-4422
                                        Fax: 617-972-7444
                        e-mail: napvi@lighthouseguild.org
                                            www.napvi.org
Lighthouse Guild is the leading not-for-profit vision + healthcare organization, with a long-standing heritage of addressing the needs of people who are blind or visually impaired as well as those with multiple disabilities or chronic medical conditions.
James A Dubin, Chairman
Susan LaVenture, Executive Director

9905 Communication Skills for Visually Impaired
Charles C Thomas Publisher
2600 S 1st Street   217-789-8980
Springfield, IL 62704-4730   Fax: 217-789-9130
                        e-mail: books@ccthomas.com
                                        www.ccthomas.com

322 pages
ISBN: 0-398066-92-2

9906 Concept Development for Visually Impaired Children: Resource Guide
AFB Press: American Foundation for the Blind
2 Penn Plaza   212-502-7600
New York, NY 10121   800-232-3044
                                        Fax: 888-545-8331
                            e-mail: literacy@afb.net
                                        www.afb.org/store
Program for integrating such concepts as body imagery, gross motor movement, posture and tactile discrimination into the curriculum from kindergarten on.
80 pages Paperback
ISBN: 0-891280-18-9
Carl R Augusto, President & CEO
Rick Bozeman, Chief Financial Officer

9907 Coping with Vision Loss
Bill Chapman, EdD, author
Hunter House Publishing
PO Box 2914   510-865-5282
Alameda, CA 94501   800-266-5592
                                        Fax: 510-865-4295
                    e-mail: ordering@hunterhouse.com
                                        www.hunterhouse.com
Maximizing what you can see and do. The Author explains the five leading causes of vision loss, and how to use new skills and vision aids.
2001 304 pages Paperback
Cristina Sverdrup, Customer Service Manager

9908 Development of Social Skills by Blind and Visually Impaired Students
AFB Press: American Foundation for the Blind
2 Penn Plaza   212-502-7600
New York, NY 10121   800-532-3044
                                        Fax: 888-545-8331
                            e-mail: literacy@afb.net
                                        www.afb.org/store
Examination of the social interactions of children with visual impairments, theory and research are combined to explore how these children can be helped to succeed socially. Innovative practical strategies are provided for educators, researchers and families on how to assist children in the development of social skills. Qualitative ethnographic approaches demonstrate how classroom teach-

ers can work effectively with individual children and present valuable insights about children's interactions.
232 pages Paperback
ISBN: 0-891282-17-3
Carl R Augusto, President & CEO
Rick Bozeman, Chief Financial Officer

9909 Early Focus: Working with Young Children Who Are Blind or Visually Impaired
AFB Press: American Foundation for the Blind
2 Penn Plaza   212-502-7600
New York, NY 10121   Fax: 888-545-8331
                            e-mail: literacy@afb.net
                                            www.afb.org/store
Early intervention has increasingly been recognized as critical in the development and growth of children with visual impairments and other disabilities. Federal regulations have mandated early indentifacation and assesment, underscoring its importance for children's well being. This revised and updated edition of Early Focus provides the important information you need to know including serving culturally diverse families with children who have multiple disabilities and practical tips.
376 pages Paperback
ISBN: 0-891282-15-7
Carl R Augusto, President & CEO
Rick Bozeman, Chief Financial Officer

9910 Encyclopedia of Blindness and Vision Impairment
Facts on File
2 Penn Plaza   212-967-8800
New York, NY 10121   800-322-8755
                                        Fax: 888-545-8331
                            e-mail: literacy@afb.net
                                            www.afb.org
Designed to provide both laymen and professionals with concise, practical information on the second most common disability in the US.
340 pages Hardcover
Carl R Augusto, President & CEO
Rick Bozeman, Chief Financial Officer

9911 Equals in Partnership: Basic Rights for Families of Children with Blindness
NAPVI
15 West 65th Street   212-769-7819
New York, NY 10023-0317   800-284-4422
                                        Fax: 617-972-7444
                        e-mail: napvi@lighthouseguild.org
                                            www.napvi.org
Lighthouse Guild is the leading not-for-profit vision + healthcare organization, with a long-standing heritage of addressing the needs of people who are blind or visually impaired as well as those with multiple disabilities or chronic medical conditions.
James A Dubin, Chairman
Susan LaVenture, Executive Director

9912 Essential Elements in Early Intervention: Visual Impairment & Multiple Disability
AFB Press: American Foundation for the Blind
2 Penn Plaza   212-502-7600
New York, NY 10121   800-232-3044
                                        Fax: 888-545-8331
                            e-mail: literacy@afb.net
                                            www.afb.org/store
Latest comprehensive resource from an outstanding early childhood specialist, this guide provides a range of information on effective early intervention with young children who are visually impaired and have other disabilities.
503 pages Paperback
ISBN: 0-891283-05-6
Carl R Augusto, President & CEO
Rick Bozeman, Chief Financial Officer

9913 Eye and Your Vision
Dr Lorrain H Marchi, author
National Association for Visually Handicapped

111 E 59th St
New York, NY 10022-6904

212-821-9497
800-284-4422
Fax: 212-727-2931
e-mail: kcampbell@lighthouse.org
lighthouse.org/navh

A large booklet offering information, with illustrations, on the eye. Includes information on protection of eyesight, how the eye works and vision disorders.
19 pages $5.00 n/members
Lorraine Marchi LHD, Founder/CEO
Cesar Gomez, Executive Director

9914   First Steps
Blind Children's Center
4120 Marathon Street
Los Angeles, CA 90029-3584

213-664-2153
Fax: 213-665-3828
e-mail: info@blindcntr.org
www.blindcntr.org

A handbook for teaching young children who are visually impaired. Designed to assist students, professionals and parents working with children who are visually impaired.
203 pages

9915   Foundations of Education
AFB Press: American Foundation for the Blind
2 Penn Plaza
New York, NY 10121

212-502-7600
800-232-3044
Fax: 888-545-8331
e-mail: literacy@afb.net
www.afb.org/store

Complete revision of landmark text. Comprehensive compilation of state-of-the-art information is the essential resource on educating visually impaired students, the essential theory forming the knowledge base, and methodology of teaching visually impaired students in all areas.
2000
ISBN: 0-891283-49-8
Carl R Augusto, President & CEO
Rick Bozeman, Chief Financial Officer

9916   Foundations of Orientation and Mobility
AFB Press: American Foundation for the Blind
2 Penn Plaza
New York, NY 10121

212-502-7600
800-232-3044
Fax: 888-545-8331
e-mail: literacy@afb.net
www.afb.org

Updated and revised, this new edition of the field's founding classics includes current research fom a variety of disiplines, an international perspective, and expanded contents on low vision, aging, multiple disabilities, accessibility, program design and adaptive technology from more than 30 eminent subject experts. Divided into four main sections, the book explores every of Orientation and Mobility learning and instruction.
800 pages Hardcover
ISBN: 0-891289-46-1
Carl R Augusto, President & CEO
Rick Bozeman, Chief Financial Officer

9917   Foundations of Rehabilitation Counseling with Persons Who Are Blind/Visually Imp.
AFB Press: American Foundation for the Blind
2 Penn Plaza
New York, NY 10121

212-502-7600
800-232-3044
Fax: 888-545-8331
e-mail: literacy@afb.net
www.afb.org/store

Rehabilitation professionals have long recognized that the needs of people who are blind or visually impaired are unique and require a special knowledge and expertise for the provision and coordination of effective rehabilitation services. Contributions to this text from more than 25 experts provide essential information on subjects as functional, medical, vocational and psychological assessments, demographic and cultural issues, pacement and employment issues, and the rehabilitation team.
464 pages Hardcover
ISBN: 0-891289-45-3
Carl R Augusto, President & CEO
Rick Bozeman, Chief Financial Officer

9918   Get a Wiggle On
American Alliance For Health, Phys. Ed. & Dance
1900 Association Drive
Reston, VA 20191-1598

703-476-3400
800-213-7193
Fax: 703-476-9527
www.aahperd.org/

Gives teachers and parents practical suggestions for helping blind and visually impaired infants grow and learn like other children.
80 pages
ISBN: 0-883140-77-2
Steve Jefferies, President
E. Paul Roetert, Chief Executive Officer

9919   Guide to Independence for the Visually Impaired and Their Families
Demos Medical Publishing
11 West 42nd Street
New York, NY 10036-8804

212-683-0072
800-532-8663
Fax: 212-683-0118
e-mail: support@demosmedical.com
www.demosmedical.com

This first comprehensive, hands-on book for the newly visually impaired and their families presents detailed instructions to deal with emotional reactions and fioght depression; contact organizations and get information; obtain federal and other types of financial aid; use the other senses more effectively; adapt their homes and do household chores; handle paperwork and become socially active.
248 pages Paperback
ISBN: 0-939957-61-2
David D'Addona, Acquisitions Editor

9920   Guidelines and Games for Teaching Efficient Braille Reading
AFB Press: American Foundation for the Blind
2 Penn Plaza
New York, NY 10121

212-502-7600
800-232-3044
Fax: 888-545-8331
e-mail: literacy@afb.net
www.afb.org/store

Based on research in the areas of rapid reading and precision teaching, these effective guidelines and games represent a unique adaptation of a general reading program to the needs of braille readers.
116 pages Paperback
ISBN: 0-891281-05-3
Carl R Augusto, President & CEO
Rick Bozeman, Chief Financial Officer

9921   Hammond Large Type World Atlas
American Map-Langensceidt Publishing Group
15 Tyger River Drive
Duncan, SC 29334

864-486-0214
800-432-6277
Fax: 888-773-7979
www.hammondmap.com

100 maps.

ISBN: 0-816159-11-4

9922   Handbook for Itinerant and Resource Teachers of Blind Students
National Federation of the Blind
200 East Wells Street
Baltimore, MD 21230-4998

410-659-9314
Fax: 410-685-5653
e-mail: nfb@nfb.org
www.nfb.org

The Handbook provides help to teachers, school administrators or other school personnel that have experience with blind or visually impaired students. The Handbook devotes 45 pages to Braille and how to teach Braille for parents and teachers; other chapters iclude law, physical education, fitting in socially, testing and evaluation, home economics, daily living skills and more.
533 pages Softcover
Mark Riccobono, President
James Gashel, Secretary

9923   Health Care Professionals Who are Blind or Visually Impaired
AFB Press: American Foundation for the Blind
2 Penn Plaza
New York, NY 10121

212-502-7600
800-232-3044
Fax: 888-545-8331
e-mail: literacy@afb.net
www.afb.org/store

Exciting career possibilities for people who are visually impaired as well as those who are sighted. Inspirational profiles of 15 sucessful role models. Written in an accesible, easy-to-read style, this book documents the stories and stategies of professionals ranging from a forensic psychiatrist to a radiology dark room technician. Information on technology and tactics that are used to perform demanding jobs are also included. Available in paperback, audio casette, or ASCII disk.

2001 166 pages
ISBN: 0-891283-88-9
Carl R Augusto, President & CEO
Rick Bozeman, Chief Financial Officer

9924 I Keep Five Pairs of Glasses in a Flower Pot
Henrietta Levner, author

National Association for Visually Handicapped
111 E 59th St   212-821-9497
New York, NY 10022-6904   800-284-4422
                                   Fax: 212-727-2931
                  e-mail: kcampbell@lighthouse.org
                                   lighthouse.org/navh

A short story, printed in 18 point type, is the saga of one womans struggle with low vision.
Lorraine Marchi LHD, Founder/CEO
Cesar Gomez, Executive Director

9925 If Blindness Comes
National Federation of the Blind
200 East Wells Street   410-659-9314
Baltimore, MD 21230-4998   Fax: 410-685-5653
                                   e-mail: nfb@nfb.org
                                            www.nfb.org

An introduction to issues relating to vision loss and provides a positive, supportive philosophy about blindness. It is a general information book which includes answers to many common questions about blindness, information about services and programs for the blind and resource listings.
Mark Riccobono, President
James Gashel, Secretary

9926 Independence Without Sight or Sound: Suggestions for Practitioners
AFB Press: American Foundation for the Blind
2 Penn Plaza   212-502-7600
New York, NY 10121   800-232-3044
                                   Fax: 888-545-8331
                        e-mail: literacy@afb.net
                                     www.afb.org/store

Written in a personal and informal style, this practical guidebook covers the essential aspects of communicating and working with deaf-blind persons. Full of valuable information on subjects such as how to talk with deaf-blind people, adapt orientation and mobility techniques for deaf-blind travelers, and interact with deaf-blind individuals socially, this useful manual also contains a substantial resource section detailing sources of information and adapted equipment. Also available in braille.
193 pages Paperback
ISBN: 0-891282-46-7
Carl R Augusto, President & CEO
Rick Bozeman, Chief Financial Officer

9927 Jewish Heritage for the Blind
1655 E 24th Street   718-338-4999
Brooklyn, NY 11229-2401   800-995-1888
                                   Fax: 718-338-0653
                  e-mail: services@jhbinternational.org
                                     www.jhbinternational.org

Offers large print traditional prayer books for the High Holy days, festivals, fast days and daily rituals for those finding it difficult or impossible to read small print.

9928 Kernel Book Series
National Federation of the Blind
200 East Wells Street   410-659-9314
Baltimore, MD 21230-4998   Fax: 410-685-5653
                                   e-mail: nfb@nfb.org
                                            www.nfb.org

A series of books written by the blind themselves. Each book is a collection of articles and stories about the real life experiences of blind persons. These books help educate the blind and the sighted alike about a positive philosophy regarding blindness.
Mark Riccobono, President
James Gashel, Secretary

9929 King James Bible: Large Print
Science Products
PO Box 888
Southeastern, PA 19399-0888   800-888-7400

24 point type easily seen with 20/200 acuity. Makes bible reading for children easier too.

9930 Knotholes are for Seeing: Therapy Through Poetry, Prose & Other Writings
Business of Living Publications
PO Box 8388   512-852-8515
Corpus Christi, TX 78468-8388

ISBN: 1-879518-08-2

9931 Large Print American Heritage Dictionary
Houghton Mifflin Harcourt
222 Berkeley Street   617-351-5000
Boston, MA 02116   800-888-7400
                                            www.hmco.com

More than 35,000 easy to read entries for those who prefer large type.

ISBN: 0-395929-32-6
Lawrence K. Fish, Director and Chairman of the Board
Sheru Chowdhry, Director

9932 Legislative Handbook for Parents
NAPVI
PO Box 317   617-972-7441
Watertown, MA 02471-0317   800-562-6265
                                   Fax: 617-972-7444
                        e-mail: napvi@perkins.org
                                         www.spedex.com

Written by parents for parents in dealing with legislative processes that ultimately affect their children's lives.
Susan LaVenture, Executive Director

9933 Library Resources for the Blind and Physically Handicapped
National Library Service for the Blind
1291 Taylor Street NW   202-707-5100
Washington, DC 20542-0002   Fax: 202-707-0712
                                   TDD: 202-707-0744
                              e-mail: nls@loc.gov
                                         www.loc.gov/nls

The mission of this web site is to provide program users, librarians, and the public a wide range of access to NLS publications, program information, and bibliographic data

9934 Low Vision: Reflections of the Past, Issues for the Future
AFB Press: American Foundation for the Blind
2 Penn Plaza   212-502-7600
New York, NY 10121   800-232-3044
                                   Fax: 888-545-8331
                        e-mail: literacy@afb.net
                                     www.afb.org/store

Research report based on a multiphase survey of professionals. Identifies important trends that will shape the field of low vision services into the next century. Designed for administrators, policy planners and university instructors, as well as for direct service providers, Low Vision includes overview papers by six eminent leaders in the low vision field.
181 pages Paperback
ISBN: 0-891282-18-1
Carl R Augusto, President & CEO
Rick Bozeman, Chief Financial Officer

9935 Madness of Usher's: Coping with Vision & Hearing Loss
Richard A. Lewis, Dorothy H. Stiefel, author

Business of Living Publications
PO Box 8388   512-852-8515
Corpus Christi, TX 78468-8388
Paperback
ISBN: 1-879518-06-6
Dorothy H Stiefel, Author

9936 Mainstreaming & the American Dream: Soc. Logical Perspectives on Parental Coping
AFB Press: American Foundation for the Blind
2 Penn Plaza   212-502-7600
New York, NY 10121   800-232-3044
                            Fax: 888-545-8331
                        e-mail: literacy@afb.net
                             www.afb.org/store
Based on in-depth interviews with parents and professionals, this research monograph presents a sociological framework for looking at the needs and aspirations of parents of blind and visually impaired children.
256 pages Paperback
ISBN: 0-891281-91-6
Carl R Augusto, President & CEO
Rick Bozeman, Chief Financial Officer

9937 Mainstreaming the Visually Impaired Child
NAPVI
15 West 65th Street   212-769-7819
New York, NY 10023-0317   800-284-4422
                            Fax: 617-972-7444
                    e-mail: napvi@lighthouseguild.org
                              www.napvi.org
Lighthouse Guild is the leading not-for-profit vision + healthcare organization, with a long-standing heritage of addressing the needs of people who are blind or visually impaired as well as those with multiple disabilities or chronic medical conditions.
James A Dubin, Chairman
Susan LaVenture, Executive Director

9938 Making Life More Livable: Adaptations for Living at Home After Vision Loss
AFB Press: American Foundation of the Blind
2 Penn Plaza   212-502-7600
New York, NY 10121   800-232-3044
                            Fax: 888-545-8331
                        e-mail: literacy@afb.net
                             www.afb.org/store
Essential guide for adults experiencing vision loss and an invaluable resource for their family and friends. Full of practical tips and illustrated by numerous photographs, this easy-to-use resource shows how people who are visually impaired can continue living independent, productive lives at home on their own. Useful general guidelines and room-by-room specifics provide simple and effective solutions for making homes accessible and everyday activities doable for visually impaired individuals.
132 pages Cassette avail.
ISBN: 0-891281-15-0
Carl R Augusto, President & CEO
Rick Bozeman, Chief Financial Officer

9939 Occupational Therapy Practice Guidelines for Adults with Low Vision
American Occupational Therapy Association
4720 Montgomery Lane   301-652-6611
Bethesda, MD 20814-1220   800-729-2682
                            Fax: 240-762-5150
                            TDD: 800-377-8555
                       e-mail: praota@aota.org.
                              www.aota.org
25 pages
ISBN: 1-569001-50-2

9940 Perkins Activity and Resource Guide: A Handbook for Teachers
Perkins School for the Blind Publications
175 N Beacon Street   617-924-3434
Watertown, MA 02472-2790   877-473-7546
                            Fax: 617-972-7334
                    e-mail: publications@perkins.org
                             www.perkins.org
This is a comprehensive, two volume guide with over 1,000 pages of activities, resources and instructional strategies for teachers and parents of students with visual and multiple disabilities.
Kathy Heydt, Author
Monica Allon, Author

9941 Preschool Learning Activities for the Visually Impaired Child
NAPVI

15 West 65th Street   212-769-7819
New York, NY 10023-0317   800-284-4422
                            Fax: 617-972-7444
                    e-mail: napvi@lighthouseguild.org
                              www.napvi.org
Lighthouse Guild is the leading not-for-profit vision + healthcare organization, with a long-standing heritage of addressing the needs of people who are blind or visually impaired as well as those with multiple disabilities or chronic medical conditions.
James A Dubin, Chairman
Susan LaVenture, Executive Director

9942 Prescriptions for Independence: Working with Older People Who Are Visually Imp.
AFB Press: American Foundation for the Blind
2 Penn Plaza   212-502-7600
New York, NY 10121   800-232-3044
                            Fax: 888-545-8331
                        e-mail: literacy@afb.net
                             www.afb.org/store
Easy-to-read manual on how older persons with visual impairments can pursue their interests and activities in community residences, senior centers, long-term care facilities and other community settings. Topics covered include signs of vision loss, recreation, personal care, orientation and mobility and modifications in the environment.
87 pages Paperback
ISBN: 0-891282-44-0
Carl R Augusto, President & CEO
Rick Bozeman, Chief Financial Officer

9943 Providing Services for People with Vision Loss: Multidisciplinary Perspective
Resources For Rehabilitation
22 Bonad Road   781-368-9080
Winchester, MA 01890   Fax: 781-368-9096
                          e-mail: info@rfr.org
                               www.rfr.org
A collection of articles by ophthalmologists and rehabilitation professionals, including chapters on operating a low vision service, starting self-help programs, mental health services, aids and techniques that help people with vision loss.
136 pages
ISBN: 0-929718-02-X
Susan L. Greenblatt, Editor

9944 Psychoeducational Assessment of Visually Impaired Students
Pro-Ed, Inc.
8700 Shoal Creek Blvd   512-451-3246
Austin, TX 78757-6897   800-897-3202
                            Fax: 800-397-7633
                       e-mail: info@proedinc.com
                             www.proedinc.com
Professional reference book that addresses the problems specific to assessment of visually impaired children. Of particular value to the practitioner are the extensive reviews of available tests, including ways to adapt those not designed for use with the visually handicapped.
140 pages Paperback
Lindy Jordaan, Marketing Coordinator

9945 Resources Family Centered Intervention for Infants, Toddlers & Preschoolers
Hope
1856 N 1200 E   435-245-2888
North Logan, UT 84341   Fax: 435-245-2888
Describes children with vision impairment in terms of characteristics, needs, and parent concerns.
Hardcover

9946 Show Me How: Manual for Parents Preschool Visually Impaired & Blind Children
AFB Press: American Foundation for the Blind
2 Penn Plaza   212-502-7600
New York, NY 10121   800-232-3044
                            Fax: 888-545-8331
                        e-mail: literacy@afb.net
                             www.afb.org/store
Practical guide for parents, teachers and others who help preschool children attain age-related goals. Includes activities for growing

and learning, building self-concept, moving around, playing, perfecting daily living skills and developing sensory awareness. It also covers such issues as observing safety precautions, choosing appropriate toys and facilitating relationships with playmates.
56 pages Paperback
ISBN: 0-891281-13-4
Carl R Augusto, President & CEO
Rick Bozeman, Chief Financial Officer

9947 Starting Points
Blind Children's Center
4120 Marathon Street   213-664-2153
Los Angeles, CA 90029-3584   Fax: 213-665-3828
Basic information for the clasroom teacher of 3 to 8 year olds whose multiple disabilities include visual impairment.
160 pages

9948 Tactile Graphics
AFB Press: American Foundation for the Blind
2 Penn Plaza   212-502-7600
New York, NY 10121   800-232-3044
                                              Fax: 888-545-8331
                                      e-mail: literacy@afb.net
                                              www.afb.org/store
Easy-to-read encyclopedia handbook on translating visual information into a three-dimensional form that the blind and visually impaired persons can understand. This heavily illustrated guide covers theory, techniques, materials and step-by-step instructions for educators, rehabilitators, graphic artists, museum and busines personnel, employers and anyone involved in producing tactile material for visually impaired persons.
544 pages Paperback
ISBN: 0-891281-94-0
Carl R Augusto, President & CEO
Rick Bozeman, Chief Financial Officer

9949 Teachers Who Are Blind or Visually Impaired
AFB Press: American Foundation for the Blind
2 Penn Plaza   212-502-7600
New York, NY 10121   800-232-3044
                                              Fax: 888-545-8331
                                      e-mail: literacy@afb.net
                                              www.afb.org/store
First volume in the Jobs That Matter series, this book profiles 18 visually impaired individuals who have successfully fulfilled their dreams of becoming teachers. These engaging individuals demonstrate how visually impaired teachers can be effective in their jobs and achieve classroom sucess and satisfaction. Available in paperback, audio cassette or braille.
1998 176 pages
ISBN: 0-891283-06-4
Carl R Augusto, President & CEO
Rick Bozeman, Chief Financial Officer

9950 Textbook Catalog
National Braille Association
95 Allens Creek Road   585-427-8260
Rochester, NY 14618   Fax: 585-427-0263
                                          www.nationalbraille.org
Lists hundreds of scholarly, college and professional textbooks offered in large print, braille or on cassette for visually impaired readers.
80 pages
Whitney Williams, President
Jana Hertz, Vice President

9951 To Love This Life: Quotations by Helen Keller
AFB Press: American Foundation for the Blind
2 Penn Plaza   212-502-7600
New York, NY 10121   800-232-3044
                                              Fax: 888-545-8331
                                      e-mail: literacy@afb.net
                                              www.afb.org/store
Beautiful and moving souvenir of one of the world's most admired women. This memorable collection of quotations from Helen Keller brings words of wisdom, courage and inspiration from a remarkable individual who above all wanted to make a difference in the lives of her fellow men and women. The thought captured here — many from unpublished letters and speeches — offer profound

statements on the meaning of being human and on life in all its complexity. Available in hardcover and audio cassette.
2000 118 pages
ISBN: 0-891283-47-1
Carl R Augusto, President & CEO
Rick Bozeman, Chief Financial Officer

9952 Unseen Minority: Social History of Blindness in the US
Frances A. Koestler, author
David McKay Company/AFB Press, Distributor
2 Penn Plaza   412-741-1398
New York, NY 10121   800-232-3044
                                              Fax: 888-545-8331
                                      e-mail: literacy@afb.net
                                              www.afb.org
Lively narrative, peppered with anecdotes, recounts how the blind overcame discrimination to gain full participation in the social, educational, economic and legislative spheres. Here are the gripping stories: Why it took a century for braille to become a universal medium in English, how america's first school for the blind began with a chance encounter on a Boston street, and how the talking book came into existence.
573 pages Hardcover
ISBN: 0-679505-39-3
Carl R Augusto, President & CEO
Rick Bozeman, Chief Financial Officer

9953 Vision and Aging: Crossroads for Service Delivery
AFB Press: American Foundation for the Blind
2 Penn Plaza   212-502-7600
New York, NY 10121   800-232-3044
                                              Fax: 888-545-8331
                                      e-mail: literacy@afb.net
                                              www.afb.org/store
This overview of the service delivery systems in the aging and blindness fields covers the essential issues concerning vision loss among older persons in this country, the growth of visual impairment among the increasing number of elderly people in the US, and the policy and service questions that will demand national attention throughout this and the coming decades.
392 pages Paperback
ISBN: 0-891282-16-5
Carl R Augusto, President & CEO
Rick Bozeman, Chief Financial Officer

9954 Visual Aids and Informational Material
National Association for Visually Handicapped
111 E 59th St   212-821-9497
New York, NY 10022-6904   800-284-4422
                                              Fax: 212-727-2931
                                  e-mail: kcampbell@lighthouse.org
                                              lighthouse.org/navh
A large reference guide offering a list of visual aids and resources for persons with visual impairments.
65 pages
Lorraine Marchi LHD, Founder/CEO
Cesar Gomez, Executive Director

9955 Visual Handicaps and Learning
Pro-Ed, Inc.
8700 Shoal Creek Blvd   512-451-3246
Austin, TX 78757-6897   800-897-3202
                                              Fax: 800-397-7633
                                      e-mail: info@proedinc.com
                                              www.proedinc.com
This text covers a range of topics associated with visual impairment, from past practices to up-to-date research, and from legal responsibilities to personal beliefs, without losing sight of the individual child.
180 pages
ISBN: 0-890795-15-0
Lindy Jordaan, Marketing Coordinator

9956 Visual Impairment: An Overview
AFB Press: American Foundation for the Blind
2 Penn Plaza   212-502-7600
New York, NY 10121   800-232-3044
                                              Fax: 888-545-8331
                                      e-mail: literacy@afb.net
                                              www.afb.org/store

Down-to-earth look at the common forms of vision loss and their impact on the individual. Explains the different aspects of visual impairment, describes adaptive techniques and devices and provides information on available resources and services in a conscise and easy-to-understand manner for professionals and visually impaired people and their families.
56 pages Paperback
ISBN: 0-891281-74-6
Carl R Augusto, President & CEO
Rick Bozeman, Chief Financial Officer

9957 Walking Alone and Marching Together
Floyd Matson, author
National Federation of the Blind
200 East Wells Street   410-659-9314
Baltimore, MD 21230-4998   Fax: 410-685-5653
e-mail: nfb@nfb.org
www.nfb.org

The history of the organized blind movement, this book spans more than 50 years of civil rights, social issues, attitudes and experiences of the blind. Published in 1990, it has been read by thousands of blind and sighted persons and is used in colleges, libraries and programs across the country as an important tool in understanding blindness and it's impact on both personal lives and the society at large.
1100 pages
Mark Riccobono, President
James Gashel, Secretary

9958 Webster Large Print Dictionary
Random House
1745 Broadway, 15-3   212-782-9000
New York, NY 10019   800-888-7400
www.penguinrandomhouse.com

They are committed to helping authors realize their very best work and to finding innovative new ways of bringing stories and ideas to audiences worldwide
880 pages
ISBN: 0-375722-32-7

9959 What Museum Guides Need to Know: Access for Blind & Visually Impaired Visitors
AFB Press: American Foundation for the Blind
2 Penn Plaza   212-502-7600
New York, NY 10121   800-232-3044
Fax: 888-545-8331
e-mail: literacy@afb.net
www.afb.org/store

Provides practical, easy-to-use guidelines on how to greet and help blind and visually impaired museum goers. With numerous photographs taken at the High School Museum of Art and the Atlanta Historical Society, this handbook also covers aesthetics and visual impairment, legal requirements for accessibility, resources, a training outline for museum requirements for accessibility, a bibliography on art and museum access for blind and visually impaired persons, and guidelines for preparing media.
64 pages Paperback
ISBN: 0-891281-58-4
Carl R Augusto, President & CEO
Rick Bozeman, Chief Financial Officer

Children's Books

9960 Belonging
Dial Books
375 Hudson Street
New York, NY 10014-3658   212-366-2000
www.penguin.com

Meg attended special schools for the blind until she was ready for high school. She decided that she wanted to go to a regular high school. She and her mother practiced her walks to school and studied the layout of the building prior to school starting, but Meg was unprepared for the trip when there were 1,500 students. She adjusted quickly to the crowds and the pace of the new school.
200 pages Hardcover
ISBN: 0-803705-30-1

9961 Beside Me
Leader Dogs For The Blind
1039 S. Rochester Road   248-651-9011
Rochester Hills, MI 48307   888-777-5332
Fax: 248-651-5812
TTY: 248-651-3713
e-mail: leaderdog@leaderdog.org
www.leaderdog.org

Marion became blind as an adult. She was totally dependent on her parents to move around and go places she wanted to be. Marion decided to go to the leader-dog program and learn to use a leader dog. Particularly she wanted the independence she would need to go to college. Marion enrolled at the Leader-Dog-For-The-Blind Program in Rochester, Michigan. After weeks of training she was given a German Shepherd named Heidi. Marion and Heidi trained together until they were a team and ready.
Films
Susan Daniels, President & CEO
Lorene Suidan, Chief Financial Officer

9962 Guide Dog Goes to School
William Morrow and Company
105 Madison Avenue   212-889-3050
New York, NY 10016-7418   800-843-9389
william-morrow-co.1.searchbook.net

Cinderena is a golden retriever. As a puppy Cindy is outgoing and not afraid of things in her environment. This disposition is ideal for a guide dog to the blind, and Cindy is selected to be in a program for guide dogs. Follow Cindy as we focus on the guide dog training.
51 pages Hardcover
ISBN: 0-688068-44-8

9963 How Do You Kiss a Blind Girl?
Charles C Thomas Publisher
2600 S First Street   217-789-8980
Springfield, IL 62704-4730   Fax: 217-789-9130
e-mail: books@ccthomas.com
www.ccthomas.com

Focuses, in a humorous way, on the attitudes toward persons with visual impairments.
126 pages
ISBN: 0-398052-62-X

9964 Living with Blindness
Franklin Watts Grolier
90 Old Sherman Turnpike   203-797-3500
Danbury, CT 06816-0001   800-621-1115
Fax: 203-797-3197
www.grolier.com

Shows how persons with visual impairments and blindness can overcome their disability and lead productive lives.
32 pages Grades 5-7
ISBN: 0-531108-43-0

9965 Man Who Sang in the Dark
Eth Clifford, author
Houghton, Mifflin & Company
1 Beacon Street   617-725-5000
Boston, MA 02108-3107
The story of a girl and a man who is blind and how they both come to an understanding about certain prejudices.
Grades 3-5

9966 Out of the Corner of My Eye
American Foundation for the Blind
15 W 16th Street   212-502-7600
New York, NY 10011-6301   Fax: 212-502-7777
A personal account of students' vision loss and subsequent adjustment that is full of practical advice and cheerful encouragement, told by an 87 year old retired college teacher who has maintained her independence and zest for life.

ISBN: 0-891281-93-2

9967 She'll Never Walk Alone
Leader Dog For The Blind
1964 Park Street   306-565-8211
Regina, SK, S4P 3G4,

Leader dogs for the blind require many weeks of training before they are ready to work with the blind individual. Two courses, basic and advanced, are provided for each dog.
Films

Magazines

9968 Access World: Technology and People with Visual Impairments
AFB Press: American Foundation for the Blind
2 Penn Plaza   212-502-7600
New York, NY 10121   800-232-3044
Fax: 888-545-8331
e-mail: literacy@afb.net
www.afb.org/store
Comprehensive and reader friendly online magazine covering every aspect of assistive technology and visual impairment.
Bimonthly
Carl R Augusto, President & CEO
Rick Bozeman, Chief Financial Officer

9969 Blind Educator
National Federation of the Blind
200 East Wells Street   410-659-9314
Baltimore, MD 21230-4998   Fax: 410-685-5653
e-mail: nfb@nfb.org
www.nfb.org
The articles in this newsletter are written by people who are blind. Blind people can teach. In fact, this newsletter captures a glimpse of the range of subjects and grade levels in which blind people are engaged.
Mark Riccobono, President
James Gashel, Secretary

9970 Braille Forum
Penny Reeder, author
American Council of the Blind
2200 Wilson Boulevard   202-467-5081
Arlington, VA 22201-2706   800-424-8666
Fax: 703-465-5085
e-mail: info@acb.org
www.acb.org
Offered in large print, braille, half speed cassette, via email and on the website.
32 pages 10x/year
Kim Charlson, President
Melanie Brunson, Executive Director

9971 Braille Monitor
National Federation of the Blind
200 East Wells Street   410-659-9314
Baltimore, MD 21230-4998   Fax: 410-685-5653
e-mail: nfb@nfb.org
www.nfb.org
The leading publication in the blindness field, with a circulation of 30,000, this publication addresses issues of concern to the blind and the philosophy and activities of the National Federation of the Blind.
100 pages Monthly
Mark Riccobono, President
James Gashel, Secretary

9972 Dialogue Magazine
Blindskills
PO Box 5181   503-581-4224
Salem, OR 97304-0181   800-860-4224
Fax: 503-518-0178
e-mail: blindsici@teleport.com
www.teleport.com
Publishes quarterly magazine in braille, large-type, cassette and disk of news items, fiction and articles of special interest.
Quarterly

9973 Future Reflections
Barbara Cheadler, author
National Federation of the Blind

200 East Wells Street   410-659-9314
Baltimore, MD 21230-4998   Fax: 410-685-5653
e-mail: nfb@nfb.org
www.nfb.org
National magazine written specifically for parents and educators of blind children. Each issue addresses various topics important to blind children, their families and to school personnel.
Quarterly
Mark Riccobono, President
James Gashel, Secretary

9974 Illinois Braille Messenger
Illinois Council of the Blind
PO Box 1336   217-523-4967
Springfield, IL 62705-1336   888-698-1862
Fax: 217-523-4302
e-mail: icb@fgi.net

Quarterly
Laura Booker, Editor

9975 Journal of Vision Rehabilitation
Media Productions & Marketing
2440 O Street   402-474-2676
Lincoln, NE 68510-1125
Multidisciplinary journal containing articles and papers dealing with low vision, its evaluation, instrumentation and rehabilitation.

9976 Journal of Visual Impairment & Blindness
AFB Press: American Foundation for the Blind
2 Penn Plaza   212-502-7600
New York, NY 10121   800-232-3044
Fax: 888-545-8331
e-mail: literacy@afb.net
www.afb.org/store
Peer-reviewed journal reporting on the cutting-edge research, innovative practice and news on all aspects of visual impairment. Available online, on cassette and ASCII disk.
10 Issues
Carl R Augusto, President & CEO
Rick Bozeman, Chief Financial Officer

9977 Recorded Periodicals
Associated Services for the Blind
919 Walnut Street   215-627-0600
Philadelphia, PA 19107-5237   Fax: 215-922-0692
e-mail: asbinfo@asb.org
www.asb.org
A subscription service of Associated Services for the Blind, this service provides 26 recorded magazines for blind and visually impaired individuals.
Audio Cassette
Patricia C Johnson, President/CEO
Brian Rusk, Public Relations Officer

9978 Review
AER
206 N Washington Street   703-823-9690
Alexandria, VA 22314-2528   Fax: 703-823-9695
The Association's practice-oriented journal.

9979 Tactic
Clovernook Ctr. for the Blind & Visually Impaired
7000 Hamilton Avenue   513-522-3860
Cincinnati, OH 45231-5240   888-224-7156
Fax: 513-728-3946
www.clovernook.org
Clovernook recognizes that each person who comes to us for services brings their own unique set of experiences and expectations. Consequently our services are never one size fits all, but individually designed to reflect your preferences and goals.
Quarterly
Jeffrey D Brasie, President

9980 Vision Enhancement Journal
Vision World Wide

5707 Brockton Drive
Indianapolis, IN 46220-5481

317-254-1332
800-733-2258
Fax: 317-251-6588
e-mail: info@visionww.org
www.visionww.org

Leading International publication providing information and resources for people with vision loss. Journal is available in large print, audio cassette and computer disk.
68-78 pages Quarterly
Patricia Price, President/Managing Editor

9981   Vision World Wide
5707 Brockton Drive
Indianapolis, IN 46220-5481

317-254-1332
800-733-2258
Fax: 317-251-6588
e-mail: info@visionww.org
www.visionww.org

Believing there is hope when vision fails. It disseminates relevant information on a variety of topics through its information and referral helpline, website, e-mail announce list and journal Vision Enhancement, all designed to encourage and support individuals with vision loss, family memebers, professionals who serve them. Aims to enhance everyday living so as to maintain an independent lifestyle. It also serves as a consumer protection against misrepresentation and fraud.
72-78 pages Quarterly
Patricia Price, President/Managing Editor

9982   Voice of the Diabetic
National Federation of the Blind
200 East Wells Street
Baltimore, MD 21230-4998

410-659-9314
Fax: 410-685-5653
e-mail: nfb@nfb.org
www.nfb.org

The leading publication in the diabetes field. Each issue addresses the problems and concerns of diabetes, with a special emphasis for those who have lost vision due to diabetes. Available in print and on cassette.
30 pages Quarterly
Mark Riccobono, President
James Gashel, Secretary

Newsletters

9983   ACB Reports
American Council of the Blind
2200 Wilson Boulevard
Arlington, VA 22201-2706

202-467-5081
800-424-8666
Fax: 703-465-5085
e-mail: info@acb.org
www.acb.org

Radio news feature program for radio information services.
Monthly
Kim Charlson, President
Melanie Brunson, Executive Director

9984   AER Report
AER
1703 N. Beauregard Street
Alexandria, VA 22311

703-671-4500
877-492-2708
Fax: 703-671-6391
e-mail: lou@aerbvi.org
www.aerbvi.org

Contains organizational news, conference dates and information concerning services to visually impaired people.
28 pages BiMonthly
Jackie Fairbarns, Assistant Director
Lou Tutt, Executive Director

9985   AFB News
American Foundation for the Blind
2 Penn Plaza
New York, NY 10121-2018

212-502-7600
800-232-3044
Fax: 888-545-8331
e-mail: literacy@afb.net
www.afb.org

National newsletter for general readership about blindness and visual impairments featuring people, programs, services and activities.
12 pages Quarterly
Carl R Augusto, President & CEO
Rick Bozeman, Chief Financial Officer

9986   Aging and Vision News
National Center for Vision and Aging
800 2nd Avenue
New York, NY 10017

212-808-0077
800-334-5497
3x Year

9987   Awareness
NAPVI
15 West 65th Street
New York, NY 10023-0317

212-769-7819
800-284-4422
Fax: 617-972-7444
e-mail: napvi@lighthouseguild.org
www.napvi.org

Lighthouse Guild is the leading not-for-profit vision + healthcare organization, with a long-standing heritage of addressing the needs of people who are blind or visually impaired as well as those with multiple disabilities or chronic medical conditions.
Quarterly
James A Dubin, Chairman
Susan LaVenture, Executive Director

9988   Braille Book Review
National Library Service for the Blind
1291 Taylor Street NW
Washington, DC 20542-0002

202-707-5100
Fax: 202-707-0712
TDD: 202-707-0744
e-mail: nls@loc.gov
www.loc.gov/nls

The mission of this web site is to provide program users, librarians, and the public a wide range of access to NLS publications, program information, and bibliographic data
BiMonthly

9989   Bulletin
National Association for Visually Handicapped
111 E 59th St
New York, NY 10022-6904

212-821-9497
800-284-4422
Fax: 212-727-2931
e-mail: kcampbell@lighthouse.org
lighthouse.org/navh

Annual report offering information on association activities and events, conferences, vision aids and resources for the visually impaired.
Lorraine Marchi LHD, Founder/CEO
Cesar Gomez, Executive Director

9990   DVH Quarterly
University of Arkansas At Little Rock
2801 S University Avenue
Little Rock, AR 72204-1000

501-569-3000
Fax: 501-663-3536
ualr.edu/www

Offers information on upcoming events, conferences and workshops on and for visual disabilities. Book reviews, information on the newest resources and technology, educational programs, want ads and more.
Quarterly
Bob Brasher, Editor

9991   Eye Research News
645 Madison Avenue
New York, NY 10022-1010

212-752-4333
800-621-0026
Fax: 212-688-6231
e-mail: inforequest@rpbusa.org
www.rpbusa.org

Newsletter on the latest development in eye research
Annual
David Weeks, Chairman
Diane S Swift, President

9992   Focus
Visually Impaired Center

1422 West Court Street
Flint, MI 48503

810-767-4014
Fax: 810-767-0020
e-mail: info@vicflint.org
www.vicflint.org

Newsletter offering information for the visually impaired person in the forms of legislative and law updates, ADA information, support groups, hotlines, and articles on the newest technology in the field.
Quarterly
Laurie MacArthur, Executive Director

9993   Gleams Newsletter
Glaucoma Research Foundation
251 Post Street
San Francisco, CA 94108

415-986-3162
800-826-6693
Fax: 415-986-3763
e-mail: question@glaucoma.org
www.glaucoma.org

It includes information about glaucoma, new treatments, updates on research findings, and more.
3x/year
Thomas M Brunner, President/CEO
Andrew L Jackson, Director Communications

9994   Guide Dog Foundation for the Blind Newsletter
371 E Jericho Turnpike
Smithtown, NY 11787-2976

631-930-9000
800-548-4337
Fax: 631-930-9009
e-mail: info@guidedog.org
www.guidedog.org

This organization relies on voluntary public contributions to provide persons with blindness the gift of second sight through the eyes of a guide dog. This nonprofit organization furnishes guide dogs, free of charge, to qualified people who seek independence, mobility and companionship.
James C. Bingham, Chair
Alphonce J. Brown, Vice Chair

9995   Guide Dog News
Guide Dogs for the Blind
PO Box 151200
San Rafael, CA 94915

415-499-4000
800-298-4050
Fax: 415-499-4035
e-mail: information@guidedogs.com
www.guidedogs.com

About graduates, volunteers and donors of Guide Dogs for the Blind.
Quarterly
Bob Burke, Board Chair
Chris Benninger, President and CEO

9996   Guideway
Guide Dog Foundation for the Blind
371 E Jericho Turnpike
Smithtown, NY 11787-2976

631-930-9000
800-548-4337
Fax: 631-930-9009
e-mail: info@guidedog.org
www.guidedog.org

Offers updates and information on the foundation's activities and guide dog programs. In print form but is also available on cassette.
6 pages Monthly
James C. Bingham, Chair
Alphonce J. Brown, Vice Chair

9997   Hearsay
Radio Information Service
600 Forbes Avenue
Pittsburgh, PA 15282

412-488-3944
Fax: 412-488-3953
e-mail: info@readingservice.org
www.readingservice.org

Newsletter for persons interested in radio reading services.
Quarterly

9998   Hub
SPOKES Unlimited
1006 Main Street
Klamath Falls, OR 97601

541-883-7547
Fax: 541-885-2469
www.spokesunlimited.org

Newsletter on rehabilitation, peer counseling, blindness, visual impairments, information and referral.
Meg Graf, Resource Librarian

9999   InSight
Foundation Fighting Blindness
7168 Columbia Gateway Dr
Columbia, MD 21046-2220

410-423-0600
800-683-5555
Fax: 410-363-2393
TDD: 800-683-5551
e-mail: info@fightblindness.org
www.blindness.org

The Foundation Fighting Blindness newsletter, delivered to members monthly. The major emphasis is to report on research and science news, and FDA approved clinical trials around retinal degenerative dieseases.
20 pages 3 per year
William T. Schmidt, CEO
Stephen M. Rose, Chief Research Officer

10000   Lion
Lions Clubs International
300 W 22nd Street
Oak Brook, IL 60523-8815

630-571-5466
www.lionsclubs.org

Publication for the blind.

10001   Listen Up
Recording for the Blind & Dyslexic (RFB&D)
20 Roszel Road
Princeton, NJ 08540-6294

609-452-0606
800-221-4792
Fax: 609-987-8116
e-mail: custserv@rfbd.org
www.learningally.org

RFB&D's bi-monthly newsletter for members.

Andrew Friedman, President & CEO
Jim Halliday, Executive Vice President

10002   Long Cane News
American Foundation for the Blind
15 West 16th Street
New York, NY 10011-6301

212-294-8301
800-232-5463
Fax: 212-502-7777
www.cjh.org

Semiannual
Amy Goldman Fowler, Chair
Kenneth J. Bialkin, Vice Chair

10003   Musical Mainstream
National Library Service for the Blind
1291 Taylor Street NW
Washington, DC 20542-0002

202-707-5100
Fax: 202-707-0712
TDD: 202-707-0744
e-mail: nls@loc.gov
www.loc.gov

Articles selected from print music magazines.
Quarterly

10004   NAVH UPDATE
National Association for Visually Handicapped
111 E 59th St
New York, NY 10022-6904

212-821-9497
800-284-4422
Fax: 212-727-2931
e-mail: kcampbell@lighthouse.org
lighthouse.org/navh

This newsletter offers vision news, medical updates, assistive device information, resources and more for the visually impaired.
4 pages Quarterly
Lorraine Marchi LHD, Founder/CEO
Cesar Gomez, Executive Director

10005   NLS News
National Library Service for the Blind
1291 Taylor Street NW
Washington, DC 20542-0002

202-707-5100
Fax: 202-707-0712
TDD: 202-707-0744
e-mail: nls@loc.gov
www.loc.gov

Newsletter on current program developments.
Quarterly

10006 NLS Update
National Library Service for the Blind
1291 Taylor Street NW   202-707-5100
Washington, DC 20542-0002   Fax: 202-707-0712
                                                   TDD: 202-707-0744
                                                   e-mail: nls@loc.gov
                                                         www.loc.gov
Newsletter on the services volunteer activities.
Quarterly

10007 NOAH News
National Organization for Albinism
PO Box 959   603-887-2310
E. Hampsted, NH 03826-0959   800-473-2310
                                                   Fax: 800-648-2310
                                                   e-mail: info@albinism.org
                                                         www.albinism.org
NOAH serves the albinism community by providing information
and support. NOAH is a not-for-profit corporation chartered in
Pennsylvania
BiAnnually

10008 Newsline for the Blind
National Federation of the Blind
200 East Wells Street   410-659-9314
Baltimore, MD 21230-4998   Fax: 410-685-5653
                                                   e-mail: nfb@nfb.org
                                                         www.nfb.org
Nation's only digital talking newspaper service for the blind. Al-
lows the blind to read the full text of leading national and local
newspapers by using a touch-tone telephone. Service is free of
charge and available 24 hours a day, 7 days per week.
Mark Riccobono, President
James Gashel, Secretary

10009 Open Windows
Sunday School Board of the Southern Baptists
127 9th Avenue N
Nashville, TN 37234-0001   800-458-2772
Guide for personal devotions on audio cassette tape, using Bible
references, devotional readings, and prayer calendar of popular
Open Windows devotional guide for visually handicapped adults.
Quarterly

10010 Personal Reader Update
Personal Reader Department
9 Centennial Drive   978-977-2000
Peabody, MA 01960-7906   800-343-0311
                                                   Fax: 978-977-2437
Offers information on new services, assistive devices and technol-
ogy for the blind.

10011 Prevent Blindness America News
Prevent Blindness America
211 West Wacker Drive   847-843-2020
Chicago, IL 60606   800-331-2020
                                                   www.preventblindness.org
Offers information and articles on eye safety, programs, and ser-
vices of the Society.
Quarterly
Parry Hugh, President & CEO
Bilazer Arzu, Creative Director

10012 RP Messenger
Texas Association of Retinitis Pigmentosa
PO Box 8388   361-852-8515
Corpus Christi, TX 78468-8388   Fax: 361-852-8515
A bi-annual newsletter offering information on Retinitis
Pigmentosa.
BiAnnual

10013 Raised Dot Computing Newsletter
Raised Dot Computing
211 S Paterson Street   608-257-9595
Madison, WI 53703-3789

Discusses braille computer techniques and devices for blind persons.

10014 SCENE
Braille Institute
741 N Vermont Avenue   213-663-1111
Los Angeles, CA 90029-3594   800-272-4553
                                                   Fax: 323-663-0867
                                                   e-mail: la@brailleinstitute.org
                                                         www.brailleinstitute.org
Offers information on the organization, question and answer col-
umn, articles on the newest technology and more for visually im-
paired persons.
Peter A. Mindnich, President
Paul J Porelli, Managing Editor

10015 Smith-Kettlewell Technical File
Smith-Kettlewell Eye Research Foundation
2318 Fillmore Street   415-345-2125
San Francisco, CA 94115-1821   Fax: 415-561-1610
                                                   www-test.ski.org/Rehab/sktf/
The Rehabilitation Engineering Research Center published the
Smith-Kettlewell Technical File, a quarterly newsletter, in braille,
large print, and recorded form, to serve as a guide to the current
technology as applied to the needs of blind and low vision people,
both electronics professionals and hobbyists. A survey of readers
showed that this narrowed the existing gaps and allowed techni-
cally-minded visually impaired people to pursue their interests.
Quarterly

10016 Student Advocate
National Alliance of Blind Students
1155 15th Street NW   202-467-5081
Washington, DC 20005   800-424-8666
                                                   e-mail: president@acbstudents.org
                                                         www.acbstudents.org
A communication forum covering issues of concern to
postsecondary students who are blind.

Cammie Vloedman, President
Olivia Norman, First Vice President

10017 Talking Book Topics
National Library Services For The Blind
1291 Taylor Street NW   202-707-5100
Washington, DC 20542-0002   Fax: 202-707-0712
                                                   TDD: 202-707-0744
                                                   e-mail: nls@loc.gov
                                                         www.loc.gov
Offers hundreds of listings of books, fiction and nonfiction, for
adults and children on cassette. Also offers listings on foreign lan-
guage books on cassette, talking magazines and reviews.
Bimonthly

10018 Tarheel Talk
North Carolina Library for the Blind
1841 Capital Boulevard   919-733-4376
Raleigh, NC 27635   888-388-2460
                                                   Fax: 919-733-6910
                                                   TDD: 919-733-1462
                                                   e-mail: nclbph@ncdcr.gov
                                                         statelibrary.ncdcr.gov/lbph

Quarterly
Carl Keehn, Director

10019 The Macula Foundation Manhattan Eye, Ear & Throat Hospital
American Macular Degeneration Foundation
P.O. Box 515   413-268-7660
Northampton, MA 01061-0515   888-622-8527
                                                   Fax: 212-605-3795
                                                   e-mail: foundation@retinal-research.org
                                                         www.macular.org/spotlite.html
Newsletter of the American Macular Degeneration Foundation, a
nationwide support group for individuals and their families to ad-
just to the restrictions and changes brought about by macular
disease.
Quarterly
Nikolai Stevenson, President
Walter Ross, VP

10020 The Pioneer Projects and Programs Periodic al
TelecomPioneers
1801 California Street 303-571-1200
Denver, CO 80202 800-872-5995
Fax: 303-572-0520
e-mail: info@pioneersvolunteer.org
www.pioneersvolunteer.org
We're a dedicated, diverse network of current and retired telecommunications employees across the US and Canada
Monthly
Gloria Pazel, Chairman
Charlene Hill, Executive Director

10021 Viva Vital News
5016 Silk Oak Drive 941-371-2153
Sarasota, FL 34232-5410
Membership service organization offering information for veterans and is an affiliate of the American Council of the Blind.

10022 Voice of Vision
GW Micro
725 Airport N Office Park 802-362-3612
Fort Wayne, IN 46825-4229 Fax: 260-489-2608
e-mail: sales@aisquared.com
www.gwmicro.com
Offers product reviews, product announcements, tips for making systems or applications more accessible, or explanations of concepts of interest to any computer user or would-be computer user. This association newsletter is available in braille, in large print, on audio cassette and on 3.5 or 5.25 IBM format diskette.
Quarterly

10023 What's Line
Alabama Regional Library for the Blind
6030 Monticello Drive 334-213-3906
Montgomery, AL 36130-6000 800-392-5671
Fax: 334-213-3993
e-mail: fzaleski@apls.state.al.us
http://statelibrary.alabama.gov
Informational 4 page newsletter in large print. Also available in braille and e-text formats.
4 pages Quarterly
Fara Zaleski, Division
Rebecca Mitchell, Director

Pamphlets

10024 About Children's Vision: Guide for Parents
National Association for Visually Handicapped
111 E 59th St 212-821-9497
New York, NY 10022-6904 800-284-4422
Fax: 212-727-2931
e-mail: kcampbell@lighthouse.org
lighthouse.org/navh
Offers a better understanding of the normal and possible abnormal development of a childs eyesight.
Lorraine Marchi LHD, Founder/CEO
Cesar Gomez, Executive Director

10025 Age Related Macular Degeneration
National Association for Visually Handicapped
111 E 59th St 212-821-9497
New York, NY 10022-6904 800-284-4422
Fax: 212-727-2931
e-mail: kcampbell@lighthouse.org
lighthouse.org/navh
Describes various conditions which affect the macular area and how to best maximize the use of residual peripheral vision.
Lorraine Marchi LHD, Founder/CEO
Cesar Gomez, Executive Director

10026 Are You Looking for a Few Good Workers?
AFB Press: American Foundation for the Blind
2 Penn Plaza 212-502-7600
New York, NY 10121 800-232-3044
Fax: 888-545-8331
e-mail: literacy@afb.net
www.afb.org/store

Helpful pamphlet explores both the importance and the advantage of hiring workers who are blind or visually impaired. Designed for human resource and other professionals responsible for hiring, it answers critical questions about hiring blind or visually impaired applicants. This enlightening guide to employment practices relating to these individuals offers insights on interviewing, job performance, tax incentives for businesses, insurance issues and more.
7 pages Pack of 20
ISBN: 0-891283-60-9
Carl R Augusto, President & CEO
Rick Bozeman, Chief Financial Officer

10027 BVA Bulletin
Blinded Veterans Association
477 H Street NW 202-371-8880
Washington, DC 20001-2694 800-669-7079
Fax: 202-371-8258
e-mail: bva@bva.org
www.bva.org
The Bulletin informs blinded veterans, their families, and those of the general public with an interest in BVA issues, about the organization. The publication includes current information relating to technology for the blind, legislation affecting blinded veterans, and news about the people who have overcome the challenges of blindness and are doing amazing work in their lives.
32 pages Quarterly
Thomas Miller, Executive Director
Stuart Nelson, Coordinator Public Relations

10028 Books are Fun for Everyone
National Library Service for the Blind
1291 Taylor Street NW 202-707-5100
Washington, DC 20542 Fax: 202-707-0712
TDD: 202-707-0744
e-mail: nls@loc.gov
www.loc.gov
The mission of this web site is to provide program users, librarians, and the public a wide range of access to NLS publications, program information, and bibliographic data

10029 Braille Alphabet and Numbers
AFB Press: American Foundation for the Blind
2 Penn Plaza 212-502-7600
New York, NY 10121 800-232-3044
Fax: 888-545-8331
e-mail: literacy@afb.net
www.afb.org/store
Embossed with the braille alphabet and numbers, this 9 x 4 inch display card includes an explanation of braille and a short history of its development.
Pack of 25
ISBN: 0-891281-98-3
Carl R Augusto, President & CEO
Rick Bozeman, Chief Financial Officer

10030 Braille Literacy: Blind Persons, Families, Prof. & Producers of Braille
AFB Press: American Foundation for the Blind
2 Penn Plaza 212-502-7600
New York, NY 10121 800-232-3044
Fax: 888-545-8331
e-mail: literacy@afb.net
www.afb.org/store
Vigorous defece of the use of braille and an explanation of the importance of positive attitudes toward it that states: Braille is an assertion of equality between blind and sighted persons with respect to written communication. For everyone who uses or teaches braille and is interested in its future.
12 pages Pack of 25
ISBN: 0-891289-28-3
Carl R Augusto, President & CEO
Rick Bozeman, Chief Financial Officer

10031 Braille: An Extraordinary Volunteer Opportunity
National Library Service for the Blind
1291 Taylor Street NW 202-707-5100
Washington, DC 20542-0002 Fax: 202-707-0712
TDD: 202-707-0744
e-mail: nls@loc.gov
www.loc.gov

The mission of this web site is to provide program users, librarians, and the public a wide range of access to NLS publications, program information, and bibliographic data

10032 Cataracts
National Eye Institute, Information Office
31 Center Drive MSC 2510   301-496-5248
Bethesda, MD 20892-2510   e-mail: 2020@nei.nih.gov
                                          www.nei.nih.gov
As part of the federal government's National Institutes of Health (NIH), the National Eye Institute's mission is to "conduct and support research, training, health information dissemination, and other programs with respect to blinding eye diseases
Paul A. Sieving, Executive Director

10033 Classification of Impaired Vision
National Association for Visually Handicapped
111 E 59th St   212-821-9497
New York, NY 10022-6904   800-284-4422
                                      Fax: 212-727-2931
                            e-mail: kcampbell@lighthouse.org
                                        lighthouse.org/navh
Describes various degrees of impaired vision.
Lorraine Marchi LHD, Founder/CEO
Cesar Gomez, Executive Director

10034 Communicating with People Who Have Trouble Hearing & Seeing: A Primer
National Association for Visually Handicapped
111 E 59th St   212-821-9497
New York, NY 10022-6904   800-284-4422
                                      Fax: 212-727-2931
                            e-mail: kcampbell@lighthouse.org
                                        lighthouse.org/navh
Line drawings that depict problems for those with both deficiencies.
Lorraine Marchi LHD, Founder/CEO
Cesar Gomez, Executive Director

10035 Dancing Cheek to Cheek
Blind Children's Center
4120 Marathon Street   213-664-2153
Los Angeles, CA 90029-3584   Fax: 213-665-3828
Discusses beginning social, play and language interactions.
33 pages

10036 Diabetes, Vision Impairment and Blindness
AFB Press: American Foundation for the Blind
2 Penn Plaza   212-502-7600
New York, NY 10121   800-232-3044
                                      Fax: 888-545-8331
                                  e-mail: literacy@afb.net
                                       www.afb.org/store
Presentation of how chronic diabetes affects vision and how diabetes can be managed at home by blind and visually impaired individuals.
32 pages
ISBN: 0-891289-02-0
Carl R Augusto, President & CEO
Rick Bozeman, Chief Financial Officer

10037 Diabetic Retinopathy
National Association for Visually Handicapped
111 E 59th St   212-821-9497
New York, NY 10022-6904   800-284-4422
                                      Fax: 212-727-2931
                            e-mail: kcampbell@lighthouse.org
                                        lighthouse.org/navh
Describes types of this disease and methods of treatment.
Lorraine Marchi LHD, Founder/CEO
Cesar Gomez, Executive Director

10038 Directory of Radio Reading Services
Radio Information Service
600 Forbes Avenue   412-488-3944
Pittsburgh, PA 15282   Fax: 412-488-3953
                            e-mail: info@readingservice.org
                                       www.readingservice.org

Annually

10039 Don't Lose Sight of Age-Related Macular Degeneration
National Eye Institute, Information Office
31 Center Drive MSC 2510   301-496-5248
Bethesda, MD 20892-2510   e-mail: 2020@nei.nih.gov
                                          www.nei.nih.gov
As part of the federal government's National Institutes of Health (NIH), the National Eye Institute's mission is to conduct and support research, training, health information dissemination, and other programs with respect to blinding eye diseases
Paul A. Sieving, Executive Director

10040 Don't Lose Sight of Cataracts
National Eye Institute, Information Office
31 Center Drive MSC 2510   301-496-5248
Bethesda, MD 20892-2510   e-mail: 2020@nei.nih.gov
                                          www.nei.nih.gov
As part of the federal government's National Institutes of Health (NIH), the National Eye Institute's mission is to conduct and support research, training, health information dissemination, and other programs with respect to blinding eye diseases
Paul A. Sieving, Executive Director

10041 Don't Lose Sight of Glaucoma
National Eye Institute, Information Office
31 Center Drive MSC 2510   301-496-5248
Bethesda, MD 20892-2510   e-mail: 2020@nei.nih.gov
                                          www.nei.nih.gov
As part of the federal government's National Institutes of Health (NIH), the National Eye Institute's mission is to conduct and support research, training, health information dissemination, and other programs with respect to blinding eye diseases
Paul A. Sieving, Executive Director

10042 Eye-Q Test
National Association for Visually Handicapped
111 E 59th St   212-821-9497
New York, NY 10022-6904   800-284-4422
                                      Fax: 212-727-2931
                            e-mail: kcampbell@lighthouse.org
                                        lighthouse.org/navh
Five questions and answers to assist in knowing more about vision.
Lorraine Marchi LHD, Founder/CEO
Cesar Gomez, Executive Director

10043 Facts: Books for Blind and Physically Handicapped Individuals
National Library Service for the Blind
101 Independence Ave, SE   202-707-5000
Washington, DC 20540-0002   Fax: 202-707-0712
                                          www.loc.gov
The Library of Congress is the nation's oldest federal cultural institution and serves as the research arm of Congress. It is also the largest library in the world, with millions of books, recordings, photographs, maps and manuscripts in its collections.
Annual
James H. Billington, Librarian

10044 Facts: Music for Blind and Physically Handicapped Individuals
National Library Service for the Blind
101 Independence Ave, SE   202-707-5000
Washington, DC 20540-0002   Fax: 202-707-0712
                                          www.loc.gov
The Library of Congress is the nation's oldest federal cultural institution and serves as the research arm of Congress. It is also the largest library in the world, with millions of books, recordings, photographs, maps and manuscripts in its collections.
Annual
James H. Billington, Librarian

10045 Facts: Playback Machines and Accessories Provided on Free Loan
National Library Service for the Blind
101 Independence Ave, SE   202-707-5000
Washington, DC 20540-0002   Fax: 202-707-0712
                                          www.loc.gov
The Library of Congress is the nation's oldest federal cultural institution and serves as the research arm of Congress. It is also the largest library in the world, with millions of books, recordings, photographs, maps and manuscripts in its collections.
James H. Billington, Librarian

10046 Facts: Sources for Purchase of Cassette & Disc Players From NLS
National Library Service for the Blind
101 Independence Ave, SE   202-707-5000
Washington, DC 20540-0002   Fax: 202-707-0712
www.loc.gov
The Library of Congress is the nation's oldest federal cultural institution and serves as the research arm of Congress. It is also the largest library in the world, with millions of books, recordings, photographs, maps and manuscripts in its collections.
James H. Billington, Librarian

10047 Family Guide to Vision Care
American Optometric Association
243 N Lindbergh Boulevard   314-991-4100
Saint Louis, MO 63141-7881   Fax: 314-991-4101
www.aoanet.org
Offers information on the early developmental years of your vision, finding a family optometrist and how to take care of your eyesight through the learning years, the working years and the mature years.

10048 Family Guide: Growth & Development of the Partially Seeing Child
National Association for Visually Handicapped
111 E 59th St   212-821-9497
New York, NY 10022-6904   800-284-4422
Fax: 212-727-2931
e-mail: kcampbell@lighthouse.org
lighthouse.org/navh
Offers information for parents and guidelines in raising a partially seeing child.
Lorraine Marchi LHD, Founder/CEO
Cesar Gomez, Executive Director

10049 General Facts and Figures on Blindness
National Society to Prevent Blindness
500 Remington Road
Schaumburg, IL 60173-5624   800-331-2020

10050 General Interest Catalog
National Braille Association
3 Townline Circle   716-427-8260
Rochester, NY 14623-2537
Lists hundreds of titles of fiction and non-fiction books offered in large print, braille or on cassette to visually impaired readers.
19 pages

10051 Glaucoma
Foundation For Glaucoma Research
490 Post Street   415-986-3162
San Francisco, CA 94102-1409
Offers information on what glaucoma is, the causes, treatments, types of glaucoma, eye exams and prevention.

10052 Glaucoma: Sneak Thief of Sight
National Association for Visually Handicapped
111 E 59th St   212-821-9497
New York, NY 10022-6904   800-284-4422
Fax: 212-727-2931
e-mail: kcampbell@lighthouse.org
lighthouse.org/navh
A pamphlet describing the disease, treatment and medications.
Lorraine Marchi LHD, Founder/CEO
Cesar Gomez, Executive Director

10053 Guide Dog Foundation Flyer
Guide Dog Foundation for the Blind
371 E Jericho Turnpike   631-930-9000
Smithtown, NY 11787-2976   800-548-4337
Fax: 631-930-9009
e-mail: info@guidedog.org
www.guidedog.org
Offers information on the programs and services provided by the foundation.
James C. Bingham, Chair
Alphonce J. Brown, Vice Chair

10054 Guidelines for Comprehensive Low Vision Care
National Association for Visually Handicapped
111 E 59th St   212-821-9497
New York, NY 10022-6904   800-284-4422
Fax: 212-727-2931
e-mail: kcampbell@lighthouse.org
lighthouse.org/navh
A description of the proper method to conduct a low vision evaluation.
Lorraine Marchi LHD, Founder/CEO
Cesar Gomez, Executive Director

10055 Guidelines for Helping Deaf/Blind Persons
Helen Keller National Center for Deaf/Blind
141 Middle Neck Road   516-944-8900
Sands Point, NY 11050-1299   Fax: 516-944-7302
TTY: 516-944-8637
e-mail: hkncinfo@hknc.com
www.hknc.org
The mission of the Helen Keller National Center for Deaf-Blind Youths and Adults is to enable each person who is deaf-blind to live and work in his or her community of choice.
Joseph McNulty, Executive Director

10056 Heart to Heart
Blind Children's Center
4120 Marathon Street   213-664-2153
Los Angeles, CA 90029-3584   Fax: 213-665-3828
Parents of blind and partially sighted children talk about their feelings.
12 pages

10057 Heartbreak of Being a Little Bit Blind
National Association for Visually Handicapped
111 E 59th St   212-821-9497
New York, NY 10022-6904   Fax: 212-727-2931
e-mail: nvah@navh.org
lighthouse.org/navh
Summary of what it means to have impaired vision with illustrations. Free for members.
Lorraine Marchi LHD, Founder/CEO
Cesar Gomez, Executive Director

10058 Helen Keller
AFB Press: American Foundation for the Blind
2 Penn Plaza   212-502-7600
New York, NY 10121   800-232-3044
Fax: 888-545-8331
www.afb.org/store
Brief biography that focuses on the major events of Helen Keller's life, from her birth in Tuscumbia, Alabama on June 27, 1880 to her death in Connecticut on June 1, 1968.
6 pages Pack of 25
ISBN: 0-891282-03-3

10059 How Does a Blind Person Get Around?
AFB Press: American Foundation for the Blind
2 Penn Plaza   212-502-7600
New York, NY 10121   800-232-3044
Fax: 888-545-8331
www.afb.org/store
Offers information on daily living as a blind person.

10060 How to Develop a Self-Help Group for Elders Losing Eyesight
National Association for Visually Handicapped
111 E 59th St   212-821-9497
New York, NY 10022-6904   Fax: 212-727-2931
e-mail: navh@navh.org
lighthouse.org/navh
The pioneer for development of self-help groups, using the NAVH model, this publication is designed to help start and facilitate self-help groups.
Lorraine Marchi LHD, Founder/CEO
Cesar Gomez, Executive Director

10061 How to Use Your Low Vision Glasses
National Association for Visually Handicapped
111 E 59th St   212-821-9497
New York, NY 10022-6904   Fax: 212-727-2931
e-mail: navh@navh.org
lighthouse.org/navh

A line drawing showing the correct way to benefit from low vision glasses.
Lorraine Marchi LHD, Founder/CEO
Cesar Gomez, Executive Director

10062 Information on Glaucoma
Foundation for Glaucoma Research
251 Post Street   415-986-3162
San Francisco, CA 94108-1409   800-826-6693
                              e-mail: question@glaucoma.org
                                        www.glaucoma.org

10063 Information on Macular Degeneration
American Council of the Blind
2200 Wilson Boulevard   202-467-5081
Arlington, VA 22201-2706   800-424-8666
                                     Fax: 202-467-5085
                                   e-mail: info@acb.org
                                             www.acb.org

Melanie Brunson, Executive Director

10064 It's All Right to Be Angry
National Association for Visually Handicapped
111 E 59th St   212-821-9497
New York, NY 10022-6904   Fax: 212-727-2931
                                  e-mail: navh@navh.org
                                      lighthouse.org/navh
A helpful pamphlet describing reactions to learning to live with vision impairment.
Lorraine Marchi LHD, Founder/CEO
Cesar Gomez, Executive Director

10065 Large Print Loan Library Catalog
National Association for Visually Handicapped
111 E 59th St   212-821-9497
New York, NY 10022-6904   Fax: 212-727-2931
                                  e-mail: navh@navh.org
                                      lighthouse.org/navh
Listing of over 9,000 commercially published and NAVH large print books available through NAVH on a loan basis. Includes a limited selection of titles available for purchase.
Lorraine Marchi LHD, Founder/CEO
Cesar Gomez, Executive Director

10066 Learning to Play
Blind Children's Center
4120 Marathon Street   213-664-2153
Los Angeles, CA 90029-3584   Fax: 323-665-3828
                       www.blindchildrenscenter.org/index.php
Discusses how to present play activities to the visually impaired preschool child.
12 pages
Susan L. Recchia, M.A., Author

10067 Let's Eat
Blind Children's Center
4120 Marathon Street   213-664-2153
Los Angeles, CA 90029-3584   Fax: 323-665-3828
                       www.blindchildrenscenter.org/index.php
Teaches competent feeding skills to children with visual impairments.
28 pages
Jill Brody, M.A., O.T.R., Co-Author
Lynne Webber, Co-Author

10068 Low Vision Questions and Answers
AFB Press: American Foundation for the Blind
2 Penn Plaza   212-502-7600
New York, NY 10121   800-232-3044
                                     Fax: 888-545-8331
                                       www.afb.org/store
What does low vision mean? What do low vision services cost? What diseases cause low vision? Answers to these and other questions are presented in a straightforward yet comprehensive format. Photographs show how objects appear to people with low vision, what low vision devices look like, and how they are used.
21 pages Pack of 25
ISBN: 0-891281-96-7

10069 Magnifier
Macular Degeneration Foundation

P.O. Box 531313   702-450-2908
Henderson, NV 89053-0752   888-633-3937
                                   e-mail: liz@eyesight.org
                                        www.eyesight.org

Large-font publication.

10070 Magnifier Highlights
Independent Living Aids
137 Rano Rd
Buffalo, NY 14207-2341   800-537-2118
                                     Fax: 516-937-3906
                               e-mail: indlivaids@aol.com
                                  www.independentliving.com
Full line of magnifiers, ranging from high-powered vision aids to instruments and accessories
Marvin Sandler, President

10071 Move with Me
Blind Children's Center
4120 Marathon Street   213-664-2153
Los Angeles, CA 90029-3584   Fax: 323-665-3828
                       www.blindchildrenscenter.org/index.php
A parent's guide to movement development for visually impaired babies.
12 pages
Doris Hug, M.S., R.P.T., Co-Author
Nancy Chernus-Mansfield, M.A., Co-Author

10072 Music Is for Everyone
National Library Service for the Blind
1291 Taylor Street NW   202-707-5100
Washington, DC 20542-0002   Fax: 202-707-0712
                                   e-mail: nls@loc.gov
                                        www.loc.gov/nls

10073 Parenting Preschoolers: Raising Young Blind & Visually Impaired Child
AFB Press: American Foundation for the Blind
2 Penn Plaza   212-502-7600
New York, NY 10121   800-232-3044
                                     Fax: 888-545-8331
                                       www.afb.org/store
Why is my baby so quiet? Why does my child seem slower than other children? What will happen when my child goes to school? This primer provides practical answers to the questions most freqently asked by parents and gives advice on what to expect, how to adapt to the child's situation and needs, and what to look for in early education programs.
28 pages Pack of 25
ISBN: 0-891289-98-4

10074 Patient's Guide to Visual Aids and Illumination
National Association for Visually Handicapped
111 E 59th St   212-821-9497
New York, NY 10022-6904   Fax: 212-727-2931
                                  e-mail: navh@navh.org
                                      lighthouse.org/navh
A reference booklet offering information on aids for the visually impaired.
Lorraine Marchi LHD, Founder/CEO
Cesar Gomez, Executive Director

10075 Puppy Walker Brochure
Guide Dog Foundation for the Blind
371 E Jericho Turnpike   631-930-9000
Smithtown, NY 11787-2976   800-548-4337
                                     Fax: 631-930-9009
                                e-mail: info@guidedog.org
                                        www.guidedog.org
Offers information on being a volunteer puppy walker family.
Wells B Jones CAE CFRE, CEO
Alphonce J. Brown, Jr., ACFRE, Vice Chair - Development

10076 Reaching, Crawling, Walking-Let's Get Moving
Blind Children's Center
4120 Marathon Street   213-664-2153
Los Angeles, CA 90029-3584   Fax: 323-665-3828
                       www.blindchildrenscenter.org/index.php

Orientation and mobility for visually impaired preschool children.
24 pages
Susan S. Simmons, Ph.D., Co-Author
Sharon O'Mara Maida, M.Ed., Co-Author

10077 Reading is for Everyone
National Library Service for the Blind
1291 Taylor Street NW
Washington, DC 20542-0002

202-707-5100
Fax: 202-707-0712
e-mail: nls@loc.gov
www.loc.gov/nls

10078 Reading with Low Vision
National Library Service for the Blind
1291 Taylor Street NW
Washington, DC 20542-0002

202-707-5100
Fax: 202-707-0712
e-mail: nls@loc.gov
www.loc.gov/nls

10079 Reference and Information Services from NLS
National Library Service for the Blind
1291 Taylor Street NW
Washington, DC 20542-0002

202-707-5100
Fax: 202-707-0712
e-mail: nls@loc.gov
www.loc.gov/nls

10080 Resource List for Persons with Low Vision
American Council of the Blind
2200 Wilson Boulevard
Arlington, VA 22201-2706

202-467-5081
800-424-8666
Fax: 202-467-5085
e-mail: info@acb.org
www.acb.org

Melanie Brunson, Executive Director

10081 Seeing Eye to Eye: An Administrator's Guide
AFB Press: American Foundation for the Blind
2 Penn Plaza
New York, NY 10121

212-502-7600
800-232-3044
Fax: 888-545-8331
www.afb.org/store

Visual impairment often has a profound impact on a child's ability to learn language and basic communication concepts. This easy-to-read booklet explains the student's needs and the practical services essential for helping them become literate and successful. An ideal tool for administrators and educators, it includes clear explanations of common terminology, the impact of visual impairment on learning, specialized services for visually impaired students, and in-service training for teachers.
72 pages Pack of 10
ISBN: 0-891283-59-5

10082 Selecting a Program
Blind Children's Center
4120 Marathon Street
Los Angeles, CA 90029-3584

213-664-2153
Fax: 323-665-3828
www.blindchildrenscenter.org/index.php
A guide for parents of infants and preschoolers with visual impairments.
28 pages
Deborah Chen, Ph.D., Co-Author
Mary Ellen McCann, M.A., Co-Author

10083 Standing on My Own Two Feet
Blind Children's Center
4120 Marathon Street
Los Angeles, CA 90029-3584

213-664-2153
Fax: 323-665-3828
www.blindchildrenscenter.org/index.php
A step-by-step guide to designing and constructing simple, individually tailored adaptive mobility devices for preschool-age children who are visually impaired.
36 pages
Lorie Lynn LaPrelle, M.A., Author

10084 Talk to Me
Blind Children's Center
4120 Marathon Street
Los Angeles, CA 90029-3584

213-664-2153
Fax: 323-665-3828
www.blindchildrenscenter.org/index.php

A language guide for parents of deaf children.
11 pages
Nancy Chernus-Mansfield, M.A., Co-Author
Linda Kekelis, M.A., Co-Author

10085 Talk to Me II
Blind Children's Center
4120 Marathon Street
Los Angeles, CA 90029-3584

213-664-2153
Fax: 323-665-3828
www.blindchildrenscenter.org/index.php
A sequel to Talk To Me, available in English and Spanish.
15 pages
Nancy Chernus-Mansfield, M.A., Co-Author
Dori Hayashi, M.A., Co-Author

10086 Talking Books for Senior Adults
National Library Service for the Blind
1291 Taylor Street NW
Washington, DC 20542-0002

202-707-5100
Fax: 202-707-0712
e-mail: nls@loc.gov
www.loc.gov/nls

10087 Touch the Baby: Blind & Visually Impaired Children as Patients
American Foundation for the Blind
2 Penn Plaza
New York, NY 10121-2018

212-502-7600
800-232-3044
Fax: 888-545-8331
www.afb.org/store

How-to manual for health care professionals working in hospitals, clinics and doctors' offices that teaches the special communication and touch-related techniques needed to prevent blind and visually impaired patients from withdrawing from healthcare staff and the outside world. includes how to talk to infants and how to signal to children that a procedure may cause discomfort.
13 pages Pack of 25
ISBN: 0-891281-97-5

10088 Volunteer at Your Braille and Talking Book Library
National Library Service for the Blind
1291 Taylor Street NW
Washington, DC 20542-0002

202-707-5100
Fax: 202-707-0712
e-mail: nls@loc.gov
www.loc.gov/nls

Brochure

10089 What Do You Do When You See a Blind Person — and What Don't You Do?
AFB Press: American Foundation for the Blind
2 Penn Plaza
New York, NY 10121

212-502-7600
800-232-3044
Fax: 888-545-8331
www.afb.org/store

Examples of real-life situations that teach sighted persons how to interact effectively with blind persons. Topics covered include how to help someone across the street, how not to distract a guide dog and how to take leave of a blind person.
8 pages Pack of 25
ISBN: 0-891281-95-9

10090 Wings for the Future
American Printing House for the Blind
1839 Frankfort Avenue
Louisville, KY 40206-3148

502-895-2405
800-223-1839
Fax: 502-899-2284
e-mail: info@aph.org
www.aph.org

This booklet offers an introduction to the American Printing House For The Blind's programs, services, tools, aids and more.
13 pages

10091 Without Sight and Sound
Helen Keller National Center for Deaf/Blind
141 Middle Neck Road
Sands Point, NY 11050-1299

516-944-8900
Fax: 516-944-7302
TTY: 516-944-8637
e-mail: hkncinfo@hknc.org
www.hknc.org

Pamphlet offering facts, causes, types and descriptions of deaf/blindness.
Joseph McNulty, Executive Director

10092 You Seem Like a Regular Kid to Me
AFB Press: American Foundation for the Blind
2 Penn Plaza   212-502-7600
New York, NY 10121   800-232-3044
                                              Fax: 888-545-8331
                                               www.afb.org/store

An interview with Jane, a blind child, allows other children to understand what it's like to be blind. Jane explains how she gets around, takes care of herself, does her school work, spends her leisure time and even pays for things when she can't see money. Photographs show Jane engaged in various activities.
16 pages Pack of 25
ISBN: 0-891289-21-6
Chrissy Cowan, M.Ed., Author

Audio & Video

10093 Adult Bible Study
Sunday School Board of the Southern Baptists
127 9th Avenue N
Nashville, TN 37234-0001   800-458-2772
Unabridged Sunday School lessons recorded on audio cassette as printed in Adult Bible Study.
Quarterly

10094 Aging and Vision: Declarations of Independence
AFB Press: American Foundation for the Blind
2 Penn Plaza   212-502-7600
New York, NY 10121   800-232-3044
                                              Fax: 888-545-8331
                                               www.afb.org/store

Very personal look at five older people who have successfully coped with visual impairment and continue to lead active, satisfying lives. Their stories are not only inspirational, they also provide paractical, down-to-earth suggestions for adapting to vision loss later in life.
18 Minutes VHS
ISBN: 0-891282-20-3

10095 Bible Alliance
PO Box 621   941-748-3031
Bradenton, FL 34206-0621   e-mail: aurora@auroraministries.org
                                             www.auroraministries.org
Offers the Christian bible on cassettes in over 52 languages for those finding it impossible to read small print.

10096 Blindness: A Family Matter
AFB Press: American Foundation for the Blind
2 Penn Plaza   212-502-7600
New York, NY 10121   800-232-3044
                                              Fax: 888-545-8331
                                               www.afb.org/store

Frank exploration of the effects of an individual's visual impairment on other members of the family and how family members can play a positive role in the rehablition process. Features three families whose success stories provide advice and encouragement, as well as interviews with newly blinded adults currently involved in a rehabilitation program. Also available in PAL.
23 Minutes VHS
ISBN: 0-891282-22-X

10097 Braille Documents
Metrolina Sight Services
P. O. Box 1830   662-323-4999
Starkville, MS 39760-2128   800-336-2232
                              e-mail: careministries@bellsouth.net
                                             www.careministries.org
This production shop creates Braille and large-print documents.

10098 Brief Encounters of the Right Kind: How to Make Your Point in 10 Minutes or Less
AFB Press: American Foundation for the Blind
2 Penn Plaza   212-502-7600
New York, NY 10121   800-232-3044
                                              Fax: 888-545-8331
                                               www.afb.org/store

Humorous and instructional tour through the do's and don'ts of lobbying at the local, state and national levels. Three seasoned lobbyists discuss how professionals, families, consumers and volunteer advocates can use their expert knowledge to influence public policy. A Toolkit for Advocates, the accompanying manual, complements the video by providing a summary of the legislative process and key points on how to meet successfully with legislators.
VHS & PAL
ISBN: 0-891282-83-1

10099 Destination Unlimited
Leader Dog For The Blind
1964 Park Street   306-565-8211
Regina, SK, S4P 3G4,
This is a documentary about Leader-Dog-For-The-Blind Program. The needs of various people and how their dog fulfills their needs are shown. In addition, the overall leader-dog program is reviewed. This training program would be of interest to many teenagers.
Films

10100 Employed Ability: Blind Persons on the Job
AFB Press: American Foundation for the Blind
2 Penn Plaza   212-502-7600
New York, NY 10121   800-232-3044
                                              Fax: 888-545-8331
                                               www.afb.org/store

Blind and visually impaired people from a wide variety of occupations talk about career opportunities and their experiences in the workplace. Employers and coworkers are also interviewed and speak openly about supervising and working alongside visually impaired employees.
14 Minutes VHS
ISBN: 0-891282-24-6

10101 Focused On: Importance and Need for Skills
AFB Press: American Foundation for the Blind
2 Penn Plaza   212-502-7600
New York, NY 10121   800-232-3044
                                              Fax: 888-545-8331
                                               www.afb.org/store

Provides an overview of the importance of social competence and details the course of social skills development in children in general and in children who are blind or visually impaired in particular. This study guide examines both the development of social skills in general and how this process applies to children who are blind or who have visual impairments.
VHS & PAL
ISBN: 0-891283-25-0

10102 Hand in Hand: It Can Be Done
AFB Press: American Foundation for the Blind
2 Penn Plaza   212-502-7600
New York, NY 10121   800-232-3044
                                              Fax: 888-545-8331
                                               www.afb.org/store

One hour introduction to working effectively with individuals who are deaf-blind. Designed as both an overview and a reinforcer of the self-study text, this video can be used as a whole or in sections for parents and regular educators, as well as in the community. Includes a discussion guide. Available in audioscribed or open captioned VHS and PAL.

ISBN: 0-891283-25-0

10103 Heart to Heart
Blind Children's Center
4120 Marathon Street   213-664-2153
Los Angeles, CA 90029-3584   Fax: 323-665-3828
                            www.blindchildrenscenter.org/index.php
Parents of blind and partially sighted children talk about their feelings.
Videotape
Nancy Chernus-Mansfield, M.A., Co-Author
Dori Hayashi, M.A., Co-Author

10104 Helen Keller in Her Story
AFB Press: American Foundation for the Blind
2 Penn Plaza   212-502-7600
New York, NY 10121   800-232-3044
                                              Fax: 888-545-8331
                                               www.afb.org/store

Patty Duke, who portrayed the young Helen Keller on stage and on screen in The Miracle Worker, introduces this Oscar-winning documentary about the extraordinary lives of Ms. Keller, her teacher Anne Sullivan Macy and her friend and companion Polly Thompson. Includes vintage still photographs as well as early movie footage and newsreel footage.
VHS & PAL
ISBN: 0-891282-25-4
Nancy Hamilton, Author

10105 Let's Eat
Blind Children's Center
4120 Marathon Street   213-664-2153
Los Angeles, CA 90029-3584   Fax: 323-665-3828
                                    www.blindchildrenscenter.org/index.php
Teaches competent feeding skills to children with visual impairments.
Videotape
Jill Brody, M.A., O.T.R., Co-Author
Lynne Webber, Co-Author

10106 Making the Most of Early Communication: Strategies for Supporting Communication
AFB Press: American Foundation for the Blind
2 Penn Plaza   212-502-7600
New York, NY 10121   800-232-3044
                                                 Fax: 888-545-8331
                                                 www.afb.org/store
Demonstrates selected interventions to assist infants and toddlers with multiple disabilities, including vision and hearing loss, in developing early communication and other skills. Emphasizing the critical importance of early intervention, this video is designed to help service providers and families create effective communication straegies that encourage cognitive development and funtional abilities in young children with multiple disabilities and those who are deaf-blind. 37 minutes.
VHS & PAL
ISBN: 0-891282-96-3
Deborah Chen, Ph.D., Co-Author
Pamela Haag Schachter, MS.Ed., Co-Author

10107 New What Do You Do When You See a Blind Person?
AFB Press: American Foundation for the Blind
2 Penn Plaza   212-502-7600
New York, NY 10121   800-232-3044
                                                 Fax: 888-545-8331
                                                 www.afb.org/store
Engaging remake of the 1971 classic brings a fresh perspective on how to interact comfortably with someone who is visually impaired. The entertaining experiences of Mark Johnson, a computer programmer who is blind, and Dave Simon, a computer salesman who is not, show the simple ways to provide assistance, if it is needed, to someone who is blind or visually impaired. 16 minutes.
VHS & PAL
ISBN: 0-891283-13-7

10108 Oh, I See
AFB Press: American Foundation for the Blind
2 Penn Plaza   212-502-7600
New York, NY 10121   800-232-3044
                                                 Fax: 888-545-8331
                                                 www.afb.org/store
Lively and entertaining video provides practical suggestions on helping students who are blind and visually impaired adapt to the mainstream classroom. The modifacations shown can easily be used by teachers, students, or anyone working with blind and visually impaired students. Seven minutes.
VHS & PAL
ISBN: 0-891282-52-1

10109 Out of Left Field
AFB Press: American Foundation for the Blind
2 Penn Plaza   212-502-7600
New York, NY 10121   800-232-3044
                                                 Fax: 888-545-8331
                                                 www.afb.org/store

Illustrates how youngsters who are blind or visually impaired are integrated with their sighted peers in a variety of recreational and athletic activites. 17 minutes.
VHS & PAL
ISBN: 0-891282-28-9

10110 Profiles in Aging and Vision
AFB Press: American Foundation for the Blind
2 Penn Plaza   212-502-7600
New York, NY 10121   800-232-3044
                                                 Fax: 888-545-8331
                                                 www.afb.org/store
Can be used on its own or in conjunction with the text, this is an informative overview of the common eye conditions that affect older people, with a detailed description of the vision-related services that help older people who are visually impaired continue to lead independent lives. Experienced professionals provide valuable information on crucial issues, and older visually impaired persons offering their own revealing perspectives. 33 minutes.
VHS
ISBN: 0-891289-48-8
Alberta L. Orr, MSW, Executive Producer

10111 Reaching Out: A Creative Access Guide for Designing Exhibits & Cultural Programs
AFB Press: American Foundation for the Blind
2 Penn Plaza   212-502-7600
New York, NY 10121   800-232-3044
                                                 Fax: 888-545-8331
                                                 www.afb.org/store
Video and accompanying manual are a creative package for making information on cultural programs and facilities accessible to people who are blind or visually impaired. Created especially for libraries, museums, historical societies, outdoor cultural facilities, corporations and everyone whose mission involves providing information to the community, this video offers practical design and program solutions. 22 minutes.
VHS & PAL
ISBN: 0-891289-49-6
Elga Joffee, Co-Author
May Ann Siller, Co-Author

10112 Seven Minute Lesson
AFB Press: American Foundation for the Blind
2 Penn Plaza   212-502-7600
New York, NY 10121   800-232-3044
                                                 Fax: 888-545-8331
                                                 www.afb.org/store
Introduction to the basic techniques used when acting as a sighted guide for a person who is blind or visually impaired.
VHS & PAL
ISBN: 0-891282-29-7

10113 Solutions for Everyday Living for Older People with Visual Impairments
AFB Press: American Foundation for the Blind
2 Penn Plaza   212-502-7600
New York, NY 10121   800-232-3044
                                                 Fax: 888-545-8331
                                                 www.afb.org/store
Presents a positive and helpful view of how older people who have lost some or all of their vision can continue to lead satisfying lives within supportive environments. This engaing video shows how staff members in continuing care communities and other living settings for older people can help residents function as independently as possible. Different types of vision loss are explained, and simple solutions are offered for carrying out everyday activities. 34 minutes.
VHS & PAL
ISBN: 0-891288-52-X
Priscilla Rogers, Author

10114 Strategies for Community Access: Braille & Raised Large Print Facility Signs
AFB Press: American Foundation for the Blind
2 Penn Plaza   212-502-7600
New York, NY 10121   800-232-3044
                                                 Fax: 888-545-8331
                                                 www.afb.org/store

Brief and effective advocacy tool that can be used to educate architects, planners, facility managers, sign makers and consumers about the value of accessible signs. Topics covered include ADA requirements for accessible signs, samples of signs designed to be compatible with an organization's interior design, demonstrations of how blind and print signs are a cost-effective way to provide access. Reproducible fact sheets on ADA signage guidelines are enclosed. Seven minutes.
VHS & PAL
ISBN: 0-891282-56-4

10115 Understanding Braille Literacy
AFB Press: American Foundation for the Blind
2 Penn Plaza   212-502-7600
New York, NY 10121   800-232-3044
                                                  Fax: 888-545-8331
                                                  www.afb.org/store
Motovational and intructional video covers all aspects of a successful braille education program. Teachers and students demonstate how braille is learned and used from preschool through high school and describes how braille skills contribute to literacy, independence, mastery of academic skills and successful education experiences in the regular classroom. Parents, classroom teachers and school administrators also speak out about the importance of braille. 25 minutes.
VHS & PAL
ISBN: 0-891282-61-0
Diane P. Wormsley, Ph.D., Author

10116 We Can Do it Together: Mobility for Students with Multiple Disabilities
AFB Press: American Foundation for the Blind
2 Penn Plaza   212-502-7600
New York, NY 10121   800-232-3044
                                                  Fax: 888-545-8331
                                                  www.afb.org/store
Illustrates a transdisiplinary team approach to teaching orientation and mobility to students with severe visual and multiple impairments, covering both adapted communication systems that are used to teach mobility skills and basic indoor mobility in the school. For mobility instructors, administrators, teachers of visually impaired and severely disabled students, occupational, physical and speech therapists and parents. Discussion guide included, 13 minutes.
VHS & PAL
ISBN: 0-891282-13-0

10117 What Can Baby See? Vision Tests & Intervention Strategies for Infants
AFB Press: American Foundation for the Blind
2 Penn Plaza   212-502-7600
New York, NY 10121   800-232-3044
                                                  Fax: 888-545-8331
                                                  www.afb.org/store
Presents common vision tests and methods of gathering information that can be used with infants and very young children to help indentify visual impairments that require early intervention services. Effective ways of working with families and early intervention strategies for encouraging infants with multiple disabilities to use their vision in functional ways are demonstrated to help families and service providers contribute to children's growth and development.
VHS & PAL
ISBN: 0-891282-99-8

Web Sites

10118 ACB Government Employees
                                                  www.acb.org
Concerns of the organization include recruitment, placement and advancement of blind and visually impaired employees.

10119 ACB Radio Amateurs
                                                  www.acb.org
A radio amateur network of blind, visually impaired and sighted members who gather and share common problems and solutions to help members improve radio amateurs in getting started, provides access to educational materials in special media and publishes a directory for the visually impaired.

10120 ACB Social Service Providers
                                                  www.acb.org
Information on blind and visually impaired social workers, social service professionals, students pursuing careers in social work, and other interested persons.

10121 American Blind Lawyers Association
                                                  www.acb.org
Information on law school admission tests and bar exams, private sector and government employment relations and specialized work techniques for the blind and visually impaired.

10122 American Council of Blind Lions
                                                  www.acb.org
Information concerning Club activities in the field of work for the blind and encourages blind people to join Lions Clubs and other civic activities.

10123 American Council of the Blind
                                                  www.acb.org
Information for the visually impaired and fully sighted individuals who are concerned about the dignity and well-being of blind people throughout America.

10124 American Foundation for the Blind
                                                  www.afb.org
Our web site unique in that it combines state-of-the-art features, an attractive visual environment and an accessible design for people with all types of disabilities. Features include a searchable database of vision services nationwide, community message boards and the largest collection of Helen Keller memorbilia on the web. It meets the stringent AAA guidelines of the Web Accessibility Initiative of the World Wide Web Consortium, established to help organizations build accessible websites.

10125 American Printing House for the Blind
                                                  www.aph.org
This organization promotes the independence of blind persons by providing special media, tools and materials needed for education and life.

10126 Blinded Veterans Association
                                                  www.bva.org
Offers two main service programs without cost to blinded veterans. Field service program provides counseling to veterans and families, and information on benefits and rehabilitation.

10127 Braille Revival League
                                                  www.acb.org
Information for people to read and write in braille, advocates for mandatory braille instruction in educational facilities for the blind, strives to make available a supply of braille materials from libraries and printing houses and more.

10128 Council of Families with Visual Impairment
                                                  www.acb.org
Offers support and outreach, shares experiences in parent/child relationships, exchanges educational, cultural and medical information about child development and more.

10129 Fidelco Guide Dog Foundation
                                                  www.fidelco.org
Fidelco breeds, raises, trains, and places German shepherd guide dogs with men and women who are visually impaired, primarily in the Northeast.

10130 Friends-In-Art
                                                  www.acb.org
Offers consultation to program planners in establishing accessible art and museum exhibits and presents Performing Arts Showcases.

10131 Guide Dog Foundation for the Blind
                                                  www.guidedog.org
Furnishes guide dogs, free of charge, to qualified people who seek independence, mobility and companionship.

10132 Guide Dog Users
                                                  www.acb.org
Promotes the acceptance of blind people and their dogs, works for enforcement and expansion of laws admitting guide dogs into public places, advocates for quality training and follow-up services.

10133 Healing Well

www.healingwell.com

An online health resource guide to medical news, chat, information and articles, newsgroups and message boards, books, disease-related web sites, medical directories, and more for patients, friends, and family coping with disabling diseases, disorders, or chronic illnesses.

10134 Health Finder

www.healthfinder.gov

Searchable, carefully developed web site offering information on over 1000 topics. Developed by the US Department of Health and Human Services, the site can be used in both English and Spanish.

10135 Healthlink USA

www.healthlinkusa.com

Health information concerning treatment, cures, prevention, diagnosis, risk factors, research, support groups, email lists, personal stories and much more. Updated regularly.

10136 Helios Health

www.helioshealth.com

Online resource for your health information. Detailed information about specific health topics, access to expert advice from our Medical Advisory Board, and up-to-date health news.

10137 Independent Visually Impaired Enterprises

www.acb.org

Information on rehabilitation facilities for all types of business enterprises and publicizes the capabilities of blind and visually impaired business persons.

10138 Library Users of America

www.acb.org

Provides for chapters in states through the US to encourage the development, acquisition and use of technology which enables blind and visually impaired persons to use printed material independently in library settings and elsewhere.

10139 Lighthouse International

www.lighthouse.org

Offers information about vision impairment and vision rehabilitation, and provides referrals to services and support groups nationwide.

10140 MedicineNet

www.medicinenet.com

An online resource for consumers providing easy-to-read, authoritative medical and health information.

10141 Medscape

www.medscape.com

Medscape offers specialists, primary care physicians, and other health professionals the Web's most robust and integrated medical information and educational tools.

10142 National Alliance of Blind Students

www.acb.org

Works to facilitate progress toward full accessibility of college programs and facilities, provides opportunities for discussion of issues important to students and assists with National Student Seminars.

10143 National Association for Visually Hand.

www.navh.org

Since 1905, Lighthouse International has led the charge in the fight against vision loss through prevention, treatment and empowerment.

10144 National Association of Blind Educators

www.nfb.org

Provides support and information regarding professional responsibilities, classroom techniques, national testing methods and career obstacles. Publishes The Blind Educator, national magazine specifically for blind educators.

10145 National Association of Blind Lawyers

www.nfb.org

Provides support and information regarding employment, techniques used by the blind, advocacy, laws affecting the blind, current information about the American Bar Association and other issues for blind lawyers.

10146 National Association of Blind Secretaries and Transcribers

www.nfb.org

Addresses issues such as technology, accomodation, career planning and job training.

10147 National Association of Blind Students

nabslink.org

The mission of the National Association of Blind Students is to promote equal access to educational and life opportunities for the blind.

10148 National Association of Blind Teachers

www.acb.org

Works to advance the teaching profession for blind and visually impaired people, protects the interest of teachers, presents discussions and solutions for special problems encountered by blind teachers and publishes a directory of blind teachers in the US.

10149 National Association of Guide Dog Users

www.nagdu.org

Provides information and support for guide dog users and works to secure high standards in guide dog training. Addresses issues of discrimination of guide dog users and offers public education about guide dog use.

10150 National Association to Promote the Use of Braille

www.nfbcal.org/napub/napub.htm

NAPUB exists to promote the use of braille.

10151 National Braille Association

www.nationalbraille.org/

National Braille Association, founded in 1945, is a non-profit organization dedicated to providing continuing education to those who prepare braille, and to providing braille materials to persons who are visually impaired.

10152 National Federation of the Blind: Blind/Deaf Division

www.nfb.org

Offers personal contact with other deaf-blind individuals knowledgeable in advocacy, education, employment, technology, discrimination and other issues surrounding deaf-blindness.

10153 National Federation of the Blind

www.nfb.org

Provides public education about blindness, support services to the newly blinded, scholarships, publications about blindness, adaptive equipment for the blind, advocacy services, Newsline for the Blind, assistive technology information and Job Opportunities for the Blind.

10154 National Federation of the Blind in Computer Science

www.nfb.org

New technologies, to secure access to current technology and to develop new ways of using current or new technologies by the blind.

10155 National Federation of the Blind: Blind Merchants Division

www.nfb.org

Provides information regarding rehabilitation, social security, tax and other issues which directly affect blind merchants. Serves as advocacy and support group.

10156 National Federation of the Blind: Human Services Division

www.nfb.org

Organization of blind persons working in counseling, personnel, psychology, social work, psychiatry, rehabilitation and other social science and human resource fields. Provides resources regarding blindness-related techniques and methods used in these fields.

10157 National Federation of the Blind: Masonic Square Club

www.nfb.org

Blind individuals committed to sharing of Masonic experiences, goals and history.

10158 National Federation of the Blind: Music Division

www.nfb.org

Offers support and information regarding copyright, publishing, promotion and other career details.

10159 National Federation of the Blind: Public Employees Division

www.nfb.org

Focuses on issues such as changes in governmental hiring and retention practices, new job skills needed for the future, government employment downsizing, new electronic means of finding public sector jobs, self-advocacy and career planning strategies.

10160 National Federation of the Blind: Science and Engineering Division

www.nfb.org

This is a strong support group to encourage blind persons in pursuit of these careers, many of which have been considered not possible for the blind in the past.

10161 National Federation of the Blind: Writers Division

www.nfb.org

Covers various aspects of this business, including selling your work, publishing, technology, motivation and discovering writing and publishing resources.

10162 National Library Service for the Blind

www.loc.gov/nls

Administers a national library service that provides braille and recorded books and magazines on free loan to anyone who cannot read standard print because of visual or physical disabilities who are eligible residents of the United States or American citizens living abroad.

10163 National Organization of Parents of Blind Children

www.nfb.org

Addresses issues ranging from help to parents of a newborn blind infant, mobility and Braille instruction, education, social and community participation, development of self-confidence and other vital factors involved in the growth of a blind child.

10164 National Organization of the Senior Blind

www.nfb.org

Provides support and information to other blind seniors. Issues include concerns such as remaining active in community and social life, maintaining private homes or living in retirement communities or nursing homes, learning the techniques used by the blind, independently caring for oneself and maintaining a positive approach to vision loss.

10165 Randolph-Sheppard Vendors of America

www.acb.org

Protects the interests of blind vendors, seeks proper implementation of the Randolph-Sheppard Act and encourages facility locations in more visible and profitable areas.

10166 Vision World Wide

www.visionww.org

Aims is to enhance everyday living so as to maintain an independent lifestyle. It also serves as a consumer protection against misrepresentation and fraud.

10167 Visually Impaired Data Processors International

www.acb.org

Provides for the exchange of work technique ideas and works with agencies to increase the availability of braille and recorded materials.

10168 Visually Impaired Piano Tuners International

www.acb.org

Works to preserve, advance and enrich the skilled professional piano tuning for competent, well-trained blind and visually impaired persons.

10169 Visually Impaired Veterans of America

www.acb.org

Promotes the rights of visually impaired veterans to receive all benefits, encourages research and development of new products for blind people.

10170 WebMD

www.webmd.com

Provides credible information, supportive communities, and in-depth reference material about health subjects. A source for original and timely health information as well as material from well known content providers.

Description

10171 War Syndromes

War syndromes have plagued soldiers for centuries. Though symptoms may vary, soldiers may become affected by various postulated physiological diseases as well as psychological illnesses. Agent Orange and the Gulf War Syndrome are two of the conditions still prevalent today.

Agent Orange is the common name for a mix of chemicals developed by the military. It was first used during the Vietnam War to destroy vegetation that concealed the enemy. During the war, soldiers were exposed heavily to this chemical; years later, many of them contracted a variety of conditions. There has been an intense controversy about whether Agent Orange caused these conditions, with medical scientists, patients, politicians and advocacy groups all involved.

Among the conditions sometimes attributed to Agent Orange exposure are a variety of cancers, an acne-like skin condition called chloracne, neurological diseases, repeated infections, sterility, and birth defects in the children of exposed persons.

To further understand this condition, the Department of Veterans Affairs has been established a registry of Vietnam veterans concerned that they may have been exposed to Agent Orange. Veterans who suspect their symptoms are related to this exposure can contact the Department's Medical Administrative Services to request the Agent Orange Registry Examination, a complete health evaluation. The Department offers service-connected compensation for those veterans who develop a condition believed to be related to exposure to Agent Orange.

Gulf War Syndrome, GWS, or Persian Gulf War Syndrome is a constellation of illnesses experienced by 5,000 to 80,000 US veterans after returning from the Persian Gulf Wars in the 1990's and 2000's. Symptoms are predominately neurologic and consist of impaired cognition, with problems of attention, memory, reasoning, insomnia, depression and headaches. Complaints of muscle and joint pain, gastrointestinal difficulties, vertigo and weakness are also common. As veterans resumed family life, various birth defects were added to the list. The cause of GWS is unknown.

A 1997 study funded by the Centers for Disease Control shows that Gulf War personnel are more likely than others to report depression, syptoms similar to post-traumatic stress disorder, chronic fatigue, cognitive difficulties, bronchitis, asthma, fibromyalgia, alcohol abuse, anxiety and sexual dysfunction.

Many causes of GWS have been suggested, but none have been definitely identified or eliminated. These include: effects of chemical and/or biological weapons; exposure to pesticides; smoke from oil well fires; air-borne contamination from munitions plants destroyed in Iraq, exposure to depleted uranium used as a material in some US munitions and exposure to volatile solvents used in the normal course of equipment maintenance. None of these exposures have been convincingly linked to a cause of the illness.

Given the range of reported GWS effects, treatment is highly individualized and symptomatic. A number of specialized support groups and websites have been established by members of the Persian Gulf War Community.

National Agencies & Associations

10172 Advocacy for the Gulf War Children
1692 6th Road   308-795-2319
St Libory, NE 68872
Gives listings of names and addresses of families with children with gulf war syndrome.

10173 Agent Orange Registry Department of Veterans Affairs
Department of Veterans Affairs
810 Vermont Avenue NW   202-233-4000
Washington, DC 20420   800-827-1000
www.va.gov
Offers a computerized index of examinations of Vietnam veterans who were worried that they may have been exposed to chemical herbicides which might be causing a variety of ill effects. Services available to any veteran, male or female, who had active military service.

10174 Centers for Disease Control
1600 Clifton Road   404-639-3311
Atlanta, GA 30333   800-232-4636
Fax: 404-639-3435
TTY: 888-232-6348
e-mail: cdcinfo@cdc.gov
www.cdc.gov
Offers reprints from the CDC Health Status of Vietnam veterans and the Journal of the American Medical Association. Also offers reports from the Centers for Disease Control Vietnam Experience Study, which was a multidimensional assessment of the health of Vietnam War veterans.
William H Gimson, Chief Operating Officer
John Tibbs, Director

10175 National Veterans Services Fund
209 West Ave   203-656-0003
Darien, CT 06820-0465   800-521-0198
Fax: 203-656-1957
e-mail: philvet@NVSF.org
www.nvsf.org
Supports and informs those who were exposed to the defoliant Agent Orange or dioxin while serving the US in the conflict in Vietnam. The organization has developed a detailed exposure survey form to collect information on exposed veterans.
Phil Kraft, President/Treasurer
Cathie Green Stansell, Vice President

10176 VA Data Processing Center
1615 E Woodward Street   512-389-5380
Austin, TX 78772-0001
Helps veterans register after receiving the Agent Orange examination.

State Agencies & Associations

Alabama

10177 Gulf War Veterans of Alabama
2344 Glendale Avenue   205-265-7723
Montgomery, AL 36107   e-mail: 76163 1323@compuserve.com
Don Reeves
Shannon Reeves

10178 Veterans Administration Medical Center: Alabama
3701 Loop Road E   205-554-2000
Tuscaloosa, AL 35404   888-269-3045
                                     Fax: 205-554-2034
                                     www.tuscaloosa.va.gov
The Tuscaloosa VA Medical Center (TVAMC) is located in West
Alabama, where the facility is situated on a beautiful campus of
125 acres with 25 major buildings. TVAMC provides primary care,
long-term health care and mental health care services to eligible
Veterans in the VA Southeast Network (Veterans Integrated Ser-
vice Network [VISN 7]. The Tuscaloosa VA Medical Center pro-
vides access to secondary and tertiary care services.
Maria R. Andrews, MS, FACHE, Director
Paula Stokes, CTRS, CPM, M.Ed,, Associate Director

10179 Veterans Association Medical Center
700 S 19th Street   205-933-8101
Birmingham, AL 35233   866-487-4243
                                     Fax: 205-933-4484
                                     www.birmingham.va.gov
The Birmingham VA Medical Center is a 313-bed acute tertiary
care facility located in the historic Southside district of the city.
The facility provides acute tertiary medical and surgical care to
veterans of Alabama and surrounding states. We provide health
care services to eligible veterans in the VA Southeast Network Vet-
erans Integrated Service Network
Thomas Smith, FACHE, Director
Phyllis Smith, MBA, FACHE, Associate Director

Alaska

10180 Alaska Gulf War Syndrome Referral Coordinator
23740 Sunny Glen Drive   907-696-8688
Eagle River, AK 99577   Fax: 907-696-8688
                                     e-mail: mcclure@alaska.net

Larry McClure

10181 Alaska VA Healthcare System
Outpatient Clinic
1201 North Muldoon Road   907-257-4700
Anchorage, AK 99504   888-353-7574
                                     Fax: 907-257-6774
                                     www.alaska.va.gov
The Alaska VA Healthcare System (AVAHS) offers primary, spe-
cialty, and mental health outpatient care. Services are provided
through a Joint Venture with the United States Air Force on nearby
Elmendorf Air Force Base, as well as through purchased care ar-
rangements with the community hospitals. The facility also fea-
tures a comprehensive Homeless Veteran Service, consisting of a
Domiciliary Residential Rehabilitation Program, Veterans Industries, Compensated Work Therapy Transitional Residence Pr
Susan M. Yeager, Director
Greg Puckett, Associate Director

Arizona

10182 Phoenix VA Healthcare System
Carl T. Hayden VA Medical Center
650 E Indian School Road   602-277-5551
Phoenix, AZ 85012   800-554-7174
                                     www.phoenix.va.gov
The Phoenix VA Health Care System proudly serves Veterans in
central Arizona at its main medical center and outpatient VA
Health Care Clinics.
Sharon Helman, Director
Lance E Robinson, MS, FACHE,, Associate Director

**10183 Veterans Adm. Medical Center: Tucson Southern Arizona VA
Health Care System**
Southern Arizona VA Health Care System
3601 S 6th Avenue   520-792-1450
Tucson, AZ 85723   800-470-8262
                                     Fax: 520-629-1818
                                     www.tucson.va.gov
The VA Medical Center located at Tucson Arizona is the "Flagship" for the Southern Arizona VA Health Care System
(SAVAHCS), which serves over 170,000 veterans located in eight
counties in Southern Arizona and one county in Western New Mexico. This 285-bed hospital provides training, primary care and
sub-specialty health care in numerous medical areas for eligible

Veterans.SAVAHCS has specialized and numerous unique treat-
ment programs to better serve its patients such as: The South
Western Blin
Jonathan Gardner, Director
Jennifer S Gutowski, MHA, FACHE, Associate Director

Arkansas

**10184 Central Arkansas Veterans Healthcare Syste Eugene J. Towbin
Healthcare Center**
Eugene J. Towbin Healthcare Center
2200 Fort Roots Drive
North Little Rock, AR 72114-1706   501-257-1000
                                     www.va.gov/directory/guide/facility.asp?
The Central Arkansas Veterans Healthcare System (CAVHS), a
flagship Department of Veterans Affairs (VA) healthcare provider,
is one of the largest and busiest VA medical centers in the country.
Its two hospitals, located in Little Rock and North Little Rock, an-
chor a broad spectrum of inpatient and outpatient healthcare services, ranging from disease prevention through primary care, to
complex surgical procedures, to extended rehabilitative care. This
System serves as a teaching facility for mor

10185 Gulf War Veterans of Arkansas
11127 Eglia Valley Drive   501-225-9347
Little Rock, AR 72212
Lydia Pace

10186 Veterans Adm. Medical Center: Fayetville
2300 Ramsey Street   910-488-2120
Fayetteville, AR 28301   800-771-6106
                                     www.fayettevillenc.va.gov
The Fayetteville Veterans Affairs Medical Center (VAMC) is a
general medicine, surgery and mental health facility. The
Fayetteville VAMC is a Complexity Level 2 Medical Center and is
authorized 58 general medical, surgical, and mental health beds. It
also maintains a 69-bed long-term care unit. The medical center
serves Veterans in 19 counties in southeastern North Carolina and
two counties in northeastern South Carolina.
Elizabeth Goolsby, Director
James Galkowski, PA-C, FACHE, Associate Director

California

10187 California Association of Persian Gulf Veterans
Santa Cruz, CA 95063   408-476-6684
                                     Fax: 415-227-0848
                                     e-mail: CAGulfVets@aol.com

Erika Lundholm

10188 Northern California Association of Persian Gulf Veterans
9141 East Stockton Boulevard   916-684-1693
Elk Grove, CA 95624   Fax: 916-684-1693
                                     e-mail: NCAPGV@aol.com

Debbie Judd

10189 Sacramento Veterans Center
1111 Howe Avenue   916-566-7430
Sacramento, CA 95825   877-927-8387
                                     Fax: 916-566-7433
                                     www.va.gov/directory/guide/facility.asp?
Michael Miracle, Team Leader
Edna Gabaldon, Counselor

10190 San Francisco VA Medical Center
4150 Clement Street   415-221-4810
San Francisco, CA 94121   877-487-2838
                                     Fax: 415-750-2185
                                     www.sanfrancisco.va.gov
SFVAMC has several National Centers of Excellence in the areas
of Epilepsy Treatment; Cardiac Surgery; Post Traumatic Stress
Disorder; HIV; and Renal Dialysis. It has many other nationally
recognized programs including: the Parkinson's Disease Re-
search, Education, and Clinical Center; the Hepatitis C Research
and Education Center; the Mental Illness Research & Education
Clinical Center; and the Western Pacemaker and AICD
Surveillance Program.
C. Diana . Nicoll, M.D., Ph.D., M.P, Acting Medical Center Director
Karen A rnold, MA, RD, Acting Associate Director

10191 Sepulveda Ambulatory Care Center
16111 Plummer Street 818-891-7711
North Hills, CA 91343 800-516-4567
Fax: 818-895-9559
www.losangeles.va.gov
The VA Greater Los Angeles Healthcare System is the largest, most complex healthcare system within the Department of Veterans Affairs. It is one component of the VA Desert Pacific Healthcare Network (VISN22) offering services to veterans residing in Southern California and Southern Nevada.
Donna M. Beiter, RN, MSN, Director
Christopher Sandles, Assistant Director

10192 VA Northern California Health Care System
10535 Hospital Way 916-843-7000
Mather, CA 95655 800-382-8387
Fax: 916-843-9001
e-mail: Robin.Jackson2@va.gov
www.northerncalifornia.va.gov
David G. Mastalski, Interim Director
Donna Iatarola, RN, MSN, Associate Director, Patient Care Service

10193 Veterans Adm. Medical Center: Livermore
4951 Arroyo Road 925-373-4700
Livermore, CA 94550 800-455-0057
Fax: 925-449-6522
www2.va.gov/directory
The VA Palo Alto Health Care System (VAPAHCS) consists of three inpatient facilities located at Palo Alto, Menlo Park, and Livermore. VAPAHCS is a teaching hospital, providing a full range of patient care services with state-of-the-art technology as well as education and research. Comprehensive health care is provided in areas of medicine, surgery, psychiatry, rehabilitation, neurology, oncology, dentistry, geriatrics, and extended care.
Elizabeth Joyce Freeman, FACHE, Director
Gloria Martinez, RN, MS, Associate Director for Patient Care & Nu

10194 Veterans Administration Medical Center: Fresno
2615 E. Clinton Avenue 559-228-6933
Fresno, CA 93703 888-826-2838
Fax: 559-487-5399
www.fresno.va.gov
VACCHCS consists of 1 inpatient facility located in Fresno (Fresno Medical Center), plus 3 outpatient clinics in Merced, Oakhurst and Tulare. We are expanding to better serve Veterans in Central California! VACCHCS mission is to honor America's Veterans by providing exceptional health care that improves their health and well-being. VACCHCS is a teaching hospital, providing a full range of services, with state-of-the-art technology as well as education and researc
Joanne Krumberger RN, FACHE, Director
Susan Shyshka FACHE, Associate Director

10195 Veterans Affairs Medical Center: Loma Linda
11201 Benton Street 909-825-7084
Loma Linda, CA 92357 800-741-8387
Fax: 909-422-3106
www.lomalinda.va.gov
Since 1977, VA Loma Linda Healthcare System has been improving the health of the men and women who have so proudly served our nation. We consider it our privilege to serve your health care needs in any way we can. Services are available to more than 67,000 Veterans living in a 2-county area of San Bernardino and Riverside.
Barbara Fallen, RD, MPA, FACHE, Director
Prachi V. Asher, FACHE, Assistant Director

10196 West Los Angeles Medical Center
11301 Willshire Boulevard 310-478-3711
Los Angeles, CA 90073 Fax: 310-268-3494
www.losangeles.va.gov
The VA Greater Los Angeles Healthcare System is the largest, most complex healthcare system within the Department of Veterans Affairs. It is one component of the VA Desert Pacific Healthcare Network (VISN22) offering services to veterans residing in Southern California and Southern Nevada.
Donna M. Beiter, RN, MSN, Director
Christopher Sandles, Assistant Director

Colorado

10197 Veterans Adm. Medical Center: Grand Junction
2121 N Avenue 970-242-0731
Grand Junction, CO 81501 866-206-6415
Fax: 970-244-1303
www.grandjunction.va.gov
The Grand Junction VA Medical Center (VAMC) serves 37,000 veterans residing on the Western Slope. The VAMC consists of one facility located in the city of Grand Junction; a Community Based Outpatient Clinic (CBOC) in Montrose, serving the southwestern Colorado counties; and a telehealth outreach clinic in Craig, serving northwestern Colorado and southwestern Wyoming. The VAMC operates 53 beds comprised of 23 acute care and 30 Transitional Care Unit beds. The VAMC provides primary and secondary c
Patricia A. Hitt, MS, Acting Director Grand Junction VA Medica
Randal France, M.D., Chief Psychiatry Service/ Int. Chf. of S

Connecticut

10198 Gulf War Veterans of Connecticut: New England Chapter
8 Frances Lane 860-623-1456
Windsor Locks, CT 6096 Fax: 860-292-1849
e-mail: DIANEDULKA@aol.com
Diane Dulka

Delaware

10199 Veterans Adm. Medical Center: Wilmington VA Medical Center
Wilmington VA Medical Center
1601 Kirkwood Highway 302-994-2511
Wilmington, DE 19805 Fax: 302-633-5591
www.va.gov/directory
The Wilmington VA Medical Center is a member of the Veterans Integrated Service Network 4 which includes 9 other facilities in Philadelphia, Coatesville, Lebanon, Wilkes-Barre, Altoona, Butler, Clarksburg, Erie, and Pittsburgh. The hospital has an approved authorized/operating bed capacity of 60. Also included within the hospital is a 60-bed Community Living Center for extended care. Both are accredited by the Joint Commission on Accreditation of Healthcare Organizations.

District of Columbia

10200 Disabled American Veterans National Service Headquarters
807 Maine Avenue SW 202-554-3501
Washington, DC 20024 Fax: 202-554-3581
www.dav.org
Serves America's disabled veterans and their families. Direct services include legislative advocacy professional counseling about compensation pension educational and job training programs and VA health care. Also offers assistance in applying for those programs.
Arthur H Wilson, National Adjutant
David G Gorman, Executive Director

10201 US Veteran's Administration
810 Vermont Avenue NW 202-273-5400
Washington, DC 20420 Fax: 202-273-4877
www2.va.gov/directory
Provides a wide range of services for those who have been in the military and their dependents as well as offering information on driver assessment and education programs.
Louise R Van Diepen MS CGP, Chief of Staff
Patricia Van MHA BS, Assistant Deputy Policy/Planning

10202 Veterans Adm. Medical Center: Washington
50 Irving Street NW 202-745-8000
Washington, DC 20422 877-328-2621
Fax: 202-754-8530
www.washingtondc.va.gov
The Washington DC VA Medical Center's employees and volunteers take great pride in serving Veterans of the national capital area. Capitol Excellence is our number one priority. From the Executive Office to the mailroom, from the canteen to the warehouse, whether offering you medical services, prosthetic devices, or a warm meal, every staff member and volunteer here is charged with

the responsibility of providing an environment of respect, courtesy and concern.

Brian A. Hawkins, MHA, Medical Center Director
Bryan C. Matthews, MBA, Associate Medical Center Director

Florida

10203 Desert Storm Justice Foundation: Florida
10 Marlow Road
Frostproof, FL 33843-9321
813-635-3261
Fax: 813-635-3261
e-mail: BillCarpenter@cjewel.com

William Carpenter

10204 Desert Storm Veterans of Florida
Titusville, FL 32782
407-269-3453
e-mail: GulfVet@Metrolink.net

Kevin Knight

10205 Veterans Adm. Medical Center: Bay Pines
10000 Bay Pines Boulevard
Bay Pines, FL 33744
727-398-6661
888-820-0230
Fax: 727-398-9442
www.baypines.va.gov

Since 1933, Bay Pines VA Healthcare System has been improving the health of the men and women who have so proudly served our nation. We consider it our privilege to serve your health care needs in any way we can. Our services are available to Veterans living in a ten county catchment area in west central Florida.

Suzanne M. Klinker, Medical Center Director
Kristine Brown, MPH, Associate Director

10206 Veterans Adm. Medical Center: Gainesville
1601 SW Archer Road
Gainesville, FL 32608-1197
352-376-1611
800-324-8387
Fax: 352-374-6113
www.northflorida.va.gov

In addition to our medical centers in Gainesville and Lake City, we offer services in three satellite outpatient clinics and several community-based outpatient clinics across North Florida and South Georgia.Patient-centered integrated health care organization for veterans providing excellent health care, research, and education; an organization where people choose to work; an active community partner; and a back-up for National emergencies..

Thomas Wisnieski, MPA, FACHE, Director
Nicklous J Ross, Associate Director

10207 Veterans Adm. Medical Center: Lake City
Lake City Veterans Administration Medical Center
619 S Marion Avenue
Lake City, FL 32025-5808
386-755-3016
800-308-8387
Fax: 386-758-3209
www.northflorida.va.gov

In addition to our medical centers in Gainesville and Lake City, we offer services in three satellite outpatient clinics and several community-based outpatient clinics across North Florida and South Georgia.Patient-centered integrated health care organization for veterans providing excellent health care, research, and education; an organization where people choose to work; an active community partner; and a back-up for National emergencies..

Thomas Wisnieski, MPA, FACHE, Director
Nicklous J Ross, Associate Director

10208 Veterans Adm. Medical Center: Miami
1201 NW 16th Street
Miami, FL 33125
305-575-7000
888-276-1785
Fax: 305-575-3232
www.miami.va.gov

The Miami VA is an accredited comprehensive medical provider, providing general medical, surgical, inpatient and outpatient mental health services, the Miami VA Healthcare System includes an AIDS/HIV center, a prosthetic treatment center, spinal cord injury rehabilitative center, and Geriatric Research, Education, and Clinical Center (GRECC). The Miami VA Healthcare System is recognized as a Center of Excellence in Spinal Cord Injury Research, Substance Abuse Treatment and is a recognized Chest

Paul M. Russo, Director
Mark E. Morgan, Associate Director

10209 Veterans Adm. Medical Center: St. Petersburg
Bay Pines VA Medical Center

10000 Bay Pines Boulevard
Bay Pines, FL 33744
727-398-6661
888-820-0230
Fax: 727-398-9442
www.baypines.va.gov

Since 1933, Bay Pines VA Healthcare System has been improving the health of the men and women who have so proudly served our nation. We consider it our privilege to serve your health care needs in any way we can. Our services are available to Veterans living in a ten county catchment area in west central Florida.

Suzanne M. Klinker, Medical Center Director
Kristine Brown, MPH, Associate Director

10210 Veterans Adm. Medical Center: Tampa
Tampa Veterans Administration Medical Center
13000 Bruce B Downs Boulevard
Tampa, FL 33612
813-972-2000
Fax: 813-972-7673
www.va.gov/visn8/tampa

Richard A Silver, Medical Center Director
Thomas E Bowen, Chief of Staff

10211 Vietnam Veterans of Brevard The Vietnam And All Veterans Of Brevard
The Vietnam And All Veterans Of Brevard
1125 W King Street
Cocoa, FL 32922-0929
321-690-0805
Fax: 321-690-0106
e-mail: BVagianos@cfl.rr.com
www.vietnamandallveteransofbrevard.com

Bill Vagianos, President
Don Wassmer, Vice President

10212 West Palm Beach VA Medical Center
7305 N Military Trail
West Palm Beach, FL 33410-6400
561-422-8262
800-972-8262
Fax: 561-422-8613
www.westpalmbeach.va.gov

The West Palm Beach VA Medical Center consists of one VHA facility located at 7305 N. Military Trail, West Palm Beach, Florida. The medical center is a general medical, psychiatric and surgical facility. It is a teaching hospital, providing a full range of patient care services, with state-of-the-art technology as well as education and limited research. Comprehensive healthcare is provided through primary care and long-term care in the areas of dentistry, extended care, medicine, neurology, onco

Charleen R. Szabo, FACHE, Medical Center Director
Cristy McKillop, FACHE, MHA, Medical Center Associate Director

Georgia

10213 Charlie Norwood VA Medical Center
950 15th Street Downtown
Augusta, GA 30904
706-733-0188
800-836-5561
Fax: 706-823-3934
www.augusta.va.gov

The Charlie Norwood VA Medical Center is a two-division Medical Center that provides tertiary care inmedicine, surgery, neurology, psychiatry, rehabilitation medicine, and spinal cord injury. The Downtown Division is authorized 155 beds (58 medicine, 37 surgery, and 60 spinal cord injury). The Uptown Division, located approximately three miles away, is authorized 315 beds (68 psychiatry, 15 blind rehabilitation and 40 medical rehabilitation. In addition, a 132-bed Restorative/Nursing Home C

Robert U. Hamilton, MHA, FACHE, Medical Center Director
Richard Toby Rose, Associate Director

10214 Gulf War Veterans of Georgia
307 Adair Street
Decatur, GA 30030
404-373-3741
Fax: 404-377-3741
e-mail: 70711 3174@compuserve.com

Paul Sullivan

10215 VA Southeast Network: Georgia
3700 Crestwood Parkway NW
Duluth, GA 30096-5585
678-924-5700
Fax: 678-924-5757
www.southeast.va.gov

The VA Southeast Network proudly serves veterans in the tri-state area which includes Alabama, Georgia, and South Carolina. Treating veterans and providing excellent health care at medical centers and community-based outpatient clinics is our focus.

10216 Veterans Adm. Medical Center: Decatur Atlanta VA Medical Center
Atlanta VA Medical Center
1670 Clairmont Road   404-321-6111
Decatur, GA 30033   Fax: 404-728-7733
www.atlanta.va.gov
The Atlanta VA Medical Center (VAMC), located on 26 acres in Decatur, is one of eight medical centers in the VA Southeast Network. It is a teaching hospital, providing a full range of patient care services complete with state-of-the-art technology, education, and research.
Leslie B. Wiggins, Medical Center Director
Thomas Grace, Associate Medical Center Director

10217 Veterans Adm. Medical Center: Dublin Carl Vinson VA Medical Center
Carl Vinson VA Medical Center
1826 Veterans Boulevard   912-272-1210
Dublin, GA 31021   800-595-5229
Fax: 912-277-2717
e-mail: Frank.Jordan@va.gov
www.dublin.va.gov
Since 1948, Carl Vinson VA Medical Center has been improving the health of the men and women who have so proudly served our nation. We consider it our privilege to serve your health care needs in any way we can. Services are available to veterans living in the Middle Georgia area.
John S. Goldman, Director
Gerald M. DeWorth, Associate Director

Hawaii

10218 Veterans Adm. Medical Centery: Honolulu VA Pacific Islands Health Care System
VA Pacific Islands Health Care System
459 Patterson Road   808-433-0600
Honolulu, HI 96819-1522   800-214-1306
Fax: 808-433-0390
www.hawaii.va.gov
The VA Pacific Islands Health Care System (VAPIHCS) Honolulu provides a broad range of medical care services, serving an estimated 127,600 veterans throughout Hawaii and the Pacific Islands. The VAPIHCS provides outpatient medical and mental health care through a main Ambulatory Care Clinic on Oahu (Honolulu) and through five Community Based Outpatient Clinics (CBOCs) on the neighboring islands including: Hawaii (Hilo and Kona), Maui, Kauai, and Guam. Traveling clinicians also provide episodi
William F. Dubbs, M.D., Acting Director
Brandon K. Yamamoto, Acting Associate Director

Idaho

10219 Idaho Persian Gulf Veterans
2055 Sotuh Colorado Street   208-344-3028
Boise, ID 83706
Vaughn Kidwell

10220 Veterans Adm. Medical Center: Boise Boise VA Medical Center
Boise VA Medical Center
500 W Fort Street   208-422-1000
Boise, ID 83702   866-437-5093
Fax: 208-422-1326
www.boise.va.gov
Boise VAMC's Primary Service Area has a radius of approximately 160 miles with an estimated veteran population of 94,000. The Boise VAMC, within VISN 20, provides highly sophisticated primary and secondary care with some tertiary services. The Boise VA Medical Center also operates a Community Based Outpatient Clinic (CBOC) in Twin Falls, Idaho and Caldwell, Idaho and an Extension Clinic in Burns, Oregon. A behavioral Health Clinic is located in Salmon, Idaho. A Vet Center and Veterans Benefits
Wayne Tippets, Director

Illinois

10221 Captain James A. Lovell Federal Health Car e Center
North Chicago VA Medical Center

3001 Green Bay Road   847-688-1900
North Chicago, IL 60064   800-393-0865
Fax: 847-578-3806
www.lovell.fhcc.va.gov
The Captain James A. Lovell Federal Health Care Center (FHCC) is a first-of-its-kind partnership between the U. S. Department of Veterans Affairs and the Department of Defense (DoD), integrating all medical care into a fully-integrated federal health care facility with a single combined VA and Navy mission.
Patrick L. Sullivan, Director
Captain Jos, Acosta, MC, USN, Director/Commanding Officer

10222 Desert Storm Justice Foundation: Illinois
Rural Route 4   618-457-2621
Carbondale, IL 62901
Shan Now

10223 Edward J Hines Jr VA Hospital
5000 South 5th Avenue   708-202-8387
Hines, IL 60141   Fax: 708-202-7998
e-mail: hineswebmaster@va.gov
www.hines.va.gov
Edward Hines, Jr. VA Hospital, located 12 miles west of downtown Chicago on a 147-acre campus, offers primary, extended and specialty care and serves as a tertiary care referral center for VISN 12. Specialized clinical programs include Blind Rehabilitation, Spinal Cord Injury, Neurosurgery, Radiation Therapy and Cardiovascular Surgery. The hospital also serves as the VISN 12 southern tier hub for pathology, radiology, radiation therapy, human resource management and fiscal services.
Joan Ricard, Director
Carol A. Gouty, M.S.N.,PhD, Associate Director for Patient Care Serv

10224 Jesse Brown VA Medical Center
820 S Damen Avenue   312-569-8387
Chicago, IL 60612   888-569-5282
www.chicago.va.gov
The Jesse Brown VA Medical Center consists of a 200-bed acute care facility and four community based outpatient clinics (CBOCs). Jesse Brown VAMC provides care to approximately 58,000 enrolled veterans who reside in the City of Chicago and Cook County, Illinois, and in four counties in northwestern Indiana. In FY10, the medical center had over 8100 inpatient admissions and 560,000 outpatient visits. A budget of over $355 million supports approximately 2,000 full-time equivalent staff, including
Michelle Y. Blakely, FACHE, Associate Director for Operations
Ronald J. Fought, RN, Associate Director for Patient Care

10225 VA Great Lakes Health Care System
11301 W. Cermak Road   708-492-3900
Hines, IL 60154-5000   Fax: 708-492-3948
www.visn12.va.gov
The VA Great Lakes Health Care System, a group of seven VA medical centers and over thirty VA clinics, is dedicated to providing a comprehensive health care package to America's veterans. VA Great Lakes serves veterans who reside in northwestern Indiana, northern Illinois, Wisconsin and the Upper Peninsula of Michigan. Our Mission is to serve the health care needs of America's veterans.

10226 VA Illinois Health Care System
1900 E Main Street   217-554-3000
Danville, IL 61832-5198   800-320-8387
Fax: 217-554-4552
www.danville.va.gov
Since 1898, our buildings, facilities, patients, and missions have changed, but remaining constant is VA Illiana Health Care System's endeavor in improving the health of the men and women who have so proudly served our nation. Being the 8th oldest VA facility, we consider it our privilege to serve your health care needs in any way we can. Services are available to more than 150,000 veterans living in the surrounding 34-county areas of Illinois and Indiana.
Emma Metcalf, MSN, RN, Director
Diana Carranza, Associate Director

10227 Veterans Adm. Medical Center: Marion Marion VA Medical Center
Marion VA Medical Center

2401 W Main Street
Marion, IL 62959 618-997-5311
www.marion.va.gov
The VA Medical Center in Marion, Illinois, is a general medical and surgical facility that operates 55 acute care beds and a 60 bed Community Living Center. Ten Outpatient Clinics that provide primary care and behavioral medicine services are located in Harrisburg; Carbondale; Effingham; and Mt. Vernon, IL; Paducah; Hanson; Owensboro; and Mayfield, Kentucky; Vincennes and Evansville, IN.
Frank Kehus, Associate Director
Rose Burke, Acting Associate Director, Patient Care/

10228 Veterans Adm. Medical Center: Northport North Chicago VA Medical Center
3001 Green Bay Road 847-688-1900
North Chicago, IL 60064 Fax: 847-578-3806
www.northchicago.va.gov

Indiana

10229 VA Northern Indiana Health Care System Marion Campus
1700 E 38th Street 765-674-3321
Marion, IN 46953-4589 800-360-8387
Fax: 765-677-3124
www.northernindiana.va.gov
Originally constructed as the Marion branch of the National Home for Disabled Volunteer Soldiers, VANIHCS Marion Campus has been improving the health of the men and woman who have so proudly served our nation since 1889. The Marion Campus has 75 acute psychiatry beds and a 150 bed nursing home care unit, as well as primary care, medical and surgical specialty care and mental health clinics. The Marion Campus also offers programs for Mental Health Intensive Case Management, Post-Traumatic Stress
Denise M. Deitzen, Medical Center Director
Helen Rhodes MPA, RN, Associate Director for Operations

10230 Veterans Adm. Medical Center: Fort Wayne
2121 Lake Avenue 260-426-5431
Fort Wayne, IN 46805 800-360-8387
Fax: 260-460-1336
www.northernindiana.va.gov
Since 1950 VANIHCS Fort Wayne Campus has been improving the health of the men and woman who have so proudly served our nation. The Fort Wayne campus has a 26 bed medical center providing acute medical and surgical services, as well as primary care, medical and surgical specialty care and mental health clinics. Fort Wayne Campus also offers programs for the treatment of disorders such as Post-Traumatic Stress Disorder (PTSD) and Substance Abuse Treatment Program (SATP).
Denise M. Deitzen, Medical Center Director
Ajay Dhawan MD FACHE, Chief of Staff

Iowa

10231 Cedar Rapids Persian Gulf Veterans, Spouses and Children
909-28th Street Southeast 1 319-366-0756
Cedar Rapids, IA 52403
Mary Shears

10232 Des Moines Division: VA Central Iowa Health Care System
3600 30th Street 515-699-5999
Des Moines, IA 50310-5774 800-294-8387
Fax: 515-699-5862
www.centraliowa.va.gov
The VA Central Iowa Health Care System (VACIHCS) operates a Veterans Health Administration (VHA) medical facility in Des Moines, with Community Based Outpatient Clinics (CBOCs) in Mason City, Fort Dodge, Knoxville, Marshalltown and Carroll. The medical center provides acute and specialized medical and surgical services, residential outpatient treatment programs in substance abuse and post-traumatic stress and a full range of mental health and long-term care services, as well as sub-acute and r
Donald Cooper, Director
Susan Martin, Associate Director for Resources and Ope

10233 Knoxville Division: VA Central Iowa Health Care System
1515 W Pleasant Street 641-842-3101
Knoxville, IA 50138 800-816-8878
Fax: 515-699-5862
www.centraliowa.va.gov/visitors/Knoxvill
Features: Primary Ambulatory Care, Mental Health, Prescriptions: Routine prescriptions processed through the mail or My HealtheVet
Donald Cooper, Director
Susan Martin, Associate Director for Resources and Ope

10234 Veterans Adm. Medical Center: Iowa City
601 Highway 6 W 319-338-0581
Iowa City, IA 52246-2208 800-637-0128
Fax: 319-339-7171
www.iowacity.va.gov
Since 1952, the Iowa City VA Health Care System has been improving the health of the men and women who have so proudly served our nation. We consider it our privelege to serve your health care needs in any way we can. Services are available to more than 184,000 veterans living in 50 counties in Eastern Iowa, Western Illinois and Northern Missouri.
Barry Sharp, Medical Center Director
Timothy McMurry, Associate Director for Operations

Kansas

10235 Veterans Adm. Medical Center: Leavenwoth Dwight D. Eisenhower VA Medical Center
Dwight D. Eisenhower VA Medical Center
4101 4th Street Trafficway 913-682-2000
Leavenworth, KS 66048-5055 800-952-8387
Fax: 913-758-4149
www.leavenworth.va.gov
Since 1886, the staff of the Dwight D. Eisenhower VA Medical Center has been serving veterans. Today, we proudly serve our nation's veterans with excellent health care as part of the VA Eastern Kansas Health Care System (VAEKHCS). We consider it our privilege to serve your health care needs in any way we can.
A. Rudy Klopfer, Director
John M Moon, Associate Director

10236 Veterans Adm. Medical Center: Topeka Colmery O'Neil VA Medical Center
Colmery O'Neil VA Medical Center
2200 SW Gage Boulevard 785-350-3111
Topeka, KS 66622 800-574-8387
Fax: 785-350-4336
www.leavenworth.va.gov
VA Eastern Kansas Health Care System's primary service area consists of 39 counties in Kansas and Missouri. Veteran population in these counties totals over 104,000. VAEKHCS provides care to approximately 36,000 veterans.
A. Rudy Klopfer, Director
John M Moon, Associate Director

10237 Veterans Adm. Medical Center: Wichita Robert J. Dole Department Of VA Medical
Robert J. Dole Department Of VA Medical Center
5500 East Kellogg Ave 316-685-2221
Wichita, KS 67218 888-878-6881
Fax: 316-651-3666
www.wichita.va.gov
For 75 years, the Dole VA Medical and Regional Office Center has been honored to serve Kansas area veterans. The Center provides a full range of primary and specialty acute and extended care services to 30,000 veterans in 59 counties of Kansas.
Kevin Inkley, MA, Interim Medical Center Director
Vicki Bondie, MBA, Associate Director

Kentucky

10238 Carol and Dr. James W Stutts
108 Whispering Hills Drive 606-986-3267
Berea, KY 40403 e-mail: cstutts@kih.net

10239 National Association of State Directors of Veterans Affairs
Kentucky Department of Veteran Affairs

107 S. West Street
Alexandria, VA 22314

334-242-5075
Fax: 334-353-5072
e-mail: les.beavers@ky.gov
www.nasdva.net

The National Association of State Directors of Veterans Affairs (NASDVA) is an organization with a history dating back to 1946. In the aftermath of World War II many veterans earned State and Federal benefits which required coordinated efforts to assure that veterans received these entitlements. Thus, states developed a Department or Agency specifically to manage veterans' affairs and carry out the responsibility for veteran services and program.

W. Clyde Marsh, President
Terry Schow, Senior Vice President

10240 Veterans Adm. Medical Center: Lexington Lexington VA Medical Center

Lexington VA Medical Center
1101 Veterans Drive
Lexington, KY 40502

859-281-4900
859-233-4511
www.lexington.va.gov

The Lexington Veterans Affairs Medical Center is a fully accredited, two-division, tertiary care medical center with an operating bed complement of 199 hospital beds. Acute medical, neurological, surgical and psychiatric inpatient services are provided at the Cooper Division, located adjacent to the University of Kentucky Medical Center. Other available services include: emergency care, medical-surgical units, acute psychiatry, ICU, progressive care unit, (includes Cardiac Cath Lab) ambulatory s

Pamala Thompson, RN, MSA, MSN,, Interim Medical Center Director
Michael M Young, Acting Associate Director

10241 Veterans Adm. Medical Center: Louisville Louisville VA Medical Center

Louisville VA Medical Center
800 Zorn Avenue
Louisville, KY 40206

502-287-4000
800-376-8387
Fax: 502-287-6225
www.louisville.va.gov

Robley Rex Veterans Affairs Medical Center improves the health of our veterans and other eligible patients by providing a continuum of care through an integrated health care delivery system.

Wayne L. Pfeffer, MHSA, FACHE, Medical Center Director
Douglas V Paxton, Sr, Associate Director / Operations

Louisiana

10242 Alexandria VA Healthcare System

Alexandria VA Medical Center
2495 Shreveport Highway
Pineville, LA 71360

318-466-4000
800-375-8387
Fax: 318-483-5029
www.alexandria.va.gov

Service Recovery is used at our facility to improve customer service and is a critical process in organizations that excel in service to their customers. It identifies a service failure, effectively resolves a service problem, classifies its root cause(s), and yields data that can be integrated with other sources of performance measurement to assess and improve the service system. It entails making a person feel whole by staff demonstrating politeness, concern and candor.

Martin J. Traxler, Medical Center Director
Yolanda Sanders-Jackson, Associate Director

10243 Southeast Louisiana Veterans Health Care S ystem

New Orleans VA Medical Center
1601 Perdido Street
New Orleans, LA 70112

504-568-0811
800-935-8387
Fax: 504-589-5210
www.neworleans.va.gov

Southeast Louisiana Veterans Health Care System (SLVHCS) provides quality, compassionate, safe health care to Veteran patients throughout 23 parishes in southeast Louisiana. In the aftermath of Hurricane Katrina, the New Orleans VAMC was devastated. SLVHCS reorganized to meet the needs of Veterans and now consists of eight community-based clinics located in New Orleans, Slidell, Hammond, St. John Parish, Houma, Franklin, Bogalusa

and Baton Rouge. Ninety percent of patients live within 30 minutes

Julie A. Catellier, Director
Jimmy Murphy, Associate Director

10244 Veterans Adm. Medical Center: Shreveport Overton Brooks VA Medical Center

Overton Brooks VA Medical Center
510 E Stoner Avenue
Shreveport, LA 71101

318-221-8411
800-863-7441
Fax: 318-424-6156
www.shreveport.va.gov

The Overton Brooks VAMC and our associated CBOC's (Community Based Outpatient Clinics) are part of the South Central Health Care Network, VISN 16. VISN stands for Veterans Integrated Service Network, and is one of 22 VISN's in the U.S. Department of Veterans Affairs. VISN 16 provides comprehensive inpatient and outpatient health care, and limited nursing home and domiciliary care, to eligible veterans of the U.S. Armed Services. health care services are provided through a network of medical cent

Shirley M. Bealer, Medical Center Director
Erik J. Glover, Associate Medical Center Director

Maine

10245 Veterans Adm. Medical Center: Augusta Togus VA Medical Center

Togus VA Medical Center
1 VA Center
Augusta, ME 4330

207-623-8411
866-590-2976
Fax: 207-623-5792
TTY: 800-829-4833
TDD: 800-829-4833
e-mail: togus.query@vba.va.gov
www.benefits.va.gov/togus

Dale Denners, Regional Office Director

Maryland

10246 Fort Howard VA Outpatient Clinic

9600 N Point Road
Fort Howard, MD 21052

410-477-1800
800-351-8387
Fax: 410-477-7177
www.maryland.va.gov/facilities/Fort_Howa

Health Care Services: Anticoagulation AC,Arthritis,Dermatology,Medication Management, Mental Health, Nutrition, Podiatry, Post Traumatic Stress, Primary Care, Pulmonary, Social Work, Telemental Health, Women's Health

Dennis H Smith, Director

10247 Loch Raven VA Community Living & Rehabilit ation Center

3900 Loch Raven Boulevard
Baltimore, MD 21218

410-605-7000
Fax: 410-605-7900
www.maryland.va.gov/facilities/LochRaven

The Loch Raven VA Community Living & Rehabilitation Center specializes in providing rehabilitation and post-acute care for patients in the VA Maryland Health Care System. The center coordinates the delivery of rehabilitation services, including physical therapy, occupational therapy, kinesiotherapy and recreation therapy, to achieve the highest level of recovery and independence for Maryland's Veterans.

10248 Maryland Group

8725 Fairhaven Place
Jessup, MD 20794

301-725-4269

Nancy Kaplan

10249 VA Capitol Health Care Network

849 International Drive
Linthicum, MD 21090

410-691-1131
Fax: 410-684-3189
www.va.gov/visn5

The VA Capitol Health Care Network (VISN 5) was established in October 1995, and serves Veterans from economically and demographically diverse areas within Maryland, the District of Columbia, and portions of Virginia, West Virginia, and Pennsylvania.

Fernando O. Rivera, MBA, FACHE, Network Director
Guy B. Richardson, MHSA, FACHE, Deputy Network Director

10250 VA Maryland Health Care System Perry Point VA Medical Center
Perry Point VA Medical Center
Perry Point, MD 21902
410-642-2411
800-949-1003
Fax: 410-642-1161
www.maryland.va.gov

The Perry Point VA Medical Center provides a broad range of inpatient, outpatient and primary care services. As the largest inpatient facility in the VA Maryland Health Care System, the medical center provides inpatient medical, intermediate and long-term care programs, including nursing home care, rehabilitation services, geriatric evaluation and management, respite care, chronic ventilator care and hospice care.
Dennis H Smith, Director
Dorothy M Snow, Chief of Staff

10251 Veterans Adm. Medical Center: Baltimore
10 N Greene Street
Baltimore, MD 21201
410-605-7000
800-463-6295
Fax: 410-605-7901
www.maryland.va.gov/facilities/Baltimore

As a modern health care facility, the Baltimore VA Medical Center offers Veterans state-of-the-art technology and clinical services. The medical center is home to the world's first filmless radiology department, which allows health care providers to have nearly instant access to patient radiology images.
Carol Nizzardini, Chief Nurse Executive
Dennis H Smith, Director

Massachusetts

10252 Persian Gulf Era Veterans
24 Beacon Street
Boston, MA 02133
617-329-8149
e-mail: jagmedic@pgev.org
www.pgev.org

The general consensus is that VA is planning to use the materials generated from the pending IOM report on Chronic Multisymptom Illness Volume 9 to create a ICD code for sick Gulf War vets. Its uncertain if this is broad sweeping or badly managed science to produce a faulty definition based on psychiatry.
VenusVal Hammack, Executive Director

10253 VA Boston Healthcare System: Jamaica Plain Jamaica Plain Campus
Jamaica Plain Campus
150 S Huntington Avenue
Jamaica Plain, MA 02130
617-232-9500
800-865-3384
Fax: 617-278-4508
www.boston.va.gov

VA Boston Healthcare System's consolidated facility consists of the Jamaica Plain campus, located in the heart of Boston's Longwood Medical Community; the West Roxbury campus, located on the Dedham line; and the Brockton campus, located 20 miles south of Boston in the City of Brockton.
Vincent Ng, Acting Director
Michael E Charness, Chief of Staff

10254 VA Boston Healthcare System: West Roxbury West Roxbury Campus
West Roxbury Campus
1400 VFW Parkway
W Roxbury, MA 02132
617-323-7700
800-865-3384
www.boston.va.gov

VA Boston Healthcare System's consolidated facility consists of the Jamaica Plain campus, located in the heart of Boston's Longwood Medical Community; the West Roxbury campus, located on the Dedham line; and the Brockton campus, located 20 miles south of Boston in the City of Brockton.
Vincent Ng, Acting Director
Susan MacKenzie, Associate Director

10255 VA New England Health Care System
200 Springs Road
Bedford, MA 01730
781-687-2000
800-838-6331
Fax: 781-687-3470
www.newengland.va.gov

Bedford VA is a long-term care facility specializing in geriatric and psychiatric care. Comprehensive health services include mental health, medicine, psychiatry, physical medicine, dentistry, geriatrics and ambulatory care.
Christine Croteau, Acting Hospital Director
Bob Colpitts, Acting Associate Director

10256 Veterans Adm. Medical Center: Brockton Brockton Campus
Brockton Campus
940 Belmont Street
Brockton, MA 02301
508-583-4500
800-865-3384
Fax: 700-885-1000
www.boston.va.gov

VA Boston Healthcare System's consolidated facility consists of the Jamaica Plain campus, located in the heart of Boston's Longwood Medical Community; the West Roxbury campus, located on the Dedham line; and the Brockton campus, located 20 miles south of Boston in the City of Brockton.
Vincent Ng, Acting Director
Michael E Charness, Chief of Staff

Michigan

10257 Detroit VA Medical Center John D. Dingell VA Medical Center
John D. Dingell VA Medical Center
4646 John R Street
Detroit, MI 48201
313-576-1000
800-511-8056
Fax: 313-576-1025
www.detroit.va.gov

Since 1939, this VA facility has been improving the health of the men and women who have so proudly served our nation. In 1996, the medical center moved from its original location in Allen Park, Michigan to the current location in Detroit. The John D. Dingell VAMC is one of the newest VA facilities in the country. It's our privilege to serve your health care needs in any way we can. Services are available to more than 330,000 Veterans living in Wayne, Oakland, Macomb, and St. Clair counties.
Pamela J Reeves, Director
Basim Dubaybo, Chief of Staff

10258 International Advocacy for Gulf War Syndrome
2297 Westfield Drive
Niles, MI 49102
616-684-5903
e-mail: DSVETERAN1@juno.com
Brian Martin

10259 Oscar G. Johnson VA Medical Center
Iron Mountain VA Medical Center
325 E H Street
Iron Mountain, MI 49801
906-774-3300
800-215-8262
Fax: 906-779-3188
www.ironmountain.va.gov

OGJVAMC is a primary and secondary level care facility with 17 acute care beds, 13 in the medical/surgical ward and 4 in the intensive care unit (ICU). The main facility provides limited emergency and acute inpatient care, and collaborates with larger VA Medical Centers in Milwaukee and Madison, WI, to provide higher-level emergency and specialty care services. OGJVAMC also provides rehabilitation and extended care, including palliative and hospice care, in its 40-bed Community Living Center.
James W. Rice, Medical Center Director
William J. Caron, PT, MHA, FACHE, Associate Director

10260 Veterans Adm. Medical Center: Ann Arbor Ann Arbor Healthcare System
Ann Arbor Healthcare System
2215 Fuller Road
Ann Arbor, MI 48105
734-769-7100
800-361-8387
Fax: 734-845-3245
www.annarbor.va.gov

The main hospital campus located in Ann Arbor serves as a referral center for specialty care and operates 105 acute care beds and 40 Community Living Center (extended care) beds. More than 500,000 outpatient visits were made at our facilities in fiscal year 2012; there were nearly 6,000 inpatient episodes of care provided in the hospital and extended care center.
Robert P. McDivitt, FACHE, Director
Randall E. Ritter, Associate Director

10261 Veterans Adm. Medical Center: Battle Creek
Battle Creek VA Medical Center

5500 Armostrong Road
Battle Creek, MI 49037

269-966-5600
888-214-1247
Fax: 269-966-5483
www.battlecreek.va.gov

The medical center offers a wide variety of health care services, which includes both inpatient and outpatient care. Once eligibility has been determined, each patient enrolling for care is assigned to a primary care provider and team, who provides continuous and coordinated care.

Mary Beth Skupien, Director
Edward Dornoff, Associate Director

10262 Veterans Adm. Medical Center: Saginaw Aleda E. Lutz VA Medical Center
Aleda E. Lutz VA Medical Center
1500 Wiess Street
Saginaw, MI 48602

989-497-2500
800-406-5143
Fax: 989-321-4903
www.saginaw.va.gov

Since 1950, the Aleda E. Lutz VA Medical Center has been improving the health of the men and women who have so proudly served our nation. We consider it our privilege to serve your health care needs in any way we can. Services are available to more than 31,000 veterans living in the Central and Northern 35 counties of Michigan's Lower Peninsula.

Peggy Kearns, Medical Center Director
Stephanie Young, Associate Director

Minnesota

10263 Desert Storm Justice Foundation: Minnesota
Buhl, MN 55713
Jeff Zakula

218-258-3685

10264 Veterans Adm. Medical Center: Minneapolis Minneapolis VA Medical Center
Minneapolis VA Medical Center
1 Veterans Drive
Minneapolis, MN 55417

612-725-2000
866-414-5058
Fax: 612-725-2049
www.minneapolis.va.gov

Minneapolis VA Health Care System (VAHCS) is a teaching hospital providing a full range of patient care services with state-of-the-art technology, as well as education and research. Comprehensive health care is provided through primary care, tertiary care and long-term care in areas of medicine, surgery, psychiatry, physical medicine and rehabilitation, neurology, oncology, dentistry, geriatrics and extended care.

Patrick J. Kelly, Director
Erik J. Stalhandske, Associate Director

10265 Veterans Adm. Regional Office: St. Paul
1 Federal Drive Fort Snelling
Saint Paul, MN 55111

612-970-5415
800-827-1000
Fax: 612-970-5415
e-mail: VBCINQ@VBA.VA.GOV
www.va.gov/directory/guide/facility.asp?

St. Paul VA Regional Office will be accessible and responsive as we provide timely, accurate, and cost-effective service to veterans and their families. We will earn the respect and trust of veteran and their families by exceeding expectations and achieving excellence in the delivery of benefits and services. May we always keep our country's promise.

Mississippi

10266 GV Montgomery VA Medical Center
1500 E Woodrow Wilson Drive
Jackson, MS 39216

601-362-4471
800-949-1009
Fax: 601-364-1359
www.jackson.va.gov

This medical center provides primary, second and tertiary medical, neurological and mental health inpatient care. Services include hemodialysis, sleep studies, substance abuse treatment, post traumatic stress disorder (PTSD), hematology/oncology, and rehabilitation programs. Both primary and specialized outpatient services are available, including such specialized programs as: ambulatory surgery, spinal cord injury, neurology, infectious disease, substance abuse, PTSD, readjustment counseling,

Joe D. Battle, Medical Center Director
Bryan C. Matthews, Acting Associate Director

10267 South Central VA Health Care Network
715 S. Pear Orchard Road,
Ridgeland, MS 39216

601-206-6900
800-639-5137
Fax: 601-206-7018
www.visn16.va.gov

This medical center provides primary, second and tertiary medical, neurological and mental health inpatient care. Services include hemodialysis, sleep studies, substance abuse treatment, post traumatic stress disorder (PTSD), hematology/oncology, and rehabilitation programs. Both primary and specialized outpatient services are available, including such specialized programs as: ambulatory surgery, spinal cord injury, neurology, infectious disease, substance abuse, PTSD, readjustment counseling,

Joe D. Battle, Medical Center Director
Bryan C. Matthews, Acting Associate Director

10268 VA Gulf Coast Veterans Health Care System
400 Veterans Avenue
Biloxi, MS 39531

228-523-5000
800-296-8872
Fax: 228-523-5719
www.biloxi.va.gov

Since 1932, VA Gulf Coast Veterans Health Care System has been improving the health of the men and women who have so proudly served our nation. The VA Gulf Coast Veterans HCS is privileged to serve over 50,000 veterans. Additionally, it provides support to readjustment counseling centers and VA National Cemeteries along the Gulf Coast. The Health Care System is a part of VISN 16, South Central VA Health Care Network.

Anthony L. Dawson, MHA, FACHE, Director
Nancy Weaver, MBA, VHA-CM, Associate Director

10269 Veterans Adm. Regional Office: Jackson
1600 E Woodrow Wilson Avenue
Jackson, MS 32916

601-364-7000
800-827-1000
Fax: 601-364-7007
www.benefits.va.gov/jackson

The Department of Veterans Affairs provides a variety of services and benefits to honorably discharged veterans of the U.S. Military and their dependents. The purpose of this Web page is to assist Mississippi veterans, their dependents and survivors, in contacting the nearest VA facility to inquire about their veterans benefits or health care services.

Missouri

10270 John J. Pershing VA Medical Center
John J. Pershing VA Medical Center
1500 N Westwood Boulevard
Poplar Bluff, MO 63901

573-686-4151
888-557-8262
Fax: 573-778-4559
www.poplarbluff.va.gov

The John J. Pershing VA Medical Center, located in Poplar Bluff, Missouri, provides primary care to veterans throughout 29 counties of Southeast Missouri and Northeast Arkansas. Approximately 50,000 veterans live in our service area and about 40 percent of them receive care at our Medical Center annually. Our facility is comprised of 18 general medicine beds and 40 extended care beds. Tertiary care support is provided by VA Medical Centers in St. Louis and Columbia, Missouri; Memphis, Tennessee;

Marj Hedstrom, Medical Center Director
Vijayachandr Nair, MD, Chief of Staff

10271 VA Heartland Network
1201 Walnut Street
Kansas City, MO 64106

816-701-3000
Fax: 816-221-0930
www.visn15.va.gov

The VA Heartland Network is one of twenty-two Veterans Integrated Service Networks (VISN) located throughout the United States. The VA Heartland Network also known as VISN 15, provides health care services to veterans in Kansas and Missouri, as well as parts of Illinois, Indiana, Kentucky and Arkansas.

10272 Veterans Adm. Medical Center: Columbia Harry S. Truman Memorial
Harry S. Truman Memorial

800 Hospital Drive
Columbia, MO 65201-5297
573-814-6000
800-349-8262
Fax: 573-814-6600
www.columbiamo.va.gov

Truman VA in Columbia, Missouri, serves 44 counties in Missouri as well as Pike County, Illinois, and is one of seven medical center facilities in the VA Heartland Network, a Veterans Integrated Service Network (VISN).
Sallie Houser-Hanfelder, FACHE, Director
Robert Ritter, FACHE, Associate Director

10273 Veterans Adm. Medical Center: Kansas City Kansas City VA Medical Center
Kansas City VA Medical Center
4801 Linwood Boulevard
Kansas City, MO 64128
816-861-4700
800-525-1483
Fax: 816-922-3303
www.kansascity.va.gov

Opening in 1952, the Kansas City VA Medical Center has a rich legacy of providing quality care to the men and women who have proudly served our nation —- America's heroes. We consider it an honor and privilege to serve the health care needs of our Veterans.
Kent D. Hill, Medical Center Director
Kevin Inkley, Associate Director

10274 Veterans Adm. Regional Office: St. Louis John Cochran Division
John Cochran Division
915 N Grand Boulevard
Saint Louis, MO 63106
314-652-4100
800-228-5459
Fax: 314-289-6557
www.stlouis.va.gov

The VA St. Louis Health Care System provides inpatient and ambulatory care in medicine, surgery, psychiatry, neurology, and rehabilitation, and many other subspecialty areas. It is a two-division facility that serves veterans and their families in east central Missouri and southwestern Illinois. The John Cochran Division, named after the late Missouri congressman, is located in midtown St. Louis and has all of the medical center's operative surgical capabilities, the ambulatory care unit, intensi
Rimaann O. Nelson, RN,, Medical Center Director
Marc A. Magill, Deputy Medical Center Director

Montana

10275 Veterans Adm. Medical Center: Fort Harrison
VA Montana Health Care System
3687 Veterans Drive
Fort Harrison, MT 59636
406-442-6410
877-468-8387
Fax: 406-477-7916
www.montana.va.gov

Fort Harrison (Helena) is a 48-bed acute care, medical-surgical facility that offers a broad range of acute, chronic, and specialized inpatient and outpatient services for both male and female veterans. Specialty care includes internal medicine, gerontology, neurology, dermatology, cardiology, palliative care, pain management, medical oncology, surgery (general, vascular, laparoscopic, endoscopic), urology, orthopedics, plastic, ophthalmology, ENT, podiatry, gynecology, chiropractic care, psych
Christine Gregory, Director
Vicki Thennis, Interim Associate Director

10276 Veterans Adm. Medical Center: Miles City
210 S Winchester
Miles City, MT 59301
406-874-5600
877-468-8387
Fax: 406-874-5696
www.va.gov/directory/guide/facility.asp?

The Miles City Division of the VA Montana Healthcare System is located in southeastern Montana in Miles City. Headquarters for the VA Montana Healthcare System is located at the Ft. Harrison facility in Helena. Services at Miles City include a community based outpatient clinic and a 30 bed Nursing Home Care Unit. Some specialty clinics are also available. The VA Montana Healthcare System provides care to over 19,000 veterans annually.

Nevada

10277 Veterans Adm. Medical Center: Las Vegas VA Southern Nevada Healthcare System
VA Southern Nevada Healthcare System (VASNHS)

6900 North Pecos Road
North Las Vegas, NV 89086
702-791-9000
877-252-4866
Fax: 702-636-3027
www.lasvegas.va.gov

Since 1972, VA Southern Nevada Healthcare System has been improving the health of the men and women who have so proudly served our nation. We consider it our privilege to serve your health care needs in any way we can. Services are available to more than 240,000 Veterans living in our catchment area.
Isabel M Duff, Acting Director
Ramu Komanduri, M.D., Chief of Staff

10278 Veterans Adm. Medical Center: Reno VA Sierra Nevada Health Care System
VA Sierra Nevada Health Care System
975 Kirman Avenue
Reno, NV 89502
775-786-7200
888-838-6256
Fax: 775-328-1464
www.reno.va.gov

The VA Sierra Nevada Health Care System (VASNHCS), Reno, Nev., provides primary and secondary care to a large geographical area that includes 20 counties in northern Nevada and northeastern California.
Kurt W Schlegelmilch, M.D., FAC, Director
Steven E Brilliant, M.D., FACP, Chief of Staff

New Hampshire

10279 Veterans Adm. Medical Center: Manchester Manchester VA Medical Center
Manchester VA Medical Center
718 Smyth Road
Manchester, NH 03104
603-624-4366
800-892-8384
Fax: 603-626-6579
www.manchester.va.gov

Mission: Honor America's Veterans by providing exceptional health care that improves their health and well-being.
Tammy A. Krueger, BS, Acting Medical Center Director
Andrew J. Breuder, MD, MPH, FACPM, Chief of Staff

New Jersey

10280 Veterans Adm. Medical Center: East Orange East Orange Campus
East Orange Campus
385 Tremont Avenue
E Orange, NJ 07018
973-676-1000
Fax: 973-395-7062
www.newjersey.va.gov

The Department of Veterans Affairs New Jersey Health Care System (VANJHCS) is a consolidated facility comprised of two main campuses, one in East Orange, the corporate office located in Northeastern New Jersey within the greater New York metropolitan area, and one in Lyons, 22 miles to the west of the East Orange Campus. The System's Diabetes Education, Pulmonary Rehabilitation, Prosthetics, Homeless Outreach Programs, and others have been recognized for outstanding achievement both within the D
Kenneth H Mizrach, Director
Steven L Lieberman, Chief of Staff

10281 Veterans Adm. Medical Center: Lyons Lyons Campus
Lyons Campus
151 Knollcroft Road
Lyons, NJ 07939
908-647-0180
Fax: 908-647-3452
www.newjersey.va.gov

Primary care is emphasized at the VANJHCS. Veterans are assigned their own health care providers whom they see on a regular basis. Access to a wide variety of specialists is available through the primary providers. In addition to general medical, psychiatry, and long-term care, a full range of medical and surgical subspecialty care is provided to veterans of the VANJHCS in a variety of special programs as listed below. Because the VANJHCS is dedicated to developing programs that meet all veteran
Kenneth H Mizrach, Director
Steven L Lieberman, Chief of Staff

New Mexico

10282 Veterans Adm. Medical Center: Albuquerque New Mexico VA Health Care System
New Mexico VA Health Care System
1501 San Pedro Drive SE 505-265-1711
Albuquerque, NM 87108-5153 800-465-8262
Fax: 505-256-2855
www.albuquerque.va.gov
The NMVAHCS is a leader in the provision of rural health care, opening its first VA-staffed community based outpatient clinic (CBOC) in Farmington, New Mexico, followed by clinics in Artesia, Gallup, Raton, Silver City, Rio Rancho and Santa Fe. In recent years, the NMVAHCS has contracted with Health Net Federal Services and Ben Archer Health Center to provide Veterans access to clinics throughout New Mexico and southwest Colorado.
George Marnell, Director
Pamela Crowell, Associate Director

New York

10283 Brooklyn Campus of the VA NY Harbor Health care System
Brooklyn Campus
800 Poly Place 718-836-6600
Brooklyn, NY 11209 Fax: 718-567-4082
www.nyharbor.va.gov
The NY Harbor Healthcare System is always improving the health of the men and women who have so proudly served our nation. We consider it our privilege to serve your health care needs in any way we can. Services are available to veterans living in the 5 boroughs of New York City.
Martina A. Parauda, Director
Veronica J. Foy, Associate Director, Facilities & Human R

10284 Gulf War Veterans of Long Island, NY
100 Robinson 516-289-1580
E Patchogue, NY 11772 Fax: 516-447-5871
e-mail: DStormMom@aol.com
Jackie Olsen

10285 Persian Gulf Veterans
212 Garfield Avenue 716-385-4097
E Rochester, NY 14445-1314 Fax: 716-924-2161
Beverly Place

10286 VA Helathcare Network: Upstate New York
113 Holland Avenue 518-626-7327
Albany, NY 12208-8980 Fax: 518-626-7333
www.visn2.va.gov
VA Health Care Upstate New York (VISN 2) is composed of five VA medical centers and 29 community based outpatient clinics. We provide comprehensive inpatient and outpatient health care to eligible Veterans.
David J. West, MSHA, FACHE, Network Director
Lawrence H Flesh, M.D., Chief Medical Officer

10287 VA NY/NJ Veterans Healthcare Network
130 W Kingsbridge Road 718-741-4110
Bronx, NY 10468 Fax: 718-741-4141
www2.va.gov/directory/guide/facility.asp
Veterans Integrated Service Network 3 serves the wide diversity of needs for the greater New York and New Jersey veteran population. The Network provides care in some of the most urban settings in the nation as well as in sprawling suburban and rural areas. A full range of services is provided with each medical center emphasizing primary care complimented by specialized care. Additional services are provided in 30 community based outpatient clinics. VA's network of facilities includes; VA Medica
Michael A Sabo, Network Director

10288 Veterans Adm. Medical Center: Albany Samuel S. Stratton: VA Medical Center
Samuel S. Stratton: VA Medical Center
113 Holland Avenue 518-626-5000
Albany, NY 12208 800-223-4810
Fax: 518-626-5500
www.albany.va.gov

The Stratton VA Medical Center opened in 1951 and serves Veterans in 22 counties of upstate New York, western Massachusetts and Vermont.
Linda W. Weiss MS, FACHE, Director
Donald W Stuart, Associate Dirctor Albany VA Medical Cent

10289 Veterans Adm. Medical Center: Batavia VA Western New York Healthcare System
VA Western New York Healthcare System at Batavia
222 Richmond Avenue 585-297-1053
Batavia, NY 14020 888-823-9656
Fax: 716-344-3305
www.buffalo.va.gov/batavia.asp
The Batavia facility opened its doors in 1933. It provides geriatric and rehabilitation services, separate residential post traumatic stress disorder units for men and women, and outpatient services. In 1995, a New York State Veterans Home was built on the Batavia grounds making additional extended care available.
Brian G. Stiller, Director
Jason C. Petti, Associate Medical Center Director

10290 Veterans Adm. Medical Center: Bath Bath VA Medical Center
Bath VA Medical Center
76 Veterans Avenue 607-664-4000
Bath, NY 14810 877-845-3247
Fax: 607-664-4511
www.bath.va.gov
The Medical Center, founded in 1878 as a Grand Army of the Republic Soldiers and Sailors Home has proudly served Veterans for more than 130 years. The facility provides a full range of patient care services. We also provide primary and mental health care through clinics in Coudersport, Elmira, Mansfield and Wellsville.
Michael J. Swartz, Medical Center Director
Kenneth P. Piazza, Associate Director

10291 Veterans Adm. Medical Center: Buffalo
3495 Bailey Avenue 716-834-9200
Buffalo, NY 14215 800-532-8387
Fax: 716-862-8759
www.buffalo.va.gov
The Buffalo VA Medical Center opened in 1950 and provides medical, surgical, mental health and long term care services through a range of inpatient and outpatient programs. It is the main referral center for cardiac surgery, cardiology and comprehensive cancer care for central and western New York and northern Pennsylvania.
Brian G. Stiller, Director
Jason C. Petti, Associate Medical Center Director

10292 Veterans Adm. Medical Center: Montrose Franklin Delano Roosevelt Campus
Franklin Delano Roosevelt Campus
2094 Albany Post Road 914-737-4400
Montrose, NY 10548 800-269-8749
Fax: 914-788-4244
e-mail: complaint@jointcommission.org
www.hudsonvalley.va.gov
Our vision is to be a patient-centered, integrated health care organization for Veterans providing excellent health care, research, and education; an organization where people choose to work; an active community partner; and a back up for national emergencies.
Gerald F Culliton, Director
Joanne J. Malina, M.D., Chief of Staff

10293 Veterans Adm. Medical Center: New York New York Campus
New York Campus
423 E 23rd Street 212-686-7500
New York, NY 10010 Fax: 718-567-4082
www.nyharbor.va.gov
The NY Harbor Healthcare System is always improving the health of the men and women who have so proudly served our nation. We consider it our privilege to serve your health care needs in any way we can. Services are available to veterans living in the 5 boroughs of New York City.
Martina A. Parauda, Director
Veronica J. Foy, Associate Director, Facilities & Human R

10294 Veterans Adm. Medical Center: Northport Northport VA Medical Center
Northport VA Medical Center

79 Middleville Road
Northport, NY 11768
516-261-4400
800-551-3996
Fax: 631-754-7933
www.northport.va.gov

The Northport Veterans Affairs Medical Center is always improving the health of the men and women who have proudly served our nation. We consider it our privilege to serve your health care needs in any way we can. Services are available to veterans living in the Long Island area of New York.
Philip C Moschitta, Director
Edward J. Mack, MD, Chief of Staff

10295 Veterans Adm. Medical Center: Syracuse Syracuse VA Medical Center
Syracuse VA Medical Center
800 Irving Avenue
Syracuse, NY 13210
315-425-4400
800-792-4334
Fax: 315-425-4375
www.syracuse.va.gov

The Syracuse VA Medical Center, part of VA Health Care Upstate New York opened its doors on June 14, 1953. The Medical Center utilizes state-of-the-art technology to provide a full range of patient care services, education and research.
Judy Hayman, Ph.D., Acting Medical Center Director
William H Marx, DO, FACS, Chief of Staff

10296 Veterans Affairs Medical Center Canandaigua
Canadaigua VA Medical Center
400 Fort Hill Avenue
Canandaigua, NY 14424
716-394-2000
800-204-9917
Fax: 716-393-8328
e-mail: Laurie.Guererri@va.gov
www.canandaigua.va.gov

The Canandaigua VA Medical Center, part of VA Health Upstate New York is located in the heart of the Finger Lakes region, 30 miles southeast of Rochester in Canandaigua, New York. Providing inpatient and outpatient care to veterans living in upstate New York since 1933, the Medical Center provides numerous health care programs and services.
Craig S. Howard, Director
Margaret Owens, Associate Director

North Carolina

10297 Charles George Veterans Affairs Medical Center
1100 Tunnel Road
Asheville, NC 28805
828-298-7911
800-932-6408
Fax: 828-299-2563
www.asheville.va.gov

The Extended Care and Rehabilitation Program at VAMC Asheville is composed of the following areas:Physical Medicine and Rehabilitation, Extended Care Center, Home and Community Care, Hospice and Palliative Care
Cynthia Breyfogle FACHE, Medical Center Director
David A Pattillo MHA FACHE, Associate Medical Center Director

10298 Desert Storm Veterans of North Carolina
739 E Haggard Avenue
Ellon College, NC 27224
910-584-5038
Kevin Treiber

10299 Veterans Adm. Medical Center: Durham Durham VA Medical Center
Durham VA Medical Center
508 Fulton Street
Durham, NC 27705
919-286-0411
888-878-6890
Fax: 919-286-6825
www.durham.va.gov

Since 1953, Durham Veterans Affairs Medical Cetner has been improving the health of the men and women who have so proudly served our nation. We consider it our privilege to serve your health care needs in any way we can. Services are available to more than 200,000 veterans living in a 26-county area of central and eastern North Carolina.
DeAnne M Seekins, Director
John D Shelburne, M.D. Ph.D, Chief of Staff

10300 Veterans Adm. Medical Center: Fayetville Fayettville VA Medical Center
Fayettville VA Medical Center

2300 Ramsey Street
Fayetteville, NC 28301
910-488-2120
800-771-6106
Fax: 910-822-7093
e-mail: james.neal@va.gov
www.fayettevillenc.va.gov

Since 1940, the Fayetteville VA Medical Center (VAMC) has improved the health of the men and women who have so proudly served our nation. We consider it our privilege to serve your health care needs in any way we can. Medical, mental health, women's health care and specialty services are available to more than 157,000 veterans living in a 21-county area of North Carolina and South Carolina.
Elizabeth Goolsby, Director
James James Galkowski, PA-C, F, Associate Director

10301 Veterans Adm. Medical Center: Salisbury W.G. Hefner VA Medical Center
W.G. Hefner VA Medical Center
1601 Brenner Avenue
Salisbury, NC 28144
704-683-9000
800-469-8262
Fax: 704-638-3395
www.salisbury.va.gov

Inpatient services include acute medicine, cardiology, surgery, psychiatry and physical medicine and rehabilitation, as well as sub-acute and extended care. Primary and specialized outpatient services are provided at the medical center complex and the community based outpatient clinics. Services are also provided at the Veterans Outreach Centers Centers in Greensboro and Charlotte. Contractual extended care is provided through an extensive residential care treatment program and a community nursi
Kaye Green, FACHE, Director
Linette Baker, MPA, Associate Director

North Dakota

10302 Fargo VA Healthcare System
Fargo VA Medical.Regional Office Center
2101 N Elm Street
Fargo, ND 58102
701-232-3241
800-410-9723
Fax: 701-239-3705
e-mail: margaret.wheelden@va.gov
www.fargo.va.gov

Since 1929, VAMC Fargo has been improving the health of the men and women who have so proudly served our nation. We consider it our privilege to serve your health care needs in any way we can. Services are available to more than 89,000 veterans living in North Dakota, Minnesota, and South Dakota.
Michael J. Murphy, FACHE, Center Director
Dale DeKrey, Associate Director for Operations and Re

Ohio

10303 Chalmers P. Wylie VA Ambulatory Care Cente r
Chalmers P. Wylie Outpatient Clinic
420 N James Road
Columbus, OH 43219-1278
614-257-5200
888-615-9448
Fax: 614-257-5460
e-mail: vhacoswebteam@va.gov
www.columbus.va.gov

The Chalmers P. Wylie VA Ambulatory Care Center (VA ACC) has been improving the health of the men and women who have so proudly served our nation. We consider it our privilege to serve your health care needs in any way we can. From surgery to diagnostics, fitness to rehabilitation, depend on us for care.
Darwin Goodspeed, Director
Laura E Ruzick, FACHE, Associate Director

10304 Persian Gulf War Veterans of Western Pennsylvania, W Virginia and NE Ohio
600 North Market Street
East Palestine, OH 44413
216-426-3203
Fax: 216-426-3309
Barry M Walker

10305 VA Healthcare System Of Ohio
11500 Northlake Drive
Cincinnati, OH 45249
513-247-4621
Fax: 513-247-4620
e-mail: visn10webmaster@med.va.gov
www.visn10.va.gov

Each VISN 10 medical facility respects the patient's right to make decisions about his or her care, treatment and services, and to involve the patient's family in care, services, and treatment decisions to the extent permitted by the patient or surrogate decision-maker.

10306 Veterans Adm. Medical Center: Chillicothe Chillicothe VA Medical Center
Chillicothe VA Medical Center
17273 State Route 104   740-773-1141
Chillicothe, OH 45601   800-358-8262
Fax: 740-773-1141
e-mail: vhacllwebmaster@va.gov
www.chillicothe.va.gov
The Chillicothe VA Medical Center provides acute and chronic mental health services, primary and secondary medical services, a wide range of nursing home care services, specialty medical services as well as specialized women Veterans health clinics. The facility is an active ambulatory care setting and serves as a chronic mental health referral center for VA Medical Centers in southern Ohio and parts of West Virginia and Kentucky.
Wendy Hepker, Medical Center Director
Keith Sullivan, FACHE, Associate Medical Center Director

10307 Veterans Adm. Medical Center: Cincinnati Cincinnati VA Medical Center
Cincinnati VA Medical Center
3200 Vine Street   513-861-3100
Cincinnati, OH 45220   888-267-7873
Fax: 513-475-6500
e-mail: vhacinwebmasters@va.gov
www.cincinnati.va.gov
Cincinnati VAMC consists of 2 divisions located in Cincinnati, Ohio and Fort Thomas, Kentucky. Provides services to 17 counties in Ohio, Kentucky, and Indiana. Cincinnati VAMC has an active affiliation with the University of Cincinnati College of Medicine. Referral site for neurosurgery. PTSD Residential Programs for Men & Women. PTSD/Traumatic Brain Injury Residential Program. Iraq/Afghanistan Clinic Veterans Mobile Health Unit
Linda D Smith, Director
David E. Ninneman, RA, Associate Director

10308 Veterans Adm. Medical Center: Cleveland Louis Stokes VA Medical Center
Louis Stokes VA Medical Center
10701 E Boulevard   216-791-3800
Cleveland, OH 44106   877-838-8262
Fax: 216-421-3217
e-mail: cleveland.webmaster@va.gov
www.cleveland.va.gov
The Louis Stokes Cleveland VA Medical Center is one of five facilities constituting the VA Healthcare System of Ohio. A full range of primary, secondary and tertiary care services are offered at the Cleveland VA Medical Center to an eligible Veteran population covering 24 counties in Northeast Ohio. Care is provided to more than 105,000 Veterans each year through an inpatient tertiary care facility (Wade Park), 13 Multi-Specialty Clinics, Vet Centers, and numerous community-based contract nursin
Susan Fuehrer, Director
Darwin Goodspeed, Associate Director

10309 Veterans Adm. Medical Center: Dayton Dayton VA Medical Center
Dayton VA Medical Center
4100 W 3rd Street   937-268-6511
Dayton, OH 45428   800-368-8262
Fax: 937-262-2179
TTY: 800-829-4833
e-mail: 552webmaster@va.gov
www.dayton.va.gov
The Dayton VAMC is a state of the art teaching facility that has been serving Veterans for 146 years, having accepted its first patient in 1867. The Dayton VA Medical Center provides a full range of health care through medical, surgical, mental health (inpatient and outpatient), home and community health programs, geriatric (nursing home), physical medicine and therapy services, neurology, oncology, dentistry, and hospice.
Glenn Costie, Medical Center Director
Mark Murdock, Associate Director

10310 Veterans and Families Support Network Ohio
5488 State Route 7   216-457-0641
New Waterford, OH 44445   Fax: 216-457-1923
e-mail: VFSN@delphi.com
Gina Brown

Oklahoma

10311 American Veterans Justice Foundation
3908 NW Santa Fe   405-355-3811
Lawton, OK 73505   e-mail: dwolf@sirinet.net
Dannie Wolf

10312 Jack C. Montgomery VA Medical Center
Dayton VA Medical Center
1011 Honor Heights Drive   918-577-3000
Muskogee, OK 74401   888-397-8387
Fax: 918-680-3648
www.muskogee.va.gov
Our Community-Based Outpatient Clinic in Tulsa is also named after a Native American. On May 27, 2008, the Tulsa Clinic was re-dedicated as the Ernest Childers VA Outpatient Clinic after Ernest Childers, a WWII Veteran and Medal of Honor recipient.
James R. Floyd, FACHE, Director
Inez Reitz, Acting Associate Medical Center Director

10313 Veterans Adm. Medical Center: Oklahoma City
Oklahoma City VA Medical Center
921 NE 13th Street   405-456-1000
Oklahoma City, OK 73104   866-835-5273
Fax: 405-270-1560
www.oklahoma.va.gov
The Oklahoma City VAMC is a tertiary care facility, classified as a Clinical Referral Level III facility (VA complexity level rating of 1b). The Oklahoma City VAMC is a teaching hospital, providing a full range of patient care services, with state-of-the-art technology as well as education and research. Comprehensive health care is provided through primary care, tertiary care, and long-term care in areas of medicine, surgery, psychiatry, physical medicine and rehabilitation, neurology, oncology
Daniel L. Marsh, Director
Debra Colombe, Acting Associate Medical Center Director

Oregon

10314 Northwest Network
3710 SW U.S. Veterans Hospital Rd.   503-220-8262
Portland, OR 97239   800-949-1004
Fax: 360-737-1405
e-mail: Daniel.Herrigstad@va.gov
www.visn20.med.va.gov
The Portland VA Medical Center (PVAMC) is a 303-bed consolidated facility with two main divisions. The medical center serves as the quaternary referral center for Oregon, Southern Washington, and parts of Idaho for the U.S. Department of Veterans Affairs. The Portland VAMC is located atop Marquam Hill on 28.5 acres overlooking the city of Portland. In addition to comprehensive medical and mental health services, the Portland VAMC supports ongoing research and medical education, including nati
John E. Patrick, MBA, Director
David Stockwell, MHA, Deputy Director of Administration and Fi

10315 Northwest Vets for Peace
811 E Burnside Street   503-656-9785
Portland, OR 97214   e-mail: NWVP@teleport.com
Marvin Simmons

10316 Veterans Adm. Medical Center: Roseburg VA Roseburg Healthcare System
VA Roseburg Healthcare System
913 NW Garden Valley Boulevard   541-440-1000
Roseburg, OR 97471   800-549-8387
Fax: 541-440-1225
e-mail: visn20webmaster@va.gov
www.roseburg.va.gov
The VA Roseburg Healthcare System (VARHS) consists of one Veterans Health Administration (VHA) facility located in Roseburg, OR, and four Community Based Outpatient Clinics (CBOC). The Roseburg campus consists of 200 acres and 32 buildings. VARHS offers primary care and hospital services in medi-

cine, surgery and mental health for the 62,000 veterans who reside in Central and Southern Oregon and Northern California.
Carol Bogedain, Director
Steven J Broskey, Associate Director

10317 Veterans Adm. Medical Center: White City VA S Oregon Rehabilitation Center
VA Southern Oregonrehabilitation Center & Clinics
8495 Crater Lake Highway   541-826-2111
White City, OR 97503   800-809-8725
                               Fax: 541-830-3500
www.va.gov/directory/guide/facility.asp?
The SORCC provides a residential program with a two-fold mission of providing bio-psychosocial rehabilitation and long-term health maintenance. The SORCC offers an appropriate level of care for Veterans who do not require acute hospitalization or nursing home care but who cannot adequately provide for themselves in the community, and therefore need residential support. The SORCC adheres to Patient Centered Care Methodologies and Philosophy and provides safety, shelter, and food in a therapeutic,
Pam Harris, Human Resources Assistant

10318 Veterans Adm. Regional Office: Portland Portland VA Medical Center
Portland VA Medical Center
3710 SW US Veterans Hospital Road   503-220-8262
Portland, OR 97239   800-949-1004
                               Fax: 503-273-5319
e-mail: Daniel.Herrigstad@va.gov
www.portland.va.gov
The Portland VA Medical Center (PVAMC) is a 303-bed consolidated facility with two main divisions. The medical center serves as the quaternary referral center for Oregon, Southern Washington, and parts of Idaho for the U.S. Department of Veterans Affairs. The Portland VAMC is located atop Marquam Hill on 28.5 acres overlooking the city of Portland. In addition to comprehensive medical and mental health services, the Portland VAMC supports ongoing research and medical education, including nati
John E. Patrick, MBA, Director
Tom Anderson, MD, Chief of Staff

10319 Veterans Administration Domicillary
8495 Crater Lake Highway   541-826-2111
White City, OR 97503   Fax: 541-830-3519
e-mail: David.Schwing@med.va.gov
www1.va.gov/domiciliary

Pennsylvania

10320 Erie VA Medical Center
135 E 38th Street Blvd.   814-868-8661
Erie, PA 16504   800-274-8387
                               Fax: 814-860-2120
e-mail: vhaeriweb@va.gov
www.erie.va.gov
Today, Erie VAMC is recognized as one of the top-performing medical centers in the delivery of high-quality health care. My goal is to assist in accelerating the improvements in service provided by our facility to the veterans we serve. These improvements are tracked in three important areas: the satisfaction veterans experience, the quality of the service we provide, and the efficiency with which we provide care and services to you. I am committed to making sure you have access to these service
Michael D Adelman MD, Director
Melissa Sundin, Associate Director

10321 Pennsylvania Gulf War Veterans
RR 3   814-226-4084
Clarion, PA 16214   e-mail: kjsmith@penn.com
Kenneth J Smith, President
Daniel J Meck, VP

10322 VA Pittsburgh Healthcare System: University Drive Division
University Drive   412-822-3578
Pittsburgh, PA 15240   866-482-7488
                               Fax: 412-688-6121
e-mail: vhapthwebmanager@va.gov
www.va.gov/pittsburgh

Terry Gerigk Wolf, Director
Rajiv Jain MD, Chief of Staff

10323 VA Stars & Stripes Healthcare Network
1010 Delafield Road   412-688-6000
Pittsburgh, PA 15240   866-482-7488
                               Fax: 412-784-3724
e-mail: vhapthwebmanager@va.gov
www.visn4.va.gov
VA Pittsburgh Healthcare System (VAPHS) is a two-campus, integrated healthcare system that proudly serves the Veteran population throughout the tri-state area of Pennsylvania, Ohio and West Virginia. VAPHS consists of two clinical care facilities in Pittsburgh as well as five community based outpatient clinics.
Michael E Moreland FACHE, Network Director
Carla Acre Sivek, MSW, Deputy Network Director

10324 Veterans Adm. Medical Center: Philadelphia
Philadelphia VA Medical Center
University & Woodland Avenues   215-823-5800
Philadelphia, PA 19104   877-626-2500
                               Fax: 215-823-6007
www.va.gov

10325 Veterans Adm. Medical Center: Coatesville
Coatesville VA Medical Center
1400 Black Horse Hill Road   610-384-7711
Coatesville, PA 19320   800-290-6172
e-mail: VHACOAWebOperations@va.gov
www.coatesville.va.gov
Coatesville VA Medical Center is an integrated health care system dedicated to providing the best in care and services to our nation's Veterans. The hospital offers health care that is continuously improving, patient-centered, data-driven and team-based and includes mental health care, primary care, geriatrics and extended care, specialty and women's health care, and pharmacy and social work services, and more for both inpatients and outpatients. Additionally, the medical center operates communi
Gary W. Devansky, MHA, Director
Jonathan Eckman, P.E, Associate Director

10326 Veterans Adm. Medical Center: Lebanon Lebanon VA Medical Center
Lebanon VA Medical Center
1700 S Lincoln Avenue   717-272-6621
Lebanon, PA 17042   800-409-8771
                               Fax: 717-228-5907
e-mail: douglas.etter@va.gov
www.lebanon.va.gov
VAMC MISSION AND VISION: Honor America's Veterans by providing exceptional health care that improves their health and well-being. To be a patient-centered integrated health care organization for Veterans providing excellent health care, research, and education; an organization where people choose to work; an active community partner; and a back-up for national emergencies.
Robert W Callahan Jr, Director
Robin C. Aube-Warren, Associate Director

10327 Veterans Adm. Medical Center: Pittsburg VA Pittsburgh Healthcare System
VA Pittsburgh Healthcare System
University Drive   412-822-3578
Pittsburgh, PA 15240   866-482-7488
                               Fax: 412-365-4213
e-mail: vhapthwebmanager@va.gov
www.pittsburgh.va.gov
VA Pittsburgh Healthcare System (VAPHS) is a two-campus, integrated healthcare system that proudly serves the Veteran population throughout the tri-state area of Pennsylvania, Ohio and West Virginia. VAPHS consists of two clinical care facilities in Pittsburgh as well as five community based outpatient clinics.
Terry Gerigk Wolf, Director
Ali Sonel, MD, Chief of Staff

10328 Wilkes-Barre VA Medical Center
1111 E End Boulevard   570-824-3521
Wilkes-Barre, PA 18711   877-928-2621
                               Fax: 570-821-7278
www.wilkes-barre.va.gov
For over 50 years, VAMC Wilkes-Barre has been improving the health of the men and women who have so proudly served our nation. We consider it our privilege to serve your health care needs in

any way we can. Services are available but not limited to veterans living in 18 counties in Pennsylvania and one county in New York.
Margaret B. Caplan, Director
Joseph F. Sharon, Interim Associate Director

Rhode Island

10329 Veterans Adm. Medical Center: Providence Providence VA Medical Center
Providence VA Medical Center
830 Chalkstone Avenue   401-273-7100
Providence, RI 02908-4799   866-363-4486
                                        Fax: 401-457-3370
                                       www.providence.va.gov
The Providence VA Medical Center is dedicated to providing high quality comprehensive outpatient and inpatient health care to Veterans residing in Rhode Island and southeastern Massachusetts. Each veteran who comes to the Medical Center for care is assured personalized care by a team of health care providers. A Primary Care Provider coordinates each patient's medical care, patient education needs and referrals to any of the medical centers 32 subspecialty clinics. The Medical Center's Ambulatory
Vincent Ng, Director
Erin Clare Sears, Associate Director

South Carolina

10330 Ralph H. Johnson VA Medical Center
109 Bee Street   843-577-5011
Charleston, SC 29401-5799   888-878-6884
                                        Fax: 843-937-6100
                                       e-mail: kevin.abel@va.gov
                                       www.charleston.va.gov
The Ralph H. Johnson VA Medical Center serves more than 53,000 Veterans in 22 counties along the South Carolina and Georgia coastline in our main medical center or one of six community-based outpatient clinics.
Carolyn L. Adams, Director
Mr. Scott R Isaacks, MBA, FAAMA, Associate Director

10331 William Jennings Bryan Dorn VA Medical Center
6439 Garners Ferry Road   803-776-4000
Columbia, SC 29209   800-293-8262
                                        Fax: 803-695-6739
                                       www.columbiasc.va.gov
The William Jennings Bryan Dorn VA Medical Center (VAMC) opened in 1932 at its current location. Dorn VAMC is a 216 authorized bed facility (204 operating as of November 2012), which includes acute medical, surgical, psychiatric, and long-term care. The hospital provides primary, secondary, and some tertiary care. In 2012, the medical center served over 73,690 uniques Veterans during FY 2012. There were 906,858 (not unique) outpatient visits and a total of 4,821 inpatient treated.
Carolyn L. Adams, MS, Interim Medical Center Director
David L. Omura, DPT, MHA, MS, Associate Director

South Dakota

10332 Sioux Falls VA Healthcare System
2501 W 22nd Street   605-336-3230
Sioux Falls, SD 57105-5046   800-316-8387
                                        Fax: 605-333-6878
                                       e-mail: daniel.deblock@va.gov
                                       www.siouxfalls.va.gov
Healthcare for eligible veterans.The Sioux Falls VA Health Care System includes a 98-bed medical center and five Community Based Outpatient Clinics. It provides inpatient and outpatient care for Veterans in eastern South Dakota, southwestern Minnesota, and northwestern Iowa. Services include primary and specialty medical care, mental health services, and rehabilitation. Affiliated with The Sanford School of Medicine of the University of South Dakota, it supports residency programs in internal me
Sandra L. Horsman, Acting Director
Sara Ackert, MS, Associate Director

10333 VA Black Hills Health Care System- Fort Meade Campus
113 Comanche Road   605-347-2511
Fort Meade, SD 57741   800-743-1070
                                        Fax: 605-347-7171
                                       e-mail: BlackHillsVAFOIA.gov@va.gov
                                       www.blackhills.va.gov
VA Black Hills Health Care System provides primary and secondary medical and surgical care, along with residential rehabilitation treatment program (RRTP) services, extended nursing home care and tertiary psychiatric inpatient services for Veterans residing in South Dakota, portions of Nebraska, North Dakota, Wyoming and Montana. Care is delivered through the Fort Meade and Hot Springs VA Medical Centers, as well as through a number of community based outpatient and rural outreach clinics.
Stephen R. DiStasio, FACHE, Director
C.B. Alexander, FACHE, Associate Director

10334 VA Black Hills Health Care System- Hot Springs Campus
500 N 5th Street   605-745-2000
Hot Springs, SD 57747   800-764-5370
                                        Fax: 605-745-2091
                                       e-mail: BlackHillsVAFOIA.gov@va.gov
                                       www.blackhills.va.gov
VA Black Hills Health Care System provides primary and secondary medical and surgical care, along with residential rehabilitation treatment program (RRTP) services, extended nursing home care and tertiary psychiatric inpatient services for Veterans residing in South Dakota, portions of Nebraska, North Dakota, Wyoming and Montana. Care is delivered through the Fort Meade and Hot Springs VA Medical Centers, as well as through a number of community based outpatient and rural outreach clinics.
Stephen R. DiStasio, FACHE, Director
C.B. Alexander, FACHE, Associate Director

Tennessee

10335 Mountain Home VA Medical Center
Corner of Lamont & Veterans Way   423-926-1171
Mountain Home, TN 37684   877-573-3529
                                        Fax: 423-979-3519
                                       e-mail: mouwebmaster@va.gov
                                       www.mountainhome.va.gov
Since 1903, James H. Quillen VA Medical Center has been improving the health of the men and women who have so proudly served our nation. We consider it our privilege to serve your health care needs in any way we can. Services are available to more than 170,000 veterans living in a 41-county area of Tennessee, Virginia, Kentucky, and North Carolina.
Charlene S. Ehret, FACHE, Director
Daniel B. Snyder III, P.E., MBA, Associate Director

10336 Persian Gulf Information Network
PO Box 10160   931-674-1518
Clarksville, TN 37042   Fax: 615-431-5222
                                       e-mail: pgin@knightwave.com
                                       www.home.att.net/~vetcenter/vetgrps.htm
Paul Lyons

10337 Tennessee Valley Healthcare System- Nashville Campus
1310 24th Avenue, South   615-327-4751
Nashville, TN 37212-2637   800-228-4973
                                        Fax: 615-321-6350
                                       www.tennesseevalley.va.gov
TVHS provides ambulatory care, primary care, and secondary care in acute medicine and surgery, specialized tertiary care, transplant services, spinal cord injury, outpatient care, and a full range of extended care and mental health services. The Nashville Campus is the only VA facility that supports all solid organ transplant programs, including total in-house kidney and bone marrow transplants. The Alvin C. York Campus is a network referral center for mental health services, geriatrics, and ext
Juan A. Morales, RN, MSN, Health System Director
Gary Trende, Chief Operating Officer, Nashville Camp

10338 Tennessee Valley Healthcare System- Alvin C. York (Murfreesboro) Campus
3400 Lebanon Pike   615-867-6000
Murfreesboro, TN 37129   800-876-7093
                                Fax: 615-225-4901
                        e-mail: TVHWebmaster@va.gov
                              www.tennesseevalley.va.gov
TVHS has active affiliations with two local institutions. The Alvin C. York Campus is primarily affiliated with Meharry Medical College, with active residency programs in oral surgery, psychiatry, general internal medicine, occupational medicine, preventive medicine, geriatric medicine, and family practice. The Nashville Campus is primarily affiliated with the Vanderbilt University School of Medicine with active residency programs in all major medical and surgical specialties and sub-specialties
Juan A. Morales, RN, MSN, Health System Director
Suzanne Jen, Chief Operating Officer, Murfreesboro

10339 VISN 9: VA Mid South Healthcare Network
1801 W End Avenue   615-695-2200
Nashville, TN 37203   Fax: 615-321-2721
                          e-mail: VISN9FOIA@va.gov
                                www.visn9.va.gov
VA MidSouth Healthcare Network (VISN 9) is committed to providing high quality, innovative, comprehensive, and compassionate care. VISN 9's goal is to ensure access for all enrolled veterans to the right care, at the right time, and at the right place to better serve Veterans in Huntington, West Virginia, Tennessee, Kentucky, and surrounding areas.

10340 Veterans Adm. Medical Center: Murfreesboro
3400 Lebanon Road   615-893-1360
Murfreesboro, TN 37130   Fax: 615-898-4872

10341 Veterans Adm. Medical Center: Memphis
1030 Jefferson Avenue   901-523-8990
Memphis, TN 38104   800-636-8262
                              www.memphis.va.gov
Since 1922, VAMC Memphis has been improving the health of the men and women who have so proudly served our nation. We consider it our privilege to serve your health care needs in any way we can. Services are available to more than 196,000 veterans living in a 53-county area of western Tennessee, northern Mississippi, and northwest Arkansas.
Jimmy H. McGlawn, MPH, Interim Medical Center Director/CEO
Douglas D. Southall, FACHE, Assistant Medical Center Director

10342 Veterans Adm. Medical Center: Muskogee
3400 Lebanon Pike   615-867-6000
Murfreesboro, TN 37129   Fax: 615-225-4901
                              www.tennesseevalley.va.gov

10343 Veterans Adm. Medical Center: Nashville
1310 24th Avenue S   615-327-4751
Nashville, TN 37212   800-228-4973
                                Fax: 901-577-7306
                              www.tennesseevalley.va.gov
TVHS has active affiliations with two local institutions. The Alvin C. York Campus is primarily affiliated with Meharry Medical College, with active residency programs in oral surgery, psychiatry, general internal medicine, occupational medicine, preventive medicine, geriatric medicine, and family practice. The Nashville Campus is primarily affiliated with the Vanderbilt University School of Medicine with active residency programs in all major medical and surgical specialties and sub-specialties
Juan A. Morales, RN, MSN, Health System Director
Gary Trende, Chief Operating Officer, Nashville Camp

10344 Veterans Affairs Medical Center
1030 Jefferson Avenue   901-523-8990
Memphis, TN 38104   800-636-8262
                                Fax: 901-577-7251
                              www.memphis.va.gov
Since 1922, VAMC Memphis has been improving the health of the men and women who have so proudly served our nation. We consider it our privilege to serve your health care needs in any way we can. Services are available to more than 196,000 veterans living in a 53-county area of western Tennessee, northern Mississippi, and northwest Arkansas.
Jimmy H. McGlawn, MPH, Interim Medical Center Director/CEO
Douglas D. Southall, FACHE, Assistant Medical Center Director

10345 Veterans Affairs Medical Center, Memphis, Tennessee
1030 Jefferson Avenue   901-523-8990
Memphis, TN 38104   Fax: 901-577-7251
                              www.memphis.va.gov
Since 1922, VAMC Memphis has been improving the health of the men and women who have so proudly served our nation. We consider it our privilege to serve your health care needs in any way we can. Services are available to more than 196,000 veterans living in a 53-county area of western Tennessee, northern Mississippi, and northwest Arkansas.
Jimmy H. McGlawn, MPH, Interim Medical Center Director/CEO
Douglas D. Southall, FACHE, Assistant Medical Center Director

Texas

10346 Amarillo VA Health Care System
6010 Amarillo Boulevard W   806-355-9703
Amarillo, TX 79106   800-687-8262
                                Fax: 806-354-7860
                        e-mail: AMARILLOFOIA@VA.GOV
                              www.amarillo.va.gov
The Amarillo VA Health Care System, a division of the Southwest VA Health Care Network (VISN 18), provides primary specialty, and extended care of the highest quality to veterans throughout the Texas and Oklahoma panhandles, eastern New Mexico, and southern Kansas. Approximately 25,000 patients are treated annually. The health care system maintains 55 acute care inpatient beds for general medical, surgical, and intensive care. Geriatric and extended care is provided in the 120-bed skilled nursin
Andrew M. Welch, MHA, FACHE, Director
Gerald Darnell, Pys.D., Associate Director

10347 Austin Outpatient Clinic
7901 Metropolis Drive   512-823-4000
Austin, TX 78744   Fax: 512-389-6545
                          www.centraltexas.va.gov/locations/Austin
The clinic is 184,000 square feet - the largest, free-standing VA outpatient clinic in the nation. The clinic will offer expanded services for oncology; chemotherapy; ear, nose and throat; orthopedic services; minor surgeries; urology; gastroenterology; an endoscopy suite, and additional space for the Women's Clinic and all current services.
Russell E Lloyd, Associate Director of Resources
William F Harper, MD, FACP, Chief of Staff

10348 Central Texas Veterans Health Care System
1901 Veterans Memorial Drive   254-778-4811
Temple, TX 76504   800-423-2111
                        e-mail: Deborah.Meyer@va.gov
                              www.centraltexas.va.gov
The Central Texas Veterans Health Care System (CTVHCS), accredited by the Joint Commission, is comprised of two large Department of Veterans Affairs (VA) medical centers located in Temple and Waco, one stand-alone outpatient clinic in Austin, four community based outpatient clinics located in Brownwood, Bryan/College Station, Cedar Park, and Palestine plus a rural outreach clinic in La Grange. The system is one of the largest integrated health care systems in the United States and provides a ful
Russell E Lloyd, Associate Director of Resources
William F Harper, MD, FACP, Chief of Staff

10349 El Paso VA Health Care Center
5001 N Piedras   915-564-6100
El Paso, TX 79930-4211   800-672-3782
                                Fax: 915-564-7920
                              www.elpaso.va.gov
The El Paso VA Health Care System serves Veterans in far Southwest Texas and Doña Ana County, New Mexico. The El Paso VA Health Care System (VAHCS) includes the main health care facility located adjacent to William Beaumont Army Medical Center (WBAMC) on Ft. Bliss, Texas, and two VA-staffed Community Based Outpatient Clinics (CBOC) - one in Las Cruces, New Mexico, the second in east El Paso. The VAHCS provides primary and

specialized ambulatory care services at its main campus with consultants

John A. Mendoza, Director
Elizabeth Lowery, Associate Director

10350 Michael E. DeBakey VA Medical Center
2002 Holcombe Boulevard   713-791-1414
Houston, TX 77030-4298   800-553-2278
                                 Fax: 713-794-7218
                    e-mail: vhahoupublicaffairs@va.gov
                                 www.houston.va.gov
Awarded re-designation for Magnet Recognition for Excellence in Nursing Services in 2008, the Michael E. DeBakey VA Medical Center serves as the primary health care provider for almost 130,000 veterans in southeast Texas. Veterans from around the country are referred to the MEDVAMC for specialized diagnostic care, radiation therapy, surgery, and medical treatment including cardiovascular surgery, gastrointestinal endoscopy, nuclear medicine, ophthalmology, and treatment of spinal cord injury and

Adam C. Walmus, M.H.A., F.A.C.H, Medical Center Director
Bryan T. Bayley, M.H.A., F.A.C.H, Deputy Medical Center Director

10351 Operation Desert Shield/Desert Storm
Odessa, TX 79760   915-368-4667
                                 Fax: 915-580-7451

Vic Sylvester

10352 Persian Gulf Veterans of America
San Antonio, TX 78280   210-666-4409
                    e-mail: KathyPGVA@aol.com

Kathy Hughes

10353 South Texas Veterans Health Care System
7400 Merton Minter   210-617-5300
San Antonio, TX 78229   877-469-5300
                                 www.southtexas.va.gov
South Texas Veterans Health Care System (STVHCS) is comprised of two inpatient campuses: the Audie L. Murphy Memorial VA Hospital in San Antonio and the Kerrville VA Hospital in Kerrville, Texas. STVHCS serves one of the largest primary service areas in the nation and is part of the VA Heart of Texas Veterans Integrated Service Network (VISN 17), with offices located in Arlington, Texas. With an FY12 budget for STVHCS of $605 million and more than 3,400 employees, South Texas provides health ca

Marie L. Weldon, Director
Wade Vlosich, Associate Director

10354 VA Heart of Texas Health Care Network Dallas VA Medical Center
Dallas VA Medical Center
4500 S Lancaster Road   214-742-8387
Dallas, TX 75216   800-849-3597
                                 Fax: 214-857-1171
                                 www.northtexas.va.gov
VANTHCS provides comprehensive health services through primary, tertiary and long-term care in many areas like medicine, surgery, mental health and rehabilitation. The 853-bed system has a Spinal Cord Injury Center, Domiciliary Care Program and Community Living Center with a dedicated hospice unit. In 2009, a Fisher House was established on the Dallas campus to provide no-cost temporary lodging in a home-like setting for families of Veterans or active duty military personnel undergoing treatment

Jeffery L. Milligan, Director
Peter Dancy, Associate Director

10355 Veterans Adm. Medical Center: Big Spring
300 Veterans Boulevard   432-263-7361
Big Spring, TX 79720-5500   800-472-1365
                                 Fax: 432-264-4834
                                 www.bigspring.va.gov
The West Texas VA Health Care System (WTVAHCS) proudly serves Veterans in 33 counties across 53,000 square miles of rural geography in West Texas and Eastern New Mexico. The George H. O'Brien, Jr. VA Medical Center is located in Big Spring, Texas and the six Community Based Outpatient Clinics (CBOC's) that comprise the remainder of the health care system are located in Abilene, TX, Stamford, TX, San Angelo, TX, Odessa, TX, Fort

Stockton, TX, and Hobbs, NM. Two Vet Centers also provide services a

Andrew M. Welch, Interim Director
Kenneth Allensworth, Associate Director

10356 Veterans Adm. Medical Center: Dallas
4500 S Lancaster Road   214-742-8387
Dallas, TX 75216   800-849-3597
                                 Fax: 214-857-1171
                                 www.northtexas.va.gov
VA North Texas Health Care System (VANTHCS) is a progressive health care provider in the heart of Texas. Poised as VA's second largest health care system, we serve over 113,000 Veterans and deliver 1.4 million outpatient episodes of care each year to Veterans in 38 Texas counties and two counties in southern Oklahoma. We have 4,700 employees and 1,700 community volunteers who are driven by the passion to serve at Dallas VA Medical Center, Sam Rayburn Memorial Veterans Center, Fort Worth Outpatie

Jeffery L. Milligan, Director
Peter Dancy, Associate Director

10357 Veterans Adm. Medical Center: Kerrville
3600 Memorial Boulevard   830-896-2020
Kerrville, TX 78028   866-487-7653
                                 www.southtexas.va.gov
The Kerrville VA Hospital (KVAH), located 65 miles northwest of San Antonio, provides primary care, some specialty care, geriatric evaluation and management, palliative care, and long-term care services with a Community Living Center. The Satellite Clinic Division (SCD) offer primary care and some specialty care while sharing resources with each other and their respective communities. When required, Veterans are referred to ALMMVAH or KVAH for specialty care including medicine, surgery, neurop

Marie L. Weldon, Director
Joe A. Perez, Assistant Director

10358 Veterans Adm. Medical Center: Marlin
1016 Ward Street   254-883-3511
Marlin, TX 76661   Fax: 254-883-9240
                                 www.southtexas.va.gov

10359 Veterans Adm. Medical Center: San Antonio
7400 Merton Minter Boulevard   210-617-5300
San Antonio, TX 78229   877-469-5300
                                 www.southtexas.va.gov
South Texas Veterans Health Care System (STVHCS) is comprised of two inpatient campuses: the Audie L. Murphy Memorial VA Hospital in San Antonio and the Kerrville VA Hospital in Kerrville, Texas. STVHCS serves one of the largest primary service areas in the nation and is part of the VA Heart of Texas Veterans Integrated Service Network (VISN 17), with offices located in Arlington, Texas. With an FY12 budget for STVHCS of $605 million and more than 3,400 employees, South Texas provides health ca

Marie L. Weldon, Director
Wade Vlosich, Associate Director

10360 Veterans Adm. Medical Center: Temple
1901 Veterans Memorial Drive   254-778-4811
Temple, TX 76504   800-423-2111
                                 Fax: 254-771-4588
                    e-mail: Deborah.Meyer@va.gov
                                 www.centraltexas.va.gov
The Central Texas Veterans Health Care System (CTVHCS), accredited by the Joint Commission, is comprised of two large Department of Veterans Affairs (VA) medical centers located in Temple and Waco, one stand-alone outpatient clinic in Austin, four community based outpatient clinics located in Brownwood, Bryan/College Station, Cedar Park, and Palestine plus a rural outreach clinic in La Grange. The system is one of the largest integrated health care systems in the United States and provides a ful

Russell E Lloyd, Associate Director of Resources
William F Harper, MD, FACP, Chief of Staff

10361 Waco VA Medical Center
4800 Memorial Drive   254-752-6581
Waco, TX 76711   800-423-2111
                    e-mail: Deborah.Meyer@va.gov
                                 www.centraltexas.va.gov

The Central Texas Veterans Health Care System (CTVHCS), accredited by the Joint Commission, is comprised of two large Department of Veterans Affairs (VA) medical centers located in Temple and Waco, one stand-alone outpatient clinic in Austin, four community based outpatient clinics located in Brownwood, Bryan/College Station, Cedar Park, and Palestine plus a rural outreach clinic in La Grange. The system is one of the largest integrated health care systems in the United States and provides a ful

Russell E Lloyd, Associate Director of Resources
William F Harper, MD, FACP, Chief of Staff

10362 West Texas VA Health Care System
300 Veterans Boulevard
Big Spring, TX 79720

432-263-7361
800-472-1365
Fax: 432-264-4834
www.bigspring.va.gov

The West Texas VA Health Care System (WTVAHCS) proudly serves Veterans in 33 counties across 53,000 square miles of rural geography in West Texas and Eastern New Mexico. The George H. O'Brien, Jr. VA Medical Center is located in Big Spring, Texas and the six Community Based Outpatient Clinics (CBOC's) that comprise the remainder of the health care system are located in Abilene, TX, Stamford, TX, San Angelo, TX, Odessa, TX, Fort Stockton, TX, and Hobbs, NM. Two Vet Centers also provide services a

Andrew M. Welch, Interim Director
Kenneth Allensworth, Associate Director

Utah

10363 VA Salt Lake City Health Care System
500 Foothill Drive
Salt Lake City, UT 84148

801-582-1565
800-613-4012
Fax: 801-584-1289
www.saltlakecity.va.gov

The George E. Wahlen Department of Veterans Affairs Medical Center is a mid-sized affiliated tertiary care facility with 121 authorized active beds. It is a teaching facility, providing a full range of patient care services, with state-of-the-art technology as well as education and research. Comprehensive health care is provided through primary care, tertiary care, and long-term care in areas of medicine, surgery, psychiatry, physical medicine and rehabilitation, neurology, oncology, dentistry,

Steven W. Young, FACHE, Director
Warren E. Hill, Associate Director

Vermont

10364 White River Junction VA Medical Center
215 N Main Street
White River Junction, VT 05009

802-295-9363
866-687-8387
Fax: 802-296-6354
www.whiteriver.va.gov

The White River Junction VA Medical Center (WRJ VAMC) is responsible for the delivery of health care services to eligible Veterans in Vermont and the 4 contiguous counties of New Hampshire. These services are delivered at the Medical Center's main campus located in White River Junction, Vermont, and at its seven Outpatient Clinics (Bennington, Brattleboro, Colchester, Newport, and Rutland, Vermont; Keene and Littleton, New Hampshire). The White River Junction VA is closely affiliated with the Ge

Deborah Amdur, Director
Danielle S Ocker, RN, BSN, Associate Director

Virginia

10365 Desert Storm Justice Foundation: Virginia
Alexandria, VA 22309

703-550-1346
Fax: 703-550-1346

10366 Gulf War Veterans of Virginia
Chesapeake, VA 23320

757-988-3PGW

Ted Myers, President

10367 Veterans Adm. Medical Center: Hampton Hampton VA Medical Center
Hampton VA Medical Center

100 Emancipation Drive
Hampton, VA 23667

757-722-9961
888-869-6060
Fax: 757-723-6620
www.hampton.va.gov

The Hampton VAMC is a tertiary care, Complexity Level 2 hospital. Hampton VAMC provides comprehensive primary and specialty care in medicine, surgery, and psychiatry. The Medical Center is geographically positioned among one of the largest DoD active duty and military retiree populations in the United States. As a result, the Medical Center has seen a 7% increase among Veterans seeking VA care. The Hampton VAMC recently opened a state-of-the-art Women's Clinic designed to provide gender speci

Michael H. Dunfee, MHA, Medical Center Director
Benita K. Miller, MHA, FACHE, Associate for Operations Director

10368 Veterans Adm. Medical Center: Richmond Hunter Holmes McGuire VA Medical Center
Hunter Holmes McGuire VA Medical Center
1201 Broad Rock Boulevard
Richmond, VA 23249

804-675-5000
800-784-8381
Fax: 804-675-5581
www.richmond.va.gov

Since 1946, the Richmond VAMC has been improving the health of the men and women who have so proudly served our nation. We consider it our privilege to serve your health care needs in any way we can. Services are available to more than 200,000 veterans coming from 52 cities and counties covering 22,515 miles of central and southern Virginia and parts of northern North Carolina.

John A. Brandecker, Director
David P. Budinger, FACHE, Associate Director for Operations

10369 Veterans Adm. Medical Center: Roanoke Roanoke Vet Center
Roanoke Vet Center
350 Albemarle Avenue SW
Roanoke, VA 24016

540-342-9726
877-927-8387
Fax: 540-857-2405
www.va.gov

Lynn McGhee, Team Leader
John Whitlock, Counselor

10370 Veterans Adm. Medical Center: Salem Salem VA Medical Center
Salem VA Medical Center
1970 Roanoke Boulevard
Salem, VA 24153

540-982-2463
888-982-2463
Fax: 540-983-1096
www.salem.va.gov

Since 1934, Salem VAMC has been improving the health of the men and women who have so proudly served our Nation. We consider it our privilege to serve your health care needs in any way we can. Services are available to more than 112,500 Veterans living in a 26-county area of southwestern Virginia.

Miguel H LaPuz, MD, MBA, Director, SAMVAMC
Rebecca J. Stackhouse, FACHE, VHA-, Associate Director

Washington

10371 Persian Gulf Veterans of Washington
13523 202nd Street E
Graham, WA 98338

360-893-2480
Fax: 360-893-3998
e-mail: amehl@ix.netcom.com

10372 VA Puget Sound Health Care Network
1660 S Columbian Way
Seattle, WA 98108

206-762-1010
800-329-8387
Fax: 206-764-2224
www.pugetsound.va.gov

With a reputation for excellence, innovation and extraordinary care of our Nation's heroes, VA Puget Sound strives to lead the nation in terms of quality, efficiency and public service through its proven record of innovation and extraordinary care of Veterans. As the primary referral site for VA's northwest region, VA Puget Sound provides care for Veteran populations encompassing Alaska, Montana, Idaho and Oregon.

Michael J. Murphy, FACHE, Director
Michael Tadych, Deputy Director

10373 Veterans Adm. Medical Center: Spokane Spokane VA Medical Center
Spokane VA Medical Center

4815 N Assembly Street
Spokane, WA 99205-6197

509-434-7000
800-325-7940
Fax: 509-434-7119
www.spokane.va.gov

The Spokane VA Medical Center is dedicated to providing quality health care services to veterans. In carrying out this mission, the VAMC focuses on providing primary and secondary care, with emphasis on preventive health and chronic disease management.

10374 Veterans Adm. Medical Center: Tacoma Tacoma Vet Center

Tacoma Vet Center
4916 Center Street
Tacoma, WA 98409

253-565-7038
877-927-8387
Fax: 253-565-4981
www.va.gov

Robert Ramsey, Team Leader
George Rippon, Counselor

10375 Veterans Adm. Medical Center: Walla Walla Johnathan M. Wainwright Memorial VA MC

Johnathan M. Wainwright Memorial VA Medical Center
77 Wainwright Drive
Walla Walla, WA 99362

509-525-5200
888-687-8863
Fax: 509-527-3452
www.wallawalla.va.gov

Since 1921, the Jonathan M. Wainwright Memorial VA Medical Center (Walla Walla VAMC) has been improving the health of the men and women who have so proudly served our nation. We consider it our privilege to serve your health care needs in any way we can. Services are available to Veterans living in eastern Washington and Oregon and western Idaho. We pride ourselves in giving the best care - anywhere!

West Virginia

10376 Veterans Adm. Medical Center: Beckley

Beckley VA Medical Center
200 Veterans Avenue
Beckley, WV 25801

304-255-2121
877-902-5142
Fax: 304-255-2431
www.beckley.va.gov

Beckley VAMC is a 40-bed general medical and surgical care facility with a 50-bed community living center. The medical center is a Joint Commission accredited, rural access facility. The community living center offers skilled nursing care, post-acute rehabilitation and restorative care, palliative care, and respite care for eligible Veterans. The medical center also operates a home based primary care program.

Karin L McGraw, Director
J. Brian Nimmo, Associate Director

10377 Veterans Adm. Medical Center: Clarksburg Louis A. Johnson VA Medical Center

Louis A. Johnson VA Medical Center
One Medical Center Drive
Clarksburg, WV 26301

304-623-3461
800-733-0512
Fax: 304-626-7026
www.clarksburg.va.gov

The Louis A. Johnson VA Medical Center exists to serve the veteran through the delivery of timely quality care by staff who demonstrate outstanding customer service, the advancement of health care through research, and the education of tomorrow's health care providers.

Beth M. Brown, MS, FACHE, VHA-C, Medical Center Director
Judy T. Finley, MBA, Associate Director

10378 Veterans Adm. Medical Center: Huntington

1540 Spring Valley Drive
Huntington, WV 25704

304-429-6741
800-827-8244
Fax: 304-429-6713
www.huntington.va.gov

Since 1932, VAMC Huntington has been improving the health of the men and women who have so proudly served our nation. We consider it our privilege to serve your health care needs in any way we can. Services are available to veterans living in southwestern West Virginia, southern Ohio, and eastern Kentucky.

Edward H Seiler, Medical Center Director
Pamela G Smith, Associate Medical Center Director

10379 Veterans Affairs Medical Center: Martinsburg

510 Butler Avenue
Martinsburg, WV 25405

304-263-0811
800-817-3807
Fax: 304-262-7448
www.martinsburg.va.gov

Since 1944, the Martinsburg VA Medical Center has been improving the health of the men and women who have so proudly served our nation. We consider it our privilege to serve your health care needs in any way we can. Services are available to more than 126,000 veterans living in 22 counties in Western Maryland, West Virginia, South Central Pennsylvania, and Northwest Virginia.

Ann R. Brown, FACHE, Medical Center Director
Timothy J. Cooke, Associate Medical Center Director

Wisconsin

10380 Clement J. Zablocki Veterans Affairs Medical Center

5000 W National Avenue
Milwaukee, WI 53295-1000

414-384-2000
Fax: 414-382-5321
e-mail: vhamiwwebmaster@va.gov
www.milwaukee.va.gov

The Clement J. Zablocki VA Medical Center is located on 125 acres on the western edge of Milwaukee and part of VA Integrated Services Network 12 (VISN 12), which includes facilities in Iron Mountain, MI; Tomah and Madison, WI, and North Chicago, Hines, and Chicago. The Medical Center delivers primary, secondary, and tertiary medical care in 168 care acute operating beds and provides over 500,000 visits annually through an extensive outpatient program. The nursing home care unit of 113 beds offer

Robert H. Beller, FACHE, Medical Center Director
James McLain, Deputy Medical Center Director

10381 Gulf War Veterans of Wisconsin

33 University Square
Madison, WI 53715

608-250-9645
e-mail: gulfwarwisc@geocities.com

Anthony Hardie

10382 MidWest Gulf War Veterans Association

Pewaukee, WI 53072

414-695-8694
Fax: 414-695-8694
e-mail: mrlbrty@execpc.com

Robert Schramm

10383 Veterans Adm. Medical Center: Tomah

500 E Veterans Street
Tomah, WI 54660

608-372-3971
800-872-8662
www.tomah.va.gov

VAMC Tomah has been improving the health of the men and women who have so proudly served our nation. We consider it our privilege to serve your health care needs in any way we can. Services are available to veterans living in a Western/Central area of Wisconsin.

Mario V. DeSanctis, FACHE, Medical Center Director
David Huffman, M.S., Associate Director

10384 William S. Middleton Memorial Veterans Hospital

2500 Overlook Terrace
Madison, WI 53705-2286

608-256-1901
888-478-8321
Fax: 608-280-7096
www.madison.va.gov

The Madison VA Hospital is one of seven facilities that comprise Veterans Integrated Services Network 12 which is administratively headquartered at Hines, IL, and includes facilities in Illinois, Wisconsin, and Michigan.

Judy K. McKee, FACHE, Director
John Rohrer, Associate Director

Wyoming

10385 Veterans Adm. Medical Center: Cheyenne

2360 E Pershing Boulevard
Cheyenne, WY 82001

307-778-7550
888-483-9127
Fax: 307-778-7336
www.cheyenne.va.gov

Cheyenne VAMC Police Service is responsible for providing a safe and secure environment for all patients, staff, and visitors to the property. The Police Service is on-duty and available for the facility/Staff 24/7/365 with professionally trained and conscientious officers.

Cynthia McCormack, RN, PhD, Medical Center Director
Paul L Roberts, Medical Center Associate Director

10386 Veterans Adm. Medical Center: Sheridan
1898 Fort Road 307-672-3473
Sheridan, WY 82801 866-822-6714
Fax: 307-672-1900
e-mail: sheridanwebmaster@va.gov
www.sheridan.va.gov
Since April 1922, the Sheridan VAMC has been a mental health care and primary care facility for men and women who have served their country. In 1898 the grounds that are now the Sheridan VAMC were set aside by President William McKinley to be a military fort. The fort was named after Brigadier General Ranald Slidell Mackenzie. The first troops to the fort in 1901 were Buffalo Soldiers who used the fort for rest and retraining. By World War I, the fort was closed and ready for demolition. Ho

Debra L. Hirschman, Director
Michele Beach, Associate Director/Chief Business Offic

Libraries & Resource Centers

10387 American GI Forum NVOP
611 N. Flores 210-212-4088
San Antonio, TX 78205 Fax: 210-223-4970
e-mail: nvopweb@agif-nvop.org
www.agif-nvop.org
Our Mision is to establish and maintain a comprehensive community service agency with a diversified funding source that will serve the needs of veterans, their families, and other needy individuals of the community.

10388 COPIN Foundation
2644 North Avenue 716-283-5622
Niagara Falls, NY 14305 Fax: 716-283-5721

10389 Kennedy-Krieger Institute
707 N Broadway 443-923-9200
Baltimore, MD 21205 800-873-3377
Fax: 443-923-9405
www.kennedykrieger.org
Kennedy Krieger Institute is an internationally recognized institution dedicated to improving the lives of individuals with disorders of the brain, spinal cord, and musculoskeletal system through Patient Care, Research and Professional Training, Special Education and Community. We at the Kennedy Krieger Institute dedicate ourselves to helping children and adolescents with disorders of the brain, spinal cord and musculoskeletal system achieve their potential and participate as fully as possible i

Jennifer Accardo, M.D., Neurologist
Adrianna Amari, Ph.D., Training and research coordinator

10390 Shriver Center University Affiliated Program
Eunice Kennedy Shriver Center
200 Trapelo Road 781-642-0001
Waltham, MA 02452-6319 e-mail: shriver.center@umassmed.edu
www.umassmed.edu/shriver
The Eunice Kennedy Shriver Center has a four-decade history of pioneering research, education, and service for people with intellectual and developmental disabilities (IDD) and their families. Founded in 1970, the Center was one of twelve original Intellectual and Developmental Disabilities Research Centers (IDDRCs) established by US Congress at that time and also one of the earliest-established University Centers of Excellence in Developmental Disabilities (UCEDD). The Center was named after Mr

William McIlvane, Director
Charles Hamad, Associate Director

10391 Veterans Benefits Clearinghouse
38 Dudley Street 617-541-8846
Roxbury, MA 02119-1707

Support Groups & Hotlines

10392 National Health Information Center
Washington, DC 20013 310-565-4167
800-336-4797
Fax: 301-984-4256
e-mail: info@nhic.org
www.health.gov/nhic
The National Health Information Center (NHIC) is a health information referral service sponsored by the Office of Disease Prevention and Health Promotion. NHIC puts health professionals and consumers who have health questions in touch with those organizations that are best able to provide answers. Using a database that contains descriptions of health-related organizations, NHIC staff refer people to the most appropriate resource. Spanish language information specialists are available.

DeSanctis, FACHE

10393 National Veterans Services Fund
Darien, CT 06820-0465 203-656-0003
800-521-0198
Fax: 203-656-1957
e-mail: NatVetSvc@aol.com
www.nvsf.org
NVSF, Inc. provides an integrated program of services managed by veterans that include the following: a national hotline for veterans and their families that responds to hundreds of inquiries each month from throughout the country; an extensive repository of free information on topics ranging from the history of the Agent Orange lawsuit to the most recent Gulf War legislation; a special fund that offers limited emergency economic assistance and relief for families in crisis; business partnership

Phil Kraft, President

Books

10394 An Assessment of Technical Issues Raised in RW Haley's Critique of Health Studies
Gus Haggstrom, author

Rand Corporation
1776 Main Street 310-393-0411
Santa Monica, CA 90407-2138 Fax: 310-393-4818
www.rand.org
The monograph/report was a product of the RAND Corporation from 1993 to 2003. RAND monograph/reports presented major research findings that addressed the challenges facing the public and private sectors.

ISBN: 0-833027-52-2
Gus Haggstrom, Author

10395 Gulf War and Health
National Academy Press
500 5th Street NW 202-334-3313
Washington, DC 20001 800-624-6242
Fax: 202-334-2793
e-mail: Customer_Service@nap.edu
www.nap.edu

Lyla M Hernandez, Editor
Merwyn R Greenlick, Editor

10396 Natural Attenuation for Groundwater Remediation
National Academy Press
500 5th Street NW 202-334-3313
Washington, DC 20001 800-624-6242
Fax: 202-334-2793
e-mail: Customer_Service@nap.edu
www.nap.edu

10397 Yes, You Can
Demos Medical Publishing
11 West 42nd Street 212-683-0072
New York, NY 10036 Fax: 212-683-0118
e-mail: support@demosmedical.com
www.demosmedical.com

112 pages
ISBN: 1-888799-48-x
Dr. Diana M Schneider

Newsletters

10398 Agent Orange Briefs
Department of Veterans Affairs
810 Vermont Avenue NW   202-233-4000
Washington, DC 20420-0002
Designed to answer questions regarding Agent Orange and related matters. This fact sheet series is prepared and updated annually.
Monthly

10399 Agent Orange Review
Department of Veterans Affairs
810 Vermont Avenue NW   202-233-4000
Washington, DC 20420-0002
Published periodically to provide information on Agent Orange to concerned veterans and their families. The most recent issues include updated information about Federal government studies and activities related to Agent Orange and the Vietnam experience.

Pamphlets

10400 Agent Orange Anxiety: The Human Response to Possable Oncogenicity and Mutagencity
National Veterans Services Fund
PO Box 2465   203-656-0003
Darien, CT 06820-0465   800-521-0198
            Fax: 203-656-1957
            e-mail: support@NVSF.org
            www.nvsf.org
Erwin R. Parson, Ph.D., Author

10401 Agent Orange Fact Sheet: A Historical Perspective
Veterans Of The Vietnam War
805 South Township Blvd   570-603-9740
Pittston, PA 18640-3327   Fax: 570-603-9741
            www.vvnw.org
Fact sheet designed to bring an awareness of Agent Orange and related herbicides to the American public, includes a bibliography for the professional.
10 pages

10402 Agent Orange and Birth Defects
Veterans Health Adminstration
810 Vermont Avenue NW   202-273-8580
Washington, DC 20420-3517   Fax: 202-273-9080
            www.tpromo2.com/usvi/index2.htm
Letters to the editor, New England Journal of Medicine articles.

10403 Agent Orange and Chloracme
National Veterans Services Fund
PO Box 2465   203-656-0003
Darien, CT 06820-0465   800-521-0198
            Fax: 203-656-1957
            e-mail: support@NVSF.org
            www.nvsf.org

10404 Agent Orange and Hodgkin's Disease
Veterans Health Administration
810 Vermont Avenue NW   203-273-8580
Washington, DC 20420-3517   Fax: 203-273-9080
            www.tpromo2.com/usvi/index2.htm

10405 Agent Orange and Mutiple Myeloma
National Veterans Services Fund
PO Box 2465   203-656-0003
Darien, CT 06820-0465   800-521-0198
            Fax: 203-656-1957
            e-mail: support@NVSF.org
            www.nvsf.org

10406 Agent Orange and Non-Hodgkin's Lymphoma
Veterans Health Administration
810 Vermont Avenue   203-273-8580
Washington, DC 20420-3517   Fax: 203-273-9080
            www.tpromo2.com/usvi/index2.htm

10407 Agent Orange and Peripheral Neuropathy
Veterans Health Administration

810 Vermont Avenue   203-273-8580
Washington, DC 20420-3517   Fax: 203-273-9080
            www.tpromo2.com/usvi/index2.htm

10408 Agent Orange and Porphyria Cutanea Tarda
National Veterans Services Fund
PO Box 2465   203-656-0003
Darien, CT 06820-0465   800-521-0198
            Fax: 203-656-1957
            e-mail: support@NVSF.org
            www.nvsf.org

10409 Agent Orange and Prostate Cancer
National Veterans Services Fund
PO Box 2465   203-656-0003
Darien, CT 06820-0465   800-521-0198
            Fax: 203-656-1957
            e-mail: support@NVSF.org
            www.nvsf.org

10410 Agent Orange and Respiratory Cancers
National Veterans Services Fund
PO Box 2465   203-656-0003
Darien, CT 06820-0465   800-521-0198
            Fax: 203-656-1957
            e-mail: support@NVSF.org
            www.nvsf.org

10411 Agent Orange and Soft Tissue Sarcomas
National Veterans Services Fund
PO Box 2465   203-656-0003
Darien, CT 06820-0465   800-521-0198
            Fax: 203-656-1957
            e-mail: support@NVSF.org
            www.nvsf.org

10412 Agent Orange and Spina Bifida
National Veterans Services Fund
PO Box 2465   203-656-0003
Darien, CT 06820-0465   800-521-0198
            Fax: 203-656-1957
            e-mail: support@NVSF.org
            www.nvsf.org

10413 Agent Orange: It is Part of Your Life
National Veterans Services Fund
PO Box 2465   203-656-0003
Darien, CT 06820-0465   800-521-0198
            Fax: 203-656-1957
            e-mail: support@NVSF.org
            www.nvsf.org

Dr. Arthur Galston, Author

10414 Brief History of the Agent Orange Lawsuit
National Veterans Services Fund
PO Box 2465   203-656-0003
Darien, CT 06820-0465   800-521-0198
            Fax: 203-656-1957
            e-mail: support@NVSF.org
            www.nvsf.org

10415 Case Control Study: Soft-Tissue Sarcomas and Exposure to Phenoxyacetic Acids
National Veterans Services Fund
PO Box 2465   203-656-0003
Darien, CT 06820-0465   800-521-0198
            Fax: 203-656-1957
            e-mail: support@NVSF.org
            www.nvsf.org

Case control study: soft-tissue sarcoma and exposure to phenoxyacetic acids or chlorophenols.
L. Hardell, Co-Author
A. Sandstrom, Co-Author

10416 Children of Vietnam Veterans: Complex Concerns and Innovative Solutions
National Veterans Services Fund

PO Box 2465
Darien, CT 06820-0465

203-656-0003
800-521-0198
Fax: 203-656-1957
e-mail: support@NVSF.org
www.nvsf.org

7 pages
Phillip R. Kraft, Author

10417 Dioxin, A Case in Point
National Veterans Services Fund
PO Box 2465
Darien, CT 06820-0465

203-656-0003
800-521-0198
Fax: 203-656-1957
e-mail: support@NVSF.org
www.nvsf.org

Luke G. Tedeschi, M.D., Author

10418 Enviromental Chloracne
National Veterans Services Fund
PO Box 2465
Darien, CT 06820-0465

203-656-0003
800-521-0198
Fax: 203-656-1957
e-mail: support@NVSF.org
www.nvsf.org

10419 History of the Agent Orange Litigation
National Veterans Services Fund
PO Box 2465
Darien, CT 06820-0465

203-656-0003
800-521-0198
Fax: 203-656-1957
e-mail: support@NVSF.org
www.nvsf.org

10420 List of Agent Orange-Related Illnesses Recognized By the VA
National Veterans Services Fund
PO Box 2465
Darien, CT 06820-0465

203-656-0003
800-521-0198
Fax: 203-656-1957
e-mail: support@NVSF.org
www.nvsf.org

10421 List of Diseases Accepted by the VA for Presumptive Service-Connection
National Veterans Services Fund
PO Box 2465
Darien, CT 06820-0465

203-656-0003
800-521-0198
Fax: 203-656-1957
e-mail: support@NVSF.org
www.nvsf.org

List of diseases accepted by the VA for presumptive service-connection that are associated with exposure to certain herbicide agents including Agent Orange.

10422 Relation of Soft-Tissue Sarcome, Malignant Lymphoma & Colon Cancer
National Veterans Services Fund
PO Box 2465
Darien, CT 06820-0465

203-656-0003
800-521-0198
Fax: 203-656-1957
e-mail: support@NVSF.org
www.nvsf.org

Relation to soft-tissue sarcomas, malignant lymphoma and colon cancer to phenoxy acids, chlorphenois and other agents.

10423 Spina Bifida Benefits Guide
National Veterans Services Fund
PO Box 2465
Darien, CT 06820-0465

203-656-0003
800-521-0198
Fax: 203-656-1957
e-mail: support@NVSF.org
www.nvsf.org

4 pages

Audio & Video

10424 Agent Orange Videotapes
Regional Learning Resources Service
915 N. Grand Boulevard
St. Louis, MO 63106

314-652-4100

Produces several Agent Orange videotape programs that explain what Agent Orange is, where, when and how it was used, why persons are concerned about exposure to it and what VA and other departments and agencies are doing in response to these concerns. These videotapes are maintained at all VA medical centers across the country.

Web Sites

10425 Gulf War Syndrome Database
www.louisville.edu/library/ekstrom
This is a substantial database of relevant documents and studies kept by University of Louisville, Ekstrom Library.

10426 Gulf War Veteran Resource Pages
www.gulfweb.org
This page is administered by Gulf War veterans and provides a great range of information on a variety of Gulf War-related items, including GWS. The site includes many links to other groups interested in GWS and to GWS studies.

10427 Healing Well
www.healingwell.com
An online health resource guide to medical news, chat, information and articles, newsgroups and message boards, books, disease-related web sites, medical directories, and more for patients, friends, and family coping with disabling diseases, disorders, or chronic illnesses.

10428 Health Finder
www.healthfinder.gov
Searchable, carefully developed web site offering information on over 1000 topics. Developed by the US Department of Health and Human Services, the site can be used in both English and Spanish.

10429 Healthlink USA
www.healthlinkusa.com
Health information concerning treatment, cures, prevention, diagnosis, risk factors, research, support groups, email lists, personal stories and much more. Updated regularly.

10430 Heatlhcentral.com
www.healthcentral.com
The HealthCentral Network has a collection of owned and operated web sites and multimedia affiliate properties providing timely, in-depth, trusted medical information, personalized tools and resources for people seeking to manage and improve their health.

10431 Helios Health
www.helioshealth.com
Online resource for your health information. Detailed information about specific health topics, access to expert advice from our Medical Advisory Board, and up-to-date health news.

10432 InteliHealth
www.intelihealth.com
InteliHealth's mission is to empower people with trusted solutions for healthier lives. They accomplish this by providing credible information fromt he most trusted sources.
Brian Berkenstock, Writer/Editor

10433 MedicineNet
www.medicinenet.com
Medicine Net is an online healthcare media publishing company. It provides easy-to-read, in-depth, authoritative medical information for consumers via its robust, user-friendly, interactive web site.

10434 Medscape
www.medscape.com
Medscape offers specialists, primary care physicians, and other health professionals the Web's most robust and integrated medical information and educational tools.

10435 National Veterans Services Fund
www.nvsf.org
Supports and informs those who were exposed to the defoliant Agent Orange, or dioxin, while serving the US in the conflict in Vietnam.

10436 Office of the Special Assistant for Gulf War Illnesses

www.gulflink.osd.mil

This is a page sponsored by the Defense Department's Special Assistant for Gulf War Illnesses. It provides information on and linkes to Federal and State-funded studies of Gulf War Illnesses.

10437 WebMD

www.webmd.com

Provides credible information, supportive communities, and in-depth reference material about health subjects. A source for original and timely health information as well as material from well known content providers.

Description

10438 Wilson's Disease

Wilson's disease is a rare genetic disorder that results from an inability to adequately excrete copper. In the United States, approximately one person in 40,000 has this condition. The resulting accumulation of copper in the body's tissues and organs leads to disease of the brain and liver, and to a lesser extent, the kidney and red blood cells. The disease is genetic; if two carriers have children, the disease would have a 1 in 4 chance of being passed on.

Build-up of copper in the liver causes a hepatitis-like illness with loss of appetite, low grade fever, abdominal discomfort and jaundice. If not detected and treated, this process can lead to cirrhosis and fatal liver failure. In 40 to 50 percent of patients, the illness affects the brain and can include unsteadiness, tremors, slurred speech and intellectual deterioration. Copper rings may appear in the eye in up to 10 percent of patients. Although they do not cause any symptoms, their appearance may help establish the diagnosis.

In untreated Wilson's, the disease is fatal, generally before the age of 30. Continual, lifelong treatment is mandatory for any patient with confirmed Wilson's disease, whether symptomatic or not. The critical therapy is to administer a drug that helps the body release its copper stores. D-penicillamine is the most common such drug. Some patients have required liver transplantation.

National Agencies & Associations

10439 American Liver Foundation

39 Broadway
New York, NY 10006

212-668-1000
212-483-8179
Fax: 212-483-8179
e-mail: info@liverfoundation.org
www.liverfoundation.org

Our mission is to facilitate, advocate and promote education, support and research for the prevention, treatment and cure of liver disease.
Rick Smith, President/CEO
Newton Guerin, COO

10440 United Liver Foundation

11646 W Pico Boulevard
Los Angeles, CA 90064

213-445-4204

Foundation offering information public awareness materials support and medical research for persons suffering from liver diseases.

10441 Wilson's Disease Association

5572 North Diversey Blvd
Milwaukee, WI 53217

414-961-0533
866-961-0533
Fax: 330-264-0974
e-mail: info@wilsonsdisease.org
www.wilsonsdisease.org

Serves as a communications support network for individuals affected by Wilson's disease; distributes information to professionals and the public; makes referrals; and holds meetings.
8 pages
Mary L. Graper, President
Stefanie F. Kaplan, Vice President

Foundations

10442 Hepatitis B Foundation

3805 Old Easton Road
Doylestown, PA 18902

215-489-4900
Fax: 215-489-4313
e-mail: info@hepb.org
www.hepb.org

We are dedicated to finding a cure and improving the quality of life for those affected by hepatitis B worldwide. Our commitment includes funding focused research, promoting disease awareness, supporting immunization and treatment initiatives, and serving as the primary source of information for patients and their families, the medical and scientific community, and the general public.

Joel Rosen, Chair
Timothy Block, PhD, Founder/President

Support Groups & Hotlines

10443 National Health Information Center

PO Box 1133
Washington, DC 20013

240-453-8280
800-336-4797
Fax: 240-453-8282
e-mail: info@nhic.org
www.health.gov/nhic

Offers a nationwide information referral service, produces directories and resource guides.

Pamphlets

10444 Wilson's Disease

American Liver Foundation
1425 Pompton Avenue
Cedar Grove, NJ 07009

800-465-4837
Fax: 973-256-3214
e-mail: info@liverfoundation.org
www.liverfoundation.org

A brochure offering information on the causes, symptoms and treatments of Wilson's Disease.
Rick Smith, President & CEO

Web Sites

10445 Healing Well

e-mail: webmaster@healingwell.com
www.healingwell.com

An online health resource guide to medical news, chat, information and articles, newsgroups and message boards, books, disease-related web sites, medical directories, and more for patients, friends, and family coping with disabling diseases, disorders, or chronic illnesses.
Peter Waite, MS, MA, Founder/Editor

10446 Health Finder

PO Box 1133
Washington, DC 20013-1133

e-mail: healthfinder@nhic.org
www.healthfinder.gov

Searchable, carefully developed web site offering information on over 1000 topics. Developed by the US Department of Health and Human Services, the site can be used in both English and Spanish.

10447 Healthlink USA

www.healthlinkusa.com

Health information concerning treatment, cures, prevention, diagnosis, risk factors, research, support groups, email lists, personal stories and much more. Updated regularly.

10448 Helios Health

www.helioshealth.com

Online resource for your health information. Detailed information about specific health topics, access to expert advice from our Medical Advisory Board, and up-to-date health news.

10449 MedicineNet

www.medicinenet.com

An online resource for consumers providing easy-to-read, authoritative medical and health information.

10450 Medscape
Corporate Headquarters
111 8th Avenue
New York, NY 10011

212-624-3700
www.medscape.com

Medscape offers specialists, primary care physicians, and other health professionals the Web's most robust and integrated medical information and educational tools.

Kate Hahn, Media Relations
Tony G Holcombe, President

10451 WebMD

www.webmd.com

Provides credible information, supportive communities, and in-depth reference material about health subjects. A source for original and timely health information as well as material from well known content providers.

National Agencies & Associations

10452 ABLEDATA
8630 Fenton Street 301-608-8998
Silver Spring, MD 20910 800-227-0216
Fax: 301-608-8958
TTY: 301-608-8912
e-mail: abledata@macrointernational.com
www.abledata.com
Provides objective information on assistive technology and reha-bilitation equipment available from domestic and international sources to consumers, organizations, professionals, and care-givers within the United States.
Katherine Belknap, Project Director
Steve Lowe, Assistant Project Manager

10453 ABLEDATA-REHAB DATA Alliance for Technology Access (ATA)
8630 Fenton Street 301-608-8998
Silver Spring, MD 20910 800-227-0216
Fax: 301-608-8958
TTY: 301-608-8912
e-mail: abledata@macrointernational.com
www.abledata.com
National organization dedicated to providing access to technology for people with disabilities through its coalition of 45 commu-nity-based resource centers in 34 states and the Virgin Islands. Each center provides information, awareness and training.
Katherine Belknap, Project Director
Juanita Hardy, Information Specialist

10454 Access Unlimited
570 Hance Road
Binghamton, NY 13903 800-849-2143
Fax: 607-669-4595
e-mail: tom@accessunlimited.com
www.accessunlimited.com
We celebrate the rich diversity of our customers' needs by creating products that allow easy access to any vehicle, from cars and vans to trucks and SUVs. We believe that adaptive equipment should be unobtrusive and should meet the needs of its user with a minimum of modification to vehicle or lifestyle. We believe every person should be able to choose the vehicle they like best, regardless of their disability. Access Unlimited products empower people with disabilities to regain control of thei
Tom Cole, Owner

10455 American Academy of Pediatrics
141 NW Point Boulevard 847-434-4000
Elk Grove Village, IL 60007-1098 800-433-9016
Fax: 847-434-8000
www.aap.org
To attain optimal physical, mental, and social health and well-be-ing for all infants, children, adolescents, and young adults.
Thomas K. McInerny, President
Errol T Alden MD FAAP, Executive Director

10456 American Association for the Advancement of Science
1200 New York Avenue NW 202-326-6400
Washington, DC 20005 Fax: 202-371-9526
e-mail: webmaster@aaas.org
www.aaas.org
The non-profit AAAS is open to all and fulfills its mission to ad-vance science and serve society through initiatives that include science policy, international programs, science education, and public understanding of science.
William Press, Chair
Phillip A. Sharp, President

10457 American Association of People with Disabilities
2013 H Street, NW 202-457-0046
Washington, DC 20006 800-840-8844
Fax: 866-536-4461
TTY: 202-457-0046
www.aapd.com
The American Association of People with Disabilities is the na-tion's largest disability rights organization. We promote equal op-portunity, economic power, independent living, and political participation for people with disabilities. Our members, including people with disabilities and our family, friends, and supporters, represent a powerful force for change.
Mark Perriello, President/CEO
Henry Claypool, Executive VP

10458 American Autoimmune Related Diseases Association
22100 Gratiot Avenue 586-776-3900
East Detroit, MI 48021 Fax: 586-776-3903
e-mail: aarda@aarda.org
www.aarda.org
Dedicated to the eradication of autoimmune diseases and the alle-viation of suffering and the socioeconomic impact of autoimmunity through fostering and facilitating collaboration in the areas of education, public awareness, research, and patient ser-vices in an effective, ethical and efficient manner.
Stanley M Finger PhD, Chairman
Virginia T Ladd, President/Executive Director

10459 American Bar Association Commission on Mental and Physical Disability Law
1050 Connecticut Ave. N.W. 202-662-1000
Washington, DC 20036 800-285-2221
Fax: 202-442-3439
e-mail: campdl@americanbar.org
www.americanbar.org
The Commission's mission is to promote the ABA's commitment to justice and the rule of law for persons with mental, physical, and sensory disabilities and to promote their full and equal participa-tion in the legal profession.
John W Parry, Director
Laurel G. Bellows, President

10460 American Camp Association
5000 State Road 67 N 765-342-8456
Martinsville, IN 46151-7902 800-428-2267
Fax: 765-342-2065
www.acacamps.org
Formerly the American Camping Association, a community of camp professionals who have joined together to share the knowl-edge and experience and to ensure the quality of camp programs.
Tisha Bolger, President
Melanie Lock Herman, Treasurer

10461 American Counseling Association
5999 Stevenson Avenue
Alexandria, VA 22304 800-347-6647
Fax: 703-823-0252
e-mail: ryep@counseling.org
www.counseling.org
A not-for-profit, professional and educational organization that is dedicated to the growth and enhancement of the counseling profes-sion. Represents professional counselors in various practice settings.
Marcheta Evans, President
Richard Yep, Executive Director

10462 American Foundation for The Blind
2 Penn Plaza 212-502-7600
New York, NY 10121 800-232-5463
Fax: 888-545-8331
e-mail: afbinfo@afb.net
www.afb.org
AFB's priorities include broadening access to technology; elevat-ing the quality of information and tools for the professionals who serve people with vision loss by providing them and their families with relevant and timely resources.
Carl R Augusto, President/CEO
Rick Bozeman, Chief Financial Officer

10463 American Institute for Preventive Medicine
30445 NW Highway 248-539-1800
Farmington Hills, MI 48334 800-345-2476
Fax: 248-539-1808
e-mail: aipm@healthylife.com
www.healthylife.com
An award winning, internationally recognized authority on th de-velopment and implementation of health promotion, wellness,

medical self-care, and disease management programs and publications.

Larry Chapman, President
Dee Edington, Director

10464 American Institute for Preventive Medicine
30445 NW Highway
Farmington Hills, MI 48334
248-539-1800
800-345-2476
Fax: 248-539-1808
e-mail: aipm@healthylife.com
www.healthylife.com

The institute provides health promotion programs disease management guides and self-care publications to hospitals HMOs corporations and government agencies. Programs are designed to lower health care costs, decrease absenteeism and improve productivity.

Larry Chapman, President
Dee Edington, Director

10465 American Organ Transplant Association
PO Box 418
Stilwell, KS 66085
713-344-2402
Fax: 281-617-4274
e-mail: aotaonline@gmail.com
www.aotaonline.org

Helps patients with free transportation to and from their transplant center, many times hundreds of miles away. Also provides transplant patients and their loved ones with resources regarding transplantation.

Pamela H Terry, Board President
Kenneth Klingensmith, Immediate Past Board President

10466 American Red Cross National Headquarters
2025 E Street NW
Washington, DC 20006
202-303-5000
800-733-2767
www.redcross.org

The nation's premier emergency response organization that aids victims of devastating natural disasters; community services that help the needy; support and comfort for military members and their families; the collection, processing and distribution of lifesaving blood and blood products; educational programs that promote health and safety; and international relief and development programs.

Gail J McGovern, President/CEO
Bonnie McElveen-Hunt, Chairman

10467 American Rehabilitation Counseling Association
5999 Stevenson Avenue
Alexandria, VA 22304-3300
800-347-6647
Fax: 800-473-2329
TTY: 703-823-6862
TDD: 7038236862
e-mail: webmaster@counseling.org
www.counseling.org

Mission of ARCA is to enhance the development of persons with disabilities throughout their life span and to promote excellence in the rehabilitation counseling professional.

Colleen Logan, President
Richard Yep, Executive Office

10468 American Society of Dermatology
Port St Lucie, FL 34984
561-873-8335
Fax: 561-344-8388
www.asd.org

The mission of this organization is to facilitate optimal dermatologic care being available to all citizens of this country by preserving, promoting and enhancing the private practice of dermatology. It shall represent its members in those scientific, educational, socioeconomic and legislative areas that affect the practice of dermatology and shall endeavor to cooperate with other organizations of similar purpose.

W Gerald Klinger MD, President
Don Printz, MD, Secretary

10469 Americas Association for the Care of Children
Boulder, CO 80306-2154
303-527-2742
www.aaccchildren.net

Americas Association for the Care of the Children (AACC) is the brain child of Deborah Young together with 2 friends that have been in the child care field for over 30 years. AACC is a non-profit, 501(c)3 and the umbrella organization for Programma Integral

Educando con Amor y Tenura (PIEAT). PIEAT is located in Nicaragua. In the United States AACC partners with Companeras, in Nepal with Hands in Nepal, in Kenya with Mama Beth's orphanage, feeding center and school, and in Bhutan with the Royal

Judi Jackson, President
Doreen Trees, Vice President

10470 Asbestos Information Association/North America
1745 Jefferson Davis Highway
Arlington, VA 22202
703-412-1150
Fax: 703-412-1586
e-mail: aiabjpigg@aol.com

Founded to represent the interests of the asbestos industry and to collect and disseminate information about asbestos and asbestos products with emphasis on safety health and environmental issues.

10471 Beach Center on Disability
University of Kansas
1200 Sunnyside Avenue
Lawrence, KS 66045
785-864-7600
Fax: 786-864-7605
e-mail: beachcenter@ku.edu
www.beachcenter.org

The Beach Center on Disability is a multi-disciplinary research and training center committed to making a significant and sustainable positive difference in the quality of life of individuals and families affected by disability and the professionals who support them. Its staff of approximately 40 professors, researchers, educators, doctoral students, and support personnel carry out research, technical assistance, and undergraduate, masters, and doctoral training. Its staff focuses on families, f

Ann Turnbull, Co-Founder, Co-Director, Distinguished P
Rud Turnbull, Co-Founder, Co-Director, Distinguished P

10472 Breaking New Ground Resource Center
2255 S University Street
W Lafayette, IN 47907
765-494-5088
800-825-4264
Fax: 765-496-1356
e-mail: bng@enc.purdue.edu
www.ninds.nih.gov/find_people/voluntary_

Has become internationally recoginzed as the primary source for information and resources on rehabilitation technology for persons working in agriculture.

Prof William Field, Project Leader

10473 Center for Children with Chronic Illness and Disability
University of Minnesota School of Public Health
2525 Chicago Avenue
Minneapolis, MN 55404
612-813-6000
e-mail: Get.Well@childrensmn.org
www.childrensmn.org

Serving as Minnesota's children's hospitalSM since 1924, we provide 347 staffed beds at our two hospital campuses in St. Paul and Minneapolis. An independent, not-for-profit health care system, Children's provides care through more than 12,000 inpatient visits and more than 200,000 emergency room and other outpatient visits each year.

Alan L. Goldbloom, MD, Chief Executive Officer
David A. Brumbaugh, SPHR, Vice President Human Resources

10474 Center for Chronic Disease Prevention and Centers for Disease Control
1600 Clifton Road
Atlanta, GA 30333
404-639-3311
800-232-4636
TTY: 888-232-6348
e-mail: cdcinfo@cdc.gov
www.cdc.gov

Chronic diseases such as heart disease cancer and diabetes are the leading causes of death and disability in the United States. These diseases account for 7 of every 10 deaths and affect the quality of life of 90 million Americans.

Richard E Besser, Director

10475 Center for Developmental Disabilities University of South Carolina
8301 Farrow Road
Columbia, SC 29208
803-935-5231
Fax: 803-935-5059
e-mail: steve.wilson@uscmed.sc.edu
www.uscm.med.sc.edu/cdrhome

The vision of The Center for Developmental Disabilities is to work as a team to create a quality environment in which the following values are embraced: Everyone is treated with dignity and respect. Individual strengths and abilities are recognized.

10476 Center for Disability Resources
University of South Carolina
8301 Farrow Road
Columbia, SC 29208
803-935-5231
Fax: 803-935-5059
e-mail: steve.wilson@uscmed.sc.edu
www.uscm.med.sc.edu/cdrhome
To enhance the well-being and quality of life of persons with disabilities and their families. Collaborates with persons with disabilities and their families to develop new knowledge and best practices, train leaders, and effect systems change.

10477 Center for Disease Control and Prevention
1600 Clifton Rd
Atlanta, GA 30333
800-232-4636
TTY: 888-232-6348
e-mail: cdcinfo@cdc.gov
www.cdc.gov
To collaborate to create the expertise, information, and tools that people and communities need to protect their health - through health promotion, prevention of disease, injury and disability, and preparedness for new health threats.
Thomas R Frieden MD MPH, Director

10478 Center for Health Research
Kaiser Permanente Northwest
3800 N Interstate Avenue
Portland, OR 97227-1098
503-335-2400
e-mail: information@kpchr.org
www.kpchr.org
Conducts professionally independent, public domain research and idsseminates its findings in the scholarly literature and scientific community.
Mary L Durham PhD, Director
Donald R Freel, Executive Director COO

10479 Center for Medical Consumers
239 Thompson Street
New York, NY 10012
212-674-7105
e-mail: centerformedicalconsumers@gmail.com
www.medicalconsumers.org
A non-profit advocacy organization that was founded with the philosophy: Whenever long-term drug therapy, elective surgery, or any other major treatment is prescribed, the question of whether the treatment has been proven safe and effective should come up.
Arthur Aaron Levin MPH, Director
Maryann Napoli, Associate Director

10480 Center for Universal Design North Carolina State University
North Carolina State University
Campus Box 7701
Raleigh, NC 27695-8613
919-515-8302
800-647-6777
Fax: 919-515-8951
e-mail: nilda_cosco@ncsu.edu
www.design.ncsu.edu
National research information and technical assistance center that evaluates develops and promotes accessible and universal design in housing buildings outdoor and urban environments and related products.
Nilda Cosco PhD, Education Specialist
Leslie Young, Director of Design

10481 Child Center
3995 Marcola Road
Springfield, OR 97477
541-726-1465
Fax: 541-726-5085
e-mail: info@thechildcenter.org
www.thechildcenter.org
To provide individualized, diagnostic, therapeutic and educational services for the emotional and behavioral problems children exhibit in the home, school and community; provide integreated community based psychiatric and support services that are child centered, family driven and culturally competent
Jeffrey Miller, President
Chris Dunnington, Vice President

10482 Children's Hospice International
1101 King Street
Alexandria, VA 22314
703-684-0330
800-242-4453
Fax: 703-684-0226
e-mail: info@chionline.org
www.chionline.org
To ensure medical, psychological, social and spiritual support to all children with life-threatening conditions and their families by providing a network of resources and care.
Ann Armstrong-Dailey, Founding Director/CEO
Richard Larkin, Secretary/Treasurer

10483 Children's National Medical Center
111 Michigan Avenue NW
Washington, DC 20010
202-476-5000
888-884-2327
TTY: 800-855-1155
e-mail: tbear@childrensnational.org
www.childrensnational.org
The only exclusive provider of pediatric care in the metropolitan Washington area and is the only freestanding children's hospital between Philadelphia, Pittsburgh, Norfolk, and Atlanta; the leader in the development and application of innovative new treatments for childhood illness and injury.
Kurt Newman MD, President/CEO
Roberta Alessi, Senior VP

10484 Christian Horizons
25 Sportsworld Crossing Road
Kitchener, N2P 0
519-650-0966
866-362-6810
Fax: 519-650-8984
e-mail: info@christian-horizons.org
www.christian-horizons.org
Empowers individuals with exceptional needs, enabling them to embrace their God-given potential and enjoy hope and opportunity in everyday living.
Nigel Wilford, Chair
Greg Wilson, Secretary

10485 Clearinghouse on Disability Information Office of Special Education & Rehab Svcs
US Department of Education
550 12th Street SW
Washington, DC 20202-2550
202-245-7307
Fax: 202-245-7636
TTY: 202-205-5637
TDD: 2022055637
e-mail: customerservice@inet.ed.gov
www.health.gov/nhic/NHICScripts/Entry.cf
Provides information to people with disabilities or anyone requesting information by doing research and providing documents in response to inquiries. Information provided includes areas of federal funding for disability-related programs.
Carolyn Corlett, Contact

10486 Council for Learning Disabilities (CLD)
11184 Antioch Road
Overland Park, KS 66210
913-491-1011
Fax: 913-491-1012
e-mail: CLDInfo@cldinternational.org
www.cldinternational.org
The Council for Learning Disabilities (CLD) is an international organization that promotes evidence-based teaching, collaboration, research, leadership, and advocacy. CLD is comprised of professionals who represent diverse disciplines and are committed to enhancing the education and quality of life for individuals with learning disabilities and others who experience challenges in learning.
Slivana Watson, President
Steve Chamberlain, President Elect

10487 Disabled & Alone: Life Services for the Handicapped
1440 Broadway
New York, NY 10018
212-532-6740
800-995-0066
Fax: 212-532-3588
e-mail: info@disabledandalone.org
www.disabledandalone.org
A non-profit organization established to help families provide a secure future for their loved ones with a disability. Also believes that no person should have to live his life in loneliness and isolation because of a disability.
Leslie D Park, Chairman
Lee Alan Ackerman, Executive Director

10488 Distance Education and Training Council
1601 18th Street NW
Washington, DC 20009
202-234-5100
Fax: 202-332-1386
e-mail: brianna@detc.org
www.detc.org

A voluntary, non-governmental, educational organization that operates a nationally recognized accrediting association, the DETC Accrediting Commission.
Michael P Lambert, Executive Director
Patrice Wall, General Information

10489 Educational Equity Center at The Academy for Educational Development
71 Fifth Avenue
New York, NY 10003
212-243-1110
Fax: 212-627-0407
e-mail: lcolon@aed.org
www.edequity.org
A national non-profit organization promoting educational excellence for children.
Merle Froschl, Co-Director
Barbara Sprung, Co-Director

10490 Equal Opportunity Employment Commission
131 M Street NE
Washington, DC 20507
202-663-4900
TTY: 202-663-4494
e-mail: info@eeoc.gov
www.eeoc.gov
The U.S. Equal Employment Opportunity Commission (EEOC) is responsible for enforcing federal laws that make it illegal to discriminate against a job applicant or an employee because of the person's race, color, religion, sex (including pregnancy), national origin, age (40 or older), disability or genetic information. It is also illegal to discriminate against a person because the person complained about discrimination, filed a charge of discrimination, or participated in an employment discrimina
Jacqueline A Berrien, Chair
Constance S. Barker, Commissioner

10491 Estate Planning for the Disabled
2232 W Avenue 133
San Leandro, CA 94577-1050
510-352-4127
Fax: 510-352-4127
e-mail: EFM@EFMOODY.com
www.efmoody.com
Counsels and assists parents of children with special needs to develop viable estate plans, letters of intent, wills and special needs trusts. EPD will work with the appropriate professionals and agencies to help put together an effective comprehensive plan.

10492 Extensions for Independence
555 Saturn Boulevard
San Diego, CA 92154
619-618-2154
866-632-7149
Fax: 866-632-7149
e-mail: info@mouthstick.net
www.mouthstick.net
Designer and manufacturer of home and office related equipment for the functional independence of the most physically challenged.
Arthur Heyer, President

10493 Favarh
225 Commerce Drive
Canton, CT 06019-1099
860-693-6662
Fax: 860-693-8662
www.favarh.org
Provides a variety of programs and services to adults with developmental, physical or mental disabilities and their families, throughout the Farmington Valley communities of Avon, Burlington and more.
Stephen Morr MPA, Executive Director

10494 Federation for Children with Special Needs
529 Main Street
Boston, MA 02129
617-236-7210
800-331-0688
Fax: 617-241-0330
e-mail: fcsninfo@fcsn.org
www.fcsn.org
Provides information, support, and assistance to parents of children with disabilities, their professional partners and their communities. Committed to listening to and learning from families, and encouraging full participation in community life by all people, especially those with disabilities.
Rich Robison, Executive Director
Sara Miranda, Associate Executive Director

10495 Florida Disabled Outdoor Association
2475 Apalachee Parkway
Tallahassee, FL 32301
850-201-2944
Fax: 850-201-2945
www.fdoa.org
Enriches lives through accessible inclusive recreation and active leisure for all.
David Jones, Director
Laurie LoRe-Gussak, Execcutive Director

10496 Goodwill Industries International
15810 Indianola Drive
Rockville, MD 20855
301-530-6500
800-741-0186
Fax: 301-530-1516
TTY: 301-530-9759
e-mail: contactus@goodwill.org
www.goodwill.org
Enhances the dignity and quality of life of individuals, families and communities by eliminating barriers to opportunity and helping people in need reach their fullest potential through the power of work.
Jim Gibbons, President/CEO
Bill J Kacal, Chair

10497 HEATH Resource Center
George Washington University
2134 G Street NW
Washington, DC 20052-0001
202-939-9329
800-544-3284
Fax: 202-994-3365
e-mail: AskHEATH@gwu.edu
www.heath.gwu.edu
Serves as a national clearinghouse on postsecondary education for individuals with disabilities.
Dr Lynda West, Principal Investigator
Dr Joel Gomez, Co-Principal Investigator

10498 Health Care For All
30 Winter Street
Boston, MA 02108
617-350-7279
Fax: 617-451-5838
TTY: 617-350-0974
e-mail: aslemmer@hcfama.org
www.hcfama.org
HCFA seeks to create a consumer-centered health care system that provides comprehensive, affordable, accessible, culturally competent, high quality care and consumer education for everyone, especially the most vulnerable.
Amy Whitcomb Slemmer, Executive Director

10499 International Association for the Study of Pain
1510 H Street NW
Washington, DC 20005-4955
202-524-5300
Fax: 202-524-5301
e-mail: iaspdesk@iasp-pain.org
www.iasp-pain.org
Brings together scientists, clinicians, health care providers, and policy makers to stimulate and support the study of pain and to translate that knowledge into improved pain relief worldwide.
Kathy Kreiter, Executive Director
Janet Brangman, Executive Assistant

10500 International Council on Disability
1012 14th Street NW
Washington, DC 20005
202-347-0102
Fax: 202-347-0315
e-mail: info@usicd.org
www.usicd.org
To promote the rights and full participation of persons with disabilities through global engagement and United States foreign affairs.
Marca Bristo, President
Barbara LeRoy, Secretary

10501 LAUNCH Department of Special Education
Department of Special Education
Commerce, TX 75428
903-886-5932
Provides resources for learning disabled individuals coordinates efforts of other local state and national LD organizations acts as a communication channel for people with learning disabilities through a monthly newsletter and provides programs.

10502 Learning Disabilities Association of America
4156 Library Road
Pittsburgh, PA 15234-1349
412-341-1515
888-300-6710
Fax: 412-344-0224
e-mail: info@ldaamerica.org
www.ldaamerica.org
To create opportunities for success for all individuals affected by learning disabilities and to reduce the incidence of learning disabilities in future generations.
Patricia Lillie, President
Andrea Turkheimer, Director Resource/Referral/Education

10503 Learning How
1583 Sulphur Spring Road
Baltimore, MD 21227
410-242-7100
Fax: 410-242-5246
e-mail: info@learninghow.com
www.learninghow.com
To provide educational materials for parents, teachers, and daycare providers that will encourage the learning process and help children reach their fullest potential.

10504 Life Development Institute
18001 N 79th Avenue
Glendale, AZ 85308
623-773-2774
866-736-7811
Fax: 623-773-2788
e-mail: info@life-development-inst.org
www.lifedevelopmentinstitute.org
LDI's mission to inspire individuals to experience success while optimizing their potential for an enhanced quality of life in a challenging and supportive learning environment. LDI is a nonprofit private organization based in Glendale Arizona.
Rob Crawford, CEO
Veronica Crawford, Vice President

10505 Lions Quest
300 W 22nd Street
Oak Brook, IL 60523-8842
630-571-5466
Fax: 630-571-5735
e-mail: matthew.kiefer@lionsclub.org
www.lions-quest.org
To empower and support adults throughout the world to nuture caring and responsibility in young people.
Matthew Kiefer, Manager
Michael Di Maria, Educational Program Specialist

10506 Lymphatic Research Foundation
40 Garvies Point Road
Glen Cove, NY 11542
516-625-9675
Fax: 516-625-9410
e-mail: lrf@lymphaticresearch.org
www.lymphaticresearch.org
A not-for-profit organization whose mission is to advance research of the lymphatic system and to find the cause of and cure for lymphatic diseases, lymphedema, and related disorders.
Roy E. Reichbach, Executive Director
Phillip Braginsky, Chair

10507 MedEscort International ABE International Airport
ABE International Airport
PO Box 8766
Allentown, PA 18105-8766
610-792-3111
800-255-7182
Fax: 610-791-9189
e-mail: service@medescort.com
www.medescort.com
Offers specially trained escorts for individuals who cannot travel alone due to age or disability.
David M Stein DO, Medical Director
Sherry L Sefcik RN/BSN, Senior Flight Nurse

10508 MedicAlert Foundation International
2323 Colorado Avenue
Turlock, CA 95382-2018
888-633-4298
Fax: 800-863-3429
e-mail: customer_service@medicalert.org
www.medicalert.org
We protect the health and well-being of more than 4 million members worldwide through our trusted emergency support network. We educate emergency responders and medical personnel - our partners in everyday emergency situations. And we communicate your health information, your wishes, and your directives to ensure you receive the best care possible
Andrew B Wigglesworth, President/CEO
Karen M. Lamoree, COO

10509 Mental Health Services Training Center
University of Maryland
3700 Koppers Street
Baltimore, MD 21227
410-646-7758
Fax: 410-646-7849
e-mail: wbaysmor@psych.umaryland.edu
www.trainingcenter.umaryland.edu
Formerly the Mental Health Services Training Collaborative, assists Mental Hygiene Administration in planning, organizing and implementing conference and training activities to support the continued growth and development of the public mental health system.
Eileen Hansen MSSW, Director
Wendy Baysmore MSHSA, Assistant Director

10510 National Association of Councils on Developmental Disabilities
1825 K Street NW
Washington, DC 20006
202-506-5813
Fax: 202-506-5846
e-mail: info@nacdd.org
www.nacdd.org
Serves as the national voice of State and Territorial Councils on Dvelopment Disabilities. Supports Councils in implementing the Developmental Disabilities Assistance and Bill of Rights Act and promoting the interests and rights of people with developmental disabilities and their familes.
Claire Mantonya, President
Brett Cunnigham, VP

10511 National Center for Family-Centered Care
695 Park Avenue
New York, NY 10021
212-772-4000
Fax: 212-452-7475
e-mail: gmallon@hunter.cuny.edu
www.hunter.cuny.edu/socwork/nrcfcpp//tra
Goals are to promote implementation of a family-centered care approach for children with special health care needs.
Karen Lawrence

10512 National Chronic Pain Outreach Association
Millboro, VA 24460
540-862-9437
Fax: 540-862-9485
e-mail: ncpoa@cfw.com
www.chronicpain.org
Purpose is to lessen the suffering of people with chronic pain by educating pain sufferers, health care professionals, and the public about chronic pain and its management.

10513 National Clearinghouse of Rehabilitation Training Materials
Utah State University
6524 Old Main Hill
Logan, UT 84322-6524
866-821-5355
Fax: 435-797-7537
e-mail: ncrtm@usu.edu
www.ncrtm.org
Offers reference materials on rehabilitation for professionals and the disabled.
Jared Schultz, Principal Investigator
Joshua Southwick, Interim Director

10514 National Council on Disability
1331 F Street NW
Washington, DC 20004
202-272-2004
Fax: 202-272-2022
TTY: 202-272-2074
e-mail: ncd@ncd.gov
www.ncd.gov
The National Council on Disability is an independent federal agency that works with the President and Congress to increase the inclusion independence and empowerment of Americans with disabilities. They are involved in policy making issues.
Jonathan Young, Ph.D., Chairman
Aaron Bishop, Executive Director

10515 National Council on Independent Living
1710 Rhode Island Avenue NW
Washington, DC 20036

202-207-0334
877-525-3400
Fax: 202-207-0341
TTY: 202-207-0340
e-mail: ncil@ncil.org
www.ncil.org

A membership organization that advanced independent living and the rights of people with disabilities through consumer-driven advocacy.
Kelly Buckland, Executive Director
Dan Kessler, President

10516 National Digestive Diseases Information Clearinghouse
2 Information Way
Bethesda, MD 20892-3570

800-891-5389
Fax: 703-738-4929
TTY: 866-569-1162
e-mail: nddic@info.niddk.nih.gov
www.digestive.niddk.nih.gov

An information dissemination service of the National Institute of Diabetes and Digestive and Kidney Diseases that was established to increase knowledge and understanding about digestive diseases among people with these conditions and their families, health care professionals, and the general public.
Griffin P Rodgers MD MACP, Director

10517 National Dissemination Center for Children
1825 Connecticut Ave NW
Washington, DC 20009

202-884-8200
800-695-0285
Fax: 202-884-8441
TTY: 202-884-8200
e-mail: nichcy@aed.org
www.nichcy.org

Provides information to the nation on: disabilities in children and youth; programs and services for infants, children, and youth with disabilities; IDEA, the nation's special education law; No Child Left Behind, the nation's general education law; and research-based information on effective practices for children with disabilities.

10518 National Endowment for the Arts: Office for Accessability
1100 Pennsylvania Avenue NW
Washington, DC 20506

202-682-5400
TTY: 202-682-5496
e-mail: webmgr@arts.endow.gov
www.nea.gov

Since 1957, the YAI Network has been providing hope and opportunity to people of all ages with developmental disabilities and their families. Our organization includes more than 450 programs and serves more than 20,000 people every day.
Stephen E. Freeman, CEO
Thomas A. Dern, COO

10519 National Institute for People with Disabil ities
460 W 34th Street
New York, NY 10001-2382

212-273-6100
www.yai.org

To create hope and opportunity for people with developmental and learning disabilities and their families.
Philip H Levy PhD, President/CEO

10520 National Institute of Child Health and Human Development
31 Center Drive
Bethesda, MD 20892

301-496-5133
800-370-2943
Fax: 866-760-5947
TTY: 888-320-6942
e-mail: NICHDInformationResourceCenter@mail.nih.
www.nichd.nih.gov

The NICHD was initially founded to realize a vision: to support the world's best minds in investigating human development throughout the entire life process, focusing on understanding developmental disabilities, including intellectual and developmental disabilities (IDDs), and illuminating important events that occur during pregnancy.
Alan E Guttmacher, Director

10521 National Institute of Disability and Rehabilitation Research
US Department of Education

400 Maryland Avenue SW
Washington, DC 20202

202-245-7640
Fax: 202-245-7323
TTY: 202-245-7316
www.ninds.nih.gov/find_people/government

provides leadership and support for a comprehensive program and research related to the rehabilitation of individuals with disabilities. All of the programmatic efforts are aimed at improving the lives of individuals with disabilities from birth through adulthood.

10522 National Job Accommodation Network
Morgantown, WV 26506-6080

304-293-7186
800-526-7234
Fax: 304-293-5407
TTY: 877-781-9403
e-mail: jan@askjan.org
www.askjan.org

The JAN is an international information service for people with disabilities and their employers. They have information about implementation of workplace accommodations as well as resources to promote an awareness of functional limitations.
Anne Hirsh, Co-Director
Louis Orslene, Co-Director

10523 National Legal Center for the Medically Dependent & Disabled
50 S Meridian Street
Indianapolis, IN 46204-3537

317-632-6245

Committed to defending the rights of vulnerable persons threatened by infanticide, euthanasia, assisted suicide, non-voluntary withdrawal/withholding of essential medical treatment and care and discrimination in health care financing.
Marilyn Bove, President

10524 National Network of Learning Disabled Adults
808 N 82nd Street
Scottsdale, AZ 85257

602-941-5112

Provides information and referral for LD adults involved with or in search of support groups and networking opportunities.

10525 National Organization for Rare Disorders
55 Kenosia Avenue
Danbury, CT 06810-1968

203-744-0100
800-999-6673
Fax: 203-798-2291
TDD: 203-797-9590
e-mail: orphan@rarediseases.org
www.rarediseases.org

The National Organization for Rare Disorders(NORD) a 501(c)3 organization is a unique federation of voluntary health organizations dedicated to helping people with rare orphan diseases and assisting the organizations that serve them.
Peter L. Saltonstall, President & CEO
Russell Teagarden, Senior Vice President of Medical and Sci

10526 National Organization on Disability
77 Water Street
New York, NY 10005

646-505-1191
Fax: 646-505-1184
e-mail: info@nod.org
www.nod.org

The National Organization on Disability (NOD) is a private, non-profit organization that promotes the full participation of America's 56 million people with disabilities in all aspects of life.
Carol Glazer, President
Aleysha Anderson, Administrative Assistant

10527 National Parent Network on Disabilities
1130 17th Street NW
Washington, DC 20036

202-434-8686
Fax: 202-638-7299
www.npnd.org

To provide a presence and national voice for all families of children, youth and adults with disabilities.
Linda Shepard, Executive Director
Jill Foss, Office Manager

10528 National Rehabilitation Information Center
8400 Corporate Drive
Landover, MD 20785

301-459-5900
800-346-2742
Fax: 301-459-4263
TTY: 301-459-5984
e-mail: naricinfo@heitechservices.com
www.naric.com

One of the three components of the office of Special Education and Rehabilitative Services. Mission is to generate, disseminate and promote new knowledge to improve the options available to disabled persons. The ultimate goal is to allow these individuals to perform their regular activities in the community and to bolster society's ability to provide full opportunities and appropriate supports for its disabled citizens.
Mark Odum, Director

10529 North American Society for Pediatric Gastroenterology, Hepatology & Nutrition
Flourtown, PA 19031
215-233-0808
Fax: 215-233-3918
e-mail: naspghan@naspghan.org
www.naspghan.org
To advance understanding of normal development, physiology and pathophysiology of diseases of the gastrointestinal tract and liver in children, improve quality of care by fostering the dissemination of this knowledge through scientific meetings, professional and public education, and policy development, and serve as an effective voice for members and the profession.
Margaret K Stallings, Executive Director
Kim Rose, Director of Membership

10530 Office of Civil Rights
US Department of Education
S/OCR, Room 7428
Washington, DC 20520-1100
202-647-9295
800-421-3481
Fax: 202-647-4969
TTY: 877-521-2172
e-mail: socr_direct@state.gov
www.state.gov/s/ocr/
To ensure equal access to education and to promote educational excellence throughout the nation through vigorous enforcement of civil rights.
Russlynn Ali, Assistant Secretary

10531 Office of Policy Planning and Legislation
200 Independence Avenue SW
Washington, DC 20201-0004
202-619-0257
877-696-6775
www.hhs.gov/about/referlst.html
Administers grants to the states for social services under Title XX of the Social Security Act to welfare recipients and others likely to become welfare recipients.
G Barry Nielsen, Director

10532 Office of Special Education Programs
Department of Education
400 Maryland Avenue SW
Washington, DC 20202
202-245-7459
www2.ed.gov/about/offices/list/osers
Dedicated to improving results for infants, toddlers, children and youth with disabilities ages birth through 21 by providing leadership and financial support to assist states and local districts.
Melody Musgrove, Director
Bill Wolf, Acting Deputy Director

10533 Office on Smoking and Health
Centers for Disease Control and Prevention
4770 Buford Highway
Atlanta, GA 30341-3717
404-639-3311
800-232-4636
TTY: 888-232-6348
e-mail: tobaccoinfo@cdc.gov
www.cdc.gov/tobacco/osh/index.htm
The leading federal agency for comprehensive tobacco prevention and control, the Office develops, conducts, and supports strategic efforts to protect the public's health from the harmful effects of tobacco use.
Tim McAfee MD MPH, Director

10534 Option Institute International Learning & Training Center
2080 S Undermountain Road
Sheffield, MA 01257
413-229-2100
800-714-2779
Fax: 413-229-8931
e-mail: participantsupport@option.org
www.option.org
Offers self improvement and personal growth workshops and seminars that provide practical tools and strategies to help people worldwide to live happier, more confident, more empowered and more fulfilling lives, and enjoy gratifying relationships and careers.
Barry Neil Kaufman, Co-Founder/Co-Director
Samahria Kaufman, Co-Founder/Co-Director

10535 Pediatric Neurology Georgetown University Hospital
Georgetown University Hospital
3800 Reservoir Road NW
Washington, DC 20007
202-444-2000
www.georgetownuniversityhospital.org
provides a wide range of consultative services, neurodiagnostic studies and therapies for children with neurodevelopmental disorders.
Cesar Santos MD, Chief

10536 People-to-People Committee for the Handicapped
Washington, DC 20036-8131
301-774-7446
Individuals concerned about the circumstances of handicapped people throughout the world. Disseminates information acts as a consultant in promoting exchange activities coordinates special assistance projects in developing countries and more.
David Brigham, Chairman

10537 President's Committee on the Employment of People with Disabilities
200 Constitution Avenue NW
Washington, DC 20210
202-693-6000
866-633-7365
Fax: 202-693-7888
TTY: 877-889-5627
e-mail: webmaster@dol.gov
www.dol.gov
Independent federal agency to facilitate the communication coordination and promotion of public and private efforts to empower Americans with disabilities through employment.
Seth D. Harris, Secretary of Labour
Ana M. Ma, Chief of Staff

10538 Rehabilitation International
25 E 21st Street
New York, NY 10010
212-420-1500
Fax: 212-505-0871
e-mail: ri@riglobal.org
www.riglobal.org
RI and its members work to protect the rights of people with disabilities, including ensuring access to and the improvement of crucial services for persons with disabilities and their families
Jan A. Monsbakken, President
Megan Brinster, Development/Program Officer

10539 Rehabilitation Services Administration
US Department of Education
1125 15th Street, NW
Washington, DC 20005-2800
202-730-1843
Fax: 202-730-1843
TTY: 202-730-1516
e-mail: dds@dc.gov
www.dc.gov/DC/DDS/Rehabilitation+Service
Oversees grant programs that help individuals with physical or mental disabilities to obtain employment and live more independently through the provision of such supports as counseling, medical and psychological services, job training and other individualized services.
Lynnae M Ruttledge, Commissioner

10540 Social Security Administration Office of Public Inquiries
Office of Public Inquiries
Windsor Park Building
Baltimore, MD 21235
800-772-1213
TTY: 800-325-0778
www.ssa.gov
Administers old age survivors and disability insurance programs under Title II of the Social Security Act. Also administers the federal income maintenance program under Title XVI of the Social Security Act. Maintains networks of local/regional offices.
Michael J Astrue, Commissioner
James A Winn, Chief of Staff

10541 US Department of Justice
950 Pennsylvania Avenue NW
Washington, DC 20530-0001
202-514-2000
e-mail: askdoj@usdoj.gov
www.usdoj.gov

To enforce the law and defend the interests of the United States according to the law; to ensure public safety against threats foreign and domestic; to provide federal leadership in preventing and controlling crime; to seek just punishment for those guilty of unlawful behavior; and to ensure fair and impartial administration of justice for all Americans.
Eric Holder, Attorney General
James Cole, Deputy Attorney General

10542 US Department of Transportation
1200 New Jersey Avenue SE
Washington, DC 20590

202-366-4000
866-377-8642
TTY: 800-877-8339
e-mail: dot.comments@dot.gov
www.dot.gov

Serves the United States by ensuring a fast, safe, efficient, accessible and convenient transportation system that meets the vital national interests and enhances the quality of life of the American people, today and into the future.
Anthony Foxx, Secretary of Transportation
John D. Porcari, Deputy Secretary of Transport

10543 US Office of Personnel Management
1900 E Street NW
Washington, DC 20415

202-606-1800
TTY: 202-606-2532
e-mail: General@opm.gov
www.opm.gov

Recruiting, retaining and honoring a world-class workforce to serve the American people.
Elaine Kaplan, Acting Director

10544 World Institute on Disability
3075 Adeline Street
Berkeley, CA 94703-1520

510-225-6400
Fax: 510-225-0477
TTY: 510-225-0478
e-mail: wid@wid.org
www.wid.org

WID's mission in communities and nations worldwide is to eliminate barriers to full social integration and increase employment, economic security, and health care for persons with disabilities
Anita Shafer Aaron, Executive Director
Rebecca Palmer, Executive Assistant

State Agencies & Associations

Alabama

10545 Division of Rehabilitation: Montgomery
Montgomery, AL 36111-0586
Marilyn Bove, President

334-281-8780

Alaska

10546 Client Assistance Program: Anchorage
3330 Arctic Boulevard
Anchorage, AK 99503

907-333-2211
800-478-1234
Fax: 907-565-1000
e-mail: akpa@dlcak.org
www.home.gci.net/~alaskacap

James Shine, President
Julie Renwick, Vice President

Arizona

10547 HPV Support Groups: Arizona
7331 E Osborn Drive
Scottsdale, AZ 85251-6422

602-994-8330
800-223-2159
e-mail: sthf@home.com

Arkansas

10548 Disability Rights Center of Arkansas
1100 N University
Little Rock, AR 72207

501-296-1775
800-482-1174
Fax: 501-296-1779
e-mail: panda@advocacyservices.org
www.arkdisabilityrights.org

Protection and advocacy system for people with disabilities in Arkansas.
Traci Perrin, President

California

10549 Disability Rights California
1831 K Street
Sacramento, CA 95811

916-504-5800
800-776-5746
Fax: 916-504-5801
TTY: 800-719-5798
e-mail: services@disabilityrightsca.org
www.disabilityrightsca.org

Mission is to advance the rights of Californians with disabilities.
Catherine Blakemore, Executive Director
Andrew Murdryk, Deputy Director

Colorado

10550 Disability Careers
5760 E Evans Avenue
Denver, CO 80222-5305

303-757-3070
Fax: 303-757-3392

This is a non profit corporation that provides employee and employer services. Founder and Executive Director Ted Pavakis is a former commercial real estate broker with multiple sclerosis.

10551 Legal Center for People with Disabilities and Older People
455 Sherman Street
Denver, CO 80203

303-722-0300
800-288-1376
Fax: 303-722-0720
TTY: 303-722-3619
e-mail: tlcmail@thelegalcenter.org
www.thelegalcenter.org

An independent public interest non-profit specializing in civil rights and discrimination issues. We protect the human, civil and legal rights of people with mental and physical disabilities, people with HIV, and older people throughout Colorado.
Mary Anne Harvey, Executive Director
Peter Lindquist, President

Connecticut

10552 Office of Protection and Advocacy for Persons with Disabilities
60B Weston Street
Hartford, CT 06120-1551

860-297-4300
800-842-7303
TTY: 860-297-4380
www.ct.gov

To advance the cause of equal rights for persons with disabilities and their families by: increasing the ability of individuals, groups and systems to safeguard rights; exposing instances and patterns of discrimination and abuse; seeking individual and systemic remediation when rights are violated; increasing public awareness of unjust situations and of means to address them; and empowering people with disabilities and their families to advocate effectively.

Delaware

10553 Client Assistance Program: Delaware
13 SW Front Street
Milford, DE 19963-1900
Marilyn Bove, President

302-422-6744

District of Columbia

10554 Client Assistance Program: District of Columbia
Rehabilitation Services Administration
605 G Street NW
Washington, DC 20001-3705
Jim Tolbert, Director

202-727-0977

10555 Information Protection & Advocacy Center for Handicapped Individuals
Center for Handicapped Individuals
4455 Connecticut Avenue NW
Washington, DC 20008-2328
Marilyn Bove, President

202-966-8081

Florida

10556 Disability Rights: Florida
2728 Centerview Drive
Tallahassee, FL 32301

850-488-9071
800-342-0823
Fax: 850-488-8640
TDD: 800-346-4127
e-mail: info@advocacycenter.org
www.disabilityrightsflorida.org

To advance the quality of life, dignity, equality, self-determination, and freedom of choice of persons with disabilities through collaboration, education, advocacy, as well, as legal and legislative issues.
Catherine Piecora, Chair
Minerva Bailey, Vice-Chair

10557 North Florida: HPV Support Group
126 Salem Court
Tallahassee, FL 32301-2810

850-877-3183

Georgia

10558 Division of Rehabilitation Service
148 Andrew Young Int'l Blvd NE
Atlanta, GA 30303-1751

404-232-3910
TTY: 404-232-3911
e-mail: rehab@dol.state.ga.us
www.vocrehabga.org

Operates five integrated and interdependent programs that share a primary goal — to help people with disabilities to become fully productive members of society by achieving independence and meaningful employment.

Hawaii

10559 Protection & Advocacy Agency
1132 Bishop Street
Honolulu, HI 96813-9607

808-949-2922
800-882-1057
Fax: 808-949-2928
TTY: 808-949-2922
e-mail: info@hawaiidisabilityrights.org
www.hawaiidisabilityrights.org

Hawaii Disability Rights Center is the State of Hawaii's designated client assistance program and designated protection and advocacy system for people with disabilities.
Gary L Smith, Executive Director

Idaho

10560 Co-Ad
4477 Emerald St
Boise, ID 83706-2017

208-336-5353
800-632-5125
Fax: 208-336-5396
TTY: 208-336-5353
e-mail: coadinc@cableone.net
www.users.moscow.com

Marilyn Bove, President

Illinois

10561 Illinois Client Assistance Program
Illinois Department of Human Services
100 N 1st Street
Springfield, IL 62702

800-641-3929
TTY: 800-447-6404
e-mail: dhs.cap@illinois.gov
www.dhs.state.il.us

Helps people with disabilities receive quality services by advocating for their interests and helping them identify resources, understand procedures, resolve problems, and protect their rights in the rehabilitation process, employment and home services.

Indiana

10562 Indiana Protection and Advocacy Services
4701 N Keystone Avenue
Indianapolis, IN 46205

800-622-4845
TTY: 800-838-1131
e-mail: kpedevilla@ipas.in.gov
www.in.gov/ipas

To protect and promote the rights of individuals with disabilities, through empowerment and advocacy.
Karen Pedevilla, Education/Training Director

Iowa

10563 Client Assistance Program: Iowa Division o n Persons with Disabilities
Division on Persons with Disabilities
Lucas State Office Building
Des Moines, IA 50310

515-281-3656
800-652-4298
Fax: 515-242-6119
TTY: 800-652-4298
e-mail: dhr.disabilities@iowa.gov
www.humanrights.iowa.gov/pd/text_version

The Division of Persons with Disabilities exists to promote the employment of Iowans with disabilities and reduce barriers to employment by providing information, referral, assessment and guidance, training, and negotiation services to employers and citizens with disabilities.
Marilyn Bove, President

Kansas

10564 Disability Rights Center of Kansas
635 SW Harrison
Topeka, KS 66603-3726

785-273-9661
877-776-1541
Fax: 785-273-9414
TTY: 877-335-3725
e-mail: rocky@drckansas.org
www.icdri.org

A public interest legal advocacy agency empowered by federal law to advocate for the civil and legal rights of Kansans with disabilities.
Rocky Nichols MPA, Executive Director
Debbie White, Deputy Director

Kentucky

10565 Client Assistance Program: Kentucky
275 E Main Street
Frankfort, KY 40621

502-564-4440
800-633-6283
e-mail: vanessa.denham@ky.gov
www.ovr.ky.gov

David Beach, Executive Director
Jane Smith, Director of Program Services

Louisiana

10566 Advocacy Center
8325 Oak Street
New Orleans, LA 70118

504-522-2337
800-960-7705
Fax: 504-522-5507
TTY: 855-861-3577
e-mail: advocacycenter@advocacyla.org
www.advocacyla.org

Serves people with disabilities and senior citizens.
Lois Simpson, Executive Director

Maine

10567 Disability Rights Center: Maine
24 Stone St
Augusta, ME 04330-2007

207-626-2774
800-452-1948
Fax: 207-621-1419
e-mail: advocate@drcme.org
www.drcme.org

To enhance and promote the equality, self-determination, independence, productivity, integration, and inclusion of people with disabilities through education, strategic advocacy and legal intervention.
Kim Moody, Executive Director
Kristin Aiello, Managing Attourney

Maryland

10568 Client Assistance Program: Maryland
Maryland State Department of Education

2301 Argonne Drive
Baltimore, MD 21218

410-554-9442
888-554-0334
Fax: 410-554-9362
TTY: 410-554-9360
e-mail: cap@dors.state.md.us
www.dors.state.md.us

Helps individuals who have concerns or difficulties when applying for or receiving rehabilitation services funded under the Rehabilitation Act.
Beth Lash, Director

Massachusetts

10569 Client Assistance Program: Massachusetts
250 Washington Street
Boston, MA 02108-1518

617-727-7440
800-322-2020
e-mail: james.aprea@state.ma.us
www.mass.gov

If you have a disability and want to work but are having trouble getting vocational rehabilitation services, or want a lifestyle which is more self-reliant but are having trouble getting independent living services, contact the Client Assistance Program (CAP).
Barbara E Lybarger Esq, Director

10570 Merrimack Valley HPV Support Group Holy Family Hospital
Holy Family Hospital
70 E Street
Methuen, MA 01844-4597

978-687-0156

10571 Neurosurgical Service
Massachusetts General Hospital
55 Fruit Street
Boston, MA 02114

617-726-2937
e-mail: Referral@Neurosurgery.MassGeneral.org
neurosurgery.mgh.harvard.edu

Uses a multidisciplinary approach to provide a complete range of services for the diagnosis, treatment and rehabilitation of patients with neurological disorders.

Michigan

10572 Client Assistance Program: Michigan
Michigan Protection and Advocacy Service
4095 Legacy Parkway
Lansing, MI 48911-7508

517-487-1755
800-292-5896
Fax: 517-487-0827
e-mail: molson@mpas.org
www.mpas.org

Assists people who are seeking or receiving services from Michigan Rehabilitation Services, Consumer Choice Programs, Michigan Commission for the Blind, Centers for Independent Living, and Supported Employment and Transition Programs.
Mark R Lezotte, President

10573 Commission for the Blind
201 N Washington 2nd Floor
Lansing, MI 48909

517-373-2062
800-292-4200
Fax: 517-335-5140
TDD: 517-373-4025
e-mail: heibeckc@michigan.gov
www.michigan.gov/mcb

To provide opportunity to individuals who are blind or visually impaired to achieve employability and/or function independently in society.
Patrick Cannon, Director

Minnesota

10574 Minnesota Disability Law Center
430 1st Avenue N
Minneapolis, MN 55401-1780

612-334-5970
Fax: 612-334-5755
TTY: 612-332-4668
www.mndlc.org

Addresses the unique legal needs of Minnesotans with disabilities. Provides free civil legal assistance to individuals with disabilities statewide on legal issues related to their disabilities.
Cathy Madouken, Executive Director
Lisa Cohen, Deputy Director of Operations

Mississippi

10575 Mississippi Client Assistance Program
Mississippi Society for Disabilities
Jackson, MS 39296

601-362-2585
800-962-2400
Fax: 601-982-1951
www.icdri.org

A federal grant to the State of Mississippi to provide advocacy services for clients and client applicants of the Office of Vocational Rehabilitation, Vocational Rehabilitation for the Blind, and the Independent Living programs.
Johnny McGinn, Director

Missouri

10576 Missouri Protection and Advocacy Services
925 S Country Club Drive
Jefferson City, MO 65109

573-893-3333
866-777-7199
Fax: 573-893-4231
TDD: 800-735-2966
e-mail: mopasjc@embarqmail.com
www.moadvocacy.org

To protect the rights of individuals with disabilities by providing advocacy and legal services.
Joe Wrinkle, Chair
Lawrence O. Daniels, Vice-Chair

Montana

10577 Disability Rights Montana
1022 Chestnut Street
Helena, MT 59601

406-449-2344
800-245-4743
Fax: 406-449-2418
TDD: 406-449-2344
e-mail: advocate@disabilityrightsmt.org
www.disabilityrightsmt.org

Protects and advocates for the human, legal, and civil rights of Montanans with disabilities while advancing dignity, equality, and self-determination.
Bernadette Franks-Ongoy, Executive Director
Alexandra Volkerts, Staff Attourney

Nebraska

10578 Client Assistance Program: Nebraska Division of Rehabilitative Services
Division of Rehabilitative Services
301 Centennial Mall S
Lincoln, NE 68509

402-471-3656
800-742-7594
e-mail: victoria.rasmussen@cap.ne.gov
www.cap.state.ne.us

The Nebraska Client Assistance Program is a free service to help you find solutions if you are having problems with any of the following programs: Vocational Rehabilitation, Nebraska Commission for the Blind and Visually Impaired or Centers for Independent Living.

10579 Omaha HPV Support Group: PP of Omaha
Planned Parenhood
4610 Dodge Street
Omaha, NE 68132-3234

402-397-2739
www.aad.org

Nevada

10580 Client Assistance Program: Nevada
2800 E Saint Louis Avenue
Las Vegas, NV 89104

775-684-3849
800-633-9879
Fax: 775-684-3850
TTY: 800-326-6868
e-mail: InternetHelp@nvdetr.org
www.detr.state.nv.us

Designed to assist individuals with disabilities resolve problems they may experience with any of Nevada's rehabilitation programs.
Maureen Cole, Rehabilitation Administrator

New Hampshire

10581 Client Assistance Program: New Hampshire
Governor's Commission for the Handicapped
57 Regional Drive   603-271-2773
Concord, NH 03301-8518   800-852-3405
Fax: 603-271-2837
e-mail: disability@nh.gov
www.nh.gov/disability/about/cap.htm
CAP provides information about vocational rehabilitation services; advises you of your rights and responsibilities; investigate your complaint; helps resolve problems with your vocational plan; and represents you at administratove reviews and fair hearings.
John Richards, Executive Director

New Jersey

10582 Disability Rights New Jersey
210 S Broad Street   609-292-9742
Trenton, NJ 08608   800-922-7233
Fax: 609-777-0187
TTY: 609-633-7106
e-mail: adocate@drnj.org
www.drnj.org
To protect, advocate for and advance the rights of persons with disabilities in pursuit of a society in hich persons with disabilities exercise self-determination and choice, and are treated with dignity.
Walter A. Woodberry, Chair
Kathleen F. Wood, Vice Chair

New Mexico

10583 Protection and Advocacy System of Alburque rque
1720 Louisiana Boulevard NE   505-256-3100
Albuquerque, NM 87110-7070   800-432-4682
Fax: 505-256-3184
e-mail: info@drnm.org
www.drnm.org
Disability Rights New Mexico - DRNM - is a private, non-profit organization whose mission is to protect, promote and expand the rights of persons with disabilities.
Marilyn Bove, President

New York

10584 Client Assistance Program: NY State Commission of Quality of Care
Advocacy Bureau
One Commerce Plaza   518-459-6422
Albany, NY 12234-2810   800-222-5627
Fax: 518-473-6296
e-mail: accesadm@mail.nysed.gov
www.acces.nysed.gov/vr/do/cap.htm
The Client Assistance Program (CAP) is a statewide network of skilled advocates that assist New Yorkers with disabilities in getting the training, equipment and services needed for employment.
Marilyn Bove, President

10585 March of Dimes Foundation
1275 Mamaroneck Avenue
White Plains, NY 10605   914-997-4488
www.marchofdimes.com
We help moms have full-term pregnancies and research the problems that threaten the health of babies
Jennifer L Howse, President/CEO

North Carolina

10586 North Carolina Client Assistance Program
805 Ruggles Drive   919-855-3600
Raleigh, NC 27603-2806   800-215-7227
Fax: 919-715-2456
e-mail: nccap@dhhs.nc.gov
www.cap.state.nc.us
Helping people understand and access rehabilitation services.
John Marens, Director
Sharon Wisner, Client Advocate

North Dakota

10587 Client Assistance Program: North Dakota
400 East Broadway   701-328-2950
Bismarck, ND 58501-1208   800-472-2670
Fax: 701-328-3934
TDD: 707-328-8968
e-mail: panda@nd.gov
www.ndpanda.org/cap
Assists clients and client applicants of North Dakota Vocational Rehabilitation services, Tribal Vocational Rehabilitation, or Independent Living services.

Ohio

10588 Cincinnati HPV Support Group: PP of Cincin nati
Planned Parenthood
PO Box 12407
Cincinnati, OH 45212-0407   513-357-7300
www.dermconsultants.com

10589 Disability Rights Center at Ohio Legal Rights Service
50 W Broad Street   614-466-7264
Columbus, OH 43215-5923   800-282-9181
TTY: 614-728-2553
www.disabilityrightsohio.org
To protect and advocate, in partnership with people with disabilities, for their human, civil and legal rights.
Kalpana Yalamanchili, Chair

10590 Richland County HPV Support Group
Mansfield, OH 44907-3881
419-525-3075
www.skinpatient.com

10591 Technology Resource Center
2140 Arbor Boulevard   937-294-8086
Dayton, OH 45439

Oklahoma

10592 Client Assistance Program: Oklahoma Office of Handicapped Concerns
Oklahoma Ofice of Handicapped Concerns
2401 NW 23rd   405-521-3756
Oklahoma City, OK 73107-5106   Fax: 405-522-6695
e-mail: Marilyn.Burr@ohc.state.ok.us
www.icdri.org

Marilyn Bove, President

10593 Oklahoma City HPV Support Group: PP of Cen tral Oklahoma
Planned Parenthood of Central Oklahoma
Oklahoma City, OK 73103-1415
405-528-0221
www.aad.org

Oregon

10594 Resources for Seniors and People with Disabilities
Department of Human Services
500 Summer Street NE   503-947-5811
Salem, OR 97301-1097   800-282-8096
Fax: 503-378-2897
TTY: 800-282-8096
e-mail: spd.web@state.or.us
www.oregon.gov
To secure economic, social, legal and political justice for individuals with disabilities through systems change
Dr Bruce Goldberg, Director
Margaret Carter, Deputy Director Human Services Program

Pennsylvania

10595 Client Assistance Program: Philadelphia
1515 Market Street   215-557-7112
Philadelphia, PA 19102   888-745-2357
Fax: 215-557-7602
TDD: 215-557-7112
e-mail: info@equalemployment.org
www.equalemployment.org

Ensuring that vocation rehabilitation is open and responsive to your needs. Provides information and advice about rehabilitation programs; to advise you of your legal rights and responsibilities; to help resolve probelms that may arise while you are seeking services from rehabilitation programs; to help you pursue administrative and legal remedies to protect your rights.
Stephen S Pennington, Executive Director
Jamie C Ray- Leonetti, Assistant Director

Rhode Island

10596 Rhode Island Disability Law Center
275 Westminster Street
Providence, RI 02903-3434
401-831-3150
800-733-5332
Fax: 401-274-5568
TTY: 401-831-5335
e-mail: info@ridlc.org
www.ridlc.org
Provides free legal assistance to persons with disabilities. Services include individual representation to protect rights or to secure benefits and services; self-help information; educational programs; and administrative and legislative advocacy.

South Carolina

10597 South Carolina Protection & Advocacy System for the Handicapped
3710 Landmark Drive
Columbia, SC 29204-4034
803-782-0639
866-275-7273
TTY: 866-232-4525
e-mail: info@pandasc.org
www.pandasc.org

Marilyn Bove, President

10598 Tri County HPV Support Group
Mt Pleasant, SC 29465-1997
843-884-7333
www.aad.org

South Dakota

10599 South Dakota Advocacy Services
221 S Central Avenue
Pierre, SD 57501
605-224-8294
800-658-4782
Fax: 605-224-5125
TTY: 800-658-4782
e-mail: sdas@sdadvocacy.com
www.sdadvocacy.com
To protect and advocate the rights of South Dakotans with disabilities through legal, administrative, and other remedies.

Tennessee

10600 Disability Law & Advocacy Center of Tennessee
2416 21st Avenue S
Nashville, TN 37212
615-298-1080
800-342-1660
Fax: 615-298-2046
e-mail: gethelp@dlactn.org
www.dlactn.org
Advocates for the rights of Tennesseans with disabilities to ensure they have an equal opportunity to be productive and respected members of the society.
Jerry Gonzalez, Chair
Shalani Rose, Vice Chair

Texas

10601 Dallas/Ft.Worth Metroplex HPV Support Group
8215 Westchester Drive
Dallas, TX 75225-6116
214-363-6733

10602 Disability Rights Texas
Advocacy Inc
2222 W Braker Lane
Austin, TX 78758-1024
512-454-4816
866-362-2851
Fax: 512-323-0902
www.advocacyinc.org
Protecting and advocating the rights of Texans with disabilities - because all people have dignity and worth.
Mary Faithfull, Executive Director

Utah

10603 Legal Center for People with Disabilities
205 North 400 West
Salt Lake City, UT 84103-3076
801-363-1347
800-662-9080
Fax: 801-363-1437
www.disabilitylawcenter.org
We enforce and strengthen laws that protect the opportunities, choices and legal rights of people with disabilities in Utah.
Kevin Murphy, President
Barbara M. Campbell, Senior VP

Vermont

10604 Citizen Advocacy of Burlington
Chase Mill 1 Mill Street
Burlington, VT 05401
802-655-0329
Marilyn Bove, President

10605 Client Assistance Program: Vermont Ladd Hall
Ladd Hall
57 N Main Street
Rutland, VT 05701-8409
802-775-0021
800-769-7459
Fax: 802-775-0022
e-mail: nbreiden@vtlegalaid.org
www.icdri.org

Marilyn Bove, President

Virginia

10606 Richmond HPV Support Group: Fan Free Clini c
Fan Free Clinic
PO Box 5669
Richmond, VA 23220-0669
804-358-6343
www.ashastd.org

10607 Virginia Office for Protection and Advocacy
1910 Byrd Avenue
Richmond, VA 23230
804-225-2042
800-552-3962
Fax: 804-662-7057
e-mail: general.vopa@vopa.virginia.gov
www.vopa.state.va.us
Helps with disability-related problems like abuse, neglect, and discrimination. Also help people with disabilities obtain services and treatment.
Coleen Miller, Executive Director
Eric Berthiaume, Administrator

Washington

10608 Seattle HPV Support Group
Seattle, WA 98103-1171
425-619-7190
www.aad.org

10609 Washington State Client Assistance Program
2531 Rainer Avenue S
Seattle, WA 98144-9510
206-721-5999
800-544-2121
Fax: 206-721-5980
TTY: 888-721-6072
e-mail: info@washingtoncap.org
www.washingtoncap.org

Jerry Johnson, Director
Bob Huven, Rehabilitation Coordinator

West Virginia

10610 Northcentral West Virginia HPV Support Group
Monongalia County Health Department
453 Van Voorhis Road
Morgantown, WV 26505-3408
304-598-5100

10611 West Virginia Advocates
1207 Quarrier Street
Charleston, WV 25301
304-346-0847
800-950-5250
Fax: 304-346-0867
e-mail: contact@wvadvocates.org
www.wvadvocates.org

Protects and advocates for the human and legal rights of persons with disabilities.
Clarice Hausch, Executive Director
Barbara Criner, Administrative Director

Wisconsin

10612 Governor's Committee for People with Disabilities
Wisconsin Department of Health Services
1 W Wilson Street
Madison, WI 53703

608-261-7816
Fax: 608-266-3386
TTY: 888-701-1251
e-mail: sarah.lincoln@wisconsin.gov
www.dhs.wisconsin.gov/Disabilities/Physi

In 1948, a Governor's Committee was established with one goal: to improve employment opportunities for people with disabilities.
Sarah Lincoln, Director

Wyoming

10613 Wyoming Protection & Advocacy System
7344 Stockman Street
Cheyenne, WY 82009

307-632-3496
Fax: 307-638-0815
e-mail: wypanda@wypanda.com
www.wypanda.com

To establish, expand, protect and enforce the human and civil rights of persons with disabilities through administrative, legal, and other appropriate remedies.
Mary Carson Barks, President
Jeanne A Thobro, CEO

Libraries & Resource Centers

Alabama

10614 Horizons Schools
2018 15th Avenue South
Birmingham, AL 35205

205-322-6606
800-822-6242
Fax: 205-322-6605
www.horizonsschool.org

The Horizons School offers a non-degree postsecondary program specifically designed to facilitate personal, social and career independence for students with mild learning disabilities and other mild handicapping conditions.
Don Lutomski, President
Bayard Tynes, Treasurer

Arizona

10615 Life Development Institute
18001 N 79th Avenue
Glendale, AZ 85308

623-773-2774
866-736-7811
Fax: 623-773-2788
e-mail: info@life-development-inst.org
www.lifedevelopmentinstitute.org

Make the special wishes of children with life-threatening or terminal illnesses come true.
Rob Crawford, CEO
Veronica Crawford, Vice President

California

10616 Center for Adaptive Learning
3227 Clayton Road
Concord, CA 94519

925-827-3863
Fax: 925-827-4080
e-mail: info@c4al.org
www.centerforadaptivelearning.org

Committed to creating and maintaining a living and working environment for neurologically impaired individuals, which will promote dignity and support a sense of community. The CAL program provides each participant with an individual program for growth. CAL is committed to maintaining the highest quality of living possible, which will allow each client to develop a sense of pride, to augment self-esteem and to foster a sense of self-worth.
Robert L. Edwards, President
Barry Chinn, VP

10617 Independence Center
3640 S Sepulveda Boulevard
Los Angeles, CA 90034

310-202-7102
Fax: 310-202-7180
e-mail: judym@independencecenter.com
www.independencecenter.com

A mainstreamed transitional residential program for young adults (18-30) with learning disabilities. Program highlights include training in independent living, social and vocational skills, counseling and more.
Judith Maizlish, Executive Director
Gloria Ogletree, Administrative Director

Connecticut

10618 Chapel Haven
1040 Whalley Avenue
New Haven, CT 06515

203-397-1714
Fax: 203-937-2466
e-mail: admissions@chapelhaven.org
www.chapelhaven.org

Providing an array of lifelong individualized support services for adults (18+) on the autism spectrum and those with developmental and social disabilities, enabling them to lead independent and productive lives.
Betsey Parlato, CEO/Executive Director

District of Columbia

10619 ERIC Clearinghouse on Disabilities and Gifted Education
ERIC Project
C/O Computer Sciences Corporation
Washington, DC 20008

800-538-3742
Fax: 703-620-4334
TTY: 703-264-9449
www.eric.ed.gov

The ERIC mission is to provide a comprehensive, easy-to-use, searchable, Internet-based bibliographic and full-text database of education research and information. The simple version of that is that it provides an enormous amount of print materials online, for easy access to important research and journal materials.
Cheryl Racey, Director

Georgia

10620 Creative Community Services (CCS)
4487 Park Drive
Norcross, GA 30093

770-469-6226
866-618-2823
Fax: 770-469-6210
e-mail: info@ccsgeorgia.org
www.ccsgeorgia.org

Provides therapeutic foster care services for children and home-based support for adults with developmental disabilities. CCS improves the quality of life for children, adults and families through its community-based support and services. CCS gives both kids and adults hope by encouraging independent living resulting in involved, engaged citizens and community members.
Nicolette Lee, President
Henri Munyengano, Secretary

Massachusetts

10621 Berkshire Center
18 Park Street
Lee, MA 01238

413-243-2576
Fax: 413-243-3351
www.berkshirecenter.org

The College Internship Program at the Berkshire Center provides individualized, post-secondary academic, internship and independent living experiences for young adults with Asperger's Syndrome and other Learning Differences.
Lucy Gosselin MSBM, Program Director

Minnesota

10622 National Resource Library on Youth with Disabilities
University of Minnesota

Minneapolis, MN 55455

612-626-3087
800-276-8642
Fax: 612-626-2134
TTY: 612-624-3939
e-mail: kdwb-var@umn.edu
www.peds.umn.edu

Offers comprehensive sources of information related to adolescents, disability and transition. The database contains bibliographic, programs, training/education and technical assistance files for the medical community, families, parents and children with chronic illnesses.
Peggy Mann Reinhart, Director
Elizabeth Latts, Resource Coordinator

New Hampshire

10623 Camp Allen
56 Camp Road
Bedford, NH 03110-6606

603-622-8471
Fax: 603-626-4295
e-mail: mary@campallennh.orgg
www.campallennh.org

Camp Allen welcomes about 600 campers each summer. They are persons of all ages with special needs and extraordinary challenges, including cerebral palsy, autism, muscular dystrophy, Down syndrome, and other developmental disabilities.
Sebastian Grasso, President & CEO
Thomas Aites, Treasurer

New Jersey

10624 HealthyWomen
157 Broad Street
Red Bank, NJ 07701

877-986-9472
Fax: 732-530-3347
e-mail: info@healthywomen.org
www.healthywomen.org

Independent health information source for women whose mission is to educate, inform and empower women to make smart health choices for themselves and their families.
Elizabeth Battaglino Cahill, RN, Executive Director
Erin Graves, Director of Marketing & Communications

New York

10625 Center for Medical Consumers
239 Thompson Street
New York, NY 10012

212-674-7105
Fax: 212-674-7100
e-mail: centersformedicalconsumers@gmail.com
www.medicalconsumers.org

A non-profit advocacy organization that was founded with the philosophy of: Whenever long-term drug therapy, elective surgery, or any other major treatment is prescribed, the question of whether the treatment has been proven safe and effective should come up. And the prescribing physician should be expected to cite the relevant studies.
Arthur Aaron Levin MPH, Director
Maryann Napoli, Associate Director

Support Groups & Hotlines

10626 Behavioral Pediatrics Program
KDWP Variety Family Center
200 Oak Street SE
Minneapolis, MN 55455-2002

612-626-4260
800-276-8642
Fax: 612-624-0997
TTY: 612-624-3939
www.peds.umn.edu/pedsadol

Behavioral Pediatrics Staff help children, teen and their families with a wide variety of behavioral concerns including adjustment to coping with chronic illness. Treatments vary depending on the age, developmental state and needs of each child and family. Often, children are taught to self-regulate their behavior.
Daniel Kohen MD, Director

10627 Childrens Hospice International
1101 King Street
Alexandria, VA 22314

703-684-0330
800-242-4453
Fax: 703-684-0226
e-mail: info@chionline.org
www.chionline.org

To ensure medical, psychological, social and spiritual support to all children with like-threatening conditions and their families by providing a network of resources and care.
Ann Armstrong Dailey, Founding Director/CEO
Richard Larkin, Secretary/Treasurer

10628 Fetal Alcohol Network
KDWP Variety Family Center
200 Oak Street SE
Minneapolis, MN 55455-2002

612-626-4260
800-276-8642
Fax: 612-624-0997
TTY: 612-624-3939
e-mail: kdwb-var@umn.edu
www.peds.umn.edu/peds-adol

Staff provide assessment, intervention and consultation regarding the physical, developmental learning, behavioral and emotional well-being of children and individuals affected by prenatal exposure to alcohol and drugs.
Daniel Kohen MD, Director

10629 Foundation for Hospice and Homecare
3801 Vanesta Drive
Manhattan, KS 66503

785-537-0688
800-748-7474
Fax: 785-537-1309
e-mail: cnolte@hcandh.org
www.homecareandhospice.org

We aim to be the premier non-profit Homecare & Hospice provider of compassionate, quality affordable health, wellness and support services. To be committed to preserving hope, dignity and independence in the sheltering embrace of a home environment.
Lowell Kohlmeier, Chair
Judine Mecseri, Director of Program Operations

10630 Friends Health Connection
New Brunswick, NJ 08903

732-418-1811
800-483-7436
Fax: 732-249-9897
e-mail: info@friendshealthconnection.org
www.friendshealthconnection.org

Enhances mind, body and soul through our personalized support network and dynamic educational and motivational programs. Works with hospitals and other nonprofit organizations to complement their program offerings and connect people with resources and support that can enrich their lives.

10631 Genetic Alliance
4301 Connecticut Avenue NW
Washington, DC 20008

202-966-5557
Fax: 202-966-8553
e-mail: info@geneticalliance.org
www.geneticalliance.org

Improves health through the authentic engagement of communities and individuals. The goal is to build capacity within the genetics community. Transform health through genetics and promote an environment of openness centered on the health of individuals, families, and communities.
Sharon F Terry, President/CEO
Greg Biggers, Entrepeneur-in-residence

10632 KDWB Family Resource Center
200 Oak Street SE
Minneapolis, MN 55455-2002

612-626-3087
800-276-8642
Fax: 612-624-0997
TTY: 612-624-3939
e-mail: kdwb-var@umn.edu
www.peds.umn.edu/peds-adol

A place families can visit to learn about their child's chronic illness or disability, identify psychological and developmental issues, and link-up with program and community resources. Information will be available by telephone and via the web site.
Elizabeth Latts, Resource Coordinator

10633 KDWB Variety Family Canter
200 Oak Street SE
Minneapolis, MN 55455-2002

612-626-3087
800-276-8642
Fax: 612-624-0997
TTY: 612-624-3939
e-mail: kdwbvar@umn.edu
www.peds.umn.edu/pedsadol/

University-Community pertnership that provides family-centered services that promote physical, emotional, psychological and social health and well being for children and youth at risk, including children and youth with disabilities. The Center is dedicated to teaching, research, outreach, and community services.
Peggy Mann Reinhart, Director
Elizabeth Latts, Resource Coordinator

10634 National Association for Home Care
228 Seventh Street SE
Washington, DC 20003

202-547-7424
Fax: 202-547-3540
e-mail: exec@nahc.org
www.nahc.org

Promotes the concepts of hospice, a philosophy of health care which is expressed through the provision of a variety of medical and nonmedical services to terminally ill patients and their families.
Val J. Halamandaris, President
Andrea Devoti, Chair

10635 National Family Caregivers Association
10400 Connecticut Avenue
Kensington, MD 20895-3944

301-942-6430
800-896-3650
Fax: 301-942-2302
e-mail: info@thefamilycaregiver.org
www.thefamilycaregiver.org

Educates, supports, empowers and speaks up for the more than 65 million Americans who care for loved ones with a chronic illness or disability or the frailties of old age. Reaches across the boundaries of diagnosis, relationships and life stages to help transform family caregivers' lives by removing barriers to health and well being
Suzanne Mintz, President/CEO

10636 National Health Information Center
Washington, DC 20013

310-565-4167
800-336-4797
Fax: 301-984-4256
e-mail: info@nhic.org
www.health.gov/nhic

Offers a nationwide information referral service, produces directories and resource guides.

10637 National Parent to Parent Support and Information System
3805 Presidential Parkway
Atlanta, GA 30340

770-451-5484
Fax: 770-458-4091
e-mail: info@p2pga.org
www.p2pusa.org

NPPSIS is a nonprofit organization established to support, strengthen, and empower families through one-on-one parent contacts. They link families nationally whose children have special health care needs and rare disorders. They provide parents with heath care information, resources and referrals to allow them to identify appropriate services.
Dana Yarbrough, President
Debra S. Tucker, Executive Director

10638 Okizu Foundation Camps
16 Digital Drive
Novato, CA 94949-6115

415-382-9083
Fax: 415-382-8384
e-mail: info@okizu.org
www.okizu.org

This foundation runs family camp programs for children who have cancer and their families, and for children who have or had a parent with cancer.
Suzie Randall, Executive Director
Heather Ferrier, Asst. Executive Director

10639 Parent to Parent of New York State
500 Balltown Road
Schenectady, NY 12304-2247

518-381-4350
800-305-8817
Fax: 518-393-9607
e-mail: staciap2p@verizon.net
www.parenttoparentnys.org

Parent to Parent programs provide informational and emotional support to parents who have a child, adolescent or adult family member with special needs. Offers an important connection for a parent who is seeking support for special disability issues, by matching him or her with a trained veteran parent who has already been there. Because the two parents share so many common concerns and interests, the support given and received is often uniquely meaningful. Also helps families locate information
Jenni Austen, Regional Coordinator
Holly Bartczak, Coordinator

10640 Pediatric Psychology
KDWP Variety Family Center
200 Oak Street SE
Minneapolis, MN 55455-2002

612-626-4260
800-276-8642
Fax: 612-624-0997
TTY: 612-624-3939
e-mail: kdwbvar@umn.edu
www.peds.umn.edu/pedsadol

Staff provide assessment, intervention and consultation regarding the physical, developmental, learning, behavioral and emotional well-being of children and individuals affected by prenatal exposure to alcohol and drugs.
Daniel Kohen MD, Director

10641 STAR Center for Family Health
KDWB University Pediatrics Family Center
200 Oak St, SE,
Minneapolis, MN 55455-2002

612-626-4260
Fax: 612-624-0997
TTY: 6126243939
e-mail: kdwb-var@umn.edu
www.peds.umn.edu/peds-adol/

Helps children, youth and families develop new and enhanced ways of coping with stress, learn strategies for adjusting to living with a chronic illness, and discover new ways of finding health, balance and well-being.
Lavon Anderson, M.A., Administrator
Linda Boche, Executive Secretary to Division Director

10642 U Special Kids
KDWB Variety Family Center
200 Oak Street SE
Minneapolis, MN 55455-2002

612-626-3081
800-276-8642
Fax: 612-624-0997
TTY: 6126243939
e-mail: uspclkid@umn.edu
www.peds.umn.edu/peds-adol/

A program that provides care coordinators for children with complex medical conditions. A team of health care providers advocates for children and their families within the health care system.
Anne Kelly MD, Director

10643 Visiting Nurse Association of America
601 Thirteenth St NW
Washington, DC 20005

202-384-1420
888-866-8773
Fax: 202-384-1444
e-mail: webadmin@vnaa.org
www.vnaa.org

The VNAA will support, promote and advance nonprofit providers of home and community-based healthcare, hospice and health promotion services to ensure quality care for their communities.
Mary B. DeVeau, Chair
Ellen Rothberg, Vice Chair

10644 Well Spouse Association
63 W Main Street
Freehold, NJ 07728

800-838-0879
e-mail: support@wellspouse.org
www.wellspouse.org

This association is a nonprofit national self-help organization serving the well spouse of the chronically ill. Members help each other develop coping and survival skills through local support

groups (including bereavement), letter and telephone networks, and personal outreach and a quarterly newsletter.
Lawrence Bocchiere, President
Gerald Bishop, Board Chair

Books

10645 A History of Childhood and Disability
Philip Safford and Elizabeth Safford, author
Teachers College Press
1234 Amsterdam Avenue
New York, NY 10027
212-678-3929
Fax: 212-678-4149
e-mail: tcpress@tc.columbia.edu
www.teacherscollegepress.com
This book presents an interdisciplinary perspective on children considered exceptional and how services have evolved in reponse to their diverse neeeds.
1996 352 pages
ISBN: 0-807734-85-3
Philip Safford, Co-Author
Elizabeth Safford, Co-Author

10646 Art of Getting Well
David Spero, RN, author
Hunter House Publishing
424 Church Street
Nashville, TN 37219
615-255-2665
800-266-5592
Fax: 615-255-5081
e-mail: ordering@hunterhouse.com
www.turnerpublishing.com
A five step plan for maximazing health when you have a chronic illness.
224 pages Paperback
David Spero, Author

10647 Assisstive Technology for Young Children: A Guide to Family-Centered Services
Sharon Lesar Judge and Howard P Parette, author
Brookline Books
8 Trumbull Rd
Northampton, MA 01060
413-584-0184
800-666-2665
Fax: 413-584-6184
e-mail: brbooks@yahoo.com
brooklinebks.com
Explores the wide range of considerations involved in evaluating children's needs, selecting and prescribing devices, and training children, families, and teachers to use the technology.
1998 Softcover
ISBN: 1-571290-51-6

10648 Awaking to Disability
Volcano Press
PO Box 270
Volcano, CA 95689-0270
209-296-7989
800-879-9636
Fax: 209-296-4995
e-mail: sales@volcanopress.com
www.volcanopress.com
From the disability activist whose columns have been avidly followed by readers of the Albuquerque Journal and Miami Herald comes this revealing compedium of her thoughts. It offers a perspective for parents of children with disabilites, or for newly disabled people.
1997 288 pages
ISBN: 1-884244-14-9

10649 Blood Pressure Book: How to Get it Down & Keep it Down
Bull Publishing
PO Box 1377
Boulder, CO 80306
303-545-6350
800-676-2855
Fax: 303-545-6354
www.bullpub.com
Provides basic information on the causes and treatment of high blood pressure includes check up charts and illustrations that will help readers find out where they stand and lead them to practical advice tailored to their own needs.
1996
ISBN: 0-923521-97-6

10650 Building Partnerships in Hospital Care
Bull Publishing
PO Box 1377
Boulder, CO 80306
303-545-6350
800-676-2855
Fax: 303-545-6354
www.bullpub.com
Aims to desensetize patients and families to their fears of illness, hospital machinery and authority figures at the same time resensitize institution weary professionals to the feelings, instincts and emotions that brought them into the field in the first place.
304 pages
ISBN: 0-923521-07-0

10651 Child of Mine: Feeding with Love and Good Sense
Bull Publishing
PO Box 1377
Boulder, CO 80306
303-545-6350
800-676-2855
Fax: 303-545-6354
www.bullpub.com
Parents need to learn how to provide a nutritionally wholesome diet, but they also need to know how to feed in a way that nurtures a child's senses of autonomy and trust in themselves and their bodies.
470 pages
ISBN: 0-923521-51-8
Ellyn Satter, Author

10652 Childhood Emergencies: What to Do A Quick Refrence Guide
Bull Publishing
PO Box 1377
Boulder, CO 80306
303-545-6350
800-676-2855
Fax: 303-545-6354
www.bullpub.com
Handy book contains clear and quick referance for most common injuries including cuts and wounds, broken bones, abdominal pain, burns, toothaches, convulsion, eye and ear injuries, abrasions, bites insect and animal, bleeding, choking, seizures, freezing and frostbite, CPR, etc.
44 pages
ISBN: 0-923521-62-3

10653 Chiropractor's Self-Help Back and Body Book
Samuel Homola, DC, author
Hunter House Publishers
424 Church Street
Nashville, TN 37219
615-255-2665
800-266-5592
Fax: 615-255-5081
e-mail: ordering@hunterhouse.com
www.turnerpublishing.com
How to relieve common aches and pains at home and on the job.
2002 320 pages Paperback
ISBN: 0-897933-76-6
Samuel Homola, Author

10654 Choose the Right Long Term Care
NOLO
950 Parker Street
Berkeley, CA 94710-2524
800-728-3555
Fax: 800-645-0895
e-mail: cs@nolo.com
www.nolo.com
You can use this book to figure out how to choose a nursing home, or find a viable alternative. Covers how to get the most out of Medicare and other benefit programs.
336 pages
ISBN: 0-873375-15-7
Chris Braun, President
Janet Portman, Executive Editor

10655 Chronic Physical Illness
S. Newman, E. Steed, K. Mulligan, author
McGraw-Hill Companies
Returns Department
Dubuque, IA 52002
877-833-5524
Fax: 609-308-4484
e-mail: pbg.ecommerce_custserv@mcgraw-hill.com
www.mcgraw-hill.com

Provides an overview of self-management in chronic physical illness, theoretical and conceptual background, and examines issues related to the delivery of self-management. Discussion of a range of chronic conditions including: asthma, coronary artery disease, heart failure, COPD, hypertension, diabetes and rheumatoid arthritis. Authored by a number of leading international experts in the diseases they discuss. Hardcover also available for $136.95.
2008 240 pages
ISBN: 0-335217-86-9

10656 Directory of Health Grants
Research Grant Guides
PO Box 1214
Loxahatchee, FL 33470-1214   561-795-6129
                                               Fax: 561-795-7794
1000 foundation profiles.
Second edition
ISBN: 0-945078-19-6

10657 Directory of Social Service Grants
Research Grant Guides
PO Box 1214
Loxahatchee, FL 33470-1214   561-795-6129
                                               Fax: 561-795-7794
1100 foundation profiles.
Second edition
ISBN: 0-945078-18-8

10658 Disabled Woman's Guide to Pregnancy and Birth
Judith Rogers OTR, author
Demos Medical Publishing
11 W 42nd Street   212-683-0072
New York, NY 10036   800-532-8663
                                               Fax: 212-683-0118
                    e-mail: support@demosmedical.com
                                  www.demosmedical.com
Based on the experiences of ninety women with disabilities who chose to have children. Contains in-depth interviews with women with 22 different types of disabilities and with a total of 143 pregnancies.
528 pages
ISBN: 1-932603-08-8
Beth Kaufman Barry, Publisher
David D'Addona, Acquisitions Editor

10659 Family Interventions Throughout Chronic Illness and Disability
Springer Publishing Company
536 Broadway   212-431-4370
New York, NY 10012-3955   Fax: 212-941-7842
                    e-mail: marketing@springerpub.com
                                    www.springerpub.com
This book provides usable methods for professionals to help families deal with the reality of chronic illness of disability of a family member. Included at the end of each section are study questions and suggested activities for those working with the disabled, as well as for students.
336 pages Hardcover
ISBN: 0-826155-80-1
Annette Imperati, Marketing Director

10660 Get Fit While You Sit: Easy Workouts From Your Chair
Charlene Torkelson, author
Hunter House Publishing
424 Church Street   615-255-2665
Nashville, TN 37219   800-266-5592
                                               Fax: 615-255-5081
                    e-mail: ordering@hunterhouse.com
                                   www.turnerpublishing.com
A total body workout that can be done right from your chair, anywhere. Perfect for office workers, travelers, and those with age-related movement limitations or special conditions.
Paperback
ISBN: 0-897932-53-0
Charlene Torkelson, Author

10661 Good Bones: Complete Guide to Building and Maintaining the Healthiest Bones
Barbara Luke, author
Bull Publishing

PO Box 1377   303-545-6350
Boulder, CO 80306   800-676-2855
                                               Fax: 303-545-6354
                                                  www.bullpub.com
Examines 17 major risks in bone health with women. Author offers nutrional advice and preventative nutritional advice and prevenative measures in this comprehensive and scientifically sound guide for woman of all ages.
192 pages
ISBN: 0-923521-44-5

10662 Grants for Organizations Serving People with Disabilities
Research Grant Guides
PO Box 1214
Loxahatchee, FL 33470-1214   Fax: 561-795-7794
800 foundation profiles, including funding for all types of nonprofits. Also two key articles on winning grant strategies.
Tenth edition
ISBN: 0-945078-17-X

10663 Habits Not Diets: Secret to Lifetime Weight Control
James M Ferguson MD, Cassandra Ferguson, author
Bull Publishing
PO Box 1377   303-545-6350
Boulder, CO 80306   800-676-2855
                                               Fax: 303-545-6354
                                                  www.bullpub.com
This sensible approach puts the emphasis on how to eat rather than what. Uses the cognitive aspects of weight management including thinking skills, stress management and problem solving to help analyze individual eating habits , break undesirable patterns and establish new ones.
352 pages
ISBN: 0-923521-70-7

10664 Health
Sage Publications
2455 Teller Road   805-499-9774
Thousand Oaks, CA 91320   800-818-7243
                                               Fax: 805-499-0871
                    e-mail: journals@sagepub.com
                                  www.sagepublications.com
A interdisciplinary and international journal committed to the social and cultural study of health, illness and medicine with a particular focus on the changing place of health matters in modern society and in public onsciousness.
Quarterly

10665 I Can't Chew Cookbook
J Randy Wilson, author
Hunter House Publishing
424 Church Street   615-255-2665
Nashville, TN 37219   800-266-5592
                                               Fax: 615-255-5081
                    e-mail: ordering@hunterhouse.com
                                   www.turnerpublishing.com
Delicious soft-diet recipes for people with chewing, swallowing and dry-mouth disorders.
224 pages Paperback
ISBN: 0-897934-00-8
J. Randy Wilson, Author

10666 Informed Woman's Guide to Breast Health
Kerry McGinn RN, author
Bull Publishing
PO Box 1377   303-545-6350
Boulder, CO 80306   800-676-2855
                                               Fax: 303-545-6354
                                                  www.bullpub.com
Covers all elements of self-examination, mammography, medical exams and tests; includes new information about the genes BRCA 1 and BRCA 2, possible early predictors of cancer

ISBN: 0-923521-61-5

10667 Insider's Guide to HMOs
Penguin Putnam

PO Box 999
Bergenfield, NJ 07621-0903   800-526-0275
                                               Fax: 800-227-9604

ISBN: 0-452276-91-8

10668 Journel to Pain Relief
Phyllis Berger, author
Hunter House Publishing
424 Church Street   615-255-2665
Nashville, TN 37219   800-266-5592
                                               Fax: 615-255-5081
                           e-mail: ordering@hunterhouse.com
                                       www.turnerpublishing.com
Hands-on guide to breakthroughs in pain treatment.
2007 288 pages Paperback
Cristina Sverdrup, Customer Service Manager

10669 Joy of Laziness
Peter Axt, PhD, Michaela Axt-Gardermann, author
Hunter House Publishing
424 Church Street   615-255-2665
Nashville, TN 37219   800-266-5592
                                               Fax: 615-255-5081
                           e-mail: ordering@hunterhouse.com
                                       www.turnerpublishing.com
Explains that every human being has a limited amount of energy at
his or her disposal.
160 pages Paperback
ISBN: 0-897934-01-5
Peter Axt, Author

10670 Just Like Everyone Else
World Institute on Disability
3075 Adeline Street   510-225-6400
Berkeley, CA 94703-1520   Fax: 510-225-0477
                                               TTY: 510-225-0478
                                          e-mail: wid@wid.org
                                                       wid.org
Provides perspective, inspiration and information about the Inde-
pendent Living Movement and the Americans with Disabilities
Act.
16 pages
Anita Shafer Aaron, Executive Director

10671 Laurel's Kitchen Caring: Recipes for Everyday Home Caregiving
Ten Speed Press
1745 Broadway   212-782-9000
New York, NY 10019-0123   800-841-2665
                                               Fax: 510-524-4588
                    e-mail: CrownOSM@penguinrandomhouse.com
                                          crownpublishing.com
A cookbook tailored to the nutritional needs of recovering patients
as well as morale booster, caregiving primer, and resource book.
1997 158 pages
ISBN: 0-898159-51-2

10672 Living a Healthy Life with Chronic Conditions
Kate Lorig, Halsted Holman, David Sobel, author
Bull Publishing
PO Box 1377   303-545-6350
Boulder, CO 80306   800-676-2855
                                               Fax: 303-545-6354
                                               www.bullpub.com
Full of tips, suggestions, and strategies to deal with chronic illness
and common symptoms, such as fatigue, pain, shortness of breath,
disability, and depression. Encourages readers to develop individ-
ual approaches to setting goals, making decisions, and finding resources and support so they are able to do the things they want, and
need, to accomplish.
292 pages
ISBN: 1-933503-01-1
Kate Lorig, DrPH, Co-Author
Halsted Holman, MD, Co-Author

10673 Maximize Your Body Potential
Joyce D Nash PhD, author
Bull Publishing

PO Box 1377   303-545-6350
Boulder, CO 80306   800-676-2855
                                               Fax: 303-545-6354
                                               www.bullpub.com
Using selftests, checklists, and fill-in forms, shows readers how to
make a committment, how to set realistic goals, and how to design
an individualized exercise and eating program.
640 pages
ISBN: 0-923521-71-4
Joyce D. Nash, Ph.D., Author

10674 Menopause Without Medicine
Linda Ojeda, author
Hunter House Publishing
424 Church Street   615-255-2665
Nashville, TN 37219   800-266-5592
                                               Fax: 615-255-5081
                           e-mail: ordering@hunterhouse.com
                                       www.turnerpublishing.com
Provides complete information on the symptoms of menopause -
hot flashes, sexual changes, deperssion and osteoporosis - and how
to alleviate them.
400 pages Paperback
ISBN: 0-897934-05-3

10675 Nolo's Guide to Soc. Security Disability: Getting and Keeping Your Benefits
David Morton MD, author
NOLO
950 Parker Street
Berkeley, CA 94710-2524   800-728-3555
                                               Fax: 800-645-0895
                                          e-mail: cs@nolo.com
                                                 www.nolo.com
The essential book for anyone dealing with a long-term or permanent disability. Written both for first-time applicants and existing
recipients of Social Security disability, this guide demystifies the
program and tells you everything you need to know about qualify-
ing and applying for benefits, maintaining your benefits, and
appealing the denial of a claim.
512 pages
ISBN: 1-413311-04-4
David Morton, M.D., Author

10676 Ostomy Book: Living Comfortably with Colostomies, Ileostomies and Urostomies
Barbara Dorr Mullen, Kerry Anne McGinn, author
Bull Publishing
PO Box 1377   303-545-6350
Boulder, CO 80306   800-676-2855
                                               Fax: 303-545-6354
                                               www.bullpub.com
For people who have a colostomy, ileostomy or urinary diversion
(utostomy), either permanent or temporary, as well as for family,
friends and health professionals.

ISBN: 0-933503-13-4

10677 Psychological Management of Chronic Pain: A Treatment Manual
Springer Publishing Company
11 West 42nd Street   212-431-4370
New York, NY 10036-3955   877-687-7476
                                               Fax: 212-941-7842
                                     e-mail: cs@springerpub.com
                                            www.springerpub.com
This volume provides the clinician with a practical guide to help
clients manage and alleviate problems associated with chronic
pain and places an emphasis on the cognitive components of treatment. The manual illustrates a time-limited, thera-
pist-guide/self-management program.
1996 80 pages Softcover
ISBN: 0-826161-12-X

10678 Self Help: Your Strategy for Living with COPD
Bull Publishing

PO Box 1377
Boulder, CO 80306

303-545-6350
800-676-2855
Fax: 303-545-6354
www.bullpub.com

Contains vital information for patients suffering from asthma, emphysema, or chronic bronchitis. Colorful charts, graphs and illustrations highlight major concepts and help make the booklet user friendly.
1997 32 pages
ISBN: 0-923521-40-2

10679 ShapeWalking
Marilyn Bach, PhD, Lorie Schleck, author
Hunter House Publishing
424 Church Street
Nashville, TN 37219

615-255-2665
800-266-5592
Fax: 615-255-5081
e-mail: ordering@hunterhouse.com
www.turnerpublishing.com

An easy low cost total fitness program that is suited for exercisers of all levels.
144 pages Paperback
ISBN: 0-897933-73-5
Marilyn L. Bach, Author

10680 Social Security, Medicare and Government Pensions
Dorothy Matthews Berman, author
NOLO
950 Parker Street
Berkeley, CA 94710-2524

800-728-3555
Fax: 800-645-0895
e-mail: cs@nolo.com
www.nolo.com

Gets you the most out of your retirement benefits
496 pages
ISBN: 1-413310-97-9
Dorothy Matthews Berman, Co-Author
Joseph Matthews, Co-Author

10681 Strength Training for Seniors
Michael Fekete, CSCS; ACE, author
Hunter House Publishing
424 Church Street
Nashville, TN 37219

615-255-2665
800-266-5592
Fax: 615-255-5081
e-mail: ordering@hunterhouse.com
www.turnerpublishing.com

How to rewind your biological clock. Reduce a person's biological age by 10-20 years.
2006 160 pages Paperback
Cristina Sverdrup, Customer Service Manager

10682 Succeeding Against the Odds: Strategies and Insights from the Learning Disabled
Jeremy P Tarcher
5858 Wilshire Boulevard
Los Angeles, CA 90036-4521

213-935-9980

Filled with information on adults with learning disabilities, including the hidden handicaps, the definition of learning disabilities, and characteristics of individuals with learning disabilities. The book also looks at the responsibility of preparing for adulthood, and includes information for parents and teachers.
Lex Frieden, Program Director

10683 Taking Care of Caregivers
D Jeanne Roberts MA, author
Bull Publishing
PO Box 1377
Boulder, CO 80306

303-545-6350
800-676-2855
Fax: 303-545-6354
www.bullpub.com

Covers the needs of caregivers; their feelings; stress management techniques; communication; grief; sharing and support

ISBN: 0-923521-09-7
D. Jeanne Roberts, M.A., Author

10684 Tax Options and Strategies for People with Disabilities
Demos Vermande

11 West 42nd Street
New York, NY 10036-8804

212-683-0072
800-532-8663
Fax: 212-683-0118
e-mail: support@demosmedical.com
www.demosmedical.com

1996 288 pages
ISBN: 0-939957-85-

10685 Teens Face to Face with Chronic Illness
Asthma and Allergy Foundation of America
8201 Corporate Drive
Landover, MD 20785-2330

202-466-7643
800-727-8462
Fax: 202-466-8940
e-mail: Info@aafa.org
www.aafa.org

Young people easily relate to this book, which uses anecdotes from teens dealing with chronic illness. Teens address issues such as peer pressure and feeling different.
129 pages Paperback

10686 The Personal Care Attendant Guide: The Art of Finding, Keeping, or Being One
Katie Rodriguez Banister, author
Program Development Associates
11 West 42nd Street
New York, NY 10036-9576

212-683-0072
800-543-2119
Fax: 315-452-0710
e-mail: support@demosmedical.com
www.demosmedical.com

To live independently, many people with chronic illness and/or disabilitiy hire a personal attendant to assist with day-to-day tasks. Finding a qualified caregiver can be challenging, but not impossible. The Guide teaches readers how to find a competent caregiver, and gives prospective attendants vital information and real-life examples to help them succeed. Includes easy-to-use forms and worksheets to make the search easy and organized, anecdotes, and resources.
2007 160 pages

10687 Time for Healing: Relaxation for Mind and Body
Bull Publishing
PO Box 1377
Boulder, CO 80306

303-545-6350
800-676-2855
Fax: 303-545-6354
www.bullpub.com

Helps and guides listeners release tension and acheive deep muscular relaxation, heightened self-awareness and total relaxation.
Catherine Regan, Ph.D., Author

10688 Understanding Addiction
Elizabeth Connell Henderson MD, author
University Press of Mississippi
3825 Ridgewood Road
Jackson, MS 39211

601-432-6205
800-737-7788
Fax: 601-432-6217
www.upress.state.ms.us

A concise overview of this complex affliction for all those affected by addiction — addicts, family members, and even employers
224 pages Paperback
ISBN: 1-578062-40-9
Elizabeth Connell Henderson, M.D., Author

10689 Understanding Anemia
Ed Uthman, MD, author
University Press of Mississippi
3825 Ridgewood Road
Jackson, MS 39211

601-432-6205
800-737-7788
Fax: 601-432-6217
www.upress.state.ms.us

Gently builds upon elementary knowledge of biology to provide the general reader with a fairly sophisticated understanding of the various causes of anemia, of the methods used to make diagnoses, and of the principles of treatment.
160 pages Paperback
ISBN: 1-578060-39-9
Ed Uthman, M.D., Author

10690 Understanding Child Sexual Abuse
Edward L Rowan, MD, author

University Press of Mississippi
3825 Ridgewood Road   601-432-6205
Jackson, MS 39211   800-737-7788
  Fax: 601-432-6217
  www.upress.state.ms.us

For those looking to comrephend and to prevent child sexual abuse, a succinct guidebook of advice and resources.
96 pages Paperback
ISBN: 1-578068-07-X
Edward L. Rowan, M.D., Author

10691 Understanding Cosmetic Laser Surgery
Robert Langdon, MD, author

University Press of Mississippi
3825 Ridgewood Road   601-432-6205
Jackson, MS 39211   800-737-7788
  Fax: 601-432-6217
  www.upress.state.ms.us

A description of the processes and procedures available in cosmetic laser surgery.
112 pages
ISBN: 1-578065-87-9
Robert Langdon, M.D., Author

10692 Understanding Dental Health
Francis G Serio, DMD; MS, author

University Press of Mississippi
3825 Ridgewood Road   601-432-6205
Jackson, MS 39211   800-737-7788
  Fax: 601-432-6217
  www.upress.state.ms.us

A user-friendly manual on the basics of dental health.
128 pages Paperback
ISBN: 1-578060-10-9
Francis G. Serio, D.M.D., M.S., Author

10693 Understanding Dietary Supplements
Jenna Hollenstein, author

University Press of Mississippi
3825 Ridgewood Road   601-432-6205
Jackson, MS 39211   800-737-7788
  Fax: 601-432-6217
  www.upress.state.ms.us

A handy guide to the evaluation and use of vitamins, minerals, herbs, botanicals, and more.
96 pages Paperback
ISBN: 1-578069-81-5
Jenna Hollenstein, MS, RD, ELS, Author

10694 Understanding Stuttering
Nathan Lavid, MD, author

University Press of Mississippi
3825 Ridgewood Road   601-432-6205
Jackson, MS 39211   800-737-7788
  Fax: 601-432-6217
  www.upress.state.ms.us

Insight into an ailment that impairs more than sixty million in the world population.
112 pages Paperback
ISBN: 1-578065-73-9
Nathan Lavid, M.D., Author

10695 Understanding Your Learning Disability
Cheri Warner, author

Ohio State University at Newark
1179 University Drive   740-366-3321
Newark, OH 43055   800-963-9275
  newark.osu.edu

Provides tips for students based on the author's experience as a Learning Disability Specialist. Offers definitions, characteristics, and suggestions related to reading, math, note taking, test taking, social interactions, and organizational strategies.

10696 Writing from Within
Bernard Selling, author

Hunter House Publishers

424 Church Street   615-255-2665
Nashville, TN 37219   800-266-5592
  Fax: 615-255-5081
  e-mail: ordering@hunterhouse.com
  www.turnerpublishing.com

A guide to creativity and life story writing
320 pages Paperback
ISBN: 0-897932-17-2

10697 Yes, You Can!: Go Beyond Physical Adversity and Live Life to Its Fullest
Janis Dietz PhD, author

Demos Medical Publishing
11 W 42nd Street   212-683-0072
New York, NY 10036   800-532-8663
  e-mail: support@demosmedical.com
  www.demosmedical.com

Based on the premise that life should be lived to the fullest extent possible, disability or no disability.
102 pages Paperback
ISBN: 1-888799-48-x

Children's Books

10698 Are You Tired Again?...I Understand: An Activities Workbook for Children
Marilyn W Deutsch PhD, author

Western Psychological Services
625 Alaska Avenue   424-201-8800
Torrance, CA 90503-1251   800-648-8857
  Fax: 424-201-6950
  e-mail: customerservice@wpspublish.com
  www.wpspublish.com

This reassuring activity and coloring book is for children with a chronically ill parent—children who often feel guilty, neglected, lonely, helpless, and afraid. It gives these youngsters the tools they need to work through their feelings, while gently explaining why Mom isn't getting better, why she's always tired, and how the family can still enjoy life and function as a family. It can be used with individuals or with support groups.

10699 In the Hospital
Peter Alsop, Bill Harley, author

Compassion Books
7036 State Highway 80 S   828-675-5909
Burnsville, NC 28714-7569   800-970-4220
  Fax: 828-675-9687
  e-mail: orders@compassionbooks.com
  www.compassionbooks.com

Wonderful songs and entertaining stories dealing with being sick, being different, being scared and finding strength and hope.
Audiotape/Book
Bruce Greene, Director

10700 Zink the Zebra

Gareth Stevens, Inc
330 West Olive Street   414-332-3520
Milwaukee, WI 53212-3952   800-542-2595
  Fax: 877-542-2596
  e-mail: customerservice@gspub.com
  www.garethstevens.com

Zink is a zebra with spots instead of stripes. Here is an inspiring and touching tale about being different in ways that don't matter and shouldn't get in the way when it comes to making friends and enjoying companionship and respect. Written by 11-year-old Kelly Weil in the last year of a battle she bravely fought, but ultimately lost, against cancer.
1997
ISBN: 0-836816-26-9

Magazines

10701 Advance: for Directors in Rehabilitation
Merion Publications

2900 Horizon Drive
King of Prussia, PA 19406-2651

215-265-7812
800-355-5627
e-mail: webmaster@advanceweb.com
www.advanceweb.com

An informational magazine designed to provide a balance of material concerning all aspects of a rehabilitation manager's job.
Scott Huelskamp, Editor
Johnathan Bassett, Senior Associate Editor

10702 Closing the Gap
526 Main Street
Henderson, MN 56044

507-248-3294
Fax: 507-248-3810
e-mail: info@closingthegap.com
www.closingthegap.com

Strives to provide parents and educators alike, the information and training necessary to locate, compare, and implement assistive technology.
BiMonthly
Budd Hagen, Co-Founder
Connie Kneip, VP/General Manager

10703 Exceptional Parent Magazine
209 Harvard Street
Brookline, MA 02446-5005

617-730-5800
800-852-2884
Fax: 617-730-8742

Lex Frieden, Program Director

Newsletters

10704 Asbestos Watch
PO Box 1483
Baltimore, MD 21203-1483

301-243-5864
Fax: 301-243-5234
www.whitelung.org

A national nonprofit organization dedicated to the education of the public to the hazards of asbestos exposure. The association developed programs of public education and consults with victims of asbestos exposure, school boards, building owners, government agencies, and others interested in identifying asbestos hazards and developing control programs.
Annual

10705 Chronic Pain Letter
Dolak
Old Chelsea Station
New York, NY 10011

718-797-0015

Brings current information on the management of chronic pain to the sufferer and the health professional.

Dorothy Fabian, Circulation Manager

10706 Health Facts
Center for Medical Consumers
237 Thompson Street
New York, NY 10012-1017

917-836-7596
Fax: 212-674-7100
e-mail: centerformedicalconsumers@gmail.com
www.medicalconsumers.org

Analyses of topics such as cancer, nutrition, depression, exercise, prescription drugs and nonmedical therapies.
6 pages Monthly

10707 In Confidence
American Health Information Management Association
233 N Michigan Avenue
Chicago, IL 60601

312-233-1100
800-335-5535
Fax: 312-233-1090
e-mail: info@ahima.org
www.ahima.org

Provides medical, legal and other professionals with a forum to exchange ideas and share knowledge about the confidentiality of health information and people's rights to privacy.
12 pages BiMonthly
Linda Kloss, Chief Executive Officer
Becky Perry, Executive Vice President & CFO

10708 Johns Hopkins Health Insider
Intelihealth

960C Harvest Drive
Blue Bell, PA 19422

800-988-1127
Fax: 800-676-3299
e-mail: service@jhinsider.com
www.jhinsider.com

Expert advice and information from America's leading health institution. The most authoritative, cutting-edge health information available today, straight from the leading specialists and experts.
David B Hellmann MD, Associate Editor
Linda A Lewandowski PhD, RN, Associate Editor

10709 Learning Disability Quarterly
Council for Learning Disabilities
11184 Antioch Road
Overland Park, KS 66210

913-491-1011
Fax: 913-491-1011
e-mail: CLDInfo@ie-events.com
www.cldinternational.org

Steve Chamberlain, President
Diane Bryant, President Elect

10710 Lifelines
Disabled & Alone/Life Services for the Handicapped
1440 Broadway
New York, NY 10018

212-532-6740
800-995-0066
Fax: 212-532-6740
e-mail: info@disabledandalone.org
www.disabledandalone.org

8 pages Quarterly
Leslie D Park, Chairman
Lee Alan Ackerman BA, Executive Director

10711 Lymphatic Research Matters
Lymphatic Research Foundation
261 Madison Avenue
New York, NY 10016

516-625-9675
Fax: 516-625-9410
e-mail: info@lymphaticnetwork.org
www.lymphaticresearch.org

Reporting information about LRF activities and current research. The newsletters are sent to registrants in our data base: patients, their families, the scientific community and health care providers.
Bi-Annual
Philip Braginsky, Esq., Chair
Kenneth R. Cerini, Treasurer

10712 Mainstay
Well Spouse Association
63 W Main Street
Freehold, NJ 7728

732-577-8899
800-838-0879
Fax: 732-577-8644
e-mail: info@wellspouse.org
www.wellspouse.org

The Well Spouse Association quarterly newsletter featuring articles written by WSA members.

10713 NHF Head Lines
National Headache Foundation
820 N Orleans
Chicago, IL 60610

312-274-2650
888-643-5552
Fax: 312-640-9049
e-mail: info@headaches.org
www.headaches.org

Up-to-date information on the latest developments in headache treatment; breaking news about newly-approved drugs; reviews of topical books; reader's mail feature, where the nation's leading medical experts answer questions about headaches; and a list of support group meetings where you can learn how to make a positive change in your life.
Bimonthly
Robert R Dalton, Executive Director

10714 National Networker
National Network of Learning Disabled Adults
808 N 82nd Street
Scottsdale, AZ 85257-3850

602-941-5112

For adults with learning disabilities.
Quarterly
Lex Frieden, Program Director

10715 Orphan Disease Update
National Organization for Rare Disorders

55 Kenosia Avenue
Danbury, CT 06810-8923

203-744-0100
800-999-6673
Fax: 203-798-2291
e-mail: orphan@rarediseases.org
www.rarediseases.org

Information about rare disorders for families with similar disorders.

10716 VSA Arts

JFK Center for the Performing Arts
1300 Connecticut Ave NW
Washington, DC 20036-1715

202-628-2600
800-933-8721
Fax: 202-737-0725
TDD: 202-737-0645
e-mail: info@vsarts.org
www.vsarts.org

VSA arts is an international, nonprofit organization dedicated to promoting artistic excellence and providing educational opportunities through the arts for children and adults with disabilities. The Creative Spirit is a quarterly newsletter that features VSA arts special events throughout the world, interviews with artistd and articles relating to disability and the arts.
8 pages
D Dixon, CEO
S Datton-Kumins, Writer/Research Coordinator

10717 Wheel Life News

University of Virginia, Rehab Engineering Centers
3363 University Station
Charlottesville, VA 22903

804-924-0311

Features tie downs and other adaptive technology for persons with disabilities.

10718 Worklife: A Publication of Employment and People with Disabilities

Office of Disability Employment Policy
200 Constitution Ave NW
Washington, DC 20210

202-693-7880
Fax: 202-693-7888
TDD: 202-376-6205

Quarterly

Pamphlets

10719 Campus Opportunities for Students with Learning Differences
Judith & Stephen Crooker, author

Octameron Associates
PO Box 2748
Alexandria, VA 22301

703-836-5480
Fax: 703-836-5650
e-mail: octameron@aol.com
www.octameron.com

Tells learning disabled students what questions to ask when selecting a school, how to prepare for the more rigorous academic schedule and when to get special assistance.
36 pages
ISBN: 1-575090-52-x
Judith Crooker, Co-Author
Stephen Crooker, Co-Author

10720 Issues in Independent Living

Independent Living Research Utilization
2323 S Shepherd Drive
Houston, TX 77019-7024

713-520-0232
Fax: 713-520-5785

This booklet is a report of the National Study Group on the Implications of Health Care Reform for Americans with Disabilities and Chronic Health Conditions.
30 pages
Lex Frieden, Program Director

10721 OSERS News in Print: Office of Special Education & Rehabilitative Services

US Department of Education
400 Maryland Avenue SW
Washington, DC 20202-0001

202-205-8241
800-872-5327
www.ed.gov

Provides information, research, and resources in the area of special learning needs.
Quarterly
Lex Frieden, Program Director

Audio & Video

10722 Assisting Parents Through the Mourning Process

Hope
5632 Van Nuys Blvd.
Van Nuys, CA 91401-4648

818-989-7221
800-405-8942
Fax: 818-989-7826
e-mail: info@childdevelopmentmedia.com
www.childdevelopmentmedia.com

Describes the mourning process experienced by some parents of children with disabilities and ways in which the professional can help them through the process.
20 minutes

10723 No Fears, No Tears
Leora Kuttner, PhD, author

Fanlight Productions
32 Court Street
Brooklyn, NY 11201-1731

718-488-8900
800-876-1710
Fax: 718-488-8642
e-mail: info@fanlight.com
www.fanlight.com

Dr. Leora Kuttner explores the effects of childrens pain management.
1985 28 Minutes

10724 No Fears, No Tears: 13 Years Later
Leora Kuttner, PhD, author

Fanlight Productions
32 Court Street
Brooklyn, NY 11201-1731

718-488-8900
800-876-1710
Fax: 718-488-8642
e-mail: info@fanlight.com
www.fanlight.com

Dr. Leora Kutner explores the effects of childrens pain management therapies 13 years after their use.
1998 47 Minutes
ISBN: 1-572952-77-6

Web Sites

10725 Access Unlimited

www.accessunlimited.com

Assists educators, health care providers and parents in discovering how personal computers help children and adults with disabilities compensate for some of the barriers imposed by their conditions.

10726 American Academy of Pediatrics

www.aap.org

Committed to the attainment of optimal physical, mental and social health and well-being for all infants, children, adolescents and yound adults.

10727 American Association for the Advancement of Science

www.aaas.org

An international non-profit organization dedicated to advancing science around the world by serving as an educators, leader, spokesperson and professional association.

10728 American Bar Association Commission

www.americanbar.org

The ABA's Commission on the Mentally Disabled was established in 1973 to respond to the advocacy needs of persons with mental disabilities.

10729 American Camp Association

www.acacamps.org

The American Camp Association (formerly known as the American Camping Association) is a community of camp professionals who, for over 100 years, have joined together to share our knowledge and experience and to ensure the quality of camp programs.

10730 American Counseling Association

www.counseling.org

Dedicated to the growth and development of the counseling profession and those who are served.

10731 American Institute for Preventive Medicine

www.healthylife.com

An award winning, internationally recognized authority on the development and implementation of health promotion, wellness, medical self-care and disease management programs and publications.

10732 American Organ Transplant Association

www.aotaonline.org

To help transplant patients lead happy, productinve lives by helping them obtain and sustain transplantation.

10733 American Red Cross

www.redcross.org

In addition to domestic disaster relief, the American Red Cross offers compassionate services in five other areas: community services that help the needy; support and comfort for military members and their families; the collection, processing and distribution of lifesaving blood and blood products; educational programs that promote health and safety; and international relief and development programs.

10734 American Self-Help Group Clearinghouse

www.selfhelpgroups.org

A keyword-searchable database of over 1,100 national, international, model and online self-help support groups for addictions, bereavement, health, mental health, disabilities, abuse, parenting, caregiver concerns and many other stressful life situations.

10735 American Society of Dermatology

www.asd.org

A non-partisan professional association of dematologists across the country whose mission is to facilitate optimal dermatologic care being available to all citizens of this country by preserving, promoting and enhancing the private practice of dermatology.

10736 Americas Association for the Care of the Children

www.aaccchildren.net

To promote support for those who are involved in early childhood care and education through educational programs and projects, including among other things, citizen exchange programs, global communication networks, and resource assistance to participating communities.

10737 Beach Center on Families and Disability

www.beachcenter.org

Makes a significant and sustainable difference in the quality of life of families and individuals affected by disability and of those who are closely involved with them.

10738 Center for Chronic Disease Prevention and Health Promotion

www.cdc.gov/nccdphp

The forefront of the nation's efforts to prevent and control chronic diseases. Leads efforts that promote health and well-being through prevention and control of chronic diseases.

10739 Center for Developmental Disabilities

www.centerfor.com

Committed to its mission of helping children and adults with differing abilities achieve their dreams by overcoming barriers to living, working, learning and enjoying recreational opportunities in the community of their choice.

10740 ChiroWeb.com

www.chiroweb.com

Chiropractic news source for chiropractors, students, patients and health care professionals. Over 7,000 articles are available.

10741 Commission on Accreditation of Rehabilitation Services

www.carf.org

CARF International, a group of companies that includes CARF Canada and CARF Europe, is an independent, nonprofit accreditor of health and human services.

10742 Disabled & Alone/Life Services for the Handicapped

www.disabledandalone.org

A non-profit organization established to help families provide a secure future for their loved ones with a disability. Believes that no person should have to live his life in loneliness and isolation because of a disability.

10743 Discovery Health

www.discoverylife.com

A large website covering various health topics; such as male and female health, senior health, children's health, mental health, alternative medicine, nutrition, fitness, and more.

10744 Educational Equity Center at AED

www.edequity.org

EEC at AED is an outgrowth of Educational Equity Concepts, a national not-for-profit organization with a 22-year history of promoting educational excellence for all children.

10745 Federation for Children with Special Needs

www.fcsn.org

Provides information, support, and assistance to parents with children with disabilities, their professional partners, and their communities.

10746 Healing Well

www.healingwell.com

A social network and support community for patients, caregivers, and families coping with the daily struggles of diseases, disorders and chronic illness.

10747 Health Care For All

www.hcfama.org

HCFA seeks to create a consumer-centered health care system that provides comprehensive, affordable, accessible, culturally competent, high quality care and consumer education for everyone, especially the most vulnerable.

10748 Health Finder

www.healthfinder.gov

A government website that contains information and tools to help you and those you care about stay healthy.

10749 Health on the Net Foundation

www.hon.ch

Promotes and guides the deployment of useful and reliable online health information, and its appropriate and efficient use.

10750 Healthcentral.com

www.healthcentral.com

Empower millions of people to improve and take control of their health and well-being.

10751 Healthlink USA

www.healthlinkusa.com

Discussion forum for treatments, symptoms and causes of 700 health conditions, diseases and topics.

10752 Helios Health

www.helioshealth.com

Online resource for your health information. Detailed information about specific health topics, access to expert advice from our Medical Advisory Board, and up-to-date health news.

10753 Life Development Institute

discoverldi.com

Serving men and women between the ages of 18-30 who have Asperger's Syndrome, ADHD, learning disabilities, anxiety, depression and other disorders

10754 MedicineNet

www.medicinenet.com

An online resource for consumers providing easy-to-read, authoritative medical and health information.

10755 Medscape

www.medscape.com

Medscape offers specialists, primary care physicians, and other health professionals the Web's most robust and integrated medical information and educational tools.

10756 Medtronic

www.medtronic.com

Medtronic is changing the face of chronic disease. By working closely with physicians around the world, they create therapies to help patients do things they never thought were possible.

10757 National Clearinghouse of Rehabilitation Training Materials

www.ncrtm.org

The mission of the NCRTM is to advocate for the advancement of best practice in rehabilitation counseling through the development, collection, dissemination, and utilization of professional knowledge, information and skill.

10758 National Council on Disability

www.ncd.gov

The National Council on Disability is an independent federal agency that works with the President and Congress to increase the inclusion, independence and empowerment of Americans with disabilities.

10759 National Organization for Rare Disorders (NORD)

www.rarediseases.org

Serves as a clearinghouse for information about rare disorders and brings together families with similar disorders for mutual support; fosters communication among rare disease voluntary agencies, Government agencies, industry, scientific researchers, academic institutions, and concerned individuals; and encourages and promotes research and education on rare disorders and orphan drugs.

10760 Office of Special Education and Rehabilitative Services

www2.ed.gov/osers

The Office of Special Education and Rehabilitative Services (OSERS) is committed to improving the results and outcomes for people with disabilities of all ages.

10761 WebMD

www.webmd.com

Provides credible information, supportive communities, and in-depth reference material about health subjects. A source for original and timely health information as well as material from well known content providers.

10762 World Institute on Disability

www.wid.org

A public policy center that is run by persons with disabilities. Conducts research, public education, and advocacy campaigns.

National Agencies & Associations

10763 A Kid Again
777-G Dearborn Park Lane   614-797-9500
Columbus, OH 43085   800-543-9735
Fax: 614-797-9600
e-mail: customerservice@akidagain.org
www.akidagain.org
Enriches the lives of children with life threatening illnesses and their families by providing year round fun-filled group activities and destination events by fostering joy, laughter, normalcy and supportive networking opportunities. Includes regional chapters.
Jeffrey Damron, CFRE, CEO
Kathy Derr, Director of Programs and Volunteers

10764 A Wish with Wings, Inc.
3817 Alamo Ave   817-469-9474
Fort Worth, TX 76107   Fax: 817-275-6005
e-mail: wish@awishwithwings.org
www.awishwithwings.org
Grants the wishes of Texas children with life-threatening diseases.
Pat Skaggs, Founder
Judy Youngs, Executive Director

10765 BASE Camp Children's Cancer Foundation
140 N Orlando Avenue   407-673-5060
Winter Park, FL 32789-3679   Fax: 407-673-5095
e-mail: email@basecamp.org
www.basecamp.org
Supports children and their families who are facing the challenge of living with cancer or other life-threatening hematological illnesses. Offers year round programs, monthly overnight camps, support groups, and weekly events.
Terri Jones, President/Founder
Cindy Whitaker, Parent & Program Coordinator

10766 Believe In Tomorrow Children's Foundation
6601 Frederick Road   410-744-1984
Baltimore, MD 21228   800-933-5470
Fax: 410-744-1984
e-mail: info@believeintomorrow.org
www.believeintomorrow.org
Formerly Grant-A-Wish Foundation, this Foundation provides exceptional hospital and retreat housing services to critically ill children and their families. The Foundation also believes that keeping families together during a child's medical crisis, and that the gentle caring environment is crucial.
Brian R Morrison, Founder
Richard E McCready, Chairman

10767 Camp Good Days
1332 Pittsford-Mendon Road   585-624-5555
Mendon, NY 14506   800-785-2135
Fax: 585-624-5799
www.campgooddays.org
A non-profit organization that provides a camping experience and more for children and adults facing the toughest challenges of life. Accepts the wishes of terminal ill children through age eighteen.
Gary Mervis, Founder/Chairman
Wendy Bleier-Mervis, Executive Director

10768 Children's Wish Foundation International
8615 Roswell Road   770-393-9474
Atlanta, GA 30350-7526   800-323-9474
Fax: 770-393-0683
e-mail: arthurs@childrenswish.org
www.childrenswish.org
Committed to bringing joy and happiness to seriously ill children throughout the world and this dedication has created special experiences for children around the globe. Our commitment is also developing hospital enrichment programs.
Linda Dozoretz, Executive Director
Jacque Niles, Director of Program Services

10769 Cure Our Children Foundation
711 S Carson Street   310-355-6046
Carson City, NV 89701   Fax: 310-454-9592
e-mail: barry@cureourchildren.org
www.cureourchildren.org

Support medical approaches to treatment of Ewings Sarcoma. Alternate and complimentary treatment information is provided only for use in conjunction with traditional approaches.
Barry Sugarman, President

10770 Dream Come True
Lehigh Valley, PA 18002   610-865-3475
Fax: 610-865-4710
e-mail: RVasko@aol.com
www.dreamcometrue.org
Seeks to fulfill the dreams of children ages 4 - 17 who are seriously, chronically and terminally ill and whom live in the Lehigh Valley area. Includes regional offices.
Rayann Vasko, Director
Jeane Hockenbury, President

10771 Dream Factory, Inc.
National Headquarters
120 W Broadway   502-561-3001
Louisville, KY 40202   800-456-7556
Fax: 502-561-3004
e-mail: dfinfo@dreamfactoryinc.org
www.dreamfactoryinc.org
Grants wishes to children and young adults ages 3 - 18 with a critical or chronic illness.
Janice Harris, President
Mark Whitworth, Vice President

10772 Dream Foundation
1528 Chapala Street   805-564-2131
Santa Barbara, CA 93101   Fax: 805-564-7002
www.dreamfoundation.org
Enhances the quality of life for individuals and families battling terminal illnesses ages 18 and over.
Thomas Rollerson, Founder/President
Carol Brown, Chief Operating Officer

10773 Fairygodmother Foundation
550 W Webster Avenue   773-388-1160
Chicago, IL 60614   Fax: 773-883-3656
e-mail: info@fairygodmother.org
www.fairygodmother.org
Our wish granting program brings joy to the lives of adults (18 and older) and loved ones in their time of greatest need by turning dreams into reality. In the process of fulfilling wishes, we create an opportunity for peace, closure and a sense of belonging.
Lena Clement, Program Director

10774 Friends of Karen
118 Titicus Road   914-277-4547
North Salem, NY 10560   e-mail: info@friendsofkaren.org
www.friendsofkaren.org
Provides financial, emotional and advocacy support to children with life-threatening illnesses and their families.
Judith Factor, Executive Director
Nancy Mariano, Regional Director

10775 Give Kids the World Village
210 S Bass Road   407-396-1114
Kissimmee, FL 34746   800-995-KIDS
Fax: 407-396-1207
e-mail: dream@gktw.org
www.gktw.org
A 70-acre non-profit resort in Central Florida that creates magical memories for children with life-threatening illnesses and their families. GKTW provides accommodations at its whimsical resort, donated attractions, tickets, meals and more for a week-long stay.
Pamela Landwirth, President
Tabrei Scott, VP

10776 High Hopes Foundation of New Hampshire, Inc.
301 Daniel Webster Highway   603-429-1010
Merrimack, NH 03054   800-639-6804
Fax: 603-429-0037
e-mail: info@highhopesnh.net
highhopesfoundation.org
Grants wishes for severely and chronically ill children and young adults ages 3-18 who live in New Hampshire.
Jacque Yinger, Founder
Rachel Camer McMeen, Director

10777 Hopes & Dreams Foundation, Inc.
517 Cedarbrook Road   215-264-2859
Southampton, PA 18966-mail: info@hopesanddreamsfoundation.org
www.hopesanddreamsfoundation.org
For children and young adults with disabilities such as down syndrome and other specific challenges. Helps to promote education
and community involvement through social activities.
Vick Franklin, President

10778 Kidd's Kids
220 E Las Colinas Boulevard   972-432-8595
Irving, TX 75039   866-541-5437
Fax: 214-853-5212
e-mail: derrick@kiddlive.com
www.kiddskids.com
Founded by nationally syndicated morning show personality Kidd
Kraddick. Provides chronically ill and/or physically challenged
children between the ages of 5 to 12 with an unforgettable
adventure.
Toby Wilson, President
Dr. Kevin Wylie, Vice President

10779 Kids Incorporated
9300 Old Keene Mill Road   703-455-5437
Burke, VA 22015-4277   Fax: 703-440-9208
www.jcambellinc.com
Grants wishes to gravely ill children 16 years and younger. Children older than 16 are sometimes eligible depending on child's situation and the availability of resources.
John Campbell, President

10780 Kids Wish Network
4060 Louis Avenue   727-937-3600
Holiday, FL 34691   888-918-9004
Fax: 727-937-3688
e-mail: info@kidswishnetwork.org
www.kidswishnetwork.org
A nationally recognized charitable organization dedicated to in-
fusing hope creating happy memories and improving the quality of
life for children. The Network also fulfills the wishes of children
ages 3 to 18 with life threatening medical conditions.
Karen Pelle, President
Andy Gottlieb, Treasurer

10781 Magic Moments
2112 11th Ave S   205-638-9372
Birmingham, AL 35205   Fax: 205-939-6717
e-mail: info@magicmoments.org
www.magicmoments.org
Grants wishes to children 4 to 19 living or being treated in Alabama
who have chronic life-threatening diseases or who have severe
trauma (burn, spinal cord or head trauma).
Joyce T. Spielberger, Executive Director
Susan J. Driggers, Director of Development

10782 Make-A-Wish Foundation of America
4742 N. 24th Street   602-279-9474
Phoenix, AZ 85016-4862   800-722-9474
Fax: 602-279-0855
e-mail: mawfa@wish.org
www.wish.org
A national organization that grants wishes for children with terminally or life threatening diseases and who are 18 years of age or
younger. Includes regional chapters.
David Williams, President/CEO

10783 Marty Lyons Foundation, Inc.
326 W 48th Street   212-977-9474
New York, NY 10036   Fax: 212-977-1752
e-mail: mac@martylyonsfoundation.org
www.martylyonsfoundation.org
A national organization that grants wishes of children between the
ages of three and seventeen who have life-threatening diseases or
terminal illnesses. Those interested can submit applications for
their wish fulfillment.
Marty Lyons, Chairman
Richard A. Miller, President

10784 New Hope for Kids Wish Program
205 E. SR 436   407-331-3059
Fern Park, FL 32730   Fax: 407-331-3063
e-mail: information@newhopeforkids.org
www.newhopeforkids.org
Grants wishes to children ages 3-18 who have been diagnosed with
a life-threatening illness.
Dave Joswick, Executive Director
Dana Duffie, Office Manager

10785 Rainbow Connection
621 W University   248-601-9474
Rochester, MI 48307   877-649-4743
Fax: 248-601-0086
e-mail: info@rainbowconnection.org
www.rainbowwishconnection.org
Make the special wishes of children with life-threatening or termi-
nal illnesses come true.
L. Brooks Patterson, Founder
Mary Grace McCarter, Executive Director

10786 Special Wish Foundation
1250 Memory Lane   614-258-3186
Columbus, OH 43209   800-486-9474
Fax: 614-258-3518
e-mail: info@spwish.org
www.spwish.org
A Special Wish Foundation Inc. is a non-profit charitable organization dedicated to granting the wishes of children under the age of
21 who have been diagnosed with a life-threatening disorder.
Laura Marchetta, Contact/Chicago Chapter
Patti Piening, Contact/Cincinnati

10787 Starlight Foundation
2049 Century Park E   310-479-1212
Los Angeles, CA 90067-1035   800-274-7827
e-mail: info@starlight.org
www.starlight.org
A non-profit organization dedicated to brightening the lives of seriously ill children and their families.
Jacqueline Hart-Ibrahim, CEO
Dvorah Waldman, VP Global Brand & Alliances

10788 Sunshine Foundation National Headquarters
1041 Mill Creek Drive   215-396-4770
Feasterville, PA 19053   Fax: 215-396-4774
e-mail: philly@sunshinefoundation.org
www.sunshinefoundation.org
Answers the dreams of seriously ill physically challenged and
abused children aged three to eighteen whose families cannot fulfill their requests due to financial strain that the child's illness may
cause.
Kate Sample, President
Pamela Vasserman, Director of Development

10789 Vision Foundation
8901 Strafford Circle   865-357-4603
Knoxville, TN 37923-1567   Fax: 865-690-9322
e-mail: gordon@visionfoundation.net
www.visionfoundation.net
Offers counseling support groups seminars and transportation for
the blind providing 600 members.
Gordon Adams, Executive Director/President
Hank Brink, Vice President

10790 Wish Upon A Star
Visalia, CA 93278   559-733-7753
800-821-6805
Fax: 559-733-0962
e-mail: info@wishuponastar.org
www.wishuponastar.org
A non-profit law enforcement effort designed to grant the wishes
of children afflicted with high-risk and life threatening illnesses.
Wally Nelson, President
Carmen Perez, Executive Director

10791 Wishing Star Foundation
139 S Sherman
Spokane, WA 99202
509-744-3411
Fax: 509-744-3414
e-mail: paulan@wishingstar.org
www.wishingstar.org
Grants wishes to children with life threatening illnesses. Ages 3-21 in Eastern Washington and all of Idaho.
Paula Nordgaarden, M.Ed. MSW, Executive Director
Sarah Carpenter, Program Director

10792 Wishing Well Foundation USA, Inc.
3000 W Esplanade Avenue
Metairie, LA 70002
504-841-0001
888-663-9474
e-mail: wellfoundation@bellsouth.net
www.wishingwellusa.org/home0.aspx
To bring joy to children with life threatening illnesses by providing them with their fondest wish in life.
Elwin Lebeau, President

Foundations

10793 Angelwish, Inc.
Rutherford, NJ 07070
201-672-0722
Fax: 201-672-0733
e-mail: info@angelwish.org
www.angelwish.org
Provides the public with an easy way to grant wishes to the millions of children that are living with HIV/AIDS around the world. Infected or affected by the disease, their opportunities for a normal childhood are virtually impossible. By harnessing the power of the Internet, Angelwish helps donors add a ray of hope to their lives.
Shimmy Mehta, Founder/CEO
Tom Fuller, Director

10794 Chef David's Kids
1100 E Oakland Park Boulevard
Fort Lauderdale, FL 33334
954-594-1024
e-mail: chefdavidmitchell@gmail.com
www.chefdavidskids.com
Helps children afflicted with any form of terminal illness such as cancer, leukemia, and pediatric HIV. Also helps neglected and abused children.
Chef David Mitchell, Founder/Director of Operations
Laurie Amber, National Hospital Events Director

10795 Children's Wish Foundation of Canada
1101 Kingston Rd
Pickering, L1V 1-7J7
905-427-5353
800-267-9474
Fax: 905-427-0536
e-mail: on@childrenswish.ca
www.childrenswish.ca
Works with the community to provide children living with high risk life threatening illnesses the opportunity to realize their most heartfelt wish.
Chris Kotsopoulos, Director
Jeannette Wakelin, Chair

10796 Dreams Come True
6803 Southpoint Parkway
Jacksonville, FL 32216
904-296-3030
Fax: 904-296-4244
www.dreamscometrue.org
Grants the dreams of children with life-threatening illnesses.
Jeffrey Conn, President
Eddie Allen, Managing Director

10797 Dreams for Seniors Charity Inc
512 Court Street
Pekin, IL 61554
309-353-7300
Fax: 309-353-7311
e-mail: info@dreamsforseniorscharity.org
www.dreamsforseniorscharity.org
Dreams for Seniors Charity (Dreams for Seniors) is a 501(c)(3) non-profit organization focused on celebrating seniors, granting their wishes and making dreams come true.
Debbie Davison, President/Founder

10798 Jason's Dreams for Kids Foundation, Inc.
20 Monmouth Street
Red Bank, NJ 07701
732-758-0060
Fax: 732-758-0070
e-mail: jasonsdreams@comcast.net
www.jasonsdreamsforkids.com

Devoted to granting wishes to children diagnosed with life-threatening illnesses. Holds a variety of fundraising events to meet the cost of fulfilling these childrens' wishes.

10799 Little Star Foundation
256 Rancho Milagro Way
Hesperus, CO 81326
800-543-6565
e-mail: info@littlestar.org
www.littlestar.org
Provides lifetime opportunities for children with cancer to enhance the quality of their lives.
Andrea Jaeger, Co-Founder & President

10800 Starlight Children's Foundation
2049 Century Park E
Los Angeles, CA 90067
310-479-1212
e-mail: info@starlight.org
www.starlight.org
Helps seriously ill children and their families cope with their pain, fear and isolation through entertainment, education and family activities.
Jacqueline Hart-Ibrahim, CEO
Dvorah Waldman, VP Global Brand & Alliances

10801 Sunshine Dreams for Kids
300 Wellington St
London, Ontario, N6B 2-5A9
519-642-0990
800-461-7935
Fax: 519-642-1201
e-mail: info@sunshine.ca
www.sunshine.ca
Grants dreams to children who are between the ages of 3 and 19 who are challenged by severe physical disabilities or life threatening illnesses.
Patrick DeMeester, MBA, President
Adam Jean, Treasurer

10802 United Special Sportsman Alliance
7864 Shotwell Lane
Pittsville, WI 54466
715-884-2256
800-518-8019
Fax: 715-884-7388
www.childswish.com
A dream wish granting charity that specializes in sending critically ill and disabled youth on the outdoor adventure of their dreams.
Brigid O'Donoghue, CEO/Founder
Ron Johnson, President

National Agencies & Associations

10803 Children's Hospice International
500 Montgomery Street
Alexandria, VA 22314
703-684-0330
800-24C-HILD
e-mail: info@chionline.org
www.chionline.org
This organization was founded to provide a network of support and care for children with life threatening conditions and their families. The hospice is a team effort which provides medical, psychological, social and spiritual expertise in the US and abroad.
Ann Armstrong-Dailey, Founding Director/CEO
Rebecca Brant, Director

10804 Childrens Hospice International
1101 King Street
Alexandria, VA 22314
703-684-0330
800-242-4453
Fax: 703-684-0226
e-mail: info@chionline.org
www.chionline.org
To ensure medical, psychological, social and spiritual support to all children with like-threatening conditions and their families by providing a network of resources and care.
Ann Armstrong Dailey, Founding Director/CEO
Richard Larkin, Secretary/Treasurer

10805 Compassionate Friends
900 Jorie Blvd
Oak Brook, IL 60523-3696
630-990-0010
877-969-0010
Fax: 630-990-0246
e-mail: nationaloffice@compassionatefriends.org
www.compassionatefriends.org
A national organization that gives support to people who have experienced the death of a child. Offers monthly support meetings to get through the difficult times and learn how to cope.
Patricia Loder, Executive Director
Terry Novy, Chapter Services Coordinator

10806 HOSPICELINK Hospice Education Institute
Hospice Education Institute
3 Unity Square
Machiasport, ME 04655-0098
207-255-8800
800-331-1620
Fax: 207-255-8008
e-mail: info@hospiceworld.org
www.hospiceworld.org
Provides educational and informational services to health professionals and the public on subjects such as hospice care, death and dying and bereavement counseling.

10807 Helping Other Parents in Normal Grief
Underwood Memorial Hospital
509 N Broad Street
Woodbury, NJ 08096
856-845-0100
www.umhospital.org
Offers support to newly bereaved parents through trained parents who have suffered a similar loss and resolved their grief.
Eileen K. Cardile, RN, MS, CNA, President/CEO
John Graham, FACHE, Executive Vice President/COO

10808 National Association for Home Care and Hospice
228 7th Street SE
Washington, DC 20003-4306
202-547-7424
Fax: 202-547-3540
e-mail: hospice@nahc.org
www.nahc.org
Promotes the concepts of hospice, a philosophy of health care which is expressed through the provision of a variety of medical and nonmedical services to terminally ill patients and their families.
Val J. Halamandaris, President
Andrea Devoti, Chair

10809 National Hospice & Palliative Care Organization
1731 King Street
Alexandria, VA 22314
703-837-1500
800-646-6460
Fax: 703-837-1233
e-mail: nhpco_info@nhpco.org
www.nhpco.org
The nation's only advocate for terminally ill patients and their families. Founded in 1978, the NHPCO is the only organization devoted to hospice in the United States. Support is included from state hospice organizations, patients, families, communities, provider program members and professional/volunteer members. Represents hospice care interests to Congress, regulatory agencies, courts, voluntary organizations and the public.
J. Donald Schumacher, PsyD, President/CEO
Galen Miller, PhD, Executive Vice President

10810 National Hospice & Palliative Care Organiz ation
1731 King Street
Alexandria, VA 22314
703-837-1500
800-646-6460
Fax: 703-837-1233
e-mail: nhpco_info@nhpco.org
www.nhpco.org
The nation's only advocate for terminally ill patients and their families. Founded in 1978, the NHPCO is the only organization devoted to hospice in the United States. Support is included from state hospice organizations, patients, families and communities.
J. Donald Schumacher, President/CEO
Galen Miller, Executive Vice President

10811 National Institute for Jewish Hospice
732 University Street
North Woodmere, NY 11581
516-791-9888
800-446-4448
Fax: 516-791-6999
e-mail: mlamm@nijh.org
www.nijh.org
Serves as a resource center that seeks to help terminal patients and their families deal with their grief by providing information on traditional Jewish views on death, dying and managing the loss of a loved one.
Shirley Lamm, Executive Director
Maurice Lamm, Founder/President

10812 Share Pregnancy and Infant Loss Support, Inc.
The National Share Office
402 Jackson Street
St. Charles, MO 63301
636-947-6164
800-821-6819
Fax: 636-947-7486
e-mail: info@nationalshare.org
www.nationalshare.org
Serving those whose lives have been touched by the tragic death of a baby through pregnancy loss, stillbirth or the first few months of life.
Cathie Lammert, Executive Director
Rose Carlson, Program Director

10813 Wrap Myself in a Rainbow Compassion Books
Compassion Books
7036 State Highway 80 S
Burnsville, NC 28714-7569
828-675-5909
800-970-4220
Fax: 828-675-9687
e-mail: bruce@compassionbooks.com
www.compassionbooks.com
This is a collection of poignant songs and sensitive guided images that validates and transforms loss with hope. Side I is guided meditation Side II delivers powerful performances of Over The Rainbow, Rainbow Connection and Bring Rainbows to Children.
Audio Cassette
Bruce Greene, Director
Karen Walker, Staff

Support Groups & Hotlines

10814 Bereavement Group for Children
Corstone Center
250 Camino Alto
Mill Valley, CA 94941-2535
415-338-6161
Fax: 415-338-6165
e-mail: info@corstone.org
www.corstone.org
The CorStone Center for Personal Resilience (CPR) develops and implements resilience-based interventions and research initiatives to improve the health, education, and self-sufficiency of marginalized adults and youth around the world.
Steve Leventhal, Executive Director
Brenda Rivas-Camarena, Program Coordinator

10815 Grief & Loss Support Group
First Love Outreach Ministries

Milwaukee, WI 53206   414-263-1323
Fax: 414-263-1148
e-mail: zelodius@aol.com
www.firstlovelifecoaching.com
Pr Zelodius Morton, CEO

10816 National Hospice Helpline
1731 King Street   703-837-1500
Alexandria, VA 22314   800-646-6460
Fax: 703-837-1233
e-mail: nhpco_info@nhpco.org
www.nhpco.org
Offers more information on hospice in general and offers referrals to a hospice program in your area.
J. Donald Schumacher, President & CEO
Galen Miller, Executive VP

10817 Rainbows for All God's Children
1360 Hamilton Parkway   847-952-1770
Itasca, IL 60143   800-266-3206
Fax: 847-952-1774
e-mail: info@rainbows.org
www.rainbows.org
A support program for children who have suffered a significant loss in their lives due to death, divorce or any other painful transition.
Bob Thomas, Executive Director
Laurie Olbrisch, Executive VP

Books

10818 A Good Death: Conversations with East Londoners
Lesley Cullen and Michael Young, author
Routledge
8th Floor, 711 3rd Avenue   212-216-7800
New York, NY 10016   800-634-7064
Fax: 212-564-7854
e-mail: orders@taylorandfrancis.com
www.routledge.com
Based on a survey in East London and provides a wide range of fascinating and helpful insights into all aspects of experiencing death and surviving grief. The voices in the book are those of people who have managed to cope despite being under the shadow of impending death. Their experience could be a comfort to anybody in a similar situation. A Good Death is intended for people who are dying, and for student doctors, nurses, and social workers.
272 pages
ISBN: 0-415137-97-3

10819 Anatomy of Bereavement
Beverly Raphael, author
Rowman & Littlefield Publishers, Inc.
15200 NBN Way   717-794-3800
Blue Ridge Summit, PA 17214   800-462-6420
Fax: 717-794-3803
e-mail: orders@rowman.com
customercare@rowman.com
In this comprehensive book, Dr. Raphael describes all the stages of mourning and healing.
454 pages Softcover
ISBN: 1-568212-70-4

10820 Bereaved Children: A Support Guide for for Parents And Professionals
Earl A. Grollman, author
Beacon Press
24 Farnsworth Street   617-742-2110
Boston, MA 02210-2824   Fax: 617-723-3097
www.beacon.org
Comprehensive guide that helps children and teens cope with the loss of a loved one.
256 pages
ISBN: 0-807023-07-5

10821 Bereaved Parent
Harriet Sarnoff Schiff, author
Penguin USA

375 Hudson Street   212-366-2372
New York, NY 10014   800-847-5515
Fax: 212-366-2933
e-mail: insidesales@us.penguingroup.com
www.penguingroup.com
Supportive advice for bereaved parents and professionals who work with them.
146 pages
ISBN: 0-140050-43-4

10822 Concerning Death: A Practical Guide for the Living
Earl A. Grollman, author
Beacon Press
24 Farnsworth Street   617-742-2110
Boston, MA 02210-2824   Fax: 617-723-3097
www.beacon.org
A guide for people to learn how to cope with death and dying, and the many decisions involved in the process.
265 pages
ISBN: 0-807027-65-0

10823 Conversations At Midnight
William Morrow & Company/Order Department
39 Plymouth Street   973-227-7200
Fairfield, NJ 07004-1633   800-821-1513
Herbert Kramer is dying of cancer. For him, as for everyone someday, death is now an unavoidable companion. This book tells how Herb learns to acknowledge this presence and come to terms with human mortality. This book is a powerful way to look at death and to deal with losing a loved one.
256 pages Hardcover
ISBN: 0-688120-84-9

10824 Death and the Quest for Meaning
Stephen Strack & Herman Feifel, author
Rowman & Littlefield Publishers, Inc.
4501 Forbes Blvd.   301-459-3366
Lanham, MD 20706   800-462-6420
Fax: 301-429-5748
rowman.com
This work covers all aspects of the study of death and dying and the care of the bereaved.
Hardcover
ISBN: 0-765700-14-x
Stephen Strack, Co-Editor
Herman Feifel, Co-Editor

10825 Death: The Final Stage of Growth
Elisabeth Kubler-Ross, author
Simon & Schuster
1230 Ave of the Americas
New York, NY 10020   212-698-7000
www.simonandschuster.com
This books shows readers how to come to terms with death as a part of human development, and how death can provide us with a key meaning of human existence.
208 pages

10826 Difference in the Family
Penguin Putnam
PO Box 999   201-387-0600
Bergenfield, NJ 07621-0903   800-526-0275
Fax: 800-227-9604
A frank chronicle of the grief, rage and guilt everyone in a family suffers after a death, and the adjustments each make to cope.
Helen Featherstone, Editor

10827 Dying and Disabled Children
Haworth Press
10 Alice Street   607-722-5857
Binghamton, NY 13904-1580   800-429-6784
Fax: 607-722-0012
www.haworthpress.com
In this sensitive and compassionate look at terminally ill and disabled children, professionals from the medical community examine the stresses faced by their parents and siblings. They address crucial element of communication in dealing with a child's serious illness. Ethical decision making, learning to recognize the child's

suffering, and talking to children about death are honestly and clearly discussed.
153 pages Hardcover
ISBN: 0-866567-59-0

10828 For Those Who Live: Helping Children Cope with Death of a Brother or Sister
Centering Corporation
7230 Maple Street
Omaha, NE 68134
402-553-1200
866-218-0101
Fax: 402-553-0507
e-mail: danni@centeringcorp.com
www.centering.org
Deals with the grieving family as a whole and offers references for further help.
122 pages
Kathy LaTour, Editor

10829 Grief, Dying and Death: Clinical Intervention for Caregivers
Research Press
2612 N Mattis Avenue
Champaign, IL 61822-1053
217-352-3273
800-519-2707
Fax: 217-352-1221
e-mail: rp@researchpress.com
www.researchpress.com
In this comprehensive manual, the author provides both the theoretical background and the practical treatment interventions necessary for working with those who are bereaved or dying. Important topics such as anticipatory grief, postdeath mourning and the stress of grief are described in detail. Grief reactions, both normal and abnormal, as well as their causes are analyzed. Special attention is given to grief caused by death of a child or spouse, death by suicide, and children's grief.
488 pages Softcover
ISBN: 0-878222-32-4
Therese A. Rando, Author

10830 Helper's Journey
Dr. Dale G. Larson, author
Research Press
2612 N Mattis Avenue
Champaign, IL 61822
217-352-3273
800-519-2707
Fax: 217-352-1221
e-mail: orders@researchpress.com
www.researchpress.com
This groundbreaking work, written for both professional and volunteer caregivers, provides exercises, activities and specific strategies for more successful caregiving, increased personal growth and effective stress management. In this thoughtfully written book, Dr. Larson explores the theory and practice of helping. He includes numerous case examples and verbatim disclosures of fellow caregivers that powerfully convey the joys and sorrows of the helpers journey.
292 pages Softcover
ISBN: 0-878223-44-4
Dale G. Larson, Author

10831 On Death & Dying
Dr. Elizabeth Kubler-Ross, author
MacMillan Publishing Company
175 Fifth Avenue
New York, NY 10010
646-307-5151
e-mail: customerservice@mpsvirginia.com
www.macmillan.com
Offers a new perspective on the terminally ill by refocusing on the patient as a human being and teacher, in hopes of learning from him or her about the final stages of life.
277 pages Paperback
Elisabeth Kubler-Ross, Author

10832 On Death and Dying
MacMillan Publishing Company
175 Fifth Avenue
New York, NY 10010
646-307-5151
A wonderful book offering information on how to deal and cope with death and dying.
Paperback

10833 Recovery from Bereavement
Rowman & Littlefield Publishers, Inc.

4501 Forbes Blvd.
Lanham, MD 20706
301-459-3366
800-462-6420
Fax: 301-429-5748
e-mail: orders@rowman.com
www.rowmanlittlefield.com
Outstanding authorities on loss and bereavement discuss the factors that play a role in successful recovery.
344 pages Softcover
ISBN: 1-568213-61-1

10834 Talking About Death - A Dialog Between Parent and Child
Earl A. Grollman, author
Beacon Press
24 Farnsworth Street
Boston, MA 02210-2824
617-742-2110
Fax: 617-723-3097
e-mail: bp_information@beacon.org
www.beacon.org
A compassionate guide for children and adults. Also includes listings of resources and organizations.
128 pages

10835 Treatment of Complicated Mourning
Dr. Therese A. Rando, author
Research Press
2612 N Mattis Avenue
Champaign, IL 61822
217-352-3273
800-519-2707
Fax: 217-352-1221
e-mail: orders@researchpress.com
www.researchpress.com
This is the first book to focus specifically on complicated mourning, often referred to as pathological, unresolved, or abnormal grief. It provides caregivers with practical therapeutic strategies with and specific interventions that are necessary when traditional grief counseling is insufficient. The author provides critically important information on the prediction, identification, assessment, classification and treatment of complicated mourning.
768 pages Hardcover
ISBN: 0-878223-29-0
Therese A. Rando, Author

10836 What Helped Me When My Loved One Died
Beacon Press
24 Farnsworth Street
Boston, MA 02210-2824
617-742-2110
Fax: 617-723-3097
www.beacon.org

Children's Books

10837 Aarvy Aardvark Finds Hope
Donna O'Toole, author
Centering Corporation
7230 Maple Street
Omaha, NE 68134
402-553-1200
866-218-0101
Fax: 402-553-0507
www.centering.org
A best selling, illustrated, read-aloud story of the pain and sadness of loss and the hope of grief recovery.
80 pages Paperback
Donna O'Toole, Author

10838 Badger's Parting Gifts
Susan Varley, author
Compassion Books, Inc.
7036 State Highway 80 S
Burnsville, NC 28714-7569
828-675-5909
800-970-4220
Fax: 828-675-9687
e-mail: orders@compassionbooks.com
www.compassionbooks.com
A story of the death of old Badger. As the animals talk about Badger they remember the gift of skills and kindnesses he taught them.
23 pages Paperback
Susan Varley, Author

10839 Compassion Books, Inc.
7036 State Highway 80 S
Burnsville, NC 28714-7569
828-675-5909
800-970-4220
Fax: 828-675-9687
e-mail: orders@compassionbooks.com
www.compassionbooks.com
Hand picked resources to help people through loss, grief and changes of all kinds. Carry over 400 books and videos on death and dying, bereavement and change, comfort and healing, hope and much more.
Bruce Greene, VP

10840 Fire in My Heart: Ice in My Veins
Enid Samuel Traisman, author
Compassion Books, Inc.
7036 State Highway 80 S
Burnsville, NC 28714-7569
828-675-5909
800-970-4220
Fax: 828-675-9687
e-mail: orders@compassionbooks.com
www.compassionbooks.com
A fill in scrapbook/journal to help teenagers experiencing a loss express feelings, sort out their thoughts and gather memories.
70 pages Paperback
Enid Samuel Traisman, Author

10841 Gentle Willow: A Story for Children About Dying
Joyce C. Mills, PhD, author
Magination Press (American Psychological Assoc.)
750 First Street NE
Washington, DC 20002-4242
202-336-5500
800-374-2721
TTY: 202-336-6123
TDD: 202-336-6123
e-mail: order@apa.org
www.apa.org
This book is written for children who may not survive their own illness or for children who know them. This tender and touching tale helps address feelings of disbelief, anger, and sadness, along with love and compassion.
2003 32 pages Hardcover
ISBN: 1-591470-71-7
Joyce C. Mills, PhD, Author
Cary Pillo, Illustration

10842 Great Change
Compassion Books, Inc.
7036 State Highway 80 S
Burnsville, NC 28714-7569
828-675-5909
800-970-4220
Fax: 828-675-9687
e-mail: orders@compassionbooks.com
www.compassionbooks.com
In this deeply moving Native American story, grandmother uses nature to explain death, the great change, to a grieving granddaughter.
32 pages Hardcover
Bruce Greene, Director

10843 Let's Talk About When A Parent Dies
Rosen Publishing Group's PowerKids Press
29 E 21st Street
New York, NY 10010
212-777-3017
800-237-9932
Fax: 888-436-4643
e-mail: customerservice@rosenpub.com
www.rosenpublishing.com
This book guides children through the grieving process in a language they can understand. Recommended for grades K-4.

ISBN: 0-823923-09-6
Elizabeth Weitzman, Author

10844 Nana Upstairs and Nana Downstairs
Compassion Books
7036 State Highway 80 S
Burnsville, NC 28714-7569
828-675-5909
800-970-4220
Fax: 828-675-9687
e-mail: orders@compassionbooks.com
www.compassionbooks.com

This charming picture book recognizes that even after a family member dies the love connections continue in heart and home.
32 pages Paperback
Bruce Greene, Director

Magazines

10845 Compassion Books Catalog
Compassion Books
7036 State Highway 80 S
Burnsville, NC 28714-7569
828-675-5909
800-970-4220
Fax: 828-675-9687
e-mail: orders@compassionbooks.com
www.compassionbooks.com
More than 400 books and videos to help with serious illness, death and dying, and losses of all kinds.
32 pages
Bruce Greene, VP

Pamphlets

10846 Approaching Grief
Richard Deitrick/Ann Armstrong Dailey, author
Children's Hospice International
500 Montgomery Street
Alexandria, VA 22314
703-684-0330
800-242-4453
e-mail: info@chionline.org
www.chionline.org
Delves into the different stages of grief, guilt, depression, fear and anger. Also tells how children approach grief and ways in which to help your children get past the sorrow.
Ann Armstrong-Dailey, Founding Director/CEO
Rebecca Brant, Director

10847 Pregnancy After a Loss
Abbott Northwestern Hospital Parent Education
800 E 28th Strt
Minneapolis, MN 55407
612-863-4000
This booklet is written by a group of parents that have experienced a pregnancy after a loss, sensitively written with suggestions for coping with the fears and anxieties of the new pregnancy.

10848 Pregnancy Heartbreak: Unfulfilled Promises
Abbott Northwestern Hospital Parent Education
800 E 28th Strt
Minneapolis, MN 55407
612-863-4000
This handbook is written for parents who had to face the reality of the diagnosis and birth of a baby with life-threatening conditions.

Audio & Video

10849 Encounters with Grief
Fanlight Productions
C/O Icarus Films
Brooklyn, NY 11201
718-488-8900
800-876-1710
Fax: 718-488-8642
e-mail: info@fanlight.com
www.fanlight.com
A mother who lost her teenage son, a woman widowed in her sixties and a man whose wife died at fifty-two discuss the emotional upheaval that followed and their moving perspectives on the process of recovery.
1992 13 Minutes
ISBN: 1-572950-91-9

10850 Grave Words: Tools for Discussing End of Life Choices
Maren Monson, MD, author
Fanlight Productions
C/O Icarus Films
Brooklyn, NY 11201
718-488-8900
800-876-1710
Fax: 718-488-8642
e-mail: info@fanlight.com
www.fanlight.com

Blends humor, music and insightful interviews to confront the issues that arise in discussions between physicians and healthcare providers and patients about end-of-life care decisions.
1996 25 Minutes
ISBN: 1-572952-24-5
Maren Monsen, MD, Author

10851 Pitch of Grief
Eric Strange, author
Fanlight Productions
C/O Icarus Films
Brooklyn, NY 11201

718-488-8900
800-876-1710
Fax: 718-488-8642
e-mail: info@fanlight.com
www.fanlight.com

Explores the process of grieving through interviews with four bereaved men and women, and is helpful to not only the grieving person, but for others within the family who have faced the loss of a loved one.
1985 28 Minutes
ISBN: 1-572950-18-8
Eric Stange, Author

10852 There Was a Child
Fred Simon, author
Fanlight Productions
C/O Icarus Film
Brooklyn, NY 11201

718-488-8900
800-876-1710
Fax: 718-488-8642
e-mail: info@fanlight.com
www.fanlight.com

Demonstrates the impact that losing a pregnancy, or the birth of a stillborn child, has had on three mothers and a father. Validates the emotions of parents who feel alone with their loss, while helping health care workers and families to give appropriate, meaningful support.
1991 32 Minutes
ISBN: 1-572950-48-X
Fred Simon, Author

10853 We Will Remember
Compassion Books, Inc.
7036 State Highway 80 S
Burnsville, NC 28714-7569

828-675-5909
800-970-4220
Fax: 828-675-9687
e-mail: orders@compassionbooks.com
www.compassionbooks.com

A video meditation that uses the beauty of natural photography, soothing music and gentle words to give permission and encouragement in using the memories of the past for healing in the present.
11 minutes
James Miller, Author

10854 When the Bough Breaks
Fanlight Productions
32 Court Street
Brooklyn, NY 11201-1731

718-488-8900
800-876-1710
Fax: 718-488-8642
e-mail: info@fanlight.com
www.fanlight.com

Based on the real story of a patient who experienced a stillbirth, these ten vignettes dramatically recreate her interactions with health care providers during the final weeks of pregnancy. Study guide included.
1992 71 Minutes
ISBN: 1-572951-08-7

Web Sites

10855 Compassionate Friends
www.compassionatefriends.org
Gives support to people who have experienced the death of a child.

10856 Hospice Association of America
www.nahc.org
Promotes the concepts of hospice, a philosophy of health care which is expressed through the provision of a variety of medical and nonmedical services to terminally ill patients and their families.

10857 National Hospice & Palliative Care Organization
www.nhpco.org
The nation's only advocate for terminally ill patients and their families. Founded in 1978, the NHPCO is the only organization devoted to hospice in the United States. Support is included from state hospice organizations, patients, families, communities, provider program members and professional/volunteer members. Represents hospice care interests to Congress, regulatory agencies, courts, voluntary organizations and the public.

10858 Share Pregnancy and Infant Loss Support, Inc.
www.nationalshare.org
Offers studies, information, statistics, help and support to parents who have suffered the loss of a child.

B

Baylor College of Medicine: General Clinical Research Center for Adults, 3862

Baylor College of Medicine: Jerry Lewis Neuromuscular Disease Research, 6592

Baylor College of Medicine: Sleep Disorder and Research Center, 7868

Baylor University Bone Marrow Transplantation Research Center, 2304

Bayou Area Chapter of the American Association of Kidney Patients, 5555

Baystate Medical Center Wesson Memorial Unit, 3052

Be BoneWise: Exercise, 6926

Be Happy, Not Sad, 4571

Be Kind to Nonsmokers, 8644

Be Smart About HIV, 510

Beach Center on Disability, 10471

Beach Center on Families and Disability, 10737

Bearly Any Fat Cookbook, 3649

Beaver County Association for the Blind, 9618

Bees-Stealy Research Foundation, 4793

Before You Take That First..., 6825

Beginning Reading and Sign Language Video, 4713

Beginning with Braille: Balanced Approach to Literacy, 9896

Beginnings for Parents of Children Who are Deaf or Hard of Hearing, 4335

Behavior Management: Collection of Articless, 7297

Behavioral Pediatrics Program, 10626

Behavioral Vision Approaches for Persons with Physical Disabilities, 9897

Behavioral and Circadian Sleep Problems of Infancy and Childhood, 2810

Behavioral and Psychosocial Sequelae of Pediatric Head Injury, 4145

Behaviors, 947

Behcet's Disease, 1220

Being Alive, 471

Being Alive Newsletter, 472

Being Close, 1372

Being in Touch, 4364

Believe In Tomorrow Children's Foundation, 10766

Belonging, 4572, 9960

Benaroya Research Institute Virginia Mason Medical Center, 3307

Bendectin Report, 1790

Benjamin B Greenfield National Alzheimer's Center, 663

Bereaved Children: A Support Guide for for Parents And Professionals, 10820

Bereaved Parent, 10821

Bereavement Group for Children, 1840, 10814

Berkshire Center, 10621

BermanGund Laboratory for the Study of Retinal Degenerations, 9839

Bernardsville Beginnings, 3569

Beside Me, 9961

Best Practices, 130

Best Practices in Educational Interpreting, 4365

Best of Public Outreach, 8645

Best of Superstuff Activity Booklet, 1339

Best of the Beacon, 7463

Bestwork Industries for the Blind, 9593

Bethy and the Mouse: God's Gifts in Special Packages, 3532

Better Breather's Clubs, 7325

Better Breathing Bulletin, 3115

Better Existence with HIV, 191

Better Hearing Institute, 4220, 4762

Better Hearing News, 4654

Between Friends, 4366

Beyond Gentle Teaching, 1668

Beyond the Loss of the Breast, 2511

Bible Alliance, 10095

Bibliography, 5453

Big Red Factor, 5015

Biliary Atresia, 5728

Bill Discusses the Twelve Traditions, 8795

Bill's Own Story, 8796

Billy's Story, 3688

Biology of Reproduction, 5442

Biology of the Autistic Syndromes, 1669

Bipolar Disorder, 6231

Birmingham VA Medical Center: Research and Development, 2198

Birth Defect News, 1796

Birth Defect Research for Children, 649, 1749

Birth Defects & Genetics: The Genetics Revolution, 1801

Birth Defects of the Female Reproductive System, 5454

Bittersweet Waltz, 3570

Black Coalition for AIDS Prevention, 192

Black Death: AIDS in Africa, 403

Black Experience, 3445

Black Lung, 5829

Black Skin, 7799

Black and Deaf in America, 4367

Black, Beautiful and Recovering, 8402, 8646

Bladder Control for Women, 5294

Blank Childrens Hospital Pediatric Pulmonology Clinic, 3040

Bleeding Disorder Foundation of Washington, 4936

Bleeding in the Digestive Tract, 9432

Blick Clinic for Developmental Disabilities, 3503

Blind Association of Western New York, 9599

Blind Childrens Center, 9682

Blind Educator, 9969

Blind Enterprises of Oregon, 9615

Blind Industries and Services of Maryland, 9571

Blind Work Association, 9600

Blinded Veterans Association, 9460, 10126

Blindness and Early Childhood Development, 9898

Blindness: A Family Matter, 10096

Blood Pressure Book: How to Get it Down & Keep it Down, 10649

Bloodlines, 5016

Blueprint for Conversational Competence, 4368

Bockus Research Institute Graduate Hospital, 4794

Body Betrayed, 3650

Body Positive HIV and AIDS Research and Re Southwest Center for HIV/AIDS, 242

Body Silent: An Anthropologist Embarks into the World of the Disabled, 8109

Body, Mind, and Spirit, 8403

Bomb in the Brain: A Heroic Tale of Science, Surgery and Survival, 7588

Bone Marrow Foundation, 2018, 2521

Bone Up on Arthritis, 1170

Boning Up on Osteoporosis, 6908

Book of Name Signs, 4369

Books are Fun for Everyone, 10028

Books for Parents of Deaf and Hard of Hearing Children, 4680

Bosma Industries for the Blind, 9559

Boston Bracing System for Idiopathic Scoliosis, 7503

Boston Hemophilia Center Fegan 5 Children's Hospital, 4943

Boston Obesity Nutrition Research Center (BONRC), 6850

Boston Sickle Cell Center Boston Medical Center, 7709

Boston University Arthritis Center, 1146

Boston University Cancer Research Center, 2251

Boston University Center for Human Genetics, 1759

Boston University Laboratory of Neuropsychology, 8331

Boston University Medical Campus General Clinical Research Center, 1147

Boston University University Medical Center, 7445

Boston University, Whitaker Cardiovascular Institute, 4795

Boulder Public Library, 9688

Bowel Cancer, 2352

Bowel Continence and Spina Bifida, 8021

Bowman Gray School of Medicine, 8170

Bowman Grey School of Medicine: Hemophilia Diagnostic Center, 4944

Boys Town National Research Hospital, 4294

Brace & Her Brace is No Handicap, 7504

Brachytherapy and IMRT, 2430

Brady Institute Jamaica Hospital Medical Center, 4051

Braille Alphabet and Numbers, 10029

Braille Book Bank: Music Catalog, 9899

Braille Book Review, 9988

Braille Documents, 10097

Braille Forum, 9970

Braille Institute Desert Center, 9840

Braille Institute Library Services, 9683

Braille Institute Orange County Center, 9841

Braille Institute Santa Barbara Center Braille Institute of Los Angeles, 9842

Braille Institute Sight Center, 9843

Braille Institute Youth Center, 9844

Braille Institute of America Library, 9461

Braille Literacy: Blind Persons, Families, Prof. & Producers of Braille, 10030

Braille Monitor, 9971

Braille Revival League, 10127

Braille Textbook Assignment Service National Braille Association, 9845

Braille: An Extraordinary Volunteer Opportunity, 10031

Brain & Behavior Research Foundation, 6266

Brain Cancer Support Group, 1913

Brain Cancer Support Group: Port Orchard, 1956

Brain Cancer Support Group: Seattle, 1957

Brain Damage is a Family Affair, 4146

Brain Injuries: A Guide for Families & Caretakers, 4147

Brain Injury Alliance of Iowa Helpline, 4079

Brain Injury Alliance of Kentucky, 4081

Brain Injury Alliance of Minnesota, 4087

Brain Injury Alliance of Montana, 4090

Brain Injury Alliance of New Jersey, 4092

Brain Injury Alliance of New Mexico, 4093

Brain Injury Alliance of Oregon, 4101

Brain Injury Alliance of Utah, 4104

Brain Injury Alliance of Wisconsin, 4110

Brain Injury Alliance of Wyoming, 4111

Brain Injury Association, 3996, 4192

Brain Injury Association of America's National Family Helpline, 4044

Brain Injury Association of Arizona, 4005, 4067

Brain Injury Association of Arkansas, 4006

Brain Injury Association of Arkansas Helpl ine, 4068

Brain Injury Association of California Hel pline, 4069

Brain Injury Association of Colorado, 4007

Brain Injury Association of Colorado Helpline, 4071

Brain Injury Association of Connecticut, 4008

Brain Injury Association of Connecticut Helpline, 4072

Brain Injury Association of Delaware, 4009

Brain Injury Association of Delaware Helpl ine, 4073

Brain Injury Association of Florida, 4010, 4074

Brain Injury Association of Hawaii, 4013, 4075

Brain Injury Association of Idaho, 4014

Brain Injury Association of Illinois, 4015

Brain Injury Association of Illinois Helpline, 4077

Brain Injury Association of Indiana, 4016

Brain Injury Association of Indiana Helpli ne, 4078

Brain Injury Association of Iowa, 4017

Brain Injury Association of Kansas and Greater Kansas City Helpline, 4018, 4080

Brain Injury Association of Kentucky, 4019

Brain Injury Association of Louisiana Help line, 4082

Brain Injury Association of Maine, 4020

Brain Injury Association of Maryland, 4021

Brain Injury Association of Maryland Helpl ine, 4083

Brain Injury Association of Massachusetts, 4022

Brain Injury Association of Massachusetts Helpline, 4084

Brain Injury Association of Michigan, 4023

Brain Injury Association of Michigan Helpline, 4086

Brain Injury Association of Minnesota, 4024

Brain Injury Association of Mississippi, 4025

Brain Injury Association of Mississippi Helpline, 4088

Brain Injury Association of Missouri, 4026

Brain Injury Association of Missouri Helpline, 4089

Brain Injury Association of Montana, 4027

Brain Injury Association of New Hampshire, 4028, 4091

Brain Injury Association of New Jersey, 4029

Brain Injury Association of New Mexico, 4030

Brain Injury Association of New York State, 4031

Brain Injury Association of New York State Helpline, 4094

Brain Injury Association of North Carolina, 4033

Brain Injury Association of North Carolina Helpline, 4097

Brain Injury Association of North Dakota, 4098

Brain Injury Association of Ohio, 4034, 4099

C

G

H

I

K

L

N

O

P

T

X

Y

Z

Alabama

AIDS Alabama, 374

Alabama Ambassador: National Ataxia Foundation, 1446

Alabama Chapter of the American Association of Kidney Patients, 5523

Alabama Chapter of the Arthritis Foundation, 1097

Alabama Council of the Blind, 9523

Alabama Department of Public Health, 239

Alabama Education of Homeless Children and Youth Program, 6118

Alabama Head Injury Foundation, 4004

Alabama Head Injury Foundation Helpline, 4066

Alabama Institute for Deaf and Blind, 4257

Alabama Organ Center, 9198

Alabama Radio Reading Service Network, 9670

Alabama Regional Library for the Blind and Physically Handicapped, 9671

Alabama Support Group: National Ataxia Foundation, 1447

Alzheimer's Association: North Alabama Chapter, 666

Alzheimer's Association: Southeast Alabama Chapter, 667

Alzheimer's Association: Southwest Alabama Chapter, 668

Alzheimer's Disease Center: University of Alabama at Birmingham, 862

American Cancer Society: Alabama, 2048

American Diabetes Association: Alabama, 3143

American Lung Association of Alabama, 5763

American Lung Association of Alabama, 9284

American Society for Reproductive Medicine, 3713

American Society for Reproductive Medicine, 5319

Arthritis and Musculoskeletal Center: UAB Shelby Interdisciplinary Biomedical Rese, 1145

Autism Society of Alabama, 1591

Autism Society of North Alabama, 1592

Birmingham VA Medical Center: Research and Development, 2198

Breast Cancer Resource Foundation of Alabama, 2199

Bureau of Family Health Services: Alabama Department of Public Health, 8840

CCFA Alabama Chapter, 2929

Cardiovascular Research and Training Center University of Alabama, 4796

Center for Neuroimmunology: University of Alabama at Birmingham, 6508

Centers for AIDS Research: University of Alabama at Birmingham, 307

Civitan International Research Center, 4298

Diabetes Research and Training Center: University of Alabama at Birmingham, 3309

Division of Mental Illness and Substance Abuse Community Programs, 8269

Division of Rehabilitation: Montgomery, 10545

General Clinical Research Center: UAB, 308

Gulf War Veterans of Alabama, 10177

Hemophilia Clinic: Childrens' Rehabilitation Service, 4964

Hemophilia and Bleeding Disorders of Alaba ma, Inc., 4893

Horizons Schools, 10614

Houston Love Memorial Library, 9672

Huntsville Subregional Library for the Blind and Physically Handicapped, 9673

Juvenile Diabetes Research Foundation: Birmingham, 3144

Knollwoodpark Hospital Sleep Disorders Cen, 7877

Knollwoodpark Hospital Sleep Disorders Center, 7876

Leukemia and Lymphoma Society: Alabama Chapter, 2049

Library and Resource Center for the Blind and Physically Handicapped, 9674

Lyme Disease Network Support Group of Alabama: Mobile Chapter, 9057

Magic Moments, 10781

NNFF Alabama Affiliate, 6741

National Alliance on Mental Illness of Alabama: NAMI Alabama, 5996

National Federation of the Blind: Alabama, 9524

National Multiple Sclerosis Society: Alabama Chapter, 6421

National Society for MVP and Dysautonomia, 4848

National Spinal Cord Injury Statistical Center, 8072

National Spinal Cord Injury Support Groups, 8108

Pediatric Brain Tumor Support Group, 1837

Pull-thru Network, 3870

Pushin On: RRTC on Secondary Conditions of Spinal, 8098

Sickle Cell Foundation of Greater Montgomery, 7708

Specialized Center of Research in Ischemic Heart Disease, 4823

Spina Bifida Association of Alabama, 7972

Stroke Research and Treatment Center UAB Medical Center, 8176

Tuscaloosa Subregional Library for the Blind & Physically Handicapped, 9675

United Cerebral Palsy of Alabama, 2599

United Cerebral Palsy of East Central Alabama, 2600

United Cerebral Palsy of Greater Birmingha m, 2601

United Cerebral Palsy of Huntsville & Tennessee Valley, 2602

United Cerebral Palsy of Mobile, 2603

United Cerebral Palsy of Northwest Alabama, 2604

United Cerebral Palsy of West Alabama, 2605

University Alzheimer Center University of Alabama at Birmingham, 883

University of Alabama At Birmingham Comprehensive Cancer Center, 2200

University of Alabama Birmingham, 7454

University of Alabama Speech and Hearing Center, 4323

University of Alabama at Birmingham Parkinsons Disease Center, 7000

University of Alabama at Birmingham: Congenital Heart Disease Center, 4825

University of Alabama at Birmingham: National Cooperative Drug/AIDS, 309

Veterans Administration Medical Center: Alabama, 10178

Veterans Association Medical Center, 10179

Alaska

AARP Alaska State Office, 32

Alaska Department of Health and Social Services: AIDS/STD Program, 240

Alaska Gulf War Syndrome Referral Coordinator, 10180

Alaska State Library Talking Book Center, 9676

Alaska VA Healthcare System, 10181

Alaskan Statewide AIDS Helpline, 378

Alzheimer's Disease Resource Agency of Alaska, 669

American Cancer Society: Alaska, 2050

American Diabetes Association: Alaska, 3145

American Lung Association of Alaska, 5764

American Lung Association of Alaska, 9285

Asthma and Allergy Foundation of America: Alaska Chapter, 1283

Client Assistance Program: Anchorage, 10546

Lupus Foundation of America: Alaska Chapter, 5856

National Alliance for the Mentally Ill (NA MI) Alaska, 6119

National Alliance on Mental Illness of Alaska, 5997

National Federation of the Blind: Alaska, 9525

National Multiple Sclerosis Society: Alaska Chapter, 6422

Office of Alcohol and Substance Abuse Department of Health and Social Services, 8270

SIDS Information and Counseling Program: Alaska Department of Health, 8841

United Cerebral Palsy of Alaska/PARENTS, 2606

Arizona

AARP Arizona: Phoenix Collier Center, 33

Alcoholism and Drug Abuse: Office of Community Behavioral Health, 8271

Alzheimer's Association: Desert Southwest Chapter, 670

Alzheimer's Association: Northern Arizona, 671

Alzheimer's Association: Northern Nevada, 672

Alzheimer's Association: Southern Arizona, 673

Alzheimer's Association: Southern Arizona Region, 674

American Cancer Society: Arizona, 2051

American Council on Alcohol Problems, 8230

American Diabetes Association: Arizona, 3146

American Diabetes Association: Arizona, Border Area, 3147

American Diabetes Association: Atlanta Met, 3148

American Diabetes Association: Northern Arizona, 3149

American Fibromyalgia Syndrome Association, 3776

American Liver Foundation Arizona Chapter, 5676

American Lung Association of Arizona, 5765

Arizona Association of the Deaf, 4258

Arizona Brain Tumor Support Group, 1838

Arizona Center for the Blind and Visually Impaired, 9526

Arizona Chapter of the ALS Association, 998

Arizona Chapter of the National Parkinson Foundation, 6963

Arizona Department of Health Services, 241

Arizona Heart Institute, 4791

Arizona Industries for the Blind, 9527

Arizona Kidney Foundation, 5524

Arizona SIDS Founation, 8842

Arizona Spinal Cord Injury Association, 8077

Arizona State Braille and Talking Book Library, 9677

Arizona Telemedicine Program, 7311

Arthritis Foundation: Central Arizona Chapter, 1098

Autism Society of Pima County, 1593

Body Positive HIV and AIDS Research and Re Southwest Center for HIV/AIDS, 242

Brain Injury Association of Arizona, 4005

Brain Injury Association of Arizona, 4067

CCFA Southwest Chapter: Arizona, 2930

Center for Neurodevelopmental Studies, 1642

Center for Neurology & Stroke Baptist Hospital Office, 2542

Central Arizona Chapter of the American Association of Kidney Patients, 5525

Child Help, 7191

Commission on Accreditation of Rehabilitation Services, 23

Cystic Fibrosis Center: Phoenix Childrens Hospital, 3015

Do it Now Foundation, 8334

Donor Network of Arizona, 9199

Eating Disorders Anonymous, 3600

Fibromyalgia Network, 3786

Flagstaff City Coconino County Public Library, 9678

HPV Support Groups: Arizona, 10547

International Holistic Center, 2052

Jim L Walker: Arizona Chapter of the Myasthenia Gravis Foundation of America, 6655

Juvenile Diabetes Research Foundation: Phoenix Chapter, 3150

Leukemia and Lymphoma Society: Mountain States Chapter, 2053

Life Development Institute, 10504

Life Development Institute, 10615

Lupus Foundation of America: Greater Arizona Chapter, 5857

Lupus Foundation of America: Southern Arizona Chapter, 5858

Make-A-Wish Foundation of America, 10782

Mayo Clinic, 7171

Mayo Clinic Scottsdale Center for Scleroderma Care & Research, 7449

Mentally Ill Kids In Distress, 5998

Mountain State Regional Hemophilia Center, 4973

Muscular Dystrophy Association, 6588

Muscular Dystrophy Association, 6597

Myasthenia Gravis Support Group of Arizona Jim L. Walker Chapter, 6684

National Alliance on Mental Illness of Arizona, 5999

National Federation of the Blind: Arizona, 9528

National Federation of the Blind: Blind/Deaf Division, 9501

National Multiple Sclerosis Society Desert Southwest Chapter, 6423

National Network of Learning Disabled Adults, 10524

National Sjogren's Syndrome Foundation NSSA, 7738

Navaho Nation K'E Project: Tuba City Children & Families Advocacy Corp, 6000
Navaho Nation K'E Project: Winslow Children & Families Advocacy Corp, 6001
Navajo Nation Office of Special Education & Rehabilitation Services (OSERS), 6120
Neurofibromatosis Association of Arizona, 6742
Northern Arizona Branch:Phoenix Area, 9286
Office of Chronic Disease Prevention and Nutrition Services, 6806
Office of Womens And Childrens Health: Alabama Department of Health, 8843
Phoenix Area Support Group: National Ataxi a Foundation, 1448
Phoenix Public Library: Special Needs Section, 9679
Phoenix VA Healthcare System, 10182
Prader-Willi Syndrome Arizona Association, 7252
Prader-Willi Syndrome Arizona Association: Phoenix Area, 7251
RESOLVE of Valley of the Sun, 5324
Ruth E Golding Clinical Pharmacokinetics Laboratory, 8357
Scleroderma Foundation: Arizona Chapter, 7416
Southern Arizona Brain Tumor Support Group, 1839
Southern Arizona Branch: Tucson Area, 9287
Southwest Association for Education in Biomedical Research, 2201
Spina Bifida Association of Arizona, 7973
St. Joseph's Hemophilia Center, 4986
Teratology OTIS, 1766
Tucson Interfaith HIV/AIDS Network (TIHAN), 243
Tucson Support Group: National Ataxia Foundation, 1449
United Cerebral Palsy of Central Arizona, 2607
United Cerebral Palsy of Southern Arizona, 2608
University of Arizona Cancer Center, 2202
Veterans Adm. Medical Center: Tucson Southern Arizona VA Health Care System, 10183

Arkansas

AARP Arkansas State Office: Little Rock, 34
Alzheimer's Arkansas Programs and Services, 675
Alzheimer's Association: Western Arkansas Chapter, 676
American Cancer Society: Arkansas, 2054
American Diabetes Association: Arkansas, 3151
American Lung Association of Arkansas, 5766
American Lung Association of Arkansas, 9288
Arkansas Association of the Deaf, 4259
Arkansas Cystic Fibrosis Center Arkansas Children's Hospital, 3016
Arkansas Department of Health AIDS Prevention Program, 244
Arkansas Department of Health: SIDS Information & Counseling Program, 8844
Arkansas FFCMH Jane Burgan, 6002
Arkansas Lighthouse for the Blind, 9530
Arkansas Regional Library for the Blind and Physically Handicapped, 9680
Arkansas Regional Organ Recovery Agency, 9200
Arthritis Foundation: Arkansas Chapter, 1099
Brain Injury Association of Arkansas, 4006
Brain Injury Association of Arkansas Helpl ine, 4068
Central Arkansas Veterans Healthcare Syste Eugene J. Towbin Healthcare Center, 10184
Disability Rights Center of Arkansas, 10548
Gulf War Veterans of Arkansas, 10185
Health Resource, 2055
Hemophilia Foundation of Arkansas, 4894
John L McClellan Memorial Veterans' Hospital Research Office, 4812
Juvenile Diabetes Research Foundation: Northwest Arkansas Branch, 3152
Library for the Blind and Handicapped, Southwest, 9681
Lions World Services for the Blind Lions Clubs International, 9480
Lupus Foundation of America: Arkansas Chapter, 5859
NAMI Arkansas, 6003
NNFF Arkansas Affilaite, 6743
National Federation of the Blind: Arkansas, 9531
National Kidney Foundation of Arkansas, 5526

National Multiple Sclerosis Society: Arkansas Chapter, 6424
Office of Alcohol and Drug Abuse Prevention, 8272
Prader-Willi Arkansas Association Prader-Willi Syndrome Association, 7253
RESOLVE Affiliate of Northwest Arkansas, 5325
Research and Training Center for Persons Who are Deaf or Hard of Hearing, 4312
United Cerebral Palsy of Central Arkansas, 2609
Veterans Adm. Medical Center: Fayetville, 10186

California

1-800-BRAILLE, 9873
AARP California State Office: Pasadena, 35
AARP California State Office: Sacramento, 36
AEGIS AIDS Education Global Information System, 373
AIDS Clinical Trials Unit CARES Clinic, 310
AIDS.ORG, 180
ALS Association Free Standing Support Groups, 1052
ALS Association: Bay Area Chapter, 999
ALS Association: Greater Los Angeles Chapter, 1000
ALS Association: Greater Sacramento Chapter, 1001
ALS Association: Greater San Diego CIO, 1002
ALS Center at UCSF, 1039
ASTHMA Hotline, 608
Adopt-A-Special-Kid America, 5317
Adult Research Opportunities, 311
Advocates 4 Health: Tick-borne Disease Self-Help Group, 9053
Aids, Medicine and Miracles, 245
Alcohol Drug Treatment Referral, 8372
Alcohol Research Group Public Health Institute, 8330
Alta Bates Summit Medical Center, 6096
Alzheimer's Association San Diego/Imperial Chapter, 677
Alzheimer's Association: California Central Chapter: Ventura County Office, 678
Alzheimer's Association: Greater North Valley Chapter, 680
Alzheimer's Association: Greater Sacramento, 679
Alzheimer's Association: Los Angeles Chapter, 681
Alzheimer's Association: Monterey County Chapter, 682
Alzheimer's Association: North Bay Chapter, 683
Alzheimer's Association: Orange County Chapter, 684
Alzheimer's Association: Riverside/San Bernardino Counties Chapter, 685
Alzheimer's Association: San Francisco Bay Area Chapter, 686
Alzheimer's Association: Santa Barbara Central Coast Chapter, 687
Alzheimer's Association: Santa Cruz County Chapter, 688
Alzheimer's Disease Center: University of California, Davis, 861
American Academy of Ophthalmology, 9447
American Association for Pediatric Ophthalmology And Strabismus, 6650
American Association of Endocrine Surgeons, 2
American Association of Gynecologic Laproscopists, 3712
American Cancer Society Santa Clara County / Silicon Valley / Central Coast Region, 2056
American Cancer Society: Central Los Angeles, 2057
American Cancer Society: East Bay/Metro Region, 2058
American Cancer Society: Fresno/Madera Counties, 2059
American Cancer Society: Inland Empire, 2060
American Cancer Society: Orange County, 2061
American Cancer Society: Sacramento County, 2062
American Cancer Society: San Diego County, 2063
American Cancer Society: San Francisco County, 2064
American Cancer Society: San Jose Prostate Cancer Support Group, 2318
American Cancer Society: Santa Maria Valley, 2065
American Cancer Society: Sonoma County, 2066
American Chronic Pain Association, 2538
American Chronic Pain Association, 2834

American Diabetes Association: California, 3153
American Liver Foundation Greater Los Angeles Chapter, 5677
American Liver Foundation Northern CA Chapter, 5678
American Liver Foundation San Diego Chapte r, 5679
American Lung Association of California, 5767
American Lung Association of California, 9289
Amyotrophic Lateral Sclerosis Toll Free Hotline, 1054
Arthritis Foundation: Northern California Chapter, 1100
Arthritis Foundation: San Diego Area Chapter, 1101
Arthritis Foundation: Southern California Chapter, 1102
Asian & Pacific Islander Wellness Center Community HIV/AIDS Services, 189
Asian and Pacific Island Wellness Center, 190
Association for the Cure of Cancer of the Prostate, 2017
Asthma and Allergy Foundation of America: Southern California Chapter, 572
Asthma and Allergy Foundation of America: Southern California Chapter, 1284
Autism Research Institute, 1584
Autism Society of California, 1594
Bay Area LE Foundation, 5860
Bay Area Turner Syndrome Society, 9370
Bees-Stealy Research Foundation, 4793
Bereavement Group for Children, 1840
Bereavement Group for Children, 10814
Blind Childrens Center, 9682
Braille Institute Desert Center, 9840
Braille Institute Library Services, 9683
Braille Institute Orange County Center, 9841
Braille Institute Santa Barbara Center Braille Institute of Los Angeles, 9842
Braille Institute Sight Center, 9843
Braille Institute Youth Center, 9844
Braille Institute of America Library, 9461
Brain Injury Association of California Hel pline, 4069
Brain Tumor Society, 1841
Brain Tumor Support Group: Fresno, 1843
Brain Tumor Support Group: Fullerton, 1844
Brain Tumor Support Group: Newport Beach, 1845
Brain Tumor Support Group: Orange, 1846
Brain Tumor Support Group: Redding, 1847
Brain Tumor Support Group: Sacramento, 1848
Brain Tumor Support Group: San Diego, 1849
Brain Tumor Support Group: San Francisco, 1850
Brain Tumor Support Group: Santa Barbara, 1851
Brain Tumor Support Group: Stanford, 1852
Brain Tumor Support Group: Westlake Village, 1853
Brain Tumor/Pituitary Patient Support Group, 1854
Breast Cancer Action, 2019
Burnham Institute Cancer Center The Burnham Institute for Medical Resear, 2203
CCFA California: Greater Los Angeles Chapter, 2931
California Ambassador: National Ataxia Foundation, 1450
California Association of Persian Gulf Veterans, 10187
California Collaborative Treatment Group CCTG Data Center, 246
California Department of Health Services Office of Aids, 247
California Institute for Medical Research, 6998
California Lyme Disease Association, 9050
California SIDS Program, 8845
California State Library Braille and Talking Book Library, 9684
California Teratogen Information Service UC San Diego School of Medicine Dept of, 1760
California Transplant Donor Network, 9201
California Women's Commission on Alcohol and Drug Dependencies, 8273
Cancer Control Society and Cancer Book House, 2067
Cancer Federation, 2194
Cancer Prevention Institute of California, 2204
Cancer Support Community, 2322
Cancervive, 2323
Canine Companions for Independence, 9462
Celiac Disease Foundation, 2563

Redding Chapter of the American Association of Kidney Patients, 5531

Region 6 of the National Association for Parents of the Visually Impaired, 9529

Regional Cancer Foundation, 2077

Research Institute of Palo Alto Medical Foundation, 600

Rosalind Russell Medical Research Center for Arthritis at UCSF, 1157

Rose Kushner Breast Cancer Advisory Center, 2078

SIDS Alliance Of Northern California, 8846

SIDS Foundation of Southern California, 8847

Sacramento Valley Chapter of the American Association of Kidney Patients, 5532

Sacramento Veterans Center, 10189

Salk Institute Cancer Center, 2211

San Diego Area Chapter National Multiple Sclerosis Society, 6431

San Diego Support Group: National Ataxia Foundation, 1454

San Francisco AIDS Foundation (SFAF), 249

San Francisco Area AIDS Education and Training Center, 250

San Francisco Clinical Research Center, 6368

San Francisco Heart & Vascular Institute, 4822

San Francisco Public Library for the Blind and Print Disabled, 9686

San Francisco VA Medical Center, 10190

San Jose State University Library, 9687

Sansum Diabetes Research Institute, 3318

Santa Barbara Breast Cancer Institute, 2212

Scleroderma Foundation: Greater San Diego Chapter, 7417

Scleroderma Foundation: Northern California Chapter, 7418

Scleroderma Foundation: Southern California Chapter, 7419

Scleroderma Research Foundation, 7452

Scripps Clinic Sleep Disorders Center Scripps Clinic, 7885

Scripps Clinic and Research Foundation: Autoimmune Disease Center, 7775

Scripps Research Institute, 601

Senior Resource, 30

Sepulveda Ambulatory Care Center, 10191

Sleep Disorders Center at California: Paci, 7894

Sleep Disorders Center at California: Pacific Medical Center, 7893

Sleep Disorders Center of Metropolitan Toronto, 7895

Smith-Kettlewell Eye Research Foundation, 9517

Smith-Kettlewell Eye Research Institute, 9865

Society of American Gastrointestinal Endoscopic Surgeons, 3856

Society of Hearing Impaired Physicians, 4253

Southern California Research Institute, 8358

Southwest Regional Training Center: Canine Companions for Independence, 9535

Spina Bifida Association of Greater San Diego, 7974

Spinal Cord Injury Network International, 8075

Stanford CF Center Packard Children's Hospital At Stanford, 3023

Stanford Center for Research in Disease Prevention, 8359

Stanford University Center for Narcolepsy Dept of Psychiatry & Behavioral Sciences, 7919

Stanford University General Clinical Research Center, 319

Stanford University National Cooperative Drug Discovery/AIDS Group, 320

Stanford University: Beckman Center for Molecular and Genetic Medicine, 2213

Starlight Children's Foundation, 10800

Starlight Foundation, 10787

Support Group for Caregivers of Brain Tumor Patients, 1862

Support Group for Parents of Children with Brain Tumors, 1867

Synergy Clinical Research Center, 7172

The Center for Culture, Trauma and Mental Health Disparities, 7173

The Sam and Rose Stein Institute for Research on the Aging, 882

Tripod, 4255

UCD Northern Central California Hemophilia Program, 4992

UCLA AIDS Clinical Research Center, 321

UCLA Anxiety Disorders Research Center, 7174

UCLA Neuropsychiatric Institute, 4060

UCSD Antiviral Research Center, 322

UCSD Comprehensive Hemophilia Treatment Center, 4993

UCSF Children's Hospital Health Library, 3520

USC Internal Medicine, 323

USC/Norris Comprehensive Cancer Center, 2214

USC: Neonatology Research Units, 8946

United Advocates for Children of California, 6005

United Cerebral Palsy of Central California, 2610

United Cerebral Palsy of Greater Sacrament o, 2611

United Cerebral Palsy of Los Angeles & Ventura Counties, 2612

United Cerebral Palsy of Orange County, 2613

United Cerebral Palsy of San Diego County, 2614

United Cerebral Palsy of San Joaquin, Calaveras & Amador Counties, 2615

United Cerebral Palsy of San Luis Obispo, 2616

United Cerebral Palsy of Santa Barbara County, 2617

United Cerebral Palsy of Santa Clara & San Mateo Counties, 2618

United Cerebral Palsy of Stanislaus County, 2619

United Cerebral Palsy of the Golden Gate, 2620

United Cerebral Palsy of the Inland Empire, 2621

United Cerebral Palsy of the North Bay, 2622

United Liver Foundation, 10440

United Organ Transplant Association (UOTA), 9197

University of California Berkeley Cancer Research Laboratory, 2215

University of California Liver Research Unit, 5710

University of California San Diego General Clinical Research Center, 4826

University of California San Francisco Center for AIDS Prevention, 324

University of California at San Francisco Women's Continence Center, 5282

University of California, San Francisco Brain Tumor Research Center, 1836

University of California: Cardiovascular Research Laboratory, 4827

University of California: Davis Gastroenterology & Nutrition Center, 3865

University of California: Institute of Health Policy Studies, 325

University of California: Irvine Brain Imaging Center, 4061

University of California: Los Angeles Alcohol Research Center, 8361

University of California: Los Angeles Bone Marrow Transplantation Program, 2216

University of California: Los Angeles Center for Ulcer Research, 3866

University of California: San Francisco Dermatology Drug Research, 7778

University of California: San Francisco Laboratory for Neurotrauma, 4062

University of California: UCLA Population Research Center, 5378

University of Southern California: Comprehensive Sickle Cell Center, 7719

University of Southern California: Coronary Care Research, 4836

University of Southern California: Division of Nephrology, 5198

VA Northern California Health Care System, 10192

Veterans Adm. Medical Center: Livermore, 10193

Veterans Administration Medical Center: Fresno, 10194

Veterans Affairs Medical Center: Loma Linda, 10195

Veterans Medical Center: Mental Health Clinical Research Center, 6115

Vital Options International, 1863

Wellness Community Cancer Support Groups, 1864

Wellness Community: South Bay Cities, 1865

Wellness Community: West Los Angeles, 1866

West Los Angeles Medical Center, 10196

Wish Upon A Star, 10790

Women Alive, 237

Women's Suffrage for Prostate Cancer Awareness, 2345

World Institute on Disability, 10544

Canada

AIDS Coalition of Cape Breton, 167

AIDS Committee of Durham, 168

AIDS Committee of London, 169

AIDS Committee of Ottawa, 170

AIDS Committee of Toronto, 171

AIDS Committee of York Region, 172

AIDS New Brunswick, 174

AIDS Niagara, 175

AIDS PEI, 176

AIDS Thunder Bay, 177

ANKORS: Kootenay & Boundary HIV/AIDS and Hepatitis C Support Services, 182

Access AIDS Network, 183

Action Autonomie, 5970

Active Healthy Kids Canada, 6794

Alberta Reappraising AIDS Society, 184

Alzheimer Society of Canada, 660

Anorexia Nervosa & Bulimia Association, 3597

Arthritis & Autoimmunity Research Centre (AARC) Foundation, 1091

Black Coalition for AIDS Prevention, 192

Breast Cancer Society of Canada, 2020

Calgary Association of Self Help, 5976

Canadian & American Spinal Research Organi zation, 7967

Canadian Adult Congenital Heart Network, 4787

Canadian Cancer Society, 2023

Canadian Cerebral Palsy Sports Association, 2594

Canadian Dermatology Association, 7412

Canadian Foundation for AIDS Research, 195

Canadian Obesity Network, 6796

Canadian Society of Allergy and Clinical Immunology, 567

Central Alberta AIDS Network Society, 196

Children's Heart Society, 4788

Children's Wish Foundation of Canada, 10795

Christian Horizons, 10484

FM-CFS Canada, 3777

Heart and Stroke Foundation of Canada, 8163

Institute for Life Course and Aging, 25

Inter-Provincial Roof Consultants, Ltd., 5072

International Federation on Aging, 26

Jessie's Hope Society, 3604

Muscular Dystrophy Canada, 6589

NF Canada, 6737

National Cancer Institute of Canada, 2035

North Bay Aids Committee, 227

Ontario HIV Treatment Network, 228

Post Polio Awareness and Support Society o f British Columbia, 7103

Rethink Breast Cancer, 2044

Rick Hansen Foundation, 8074

Scleroderma Society of Ontario, 7415

Sickle Cell Association of Ontario, 7702

Society for Muscular Dystrophy Information International, 6591

Spina Bifida and Hydrocephalus Association of Canada, 7971

Stroke Recovery Canada, 8168

Sunshine Dreams for Kids, 10801

Thyroid Federation International, 9024

Thyroid Foundation of Canada, 9025

Tourette Syndrome Foundation of Canada, 9104

Turner's Syndrome Society of Canada, 9368

World Federation of Hemophilia, 4892

Colorado

AARP Colorado State Office: Denver, 37

ALS Association: Rocky Mountain Chapter, 1004

AMC Cancer Research Center, 2217

Aging Support Group, 87

Alcohol and Drug Abuse Division Department of Human Services, 8275

Alzheimer's Association: Greater Grand Junction Area Chapter, 689

Alzheimer's Association: Rocky Mountain Chapter, 690

American Cancer Society: Colorado, 2079

American Diabetes Association: Denver, 3161

American Homes for the Aging: Western, 691

American Liver Foundation Rocky Mountain Division, 5680
American Lung Association of Colorado, 5768
American Lung Association of Colorado, 9290
Americas Association for the Care of Children, 10469
Americas Association for the Care of the Children, 2015
Arthritis Foundation: Rocky Mountain Chapter, 1103
Autism Society of Colorado, 1595
BACCHUS of the US, 8234
Barbara Davis Center for Childhood Diabetes, 3305
Boulder Public Library, 9688
Brain Injury Association of Colorado, 4007
Brain Injury Association of Colorado Helpline, 4071
Brain Tumor Resource and Vital Encouragement, 1868
CCFA Rocky Mountain Chapter, 2932
CO Center for AIDS Research: University Colorado Health Sciences Center/CFAR, 251
Centers for AIDS Research: University of Colorado Health Sciences Center, 326
Colorado Brain Tumor Support Group, 1869
Colorado Cancer Research Program, 2218
Colorado Chapter National Hemophilila Foun dation, 4899
Colorado Chapter of the American Association of Kidney Patients, 5533
Colorado FFCMH, 6006
Colorado Parkinson Foundation, 6970
Colorado SIDS Program, 8848
Colorado Talking Book Library, 9689
Colordao Department of Health and Environment, 8849
Denver Childrens Hospital, 3024
Denver Support Group: National Ataxia Foundation, 1455
Disability Careers, 10550
Donor Alliance, 9205
FFCMH: Denver/Aurora Chapter, 6007
International Hearing Dog, 4239
Jimmie Heuga Center, 6509
Juvenile Diabetes Research Foundation: Colorado Springs Chapter, 3162
Juvenile Diabetes Research Foundation: Roc ky Mountain Chapter, 3163
Laradon Services for Children and Adults w ith Developmental Disabilities, 6121
Legal Center for People with Disabilities and Older People, 10551
Little Star Foundation, 10799
Lung Facts, 5821
Lupus Foundation of Colorado, 5862
Mile High Down Syndrome Association, 3475
Mountain-Plains AIDS Education and Training Center (MPAETC), 252
NNFF Colorado Chapter, 6744
National Alliance for the Mentally Ill of Colorado, 6008
National Association of Blind Lawyers Scott LaBarre, 9487
National Federation of the Blind: Blind Merchants Division, 9522
National Federation of the Blind: Colorado, 9536
National Jewish Center for Immunology, 5817
National Jewish Center for Immunology and Respiratory Medicine, 599
National Jewish Division of Immunology, 1314
National Jewish Medical and Research Center, 5757
National Kidney Foundation of Colorado, Idaho, Montana, and Wyoming, 5548
National Kidney Foundation of Colorado/Idaho/Montana/Wyoming, 5564
National Kidney Foundation of Colorado/Idaho/Montana/Wyoming, 5602
National Kidney Foundation of Colorado: Idaho, Montana, and Wyoming, 5534
National MS Society: Colorado Chapter, 6432
National Native American AIDS Prevention Center, 223
National Stroke Association, 5188
National Stroke Association, 8167
Neurofibromatosis Foundation: Colorado, 6771
No. Colorado FFCMH, 6009
Prader-Willi Colorado Association, 7255
RESOLVE of Colorado, 5329

Rocky Mountain CFIDS/FMS Association, 3789
Scleroderma Foundation: Colorado Chapter, 7420
Spina Bifida Association of Colorado, 7975
Turner's Syndrome Society of Rocky Mountain, 9371
United Cerebral Palsy of Colorado, 2623
United States Association for Blind Athletes, 9519
University of Colorado Cancer Center, 2219
University of Colorado: General Clinical Research Center, Pediatric, 3320
Veterans Adm. Medical Center: Grand Junction, 10197
Western Slope Chapter of the American Association of Kidney Patients, 5535

Connecticut

Alzheimer's Association: Connecticut Chapter, 692
Alzheimer's Association: South Central Connecticut Chapter, 693
American Cancer Society: Connecticut, 2080
American Diabetes Association: Connecticut, 3164
American Epilepsy Society, 7551
American Liver Foundation: Connecticut Chapter, 5681
American Lung Association of Connecticut, 5769
American Lung Association of Connecticut, 9291
American Lyme Disease Foundation, 9054
Arthritis Foundation: Southern New England Chapter, 1104
Arthritis Foundation: Southern New England Chapter, 1135
Autism Society of Connecticut, 1596
Brain Injury Association of Connecticut, 4008
Brain Injury Association of Connecticut Helpline, 4072
CCFA Central Connecticut Chapter, 2933
CCFA Northern Connecticut Affiliate Chapter, 2934
Chapel Haven, 10618
Connecticut Alcohol and Drug Abuse Commission, 8276
Connecticut Brain Tumor Support Group, 1870
Connecticut Chapter of the ALS Association, 1005
Connecticut Chapter of the Myasthenia Gravis Foundation of America, 6656
Connecticut Chapter of the Myasthenia Gravis Foundation of America, 6664
Connecticut Chapter of the Myasthenia Gravis Foundation of America, 6676
Connecticut Chapter of the Myasthenia Gravis Foundation of America, 6679
Connecticut Department of Health Services AIDS Programs, 253
Connecticut Down Syndrome Congress, 3476
Connecticut Pregnancy Exposure Information Service, 1774
Connecticut SIDS Alliance, 8850
Connecticut State Library for the Blind and Physically Handicapped, 9690
Cornelia de Lange Syndrome Foundation, 1752
Exceptional Cancer Patients/ECaP, 2328
Families United For CMH, Inc., 6010
Favarh, 10493
Fidelco Guide Dog Foundation, 9467
Gulf War Veterans of Connecticut: New England Chapter, 10198
International Lawyers in Alcoholics Anonymous, 8377
Juvenile Diabetes Research Foundation: Fai rfield County Chapter, 3166
Juvenile Diabetes Research Foundation: Greater New Haven Chapter, 3165
Juvenile Diabetes Research Foundation: Nor th Central CT and Western MA, 3167
Leukemia and Lymphoma Society: Connecticut Chapter, 2081
Leukemia and Lymphoma Society: Fairfield County Chapter, 2082
Lupus Foundation of America: Connecticut Chapter, 5863
Lupus Network, 5855
Lyme Disease Foundation, 9047
Motor Neuron Disease Clinic University of Connecticut Health Center, 1045

Myasthenia Gravis Support Group of Connect icut (Nutmeg Group), 6685
NNFF Connecticut Chapter, 6745
National Alliance for the Mentally Ill of Connecticut, 6011
National Federation of the Blind: Connecticut, 9537
National Kidney Foundation of Connecticut, 5536
National MS Society: Greater Connecticut Chapter, 6433
National Organization for Rare Disorders, 8988
National Organization for Rare Disorders, 10525
National Organization for Rare Disorders (NORD), 3756
National Organization for Rare Disorders (NORD), 3944
National Organization for Rare Disorders (NORD), 8835
National Spinal Cord Injury Association: Connecticut Chapter, 8080
National Veterans Services Fund, 10175
National Veterans Services Fund, 10393
NorthEast Organ Procurement Organization, 9206
Northwestern Connecticut AIDS Project, 254
Office of Protection and Advocacy for Persons with Disabilities, 10552
Prader-Willi Connecticut Association, 7256
Prevent Blindness Tri-State, 9538
RESOLVE of Fairfield County, 5330
RESOLVE of Greater Hartford, 5331
Raynaud's Association, 7413
Raynaud's Foundation, 7309
Reflex Sympathetic Dystrophy Syndrome Association (RSDSA), 2842
Renfrew Center of Connecticut, 3611
SIDS Program: Connecticut Department of Health, 8851
Spina Bifida Association of Connecticut, 7976
Sudden Infant Death Syndrome (SIDS) Network, 8838
Terri Gotthelf Lupus Research Institute, 5931
Tourette Syndrome Clinic Yale Child Study Center, 9105
United Cerebral Palsy of Eastern Connecticut, 2624
United Cerebral Palsy of Greater Hartford, 2625
United Cerebral Palsy of Southern Connecticut, 2626
University of Connecticut Health Center, 3025
University of Connecticut Osteoporosis Center, 6901
Yale Child Study Center, 7175
Yale University Comprehensive Cancer Center, 2220
Yale University Cystic Fibrosis Research Center, 3026
Yale University: Behavioral Medicine Clinic, 6276
Yale University: Ribicoff Research Facilities/CT Mental Health Center, 6277
Yale University: Vision Research Center, 9871

Delaware

Alliance for the Mentally Ill in Delaware (AMID), 6012
Alzheimer's Association: Delaware Chapter, 694
American Cancer Society: Delaware, 2083
American Diabetes Association: Delaware, 3168
American Lung Association of Delaware, 5770
American Lung Association of Delaware, 9292
Autism Society of Delaware, 1597
Brain Injury Association of Delaware, 4009
Brain Injury Association of Delaware Helpl ine, 4073
Client Assistance Program: Delaware, 10553
Delaware Assocation for the Blind Department of Health & Social Services, 9539
Delaware Department of Health and Social Services, 255
Delaware Division of Alcoholism, Drug Abuse and Mental Health, 8277
Delaware Division of Libraries: Library for the Blind and Physically Handicapped, 9691
Delaware FFMCH, 6013
Juvenile Diabetes Research Foundation: Del aware, 3169
Leukemia and Lymphoma Society: Delaware Chapter, 2084
Lupus Foundation of America: Delaware Chapter, 5864

Mental Health Association of Delaware, 6014
National Federation of the Blind: Delaware, 9540
National MS Society: Delaware Chapter, 6434
Pediatric Brain Tumor Support Group, 1871
Prader-Willi Delaware Association, 7257
SIDS Information & Counseling: Division of Public Health, 8852
Sarcoidosis Support Group Delaware, 7335
Spina Bifida Association of Delaware, 7977
United Cerebral Palsy of Delaware, 2627
Veterans Adm. Medical Center: Wilmington VA Medical Center, 10199

District of Columbia

AAA Foundation for Traffic Safety, 8224
AIDS United, 179
ALS Association National Office, 995
ARC The ARC of the United States, 3466
Administration for Children and Families, 1285
Administration for Children and Families, 3477
Administration for Children and Families, 3612
Administration for Children and Families, 4260
Administration for Children and Families, 5682
Administration for Children and Families, 7140
Administration for Children and Families, 7556
Administration for Community Living, 7141
Agent Orange Registry Department of Veterans Affairs, 10173
Alliance for Aging Research, 9446
Alzheimer's Association: Greater Washington DC Chapter, 695
American Academy of Child & Adolescent Psychiatry, 5971
American Academy of Child and Adolescent Psychiatry, 7122
American Association for the Advancement of Science, 10456
American Association of People with Disabilities, 10457
American Association of Retired Persons, 22
American Association of Spinal Cord Injury Nurses, 8060
American Association on Intellectual and D evelopmental Disabilities, 5973
American Bar Association Commission on Mental and Physical Disability Law, 10459
American Cancer Society: District of Columbia, 2085
American Coucnil of the Blind Impairment, 9449
American Diabetes Association: District of Columbia, 3170
American Federation of Teachers HIV/AIDS Education Project, 187
American Foundation for the Blind: Governmental Relations, 9541
American Hellenic Educational Progressive Association, 2882
American Institute for Cancer Research, 2086
American Institute for Cancer Research, 2320
American Lung Association, 1278
American Lung Association, 5755
American Lung Association, 9279
American Lung Association of Washington, 9293
American Lung Association of the District of Columbia, 5771
American Lung Association of the District of Columbia, 9294
American Obesity Association, 6795
American Paraplegic Society, 8061
American Pseudo-Obstruction and Hirschsprung's Disease Society, 3842
American Psychological Association, 5975
American Psychological Association, 7125
American Public Health Association, 7126
American Red Cross Blood Services, 4887
American Red Cross Hemophilia Center, 4942
American Red Cross National Headquarters, 10466
American Sleep Apnea Association, 7861
American Society for Bone and Mineral Research, 6865
American Society for Deaf Children, 4215
American Society of Hematology, 2883
Arthritis Foundation: Metropolitan Washington Chapter, 1105

Associate Administrator for Alcohol Prevention and Treatment Policy, 8232
Association of Spinal Cord Injury Psychologists and Social Workers, 8064
Asthma and Allergy Foundation of America, 1308
Asthma and Allergy Foundation of America, 1319
Asthma and Allergy Foundation of America: Washington Chapter, 1286
Autism Society of District Columbia, 1598
Better Breather's Clubs, 7325
Better Hearing Institute, 4220
Blinded Veterans Association, 9460
Brain Research Center Children s Hospital National Medical Cen, 1832
Center for Mental Health Services: Knowledge Exchange Network, 5979
Center for Mind-Body Medicine, 7176
Center for Science in the Public Interest, 2087
Children's AIDS Fund, 198
Children's National Medical Center, 10483
Children's Rights Program, 4337
Clearinghouse on Disability Information Office of Special Education & Rehab Svcs, 10485
Client Assistance Program: District of Columbia, 10554
Cochlear Implant Association, 4224
Columbia Lighthouse for the Blind, 9542
Committee of Ten Thousand, 200
Council of Citizens with Low Vision International, 9466
Council of Families with Visual Impairment, 9692
DC Department of Health Maternal and Family Health Administration, 8853
DC Public Library Adaptive Services Division, 9693
DC Threshold Alliance for the Mentally Ill, 6015
Deaf REACH, 4228
Deafness and Communicative Disorders Branch, 4230
Department of Health and Human Services, 8854
Digestive Disease National Coalition, 3848
Disabled American Veterans National Service Headquarters, 10200
Distance Education and Training Council, 10488
District of Columbia Public Library Librarian for the Deaf Community, 9669
ERIC Clearinghouse on Disabilities and Gifted Education, 10619
Eating Disorders Coalition for Research, Policy and Action, 3601
Elizabeth Glaser Pediatric AIDS Foundation, 203
Equal Opportunity Employment Commission, 10490
Family Advocacy and Support Association, 6016
Federal Emergency Management Agency, 7142
Food Safety and Inspection Service, 573
Gallaudet University: Center for Auditory and Speech Sciences, 4302
Genetic Alliance, 1650
Genetic Alliance, 3964
Genetic Alliance, 10631
George Washington National Cooperative: Drug Discovery/AIDS Treatment, 327
Georgetown University Center for Hypertension and Renal Disease Research, 5537
Georgetown University Child Development Center, 1763
Georgetown University Hospital Transplant Institute, 9250
Georgetown University Hospital: Department of Rheumatology, 7447
Georgetown University: Vincent T Lombardi Cancer Research Center, 2221
Gerontological Society of America, 24
HEATH Resource Center, 1530
HEATH Resource Center, 10497
Health Planning and Development, 8278
Hemophilia Treatment Center at Children's National Medical Center, 4965
Howard University Cancer Center, 2222
Howard University Center for Sickle Cell Disease, 7712
Information Protection & Advocacy Center for Handicapped Individuals, 10555
International Association for the Study of Pain, 10499
International Council on Disability, 10500
Juvenile Diabetes Research Foundation: Cap itol Chapter, 3171

Leading Age, 27
Library Services to the Deaf Community, 4291
Listening and Spoken Knowledge Center, 4292
Listening and Spoken Language Knowledge Ce nter, 4242
Lung Association, 7863
Lung Cancer Alliance Support Group, 2337
Lupus Foundation of America, 5854
Lupus Foundation of America: DC, Maryland and Central & Northern Virginia, 5883
Medstar Georgetown University Hospital Facility, 4815
Melanoma Research Foundation, 2223
Metropolitan DC Cystic Fibrosis Center Children s Hospital National Medical Cen, 3027
National AIDS Fund, 218
National Alliance for Hispanic Health, 5984
National Association for Home Care, 10634
National Association for Home Care and Hospice, 10808
National Association of Councils on Developmental Disabilities, 10510
National Association of Nurse Practitioners In Women's Health, 6896
National Association of Social Workers, 7137
National Association of Special Education Teachers, 2885
National Center for Education in Maternal and Child Health, 8834
National Center for Victims of Crime, 7160
National Coalition on Immune System Disorders, 220
National Council for Community Behavior Healthcare, 5988
National Council on Aging, 28
National Council on Aging, 5276
National Council on Disability, 10514
National Council on Independent Living, 10515
National Dissemination Center for Children, 4247
National Dissemination Center for Children, 10517
National Dissemination Center for Children with Disabilities, 1529
National Dissemination Center for Children with Disabilities, 3470
National Endowment for the Arts: Office for Accessability, 10518
National Federation of the Blind: DC, 9543
National Health Information Center, 8
National Health Information Center, 89
National Health Information Center, 388
National Health Information Center, 609
National Health Information Center, 892
National Health Information Center, 1056
National Health Information Center, 1162
National Health Information Center, 1320
National Health Information Center, 1445
National Health Information Center, 1533
National Health Information Center, 1652
National Health Information Center, 1778
National Health Information Center, 1872
National Health Information Center, 2339
National Health Information Center, 2545
National Health Information Center, 2564
National Health Information Center, 2722
National Health Information Center, 2759
National Health Information Center, 2843
National Health Information Center, 2900
National Health Information Center, 2970
National Health Information Center, 3109
National Health Information Center, 3338
National Health Information Center, 3645
National Health Information Center, 3725
National Health Information Center, 3788
National Health Information Center, 3869
National Health Information Center, 3949
National Health Information Center, 3975
National Health Information Center, 4001
National Health Information Center, 4341
National Health Information Center, 4847
National Health Information Center, 5000
National Health Information Center, 5078
National Health Information Center, 5143
National Health Information Center, 5201
National Health Information Center, 5247
National Health Information Center, 5280
National Health Information Center, 5382

Florida

Georgia

Centers for Disease Control and Prevention Hepatitis Branch, 5068

Centers for Disease Control and Prevention National Center for Prevention Services, 9280

Charlie Norwood VA Medical Center, 10213

Children's Wish Foundation International, 10768

Columbus Library for Accessible Services (CLASS), 9711

Comprehensive Sickle Cell Center, 7700

Creative Community Services (CCS), 10620

Department of Pediatrics Medical College of Georgia, 3031

Division of Adolescent and School Health, 578

Division of Adolescent and School Health, 1289

Division of Adolescent and School Health, 3481

Division of Adolescent and School Health, 3616

Division of Diabetes Translation, 3298

Division of Rehabilitation Service, 10558

Down Syndrome Association of Atlanta, 3482

Educational Materials Database Centers for Disease Control, 334

Emory Autism Resource Center, 1640

Emory Brain Tumor Support Group, 1883

Emory University: Cystic Fibrosis Center, 3032

Emory University: Georgia Center for Cancer Statistics, 2226

Emory University: Laboratory for Ophthalmic Research, 9850

Emory University: National Cooperative Drug Discovery for AIDS Treatment, 335

Emory University: Winship Cancer Institute, 2227

Families in Action National Drug Information Center, 8242

Fertility Clinic at the Shepherd Spinal Center, 5375

Funding Database Centers for Disease Control, 336

Georgia Alliance for the Mentally Ill, 6019

Georgia Association of the Deaf, 4264

Georgia Atlanta Turner Syndrome Society, 9374

Georgia Chapter of the Myasthenia Gravis Foundation of America, 6660

Georgia Department of Human Resources: Center for Family Resource Planning, 8862

Georgia Department of Human Resources: Division of Public Health, 259

Georgia Department of Human Resources: Infant and Child Health, 8863

Georgia Industries for the Blind, 9548

Georgia Library for Accessible Services (GLASS), 9712

Georgia National Spinal Cord Injury Association Support Group Network, 8100

Georgia Parent Support Network (GPSN), 6124

Georgia SIDS Project, 8864

Georgia Support Group: National Ataxia Foundation, 1459

Gulf War Veterans of Georgia, 10214

HIV/AIDS Prevention Program, 384

Hall County Library System: East Hall Branch and Special Needs Library, 9713

Hearts and Minds, 1884

Hemophilia Foundation of Georgia, 4901

I Can Cope, 2333

Immunization Division Centers for Disease Control, 385

Impotence Resource Center of the Geddings Osbon Sr Foundation, 5240

Juvenile Diabetes Research Foundation: Georgia Chapter, 3183

Kids on the Block Arthritis Programs, 1161

Kidscope, 2095

Leukemia and Lymphoma Society: Georgia Chapter, 2096

LifeLink of Georgia, 9210

Look Good... Feel Better, 2336

Lupus Foundation of America: Columbus Chapter, 5871

Lupus Foundation of America: Greater Atlanta Chapter, 5872

Marcus Institute for Development and Learning, 3516

Medical College of Georgia Alzheimers Research Center, 875

Medical College of Georgia: Sickle Cell Center, 7713

Middle Georgia Subregional Library for the Blind and Physically Handicapped, 9714

Mood and Anxiety Disorders Program of Emory University, 7178

Myasthenia Gravis Support Group of Atlanta, 6686

NAMES Project Foundation AIDS Memorial Quilt, 217

NNFF Georgia Affiliate, 6747

National Association of Chronic Disease Directors, 6893

National Down Syndrome Congress, 3471

National Down Syndrome Congress, 3527

National Families in Action, 8256

National Federation of the Blind: Georgia, 9549

National Gaucher Disease Foundation, 3759

National Gaucher Foundation, 3943

National Gaucher Foundation (NGF), 5715

National Kidney Foundation of Georgia, 5545

National MS Society: Georgia Chapter, 6441

National Parent to Parent Support and Information System, 10637

National Spinal Cord Injury Support Groups, 8106

Northwest Georgia Parkinson Disease Association, 6977

Oconee Regional Library for the Blind and Physically Handicapped, 9715

Office on Smoking and Health, 10533

Office on Smoking and Health: CDCP, 8261

Prader-Willi Georgia Association, 7259

RESOLVE of Georgia, 5336

Reach to Recovery, 2342

Resources and Services Database Centers for Disease Control, 232

Rome Georgia Chapter of the American Association of Kidney Patients, 5546

Rome Subregional Library for People with Disabilities, 9716

SBTF Brain Tumor Support Group, 1885

Scleroderma Foundation: Georgia Chapter Scleroderma Foundation, 7423

Shepherd Center, 8082

Sickle Cell Foundation of Georgia, 7707

Sickle Cell Information Center Grady Memorial Hospital, 7704

Southeastern Region: Helen Keller National Center, 9550

Special Needs Library of Northeast Georgia, 9717

Spina Bifida Association of Georgia, 7981

Subregional Library for the Blind and Physically Handicapped, 9718

Three Rivers Regional Library, 9719

United Cerebral Palsy of Georgia, 2640

VA Southeast Network: Georgia, 10215

Valdosta Talking Book Library, 9720

Veterans Adm. Medical Center: Decatur Atlanta VA Medical Center, 10216

Veterans Adm. Medical Center: Dublin Carl Vinson VA Medical Center, 10217

Well Project, 236

Hawaii

AARP Hawaii State Office: Honolulu, 41

Alcohol and Drug Abuse Division Department of Health, 8281

Alzheimer's Association: Honolulu Chapter, 716

Alzheimer's Association: West Hawaii Chapter, 717

American Cancer Society: Hawaii, 2097

American Diabetes Association: Hawaii, 3184

American Lung Association of Hawaii, 5775

American Lung Association of Hawaii, 9297

Autism Society of Hawaii, 1601

Brain Injury Association of Hawaii, 4013

Brain Injury Association of Hawaii, 4075

Division of Vocational Rehabilitation and Services for the Blind, 9551

Hawaii Department of Health: Communicable Disease Division, 260

Hawaii Department of Health: Family Health Division, 8865

Hawaii Down Syndrome Congress, 3483

Hawaii Families As Allies (HFAA), 6125

Hawaii Lupus Foundation, 5873

Hawaii Parkinson Association Gwendolyn A Montibon President, 6978

Hawaii State Library for the Blind and Physically Handicapped, 9721

Hemophilia Foundation of Hawaii Kapiolani Medical Center, 4902

Ho'opono Workshop for the Blind, 9552

Juvenile Diabetes Research Foundation: Hawaii Chapter, 3185

Kuakini Parkinson Disease (PD) Information & Referral, 7006

NAMI: The Local Affiliate of the National Alliance for the Mentally Ill, 6020

National Federation of the Blind: Hawaii, 9553

National Kidney Foundation of Hawaii, 5547

National MS Society: Hawaii Chapter, 6442

Organ Donor Center of Hawaii, 9211

Pacific Health Research Institute, 2228

Prader-Willi Hawaii Association, 7260

Protection & Advocacy Agency, 10559

RESOLVE of Hawaii, 5337

United Cerebral Palsy of Hawaii, 2641

University of Hawaii: Cancer Research Center, 2229

Veterans Adm. Medical Centery: Honolulu VA Pacific Islands Health Care System, 10218

Idaho

AARP Idaho State Office: Meridian, 42

Alzheimer's Association: Greater Idaho Chapter, 718

Alzheimer's Association: Northern Idaho Chapter, 719

American Cancer Society: Idaho, 2098

American Lung Association of Idaho, 5776

Autism Society of Treasure Valley, 1602

Brain Injury Association of Idaho, 4014

Co-Ad, 10560

Department of Health and Welfare Department Of Health And Welfare, 8282

FFCMH: Idaho Chapter, 6021

Hemophilia Foundation of Idaho, 4903

Idaho Alliance for the Mentally Ill, 6022

Idaho Commission for Libraries Talking Book Service, 9722

Idaho Department of Health and Welfare, 8866

Idaho Department of Health and Welfare The STD/AIDS Program, 261

Idaho Persian Gulf Veterans, 10219

NNFF Idaho Chapter, 6748

National Federation of the Blind: Idaho, 9554

National MS Society: Idaho Division, 6443

Prader-Willi Idaho Association, 7261

United Cerebral Palsy of Idaho, 2642

Veterans Adm. Medical Center: Boise Boise VA Medical Center, 10220

Illinois

AARP Illinois State Office: Chicago, 43

AIDS Legal Council of Chicago, 262

ARRISE, 1583

Academy for Eating Disorders, 3594

Academy for Eating Disorders, 3633

Adult Down Syndrome Center of Lutheran General Hospital, 3501

Aid to the Aged, Blind or Disabled, 9555

Alzheimer's Association: Central Illinois Chapter, 720

Alzheimer's Association: East Central Illinois Chapter, 721

Alzheimer's Association: Four Rivers Chapter, 722

Alzheimer's Association: Greater Illinois Chapter, 723

Alzheimer's Association: Greater Illinois Chapter: Carbondale Office, 724

Alzheimer's Association: Land of Lincoln Chapter, 725

Alzheimer's Disease and Related Disorders Association, 662

American Academy of Dermatology, 7756

American Academy of Orthopaedic Surgeons, 2537

American Academy of Orthopaedic Surgeons, 7484

American Academy of Pediatrics, 10455

American Academy of Sleep Medicine, 2750

American Association of Diabetes Educators, 3136

American Board of Dermatology American Society for Dermatologic Surger, 7757
American Brain Tumor Association, 1824
American Brain Tumor Association, 3995
American Brain Tumor Association Patient Line, 4076
American Cancer Society: Illinois, 2099
American College of Allergy, Asthma & Immunology, 563
American Dental Association Department of Library Services, 8231
American Dermatological Association University of Iowa Hospital and Clinics, 7758
American Diabetes Association: Greater Ill inois, 3186
American Diabetes Association: Northern Il linois, 3187
American Dietetic Association, 564
American Dietetic Association, 3595
American Dietetic Association, 3837
American Hearing Research Foundation, 4214
American Homes for the Aging: Midwest Regional Office, 726
American Liver Foundation Illinois Chapter, 5686
American Lung Association Help Line, 5820
American Lung Association of Illinois, 5777
American Lung Association of Illinois-Iowa, 9298
American Medical Association, 7123
American Osteopathic Association, 2835
American Pain Society, 2836
American Society for Dermatologic Surgery, 7759
American Society for Gastrointestinal Endoscopy, 3843
American Society for Surgery of the Hand, 2539
American Society of Colon and Rectal Surgeons, 2014
American Society of Plastic and Reconstructive Surgeons, 7760
Arthritis Foundation: Greater Chicago Chapter, 1108
Arthritis Foundation: Greater Illinois Chapter, 1109
Arthritis Foundation: Northwestern Ohio Chapter, 1130
Association of Halfway House Alcoholism Programs of North America, 8233
Association of Late-Deafened Adults, 4218
Association of Professional Sleep Societies, 7862
Autism Society of Illinois, 1603
Baxter Hyland Division, 4888
Benjamin B Greenfield National Alzheimer's Center, 663
Better Existence with HIV, 191
Brain Injury Association of Illinois, 4015
Brain Injury Association of Illinois Helpline, 4077
Brain Research Foundation, 1833
Brain Tumor Support Group, 1886
CANDU Parent Group, 6126
CCFA Illinois: Carol Fisher Chapter, 2937
Cancer and Leukemia Group B, 2230
Captain James A. Lovell Federal Health Car e Center, 10221
Catholic Guild for the Blind, 9723
Catholic Guild for the Blind Catholic Charities of the Archdiocese of, 9464
Center for Digestive Disorders: Central, 3846
Center for Narcolepsy Research at the University of Illinois at Chicago, 7870
Central Brain Tumor Registry of the US, 1835
Chicago Area Support Group: National Ataxia Foundation, 1460
Chicago Department of Health, 263
Chicago Lighthouse for People Who are Blind and Visually Impaired, 9556
Chicago Metro Support Group: National Ataxia Foundation, 1461
Chicagoland Chapter of the American Association of Kidney Patients, 5549
Citizens Alliance for VD Awareness, 7663
Clinical Research Center Northwestern Center for Clinical Researc, 337
Cognitive Neurology and Alzheimer's Disease Center, 866
Comer Children's Hospital at the Universit, 3034
Comer Children's Hospital at the University of Chicago, 3033
Compassionate Friends, 8833

Compassionate Friends, 10805
Cooley's Anemia Foundation (CAF): Illinois Oakbrook Towers, 2887
Cystic Fibrosis Center: Childrens Memorial Hospital, 3035
Cystic Fibrosis Center: Park Ridge Lutheran General Children's Hospital, 3036
David T Siegel Institute for Communicative Disorders, 4300
Department of Alcoholism and Substance Abuse, 8283
Department of Ophthalmology Information Line, 9878
Depression and Bipolar Support Alliance, 6278
Depression and Bipolar Support Alliance, 7132
Dermatology Foundation, 2192
Dermatology Foundation, 7761
Desert Storm Justice Foundation: Illinois, 10222
Division on Endocrinology Northwestern University Feinberg School, 3310
Dreams for Seniors Charity Inc, 10797
Easter Seals, 1753
Easter Seals, 2595
Easter Seals, 7968
Edward J Hines Jr VA Hospital, 10223
Fairygodmother Foundation, 10773
Gastro-Intestinal Research Foundation, 3860
Gastrointestinal Research Foundation, 3864
Hands Organization: Advocacy Network for the Deaf and Hearing Impaired, 4233
Helen Keller National Center Regional Representatives, 9557
Hemophilia Foundation of Illinois, 4904
Ileitis and Colitis Educational Foundation, 2922
Illinois Alliance for the Mentally Ill, 6023
Illinois Association of the Deaf, 4265
Illinois Church Action on Alcohol Problems, 8284
Illinois Client Assistance Program, 10561
Illinois Department of Public Health: Division of Infectious Diseases, 264
Illinois Federation of Families, 6024
Illinois Midwest Neurofibromatosis, 6749
Illinois Spina Bifida Association, 7982
Illinois State Library Talking Book and Braille Service, 9724
Illinois Teratogen Information Service (IT IS), 1775
International Association for Chronic Fatigue, 2751
International Association of Eating Disorders Professionals, 3603
International Pelvic Pain Society Women's Medical Plaza, 2839
International Pelvic Pain Society Women's Medical Plaza, 3717
International Society for Traumatic Stress Studies, 7134
International Society for Traumatic Stress Studies, 7179
Jesse Brown VA Medical Center, 10224
Juvenile Diabetes Research Foundation: Gre ater Chicago Chapter, 3188
KALEIDOSCOPE, 6127
Kellogg Cancer Care Center Evanston Hospital, 2231
LaRabida Children's Hospital: Developmental Disabilities & Delays, 3515
Les Turner Amyotrophic Lateral Sclerosis Foundation, 1055
Les Turner Research Laboratory Northwestern University Medical School, 1043
Let's Breathe Sarcoidosis Support Group, 7326
Leukemia Research Foundation, 2232
Leukemia and Lymphoma Society: Illinois Chapter, 2100
Lions Quest, 10505
Lois Insolia ALS Center at Northwestern Memorial Hospital, 1010
Loyola University Medical Center: Department of Pediatrics, 3037
Loyola University of Chicago Cardiac Transplant Program, 4814
Loyola University of Children: Parmly Hearing Institute, 4305
Lupus Foundation of America: Illinois Chapter, 5874
MAGIC Foundation for Children's Growth, 3969
MAGIC Foundation for Children's Growth: Turner's Syndrome Division, 9367

Male Sexual Dysfunction Clinic, 5243
Medical Library Association, 215
Metro Chicago Turner Syndrome Society, 9375
Mid-Illinois Talking Book Center, 9725
NF Center: North Broward Medical Center Neurofibromatosis, 6750
NNFF Illinois Chapter: Chicago Area, 6751
NNFF Illinois Chapter: Silvis Area, 6752
NNFF Illinois Chapter: Springfield Area, 6753
NNFF Illinois Chapter:Peoria Region, 6754
National Association for Down Syndrome, 3469
National Association of Anorexia Nervosa and Associated Disorders, 3605
National Center for Sight, 9881
National Certification Board for Diabetes Educators, 3140
National Eye Health Education Program, 9882
National Federation of the Blind: Illinois, 9558
National Headache Foundation, 6366
National Headache Foundation, 7161
National Kidney Foundation of Illinois, 5550
National MS Society: Chicago, Greater Illinois Chapter, 6444
Nevada Kidney Disease & Hypertension Cente rs, 5606
Northern Illinois University Research and Training Center, 4306
Northwestern University: Division of Allergy and Immunology, 1315
Oncology Hematology Associates of Central Illinois, 2233
Parents Information Network FFCMH, 6128
Parents of Children with Brain Tumors PCBT, 1887
Parkside Medical Services Corporation, 8285
Prader-Willi Illinois Association, 7262
Prevent Blindess America, 9512
Pulmonary Fibrosis Association, 5758
Pulmonary Fibrosis Foundation, 5759
RESOLVE of Illinois, 5338
Rainbow House, 4002
Rainbows for All God's Children, 10817
Recovery International, 7203
Regional Organ Bank of Illinois, Inc., 9212
Rehabilitation Institute of Chicago, 1156
Robert H Lurie Comprehensive Cancer Center of Northwestern University, 2234
Rockford Parkinson's Support Group, 7007
Rush University Multiple Sclerosis Center, 6511
SIDS of Illinois, 8867
Saint Francis Medical Center Peoria Pulmonary Association, 3038
Scleroderma Foundation: Greater Chicago Chapter, 7424
Sentry Health Monitors, 5190
Shawnee Library System: Southern Illinois Talking Book Center, 9726
Shriners Hospital for Crippled Children Chicago Unit, 7489
Simon Foundation Helpline for Incontinence Information, 5281
Simon Foundation for Continence, 5277
Skokie Accessible Library Services, 9727
Sleep Research Society American Academy of Sleep Medicine, 7867
Society of Gastroenterology Nurses and Associates, 3857
Society of Mitral Valve Prolapse Syndrome, 4850
Spinal Cord Injury Association of Illinois, 8083
Statewide SIDS Program: Illinois Department of Public Health, 8868
Sulzberger Institute for Dermatologic Educ, 7777
Sulzberger Institute for Dermatologic Education, 7776
Test Positive Aware Network (TPAN), 265
Thresholds Psychiatric Rehabilitation, 6109
United Cerebral Palsy Land of Lincoln, 2643
United Cerebral Palsy of East Central Illinois, 2644
United Cerebral Palsy of Greater Chicago, 2645
United Cerebral Palsy of Illinois, 2646
United Cerebral Palsy of Southern Illinois, 2647
United Cerebral Palsy of Will County, 2648
United Cerebral Palsy of the Blackhawk Region, 2649
United Cerebral Palsy: Eastern Seals, 2650
University of Chicago Cancer Research Center, 2235

University of Chicago Center for Advanced Medicine Duchossis Center, 7455
University of Chicago Committee on Virology, 7668
University of Chicago Dept of Neurology University of Chicago Hospital, 885
University of Chicago: Clinical Nutrition Research Unit, 2236
University of Chicago: Comprehensive Diabetes Center, 3319
University of Chicago: Temporal Bone Laboratory for Ear Research, 4324
University of Illinois Eye and Ear Infirma ry, 9866
University of Illinois Health Services Research, 886
University of Illinois at Chicago Consultation Clinic for Epilepsy, 7582
University of Illinois at Chicago Craniofacial Center, 1768
University of Illinois at Chicago Lions, 9332
University of Illinois at Chicago Lions of Illinois Eye Research Institute, 9867
University of Illinois at Chicago Medical Center Outpatient Clinical Center, 7456
University of Illinois at Chicago: Institute for Tuberculosis Research, 9333
VA Great Lakes Health Care System, 10225
VA Illinois Health Care System, 10226
Veterans Adm. Medical Center: Marion Marion VA Medical Center, 10227
Veterans Adm. Medical Center: Northport North Chicago VA Medical Center, 10228
Voices of Vision Talking Book Center, 9728
Y-ME National Breast Cancer Organization, 2047

Indiana

AARP Indiana State Office: Indianapolis, 44
ALS Association: Indiana Chapter, 1011
Alzheimer's Association: Central Indiana Chapter, 727
Alzheimer's Association: Northern Indiana Chapter, 728
Alzheimer's Support Group, 891
American Camp Association, 10460
American Cancer Society: Indiana, 2101
American Diabetes Association: Northern In diana/Northern Ohio, 3189
American Liver Foundation Indiana Chapter, 5687
American Lung Association of Indiana, 5778
American Lung Association of Indiana: State Office & Support Office, 9299
Ann Whitehill Down Syndrome Program, 3502
Arthritis Foundation: Indiana Chapter, 1110
Autism Society of Indiana, 1604
Ball State University Public Health Entomology Laboratory, 9051
Bartholomew County Public Library, 9729
Bosma Industries for the Blind, 9559
Brain Injury Association of Indiana, 4016
Brain Injury Association of Indiana Helpli ne, 4078
Brain Tumor Support Group, 1888
Breaking New Ground Resource Center, 10472
CCFA Indiana Chapter, 2938
Children's Organ Transplant Association (COTA), 9188
Chronic Fatigue Syndrome & Fibromyalgia Support, 2757
Diabetes Youth Foundation of Indiana, 3190
Division of Addiction Services Department of Mental Health, 8286
Evansville-Vanderburgh County Public Library, 9730
FFCMH: Indiana Chapter, 6025
Family Action Network, 6026
GoldPoint Clinical Research, 7180
Greater Indianapolis Chapter of the Myasthenia Gravis Foundation of America, 6663
Hemophilia Foundation of Indiana, 4905
Indiana Chapter Turner Syndrome Society, 9376
Indiana Down Syndrome Foundation, 3484
Indiana Organ Procurement Organization,, 9213
Indiana Protection and Advocacy Services, 10562
Indiana Resource Center for Autism (IRCA), 1641
Indiana State Department of Health Maternal And Child Health Services, 8869
Indiana Talking Book & Braille Library, 9731

Indiana Teratogen Information Service, 1776
Indiana University Center for Aging Research, 870
Indiana University: Area Health Education Center, 3312
Indiana University: Center for Diabetes Research, 3313
Indiana University: Human Genetics Center of Medical & Molecular Genetics, 871
Indiana University: Hypertension Research Center, 5194
Indiana University: Pharmacology Research Laboratory, 3314
International Academy of Proctology, 3849
Juvenile Diabetes Research Foundation: Ind iana State Chapter, 3191
Juvenile Diabetes Research Foundation: Nor thern Indiana Chapter, 3192
Krannert Institute of Cardiology, 4813
Lake County Public Library, 9732
Leukemia and Lymphoma Society: Indiana Chapter, 2102
Lupus Foundation of America: Northeast Indiana Chapter, 5875
Lupus Foundation of America: Northwest Indiana Lupus Chapter, 5876
Lupus Foundation of Indiana, 5877
Mary Margaret Walther Program Walther Cancer Institute, 2237
MidWest Medical Center: Sleep Disorders Center, 7880
Multipurpose Arthritis and Musculoskeletal Disease Center, 1154
NAMI Indiana, 6027
NAMI Indiana - National Alliance on Mental Illness, 6129
NNFF Indiana Chapter, 6755
National Federation of the Blind: Indiana, 9560
National Kidney Foundation of Indiana, 5551
National Legal Center for the Medically Dependent & Disabled, 10523
National MS Society: Indiana State Chapter, 6445
National Spinal Cord Injury Association: Central Indiana Chapter, 8084
Parent Care, 8836
Prader-Willi Indiana Association, 7263
Primary Brain Cancer Support Group, 1889
Purdue Cancer Center Purdue University, 2197
Purdue University Center for AIDS Research, 338
Purdue University William A Hillenbrand Biomedical Engineering Center, 4820
Purdue University: Center for Research on Aging, 84
RESOLVE of Indiana, 5339
Riley Hemophilia & Hemophilia Center Riley Hospital for Children, 4983
SIDS Center of Indiana, 8870
Sleep Alertness Center: Lafayette Home Hospital, 7886
Sleep/Wake Disorders Center: Community Hospitals of Indianapolis, 7917
Southern Indiana Support Group: National Ataxia Foundation, 1462
Spina Bifida Association of Central Indiana, 7983
The Riley Cystic Fibrosis Center, 3039
United Cerebral Palsy Association of Indiana, 2651
United Cerebral Palsy Associations, 2652
United Cerebral Palsy of the Wabash Valley, 2653
VA Northern Indiana Health Care System Marion Campus, 10229
Veterans Adm. Medical Center: Fort Wayne, 10230
Vision World Wide, 9520

Iowa

AARP Iowa State Office: Des Moines, 45
Alzheimer's Association: Big Sioux Chapter, 729
Alzheimer's Association: East Central Iowa Chapter, 730
Alzheimer's Association: Greater Iowa Chapter, 731
Alzheimer's Association: Heart of Iowa Chapter, 732
American Cancer Society: Iowa, 2103
American Diabetes Association: Cedar Rapid s District, 3193
American Lung Association of Iowa, 5779
Arthritis Foundation: Iowa Chapter, 1111

Association for Glycogen Storage Disease, 5673
Autism Society of Iowa, 1605
Blank Childrens Hospital Pediatric Pulmonology Clinic, 3040
Brain Injury Alliance of Iowa Helpline, 4079
Brain Injury Association of Iowa, 4017
CCFA Iowa Chapter, 2939
Cedar Rapids Persian Gulf Veterans, Spouses and Children, 10231
Center for Disabilities and Development, 3504
Client Assistance Program: Iowa Division o n Persons with Disabilities, 10563
Department of Public Health: Division of Substance Abuse and Health, 8287
Des Moines Division: VA Central Iowa Health Care System, 10232
FFCMH: Iowa Chapter, 6028
Gilda's Club: Quad Cities, 2331
Great Plains Regional Hemophilia Center University of Iowa Hospitals, 4953
Greater Iowa Chapter Alzheimer's Association Quadcity Office, 733
Iowa Brain Tumor Support Group, 1890
Iowa Chapter of the Association of Kidney Patients, 5552
Iowa Department for the Blind, 9733
Iowa Donor Network, 9214
Iowa Federaion of Families for Children's Mental Health (FFCMH), 6130
Iowa Oncology Research Association, 2238
Iowa SIDS Alliance, 8871
Iowa SIDS Program Iowa Department of Public Health, 8872
Juvenile Diabetes Research Foundation: Eas tern Iowa Chapter, 3194
Juvenile Diabetes Research Foundation: Gre ater Iowa Chapter, 3195
Kidneeds, 5613
Knoxville Division: VA Central Iowa Health Care System, 10233
Lupus Foundation of America: Iowa Chapter, 5878
Myasthenia Gravis Support Group of Ames, 6687
NAMI Iowa: National Alliance on Mental Illness, 6029
NNFF Iowa Chapter, 6756
National Center for Voice and Speech: Univ ersity of Iowa, 4245
National Federation of the Blind in Computer Science, 9500
National Federation of the Blind: Iowa, 9561
National MS Society: Iowa Chapter, 6446
Neurological Center of Iowa, 1891
Orthopaedic Biomechanics Laboratory Shriners Hospital for Crippled Children, 2720
Pediatric Allergy & Pulmonary Division University of Iowa Healthcare, 3041
People Against Cancer, 2104
Prader-Willi Iowa Association, 7264
Quad Cities Brain Tumor Support Group, 1892
RESOLVE Affiliate of Iowa, 5340
Spina Bifida Association of Iowa, 7984
Turner's Syndrome Society of Iowa, 9377
University of Iowa Birth Defects and Genetic Disorders Unit, 1769
University of Iowa College of Medicine, 8177
University of Iowa Mental Health Clinical Research Center, 6336
University of Iowa Teratogen Information Service, 1787
University of Iowa: Diabetes Research Center, 3321
University of Iowa: Holden Comprehensive Cancer Center, 2239
University of Iowa: Iowa Cardiovascular Center, 4829
Veterans Adm. Medical Center: Iowa City, 10234

Kansas

AARP Kansas State Office: Topeka, 46
ALS Association: Keith Worthington Chapter, 1012
ALS Association: Keith Worthington Chapter Central/Western Kansas Branch, 1013
Alcohol and Drug Abuse Services, 8288
Alzheimer's Association: Heart of America Chapter, 734

Alzheimer's Association: Sunflower Chapter, 735
American Academy of Environmental Medicine, 562
American Cancer Society: Kansas City, 2105
American Diabetes Association: Kansas, 3196
American Lung Association of Kansas, 5780
American Lung Association of Kansas, 9300
American Lung Association of Missouri, 5789
American Organ Transplant Association, 10465
American Stroke Foundation, 8169
Arthritis Foundation: Kansas Chapter, 1112
Arthritis Foundation: Western Missouri, Greater Kansas City, 1120
Association for Neuro-Metabolic Disorders, 3752
Autism Society of Kansas Autism Society of America, 1606
Beach Center on Disability, 10471
Brain Injury Association of Kansas and Greater Kansas City, 4018
Brain Injury Association of Kansas and Greater Kansas City Helpline, 4080
CKLS Headquarters, 9734
Council for Learning Disabilities (CLD), 10486
Disability Rights Center of Kansas, 10564
Foundation for Hospice and Homecare, 10629
Gray Matters Support: Kansas City, 1893
Headstrong Brain Tumor Support Group, 1894
Kansas Association of the Deaf, 4266
Kansas Department of Health & Environment Bureau of Family Health, 8873
Kansas Department of Health & Environment Epidemiology & Disease Prevention: HIV, 266
Kansas Industries for the Blind, 9562
Kansas Services for the Blind and Visually Impaired, 9872
Kansas State University: Terry C Johnson Center for Basic Cancer Research, 2240
Kansas University Medical Center: Cystic Fibrosis Center, 3042
Keys for Networking: Kansas FFCMH, 6030
Landon Center on Aging University of Kansas Medical Center, 83
Leukemia and Lymphoma Society: Mid-America Chapter, 2106
Leukemia and Lymphona Society: Kansas Chapter, 2107
Lupus Foundation of America: Heartland Chapter, 5879
Manhattan Subregional Library of the Kansas Talking Books Service, 9735
Midwest Transplant Network & Organ Bank, 9215
NAMI Kansas: Kansas' Voice on Mental Illness, 6031
National Federation of the Blind: Kansas, 9563
National Kidney Foundation of Kansas and Western Missouri, 5553
National MS Society: Mid-America Chapter, 6447
National MS Society: South Central & West Kansas Division, 6448
Neurofibromatosis Kansas and Central Plains, 6758
Northeast Kansas Parkinson Association, 6979
Northwest Kansas Library System, 9736
Parkinson Association of Greater Kansas City, 6980
Region VII Office Program: Consultants for Maternal and Child Health, 8894
SIDS Network of Kansas, 8874
South Central Kansas Library System, 9737
St. Joseph Medical Center Cystic Fibrosis Care and Teaching Center, 3043
Talking Books Service, 9738
United Cerebral Palsy of Kansas, 2654
University of Kansas Allergy and Immunology Clinic, 604
University of Kansas Cray Diabtetes Center, 3322
University of Kansas Kidney and Urology Research Center, 5608
Veterans Adm. Medical Center: Leavenwoth Dwight D. Eisenhower VA Medical Center, 10235
Veterans Adm. Medical Center: Topeka Colmery O'Neil VA Medical Center, 10236
Veterans Adm. Medical Center: Wichita Robert J. Dole Department Of VA Medical, 10237
Wichita Medical Research & Education Foundation, 1772
Wichita Public Library, 9739

Kentucky

AARP Kentucky State Office: Louisville, 47
ALS Association: Kentucky CIO, 1014
Academy of Doctors of Audiology, 4208
Alzheimer's Association: Lexington/ Bluegrass Chapter, 736
Alzheimer's Association: Louisville Chapter, 737
Alzheimer's Disease Center Kentucky University, 856
American Cancer Society: Kentucky, 2108
American Council of Blind Lions, 9450
American Diabetes Association: Kentucky, 3197
American Lung Association of Kentucky, 5781
American Lung Association of Kentucky, 9301
American Printing House for the Blind, 9456
Arthritis Foundation: Kentucky Chapter, 1113
Autism Chapter of Bluegrass Chapter, 1607
Autism Society of Western Kentucky, 1608
Brain Injury Alliance of Kentucky, 4081
Brain Injury Association of Kentucky, 4019
Carol and Dr. James W Stutts, 10238
Client Assistance Program: Kentucky, 10565
Department of Public Health: Adult and Child Health Division, 8875
Diabetes Exercise and Sports Association, 3138
Division of Substance Abuse: Department of Mental Health, 8289
Dream Factory, Inc., 10771
Henry Vogt Cancer Research Institute James Graham Brown Cancer Center, 2241
Jewish Hospital Transplant Center, 9191
Juvenile Diabetes Research Foundation: Kentuckiana Chapter, 3198
KY Partnership For Families and Children, 6032
Kentucky Alliance for the Mentally Ill, 6033
Kentucky Association of the Deaf, 4267
Kentucky Cancer Program, 2242
Kentucky Hemophilia Foundation, 4906
Kentucky IMPACT, 6131
Kentucky Industries for the Blind, 9564
Kentucky Organ Donor Affiliates, 9216
Kentucky Talking Book Library, 9740
Kentucky University: Cystic Fibrosis Center, 3044
Kosair Childrens Cystic Fibrosis Center, 3045
Leukemia and Lymphoma Society: Kentucky Chapter, 2109
Louisville Talking Book Library for the Blind and Physically Handicapped, 9741
Lovelace Respiratory Research Institute, 5605
Meningioma/Benign Brain Tumor Support Group, 1895
Myasthenia Gravis Support Group of Louisvi lle, 6688
National Anxiety Foundation, 6269
National Federation of the Blind: Kentucky, 9565
National Kidney Foundation of Kentucky, 5554
National MS Society: Kentucky Chapter, 6449
National Spinal Cord Injury Association: Derby City Area Chapter, 8085
Northern Kentucky Talking Book Library, 9742
Parents Resource Institute for Drug Education, 8328
Prader-Willi Kentucky Association, 7265
RESOLVE of Kentucky, 5341
SIDS Network of Kentucky, 8876
Spina Bifida Association of Kentucky, 7985
USA Deaf Sports Federation, 4256
University of Kentucky: Children Cancer Study Group, 2243
University of Kentucky: Lucille Parker Markey Cancer Center, 2244
Veterans Adm. Medical Center: Lexington Lexington VA Medical Center, 10240
Veterans Adm. Medical Center: Louisville Louisville VA Medical Center, 10241
Wellness Community: Kentucky, 1896

Louisiana

AARP Louisiana State Office: Baton Rouge, 48
Advocacy Center, 10566
Alexandria VA Healthcare System, 10242
Alzheimer's Association: Greater New Orleans Chapter, 739
Alzheimer's Association: Northeast/Central Louisiana Chapter, 738
Alzheimer's Services of the Capital Area, 740
American Bone Marrow Donor Registry, 2011
American Cancer Society: Louisiana, 2110
American Celiac Society, 2558
American Celiac Society Hotline, 2562
American Diabetes Association: Louisana, 3199
American Lung Association of Louisiana, 5782
American Lung Association of Louisiana, 9302
Autism Society of Louisiana, 1609
Baton Rouge Regional Tumor Registry Mary Bird Perkins Cancer Center, 2245
Bayou Area Chapter of the American Association of Kidney Patients, 5555
Brain Injury Association of Louisiana Help line, 4082
Brain Tumor Support Group, 1897
CCFA Louisiana Chapter, 2941
Central Louisiana State Hospital Medical and Professional Library, 6097
Clinical Immunology, Allergy, and Rheumatology, 1311
Eljay Foundation for Parkinson Syndrome Awareness, 6981
Ernest N Morial Asthma, Allergy & Respiratory Disease Center, 3046
Industries for the Blind and Visually Impaired of Louisiana, 9566
Juvenile Diabetes Research Foundation: Bat on Rouge Chapter, 3200
Juvenile Diabetes Research Foundation: Lou isiana Chapter, 3201
Juvenile Diabetes Research Foundation: Shr eveport Chapter, 3202
Louisiana Alliance for the Mentally Ill, 6034
Louisiana Association for the Blind, 9567
Louisiana Association of the Deaf, 4268
Louisiana Chapter of the National Hemophilia Foundation, 4907
Louisiana Comprehensive Hemophilia Care Center, 4967
Louisiana Department of Health & Hospitals : Office of Public Health, 267
Louisiana Lupus Foundation, 5881
Louisiana Organ Procurement Agency, 9217
Louisiana State University Genetics Section of Pediatrics, 1764
Louisiana Support Group: National Ataxia Foundation, 1463
Myasthenia Gravis Support Group of Louisia na, 6689
NNFF Louisiana Chapter, 6759
National Federation of the Blind: Louisana, 9568
National Kidney Foundation of Louisiana, 5556
National Multiple Sclerosis Society: Louisiana, 6450
National Spinal Cord Injury Association: Louisiana Chapter, 8086
Northeast Louisiana Sickle Cell Anemia Foundation, 7706
Office of Human Services: Division of Alcohol and Drug Abuse, 8290
Office of Public Health, 8877
Public Health Services of Louisiana, 8878
RESOLVE of Louisiana, 5342
Randolph-Sheppard Vendors of America, 9513
Southeast Louisiana Veterans Health Care S ystem, 10243
Spina Bifida Association of Greater New Orleans, 7986
State Library of Louisiana, 9743
Tulane University Pulmonary Diseases Critical Care and Enviromental Medicine, 2246
Tulane University: US-Japan Biomedical Research Laboratories, 4059
United Cerebral Palsy of Baton Rouge McMains Children's Developmental Center, 2655
United Cerebral Palsy of Greater New Orleans, 2656
Veterans Adm. Medical Center: Shreveport Overton Brooks VA Medical Center, 10244
Wishing Well Foundation USA, Inc., 10792

Maine

AARP Maine State Office: Portland, 49

Alzheimer's Association: Maine Chapter, 741
American Cancer Society: Maine, 2111
American Diabetes Association: Maine, 3203
American Lung Association of Maine, 5783
American Lung Association of Maine, 9303
Autism Society of Maine, 1610
Bangor Public Library, 9744
Brain Injury Association of Maine, 4020
Brain Tumor Support Group of Maine, 1898
Cary Library, 9745
Central Maine Cystic Fibrosis Center, 3047
Department of Human Services, 8879
Disability Rights Center: Maine, 10567
Gift From Within, 7157
HOSPICELINK Hospice Education Institute, 10806
Juvenile Diabetes Research Foundation: New
    England/Maine Chapter, 3204
Lewiston Public Library, 9746
Lupus Group of Maine, 5882
Maine Alliance for the Mentally Ill, 6035
Maine Alzheimer's Care Center, 742
Maine Bureau of Health: Division of Disease Control,
    268
Maine Center for the Blind and Visually Impaired,
    9569
Maine Hemophilia Treatment Center, 4968
Maine Medical Center: Cystic Fibrosis Clin, 3049
Maine Medical Center: Cystic Fibrosis Clinical
    Center, 3048
Maine SIDS Foundation, 8880
Maine SIDS Program Department Of Human
    Services, 8881
Maine State Library, 9747
Maine Support Group: National Ataxia Foundation,
    1464
National Federation of the Blind: Maine, 9570
National Kidney Foundation of Maine, 5557
National MS Society: Maine Chapter, 6451
Office of Alcohol and Drug Abuse Prevention, 8291
Portland Public Library, 9748
Sleep Laboratory, Maine Medical Center, 7911
United Cerebral Palsy of Northeastern Maine, 2657
United Families for Children's Mental Health, 6036
University of Maine: Communication Science s &
    Disorders, 4325
Veterans Adm. Medical Center: Augusta Togus VA
    Medical Center, 10245
Waterville Public Library, 9749

Maryland

ABLEDATA, 4206
ABLEDATA, 10452
ABLEDATA-REHAB DATA Alliance for Technology
    Access (ATA), 10453
ADARA, 4207
AIDSinfo, 181
AIDSinfo, 377
ALS Association: National Capital Area Chapter,
    1006
AMSUS, 7120
Agency for Healthcare Research and Quality, 579
Agency for Healthcare Research and Quality, 1290
Agency for Healthcare Research and Quality, 3485
Agency for Healthcare Research and Quality, 3617
Agency for Healthcare Research and Quality, 4269
Agency for Healthcare Research and Quality, 5688
Agency for Healthcare Research and Quality, 7145
Agency for Healthcare Research and Quality, 7566
Alabama Kidney Foundation, 5518
Alzheimer's Association: Central Maryland Chapter,
    743
Alzheimer's Association: Eastern Shore Chapter, 744
Alzheimer's Association: Western Maryland Chapter,
    745
Alzheimer's Disease Center: Johns Hopkins
    University School of Medicine, 860
Alzheimer's Disease Education and Referral Center,
    661
American Action Fund for Blind Children and Adults,
    9750
American Association of the Deaf-Blind, 4212
American Association of the Deaf-Blind, 9448
American Cancer Society: Maryland, 2112

American College of Gastroenterology, 3836
American Diabetes Association: Maryland, 3205
American Foundation for Urologic Disease: Us Too
    Line, 2319
American Gastroenterological Association, 9419
American Gastroenterological Association National
    Office, 3838
American Lung Association of Maryland, 5784
American Lung Association of Maryland, 9304
American Medical Directors Association, 6891
American Prostate Society, 2013
American Society for Parenteral and Enteral Nutrition
    (ASPEN), 3844
American Society of Human Genetics, 1053
American Speech-Language-Hearing Association,
    4216
American Urlogical Association American
    Foundation for Urologic Disease, 5238
American Venereal Disease Association, 7661
Anxiety Disorders Association of America, 6265
Anxiety Disorders Association of America, 7128
Anxiety and Depression Association of America,
    7129
Arthritis Foundation: Maryland Chapter, 1114
Asthma and Allergy Foundation of America, 566
Asthma and Allergy Foundation of America:
    Maryland/Greater Washington, DC, 580
Asthma and Allergy Information Association, 1281
Autism Society of America, 1586
Autism Society of America, 1649
Autism Society of Baltimore-Chesapeake, 1611
Baltimore Headache Institute, 6367
Believe In Tomorrow Children's Foundation, 10766
Blind Industries and Services of Maryland, 9571
Brain Injury Association of Maryland, 4021
Brain Injury Association of Maryland Helpl ine, 4083
Brain Tumor Networking Group, 1899
Brain Tumor Support Group: Maryland, 1900
Brainiacs, 1901
CCFA Maryland Chapter, 2942
CDC National Prevention Information Network
    (NPIN), 194
CDC National Prevention Information Network
    (NPIN), 306
CSAP State Liason Program CSAP Division of
    Communications Programs, 8235
Cancer Information Service, 2195
Candlelighters Childhood Cancer Foundation, 2025
Captioned Films/Videos, 4288
Captioned Media Program, 4289
Center for AIDS Research: Johns Hopkins University
    School of Medicine, 339
Center for Mental Health Services, 7146
Center for Research for Mothers & Children, 8832
Center for Substance Abuse Prevention, 8236
Center for the Study of Traumatic Stress, 7156
Center for the Study of Traumatic Stress, 7181
Centers for Medicare & Medicaid Services, 581
Centers for Medicare & Medicaid Services, 7147
Centers for Medicare and Medicaid Services, 1291
Centers for Medicare and Medicaid Services, 3486
Centers for Medicare and Medicaid Services, 3618
Centers for Medicare and Medicaid Services, 4270
Centers for Medicare and Medicaid Services, 5689
Centers for Medicare and Medicaid Services, 7567
Chesapeake Area Support Group: National Ataxia
    Foundation, 1465
Children & Adults with Attention Deficit Disorders,
    1524
Client Assistance Program: Maryland, 10568
Clinical Focus on Primary Immune Deficiency
    Diseases, 199
Community Services for Autistic Adults & Children,
    1589
Cooley's Anemia Foundation (CAF): Capital Area,
    2888
Cystic Fibrosis Center: National Institute of Health
    NIDDK, 3050
Cystic Fibrosis Foundation, 3013
Cystic Fibrosis Foundation, 3051
Deaf AIDS Project Family Service Foundation, 202
Digestive Disorders Associates Ridgely Oaks
    Professional Center, 3863
Disability Resource Center of Montgomery County
    Public Libraries, 9751

Drug Free Workplace Hotline, 8374
Endocrine Society, 3
Epilepsy Foundation, 7552
Epilepsy Foundation of America Helpline, 7585
Federation of Families for Children's Mental Health,
    5981
First Candle, 8882
Fort Howard VA Outpatient Clinic, 10246
Foundation Fighting Blindness, 9469
Foundation Fighting Blindness, 9667
Frederick Cancer Research Center, 2247
Friends Medical Science Research Center, 8338
Friends of Libraries for Deaf Action USA, 4290
Genetic and Rare Diseases Information Center, 3753
Goodwill Industries International, 10496
Health Resources and Services Administration
    (HRSA), 9190
Hearing Loss Association of America, 4236
Hemophilia Foundation of Maryland, 4908
Hepatitis Foundation International, 5070
Hydrocephalus Association, 5136
Hydrocephalus Association Hydrocephalus
    Association, 5129
Immune Deficiency Foundation, 211
Immune Deficiency Foundation, 570
Impotents Anonymous, 5246
Indian Health Service, 8244
Institute of Psychiatry and Human Behavior:
    University of Maryland, 6101
International Agency for the Prevention of Blindness,
    9477
International Braille and Technology Center for the
    Blind, 9752
Job Opportunities for the Blind, 9879
Johns Hopkins Brain Tumor Education Group, 1902
Johns Hopkins University: Asthma and Allergy
    Center, 1313
Johns Hopkins University: Behavioral Pharmacology
    Research Unit, 8342
Johns Hopkins University: Center for Communication
    Programs, 340
Johns Hopkins University: Dana Center for
    Preventive Ophthalmology, 9860
Johns Hopkins University: Scleroderma Center, 7448
Johns Hopkins University: Sleep Disorders Francis
    Scott Key Medical Center, 7875
Johns Hopkins University: Sydney Kimmel
    Comprehensive Cancer Center, 2248
Joslin Center at University of Maryland Medicine,
    3300
Juvenile Diabetes Research Foundation: Mar yland
    Chapter, 3206
Kennedy Krieger Institute, 3514
Kennedy Krieger Institute - Down Syndrome, 3524
Kennedy-Krieger Institute, 10389
Learning How, 10503
Leukemia and Lymphoma Society: Maryland Chapter,
    2113
Little People's Research Fund (LPRF), 3966
Loch Raven VA Community Living & Rehabilit ation
    Center, 10247
MD/DC/Delaware Chapter of Myasthenia Gravis
    Foundation of America, 6657
MD/DC/Delaware Chapter of Myasthenia Gravis
    Foundation of America, 6658
MD/DC/Delaware Chapter of Myasthenia Gravis
    Foundation of America, 6665
Maryland Group, 10248
Maryland National Spinal Cord Injury Association
    Support Group Network, 8102
Maryland Psychiatric Research Center, 6332
Maryland SIDS Information & Counseling Program,
    8883
Maryland State Alcohol and Drug Abuse
    Administration, 8292
Maryland State Library for the Blind and Physically
    Handicapped, 9753
Mental Health America, 6267
Mental Health Services Training Center, 10509
Mt. Washington Pediatric Clinic, 3518
NIH Clinical Center, 6107
NIH Osteoporosis and Related Bone Diseases -
    National Resource Center, 6861
NIH Osteoporosis and Related Bone Diseases -
    National Resource Center, 6864

Urban Cardiology Research Center, 4841
Urology Care Foundation, 5278
VA Capitol Health Care Network, 10249
VA Maryland Health Care System Perry Point VA Medical Center, 10250
Veterans Adm. Medical Center: Baltimore, 10251
Warren Grant Magnuson Clinical Center, 607
Warren Grant Magnuson Clinical Center, 1159
Warren Grant Magnuson Clinical Center, 2250
Warren Grant Magnuson Clinical Center, 3333
Warren Grant Magnuson Clinical Center, 4842
Warren Grant Magnuson Clinical Center, 5611
Warren Grant Magnuson Clinical Center, 5819
Warren Grant Magnuson Clinical Center National Institute of Health, 9870
Washington DC Metropolitan Area Brain Tumor Support Group, 1903
Washington Ear, 9521
Weight-Control Information Network National Institutes of Health, 3610
Weight-control Information Network, 6800
White Lung Association, 5762
Workplace Program CSAP Division of Communication Programs, 8268

Massachusetts

AARP Massachusetts State Office: Boston, 50
AIDS Support Group of Cape Cod, 376
ALS Association: Massachusetts Chapter, Wakefield Office, 1015
Affiliated Children's Arthritis Centers of New England, 1144
Alzheimer's Association: Massachusetts Chapter, 746
Alzheimer's Association: Western Regional Office: Massachusetts Chapter, 747
Alzheimer's Disease Center: Boston University, 859
American Cancer Society: Boston, 2114
American Cancer Society: Central New England Region-Weston MA, 2115
American Diabetes Association: Boston, 3207
American Lung Association of Massachusetts, 5785
American Lung Association of Massachusetts, 9305
American Society of Adults with Pseudo-Obstruction, 3845
Arthritis Foundation: Massachusetts Chapter, 1115
Association of Gastrointestinal Motility D isorders, 3639
Asthma and Allergy Foundation of America: New England Chapter, 587
Asthma and Allergy Foundation of America: New England Chapter, 1298
Attention Deficit Information Network, 1531
Autism Society of Massachusetts, 1612
Autism Treatment Center of America, 1587
Autism Treatment Center of America: Son-Rise Program, 1588
Baystate Medical Center Wesson Memorial Unit, 3052
Berkshire Center, 10621
BermanGund Laboratory for the Study of Retinal Degenerations, 9839
Boston Hemophilia Center Fegan 5 Children's Hospital, 4943
Boston Sickle Cell Center Boston Medical Center, 7709
Boston University Arthritis Center, 1146
Boston University Cancer Research Center, 2251
Boston University Center for Human Genetics, 1759
Boston University Laboratory of Neuropsychology, 8331
Boston University Medical Campus General Clinical Research Center, 1147
Boston University University Medical Center, 7445
Boston University, Whitaker Cardiovascular Institute, 4795
Brain Injury Association of Massachusetts, 4022
Brain Injury Association of Massachusetts Helpline, 4084
Brain Tissue Resource Center McLean Hospital, 1834
Brain Tumor Patient and Caregiver Support Group, 1904
Brain Tumor Society, 1825
Brain Tumor Support Group: Duarte, 1842

Brain Tumor Support Group: Lahey, 1905
Brain Tumor Support Group: Worcester, 1906
Brigham and Women's Hospital: Center for Neurologic Diseases, 6507
Brigham and Women's Hospital: Rheumatology Immunology, and Allergy Division, 1309
Brigham and Women's Orthopedica and Arthritis Center, 1148
CAPP National Parent Resource Center, 1750
CCFA New England Chapter: Massachusetts, 2943
California Center for Population Research, 5374
Cape Cod Chapter National Parkinson Foundation, 6982
Caption Center, 9755
Carroll Center for the Blind, 9573
Carroll Center for the Blind, 9846
Carroll Center for the Blind, 9877
Center for AIDS Research: Harvard Medical School, Division of AIDS, 344
Center for Anxiety and Related Disorders at Boston University, 7183
Center for Blood Research Harvard Medical School/CBR, 345
Centers for AIDS Research: University of Massachusetts Medical School, 346
Childrens Hospital Immunology Division Children's Hospital, 1310
Childrens Hospital Medical Center Cystic Fibrosis Center, 3053
Client Assistance Program: Massachusetts, 10569
Cooley's Anemia Foundation (CAF): Massachusetts Chapter, 2889
Cystic Fibrosis Worldwide, 3012
Cystic Firbrosis Center: Tufts New England Medical Center, 3054
Dana Farber Cancer Institute National Drug Discovery Group for AIDS Treatment, 347
Dana-Farber Institute: Department of Biostatistics and Computational Biology, 2252
David H. Koch Institute for Integrative Ca ncer Research, 2253
Developmental Medicine Center (DMC), 3509
Developmental Medicine Center Children's Hospital Boston, 348
Division of Substance Abuse, 8293
Eaton-Peabody Laboratory of Auditory Physiology, 4301
Facioscapulohumeral Muscular Dystrophy Soc iety (FSH Society), 6599
Federation for Children with Special Needs, 1754
Federation for Children with Special Needs, 10494
Fertility and Women's Health Care Center, 5376
Framingham Heart Study, 4804
General Clinical Research Center at Beth Israel Hospital, 4805
Harris Center for Education and Advocacy in Eating Disorders, 3636
Harvard Clinical Nutrition Research Center, 6801
Harvard Cocaine Recovery Project, 8340
Harvard Throndike Laboratory Harvard Medical Center, 4808
Harvard University Howe Laboratory of Ophthalmology, 9854
Health Care For All, 10498
Hydrocephalus Foundation, 5130
Joslin Diabetes Center, 3316
Juvenile Diabetes Research Foundation: New England/Bay State Chapter, 3208
Laboure College Library, 9756
Lupus Foundation of America: Massachusetts Chapter, 5884
Macular Degeneration Foundation, 9481
Mass./New Hampshire Chapter of the Myasthenia Gravis Foundation of America, 6666
Mass./New Hampshire Chapter of the Myasthenia Gravis Foundation of America, 6670
Massachusetts Alliance for the Mentally Ill, 6039
Massachusetts Alzheimers Disease Research Center, 874
Massachusetts Commission for the Blind, 9574
Massachusetts Department of Health HIV/AIDS Bureau, 269
Massachusetts Down Syndrome Congress, 3491
Massachusetts Eating Disorder Association, 3623

Massachusetts General Departments of Neurology and Neurosurgery, 8175
Massachusetts General Hospital, 3055
Massachusetts General Hospital: Harvard Cutaneous Biology Research Center, 7770
Massachusetts State Association of the Deaf, 4274
Massachusetts Sudden Infant Death Syndrome Boston City Hospital, 8943
Merrimack Valley HPV Support Group Holy Family Hospital, 10570
Myasthenia Gravis Support Group of Eastern Massachusetts and New Hampshire, 6690
Myasthenia Gravis Support Group of Eastern Massachusetts and New Hampshire, 6695
Myasthenia Gravis Support Group of Western Massachusetts and New Hampshire, 6691
Myasthenia Gravis Support Group of Western Massachusetts and New Hampshire, 6696
National Association for Parents of the Visually Impaired, 9483
National Association for Parents of the Visually Impaired, 9880
National Braille Press, 9494
National CFIDS Foundation, 2755
National Eating Disorders Screening Program, 3608
National Federation of the Blind: Massachusetts, 9575
National Kidney Foundation of MA/RI/NH/VT, 5559
National Kidney Foundation of MA/RI/NH/VT, 5566
National Kidney Foundation of MA/RI/NH/VT, 5585
National Kidney Foundation of MA/RI/NH/VT, 5599
National MS Society: Central New England Chapter, 6462
National MS Society: Massachusetts Chapter, 6453
National Parkinson Foundation:Cape Cod Chapter, 6983
National Scoliosis Foundation, 7486
National Spinal Cord Injury Association, 8087
National Spinal Cord Injury Association: Greater Boston Chapter, 8088
National Tay-Sachs and Allied Disease Association, 3757
National Tay-Sachs and Allied Diseases Association (NTSAD), 8989
National Tay-Sachs and Allied Diseases Association (NTSAD), 8990
National TaySachs & Allied Diseases, 8993
Neurofibromatosis: New England, 6761
Neurological Support Group of St. Luke's Hospital, 1907
Neurosurgical Service, 10571
New England AIDS Education & Training Center (NEHEC), 270
New England AIDS Education and Training Center, 226
New England Area Support Group: National Ataxia Foundation, 1466
New England Hemophilia Association, 4909
New England Medical Center: ALS Laboratory, 1048
New England Organ Bank Massachusetts, 9219
New England Region: Helen Keller National Center, 9576
New England Regional Genetics Group, 1765
Northeast Parkinson's and Caregivers, 6984
Option Institute, 2754
Option Institute, 3784
Option Institute, 6272
Option Institute International Learning & Training Center, 10534
Option Istitute Learning and Training Center, 5992
PALS Support Groups, 1781
Parent Education/Support Group, 1908
Parent Professional Advocacy League, 1758
Parent Professional Advocacy League, 6132
Pediatric Crohn's and Colitis Association, 2925
Pediatric Pulmonary Unit Massachusetts General Hospital, 8944
Perkins Braille and Talking Book Library, 9757
Persian Gulf Era Veterans, 10252
Prader-Willi New England Association, 7266
RESOLVE of the Bay State, 5343
Region 1 of the National Association for Parents of the Visually Impaired, 9577
Region I Office Program: Consultants for Maternal and Child Health, 8884

Rhode Island Hemophilia Foundation, 4928
SIDS Support Group, 8951
Safe Homes, 8265
Scleroderma Foundation, 7414
Scleroderma Foundation: New England Chapter, 7425
Scleroderma Foundation: New England Chapter, 7426
Scleroderma Foundation: New England Chapter, 7431
Scleroderma Foundation: New England Chapter, 7437
Scleroderma Foundation: New England Chapter, 7441
Scleroderma Support Groups, 7462
Screening For Mental Health, 6273
Shriver Center University Affiliated Program, 10390
Sleep Disorders Unit Beth Israel Deaconess Medical Center, 7909
Sleep Research Foundation, 7913
Society for Surgery of the Alimentary Tract, 3855
Southern New England Turner Syndrome Society, 9378
Spina Bifida Association of Massachusetts, 7989
Students Against Destructive Decisions, 8266
Suicide Prevention Resource Center, 7166
Talking Book Library at Worcester Public Library, 9758
Traditional Tibetan Healing, 6516
Trauma Center, 7167
Trauma Center, 7184
Tufts Medical Center, 4991
United Cerebral Palsy of Berkshire County, 2661
United Cerebral Palsy of MetroBoston, 2662
United Scleroderma Foundation, 7310
University of Massachusetts Memorial Medical Center, 3056
University of Massachusetts: Diabetes and Endocrinology Research Center, 3323
VA Boston Healthcare System: Jamaica Plain Jamaica Plain Campus, 10253
VA Boston Healthcare System: West Roxbury West Roxbury Campus, 10254
VA New England Health Care System, 10255
VALT Support Group (Vital Active Life After Trauma), 4085
Veterans Adm. Medical Center: Brockton Brockton Campus, 10256
Veterans Benefits Clearinghouse, 10391
Vision Use in Employment, 9888

Michigan

AARP Michigan State Office: Lansing, 51
ALS Association: Michigan Chapter, 1016
ALS Association: West Michigan Chapter, 1017
Alzheimer's Association: East Central Michigan Chapter, 748
Alzheimer's Association: Greater Michigan Chapter, 749
Alzheimer's Association: Greater Michigan Chapter: Upper Peninsula Region, 750
Alzheimer's Association: Michigan Great Lakes Chapter: West Shore Region, 751
Alzheimer's Association: Mid-Michigan Chapter, 752
Alzheimer's Association: Northeast Michigan Chapter, 753
Alzheimer's Association: Northwest Michigan Chapter, 754
American Autoimmune Related Diseases Association, 185
American Autoimmune Related Diseases Association, 4844
American Autoimmune Related Diseases Association, 10458
American Diabetes Association: Michigan, 3209
American Institute for Preventive Medicine, 10463
American Institute for Preventive Medicine, 10464
American Liver Foundation Michigan Chapter, 5697
American Lung Association of Michigan, 5786
American Lung Association of Michigan, 9306
American Motility Society, 3840
Anxiety Resource Center, 7153
Apnea Identification Program Children's Ho spital of Michigan, 8885
Arthritis Foundation: Michigan Chapter Chapter and Metro Detroit, 1116
Association for Children's Mental Health, 6040
Association for the Blind & Visually Impaired, 9578

Asthma and Allergy Foundation of America: Michigan Chapter, 588
Asthma and Allergy Foundation of America: Michigan Chapter, 1299
Autism Society of Michigan, 1613
Autoimmune Diseases Association, 5853
Brain Injury Association of Michigan, 4023
Brain Injury Association of Michigan Helpline, 4086
Brain Tumor Networking Club, 1909
Brain Tumor Support Group for Patients & Families, 1910
Brain Tumor Support Group: Ann Arbor, 1911
Brain Tumor Support Group: West Bloomfield, 1912
CCFA Michigan Chapter: Farmington Hills, 2944
Childhood Liver Disease Research Network, 3011
Client Assistance Program: Michigan, 10572
Commission for the Blind, 10573
Council on Education of the Deaf College of Education, 4226
Detroit Subregional Library for the Blind and Physically Handicapped, 9759
Detroit Support Group: National Ataxia Foundation, 1467
Detroit VA Medical Center John D. Dingell VA Medical Center, 10257
Dynamic Rehab, 3997
East Lansing Cystic Fibrosis Center Michigan State University, 3057
Eastern Michigan Hemophilia Center St. Joseph Hospital, 4950
Genesee County Health Department, 8886
Gershenson Radiation Oncology Center Barbara Ann Karmanos Cancer Institute, 2254
Gilda's Club: Grand Rapids, 2329
Glaucoma Laser Trabeculoplasty Study Sinai Hospital of Detroit, 9852
Grand Traverse Area Library for the Blind and Physically Handicapped, 9760
Great Lakes Chapter of the Myasthenia Gravis Foundation of America, 6667
Greater Detroit Agency for the Blind and Visually Impaired, 9579
Greater Grand Rapids Pediatric Hemophilia Program, 4954
Hemophilia Foundation of Michigan, 4910
Henry Ford Hospital: Hypertension and Vascular Research Division, 5193
Hydrocephalus Support Group of Michigan Children's Hospital of Michigan, 5137
International Advocacy for Gulf War Syndrome, 10258
International Hearing Society, 4240
International Hearing Society, 4339
JIMHO Affiliated Centers (Justice in Mental Health Organization), 6041
Juvenile Diabetes Research Foundation: Metropolitan Detroit/SE Michigan, 3210
Juvenile Diabetes Research Foundation: Wes t Michigan Chapter, 3211
Kalamazoo Center for Medical Studies Michigan State University, 3058
Kent County Health Department, 8887
Kent County Library for the Blind, 9761
Leukemia and Lymphoma Society: Michigan Chapter, 2116
Library of Michigan Service for the Blind, 9762
Lupus Foundation of America: Michigan Lupus Foundation, 5885
Lyme Alliance, 9055
Macomb Library for the Blind and Physically Handicapped, 9763
Meyer L Prentis Comprehensive Cancer Cente Barbara Ann Karmanos Cancer Institute, 2256
Meyer L Prentis Comprehensive Cancer Center of Metropolitan Detroit, 2255
Michigan Alliance for the Mentally Ill, 6042
Michigan Alzheimer's Disease Research Center, 876
Michigan Chapter: Southeast, 9379
Michigan Deaf Association, 4275
Michigan Department of Community Health, 8888
Michigan Department of Community Health HIV/AIDS Prevention & Intervention Secti, 271
Michigan Hand Center, 2543
Michigan Kidney Foundation, 5560

Michigan State University Hemophilia Comprehensive Care Clinic, 4971
Midwestern Michigan Library Cooperative, 9764
Motor Neuron Disease Program University of Michigan Health System, 1046
Muskegon County Library for the Blind, 9765
NF Support Group of West Michigan, 6768
National Federation of the Blind: Michigan, 9580
National MS Society: Michigan Chapter, 6454
Northland Library Cooperative, 9766
Oakland County Health Division: SIDS Project, 8889
Oakland County Library for the Visually and Physically Impaired, 9767
Office of Substance Abuse Services Department of Public Health, 8294
Oscar G. Johnson VA Medical Center, 10259
PRIDE Youth Programs, 8262
Patient Advocates for Advanced Cancer Treatments (PAACT), 2196
Prader-Willi Michigan Association, 7267
RESOLVE of Michigan, 5344
Rainbow Connection, 10785
Regional Hemophilia Treatment Center Children's Hospital of Michigan, 4981
Rehabilitation Institute of Michigan, 4056
SIDS LEAD: Children's Special Health Care Services, 8890
Scleroderma Foundation: Michigan Chapter, 7427
Spina Bifida Association of Grand Rapids, 7990
Spina Bifida Association of Upper Peninsula Michigan, 7991
Spina Bifida and Hydrocephalus Association of Southwestern Michigan, 7992
St. Clark County Library for the Blind and Physically Handicapped, 9768
Transplantation Society of Michigan, 9220
United Cerebral Palsy of Metropolitan Detroit, 2663
United Cerebral Palsy of Michigan, 2664
University of Michigan Communicative Disorders Clinic, 4326
University of Michigan Hemophilia Center, 4997
University of Michigan Michigan Gastrointestinal Peptide Research Ctr., 3867
University of Michigan Montgomery: John M. Sheldon Allergy Society, 605
University of Michigan Nephrology Division, 5609
University of Michigan Pulmonary and Critical Care Division, 4830
University of Michigan Reproductive Sciences Program, 5379
University of Michigan: Alcohol Research Center, 8362
University of Michigan: Cancer Center Cancer Research Committee, 2257
University of Michigan: Cardiovascular Med icine, 4831
University of Michigan: Cystic Fibrosis Center, 3059
University of Michigan: Division of Hypertension, 5196
University of Michigan: Kresge Hearing Research Institute, 4327
University of Michigan: Mental Health Research Institute, 6110
University of Michigan: National Cooperative Drug/AIDS Group, 349
University of Michigan: Orthopaedic Research Laboratories, 1158
University of Michigan: Psychiatric Center, 8363
Upper Peninsula Library for the Blind and Physically Handicapped, 9769
Veterans Adm. Medical Center: Ann Arbor Ann Arbor Healthcare System, 10260
Veterans Adm. Medical Center: Battle Creek, 10261
Veterans Adm. Medical Center: Saginaw Aleda E. Lutz VA Medical Center, 10262
Visually Impaired Center, 9869
Washtenaw County Library for the Blind and Physically Disabled, 9770
Wayne County Regional Library for the Blind and Physically Handicapped, 9771
Wayne State University Center for Health Research, 350
Wayne State University Center for Molecular Medicine and Genetics, 2258

Wayne State University: CS Mott Center for Human Growth and Development, 1771
Wayne State University: Comprehensive Sickle Cell Center, 7721
Wayne State University: Gurdjian-Lissner Biomechanics Laboratory, 4065
Wayne State University: University Women's Care, 5381
William T Gossett Parkinson's Disease Center, 7001

Minnesota

AARP Minnesota State Office: Saint Paul, 52
ALS Association: Minnesota Chapter, 1018
African American Family Services, 8225
Alzheimer's Association: Minnesota/Dakotas, 755
Alzheimer's Disease Center Mayo Clinic Mayo Medical School, 857
American Academy of Neurology, 6360
American Academy of Neurology: Tourette Syndrome, 9101
American Association of Neuromuscular & Electrodiagnostic Medicine, 996
American Association of Neuromuscular & Electrodiagnostic Medicine, 6651
American Association of Neuromuscular & Electrodiagnostic Medicine, 7099
American Cancer Society: Duluth, 2117
American Cancer Society: Mendota Heights Mendota Heights, 2118
American Cancer Society: Rochester, 2119
American Cancer Society: Saint Cloud, 2120
American Diabetes Association: Minnesota, 3212
American Liver Foundation Minnesota Chapte r, 5698
American Lung Association of Minnesota, 5787
American Lung Association of Minnesota, 9307
American Pancreatic Association, 3841
Anna Westin Foundation, 3596
Arthritis Foundation: North Central Chapter, 1117
Autism Society of Minnesota, 1614
Behavioral Pediatrics Program, 10626
Brain Injury Alliance of Minnesota, 4087
Brain Injury Association of Minnesota, 4024
CCFA Minnesota Chapter, 2945
Center for Children with Chronic Illness and Disability, 10473
Chemical Dependency Program Division Department of Human Services, 8295
Dads and Daughters, 3598
Dentists Concerned for Dentists, 8296
Desert Storm Justice Foundation: Minnesota, 10263
Down Syndrome Association of Minnesota, 3492
Duluth Lighthouse for the Blind, 9581
Duluth Public Library, 9772
Emotional Health Anonymous, 6133
Fairview-University Hemophilia & Thrombosis Center, 4952
Fetal Alcohol Network, 10628
Hazelden, 8243
Hear Now: Starkey Hearin Foundation, 4234
Hemophilia Foundation of Minnesota and the Dakotas, 4911
Immunization Action Coalition, 5071
Impotence Information Center, 5245
International Diabetes Center at Nicollet, 3315
Juvenile Diabetes Research Foundation: Min nesota Chapter, 3213
KDWB Family Resource Center, 10632
KDWB Variety Family Canter, 10633
Lawyers Concerned for Lawyers, 8245
Leukemia and Lymphoma Society: Minnesota Chapter, 2121
LifeSource, Upper Midwest Organ Procurement Organization, Inc., 9221
Lupus Foundation of America: Minnesota Chapter, 5886
MN Chapter of the Turner Syndrome Society, 9380
Mayo Clinic and Foundation Mayo Foundation, 6596
Mayo Clinic and Foundation: Division of Allergic Diseases, 598
Mayo Clinic: Department of Neurology, 1044
Mayo Comprehensive Cancer Center, 2259
Mayo Comprehensive Hemophilia Center Mayo Clinic, 4969

Melpomene Institute for Women's Health Research, 5377
Minnesota AIDS Project AIDSLine, 387
Minnesota Alliance for the Mentally Ill, 6043
Minnesota Ambassador: National Ataxia Foundation, 1468
Minnesota Association for Children's Mental Health, 6044
Minnesota Department of Health: AIDS/STD Prevention Service, 272
Minnesota Disability Law Center, 10574
Minnesota Library for the Blind, 9773
Minnesota Obesity Center, 6802
Minnesota State Chapter of the Myasthenia Gravis Foundation of America, 6668
Minnesota Sudden Infant Death Center Minneapolis Children's Medical Center, 8891
Myasthenia Gravis Support Group of Mid-Min n, 6692
Myasthenia Gravis Support Group of South East Minnesota, 6693
Myasthenia Gravis Support Group of the Twin Cities, 6694
National Association of Blind Educators Sheila Koenig, 9486
National Association of Epilepsy Centers, 7553
National Association to Promote the Use of Braille, 9492
National Ataxia Foundation, 1444
National Federation of the Blind: Minnesota, 9582
National Kidney Foundation Serving Minneso ta, Dakotas & Iowa Division Office, 5587
National Kidney Foundation of Minnesota, 5561
National MS Society: Minnesota Chapter, 6455
National Marrow Donor Program, 2041
National Resource Library on Youth with Disabilities, 10622
Neurofibromatosis, 6738
Neurofibromatosis: Minnesota, 6762
Orthopaedic Rehabilitation Association, 7101
PACER Center, 6134
Parkinson Association of Minnesota, 6985
Pediatric Psychology, 10640
Prader-Willi Minnesota Association, 7268
RESOLVE of Minnesota, 5345
STAR Center for Family Health, 10641
Schulze Diabetes Institute, 3303
Scleroderma Foundation: Minnesota Chapter, 7428
Spina Bifida Association of Minnesota, 7993
Spinal Cord Society, 8076
Twin Cities Area Support Group: National Ataxia Foundation, 1469
U Special Kids, 10642
United Cerebral Palsy of Central Minnesota, 2665
United Cerebral Palsy of Minnesota, 2666
United Ostomy Association, 2927
United Ostomy Association, 3858
United Ostomy Association, 9423
United Ostomy Associations of America Advocacy Hotline, 2343
University of Minnesota Department of Psychiatry, 6111
University of Minnesota Masonic Cancer Center, 2260
University of Minnesota: Cystic Fibrosis Center, 3060
University of Minnesota: Hypertensive Research Group, 5197
University of Minnesota: Program on Alcohol/Drug Control, 8364
Veterans Adm. Medical Center: Minneapolis Minneapolis VA Medical Center, 10264
Veterans Adm. Regional Office: St. Paul, 10265

Mississippi

Alzheimer's Association: Mississippi Chapter, 756
Alzheimer's Foundation of the South: Mississippi Division, 757
American Cancer Society: Jackson, 2122
American Diabetes Association: Mississippi, 3214
American Lung Association of Mississippi, 5788
American Lung Association of Mississippi, 9308
Arthritis Foundation: Mississippi Chapter, 1118
Brain Injury Association of Mississippi, 4025

Brain Injury Association of Mississippi Helpline, 4088
Christian Resource for People Who Are Blind, 9774
Division of Alcohol & Drug Abuse: Mississippi, 8297
Division of Alcohol & Drug Abuse: South Department of Mental Health, 8298
G.V Montgomery VA Medical Center, 10266
Leukemia and Lymphoma Society: Mississippi Chapter, 2123
Lupus Foundation of America: Mississippi Chapter, 5887
Mississippi Alliance for the Mentally Ill, 6045
Mississippi Area Support Group: National Ataxia Foundation, 1470
Mississippi Client Assistance Program, 10575
Mississippi Department of Public Health: STD/HIV Prevention Program, 273
Mississippi Families as Allies, 6046
Mississippi Hemophilia Foundation, 4912
Mississippi Industries for the Blind, 9583
Mississippi Library Commission, 9775
Mississippi Organ Recovery, 9222
Mississippi SIDS Alliance, 8892
Mississippi State Department of Health and Child Health Services, 8893
National Federation of the Blind: Mississippi, 9584
National Kidney Foundation of Mississippi, 5562
National Multiple Sclerosis Society: Alaba ma-Mississippi Chapter, 6456
South Central VA Health Care Network, 10267
University of Mississippi Medical Center, 3061
VA Gulf Coast Veterans Health Care System, 10268
Veterans Adm. Regional Office: Jackson, 10269

Missouri

AARP Missouri State Office: Kansas City, 53
ALS Association: Keith Worthington Chapter Central Missouri Branch Office, 1019
ALS Association: St. Louis Regional Chapter, 1020
APDA Center for Advanced Parkinson Disease Research, 7009
Adriene Resource Center for Blind Children, 9776
Alphapointe Association for the Blind, 9585
Alzheimer's Association: Mid-Missouri Chapter, 758
Alzheimer's Association: Northwest Missouri-Chapter, 759
Alzheimer's Association: Southwest Missouri Chapter, 760
Alzheimer's Association: St. Louis Chapter, 761
Alzheimer's Disease Research Center Washington University School of Medicine, 864
American Cancer Society: Saint Louis, 2124
American Diabetes Association: Missouri, 3215
American Liver Foundation Greater Kansas City Chapter, 5699
American Lung Association of Eastern Missouri, 5790
American Lung Association of Missouri, 9309
American Lung Association: Kansas City Office, 5791
American Optometric Association, 9455
Arthritis Foundation: Eastern Missouri Chapter, 1119
Assemblies of God National Center for the Blind, 9777
Asthma and Allergy Foundation of America: Greater Kansas City Chapter, 1300
Asthma and Allergy Foundation of America: St. Louis Chapter, 589
Asthma and Allergy Foundation of America: St. Louis Chapter, 1301
Autism Society of Gateway Chapter, 1615
Brain Cancer Support Group, 1913
Brain Injury Association of Missouri, 4026
Brain Injury Association of Missouri Helpline, 4089
Brain Tumor Support Group: Kansas City, 1914
Brain Tumor Support and Networking Group, 1915
CCFA Mid-America Chapter: Kansas, 2940
CCFA Mid-America Chapter: Missouri, 2946
Cancer Research Center, 2261
Canine Assistance for the Disabled CADI, 4222
Central Institute for the Deaf, 4296

Montana

Nebraska

Nevada

New Hampshire

Alzheimer's Association of Vermont and New Hampshire, 768

American Cancer Society: New Hampshire Gail Singer Memorial Building, 2129

American Diabetes Association: New Hampshire, 3224

American Lung Association of New Hampshire, 5795

American Lung Association of New Hampshire, 9313

Arthritis Foundation: Northern New England Chapter, 1139

Autism Society of New Hampshire, 1618

Brain Injury Association of New Hampshire, 4028

Brain Injury Association of New Hampshire, 4091

Brain Injury/Brain Tumor Support Group, 1917

Camp Allen, 10623

Client Assistance Program: New Hampshire, 10581

Dartmouth Medical School: Microbiology Department, 3721

Dartmouth-Hitchcock Medical Center - Genetics and Development, 3507

Granite State FFCMH, 6054

High Hopes Foundation of New Hampshire, Inc., 10776

Juvenile Diabetes Research Foundation: New England/New Hampshire Chapter, 3225

National Alliance for the Mentally Ill: New Hampshire, 6055

National Alliance for the Mentally Ill: New Hampshire, 6138

National Federation of the Blind: New Hampshire, 9592

New Hampshire Cancer Pain Initiative, 2130

New Hampshire Chapter NSCIA, 8089

New Hampshire Cystic Fibrosis Care Teaching and Research Center, 3067

New Hampshire Department of Health and Human Services, 278

New Hampshire Lupus Foundation, 5893

New Hampshire SIDS Program, 8901

New Hampshire State Library, 9787

Norris Cotton Cancer Center Dartmouth-Hitchcock Medical Center, 2264

Northern New England Turner Society, 9383

Office of Alcohol and Drug Abuse Prevention, 8303

RESOLVE of New Hampshire, 5348

Sleep Disorders Center Dartmouth Hitchcock Medical Center, 7890

Sleep/Wake Disorders Center: Hampstead Hospital, 7918

Veterans Adm. Medical Center: Manchester Manchester VA Medical Center, 10279

Voices for the Blind, 9788

New Jersey

AARP New Jersey State Office: Princeton, 58

Alcohol Disease Foundation, 8329

All Access Mental Health, 6056

Alzheimer's Association: Greater New Jersey Chapter, 769

Alzheimer's Association: South Jersey Chapter, 770

American Anorexia Bulimia Association: New Jersey Chapter, 3624

American Auditory Society, 4213

American Cancer Society: New Jersey, 2131

American Council for Headache Education, 6361

American Diabetes Association: New Jersey, 3226

American Headache Society, 6362

American Lung Association of New Jersey, 5796

American Lung Association of New Jersey, 9314

American Society of Transplantation (AST), 9186

Angelwish, Inc., 10793

Arthritis Foundation: New Jersey Chapter, 1122

Asthma and Allergy Foundation of America: Southeast Pennsylvania Chapter, 1302

Asthma and Allergy Foundation of America: Southern Pennsylvania Chapter, 592

Autism Society of Southwest New Jersey, 1619

Bestwork Industries for the Blind, 9593

Brain Injury Alliance of New Jersey, 4092

Brain Injury Association of New Jersey, 4029

Brain Tumor Support Group: New Jersey, 1918

Brain Tumor Support Group: Toms River, 1919

CCFA New Jersey Chapter, 2947

COPLINE, 7190

CanHelp, 2132

Central New Jersey Brain Tumor Support Group, 1920

Christ Hospital Hepatitis C Support Group, 5076

Christopher & Dana Reeve Foundation Paralysis Resource Center, 8065

Community Mental Health Foundation, 6057

Congenital Heart Information Network, 2874

Cooley's Anemia Foundation (CAF): New Jersey Chapter, 2890

Department of Health, 8304

Disability Rights New Jersey, 10582

Division of Narcotic and Drug Abuse Control, 8305

Eating Disorders Association of New Jersey, 3642

Epilepsy Foundation of New Jersey, 7573

Friends Health Connection, 10630

Garden State Chapter of the Myasthenia Gravis Foundation of America, 6671

Garrett Mountain Chapter of the American Association of Kidney Patients, 5567

Greater New York Pull-Thru Network, 5279

HealthyWomen, 10624

Helping Other Parents in Normal Grief, 10807

Huxley Insititute-American Schizophrenic Association, 6331

Hydrocephalus Parents Support Group, 5142

Institute of Ophthalmology and Visual Scie nce New Jersey Medical School, 9858

Jason's Dreams for Kids Foundation, Inc., 10798

Juvenile Diabetes Research Foundation: Cen tral Jersey Chapter, 3228

Juvenile Diabetes Research Foundation: Mid -Jersey Chapter, 3229

Juvenile Diabetes Research Foundation: Roc kland County/Northern New Jersey, 3230

Juvenile Diabetes Research Foundation: South Jersey Chapter, 3227

Leukemia and Lymphoma Society: Northern New Jersey Chapter, 2133

Leukemia and Lymphoma Society: Southern New Jersey Chapter, 2134

Lupus Foundation of America: New Jersey Chapter, 5894

Lupus Foundation of America: South Jersey Chapter, 5895

Lyme Disease Association, 9046

Lyme Disease Network, 9056

Lyme Disease Network of New Jersey, 9058

Meadowlands Chapter of the American Association of Kidney Patients, 5568

Monmouth Medical Center: Cystic Fibrosis & Monmouth Medical Center, 3069

Monmouth Medical Center: Cystic Fibrosis & Pediatric Pulmonary Center, 3068

Multiple Sclerosis Association of America, 6416

Musculoskeletal Transplant Foundation, 9249

Nadeene Brunini Comprehensive Hemophilia Care Center, 4974

National Federation of the Blind: New Jersey, 9594

National MS Society: Greater North Jersey Chapter, 6463

National MS Society: Mid-Jersey Chapter, 6464

National Sarcoidosis Resource Center, 7321

National Women's Health Resource Center, 5373

National Women's Health Resource Center, 9023

National Womens Health Resource Center, 3720

Neuromuscular and ALS Center The Clinical Academic Building, 1047

New Eyes for the Needy, 9511

New Jersey Alliance for the Mentally Ill, 6058

New Jersey Department of Health: Child Health Program, 8902

New Jersey Department of Health: Division of AIDS Prevention & Control, 279

New Jersey Institute of Technology Center for Biomedical Engineering, 3973

New Jersey Library for the Blind and Handicapped, 9789

New Jersey Medical School, 3070

New Jersey Medical School: National Tuberculosis Center, 9282

New Jersey Metroplitan Turner Syndrome Society Association, 9384

New Jersey Parkinson's Disease Information Center, 7011

New Jersey Pregnancy Risk Information Service, 1780

New Jersey SIDS Alliance, 8903

New Jersey Woman AIDS Network, 280

Northern New Jersey Chapter of the American Association of Kidney Patients, 5569

Parent Project: Muscular Dystrophy, 6590

Parkinson Alliance, 6986

Prader-Willi New Jersey Association, 7271

RESOLVE of New Jersey, 5349

Recording for the Blind Helpline, 9887

Recording for the Blind and Dyslexic, 9514

Renfrew Center of Northern New Jersey, 3625

Rutgers University Center of Alcohol Studies, 8355

Rutgers University: Controlled Drug- Delivery Research Center, 8356

SIDS Center of New Jersey, 8904

Sarcoidosis Support Group: New Jersey, 7336

Seeing Eye, 9516

Sharing Network Organ Tissue Donation Services, 9226

Sleep Disorders Center: Newark Beth Israel Medical Center, 7904

Spina Bifida Association of the Tri-State Region, 7996

United Cerebral Palsy of Hudson County, 2672

United Cerebral Palsy of Morris-Somerset, 2673

United Cerebral Palsy of New Jersey, 2674

Veterans Adm. Medical Center: East Orange East Orange Campus, 10280

Veterans Adm. Medical Center: Lyons Lyons Campus, 10281

Well Spouse Association, 10644

Women's AIDS Network Women and Children's Service Program, 238

World Ostomy and Continence Nurses Society, 2928

New Mexico

AARP New Mexico State Office: Sante Fe, 59

ALS Association: New Mexico CIO, 1023

Alzheimer's Association: New Mexico Chapter, 771

American Cancer Society: New Mexico, 2135

American Diabetes Association: New Mexico, 3231

American Lung Association of New Mexico, 5797

Autism Society of New Mexico, 1620

Brain Injury Alliance of New Mexico, 4093

Brain Injury Association of New Mexico, 4030

Hemophilia Foundation of New Mexico, 4916

Juvenile Diabetes Research Foundation: Albuquerque, 3232

Leukemia and Lymphoma Society: Mountain States Chapter, 2136

Lovelace Medical Foundation, 5604

Lupus Foundation of America: New Mexico Chapter, 5896

Myasthenia Gravis Support Group of New Mex ico, 6697

National Federation of the Blind: New Mexico, 9595

National Kidney Foundation of New Mexico, 5570

National MS Society: Rio Grande Division, 6465

Navaho Nation K'E Project Children and Families Advocacy Corp, 6059

Navajo Nation K'E Project: Shiprock Children & Families Advocacy Corp, 6060

Navajo Nation Office Special Education & R ehabilitation Services, 6139

New Mexico Alliance for the Mentally Ill, 6061

New Mexico Branch, 9315

New Mexico Donor Services, 9227

New Mexico Health Department: Public Health Division, 281

New Mexico Industries for the Blind, 9596

New Mexico SIDS Information and Counseling Program, 8905

New Mexico State Library for the Blind and Physically Handicapped, 9790

Overeaters Anonymous World Service Office, 6798

People Living Through Cancer Support Groups, 1921

Protection and Advocacy System of Alburque rque, 10583

RESOLVE of New Mexico, 5350

Spina Bifida Association of New Mexico, 7997
State of New Mexico Commission for the Blind, 9597
Substance Abuse Bureau, 8306
Ted R Montoya Hemophilia Program University of New Mexico, 4987
University of New Mexico General Clinical Research Center, 3325
University of New Mexico: Cancer Research and Treatment Center, 2265
University of New Mexico: Center for Non-Invasive Diagnosis, 2266
Veterans Adm. Medical Center: Albuquerque New Mexico VA Health Care System, 10282

New York

AARP New York State Office: Albany, 60
AARP New York State Office: New York City, 61
AFB Toll-Free Hotline, 9874
AIDS Hotline of Central New York, 375
AIDS Treatment Data Network, 178
ALS Association: Greater New York Chapter, 1024
ALS Association: Upstate New York CIO, 1025
Aaron Diamond AIDS Research Center, 351
Access Unlimited, 10454
Ackerman Institute for the Family, 2267
Aging In America/Morningside House Nursing, 78
Albany Medical College Joint Center for Cancer and Blood Disorders, 2268
Albany Medical College Pediatric Pulmonary & Cystic Fibrosis Center, 3071
Albany Medican Center, 4940
Albert Einstein Cancer Center Albert Einstein College of Medicine, 2269
Alcoholics Anonymous General Service Office/Grand Central Sta, 8228
Alcoholics Anonymous World Services, 8373
Aleh Foundation Aleh Institustions USA, 3467
Alliance for Lupus Research, 5929
Alzheimer's Association: Central New York Chapter, 773
Alzheimer's Association: Hudson Valley/ Rockland/Westchester NY Chapter, 774
Alzheimer's Association: Long Island Chapter, 775
Alzheimer's Association: New York City Chapter, 776
Alzheimer's Association: Northeastern New York Chapter, 777
Alzheimer's Association: Putnam County Chapter, 778
Alzheimer's Association: Rochester Chapter, 779
Alzheimer's Association: Southern Tier Chapter, 780
Alzheimer's Association: Sullivan/Delaware Chapter, 772
Alzheimer's Association: Western New York Chapter, 781
Alzheimer's Foundation of Staten Island, 782
American Cancer Society: Central New York Region/East Syracuse, 2137
American Cancer Society: Long Island, 2138
American Cancer Society: New York City, 2139
American Cancer Society: Queens Region / Rego Park, 2140
American Cancer Society: Westchester Region/White Plains, 2141
American Civil Liberties Union AIDS Project, 186
American Council for Drug Education, 8229
American Diabetes Association: New York, 3233
American Fertility Association, 5318
American Foundation for AIDS Research, 188
American Foundation for The Blind, 10462
American Foundation for the Blind, 9452
American Foundation for the Blind Information Center, 9875
American Foundation for the Blind: National Employment Center, 9453
American Foundation for the Prevention of Venereal Disease, 7659
American Hepatitis Association, 5067
American Liver Foundation, 5672
American Liver Foundation, 10439
American Liver Foundation Greater New York Chapter, 5700

American Liver Foundation Western New York Chapter, 5701
American Lung Association of Mid New York, 9316
American Lung Association of New York State, 5798
American Parkinson Disease Association, 6954
American Parkinson Disease Association Hotline, 7012
American Skin Association, 6939
American Society of Hypertension, 5185
Armond V Mascia Cystic Fibrosis Center NY Medical College, 3072
Arthritis Foundation: Central New York Chapter, 1123
Arthritis Foundation: Long Island Chapter, 1124
Arthritis Foundation: New York Chapter, 1125
Arthritis Foundation: Rockland/Orange Unit, 1126
Association for Behavioral and Cognitive Therapies, 7130
Association for Children with Down Syndrome, 3493
Association for Macular Diseases, 9459
Association for Research of Childhood Cancer, 2016
Association for Research of Childhood Cancer, 2270
Association for the Blind & Visually Impaired Greater Rochester, 9598
Association of Cancer Online Resources, 5674
Aurora of Central New York, 4334
Aurora of Central New York, 9876
Autism Society of Albany, 1621
Bassett Research Institute, 2271
Blind Association of Western New York, 9599
Blind Work Association, 9600
Bone Marrow Foundation, 2018
Brady Institute Jamaica Hospital Medical Center, 4051
Braille Textbook Assignment Service National Braille Association, 9845
Brain & Behavior Research Foundation, 6266
Brain Injury Association of New York State, 4031
Brain Injury Association of New York State Helpline, 4094
Brain Trauma Foundation, 4050
Brain Tumor Support Group for Patients and Families, 1922
Brain Tumor Support Group: Long Island, 1923
Brooklyn Campus of the VA NY Harbor Health care System, 10283
CCFA Camps Across America Crohn's & Colitis Foundation of America, 2920
CCFA Greater New York Chapter: National Headquarters, 2948
CCFA Long Island Chapter, 2949
CCFA Rochester/Southern Tier Chapter, 2950
CCFA Upstate/Northeastern New York Chapter, 2951
CCFA Western New York Chapter, 2952
CF & Pediatric Pulmonary Care Center, 3073
COMPASS Program, 380
COPIN Foundation, 10388
CUNY: Teratogen Information Service, 1773
Cafe Plus, 4095
Camp Good Days, 10767
Cancer Institute of Brooklyn, 2272
Cancer Research Institute: New York, 2273
CancerCare, 2024
Canine Helpers for the Disabled, 9463
Capital Regional Sleep-Wake Disorders Center, 7869
Center for Donation & Transplantation, 9228
Center for Hearing and Communication, 4276
Center for Medical Consumers, 10479
Center for Medical Consumers, 10625
Center for Rheumatology, 7446
Center for Sleep Medicine of the Mount Sinai Medical Center, 7873
Center for the Disabled, 2675
Center for the Study of Aging, 80
Center for the Study of Anorexia and Bulimia, 3634
Center on Employment: Rochester Institute of Technology, 4223
Centers for AIDS Research: Albert Einstein College of Medicine, 352
Centers for AIDS Research: Columbia University College of Physicians, 353
Centers for AIDS Research: NYU School of Medicine, 354
Central Association for the Blind and Visually Impaired, 9601

Central NY Area Support Group: National Ataxia Foundation, 1473
Central New York Male Sexual Dysfunction Center, 5242
Central Texas Brain Tumor Support Group, 1950
Cerebral Palsy Associations of New York State, 2676
Chemotherapy Foundation, 2191
Children's Brain Tumor Foundation, 1830
Children's Mental Health Coalition of WNY, Inc., 6062
Children's Tumor Foundation, 6736
Children's Tumor Foundation, 6767
Childrens Lung and Cystic Fibrosis Center, 3074
Choice Magazine Listening, 9791
City University of New York Center for Research in Speech and Hearing, 4297
Client Assistance Program: NY State Commission of Quality of Care, 10584
Columbia Presbyterian Medical Center Neurological Institute, 6593
Columbia University Center for Geriatrics Gerontology, 81
Columbia University Clinical Research Center for Muscular Dystrophy, 6594
Columbia University Comprehensive Cancer Center, 2274
Columbia University Irving Center for Clinical Research Adult Unit, 4799
Columbia University: Comprehensive Sickle Cell Center, 7710
Community Access, 5980
Cooley's Anemia Foundation (CAF): Buffalo, 2892
Cooley's Anemia Foundation (CAF): Long Island, 2893
Cooley's Anemia Foundation (CAF): Queens, 2894
Cooley's Anemia Foundation (CAF): Staten Island, 2895
Cooley's Anemia Foundation (CAF): Suffolk Chapter Office, 2896
Cooley's Anemia Foundation (CAF): Westches ter/Rockland Chapter, 2897
Cooleys Anemia Foundation, 2899
Cornell University: Winifred Masterson Burke Medical Research-Dementia, 867
Cornerstone Medical Arts Center Hospital, 8333
Corporate Angel Network, 2327
Crohn's & Colitis Foundation of America, 2921
Crohn's & Colitis Foundation of America, 9420
Crohn's & Colitis Foundation of America Hotline, 2969
Cystic Fibrosis Center St. Vincent's Hospital & Medical Center, 3075
Dana Alliance for Brain Initiatives, 4052
Deaf Artists of America, 4227
Deafness Research Foundation, 4229
Developmental Evaluation Clinic, 3508
Disabled & Alone: Life Services for the Handicapped, 10487
Division of Digestive & Liver Diseases of Cloumbia University, 3635
Division of Substance Abuse Services, 8307
Drugs Anonymous, 8240
ENCORE YWCA-National Board, 2028
Eastern Paralyzed Veterans Association of America, 8066
Eating Disorder Resource Center, 3641
Educational Equity Center at The Academy for Educational Development, 10489
Endocrinology Research Laboratory Cabrini Medical Center, 3311
Epilepsy Foundation of Long Island, 7574
Families Together in New York State, 6063
Feingold Association of the US, 1526
Fertility Research Foundation, 3719
Fertility Research Foundation, 5372
Fibromyalgia Resources Group, 3785
Fight for Sight, 9468
Finger Lakes Donor Recovery Network, 9229
First Presbyterian Church in the City of New York Support Groups, 3643
Foundation for Advancement in Cancer Therapy, 2142
Freedom From Fear, 7133
Friends of Karen, 10774

Reach Out for Youth with Ileitis and Colitis, 2926
Reach Out for Youth with Ileitis and Colitis, 9422
Reader-Transcriber Registry National Braille
    Association, 9864
Region II Office Program: Consultants for Maternal
    and Child Health, 8909
Regional Bone Center Helen Hayes Hospital, 6900
Rehabilitation International, 10538
Remove Intoxicated Drivers (RID-USA), 8264
Renfrew Center of New York, 3626
Research Institute on Alcoholism State University of
    New York at Buffalo, 8353
Research to Prevent Blindness, 9515
Rochester Institute of Technology: Nationa l
    Technical Institute for the Deaf, 4313
Rockefeller University Laboratory for Investigative
    Dermatology, 7773
Rockefeller University Laboratory of Biology, 8354
Rockefeller University Laboratory of Cardiac
    Physiology, 4821
Rockefeller University, Laboratory for Investigative
    Dermatology, 7774
Roswell Park Cancer Institute National Cancer
    Institute, 2278
SLE Foundation, 5904
SLE Lupus Foundation, 5928
SUNY Health Science Center at Brooklyn Sickle Cell
    Center, 7715
SUNY at Buffalo National Cooperative Drug
    Discovery Group for AIDS Treatment, 358
Sarcoidosis HelpNet, 7331
Sarcoidosis Self-Help Group: New York, 7333
Schneeweiss Adult Congenital Heart Disease Center,
    2876
Scleroderma Clinical & Research Center State
    University of New York at Stonybro, 7451
Scleroderma Foundation: Tri-State Chapter, 7432
Scleroderma Foundation: Western New York Chapter,
    7433
Skin Cancer Foundation, 2045
Sleep Center: Community General Hospital, 7887
Sleep Disorders Center Columbia Presbyterian
    Medical Center, 7889
Sleep Disorders Center of Rochester: St. Mary's
    Hospital, 7896
Sleep Disorders Center of Western New York Millard
    Fillmore Hospital, 7897
Sleep Disorders Center: University Hospital, SUNY
    at Stony Brook, 7907
Sleep Disorders Center: Winthrop, University
    Hospital, 7908
Sleep Laboratory St Joseph's Hospital, 7910
Sleep Wake Disorders Center Montefiore Sleep
    Disorders Center, 7914
Sleep-Wake Disorders Center: New York
    Hospital-Cornell Medical Center, 7916
Southern Tier Association for the Visually Impaired,
    9604
Southern Tier Hemophilia Center United Health
    Services-Wilson Hospital, 4985
Spellman Center for HIV Related Disease The
    Spellman Center, 359
Spina Bifida Association of Albany/Capital District,
    7998
Spina Bifida Association of Greater Rochester, 7999
Spina Bifida Association of Nassau County, 8000
St. Agnes Hospital Medical: Health Science Library,
    6506
St. John's Episcopal Hospital, 7015
State University College at Fredonia Youngerman
    Clinic, 4316
State University College at Plattsburgh Auditory
    Research Laboratory, 4317
State University of NY Hospital: Upstate Medical
    Center, 3077
State University of New York At Stony Brook:
    Mental Health Research, 6108
State University of New York Health Science Center
    At Brooklyn, 2279
State University of New York Health Sciences Center,
    1647
State University of New York at Buffalo Toxicology
    Research Center, 8360
State University of New York: SUNY Stony HIV
    Treatment Development Center, 360

Suffolk Cooperative Library System, 9795
Support for Asthmatic Youth, 1322
Support for People with Oral and Head and Neck
    Cancer, 2046
Syracuse University Institute for Sensory Research,
    4318
Taub Institute for Research on Alzheimers Disease
    and the Aging Brain, 880
The Coalition of Behavioral Health Agencies, 5994
The Dana Foundation, 7185
Tick-Borne Disease Alliance, 9049
Tourette Syndrome Association, 9103
Tri-State Area Support Group: National Ataxia
    Foundation, 1475
Turner Syndrome Support Group of Central New
    York, 9385
Turner's Syndrome Society New York - Metro, 9386
UNICEF USA, 235
United Cerebral Palsy of Chemung County, 2679
United Cerebral Palsy of Fulton & Montgomery
    Counties, 2680
United Cerebral Palsy of Greater Suffolk, 2681
United Cerebral Palsy of Nassau County, 2682
United Cerebral Palsy of New York City, 2683
United Cerebral Palsy of Putnam & Southern
    Dutchess Counties, 2684
United Cerebral Palsy of Queens: Queens Centers for
    Progress, 2685
United Cerebral Palsy of Westchester County, 2686
United Cerebral Palsy of Western New York, 2687
United Cerebral Palsy of the North Country, 2688
University of Rochester, 7016
University of Rochester: Clinical Research Center,
    4835
University of Rochester: James P Wilmot Cancer
    Center, 2280
University of Rochester: Nephrology Research
    Program, 5610
Upstate NY Chapter of the Myasthenia Gravis
    Foundation of America, 6672
Upstate New York Transplant Services, Inc., 9231
VA Helathcare Network: Upstate New York, 10286
VA NY/NJ Veterans Healthcare Network, 10287
Veterans Adm. Medical Center: Albany Samuel S.
    Stratton: VA Medical Center, 10288
Veterans Adm. Medical Center: Batavia VA Western
    New York Healthcare System, 10289
Veterans Adm. Medical Center: Bath Bath VA
    Medical Center, 10290
Veterans Adm. Medical Center: Buffalo, 10291
Veterans Adm. Medical Center: Montrose Franklin
    Delano Roosevelt Campus, 10292
Veterans Adm. Medical Center: New York New York
    Campus, 10293
Veterans Adm. Medical Center: Northport Northport
    VA Medical Center, 10294
Veterans Adm. Medical Center: Syracuse Syracuse
    VA Medical Center, 10295
Veterans Affairs Medical Center Canandaigua, 10296
WE MOVE, 6962
WNYS Center for SIDS, 8910
Wainwright House Cancer Support Programs, 2344
Wallace Memorial Library, 4293
Westchester Task Force on Eating
    Disorders/American Anorexia Bulimia, 3627
Xavier Society for the Blind, 9796
Yeshiva University General Clinical Research Center,
    4843
Yeshiva University Marion Bessin Liver Research
    Center, 5713
Yeshiva University: Institute of Communication
    Disorders, 4333
Yeshiva University: Resnick Gerontology Center, 889
Yeshiva University: Soundview-Throgs Neck
    Community Mental Health Center, 6116

North Carolina

AARP North Carolina State Office: Raleigh, 62
ALS Association: Jim (Catfish) Hunter Chapter, 1031
Alcohol and Drug Abuse Section, 8308
Alzheimer's Association: Eastern North Carolina
    Chapter, 783

Alzheimer's Association: Western North Car olina
    Chapter, 784
Alzheimer's Disease Research Center Duke
    University, 865
American Cancer Society: North Carolina, 2150
American Diabetes Association: North Carolina, 3242
American Lung Association of North Carolina, 5799
American Lung Association of North Carolina, 9317
American Social Health Association, 7660
Arthritis Foundation: Carolinas Chapter, 1127
Autism Society of North Carolina, 1622
Beginnings for Parents of Children Who are Deaf or
    Hard of Hearing, 4335
Bowman Gray School of Medicine, 8170
Bowman Grey School of Medicine: Hemophilia
    Diagnostic Center, 4944
Brain Injury Association of North Carolina, 4033
Brain Injury Association of North Carolina Helpline,
    4097
Brain Tumor Support Group: Raleigh Area, 1927
CCFA Carolinas Chapter, 2953
CCFA South Carolina Chapter, 2954
Cancer Center of Wake Forest University at Bowman
    Gray School of Medicine, 2281
Carolinas Chapter of the Myasthenia Gravis
    Foundation of America, 6673
Carolinas Chapter of the Myasthenia Gravis
    Foundation of America, 6677
Center for Universal Design North Carolina State
    University, 10480
Centers for AIDS Research: Univeristy of North
    Carolina at Chapel Hill, 361
Charles George Veterans Affairs Medical Center,
    10297
Chronic Syndrome Support Association, 7100
Cleft Palate Foundation, 1751
Comprehensive Hemophilia Diagnostic and
    Treatment Center, 4948
Department of Pediatrics, Division of Rheumatology,
    1150
Desert Storm Veterans of North Carolina, 10298
Division TEACCH University of North Carolina at
    Chapel H, 1643
Dorothea Dix Hospital Clinical Research Unit, 8335
Duke Asthma, Allergy and Airway Center, 1312
Duke Comprehensive Cancer Center, 2282
Duke Pediatric Brain Tumor Family Support
    Program, 1928
Duke University Center for the Advanced Study of
    Epilepsy, 7580
Duke University Center for the Study of Aging and
    Human Development, 868
Duke University Clinical Research Institute, 869
Duke University Pediatric Cardiac Catheterization
    Laboratory, 4802
Duke University Plastic Surgery Research
    Laboratories, 7768
Easter Seals UCP North Carolina & Virginia, 2689
Families in Action National Drug Abuse Center, 8337
Hemophilia Foundation of North Carolina, 4919
Herpes Resource Center, 7664
Herpes Resource Center, 7666
International Federation of Spine Associations, 7485
Juvenile Diabetes Research Foundation: Cha rlotte
    Chapter, 3244
Juvenile Diabetes Research Foundation: Pie dmont
    Triad Chapter, 3245
Juvenile Diabetes Research Foundation:
    Triangle/Eastern North Carolina Chapter, 3243
Leukemia and Lymphoma Society: Eastern North
    Carolina Chapter, 2151
Leukemia and Lymphoma Society: North Carolina
    Chapter, 2152
Life Share of the Carolinas, 9232
Lions Industries for the Blind, 9605
Lupus Foundation of America: North Carolin a
    Chapter, 5906
Lupus Foundation of America: Winston-Triad Lupus
    Chapter NCLF, 5905
Myasthenia Gravis Support Group of Central North
    Carolina, 6701
Myasthenia Gravis Support Group of Charlotte, 6700
Myasthenia Gravis Support Group of Durham/
    Chapel Hill, 6702

North Dakota

Ohio

National Association of Blind Office Professionals, 9489

National Federation of the Blind: Ohio, 9612

National Kidney Foundation of Ohio, 5579

National MS Soceity: Western Ohio Chapter The Woolpert Building, 6478

National MS Society: Northeast Ohio Chapter, 6480

National MS Society: Northwest Ohio Chapter, 6481

National MS Society: Southwestern Ohio/Northern Kentucky, 6479

National Reye's Syndrome Foundation, 5717

North East Ohio Support Group National Ataxia Foundation, 1477

Northern Ohio Chapter of the National Hemophilia Foundation, 4921

Northwest Ohio Hemophilia Association, 4922

Northwest Ohio Hemophilia Treatment Center, 4978

Northwest Ohio Sleep Disorders Center Toledo Hospital, 7881

Ohio Alliance for the Mentally Ill, 6069

Ohio Ambassador: National Ataxia Foundation, 1478

Ohio Department of Health, 8915

Ohio Department of Health: Division of Preventive Medicine, 284

Ohio Regional Library for the Blind and Physically Handicapped, 9801

Ohio Sleep Medicine Institute, 7882

Ohio State University Clinical Pharmacology Division, 8351

Ohio State University Comprehensive Cancer Center, 2287

Ohio State University General Clinical Research Center, 2288

Ohio State University Laboratory of Psychobiology, 4055

Ohio State University Neuroscience Program, 879

Ohio State University Otological Research Laboratories, 4307

Ohio University Therapy Associates: Hearing, Speech and Language Clinic, 4308

Ohio Valley LifeCenter, 9236

Pediatric Pulmonary Center The Children's Medical Center of Dayton, 3084

Persian Gulf War Veterans of Western Pennsylvania, W Virginia and NE Ohio, 10304

Prader-Willi Ohio Association, 7275

RESOLVE of Ohio, 5355

Rainbow Alliance of the Deaf, 4251

Richland County HPV Support Group, 10590

SIDS Network of Ohio, 8916

Scleroderma Foundation: Ohio Chapter, 7434

Sleep Disorders Center Bethesda Oak Hospital, 7888

Sleep Disorders Center Ohio State University Medical Center, 7892

Sleep Disorders Center: Cleveland Clinic Foundation, 7898

Sleep Disorders Center: Kettering Medical Center, 7902

Sleep Disorders Center: St. Vincent Medical Center, 7906

Southwest Ohio Brain Tumor Support Group, 1931

Southwestern Ohio Chapter of the National Hemophilia Foundation, 4923

Special Wish Foundation, 10786

Spina Bifida Association of Canton, 8002

Spina Bifida Association of Central Ohio, 8003

Spina Bifida Association of Cincinnati, 8004

Spina Bifida Association of Greater Dayton, 8005

Spina Bifida Association of Northwest Ohio, 8006

State Library of Ohio Talking Book Program, 9802

Support Group for Parents of Children with Brain Tumors, 1932

Technology Resource Center, 10591

The Cancer Prevention Institute, 2289

Turner Syndrome Chapter of Ohio, 9388

United Cerebral Palsy of Central Ohio, 2690

United Cerebral Palsy of Cincinnati, 2691

United Cerebral Palsy of Greater Cleveland, 2692

United Cerebral Palsy of Greater Dane, 2693

University Alzheimer Center UHC: Case Western Reserve University, 884

University Treatment Center of University Hospitals of Cleveland, 4995

University of Cincinnati Adult Hemophilia Treatment Program, 4996

University of Cincinnati College of Medicine Division of Pediatrics, 3085

University of Cincinnati Department of Pathology & Laboratory Medicine, 4828

VA Healthcare System Of Ohio, 10305

Veterans Adm. Medical Center: Chillicothe Chillicothe VA Medical Center, 10306

Veterans Adm. Medical Center: Cincinnati Cincinnati VA Medical Center, 10307

Veterans Adm. Medical Center: Cleveland Louis Stokes VA Medical Center, 10308

Veterans Adm. Medical Center: Dayton Dayton VA Medical Center, 10309

Veterans and Families Support Network Ohio, 10310

West Central Ohio Hemophilia Center Childens Medical Center, 4999

World Hypertension League, 5135

Oklahoma

AARP Oklahoma State Office: Edmond, 65

Alzheimer's Association: Oklahoma Chapter, 795

American Association of Kidney Patients: Tulsa Chapter, 5580

American Cancer Society: Oklahoma, 2158

American Diabetes Association: Oklahoma, 3254

American Lung Association of Oklahoma, 5802

American Lung Association of Oklahoma, 9320

American Veterans Justice Foundation, 10311

Arthritis Foundation: Oklahoma Chapter, 1133

Autism Society of Central Oklahoma, 1626

Brain Injury Association of Oklahoma, 4035

Brain Injury Association of Oklahoma Helpl ine, 4100

CCFA Oklahoma Chapter, 2958

Client Assistance Program: Oklahoma Office of Handicapped Concerns, 10592

Dean A McGee Eye Institute, 9849

Jack C. Montgomery VA Medical Center, 10312

Juvenile Diabetes Research Foundation: Cen tral Oklahoma Chapter, 3255

Juvenile Diabetes Research Foundation: Tul sa Green County Chapter, 3256

Leukemia and Lymphoma Society: Oklahoma Chapter, 2159

Myasthenia Gravis Support Group of Tulsa and Oklahoma City, 6706

Natalie Warren Bryant Cancer Center St. Francis Hospital, 2290

National Federation of the Blind: Oklahoma, 9613

National Kidney Foundation of Oklahoma, 5581

National MS Society: Oklahoma Chapter, 6482

Neuroscience Institute at Mercy Hospital, 6773

Oklahoma Alliance for the Mentally Ill, 6070

Oklahoma Ambassador: National Ataxia Foundation, 1479

Oklahoma Association of the Deaf, 4280

Oklahoma Chapter of the Myasthenia Gravis Foundation of America, 6674

Oklahoma Chapter of the National Hemophilia Foundation, 4924

Oklahoma City HPV Support Group: PP of Cen tral Oklahoma, 10593

Oklahoma Comprehensive Hemophilia Diagnostic Treatment Center, 4979

Oklahoma Department of Health: AIDS Division, 285

Oklahoma Department of Mental Health and Substance Abuse Services, 8312

Oklahoma League for the Blind, 9614

Oklahoma Library for the Blind and Physically Handicapped, 9803

Oklahoma Lupus Association, 5908

Oklahoma Medical Research Foundation, 1155

Oklahoma Medical Research Foundation Immunobiolgy & Cancer Research, 2291

Oklahoma Medical Research Foundation: Cardiovascular Research Program, 4817

Oklahoma Organ Sharing Network, 9237

Oklahoma State Department of Health: Maternal and Child Health Services, 8917

Parkinson Foundation of the Heartland Oklahoma Branch, 6989

Prader-Willi Oklahoma Association, 7276

RESOLVE of Oklahoma, 5356

Samuel Roberts Noble Foundation Biomedical Division, 2292

Tulsa City: County Library System, 9804

Tulsa Unified FFCMH, 6071

Turner Syndrome Chapter of Oklahoma, 9389

United Cerebral Palsy of Oklahoma, 2694

University of California Northern Comprehensive Sickle Cell Center, 7718

University of Oklahoma: Cystic Fibrosis Center, 3086

University of Oklahoma: Health Sciences Ce nter, 4330

Veterans Adm. Medical Center: Oklahoma City, 10313

Oregon

AARP Oregon State Office: Clackamas, 66

ALS Association: Oregon & SW Washington CIO, 1028

ALS Association: Oregon & SW Washington CIO, 1037

Aging and Alzheimer's Disease Center Oregon Health Sciences University, 854

Alzheimer's Association: Cascade/Coast Chapter, 797

Alzheimer's Association: Columbia-Willamet Chapter, 796

Alzheimer's Association: Mary's Peak Chapter, 798

Alzheimer's Association: Mid-Willamette Chapter, 799

American Cancer Society: Oregon, 2160

American Diabetes Association: Oregon, 3257

American Lung Association of Oregon, 5803

American Lung Association of Oregon, 9321

American Tinnitus Association, 4217

Asthma and Allergy Foundation of America: Oregon Chapter, 591

Asthma and Allergy Foundation of America: Oregon Chapter, 1304

Autism Society of Oregon, 1627

Blind Enterprises of Oregon, 9615

Brain Injury Alliance of Oregon, 4101

Brain Injury Association of Oregon, 4036

Brain Tumor Education & Support Group, 1933

Cascade AIDS Project Hotline, 381

Center for Health Research, 10478

Central Oregon Brain Tumor Support Group, 1934

Child Center, 10481

Comprehensive Stroke Center of Oregon University of Oregon Health Sciences Cen, 8172

Dogs for the Deaf, 4231

Fanconi Anemia Research Foundation, 2884

Hemophilia Foundation of Oregon, 4925

Juvenile Diabetes Research Foundation: Ore gon/SW Washington Chapter, 3258

Leukemia and Lymphoma Society: Oregon Chapter, 2161

NAMI-Oregon, 6072

NNFF Oregon Affiliate Kaiser Permanente Northwest, 6764

National Consortium on Deaf-Blindness, 4246

National Federation of the Blind: Oregon, 9616

National MS Society: Oregon Chapter, 6483

National Psoriasis Foundation, 7766

Northwest Network, 10314

Northwest Vets for Peace, 10315

Office of Alcohol and Drug Abuse Programs, 8313

Oregon Association of the Deaf, 4281

Oregon Department of Human Resources Health Division HIV Program, 286

Oregon Department of Human Services, 8918

Oregon Family Support Network, 6073

Oregon Health & Science University, 3087

Oregon Health Sciences University, 7017

Oregon Health Sciences University Oregon Hearing Research Center Tinnitus Clinic, 4309

Oregon Health Sciences University: Elk's Children's Eye Clinic, 9863

Oregon State Library, 9805

Pacific NW Transplant Bank, 9238

Parkinsons Resources of Oregon, 6990

Prader-Willi Oregon Association, 7277

Psoriasis Research Institute, 7772

RESOLVE of Oregon, 5357

Regional Resource Center on Deafness Western Oregon State College, 4310

Resources for Seniors and People with Disabilities, 10594

Sarcoid Networking Association, 7322

Scleroderma Foundation: Oregon Chapter, 7435

United Cerebral Palsy of Oregon & SW Washington, 2695

Veterans Adm. Medical Center: Roseburg VA Roseburg Healthcare System, 10316

Veterans Adm. Medical Center: White City VA S Oregon Rehabilitation Center, 10317

Veterans Adm. Regional Office: Portland Portland VA Medical Center, 10318

Veterans Administration Domicillary, 10319

Willamette Valley Support Group: National Ataxia Foundation, 1480

Pennsylvania

AARP Pennsylvania State Office: Harrisburg, 67

AIDS Library of Philadelphia, 304

ALS Association: Greater Philadelphia Chapter, 1029

ALS Association: Western Pennsylvania Chapter, 1030

ALS Clinic at Penn Neurological Institute ALS Association Greater Philadelphia Cha, 1040

Abramson Cancer Center of the University of Pennsylvania, 2293

Adult Congenital Heart Association, 2873

Albert Einstein Medical Center Hemophilia Program, 4941

Allegheny Singer Research Institute West Penn Allegheny Health System, 2294

Alzheimer's Association: Delaware Valley Chapter, 800

Alzheimer's Association: Greater Mid-Ohio, 802

Alzheimer's Association: Greater Pennsylvania Chapter: SW Regional Office, 801

Alzheimer's Association: Laurel Mountains Chapter, 803

Alzheimer's Association: Northeast Pennsylvania Chapter, 804

Alzheimer's Association: Northwest Pennsylvania Chapter, 805

Alzheimer's Association: South Central Pennsylvania Chapter, 806

Alzheimer's Disease Center Pennsylvania University School of Medicine, 858

American Anorexia Bulimia Association of Philadelphia, 3629

American Cancer Society: Harrisburg Capital Area Unit, 2162

American Cancer Society: Philadelphia, 2163

American Cancer Society: Pittsburgh, 2164

American Diabetes Association: Pennsylvania, 3259

American Diabetes Association: Western Pennsylvania, 3260

American Liver Foundation Delaware Valley Chapter, 5703

American Liver Foundation Western Pennsylv ania, 5704

American Lung Association of Pennsylvania, 9322

American Respiratory Alliance of Western Pennsylvania, 5804

Arthritis Foundation: Central Pennsylvania Chapter, 1134

Associated Services for the Blind, 9458

Association for the Blind & Visually Impaired of Lehigh County, 9617

Association of Hydrocephalus Education Advocacy & Discussion (AHEAD), 5127

Autism Society of Greater Harrisburg, 1628

Beaver County Association for the Blind, 9618

Bockus Research Institute Graduate Hospital, 4794

Brain Injury Association of Pennsylvania, 4037

Brain Tumor Community Group, 1935

Brain Tumor Support Group: Johnstown, 1936

Brain Tumor Support Group: Philadelphia, 1937

Brain Tumor Support Group: Pittsburgh, 1938

Breathe Pennsylvania, 5805

Burger King Cancer Caring Center, 2021

CCFA Philadelphia/Delaware Valley Chapter, 2959

CCFA Western Pennsylvania/West Virginia Chapter, 2960

Cambria County Association for the Blind and Handicapped, 9619

Carnegie Library of Pittsburgh, 9806

Center for Organ Recovery & Education, 9239

Centers for AIDS Research: University of Pennsylvania, 363

Chemical People Project Public Television Outreach Alliance, 8237

Chester County Association for the Blind, 9620

Children of Aging Parents, 88

Children's Hospital of Philadelphia, 3505

Childrens Hospital of Philadelphia Hemophilia Program, 4946

Client Assistance Program: Philadelphia, 10595

Cystic Fibrosis Center: Polyclinic Medical Center, 3088

Delaware County Branch of the Pennsylvania Association for the Blind, 9621

Delaware Valley Chapter of the National Hemophilia Foundation, 4926

Delware Valley Brain Tumor Support Group at Jefferson, 1939

Department of Reproductive Genetics: Magee Women's Hospital, 1761

Diabetes Education and Research Center The Franklin House, 3308

Dial-a-Hearing Screening Test, 4338

Down Syndrome Center of Western Pennsylvania, 3510

Dr. Gertrude A Barber National Institute, 3512

Dream Come True, 10770

Drug and Alcohol Programs Department Of Health, 8314

Eastern Cooperative Oncology Group, 2295

Epilepsy Foundation of Western Pennsylvania, 7576

Erie VA Medical Center, 10320

Foundation for Children with AIDS, 205

Foundation for Dignity, 2029

Fox Chase Cancer Center, 2296

Free Library of Philadelphia, 9807

Geisinger Wyoming Valley Medical Center: Sleep Disorders Center, 7874

Gift of Life Donor Program Pennsylvania, 9240

Greater Wilkes-Barre Association for the Blind, 9622

Hahnemann University Hospital, Orthopedic Wellness Center, 1151

Hahnemann University Laboratory of Human Pharmacology, 8339

Hahnemann University Likoff Cardiovascular Institute, 4807

Hahnemann University Lupus Study Center Hahnemann University Medical Center, 5930

Hahnemann University, Krancer Center for Inflammatory Bowel Disease Research, 2968

Hahnemann University: Division of Surgical Research, 5192

Hemophilia Center of Central Pennsylvania Penn State Milton S Hershey Medical Cent, 4959

Hepatitis B Foundation, 5074

Hepatitis B Foundation, 10442

Hopes & Dreams Foundation, Inc., 10777

Hospital of the University of Pennsylvania, 8174

Hospital of the University of Pennsylvania University of Pennsylvania, 6595

Hydrocephalus Association of Philadelphia, 5138

Hysterectomy Educational Resources & Services (HERS) Foundation, 3716

Hysterectomy Educational Resources & Services (HERS) Foundation, 5320

Independent Visually Impaired Enterprises, 9476

Indiana County Association for the Blind, 9623

Intestinal Disease Foundation, 5274

Juvenile Diabetes Research Foundation: Ber ks County Chapter, 3262

Juvenile Diabetes Research Foundation: Central Pennsylvania Chapter, 3261

Juvenile Diabetes Research Foundation: Nor thwestern Pennsylvania Chapter, 3263

Juvenile Diabetes Research Foundation: Phi ladelphia Chapter, 3264

Juvenile Diabetes Research Foundation: Wes tern Pennsylvania, 3265

Keystone Blind Association, 9624

Lancaster County Association for the Blind, 9625

Learning Disabilities Association of America, 1527

Learning Disabilities Association of America, 10502

Lehigh Valley Chapter of the American Association of Kidney Patients, 5582

Lehigh Valley Sickle Cell Support Group, 7723

Leukemia and Lymphoma Society: Central Pennsylvania Chapter, 2165

Leukemia and Lymphoma Society: Eastern Pennsylvania Chapter, 2166

Leukemia and Lymphoma Society: Western Pennsylvania/West Virginia Chapter, 2167

Lupus Foundation of America: Central Pennsylvania Chapter, 5909

Lupus Foundation of America: Northeast Pennsylvania Chapter, 5910

Lupus Foundation of America: Northwestern Pennsylvania Chapter, 5911

Lupus Foundation of America: Western Pennsylvania Chapter, 5912

Lupus Foundation of Philadelphia, 5913

Lysosomal Disease Center at the University of Pittsburgh, 3758

MedEscort International ABE International Airport, 10507

Medical College of Pennsylvania Center for the Mature Woman, 6898

Medical College of Pennsylvania: Eastern Psychiatric Institute, 6104

Montgomery County Association for the Blind, 9626

Myasthenia Gravis Support Group of Scranto n, 6707

National Federation of the Blind: Pennsylvania, 9627

National Kidney Foundation of Delaware Valley, 5583

National Kidney Foundation of Western Pennsylvania, 5584

National MS Society: Central Pennsylvania Chapter, 6484

National MS Society: Greater Delaware Valley Chapter, 6485

National Mental Health Consumer's Self-Help Clearinghouse, 6098

National Mental Health Consumers' Self- Help Clearinghouse, 6099

National Organization for Hearing Research, 4250

National Sexual Violence Resource Center, 7162

National Tay-Sachs Association: Delaware Valley (NTSAD-DV), 8992

National Transplant Assistance Fund (NTAF), 9194

North American Society for Pediatric Gastroenterology and Nutrition, 3853

North American Society for Pediatric Gastroenterology, Hepatology & Nutrition, 10529

North Central Sight Services, 9628

Parents Involved Network, 6074

Parkinson Chapter of Greater Pittsburgh, 6991

Parkinson Council, 6992

Pediatric Cancer Foundation of the Lehigh Valley, 1940

Pediatric Pulmonary and Cystic Fibrosis Center, 3089

Penn Center for Sleep Disorders: Hospital of the University of Pennsylvania, 7883

Pennsylvania Alliance for the Mentally Ill, 6075

Pennsylvania Department of Health Bureau of Family Health, 8919

Pennsylvania Department of Health: Bureau of HIV/AIDS, 287

Pennsylvania Educational Network for Eating Disorders, 3630

Pennsylvania Gulf War Veterans, 10321

Pennsylvania State University Artificial Heart Research Project, 4818

Philadelphia Biomedical Research Institute, 7714

Philadelphia Department of Public Health: AIDS Program, 288

Philadelphia Turner Syndrom Society, 9390

Pittsburgh Vision Services, 9629

Prader-Willi Pennsylvania Association, 7278

Pregnancy Healthline: Pennsylvania Hospital, 1782

Pregnancy Safety Hotline, 1784

Presbyterian-University Hospital: Pulmonary Sleep Evaluation Center, 7884

RESOLVE of Philadelphia, 5358

RESOLVE of Pittsburgh, 5359

RESOLVE of Southcentral Pennsylvania, 5360

Recorded Periodicals, 9886
Renfrew Center of Bryn Mawr, 3631
Renfrew Center of Philadelphia, 3632
SIDS of Pennsylvania, 8920
SW Pennsylvania Turner Syndrome Support Gr oup, 9391
Sarcoidosis Treatment and Research Center Thomas Jefferson University Hospital, 7324
Scleroderma Foundation: Western Pennsylvania Chapter, 7436
Shriners Hospital for Children, 8092
Sickle Cell Disease Association of America Philadelphia/Delaware Valley Chapter, 7726
Sleep Disorders Center Lankenau Hospital, 7891
Sleep Disorders Center: Community Medical Center, 7899
Sleep Disorders Center: Crozer-Chester Medical Center, 7900
Sleep Disorders Center: Good Samaritan Medical Center, 7901
Sleep Disorders Center: Medical College of Pennsylvania, 7903
Sleep and Chronobiology Center: Western Psychiatric Institute and Clinic, 7915
Somerset County Blind Center, 9630
Spina Bifida Association of Central Pennsylvania, 8007
Spina Bifida Association of Delaware Valley, 8008
Spina Bifida Association of Greater Pennsylvania, 8009
Spinal Cord Injury Program at Harmarville Rehabilitation Center, 8093
Sunshine Foundation National Headquarters, 10788
Temple University Clinical Research Center Office of Clinical Research, 364
Temple University FELS Institute for Cancer Research, 2297
Temple University Speech and Hearing Science Laboratories, 4319
Temple University: Section of Auditory Research, 4320
The International Alliance of ALS/MND Associations, 997
Thomas Jefferson University Hospital, 7453
Thomas Jefferson University Ischemia-Shock, 4058
Thomas Jefferson University Ischemia-Shock Research Center, 4057
Thomas Jefferson University: Sleep Disorders Center, 7920
Thomas Jefferson University: Cardenza Foundation for Hematologic Research, 4990
Thomas Jefferson University: Center for Research in Medical Education, 365
Thomas Jefferson University: Daniel Baugh Institute, 1767
ToughLove International, 8379
Tri-County Association for the Blind, 9631
United Cerebral Palsy Central PA, 2696
United Cerebral Palsy of Beaver, Butler & Lawrence Counties, 2697
United Cerebral Palsy of Northwestern Pennsylvania, 2698
United Cerebral Palsy of Pennsylvania, 2699
United Cerebral Palsy of Philadelphia Vicinity, 2700
United Cerebral Palsy of Pittsburgh, 2701
United Cerebral Palsy of South Central Pennsylvania, 2702
United Cerebral Palsy of Southern Alleghenies Region, 2703
United Cerebral Palsy of Southwestern Pennsylvania, 2704
United Cerebral Palsy of Western Pennsylvania, 2705
University of Pennsylvania Diabetes and Endocrinology Research Center, 3326
University of Pennsylvania Institute on Aging, 86
University of Pennsylvania Muscle Institut e, 4833
University of Pennsylvania: Depression Research Unit, 6274
University of Pennsylvania: Harrison Department of Surgical Research, 3868
University of Pennsylvania: Penn Lung Center, 3090
University of Pittsburgh, 7018
University of Pittsburgh, 7457
University of Pittsburgh Cancer Institute, 2298

University of Pittsburgh Cystic Fibrosis Center: Children's Hospital, 3091
University of Pittsburgh: Department of Molecular Genetics and Biochemistry, 3327
University of Pittsburgh: Human Energy Research Laboratory, 4834
University of Pittsburgh: Western Psychiatric Institute & Clinic, 6113
VA Pittsburgh Healthcare System: University Drive Division, 10322
VA Stars & Stripes Healthcare Network, 10323
VIABL Services of Northampton County, 9632
Veterans Adm. Medical Center: Philadelphia, 10324
Veterans Adm. Medical Center: Coatesville, 10325
Veterans Adm. Medical Center: Lebanon Lebanon VA Medical Center, 10326
Veterans Adm. Medical Center: Pittsburg VA Pittsburgh Healthcare System, 10327
WFS' New Life Program, 8380
WM Krogman Center for Research in Child Growth and Development, 3974
Washington-Greene County Branch for the Pennsylvania Association for Blind, 9633
Western Pennsylvania Chapter of the National Hemophilia Foundation, 4927
Wilkes-Barre VA Medical Center, 10328
Women's Resource Center, 7168
York Industries for the Blind: Division of York County Blind Center, 9634

Rhode Island

Alzheimer's Association: Rhode Island Chapter, 807
American Cancer Society: Rhode Island, 2168
American Diabetes Association: Rhode Island, 3266
American Lung Association of Rhode Island, 5806
American Narcolepsy Association, 7860
Autism Society of Rhode Island, 1629
Brain Injury Association of Rhode Island, 4038
Brain Injury Association of Rhode Island H elpline, 4102
Brain Tumor Support Group: Providence, 1941
Brown University Division of Biology and Medicine, 2299
Center for Alcohol & Addiction Studies Brown University, 8332
Centers for AIDS Research: Brown University, 366
Children's Neurodevelopment Center, 3506
Division of Substance Abuse: Department of Mental Health and Hospitals, 8315
Hemophilia Center of Rhode Island Rhode Island Hospital, 4960
Hydrocephalus Association of Rhode Island, 5139
IN-SIGHT, 9635
Leukemia and Lymphoma Society: Rhode Island Chapter, 2169
Lupus Foundation of America: Rhode Island Chapter, 5914
Narcolepsy Network, 7923
National Alliance for the Mentally Ill of Rhode Island (NAMI), 6076
National Federation of the Blind: Rhode Island, 9636
National MS Society: Rhode Island Chapter, 6486
Parent Support Network of Rhode Island, 6147
RESOLVE of the Ocean State, 5361
Rhode Island Association of the Deaf, 4282
Rhode Island Brain & Spine Tumor Foundation, 1942
Rhode Island Department of Health, 8921
Rhode Island Department of Health: Division of Disease Prevention & Control, 289
Rhode Island Department of State Library for the Blind and Physically Handicapped, 9808
Rhode Island Disability Law Center, 10596
Rhode Island Hospital: Cystic Fibrosis Center, 3092
Rhode Island Scleroderma Support Group, 7461
Rhode Island Turner Syndrome Society, 9392
Roger Williams Clinical Cancer Research Center, 2300
Sleep Disorders Center: Rhode Island Hospital, 7905
Spina Bifida Association of Rhode Island, 8010
United Cerebral Palsy of Rhode Island, 2706
Veterans Adm. Medical Center: Providence Providence VA Medical Center, 10329

South Carolina

AARP South Carolina Office: Columbia, 68
Agromedicine Program Medical University of South Carolina, 7767
Alzheimer's Association: Low Country Chapter, 808
Alzheimer's Association: Mid-State South Carolina Chapter, 809
Alzheimer's Association: Upstate South Carolina Chapter, 810
American Cancer Society: South Carolina, 2170
American Diabetes Association: South Carolina, 3267
American Lung Association of South Carolina, 5807
American Lung Association of South Carolina, 9323
Association for Traumatic Stress Specialists, 7131
Autism Society of South Carolina, 1630
Brain Injury Association of South Carolina, 4039
Brain Tumor Support Group: Charleston, 1943
Brain Tumor Support Group: Florence, 1944
Carolinas Support Group: National Ataxia National Ataxia Foundation, 1481
Center for Developmental Disabilities University of South Carolina, 10475
Center for Disability Resources, 10476
Children's Center for Cancer and Blood Disorders, 2301
Division of Perinatal Systems Mills Jarret Complex, 8922
Federation of Families of South Carolina, 6148
Hemophilia Association of South Carolina, 4929
Interdisciplinary Program in Cell and Molecular Pharmacology, 8341
James R Clark Memorial Sickle Cell Foundation, 7705
Juvenile Diabetes Research Foundation: Low Country Chapter, 3269
Juvenile Diabetes Research Foundation: Palmetto Chapter, 3268
The Kidney Foundation of Canada, 5134
Leukemia and Lymphoma Society: South Carolina Chapter, 2171
Leukemia and Lymphoma Society: South/West, 2172
Lupus Foundation of America: South Carolina Chapter, 5915
Lyme Disease Network of South Carolina, 9059
Medical University of South Carolina, 1152
Medical University of South Carolina Health Services Administration, 367
Medical University of South Carolina Medical University of South Carolina, 7450
Medical University of South Carolina: Cystic Fibrosis Center, 3093
Medical University of South Carolina: Division of Rheumatology & Immunology, 1153
Myasthenia Gravis Support Group of Low Country, 6708
Myasthenia Gravis Support Group of the Mountain and Up Country, 6709
NAMI-SC: National Alliance on Mental Illness: South Carolina, 6077
NNFF South Carolina Chapter, 6765
National Association for Continence, 5275
National Federation of the Blind: South Carolina, 9637
National Kidney Foundation of South Carolina, 5586
National MS Society: South Carolina Branch, 6487
Prader-Willi South Carolina Association, 7279
RESOLVE of South Carolina, 5362
Ralph H. Johnson VA Medical Center, 10330
Richland Memorial Comprehensive Pediatric Hemophilia Center, 4982
Scleroderma Foundation: South Carolina Chapter, 7438
South Carolina Commission on Alcohol and Drug Abuse, 8316
South Carolina Department of Health & Environmental Control, 290
South Carolina Palmetto Turner Syndrome So ciety, 9393
South Carolina Protection & Advocacy System for the Handicapped, 10597
South Carolina State Library, 9809
Tri County HPV Support Group, 10598
William Jennings Bryan Dorn VA Medical Center, 10331

South Dakota

American Cancer Society: South Dakota, 2173
American Lung Association of South Dakota, 5808
American Lung Association of South Dakota, 9324
Autism Society of Black Hills, 1631
Cancer Support Group, 1945
Division of Alcohol & Drug Abuse: South Dakota, 8317
Juvenile Diabetes Research Foundation: Sio ux Falls Chapter, 3270
NAMI South Dakota, 6078
National Federation of the Blind: South Dakota, 9638
Parkinson Association of South Dakota, 6993
Sioux Falls VA Healthcare System, 10332
South Dakota Advocacy Services, 10599
South Dakota Department of Health, 8923
South Dakota State Library, 9810
Teratogen and Birth Defects Information Project, 1786
VA Black Hills Health Care System- Fort Meade Campus, 10333
VA Black Hills Health Care System- Hot Springs Campus, 10334

Tennessee

AARP Tennessee State Office: Nashville, 69
ALS Association: Middle Tennessee Chapter, 1032
Alzheimer's Association: Eastern Tennessee Chapter, 811
Alzheimer's Association: Highland Rim Chapter, 812
Alzheimer's Association: Memphis Area Office, 813
Alzheimer's Association: Middle Tennessee Chapter, 814
Alzheimer's Association: Northeast Tennessee Chapter, 815
Alzheimer's Association: Southeast Tennessee Chapter, 816
American Cancer Society: Tennessee, 2174
American Diabetes Association: Nashville, 3271
American Diabetes Association: Tennessee, 3272
American Liver Foundation Midsouth Chapter, 5705
American Lung Association of Tennesse, 9325
American Lung Association of Tennessee, 5809
Arthritis Foundation: Southeast Region, 1136
Arthritis Trust of America, 2540
Autism Society of East Tennessee, 1632
Brain Injury Association of Tennessee, 4040
Brain Injury Association of Tennessee Help line, 4103
CCFA Tennessee Chapter, 2961
Cancer Support Group: Knoxville, 1946
Cancer Support Group: Nashville, 1947
Centers for AIDS Research: Vanderbilt University Medical Center, 368
Department of Mental Health and Mental Retardation, Alcohol & Drug Service, 8318
Disability Law & Advocacy Center of Tennessee, 10600
Down Syndrome Association of Middle Tennessee, 3496
EAR Foundation, 4232
Ed Lindsey Industries of the Blind, 9639
Endometriosis Association Research Program : Vanderbuilt University, 3722
Hemophilia Health Services, 4890
Impotence Institute of America, 5239
Juvenile Diabetes Research Foundation: East Tennessee Chapter, 3273
Juvenile Diabetes Research Foundation: Mid dle Tennessee Chapter, 3274
LRC for Students with Disabilities, 9811
Leukemia & Lymphoma Society: Tennessee Chapter, 2175
Lupus Foundation of America Memphis Area Chapter, 5916
Lupus Foundation of America: East Tennessee Chapter, 5917
Lupus Foundation of America: Mid-South Area Chapter, 5918
Lupus Foundation of Kentuckiana, 5880
Memphis Cystic Fibrosis Center LeBonheur Children's Medical Center, 3094

Memphis Regional Brain Tumor Survivors Group, 1948
Mid-South Transplant Foundation, Inc. Tennessee, 9241
Middle Tennessee Sarcoidosis Support Group, 7327
Mountain Home VA Medical Center, 10335
National Federation of the Blind: Tennessee, 9640
National Foundation for Transplants, 9192
National Kidney Foundation of East Tennessee, 5588
National Kidney Foundation of West Tennessee, 5589
National MS Society: Mid-South Chapter, 6489
National MS Society: Mid-South Chapter, Nashville Office, 6490
National MS Society: Southeast Tennessee/North Georgia Chapte, 6488
Persian Gulf Information Network, 10336
Prader-Willi Tennessee Association, 7280
RESOLVE of Tennessee, 5363
Sarcoidosis Center, 7323
Sarcoidosis Research Institute (SRI), 7332
Scleroderma Foundation: Tennessee Chapter, 7439
Spina Bifida Association of Tennessee, 8011
St. Jude Children's Research Hospital, 2302
Support4Hope, 7205
Tenessee Department of Health, 8924
Tennessee Alliance for the Mentally Ill, 6079
Tennessee Department of Health: AIDS Program, 291
Tennessee Donor Services, 9242
Tennessee Hemophilia & Bleeding Disorder Foundation, 4930
Tennessee Hemophilia and Bleeding Disorder Foundation, 4988
Tennessee Kidney Foundation, 5591
Tennessee Library for the Blind and Physically Handicapped, 9812
Tennessee Neuropsychiatric Institute Middle Tennessee Mental Health Institute, 6335
Tennessee SIDS Alliance, 8925
Tennessee Valley Healthcare System- Alvin C. York (Murfreesboro) Campus, 10338
Tennessee Valley Healthcare System- Nashville Campus, 10337
Tennessee Voices for Children, 6149
The University of Memphis: School of Commu nication Sciences and Disorders, 4321
The Vanderbilt Hemostasis Clinic, 4989
United Cerebral Palsy of Middle Tennessee, 2707
United Cerebral Palsy of the Mid-South, 2708
University of Memphis: Department of Psych ology, 4063
University of Tennessee Drug Information Center, 8366
University of Tennessee Medical Group, 7458
University of Tennessee Memphis: Cancer Center, 2303
University of Tennessee: Center for Neuroscience, 7583
University of Tennessee: Division of Cardiovascular Diseases, 4837
University of Tennessee: Division of Reproductive Endocrinology, 3724
University of Tennessee: General Clinical Research Center, 3328
VISN 9: VA Mid South Healthcare Network, 10339
Vanderbilt Children's Hospital, 3095
Vanderbilt Kennedy Center, 6114
Vanderbilt University Diabetes Center, 3331
Vanderbilt University: Center for Fertility and Reproductive Research, 5380
Veterans Adm. Medical Center: Murfreesboro, 10340
Veterans Adm. Medical Center: Memphis, 10341
Veterans Adm. Medical Center: Muskogee, 10342
Veterans Adm. Medical Center: Nashville, 10343
Veterans Affairs Medical Center, 10344
Veterans Affairs Medical Center, Memphis, Tennessee, 10345
Vision Foundation, 10789
West Tennessee Sarcoidosis Support Group, 7341

Texas

A Wish with Wings, Inc., 10764
AARP Texas State Office: Austin, 70
AIDS Outreach Center (AOC), 292

ALS Association: Greater Houston CIO, 1033
ALS Association: North Texas Chapter, 1034
ALS Association: South Texas Chapter, 1035
Academy of Rehabilitative Audiology, 4209
Alzheimer's Alliance: Texarkana Area, 817
Alzheimer's Association: Capital of Texas Chapter, 818
Alzheimer's Association: El Paso Chapter, 819
Alzheimer's Association: Greater Beaumont Area Chapter, 820
Alzheimer's Association: Greater Dallas Chapter, 821
Alzheimer's Association: Greater East Texas Chapter, 822
Alzheimer's Association: Greater Wichita Falls Chapter, 823
Alzheimer's Association: Houston and Southeast Texas Chapter, 824
Alzheimer's Association: Northeast Texas Chapter, 825
Alzheimer's Association: Rio Grande Valley Region, 826
Alzheimer's Association: STAR Chapter, Midland Region, 827
Alzheimer's Association: South Central Texas, 828
Alzheimer's Association: Tarrant County Chapter, 829
Amarillo VA Health Care System, 10346
American Association for Respiratory Care, 5754
American Association of Kidney Patients: Piney Woods Chapter, 5592
American Cancer Society: Texas, 2176
American Diabetes Association: Texas, 3275
American Foundation for the Blind, 9641
American Foundation for the Blind: National Aging Center, 9642
American GI Forum NVOP, 10387
American Heart Association, 4786
American Heart Association, 8161
American Lung Association of Texas, 5810
American Lung Association of Texas, 9326
American Porphyria Foundation, 3859
American Stroke Association, 8162
Arthritis Foundation: North Texas Chapter, 1137
Asthma and Allergy Foundation of America, 1305
Asthma and Allergy Foundation of America: North Texas Chapter, 593
Asthma and Allergy Foundation of America: North Texas Chapter, 1306
Austin Outpatient Clinic, 10347
Autism Society of Dallas, 1633
Baylor College of Medicine: Children's General Clinical Research Center, 3306
Baylor College of Medicine: Cullen Eye Institute, 9838
Baylor College of Medicine: Debakey Heart Center, 4792
Baylor College of Medicine: Epilepsy Research Center, 7579
Baylor College of Medicine: General Clinical Research Center for Adults, 3862
Baylor College of Medicine: Jerry Lewis Neuromuscular Disease Research, 6592
Baylor College of Medicine: Sleep Disorder and Research Center, 7868
Baylor University Bone Marrow Transplantation Research Center, 2304
Brain Injury Association of Texas, 4041
Brain Tumor Support Group: El Paso, 1949
CCFA Houston Gulf Coast/South Texas Chapter, 2962
CCFA North Texas Chapter, 2963
Cancer Therapy and Research Center, 2305
Centers for AIDS Research: Baylor College of Medicine, 369
Central Texas FFCMH, 6080
Central Texas Veterans Health Care System, 10348
Cerebral Blood Flow Laboratories Veterans Administration Medical Center, 8171
Children's Heart Institute of Texas, 4797
Christus Santa Rosa Health System, 4947
Convention of American Instructors of the Deaf, 4225
Cook Children's Medical Center: Cystic Fibrosis Clinic, 3096
Cooley's Anemia Foundation (CAF): Texas, 2898

Utah

University of Utah: Artificial Heart Research Laboratory, 4839

University of Utah: Cardiovascular Genetic Research Clinic, 4840

University of Utah: Center for Human Toxicology, 8369

Utah Alliance for the Mentally Ill, 6085

Utah Chapter of the National Hemophilia Foundation, 4933

Utah Department of Health, 8931

Utah Department of Health: Bureau of Communicable Disease Control, 295

Utah Industries for the Blind, 9654

Utah SIDS Alliance, 8932

Utah State Library Division, 9816

Utah Support Group: National Ataxia Foundation, 1485

VA Salt Lake City Health Care System, 10363

Veterans Affairs Medical Center: Research Service, 3332

Vermont

AARP Vermont State Office: Montpelier, 72

ALS Clinical Department of Neurology, 1041

Alcohol and Drug Abuse Programs of Vermont Department Of Health, 8321

Alzheimer's Association: Vermont Chapter, 831

American Cancer Society: Vermont, 2181

American Diabetes Association: Vermont, 3282

American Lung Association of Vermont, 9328

Autism Society of Vermont Autism Society of America, 1634

Brain Injury Association of Vermont, 4043

Brain Injury Association of Vermont Helpli ne, 4105

Citizen Advocacy of Burlington, 10604

Client Assistance Program: Vermont Ladd Hall, 10605

Lupus Foundation of America: Vermont Chapter, 5924

Medical Center Hospital of Vermont Cystic Fibrosis Center, 3102

National Federation of the Blind: Vermont, 9655

National MS Society: Vermont Division, 6497

RESOLVE of Vermont, 5369

University of Vermont Cancer Center University of Vermont, 2312

University of Vermont: Office of Health Promotion Research, 370

Vermont Alliance for the Mentally Ill, 6086

Vermont Department of Health: Health Surveillance HIV/AIDS/STD/TB Program, 296

Vermont Department of Health: SIDS Information and Counseling Program, 8933

Vermont Department of Libraries Special Services Unit, 9817

Vermont FFCMH, 6087

Vermont FFCMH, 6152

Vermont Pregnancy Risk Information Service, 1789

Vermont Regional Hemophilia Center, 4998

White River Junction VA Medical Center, 10364

Virginia

AABA Support Group, 3637

AARP Virginia State Office: Richmond, 73

ACB Radio Amateurs, 9445

Al-Anon Alateen Family Group Hotline, 8371

Al-Anon Family Group Headquarters, 8226

Alateen Al-Anon Family Group Headquarters, 8227

Allergy & Asthma Network Mothers of Asthmatics, 559

Allergy & Asthma Network Mothers of Asthmatics, 1276

Allergy & Asthma Networks Hotline, 1318

Alzheimer's Association: Central Virginia Chapter, 832

Alzheimer's Association: Greater Richmond Chapter, 833

Alzheimer's Association: National Capital Area Chapter, 834

Alzheimer's Association: Piedmont-Valley Area Chapter, 835

Alzheimer's Association: Roanoke Salem Chapter, 836

Alzheimer's Association: Southeastern Virginia Chapter, 837

Alzheimer's Association: Southside Virginia Chapter, 838

American Academy of Audiology, 4210

American Academy of Otolaryngology: Head, 4211

American Association for the Study of Liver Diseases, 5671

American Cancer Society: Virginia, 2182

American Council of the Blind, 9451

American Counseling Association, 6263

American Counseling Association, 10461

American Diabetes Association, 3137

American Diabetes Association National Center, 3335

American Diabetes Association: Richmond, 3283

American Diabetes Association: Virginia, 3284

American Lung Association of Virginia, 5812

American Lung Association of Virginia, 9329

American Physical Therapy Association, 2837

American Physical Therapy Association, 6892

American Psychiatric Association, 5974

American Psychiatric Association, 6264

American Psychiatric Association, 7124

American Rehabilitation Counseling Association, 10467

American Thyroid Association, 9022

American Trauma Society, 7127

Arlin J Brown Information Center, 2183

Arlington County Department of Libraries, 9818

Arthritis Foundation: Virginia Chapter, 1140

Asbestos Information Association/North America, 10470

Assoc. for Education & Rehabilitation of the Blind & Visually Impaired, 9457

Association of Organ Procurement Organizations (AOPO), 9187

Auditory-Verbal International, 4219

Autism Society of Northern Virginia, 1635

Brain Injury Association, 3996

Brain Injury Association of America's National Family Helpline, 4044

Brain Injury Association of Virginia, 4045

Brain Injury Association of Virginia Helpline, 4106

Brain Tumor Support Group: Richmond, 1954

BrainLine.org, 7155

CAPCOM, 4221

CCFA Greater Washington DC/Virginia Chapter, 2964

Cancer Research Foundation of America, 2313

Central Rappahannock Regional Library, 9819

Cerebral Palsy of Virginia, 2714

Children's Hospice International, 10482

Children's Hospice International, 10803

Childrens Hospice International, 10627

Childrens Hospice International, 10804

Council for Exceptional Children, 1525

Council for Exceptional Children, 9465

Desert Storm Justice Foundation: Virginia, 10365

Division for the Visually Handicapped, 9820

Donate Life America, 9189

Down Syndrome Association of Hampton Roads, 3499

Eastern Virginia Medical School Children's Hospital of The King's Daught, 3103

Fairfax County Public Library, 9821

Food Allergy and Anaphylaxis Network, 569

Gulf War Veterans of Virginia, 10366

Hampton Subregional Library for the Blind, 9822

Hemophilia Association of the Capital Area, 4934

Infections Disease Society of America, 9045

International Brain Injury Association, 4000

International Council on Infertility Information Dissemination, 5321

International Society for the Study of Dissociation, 6328

International Society for the Study of Trauma And Dissociation, 7135

Juvenile Diabetes Research Foundation: Gre ater Blue Ridge Chapter, 3285

Keon Paschal Perry Sickle Cell Anemia Disease Awareness, 7722

Kids Incorporated, 10779

Leukemia and Lymphoma Society: National Capital Area Chapter, 2184

Library Users of America, 9478

LifeNet, 9244

Lupus Foundation of America: Eastern Virginia Chapter, 5925

Mental Health America, 5982

Mental Health America, 7195

Mental Health America Resource Center, 5983

Migraine Awareness Group: A National Understanding for Migraineurs, 6365

Myasthenia Gravis Support Group of Manassa s, 6710

Myositis Association, 1094

National Alliance On Mental Illness, 6268

National Alliance for the Mentally Ill, 5985

National Alliance for the Mentally Ill, 6330

National Alliance of Blind Students, 9482

National Alliance on Mental Illness, 7136

National Association of Alcoholism and Drug Abuse Counselors, 8251

National Association of State Directors of Veterans Affairs, 10239

National Association of State Mental Health Program Directors, 5986

National Capital Lyme Disease Association, 9048

National Captioning Institute, 4244

National Chronic Pain Outreach Association, 10512

National Crime Prevention Council, 8255

National Federation of the Blind: Virginia, 9656

National Fibromyalgia Partnership (NFP), 3781

National Hospice & Palliative Care Organiz ation, 10810

National Hospice & Palliative Care Organization, 10809

National Hospice & Palliative Care Organization (NHPCO), 221

National Hospice & Palliative Care Organization (NHPCO), 2038

National Hospice Helpline, 2340

National Hospice Helpline, 10816

National Industries for the Blind, 9508

National Kidney Foundation of Virginia, 5600

National MS Society: Blue Ridge Chapter, 6498

National MS Society: Central Virginia Chapter, 6499

National MS Society: Hampton Roads Chapter, 6500

National Mental Health Association, 6270

National Mental Health Information Center, 6271

National Science Foundation, 1307

National Science Foundation, 4284

National Science Foundation, 5706

National Science Foundation, 7152

National Science Foundation, 7577

National Women's Health Information Center, 3609

Newport News Public Library System, 9823

Old Dominion Area Chapter: NSCIA, 8095

Organ Procurement and Transplantation Network (OPTN), 9195

PACCT, 6153

PACCT of Roanoke Valley, 6154

PTSD Family Support Group, 7197

Parkinson Foundation of the National Capitol Area, 6994

Pediatric Endocrine Society, 7

RESOLVE Helpline, 3726

RESOLVE of Alabama, 5323

RESOLVE of the Washington Metro Area, 5332

RESOLVE: The National Infertility Association, 5322

Registry of Interpreters for the Deaf, 4252

Richmond HPV Support Group: Fan Free Clini c, 10606

Richmond Support Group, 3647

Roanoke City Public Library System, 9824

SIDS Mid-Atlantic, 8934

Samueli Institute, 7186

Sarcoidosis Self-Help Group: Virginia, 7334

Scleroderma Foundation: Greater Washington DC Chapter, 7421

Scleroderma Foundation: Greater Washington DC Chapter, 7442

Sickle Cell Anemia Research Foundation, 7716

Speech Simulation Research Foundation, 4315

Substance Abuse Services Office of Virginia, 8322

United Network for Organ Sharing (UNOS), 9196

United Virginia Chapter of the National Hemophilia Foundation, 4935
University Library Services, 9826
University of Virginia School of Medicine Cystic Fibrosis Center, 3104
University of Virginia: General Clinical Research Center, 1316
University of Virginia: Hypertension and Atherosclerosis Unit, 5199
Valley Brain Tumor Support Group, 1955
Veterans Adm. Medical Center: Hampton Hampton VA Medical Center, 10367
Veterans Adm. Medical Center: Richmond Hunter Holmes McGuire VA Medical Center, 10368
Veterans Adm. Medical Center: Roanoke Roanoke Vet Center, 10369
Veterans Adm. Medical Center: Salem Salem VA Medical Center, 10370
Virginia Alliance for the Mentally Ill, 6088
Virginia Association of the Deaf, 4285
Virginia Beach Public Library, 9827
Virginia Commonwealth University: Massey Cancer Center, 2314
Virginia Commonwealth University: Rehab Research and Training Center, 4064
Virginia Department of Health: Division of HIV, STD, and Pharmacy Services, 297
Virginia Industries for the Blind, 9657
Virginia Office for Protection and Advocacy, 10607
Virginia SIDS Alliance, 8935
Virginia SIDS Program: Virginia Department of Health, 8936
Washington Regional Transplant Consortium, 9245
World Federation for Mental Health, 5995

Washington

AARP Washington State Office: Seattle, 74
ALS Association: Evergreen Chapter, 1036
African American Post Traumatic Stress Disorder Association, 7121
Alzheimer's Association Autopsy Assistance Network, 890
Alzheimer's Association: Inland Northwest Chapter, 839
Alzheimer's Association: Western & Central Washington Chapter, 840
Alzheimer's Disease Center: Washington University, 863
American Cancer Society: Washington, 2185
American Diabetes Association: Seattle, 3286
American Diabetes Association: Washington, 3287
American Liver Foundation Pacific Northwest Chapter, 5707
American Lung Association of Washington, 5813
Arthritis Foundation: Washington/Alaska Chapter, 1141
Asthma and Allergy Foundation of America: Washington State Chapter, 594
Autism Society of Washington, 1636
BABES Network-YWCA, 379
Benaroya Research Institute Virginia Mason Medical Center, 3307
Bleeding Disorder Foundation of Washington, 4936
Brain Cancer Support Group: Port Orchard, 1956
Brain Cancer Support Group: Seattle, 1957
Brain Injury Association of Washington, 4046
Brain Injury Association of Washington Hel pline, 4107
Brain Injury Resource Center, 4108
Brain Injury Resource Center, 7154
CCFA Washington State Chapter, 2965
Cancer Information Service, 2321
Center for Anxiety and Traumatic Stress, 7187
Centers for AIDS Research: University of Washington, Harborview Medical Center, 371
Children's Hydrocephalus Support Group, 5141
Common Voice for Pierce County Parents, 6155
Dunshee House, 382
Epilepsy Foundation of North West Washington, 7578
Fred Hutchinson Cancer Research Center, 2315
Gluten Intolerance Group: GIG, 2561
HIV Prevention Trials Unit University of Washington/Seattle HPTU Si, 372

Health Information Network, 208
Health Information Network for Women and AIDS, 209
Hepatitis Education Project, 5075
Hepatitis Education Project, 5077
Hope Heart Institute, 4811
Inland Empire Bleeding Disorders, 4937
International Association for the Study of Pain, 2838
Juvenile Diabetes Research Foundation: Sea ttle Chapter, 3289
Juvenile Diabetes Research Foundation: Seattle Guild, 3288
Juvenile Diabetes Research Foundation: Spo kane County Area Chapter, 3290
King County Crisis Clinic, 386
LifeCenter Northwest, 9246
Lighthouse for the Blind of Washington, 9658
Lupus Foundation of America: Pacific Northwest Chapter, 5926
Mental Illness Research and Education Institute, 6106
Multifaith Works, 216
Myasthenia Gravis Support Group of Seattle , Olympia and Poulsbo, 6711
Myasthenia Gravis Support Group of Spokane, 6712
NAMI Washington (National Alliance for the Mentally Ill of Washington), 6089
National Association for Native American Children of Alcoholics, 8250
National Eating Disorders Association, 3607
National Federation of the Blind: Public Employees Division, 9505
National MS Society: Greater Washington Chapter, 6501
National MS Society: Inland Northwest Chapter, 6502
National Service Dog Center, 9884
Northwest AIDS Education and Training Center (AETC), 298
Northwestern Region: Helen Keller National Center, 9659
Pacific NW Support Group, 7330
Pacific Northwest Chapter of the Myasthenia Gravis Foundation of America, 6654
Pacific Northwest Chapter of the Myasthenia Gravis Foundation of America, 6661
Pacific Northwest Chapter of the Myasthenia Gravis Foundation of America, 6662
Pacific Northwest Chapter of the Myasthenia Gravis Foundation of America, 6669
Pacific Northwest Chapter of the Myasthenia Gravis Foundation of America, 6675
Pacific Northwest Chapter of the Myasthenia Gravis Foundation of America, 6680
Pacific Northwest Chapter of the Myasthenia Gravis Foundation of America, 6682
Persian Gulf Veterans of Washington, 10371
Prader-Willi Washington Association, 7283
Puget Sound Blood Center, 4980
Region X Office Program Consultants for Maternal and Child Health, 8937
SIDS Foundation of Washington, 8938
SIDS Northwest Regional Center, 8939
Scleroderma Foundation: Evergreen Chapter, 7443
Seattle HPV Support Group, 10608
Seattle Support Group: National Ataxia Foundation, 1486
Solomon Park Research Institute, 1049
Spina Bifida Association of Washington State, 8015
United Cerebral Palsy of Pierce County, 2715
University of Washington, 7021
University of Washington Department of Speech & Hearing Sciences, 4332
University of Washington Diabetes: Endocrinology Research Center, 3330
University of Washington: Cystic Fibrosis Center, 3105
University of Washington: Experimental Education Unit, 3522
VA Puget Sound Health Care Network, 10372
Veterans Adm. Medical Center: Spokane Spokane VA Medical Center, 10373
Veterans Adm. Medical Center: Tacoma Tacoma Vet Center, 10374

Veterans Adm. Medical Center: Walla Walla Johnathan M. Wainwright Memorial VA MC, 10375
Virginia Mason Brain Tumor Support Group, 1958
Virginia Mason Medical Center Neuroscience Institute, 1051
Washington Ambassador National Ataxia Foundation, 1487
Washington Department of Health: Division of HIV/AIDS Prevention Services, 299
Washington Department of Social and Health Services, Alcohol and Drug Prog., 8323
Washington FFCMH, 6090
Washington Leukemia and Lymphoma Society: Alaska Chapter, 2186
Washington Puget Sound Turner Syndrome Society, 9396
Washington State Client Assistance Program, 10609
Washington State Department of Services for the Blind, 9660
Washington Talking Book & Braille Library, 9828
Wenatchee Valley Brain Tumor Support Group, 1959
Wishing Star Foundation, 10791

West Virginia

AARP West Virginia Office: Charleston, 75
AFB Technology & Employment Center, 9661
Alzheimer's Association: Greater Mid-Ohio Valley Chapter, 841
Alzheimer's Association: N Central West Virginia Chapter, 842
Alzheimer's Association: South West Virginia Chapter, 843
American Cancer Society: West Virginia, 2187
American Diabetes Association: West Virginia, 3291
American Lung Association of West Virginia, 5814
American Lung Association of West Virginia, 9330
Autism Services Center, 1585
Autism Services Center, 1639
Autism Socity of West Virginia, 1637
Brain Injury Association of West Virginia, 4047
Brain Injury Association of West Virginia Helpline, 4109
Brain Tumor Support Group: Southern West Virginia, 1960
Cabell County Public Library, 9829
Health Science Library, 3299
Hemophilia Association of the Huntington Area, 4958
Hemophilia Center of West Virginia University Health Sciences Center, 4961
Juvenile Diabetes Research Foundation: Hun tington Chapter, 3292
Kanawha County Public Library, 9830
Mountain State/Parents/Children/ Adolescents Network, 6091
NAMI West Virginia, 6092
National Association of Therapeutic Wilderness Camps, 5987
National Autism Hotline Autism Services Center, 1651
National Federation of the Blind: West Virginia, 9662
National Job Accommodation Network, 10522
Northcentral West Virginia HPV Support Group, 10610
Office of Maternal, Child & Family Health, 8940
Ohio County Public Library Services for the Blind and Physically Handicapped, 9831
Parkersburg and Wood County Public Library, 9832
The West Virginia Autism Training Center Marshall University, 1648
Veterans Adm. Medical Center: Beckley, 10376
Veterans Adm. Medical Center: Clarksburg Louis A. Johnson VA Medical Center, 10377
Veterans Adm. Medical Center: Huntington, 10378
Veterans Affairs Medical Center: Martinsburg, 10379
West Virginia Advocates, 10611
West Virginia Department of Health & Human Resources, 300
West Virginia Division of Alcohol & Drug Abuse, 8324
West Virginia Library Commission, 9833
West Virginia School for the Blind, 9834
West Virginia University Cystic Fibrosis Center, 3106

West Virginia University: Mary Babb Randolph Cancer Center, 2316

Wisconsin

AARP Wisconsin State Office: Madison, 76
AIDS Network, 173
ALS Association: Southeast Wisconsin Chapter, 1038
About Kids GI Disorders, 3638
Alzheimer's Association: Greater Wisconsin Chapter, 844
Alzheimer's Association: Indianhead Chapter, 845
Alzheimer's Association: Lake Superior Chapter, 846
Alzheimer's Association: Midstate Wisconsin Chapter, 847
Alzheimer's Association: North Central Wisconsin Chapter, 848
Alzheimer's Association: Northeast Wisconsin Chapter, 849
Alzheimer's Association: South Central Wisconsin Chapter, 850
Alzheimer's Association: Southeast Wisconsin Chapter, 851
American Academy for Cerebral Palsy and Developmental Medicine, 2593
American Academy of Allergy, Asthma & Immunology, 561
American Academy of Allergy, Asthma & Immunology, 1277
American Association of Children's Residential Centers, 5972
American Cancer Society: Wisconsin, 2188
American Diabetes Association: Wisconsin, 3293
American Liver Foundation Wisconsin Chapter, 5708
American Lung Association of Wisconsin, 5815
American Lung Association of Wisconsin, 9331
Anxiety Disorders Center University of Wisconsin, 6100
Arthritis Foundation: Wisconsin Chapter Foundation, 1142
Autism Society of Wisconsin, 1638
Brain Injury Alliance of Wisconsin, 4110
Brain Injury Association of Wisconsin, 4048
Brain Tumor Support Group: John Sierzant Lutheran Hospital, Gunderson Clinic, 1961
Brown County Library, 9835
CCFA Wisconsin Chapter, 2966
Children's Brittle Bone Foundation, 6866
Clement J. Zablocki Veterans Affairs Medical Center, 10380
Cyclic Vomiting Syndrome Association, 3847
Down Syndrome Association of Wisconsin, 3500
Eau Claire Hemophilia Center, 4951
Endometriosis Association International, 3715
FASST, Friends & Survivors Standing Together, 3998
Governor's Committee for People with Disabilities, 10612
Great Lakes Hemophilia Foundation, 4938
Grief & Loss Support Group, 10815

Gulf War Veterans of Wisconsin, 10381
Gundersen Clinic Comprehensive Hemophilia Treatment Center, 4956
Hematology Treatment Center of the Great Lakes Hemophilia Foundation, 4957
Infant Death Center of Wisconsin, 8941
Injury Research Center, 7188
International Foundation for Functional Gastrointestinal Disorders (IFFGD), 2923
International Foundation for Functional Gastrointestinal Disorders, 3850
International Foundation for Functional Gastrointestinal Disorders (IFFGD), 5273
International Parkinson and Movement Disorder Society, 1443
Juvenile Diabetes Research Foundation: Gre ater Madison Chapter, 3295
Juvenile Diabetes Research Foundation: Nor theast Wisconsin Chapter, 3296
Juvenile Diabetes Research Foundation: Southeastern Chapter, 3294
Kids with Heart National Association for Children's Heart Disorders, 2875
LODAT: Brain Tumor Support Group, 1962
Leukemia and Lymphoma Society: Wisconsin Chapter, 2189
Lupus Foundation of America: Wisconsin Chapter, 5927
Medical College of Wisconsin: Cystic Fibrosis Clinic, 3107
MidWest Gulf War Veterans Association, 10382
Myasthenia Gravis Support Group of Fox Valley, 6713
Myasthenia Gravis Support Group of Milwauk ee, 6714
NNFF Wisconsin Chapter, 6766
National Federation of the Blind: Wisconsin, 9663
National Federation of the Blind: Writers, 9664
National Kidney Foundation of Wisconsin, 5601
National MS Society: Wisconsin Chapter, 6503
Obsessive Compulsive Information Center Dean Foundation, 5991
Office of Alcohol and Other Drug Abuse, 8325
Physician Referral and Information Line, 1321
Prader-Willi Wisconsin Association, 7284
RESOLVE of Wisconsin, 5370
Scoliosis Research Society, 7488
Society for the Study of Reproduction, 5371
Southeastern Wisconsin Chapter of the Nati onal Spinal Cord Injury Association, 8096
Spina Bifida Association of Northern Wisconsin, 8016
Spina Bifida Association of Southeastern Wisconsin, 8017
Spina Bifida Association of the Greater Fox Valley, 8018
Stem Cell Research Program University of Wisconsin-Madison, 1050
Trace Center University of Wisconsin: Madison, 4322
United Cerebral Palsy of Greater Dane County, 2716

United Cerebral Palsy of North Central Wisconsin, 2717
United Cerebral Palsy of Southeastern Wisconsin, 2718
United Cerebral Palsy of Wisconsin, 2719
United Special Sportsman Alliance, 10802
University of Wisconsin Madison Neurophysiology Laboratory, 7584
University of Wisconsin Milwaukee Medicinal Chemistry Group, 8370
University of Wisconsin Organ Procurement Organization, 9247
University of Wisconsin Paul P Carbone Comprehensive Cancer Center, 2317
University of Wisconsin-Madison: Cystic Fibrosis/Pulmonary Center, 3108
University of Wisconsin: Asthma, Allergy and Pulmonary Research Center, 1317
Veterans Adm. Medical Center: Tomah, 10383
We Are the Children's Hope/Support Group, 6156
William S. Middleton Memorial Veterans Hospital, 10384
Wilson's Disease Association, 5718
Wilson's Disease Association, 10441
Wisconsin Alliance for the Mentally Ill, 6093
Wisconsin Association of the Deaf, 4286
Wisconsin Chapter of the Myasthenia Gravis Foundation of America, 6681
Wisconsin Department of Health and Social Services: Division of Health, 301
Wisconsin Family Ties, 6094
Wisconsin Parkinson Association, 6995
Wisconsin Regional Library for the Blind Talking Book Program, 9836
Wiscraft: Wisconsin Enterprises for the Blind, 9665
Wisonsin Donor Network, 9248

Wyoming

AARP Wyoming State Office: Cheyenne, 77
Alcohol & Drug Abuse Programs of Wyoming Department Of Health, 8326
Alzheimer's Wyoming, 852
American Cancer Society: Wyoming, 2190
Brain Injury Alliance of Wyoming, 4111
Brain Injury Association of Wyoming, 4049
Concerned Parent Coalition, 6157
Deaf Association of Wyoming, 4287
National Federation of the Blind: Wyoming, 9666
National MS Society: Wyoming Chapter, 6504
Uplift, 6158
Veterans Adm. Medical Center: Cheyenne, 10385
Veterans Adm. Medical Center: Sheridan, 10386
Wyoming Alliance for the Mentally Ill, 6095
Wyoming Department of Health, 8942
Wyoming Department of Health HIV/AIDS/Hepatitis Program, 302
Wyoming Protection & Advocacy System, 10613
Wyoming Services for the Visually Disabled, 9837

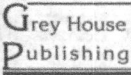
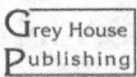

2015 Title List

Visit www.GreyHouse.com for Product Information, Table of Contents, and Sample Pages.

General Reference

An African Biographical Dictionary
America's College Museums
American Environmental Leaders: From Colonial Times to the Present
Encyclopedia of African-American Writing
Encyclopedia of Constitutional Amendments
Encyclopedia of Gun Control & Gun Rights
An Encyclopedia of Human Rights in the United States
Encyclopedia of Invasions & Conquests
Encyclopedia of Prisoners of War & Internment
Encyclopedia of Religion & Law in America
Encyclopedia of Rural America
Encyclopedia of the Continental Congress
Encyclopedia of the United States Cabinet, 1789-2010
Encyclopedia of War Journalism
Encyclopedia of Warrior Peoples & Fighting Groups
The Environmental Debate: A Documentary History
The Evolution Wars: A Guide to the Debates
From Suffrage to the Senate: America's Political Women
Global Terror & Political Risk Assessment
Media & Communications 1900-2020
Nations of the World
Political Corruption in America
Privacy Rights in the Digital Era
The Religious Right: A Reference Handbook
Speakers of the House of Representatives, 1789-2009
This is Who We Were: 1880-1900
This is Who We Were: A Companion to the 1940 Census
This is Who We Were: In the 1910s
This is Who We Were: In the 1920s
This is Who We Were: In the 1940s
This is Who We Were: In the 1950s
This is Who We Were: In the 1960s
This is Who We Were: In the 1970s
U.S. Land & Natural Resource Policy
The Value of a Dollar 1600-1865: Colonial Era to the Civil War
The Value of a Dollar: 1860-2014
Working Americans 1770-1869 Vol. IX: Revolutionary War to the Civil War
Working Americans 1880-1999 Vol. I: The Working Class
Working Americans 1880-1999 Vol. II: The Middle Class
Working Americans 1880-1999 Vol. III: The Upper Class
Working Americans 1880-1999 Vol. IV: Their Children
Working Americans 1880-2015 Vol. V: Americans At War
Working Americans 1880-2005 Vol. VI: Women at Work
Working Americans 1880-2006 Vol. VII: Social Movements
Working Americans 1880-2007 Vol. VIII: Immigrants
Working Americans 1880-2009 Vol. X: Sports & Recreation
Working Americans 1880-2010 Vol. XI: Inventors & Entrepreneurs
Working Americans 1880-2011 Vol. XII: Our History through Music
Working Americans 1880-2012 Vol. XIII: Education & Educators
World Cultural Leaders of the 20th & 21st Centuries

Education Information

Charter School Movement
Comparative Guide to American Elementary & Secondary Schools
Complete Learning Disabilities Directory
Educators Resource Directory
Special Education: A Reference Book for Policy and Curriculum Development

Health Information

Comparative Guide to American Hospitals
Complete Directory for Pediatric Disorders
Complete Directory for People with Chronic Illness
Complete Directory for People with Disabilities
Complete Mental Health Directory
Diabetes in America: Analysis of an Epidemic
Directory of Drug & Alcohol Residential Rehab Facilities
Directory of Health Care Group Purchasing Organizations
Directory of Hospital Personnel
HMO/PPO Directory
Medical Device Register
Older Americans Information Directory

Business Information

Complete Television, Radio & Cable Industry Directory
Directory of Business Information Resources
Directory of Mail Order Catalogs
Directory of Venture Capital & Private Equity Firms
Environmental Resource Handbook
Food & Beverage Market Place
Grey House Homeland Security Directory
Grey House Performing Arts Directory
Grey House Safety & Security Directory
Grey House Transportation Security Directory
Hudson's Washington News Media Contacts Directory
New York State Directory
Rauch Market Research Guides
Sports Market Place Directory

Statistics & Demographics

American Tally
America's Top-Rated Cities
America's Top-Rated Smaller Cities
America's Top-Rated Small Towns & Cities
Ancestry & Ethnicity in America
The Asian Databook
Comparative Guide to American Suburbs
The Hispanic Databook
Profiles of America
"Profiles of" Series - State Handbooks
Weather America

Financial Ratings Series

TheStreet Ratings' Guide to Bond & Money Market Mutual Funds
TheStreet Ratings' Guide to Common Stocks
TheStreet Ratings' Guide to Exchange-Traded Funds
TheStreet Ratings' Guide to Stock Mutual Funds
TheStreet Ratings' Ultimate Guided Tour of Stock Investing
Weiss Ratings' Consumer Guides
Weiss Ratings' Guide to Banks
Weiss Ratings' Guide to Credit Unions
Weiss Ratings' Guide to Health Insurers
Weiss Ratings' Guide to Life & Annuity Insurers
Weiss Ratings' Guide to Property & Casualty Insurers

Bowker's Books In Print® Titles

American Book Publishing Record® Annual
American Book Publishing Record® Monthly
Books In Print®
Books In Print® Supplement
Books Out Loud™
Bowker's Complete Video Directory™
Children's Books In Print®
El-Hi Textbooks & Serials In Print®
Forthcoming Books®
Large Print Books & Serials™
Law Books & Serials In Print™
Medical & Health Care Books In Print™
Publishers, Distributors & Wholesalers of the US™
Subject Guide to Books In Print®
Subject Guide to Children's Books In Print®

Canadian General Reference

Associations Canada
Canadian Almanac & Directory
Canadian Environmental Resource Guide
Canadian Parliamentary Guide
Canadian Venture Capital & Private Equity Firms
Financial Services Canada
Governments Canada
Health Guide Canada
The History of Canada
Libraries Canada
Major Canadian Cities

Grey House Publishing | Salem Press | H.W. Wilson | 4919 Route, 22 PO Box 56, Amenia NY 12501-0056

2015 Title List
Visit www.SalemPress.com for Product Information, Table of Contents, and Sample Pages.

Science, Careers & Mathematics

Ancient Creatures: Unearthed
Applied Science
Applied Science: Engineering & Mathematics
Applied Science: Science & Medicine
Applied Science: Technology
Biomes and Ecosystems
Careers in Business
Careers in Chemistry
Careers in Communications & Media
Careers in Environment & Conservation
Careers in Healthcare
Careers in Hospitality & Tourism
Careers in Human Services
Careers in Law, Criminal Justice & Emergency Services
Careers in Physics
Careers in Technology Services & Repair
Computer Technology Innovators
Contemporary Biographies in Business
Contemporary Biographies in Chemistry
Contemporary Biographies in Communications & Media
Contemporary Biographies in Environment & Conservation
Contemporary Biographies in Healthcare
Contemporary Biographies in Hospitality & Tourism
Contemporary Biographies in Law & Criminal Justice
Contemporary Biographies in Physics
Earth Science
Earth Science: Earth Materials & Resources
Earth Science: Earth's Surface and History
Earth Science: Physics & Chemistry of the Earth
Earth Science: Weather, Water & Atmosphere
Encyclopedia of Energy
Encyclopedia of Environmental Issues
Encyclopedia of Environmental Issues: Atmosphere and Air Pollution
Encyclopedia of Environmental Issues: Ecology and Ecosystems
Encyclopedia of Environmental Issues: Energy and Energy Use
Encyclopedia of Environmental Issues: Policy and Activism
Encyclopedia of Environmental Issues: Preservation/Wilderness Issues
Encyclopedia of Environmental Issues: Water and Water Pollution
Encyclopedia of Global Resources
Encyclopedia of Global Warming
Encyclopedia of Mathematics & Society
Encyclopedia of Mathematics & Society: Engineering, Tech, Medicine
Encyclopedia of Mathematics & Society: Great Mathematicians
Encyclopedia of Mathematics & Society: Math & Social Sciences
Encyclopedia of Mathematics & Society: Math Development/Concepts
Encyclopedia of Mathematics & Society: Math in Culture & Society
Encyclopedia of Mathematics & Society: Space, Science, Environment
Encyclopedia of the Ancient World
Forensic Science
Geography Basics
Internet Innovators
Inventions and Inventors
Magill's Encyclopedia of Science: Animal Life
Magill's Encyclopedia of Science: Plant life
Notable Natural Disasters
Principles of Chemistry
Science and Scientists
Solar System
Solar System: Great Astronomers
Solar System: Study of the Universe
Solar System: The Inner Planets
Solar System: The Moon and Other Small Bodies
Solar System: The Outer Planets
Solar System: The Sun and Other Stars
World Geography

Literature

American Ethnic Writers
Classics of Science Fiction & Fantasy Literature
Critical Insights: Authors
Critical Insights: New Literary Collection Bundles
Critical Insights: Themes
Critical Insights: Works
Critical Survey of Drama
Critical Survey of Graphic Novels: Heroes & Super Heroes
Critical Survey of Graphic Novels: History, Theme & Technique
Critical Survey of Graphic Novels: Independents/Underground Classics
Critical Survey of Graphic Novels: Manga
Critical Survey of Long Fiction
Critical Survey of Mystery & Detective Fiction
Critical Survey of Mythology and Folklore: Heroes and Heroines
Critical Survey of Mythology and Folklore: Love, Sexuality & Desire
Critical Survey of Mythology and Folklore: World Mythology
Critical Survey of Poetry
Critical Survey of Poetry: American Poets
Critical Survey of Poetry: British, Irish & Commonwealth Poets
Critical Survey of Poetry: Cumulative Index
Critical Survey of Poetry: European Poets
Critical Survey of Poetry: Topical Essays
Critical Survey of Poetry: World Poets
Critical Survey of Shakespeare's Sonnets
Critical Survey of Short Fiction
Critical Survey of Short Fiction: American Writers
Critical Survey of Short Fiction: British, Irish, Commonwealth Writers
Critical Survey of Short Fiction: Cumulative Index
Critical Survey of Short Fiction: European Writers
Critical Survey of Short Fiction: Topical Essays
Critical Survey of Short Fiction: World Writers
Cyclopedia of Literary Characters
Holocaust Literature
Introduction to Literary Context: American Poetry of the 20th Century
Introduction to Literary Context: American Post-Modernist Novels
Introduction to Literary Context: American Short Fiction
Introduction to Literary Context: English Literature
Introduction to Literary Context: Plays
Introduction to Literary Context: World Literature
Magill's Literary Annual 2015
Magill's Survey of American Literature
Magill's Survey of World Literature
Masterplots
Masterplots II: African American Literature
Masterplots II: American Fiction Series
Masterplots II: British & Commonwealth Fiction Series
Masterplots II: Christian Literature
Masterplots II: Drama Series
Masterplots II: Juvenile & Young Adult Literature, Supplement
Masterplots II: Nonfiction Series
Masterplots II: Poetry Series
Masterplots II: Short Story Series
Masterplots II: Women's Literature Series
Notable African American Writers
Notable American Novelists
Notable Playwrights
Notable Poets
Recommended Reading: 500 Classics Reviewed
Short Story Writers

Grey House Publishing | Salem Press | H.W. Wilson | 4919 Route, 22 PO Box 56, Amenia NY 12501-0056

2015 Title List
Visit www.SalemPress.com for Product Information, Table of Contents, and Sample Pages.

History and Social Science
The 2000s in America
50 States
African American History
Agriculture in History
American First Ladies
American Heroes
American Indian Culture
American Indian History
American Indian Tribes
American Presidents
American Villains
America's Historic Sites
Ancient Greece
The Bill of Rights
The Civil Rights Movement
The Cold War
Countries, Peoples & Cultures
Countries, Peoples & Cultures: Central & South America
Countries, Peoples & Cultures: Central, South & Southeast Asia
Countries, Peoples & Cultures: East & South Africa
Countries, Peoples & Cultures: East Asia & the Pacific
Countries, Peoples & Cultures: Eastern Europe
Countries, Peoples & Cultures: Middle East & North Africa
Countries, Peoples & Cultures: North America & the Caribbean
Countries, Peoples & Cultures: West & Central Africa
Countries, Peoples & Cultures: Western Europe
Defining Documents: American Revolution (1754-1805)
Defining Documents: Civil War (1860-1865)
Defining Documents: Emergence of Modern America (1868-1918)
Defining Documents: Exploration & Colonial America (1492-1755)
Defining Documents: Manifest Destiny (1803-1860)
Defining Documents: Post-War 1940s (1945-1949)
Defining Documents: Reconstruction (1865-1880)
Defining Documents: The 1920s
Defining Documents: The 1930s
Defining Documents: The American West (1836-1900)
Defining Documents: The Ancient World (2700 B.C.E.-50 C.E.)
Defining Documents: The Middle Ages (524-1431)
Defining Documents: World War I
Defining Documents: World War II (1939-1946)
The Eighties in America
Encyclopedia of American Immigration
Encyclopedia of Flight
Encyclopedia of the Ancient World
The Fifties in America
The Forties in America
Great Athletes
Great Athletes: Baseball
Great Athletes: Basketball
Great Athletes: Boxing & Soccer
Great Athletes: Cumulative Index
Great Athletes: Football
Great Athletes: Golf & Tennis
Great Athletes: Olympics
Great Athletes: Racing & Individual Sports
Great Events from History: 17th Century
Great Events from History: 18th Century
Great Events from History: 19th Century
Great Events from History: 20th Century (1901-1940)
Great Events from History: 20th Century (1941-1970)
Great Events from History: 20th Century (1971-2000)
Great Events from History: Ancient World
Great Events from History: Cumulative Indexes
Great Events from History: Gay, Lesbian, Bisexual, Transgender Events
Great Events from History: Middle Ages
Great Events from History: Modern Scandals
Great Events from History: Renaissance & Early Modern Era

Great Lives from History: 17th Century
Great Lives from History: 18th Century
Great Lives from History: 19th Century
Great Lives from History: 20th Century
Great Lives from History: African Americans
Great Lives from History: Ancient World
Great Lives from History: Asian & Pacific Islander Americans
Great Lives from History: Cumulative Indexes
Great Lives from History: Incredibly Wealthy
Great Lives from History: Inventors & Inventions
Great Lives from History: Jewish Americans
Great Lives from History: Latinos
Great Lives from History: Middle Ages
Great Lives from History: Notorious Lives
Great Lives from History: Renaissance & Early Modern Era
Great Lives from History: Scientists & Science
Historical Encyclopedia of American Business
Immigration in U.S. History
Magill's Guide to Military History
Milestone Documents in African American History
Milestone Documents in American History
Milestone Documents in World History
Milestone Documents of American Leaders
Milestone Documents of World Religions
Musicians & Composers 20th Century
The Nineties in America
The Seventies in America
The Sixties in America
Survey of American Industry and Careers
The Thirties in America
The Twenties in America
United States at War
U.S.A. in Space
U.S. Court Cases
U.S. Government Leaders
U.S. Laws, Acts, and Treaties
U.S. Legal System
U.S. Supreme Court
Weapons and Warfare
World Conflicts: Asia and the Middle East

Health
Addictions & Substance Abuse
Adolescent Health
Cancer
Complementary & Alternative Medicine
Genetics & Inherited Conditions
Health Issues
Infectious Diseases & Conditions
Magill's Medical Guide
Psychology & Behavioral Health
Psychology Basics

Grey House Publishing | Salem Press | H.W. Wilson | 4919 Route, 22 PO Box 56, Amenia NY 12501-0056

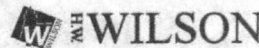 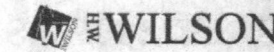
Current Biography
Current Biography Cumulative Index 1946-2013
Current Biography Monthly Magazine
Current Biography Yearbook: 2003
Current Biography Yearbook: 2004
Current Biography Yearbook: 2005
Current Biography Yearbook: 2006
Current Biography Yearbook: 2007
Current Biography Yearbook: 2008
Current Biography Yearbook: 2009
Current Biography Yearbook: 2010
Current Biography Yearbook: 2011
Current Biography Yearbook: 2012
Current Biography Yearbook: 2013
Current Biography Yearbook: 2014
Current Biography Yearbook: 2015

Core Collections
Children's Core Collection
Fiction Core Collection
Middle & Junior High School Core
Public Library Core Collection: Nonfiction
Senior High Core Collection

The Reference Shelf
Aging in America
American Military Presence Overseas
The Arab Spring
The Brain
The Business of Food
Conspiracy Theories
The Digital Age
Dinosaurs
Embracing New Paradigms in Education
Faith & Science
Families: Traditional and New Structures
The Future of U.S. Economic Relations: Mexico, Cuba, and
Venezuela
Global Climate Change
Graphic Novels and Comic Books
Immigration in the U.S.
Internet Safety
Marijuana Reform
The News and its Future
The Paranormal
Politics of the Ocean
Reality Television
Representative American Speeches: 2008-2009
Representative American Speeches: 2009-2010
Representative American Speeches: 2010-2011
Representative American Speeches: 2011-2012
Representative American Speeches: 2012-2013
Representative American Speeches: 2013-2014
Representative American Speeches: 2014-2015
Revisiting Gender
Robotics
Russia
Social Networking
Social Services for the Poor
Space Exploration & Development
Sports in America
The Supreme Court
The Transformation of American Cities
U.S. Infrastructure
U.S. National Debate Topic: Surveillance
U.S. National Debate Topic: The Ocean
U.S. National Debate Topic: Transportation Infrastructure
Whistleblowers

Readers' Guide
Abridged Readers' Guide to Periodical Literature
Readers' Guide to Periodical Literature

Indexes
Index to Legal Periodicals & Books
Short Story Index
Book Review Digest

Sears List
Sears List of Subject Headings
Sears: Lista de Encabezamientos de Materia

Facts About Series
Facts About American Immigration
Facts About China
Facts About the 20th Century
Facts About the Presidents
Facts About the World's Languages

Nobel Prize Winners
Nobel Prize Winners: 1901-1986
Nobel Prize Winners: 1987-1991
Nobel Prize Winners: 1992-1996
Nobel Prize Winners: 1997-2001

World Authors
World Authors: 1995-2000
World Authors: 2000-2005

Famous First Facts
Famous First Facts
Famous First Facts About American Politics
Famous First Facts About Sports
Famous First Facts About the Environment
Famous First Facts: International Edition

American Book of Days
The American Book of Days
The International Book of Days

Junior Authors & Illustrators
Tenth Book of Junior Authors & Illustrations

Monographs
The Barnhart Dictionary of Etymology
Celebrate the World
Guide to the Ancient World
Indexing from A to Z
The Poetry Break
Radical Change: Books for Youth in a Digital Age

Wilson Chronology
Wilson Chronology of Asia and the Pacific
Wilson Chronology of Human Rights
Wilson Chronology of Ideas
Wilson Chronology of the Arts
Wilson Chronology of the World's Religions
Wilson Chronology of Women's Achievements

Grey House Publishing | Salem Press | H.W. Wilson | 4919 Route, 22 PO Box 56, Amenia NY 12501-0056